Sixth Edition

CAMPBELL'S UROLOGY

W. B. SAUNDERS COMPANY

A Division of Harcourt Brace & Company

Philadelphia   London   Toronto   Montreal   Sydney   Tokyo

W. B. SAUNDERS COMPANY
A Division of
Harcourt Brace & Company

The Curtis Center
Independence Square West
Philadelphia, PA 19106

Library of Congress Cataloging-in-Publication Data

Campbell's Urology—6th ed. / [edited by] Patrick C. Walsh
. . . [et al.]

    p.   cm.

Includes bibliographical references and index.

ISBN 0–7216–3059–6 (set)

1. Urology.   I. Campbell, Meredith F. (Meredith
    Fairfax),   . II. Walsh, Patrick C.,   . III. Title:
    Urology.
    [DNLM: 1. Urologic Diseases.   WJ 100 C192]

RC871.C33 1992   616.6—dc20   90–9237
DNLM/DLC

Listed here are the latest translated editions of this book together with the language of the translation
and the publisher.

Italian (3rd Edition)   Casa Editricc Universo,
                    Rome, Italy

Portuguese (1st Edition)   Editora Guanabara Koogan,
                    Rio de Janeiro, Brazil

Editor: W. B. Saunders Staff
Developmental Editor: Rosanne Hallowell
Designer: Maureen Sweeney
Production Manager: Carolyn Naylor
Manuscript Editors: Mary Anne Folcher, Carol Robins,
                     Mary Ellen Ford, and Terry Belanger
Illustration Coordinator: Walter Verbitski
Indexers: Angela Holt and Julie Figures
Cover Designer: Michelle Maloney

Volume 1 ISBN 0–7216–4048–6
Volume 2 ISBN 0–7216–4049–4
Volume 3 ISBN 0–7216–4050–8
Set ISBN 0–7216–3059–6

Campbell's Urology, 6th edition

Printed in the United States of America.

Last digit is the print number: 9   8   7   6   5   4   3

CAMPBELL'S UROLOGY

■

Edited by

Patrick C. Walsh, M.D.

David Hall McConnell Professor
The Johns Hopkins University School of Medicine
Urologist-in-Chief
Brady Urological Institute
The Johns Hopkins Hospital
Baltimore, Maryland

Alan B. Retik, M.D.

Professor of Surgery (Urology)
Harvard Medical School
Chief, Division of Urology
Children's Hospital
Boston, Massachusetts

Thomas A. Stamey, M.D.

Professor and Chairman
Department of Urology
Stanford University School of Medicine
Stanford, California

E. Darracott Vaughan, Jr., M.D.

James J. Colt Professor of Urology
Cornell University Medical College
Urologist-in-Chief
The New York Hospital–Cornell Medical Center
New York, New York

■

CONTRIBUTORS

Mark C. Adams, M.D.
Assistant Professor of Urology, Indiana University School of Medicine, Indianapolis, Indiana. Attending Physician, Department of Urology, James Whitcomb Riley Hospital for Children, Indianapolis.
> AUGMENTATION CYSTOPLASTY IMPLANTATION OF ARTIFICIAL URINARY SPHINCTER IN MEN AND WOMEN AND RECONSTRUCTION OF THE DYSFUNCTIONAL URINARY TRACT

John M. Barry, M.D.
Professor of Surgery, and Chairman, Division of Urology and Renal Transplantation, Oregon Health Sciences University, Portland, Oregon. Staff Surgeon, University Hospital; and Consultant, Veterans Hospital, Portland.
> RENAL TRANSPLANTATION

Stuart B. Bauer, M.D.
Associate Professor of Surgery (Urology), Harvard Medical School, Boston, Massachusetts. Associate in Surgery (Urology), Children's Hospital, Boston.
> ANOMALIES OF THE UPPER URINARY TRACT
> NEUROGENIC VESICAL DYSFUNCTION IN CHILDREN

Arie Belldegrun, M.D.
Associate Professor of Surgery/Urology, University of California School of Medicine, Los Angeles, California. Attending Physician, UCLA Medical Center; Chief, Division of Urology, Olive View/UCLA Medical Center; and Clinical Director, Adoptive Immunotherapy Core Laboratory, Jonsson Comprehensive Cancer Center, Los Angeles.
> RENAL TUMORS

Mitchell C. Benson, M.D.
Associate Professor of Clinical Urology, Columbia University College of Physicians and Surgeons, New York, New York. Director, Urologic Oncology, Columbia–Presbyterian Medical Center, New York.
> URINARY DIVERSION

Richard E. Berger, M.D.
Associate Professor of Urology, University of Washington, Seattle, Washington. Attending Physician, University of Washington Affiliated Hospitals, Seattle.
> SEXUALLY TRANSMITTED DISEASES: THE CLASSIC DISEASES

Jon David Blumenfeld, M.D.
Assistant Professor of Medicine, Cornell University Medical College, New York, New York. Assistant Attending Physician in Medicine, The New York Hospital, New York.
> THE ADRENALS

Charles B. Brendler, M.D.
Associate Professor of Urology, The Johns Hopkins University School of Medicine, Baltimore, Maryland. Attending Physician, The Johns Hopkins Hospital, Baltimore.
> EVALUATION OF THE UROLOGIC PATIENT: HISTORY, PHYSICAL EXAMINATION, AND URINALYSIS
> URETHRECTOMY
> PERIOPERATIVE CARE

Peter N. Burns, Ph.D.
Associate Professor of Medical Biophysics and Radiology, University of Toronto, Toronto, Ontario, Canada. Senior Scientist, Sunnybrook Health Science Centre, Toronto.
> IMAGING OF THE URINARY TRACT:
> ULTRASONOGRAPHY OF THE URINARY TRACT

H. Ballentine Carter, M.D.
Assistant Professor of Urology, The Johns Hopkins University School of Medicine, Baltimore, Maryland. Department of Urology, The Johns Hopkins Hospital and Francis Scott Key Hospital, Baltimore.
> EVALUATION OF THE UROLOGIC PATIENT: INSTRUMENTATION AND ENDOSCOPY

William J. Catalona, M.D.
Professor of Surgery/Urology, Washington University School of Medicine, St. Louis, Missouri. Attending Physician, Barnes Hospital, The Jewish Hospital of St. Louis, and St. Louis Children's Hospital, St. Louis.
UROTHELIAL TUMORS OF THE URINARY TRACT

Thomas S. K. Chang, Ph.D.
Associate Professor, Department of Urology, The Johns Hopkins School of Medicine, Baltimore, Maryland.
PHYSIOLOGY OF MALE REPRODUCTION: THE TESTIS, EPIDIDYMIS, AND DUCTUS DEFERENS

Robert L. Chevalier, M.D.
Professor and Vice-Chairman, Department of Pediatrics, University of Virginia School of Medicine, Charlottesville, Virginia. Attending Pediatrician, and Chief, Division of Pediatric Nephrology, University of Virginia Health Sciences Center, Charlottesville.
RENAL FUNCTION IN THE FETUS AND NEONATE

Robert J. Churchill, M.D.
Professor and Chairman of Radiology, University of Missouri School of Medicine, Columbia, Missouri. Chairman, Department of Radiology, University of Missouri Hospital and Clinics, Columbia.
IMAGING OF THE URINARY TRACT: COMPUTED TOMOGRAPHY OF THE URINARY TRACT

Ralph V. Clayman, M.D.
Professor of Urologic Surgery and Radiology, Washington University School of Medicine, St. Louis, Missouri. Attending Physician, Barnes Affiliated Hospitals, Barnes Hospital, Veterans Administration Hospital, The Jewish Hospital of St. Louis, and St. Louis Children's Hospital, St. Louis.
ENDOSURGICAL TECHNIQUES FOR THE DIAGNOSIS AND TREATMENT OF NONCALCULOUS DISEASE OF THE URETER AND KIDNEY

Donald S. Coffey, Ph.D.
Professor, The Johns Hopkins University School of Medicine, Baltimore, Maryland.
PHYSIOLOGY OF MALE REPRODUCTION: THE MOLECULAR BIOLOGY, ENDOCRINOLOGY, AND PHYSIOLOGY OF THE PROSTATE AND SEMINAL VESICLES

Giulio J. D'Angio, M.D.
Professor of Radiation Oncology, Radiology, and Pediatric Oncology, University of Pennsylvania School of Medicine, Philadelphia, Pennsylvania. Vice-Chairman, Department of Radiation Oncology, Hospital of the University of Pennsylvania, Philadelphia.
PEDIATRIC ONCOLOGY

Jean B. deKernion, M.D.
Professor of Surgery/Urology, and Chief, Division of Urology, University of California School of Medicine, Los Angeles, California. Professor of Surgery/Urol-
ogy—UCLA School of Medicine, and Chief, Division of Urology, Los Angeles.
RENAL TUMORS

Francesco Del Greco, M.D.
Professor of Medicine, Northwestern University Medical School, Chicago, Illinois. Attending Physician and Medical Director, Dialysis Center, Northwestern Memorial Hospital, Chicago. Visiting Attending Physician, Veterans Administration Lakeside Hospital, Chicago.
OTHER RENAL DISEASES OF UROLOGIC SIGNIFICANCE

Charles J. Devine, Jr., M.D.
Professor of Urology, Eastern Virginia Medical School, Norfolk, Virginia. Attending Physician, The Devine Center for Genitourinary Reconstructive Surgery, Sentara Norfolk General Hospital, Sentara Leigh Memorial Hospital, and Children's Hospital of the King's Daughters, Norfolk.
SURGERY OF THE PENIS AND URETHRA

William C. DeWolf, M.D.
Associate Professor of Surgery, Harvard Medical School, Boston, Massachusetts. Urologist-in-Chief, Beth Israel Hospital, Boston.
GENETIC DETERMINANTS OF UROLOGIC DISEASE

George W. Drach, M.D.
Professor of Surgery, and Chief of Urology, University of Arizona, Tucson, Arizona. Attending Urologist, University Medical Center; and Consultant in Urology, Veterans Administration Medical Center, Tucson.
URINARY LITHIASIS: ETIOLOGY, DIAGNOSIS, AND MEDICAL MANAGEMENT

John W. Duckett, M.D.
Professor of Urology in Surgery, University of Pennsylvania School of Medicine, Philadelphia, Pennsylvania. Director, Division of Urology, Children's Hospital of Philadelphia, Philadelphia.
HYPOSPADIAS

J. S. Dunbar, M.D.
Professor Emeritus, Department of Radiology, University of Toronto, Toronto, Ontario, Canada. Consultant in Radiology, Hospital for Sick Children, Toronto.
IMAGING OF THE URINARY TRACT: EXCRETORY UROGRAPHY IN INFANTS AND CHILDREN

Jack S. Elder, M.D.
Associate Professor of Urology and Pediatrics, Case Western Reserve University School of Medicine, Cleveland, Ohio. Director of Pediatric Urology, Rainbow Babies and Children's Hospital and MetroHealth Hospital, Cleveland.
CONGENITAL ANOMALIES OF THE GENITALIA

Audrey E. Evans, M.D.
Professor of Pediatrics and Human Genetics, University of Pennsylvania School of Medicine, Philadelphia, Pennsylvania. Professor of Pediatric Oncology, Children's Hospital of Philadelphia, Philadelphia.
PEDIATRIC ONCOLOGY

William R. Fair, M.D.
Professor of Surgery/Urology, Cornell University Medical College, New York, New York; and Member, Sloan–Kettering Institute, New York. Chief, Urology Service, Memorial Sloan–Kettering Cancer Center; and Attending Surgeon, Memorial Hospital and New York Hospital, New York.
OVERVIEW OF CANCER BIOLOGY AND PRINCIPLES OF ONCOLOGY

Fuad S. Freiha, M.D.
Professor of Urology, Stanford University School of Medicine, Stanford, California. Chief, Urologic Oncology, Stanford University Medical Center, Stanford.
OPEN BLADDER SURGERY

Richard M. Friedenberg, M.D.
Professor and Chairman, Department of Radiological Sciences, University of California, Irvine, California. Chairman, Department of Radiological Sciences, University of California, Irvine Medical Center, Orange, California.
IMAGING OF THE URINARY TRACT: EXCRETORY UROGRAPHY IN THE ADULT

John P. Gearhart, M.D.
Associate Professor of Pediatric Urology and Pediatrics, The Johns Hopkins University School of Medicine, Baltimore, Maryland. Director of Pediatric Urology, The Johns Hopkins Hospital; and Consultant in Pediatric Urology, Francis Scott Key Hospital, The University of Maryland Hospital, and John F. Kennedy Hospital, Baltimore.
EXSTROPHY OF THE BLADDER, EPISPADIAS, AND OTHER BLADDER ANOMALIES

Fredrick W. George, Ph.D.
Assistant Professor of Internal Medicine, Department of Internal Medicine, University of Texas Southwestern Medical Center, Dallas, Texas.
EMBRYOLOGY OF THE GENITAL TRACT

Bruce R. Gilbert, M.D., Ph.D.
Clinical Instructor in Surgery (Urology), The New York Hospital–Cornell Medical Center, New York, New York. Assistant Attending Surgeon (Urology), The New York Hospital, New York.
NORMAL RENAL PHYSIOLOGY

Jay Y. Gillenwater, M.D.
Professor and Chairman of Urology, University of Virginia Medical School, Charlottesville, Virginia. Chairman of Urology, University of Virginia Hospital, Charlottesville.
THE PATHOPHYSIOLOGY OF URINARY TRACT OBSTRUCTION

Kenneth I. Glassberg, M.D.
Professor of Urology, State University of New York Health Science Center, Brooklyn, New York. Director, Division of Pediatric Urology, University Hospital of Brooklyn, Kings County Hospital Center, and Long Island College Hospital; Attending Physician in Urology at Maimonides Medical Center, Brooklyn.
RENAL DYSPLASIA AND CYSTIC DISEASE OF THE KIDNEY

Irwin Goldstein, M.D.
Professor of Urology, Boston University School of Medicine, Boston, Massachusetts. Visiting Surgeon, University Hospital, Boston.
DIAGNOSIS AND THERAPY OF ERECTILE DYSFUNCTION

Marc Goldstein, M.D.
Associate Professor of Surgery (Urology), Cornell University Medical College; and Staff Scientist, Center for Biomedical Research, The Population Council, New York, New York. Associate Attending Surgeon and Director, The Male Reproduction and Microsurgery Unit, The James Buchanan Brady Foundation, Department of Surgery, Division of Urology, The New York Hospital–Cornell Medical Center, New York.
SURGERY OF MALE INFERTILITY AND OTHER SCROTAL DISORDERS

Edmond T. Gonzales, Jr., M.D.
Professor of Urology, Scott Department of Urology, Baylor College of Medicine, Houston, Texas. Chief, Urology Service, and Head, Department of Surgery, Texas Children's Hospital, Houston.
POSTERIOR URETHRAL VALVES AND OTHER URETHRAL ANOMALIES

Rafael Gosalbez, M.D.
Fellow, Pediatric Urology, Emory University School of Medicine, Atlanta, Georgia.
NEONATAL AND PERINATAL EMERGENCIES

James G. Gow, M.D., Ch.M., F.R.C.S.
Former Clinical Lecturer, University of Liverpool, Liverpool, United Kingdom. Attending Physician, Lourdes Private Hospital, Liverpool.
GENITOURINARY TUBERCULOSIS

Damian R. Greene, M.B., F.R.C.S.I.
Post-Doctoral Research Fellow in Urologic Oncology, Baylor College of Medicine, Houston, Texas.
UROLOGIC ULTRASONOGRAPHY

Alexander Greenstein, M.D.
Assistant Professor of Urology, Department of Urology, Sourasky Medical Center, Ichilov Hospital, Tel-Aviv University, Tel-Aviv, Israel.
SURGERY OF THE URETER

James E. Griffin, M.D.
Professor of Internal Medicine, University of Texas Southwestern Medical Center, Dallas, Texas. Attending Physician, Parkland Memorial Hospital, Dallas.
DISORDERS OF SEXUAL DIFFERENTIATION

John Hale, Ph.D.
Professor Emeritus, Radiological Physics, University of Pennsylvania School of Medicine, Philadelphia, Pennsylvania.
IMAGING OF THE URINARY TRACT: RADIATION PROTECTION

W. Hardy Hendren, M.D.
Robert E. Gross Professor of Surgery, Harvard Medical School, Boston, Massachusetts. Chief of Surgery, Children's Hospital, and Visiting Surgeon, Massachusetts General Hospital, Boston.
CLOACAL MALFORMATIONS
URINARY UNDIVERSION: REFUNCTIONALIZATION OF THE PREVIOUSLY DIVERTED URINARY TRACT

Harry W. Herr, M.D.
Associate Professor of Surgery, Cornell University Medical College, New York, New York. Associate Attending Surgeon, Memorial Sloan–Kettering Cancer Center, New York.
SURGERY OF PENILE AND URETHRAL CARCINOMA

Marjorie Hertz, M.D.
Professor of Radiology and Head, Section of Imaging, Sackler Faculty of Medicine, Tel-Aviv University, Ramat Aviv, Israel. Senior Radiologist, Imaging Department, Sheba Medical Center, Tel-Hashomer, Israel.
IMAGING OF THE URINARY TRACT: CYSTOURETHROGRAPHY

Warren D. W. Heston, Ph.D.
Associate Member and Director of Urologic Oncology Research, Memorial Sloan–Kettering Cancer Center, New York, New York.
OVERVIEW OF CANCER BIOLOGY AND PRINCIPLES OF ONCOLOGY

Stuart S. Howards, M.D.
Professor of Urology and Physiology, University of Virginia Health Sciences Center, Charlottesville, Virginia. Staff Urologist, University of Virginia Hospital, Charlottesville.
MALE INFERTILITY
SURGERY OF THE SCROTUM AND TESTIS IN CHILDHOOD

Jeffry L. Huffman, M.D.
Associate Professor of Urology, University of Southern California School of Medicine, Los Angeles, California. Attending Physician, USC University Hospital, Los Angeles.
URETEROSCOPY

Robert D. Jeffs, M.D., F.R.C.S.(C.)
Professor of Pediatric Urology, The Johns Hopkins University School of Medicine, Baltimore, Maryland. Director Emeritus of Pediatric Urology, The Johns Hopkins Hospital; and Consultant in Pediatric Urology, Francis Scott Key Medical Center, University of Maryland Hospital, and John F. Kennedy Institute, Baltimore.
EXSTROPHY OF THE BLADDER, EPISPADIAS, AND OTHER BLADDER ANOMALIES

Gerald H. Jordon, M.D.
Associate Professor, Department of Urology, Eastern Virginia Medical School, Norfolk, Virginia. Attending Physician, Sentara Hospitals, Norfolk General and Leigh Memorial, The Children's Hospital of the King's Daughters, and DePaul Medical Center, Norfolk.
TUMORS OF THE PENIS
SURGERY OF THE PENIS AND URETHRA

Saad Juma, M.D.
Assistant Clinical Professor, Division of Urology, University of California School of Medicine, San Diego, California.
FEMALE UROLOGY

John N. Kabalin, M.D.
Assistant Professor of Urology, Stanford University School of Medicine, Stanford, California. Chief, Urology Section, Veterans Administration Medical Center, Palo Alto, California.
SURGICAL ANATOMY OF THE GENITOURINARY TRACT: ANATOMY OF THE RETROPERITONEUM AND KIDNEY

Louis R. Kavoussi, M.D.
Assistant Professor, Harvard Medical School, Boston, Massachusetts. Head, Section of Endourology, Division of Urologic Surgery, Brigham and Women's Hospital, Boston.
ENDOSURGICAL TECHNIQUES FOR THE DIAGNOSIS AND TREATMENT OF NONCALCULOUS DISEASE OF THE URETER AND KIDNEY

Lowell R. King, M.D.
Professor of Urology, Associate Professor of Pediatrics, and Head, Section on Pediatric Urology, Duke University, Durham, North Carolina. Attending Urologist, Duke University Medical Center, Durham.
VESICOURETERAL REFLUX, MEGAURETER, AND URETERAL REIMPLANTATION

Saulo Klahr, M.D.
John E. and Adaline Simon Professor of Medicine, Washington University School of Medicine, St. Louis, Missouri. Physician-in-Chief, The Jewish Hospital of St. Louis, and Physician, Barnes Hospital, St. Louis.
RENAL ENDOCRINOLOGY

Stephen A. Koff, M.D.
Professor of Surgery, Ohio State University College of Medicine, Columbus, Ohio. Chief, Division of Pediatric Urology, Children's Hospital, Columbus.
ENURESIS

Warren W. Koontz, Jr., M.D.
Professor and Chairman, Division of Urology, Medical College of Virginia, Virginia Commonwealth University, Richmond, Virginia.
SURGERY OF THE URETER

Robert J. Krane, M.D.
Professor and Chairman, Department of Urology, Boston University School of Medicine, Boston, Massachusetts.
DIAGNOSIS AND THERAPY OF ERECTILE
DYSFUNCTION

Herbert Y. Kressel, M.D.
Professor of Radiology, University of Pennsylvania School of Medicine, Philadelphia, Pennsylvania. Chief of MRI, Hospital of the University of Pennsylvania, Philadelphia.
IMAGING OF THE URINARY TRACT: MAGNETIC
RESONANCE IMAGING

John N. Krieger, M.D.
Associate Professor, Department of Urology, University of Washington School of Medicine, Seattle, Washington.
SEXUALLY TRANSMITTED DISEASES: THE ACQUIRED
IMMUNODEFICIENCY SYNDROME AND RELATED
CONDITIONS

Elroy D. Kursh, M.D.
Associate Professor of Urology, Case Western Reserve University School of Medicine, Cleveland, Ohio. Attending Urologist, University Hospitals of Cleveland, MetroHealth Medical Center, and Veterans Administration Medical Center, Cleveland.
EXTRINSIC OBSTRUCTION OF THE URETER

Elliott C. Lasser, M.D.
Professor, Department of Radiology, University of California, San Diego, California. Attending Physician, UCSD Medical Center, San Diego.
IMAGING OF THE URINARY TRACT: CONTRAST MEDIA
FOR UROGRAPHY

Jay Stauffer Lehman, M.D.*
Formerly, Assistant Director, The Edna McConnell Clark Foundation, New York, New York.
PARASITIC DISEASES OF THE GENITOURINARY
SYSTEM

Bruce R. Leslie, M.D.
Staff Physician, Division of Hypertensive Diseases, Ochsner Medical Institutions, New Orleans, Louisiana.
NORMAL RENAL PHYSIOLOGY

John A. Libertino, M.D.
Associate Clinical Professor of Surgery, Harvard Medical School, Boston, Massachusetts. Chief of Surgery, Lahey Clinic Medical Center, Burlington, Massachusetts.
RENOVASCULAR SURGERY

Nancy A. Little, M.D.
Assistant Clinical Professor, Division of Urology, University of Texas Health Science Center at San Antonio, Texas.
FEMALE UROLOGY

*Deceased.

Leon Love, M.D.
Professor of Radiology, and Acting Chairman, Loyola University Medical Center, Maywood, Illinois. Chairman, Department of Radiology, Cook County Hospital, Chicago.
IMAGING OF THE URINARY TRACT: COMPUTED
TOMOGRAPHY OF THE URINARY TRACT

Franklin C. Lowe, M.D.
Assistant Professor of Clinical Urology, Columbia College of Physicians and Surgeons, New York, New York. Associate Director, Department of Urology, St. Luke's–Roosevelt Hospital Center, New York.
EVALUATION OF THE UROLOGIC PATIENT: HISTORY,
PHYSICAL EXAMINATION, AND URINALYSIS

Tom F. Lue, M.D.
Associate Professor of Urology, University of California School of Medicine, San Francisco, California.
PHYSIOLOGY OF ERECTION AND PATHOPHYSIOLOGY
OF IMPOTENCE

Peter J. Lynch, M.D.
Professor and Head, Department of Dermatology, University of Minnesota Medical School, Minneapolis, Minnesota. Attending Physician, University of Minnesota Hospital and Clinic, Minneapolis.
CUTANEOUS DISEASES OF THE EXTERNAL GENITALIA

Max Maizels, M.D.
Associate Professor of Urology, Northwestern University Medical School, Chicago, Illinois. Attending Physician, Children's Memorial Hospital and Northwestern Memorial Hospital, Chicago.
NORMAL DEVELOPMENT OF THE URINARY TRACT

James Mandell, M.D.
Associate Professor of Surgery, Harvard Medical School, Boston, Massachusetts. Associate in Surgery, Children's Hospital, Boston.
RENAL FUNCTION IN THE FETUS AND NEONATE
PRENATAL AND POSTNATAL DIAGNOSIS AND
MANAGEMENT OF CONGENITAL ABNORMALITIES

David L. McCullough, M.D.
William H. Boyce Professor and Chairman, Department of Urology, Bowman Gray School of Medicine of Wake Forest University, Winston-Salem, North Carolina. Chairman, Department of Urology, North Carolina Baptist/Wake Forest University Medical Center, Winston-Salem.
EXTRACORPOREAL SHOCK WAVE LITHOTRIPSY

W. Scott McDougal, M.D.
Professor of Surgery (Urology), Harvard Medical School, Boston, Massachusetts. Chief, Department of Urology, Massachusetts General Hospital, Boston.
USE OF INTESTINAL SEGMENTS IN THE URINARY
TRACT: BASIC PRINCIPLES

John E. McNeal, M.D.
Clinical Professor of Urology (Surgery), Stanford University School of Medicine, Stanford, California.
ADENOCARCINOMA OF THE PROSTATE

Edwin M. Meares, Jr., M.D.
Charles M. Whitney Professor and Chairman, Division of Urology, Tufts University School of Medicine, Boston, Massachusetts. Chairman, Department of Urology, New England Medical Center Hospitals, Boston.
PROSTATITIS AND RELATED DISORDERS

Winston K. Mebust, M.D.
Professor of Surgery/Urology, University of Kansas School of Medicine, Kansas City, Kansas. Professor and Chairman, Section of Urology, University of Kansas Medical Center, Kansas City.
TRANSURETHRAL SURGERY

Edward M. Messing, M.D.
Associate Professor of Surgery and Human Oncology, Division of Urology, University of Wisconsin School of Medicine, Madison, Wisconsin. Attending Urologist, University Hospital; and Consulting Urologist, Middleton Veterans Administration Hospital, Madison.
INTERSTITIAL CYSTITIS AND RELATED SYNDROMES

Michael E. Mitchell, M.D.
Professor of Urology, University of Washington School of Medicine, Seattle, Washington. Chief, Division of Pediatric Urology, Children's Hospital and Medical Center, Seattle.
AUGMENTATION CYSTOPLASTY IMPLANTATION OF ARTIFICIAL URINARY SPHINCTER IN MEN AND WOMEN AND RECONSTRUCTION OF THE DYSFUNCTIONAL URINARY TRACT

Andrew C. Novick, M.D.
Chairman, Department of Urology, Cleveland Clinic Foundation, Cleveland, Ohio.
SURGERY OF THE KIDNEY

Carl A. Olsson, M.D.
Professor and Chairman, Department of Urology, Columbia University College of Physicians and Surgeons, New York, New York. Chairman, Department of Urology, Columbia–Presbyterian Medical Center, New York.
URINARY DIVERSION

Olle Olsson, M.D.
Professor Emeritus, Consulting Radiologist, Department of Diagnostic Radiology, University Hospital, Lund, Sweden.
IMAGING OF THE URINARY TRACT: AN OVERVIEW OF URORADIOLOGY

David F. Paulson, M.D.
Professor of Surgery, Duke University School of Medicine, Durham, North Carolina. Chief of Urologic Surgery, Duke University Medical Center, Durham.
PERINEAL PROSTATECTOMY

Alan D. Perlmutter, M.D.
Professor of Urology, Wayne State University School of Medicine, Detroit, Michigan. Chief, Department of Pediatric Urology, Children's Hospital of Michigan, Detroit.
ANOMALIES OF THE UPPER URINARY TRACT
SURGICAL MANAGEMENT OF INTERSEXUALITY

Craig A. Peters, M.D.
Assistant Professor in Surgery, Harvard Medical School, Boston, Massachusetts. Assistant in Surgery, Children's Hospital, Boston.
PRENATAL AND POSTNATAL DIAGNOSIS AND MANAGEMENT OF CONGENITAL ABNORMALITIES
ECTOPIC URETER AND URETEROCELE

Paul C. Peters, M.D.
E.E. and Greer Garson Fogelson Distinguished Professor of Urology, The University of Texas Southwestern Medical School, Dallas, Texas. Chief of Service, Parkland Memorial Hospital; and Attending Physician, Dallas Veterans Administration Medical Center, Baylor University Medical Center, Children's Medical Center, Zale Lipshy University Hospital, Dallas, and John Peter Smith Hospital, Fort Worth.
GENITOURINARY TRAUMA

Howard M. Pollack, M.D.
Professor of Radiology and Urology, University of Pennsylvania School of Medicine, Philadelphia, Pennsylvania. Chief, Section of Uroradiology, Department of Radiology, Hospital of the University of Pennsylvania, Philadelphia.
IMAGING OF THE URINARY TRACT

Jacob Rajfer, M.D.
Professor of Surgery/Urology, University of California School of Medicine, Los Angeles, California. Chief, Division of Urology, Harbor–UCLA Medical Center, Los Angeles.
CONGENITAL ANOMALIES OF THE TESTIS

R. Beverly Raney, M.D.
Professor and Chairman, Department of Clinical Pediatrics, Non-Neuro Solid Tumor Section, M.D. Anderson Cancer Center, Houston, Texas. Deputy Head, Division of Pediatrics, M.D. Anderson Cancer Center, Houston.
PEDIATRIC ONCOLOGY

Shlomo Raz, M.D.
Professor of Surgery/Urology, Center for Health Sciences, University of California School of Medicine, Los Angeles, California.
FEMALE UROLOGY

Claude Reitelman, M.D.
Assistant Professor of Urology, Wayne State University School of Medicine, Detroit, Michigan. Associate Attending Physician, Department of Pediatric Urology, Children's Hospital of Michigan, Detroit.
SURGICAL MANAGEMENT OF INTERSEXUALITY

Martin I. Resnick, M.D.
Lester Persky Professor of Urology, Case Western Reserve University School of Medicine, Cleveland, Ohio. Director of Urology, University Hospitals of Cleveland; and Attending Urologist, Veterans Administration Medical Center, Cleveland.
EXTRINSIC OBSTRUCTION OF THE URETER

Neil M. Resnick, M.D.
Assistant Professor of Medicine, Harvard Medical School, Boston, Massachusetts. Chief of Geriatrics and Director of the Continence Center, Brigham and Women's Hospital; and Geriatric Research and Education Clinical Center, Brockton/West Roxbury Veterans Administration Medical Center, Boston.
EVALUATION AND MEDICAL MANAGEMENT OF
    URINARY INCONTINENCE

Alan B. Retik, M.D.
Professor of Surgery (Urology), Harvard Medical School, Boston, Massachusetts. Chief, Division of Urology, Children's Hospital, Boston.
ANOMALIES OF THE UPPER URINARY TRACT
PRENATAL AND POSTNATAL DIAGNOSIS AND
    MANAGEMENT OF CONGENITAL ABNORMALITIES
ECTOPIC URETER AND URETEROCELE

Jerome P. Richie, M.D.
Elliott C. Cutler Professor of Urologic Surgery, Harvard Medical School, Boston, Massachusetts. Chairman, Harvard Program in Urology (Longwood area); and Chief of Urology, Brigham and Women's Hospital, Boston.
NEOPLASMS OF THE TESTIS

Christopher M. Rigsby, M.D.
Attending Radiologist, Fairfax Hospital, Falls Church, Virginia.
IMAGING OF THE URINARY TRACT:
    ULTRASONOGRAPHY OF THE URINARY TRACT

Richard C. Rink, M.D.
Associate Professor of Urology, Indiana University School of Medicine, Indianapolis, Indiana. Chief, Pediatric Urology, James Whitcomb Riley Hospital for Children, Indianapolis.
AUGMENTATION CYSTOPLASTY IMPLANTATION OF
    ARTIFICIAL URINARY SPHINCTER IN MEN AND
    WOMEN AND RECONSTRUCTION OF THE
    DYSFUNCTIONAL URINARY TRACT

Roberto Romero, M.D.
Associate Professor, and Director of Perinatal Research, Department of Obstetrics and Gynecology, Yale University Medical School, New Haven, Connecticut.
IMAGING OF THE URINARY TRACT:
    ULTRASONOGRAPHY OF THE URINARY TRACT

Arthur T. Rosenfield, M.D.
Professor of Diagnostic Radiology and Surgery (Urology), Yale University School of Medicine, New Haven, Connecticut. Attending Radiologist, and Director of Computed Tomography, Yale–New Haven Hospital, New Haven.
IMAGING OF THE URINARY TRACT:
    ULTRASONOGRAPHY OF THE URINARY TRACT

Daniel B. Rukstalis, M.D.
Instructor in Surgery, University of Chicago Medical School, and University of Chicago Hospital, Chicago, Illinois.
GENETIC DETERMINANTS OF UROLOGIC DISEASE

Arthur I. Sagalowsky, M.D.
Professor of Urology, University of Texas Southwestern Medical School, Dallas, Texas. Attending Physician, Parkland Memorial Hospital, Baylor University Medical Center, Veterans Administration Medical Center, and Zale Lipshy University Hospital, Dallas.
GENITOURINARY TRAUMA

Peter T. Scardino, M.D.
Russell and Mary Hugh Scott Professor and Chairman, Scott Department of Urology, Baylor College of Medicine, Houston, Texas. Chief of Urology Service, The Methodist Hospital and Harris County Hospital District, Houston.
UROLOGIC ULTRASONOGRAPHY

Anthony J. Schaeffer, M.D.
Professor and Chairman, Department of Urology, Northwestern University Medical School, Chicago, Illinois. Attending Physician, Northwestern Memorial Hospital, Children's Memorial Hospital, and Veterans Administration Lakeside Hospital, Chicago.
INFECTIONS OF THE URINARY TRACT
OTHER RENAL DISEASE OF UROLOGIC SIGNIFICANCE

Paul F. Schellhammer, M.D.
Professor and Chairman, Department of Urology, Eastern Virginia Medical School, Norfolk, Virginia. Attending Physician, Sentara Hospitals, Norfolk General and Leigh Memorial, The Children's Hospital of the King's Daughters, and DePaul Medical Center, Norfolk.
TUMORS OF THE PENIS

Peter N. Schlegel, M.D.
Assistant Professor of Surgery (Urology), Cornell University Medical College, New York, New York. Staff Scientist, The Population Council, Center for Biomedical Research, New York. Assistant Attending Surgeon, The New York Hospital, New York.
PHYSIOLOGY OF MALE REPRODUCTION: THE TESTIS,
    EPIDIDYMIS, AND DUCTUS DEFERENS

Steven M. Schlossberg, M.D.
Associate Professor, Departments of Urology and Anatomy, Eastern Virginia Medical School, Norfolk, Virginia. Attending Physician, Sentara Hospitals, Norfolk General and Leigh Memorial, The Children's Hospital of the King's Daughters, and DePaul Medical Center, Norfolk.
TUMORS OF THE PENIS
SURGERY OF THE PENIS AND URETHRA

Robert W. Schrier, M.D.
Professor and Chairman, Department of Medicine, University of Colorado School of Medicine, Denver, Colorado. Chief, Renal Division, University Hospital at the University of Colorado Health Sciences Center, Denver.
ETIOLOGY, PATHOGENESIS, AND MANAGEMENT OF RENAL FAILURE

Joseph W. Segura, M.D.
Carl Rosen Professor of Urology, Mayo Medical School, Mayo Clinic, Rochester, Minnesota. Staff Consultant, St. Mary's Hospital and Rochester Methodist Hospital, Rochester.
PERCUTANEOUS MANAGEMENT

Ridwan Shabsigh, M.D.
Assistant Professor of Urology, Department of Urology, Columbia University, New York, New York. Attending Physician, Columbia–Presbyterian Hospital, New York.
UROLOGIC ULTRASONOGRAPHY

Joseph I. Shapiro, M.D.
Assistant Professor of Medicine and Radiology, University of Colorado School of Medicine, Denver, Colorado. Co-Director, NMR Spectroscopy, and Director, Chronic Dialysis, University Hospital at the University of Colorado Health Sciences Center, Denver.
ETIOLOGY, PATHOGENESIS, AND MANAGEMENT OF RENAL FAILURE

Linda M. Dairiki Shortliffe, M.D.
Associate Professor of Urology, Stanford University School of Medicine, Stanford, California. Chief of Pediatric Urology, Lucile Salter Packard Children's Hospital at Stanford.
URINARY TRACT INFECTIONS IN INFANTS AND CHILDREN

Mark Sigman, M.D.
Assistant Professor of Urology, Division of Urology, Brown University, Providence, Rhode Island. Staff Urologist, Rhode Island Hospital and Veterans Administration Hospital, Providence.
MALE INFERTILITY

Donald G. Skinner, M.D.
Professor and Chairman, Department of Urology, University of Southern California, Los Angeles, California. Chief of Surgery and Urology, Kenneth Norris Jr. Cancer Hospital; and Chairman, Department of Urology, USC/LAC Medical Center, Los Angeles.
SURGERY OF TESTICULAR NEOPLASMS

Eila C. Skinner, M.D.
Assistant Professor of Urology, University of Southern California, Los Angeles, California. Provisional Staff Physician, Norris Cancer Hospital and Hospital of Good Samaritan, Los Angeles.
SURGERY OF TESTICULAR NEOPLASMS

Jerome Hazen Smith, M.D.
Professor of Pathology, University of Texas Medical Branch, Galveston, Texas. Attending Physician, University of Texas Medical Branch Hospitals, Galveston.
PARASITIC DISEASES OF THE GENITOURINARY SYSTEM

Joseph A. Smith, Jr., M.D.
Professor and Chairman, Department of Urology, Vanderbilt University, Nashville, Tennessee. Chief of Urologic Surgery, Vanderbilt University Hospital, Nashville.
UROLOGIC LASER SURGERY

M. J. Vernon Smith, M.D., Ph.D.
Professor of Urology, Medical College of Virginia, Virginia Commonwealth University, Richmond, Virginia.
SURGERY OF THE URETER

Howard M. Snyder III, M.D.
Associate Professor of Urology, Department of Surgery, University of Pennsylvania School of Medicine, Philadelphia, Pennsylvania. Associate Director, Division of Pediatric Urology, Children's Hospital of Philadelphia, Philadelphia.
PEDIATRIC ONCOLOGY

R. Ernest Sosa, M.D.
Assistant Professor of Surgery, Division of Urology, Cornell University Medical College, New York, New York. Assistant Attending Surgeon, New York Hospital–Cornell Medical Center, New York.
RENOVASCULAR HYPERTENSION

Thomas A. Stamey, M.D.
Professor and Chairman, Department of Urology, Stanford University School of Medicine, Stanford, California.
ADENOCARCINOMA OF THE PROSTATE
URINARY INCONTINENCE IN THE FEMALE: THE STAMEY ENDOSCOPIC SUSPENSION OF THE VESICAL NECK FOR STRESS URINARY INCONTINENCE

William D. Steers, M.D.
Assistant Professor of Urology, University of Virginia Health Science Center, Charlottesville, Virginia. Attending Physician, University of Virginia Hospital, Charlottesville.
PHYSIOLOGY OF THE URINARY BLADDER

Stevan B. Streem, M.D.
Head, Section of Stone Disease and Endourology, Department of Urology, Cleveland Clinic Foundation, Cleveland, Ohio.
SURGERY OF THE KIDNEY

Ray E. Stutzman, M.D.
Associate Professor of Urology, The Johns Hopkins University School of Medicine, Baltimore, Maryland.

Staff Physician, The Johns Hopkins Hospital; and Chief of Urology, Francis Scott Key Medical Center, Baltimore.
SUPRAPUBIC AND RETROPUBIC PROSTATECTOMY

Ronald S. Swerdloff, M.D.
Professor of Medicine, University of California School of Medicine, Los Angeles, California. Chief, Division of Endocrinology, Harbor–UCLA Medical Center, Los Angeles.
PHYSIOLOGY OF MALE REPRODUCTION:
HYPOTHALAMIC-PITUITARY FUNCTION

Emil A. Tanagho, M.D.
Professor and Chairman, Department of Urology, University of California School of Medicine, San Francisco, California.
SURGICAL ANATOMY OF THE GENITOURINARY
TRACT: ANATOMY OF THE LOWER URINARY TRACT

E. Darracott Vaughan, Jr., M.D.
James J. Colt Professor of Urology, Cornell University Medical College, New York, New York. Urologist-in-Chief, The New York Hospital–Cornell Medical Center, New York.
NORMAL RENAL PHYSIOLOGY
RENOVASCULAR HYPERTENSION
THE ADRENALS

Franz von Lichtenberg, M.D.
Professor of Pathology, Harvard Medical School, Boston, Massachusetts. Pathologist, Peter Bent Brigham Hospital, Boston.
PARASITIC DISEASES OF THE GENITOURINARY
SYSTEM

Patrick C. Walsh, M.D.
David Hall McConnell Professor, The Johns Hopkins University School of Medicine, Baltimore, Maryland. Urologist-in-Chief, Brady Urological Institute, The Johns Hopkins Hospital, Baltimore.
BENIGN PROSTATIC HYPERPLASIA
SUPRAPUBIC AND RETROPUBIC PROSTATECTOMY
RADICAL RETROPUBIC PROSTATECTOMY

Christina Wang, M.D.
Professor of Medicine, University of California Medical Center, Los Angeles, California. Director of Andrology, Division of Endocrinology/Metabolism and Division of Reproductive Endocrinology/Infertility, Cedars–Sinai Medical Center, Los Angeles.
PHYSIOLOGY OF MALE REPRODUCTION:
HYPOTHALAMIC-PITUITARY FUNCTION

Alan J. Wein, M.D.
Professor and Chairman, Division of Urology, University of Pennsylvania School of Medicine, Philadelphia, Pennsylvania. Chief of Urology, Hospital of the University of Pennsylvania, Philadelphia.
NEUROMUSCULAR DYSFUNCTION OF THE LOWER
URINARY TRACT

Robert M. Weiss, M.D.
Professor and Chief, Section of Urology, Yale University School of Medicine, New Haven, Connecticut. Professor and Chief, Section of Urology, Yale–New Haven Hospital, New Haven.
PHYSIOLOGY AND PHARMACOLOGY OF THE RENAL
PELVIS AND URETER

Richard D. Williams, M.D.
Professor and Head, Department of Urology, University of Iowa, Iowa City, Iowa. Chief of Urology, University of Iowa Hospitals and Clinics; and Consultant, Iowa City Veterans Affairs Medical Center, Iowa City.
SURGERY OF THE SEMINAL VESICLES

Jean D. Wilson, M.D.
Professor of Internal Medicine, University of Texas Southwestern Medical Center, Dallas, Texas. Attending Physician, Parkland Memorial Hospital, Dallas.
EMBRYOLOGY OF THE GENITAL TRACT
DISORDERS OF SEXUAL DIFFERENTIATION

Gilbert J. Wise, M.D.
Clinical Professor, Department of Urology, State University of New York Health Science Center, Brooklyn, New York. Director, Division of Urology, Maimonides Medical Center, Brooklyn.
FUNGAL INFECTIONS OF THE URINARY TRACT

John R. Woodard, M.D.
Clinical Professor of Surgery (Urology) and Director of Pediatric Urology, Emory University School of Medicine, Atlanta, Georgia. Chief, Urology Section, Egleston Hospital for Children at Emory University; Attending Physician, Scottish Rite Children's Medical Center, Atlanta.
NEONATAL AND PERINATAL EMERGENCIES
PRUNE-BELLY SYNDROME

Subbarao V. Yalla, M.D.
Associate Professor of Surgery (Urology), Harvard Medical School, Boston, Massachusetts. Chief of Urology, Brockton/West Roxbury Medical Center of Veterans Affairs; and Associate Surgeon, Brigham and Women's Hospital, Boston.
EVALUATION AND MEDICAL MANAGEMENT OF
URINARY INCONTINENCE

PREFACE

In the six years that have elapsed since the last edition was published, the field of urology has undergone a major transformation. Today, advances in basic science, pharmacology, diagnostic imaging, instrumentation, and surgical technique have expanded the field and added to the complexity of patient management. In response to these changes, the Sixth Edition of *Campbell's Urology* has been expanded and rewritten. The authors of each chapter were challenged to take a scholarly, encyclopedic approach to each topic rather than provide merely a personal viewpoint. In doing so, we hope to maintain the reputation of this book as "the bible of urology." Also, to keep pace with these rapid advances in the future, an "Update" series is planned. These Updates will complement *Campbell's Urology* and will cover the latest advances in urology. This will enable the reader to maintain a contemporary grasp of the field until the next edition is published.

More than half of the three-volume Sixth Edition is new, with 22 new chapters and 27 new contributors. To provide a completely fresh approach to all topics, there are two new editors: Dr. Alan B. Retik, Professor and Chairman of Pediatric Urology, Boston Children's Hospital and Harvard Medical School; and Dr. E. Darracott Vaughan, Jr., Professor and Chairman of Urology, Cornell Medical Center, The New York Hospital.

The Sixth Edition begins with a new chapter, "Surgical Anatomy of the Genitourinary Tract," complete with full-page color illustrations of the gross anatomy correlated with cross-sections of whole body tomography. The topic of renal physiology has been expanded by the addition of two new chapters: "Renal Endocrinology" and "Renal Function in the Fetus and Neonate." Recognizing the importance of office ultrasound procedures, we have added a new chapter, "Urologic Ultrasonography." The coverage of male sexual dysfunction has been expanded by the development of two new chapters: "Physiology of Erection and Pathophysiology of Impotence" and "Diagnosis and Therapy of Erectile Dysfunction." These two chapters complement one another and provide a comprehensive approach to the understanding of male sexual dysfunction, its pathophysiology, and its management. Similarly, because of increased interest in female urology, we have also added two new chapters: "Evaluation and Medical Management of Urinary Incontinence" and "Female Urology."

The section on pediatric urology has been expanded to include "Prenatal and Postnatal Diagnosis and Management of Congenital Abnormalities," "Posterior Urethral Valves and Other Urethral Anomalies," "Congenital Anomalies of the Genitalia," and "Surgery of the Scrotum and Testis in Childhood." The topic of renal calculus disease and related disorders is described in separate chapters: "Extracorporeal Shock Wave Lithotripsy," "Percutaneous Management," "Ureteroscopy," and "Endosurgical Techniques for the Diagnosis and Treatment of Noncalculous Disease of the Ureter and Kidney."

Recognizing the expanded role of reconstruction of the lower urinary tract in urology, we have created three new complementary chapters: "Use of Intestinal Segments in the Urinary Tract: Basic Principles"; "Augmentation Cystoplasty Implantation of Artificial Sphincter in Men and Women and Reconstruction of the Dysfunctional Urinary Tract"; and "Urinary Diversion," with a major emphasis on continent urinary diversion. In addition, we have added new chapters on laser surgery and the surgery of male infertility.

We wish to thank the editors and authors of prior editions, since this new edition has been built upon the solid foundation they laid. Our gratitude is greatest for the contingent of contributing authors who collectively represent the best scientists and clinicians associated with the field of urology. A work of this scope and magnitude cannot be accomplished without the assistance of a great number of persons whose effort may not be specifically attributed within this book. Specifically, we wish to express our thanks to Martin J. Wonsiewicz, William J. Lamsback, Rosanne Hallowell, Carolyn Naylor, Carol Robins, Mary Anne Folcher, Walter Verbitski, Maureen Sweeney, and the staff of the W. B. Saunders Company for their patience and help in bringing this ambitious undertaking to publication.

PATRICK C. WALSH
For the Editors

CONTENTS

VI
SEXUAL FUNCTION

16
PHYSIOLOGY OF ERECTION AND PATHOPHYSIOLOGY OF IMPOTENCE
Tom F. Lue, M.D.

VII
INFECTIONS AND INFLAMMATION OF THE GENITOURINARY TRACT

17
INFECTIONS OF THE URINARY TRACT
Anthony J. Schaeffer, M.D.

21

PARASITIC DISEASES OF THE GENITOURINARY SYSTEM 883

Jerome Hazen Smith, M.D., Franz von Lichtenberg, M.D.
and Jay Stauffer Lehman, M.D.

22

FUNGAL INFECTIONS OF THE URINARY TRACT 928

Gilbert J. Wise, M.D.

23

GENITOURINARY TUBERCULOSIS 951

James G. Gow, M.D.

33

RENAL FUNCTION IN THE FETUS AND NEONATE 1344
Robert L. Chevalier, M.D. and James Mandell, M.D.

34

ANOMALIES OF THE UPPER URINARY TRACT 1357
Stuart B. Bauer, M.D., Alan D. Perlmutter, M.D. and Alan B. Retik, M.D.

35

RENAL DYSPLASIA AND CYSTIC DISEASE OF THE KIDNEY 1443
Kenneth I. Glassberg, M.D.

Volume 3

XIII
URINARY LITHIASIS 2083

62

ENDOSURGICAL TECHNIQUES FOR THE DIAGNOSIS AND TREATMENT OF NONCALCULOUS DISEASE OF THE URETER AND KIDNEY

Ralph V. Clayman, M.D. and Louis R. Kavoussi, M.D.

XIV

UROLOGIC SURGERY

63

PERIOPERATIVE CARE

Charles B. Brendler, M.D.

67
RENOVASCULAR SURGERY 2521
John A. Libertino, M.D.

68
SURGERY OF THE URETER 2552
Alexander Greenstein, M.D., M. J. Vernon Smith, M.D., Ph.D.
and Warren W. Koontz, Jr., M.D.

69
GENITOURINARY TRAUMA 2571
Paul C. Peters, M.D. and Arthur I. Sagalowsky, M.D.

70

USE OF INTESTINAL SEGMENTS IN THE URINARY TRACT: BASIC PRINCIPLES
W. Scott McDougal, M.D.

71

AUGMENTATION CYSTOPLASTY IMPLANTATION OF ARTIFICIAL URINARY SPHINCTER IN MEN AND WOMEN AND RECONSTRUCTION OF THE DYSFUNCTIONAL URINARY TRACT
Michael E. Mitchell, M.D., Richard C. Rink, M.D. and Mark C. Adams, M.D.

72

URINARY DIVERSION
Mitchell C. Benson, M.D. and Carl A. Olsson, M.D.

73

URINARY UNDIVERSION: REFUNCTIONALIZATION OF THE PREVIOUSLY DIVERTED URINARY TRACT

W. Hardy Hendren, M.D.

74

OPEN BLADDER SURGERY

Fuad S. Freiha, M.D.

IX
TUMORS OF THE GENITOURINARY TRACT IN THE ADULT

26
OVERVIEW OF CANCER BIOLOGY AND PRINCIPLES OF ONCOLOGY

William R. Fair, M.D.
Warren D. W. Heston, Ph.D.

Cancerous cells reflect a broad spectrum of altered biologic behavior relative to their cell of origin. In the least, this alteration is barely discernible. In the extreme, the anaplastic cell no longer possesses distinguishing features that allow one to characterize its tissue of origin. In the steady-state maintenance of normal adult tissue, there is an invariant routine of stem cell division, differentiation, and cell death so that the tissue is maintained at a fairly constant mass and configuration. This steady state is the result of a complex interplay of extracellular signals and intracellular signal transduction, and the response of the genomic DNA to these signals. The final arbiter of interpretation and response to these signals is the genomic DNA itself. In normal somatic cells this is a constant. The DNA of cancer cells is unstable, and any chromosomal alterations tend to accumulate and become more frequent. This effect leads to abnormal responses to intracellular and extracellular signals and to tumor progression from a well-differentiated to an anaplastic state (Heim et al., 1988; Pienta et al., 1989; Pierce and Speers, 1988).

TUMOR CELL GROWTH

Stem Cell Concept

A stem cell is defined operationally as a cell that has the characteristics of the extended capacity for self-renewal and the capacity to mature into one or more differentiated forms (Buick, 1986; Hall, 1989; Mauch et al., 1989; Pierce and Speers, 1988). The classic example of a stem cell population is the bone marrow with the pluripotent hematopoietic stem cell. This represents the most primitive cell within the normal tissue and can reproduce itself as well as provide for the generation of differentiated cell populations. Thus, the pluripotent progenitor can not only reproduce itself but can also form all the differentiated blood cellular elements of red blood cell, platelets, eosinophils, macrophages, granulocytes, T and B lymphocytes, and so forth. The number of pluripotent hematopoietic stem cells can be approximated by bioassays. Different numbers of bone marrow cells are injected into lethally irradiated animals, and the number of hematologic colonies found in the spleen is used to approximate the number of progenitor cells (Till and McCulloch, 1967). Similarly, the cells can be plated in agar in Petri dishes and the number of colony-forming units per number of cells plated, can be used to determine the number of stem cells. The number of stem cells determined is often quite low—one stem cell per 10^4 bone marrow cells (Hall and Watt, 1989). These assays also make it possible to purify growth factors that specifically stimulate the pathways of stem cell differentiation, resulting in agents such as erythropoietin (EPO), granulocyte growth factor (G-CSF), and granulocyte-macrophage colony stimulating factor (GM-CSF). These are genetically cloned, produced, and made available in pharmaceutic quantities.

T and B cells are committed cells, not stem cells, yet they can be maintained and their numbers increased by specific growth factors. This characteristic has led to the speculation that given the right growth factors, any cell can be made to reproduce. However, some cells are committed to terminal differentiation. The maturing red blood cell will eventually produce principally hemoglobin and shed its nucleus, becoming incapable of reproduction. In these terminal cells, the changes associated with differentiated phenotypes are not reversible.

Tumor Stem Cells

Tumor stem cells are the subset of tumor cells responsible for repopulating the tumor following therapy (Steel, 1977). Tumor stem cells can be considered to be developmentally based in the tissue cell of origin in which they arose. Therefore, kidney tumor stem cells are derived from the proximal tubular cells, bladder carcinomas from the basal cells, prostatic carcinoma cells from the region of the end buds of the terminal ducts of the outer region of the prostate, and testicular carcinomas from the germinal epithelium.

Three theories regarding the origin of tumors from differentiating tissue are depicted in Figure 26–1. In the first theory, the initiating event, the carcinogenic insult, renders the cell proliferative, although it might maintain its ability to produce differentiated features. If this occurs in a totally differentiated cell, it requires an assumption of *de-differentiation*. A second theory proposes the process of transformation at various stages of differentiation but with terminal differentiation blocked. The third theory requires that the transforming event (initiation) occur in the stem cell. In this group there is no need to explain proliferation. It is necessary only to explain the relationship among the initiating event, the subsequent loss of growth control, and the reduced ability to terminally differentiate. Evidence of the pluripotent nature of the tumor stem cell is provided by the observation that a single human colonic adenocarcinoma cell can differentiate into columnar, goblet, and enteroendocrine cells in culture (Kirkland, 1988). The altered ability to differentiate can be viewed as a spectrum, with greater DNA damage associated with a lesser capacity to terminally differentiate. In many cases, the tumors resemble the tissue of origin and immunohisto-chemically display many of the antigens of the normal tissue (Buick, 1986; Hall and Watt, 1989; Pierce and Speers, 1988).

Tumor stem cells can also be viewed as developmentally blocked so that markers associated with division of the precursor cell, such as transferrin receptor or epidermal growth factor receptor (EGFr), are maintained or increased as a result of the fact that most cells do not proceed to differentiate. Expansion of the precursor/stem cell population leads to increases in phenotypic markers. Consequently, markers or differentiated cells, such as prostatic acid phosphatase or prostate-specific antigen (PSA), decrease. The concept that the tumor represents a defect in differentiation is supported by the observation that teratocarcinoma cells implanted into a developing embryo can undergo differentiation and behave as normal cells (Illmensee and Mintz, 1976).

Assays of Tumor Stem Cells

Cells may be separated based on cell density; the different populations may be examined for their ability to form colonies in soft agar, because many normal cells do not grow in soft agar (Hall and Watt, 1989). Some cells were able to form very large colonies resulting from many rounds of division, whereas other cells formed only small colonies (Hall and Watt, 1989). This finding suggests that the smaller colonies arose from committed cells with limited reproductive capacity and that the larger colonies arose from true stem cells with unlimited reproductive capacity.

A number of assays approximate the stem cell population of a tumor. Growth in semisolid agar is one method. A unique feature of tumor cells is that if they

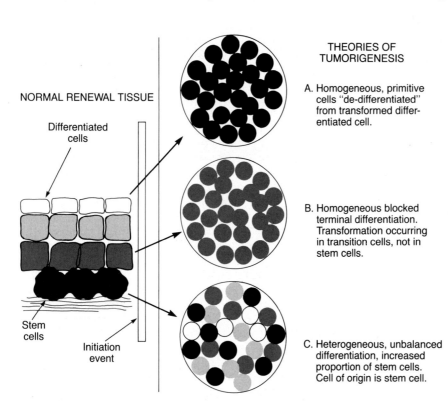

THEORIES OF
TUMORIGENESIS

A. Homogeneous, primitive cells "de-differentiated" from transformed differentiated cell.

B. Homogeneous blocked terminal differentiation. Transformation occurring in transition cells, not in stem cells.

C. Heterogeneous, unbalanced differentiation, increased proportion of stem cells. Cell of origin is stem cell.

NORMAL RENEWAL TISSUE

Differentiated cells

Stem cells

Initiation event

Figure 26–1. Normal tissue renewal involves the progressive maturation of cells from stem cells to transitional cells to terminally differentiated cells. Tumor initiation may occur in each area. The results of the transformation event occurring in each of the different cell types are depicted.

are transplanted into a suitable host they will grow, whereas normal cells will not grow. In tumor models, such as L1210 leukemia, it takes the transplantation of only a single tumor cell for the animal to develop a tumor and die. Thus, in the L1210 leukemia model system, every tumor cell is a tumor stem cell. In most solid tumors, true "stem cells" constitute a small percentage of the total tumor cell population. Because the number of cells required to form a tumor is often used as an indicator of the number of tumor stem cells present within the tumor, one technique to determine stem cell number is to implant different numbers of tumor cells and calculate the number of tumor cells required to achieve tumor growth ("take") in 50 per cent of the implanted animals. This technique is referred to as the limiting dilution assay. Within the region of cell concentrations achieving 1 to 99 per cent takes, the number of tumor stem cells can be calculated based on Poisson distribution.

Tumor Stem Cell Assay: An Example of The Effect of Androgen Withdrawal on Tumor Stem Cell Content

The limiting dilution assay was used to demonstrate the relative hormonal sensitivity of malignant cells and the effect of castration on the stem cell population by Bruchovsky and colleagues (1990), with the androgen-dependent mammary tumor line. In *androgen-dependent* tumors, androgen withdrawal leads to the death of the tumor cell. Conversely, *androgen-sensitive* tumors do not die in the absence of androgen, but androgens stimulate their growth. *Androgen-insensitive* cells are unaffected by androgen levels.

These investigators transplanted the tumor into nude mice and found a normal growth pattern, with the average tumor attaining the weight of approximately 6 g, 20 days after transplantation. Following castration, the tumor lost approximately 90 per cent of its total weight and reached a nadir on approximately day 35. After a short dormant period, the remaining cells again started to grow and by day 80 approximated the tumor weight prior to castration (Fig. 26–2). In an elegant set of experiments, these investigators took cells from the parent tumor (the rapidly growing tumor prior to castration) and from the "castrate" tumor (at the time of maximum tumor regression following orchiectomy) and they sampled the cell population from the "recurrent" tumor (at the time when the tumor weight approximated the weight of the parent tumor). The stem cell ratios were then calculated in each population by determining the number of tumors that developed compared with the number of cells inoculated into the animal.

Using this ingenious in vivo clonogenic assay, these workers calculated that in the male host, one new tumor developed per 4000 cells inoculated, but it took almost 100 times more cells to develop a single tumor take in a female host, indicating the marked effect of hormonal manipulation in the cells derived from the parent tumor (Table 26–1). When the cells from the recurrent tumor, which grew following castration, were injected there was

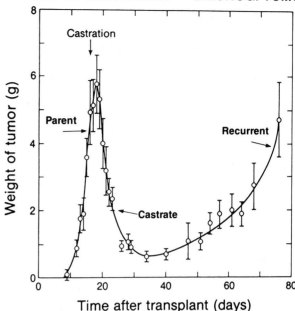

EFFECT OF CASTRATION — SHIONOGI TUMOR

Figure 26–2. Experimental system for obtaining tumor tissue for stem cell quantitation before castration (parent), following castration during tumor regression (castrate), and during tumor regrowth (recurrent). (Adapted from Bruchovsky, N., Rennie, P. S., Coldman, A. J., Goldenberg, J. L., To, M., and Lawson, D.: Cancer Res. 50:2275–2287, 1990.)

a marked enrichment of the stem cell ratio. Injecting the recurrent cells into the male host resulted in one tumor take per 200 cells inoculated and in the female host one per 800 cells.

Despite the enrichment of the stem cell population in both the male and female hosts, the hormonal sensitivity (the increased propensity for the tumor to develop in the male host) was evident. It required four times more cells to develop a tumor in the female host as opposed to the male host using this population of cells that grew following castration and that, presumably, were androgen "resistant."

The greatest stem cell ratios occurred utilizing the cell population obtained at the time of maximum tumor regression. In these cells, which were obtained 7 days following castration, it took approximately 70,000 cells to form a single tumor when injected into the male host and 2,200,000 cells to form a single tumor when cells from the same population were injected into the female host. These data show a marked depletion of the stem

Table 26–1. HORMONAL INFLUENCE ON THE CLONOGENIC CELL CONTENT OF THE SHIONOGI ANDROGEN-DEPENDENT TUMOR

	Tumor Stem Cell Content	
Tumor Growth Status	*Males*	*Females*
Parent	1 per 4000	1 per 370,000
Castrate	1 per 70,000	1 per 2,200,000
Recurrent	1 per 200	1 per 800

cell population 7 days following castration at the time of maximum tumor regression. Thus, if one were planning additional therapy to augment hormonal manipulation, it seems reasonable that the ideal time to administer the therapy is when the ratio of stem cells to all cells is at its lowest level. The results also indicate that despite injecting cells obtained after castration and at the time of maximum tumor regression, there was a 30-fold difference in tumor cell take in the male host compared with the female host. This reflects a sex hormone sensitivity is still present and indicates the relative nature of the terms hormone sensitive and hormone resistant.

In summary, these animal studies revealed the following:

1. Not every tumor cell can produce a tumor, that is, not every cell is a stem cell.

2. The hormonal milieu is important, and thus the terms hormone sensitive and resistant should be considered relative terms indicating the differential growth in environments containing androgens or estrogens.

3. Hormone "resistant" cells surviving after castration still show differential growth when exposed to androgens or estrogens, indicating that the hormone resistance is relative.

4. The "recurrent" tumor, that is, the tumor occurring following castration, appears to be the more aggressive tumor with the highest percentage of stem cells noted. The clinical parallel to this observation would be the apparent increased aggressiveness of prostate cancer recurring following castration or estrogen treatment.

5. The lowest stem cell ratio was observed at the time of maximal regression following castration. Hence, theoretically, this would be the optimal time when surgical extirpation of the residual tumor is most likely to be effective in removing all the remaining stem cells.

Although this experiment is an example of the effect of hormonal manipulation, other effects can be similarly studied following chemotherapy or radiation therapy. The maximum effect of hormone deprivation (castrate population in the female) represents a decrease in stem cells of nearly 99.9 per cent and may be thought of as reasonable monotherapy, considering the minimal toxicity. However, unless all stem cells are eradicated, tumor regrowth is likely. Also, if the stem cell is responsible for tumor regrowth and if only the stem cell represents the true reproductive component of the tumor, one does not have to kill every tumor cell to eradicate the tumor, just eliminate the tumor stem cell. If the tumor stem cell theory is correct, we need to be able to identify and destroy the tumor stem cell. The limiting dilution assay is one of many assays designed to address the issue of determining the number of stem cells in a tumor. Tumor cells can also be administered intravenously and the number of lung colonies determined. An in vitro assay is performed by dispersing a tumor into single cells, plated in soft agar in tissue culture dishes. After incubation, the number of colonies is determined. In examining a variety of primary human solid tumors for the number of stem cells, it was found by clonogenic assay that the number was in the range

of one per 10,000 to 100,000 cells (Fleischmann et al., 1984).

The role of other factors in determining the apparent stem cell population can be dramatic. Revesz (1958) observed that mixing other cells that could not form tumors with the tumor cells made the viable tumor cells grow more frequently and kill the host more quickly. Many factors are thought to play a role in the Revesz phenomenon, such as growth factor production by the passenger cells, or to provide a means to maximally retain the implanted cells. The finding demonstrates the need for caution in the interpretation of stem cell assays and the need to consider every tumor cell as potentially lethal.

The stem cell concept has led to an attempt to predict which drugs will be useful in the treatment of a patient's malignancy, the development of methods to circumvent resistance, the assessment of tumor stem cell number as an indicator of a patient's prognosis, the development of new agents, and the determination of the impact of stem cell number on curability. These efforts have had varying degrees of success because of the limitations in our understanding of the optimal methods for mimicking in vivo growth conditions.

PROLIFERATION AND CELL CYCLE KINETICS

A major feature of the stem cell is its ability to proliferate. Many investigations have centered on tumor cell proliferation as a prognosticator of malignant potential and therapeutic opportunity. Studies of cell proliferation were greatly enhanced by the development of radiolabeled derivatives of thymidine. This method enables by autoradiographic means the detection of cells that had incorporated the label into their DNA. Mitosis can be determined by visualization of the condensed chromosomes at metaphase and anaphase. This visualization allowed the division of cells into four phases (Fig. 26–3). G_1 is a gap between mitosis and DNA synthesis; S is the period of incorporation of radiolabeled thymidine or thymidine analogue in DNA synthesis; G_2 is the gap between the S phase and mitosis; and M is the phases of mitosis. This cycle can be viewed as a clock or cell history in that it moves only one way once the cell commits to division. It proceeds through S, G_2, and M and produces two daughter cells. Differences occur in the duration of time spent in the phases of S, G_2, and M, but the greatest difference in time is in G_1. Some workers have suggested that cells can leave the cell cycle and enter a totally quiescent period called G_0. The question of controls and regulation have focused on the G_1 phase of the cell cycle. Studies on fibroblasts have suggested that certain growth factors can make a cell competent to commit to cell cycle and others make a cell progress through the cell cycle following the commitment step (Beserga, 1990; Gouston et al., 1986; Touchette, 1990a).

Once the threshold for cell division is reached, the cell is committed to divide. The end result of the division is two cells either or both of which can further divide,

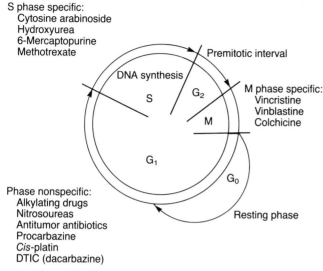

S phase specific:
Cytosine arabinoside
Hydroxyurea
6-Mercaptopurine
Methotrexate

DNA synthesis

Premitotic interval

M phase specific:
Vincristine
Vinblastine
Colchicine

Phase nonspecific:
Alkylating drugs
Nitrosoureas
Antitumor antibiotics
Procarbazine
Cis-platin
DTIC (dacarbazine)

Resting phase

Figure 26–3. The phases of the cell cycle and the cytotoxic agents that are active in the cycling cells or in the specific phases.

commit to terminal differentiation, or enter a noncycling state from which it may enter the cell cycle at a later time.

Cell Cycle Detection Methods

MITOTIC INDEX. The mitotic index is the number of mitoses as a percentage of the cells counted. It is a direct measure. The mitotic index is a reliable direct proportional indication of proliferation rate. Alison and Wright (1981) reported on the mitotic index in human prostatic adenocarcinomas of differing histopathologic type as shown in Table 26–2.

If there is no cell loss, if the cell production rate remains constant in relation to population size, and if growth is exponential, the potential doubling time (T_{pot}) is a fraction (.693) of the turnover time. Turnover time in the population or (T_t) = t_m/MI is equal to the time required to replace all of the cells (double), where t_m is the duration of mitosis and MI is the mitotic index (T_{pot} = .693 t_m/MI). Usually, the time cells spend in mitosis is 1 to 2 hours. If exponential growth is assumed, the poorly differentiated cells have a potential population doubling time of 1.6 days with no cell loss fraction (Alison and Wright, 1981; Steel, 1977). Obviously, even poorly differentiated prostatic cancer does not grow with

Table 26–2. RELATIONSHIP OF HISTOLOGIC PATTERN AND MITOTIC INDEX IN PROSTATIC CANCER

Histologic Pattern	Mitotic Index*
Well-differentiated (N = 10)	0.9 ± 0.3
Moderately Differentiated (N = 16)	2.3 ± 1.3
Poorly Differentiated (N = 28)	3.6 ± 0.8
Anaplastic (N = 4)	12.1 ± 5.5

*Determined by counting 6000 cells of similar histologic type within each tumor. Values represent mean ± SEM
Adapted from Alison, M. R., and Wright, N. A.: Growth kinetics. Recent Results Cancer Res., 78:29–43, 1981.

such a rapid doubling time. These and other data suggest a high rate of cell loss from these tumors, an observation common to most adenocarcinomas.

Although metaphase and anaphase are recognized without difficulty, prophase and telophase are not. Agents such as colchicine arrest metaphase. Such agents can be used to determine the rate at which cells accumulate in metaphase as an index of the rate of entry into mitosis, provided they have no effect on other phases of the cell cycle. This procedure is referred to as the stathmokinetic method (Alison and Wright, 1981; Steel, 1977). Fulker and co-workers (1971) used the stathmokinetic method to determine potential growth rates of bladder cancer. They obtained mitotic indices of 1.3, 4.8, and 13.1 and potential doubling times of 22, 6, and 2.2 days for well-differentiated, poorly differentiated, and undifferentiated tumors, in order. These investigators also point out that the true doubling times observed clinically are much longer, suggesting a substantial cell loss fraction.

THYMIDINE-LABELING INDEX. The thymidine-labeling index refers to the percentage of cells labeled following administration of radiolabeled thymidine. The majority of labeling studies are performed on tumors or biopsy samples by incubation. Radiolabeled thymidine is in tissue culture media in vitro to avoid the toxicity associated with giving radiolabeled thymidine to patients. The advantage of the thymidine-labeling index is that it provides another parameter to determine the potential tumor doubling time and to calculate the amount of cell loss without giving the patient a metaphase-blocking agent. If one assumes that the mitotic rate is constant in relation to the population size and that growth is therefore exponential, one can calculate the potential tumor doubling time for mitosis as follows:

$$T_{pot} = .693\ T_s/LI$$

LI is the labeling index, and T_s is the duration of S phase.

The cell loss factor can be calculated as follows:

$$\text{Cell loss factor (LF)} = K_L/K_P$$

K_L is the rate constant for cells lost per time, and K_P is the rate constant for cell production. Tumor growth is the competition between cell production and cell death (tumor growth = cell production − cell death).

Thus, the cell loss factor is related to the actual and potential doubling times by the following equation:

$$LF = 1 - T_{pot}/T_d$$

The T_d doubling time refers to the cellular doubling time, which is often less than the volume doubling time because of the tendency for acellular products of tumor growth (e.g., necrosis, keratin) to increase with greater tumor volume. In solid tumors, such as lymphomas, the thymidine-labeling index has been reported to be 3 per cent, whereas that for colorectal tumors has been reported to be 15 per cent. The cell loss factor for lymphomas is only 29 per cent, whereas that for colo-

Table 26–3. S-INDEX IN PRIMARY (Prim) AND METASTATIC (Met) UROLOGIC SOLID TUMORS

Diagnosis	Site	DNA Ploidy	Median S-index (%)
Renal CA	Prim	Diploid	5.7
	Met	Diploid	18.9
	Prim	Aneuploid	13.4
	Met	Aneuploid	19.6
Bladder	Prim	Diploid	6.9
	Met	Diploid	9.3
	Prim	Aneuploid	22.6
	Met	Aneuploid	26.5
Prostate	Prim	Diploid	6.3
		Aneuploid	11.9

Adapted from Frankfurt, O. S., Greco, W. R., Slocum, H. K., Arbuck, S. G., Gonarra, M., Pavelic, Z. P., and Rustum, Y. M.: Proliferative characteristics of primary and metastatic human solid tumors by DNA flow cytometry. Cytometry, 5:629–635, 1984.

rectal cancer is nearly 100 per cent. This finding demonstrates the difficulty of relying strictly on the apparent proliferation rate as an index for tumor growth. The importance of cell loss in urologic tumors is emphasized by the studies on the Dunning R3327G prostatic tumor (Humphries and Isaacs, 1982). Following castration, it was not proliferation that was affected but an increase in cell loss. Although studies with radiolabeled thymidine have been useful, flow cytometry can determine cell cycle parameters and can be used to evaluate the aforementioned parameters (Melamed and Staianco-Coico 1990; Raber and Barlogie, 1990). S phase has been examined in a number of urologic tumors by Frankfurt and co-workers (1984) (Table 26–3).

The labeling index determined by flow cytometry is often greater than that determined by thymidine incorporation. New methods have been developed that allow flow to be combined with bromodeoxyuridine (BrdU) incorporation; DNA synthesis is followed directly into the various normal diploid, aneuploid, and tetraploid populations (Nemoto et al., 1990). BrdU can also be given with less risk to patients than radiolabeled thymidine. Actual incorporation into the tumor, as it is available in the patient, is more readily achievable. In the study by Frankfurt's group and in other studies, it is not always possible to correlate the apparent degree of differentiation and the proliferation index. Some well-differentiated tumors can have high proliferation rates, and some poorly differentiated tumors can have low proliferation rates (Frankfurt et al., 1984). Although aneuploidy is associated with a higher proliferation rate, it does not always correlate with survival (Raber and Borlogie, 1990). In studies involving prostatic cancer patients with microscopic lymph node metastases, those with aneuploid metastatic lesions survived only half as long as those with diploid or tetraploid tumors (Stephenson et al., 1987).

Tumor Heterogeneity and Volume

The concept of a tumor stem cell is useful in theoretic discussions of tumor lineage and the impact of therapy required to eradicate the tumor. However, tumors are heterogeneous. The *genome of the transformed cell is unstable,* and *increasing changes occur with each cell division.* These changes have an impact on subsequent cell behavior. The cells become increasingly *heterogeneous,* resembling less and less the stem cell of origin or the differentiated phenotype of that cell line. The progression of a tumor to a more aggressive phenotype can be attenuated or enhanced, based on predisposing factors of the individual's genotype and exposure to environmental factors. Within a tumor, considerable heterogeneity exists. Cells are found that are resistant to cytotoxics, hormones, or radiation de novo, while the surrounding normal tissue remains uniform in its response (Goldie and Coldman, 1984; Pienta, 1988; Poste, 1983). *The likelihood of heterogeneity increases with cell division.*

It becomes more likely that cells resistant to therapy will be found with greater frequency, as the tumor size increases. Not every cell division leads to an increase in tumor size. Most tumors have a large fraction of cells dying or leaving (cell loss) the reproductive pool of cells. This cell loss requires more cell division to reach the same tumor volume as neoplasms without a large cell loss fraction. This finding may help explain the difference in resistance to cytotoxic therapy seen with many solid tumors. These tumors have undergone many more divisions to reach the same size as tumors with high growth fractions, such as testicular cancer and leukemias (Goldie and Coldman, 1984).

Tumor Cell Growth Kinetics

At the time of the initial presentation of a patient with a tumor, the clinician has little in the way of guidance to approximate the growth rate of a particular tumor. In general, some nonspecific observations, such as histologic grade, stage, and DNA ploidy status, roughly correlate with clinical progression, but the actual growth rate of an individual tumor can be approximated only by serial measurements over time. For obvious reasons, the data relative to tumor doubling times in humans is limited, but Steel (1977) in a review of 780 patients not receiving treatment observed that most common tumors have a doubling time of 2 to 4 months, although a wide variation was noted even among tumors of the same histologic type. Testicular cancer has a doubling time that approximates 1 month, whereas a slow growing tumor, such as prostate cancer, may have a doubling time longer than 12 months (Steel, 1977). A 1-g tumor mass contains approximately 1 billion (10^9) cells and occupies a volume of 1 cm^3 (Table 26–4). To the clinician, a 1-cm tumor is frequently thought of as a small "early" tumor. Yet, if one assumes that the tumor develops initially from a single malignant cell, we can calculate that it has already completed 30 cell doublings to reach 1 g (1 cm^3).

A further ten doublings (total of 40) would result in a kilogram mass (10^{12} cells), which is frequently the maximum tumor burden compatible with life. Thus, at the earliest time of clinical detection, this "small" 1-cm tumor has already completed three fourths of its life

Table 26–4. RELATIONSHIP BETWEEN TUMOR DOUBLINGS, CELL NUMBER, AND TUMOR SIZE

Tumor Doublings	Cell Number	Grams of Tumor	Detection
0	1	Nanogram	—
10	10^3	Microgram	—
20	10^6	Milligram	Microscopic
30	10^9	Gram	Palpable
40	10^{12}	Kilogram	Debilitation Death

Assumes every cell produced proliferates and no cell loss.

span, and considerable opportunity for cell heterogeneity and metastatic potential may have already occurred. To further illustrate, a human breast tumor with a doubling time of 3 months would take apparently 7½ years to reach 1 cm³, assuming an origin from a single cell. Furthermore, even assuming some slowing in the growth rate with increased size resulting in tumor vascularity and necrosis, it can reach a lethal size of approximately 1 kg in just an additional 2½ years assuming no effective treatment is administered (Tannock, 1989). This example amply illustrates the difficulty facing the clinician in that, despite the small size of a given lesion, the tumor already is "old" with respect to its overall life span. The tumor also may have already spawned distant unrecognized micrometastasis that will eventually lead to the death of the patient despite therapy that eradicates the primary tumor.

Stem Cells and Cell-Cell Interactions

Cells of solid tumors grow in an environment of other cells. They not only interact with other tumor cells but with diffusible factors from the surrounding stroma. The cells are altered in their activity by contact with basement membranes and the development of support from vascular endothelial cells. These interactions are a composite of growth stimulatory and inhibitory signals.

The importance of the stroma in cell interactions is emphasized in the investigations of Cunha and coworkers (1983, 1987). The stroma of animals with testicular feminization syndrome was responsible for the lack of development of the prostatic epithelial cells. Manipulation of the stroma and epithelium during normal development demonstrated that if neonatal stroma from the prostate is grown with neonatal bladder epithelial cells, the bladder epithelia become prostate like. If neonatal prostate epithelial cells are grown on bladder mesenchyme the prostate epithelium becomes bladder epithelium. The importance of the stroma in tumor development is emphasized by the finding that fully transformed prostatic adenocarcinoma cells are stimulated in their growth by prostatic stroma. As described for the Revesz effect, the addition of these stromata to prostatic adenocarcinoma cells implanted into the flank of animals enhances their ability to form rapidly growing tumors (Camps et al., 1990). Others have shown that prostatic cancer cells are stimulated to grow by diffusible factors produced by bone marrow stromal cells

(Chackal-Roy et al., 1989). It is expected that these are interactive systems. Indeed, in a number of carcinomas, the presence of cancer induces a change in the stroma. This is detected by the expression of new protein by the stroma, which is not normally present except during wound healing (Garin-Chesa et al., 1990).

MOLECULAR BASIS FOR TUMOR STEM CELL FORMATION: POSITIVE-ACTING ONCOGENES AND NEGATIVE-ACTING TUMOR SUPPRESSOR GENES

The molecular mechanisms of tumor initiation and progression are now understood at the level of the DNA. The process involving (1) DNA extraction from a cell, (2) precipitation with calcium phosphate, (3) introduction of the precipitated DNA into another cell, and (4) integration into and expression by the recipient cell's genome is called *transfection*. Versions of this technique have been employed to identify DNA that is *oncogenic* (it can cause the formation of tumors) or DNA that can block a tumor cell's ability to grow (antioncogene, tumor suppressor gene).

The first DNA changes identified in human tumors were also observed in retrovirus- and carcinogen-induced tumors (*ras*). This observation briefly raised the hope that one change might be responsible for malignant transformation. Such was not the case, however, because many oncogenes and suppressor genes have subsequently been identified. The common denominator is that the oncogenic changes reduce the cell's ability to suppress growth and respond to growth control signals. There are many oncogenes and tumor suppressor genes. Only a few are addressed in this chapter, but they have been reviewed in detail elsewhere (Chung et al., 1990; De Vita et al., 1989; Studzinski, 1989).

Dominant Acting Oncogenes

Ras PROTEINS. DNA extracted from human bladder carcinoma cell lines, T-24 or EJ, and transfected into nontumorigenic cells, such as the contact-inhibited Balb/c 3T3 fibroblasts, can make the fibroblast "transform" (Pulciani et al., 1982; Shih and Weinburg, 1982). The transformed cells are no longer contact inhibited and continue to grow and form discrete colonies, which can be separated and grown as clones of the transformed cells. This transfection assay was utilized to isolate tumor-genomic DNA capable of transforming cells, i.e., an *oncogene*.

To isolate and identify the oncogene from the T-24 bladder carcinoma cell line, the cells are grown on tissue culture plates. The DNA is extracted, precipitated, sheared (made smaller), and dissolved in phosphate buffer. Calcium chloride is then added, and the precipitate is added to NIH/3T3 mouse fibroblasts. The fibroblast cells are allowed to grow for 2 to 3 weeks. The cells are checked for the transformed phenotype (continue growing, not contact inhibited). The transformants are isolated and the DNA extracted, and the process is repeated. By multiple serial transfections and selection for the transformed cell phenotype, one can be confident that only the DNA fragment containing the oncogenic sequence is present. Although this DNA may contain other information adjacent to the transforming gene, the repeated transfections from the transformed NIH/3T3 cells reduce the likelihood of inclusion of nononcogenic DNA. The total cell DNA is then extracted and digested ("cut") into smaller sequence fragments with *restriction enzymes,* which have specificity for certain regions of DNA. These enzymes are isolated from bacteria, thus their names reflect their origin: *Eco*RI, *E. coli* strain RY13; *Hin*dIII, *Haemophilus influenzae* strain Rd; and so forth. These enzymes help protect the host bacteria from foreign DNA.

Following enzyme digestion, the DNA is examined for its electrophoretic migration through agarose gel that separates the DNA, based on size. The greater the number of nucleotide bases, the slower the DNA fragments move through the agarose gel. During probing for the DNA of interest, one uses a complementary fragment to the nucleotide sequence of interest: **G**uanine bonds to **C**ytosine, and **A**denine bonds to **T**hymidine (DNA) or **U**racil (RNA). Thus, if the nucleotide sequence to be probed is **GCCATAGCGAATC,** then the sequence used to probe should be **CGGTATCGCT-TAG.**

The initial problem in the identification of the T-24 oncogene was determining what sequence to use as a probe, because the oncogenic sequence was unknown. Fortunately, genomic DNA contains highly repetitive sequences scattered and interspersed throughout. This repetitive DNA differs between species so it can identify human DNA inserted into the mouse genome. Human repetitive DNA sequences are referred to as *alu* sequences. It was the *alu* sequences that were employed to probe for and aid in identifying the oncogenic transfected DNA.

When DNA sequences are being probed the procedure is referred to as *Southern* analysis after the investigator who established the method. When RNA is being probed, it is referred to as *Northern* analysis. Protein probing is called *Western* analysis. Probing is accomplished by bonding the nucleic acid of interest to a membrane, usually of nylon or nitrocellulose. The nucleic acid is eluted from the agarose gel onto the membrane. The attachment is made permanent by baking the membrane (Sambrook et al., 1989).

The probe sequence is radiolabeled to a high-specific activity with ^{32}P-nucleotide triphosphates and DNA polymerase. The radiolabeled probe is then incubated with the membrane and bonds with its complementary sequences on the membrane. The bound probe is visualized by autoradiography. The position and intensity of the signal are directly proportional to the type and amount of the nucleic acid being probed. This information can then be utilized to remove the DNA of interest for further study (Sambrook et al., 1989).

To investigate the oncogene in bladder tissue, the DNA was incorporated into a bacteriophage so that it could be grown. This increases the amount of DNA extracted. This cellular DNA (cDNA) was radiolabeled and used to probe normal nontransformed bladder cells to determine whether similar DNA sequences were present. The nontransforming DNA and the oncogenic DNA were then cut with restriction enzymes and the size of the fragments compared. If the oncogene was substantially different from the normal DNA, the restriction digests should produce different size fragments between the two types of DNA. In fact, all of the restriction fragments were the same size. This finding meant that whatever change made the difference between the normal cell DNA and the transforming oncogene had to be a very small one (Shih and Weinburg, 1982).

Indeed, the oncogenes of EJ and T-24 bladder cancer cells have both been sequenced and found to be the same as the normal cell's c-H-*ras*-1 gene except for a *single nucleic acid substitution.* A guanine had been changed to an adenine, and the 12th amino acid was changed from a glycine to a valine (Capon et al., 1983; Parada et al., 1982). These changes do not cause a major effect in the physical characteristics of the amino acid sequence. The normal cellular homologue of *ras*, p-21, is a GTP-binding protein. Its normal function is unknown.

The GTP-binding proteins often are active when they bind GTP but are inactive when the GTP is hydrolyzed to GDP. The single base pair substitution greatly reduces the GTPase activity of the c-H-*ras*-1 gene, which may result in the p-21 protein remaining in the "switched-on" position (Hall, 1990). The *ras* oncogene product, when injected into a single cell, stimulates cell division. Antibodies to *ras* co-injected into cells reduces cell division. Oncogenic *ras* causes cells to change their shape and become much more motile. When cells are transfected with normal *ras* so that the cell overexpresses the normal cellular c-H-*ras*-1 gene, they grow a little faster and may exhibit some structural alterations, but when they are injected into animal hosts they do not form tumors as their oncogenic counterparts do. In this case, an oversupply of the normal gene product is not transforming (Hall, 1990). A number of *ras*-like proteins have been identified (H-*ras*, K-*ras*, and N-*ras*). The protein products of the *ras* oncogenes are the p-21 proteins.

Current research focused on the *ras* protein has shown it to bind to the inner cytoplasmic side of plasma membrane. It is covalently bound to the fatty acids palmitate and farnesyl, the cholesterol precursors. Because *ras* activity requires a membrane location, it may be possible to block this activity by blocking the covalent attachment of palmitate or farnesyl (Gibbs, 1990; Reiss, 1990). Modifications of the p-21 proteins by different techniques have identified regions associated with transformation. In all cases, the modifications are associated with reduced GTPase activity. The *ras,* p-21 protein may not be solely responsible for these changes, because other proteins that associate with *ras* and help modify GTPase activity have also been reported (Gibbs, 1990). One of the proteins that has been found to enhance *ras* GTPase activity is called GAP (GTPase activating protein). It is been hypothesized that the *ras*/GAP complex is responsible for transformation rather than p-21 alone. This possibility has been given support with the observation that the gene that codes for the abnormal growth condition, neurofibromatosis, is a GAP-like protein (Xu, 1990).

Ras oncogenes have been reported in approximately 50 per cent of colon and 100 per cent of pancreatic cancers. Although it is the most common oncogene associated with human cancer and was originally isolated from bladder cancer cell lines, *ras* oncogenes are identified in only a small percentage of urologic malignancies (Carter, 1990; Wood et al., in press; Yao, 1988). It remains to be determined whether this represents the more aggressive aneuploid anaplastic malignancies associated with metastatic disease and decreased survival.

The expression of *ras* represents a somatic activation of the cellular oncogene by a point mutation. Other mechanisms of activation of oncogenes include rearrangements where the normal cellular gene becomes active and/or amplified (Carroll and Chiganti, 1990).

GROWTH FACTORS AND THEIR RECEPTORS.
Characteristic of a number of cancer cells is their ability to grow in tissue culture under conditions of reduced serum supplementation. This observation suggests the possibility that they may be producing their own growth factors. The growth factors are released by the tumor cell and bind to a cell surface receptor. This leads to growth of the tumor cell. This form of uncontrolled self-stimulation is referred to as *autocrine* growth (Sporn and Roberts, 1985). Two growth factors that have been isolated based on their ability to cause fibroblasts to grow in soft agar, a characteristic of transformed cells, were named *transforming growth factors,* alpha and beta, or *TGF-α* and *TGF-β*. Both of these factors together are required to enable fibroblasts to form colonies in agar.

TGF-β causes growth of mesenchyme, but this growth is suppressive to epithelium. Thus, although associated with growth factor potential for sarcomas, it has been shown to inhibit the growth of carcinomas. In tissues such as the breast and normal prostatic epithelial cells, TGF-β is growth suppressive. Thus, TGF-β may be a regulator of normal epithelial tissue and adenocarcinoma growth (Roberts et al., 1985).

The other TGF isolated by bioassay and protein purification procedure, TGF-α, has been found to bind and activate EGFrs. TGF-α has been found to be produced by a number of carcinoma cells. Originally, it was thought that TGF-α was specifically associated with transformation of epithelial cells. Many fetal epithelial cells produce TGF-α, and it was believed that TGF-α represented the fetal form of EGF. A more thorough examination has revealed that TGF-α could be detected in a few normal adult tissues, particularly keratinocytes. Increased TGF-α is observed in both kidney and transitional cell carcinomas (Derynck et al., 1987; Mydlo et al., 1989).

Another family of growth factors thought to play an important role in tumor formation is the fibroblast (heparin-binding) growth factor (FGF) (Goldfarb, 1990). Indeed, FGFs not only stimulated fibroblasts but

also increased the growth of some epithelial cells, such as those of the prostate (Mannson et al., 1989; Mydlo et al., 1988; Story et al., 1987). FGFs probably are involved in the stromal reactivity and angiogenic activity associated with carcinoma growth.

In some cases, overproduction or unregulated production of a growth factor is responsible for transformation. In others, it is the growth factor receptors that have been subverted, causing the oncogenic transformation. The EGFr is an example: EGFr is a transmembrane-spanning protein that undergoes phosphorylation on tyrosine residues when stimulated with EGF or TGF-α (Yarden and Ulrich, 1988). Overexpression of the normal EGFr can lead to transformation. A number of tumors contain increased levels of EGFr. Many urologic tumors with increased levels of EGFr have been reported, especially in renal cancers and bladder carcinomas (Freeman et al., 1989; Neal et al., 1990; Yao et al., 1988).

A mutated receptor can also be transforming, as in the case of the oncogene *erb* B; v-*erb* B resembles the normal EGFr but lacks the external portion of the receptor, which normally binds to EGF. Thus, the *erb* B truncated receptor is not under normal regulatory control by growth factor but is in a constant "activated" state. Many of these kinases phosphorylate proteins on serine or threonine amino acid residues. Phosphotyrosine is a minor species for amino acid side chain phosphorylation but is a major site of phosphorylation by growth factor receptors associated with oncogenic activity.

It is common to find increased levels of phosphotyrosine in transformed cells. Although increased levels of tyrosine kinase active growth factors are found in tumors, decreased levels of tyrosine phosphatases are also found. Prostatic acid phosphatase is a tyrosine phosphatase, and this may account for the observation that the individual cell content of acid phosphatase is decreased in prostate cancer cells compared with normal prostate cells (Nguyen et al., 1990). The transforming activity of growth factors can be increased by the simultaneous action of other oncogenes. Overexpression of EGFr itself is not sufficient to express a transformed phenotype nor is transfection with the *neu* growth factor receptor. The *neu* shares homology with the EGFr, but the ligand for the *neu* receptor has not yet been isolated. Most growth factor receptors can "cross-talk," so that stimulation of one receptor will often result in the phosphorylation of another (Kokai et al., 1988). EGF binding to the EGFr results not only in the phosphorylation of its own receptor but also that of the *neu* receptor. If cells are co-transfected with both EGFr and *neu*, the cells become fully transformed and are capable of forming tumors in nude mice (Kokai et al., 1989). Although an increase in the number of EGF receptors is observed in urologic tumors such as kidney and bladder carcinomas, the demonstration of a receptor-like *neu*, which is found in tumor but not in normal tissue, presents a better target for therapy than the EGFr, which is expressed in many tissues.

NUCLEAR TRANSCRIPTIONAL ONCOGENES.
An oncogene of the avian erythroblastosis virus is the

v-*erb* A, which like *erb* B lacks the ability to bind ligand. However, the ligand for *erb* A is also the intracellular receptor for thyroxin (T$_4$). The *erb* A itself is considered capable of completely transforming cells (Zenke et al., 1990). However, *erb* A can act in concert with any of a number of other oncogenes to cause erythroid cell transformation. The sequence of *erb* A was used to isolate and characterize a large "super family" of steroid/thyroid receptor–like proteins. This super family consists of the receptors for T$_4$; steroids, such as estrogen, androgen, progestin, glucocorticoid, and mineralocorticoid; and vitamin D and retinoid (Carson-Jurica et al., 1990; Evans, 1988; Sluyser, 1990; Touchette, 1990b). Each has three different domains that share significant degrees of homology. The highest degree of homology is found in the DNA-binding region (Carson-Jurica et al., 1990, Evans, 1988, Sluyser, 1990; Touchette, 1990).

A unique characteristic of this DNA-binding region is that the protein forms a region that juts out like a finger. This configuration is held together partly by disulfide bridges between four cysteine residues coordinated with zinc and is given the name "zinc finger." There are two zinc fingers per receptor. Two receptors bind in the same region of DNA during their mediation of transcription. The affinity of the zinc-binding region for DNA is either enhanced or reduced by binding of the various ligands. The *erb* A lacks the ability to bind T$_3$, which interferes with the normal activity of the T$_3$ in erythroid cells. When T$_3$ binds to the normal cellular receptor, it removes (1) the transcriptional inhibition of the major genes of erythrocyte differentiation, (2) the erythrocyte-specific carbonic anhydrase, (3) the erythrocyte anion transporter band 3, and (4) the enzyme γ-aminolevulinate synthase (the rate-limiting enzyme of heme synthesis). Thus, the presence of *erb* A product inhibits transcription and normal differentiation.

Most tissues of interest to the urologist contain one or more members of the thyroid/steroid super gene family. Mutations in these receptors, like those of *erb* A, can lead to an inability of these tissues to undergo differentiation and can allow for a greater susceptibility to the influence of other oncogenes. Indeed, cancer is often thought of in terms of a "block in differentiation" with a corresponding proliferation of the precursor cell type.

When probing DNA for its similarity to a known sequence, the "stringency" of the hybridization conditions can be adjusted such that the probe can pick up either sequences that match exactly (homologous) or those that are similar but not exactly the same. By loosening the stringency, a number of "orphan receptors" of the thyroid/steroid super gene family have been identified. Following castration, some of these orphan receptors are increased (up regulated). The ligands for many of these orphan receptors have not been identified.

Other oncogenic proteins, like the thyroid/steroid super family, are transcriptional regulators and have an intracellular nuclear location. The more classic examples are the oncogenes *jun, fos,* and *myc.* All of these oncogenes are derived from normal cellular proteins involved in control of cell growth, differentiation, and function. These cellular oncogenes (c-*onc* or proto-oncogenes) are normal cellular constituents, which serve as major positive control elements in the signal transduction mechanisms regulating cell metabolism. The oncogenes described so far are considered to be dominant acting, because the genetic alteration resulting in oncogenic change has to occur only in one of the two chromosomal alleles to be fully expressed.

The dominant-acting oncogenes often have a higher transformation capability when expressed in concert with other oncogenes or with overexpressed proto-oncogenes. Often, the transformed state is reversed when a transformed cell is fused with a nontransformed cell. This finding led to the proposal that antioncogenes, as well as proto-oncogenes, are present in the cell. Such controlling sequences have been clearly demonstrated and are referred to as the antioncogenes or suppressor genes (Harris, 1988; Peehl et al., 1990; Sager, 1989; Touchette, 1990b; Weinberg, 1989).

Tumor Suppressor Genes (Antioncogenes)

In addition to genes that code for positive regulators of growth (accelerators), there are genes that code for inhibition of growth (brakes). These genes have been designated by various names, including antioncogenes, recessive oncogenes, growth suppressor genes, and tumor suppressor genes (Sager, 1989; Touchette, 1990b). Unlike the dominant-acting oncogenes, which require that one chromosomal allele be affected in order to exhibit the change, in the recessive-acting suppressor genes both alleles need to be inactivated to cause loss of growth control. Tumor suppressor genes have received widespread attention following the isolation of the retinoblastoma gene in 1985.

Retinoblastoma Suppressor Genes

Retinoblastoma is a rare hereditary form of cancer. Knudson used Poisson statistics to develop a "two-hit" theory to explain the distribution of retinoblastoma. In the hereditary form, the patient inherits one bad copy (one hit) of the retinoblastoma gene. Cancer results when the other good copy is inactivated by a somatic mutation (second hit). In contrast, the sporadic form of retinoblastoma is the result of inactivation of both good copies by somatic mutation (Knudson, 1971).

The retinoblastoma gene (*Rb*) is located on the long arm of chromosome (13q14) and resides in the nucleus where it is thought to play a role in controlling cell growth. This protein is modified by phosphorylation; the degree of its phosphorylation is associated with cell cycle status (Freeman et al., 1990). As the cellular DNA undergoes replication in S phase, *Rb* is fully phosphorylated. At mitosis, *Rb* undergoes dephosphorylation. A number of transforming viral proteins (T-antigen, E1A, E7) can bind to *Rb* in the underphosphorylated form (Whyte et al., 1988). A major regulator of growth and repair in adjacent tissues, TGF-β functions as a *paracrine* growth factor (Fig 26–4). TGF-β inhibits the growth of many types of epithelial cells and has been

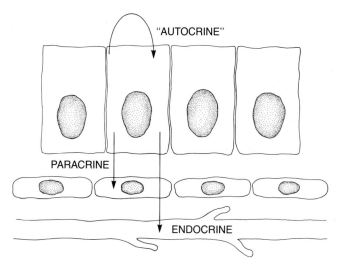

Figure 26–4. Depiction of "autocrine" (self), paracrine (nearby), and endocrine (distant) action of growth factors.

shown to inhibit the phosphorylation of *Rb* (Laiho et al., 1990). TGF-β prevents the phosphorylation of *Rb* during mid/late G$_1$ and inhibits entry of the cell into S phase. Although the experimental evidence implicates *Rb* controlling the cell cycle, the exact mechanism remains to be determined. It may be the substrate for the cdc2 kinase/cycline complex, which regulates phosphorylation during the cell cycle (Lewin, 1990). Another intranuclear suppressor gene bound by transforming viral proteins and differentially phosphorylated in various phases of the cell cycle is *p53* (Raycroft et al., 1990). Loss of *p53* is observed in aggressive bladder carcinomas (Olumni et al., 1990).

Wilms' Tumor Suppressor Gene

Of particular interest to urologists is the hereditary form of Wilms' tumor—an embryonic kidney tumor thought to arise through aberrant mesenchymal stem cell differentiation by loss of a tumor suppressor gene. Deletional analysis of individuals with WAGR syndrome (Wilms' tumor, aniridia, genitourinary abnormalities, mental retardation) revealed that a Wilms' tumor gene is located on chromosome 11p13 (Call et al., 1990). This finding is in keeping with the observation reported by Stanbridge and co-workers that insertion of chromosome 11 into the G401WT Wilms' tumor cell line reverses the malignant phenotype (Weissman et al., 1987). To isolate the gene, large fragments of DNA were generated by cutting the 11p13 region with restriction enzymes to obtain rare sequences and analyzing for the presence of CpG islands. These are regions of DNA preceding the 5' ends of expressed sequences of housekeeping and tissue-specific genes. A gene was identified that showed deletions in Wilms' tumor (Call et al., 1990; Gessler et al., 1990; Pritchard-Jones et al., 1990). The gene codes for a transcriptional regulatory DNA binding protein, and the highest level of expression is in the embryonic kidney. This is probably not the only gene implicated in Wilms' tumor, as other genetic and restriction fragment length polymorphism data suggest that multiple loci may be involved.

In carcinoma of the kidney, a common deletion, found by either cytogenetics or restriction fragment length polymorphism (RFLP) is on chromosome 3. Evidence that chromosome 3 contains a suppressor gene comes from Shimizu and co-workers (1990) who found that transfection with material from a normal human chromosome 3 suppressed the tumorigenicity of the human renal cell carcinoma line YCR. Transferred chromosomal material from chromosome 11 or the X chromosome was not tumor suppressive. Because of this useful model system and readily available probes for the region of interest on chromosome 3, it is likely that a tumor suppressor gene will be identified on this chromosome.

Tumor Progression and Aneuploidy

Although we have emphasized individual chromosomal or molecular changes that can occur during tumor formation and progression, more commonly multiple changes occur. These multiple changes can be crudely approximated by measuring the DNA content of the cell. The change in amount of DNA can be approximated by flow cytometry or Feulgen staining of fixed tissue. The normal diploid DNA content is designated 2n. Polyploidy of the DNA content can occur with 4n DNA, which represents a doubling of the normal cellular DNA. Aneuploidy represents an uneven multiple of the normal cellular DNA content not related to DNA replication. Flow cytometers record the number of cells and the amount of DNA stain per cell relative to a known 2n standard, such as that of blood lymphocytes. By counting many thousands of cells, a statistically relevant DNA population distribution is calculated. If a normal population is 2n, a population with a distribution of 3.2 n would be an example of an aneuploid population and would represent an unbalanced 60 per cent increase in DNA content.

Fixed-section Feulgen staining can identify individual cell types in relation to DNA content. In both flow cytometry and staining techniques the change in DNA content has to be fairly significant to be detected. To identify actual individual chromosomal changes, cytogenic analysis has been the "gold standard," but it is extremely intensive and requires growing cells and obtaining metaphase spreads for adequate evaluation. An exciting development is the identification of probes for the highly repetitious DNA regions near the centromeric region of the various chromosomes. These paracentromeric probes make possible in situ hybridization on an individual chromosome's DNA. Thus, this technique theoretically can detect hyperdiploidy of a single chromosome, as opposed to flow cytometry that measures the total DNA content. Probes can be used on cells in any phase of the cell cycle and with attached biotin can be visualized with fluorescent avidin.

Preliminary studies employing fluorescent in situ hybridization (FISH) technique have demonstrated that DNA flow patterns, which appear to be diploid, may actually contain an increase of one chromosome and the deletion of another. The technique has also been modified to analyze paraffin-embedded tissue and promises to be a powerful tool for the evaluation of chromosomal aberrations in solid tumors. Current limitations are related to the lack of probes for all the chromosomes and their restriction to the paracentromeric region (Van Dekken et al., in press). The rapid development of probes suggests that this will not be a permanent limitation and that probes (telemetric) for the ends of the chromosomes will be developed.

In general, studies on DNA content suggest that increasing DNA derangement and aneuploidy are associated with poor prognosis. This type of genetic event has been best characterized in colon cancer by Vogelstein and colleagues (1988; 1989). These investigators screened for heterozygotic deletions by restriction fragment length polymorphism (RFLP) analysis. Probes were utilized for every nonacrocentric autosomal arm in a large series of paired colorectal tumors and adjacent normal colon. Allelic deletions were common with a substantial loss of heterogeneity in most of the tumors. Allelic loss was especially prevalent on chromosomes 17 and 18 where RFLP analysis detected a loss in 70 per cent of the tumor specimens examined. To be scored as a loss, the restriction enzyme digest had to exhibit a different size banding pattern when probed, which suggests an allelic shift from the parents. These were considered informative. A patient's chromosome was not considered informative if it was homozygous at the probed locus. A loss was scored if an RFLP fragment present in the normal DNA was absent or decreased by at least 80 per cent in the tumor as determined by densitometric quantitation of the autoradiogram. The number of chromosomal arms on which allelic loss was observed was divided by the number of chromosomal arms for which allelic markers were informative. This was recorded as the fractional allelic loss (FAL). The median FAL was 0.2, which meant that alleles were lost from 20 per cent of the evaluable chromosomal arms.

The investigators determined whether there was any clinical correlation with the degree of allelic loss by splitting the group into those with an FAL of less than 20 per cent (mean 0.11) and greater than 20 per cent (mean 0.32). The groups were equivalent in terms of age, number of patients, tumor size (5.3 cm), follow-up period (38 months), per cent with a *ras* mutation (52%), and Dukes class (2.3) but did differ significantly in terms of tumor recurrence (30% versus 68%) and death (26% versus 64%). This was a conservative estimate of allelic loss because not all foci were evaluable. This value represents a higher estimate than others have reported, because the DNA was isolated from cryostat sections, providing a better preparation of normal and tumor fractions. The allelic loss can be determined at the molecular level for multiple chromosomes and further demonstrates the underlying heterogeneous nature of tumors and the inverse correlation of genetic alteration with survival.

In this study of colon cancers, allelic losses on chromosomes 17 and 18 approached 70 per cent. Because these chromosomal losses are suggestive of the loss of a tumor suppressor gene, these two chromosomal regions may be critical for suppression of the development of colon cancer (Fearon et al., 1990a). As previously described, chromosome 17 contains the p53 suppressor gene locus and represents the site often associated with abnormalities on this chromosome. A clever linking of the polymerase chain reaction for gene amplification and an exon connection to identify the suppressor gene on chromosome 18 was titled the "deleted in colon carcinoma (DCC) gene" (Fearon et al., 1990a; Fearon and Vogelstein, 1990b). When the sequence of the cloned gene was determined, a surprising homology was observed with neural cell adhesion molecules (N-CAMs) in a region of Ig-like domains. Cancerous changes are often associated with alterations in cell surface interactions along with structural disorganization, diminished cell adhesion, and loss of growth control by cell-cell contact. Intracellular adhesion mediated by CAMs has been shown to affect differentiation. Loss of differentiated functions is a common feature of malignancy. These data suggest that the loss of this suppressor gene may identify one of the molecular-based explanations for this altered cellular behavior.

METASTASIS

The Metastatic Process

The most clinically devastating biologic alteration of malignant tumors is related to their ability to metastasize and colonize different organs. Many forms of locoregional control are effective, but for the majority of urologic tumors once they have metastasized the result is death. This is directly related to the low activity of standard cytotoxic chemotherapy in urologic tumors, testicular tumors being the exception. Some tumors are able to spread by direct extension, i.e., abdominal ovarian carcinomatosis. But invasion and metastatic spread, either hematogenous or vascular, represent the usual mechanisms of tumor spread. Liotta and co-workers (1985) have identified the steps involved in the metastatic cascade.

First, the tumor cells need to invade and penetrate the vasculature and include the extracellular matrix (Liotta et al., 1985). Tumor cell surface receptors attach to specific components in the matrix, such as fibronectin or laminin. Laminin is a large glycoprotein found predominantly in the basement membrane where one end of the molecule binds to type IV collagen. High concentrations of laminin receptors have been demonstrated in several neoplastic cell lines (Liotta et al., 1985). Interference with the laminin receptors' ability to bind matrix has been associated with diminished metastasis in a melanoma model system (Barsky et al., 1984). Normal cells possess laminin receptors, but they appear to be fewer in number compared with homologous cancer cells, such as colon (Liotta, 1986).

Second, the matrix needs to be dissolved. This is done by the elaboration of a variety of proteolytic enzymes. These include collagenase, in particular type IV collagenase. Type IV collagen is a major structural component of the basement membrane (Liotta et al., 1980). The implication is that the malignant cell has the ability to degrade the matrix of the endothelial membrane, facilitating its entry into the blood stream. Plasminogen activator activates other proteolytic enzymes and has been proposed to play a major role in the plasminogen activator-plasmin-collagenase cascade. Tumor plasminogen activator activates plasmin, which in turn activates collagenase that degrades the matrix (Mignatti et al., 1986). This proteolytic activity can be balanced by tissue-specific proteolytic inhibitors that block invasive behavior (Thorgeirsson, 1982).

The third step in the invasion process is movement of the cells through the attenuated matrix. Laminin itself maybe chemotactic for some tumor cells (McCarthy et al., 1985). Because tumor cells lack lymphatics, the hydrostatic pressure of edema may force tumor cells into the interstitium (Butler et al., 1975). However, this movement may also be a characteristic associated with the heterogeneity of the transformed cell. Several investigators have examined a series of prostatic tumor cell variants, which differed in their metastatic activity, by using a video camera to record cell movement in vitro. They demonstrated that the most highly motile cells were the most metastatic (Mohler et al., 1987; Partin et al., 1989). As noted, *ras* oncogenic transformation is often associated with increased motility and metastatic aggressiveness (Partin et al., 1988). Liotta and Schiffmann (1988) were able to purify a secreted factor from metastatic melanomas that stimulates motility in tumor cells. Because the factor is produced by tumors and stimulates motility in the same cells that produced it, they called it the tumor *autocrine motility factor* (*AMF*). Similar to many factors that bind to the cell, AMF stimulates the cell's signal transduction pathways by increasing inositol triphosphate. AMF activation is significantly inhibited by pertussis toxin, which suggests a G_i protein–mediated intracellular signalling pathway (Kohn and Liotta, 1990).

Once the tumor successfully penetrates the endothelial basement membrane, it gains access to the systemic circulation. However, not all tumor cells reaching the circulation survive. Indeed, even with a highly metastatic melanoma tumor model, only 1 per cent of the injected tumor cells can reach the circulatory system and retain viability (Fidler, 1990). The tumor cell must also have the ability to leave the circulation and evolve into a metastatic deposit. A cell simply gaining entrance into the circulation does not guarantee metastases. A clinical example of this fact is in the patient with ovarian carcinomatosis and in whom ascites is often palliated by peritovenous shunting.

Despite the millions of tumor cells passing through the circulation daily, metastases are rarely seen at autopsy (Tarin et al., 1984). The metastatic tumor cell may finally undergo arrest in the capillaries of remote organs. The "mechanical theory" of metastasis suggests that filtration can account for entrapment of large emboli and the eventual generation of metastatic deposits. Indeed, in some situations it would appear that a metastatic lesion was a passive result with regard to the lymphatic and venous drainage systems (mechanical). However, when B16 tumor cells are injected and followed to determine where they lodge, a significant number settle in the liver and spleen. Yet, invariably, it

is in the lung that the cells take hold and grow. Such data have provided evidence for the "seed and soil" hypothesis of metastasis first proposed by Paget in 1989 (Zetter, 1990).

Sugarbaker and associates (1971) demonstrated the tissue-specific nature of metastasizing cells when ectopic organ grafts were transplanted and sarcomas implanted that metastasized strictly to the lungs. The only tissue in which metastatic deposits were observed were in the lung and the ectopic lung tissue. None of the other ectopic tissues demonstrated metastases.

Metastatic site selection can often be determined by cell surface components. Experiments in which the plasma membrane components of cells with different rates of metastases were reversed show a change to the opposite rate at which they metastasize (Poste and Nicolson, 1980). Factors from the tissue to which a tumor metastasizes (soil) also affect selection. Substances have been isolated from tissues that enhance the rate of metastasis to that site. Terranova and colleagues (1986) demonstrated that a variety of malignancies were selectively influenced by extracts from the specific organs to which they metastasize. In some cases, inhibitory factors are produced, which prevent growth of metastatic cells. In others, growth stimulatory factors are produced, such as bone marrow stroma, which may stimulate the growth of prostatic cancer cells (Chackal-Roy et al., 1989).

It should not be surprising that tumors vary in their metastatic capability. When a number of highly metastatic tumors were cloned and the clones examined for metastatic potential, there was an incredible range of metastatic expression even in the original tumors (Fidler, 1990). One can also isolate cells that metastasize to different tissues and maintain this feature on repassage and cloning (Fidler, 1990). Primary tumors are also heterogeneous with respect to their organ specificity. Individual cells within a primary tumor exhibit different abilities not only to metastasize but also preferences as to the organ that they colonize (Zetter, 1990). By recognizing the heterogeneous nature of tumors with respect to cellular composition and metastatic propensity, the physician is able to appreciate the marked variability in clinical behavior observed in human tumors. This also underscores the magnitude of the difficulties that need to be surmounted to effectively control the cancer process.

Antimetastatic Genes

Autocrine motility factor is a positive-acting factor for tumor motility and metastatic tumor spread. As with positive oncogenes versus tumor suppressor genes, a described antimetastatic factor appears to be expressed at high levels in nonmetastatic tumors and lost or nearly absent in metastatic tumors. Steeg and colleagues (1988) utilized a series of related rodent melanoma cell lines derived from the K1735 line that differed greatly in their metastatic potential but not in their response to host immune factors. This finding suggests that there were nonimmunologic reasons for differential metastatic capability.

They isolated 24 clones differentially expressed between the high and low metastatic cells. In two nonmetastatic clones, the pNM23 cDNA insert exhibited a consistently greater level of mRNA than that found in five highly metastatic clones. These investigators also observed gene expression in several nonmetastatic breast tumors. Greatly reduced amounts were noted in metastatic breast tumors. In c-Harvey *ras* transfected rat embryo fibroblasts, which were co-transfected with adenovirus 2 E1A, it was observed that E1A transfection eliminated metastatic ability and increased NM23 expression. In primary human breast biopsy samples, 75 per cent of node-negative tumors expressed high levels of NM23. Low level node-negative tumors were also poorly differentiated and had a low content of nuclear receptors, characteristically predictive of eventual metastatic spread. Indeed, at the time of the report, two of the low level NM23 tumors had metastasized, whereas none of the high level NM23 tumors had metastasized (Bevilacqua et al., 1989).

The NM23 gene has been definitively established as a nucleotide diphosphate kinase (NDP). The function of this enzyme is to take a compound, such as guanine diphosphate (GDP), and add a phosphate to make guanine triphosphate (GTP). This can happen while the GDP is still bound to the G-binding protein. Similar to the prior discussion on GTP binding proteins, such as *ras* and p-21, which hydrolyze GTP to GDP and which may be modulated by GTPase-activating proteins, this protein has the opposite action of taking the inactive GDP to GTP. Erythrocyte NDP kinase has been sequenced and found to be identical to NM23. The NDP kinases have been shown to form complexes with GTP-binding proteins, and their association with the $G_{\alpha}s$ subunit indicates a role in adenylate cyclase regulation. Interaction with GTP-binding proteins and in GTP metabolism (converting GDP to GTP) may prove to be the major function of this enzyme in growth control, oncogenic transformation, and metastases (Wallet et al., 1990).

ANGIOGENESIS

A feature common to many malignancies is the formation of new blood vessels, called angiogenesis. Tumor growth obviously requires a vascular supply. The normal vascular endothelium can be induced to grow in response to injury or to the normal growth processes associated with menstruation or pregnancy. Thus, angiogenesis does not always imply malignancy. The term angiogenesis was coined in 1935 to describe the formation of new blood vessels in the placenta (Hertig, 1935). Also, angiogenesis may not always appear as the initial step in tumor formation. In cervical neoplasia, angiogenesis typically occurs prior to the gross appearance of tumor: in breast and bladder, a marked increase in angiogenesis occurs coincidentally with tumor development; and in melanoma and ovarian carcinoma, angiogenesis occurs after tumor formation (Folkman, 1990).

Basic fibroblast growth factor (bFGF) may be involved in tumor growth and stimulated the growth of colon tumors when administered to animals that were receiving implants of tumor cells that lacked FGF acceptors. The same cells did not produce tumors in the absence of FGF, and this finding represents further evidence for the importance of angiogenesis in the growth of tumor (Folkman, 1990).

Folkman (1990) has summarized a great amount of evidence for the angiogenic dependence of tumors as follows:

1. Tumors grown in isolated perfused organs in which blood vessels do not proliferate are limited in size to 2 mm^3 but expand rapidly to cm^3 when transplanted into mice and vascularized.
2. The growth of experimental tumors implanted in the avascular cornea is limited until after vascularization, when growth rapidly accelerates.
3. Within a solid tumor, the [^{3}H]thymidine-labeling index of tumor cells, which indicates cell growth, decreases with the increasing distance of the cell from the nearest open capillary.
4. Carcinoma of the ovary metastasizes to the peritoneal membrane as tiny avascular seeds, which rarely grow beyond a limited size until after vascularization.
5. Angiogenic inhibitors that are not growth suppressive in tissue cultures are in animal models.
6. In transgenic animals that develop carcinoma, large tumors arise from preneoplastic hyperplastic areas that are vascularized.

The identification of angiogenic factors requires the development of reproducible bioassay systems. These systems have focused on visualization and quantitation of the ingrowth of capillaries. The bioassays include (1) the implantation of tumor or biopolymer containing angiogenic molecules into the cornea of the rabbit, rat, or mouse or into the chorioallantoic membrane of chick eggs and (2) the tissue culture growth of vascular endothelial cells (Folkman, 1987). Based on these assays, a number of agents with angiogenic as well as antiangiogenic activity have been found and are summarized by Bouck (Bouck, 1990).

A number of inducers and inhibitors of angiogenesis are found in tissue. In this tightly regulated system it appears that there are many possible areas where positive-acting or negative-acting factors could be subverted as part of tumor progression. The isolation of angiogenic factors was helped by the development of in vitro culturing of endothelial cells to study their growth and motility. Those found especially potent were the fibroblast growth factors. In many tissues, the concentrations of FGFs are higher than would be anticipated from the degree of angiogenesis normally found.

It appears that bFGF is bound to both the cytosolic and extracellular forms of heparan sulfate, which eventually become part of the cell matrix. Because it is unlikely that the bound form of FGF is active in angiogenesis, the bFGF must be released from the extracellular matrix. Heparan sulfate is degraded by heparinase, and the matrix core proteins are degraded by proteinases. Folkman and Klagsburn (1987) observed that the basement membrane bFGF can be released by heparinase and can induce endothelial cell growth. Heparinase may serve two purposes. First it may serve to release FGF that diffuses to the endothelial cell and induces chemotaxis toward the site of matrix degradation. Second, the residual heparan fragment bound to FGF protects the FGF from degradation by proteolytic enzymes, such as plasmin. Although FGF is bound to the heparan fragment, it is still able to activate endothelial cell growth and plasminogen activator production (Folkman and Klagsburn, 1987).

Other potent angiogenic factors beside FGF include TGF-α, angiogenin, and copper. TGF-α stimulates the growth of microvascular endothelial cells in vitro but is less effective in vivo. Angiogenin is a polypeptide isolated from a human colon carcinoma cell line. It is potent in stimulating angiogenesis in the rabbit corneal assay but is ineffective in stimulating the growth of endothelial cells in vitro. The other factor that exhibits angiogenic activity in vivo is copper (Folkman and Klagsburn, 1987).

As with the other physical features of cancer, it can be surmised that the angiogenic cells in a tumor arise from normal nononcogenic cells by the accumulation of genetic changes that activate oncogenes and inactivate suppressor genes (Bouck, 1990).

Experimentally, a transfected oncogene can make a cell angiogenic. Thompson and colleagues (1989) have introduced *ras* and *myc* oncogenes into normal epithelial and stromal cells and reconstituted the prostate. They observed a tenfold increase in the number of new blood vessels within the prostate. Neoangiogenesis, therefore, may be due to *ras*-induced synthesis of growth factors. The secreted medium of *ras*-transformed cells has been shown to contain mitogens, which stimulate the *neu*-receptor (Yarden and Weinberg, 1989). Suppressor gene loss can also influence angiogenesis. A suppressor gene was isolated from hamster fibroblasts (Moroco et al., 1990). Its inactivation leads to an increase in angiogenic activity that parallels its increase in tumorigenicity. This inhibitor of angiogenic activity turns out to be the extracellular protein thrombospondon (Moroco et al., 1990). Loss of suppressor genes has been correlated with angiogenic activity in many cell systems (Yarden and Weinberg, 1989).

Once the tumor has metastasized, the role of locoregional management becomes minimal except for local palliation of symptoms. Currently, nonspecific cytotoxic therapies are utilized for metastatic disease.

PRINCIPLES OF CHEMOTHERAPY

Basic Principles

The word chemotherapy was first applied by Paul Ehrlich to systemic therapy for infectious disease. Of particular interest to the urologist were the landmark contributions of Charles Brenton Huggins and others who first utilized hormonal manipulation by castration or estrogen administration in the therapy of metastatic prostatic cancer (Huggins and Hodges, 1941). This ob-

servation, the significance of which was recognized by the awarding of the Nobel Prize, justifies Huggins as the father of the modern era of cancer chemotherapy. He was the first to demonstrate the significant clinical response of metastatic cancer to systemic therapy.

The work of Skipper and colleagues (1964), with the L1210 leukemia model, served to establish guidelines for systemic therapy. The L1210 leukemia system is particularly useful for tumor kinetic studies, because in this model basically all the tumor cells are stem cells—the injection of a single cell in an appropriate animal will lead to tumor formation. Eventually, death of the animal occurs when the tumor volume reaches 1 billion (10^9) cells. The growth rate of the tumor thus established can be accurately determined by measuring the length of survival of the animal following the injection of various cell numbers. The L1210 cells have a doubling time of approximately 12 hours; therefore, the injection of a single cell will lead to death of the animal with a tumor containing 10^9 cells in 19 days. Injection of 10^5 cells will kill the animal in 10 days and 10^8 cells in 5 days. The effect of chemotherapy in delaying the time to death of the animals can then by extrapolation be employed as a measurement of cell kill. Thus, an increase of 5 days in survival would be the equivalent of a 3 log cell kill or destruction of 99.9 per cent of the tumor cells. However, a cell kill from 10^8 to 10^5 cells will not be curative. In these experiments, the magnitude of cell kill followed log kill kinetics. A particular drug dose will kill the same log number of cells, regardless of the initial tumor population. Thus, the likelihood of cure with a given drug depends on the initial cell volume treated. This led to one of the principal maxims of chemotherapy in that the possibility of cure is inversely related to the volume of the tumor (De Vita, 1989).

The data derived from experiments involving log kill kinetics are applicable only in cell systems with exponential tumor growth. In contrast to animal models, most human tumors appear to more closely approximate a Gompertz model of tumor growth, in which the growth fraction is not constant but declines with increasing tumor volume. As a result, with larger tumor volumes, the growth rate of the tumor slows and the effect of chemotherapy is less pronounced. In accord with the kinetics of Gompertz, small tumor volumes, such as those remaining after surgical therapy, would be expected to have higher growth fractions. In this setting, a specific dose of chemotherapy may have a greater cell kill effect than if given to a larger tumor volume. However, a small volume of residual tumor remaining after surgical ablation of a much larger tumor volume will reflect the same heterogeneity as existed in the original larger tumor. As a result, the likelihood that cell changes leading to the development of resistance to chemotherapy or irradiation has occurred is higher in small volume disease resulting from incomplete surgical excision of bulky tumor than in the same small volume tumor arising de novo. The majority of currently available chemotherapeutic agents are more active against proliferating cells. Many act against cells in a specific phase of the cell cycle (see Fig. 26–3).

Cytotoxic Chemotherapy

1. Induction chemotherapy is the term used to indicate the selection of chemotherapy as the sole therapy in patients with advanced disease (Steel, 1977).

2. "Salvage" chemotherapy is employed in the attempt to treat those patients who have failed initial attempts with induction chemotherapy.

3. Adjuvant chemotherapy implies systemic chemotherapy *after* treatment of the primary tumor by surgery and/or radiation. Adjuvant chemotherapy is used in a patient with high potential for recurrence after local treatment. It does not denote the chemotherapy after surgery in a patient whose tumor is incompletely resected with viable gross disease still present.

4. Neoadjuvant (*primary*) chemotherapy is the chemotherapy used as the initial therapy prior to definitive surgery or radiation therapy in a patient with apparently localized cancer. Although the name neoadjuvant or "up-front" chemotherapy has been applied to drugs given in this manner, the term primary chemotherapy is more appropriate (DeVita, 1989).

Conceptually, primary chemotherapy is appealing because, in most cases, the major problem facing the clinician in attempting to cure the patient with cancer is the presence of unrecognized distant micrometastases at the time of the definitive treatment of the local lesion. Most patients with malignancies die of the distant disease, rather than an uncontrollable local lesion; therefore, combined treatment, encompassing systemic treatment of both local and distant malignant disease, is theoretically ideal. Indeed, the tremendous improvement in overall survival rates in patients with testicular cancer is, in large measure, due to the more frequent and effective administration of multimodal therapy. Encouraging early results with primary MVAC (methotrexate, vinblastine, adriamycin, and *cis*-platinum) in patients with transitional cell urothelial tumors have been reported in nonrandomized trials (Scher et al., 1988) and warrant further investigation.

The theoretic advantages of primary chemotherapy include the ability to assess the effectiveness of therapy by having a "marker lesion" in place at the time the chemotherapy is given. In the absence of a demonstrable effect of the therapy on the local lesion, primary chemotherapy can be discontinued, thus avoiding unnecessary toxicity in some patients who are unresponsive to therapy. This "in vivo chemosensitivity test" will indicate those patients in whom chemotherapy is effective and guide the clinician to the proper dosage and number of cycles necessary to achieve maximal effect. This observation is not possible when all visible tumor is removed prior to the initiation of therapy. The potential for tumor "downstaging" with significant reduction in tumor volume, thus making it possible to reduce the extent and severity of subsequent surgery, also makes primary chemotherapy appealing. This is especially true when radical surgery carries with it a significant impact on the quality of life, such as a patient requiring cystectomy.

Another theoretic advantage of primary chemotherapy is the likelihood of fewer resistant cells being present as a result of the initiation of treatment before surgery or radiation. Presumably, the tumor will have less opportunity to be differentiated as opposed to later in the tumor's life span.

Despite the potential advantages, significant negative aspects to primary therapy exist. Practically, chemotherapy may delay the timing and impair the effectiveness or increase the side effects of subsequent surgery or irradiation. In addition, it exposes those patients who would be cured by definitive treatment alone to unnecessary toxicity and death. Although the primary tumor and micrometastases may exhibit similar responses to chemotherapy, the initial lesion, by virtue of being the oldest, is the most likely to contain drug-resistant cell lines and has the least favorable cell kinetics. As mentioned, animal experiments indicate that chemotherapy may be more effective when the tumor volume is less. This would support the idea of definitive treatment to lessen cell volume before initiating chemotherapy. Additionally, resection of the initial tumor appears to favorably alter the cell kinetics of tumor proliferation on residual micrometastatic disease (DeVita, 1989).

Principles of Combination Chemotherapy

With the exception of choriocarcinoma and Burkitt's lymphoma, combination chemotherapy is required to cure *all* chemotherapy-sensitive human tumors (DeVita, 1989). Combination therapy has the advantage over single agent therapy in that it may provide maximum cell kill with a toxicity that can be safely tolerated by the patient. Because tumors are heterogeneous, combination therapy may provide broader coverage and decrease the likelihood of resistance. Such therapy may also prevent or retard the development of resistant cell lines. DeVita (1989) has outlined principles useful in selecting drugs for combination therapy as follows:

1. If a drug is ineffective when used as a single agent it is unlikely to be effective in combination. Ideally, drugs that will induce some complete remissions are preferable to those that cause only partial tumor regressions.

2. When several drugs of the same class are available, a drug should be selected to minimize overlapping toxicity with other drugs in the combination. Such selection may lend itself to a greater range of side effects in those patients; it lessens the risk of any single side effect and minimizes the possibility of a lethal toxicity as a result of multiple insults to the same organ system by multiple agents.

3. Drugs should be used at the optimum dosage and schedule.

4. Combination chemotherapy should be given cyclically and at constant intervals. The time between cycles should be the shortest possible necessary for recovery of the most sensitive normal target tissue—usually the bone marrow. Minimizing the time between cycles also will reduce the chance of regrowth of residual tumor cells between cycles.

Because the bone marrow storage can continue to supply mature cells to the peripheral blood for 8 to 10 days after the stem cell pool has been depleted, the peripheral blood counts are generally a week or so behind the events in the marrow. In most patients, nadir blood counts are noted between day 14 and 18 following therapy, with recovery between day 21 and 28. Hence, many chemotherapy regimens employ 21- to 28-day cycles.

As previously described, tumors are heterogeneous. In general, the greater the number of tumor doublings the more likely the tumor will have cytotoxic-resistant tumor cells present. Many biochemical reasons for tumor resistance are known: the drug is poorly transported into the cell or is actively transported out of the cell (multidrug resistance); the tumor is unable to activate a drug to the cytotoxic metabolite; the drug is inactivated by the tumor; the tumor cell has increased DNA damage repair enzymes; the genes are amplified for drug resistance; the cell uses alternate pathways and circumvents the drug's inhibition; and the cell makes an altered form of the protein inhibited by the drug so that the drug is less effective. Any or all of these pharmacologic and biochemical reasons for resistance may obtain (DeVita, 1989).

The dramatic potential for cancer cure by cytotoxic chemotherapy is emphasized by the response to treatment of testicular carcinoma. The damage to normal host tissue by these cytotoxic agents and the resistance of urologic neoplasms other than testicular carcinomas to current chemotherapeutic agents require new therapeutic approaches (Dmitrovsky et al., 1990; Eastman, 1990; Fitzgerald and Pastan, 1989; Tritton and Hickman, 1990).

NEWER THERAPEUTIC APPROACHES

Nutrition and Lifestyle Changes

Numerous reports of increased risk for the development of cancer from various environmental and lifestyle factors are reported (Lerman et al., 1989). Elimination of tobacco products and alterations in nutritional habits, such as decreasing overall caloric intake, especially in fats; eating more vegetables, especially broccoli and carrots; and increasing fiber intake have all been recommended (Greenberg, 1990; Lerman et al., 1989; Newmark et al., 1990). These recommendations are not based on the results of large prospective randomized trials but do have support from numerous retrospective studies, which requires cautious interpretation (Prentice et al., 1989).

The task here is to identify models that would be useful in predicting the agents that would decrease if not eliminate the progression of cancer. For instance, in the study of breast cancer the *neu* and *ras* oncogenes have been transfected into embryonic tissue that is then maintained in the germ line of descendants in model systems referred to as *transgenic* animals. These the animals develop breast tumors as they mature (Muller et al., 1988). Development of such models for urologic

tumors should provide a tool for identifying effective dietary intervention strategies and chemoprevention agents.

Circumventing Host Toxicity

Although our understanding of cancer has substantially increased with the current molecular biologic approach, the treatment approach is largely unchanged. In cancer therapy, one strives to increase the activity of the therapy against the tumor and to decrease the toxicity to the host. The ability to deliver an effective dose of a given chemotherapeutic agent is largely determined by the toxicity of the therapy. In an effort to reduce systemic toxicity, the dose of a given drug may be decreased to an amount in which its tumoricidal effect in diminished. Thus, as stated by DeVita (1989) "the most toxic effect of treatment may be premature death from insufficient dosing."

The introduction of hematopoietic growth factors (G-CSF-CSF) has significantly reduced the toxicity associated with some types of combination chemotherapy. Reduction in toxicity may permit dose intensification of chemotherapy with a subsequent increase in efficacy (Gabrilove, 1988).

Toxin Targeting

ANTIBODY TOXIN TARGETING. The concept of linking cytotoxic agents, such as ricin, to deliver a "magic bullet" to tumor cells while sparing normal cells is appealing. Pharmacologic amounts of toxin and the chemical means for linking the toxin to an antibody are currently not available as are antibodies specific to various tissues. These antibodies are monoclonal and produced from the fusion of a myeloma cell and an antibody-producing cell (Kohler and Milstein, 1975). A number of potentially useful antibodies have been identified with specificity for bladder, kidney, and prostatic carcinoma (Bander, 1987; Olsnes and Sandvig, 1988; Rowland et al., 1990; Sheinfeld et al., 1990).

Potent toxins, such as ricin and *Pseudomonas* exotoxin, are also readily available. These toxins are manipulated so that the regions responsible for binding to the cell and allowing nonspecific cytotoxicity are eliminated. These toxins are then linked to the targeting antibody to permit selective killing of tumor cells. Most of the available toxins are protein synthesis inhibitors. When taken up by the cell, they ribosylate the ribosomal initiation factors, leaving them unable to synthesize proteins. This results in cell death. Because these toxins are also enzymes, it requires as little as one molecule per cell to kill the cell (Bander, 1987; Frankel, 1988; Kohler and Milstein, 1975; Olsnes and Sandvig, 1988).

GROWTH FACTOR RECEPTOR TARGETING. Some tumors exhibit increased levels of receptors on their cell surfaces. Increased levels of EGFrs have been reported on renal and bladder cancer cells. This finding implies that these receptors could serve as targets for specific blockades. Antibodies against the EGFr have been shown to block the growth of some tumors, i.e., xenografts in nude mice (Masui et al., 1986).

TGF-α is a growth factor expressed in many epithelial cancers and is a ligand for the EGFr. Molecular engineering has created some molecules that combine the TGF-α binding region and the toxic portion of the *Pseudomonas* exotoxin (Heimbrook et al., 1990). This molecule uses the EGFr for its uptake into cells, and the exotoxin very efficiently kills those cells. Although targeting cells in this way is appealing, many nontumor cells also have EGFrs. The *neu* receptor appears to be restricted to malignant cells, and compounds designed to attach to *neu* receptors may provide effects that are united to tumor cells (Hellstrom and Hellstrom, 1989).

Many of the GFRs have tyrosine kinase activation as part of their action. This has become an area of development for specific tyrosine kinase inhibitors for the growth factors associated with tumor development (Levitzki, 1990). Many membrane-associated oncogenes, such as *ras*, need to be anchored to the membrane to be active. A number of agents are being investigated, including the cholesterol synthesis antagonists, as a means to block the cell membrane–anchoring mechanism (Gibbs, 1990).

Cell Transfection

The loss of suppressor genes is associated with the development of malignancies in some systems. The reinsertion of the suppressor gene function with retroviral vectors has been shown to normalize the cell and represents another therapeutic approach under investigation (Baker et al., 1990; Bookstein et al., 1990). Another approach is using genetically manipulated cells to produce agents that can kill tumor cells, such as tumor necrosis factor (TNF) or interleukin-2 (IL2), which activates immunotherapeutic responses (Rosenberg et al., 1990).

Differentiation Agents

Cancer may also be thought of as a block in the cell's ability to differentiate. Methods to stimulate the differentiation signal may prove useful in treatment, such as the possibility of restoring androgen dependency to the hormone refractory prostatic tumor. Examples of differentiation treatment activity have been observed in model systems, but to date agents tested clinically, such as hexamethylene-bis-acetamide (HMBA), still suffer from toxicity without providing a demonstrable survival benefit. New derivatives of retinoids are less toxic, and identification of ligands for the orphan receptors found in tumors may provide further approaches in this area (Russo et al., 1987).

Antimetastatic Agents

Agents that interfere with a cell's ability to metastasize are being identified. Because of the importance of the cell's ability to extravasate and intravasate and the involvement of the tumor cell's attachment to and degradation of the matrix in the metastatic process, identification of a number of important cell attachment factors is an area of focus. Some workers have demonstrated that fragments of adhesion molecules, integrins, and others may be able to block metastasis (Albeda and Buck, 1990). Other agents that show potential as antimetastatic agents are being tested as are unique methods to deliver them (Kohn and Liotta, 1990; Roedink, 1989).

Cachexia and Well-Being

Cancer can be debilitating with the patient becoming cachectic during the course of the disease. This effect decreases the patient's quality of life and makes treatment interventions more difficult. Tumor necrosis factor is thought to play a role in cachexia. In one report, pentoxifylline was found to reverse these negative aspects of cancer with improvement in appetite, sense of well-being, and performance status (Dezube et al., 1990). This treatment was shown to decrease TNF production but not IL-6 production (Dezube et al., 1990; Waage et al., 1990). This improvement was achieved at nontoxic doses of pentoxifylline.

Although these potential approaches to therapy are novel and exciting, it is likely that, at least in the near term, the highest probability of success in solid tumor chemotherapy lies in dose-intensification strategies to enable maximum cytotoxic therapy at a morbidity that is tolerable.

REFERENCES

Alison, M. R., and Wright, N. A.: Growth kinetics. Recent Results Cancer Res., 78:29–43, 1981.

Albeda, S. M., and Buck, C. A.: Integrins and other cell adhesion molecules. FASEB J, 4:2868–2880, 1990.

Baker, S. J., Markowitz, S., Fearon, E. R., Wilson, J. K. V., and Vogelstein, B.: Suppression of human colorectal carcinoma cell growth by wild type p53. Science, 249:912–915, 1990.

Bander, N. H.: Monoclonal antibodies:state of the art. J. Urol., 137:603–612, 1987.

Barsky, S. H., Rao, C. N., Williams, J. E., and Liotta, L. A.: Laminin molecular domains which alter metastasis in a murine model. J. Clin. Invest., 74:843–848, 1984.

Beserga, R.: The cell cycle: myths and reality. Cancer Res., 50:6769–6771, 1990.

Bevilacqua, G., Sobel, M. E., Liotta, L. A., and Steeg, P. S.: Association of low nm23 RNA levels in human primary infiltrating ductal breast carcinomas with lymph node involvement and other histopathological indicators of high metastatic potential. Cancer Res., 49:5185–5190, 1989.

Bookstein, R., Shew, J. Y., Chen, P. L., Scully, P., and Lee, W. H.: Suppression of tumorigenicity of human prostate carcinoma cells by replacing a mutated RB gene. Science, 247:712–715, 1990.

Bouck, N.: Tumor angiogenesis:the role of oncogenes and tumor suppressor genes. Cancer Cells, 2:179–185, 1990.

Bruchovsky, N., Rennie, P. S., Coldman, A. J., Goldenberg, J. L., To, M., and Lawson, D.: Effects of androgen withdrawal on the stem cell composition of the Shionogi carcinoma. Cancer Res., 50:2275–2287, 1990.

Buick, R. N.: Biological and clinical implications of the tumor stem cell concept in human malignancy. *In* Cory, J. G., and Szentireny, A. (Eds.): Cancer Biology and Therapeutics. New York, Plenum Press, 1986, pp. 65–77.

Butler, T. P., Grantham, F. H., and Gullino, P. M.: Bulk transfer of fluid in the interstitial compartment of mammary tumors. Cancer Res., 35:3084–3088, 1975.

Call, K. M., Glaser, T., Ito, C. Y., Buckler, A. J., Pelletier, J., Haber, D. A., Rose, E. A., Kral, A., Yeger, H., Lewis, W. H., Jones, C., and Housman, D. E.: Isolation and characterization of a zinc finger polypeptide gene at the human chromosome 11 Wilms' tumor locus. Cell, 60:509–520, 1990.

Camps, J. L., Chang, S.-M., Hsu, T. C., Freeman, M. R., Hong, S.-J., Zhou, H. Y., Eschenbach, A. C., and Chung, L. W. K.: Fibroblast-mediated acceleration of human epithelial tumor growth in vivo. Proc. Natl. Acad. Sci. U S A, 87:75–79, 1990.

Capon, D. J., Chen, E. Y., Levinson, A. D., Seeburg, P. H., and Goeddel, D. V.: Complete nucleotide sequences of the T-24 human bladder carcinoma oncogene and its normal homologue. Nature, 302:33–37, 1983.

Carroll, P. R., and Chiganti, R. S. V.: Cytogenetics: Chromosomal abnormalities in urologic tumors. *In* Chisholm, G. D., and Fair, W. R. (Eds.): Scientific Foundations of Urology. Oxford, Heinemann Medical Books, 1990, pp. 481–489.

Carson-Jurica, M. A., Schrader, W. T., and O'Malley, B. W.: Steroid receptor family: structure and function. Endocr. Res., 11:201–220, 1990.

Carter, B. S., Epstein, J. I., and Isaacs, W. B.: *ras* gene mutations in human prostate cancer. Cancer Res., 50:6830–6832, 1990.

Chackal-Roy, M., Niemeyer, C., Moore, M., and Zetter, B. R.: Stimulation of prostatic carcinoma cell growth by factors present in human bone marrow. J. Clin. Invest., 84:43–50, 1989.

Chung, L. W. K., Camps, J. L., and Von Eschenbach, A. C.: Cancer Biology II. *In* Chisholm, G. D., and Fair, W. R. (Eds.): Scientific Foundations of Urology. Oxford, Heinemann Medical Books, 1990, pp. 459–473.

Cunha, G. R., Chung, L. W. K., Shannon, J. M., Taguchi, O., and Fuji, H.: Hormone-inducing morphogenesis and growth: role of mesenchymal epithelial interactions. Recent Prog. Horm. Res., 39:559–598, 1983.

Cunha, G. R., Donjacour, A. A., Cooke, P. S., Mee, S., Bigsby, R. M., Higgins, S. J., and Sugimura, Y.: The endocrinology and developmental biology of the prostate. Endocr. Rev., 8:338–362, 1987.

Derynck, R., Goeddel, D. V., Ulrich, A., Gutterman, J. U., Williams, R. D., Bringman, T. S., and Berger, W. H.: Synthesis of messenger RNAs for TGFα, TGFβ, and EGF receptor in human tumors. Cancer Res., 47:707–712, 1987.

DeVita, V. T.: Principles of chemotherapy. *In* DeVita, V. T., Hellman, S., and Rosenberg, S. A. (Eds.): Cancer: Principles and Practice of Oncology. Philadelphia, J. B. Lippincott, Co., 1989, pp. 276–290.

DeVita, Jr., V. T., Hellman, S., and Rosenberg, S. A. (Eds.): Cancer: Principles and Practice of Oncology, vol. 1. Philadelphia, J. B. Lippincott Co., 1989.

Dezube, B. J., Fridovich-Keil, J. L., Bouvard, I., Lange, R. F., and Pardee, A. B.: Pentoxifylline and well-being in patients with cancer. Lancet, 335:662, 1990.

Dmitrovsky, E., Markman, M., and Marks, P. A.: Clinical use of differentiating agents in cancer therapy. *In* Pineto, H. M., Chabner, B. A., Longo, D. L. (Eds.): Cancer Chemotherapy and Biologic Response Modifiers. New York, Elsevier, 1990, pp. 303–320.

Eastman, A.: Activation of programmed cell death by anticancer agents: *cis*-platin as a model system. Cancer Cells, 2:275–280, 1990.

Evans, R. M.: The steroid and thyroid hormone receptor super family. Science, 240:889–895, 1988.

Fearon, E. R., Cho, K. R., Nigro, J. M., Kern, S. E., Simons, J. W., Ruppert, J. M., Hamilton, S. R., Preisinger, A. C., Thomas, G., Kinzler, K. W., and Vogelstein, B.: Identification of a chromosome 18q gene that is altered in colorectal cancers. Science, 247:49–56, 1990a.

Fearon, E. R., and Vogelstein, B.: A genetic model for colorectal tumorigenesis. Cell, 61:759–767, 1990b.

Fidler, I. J.: Critical factors in the biology of human cancer metastasis:Twenty-eighth G.H.A. Clowes Award Memorial Lecture. Cancer Res., 50:6130–6138, 1990.

Fitzgerald, D., and Pastan, I.: Targeted toxin therapy for the treatment of cancer. J. Natl. Cancer Inst., 81:1455–1462, 1989.

Fleischmann, J., Heston, W. D. W., and Fair, W. R.: In-vitro assays for directing therapy of genitourinary tumors. *In* Ratliff, T. L., and Catalona, W. J. (Eds.): Urologic Oncology. Boston, Martinus Nijhoff, 1984, pp. 89–108.

Folkman, J.: What is the evidence that tumors are angeogenesis dependent? J. Natl. Cancer Inst., 82:4–6, 1990.

Folkman, J., and Klagsburn, M.: Angiogenic factors. Science, 235:442–447, 1987.

Frankel, A. E. (Ed.): Immunotoxins. Norwell, MA, Kluwer Acad. Publ., 1988.

Frankfurt, O. S., Greco, W. R., Slocum, H. K., Arbuck, S. G., Gamarra, M., Pavelic, Z. P., and Rustum, Y. M.: Proliferative characteristics of primary and metastatic human solid tumors by DNA flow cytometry. Cytometry, 5:629–635, 1984.

Freeman, C. S., Martin, M. R., and Marks, C. L.: An overview of tumor biology. Cancer Invest., 8:71–90, 1990.

Freeman, M. R., Washecka, R., and Chung, L. W. K.: Aberrant expression of epidermal growth factor receptor and her-2 (erb B-2) messenger RNAs in human renal cancers. Cancer Res., 49:6221–6225, 1989.

Fulker, M. J., Cooper, E. H., and Tanaka, T.: Proliferation and ultrastructure of papillary transitional cell carcinoma of the human bladder. Cancer, 27:71–82, 1971.

Gabrilove, J. L., Jakubowski, A., Scher, H., Sternberg, C., Wong, J., Grous, J., Yagoda, A., Fain, K., Moore, M., Clarkson, B., Oettgen, H. F., Alton, K., Welte, K., and Souza, L.: Effect of granulocyte-colony stimulating on neutropenia and associated morbidity due to chemotherapy for transitional cell carcinoma of the urothelium N. Engl. J. Med., 318:1414–1422, 1988.

Garin-Chesa, P., Old, L. J., and Rettig, W. J.: Cell surface glycoprotein of reactive stromal fibroblasts as a potential target in human epithelial cancers. Proc. Natl. Acad. Sci. U S A, 87:7235–7239, 1990.

Gessler, M., Poustka, A., Cavenee, W., Neve, R. L., Orkin, S. H., and Bruns, G. A. P.: Homozygous deletion in Wilms' tumours of a zinc-finger gene identified by chromosome jumping. Nature, 343:774–778, 1990.

Gibbs, J. B.: Toward the function of *ras*:Filling in the GAPs. Cancer Cells, 2:291–293, 1990.

Goldfarb, M.: The fibroblast growth factor family. Cell Growth Differ., 1:439–445, 1990.

Goldie, J. H., and Coldman, A. J.: The genetic origin of drug resistance in neoplasms: implications for systemic therapy. Cancer Res., 44:3643–3563, 1984.

Gouston, A. S., Leof, E. B., Shipley, G. D., and Moses, H. L.: Growth factors and cancer. Cancer Res., 46:1015–1028, 1986.

Greenberg, E. R., et al.: A clinical trial of beta carotene to prevent basal-cell and squamous-cell cancers of the skin. N. Engl. J. Med., 323:789–795, 1990.

Hall, A.: The cellular function of small GTP-binding proteins. Science, 249:635–640, 1990.

Hall, P. A., and Watt, F. M.: Stem cells: the generation and maintenance of cellular diversity. Development, 106:619–633, 1989.

Harris, H.: The analysis of malignancy by cell fusion: the position in 1988. Cancer Res., 48:3302–3306, 1988.

Heim, S., Mandahl, N., and Mitelman, F.: Genetic convergence and divergence in tumor progression. Cancer Res., 48:5911–5916, 1988.

Heimbrook, D. C., Stirdivant, S. M., Ahern, J. D., Balishin, N. L., Patrick, D. R., Edwards, G. M., Defoe-Jones, D., Fitzgerald, D. J., Pastan, I., and Oliff, A.: Transforming growth factor α–*Pseudomonas* exotoxin fusion protein prolongs survival of nude mice bearing tumor xenografts. Proc. Natl. Acad. Sci. U S A, 87:4687–4701, 1990.

Hellstrom, K. E., and Hellstrom, I.: Oncogene-associated tumor antigens as targets for immunotherapy. FASEB J, 3:1715–1722, 1989.

Hertig, A. T.: Contrib. Embryol., 25:37, 1935.

Huggins, C., and Hodges, C. V.: Studies on prostatic cancer. I. The effect of castration, of estrogen and of androgen injection on serum phosphatases in metastatic carcinoma of the prostate. Cancer Res., 1:293–297, 1941.

Humphries, J. E., and Isaacs, J. T.: Unusual androgen sensitivity of the androgen-independent Dunning R3327G rat prostatic adenocarcinoma: Androgen effect on tumor cell loss. Cancer Res., 42:3148–3156, 1982.

Illmensee, K., and Mintz, B.: Totoipotency and normal differentiation of single teratocarcinoma cells by injection into blastocysts. Proc. Natl. Acad. Sci. U S A, 73:549–553, 1976.

Jones, R. J., Wagner, J., Celano, P., Zicha, M. I., and Sharkas, S. J.: Separation of pluripotent haematopoietic stem cells from colony-forming cells. Nature, 347:188–189, 1990.

Kirkland, S. C.: Clonal origins of columnar, mucous, and endocrine cell lineages in human colorectal epithelium. Cancer, 61:1359–1363, 1988.

Knudson, A. G.: Mutation and cancer: statistical study of retinoblastoma. Proc. Natl. Acad. Sci. U S A, 68:820–823, 1971.

Kohler, G., and Milstein, C.: Continuous cultures of fused cells secreting antibody of predefined specificity. Nature, 256:495–497, 1975.

Kohn, E. C., and Liotta, L. A.: L651582: A novel antiproliferative and antimetastasis agent. J. Natl. Cancer Inst., 82:54–60, 1990.

Kokai, Y., Dobaski, K., Myers, J. N., Nowell, P. C., and Greene, M. I.: Phosphorylation induced by epidermal growth factor alters cellular and oncogenic *neu* gene products. Proc. Natl. Acad. Sci. U S A, 85:5389–5393, 1988.

Kokai, Y., Myers, J. N., Wada, T., Brown, V. I., LeVea, C. M., Davis, S. G., Dobaski, K., and Greene, M. I.: Synergistic interaction of p185e-*neu* and the EGF receptor leads to transformation of rodent fibroblasts. Cell, 58:287–292, 1989.

Laiho, M., DeCaprio, J. A., Ludlow, J. W., Livingston, D. M., and Massague, J.: Growth inhibition by TGF-β linked to suppression of retinoblastoma protein phosphorylation. Cell, 62:175–185, 1990.

Lerman, C., Rimer, B., and Engstrom, P. F.: Reducing avoidable cancer mortality through prevention and early detection regimens. Cancer Res., 49:4955–4962, 1989.

Levitzki, A.: Tryphostins-potential antiproliferative agents and novel molecular tools. Biochem. Pharmacol., 40:913–918, 1990.

Lewin, B.: Driving the cell cycle: M phase kinase, its partners and substrates. Cell, 61:743–752, 1990.

Liotta, L. A.: Tumor invasion and metastasis: role of the extracellular matrix. Rhoads Memorial Award Lecture. Cancer Res., 46:1–7, 1986.

Liotta, L. A., Horan Hand, P., Rao, C. N., Bryant, G., Barsky, S. H., and Schlom, J.: Monoclonal antibodies to the human laminin receptor recognize structurally distinct sites. Exp. Cell Res., 156:117–126, 1985.

Liotta, L. A. and Schiffmann, E.: Tumor autocrine motility factors. *In* DeVita, V. T., Jr., Hellman, S., and Rosenberg, S. A. (Eds.): Important Advances in Oncology. Philadelphia, J. B. Lippincott, 1988, pp. 17–30.

Liotta, L. A., Tryggvason, K., Garbisa, S., Hart, I., Foltz, C. M., and Shafie, S.: Metastatic potential correlates with enzymatic degradation of basement membrane collagen. Nature, 284:67–68, 1980.

Mackillop, W. J., Bizarri, J. P., and Ward, G. K.: Cellular heterogeneity in normal and neoplastic urothelium. Cancer Res., 45:4360–4365, 1985.

Mannson, P. F., Adams, P., Kan, M., and McKeehan, W. L.: Heparin binding growth factor gene expression and receptor characteristics in normal rat prostate and two transplantable rat prostate tumors. Cancer Res., 49:1485–1494, 1989.

Masui, H., Moroyama, T., and Mendelsohn, J.: Mechanism of anti-tumor activity in mice for anti-epidermal growth factor receptor monoclonal antibodies with different isotypes. Cancer Res., 46:5592–5598, 1986.

Mauch, P., Ferra, J., and Hellman, S.: Stem cell self-renewal considerations in bone marrow transplantation. Bone Marrow Transplant., 4:601–607, 1989.

McCarthy, J. B., Basara, M. J., Palm, S. L., Sas, D. F., and Furcht, L. T.: The role of cell adhesion proteins—laminin and fibronectin—in the movement of malignant and metastatic cells. Cancer Metastasis Rev., 4:125–152, 1985.

Melamed, M. R., and Staianco-Coico, L.: Flow cytometry in clinical cytology. *In* Melamed, M. R., Lindmore, T., and Mendelsohn, M. L. (Eds.): Flow Cytometry and Sorting. New York, Wiley-Liss, 1990, pp. 755–772.

Mignatti, P., Robbins, E., and Rifkin, D. B.: Tumor invasion through the human amniotic membrane: requirement for a proteinase cascade. Cell, 47:487–498, 1986.

Mohler, J. L., Partin, A. W., and Coffey, D. S.: Prediction of metastatic potential by a new grading system of cell motility: validating in the Dunning r3327 prostatic adenocarcinoma model. J. Urol., 138:168–170, 1987.

Moroco, J. R., Solt, D. B., and Polverini, P. S.: Sequential loss of suppressor genes for three specific functions during *in vivo* carcinogenesis. Lab. Invest., 63:298–306, 1990.

Muller, W. J., Simm, E., Pattengale, P. K., Wallace, R., and Leder, P.: Single-step induction of mammary adenocarcinoma in transgenic mice bearing the activated c-*neu* oncogene. Cell, 54:105–115, 1988.

Mydlo, J. H., Bulbul, M. A., Richon, V. M., Heston, W. D. W., and Fair, W. R.: Heparin-binding growth factors isolated from human prostatic extracts. Prostate, 12:343–355, 1988.

Mydlo, J. H., Michaeli, J., Cordon-Cardo, C., Goldenberg, A. S., Heston, W. D. W., and Fair, W. R.: Expression of transforming growth factor receptor messenger RNA in neoplastic and non-neoplastic human kidney tissue. Cancer Res., 49:3407–3411, 1989.

Neal, D. E., Sharples, L., Smith, K., Fennelly, J., Hall, R. R., and Harris, A. L.: The epidermal growth factor receptor and the prognosis of bladder cancer. Cancer, 65:1619–1625, 1990.

Nemoto, R., Hattori, K., Uchida, K., Shimazui, T., Nishijima, Y., Koiso, K., and Harada, M.: S phase fraction of human prostate adenocarcinoma studied with in vivo bromodeoxyuridine labeling. Cancer, 66:509–514, 1990.

Newmark, H. L., Lipkin, M., and Maheshwari, N.: Colonic hyperplasia and hyperproliferation induced by a nutritional stress diet with four components of Western-style diet. J. Natl. Cancer Inst., 82:491–496, 1990.

Nguyen, L., Chapdelaine, A., and Chevalier, S.: Prostatic acid phosphatase in serum of patients with prostatic cancer is a specific phosphotyrosine acid phosphatase. Clin. Chem., 36:1450–1455, 1990.

Olsnes, S., and Sandvig, K.: How protein toxins enter and kill cells. *In* Frankel, A. E. (Ed.): Immunotoxins. Norwell, MA, Kluwer Acad. Publ., 1988, pp. 39–73.

Olumni, A. F., Tsai, Y. C., Nichols, P. W., Skinner, D. G., Cain, D. G., Cain, D. R., Bender, L. I., and Jones, P. A.: Allelic loss of chromosome 17p distinguishes high-grade from low-grade transitional cell carcinomas of the bladder. Cancer Res., 50:7081–7083, 1990.

Parada, L. F., Tabin, C. J., Shih, C., and Weinberg, R. A.: Human EJ bladder carcinoma oncogene is homologue of Harvey sarcoma virus *ras* gene. Nature, 297:474–478, 1982.

Partin, A. W., Isaacs, J. T., Treiger, B., and Coffey, D. S.: Early cell motility changes associated with an increase in metastatic ability in rat prostatic cancer cells transfected with the v-Harvey-*ras* oncogene. Cancer Res., 48:6050–6053, 1988.

Partin, A. W., Schoenigen, J. S., Mohler, J. L., and Coffey, D. S.: Fourier analysis of cell motility with metastatic potential. Proc. Natl. Acad. Sci. U S A, 86:1254–1258, 1989.

Peehl, D. M., Wong, S. T., McNeal, J. E., and Stamey, T. A.: Analysis of somatic cell hybrids derived from normal human prostatic epithelial cells fused with HELA cells. Prostate, 17:123–136, 1990.

Pienta, K. J., Partin, A. W., and Coffey, D. S.: Cancer as a disease of DNA organization and dynamic cell structure. Cancer Res., 49:2525–2532, 1989.

Pierce, G. B., and Speers, W. C.: Tumors as caricatures of the process of tissue renewal: Prospects for therapy by directing differentiation. Cancer Res., 48:1996–2004, 1988.

Poste, G., and Greig, R.: The experimental and clinical implications of cellular heterogeneity in malignant tumors. J. Cancer Res. Clin. Oncol., 106:159–170, 1983.

Poste, G., and Nicolson, G. L.: Arrest and metastasis of blood-borne tumor cells are modified by fusion of plasma membrane vesicles from highly metastatic cells. Proc. Natl. Acad. Sci. U S A, 77:399–403, 1980.

Prentice, R. L., Pepe, M., and Self, S. G.: Dietary fat and breast cancer: a quantitative assessment of the epidemiological literature and a discussion of methodological issues. Cancer Res., 49:3147–3156, 1989.

Pritchard-Jones, K., Fleming, S., Davidson, D., Bickmore, W., Porteous, D., Gosden, C., Bard, J., Buckler, A., Pelletier, J., Housman, D., van Heyningen, V., and Hastie, N.: The candidate Wilms' tumor gene is involved in genitourinary development. Nature, 346:194–196, 1990.

Pulciani, S., Santos, E., Lauver, A. O., Long, L. K., Robbins, K.

C., and Barbacid, M.: Oncogenes in human tumor cell lines: Molecular cloning of a transforming gene from human bladder carcinoma cells. Proc. Natl. Acad. Sci. U S A, 79:2845–2849, 1982.

Raber, M., and Barlogie, B.: DNA flow cytometry of human solid tumors. *In* Melamed, M. R., Lindmore, T., Mendelsohn, M. L. (Eds.): Flow Cytometry and Sorting. New York, Wiley-Liss, 1990, pp. 745–754.

Raycroft, L., Wu, H., and Lozano, G.: Transcriptional activation by wild-type but not transforming mutants of the p53 antioncogene. Science, 249:649–651, 1990.

Reiss, Y., Goldstein, J. L., Seabra, M. C., Casey, P. J., and Brown, M. S.: Inhibition of purified p21^{ras} farnesyl: Protein transferase by Cys-AAX tetrapeptides. Cell, 62:81–88, 1990.

Revesz, L.: Effect of lethally damaged tumor cells upon the development of admixed viable cells. J. Natl. Cancer Inst., 20:1157–1186, 1958.

Roberts, A. B., Anzano, M. A., Walsefield, L. M., Roche, N. S., Stern, D. F., and Sporn, M. B.: Type B transforming growth factor: bifunctional regulator of cell growth. Proc. Natl. Acad. Sci. U S A, 82:119–123, 1985.

Roedink, F. H., and Kroon, A. M. (Eds.): Drug Carrier Systems. New York, John Wiley & Sons, 1989.

Rosenberg, S. A., Aebersold, P., Cornetta, K., Kasid, A., Morgan, R. A., Moen, R., Karson, E. M., Lotze, M. T., Yang, J. C., Topalian, S. L., Merino, M. J., Culver, K., Miller, A., Blaese, R. M., and Anderson, W. F.: Gene transfer into humans—Immunotherapy of patients with advanced melanoma using tumor-infiltrating lymphocytes modified by retroviral gene transduction. N. Engl. J. Med., 323:570–578, 1990.

Rowland, A. J., Harper, M. E., Wilson, D. W., and Griffiths, K.: The effect of an anti-membrane antibody-methotrexate conjugate on the human prostatic tumor line PC3. Br. J. Cancer, 61:702–708, 1990.

Russo, P., Sheinfeld, J., Cordon-Cardo, C., Fair, W. R., Marks, P. A., and Rifkind, R. A.: Changes in phenotype and growth induced by hexamethylene *bis*-acetamide and *cis*-retinoic acid in human urothelial carcinoma cells obtained from bladder washings. Surg. Forum, 38:685–688, 1987.

Sager, R.: Tumor suppressor genes: the puzzle and the promise. Science, 246:1406–1412, 1989.

Sambrook, J., Fritsch, E. F., and Maniatis, T. (Eds.): Molecular Cloning. Cold Spring Harbor, NY, Cold Spring Harbor Press, 1989.

Scher, S.: Chemotherapy for bladder cancer: neoadjuvant versus adjuvant. Semin. Oncol., 17:555–565, 1990.

Scher, H. I., Yagoda, A., Herr, H. W., Sternberg, C. N., Morse, M. J., Sogani, P. C., Watson, R. C., Reuter, V., Whitmore, W. F., Jr., and Fair, W. R.: Neoadjuvant M-VAC (methotrexate, vinblastine, doxorubicin and *cis*-platin) for extravesical urinary tract tumors. J. Urol., 139:475–477, 1988.

Sheinfeld, J., Reuter, V. E., Melamed, M. R., Fair, W. R., Morse, M., Sogani, P., Herr, H. W., Whitmore, W. F., Jr., and Cordon-Cardo, C.: Enhanced bladder cancer detection with the Lewis x antigen as a marker of neoplastic transformation. J. Urol., 143:285–288, 1990.

Shih, C., and Weinburg, R. A.: Isolation of a transforming sequence from a human bladder carcinoma cell line. Cell, 29:161–169, 1982.

Shimizu, M., Yokota, J., Mori, N., Shinoda, M., Terada, M., and Oshimura, M.: Introduction of normal chromosome 3p modulates tumorigenicity of a human renal cell carcinoma cell line YCR. Oncogene, 5:185–194, 1990.

Skipper, H. E., Schabel, F. M., Jr., and Wilcox, W. S.: Experimental evaluation of potential anticancer agents. XII. On the criteria and kinetics associated with 'curability' of experimental leukemia. Cancer Chemother. Rep., 35:1–111, 1964.

Sluyser, M.: Steroid/thyroid receptor–like proteins with oncogenic potential: A review. Cancer Res., 50:451–458, 1990.

Sporn, M. B., and Roberts, A. B.: Autocrine growth factors and cancer. Nature, 313:747–751, 1985.

Steeg, P. S., Bevilacqua, G., Kopper, L., Thorgeirsson, U. P., Talmadge, J. E., Liotta, L. A., and Sobel, M. E.: Evidence for a novel gene associated with low tumor metastatic potential. J. Natl. Cancer Inst., 80:200–204, 1988.

Steel, G. G.: Growth Kinetics of Tumors. London, Oxford University Press, 1977, p. 217.

Stephenson, R. A., James, B. C., Gay, H., Fair, W. R., Whitmore, W. F., and Melamed, M. R.: Flow cytometry of prostatic cancer: relationship of DNA content to survival. Cancer Res., 47:2504–2509, 1987.

Story, M. T., Esch, F., Shimasaki, S., Sasse, J., Jacobs, S. C., and Lawson, R. K.: Aminoterminal signal of a large form of basic fibroblast growth factor isolated from human BPH. Biochem. Biophys. Res. Commun., 142:702–709, 1987.

Studzinski, G. P.: Oncogenes, growth and the cell cycle: an overview. Cell Tissue Kinet., 22:495, 1989.

Sugarbaker, E. V., Cohen, A. M., and Ketcham, A. S.: Do metastases metastasize? Ann. Surg., 174:161–166, 1971.

Tannock, I. F.: Principles of cell proliferation: Cell kinetics. *In* DeVita, Jr., V. T., Hellman, S., and Rosenberg, S. A. (Eds.): Cancer: Principles and Practice of Oncology. Philadelphia, J. B. Lippincott Co., 1989, pp. 3–13.

Tarin, D., Vass, A. C. R., Kettlewell, M. G. W., and Price, J. E.: Absence of metastatic sequelae during long-term treatment of malignant ascites by peritoneo-venous shunting. Invasion Metastasis, 4:1–12, 1984.

Terranova, V. P., Hujanen, E. S., and Martin, G. R.: Basement membrane and the invasive activity of metastatic tumor cells. J. Natl. Cancer Inst., 77:311–316, 1986.

Thompson, T. C., Southgate, J., Kitchener, G., and Land, H.: Multistage carcinogenesis induced by *ras* and *myc* oncogenes in reconstituted organ. Cell, 56:917–930, 1989.

Thorgeirsson, U. P., Liotta, L. A., Kalebic, T., Margulies, I. M., Thomas, K., Rios-Candelore, M., and Russo, R. G.: Effect of neutral protease inhibitors and a chemoattractant on tumor cell invasion in vitro. J. Natl. Cancer Inst. 69:1049–1054, 1982.

Till, J. E., and McCulloch, E. A.: A direct measurement of the radiation sensitivity of the normal mouse bone marrow. Radiat. Res., 18:96–102, 1967.

Touchette, N.: The cell cycle comes full circle. J. NIH Res. 2:53–57, 1990a.

Touchette, N.: Tumor suppressors: A new arena in the war against cancer. J. NIH Res. 2:62–66, 1990b.

Tritton, T. R., and Hickman, J. A.: How to kill cancer cells: membranes and cell signaling as targets in cancer chemotherapy. Cancer Cells, 2:95–105, 1990.

Van Dekken, H., Schervish, E. W., Pizzolo, J. G., Fair, W. R., and Melamed, M. R.: Simultaneous detection of fluorescent in situ hybridization and in vivo incorporated BRDU in a human bladder tumor. J. Pathol. In press.

Vogelstein, B., Fearon, E. R., Hamilton, S. R., Kern, S. E., Preisinger, A. C., Leppert, M., Nakamura, Y., White, R., Smits, A., and Bos, J. L.: Genetic alterations during colorectal tumor development. N. Engl. J. Med. 319:525–532, 1988.

Vogelstein, B., Fearon, E. R., Kern, S. E., Hamilton, S. R., Preisinger, A. C., Nakamura, Y., and White, R.: Allelotype of colorectal carcinomas. Science, 244:207–211, 1989.

Waage, A., Sorensen, M., and Stordal, B.: Differential effect of oxypentifylline on tumor necrosis factor and interleukin-6 production. Lancet, 335:543, 1990.

Wallet, V., Mutzel, R., Troll, H., Barzu, O., Wurster, B., Veron, M., and Lacombe, M. L.: *Dictyostelium* nucleoside diphosphate kinase highly homologous to nm23 and awd proteins involved in mammalian tumor metastasis and *Drosophila* development. J. Natl. Cancer Inst., 82:1199–1202, 1990.

Weinberg, R. A.: Oncogenes, antioncogenes, and the molecular basis for multi-step carcinogenesis. Cancer Res., 49:3713–3721, 1989.

Weissman, B. E., Saxon, P. S., Pasquale, S. R., Jones, G. R., Geiser, A. G., and Stanbridge, E. J.: Introduction of a normal human chromosome 11 into a Wilms' tumor cell line controls its tumorigenic expression. Science, 236:175–180, 1987.

Whyte, P., Buchovich, K. J., Horowitz, J. M., Friend, S. H., Raybuck, M., Weinberg, R. A., and Harlow, E.: Association between an oncogene and an antioncogene: the adenovirus E1A proteins bind to the retinoblastoma gene product. Nature, 334:124–129, 1988.

Wood, D. P., Anderson, A. E., Klein, E., Fair, W. R., and Chaganti, R. S. K.: Metallothionein gene expression and *ras* point mutations in bladder cancer resistant to *cis*-platin. J. Urol. In press.

Xu, G., O'Connell, P., Viskochil, D., Cawthon, R., Robertson, M.,

Culver, M., Dunn, D., Stevens, J., Gesteland, R., White, R., and Weiss, R.: The neurofibromatosis type 1 gene encodes a protein related to GAP. Cell, 62:599–608, 1990.

Yao, M., Shuin, T., Misaki, H., and Kubata, Y.: Enhanced expression of c-myc and epidermal growth factor receptor (c-*erb* B-1) genes in primary human renal cancer. Cancer Res., 48:6753–6757, 1988.

Yarden, Y., and Ulrich, A.: Growth factor receptor tyrosine kinases. Ann. Rev. Biochem., 57:443–478, 1988.

Yarden, Y., and Weinberg, R. A.: Experimental approaches to hypothetical hormones: Detection of a candidate ligand of the *neu* proto-oncogene. Proc. Natl. Acad. Sci. U S A, 86:3179–3183, 1989.

Zenke, M., Munoz, A., Sap, J., Vennstrom, B., and Beug, H.: V-Erb-A oncogene activation entails the loss of hormone-dependent regulatory activity of C-Erb-A. Cell, 61:1031–1049, 1990.

Zetter, B. R.: The cellular basis of site-specific metastasis. N. Engl. J. Med., 322:605–612, 1990.

27
RENAL TUMORS

Jean B. deKernion, M.D.
Arie Belldegrun, M.D.

HISTORICAL CONSIDERATIONS

The evolution of knowledge about renal tumors is in actuality the history of surgical daring in a microcosm. Autopsy information relative to renal disorders was scant. The introduction of nephrectomy and other subsequent surgical interventions for renal diseases provided the clinical information and histopathologic insight that form the bases of our current concepts of renal tumors. Thus, the historical data available to us date back little more than 100 years.

Harris (1882) reported on 100 surgical extirpations of the kidney, a sufficient number to permit some sort of analysis of clinical, surgical, and pathologic features of renal disorders that require surgery. The first documented nephrectomy was apparently accomplished by Wolcott in 1861, who operated with the mistaken assumption that the tumor mass was a hepatoma. In 1867, Spiegelberg removed a kidney incidentally in the course of excising an echinococcus cyst. The first planned nephrectomy was performed by Gustav Simon in 1869 for persistent ureteral fistula, and this patient survived with cure of the fistula. It was only 1 year later (1870) that the first planned nephrectomy was successfully accomplished in the United States, by John Gilmore of Mobile, Alabama—on this occasion as treatment for atrophic pyelonephritis and persistent urinary infection (Glenn, 1980).

With surgical intervention, tissue became available to pathologists for histologic interpretation. Unfortunately, such interpretation was not always accurate, and there were often serious professional differences of opinion. According to Carson (1928), the first accurate gross description of kidney tumors dates to 1826, with König's observations. In 1855, Robin examined solid tumors apparently arising in the kidney and concluded that renal carcinoma arose from renal tubular epithelium. This interpretation was confirmed by Waldeyer in 1867. Unfortunately, theoretical and practical considerations of renal tumors were confused by Grawitz (1883), who contended that such apparent renal tumors arose from adrenal rests within the kidney. He introduced the terminology "struma lipomatodes aberrata renis" as descriptive nomenclature for the tumors of clear cells that he believed were derived from the adrenal glands. He based his conclusions not only on the fatty content of the tumors, analogous to that seen in the adrenal glands, but also on the location of the tumors beneath the renal capsule, the approximation to the adrenal glands, the lack of similarity of the cells to uriniferous tubules, and the demonstration of amyloid not unlike that seen with adrenal degeneration.

This histogenetic concept was adopted by subsequent investigators, and pathologists of the era readily embraced the idea that renal tumors truly arose from the adrenal glands. In 1894, Lubarch endorsed the idea of a suprarenal origin of renal tumors, and the term "hypernephroid tumors," indicating origin above the kidneys, was advocated by Birch-Hirschfeld (Birch-Hirschfeld and Doederlein, 1894.) This semantic and conceptual mistake led to the introduction of the term "hypernephroma," which predominates in the literature describing parenchymal tumors of primary renal origin.

Weichselbaum and Greenish (1883) described renal adenomas containing both papillary and alveolar cell types. Some clarification of the histopathology of renal tumors is derived from the work of Albarran and Imbert (1903), and the four-volume contribution of Wolff (1883), written between 1883 and 1928, adds further historical significance to our understanding of renal tumors today (Glenn, 1980).

CLASSIFICATION

An appropriate, simple, and all-inclusive classification of renal tumors has eluded surgical pathologists and urologic surgeons alike over the past century. Even with the elimination of hydronephrosis and various inflammatory tumefactions of the kidney, such as xanthogranulomatous pyelonephritis, from the category, the spectrum of renal tumors remains extremely broad. Various classifications have been adopted in an effort to acknowledge and include the various new growths of diverse causes that can afflict the human kidney.

Certainly, the most comprehensive classification of renal tumors is that offered by Deming and Harvard (1970) in a previous edition of this text. They established 11 categories of renal tumors, with multiple subdivisions embracing virtually every known new growth that may involve the kidney—common, uncommon, or rare—including the various renal cystic disorders as well as the perirenal retroperitoneal tumors that may involve the kidney secondarily. This classification is reproduced here (Table 27–1) because it provides the most succinct presentation of renal tumors, yet retains accuracy and inclusiveness.

Another approach has been taken by other investigators. Only new solid parenchymal growths arising primarily in the kidney have been considered. Lakey (1975), for example, subdivides the renal neoplasms into benign and malignant tumors, classifying these neoplasms as shown in Table 27–2. When one considers that the majority of benign renal tumors represent the various cystic disorders, with few solid lesions, one can

Table 27–2. LAKEY'S CLASSIFICATION OF RENAL TUMORS

Benign Tumors	Malignant Tumors
Adenoma	Nephroblastoma (Wilms' tumor)
Fibroma	Adenocarcinoma, renal cell carcinoma
Lipoma	Sarcomas
Leiomyoma	Fibrosarcoma
Angioma	Liposarcoma
Rhabdomyoma	Leiomyosarcoma
Neurofibroma	Osteogenic sarcoma
Dermoid	Lymphoblastoma
Endometriosis	Lymphomas, myeloma
Angiomyolipoma (hamartoma)	Secondary malignant tumors

Adapted from Lakey, W. H.: Tumors of the kidney. In Karafin, L., and Kendall, A. R. (Eds.): Urology, Vol. 2. New York, Harper & Row, 1975.

focus attention on the category of renal malignancies. Within the past decade, arguments have been made for the classification of malignant renal neoplasms into four categories: (1) nephroblastoma and other embryonic renal malignancies; (2) nephrocarcinoma, the generic term for adult renal parenchymal malignancies; (3) urothelial malignancies of the renal pelvis; and (4) other malignancies of the renal substance, capsule, or perirenal structures. Such a simplistic subcategorization of renal malignancies offers considerable appeal.

An effort must be made, however, to provide a classification that is both complete and uncomplicated, embracing all the lesions that predispose an individual to renal mass or new growth. Such a simplified classification was proposed by Glenn (1980) (Table 27–3). Benign tumors include those of the renal capsule (such as fibroma), renal parenchymatous adenomas, vascular tumors, various cystic lesions and dysplasias, heteroplastic and mesenchymal tumors, and even various hydronephroses. Tumors of the renal pelvis, not a primary consideration here, include the benign papillomas as well as transitional, squamous, and adenocarcinomatous malignancies. Perirenal tumors are those that involve

Table 27–1. CLASSIFICATION OF RENAL TUMORS

Tumors of the Renal Capsule	**Neurogenic Tumors**
Fibroma	Neuroblastoma
Leiomyoma	Sympathicoblastoma
Lipoma	Schwannoma
Mixed	**Heteroplastic Tissue Tumors**
Tumors of the Mature Renal	Adipose
Parenchyma	Smooth muscle
Adenoma	Adrenal rests
Adenocarcinoma	Endometriosis
Hypernephroma	Cartilage
Renal cell cancer	Bone
Alveolar carcinoma	**Mesenchymal Derivatives**
Tumors of the Immature Renal	Connective tissue
Parenchyma	Fibroma
Nephroblastoma (Wilms')	Fibrosarcoma
Embryonic carcinoma	Osteogenic sarcoma
Sarcoma	Adipose tissue
Epithelial Tumors of the Renal	Lipoma
Pelvis	Liposarcoma
Transitional cell papilloma	Muscle tissue
Transitional cell carcinoma	Leiomyoma
Squamous cell carcinoma	Leiomyosarcoma
Adenocarcinoma	Rhabdomyosarcoma
Cysts	**Pararenal/Perirenal Solid Tumors**
Solitary	Lipoma
Unilateral multiple	Sarcoma
Calyceal	Liposarcoma
Pyogenic	Fibrosarcoma
Calcified	Lymphangiosarcoma
Tubular ectasia	Cancer
Tuberous sclerosis	Teratoma
Cystadenoma	Lymphoblastoma
Papillary cystadenoma	Neuroblastoma
Dermoid	Hodgkin's disease
Pararenal/Perirenal cysts	**Secondary Tumors**
Hydrocele renalis	Cancer
Lymphatic	Sarcoma
Wolffian	Blastoma
Malignant	Granuloma
Vascular Tumors	Thymoma
Hemangioma	Testicular
Hamartoma	Renal
Lymphangioma	

Table 27–3. SIMPLIFIED CLASSIFICATION OF RENAL TUMORS

Benign Tumors
Renal capsule
Renal parenchyma
Vascular tumors
Cystic lesions, dysplasia, hydronephrosis
Heteroplastic, mesenchymal tumors
True oncocytoma
Tumors of Renal Pelvis
Benign papilloma
Transitional and squamous cell carcinomas, adenocarcinomas
Pararenal Tumors
Benign
Malignant
Embryonic Tumors
Nephroblastoma (Wilms' tumor)
Embryonic, mesotheliomatous tumors
Sarcomas
Nephrocarcinoma
Renal cell carcinoma, adenocarcinoma, "hypernephroma"
Papillary cystadenocarcinoma
Other Malignancies
Primary: mesenchymal, hemangiopericytoma, myeloma
Secondary: metastatic lesions

the kidney by extension and invasion, and they may be either benign or malignant. Embryonic tumors include predominantly nephroblastoma (Wilms' tumor) and the embryonic or mesotheliomatous carcinomas and sarcomas of childhood. Nephrocarcinoma is the generic category that includes adult renal parenchymatous malignancies, primarily the classic "hypernephroma" and papillary adenocarcinoma. The category of other malignancies embraces the relatively rare mesenchymal malignancies, such as the various sarcomas, hemangiopericytomas, infiltrative malignancies like myeloma, and secondary or metastatic malignancies manifesting within the renal substance. To Glenn's original classification has been added the oncocytoma.

The true oncocytoma has now been established to be a specific entity with a cell of origin different from that for renal cell carcinoma, and it is invariably benign (see following discussion). This lesion must be carefully distinguished from renal lesions that have the appearance of oncocytoma, both grossly and microscopically, but which have foci of other than grade I cells.

Wilms' tumor, the common renal malignancy of childhood, is addressed elsewhere in this book, as are neuroblastoma, renal cystic disorders, and primary retroperitoneal tumors. These entities, therefore, are beyond the scope of discussion in this chapter.

BENIGN RENAL TUMORS

Benign renal tumors may arise from any of the multiple cells types within and around the kidney. Renal cysts are perhaps the most common benign renal mass lesions. Approximately 70 per cent of asymptomatic renal mass lesions are simple cysts and are of no clinical significance (Lang, 1973). The major import of most benign lesions lies in either their growth to a large size, creating clinical symptoms, or their differential diagnosis from malignant renal tumors (see following discussion) (Fig. 27–1). Cysts may be single or multiple and unilateral or bilateral.

As discussed later, modern uroradiographic tech-

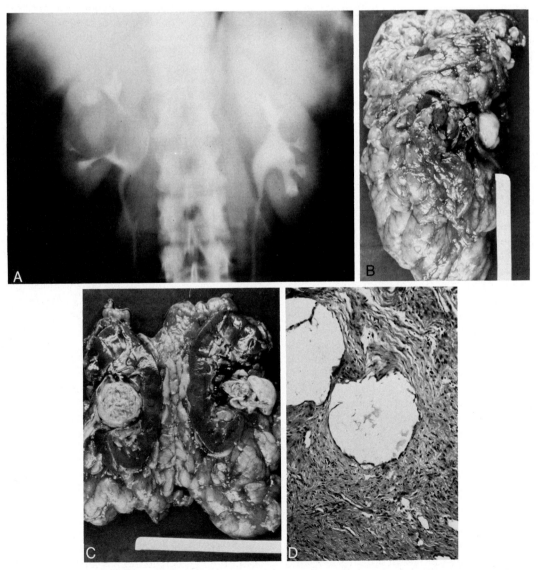

Figure 27–1. *A,* Pyelogram demonstrating a large parapelvic filling defect, which was compound on ultrasonic examination. *B,* A smooth glistening wall of cyst protruding through renal pelvis. *C,* Sagittal section demonstrating laminated, compound cyst. *D,* Microscopic section showing pure cystic nature of the mass.

niques can distinguish renal carcinoma from simple cysts with great accuracy. Occasionally, especially in the case of complex cysts, the true nature of the lesion may be determined only at surgery. It is beyond the scope of this discussion to cite each case report associated with the myriad rare benign tumors; we concentrate here on those that are found more commonly and those that are associated with symptoms or bear similarities to malignant tumors.

Cortical Adenoma

Renal cortical adenomas are commonly encountered at autopsy and are benign tumors both clinically and histologically. Bell (1950) found a direct correlation between size and malignant potential, noting that tumors less than approximately 3 cm in size had little propensity for metastasis. However, in his series of 62 tumors less than 3 cm in diameter, three had metastasized. Murphy and Mostofi (1970) concluded that renal adenomas are benign tumors, distinguishable from true adenocarcinomas. An alternative view was presented by Bennington and Beckwith (1975), who argued that all tubular cell adenomas are malignant, simply representing an early stage of renal carcinoma growth.

The etiology of renal cortical adenomas is unclear. Because of the frequency with which they are encountered in autopsy specimens as well as their frequency in males, an endocrine relationship has been suggested. No definite etiologic factor has been recognized, however, and no absolute association with the presence of frank renal cell carcinoma has been established.

The renal adenoma is characterized by uniform acidophilic or clear cells, with monotonous nuclear and cellular characteristics. Symptoms are unusual and are observed only when the tumor erodes the collecting system or adjacent vessels. Most renal adenomas are discovered incidentally. The computed tomography and arteriography characteristics are often indistinguishable from those of small renal adenocarcinomas, except for the general absence of arteriovenous fistulae, venous pooling, and calcification.

The clinician is often faced with a dilemma when a small, 3-cm renal parenchymal tumor is diagnosed. Although segmental resection or wedge resection may be appropriate, the true tendency for multiplicity is uncertain, and the final characterization of the mass as an adenoma usually awaits careful tissue sectioning. For this reason, most diagnosed renal parenchymal tumors are treated as true renal cell carcinomas.

Renal Oncocytoma

Renal oncocytoma has become a recognized clinical and pathologic entity with almost invariably benign clinical behavior. This tumor is characterized by a histologic pattern of large eosinophilic cells with a granular cytoplasm and typical polygonal form. Mitoses are rare, and the cells have a benign ultrastructure characterized by a profusion of mitochondria. Electron microscopy demonstrates the abundance of mitochondria with endoplasmic reticulum or Golgi apparatus, distinguishing this cell type from the low-grade renal carcinoma cell (Landier et al., 1979). It is important to remember that many renal cell carcinomas have typical oncocytic features and contain eosinophilic granular cells, either alone or in combination with cell-cell neoplastic elements. Differentiation between a typical renal oncocytoma and oncocytic renal cell carcinoma can, therefore, be a somewhat difficult pathologic task based on nuclear morphology. The term "renal oncocytoma" refers only to tumors that contain a population of highly differentiated eosinophilic granular cells or oncocytes.

Grossly, the tumors have a typical appearance, usually tan or light brown in color, well-circumscribed, round, encapsulated, and containing a central dense fibrous band with fibrous trabeculae extending out in a stellate pattern. The characteristic central scar is often imaged preoperatively by a computed tomographic (CT) or magnetic resonance imaging (MRI) examination of the tumor, sometimes even by ultrasound examination, and can serve to suggest the diagnosis of oncocytoma preoperatively. Necrosis and hypervascular areas are absent (Fig. 27–2). The typical cell appearance suggests an origin from the distal renal tubules, in particular from the interrelated cells of the collecting tubules (Nogueira and Bannasch, 1988; Zerban et al., 1987).

The exact incidence of oncocytoma compared with other renal tumors is unknown; however, current series suggest that 3 to 7 per cent of solid renocortical tumors previously classified as renal cell carcinomas are, in fact, typical renal oncocytomas (Lieber et al., 1981, 1986; Lieber, 1990). Renal oncocytomas occur more commonly in males than in females and have generally the same age incidence as that of renal cell carcinoma.

Oncocytomas vary in size and may be quite large. In collected series, the median size was 6 cm in diameter. They can be found throughout the body and are not necessarily limited to the kidneys. These tumors are typically unifocal, but it is important to remember that, in approximately 6 per cent of cases, bilateral oncocytomas can be found. Both synchronous and asynchronous bilateral renal oncocytomas have been reported.

Warfel and Eble (1982) reported a case in which more than 200 small renal oncocytomas were found in bilateral distribution; the specific term "oncocytomastosis" has thus been used to describe this typical entity. Multifocality of renal oncocytomas should be borne in mind when attempting a more conservative surgery, i.e., enucleation or partial nephrectomy. Careful search by radiologic imaging techniques and by direct examination at time of surgery should thus be performed, so that all tumors can be removed during the same operative procedure.

Oncocytomas are usually asymptomatic with the majority of tumors being discovered incidentally. Gross hematuria, abdominal pain, flank mass, and microscopic hematuria have all been infrequent findings. Because more ultrasound, CT, and MRI scans are being performed for unrelated conditions, it is anticipated that both renal cell carcinomas and oncocytomas will be discovered earlier, in the asymptomatic stages.

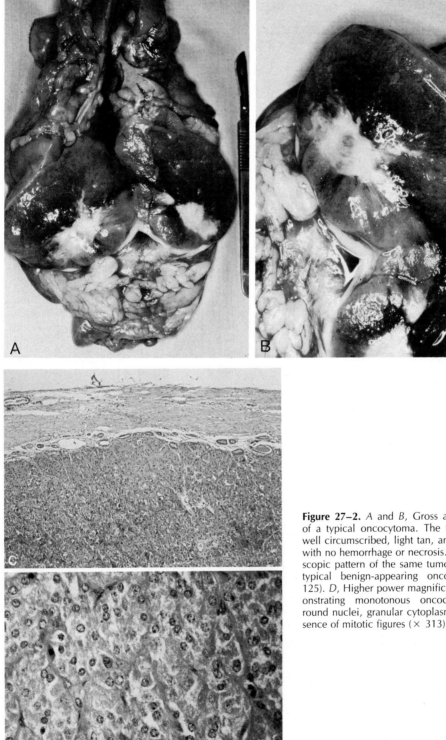

Figure 27–2. *A* and *B*, Gross appearance of a typical oncocytoma. The tumor was well circumscribed, light tan, and smooth, with no hemorrhage or necrosis. *C*, Microscopic pattern of the same tumor showing typical benign-appearing oncocytes (× 125). *D*, Higher power magnification demonstrating monotonous oncocytes with round nuclei, granular cytoplasm, and absence of mitotic figures (× 313).

The typical radiographic appearance of the renal oncocytoma has been largely responsible for its identification as a specific clinical entity. The pyelographic appearance is one of a circumscribed solid mass of varying size and location in the kidney. The arterial phase of the angiogram reveals a typical "spoke-wheel" or stellate pattern seldom associated with venous pooling or arteriovenous fistulae (Bonavita et al., 1981). However, the typical angiographic picture is not always identified, and the angiogram may be indistinguishable from that of a hypovascular renal cell carcinoma. No typical CT scan or specific radionuclide scan has been identified. Nuclear DNA ploidy cannot be used to distinguish between benign and malignant neoplasms in the kidney because certain typical oncocytomas will have abnormal—tetraploidy or aneuploidy—patterns (Rainwater et al., 1986).

The management of renal oncocytomas, therefore, must be influenced by two characteristic features: (1) the unreliability and nonspecificity of current radiographic studies and (2) the presence of malignant elements and oncocytoma cells in the same tumor. Clearly, a reliable preoperative diagnosis of renal oncocytoma merits an attempt at more conservative surgery, i.e., partial nephrectomy with frozen section control of the margins of resection. Radical nephrectomy is still the safest method of therapy unless contraindicated by other factors (e.g., solitary kidney, small size, poor renal function). For very elderly patients or patients who are otherwise very poor operative risks because of extensive medical problems, "observation treatment" of oncocytomas might be appropriate (Lieber, 1990).

Renal Hamartoma (Angiomyolipoma)

Renal hamartomas (Fig. 27–3) are benign tumors that may occur as an isolated phenomenon or as part of the syndrome associated with tuberous sclerosis. Approximately 80 per cent of patients with the diagnosis of hamartoma have some or all of the other stigmata of tuberous sclerosis. This is a disease that is both hereditary and familial and is characterized by mental retardation, epilepsy, and adenoma sebaceum. In these patients, hamartomas may also be found in the brain, eye, heart, lung, and bone (McCullough et al., 1971). Patients with tuberous sclerosis require careful screening for the presence of renal tumors (Stillwell et al., 1987).

Renal hamartomas are frequently bilateral. They are often yellow and gray and have a propensity for profuse hemorrhage, large size, and multiplicity. Microscopically, the tumor is named for the three primary components—unusual abdominal blood vessels, clusters of adipocytes, and sheets of smooth muscle. Pleomorphism is common, and mitotic figures, although rarely seen, can be prominent (Colvin and Dickersin, 1978). Although no case of widespread metastases has been reported, involvement of regional lymph nodes has been documented (Taylor et al., 1989).

Because of the multiplicity of these tumors and their propensity for bilaterality, conservative surgery is often imperative. The angiographic pattern of the tumor is not sufficiently typical to reliably separate it from renal carcinoma. However, the high fat content allows for a distinctive pattern on CT scan, with areas having density corresponding to fatty tissue (DaPonte et al., 1983). This typical CT picture (Fig. 27–4) accurately defines the presence of angiomyolipoma in most cases (Lingeman et al., 1982); however, reports by Taylor and co-workers (1989) and Blute and co-workers (1988) document the occasional presence of renal carcinoma in patients with proven angiomyolipoma. It therefore seems prudent to surgically excise tumors that are multiple, that do not have all of the classic characteristics of angiomyolipoma, and that contain calcifications.

Angiomyolipomas present clinically in several ways.

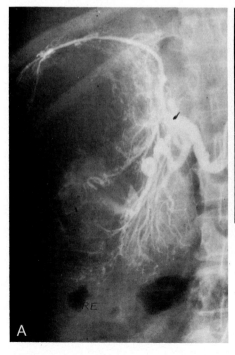

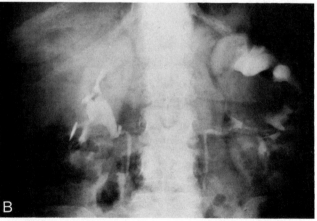

Figure 27–3. *A,* A 60-year-old woman with no evidence of tuberous sclerosis presented with hemorrhage into a large right flank tumor. Exploration and biopsy revealed hamartoma. *B,* One year after percutaneous angioinfarction of right renal hamartoma, also demonstrating central hamartoma in left kidney, is unchanged in 1 year.

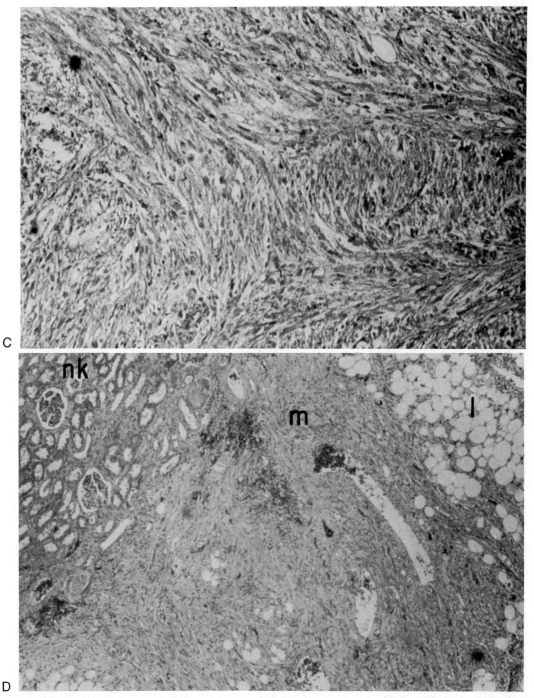

Figure 27–3 *Continued C,* Histologic appearance of fibromyomatous elements of tumor. *D* Normal kidney *(nk)* is seen with adjacent myomatous *(m)* and lipomatous *(l)* elements of intrinsic tumor, diagnosed as angiofibromyolipoma (hamartoma).

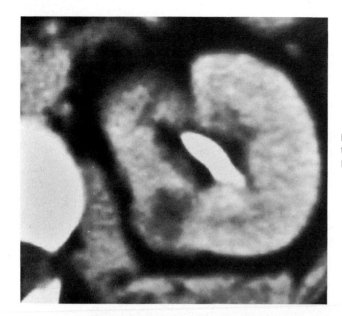

Figure 27–4. Small angiomyolipoma in the left kidney discovered incidentally. Contrast computed tomography scan shows that the mass is composed predominantly of fat.

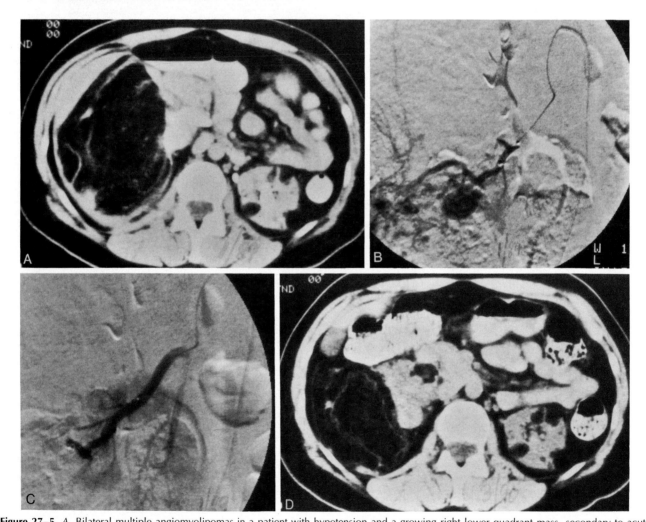

Figure 27–5. *A*, Bilateral multiple angiomyolipomas in a patient with hypotension and a growing right lower quadrant mass, secondary to acute hemorrhage. Computed tomography scan shows a large hematoma in the right perinephric space displacing the kidney anteriorly and medially.

B, Selective right renal arteriogram shows a large hypervascular mass arising from the lower pole of the right kidney and identifies the bleeding site. Note the multiple tortuous irregular vessels that form the bleeding aneurysms.

C, Subtraction renal arteriogram following a successful transcatheter, supraselective embolization of the lower pole branch, using steel coils. The upper pole branch was successfully embolized, 2 days later.

D, One-year follow-up postembolization. The right renal angiomyolipoma has only slightly decreased in size, but the hemorrhage at the periphery of the tumor has demonstrated significant reabsorption. Both kidneys are functioning well. The patient resumed normal activity and had no further bleeding episodes.

First, they often are detected incidentally in patients who undergo CT scans for unrelated abdominal problems, or in patients with tuberous sclerosis. Second, very large tumors may cause local discomfort and gastrointestinal symptoms by compression of the duodenum and stomach. Third, patients may present with sudden pain or hypotension due to massive hemorrhage within the lesions.

The management of angiomyolipoma is controversial, but several generalizations can be made. In their review, Oesterling and associates (1986) noted that the size of the lesions was usually associated with propensity for symptoms, especially hemorrhage. Accordingly, based on the literature and on the review of 13 patients at their institution, they concluded that asymptomatic lesions smaller than 4 cm in diameter may not require therapy but must be observed. Many of these tumors do not increase in size even after many years of follow-up. For persistently symptomatic tumors of any size, these same investigators recommend angiography and selective arterial embolization if possible or surgical or conservative surgical therapy if embolization is not practical. They advocate frequent monitoring of asymptomatic lesions larger than 4 cm.

Angioinfarction should be the first attempted therapy in any patient having hemorrhage into an angiomyolipoma. However, our experience has shown that very large tumors will not decrease in size after angioinfarction, although bleeding may be prevented (Fig. 27–5). Therefore, patients with very large lesions who can undergo excision with preservation of functioning renal tissue should be strongly considered for this approach. Symptomatic lesions that cannot be managed by angioinfarction, multiple lesions that are not all characteristic of angiomyolipoma, and calcification also require exploration and conservative surgical excision when possible.

Fibroma

Fibrous tissue is found in the renal parenchyma, the perinephric tissues, and the renal capsule, and fibromas may arise from any of these structures. Glover and Buck (1982) reviewed the eight reported cases of medullary fibroma and noted that most occurred in women. These are rare tumors that are uniformly benign and occasionally are difficult to distinguish from fibrosarcomas of the retroperitoneum. They are often on the periphery of the kidney and may have to grow to a large size before becoming clinically obvious. Symptoms are rare and are usually associated with either distortion of the collecting system or growth outside the confines of the renal fossa, although hematuria is common in patients with medullary fibromas.

These tumors are large, adherent to the kidney, and often resemble uterine fibroids. They are microscopically benign, with sheets of fibroblasts or a loose, myxomatous stroma. Angiographically, they are generally hypovascular but have no specific radiographic characteristics to distinguish them from hypovascular malignant tumors. A radical nephrectomy is usually performed because of the uncertainty of the diagnosis,

but awareness of their benign nature warrants partial nephrectomy in selected cases.

Lipoma

Renal lipomas are among the rarest of renal tumors. Their origin is unclear, but they probably originate from fat cells within the renal capsule or parenchyma (Robertson and Hand, 1941). Dineen and colleagues (1983) reported a case of lipoma and reviewed the literature, documenting 18 cases of proven intrarenal lipoma. This tumor typically occurs in middle-aged women, grows to a large size, and has pain as its presenting symptom, with hematuria occurring in some patients. A malignant potential has been suggested but has not been proved.

The gross characteristics are the same as those of any lipoma. Renal lipomas are confined within the renal capsule, in contrast to perirenal lipomas, which are extracapsular. These tumors have the greasy feeling of all lipomas, pale lobules being interposed with streaks consisting of blood vessels. Microscopically, the cells are uniform fat cells with peripherally placed nuclei surrounded by plasma membranes. The treatment is surgical excision, usually requiring total nephrectomy.

Commonly, these lipomas have other cellular elements (Robertson and Hand, 1941) and can be classified as variants of angiomyolipoma. They should not be classified as pure lipomas, but they have the same clinical significance and the same benign course.

Perinephric lipomas are difficult or impossible to separate from intrarenal lipomas and may arise from perinephric fat or adjacent areas of the retroperitoneum (Pfeiffer and Gandin, 1946). These tumors are often huge, and excision without nephrectomy is seldom possible. CT scan should show the typical fat density, allowing preoperative consideration of conservative excision.

Other Benign Tumors

Because the kidney is a complex organ consisting of many cell types within and surrounding the renal capsule, virtually every classification of benign tumor has been reported. Myomas, lymphangiomas, and hemangiomas have been found.

One of the rarest but most fascinating tumors is the functional renin-secreting juxtaglomerular tumor. It was first described by Robertson and co-workers (1967), and approximately ten cases have been described in the literature. These tumors arise from the juxtaglomerular cells in young patients (Orjauvik et al., 1975), who present typically with hypertension, elevated serum renin levels, and hyperaldosteronism. Presence of the tumor is suspected in individuals with an extremely high differential renal vein/renin ratio with no other obvious cause for hypertension.

Functional renin-secreting juxtaglomerular tumors are typically very small, seldom more than 2 or 3 cm in diameter, and often are not detectable radiographically. Occasionally, the segments of the kidney harboring the tumor can be identified by selective renal vein sampling (Bonnin et al., 1977). Grossly, the tumors are gray-yellow with hemorrhagic areas; microscopically, they are typical hemangiopericytomas. Electron microscopic studies reveal the characteristics of the juxtaglomerular cells, and tumor extracts may be shown to contain high concentrations of renin (Colvin and Dickersin, 1978).

This tumor is always benign and should be distinguished from the generally larger, nonfunctional, and sometimes malignant typical renal hemangiopericytoma.

MALIGNANT RENAL TUMORS

Renal Cell Carcinoma

Incidence

Renal cell carcinoma is a relatively rare tumor, accounting for approximately 3 per cent of adult malignancies. In a report from the National Cancer Institute, approximately 24,000 new cases of renal carcinoma were predicted to occur in 1990 (Silverberg et al., 1990). Little evidence suggests that the tumor is increasing in incidence, although it may be detected in earlier stages than previously.

Renal cell carcinoma is more common among urban dwellers and is more common in males, with a male-to-female ratio of approximately 2:1. Familial renal carcinoma has been reported, affecting as many as five family members. Patients with von Hippel-Lindau disease have a higher incidence of carcinoma (Lauritsen, 1975). Patients with polycystic kidney disease appear to have a predisposition for development of the tumor, although this has not been firmly established. Renal carcinoma is a tumor of adults, occurring primarily in the 5th to 7th decades of life, but it may occasionally occur in younger age groups.

Etiology

Renal cell carcinomas seem to arise from the proximal convoluted tubule, the same cell of origin as that of renal adenomas (Tannenbaum, 1971). Although a number of etiologic agents have been identified in animal models (Bennington and Beckwith, 1975), no specific agent has been definitely incriminated as being causative of human renal carcinoma. Epidemiologic studies have incriminated tobacco, although the specific carcinogen has not been described (Kantor, 1977; Weir and Dunn, 1970). A high incidence of renal carcinoma has been noted in men who smoke pipes or cigars (Kantor, 1977).

In one study, La Vecchia and associates (1990) found a 1.7-fold increase in the incidence of renal cell carcinoma among ex-smokers compared with those who never smoked. A direct and significant dose-risk relationship was observed among current smokers, with a relative risk of 1.1, 1.9, and 2.3 for moderate, intermediate, and heavy smokers, respectively. This trend in risk was statistically significant. The risk was directly related to duration of smoking and inversely related to age at starting. Among ex-smokers, risk was inversely related to time elapsed since stopping. The typical renal cell carcinoma can be produced in the adult Syrian hamster by long-term treatment with diethylstilbestrol (Kirkman and Bacon, 1949), but this hormone has not been shown to cause renal carcinoma in humans.

No definitive relationship between occupational and industrial carcinogens and renal carcinoma has been documented. Male cigarette smokers exposed to industrial contaminants of cadmium have been reported to have a slightly increased risk of developing the tumor (Kolonel, 1976). No other relationship has been reported, although research in this area has been limited. The radiographic agent colloidal thorium diozide was reported to be associated with a high incidence of renal carcinoma in one study (Wenz, 1967). At the present time, there is a paucity of studies regarding the cause of renal carcinoma, and few hypotheses seem to warrant extensive investigation (Dayal and Wikinson, 1989).

Molecular Biology and Immunology

CYTOGENETICS

The most consistent chromosomal changes observed in renal cell carcinoma are deletions and translocation involving the short arm of chromosome 3 (3p). In two families, each member carrying a germ-line chromosomal mutation in the form of translocation (3;8) (Cohen et al., 1979) and translocation (3;6) (Kovacs et al., 1989) developed multiple and/or bilateral renal cancers at an earlier age of onset (40 to 50 years) than patients with sporadic renal cell carcinoma (60 to 70 years). The breakpoint on chromosome 3 was localized at the same region (3p13–14.2).

Chromosomal analysis by Carroll and associates (1987) of nonfamilial renal cell carcinoma led to subsequent studies in which restriction fragment length polymorphism (RFLP) analysis of normal tumor tissues from patients with sporadic renal cell carcinoma was used. One allele of a particular DNA probe for chromosome 3 (pH3H2) was consistently found to be deleted in most tumor tissues (Kovacs et al., 1988; Zbar et al., 1987). These findings support the hypothesis that a suppressor cancer gene may be located on the 3p segment and that a loss of this locus is likely to be indicative of the development of renal cell carcinoma.

Molecular activation of proto-oncogenes has also been proposed to explain the observed cytogenetic findings. However, no single oncogene abnormality has been identified as characteristic of renal cell carcinoma. Overexpression of c-myc and epidermal growth factor receptor (EGFR) (c-erb B-1) mRNA, and underexpression of HER-2 (erb B-2) mRNA can be found in the majority of patients with renal cell carcinoma (Freeman et al., 1989; Weidner et al., 1990; Yao et al., 1988). c-Ha-ras, c-fos, c-fms, and f-raf-1 expression is elevated in some tumors as well (Karthaus et al., 1987; Slamon et al., 1984; Teyssier et al., 1986; Yao et al., 1988). The significance of these altered patterns of proto-oncogene expression in renal cell carcinoma remains incompletely understood.

GROWTH FACTORS

Transforming growth factors (TGFs) alpha and beta are two tumor-produced regulatory growth factors that may be related to the development of renal cell carcinoma (Gomella et al., 1989; Linehan et al., 1989). TGF-alpha is known to bind to EGFR, and because TGF-alpha and EGFR are both overexpressed in kidney tumor tissue, it is possible that interaction between TGF-alpha and EGFR plays a role in promoting transformation and/or proliferation of kidney neoplasms, perhaps by an autocrine mechanism (Mydlo et al., 1989). TGF-beta is produced in a biologically latent form by human renal cell carcinoma lines in culture, and the addition of exogenous TGF-beta to these cells inhibits their proliferation (Sargent et al., 1989). It appears, therefore, that changes in the production of, and response to, these stimulatory and inhibitory growth factors may lead to an imbalance of growth control, loss of autocrine growth inhibition, and cancer formation.

MULTIDRUG RESISTANCE

Renal cell carcinoma remains resistant to currently available chemotherapeutic agents. The basis for this multidrug resistance (MDR) in renal cell carcinoma appears to be related to a 170-kilodalton transmembrane glycoprotein (P-glycoprotein, P170) encoded by the MDR1 gene that functions as an energy-dependent drug efflux pump (Fojo et al., 1987; Kakehi et al., 1988). This action results in decreased accumulation within cells of multiple structurally unrelated naturally occurring products used as chemotherapeutic agents (Moscow and Cowan, 1988). Cells resistant to chemotherapeutic drugs by virtue of P-glycoprotein expression can be made more sensitive by agents, such as verapamil, amiodarone, quinidine, and cyclosporines, that inhibit the function of the efflux pump and result in increased intracellular concentrations of chemotherapeutic drugs (Kanamaru et al., 1989; Mickisch et al., 1990a; Tsuruo et al., 1984).

A second independent mechanism associated with renal cell carcinoma MDR is the glutathione redox cycle, which is involved in the intracellular binding and detoxification of chemotherapeutic agents and can be inactivated by buthionine sulfoximine (Mickisch et al., 1990b). Further investigation of these mechanisms of MDR may provide the understanding necessary to develop means for overcoming resistance to chemotherapy in renal cell carcinoma.

Pathology

Renal cell carcinomas are typically round, varying in size from tumors several centimeters in diameter to tumors that almost fill the abdomen (Fig. 27–6). They generally do not have a true histologic capsule but almost always have a pseudocapsule composed of compressed parenchyma and fibrous tissue. The amount of hemorrhage and necrosis varies greatly, but few tumors are uniform in gross appearance. Areas of yellowish or brownish soft tumor are usually interposed between sclerotic bifrontal areas and patches of hemorrhage and necrosis. Multiple cysts are found not infrequently, probably resulting from segmental necrosis and resorption. The collecting system is generally displaced and is

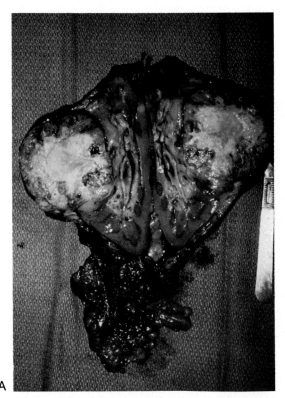
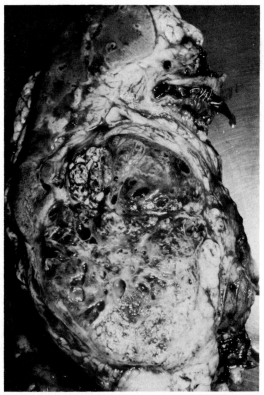

A

B

Figure 27–6. *A,* Specimen opened to reveal massive tumor. *B,* Typical renal cell carcinoma with thick pseudocapsule.

often invaded. Gerota's fascia seems to provide a barrier against local spread, but it may be compressed and invaded. Calcification can occur and may be stifled or may occur in a plaque-like arrangement.

Renal carcinoma is typically unilateral, but bilaterality, either synchronous or asynchronous, occurs in approximately 2 per cent of cases (Moertel et al., 1961). Von Hippel-Lindau disease is characteristically associated with the presence of multiple and bilateral renal carcinomas (Fig. 27–7) (Glenn et al., 1990). As noted further on, the tumor frequently extends into the renal vein as a thrombus, which may be propagated for varying distances into the inferior vena cava. The more malignant and larger tumors can invade locally, with extension into the surrounding muscles and direct invasion into adjacent organs.

Electron microscopic studies have identified the proximal tubular cell as the origin of renal cell carcinoma. The proximal tubular cell has multiple surface microvilli, giving the brush border characteristic, and contains a more complex cytoplasm than the more distal tubular cells. The ultrastructural characteristics of the proximal cell are found in varying degrees in most renal carcinomas. However, brush borders are usually not fully developed and are present on only some cells.

The origin of the tumor from proximal tubular cells has been supported by a number of investigators (Fisher and Horvat, 1972; Sun et al., 1977; Tannenbaum, 1971). Bander and colleagues (1989) further refined the derivation of renal cell carcinoma cells by subclassifying the proximal tubular cells using monoclonal antibody (Mo Ab) probes. They found that, in the normal adult kidney, cells of the convoluted portion are URO10+/URO8−; those of the straight portion are URO10−/URO8+. Whereas adult proximal tubular cells demonstrate reciprocal expression of URO10 and URO8, fetal kidney proximal tubule progenitor cells coexpress both antigens (URO10+/URO8+). In renal cell carcinoma specimens, 30 per cent of the cells are derived from the proximal convoluted tubule, 18 per cent are derived from the proximal straight tubule, and 50 per cent are derived from proximal tubule progenitor cells (URO10+/URO8+). The ultrastructure of the various cell types composing the classic renal carcinoma has been carefully detailed by Colvin and Dickersin (1978).

Although it is unusual to find absolutely pure examples, renal cell carcinomas can be broadly grouped into four histologic types: clear cell, granular cell, tubulopapillary, and sarcomatoid (Murphy, 1989). The clear cell variant of renal cell carcinoma is microscopically characterized by sheets, acini, or alveoli of neoplastic cells bounded by a network of delicate vascular sinusoids and reticulin fibers. The clear cells are rounded or polygonal with abundant cytoplasm (Fig. 27–8), which contains cholesterol, cholesterol esters, phospholipids, and glycogen; these substances are largely extracted by the solvents used in routine histologic preparations.

Few tumors contain only clear cells, however; a granular cell (dark cell) component is usually present in varying degrees and may actually compose the major portion of the tumor (Fig. 27–9). Granular cells have eosinophilic cytoplasm and abundant mitochondria. The tubulopapillary variant appears to be a histologically distinctive tumor. Macroscopically, this tumor is small, nearly completely encapsulated, and confined to the cortex. In purely papillary neoplasms, significant nuclear anaplasia is uncommon. The sarcomatoid variant (carcinosarcoma, mixed tumor) of renal cell carcinoma is characterized by a predominantly spindle cell pattern, aggressive behavior, and poor prognosis (Tomera et al., 1983). Spindle cells may resemble pleomorphic mesenchymal cells (Fig. 27–10), and differentiation from fibrosarcoma may be difficult.

Thoenes and colleagues (1988) have provided evidence for a new type of renal cell carcinoma—the

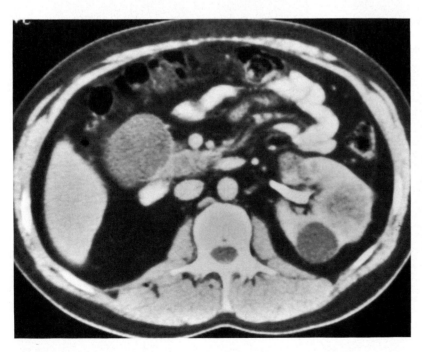

Figure 27–7. Computed tomography scan in a patient with von Hippel-Lindau disease showing multiple pancreatic cysts, posterior renal cyst, and two solid renal tumors in the lateral and anterior aspects (isointense to the cortex representing two renal carcinomas). (Courtesy of Dr. Sachiko Cochran.)

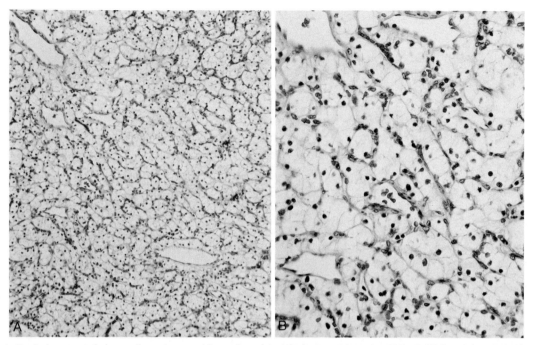

Figure 27–8. *A*, Typical pattern of clear cell carcinoma with small nuclei and clear cytoplasm (× 125). *B*, Higher power magnification showing pure clear cell pattern (× 313).

chromophobe type—which exhibits morphologic and immunohistochemical features of the cortical collecting-duct epithelia. Chromophobe cells are characterized by their light (transparent) cytoplasm with a finely reticular, but not empty, appearance. Sometimes, a moderately intense eosinophilia is observed. In electron micrographs, the cytoplasm displays abundant reticular struc-

tures poor in glycogen. Preliminary data suggest better survival in patients with the chromophobe rather than the clear cell type of renal cell carcinoma.

A number of investigators have related various types of grading systems to prognosis, perhaps the first being Hand and Broders (1932). Within a given stage, however, the microscopic grading seems to have less signif-

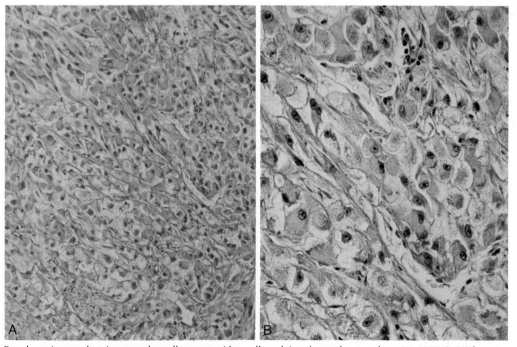

Figure 27–9. *A*, Renal carcinoma showing granular cell pattern with small nuclei and granular cytoplasm (× 125). *B*, Higher power magnification emphasizing typical granular cell pattern (× 313).

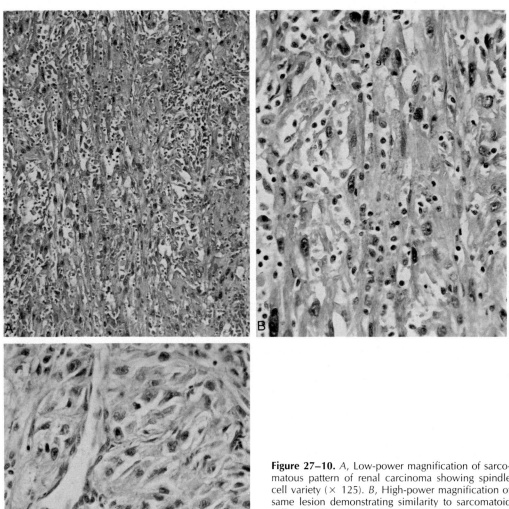

Figure 27–10. *A,* Low-power magnification of sarcomatous pattern of renal carcinoma showing spindle cell variety (× 125). *B,* High-power magnification of same lesion demonstrating similarity to sarcomatoid cells (× 313). *C,* Similar pattern in another renal carcinoma (× 313).

icance than in some tumors. Nonetheless, tumors with nuclei resembling those of normal cells demonstrate a low malignant potential in contrast to the bizarre heterogeneous nuclei typical of spindle cell tumors, which are associated with a worse prognosis. A great disparity in survival has not been demonstrated between patients whose tumors contain clear cells and patients whose tumors contain granular cells. However, tumors composed mainly of spindle cells seem to indicate a worse prognosis for the patient (Colvin and Dickersin, 1978).

Nuclear DNA content as measured by image cytometry or flow cytometry has been shown to correlate with tumor behavior (Rainwater et al., 1987). Most reports have confirmed a general relationship between DNA ploidy and nuclear grade with a high percentage of anaplastic tumors harboring aneuploid cells. Similar correlations have been made between DNA ploidy and the prognoses of patients with various stages of renal cell carcinomas (Grignon et al., 1989). Although measurements of DNA ploidy may be the reflection of tumor heterogeneity and an indication of biologic potential, the clinical value of this technique remains to be determined for renal cell carcinoma (Murphy, 1989).

Clinical Presentation

Nature has provided a well-protected environment for the human kidney, and its only expression to the outside environment is through its primary product, the urine. Pain cannot be expected to occur unless the tumor invades surrounding areas or obstructs the outflow of urine owing to hemorrhage and subsequent formation of blood clots. Therefore, it is not surprising that the presenting signs and symptoms are often those related to local invasion or distant metastases.

The classic triad of pain, hematuria, and flank mass is certainly a reliable clinical symptom complex, but it is found in few patients and generally indicates advanced disease. One or two of these symptoms or signs are commonly associated with renal carcinoma (Table 27–4). The most frequent findings are pain or hematuria secondary to the primary tumor, but symptoms due to metastatic disease probably occur more frequently. Weight loss, fever, night sweats, and the sudden development of a varicocele in the male patient are not uncommon findings. Hypertension is due to segmental renal artery occlusion or to elaboration of renin or renin-like substances.

Few tumors are associated with such a diversity of paraneoplastic syndromes, some of which may represent the presenting symptoms in patients with renal carcinoma (Sufrin et al., 1989). The normal kidney is involved in the production of prostaglandins, 1,25-dihydroxycholecalciferol, renin, and erythropoietin. Renal malignancies may elaborate these substances in amounts greater than normal and may elaborate parathormone-like factors, glucagon, human chorionic gonadotropin (hCG), and insulin (Mangin et al., 1988; Pavelic and Popovic, 1981).

The most dramatic syndrome is associated with non-metastatic hepatic dysfunction and is referred to as Staufer syndrome. Patients with this syndrome have abnormal liver function tests, white blood cell loss, fever, and areas of hepatic necrosis without hepatic metastases (Boxer et al., 1978). Renal function returns to normal after nephrectomy in many patients; this is an important prognostic sign because 88 per cent of such patients have survival at least greater than 1 year. Persistence or recurrence of this syndrome is almost invariably associated with recurrence of the tumor.

Hypercalcemia has been reported in up to 10 per cent of patients with renal carcinoma, and the etiology is rather obscure. A peptide produced by the tumor that is analogous to the amino-terminal regions of a parathyroid hormone–related protein may be the causative agent (Goldberg et al., 1964; Kemp et al., 1987). Removal of the primary tumor is often associated with a

Table 27–5. INCIDENCE OF SYSTEMIC SYNDROMES IN PATIENTS WITH RENAL CELL CARCINOMA

Effect	Ratio	Per Cent
Raised erythrocyte sedimentation rate	362/651	55.6
Hypertension	89/237	37.5
Anemia	473/1300	36.3
Cachexia, weight loss	338/979	34.5
Pyrexia	164/954	17.2
Abnormal liver function	65/450	14.4
Raised alkaline phosphatase	64/434	10.1
Hypercalcemia	44/886	4.9
Polycythemia	43/1212	3.5
Neuromyopathy	13/400	3.2
Amyloidosis	12/573	2.0

Adapted from Chisholm, G. D.: Ann. N.Y. Acad. Sci., 230:403, 1974.

fall in the serum calcium level, although the metastatic sites may elaborate the factor and eventually cause recurrent hypercalcemia. Hypercalcemia may be associated with skeletal metastases.

Hypertension has been associated with renal carcinoma, and elevated renin serum levels were reported in patients with high-stage renal tumors. The levels often fall to normal after nephrectomy (Sufrin et al., 1989). Hypertension in these patients may also be secondary to arterial venous fistulae within the tumor, hypercalcemia, ureteral obstruction, cerebral metastases, and polycythemia.

Erythropoietin, a glycoprotein elaborated by the renal cortex in response to hypoxia is a major regulator of erythropoiesis and induces erythrocyte differentiation. Increased levels have been detected in many patients with renal carcinoma, but the mechanism is unclear. This substance may be elaborated by the tumor cells or by the normal renal cells in response to relative hypoxia induced by the tumor (Erslev and Caro, 1986).

The myriad of syndromes and their relative incidences are listed in Table 27–5 (Chisholm, 1974).

Radiographic Diagnoses

The rapid evolution of uroradiography has provided the urologist with a number of diagnostic tests designed primarily to determine whether a renal mass lesion exists and to distinguish solid renal mass lesions from the more common benign renal cysts (Fig. 27–11). Controversy exists regarding the reliability of each method and its place in the decision-making process as well as the extent to which each can provide the most cost-effective preoperative information.

With greater use of ultrasound, CT, and MRI, the ability to detect renal tumors earlier and in lower stages has now significantly increased, resulting in better patient survival. Estimates are that approximately two thirds of all locally confined renal tumors are found serendipitously (Levine et al., 1989; Thompson and Peek, 1988). Although the traditional intravenous pyelography with infusion nephrotomography remains the primary diagnostic step in most medical institutions, it is not surprising that many more renal masses are being demonstrated with ultrasound and CT than with urog-

Table 27–4. INCIDENCE OF SYMPTOMS IN 180 PATIENTS WITH RENAL CELL CARCINOMA

Symptom	Per Cent
Classic triad	10
Pain	41
Hematuria	38
Mass	24
Weight loss	36
Fever	18
Hypertension	22
Hypercalcemia	6

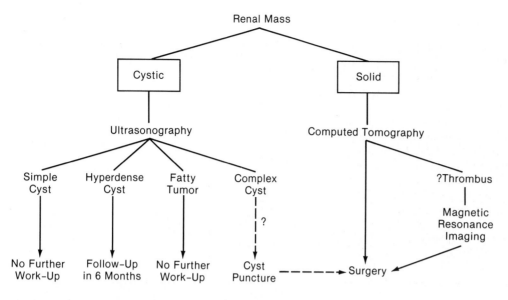

Figure **27–11.** Work-up of a renal mass. (Modified from Barbaric, Z. L.: Principles of Genitourinary Radiology. New York, Thieme Medical Publishers Inc., 1991. With permission.)

raphy (Fig. 27–12). Renal tumors that may not be detected with urography because of location, size, or coexisting anatomic abnormality can be detected with increased accuracy with the cross-sectional imaging afforded by CT or the multiple methods of display available with ultrasound (Smith et al., 1989).

Ultrasound evaluation has the advantage of being able to distinguish among solid, cystic, and complex masses. The sonographic criteria for a simple benign cyst include an absence of internal echoes, a smooth and well-defined wall, a good sound transmission, a round or oval shape, and an acoustic shadow arising from the edges of the cyst. Any lesion that on ultrasound is not clearly a simple cyst must be studied further by CT scan.

Solid renal masses have variable echogenicity, ranging from very bright echoes to less echogenic than the normal renal parenchyma, no or little through transmission, poorly demarcated walls, and irregular shape. Small renal parenchymal tumors, however, usually have smooth, well-defined margins and do not cause displacement of the renal sinus or calyces, or project significantly beyond the renal contour. Such tumors may simulate normal renal parenchyma, such as a prominent renal column of Bertin or fetal lobation. In these cases, additional studies, such as radionuclide scan or CT scan, help in differentiation (Bosniak and Subramanyam, 1990). Highly echogenic malignant renal masses are rare; most are angiomyolipomas or hemangiomas, which are discussed further in this chapter.

Very few purely cystic lesions will prove to harbor renal carcinoma. This small group of cystic tumors can be identified in almost every case by CT or by cyst aspiration and injection of contrast material (Bosniak and Subramanyam, 1990). Clear fluid that has no malignant cells, low fat and protein content, and low lactic acid dehydrogenase levels, aspirated from a cyst with smooth walls, is almost absolute evidence of the absence of malignancy (see Fig. 27–12) (Lang, 1977). The only consistent difference between a cyst containing a tumor and a hemorrhagic benign cyst is the presence of malignant cells. Because detection of low-grade tumors may be difficult in aspirated old blood, the presence of blood in a cyst must raise the index of suspicion sufficiently to prompt further diagnostic tests.

The development of CT, which offers a number of specific advantages over other methods, has demanded a complete re-evaluation of the traditional approaches to diagnosis (Fig. 27–13). Although infusion of contrast material and ingestion of contrast material are important components, the procedure is less invasive than angiography. Cyst density of the mass lesions can now be accurately measured, usually obviating the need for cystography or cyst puncture. The CT scan is performed as an outpatient procedure, in contrast to angiography, which requires hospitalization. In addition, more thorough staging information is obtained from CT scanning than from any of the other diagnostic methods (Figs. 27–14 through 27–16).

Jaschke and colleagues (1982) correlated preoperative staging of 125 renal carcinomas with the angiographic and pathologic findings. The CT scan allows the correct diagnosis of renal vein involvement in 91 per cent, vena

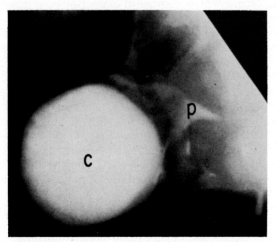

Figure **27–12.** Simple renal cyst (c) after needle puncture, aspiration, and instillation of contrast material with simultaneous intravenous pyelogram to opacify renal collecting system (p).

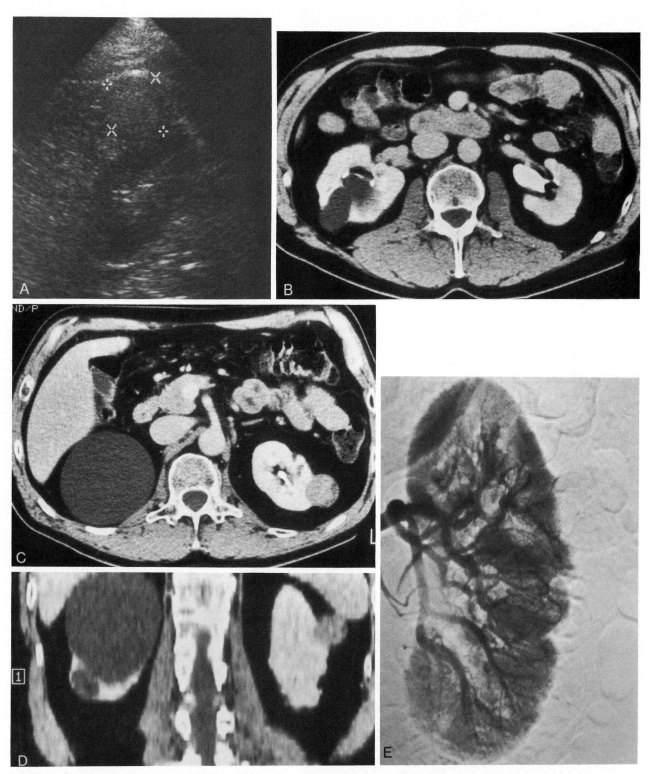

Figure 27–13. Incidental finding of a tumor (left).

A, Transverse ultrasound scan shows a well-circumscribed solid mass of equal echogenicity to adjacent cortex.

B, Computed tomography scan reveals small renal calculi and multiple renal cysts in the right kidney. Patient presented with hematuria and right flank pain.

C, D, Different computed tomography cuts of the same patient demonstrating a large right renal cyst and a 3 × 3–cm complex renal mass in the lateral aspect of the left kidney.

E, Selective left renal angiogram reveals an avascular lesion with no evidence of neovascularity. Partial nephrectomy confirmed the mass to be an oncocytoma.

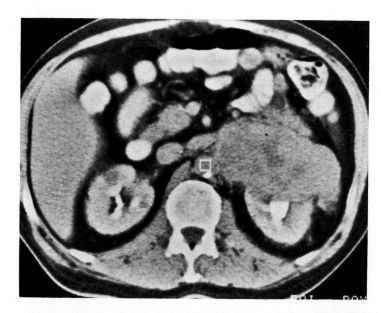

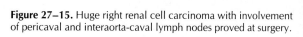

Figure 27–14. Computed tomography scan demonstrating two small cysts in the right kidney and a large solid mass in the left kidney extending over the aorta and filling the left renal vein.

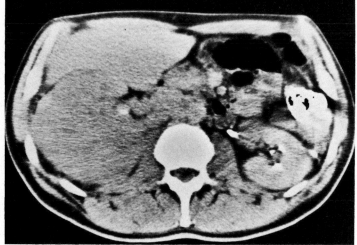

Figure 27–15. Huge right renal cell carcinoma with involvement of pericaval and interaorta-caval lymph nodes proved at surgery.

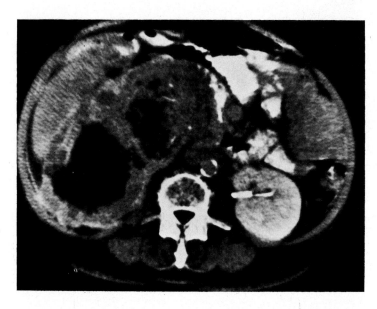

Figure 27–16. Large right renal mass, mixed solid and cystic on ultrasound. Computed tomography scan demonstrates a renal cell carcinoma with extensive central necrosis and involvement of adjacent lymph nodes.

caval extension in 97 per cent, perirenal extension in 79 per cent, lymph node metastases in 87 per cent, and extension to adjacent organs in 96 per cent of patients. Richie and co-workers (1983) studied not only the staging accuracy but also the diagnostic reliability of CT scan in 45 patients compared with that of the angiogram. The tests were similar in diagnostic accuracy (95 per cent versus 85 per cent) and detection of renal vein extension, but CT scan was more accurate in detection of regional lymph node metastases. The sensitivity of the CT scan was further supported by Raval and Lamki (1983). The CT scan detected occult renal carcinoma in five patients whose tumors were not found by other diagnostic tests.

In the excellent article by Lang (1984), the relative accuracy of enhanced CT scan compared with other diagnostic studies was determined in a prospective fashion. In addition to accurately separating cystic from solid lesions, properly performed, enhanced CT can detect tumor extension through the capsule or into surrounding structures. Extension to the renal vein and vena cava can be determined with great accuracy, obviating the need for the traditional venacavography. Extension to the regional lymph nodes is a poor prognostic sign, and few patients are cured surgically. CT can detect extensive regional lymph node involvement in many patients.

From the data presented by Lang (1984), it appears that, as a single diagnostic study, CT is the most cost-effective method of evaluating a suspected renal mass lesion and should be the first-line technique for that purpose. Utilizing the rapid-enhancement method suggested by Lang, further staging information seems plausible. However, certain pitfalls of CT have also become apparent. Although extension through the capsule is often accurately diagnosed, a number of false-positive findings will occur. The test will not detect limited lymph node involvement, and a small but disconcerting number of patients will seem to have involved lymph nodes, which prove to be normal at surgery. One must be careful not to deny patients the potential for surgical cure on the basis of these false-positive readings. None-

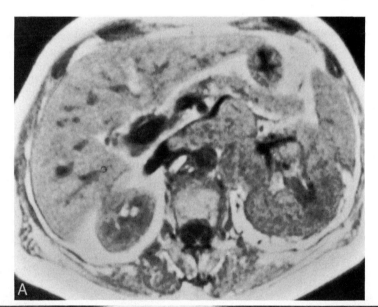

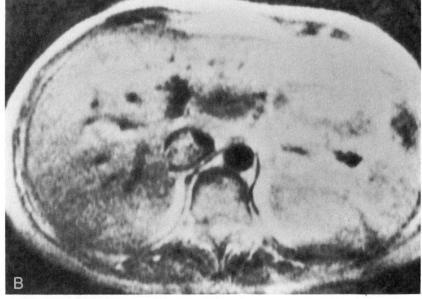

Figure 27–17. *A* and *B*, T1-weighted magnetic resonance spin-echo image displays a large left renal carcinoma extending into the enlarged renal vein and inferior vena cava. (Courtesy of Dr. Sachiko Cochran.)

theless, the new-generation CT scanners have provided us with a single test for diagnosis and staging of renal tumors that is minimally invasive and cost-effective.

The role of MRI in the diagnosis and staging of renal cell carcinoma is currently under investigation. Initially, MRI held promise as a means of distinguishing different types of solid renal masses. Subsequent reports have shown that MRI is less sensitive than CT for the discovery of solid lesions less than 3 cm in diameter (Amendola et al., 1988; Hricak et al., 1988; Quint et al., 1988). However, MRI provides useful information about neoplastic invasion of the renal vein or inferior vena cava without the need for contrast material, and in cases of large, bulky tumors, MRI adds a multidimensional assessment of the tumor extent (Fig. 27–17) (Horan et al., 1989; Hricak et al., 1985; Stewart and Dunnick, 1990). Like CT, MRI cannot reliably distinguish between bland and tumor thrombus, stage I and II disease, or hyperplastic and malignant adenopathy.

Selective renal arteriography was the final and definitive diagnostic step in evaluation of renal masses for decades (Fig. 27–18). However, the emergence of CT has resulted in a marked narrowing of indications for angiography. Because CT gives no information regarding renal vasculature, angiography remains the primary diagnostic test in the patient with a suspected tumor in the solitary kidney, when parenchymal-sparing procedures are anticipated. Also, although differentiation of primary versus metastatic lesions to the kidney is difficult even with angiography, metastatic lesions are typically hypovascular. This feature can be helpful in selected patients for planning therapy when a metastatic lesion

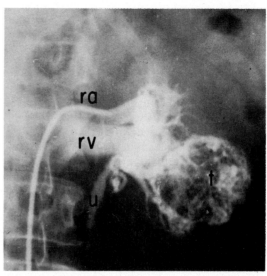

Figure 27–19. Selective renal arteriogram *(ra)* demonstrating neovascularization of renal tumor *(t)*, early filling of renal vein *(rv)*, and opacification of renal pelvis and ureter *(u)*.

to the kidney is suspected. Lastly, interpretation of some lesions by CT scan may be unclear; angiography, with demonstration of small tumor vessels and other characteristic findings, may assist in ensuring the proper diagnosis.

The classic angiographic picture of renal carcinoma is illustrated in Figure 27–19. Neovascularity, arteriovenous fistulae, pooling of contrast media, and accentuation of capsular vessels are the hallmarks of these tumors. However, all variations of this angiographic picture may exist, and vast hypovascular tumors impose a difficult diagnostic problem. The addition of epinephrine infusion to constrict normal vessels, without constricting tumor vessels, may obviate this difficulty. Properly performed, selected renal arteriography remains an important part of the diagnosis of renal carcinoma in these selected circumstances.

Staging

The staging system most commonly employed in the United States is Robson's modification of the system of Flocks and Kadesky (Fig. 27–20) (Robson et al., 1968). The limitations of this system become obvious when it is noted that survival of patients with stage II tumor is equal to that of patients with stage III tumor in some series, indicating an inappropriate assignment of prognostic factors. The placement of renal vein, vena cava, and lymph node involvement into the stage III group accounts for this apparent contradiction because of the inclusion of all levels of renal vein extension. Furthermore, the extent of lymphatic metastases is not considered.

Several tumor, node, and metastases (TNM) systems have been proposed, and none has thus far satisfied all of the issues related to staging of renal cancer. However, the system proposed by the International Union Against Cancer is an improvement over older systems in that size of the primary tumor, extent of local invasion,

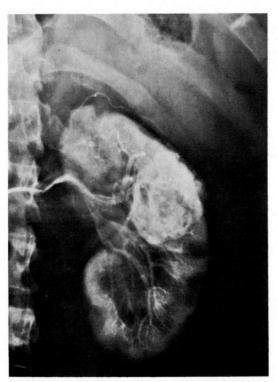

Figure 27–18. Typical arterial phase of selective renal angiogram demonstrating renal carcinoma in solitary kidney as well as multiple small cysts. Typical pattern of puddling of contrast material is noted.

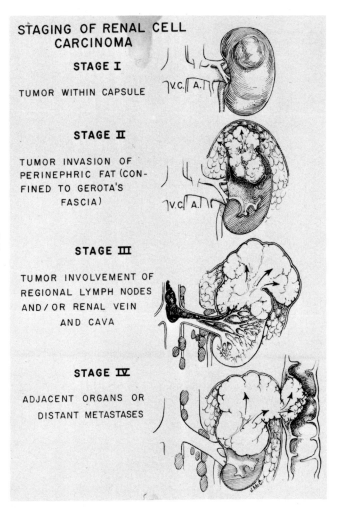

STAGING OF RENAL CELL
CARCINOMA

STAGE I

TUMOR WITHIN CAPSULE

STAGE II

TUMOR INVASION OF
PERINEPHRIC FAT (CON-
FINED TO GEROTA'S
FASCIA)

STAGE III

TUMOR INVOLVEMENT OF
REGIONAL LYMPH NODES
AND/OR RENAL VEIN
AND CAVA

STAGE IV

ADJACENT ORGANS OR
DISTANT METASTASES

Figure 27–20. Staging of nephrocarcinoma as proposed by Holland, in accord with schemes of Robson, Murphy, and Flocks and Kadesky. (From Holland, J. M.: Cancer, 32:1030, 1973.)

degree of extension into the vein, and extent of lymph node metastases are all considered (Hermanek and Schrott, 1990). Table 27–6 includes a comparison of the TNM and the Robson systems.

Clinical staging of renal carcinoma has been alluded to in the discussion of diagnosis. Regional staging with CT is valuable but sometimes misleading, and the true local and regional extent of the tumor is most accurately determined by the pathologist. Evaluation for the presence of distant metastases is important in light of the recognized incurability of patients with metastatic disease. Renal carcinoma bloodborne metastases may be manifested in any organ system, but the most common sites are the lung, liver, subcutaneous tissue, and central nervous system.

The extent of the preoperative evaluation in the asymptomatic patient must emphasize cost-effectiveness. In a study at our institution, no patient with normal liver function tests and a nonpalpable liver was found to have metastases on the radionuclide liver-spleen scan (Lindner et al., 1983). Similarly, no patient without symptoms of skeletal involvement and with normal alkaline phosphatase and serum calcium values had detectable skeletal metastases on radionuclide bone scan. An appropriate preoperative evaluation, therefore, seems to comprise a routine chest radiograph, liver function tests, serum calcium measurement, history, and physical examination.

Prognostic Factors

The factors that have been associated with a poor prognosis in renal cell carcinoma are renal vein involvement, extension to regional lymph nodes, extension through Gerota's fascia, involvement of contiguous organs, and distant metastases (deKernion and Berry, 1980; Maldazys and deKernion, 1986). Although renal vein extension has long been thought to be associated with a poor prognosis (Myers et al., 1968), some studies have failed to show this correlation (Selli et al., 1983; Skinner et al., 1972). This finding may be due to the emphasis on complete excision of the renal veins and on preoperative identification of renal vein extension.

Hoehn and Hermanek (1983) quantitated renal vein extension according to whether the main renal vein was involved or whether only microscopic extension was present. They found a significant increase in local recurrence and metastases in patients with extension into the main renal vein, but no prognostic importance could be attributed to microscopic vein involvement. In future development of staging systems, this important distinction must be considered.

Table 27–6. COMPARISON OF STAGING SYSTEMS*

TNM Clinical Classification

T	Primary tumor
TX	Primary tumor cannot be assessed
TO	No evidence of primary tumor
T1	Tumor 2.5 cm or less in greatest dimension, limited to the kidney
T2	Tumor more than 2.5 cm in greatest dimension, limited to the kidney
T3	Tumor extends into major veins or invades adrenal gland or perinephric tissues but not beyond Gerota's fascia
T3a	Tumor invades adrenal gland or perinephric tissues but not beyond Gerota's fascia
T3b	Tumor grossly extends into renal vein(s) or vena cava
T4	Tumor invades beyond Gerota's fascia
N	Regional lymph nodes
NO	No identifiable nodes in a specified clinical assessment
N1	Metastasis in single lymph node, 2 cm or less in greatest dimension
N2	Metastasis in single lymph node, 2 cm but not more than 5 cm in greatest dimension; in multiple lymph nodes, none more than 5 cm in greatest dimension
N3	Metastasis in a lymph node more than 5 cm in greatest dimension
M	Distant metastasis
MO	Tumors without distant metastasis
M1	Tumors with distant metastasis
G	Histopathologic grading
G1	Well differentiated
G2	Moderately differentiated
G3–G4	Undifferentiated, anaplastic

Stage Grouping

Stage I	T1	NO	MO
Stage II	T2	NO	MO
Stage III	T1	N1	MO
	T2	N1	MO
	T3a	NO,N1	MO
	T3b	NO,N1	MO
Stage IV	T4	Any N	MO
	Any T	N2,N3	MO
	Any T	Any N	M1

*The regional lymph nodes are the hilar, abdominal para-aortic, and paracaval nodes. Laterality does not affect the N categories.

Adapted from International Union Against Cancer: Hermanek, P., Sobin, L. H. (Eds.): TNM Classification of Malignant Tumors, Ed 4. Berlin, Springer-Verlag, 1987.

Involvement of the regional lymph nodes draining the renal parenchyma is a dire prognostic sign, associated with a 5-year survival rate of 0 to 30 per cent (deKernion, 1980a). The extent of lymphatic dissemination is no doubt important, and those who survive seem to be patients with very limited early lymphatic involvement. The implications with respect to the extent of the surgical procedure are discussed later. Invasion through Gerota's fascia and into the perinephric fat decreases the 5-year survival rate to approximately 45 per cent (Siminovitch et al., 1983; Skinner et al., 1972). Tumor extension to contiguous organs is rarely associated with 5-year survival even after radical surgical excision.

The significance of local tumor persistence or recurrence is reflected in our study of patients with metastatic renal carcinoma (deKernion et al., 1978). Those who had incomplete tumor excision because of extension into Gerota's fascia had a much poorer prognosis than even

those who developed distant metastases without local tumor recurrence. The size of the renal tumor is only indirectly correlated with survival (Böttiger, 1970). Size is perhaps important only in discerning renal adenomas from true renal carcinomas, a subject discussed previously.

Preliminary DNA flow cytometry data suggest that both prognosis and tumor progression rate may well correlate with nondiploid tumor patterns. Frignon and co-workers (1989) observed 37 per cent mortality within 10 years from tumor progression in 19 patients with stage I disease whose tumor was nondiploid, versus 8 per cent mortality in 25 patients with diploid renal cell carcinomas. Studies from UCLA and from the Mayo Clinic confirm these data, showing a markedly improved survival in patients with metastases whose tumors are diploid compared with those who have aneuploid tumors (deKernion and Huland, 1990).

Surgical Treatment of Localized Renal Carcinoma

RADICAL NEPHRECTOMY

Surgery remains the only effective method of treatment of primary renal carcinoma, and the objective of the procedure must be to excise all tumor with an adequate surgical margin. Simple nephrectomy was practiced for decades but has been supplanted by radical nephrectomy, which is presumed, although not absolutely proved, to increase the surgical cure rate (Patel and Lavengood, 1978; Robson, 1963).

Although the definition varies, radical nephrectomy generally implies the excision of Gerota's fascia and its contents, including the kidney and the adrenal gland. This approach accomplishes several objectives: (1) the adrenal gland, which is not infrequently involved, is excised; (2) lymphatic metastases, which may diffuse through the perirenal fat, are removed; and (3) a more adequate margin away from the tumor is achieved, especially when the tumor invades the perirenal fat. More adequate renal vein division is also accomplished. Because these appear to be important factors in determining survival, especially invasion of the perinephric fat, cure can be expected to be seriously compromised if microscopic or gross tumor is left in Gerota's fascia. Although the true increase in survival realized by radical nephrectomy versus simple nephrectomy is often debated, the radical nephrectomy has become the standard method of surgical therapy.

Regional lymphadenectomy is often added to radical nephrectomy, and increased survival has been attributed to removal of involved lymph nodes (Peters, 1980; Robson, 1963). As noted earlier, regional node extension is an important prognostic factor seldom associated with long-term cure. It is generally impossible to assess the impact of lymph node involvement on survival, because other factors usually exist. Survival in patients who have unresectable lymph nodes approaches zero, but some investigators have reported survival when limited lymph node involvement is successfully resected.

Skinner and colleagues (1972) found a 17 per cent 10-

year survival in those with lymph node involvement. The greatest survival—30 per cent of patients alive at 10 years following extensive lymphadenectomy—was reported by Robson (1963). However, Hulten and co-workers (1969) found no survivors when involved regional lymph nodes were excised. Pizzocaro (1990) reported an improved disease-free survival in patients undergoing extensive regional lymphadenectomy. Approximately 20 per cent of patients with positive nodes survived 5 years. However, patients were not randomized and the extent and location of the lymph node metastases were not clearly defined. The data, however, do suggest that some patients benefited by regional lymphadenectomy.

Interpretation of the literature is difficult, because the number and location of involved lymph nodes are often not stated as fully as other important factors, such as the type of primary operation performed. However, it is possible that the improved survival that has occurred since the advent of radical nephrectomy with lymphadenectomy stems from the complex excision of the primary tumor rather than from excision of the regional nodes.

Several characteristics of renal carcinoma argue against a therapeutic role for lymphadenectomy. First, the tumor metastasizes through the bloodstream and the lymphatic system with equal frequency, and most patients with positive lymph nodes eventually have blood-borne metastases. Second, the lymphatic drainage of renal carcinoma is variable and may occur anywhere in the retroperitoneum. Third, many patients without metastases to regional lymph nodes develop disseminated metastases (deKernion, 1980a). However, as pointed out by Marshall and Powell (1982) and confirmed by our own experience, most tumors initially metastasize to lymph nodes in the renal hilum or in the paracaval or para-aortic area immediately adjacent to the hilum. Although an occasional patient will have distant retroperitoneal lymph nodes as the first site of metastases, one can encompass the most probable first and second drainage areas by performing a limited lymph node dissection—paracaval and interaortacaval for right-sided tumors, and para-aortic and interaortacaval for left-sided tumors.

Golimbu and associates (1986) were able to show a 10 to 15 per cent increase in the 5-year survival with lymphadenectomy for microscopic disease in patients with stage II cancers and in those with renal vein involvement. They evaluated 52 patients who underwent a lymphadenectomy in whom no lymphatic disease was identified and compared their survival with that of 141 patients who had palpably normal retroperitoneal lymph nodes and underwent a radical nephrectomy alone. Lymphadenectomy did not improve survival in their patients with stage I disease. Although the practical therapeutic value of lymphadenectomy is still uncertain because of the factors mentioned, it can be accomplished simply and provides valuable staging information.

The surgical technique of radical nephrectomy has been described by a number of investigators (deKernion, 1980b; Stewart, 1975). The surgical approach is guided more by individual preference than by necessity. The transperitoneal approach through a subcostal incision allows early ligation of the renal artery and vein prior to tumor manipulation. This is an essential technical consideration in the management of renal carcinoma (i.e., early ligation of the artery and vein), and, to be acceptable, any approach must incorporate it. Other transabdominal incisions have also been employed with a similar intent of early ligation of the vessels.

The thoracoabdominal incision described by Chute and colleagues (1949) is commonly practiced and is especially suitable for large tumors in the upper pole of the kidney. This technique may include extraperitoneal or intraperitoneal incision as a disadvantage and perhaps an increased postoperative morbidity and increased recovery time. The dorsolumbar osteoplastic flap described by Nagamatsu (1950) also provides excellent exposure. In many cases, a flank incision through the 11th intercostal space or a supracostal incision allows excellent exposure without entering the pleural cavity and can be performed extraperitoneally. We have employed this approach for many small tumors and tumors in the lower pole and have found it to be associated with minimal postoperative morbidity, provided that the costovertebral ligaments of the 11th rib are divided adequately, allowing the rib to be deflected downward (deKernion, 1980b). The urologic surgeon should be skilled in a number of approaches, tailoring the incision to the body habitus of the patient and the size and position of the renal tumor.

Since the advent of sophisticated angiographic methods, preoperative occlusion of the renal artery has been advocated as an adjunct to the surgical procedure. Hemorrhage is reduced, especially in patients with very large tumors supplied by many parasitized vessels. The renal vein can be ligated prior to dissection of the renal artery, and a host immune stimulation has been attributed to renal infarction (Hirsh et al., 1979). However, a salutary effect on survival has not been demonstrated, and the procedure can be associated with complications that may compromise the ability of the patient to tolerate surgery, including pain, ileus, sepsis, and dislocation of the infarcting coil. Early ligation of the renal artery and vein can be safely performed without preoperative infarction, and little evidence suggests that the latter is an appropriate preoperative measure. However, it may be a reasonable adjunct in patients with large vascular tumors, especially in patients with large caval thrombi.

The long-term outcome following surgical therapy for renal carcinoma depends on many factors, including the tumor stage, grade, and histologic type, and the surgical procedure. Data, therefore, are difficult to compare, and the use of various staging systems compounds the problem. Some general statements, however, can be made with respect to the efficacy of radical nephrectomy.

After radical nephrectomy for stage I renal carcinoma, 5-year survival ranges from 60 to 82 per cent, compared with 5-year survival for stage II of 47 to 80 per cent (McNichols et al., 1981; Robson et al., 1968; Skinner et al., 1972). In the series reported by Robson (1963), in which all patients underwent radical nephrectomy and extensive lymphadenectomy after careful preoperative selection, the survival of patients with stage II tumors (extension through the capsule) was identical to that for those with stage I disease, presumably because of a more thorough excision of the tumor and a decreased local tumor recurrence. Individuals with stage III tumors have an expected survival of between 35 and 51 per cent, depending on the number of patients included in the category because of renal vein involvement without lymph node extension or extracapsular extension. As mentioned, patients with extension to the contiguous organs have a very poor prognostic outlook, and those with distant metastases have virtually no chance of surviving 2 years (Best, 1987).

Radiation therapy has been employed as a preoperative or postoperative surgical adjunct. Several reports showed an increased survival with preoperative radiotherapy (Cox et al., 1970; Richie, 1966). A randomized study conducted by van der Werf-Messing (1973) compared the results of 3000 rads of preoperative therapy with those of no therapy. Five-year survival was not improved, although the onset of local recurrence was postponed. Thus far, no study has demonstrated effectiveness of preoperative radiotherapy for renal carcinoma.

The purpose of postoperative radiotherapy is to sterilize any existing microscopic or gross tumor. A number of studies have used varying doses of radiotherapy to the renal fossa following nephrectomy but have not shown a significantly improved survival (Peeling et al., 1969). Indeed, survival after postoperative radiotherapy was diminished in the study by Finney (1973). For similar reasons, radiotherapy for regional lymph node extension was not proved to be of significant value. Although occasionally a large tumor may be reduced in size by preoperative radiotherapy, no evidence currently exists to support the routine use of radiotherapy in renal carcinoma other than for palliative treatment of skeletal metastases.

Tumor in the Solitary Kidney and Bilateral Renal Tumors

Renal cell carcinoma may occur in the patient who has a solitary kidney, the other kidney either being congenitally absent or having been removed for benign disease. Bilateral neoplasms may also occur, either synchronously or asynchronously (Fig. 27–21). A clearer understanding of the renal vasculature and more sophisticated surgical approaches now usually make it possible to excise the tumor, leaving the patient with sufficient parenchyma to maintain life without dialysis. The standard partial nephrectomy in vivo, combined with regional hypothermia, is the most common approach. Autotransplantation following ex vivo excision is now commonplace in many large medical centers. However, the enthusiasm for this approach has diminished considerably, and most tumors are now excised from the solitary kidney without the need for the "workbench" approach.

Excision of tumor in the solitary kidney is associated with excellent short-term results (Marberger et al., 1981;

Zincke and Swanson, 1982). Initial studies suggested that survival was significantly better in patients with tumor in the solitary kidney than in those with synchronous or asynchronous tumor in the opposite kidney (approximately 70 per cent versus 50 per cent) (Wickham, 1975). A report by Topley and co-workers (1983), however, suggested that 5-year survival was poor only in those with asynchronous bilateral tumors (38 per cent) compared with unilateral tumors in a solitary kidney (71 per cent) and bilateral synchronous tumors (71 per cent). This conclusion was supported by the cumulative experience from this institution (Smith et al., 1984). Twenty patients with tumor in the solitary kidney and 18 patients with bilateral renal carcinoma were treated by partial nephrectomy in vivo (21) or ex vivo incision and autotransplantation (17). Radical nephrectomy with dialysis was the treatment in three patients. A number of conclusions were possible from this study. First, complete removal of the tumor, whether tumor in the solitary kidney or bilateral renal tumors, was associated with a 72 per cent tumor-free survival at 3 years. Second, the survival was independent of whether the patient had tumor in the opposite kidney. Third, overall crude survival for patients with bilateral renal tumors that were completely excised was 57 per cent. Fourth, survival was dependent on the stage of the local tumor. Of patients with stage I tumors, 80 per cent have survived 3 years, versus 50 per cent with stage II tumors. Fifth, ex vivo surgery is seldom necessary, and most patients can be adequately managed with regional hypothermia. Lastly, although bilateral nephrectomy with dialysis is seldom necessary, it should be an option offered to selected patients in this modern era of hemodialysis and transplantation.

Conservative surgery with enucleation or partial nephrectomy as a treatment for renal cell carcinoma remains controversial despite good results in terms of local control and disease-free survival (Marshall et al., 1986; Novick et al., 1986, 1989). Although long-term follow-up has not been achieved in most studies, the experience of Novick and associates (1986, 1989), in which a large number of patients have been followed for at least 3 to 4 years, indicates that the majority can be cured by conservative surgery. The cause-specific predicted 5-year survival was 100 per cent for patients with unilateral tumors, 79 per cent for bilateral synchronous tumors, and 82 per cent for bilateral asynchronous tumors. Cause-specific survival was 90 per cent for patients with stage I tumors versus 76 per cent for patients with stage III tumors. Only 5 of the 100 patients followed developed local recurrence in the renal remnant without other sites of recurrence. However, others developed concomitant local recurrence and distant metastases.

This study confirmed that most tumors can be successfully excised in situ and that excellent short-term results can be achieved by conservative surgery. In the opinion of the investigators, partial nephrectomy may be an option for some patients with a solitary, peripheral, small lesion. Enucleation may be indicated only when partial nephrectomy with a margin of normal tissue is not feasible, as in the patient with multiple small tumors in a solitary kidney.

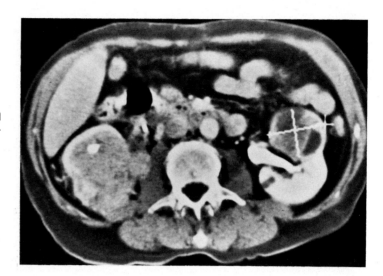

Figure 27–21. Bilateral renal cell carcinoma in a 61-year-old man with microhematuria. Patient underwent partial left nephrectomy and, subsequently, right radical nephrectomy.

Inferior Vena Cava Extension

Propensity for renal carcinoma to invade the renal veins and extend into the main renal vein as a tumor thrombus is well recognized. Continued growth of the thrombus into the vena cava occurs in a small number of cases, usually without direct invasion of the vessel. The importance of delineating the extent of venous involvement is therefore obvious, and inferior venacavogram, CT, or MRI (Fig. 27–22) is essential in preoperative evaluation of renal tumors. Vena cava extension was considered to be a dire prognostic sign in the past, associated with little prospect for surgical cure. However, since the recognition of the importance of caval extension and aggressive surgical treatment, it is realized that most patients can still be cured surgically (Shefft et al., 1978).

The anatomic and surgical considerations in the patient with vena caval extension have been reviewed by Clayman and associates (1980). In this excellent review, 1-year survival of patients following surgical removal of vena cava extension was 75 per cent. This study and others attest to the wisdom of surgical removal of the vena cava thrombus, even when the tumor extends into the right atrium. The surgical approaches to accomplish vena caval thrombus excision have been thoroughly described (Cummings, 1982; Marshall et al., 1984). A limited infracaval extension, once recognized, is managed without difficulty (deKernion and Smith, 1984). However, supradiaphragmatic and right atrial extension require an extended operation, often with cardiopulmonary bypass. Although this procedure has been accomplished and is technically feasible, little is known about the long-term survival of these patients.

A number of studies have described refinements in the surgical technique for management of caval thrombi and the expectations after excision. Libertino and colleagues (1987) reported a 10-year survival of 60 per cent in 32 patients who had no regional or metastatic disease. Most of the patients had infradiaphragmatic extension, but 21 per cent had either supradiaphragmatic or atrial extension. Survival did not differ significantly according to extent of the thrombus. Operative mortality was 4.5 per cent. In contrast, the medium survival time for 12 patients with either regional or distant metastases undergoing excision of caval thrombi was 1.2 years, with no patient living 5 years.

The feasibility of resection of extensive caval thrombi and successful short-term outcome has been improved by collaboration with cardiac surgeons. As described in a report by Montie and co-workers (1988), cardiac bypass and circulatory arrest were implemented in 15 patients with thrombi above the hepatic veins. One intraoperative death occurred, and nine of 12 patients were free of disease after a short follow-up. Marshall and associates (1988) advocated hypothermia and exsanguination for patients with intracaval extension of thrombi. Nine patients were treated, and one postoperative death was reported. However, many patients had local extension, and most developed metastatic disease. Foster and colleagues (1988) proposed a more simple caval-atrial shunt for extensive thrombi, but little experience has thus far been reported with this technique.

The current experience indicates that excision of renal carcinoma with caval extension remains the treatment of choice and can be safely performed, even with extension into the right atrium. However, as reported previously (Cherrie et al., 1982) and confirmed by later studies, patients with regional and distant metastases seldom are helped by the radical extension. Long-term survival of a patient who has supradiaphragmatic extension is still uncertain, although some have survived several years. Application of modern cardiac surgical techniques to minimize intraoperative hemorrhage and to facilitate tumor removal has further improved expected survival following surgery.

Occasionally, the tumor may invade the wall of the vena cava. Resection of the vena cava is feasible, with preservation of a sleeve to accommodate venous drainage. This technique is most practical in patients with right-sided renal tumors, because the left renal vein can drain through the spermatic vein. The anatomic considerations and surgical approaches have been described (Clayman et al., 1980; McCullough and Gittes, 1975), but the procedure is rarely indicated.

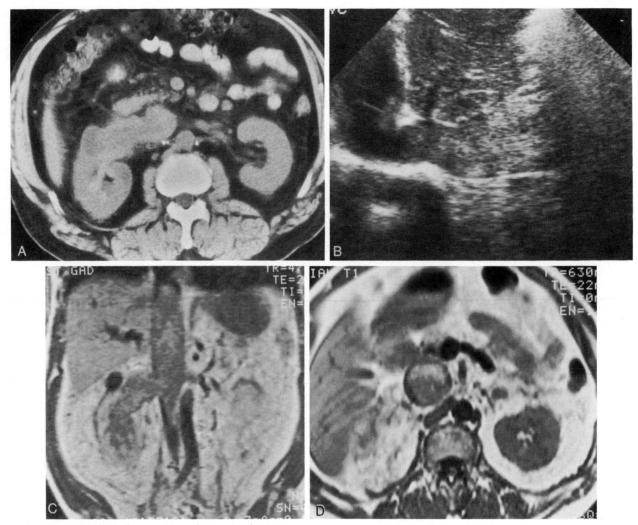

Figure 27–22. Right renal cell carcinoma with vena caval extension.

A, Computed tomography shows a tumor with intensity similar to that of the normal right kidney. Tumor extends into the enlarged right renal vein and inferior vena cava (IVC).

B, Longitudinal sonogram displays echogenic tumor in the lumen of the enlarged IVC.

C, Coronal spin-echo image demonstrated intracaval tumor. The tumor extends proximally as far as the diaphragm but does not enter the thoracic segment of the IVC.

D, Axial magnetic resonance image. Tumor thrombus is in the IVC.

Locally Invasive Renal Carcinoma

The propensity for renal carcinoma to grow to large size locally and to disseminate prior to diagnosis results in many patients presenting with large primary tumors that invade adjacent structures. Such patients usually present with pain, generally from invasion of the posterior abdominal wall, nerve roots, or paraspinous muscles. Liver extension is uncommon, and intrahepatic metastases occur more often than local extension. The capsules of large tumors may indent and compress adjacent liver parenchyma but seldom actually grow by direct extension into the liver. Duodenal and pancreatic invasion is an extremely poor prognostic sign, and we are not aware of any such patients being surgically cured. The propensity for the tumors to parasitize vessels accounts for the frequent extension into the large bowel, mesentery, and colon.

Because surgical therapy is the only effective manage-

ment for this type of tumor, extended operations are sometimes indicated. Complete excision of the tumor, including excision of the involved bowel, spleen, or abdominal wall muscles, is essential. En bloc partial hepatectomy is rarely curative but may occasionally be worthwhile because no other therapeutic options exist.

Partial excision of the large primary tumor, or "debulking," is seldom, if ever, indicated. Only 12 per cent of patients who underwent incomplete excision of locally extensive tumor were alive at 12 months in a report from this institution (deKernion et al., 1978). Most reports suggest that less than 5 per cent of patients with extension into adjacent viscera survive 5 years after surgery. However, it is unclear in these reports which patients underwent complete excision, and the extent of involvement is often not stated. It is appropriate, therefore, to individualize when choosing patients for such extended radical nephrectomy. Preoperative staging by CT scanning may spare the patient an unnecessary operation that is incapable of removing all or even most of the invasive tumor.

The role of radiation therapy in the treatment of locally extensive carcinoma has been debated. Standard preoperative adjunctive radiotherapy has been shown in several early series to improve survival (Cox et al., 1970; Richie, 1966). However, a subsequent study by van der Werf-Messing (1973) compared results for preoperative therapy of 3000 rads with results for no preoperative therapy. Survival was not influenced at 5 years, although the radiotherapy seemed to delay the time to local renal fossa recurrence. Large tumors may sometimes be decreased in size by radiotherapy, and nonresectable left-sided renal tumors may occasionally become resectable after such therapy, but delivery of effective radiotherapy to right renal tumors is difficult given the proximity to the liver.

As noted previously, routine postoperative radiotherapy, although an attractive concept for sterilizing minimal residual tumor, has not been shown to influence overall survival. However, it still seems appropriate to use postoperative radiotherapy in selected patients after excision of locally invasive tumors. When tumor is known to have been left behind in the renal fossa or adjacent structures, postoperative radiotherapy may occasionally retard regrowth of tumor mass. The involved area should be carefully marked with metal clips to direct the radiotherapy. The frequency with which this postoperative therapy will be effective is uncertain, and the specter of distant dissemination dampens enthusiasm for all such local-regional therapies.

Many tumors are very extensive and involve the retroperitoneum extensively as well as adjacent viscera. As noted, debulking seems to have little beneficial effect. Chemotherapeutic or hormonal agents have not been successful.

Symptomatic therapy to control pain and bleeding by angioinfarction and modern pain management techniques is perhaps the most that can be accomplished. However, some patients are occasionally suitable for the new experimental biologic response modifier therapies (Belldegrun et al., 1990). Local recurrence of renal cell carcinoma often follows nephrectomy, especially for tumors that have invaded through the capsule. Surgical excision of local recurrence is the only known successful method of therapy, but this is only of value when the recurrence can be completely excised, which is a rare circumstance. When this is not feasible, palliative radiotherapy and inclusion in experimental studies are the only reasonable options.

Treatment of Metastatic Renal Carcinoma

CHEMOTHERAPY

The traditional modern management of advanced solid tumors has been with cytotoxic agents. In spite of the remarkable advances realized with other tumors, renal cell carcinoma has remained refractory to these agents. A number of drugs have been used as single agents (deKernion and Lindner, 1982). These drugs have been utilized in various dosage schedules, and responses have been measured by disparate criteria. The lack of therapeutic efficacy, however, is apparent. A major complicating factor in interpretation of these and other trials is the unusual natural history of renal cell carcinoma, which may remain stable for varying intervals. Partial regress and stabilization of previously growing lesions are not uncommon, regardless of the therapeutic intervention, and natural history factors are often impossible to separate from results of therapy.

Vinblastine appears to be the most commonly employed single agent. Hrushesky and Murphy (1977) reported a 25 per cent objective response, superior to any other single agent or combination of agents. We have noted partial regression in only one of 16 patients treated with vinblastine.

Because single agents have generally not been proven to be effective, and because combination therapy depends on the combined efficacy of the agents, responses to combination chemotherapy have been expectedly low (deKernion and Lindner, 1982). Yagoda (1989) summarized the results of 39 agents evaluated in 2120 patients and found a total of 93 or 8.77 per cent complete plus partial responses, mostly of short duration, i.e., 5 months. This "background noise" of response clearly documents that renal cell carcinoma is a chemotherapeutically resistant tumor. At this time, new drugs need to be evaluated in carefully constructed prospective clinical trials with the hope of identifying more effective treatment regimens.

HORMONAL THERAPY

The basis for hormone treatment of advanced renal carcinoma was the demonstration of its efficacy against an estrogen-induced clear cell tumor in the adult Syrian hamster (Kirkman and Bacon, 1949). A review of the clinical literature by Bloom (1973) showed an objective response of approximately 15 per cent in patients with metastatic renal carcinoma. However, this represented a summary of phase II trials with various methods of patient selection and criteria of response. In a review of 110 patients at our institution, no patient had a response to progestational agents (deKernion et al., 1978). Although no reports have substantiated the role of progesterones, the paucity of side effects and the lack of effective cytotoxic treatment have prompted propagation of its use as the agent of choice. Side effects include nausea, vomiting, breast tenderness, and uterine bleeding, but these are seldom sufficient to cause cessation of therapy.

The variability of response has been attributed to varying dosage schedules. Although no good study has compared the types of progesterones or the dosage schedules, an orally administered divided dose of 160 mg per day of Provera is well tolerated and is the frequent choice. Medroxyprogesterone acetate (Provera) is administered twice weekly and is well tolerated.

In summary, progesterone therapy continues to be a method of management in the absence of more effective agents. However, no proper study has proved the efficacy of these agents in the management of advanced renal carcinoma.

IMMUNOTHERAPY

The theory supporting immunotherapy for metastatic renal carcinoma is that host immune functions play a role in tumor control, and that these immune functions can be further stimulated. Immunotherapy can be classified into active and passive categories. Active immunotherapy refers to the immunization of the tumor-bearing host with materials that attempt to induce in the host a state of immune responsiveness to the tumor. Passive (adoptive) immunotherapy involves the transfer to the tumor-bearing host of active immunologic reagents, such as cells with antitumor reactivity, that can mediate, either directly or indirectly, antitumor effects (Fig. 27–23). The unusual natural history of renal carcinoma, including spontaneous regression, delayed growth of metastatic lesions, and varying tumor doubling times, suggests that host immune factors may be important in the immune surveillance of this tumor.

Most attempts at immunotherapy in the last several decades have involved active immunotherapy utilizing nonspecific immune stimulators, such as bacillus Calmette-Guérin (BCG), *Corynebacterium parvum*, and levamisole, with the hope that a nonspecific increase in human reactivity would concomitantly result in an augmentation of the putative antitumor immunologic response of the tumor-bearing host. Several reports of small numbers of patients treated with BCG (Minton et al., 1976; Montie et al., 1982; Morales et al., 1982), *C. parvum* (McCune et al., 1981), or transfer factor (Bukowski et al., 1979) have noted some benefit. Subsequent randomized trials confirming such benefit have yet to be published.

Xenogeneic immune RNA (probably a stimulator of interferon production) showed initial promise in uncontrolled studies at University of California, Los Angeles (UCLA) (Ramming and deKernion, 1977). Subsequent studies, however, revealed no significant improvement in survival time over controls and, by 4 years, all patients had died of metastatic disease (deKernion and Ramming, 1980). Although Steele and colleagues (1981) and Richie and colleagues (1981) have reported some responses in patients infused with in-vitro, RNA-treated, autologous lymphocytes, the efficacy of RNA administered by any route remains questionable.

Coumarin (1,2-benzopyrone) and cimetidine have also been shown to mediate antitumor activity in patients with metastatic renal cell carcinoma (Marshall et al., 1987). A 33 per cent response without any toxicity was achieved in 45 patients treated in a pilot study. Subsequent phase II studies (50 patients) using the same drug and schedule, however, were associated with only a 6 per cent response (Dexeus et al., 1990).

In the past decade, development of recombinant DNA techniques has enabled the production of large quantities of purified lymphokines (cytokines), which are biologic substances involved in the regulation of the immune system. The first of these lymphokines to receive clinical use was *interferon*. The interferons are a family of secreted proteins that were originally characterized by their ability to induce an antiviral state. It has been established that the same proteins that have antiviral activities also have potent antiproliferative and immunomodulatory activities.

The interferons have been divided into antigenically distinct types and classified according to their primary

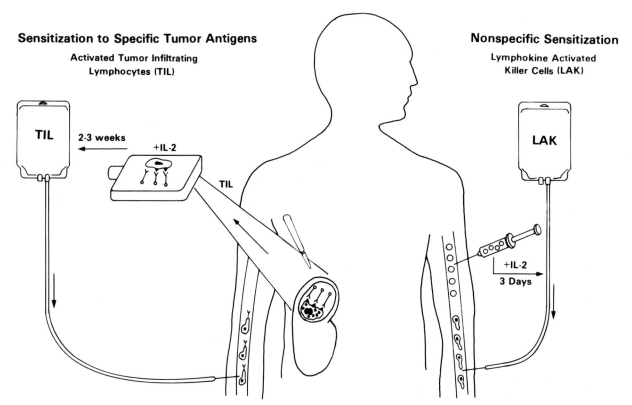

Sensitization to Specific Tumor Antigens

Activated Tumor Infiltrating Lymphocytes (TIL)

Nonspecific Sensitization

Lymphokine Activated Killer Cells (LAK)

Figure 27–23. Two approaches to the adoptive immunotherapy of patients with advanced renal cell carcinoma (IL-2, interleukin-2).

cell of origin or the stimulus for induction. Type I interferons are induced by virus infection in many cell types and include interferon alpha, produced by leukocytes, and interferon beta, produced by fibroblasts. Type II interferon (interferon gamma) is induced by antigen or mitogen in T lymphocytes. In humans, there are over 30 interferon alpha subspecies, the most important of which is interferon alpha-2.

Recombinant molecular technology has led to the insertion of human DNA sequences coding for interferon alpha-2 into *Escherichia coli*. The *E. coli* then express large quantities of the molecule, which is purified by chromatography (Roferon-A, interferon alpha-2a, Hoffman LaRoche; Intron-A, interferon alpha-2b, Schering-Plough). A human lymphoblastoid cell line can also be stimulated in vitro to produce a combination of interferon alpha subtypes, which are then purified (Wellferon, Wellcome). Recombinant interferons, unlike the natural interferons, are not glycosylated. This does not affect their activity, but it may make them more antigenic.

The interferons have shown some efficacy against a number of human malignancies, including hairy cell leukemia, chronic myelogenous leukemia, T cell lymphoma, and malignant melanoma (Gutterman, 1988). Several studies have been conducted in patients with renal cell carcinoma. In independent studies, deKernion and co-workers (1983) and Quesada and co-workers (1982) reported on the regression of metastatic renal cell carcinoma with a partially purified human interferon alpha preparation. Objective responses, complete and partial responses, occurred in 16.5 per cent and 26 per cent of patients treated, respectively. Following this initial report, numerous phase II trials with interferon alpha were conducted with a reproducible objective response rate of 15 to 20 per cent and a complete response rate of 1 per cent (Figlin et al., 1988; Kirkwood et al., 1985; Muss et al., 1987; Umeda and Niijima, 1986; Vugrin et al., 1986). Responses appear independent of the interferon alpha preparation used and correlate with those patients who have undergone previous nephrectomy and with those who have had good performance status, a long disease-free interval, and lung-predominant disease.

The survival rate of 84 evaluable patients treated at UCLA was 49 weeks. Patients with the favorable prognostic variables scored best with slightly higher response rates and a median survival of 155 weeks (Sarna et al., 1987). Combination of interferon with vinblastine resulted in an overall efficacy similar to that achieved by interferon alone, and vinblastine, with its added toxicity, seemed to be unrelated to clinical gain (Figlin et al., 1985). Although interferons have unquestionable activity against renal cell carcinoma, most patients who respond are those with limited metastases, and especially limited pulmonary metastases. This low level of clinical response indicates the need for further trials with combination interferons and with interferons combined with other agents.

The combination of interferon alpha and interferon gamma demonstrates synergistic activity in vitro and in a murine renal cancer (Renca) model in vivo (Sayers et al., 1990). Because some activity of interferon gamma against human renal cell carcinoma has been documented (Aulitzky et al., 1989), this combination of interferons is currently being tested in clinical trials. Initial reports demonstrate activity, but no definite synergism, and it is still too soon to determine any superiority over single-agent interferon alpha therapy (Ernstoff et al., 1990; Foon et al., 1988; Geboers et al., 1988; Quesada et al., 1988).

The discovery in 1976 by Morgan and colleagues of the T-cell growth factor (TCGF) *interleukin-2* (IL-2) revolutionized the field of cancer immunotherapy and altered substantially the prospects for the treatment of renal cell carcinoma. IL-2 is a 15,000-dalton glycoprotein produced in minute quantities by helper T lymphocytes upon antigen or antigen-induced activation of resting T cells. In vivo, IL-2 has been shown to generate lymphokine-activated killer (LAK) cells (Belldegrun et al., 1988b), enhance natural killer (NK) cell function, augment alloantigen responsiveness, stimulate growth of T cells with antitumor reactivity, and mediate regression of cancer in experimental animals and in selected patients with advanced cancer (Rosenberg, 1986, 1988a).

In 1985, Rosenberg and co-workers reported the initial National Cancer Institute (NCI) results of adoptive cellular therapy with LAK cells plus IL-2 in 25 patients with advanced cancer. The study was extended to include 139 patients by 1988 (Rosenberg et al., 1985; Rosenberg, 1988b). Of 54 patients with renal cell carcinoma who were treated, seven patients experienced complete response and ten patients had a partial response, for a total of 33 per cent response. Of 38 patients with renal cell carcinoma treated with high-dose bolus IL-2 alone, four complete responses and three partial responses were achieved, for a total of 18.4 per cent response. Responses occurred at a number of different sites, including lung, liver, soft tissue, subcutaneous tissue, and bone.

Fisher and associates (1988), performing a phase II NCI-sponsored extramural study of the same regimen, reported a 16 per cent objective response in 35 patients with metastatic or unresectable renal cell carcinoma. Two patients had complete regression of all tumor, and three additional patients had partial responses with greater than 50 per cent reduction in the total tumor burden. In other studies, the objective responses obtained with IL-2–based immunotherapy were significantly lower than those reported by the NCI (Parkinson, 1990). Nonetheless, there can be no doubt that, in some patients with renal cell carcinoma, IL-2 treatment can produce remarkable changes in the natural history of the disease. However, this group represents the minority of patients treated. Only 5 per cent of patients treated with IL-2 respond completely, and an additional 10 to 15 per cent respond partially. These numbers so far are small enough that it has been difficult to demonstrate overall survival benefit for IL-2–treated patients as a group.

Side effects of IL-2 therapy have been well documented and include fever, chills, malaise, nausea, vomiting, diarrhea, and other constitutional symptoms. The most common serious side effects, however, are primar-

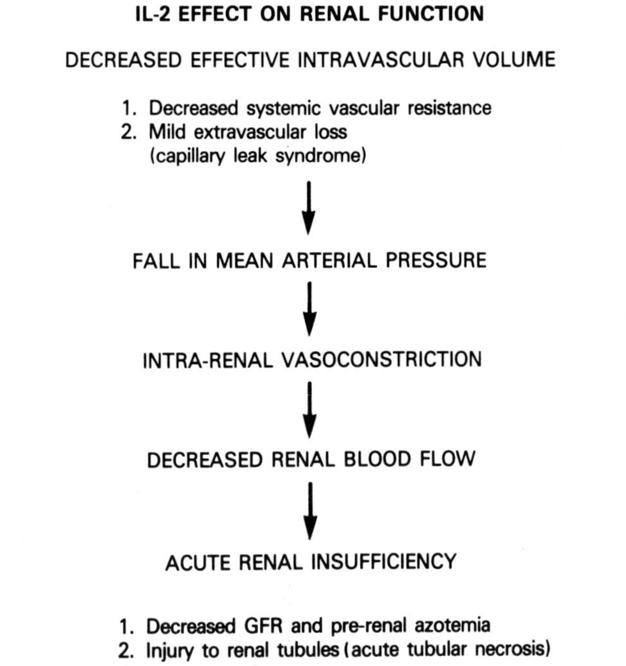

IL-2 EFFECT ON RENAL FUNCTION

DECREASED EFFECTIVE INTRAVASCULAR VOLUME

1. Decreased systemic vascular resistance
2. Mild extravascular loss
   (capillary leak syndrome)

↓

FALL IN MEAN ARTERIAL PRESSURE

↓

INTRA-RENAL VASOCONSTRICTION

↓

DECREASED RENAL BLOOD FLOW

↓

ACUTE RENAL INSUFFICIENCY

1. Decreased GFR and pre-renal azotemia
2. Injury to renal tubules (acute tubular necrosis)

Figure 27–24. Effects of interleukin-2 (IL-2) on renal function (GFR, glomerular filtration rate).

ily renal and cardiopulmonary (Rosenberg et al., 1985). IL-2 therapy induces a prerenal azotemia with hypotension, fluid retention, respiratory distress syndrome, oliguria, and low fractional sodium excretion (Fig. 27–24). Importantly, cessation of IL-2 administration results in a rapid recovery and reversal of almost all side effects. Renal function values return to baseline levels within 7 days in 62 per cent of patients and within 30 days in 95 per cent of patients (Belldegrun et al., 1987, 1989). Treatment-related mortality is low at less than 2 per cent.

In an attempt to achieve better response and lower toxicity, there has been interest in combining interferon with IL-2. In experimental murine models, this combination of IL-2 and interferon alpha can result in better antitumor effects than the administration of either agent alone (Brunda et al., 1987; Cameron et al., 1988). In our own institution, 30 patients with measurable renal cell carcinoma were treated in an outpatient setting with rIL-2 (2 million units m²), by continuous infusion on days 1 through 4, and Roferon-A (6 million units m²), by intramuscular (IM) or subcutaneous (SC) administration on days 1 and 4 of each week. Each 4-week treatment period (one course) was followed by a 2-week rest. One complete (3.3 per cent) response and eight (27 per cent) partial responses were observed for a total objective response rate of 30 per cent. Two patients had a surgical complete response following a salvage nephrectomy. In a very similar regimen, Hirsh and colleagues (1990) reported objective responses in 6 of 12 assessable (three complete responses and three partial responses) patients with metastatic renal cell carcinoma who received the bulk of treatment as outpatients at home. Atzpodien and co-workers (1990) observed partial tumor regression in 40 per cent of patients receiving long-term SC administration of IL-2 and interferon alpha.

The most promising new application of IL-2 is with tumor-infiltrating lyphocytes (TIL) (see Fig. 27–23). TIL are grown selectively from single-cell tumor suspensions cultured in IL-2. After a short period of culture, renal cell carcinoma cells die and the culture is overgrown by T lymphocytes. This cell population may be expanded in long-term cultures with IL-2 so that about 2 to 3 × 10¹¹ lymphocytes may be reinfused into the patients (Belldegrun et al., 1988a, 1989).

Whereas LAK cells are mainly activated NK cells, TIL are activated cytotoxic T cells, which show greater specificity in their targets and recirculate and home to tumor masses in a way that LAK cells do not. In experimental systems, TIL are 50 to 100 times as powerful as LAK cells. In addition, TIL, when administered in combination with cyclophosphamide and IL-2, are capable of eradicating advanced bulky tumors against which LAK cells are not effective (Rosenberg et al., 1986a).

In a pilot study using TIL, IL-2, and cyclophosphamide to treat 12 patients with metastatic disease, two partial responses to therapy were observed. Pulmonary and mediastinal masses regressed in a patient with melanoma, and a lymph node mass regressed in a patient with renal cell carcinoma (Topalian et al., 1988). In a subsequent study involving 20 patients with metastatic melanoma, Rosenberg (1988d) observed objective responses in 11 patients (55 per cent), including one complete remission. Two of the patients who responded had previously shown no response to LAK cell therapy.

Current efforts are in progress to enhance the therapeutic efficacy of TIL. At UCLA, we have just begun a clinical study testing the antitumor activity of a combination of TIL primed in vivo with interferon, continuous infusion of IL-2, and SC interferon alpha in patients with advanced renal cell carcinoma. The successful introduction of genes coding for neomycin resistance or for other lymphokine genes into human TIL raises the possibility of introducing other programmed genetic materials into TIL that would augment their antitumor properties and be delivered directly to the tumor site. Given this small and preliminary body of clinical and experimental data, further studies will focus on various forms of combination immunotherapy, which may evolve to be one of the most promising areas of cancer treatment.

PALLIATIVE OR ADJUNCTIVE NEPHRECTOMY

Approximately 30 per cent of patients have metastases at the time the diagnosis of renal carcinoma is first made, and early reports suggested that removal of the primary lesion induces regression of the metastases. This approach has been widely embraced by urologists and performed both for the purpose of control of symptoms and for the purpose of regression of metastatic sites.

The term "palliative nephrectomy" is best reserved for an operation performed for the control of severe symptoms. This procedure seems to be most effective in patients with severe hemorrhage, severe pain, paraneoplastic syndromes, and compression of adjacent viscera. The frequency with which each of these specific symptoms is controlled, however, is unclear, and modern methods, including angioinfarction, seldom make this the only palliative alternative. Patients with metastases at the time of presentation have an average survival of approximately 4 months, and only 10 per cent can be expected to survive 1 year (deKernion et al., 1978). The surgical mortality from the operation must also be superimposed on the potential benefits (Fowler, 1987). Nonetheless, palliative nephrectomy is occasionally warranted for control of severe symptoms, especially profuse hemorrhage.

The term "adjunctive nephrectomy" has been adopted to describe removal of the primary tumor in the patient with metastases, for the purpose of either prolonging survival or causing regression of metastatic lesions. Although a common practice for many years, the procedure has come under more careful scrutiny. The known spontaneous regression of renal tumors has been cited as support for the practice of adjunctive nephrectomy. Regression occurs in renal tumors only rarely, in perhaps 0.4 per cent of patients, or one in 250 (Montie et al., 1977). Some reports are even more pessimistic, such as that from the Mayo Clinic, in which no patient underwent regression in the 533 patients reviewed (Myers et al., 1968).

Following adjunctive nephrectomy, regression can be expected to occur in less than 1 per cent of patients (Montie et al., 1977). Such regressions are often short-lived, and the mortality rate ranges from 2 to 15 per cent, mainly dependent on patient selection. Furthermore, Oliver (1989) found a 6 per cent spontaneous tumor regression rate despite the absence of any therapeutic intervention in 73 patients with renal cell carcinoma followed systematically for 5 years. On the basis of this information, it seems difficult to support routine practice of adjunctive nephrectomy.

Improvement of patient survival by removal of a large primary tumor has also been cited in support of adjunctive nephrectomy. No study has thus far been reported in which patients are properly stratified and then randomized to undergo adjunctive nephrectomy versus no nephrectomy. However, in a study from this institution, survival of patients undergoing nephrectomy was identical to the survival for the general population of patients with renal carcinoma, suggesting that the nephrectomy had minimal impact on the outcome (deKernion et al., 1978).

Adjunctive nephrectomy is, therefore, no longer practiced in many treatment centers on a routine basis, although some investigators still support its application in selected patients (Freed, 1977). Indeed, the procedure may have application in certain clinical settings. Five-year survival seems to be improved in patients who have excision of solitary renal metastases (Middleton, 1967; O'Dea et al., 1978). It may be appropriate, therefore, to recommend nephrectomy with excision of solitary metastasis in this select group of patients, although micrometastases are likely to be present at other sites. Similarly, as part of an experimental study, adjunctive nephrectomy may be appropriate.

In conclusion, the heterogeneity of renal cell carcinoma and its variable natural history defy therapeutic generalizations. Patients with limited pulmonary metastases, a resectable primary lesion, and a normal performance status seem to have a survival greater than that for others with metastatic disease. In a review of patients at this institution, those in the aforementioned category had a 5-year survival of approximately 30 per cent following adjunctive nephrectomy and various postoperative treatment programs. The impact of the postoperative treatment programs is unclear, but the data indicated that some effect was independent of these systemic therapies.

The impact of the adjunctive nephrectomy can also be questioned because a similar group of patients who did not undergo nephrectomy has not been followed. However, in young healthy patients who meet these specific criteria, adjunctive nephrectomy may be appropriate, especially if it is part of a planned treatment program. The role of adjunctive nephrectomy must constantly be reassessed in careful clinical studies (Flanigan, 1989).

Angioinfarction followed by adjunctive nephrectomy was advocated in the past. However, review of a large experience using this appraoch (Flanigan, 1987; Gottesman et al., 1985; Kurth et al., 1987; Swanson et al., 1983), does not substantiate its benefit, and it is not indicated as a treatment modality in patients with metastatic disease.

The performance of adjunctive nephrectomy for the purpose of facilitating or instituting experimental immunotherapy is currently an important issue. This indication represents the most valid reason for adjunctive nephrectomy in the presence of metastatic disease. It should be stressed, however, that patients with metastatic renal cell carcinoma who are potential candidates for biologic therapy should be referred to an immunotherapy center for review prior to the time of nephrectomy. Removing the kidney might result in unnecessary procedures in a patient who is not eligible for this type of therapy.

Of the first nine metastatic renal cell carcinoma patients treated with either IL-2 or IL-2 plus LAK cells at the Surgery Branch of the NCI, no responses were seen (Robertson et al., 1990). Strategy was then developed to remove the primary kidney tumor before adoptive immunotherapy if the bulk of the primary kidney tumor was greater than that of the metastatic tumor. The goal was to decrease tumor bulk and to achieve maximum therapeutic response to therapy. The beneficial effect of prior nephrectomy on response to immunotherapy has not been consistently demonstrated, and it remains unclear what influences other factors (performance status, sites of metastases) may have on this effect. However, several trials of interferon alpha in metastatic renal cell carcinoma, when retrospectively analyzed, have suggested that prior nephrectomy was an independent variable in determining patient response to interferon (Muss et al., 1987; Umeda and Niijima, 1986).

Muss and co-workers (1987), for example, found a 23 per cent response rate in patients with prior nephrectomy as compared with an 8 per cent response rate in the entire patient population. In a large multicenter study in Japan, Umeda and Niijima (1986) demonstrated a significantly higher response rate for patients who had undergone radical or palliative nephrectomy. These two studies were summaries of different clinical trials using varying doses, schedules, and types of interferons.

Current analysis of our combined UCLA data suggests a better response rate in the group of patients who underwent nephrectomy within 1 year prior to the initiation of immunotherapy (Belldegrun et al., 1990). Of 84 evaluable patients, 45 patients were started on interferon therapy within 1 year of the initial diagnosis/nephrectomy. The two groups of patients (nephrectomy versus no nephrectomy) were similar with regard to performance status and lung metastases. Of patients who underwent nephrectomy prior to immunotherapy 24.3 per cent responded to interferon compared with 8.3 per cent who did not have prior nephrectomy. The difference was not statistically significant; however, the power of statistical testing was limited by the small number of patients in the no nephrectomy group.

At this relatively early stage of clinical investigation, little information can be extracted from the literature with regard to the role of nephrectomy in IL-2 therapy. One can perhaps see an early trend of more favorable therapeutic response in patients with prior nephrectomy who undergo IL-2 treatment. Fisher and associates (1988), for example, have reported only one objective response in 14 patients with an intact renal primary (7 per cent response rate) as compared with a 26 per cent response rate for all patients. Krigel and colleagues (1990) noted that five of ten patients who had a prior nephrectomy responded to a combination of IL-2 and interferon beta, as compared with only 1 of 12 patients who had not had a prior nephrectomy (p = .04). Thus, with the advent of promising immunotherapy, prospective analysis is needed to evaluate the role of nephrectomy in metastatic renal cell carcinoma, as part of a multimodality therapeutic protocol.

Sarcomas of the Kidney

Sarcomas constitute only about 2 to 3 per cent of malignant tumors of the kidney but increase in incidence with advancing age (Farrow et al., 1968; Saitoh et al., 1982). Differentiation from renal cell carcinoma is usu-

ally difficult or impossible. The most common presenting signs and symptoms are essentially those of a large renal carcinoma, e.g., pain, a flank mass, and hematuria (Fig. 27–25).

CT may be helpful in delineating whether a renal mass is parenchymal in origin or whether it originates in the renal sinus or capsule. Otherwise, the density of these tumors mimics that of soft tissue, with the exception of the fat density seen in liposarcoma or osteosarcoma, in which bone may be seen. The findings of tumor originating from renal sinus or capsule or the presence of a mass with fat or bone would be highly suggestive of a renal sarcoma. Absence of retroperitoneal lymphadenopathy in a patient with a large renal tumor is also more compatible with sarcoma than carcinoma (Pollack et al., 1987). Angiographically, these tumors are hypovascular without arteriovenous fistulae (Shirkhoda and Lewis, 1987).

Leiomyosarcomas, originating from smooth muscle cells, are the most common variety, composing about 60 per cent of the total incidence of sarcomas. Sixty-six cases were identified by Niceta and co-workers (1974) and were most common in women in the 4th to 6th decades of life. These tumors tend to compress and displace the kidney rather than invade it. They usually attain large size and metastasize early and widely throughout the body. Leiomyosarcomas are generally well encapsulated, firm, and multinodular, and they tend to recur locally after resection.

Treatment for leiomyosarcoma, as with any sarcoma, is radical nephrectomy. This approach is especially important because these tumors can seldom be definitely differentiated from renal adenocarcinoma. The prognosis is generally poor when patients are treated with surgery alone. Adjuvant chemotherapy may be beneficial (Rakowsky et al., 1987; Taniguchi et al., 1987). Beccia and associates (1979) treated a patient with adjuvant chemotherapy, and the individual survived for 4 years without evidence of recurrence. Two patients were treated by Helmbrecht and Cosgrove (1974) with adjuvant radiation therapy and chemotherapy in addition to surgery. In view of the experience with other sarcomas, doxorubicin is perhaps the most logical agent for adjuvant therapy and definitive treatment.

Osteogenic sarcomas are extremely rare tumors of the kidney. The genesis of such tumors is problematic, and osteogenic differentiation may occur in various sarcom-

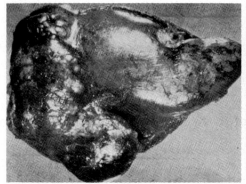
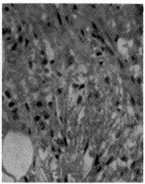

Figure 27–25. Sarcoma of renal capsule. *A*, Massive tumor arising from renal capsule. *B*, Histologic specimen diagnostic of fibrosarcoma.

A   B

atoid renal cell tumors (Micolonghi et al., 1984; Moon et al., 1983). These tumors contain calcium and are rock-hard or may have sunburst calcification. The presence of extensive calcification in a rather hypovascular tumor should suggest the presence of this rare lesion. The tumor may metastasize to bone and pose a problem as to whether the tumor in the kidney is a metastasis or truly a primary lesion. Biggers and Stewart (1979) reviewed the literature and recorded seven cases, detailing the clinical and pathologic features of the tumor. The poor prognosis was emphasized and, although radical nephrectomy is the treatment of choice, few patients are cured.

Virtually every other variety of sarcoma has been described in the kidney. *Liposarcomas* represent about 19 per cent of renal sarcomas and are often confused with angiomyolipomas or with very large, benign primary lipomas. These tumors occur generally in the 5th and 6th decades of life and are usually of large size (Economou et al., 1987). They frequently recur locally, and re-excision is usually feasible. Postoperative adjuvant therapy is appropriate when margins are positive, and we have seen responses to a combination of radiotherapy, *cis*-platinum, and phosphamide. *Carcinosarcoma* of the kidney has been described in several cases and is composed of classic renal cell carcinoma components in addition to fibrosarcomatous elements (Rao et al., 1977). *Fibrosarcoma* has been described and is easily mistaken for leiomyoma or leiomyosarcoma (Kansara and Powell, 1980). Fibroxanthosarcoma (Chen, 1979) and *angiosarcoma* (Allred et al., 1981) have also been described.

Rhabdomyosarcoma of the adult, one of the rarest and most malignant renal neoplasms, arises from striated muscle. These tumors are usually large and multinodular with a well-defined capsule. One patient with rhabdomyosarcoma, who was treated in recent years at our institution, succumbed to metastatic disease 14 months after radical nephrectomy.

One of the most thorough studies of the incidence and metastatic pattern of sarcomas was made by Saitoh and colleagues (1982). In 2651 cases of renal tumors, they reported an incidence of sarcomas of 1 per cent; nine were leiomyosarcoma, five were rhabdomyosarcoma, and five were fibrosarcoma. The most common sites of metastases were the liver, lymph nodes, and lung.

Surgery is the only potentially curative method of treating these rare tumors. The survival following surgery alone, however, is extremely poor. The success that has been realized by intra-arterial doxorubicin therapy combined with radiation provides at least a testable hypothesis for the adjuvant treatment of these tumors. The patient illustrated in Figure 27–26 had a poorly differentiated sarcoma of the kidney that completely regressed following doxorubicin and external radiotherapy, and the residual fibrous mass was subsequently excised. The patient is free of disease 2 years after surgery. Although adjuvant intravenous doxorubicin following nephrectomy has not been proven to be of value, the current experience suggests that this may be a reasonable approach.

Malignant fibrous histiocytoma is the most common soft tissue sarcoma of late adult life and often occurs in the retroperitoneal space (Goldman et al., 1986). Eight such tumors arising in the kidney have been reported (Scriven et al., 1984). The tumors usually grow to large size and may be clinically and angiographically indistinguishable from renal cell carcinoma. The histology is similar to that of histiocytomas arising in other areas. Therapy is radical nephrectomy, but local recurrence is frequent. Radiotherapy may be effective (Osamura et al., 1978; Raghavaiah et al., 1980).

Hemangiopericytomas, renin-secreting tumors of the kidney, are usually small, benign tumors that produce severe hypertension. These tumors are often histologically hemangiopericytomas (Weiss et al., 1984). However, renal and perirenal hemangiopericytoma may exist, may grow to large size, and may develop a malignant potential. Most investigators consider it to be a true sarcomatous lesion.

Local or distant metastases have been reported in approximately 15 per cent of patients (Glenn, 1980). Ordonez and co-workers (1982) described a hemangiopericytoma extending into the vena cava as a thrombus. DiEsidio and associates (1980) reported a retroperitoneal hemangiopericytoma that metastasized to the liver, kidney, and abdominal cavity. A major concern with these tumors is their profuse vascularity. Smullens and colleagues (1979) described catheter embolization of hemangiopericytoma of the retroperitoneum in two cases, which greatly facilitated safe removal. When these tumors are confined to the kidney, the most appropriate treatment is radical nephrectomy.

Lymphoblastoma

Malignancies of the lymphoma type, including reticulum cell sarcoma, lymphosarcoma, and leukemia, are uncommon and generally occur in the kidney as only one manifestation of the systemic disease. Knoepp (1956) identified a primary lymphosarcoma of the kidney treated, apparently successfully, with radical nephrectomy. Silber and Chang (1973) also reported a primary lymphoma of the kidney. Leukemia generally involves the kidney in an infiltrative pattern; it can be silent or can produce hematuria, enlarged kidneys, and progressive renal failure. At autopsy, up to 50 per cent of cases with leukemia have renal involvement.

The treatment of these processes is generally the indicated systemic treatment of that particular disease. Nephrectomy is seldom, if ever, indicated, except in the case of a solitary lesion or in the patient with severe symptoms, such as uncontrollable hemorrhage.

Because the treatment of these lesions is not the primary purview of the urologist, major concern rests in the diagnosis of renal involvement by these systemic diseases and in their distinction from other renal mass lesions. Hartman and co-workers (1982) related pathologic findings with radiologic findings in 21 patients with renal lymphoma. The radiographic picture depended on the pattern of involvement and the size, number, and distribution of the lesions. These workers concluded that

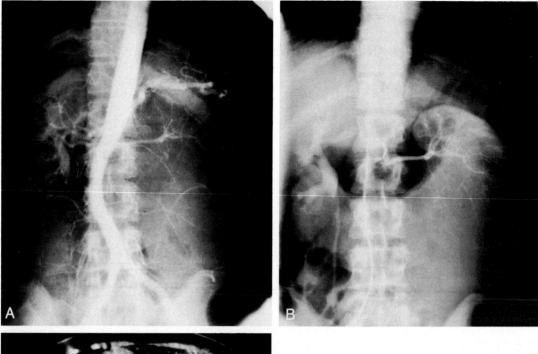

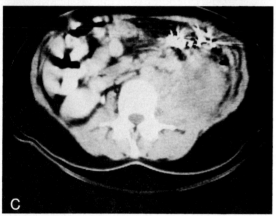

Figure 27–26. *A*, Aortic flush phase demonstrating huge left flank mass in a 36-year-old woman with flank pain. Note aortic displacement. *B*, Selective left renal arteriogram showing typical hypovascular pattern associated with sarcomas. *C*, Computed tomography scan demonstrating the large tumor fixed to the posterior abdominal wall and paraspinous muscles proved to be a poorly differentiated sarcoma by biopsy.

the lymphoma initially grows between the nephrons and subsequently expands and produces the typical lymphomatous masses.

CT appears to be the method of choice in diagnosing renal lymphoma (Heiken et al., 1983). The initial nodular lesions, which later become confluent, are best detected with contrast medium administration. Four patterns of involvement were documented with CT by Heiken and associates (1983): (1) multiple intraparenchymal nodules, (2) direct contiguous lymph node masses, (3) solitary renal lesions, and (4) diffuse infiltration. Jafri and associates (1982) described similar findings in 16 patients with non-Hodgkin's lymphomas of the kidney.

CT was accurate in determining the size and location of the tumor and was useful in evaluating the response to systemic therapy. Various patterns of involvement, including solitary nodules, multiple nodules, focal infiltration, diffuse infiltration, contiguous extension, and renal enlargement, were noted. Retroperitoneal adenopathy was identified by CT scan in all of the patients. Others have suggested that the findings of renal infiltration and multiple intraparenchymal nodules associated

with retroperitoneal adenopathy should raise the possibility of renal lymphoma. At the present time, CT appears to be the most reliable way to diagnose renal involvement by lymphoma and to monitor the progress of therapy.

The major diagnostic problem is differentiating a renal lymphoma mass from a renal cell carcinoma. Aspiration

Table 27–7. RADIOLOGIC FINDINGS IN RENAL LYMPHOMA

Computed Tomography	Sonography	Angiography
Multiple renal masses (45%)	Hypoechoic Anechoic	Hypovascular Capsular artery displacement
Solitary mass (15%)		
Invasion from outside (25%)	No through transmission	
Diffuse infiltration (10%)	Diminished central sinus echoes	Fuzzy renal outline
Perinephric involvement (5%)		

Adapted from Barbaric, Z. L.: Principles of Genitourinary Radiology. New York, Thieme Medical Publishers, Inc., 1991, p. 181. With permission.

biopsy under CT guidance may help in arriving at a histologic diagnosis. Radiologic findings are summarized in Table 27–7 (Barbaric, 1991).

Metastatic Tumors

The kidney is a frequent site of metastatic deposits from a variety of solid tumors and hematologic malignancies. The high blood flow, profuse vascularity, and "fertile soil" of the renal parenchyma provide a hospitable environment for deposition and growth of malignant cells.

Metastases to the kidney are seldom clinically identified and are most often discovered at autopsy. They are, in that sense, often clinically inconsequential, because the nature of the metastatic disease militates against the removal of an isolated renal metastasis. In a review of 5000 autopsies, Klinger (1951) found 21 cases of metastases from lung carcinoma (Fig. 27–27). Olsson (1971) reported that 20 per cent of patients dying of lung cancer had renal metastases, 40 per cent of which were bilateral. These tumors are often small and multiple, and it has been estimated that as many as 19,000 persons annually may have lung cancer with secondary renal metastases. Although these tumors seldom are associated with clinical symptoms, massive hemorrhage has

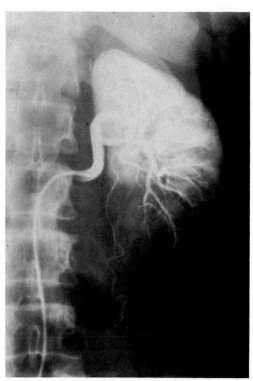

Figure 27–28. Arteriogram demonstrating hypovascular mass in left kidney. A solitary metastasis of lymphoblastoma was confirmed.

been reported (Walther et al., 1979). Virtually every other solid neoplasm may metastasize to the kidney, including ovarian, bowel, and breast malignancies. Lymphoma and lymphoblastoma are among the most common metastatic lesions of the kidney. These tumors usually appear as multiple nodules but, occasionally, single nodules and diffuse infiltration have been reported (Kyaw and Koehler, 1969).

Metastatic or secondary lesions within the kidney generally produce few symptoms. Flank pain and hematuria may occur. With pyelographic or ultrasonographic identification, it is difficult to distinguish metastatic tumors from primary renal neoplasms. The principal method of detection is CT, and identification often requires a CT-guided aspiration biopsy. The mass on the precontrast scan is almost isodense to the kidney and enhances only slightly on the postcontrast scan (Barbaric, 1991; Choyke et al., 1982). Arteriographically, these tumors are usually round and hypovascular, without the discrete neovascularity and other angiographic characteristics associated with primary renal cell carcinoma (Fig. 27–28).

Whether renal carcinoma frequently metastasizes to the opposite kidney is controversial. The same malignant propensity that caused a tumor in one kidney could be reasonably expected to give rise to another primary lesion in the opposite kidney. The short-term results (cited previously) following excision of tumor in the contralateral kidney (synchronously or asynchronously) seem to be better than survival following excision of a solitary metastasis. However, no serologic or histologic method has been devised to accurately determine whether such tumors are metastatic or de novo lesions.

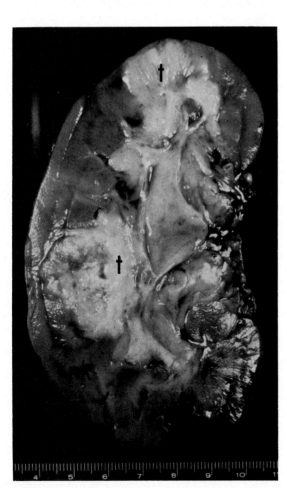

Figure 27–27. Metastatic carcinoma of the kidney from the lung demonstrating the diffuse invasive character of metastatic tumor *(t)* in normal renal substance *(nk)*.

REFERENCES

Albarran, J., and Imbert, L.: Les Tumeurs du Rein. Paris, Masson et Cie, 1903.

Allred, C. D., Cathey, W. J., and McDivitt, R. W.: Primary renal angiosarcoma: A case report. Hum. Pathol., 12:665, 1981.

Amendola, M. A., Bree, R. L., et al.: Small renal cell carcinomas: Resolving a diagnostic dilemma. Radiology, 166:637, 1988.

Atzpodien, J., and Kirchner, H.: Cancer, cytokines, and cytotoxic cells: Interleukin-2 in the immunotherapy of human neoplasms. Klin. Wochenschr., 68:1, 1990.

Aulitzky, W., Gastl, G., Aulitzky, W. E., Herold, M., Kemmler, J., Mull, B., Frick, J., and Huber, Ch.: Successful treatment of metastatic renal cell carcinoma with a biologically active dose of recombinant interferon-gamma. J. Clin. Oncol., 7:1875, 1989.

Bander, N. H., Finstad, C. L., Cordon-Cardo, C., Ramsawak, R. D., Vaughn, E. D., Jr., Whitmore, W. F., Jr., Oettgen, H. F., Melamed, M. R., and Old, L. J.: Analysis of mouse monoclonal antibody that reacts with a specific region of the human proximal tubule and subsets renal cell carcinomas. Cancer Res., 49:6774, 1989.

Barbaric, Z. L.: Genitourinary Radiology. New York, Thieme Medical Publishers, Inc., 1991, p. 171.

Barnes, C. A., and Beckman, E. N.: Renal oncocytoma and its cocongeners. Am. J. Clin. Pathol., 79:312, 1983.

Beccia, D. J., Elkurt, R. J., and Rane, R. J.: Adjuvant chemotherapy in renal leiomyosarcoma. Urology, 13:652, 1979.

Bell, E. T.: Renal Disease, Ed. 2. Philadelphia, Lea & Febiger, 1950, p. 435.

Belldegrun, A., Koo, A. S., Bochner, B., Figlin, R., and deKernion, J. B.: Immunotherapy for advanced renal cell cancer: The role of radical nephrectomy. Eur. Urol., 18(Suppl. 2):42, 1990.

Belldegrun, A., Muul, L. M., and Rosenberg, S. A.: Interleukin-2 expanded tumor infiltrating lymphocytes in human renal cell cancer: Isolation, characterization and antitumor activity. Cancer Res., 48:206, 1988a.

Belldegrun, A., and Rosenberg, S. A.: Adoptive immunotherapy of urologic tumors. In Lepor, H., and Ratliff, T. L. (Eds.): Urologic Oncology. Boston, Kluwer Academic Publishers, 1989, p. 213.

Belldegrun, A., Uppenkamp, I., and Rosenberg, S. A.: Antitumor reactivity of human lymphokine activated killer (LAK) cells against fresh and cultured preparations of renal cell cancer. J. Urol., 139:150, 1988b.

Belldegrun, A., Webb, D. E., Austin, H. A., et al.: Effects of interleukin-2 in renal function in patients receiving immunotherapy for advanced cancer. Ann. Intern. Med., 106:817, 1987.

Belldegrun, A., Webb, D. E., Austin, H. A., et al.: Renal toxicity of interleukin-2 administration in patients with metastatic renal cell cancer: Effect of pretherapy nephrectomy. J. Urol., 141:499, 1989.

Bennington, J. L., and Beckwith, J. B.: Tumors of the kidney, renal pelvis and ureter. In Atlas of Tumor Pathology. Washington, D.C., Armed Forces Institute of Pathology, 1975, Facs. 12.

Best, B. G.: Renal carcinoma: A ten-year review 1971–1980. Br. J. Urol., 60:100, 1987.

Biggers, R., and Stewart, J.: Primary renal osteosarcoma. Urology, 13:674, 1979.

Birch-Hirschfeld, F. V., and Doederlein, A.: Zentralbl. Krankh. Horn. Sex Org., Vol. 3, 1894.

Bloom, H. J.: Hormone induced and spontaneous regression of metastatic renal cancer. Cancer, 32:1006, 1973.

Blute, M. L., Malek, R. S., and Segura, J. W.: Angiomyolipoma: Clinical metamorphosis and concepts for management. J. Urol., 139:20, 1988.

Bonavita, J. A., Pollack, H. M., and Banner, M. P.: Renal oncocytoma: Further observations and literature review. Urol. Radiol., 2:229, 1981.

Bonnin, J. M., Cain, M. D., Jose, J. S., Mukherjee, T. M., Perrett, L. V., Scroop, G. C., and Seymour, A. E.: Hypertension due to renin-secreting tumor localized by segmental renal vein sampling. Aust. N.Z. J. Med., 7:630, 1977.

Bosniak, M. A., and Subramanyam, B. R.: Renal parenchymal and capsular tumors in adults. In Taveras, J. M., and Ferrucci, J. T. (Eds.): Radiology—Diagnosis, Imaging, Intervention, Vol. 4. Philadelphia, J. B. Lippincott Co., 1990, p. 1.

Böttiger, L. E.: Prognosis in renal carcinoma. Cancer 26:780, 1970.

Boxer, R. J., Waisman, J., Lieber, M. M., Mampaso, F. M., and Skinner, D. G.: Non-metastatic hepatic dysfunction associated with renal carcinoma. J. Urol., 119:468, 1978.

Brunda, M. J., Bellantoni, D., and Sulich, V.: In vivo antitumor activity of combinations of interferon-α and interleukin-2 in a murine model: Correlation of efficacy with the induction of cytotoxic cells resembling natural killer cells. Int. J. Cancer, 40:365, 1987.

Bukowski, R. M., Groppe, D., Reimer, R., Weick, J., and Hewlett, J. S.: Immunotherapy (IT) of metastatic renal cell carcinoma [Abstract C-457]. Proc. Am. Assoc. Cancer Res./Am. Soc. Clin. Oncol., 20:402, 1979.

Cameron, R. B., McIntosh, J. K., and Rosenberg, S. A.: Synergistic antitumor effects of combination immunotherapy with recombinant interleukin-2 and a recombinant hybrid alpha-interferon in the treatment of established murine hepatic metastases. Cancer Res., 48:5810, 1988.

Carroll, P. R., Murty, V. V. S., Reuter, V., Jhanwar, S., Fair, W. R., Whitmore, W. F., and Chaganti, R. S.: Abnormalities at chromosome region 3p12014 characterize clear cell renal carcinoma. Cancer Genet. Cytogenet., 27:253, 1987.

Carson, W. J.: Tumors of the kidney: Histologic study. Trans. Sect. Urol. A.M.A., 1928.

Chen, K. T.: Fibroxanthosarcoma of the kidney. Urology, 13:439, 1979.

Cherrie, R. J., Goldman, D. G., Lindner, A., and deKernion, J. B.: Prognostic implications of vena caval extension of renal cell carcinoma. J. Urol., 128:910, 1982.

Chisholm, G. D.: Nephrogenic ridge tumors and their syndromes. Ann. N.Y. Acad. Sci., 230:403, 1974.

Choyke, P. L., White, E. M., Zeman, R. K., et al.: Renal metastases: Clinicopathologic and radiologic correlation. Radiology, 162:359, 1982.

Chute, R., Soutter, L., and Kerr, W.: The value of thoracoabdominal incision in the removal of kidney tumors. N. Engl. J. Med., 241:951, 1949.

Clayman, R. V., Gonzalez, R., and Fraley, E. E.: Renal cell carcinoma invading the inferior vena cava: Clinical review and anatomical approach. J. Urol., 123:157, 1980.

Cohen, A. J., Li, F. P., Berg, S., Marchetto, D. J., Tsai, S., Jacobs, S. C., and Brown, R. S.: Hereditary renal cell carcinoma associated with a chromosomal translocation. N. Engl. J. Med., 301:592, 1979.

Colvin, R. B., and Dickersin, G. R.: Pathology of renal tumors. In Skinner, D. G., and deKernion, J. B. (Eds.): Genitourinary Cancer. Philadelphia, W. B. Saunders Co., 1978, p. 84.

Cox, C. E., Lacy, S. S., Montgomery, W. G., and Boyce, W. H.: Renal adenocarcinoma: A 28-year review with emphasis on rationale and feasibility of preoperative radiotherapy. J. Urol., 105:51, 1970.

Cummings, K. B.: Surgical management of renal cell carcinoma with extension into the vena cava. In Crawford, E. E., and Borden, T. A. (Eds.): Genitourinary Cancer Surgery. Philadelphia, Lea & Febiger, 1982, p. 70.

Daponte, D., Zungri, E., Algaba, F., and Sole-Balcells, F.: Angiomyolipome renal isole—etude de 10 cas. J. Urol. (Paris), 89:267–271, 1983.

Dayal, H. H., and Wikinson, G. S.: Epidemiology of renal cell cancer. Semin. Urol., 3:139, 1989.

deKernion, J. B.: Lymphadenectomy for renal cell carcinoma: Therapeutic implications. Urol. Clin. North Am., 7:697, 1980a.

deKernion, J. B.: Radical nephrectomy. In Ehrlich, R. E. (Ed.): Modern Techniques in Surgery. New York, Futura, 1980b, p. 1.

deKernion, J. B., and Berry, D.: The diagnosis and treatment of renal cell carcinoma. Cancer, 45:1947, 1980.

deKernion, J. B., and Huland, H.: The operable renal cell carcinoma: Summary and conclusions. Eur. Urol., 18(Suppl. 2):48, 1990.

deKernion, J. B., and Lindner, A.: Treatment of advanced renal cell carcinoma. In Kuss, R., Murphy, G., Khoury, S., and Karr, J. (Eds.): Proceedings of the First International Symposium on Kidney Tumors. New York, Alan R. Liss, 1982, p. 614.

deKernion, J. B., and Ramming, K. P.: The therapy of renal adenocarcinoma with immune RNA. Invest. Urol., 17:378, 1980.

deKernion, J. B., Ramming, K. P., and Smith, R. B.: Natural history of metastatic renal cell carcinoma: A computer analysis. J. Urol., 120:148, 1978.

deKernion, J. B., and Smith, R. B.: The kidney and adrenal glands. In Paulson, D. F. (Ed.): Genitourinary Surgery, Vol. 1. New York, Churchill Livingstone, 1984, p. 1.

Deming, C. L., and Harvard, B. M.: Tumors of the kidney. *In* Campbell, M. F., and Harrison, J. H. (Eds.): Urology, Vol. 2, Ed. 3. Philadelphia, W. B. Saunders Co., 1970, p. 884.

Dexeus, F., Logothetics, C., Sella, A., et al.: Phase II study of coumarin and cimetidine in metastatic renal cell carcinoma. J. Clin. Oncol., 8:325, 1990.

DiEsidio, M., Gadaleta, A., Monina, M., and Cappelletti, V.: Retroperitoneal hemangiopericytoma: Presentation of a case with recurrence and multiple metastases. Radiol. Med. (Torino), 66:331, 1980.

Dineen, M. K., Venable, D. D., and Misra, R. P.: Pure intrarenal lipoma—report of a case and review of the literature. Presented at the Annual Meeting, Southeastern Section of the American Urologic Association. Florida, 1983.

Economou, J. S., Lindner, A., and deKernion, J. B.: Sarcomas of the genitourinary tract. *In* Eilber, F. R., et al. (Eds.): The Soft Tissue Sarcomas. Orlando, Grune & Stratton, 1987, p. 219.

Ernstoff, M. S., Nair, S., Bahnson, R. R., et al.: A phase Ia trial of sequential administration recombinant DNA–produced interferons: Combination recombinant interferon gamma and recombinant interferon alpha in patients with metastatic renal cell carcinoma. J. Clin. Oncol., 8:1637, 1990.

Erslev, A. J., and Caro, J.: Physiologic and molecular biology of erythropoietin. Med. Oncol. Tumor Pharmacother., 3:159, 1986.

Farrow, G. M., Harrison, E. G., Utz, D. C., and Remine, W. H.: Sarcomas and sarcomatoid and mixed malignant tumors of the kidney in adults. Cancer, 22:545, 1968.

Figlin, R. A., deKernion, J. B., Maldazys, J., et al.: Treatment of renal cell carcinoma with alpha (human leukocyte) interferon and vinblastine in combination: A phase I-II trial. Cancer Treat. Rep., 69:263, 1985.

Figlin, R. A., deKernion, J. B., Mukamel, E., et al.: Recombinant interferon alpha-2a in metastatic renal cell carcinoma: Assessment of antitumor activity and anti-interferon antibody formation. J. Clin. Oncol., 6:1604, 1988.

Finney, R.: The value of radiotherapy in the treatment of hypernephroma—a clinical trial. Br. J. Urol., 45:258, 1973.

Fisher, E. R., and Horvat, B.: Comparative ultrastructural study of so-called renal adenoma and carcinoma. J. Urol., 108:382, 1972.

Fisher, R. I., Coltman, C. A., Jr., Doroshow, J. H., et al.: Metastatic renal cancer treated with interleukin-2 and lymphokine-activated killer cells: A phase II clinical trial. Ann. Intern. Med., 108:518, 1988.

Flanigan, R. C.: The failure of infarction and/or nephrectomy in stage IV renal cell cancer to influence survival or metastatic regression. Urol. Clin. North Am., 14:757, 1987.

Flanigan, R. C.: Role of surgery in metastatic renal cell carcinoma. Semin. Urol., 7:191, 1989.

Fojo, A. T., Shen, D. W., Mickley, L. A., Pastan, I., and Gottesman, M. M.: Intrinsic drug resistance in kidney cancers is associated with expression of a human multidrug resistance gene. J. Clin. Oncol., 5:1922, 1987.

Foon, K., Doroshow, J., Bonnem E., et al.: A prospective randomized trial of alpha 2b-interferon/gamma-interferon or the combination in advanced metastatic renal cell carcinoma. J. Biol. Response Mod., 7:540, 1988.

Foster, R. S., Mahomed, Y., Bihrle, R., and Strup, S.: Use of a caval-atrial shunt for resection of a caval tumor thrombus in renal cell carcinoma. J. Urol., 140:1370, 1988.

Fowler, J. E., Jr.: Nephrectomy in metastatic renal cell carcinoma. Urol. Clin. North Am., 14:749, 1987.

Freed, S. Z.: Nephrectomy for renal cell carcinoma with metastases. Urology, 9:613, 1977.

Freeman, M. R., Washecka, R., and Chung, L. W. R.: Aberrant expression of epidermal growth factor receptor and HER-2 (erb B-2) messenger RNAs in human renal cancers. Cancer Res. 49:6221, 1989.

Frignon, D. J., El-Naggar, A., Green, L. K., et al.: DNA flow cytometry as a predictor of outcome of stage I renal cell carcinoma. Cancer, 6:1161, 1989.

Geboers, A. D., deMulder, P. H., Debruyne, F. M., et al.: Alpha and gamma interferon in the treatment of advanced renal cell carcinoma. Semin. Surg. Oncol., 4:191, 1988.

Glenn, G. M., Choyke, P. L., Zbar, B., and Linehan, W. M.: Von Hippel-Lindau disease: Clinical review and molecular genetics. Probl. Urol., 4:312, 1990.

Glenn, J. F.: Renal tumors. *In* Harrison, J. H., Gittes, R. F., Perlmutter, A. D., et al. (Eds.): Campbell's Urology, Ed. 4. Philadelphia, W. B. Saunders Co., 1980.

Glover, S. D., and Buck, A. C.: Renal medullary fibroma: A case report. J. Urol., 127:758, 1982.

Goldberg, M. F., Tashjian, A. H., Order, S. C., and Dammin, G. J.: Renal adenocarcinoma containing a parathyroid hormone–like substance and associated with marked hypercalcemia. Am. J. Med., 36:805, 1964.

Goldman, S. M., Hartman, D. S., and Weiss, S. W.: The varied radiographic manifestations of retroperitoneal malignant fibrous histiocytoma revealed through 27 cases. J. Urol., 132:337, 1984.

Golimbu, M., Joshi, P., Sperber, A., et al.: Renal cell carcinoma: Survival and prognostic factors. Urology, 27:291, 1986.

Gomella, L. G., Sargent, E. R., Wade, T. P., Anglard, P., Linehan, W. M., and Kasid, A.: Expression of transforming growth factor α in normal human adult kidney and enhanced expression of transforming growth factors α and β1 in renal cell carcinoma. Cancer Res., 49:6972, 1989.

Gottesman, J. E., Crawford, E. D., Grossman, H. B., et al.: Infarction-nephrectomy for metastatic renal carcinoma. Urology, 25:248, 1985.

Grawitz, P.: Die sogenannten Lipome der Niere. Virchows Arch. [A], 93:39, 1883.

Greene, L. F., and Rosenthal, M. H.: Multiple hypernephromas of the kidney in association with Lindau's disease. N. Engl. J. Med., 244:633, 1951.

Grignon, D. J., Ayala, A. G., El-Naggar, A., Wishnow, K. I., Ro, J. Y., Sawnson, D. A., McLemore, D., Giacco, G. G., and Guinee, V. F.: Renal cell carcinoma: A clinicopathologic and DNA flow cytometric analysis of 103 cases. Cancer, 64:2133, 1989.

Gutterman, J.: Overview of advances in the use of biological proteins in human cancer. Semin. Oncol., 15(Suppl.):2, 1988.

Hand, J. R., and Broders, A. C.: Carcinoma of the kidney: The degree of malignancy in relation to factors bearing on prognosis. J. Urol., 28:199, 1932.

Harris, R. P.: An analytical examination of 100 cases of extirpations of the kidney. Am. J. Med. Sci., 84:109, 1882.

Hartman, D. S., Davis, C. J., Goldman, S. M., Friedman, A. C., and Fritzsche, P.: Renal lymphoma: Radiologic-pathologic correlation of 21 cases. Radiology, 144:759, 1982.

Heiken, J. P., Gold, R. P., Schnur, M. J., King, M. J., Bashist, B., and Glazer, H. S.: Computed tomography of renal lymphoma with ultrasound correlation. J. Comput. Assist. Tomogr., 7:245, 1983.

Helmbrecht, L. J., and Cosgrove, M. D.: Triple therapy for leiomyosarcoma of the kidney. J. Urol., 112:581, 1974.

Hermanek, P., and Schrott, K. M.: Evaluation of the new tumor, nodes and metastases classification of renal cell carcinoma. J. Urol., 144:238, 1990.

Hirsh, E. M., Wallace, S., Johnson, D. E., and Bracken, R. B.: Immunological studies in human urological cancer. *In* Johnson, D. E., and Samuels, M. L. (Eds.): Cancer of the Genitourinary Tract. New York, Raven Press, 1979, p. 47.

Hirsh, M., Lipton, A., Harvey, H., Givant, E., Hopper, K., Jones, G., Zeffren, J., and Levitt, D.: Phase I study of interleukin-2 and interferon alpha-2a as outpatient therapy for patients with advanced malignancy. J. Clin. Oncol., 8:1657, 1990.

Hoehn, W., and Hermanek, P.: Invasion of veins in renal cell carcinoma—frequency, correlation and prognosis. Eur. Urol., 9:276, 1983.

Horan, J., Robertson, C., Choyke, P., et al.: The detection of renal carcinoma extension into the renal vein and inferior vena cava: A prospective comparison of venacavography and magnetic resonance imaging. J. Urol., 142:943, 1989.

Hricak, H., Demas, B. E., et al.: Magnetic resonance imaging in the diagnosis and staging of renal and perirenal neoplasms. Radiology, 154:709, 1985.

Hricak, H., Thoeni, R. F., et al.: Detection and staging of renal neoplasms: A reassessment of MR imaging. Radiology, 166:643, 1988.

Hrushesky, W. J., and Murphy, G. P.: Current status of the therapy of advanced renal carcinoma. J. Surg. Oncol., 9:277, 1977.

Hulten, L., Rosencrantz, T., Seeman, L., Wahlquist, L., and Ahren, C.: Occurrence and localization of lymph node metastases in renal cell carcinoma. Scand. J. Urol. Nephrol., 3:129, 1969.

Jafri, S. Z., Bree, R. L., Amendola, M. A., Glazer, G. N., Schwab,

R. E., Francis, I. R., and Borlaza, G.: CT of renal and perirenal non-Hodgkin lymphoma. Am. J. Radiol., 138:1101, 1982.

Jaschke, W., van Kaick, G., Peter, S., and Palmtas, H.: Accuracy of computed tomography in staging of kidney tumors. Acta. Radiol. Diagn. (Stockh.), 23:593, 1982.

Kakehi, Y., Kanamaru, H., Yoshida, O., Ohkubo, H., Nakanishi, S., Gottesman, M. M., and Pastan, I.: Measurement of multidrug resistance messenger RNA in urogenital cancers; elevated expression in renal cell carcinoma is associated with intrinsic drug resistance. J. Urol., 139:862, 1988.

Kanamaru, H., Kakehi, Y., Yoshida, O., Nakanishi, S., Pastan, I., and Gottesman, M. M.: MDR1 RNA levels in human renal cell carcinomas: Correlation with grade and prediction of reversal of doxorubicin resistance by quinidine in tumor explants. JNCI, 81:844, 1989.

Kansara, V., and Powell, I.: Fibrosarcoma of the kidney. Urology, 16:419, 1980.

Kantor, A. F.: Current concepts in the epidemiology and etiology of primary renal cell carcinoma. J. Urol., 117:415, 1977.

Karthaus, H. F. M., Bussemakers, M. J. G., Schalken, J. A., et al.: Expression of proto-oncogenes in xenografts of human renal cell carcinomas. Urol. Res., 15:349, 1987.

Kemp, B. E., Moseley, J. M., Rodda, C. P., et al.: Parathyroid hormone–related protein of malignancy: Active synthetic fragments. Science, 238:1568, 1987.

Kirkman, H., and Bacon, R. L.: Renal adenomas and carcinomas in diethylstilbestrol-treated male golden hamsters. Anat. Rec., 103:475, 1949.

Kirkwood, J. M., Harris, J. E., Vera, R., et al.: A randomized study of low and high doses of leukocyte alpha-interferon in metastatic renal cell carcinoma: The American Cancer Society Collaborative Trial. Cancer Res., 45:863, 1985.

Klinger, M. E.: Secondary tumors of the genitourinary tract. J. Urol., 65:144, 1951.

Knoepp, L. F.: Lymphosarcoma of the kidney. Surgery, 39:510, 1956.

Kolonel, L. N.: Association of cadmium with renal cancer. Cancer, 37:1782, 1976.

Konnak, J. W., and Grossman, H. B.: Renal cell carcinoma as an incidental finding. J. Urol., 134:1094, 1985.

Kovacs, G., Brusa, P., and DeRiese, W.: Tissue-specific expression of a constitutional 3;6 translocation: Development of multiple bilateral renal cell carcinomas. Int. J. Cancer, 43:422, 1989.

Kovacs, G., Erlandsson, R., Boldog, F., Ingvarsson, S., Muller-Brechlin, R., Klein, G., and Sumegi, J.: Consistent chromosome 3p deletion and loss of heterozygosity in renal cell carcinoma. Proc. Natl. Acad. Sci. USA, 85:1571, 1988.

Krigel, R. L., Padavic-Shaller, K. A., Rudolph, A. R., Konrad, M., Bradley, E. C., and Comis, R. L.: Renal cell carcinoma: Treatment with recombinant interleukin-2 plus beta-interferon. J. Clin. Oncol., 8:460, 1990.

Kurth, K. H., Debruyne, F. M., Hall, R. R., et al.: Embolization and postinfarction nephrectomy in patient with primary metastatic renal adenocarcinoma. Eur. Urol., 13:251, 1987.

Kyaw, M., and Koehler, P. R.: Renal and perirenal lymphoma: Arteriographic findings. Radiology, 93:1055, 1969.

Lakey, W. H.: Tumors of the kidney. In Karafin, L., and Kendall, A. R. (Eds.): Urology, Vol. 2. New York, Harper & Row, 1975.

Landier, J. F., Desligneres, S., Boccon-Gibod, L., and Steg, A.: Renal oncocytomas. Sem. Hop. Paris, 55:1275, 1979.

Lang, E. K.: Roentgenographic assessment of asymptomatic renal lesions. Radiology, 109:257, 1973.

Lang, E. K.: Asymptomatic space occupying lesions of the kidney: A programmed sequential approach and its impact on quality and cost of health care. South. Med. J., 70:277, 1977.

Lang, E.: Comparison of dynamic and conventional computed tomography, angiography and ultrasonography in the staging of renal cell carcinoma. Cancer, 54:2205, 1984.

Lang, E., and deKernion, J. B.: Transcatheter embolization of advanced renal cell carcinoma with radioactive seeds. J. Urol., 126:581, 1981.

Lauritsen, J. G.: Lindau's disease: A study of one family through six generations. Acta Chir. Scand., 139:482, 1975.

La Vecchia, C., Negri, E., D'Avanzo, B., and Franceschi, S.: Smoking and renal cell carcinoma. Cancer Res., 50:5231, 1990.

Levine, E., Huntrakoon, M., and Wetzel, L. H.: Small renal neo-

plasms: Clinical, pathologic, and imaging findings. Am. J. Radiol., 153:69, 1989.

Libertino, J. A., Zinman, L., and Watkins, E., Jr.: Long-term results of resection of renal cell cancer with extension into inferior vena cava. J. Urol., 137:21, 1987.

Lieber, M. M.: Renal oncocytoma: Prognosis and treatment. Eur. Urol., 18(Suppl. 2):17, 1990.

Lieber, M. M., Tomera, K. M., and Farrow, G. M.: Renal oncocytomas. J. Urol., 125:481, 1981.

Lieber, M. M., and Tsukamoto, T.: Renal oncocytoma. In deKernion, J. B., Pavone-Macaluso, M. (Eds.): Tumors of the Kidney. Baltimore, Williams & Wilkins, 1986, p. 257.

Lieberman, S. F., Keller, F. S., Pearse, H. D., Fuchs, E. F., Rosch, J., and Barry, J. M.: Percutaneous vaso-occlusion for non-malignant renal lesions. J. Urol., 129:805, 1983.

Lindner, A., Goldman, D. G., and deKernion, J. B.: Cost effective analysis of prenephrectomy radioisotope scans in renal cell carcinoma. Urology, 22:566, 1983.

Linehan, W. M., Robertson, C. N., Anglard, P., Gomella, E. R., Sargent, E. R., Wade, T., Ewing, M. W., and Kasid, A.: Clinical perspective—renal cell carcinoma: Potential biologic and molecular approaches to diagnosis and therapy. In Cancer Cells 7, Molecular Diagnostics of Human Cancer. Cold Spring Harbor Laboratory, 1989, p. 59.

Lingeman, J. E., Donohue, J. P., Madrua, J. A., and Selke, F.: Angiomyolipoma: Emerging concepts in management. Urology, 20:566, 1982.

Lingeman, J. E., Eble, J. N., and Donohue, J. P.: Renal oncocytomas: Clinical and pathologic features. Presented at the American Urologic Association Meeting. Las Vegas, 1983.

Maldazys, J. D., and deKernion, J. B.: Prognostic factors in metastatic renal carcinoma. J. Urol., 136:376, 1986.

Mangin, M., Webb, A. C., Dreyer, B. E., et al.: Identification of a cDNA encoding a parathyroid hormone–like peptide from a human tumor associated with humoral hypercalcemia of malignancy. Proc. Natl. Acad. Sci. USA, 85:597, 1988.

Marberger, M., Pugh, R. C. B., Auvert, J., Bertermann, H., Costantini, A., Gammelgaard, P. A., Petterson, S., and Wickham, J. E. A.: Conservative surgery of renal carcinoma: The EIRSS experience. Br. J. Urol., 53:528, 1981.

Marshall, F. F., Dietrick, D. D., Baumgartner, W. A., and Reitz, B. A.: Surgical management of renal cell carcinoma with intracaval neoplastic extension above the hepatic veins. J. Urol., 139:116, 1988.

Marshall, F., and Powell, K. C.: Lymphadenectomy for renal cell carcinoma: Anatomical and therapeutic considerations. J. Urol., 128:677, 1982.

Marshall, F. F., Reitz, B. A., and Diamond, D. A.: New technique for management of renal cell carcinoma involving right atrium: Hypothermia and cardiac arrest. J. Urol., 131:103, 1984.

Marshall, F. F., Taxy, J. B., Fishman, E. K., and Chang, R.: The feasibility of surgical enucleation for renal cell carcinoma. J. Urol., 135:231, 1986.

Marshall, M. E., Mendelsohn, L., Butler, K., et al.: Treatment of metastatic renal cell carcinoma with coumarin (1,2-benzopyrone) and cimetidine: A pilot study. J. Clin. Oncol., 6:682, 1987.

Mauro, M. A., Wadsworth, D. E., Stanley, R. J., and McClennan, B. L.: Renal cell carcinoma: Angiography in the CT era. Am. J. Radiol., 139:1135, 1982.

McCullough, D. L., and Gittes, R. F.: Ligation of the renal vein in solitary kidney: Effects on renal function. J. Urol., 113:295, 1975.

McCullough, D. L., Scott, R., Jr., and Seybold, H. M.: Renal angiomyelolipoma (hamartoma): Review of the literature and report of 7 cases. J. Urol., 105:32, 1971.

McCune, C. S., Schapira, D. V., and Henshaw, E. C.: Specific immunotherapy of advanced renal carcinoma: Evidence for the polyclonality of metastases. Cancer, 47:1984, 1981.

McNichols, D. W., Segura, J. W., and deWeerd, J. H.: Renal cell carcinoma: Long-term survival and late recurrence. J. Urol., 126:17, 1981.

Mickisch, G. H., Kossig, J., Keilhauer, G., Schlick, E., Tschada, R. K., and Alken, P. M.: Effects of calcium antagonists in multidrug resistant primary human renal cell carcinomas. Cancer Res., 50:3570, 1990a.

Mickisch, G. H., Roehrich, K., Koessig, J., Forster, S., Tschada, R.

K., and Alken, P. M.: Mechanisms and modulation of multidrug resistance in primary human renal cell carcinoma. J. Urol., 144:744, 1990b.

Micolonghi, T. S., Liang, D., and Schwartz, S.: Primary osteogenic sarcoma of the kidney. J. Urol., 131:1164, 1984.

Middleton, R. G.: Surgery for metastatic renal cell carcinoma. J. Urol., 97:973, 1967.

Minton, J. P., Pennline, K., Nawrocki, J. F., Kibbey, W. E., and Dodd, M. C.: Immunotherapy of human kidney cancer [Abstract C-258]. Proc. Am. Assoc. Cancer Res. Am. Soc. Clin. Oncol., 17:301, 1976.

Moertel, C. G., Dockerty, M. B., and Baggenstoss, A. H.: Multiple primary multiple malignant neoplasms: III. Tumors of multicentric origin. Cancer, 14:238, 1961.

Montie, J. D., Bukowski, R. M., James, R. E., et al.: A critical review of immunotherapy of disseminated renal adenocarcinoma. J. Surg. Oncol., 21:5, 1982.

Montie, J. E., Jackson, C. L., Cosgrove, D. M., Streem, S. B., Novick, A. C., and Pontes, J. E.: Resection of large inferior vena cava thrombi from renal cell carcinoma with the use of circulatory arrest. J. Urol., 139:25, 1988.

Montie, J. E., Stewart, B. H., Straffon, R. A., et al.: The role of adjunctive nephrectomy in patients with metastatic renal cell carcinoma. J. Urol., 117:272–275, 1977.

Moon, T. D., Dexter, D. F., and Morales, A.: Synchronous independent primary osteosarcoma and adenocarcinoma of the kidney. Urology, 21:608, 1983.

Morales, A., Wilson, J. L., Pater, J. L., and Loeb, M.: Cytoreductive surgery and systemic bacillus Calmette-Guérin therapy in metastatic renal cancer: A phase II trial. J. Urol., 127:230, 1982.

Morgan, D. A., Ruscetti, F. W., and Gallo, R. G.: Selective in vitro growth of T lymphocytes from normal human bone marrows. Science, 193:1007, 1976.

Moscow, J. A., and Cowan, K. H.: Multidrug resistance. JNCI, 80:14, 1988.

Murphy, G. P., and Mostofi, F. K.: Histologic assessment and clinical prognosis of renal adenoma. J. Urol., 103:31, 1970.

Murphy, W. M.: Diseases of the kidney. In Urological Pathology. Philadelphia, W. B. Saunders, 1989, p. 409.

Muss, H. B., Costanzi, J. J., Leavitt, R., et al.: Recombinant interferon alpha in renal cell carcinoma: A randomized trial of two routes of administration. J. Clin. Oncol., 5:286, 1987.

Mydlo, J. H., Michaeli, J., Cordon-Cardo, C., Goldenberg, A. S., Heston, W. D. W., and Fair, W. R.: Expression of transforming growth factor α and epidermal growth factor receptor messenger RNA in neoplastic and nonneoplastic human kidney tissue. Cancer Res., 49:3407, 1989.

Myers, G. H., Fehrenbaker, L. G., and Kellais, P. P.: Prognostic significance of renal vein invasion by hypernephroma. J. Urol., 100:420–423, 1968.

Nagamatsu, G.: Dorso-lumbar approach to kidney and adrenal with osteoplastic flap. J. Urol., 63:569, 1950.

Niceta, T., Lavengood, R. W., Jr., and Fernandes, M.: Leiomyosarcoma of kidney. Review of the literature. Urology, 3:270, 1974.

Nogueira, E., and Bannasch, P.: Cellular origin of rat renal oncocytoma. Lab. Invest., 59:337, 1988.

Novick, A. C., Streem, S., Montie, J. A., Pontes, J. E., Siegel, S., Montague, D. K., and Goormastic, M.: Conservative surgery for renal cell carcinoma: A single-center experience with 100 patients. J. Urol., 141:835, 1989.

Novick, A. C., Zincke, H., Neaves, R. J., and Topley, H. M.: Surgical enucleation for renal cell carcinoma. J. Urol., 135:235, 1986.

O'Dea, M. J., Zincke, H., Utz, D. C., and Bernatz, P. E.: The treatment of renal cell carcinoma with solitary metastases. J. Urol., 120:540, 1978.

Oesterling, J. E., Fishman, E. K., Goldman, S. M., and Marshall, F. F.: The management of renal angiomyolipoma. J. Urol., 135:1121, 1986.

Oliver, R. T. D.: Surveillance as a possible option for management of metastatic renal cell carcinoma. Semin. Urol., 7:149, 1989.

Olsson, C. A.: Pulmonary cancer metastatic to the kidney: A common renal neoplasm. J. Urol., 105:492, 1971.

Ordonez, N. G., Bracken, R. B., and Strohlein, K. B.: Hemangiopericytoma of the kidney. Urology, 20:191, 1982.

Orjauvik, O. S., Aas, M., Fauchald, P., Hovig, T., Oystese, B., Brodwall, E. K., and Flatmark, A.: Renin-secreting renal tumor with severe hypertension. Acta Med. Scand., 197:329, 1975.

Osamura, R. Y., Watanabe, K., Yoneyama, L., and Hayashi, T.: Malignant fibrous histiocytoma of the renal capsule: Light and electron microscopic study of a rare tumor. Virchows Arch. [A], 380:377, 1978.

Otto, U., Baisch, H., Kloeppel, G., and Huland, H.: Tumor heterogeneity of renal cell carcinoma. Eur. Urol., 18(Suppl. 2):38, 1990.

Parkinson, D. R.: Interleukin-2: Further progress through greater understanding. JNCI, 82:1374, 1990.

Patel, N. P., and Lavengood, R. W.: Renal cell carcinoma: Natural history and results of treatment. J. Urol., 119:722, 1978.

Pavelic, K., and Popovic, M.: Insulin and glucagon secretion by renal adenocarcinoma. Cancer, 48:98, 1981.

Peeling, W. B., Martell, B., and Shepheard, B. G.: Postoperative irradiation in the treatment of renal cell carcinoma. Br. J. Urol., 41:23, 1969.

Peters, P.: The role of lymphadenectomy in the management of renal cell carcinoma. Urol. Clin. North Am., 7:705, 1980.

Pfeiffer, G. E., and Gandin, M. M.: Massive perirenal lipoma with report of a case. J. Urol., 56:12, 1946.

Pizzocaro G., and Piva, L.: Pros and cons of retroperitoneal lymphadenectomy in operable renal cell carcinoma. Eur. Urol., 18 (Suppl.):22, 1990.

Pollack, H. M., Banner, M. P., and Amendola, M. A.: Other malignant neoplasms of the renal parenchyma. Semin. Roentgenol., 22:260, 1987.

Quesada, J. R., Evans, L., Saks, S. R., et al.: Recombinant interferon alpha and gamma combination as treatment in metastatic renal cell carcinoma. J. Biol. Response Mod., 7:234, 1988.

Quesada, J. R., Swanson, D. A., Trinidade, A., et al.: Renal cell carcinoma: Antitumor effects of leukocyte interferon. Cancer Res., 43:940, 1983.

Quint, L. E., Glazer, G. M., Chenevert, T. L., et al.: In vivo and in vitro MR imaging of renal tumors: Histopathologic correlation and pulse sequence optimization. Radiology, 169:359, 1988.

Raghavaiah, N. V., Mayer, R. F., Hagitt, R., and Soloway, M. S.: Malignant fibrous histiocytoma of the kidney. J. Urol., 123:951, 1980.

Rainwater, L. M., Farrow, G. M., and Lieber, M. M.: Flow cytometry of renal oncocytoma: Common occurrence of deoxyribonucleic acid polyploidy and aneuploidy. J. Urol., 135:1167, 1986.

Rainwater, L. M., Hosaka, Y., Farrow, G. M., and Lieber, M. W.: Well-differentiated clear cell renal carcinoma: Significance of nuclear deoxyribonucleic acid patterns studied by flow cytometry. J. Urol., 137:15, 1987.

Rakowsky, E., Barzilay, J., Schujman, E., and Servadio, C.: Leiomyosarcoma of kidney. Urology, 29:68, 1987.

Ramming, K. P., and deKernion, J. B.: Immune RNA therapy for renal cell carcinoma: Survival and immunologic monitoring. Ann. Surg., 186:459, 1977.

Rao, M. S., Lotuaco, L. G., and McGregor, D. H.: Carcinosarcoma of the adult kidney. Postgrad. Med., J. 53:408, 1977.

Raval, B., and Lamki, N.: Computer tomography in detection of occult hypernephroma. CT, 7:199, 1983.

Richie, E. W.: The place of radiotherapy in the management of parenchymal carcinoma. J. Urol., 95:313, 1966.

Richie, J. P., Garnick, M. B., Seltzer, S., and Bettman, M. A.: Computerized tomography scan for diagnosis and staging of renal cell carcinoma. J. Urol., 129:1114, 1983.

Richie, J. P., Wang, B. S., Steele, G. D., Jr., Wilson, R. E., and Mannick, J. A.: In vivo and in vitro effects of xenogeneic immune ribonucleic acid in patients with advanced renal cell carcinoma: A phase I study. J. Urol., 126:24, 1981.

Ro, J. Y., Ayala, A. G., Sella, A., Samuels, M., and Swanson, D. A.: Sarcomatoid renal cell carcinoma: Clinicopathologic. Cancer, 59:516, 1987.

Robertson, D. N., Linehan, W. M., Pass, H. I., Gomella, L. G., Haas, G. P., Berman, A., Merino, M., and Rosenberg, S. A.: Preparative cytoreductive surgery in patients with metastatic renal cell carcinoma treated with adoptive immunotherapy with interleukin-2 or interleukin-2 plus lymphokine activated killer cells. J. Urol., 144:614, 1990.

Robertson, P. W., Klidjiian, A., Harding, L. K., Walters, G., Lee,

M. R., and Robb-Smith, A. H.: Hypertension due to a renin-secreting renal tumor. Am. J. Med., 43:963, 1967.

Robertson, T. D., and Hand, J. R.: Primary intrarenal lipoma of surgical significance. J. Urol., 46:458, 1941.

Robson, C. J.: Radical nephrectomy for renal cell carcinoma. J. Urol., 89:37, 1963.

Robson, C. J., Churchill, B. M., and Anderson, W.: The results of radical nephrectomy for renal cell carcinoma. Trans. Am. Assoc. Genitourin., Surg., 60:122, 1968.

Rosenberg, S. A.: Adoptive immunotherapy of cancer using lymphokine activated killer cells and recombinant interleukin-2. In DeVita, V. T., Hellman, S., and Rosenberg, S. A. (Eds.): Important Advances in Oncology. New York, J. B. Lippincott Co., 1986, p. 55.

Rosenberg, S. A.: Immunotherapy of patients with advanced cancer using interleukin-2 alone or in combination with lymphokine activated killer cells. In DeVita, V. T., Hellman, S., and Rosenberg, S. A. (Eds.): Important Advances in Oncology. New York, J. B. Lippincott Co., 1988a, p. 217.

Rosenberg, S. A.: Immunotherapy of cancer using interleukin-2: Current status and future prospects. Immunol. Today, 9:58, 1988b.

Rosenberg, S. A.: The development of new immunotherapies for the treatment of cancer using interleukin-2. Ann. Surg., 208(2):121, 1988c.

Rosenberg, S. A.: Use of tumor-infiltrating lymphocytes and interleukin-2 in the immunotherapy of patients with metastatic melanoma: A preliminary report. N. Engl. J. Med., 319:1676, 1988d.

Rosenberg, S. A., Lotze, M. T., Muul, L. M., Leitman, S., Chang, A. E., Ettinghausen, S. E., Matory, Y. L., Skibber, J. M., Shiloni, E., Vetto, J. T., Seipp, C. A., Simpson, C., Reichert, C. M.: Observations on the systemic administration of autologous lymphokine-activated killer cells and recombinant interleukin-2 to patients with metastatic cancer. N. Engl. J. Med., 313:1485, 1985.

Rosenberg, S. A., Spiess P., and Lafreniere, R.: A new approach to the adoptive immunotherapy of cancer using tumor infiltrating lymphocytes. Science, 233:1318, 1986.

Saitoh, H., Shimbo, T., Wakabayashi, T., Takeda, M., and Ogishima, K.: Metastases of renal sarcoma. Tokai J. Exp. Clin. Med., 7:365, 1982.

Sargent, E. R., Gomella, L. G., Wade, T. P., Ewing, M. W., Kasid, A., and Linehan, W. M.: Expression of mRNA for transforming growth factors-alpha and -beta and secretion of transforming growth factor-B in renal cell carcinoma cell lines. Cancer Communications, 1:317, 1989.

Sarna, G., Figlin, R., and deKernion, J.: Interferon in renal cell carcinoma: The UCLA experience. Cancer, 59:610, 1987.

Sayers, T. J., Wiltrout, T. A., McCormick, K., Husted, C., and Wiltrout, R. H.: Antitumor effects of alpha-interferon and gamma-interferon on a murine renal cancer (Renca) in vitro and in vivo. Cancer Res., 50:5414, 1990.

Scriven, R. R., Thrasher, T. V., Smith, D. C., and Stewart, S. C.: Primary renal malignant fibrous histiocytoma: A case report and literature review. J. Urol., 131:948, 1984.

Selli, C., Hinshaw, W. M., Woodard, B. H., and Paulson, D. F.: Stratification of risk factors in renal cell carcinoma. Cancer, 52:899, 1983.

Shefft, P., Novick, A. C., Straffon, R. A., and Stewart, B. H.: Survey for renal cell carcinoma extending into the inferior vena cava. J. Urol., 120:28, 1978.

Shirkhoda, A., and Lewis, E.: Renal sarcoma and sarcomatoid renal cell carcinoma: CT and angiographic features. Radiology, 162:353, 1987.

Silber, S. J., and Chang, C. Y.: Primary lymphoma of the kidney. J. Urol., 110:282, 1973.

Silverberg, E., Boring, C. C., and Squires, T. S.: Cancer statistics, 1990. Cancer, 40:9, 1990.

Siminovitch, J. M., Montie, J. E., and Straffon, R. A.: Prognostic indicators in renal adenocarcinoma. J. Urol., 130:20, 1983.

Skinner, D. G., Pfister, R. F., and Colvin, R.: Extension of renal cell carcinoma into the vena cava: The rationale for aggressive surgical management. J. Urol., 107:711, 1972.

Slamon, D. J., deKernion, J. B., Verma, I. M., et al.: Expression of cellular oncogenes in human malignancies. Science, 224:256, 1984.

Smith, R. B., deKernion, J. B., Ehrlich, R. M., Skinner, D. G., and Kaufman, J. J.: Bilateral renal cell carcinoma and renal cell carcinoma in the solitary kidney. J. Urol., 132:450, 1984.

Smith, S. J., Bosniak, M. A., Megibow, A. J., et al.: Renal cell carcinoma: Earlier discovery and increased detection. Radiology, 170:699, 1989.

Smullens, S. N., Scotti, D., Osterholm, J., and Weiss, A.: Preoperative embolization of retroperitoneal angiopericytomas as an aid in their removal. Proc. Am. Assoc. Cancer Res., 20:394, 1979.

Steele, G., Jr., Wang, B. S., Richie, J. P., et al.: Results of oncogenic I-RNA therapy in patients with metastatic renal cell carcinoma. Cancer, 47:1286, 1981.

Stewart, B. H.: Radical nephrectomy. In Stewart, B. H. (Ed.): Operative Urology: The Kidney, Adrenal Gland and Retroperitoneum. Baltimore, Williams & Wilkins, 1975, p. 114.

Stewart, R. R., and Dunnick, N. R.: Imaging renal neoplasms. Prob. Urol., 4:175, 1990.

Stillwell, T. J., Gomez, M. R., and Kelalis, P. P.: Renal lesions in tuberous sclerosis. J. Urol., 138:477, 1987.

Sufrin, G., Chasan, S., Golio, A., and Murphy, G. P.: Paraneoplastic and serologic syndromes of renal adenocarcinoma. Semin. Urol., 7:158, 1989.

Sun, C. N., Bissada, N. K., White, H. J., and Redman, J. F.: Spectrum of ultrastructural patterns of renal cell carcinoma. Urology, 9:195, 1977.

Swanson, D. A., et al.: Angioinfarction plus nephrectomy for metastatic renal cell carcinoma—an update. J. Urol., 130:449, 1983.

Taniguchi, H., Takahashi, T., Fujita, Y., et al.: Leiomyosarcoma of the kidney: Report of a patient with favorable response to doxorubicin and cisplatin suspended in a lipid contrast medium and cyclophosphamide. Med. Pediatr. Oncol., 15:285, 1987.

Tannenbaum, M.: Ultrastructural pathology of human renal cell tumors. Pathol. Annu., 6:259, 1971.

Taylor, R. S., Joseph, D. B., Kohaut, E. C., Wilson, E. R., and Bueschen, A. J.: Renal angiomyolipoma associated with lymph node involvement and renal cell carcinoma in patients with tuberous sclerosis. J. Urol., 141:930, 1989.

Teyssier, J. R., Dozier, H. C., Ferre, D., et al.: Recurrent deletion of the short arm of chromosome 3 in human renal cell carcinoma: Shift with the c-raf 1 locus. JNCI, 7:1187, 1986.

Thoenes, W., Storkel, S., Rumpelt, H. J., Mell, R., Baum, H. P., and Werner, S.: Chromophobe cell renal carcinoma and its variants: A report on 32 cases. J. Pathol., 155:277, 1988.

Thompson, I. M., and Peek, M.: Improvement in survival of patients with renal cell carcinoma: The role of the serendipitously detected tumor. J. Urol., 140:487, 1988.

Tomera, K. V., Farrow, G. M., and Lieber M. M.: Sarcomatoid renal carcinoma. J. Urol., 130:657, 1983.

Topalian, S. L., Solomon, D., Avis, F. P., et al.: Immunotherapy of patients with advanced cancer using tumor infiltrating lymphocytes and recombinant interleukin-2: A pilot study. J. Clin. Oncol., 6:839, 1988.

Topley, M., Novick, A. C., and Montie, J. E.: Long-term results following partial nephrectomy for localized renal adenocarcinoma. Presented at the American Urologic Association Annual Meeting. Las Vegas, 1983.

Tsuruo, T., Iida, H., Kitatani, Y., and Tsukagoshi, S.: Effects of quinidine and related compounds on cytotoxicity and cellular accumulation of vincristine and adriamycin in drug-resistant tumor cells. Cancer Res., 44:4303, 1984.

Umeda, T., and Niijima, T.: Phase II study of alpha interferon on renal cell carcinoma. Cancer, 58:1231, 1986.

van der Walt, J. D., Reid, H. A., Rigdon, R. A., and Shaw, J. H.: Renal oncocytoma: A review of the literature and report of an unusual multicentric case. Virchows Arch. [A], 398:291, 1983.

van der Werf-Messing, B.: Carcinoma of the kidney. Cancer, 32:1056, 1973.

Van Moorselaar, R. J., Beniers, A. J., Hendriks, B. T., van der Meide, P. H., Schellekens, H., Debruyne, F. M., and Schalken, J. A.: In vivo antiproliferative effects of gamma-interferon and tumor necrosis factor alpha in a rat renal cell carcinoma model system. J. Urol., 143:1247, 1990.

Vugrin, D., Hood, L., and Laszlo, J.: A phase II trial of high-dose human lymphoblastoid alpha interferon in patients with advanced renal carcinoma. J. Biol. Response Mod., 5:309, 1986.

Wallace, A. C., and Nairn, R. C.: Renal tubular antigens in kidney tumors. Cancer, 29:977, 1972.

Walther, P. J., Marks, L. S., Stern, D., and Smith, R. B.: Renal metastasis of adenocarcinoma of the lung: Massive hematuria managed by therapeutic embolization. J. Urol., 122:398, 1979.

Warfel, K. A., and Eble, J. N.: Renal oncocytomatosis. J. Urol., 127:1179, 1982.

Weichselbaum, A., and Greenish, R. W.: Pasadenome der Neire. Med. Jahrb. Vien., Vol. 213, 1883.

Weidner, U., Peter, S., Strohmeyer, T., Hussnatter, R., Ackermann, R., and Sies, H.: Inverse relationship of epidermal growth factor receptor and HER2/neu gene expression in human renal cell carcinoma. Cancer Res., 50:4504, 1990.

Weir, J. M., and Dunn, J. E., Jr.: Smoking and mortality: A prospective study. Cancer, 25:105, 1970.

Weiss, J. P., Pollack, H. M., McCormick, J. F., et al.: Renal hemangiopericytoma: Surgical, radiological and pathological implications. J. Urol., 132:337, 1984.

Wenz, W.: Tumors of the kidney following retrograde pyelography with colloidal thorium diozide. Ann. N.Y. Acad. Sci., 145:806, 1967.

West, W., Tauer, K., Yannelli, J., Marshall, G., Orr, D., Thurman, G., and Oldham, R.: Constant infusion recombinant interleukin-2 in adoptive immunotherapy of advanced cancer. N. Engl. J. Med., 316:898, 1987.

Wickham, J. E. A.: Conservative renal surgery for adenocarcinoma: The place of bench surgery. Br. J. Urol., 47:25, 1975.

Wolff, J.: Die Lehre von der Krebskronsheit: Von den altesten Zeiten bis zur Gagenwart. *In* Adenome der Neire. Med. Jahrb. Vien, Vol. 213, 1883.

Yagoda A.: Chemotherapy of renal cell carcinoma: 1983–1989. Semin. Urol., 7:199, 1989.

Yao, M., Shuin, T., Misaki, H., et al.: Enhanced expression of c-*myc* and epidermal growth factor receptor (c-*erb*B-1) genes in primary human renal cancer. Cancer Res., 48:6753, 1988.

Zbar, B., Brauch, H., Talmadge C., and Linehan, M.: Loss of alleles of loci on the short arm of chromosome 3 in renal cell carcinoma. Nature, 327:721, 1987.

Zerban, H., Nogueira, E., Riedasch, G., and Bannasch, P.: Renal oncocytoma: Origin from the collecting duct. Virchows Arch., 52:375, 1987.

Zincke, H., and Swanson, S. K.: Bilateral renal cell carcinoma: Influence of synchronous and asynchronous occurrence on patient survival. J. Urol., 128:913, 1982.

28
UROTHELIAL TUMORS OF THE URINARY TRACT

William J. Catalona, M.D.

BLADDER CANCER

Bladder cancer is one of the most common diseases treated by urologists. Most bladder cancers are transitional cell carcinomas. Bladder cancers exhibit the entire spectrum of biologic aggressiveness from the virtually benign superficial low-grade papilloma to the highly malignant anaplastic carcinoma. In practice, however, bladder cancers tend to occur in two principal forms: low-grade superficial tumors and high-grade invasive cancer.

BASIC BIOLOGY

Most evidence favors a strong role for chemical carcinogens in the etiology of bladder cancer, but many cases involve no obvious chemical carcinogen to explain the cancer. All cancers are genetic diseases in which the normal mechanisms regulating cell differentiation and proliferation are deficient or have gone awry. It is currently popular to ascribe these derangements to inherited or acquired lesions in the host's genetic material or to the induction of so-called oncogenes by viruses or chemical carcinogens. In fact, relatively little is known about the etiology of bladder cancer.

Bladder cancer usually behaves as a field change disease in which the entire urothelium from the renal pelvis to the urethra may be susceptible to malignant transformation. The demonstrated tendency for transitional cell carcinoma cells to implant often makes it difficult to distinguish among multifocal carcinogenesis, recurrence of inadequately treated tumor, and tumor cell implantation. Evidence exists, based on the presence of chromosomal abnormalities in grossly unaffected urothelium in bladder cancer patients, of a true multifocal etiology of bladder cancer.

EPIDEMIOLOGY

Incidence and Mortality Rates

Incidence—Sex and Race

The *incidence* rate of a cancer is defined as the number of new cases diagnosed per 100,000 persons per year. The bladder is the most common site of cancer in the urinary tract. It is estimated that in 1990, 47,100 new cases of bladder cancer will have been diagnosed in the United States. Bladder cancer is 2.7 times more common among men (34,500) than women (12,600) (Table 28–1). In men, it is the fourth most common cancer after prostate, lung, and colorectal cancer, accounting for 10 per cent of all cancer cases (Silverberg et al., 1990). In women, it is the eighth most common cause of cancer, accounting for 4 per cent of all cancers (Silverberg et al., 1990). The incidence of bladder cancer among whites (31.5 per cent in men and 7.8 per cent in women) is higher than among blacks (16.2 per cent in men and 5.0 per cent in women) (1987 Annual Cancer Statistics Review; Morrison, 1984); however, the increased risk in whites appears to be limited to patients with noninvasive tumors (Schairer et al., 1988). This observation suggests that some superficial tumors diagnosed in whites may go undetected in blacks.

Mortality—Sex and Race

The *mortality* rate of a cancer is the number of deaths occurring per 100,000 persons per year. It is estimated that in 1990, there will have been 10,200 bladder cancer deaths, including 6900 men and 3300 women (1987 Annual Cancer Statistics Review). This makes bladder cancer the fourth most common cause of cancer deaths

Table 28–1. 1985 AGE-ADJUSTED BLADDER CANCER INCIDENCE RATES*: SEER PROGRAM—RACE AND SEX DIFFERENCES

	Black	White	Total
Males	15.4	30.4	28.5
Females	6.0	8.1	7.8
Total	9.9	17.5	16.5

*Rates are per 100,000 and are age-adjusted to the 1970 U.S. standard population.
From 1987 Annual Cancer Statistics Review: Including Cancer Trends: 1950–1985. Bethesda, Maryland, National Cancer Institute, pp. III 12–III 20.

in men after lung, prostate, and colorectal cancer, accounting for 5 per cent of all cancer deaths in men (Silverberg et al., 1990). Bladder cancer accounts for about 3 per cent of all cancer deaths in women (Silverberg, et al., 1990). The mortality rates in whites (6.0 per cent for men and 1.7 per cent for women) are comparable to those in blacks (4.2 per cent for men and 2.4 per cent for women), providing further evidence that the differences in the incidence rates between races is due mainly to differences in diagnosis and reporting of superficial tumors (Table 28–2).

Blacks have significantly lower 5-year survival rates than whites, stage-for-stage. In patients with localized tumors, the 5-year survival rate is 88 per cent for whites as compared with 74 per cent for blacks. In patients with regional tumors, the 5-year survival is 44 per cent for whites and 30 per cent for blacks. In those with distant metastases, the 5-year survival is 9 per cent for whites and 8 per cent for blacks. Part of the reason for this difference may be that black patients are more likely to go untreated (Mayer and McWhorter, 1989). Overall, approximately 72 per cent of patients present with localized disease, 20 per cent with regional disease, and 3 per cent with distant metastases (Silverberg et al., 1990). In general, the mortality rates from bladder cancer are about 20 per cent of the incidence rates, indicating that most patients with bladder cancer die of other causes.

Since the 1950s, the incidence of bladder cancer has steadily increased at an annual rate of 0.8 per cent per year for an overall increase of approximately 50 per cent (1987 Annual Cancer Statistics Review). It is to be anticipated with aging of the United States population that this trend will continue. In addition, improved diagnostic techniques and increased availability of these techniques have contributed to the increased incidence rates. In comparison, there has been a steady decrease

Table 28–2. 1985 AGE-ADJUSTED BLADDER CANCER MORTALITY RATES*: SEER PROGRAM—RACE AND SEX DIFFERENCES

	Black	White	Total
Males	4.9	6.2	6.0
Females	2.2	1.7	1.7
Total	3.3	3.4	3.4

*Rates are per 100,000 and are age-adjusted to the 1970 U.S. standard population.
From 1987 Annual Cancer Statistics Review: Including Cancer Trends: 1950–1985. Bethesda, Maryland, National Cancer Institute, pp. IV 8–IV 16.

in the mortality rates from bladder cancer during the same interval for an overall decrease of approximately 33 per cent (1987 Annual Cancer Statistics Review). This decrease in mortality is due primarily to shifts in the proportion of patients diagnosed with early disease but also, to some extent, to improved treatment.

Age

Although bladder cancer can occur at any age—even in children—it is generally a disease of the elderly with the median age of diagnosis being approximately 67 to 70 years old. In the National Cancer Institute Surveillance, Epidemiology, and End Results Survey, the average annual incidence rates were less than 1.0 for people younger than age 35, 9.9 to 19.1 for those in their 40s, 31.5 to 53.8 for those in their 50s, 82.1 to 111.5 for those in their 60s, 140.3 to 170.9 for those in their 70s, and as high as 194.4 in those 80 and older (1987 Annual Cancer Statistics Review, 1989). In patients younger than age 30, bladder cancer tends to express a well-differentiated histology and behave in a more indolent fashion (Benson, et al., 1983b). Younger patients appear to have a more favorable prognosis because they present more frequently with superficial, low-grade tumors; however, the risk for disease progression is the same grade-for-grade in young patients as in older patients (Wan and Grossman, 1989). All patients should be treated on the basis of tumor stage and grade regardless of patient age (Kurz et al., 1987).

Regional and National Differences

The incidence rates of bladder cancer have been reported to be 30 to 50 per cent higher in the northern region of the United States than in the southern region (Cutler and Young, 1975; Morrison, 1984).

Significant national differences exist in the incidence of bladder cancer. For example, the reported incidence of bladder cancer is higher in the United States and England than in Japan and Finland (Morrison, 1984). In Hawaii, the incidence is more than twice as high in whites as in Japanese (Waterhouse et al., 1982). Jewish people also have been reported to have a higher incidence of bladder cancer (Sullivan, 1982).

These differences are probably related to the combined effects of environmental and hereditary factors.

ETIOLOGY

Factors reported to be causally related to bladder cancer include occupational exposure to chemicals, cigarette smoking, coffee drinking, analgesics, artificial sweeteners, bacterial and parasitic infections, bladder calculi, pelvic irradiation, and cytotoxic chemotherapeutic agents. Much data suggest that many bladder cancers are carcinogen induced. Carcinogens produce lesions in the genome of the transitional epithelial cells, initiating the process of carcinogenesis. It is likely that multiple lesions are required to cause malignant transformation of the cell. Abnormalities of chromosomes 1, 5, 7, 9, 11, 17, 18, and 21 have been reported in bladder cancer (Atkin and Fox, 1990; Babu et al., 1989; Hopman et al., 1989; Tsai et al., 1990; Vanni et al., 1987). Many tumors show multiple deletions of alleles. Some genetic losses may be a common feature of more than one type of cancer, whereas others may be specific for certain types of cancer. It has been proposed that deletions on chromosome 9 may be a specific defect associated with bladder cancer (Tsai et al., 1990). The cancer does not become clinically apparent until the altered genome is expressed or, in the case of deleted cancer suppressor genes, not expressed. Promoters stimulate the expression of the altered genome.

Currently, several different potential mechanisms could account for carcinogenesis. One involves the induction of oncogenes. Oncogenes are altered genes that encode for the malignant phenotype. Several oncogenes in the *ras* gene family located on chromosomes 1, 11, and 12 have been demonstrated in bladder cancer (Parada et al., 1982; Santos et al., 1982). These genes can acquire transforming potential by single point mutations. The encoded *ras* protein may behave like one of the guanine nucleotide–binding proteins that transduce signals from growth factors at the cell surface to induce proliferation. The nature of the interaction between the *ras*-guanosine triphosphate complex growth factors and other cytosolic proteins determines whether cells proliferate. Other oncogenes have been demonstrated in bladder cancer cell lines (Fujita et al., 1984). One of these, the p21 *ras* oncogene (Meyers et al., 1989; Visvanathan et al., 1988), has been shown to be insufficient alone to produce the malignant phenotype (Dunn et al., 1988). Viola and co-workers (1985) have reported a correlation between expression of p21 *ras* protein and histologic grade. Masters and colleagues (1988) found a correlation between the expression of c-*myc* oncogene and recurrence or invasion in superficial bladder cancer. The level of methylation of the c-*myc* oncogene may correlate with the stage and grade of bladder cancer (Del Senno et al., 1989).

Another possible mechanism of carcinogenesis involves the deletion or inactivation of so-called cancer suppressor genes. These genes, whose expression normally regulates cellular growth and differentiation, prevent the uncontrolled proliferation that is characteristic of cancer cells. In this regard, familial bladder cancer has been reported in association with retinoblastoma and osteosarcoma, two tumors that may be caused by deletion of the retinoblastoma tumor suppressor gene on chromosome 13 (Aherne, 1974; Chan and Pratt, 1977).

A third type of carcinogenic mechanism includes amplification of the expression of genes that encode for growth factors or growth factor receptors, which normally regulate the growth and differentiation of cells. Overactivity of these genes could result in chronic cellular proliferation, leading to cancer (Messing, 1990; Neal et al., 1985, 1990).

Some evidence implicates each of these mechanisms in the etiology of bladder cancer, but in all cases the data are insufficient to prove a causal relationship.

Occupational Exposure

Aniline dyes, introduced in the mid-1800s to color fabrics, are urothelial carcinogens (Rehn, 1895). Other chemicals that have been shown to be carcinogens for bladder cancer include 2-naphthylamine, 4-aminobiphenyl (xenylamine), 4-nitrobiphenyl, 4,4-diaminobiphenyl (benzidine), and 2-amino-1-naphthol (Morrison and Cole, 1976); combustion gases and soot from coal; and, possibly, chlorinated aliphatic hydrocarbons (Steinbeck et al., 1990).

It is estimated that occupational exposure accounts for one fourth to one third of bladder cancer cases in the United States (Cole et al., 1972). The latent period may be as long as 40 to 50 years, but more intensive exposure to the carcinogen may shorten the latent period (Case et al., 1954).

Most bladder carcinogens are aromatic amines. Another potential source of such compounds is dietary nitrites and nitrates that are acted upon by intestinal bacterial flora (Chapman et al., 1981). Metabolites of the amino acid, tryptophan, have been reported—but not proved—to be potentially carcinogenic.

Occupations reported to be associated with an increased risk of bladder cancer include those of auto workers, painters, truck drivers, drill press operators, leather workers, and metal machiners and those that involve organic chemicals, such as dry cleaners, paper manufacturers, rope and twine makers, dental technicians, barbers and beauticians, physicians, workers in apparel manufacturing, and plumbers (Malker et al., 1987; Morrison, 1984; Silverman, et al., 1989a, 1989b).

Cigarette Smoking

Cigarette smokers have up to a fourfold higher incidence of bladder cancer than nonsmokers (Burch et al., 1989; Clavel et al., 1989; Morrison et al., 1984). The risk correlates with the number of cigarettes smoked, the duration of smoking, and the degree of inhalation of the smoke. This risk has been observed in both sexes. Ex-cigarette smokers have a reduced incidence of bladder cancer compared with smokers (Augustine et al., 1988). Other forms of tobacco are associated with only a slightly higher risk for bladder cancer (Burch et al., 1989; Harge et al., 1985). An estimated one third of bladder cancer cases may be related to cigarette smoking (Howe et al., 1980).

The specific chemical carcinogen responsible for bladder cancer in cigarette smoke has not been identified. Nitrosamines as well as 2-naphthylamine are known to be present. Increased urinary tryptophan metabolites also have been demonstrated in cigarette smokers (Hoffman et al., 1969).

Coffee and Tea Drinking

Coffee drinking has been implicated in some—but not all—studies in the etiology of bladder cancer (Ciccone and Vineis, 1988; Morrison, 1984; Slattery et al., 1988). This association is complicated because of the widespread consumption of coffee and the fact that coffee drinking, use of artificial sweeteners, and cigarette smoking are often associated. An increased risk of bladder cancer also has been reported in association with tea drinking (Slattery et al., 1988).

Analgesic Abuse

Consumption of large quantities (5 to 15 kg over a 10-year period) of the analgesic, phenacetin, which has a chemical structure similar to that of the aniline dyes, is associated with an increased risk for transitional cell carcinoma of the renal pelvis and bladder (Piper et al., 1985). The latency period may be longer for bladder tumors than renal pelvis tumors, which may be as long as 25 years (Steffens and Nagel, 1988). A correlation with the use of other analgesics has not been clearly demonstrated (McCredie et al., 1983; Wahlqvist, 1980).

Artificial Sweeteners

Large doses of artificial sweeteners, including saccharin and cyclamate, have been shown in experimental studies to be bladder carcinogens in rodents. These studies are controversial because of the extremely high doses of sweeteners given and the fact that cancer occurred only in animals exposed in utero or in the neonatal period (Sontag, 1980). In contrast, case-control epidemiologic studies in humans show little evidence for an increased risk of bladder cancer in consumers of artificial sweeteners (Morrison, 1984; Risch et al., 1988). Some investigators report that nonsmoking women and heavy-smoking men may have some increased risk associated with the consumption of artificial sweeteners (Hoover and Strasser, 1980).

Chronic Cystitis

Chronic cystitis in the presence of indwelling catheters or calculi is associated with an increased risk for squamous cell carcinoma of the bladder (Kunter et al., 1984; Locke et al., 1985). Between 2 and 10 per cent of paraplegics with long-term indwelling catheters develop bladder cancer. Approximately 80 per cent of these are squamous cell carcinomas.

Similarly, *Schistosoma haematobium* cystitis is causally related to the development of squamous cell cancer (Lucas, 1982). In Egypt, where schistosomiasis is endemic, squamous cell carcinoma of the bladder (bilharzial bladder cancer) is the most common cancer. Cystitis-induced bladder cancer from all causes is usually associated with severe, long-term infections. The mechanisms of carcinogenesis are not understood but may involve formation of nitrite and N-nitroso compounds in the bladder (Tricker et al., 1989).

A viral etiology of transitional cell carcinoma has been investigated but not established (Fraley et al., 1976).

Pelvic Irradiation

Women treated with radiation therapy for carcinoma of the uterine cervix have a twofold to fourfold increased risk of developing transitional cell carcinoma of the bladder (Duncan et al., 1977; Sella et al., 1989). These tumors are characteristically high-grade and locally advanced at the time of diagnosis (Quilty and Kerr, 1987).

Cyclophosphamide

Patients treated with cyclophosphamide have an up to ninefold increased risk of developing bladder cancer, although the relationship has not yet been formally demonstrated in case-controlled epidemiologic studies (Morrison, 1984; O'Keane, 1988; Tuttle et al., 1988). The cumulative risk is 3.5 per cent at 8 years and 10.7 per cent at 12 years (Pedersen-Bjergaard et al., 1988). Most of these tumors are muscle infiltrating at the time of diagnosis (Durkee and Benson, 1980). The urinary metabolite of Cytoxan, acrolein, is believed to be responsible for both hemorrhagic cystitis and bladder cancer; however, the development of hemorrhagic cystitis does not necessarily correlate with the development of bladder cancer. There does not appear to be an increased incidence of bladder cancer in patients treated with intermittent Cytoxan therapy (Pedersen-Bjergaard et al., 1988). The latent period for cyclophosphamide-induced bladder cancer is relatively short, ranging from 6 to 13 years. Experimental animal studies suggest that the administration of sulfhydryl-containing uroprotectors, such as Mesna (2-mercaptoethanesulfonic acid), may reduce the risk of bladder cancer (Habs and Schmahl, 1983).

Endogenous Tryptophan Metabolites

Bladder cancer patients have been reported to have increased urinary tryptophan metabolite levels (Brown et al., 1969; Wolf, 1973). High levels have been reported to correlate with tumor recurrence rates (Brown et al., 1969; Teulings et al., 1978). Pyridoxine administration normalized urinary tryptophan metabolite levels in some patients. Moreover, a controlled clinical trial showed that pyridoxine significantly reduced early tumor recurrence rates in patients with superficial bladder cancer (Byar and Blackhard, 1977). In this trial, however, tryptophan metabolite levels were not measured.

In contrast, current studies suggest that endogenous tryptophan metabolites do *not* contribute significantly to the development of bladder cancer (Renwick et al., 1988). Tryptophan metabolites have failed to induce bladder cancer in experimental animals; however, the combination of tryptophan plus 2-acetylaminofluorine or tryptophan plus a pyridoxine-deficient diet induced bladder tumors in experimental animals (Bryan, 1971, 1977; Wolf, 1973). Thus, the role, if any, of endogenous metabolites in the etiology of bladder cancer remains controversial.

Heredity

Little evidence exists for a hereditary cause of most cases of bladder cancer. Familial clusters of bladder cancer have been reported (Aherne, 1974; Fraumeni and Thomas, 1967; McCullough et al., 1975). An alternative explanation for these familial clusters may be similar exposure to the same environmental factors. An increased incidence of HLA-B5 and CW4 also was reported in bladder cancer patients (Arce et al., 1978).

Genetic polymorphisms relating to liver arylamine acetyltransferase activity have been reported. Patients who tested as slow acetylators were reported to be more susceptible to develop bladder cancer than fast acetylators (Lower et al., 1979). Other studies have not confirmed this observation (Horai et al., 1989; Miller and Cosgriff, 1983).

Quantification of molecular adducts of aromatic amines to test for genetic susceptibility to bladder cancer may prove useful in the future (Kadlubar et al., 1988).

Two different patterns of genetic involvement have been suggested for bladder cancer: an autosomal dominant pattern that accounts for a small number of cases and a multifactorial, polygenic pattern that involves genetic and environmental interactions (Schulte, 1988).

PATHOLOGY

Normal Bladder Urothelium

The urothelium of the normal bladder is a transitional cell epithelium three to seven cell layers thick. There is a basement cell layer upon which rests one or more layers of intermediate cells. The most superficial layer is composed of the large flat umbrella cells. The cells of the urothelium are oriented with the long axis of the oval nuclei being perpendicular to the basement membrane, giving the urothelium its normal appearance of cellular polarity (Koss et al., 1974). The urothelium rests upon a lamina propria basement membrane (Zuk et al., 1989). In the lamina propria is a tunica muscularis mucosa containing scattered muscle fibers, which are irregularly arranged (Keep et al., 1989; Ro et al., 1987).

Epithelial Hyperplasia

The term *epithelial hyperplasia* is used to describe an increase in the number of cell layers without nuclear or architectural abnormalities.

Urothelial Dysplasia

Preneoplastic Proliferative Abnormalities

A variety of changes can occur in the urothelium in response to inflammation, irritation, or carcinogens. These changes may be proliferative, metaplastic, or both (Fig. 28–1).

Atypical hyperplasia is similar to epithelial hyperplasia, except that there are also nuclear abnormalities and partial derangement of the umbrella cell layer (Koss et al., 1974). In patients with superficial bladder cancer, the presence of atypia in adjacent urothelium is associated with a 35 to 40 per cent risk of developing invasive disease (Althausen et al., 1976).

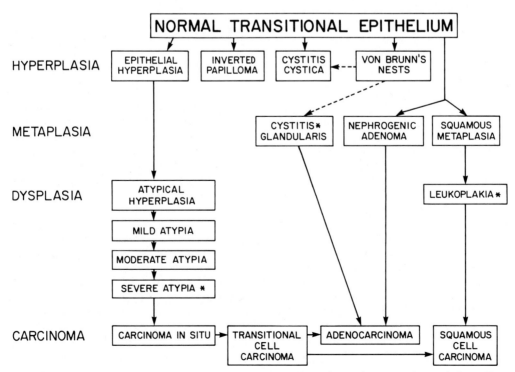

Figure 28–1. Interrelationships among hyperplastic, metaplastic, dysplastic, and neoplastic changes in the urothelium. (From Catalona, W. J.: Bladder cancer. *In* Gillenwater, J. Y., Grayhack, J. T., Howards, S. S., and Duckett, J. W. (Eds.): Adult and Pediatric Urology. Chicago, Year Book Medical Publishers, Inc., 1987, p. 1000.)

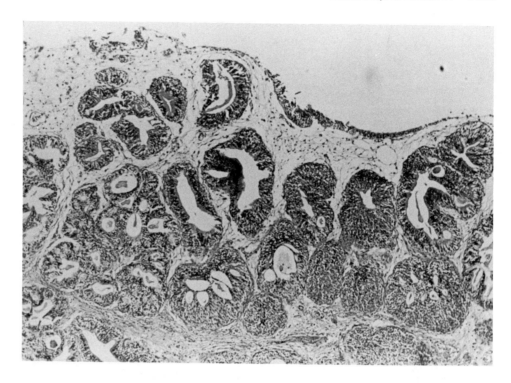

Figure 28–2. The von Brunn's nests. (From Mostofi, F. K., Sobin, L. H., and Torloni, H.: Histological Typing of Urinary Bladder Tumors, no. 10. International Histological Classification of Tumors. Geneva, World Health Organization, 1973.)

Von Brunn's nests are islands of benign-appearing urothelium situated in the submucosa (Fig. 28–2). They are believed to result from *inward* proliferation of the basal cells (Patch and Rhea, 1935). These nests have been reported to be a normal urothelial variant in the supramontanal prostatic urethra (Kierman and Gafney, 1987) and occur in 89 per cent of normal bladders at autopsy (Wiener et al., 1979).

Cystitis cystica is similar to von Brunn's nests except that the center of the nests of urothelium have undergone eosinophilic liquefaction (Kunze et al., 1983) (Fig. 28–3). Cystitis cystica also occurs in 60 per cent of

normal bladders at autopsy (Wiener et al., 1979). Cystitis cystica should be distinguished from *cystitis follicularis,* a non-neoplastic response to chronic bacterial infection. Histologically, cystitis follicularis is composed of submucosal lymphoid follicles. Grossly, it appears as punctate yellow submucosal nodules, which have been given the descriptive apellation, "bacteruric bumps."

Cystitis glandularis is similar to cystitis cystica except that the transitional cells have undergone glandular metaplasia. It appears histologically as submucosal nests of columnar epithelial cells surrounding a central liquefied region of cellular degeneration (Mostofi, 1954) (Fig.

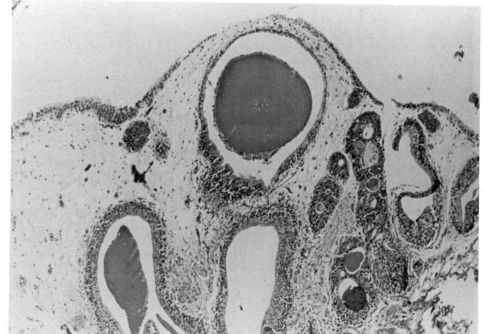

Figure 28–3. Cystitis cystica. (From Mostofi, F. K., Sobin, L. H., and Torloni, H.: Histological Typing of Urinary Bladder Tumors, no. 10. International Histological Classification of Tumors. Geneva, World Health Organization, 1973.)

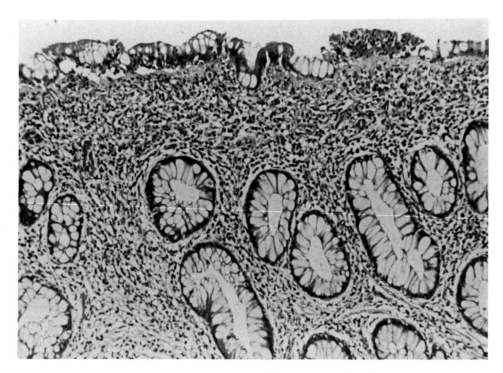

Figure 28–4. Cystitis glandularis. (From Mostofi, F. K., Sobin, L. H., Torloni, H.: Histological Typing of Urinary Bladder Tumors, no. 10. International Histological Classification of Tumors. Geneva, World Health Organization, 1973.)

28–4). Cystitis glandularis may be a precursor of adenocarcinoma (Edwards et al., 1972). It has been reported to occur frequently in patients with pelvic lipomatosis (Gordon et al., 1990; Johnson et al., 1980; Yalla et al., 1975). Cystoscopically, cystitis glandularis may appear as a papillary lesion.

Dysplasia

The term *dysplasia* denotes epithelial changes that are intermediate between normal urothelium and carcinoma in situ. There are three categories of dysplasia: mild, moderate, and severe. Dysplastic cells have large, round, notched, basally situated nuclei that do not exhibit the normal epithelial polarity. Dysplastic epithelium does not have an increased number of cell layers or mitotic figures (Murphy and Soloway, 1982). It is difficult to make a sharp distinction between severe dysplasia and carcinoma in situ (Friedell et al., 1986).

Inverted Papilloma

An inverted papilloma is a benign proliferative lesion caused by chronic inflammation or bladder outlet obstruction. Most commonly, it occurs in the trigone and bladder neck areas in men with prostatism (DeMeester et al., 1975).

Papillary fronds project into the fibrovascular stroma of the bladder rather than into the bladder lumen. The lesion is usually covered by a layer of normal urothelium (Fig. 28–5). Inverted papillomas may contain areas of cystitis cystica or squamous metaplasia.

Two different types of inverted papilloma occur: trabecular and glandular. The trabecular type arises from proliferation of the basal cells. The glandular type is a form of cystitis glandularis arising in the intermediate cells and as such is considered to be potentially a preneoplastic lesion (Kunze et al., 1983).

Rare cases of malignant transformation of inverted papillomas have been reported (Lazarevic and Garret, 1978).

Nephrogenic Adenoma

Nephrogenic adenoma is a rare lesion that histologically resembles primitive renal collecting tubules (Fig. 28–6). It is a metaplastic response of urothelium to trauma, infection, or radiation therapy. Edema and inflammatory cell infiltration are common, but there is little nuclear atypia or mitotic activity (Navarre et al., 1982). Nephrogenic adenoma is more common in men and often is associated with symptoms of dysuria and urinary frequency. Nephrogenic adenoma also has been reported in children (Kay and Lattanzi, 1985).

Mesonephric adenocarcinoma is the malignant counterpart of nephrogenic adenoma (Schultz et al., 1984). This lesion usually invades through the lamina propria. Radical cystectomy is indicated for muscle-invasive tumors.

Squamous Metaplasia

Squamous metaplasia is a proliferative lesion in which the urothelium is replaced by a mature, nonkeratinizing squamous epithelium. It occurs most commonly in the bladder neck and trigone area (Fig. 28–7). Although some workers have reported that it may be precancerous (Mostofi, 1954), others have reported that squamous metaplasia of the vaginal type on the trigone of women is a normal variant occurring under hormonal influence (Tyler, 1962). Autopsy studies have shown that squamous metaplasia occurs in the bladder of nearly half of women and in fewer than 10 per cent of men (Wiener et al., 1979). Squamous metaplasia in the absence of cellular atypia or marked keratinization is probably a benign condition in either sex.

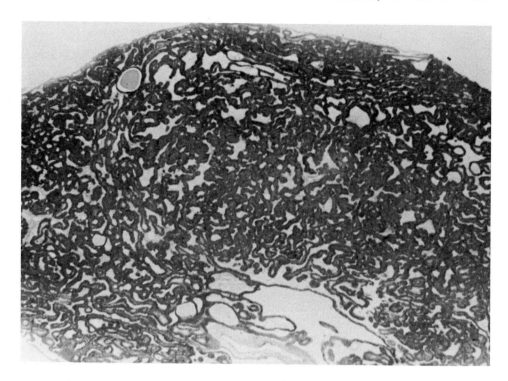

Figure 28–5. Inverted papilloma. (From Mostofi, F. K., Sobin, L. H., and Tortoni, H.: Histological Typing of Urinary Bladder Tumors, no. 10. International Histological Classification of Tumors. Geneva, World Health Organization, 1973.)

Vesical Leukoplakia

Leukoplakia is defined as cornification of a normally noncornifying membrane. The histopathologic criteria include squamous metaplasia with marked keratinization, downward growth of the rete pegs (acanthosis), cellular atypia, and dysplasia (Fig. 28–8) (Benson et al., 1984). Leukoplakia is believed to be a response of the normal urothelium to noxious stimuli and generally is considered a premalignant lesion or a lesion that heralds the presence of malignant disease elsewhere in the bladder (Benson et al., 1984). Vesical leukoplakia may progress to squamous cell carcinoma in up to 20 per cent of patients (Benson et al., 1984; DeKock et al.,

1981). Leukoplakia is frequently found in patients with chronic cystitis, bladder calculi, long-term indwelling catheters, or schistosomiasis.

Pseudosarcoma (Postoperative Spindle Cell Nodule)

Postoperative spindle cell nodule is a rare lesion resembling a sarcoma of the bladder. It consists of reactive proliferation of spindle cells occurring several months after a lower urinary tract procedure or infection (Fig. 28–9). These lesions have been misinterpreted as being malignant, and radical surgery has been performed

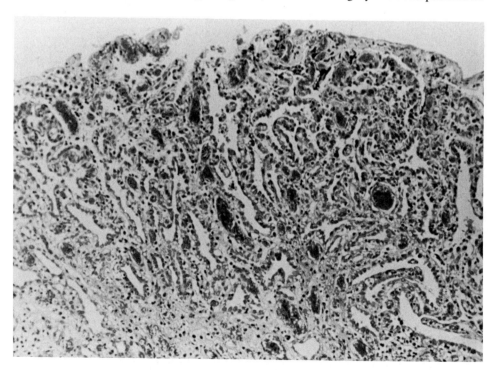

Figure 28–6. Nephrogenic adenoma. (From Mostofi, F. K., Sobin, L. H., and Torloni, H.: Histological Typing of Urinary Bladder Tumors, no. 10. International Histological Classification of Tumors. Geneva, World Health Organization, 1973.)

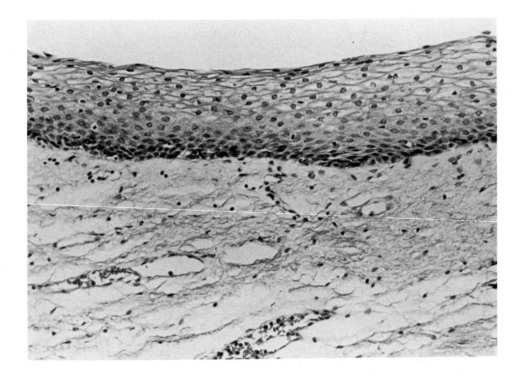

Figure 28–7. Squamous metaplasia. (From Mostofi, F. K., Sobin, L. H., and Torloni, H.: Histological Typing of Urinary Bladder Tumors, no. 10. International Histological Classification of Tumors. Geneva, World Health Organization, 1973.)

inappropriately. Usually, they are confused with a leiomyosarcoma (Huang et al., 1990; Stark et al., 1989; Vekemans et al., 1990; Wick et al., 1988; Young and Scully, 1987).

Urothelial Carcinoma

Carcinoma in Situ

Carcinoma in situ appears as a velvety patch of erythematous mucosa on cystoscopic examination. His-

tologically, it consists of poorly differentiated transitional cell carcinoma confined to the urothelium (Fig. 28–10). Carcinoma in situ may be asymptomatic or may produce severe symptoms of urinary frequency, urgency, and dysuria (Utz et al., 1970; Utz and Farrow, 1984). Urine cytopathology study results are positive in 80 to 90 per cent of patients with carcinoma in situ because of the poor cohesiveness of the tumor cells. Carcinoma in situ occurs more commonly in men. Its symptoms may be mistaken for prostatism, urinary tract infection, or neurogenic bladder.

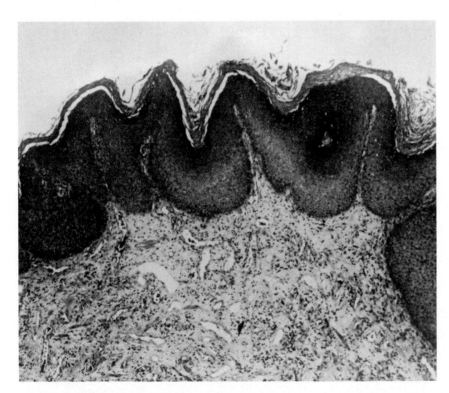

Figure 28–8. Vesical leukoplakia. (From Farrow, G. M.: Relationship of leukoplakia to urothelial malignancy. J. Urol., 131:507, 1985.)

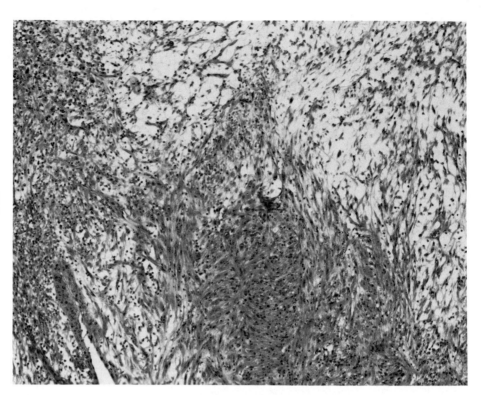

Figure 28–9. Postoperative spindle cell nodule. (Courtesy of F. K. Mostofi, M.D.)

Carcinoma in situ occurs only rarely in patients with well-differentiated, superficial bladder tumors, but it is present in one fourth or more of patients with high-grade tumors (Flamm and Dona, 1989; Koss et al., 1974). It portends a poor prognosis. Patients with carcinoma in situ have higher tumor recurrence rates (Flamm and Dona, 1989); between 40 and 83 per cent progress to invasive cancer (Althausen et al., 1976). Carcinoma in situ occurs in 20 to 75 per cent of high-grade muscle-invasive cancers (Prout et al., 1983). It is also more common in patients with multiple tumors.

The natural history of carcinoma in situ is not clearly understood. Early in its clinical evolution, it may be asymptomatic; later, it may produce severe symptoms of bladder irritability. Some patients have a protracted course lasting for more than a decade without developing invasive bladder cancer (Riddle et al., 1976; Weinstein et al., 1979). Others progress rapidly to invasive bladder cancer that has a poor prognosis despite definitive therapy (Utz et al., 1970).

In the early 1970s, radical cystectomy was recommended for carcinoma in situ (Utz et al., 1970; Utz and Farrow, 1984). Later studies documented the possibly protracted clinical course and responsiveness to intravesical therapy.

Some investigators have characterized carcinoma in situ as a peculiar cancer expressing sinister morphologic features but having a limited capacity to invade and metastasize (Weinstein et al., 1980). Patients with marked urinary symptoms generally have a shorter interval preceding the development of invasive cancer. About 20 per cent of patients treated with cystectomy for diffuse carcinoma in situ are found to have microinvasive cancer (Farrow et al., 1976).

In current years, intravesical therapy has become the preferred primary treatment for carcinoma in situ. Chemotherapeutic agents used include triethylenethiophosphoramide (thiotepa), etoglucid (Epodyl), mitomycin C, and doxorubicin (Adriamycin). These agents are effective in eradicating carcinoma in situ in approximately one third of patients (Soloway, 1984). The most effective intravesical therapy for carcinoma in situ is intravesical bacille Calmette-Guérin (BCG) therapy, producing complete regression in approximately 50 to 65 per cent of patients (Coplen et al., 1990). Radiation therapy and systemic chemotherapy are not effective in eradicating carcinoma in situ (Whitmore et al., 1977).

Transitional Cell Carcinoma (Papillary or Solid)

More than 90 per cent of bladder cancers are transitional cell carcinomas (Figs. 28–10 through 28–12). These tumors differ from normal urothelium by having an increased number of epithelial cell layers with papillary folding of the mucosa, loss of cell polarity, abnormal cell maturation from the basal to superficial layers, giant cells, nuclear crowding, increased nuclear-cytoplasmic ratio, prominent nucleoli, clumping of chromatin, and increased number of mitoses (Koss, 1975). The most significant criteria are the prominent nucleoli, clumping of chromatin, increased cell layers, and loss of cell polarity (Melamed et al., 1960). Some of these same changes can occur in inflammatory, reactive, or regenerative conditions (Mostofi, 1954).

Transitional cell carcinomas manifest a variety of patterns of tumor growth including papillary, sessile infiltrating, nodular, mixed, and flat intraepithelial

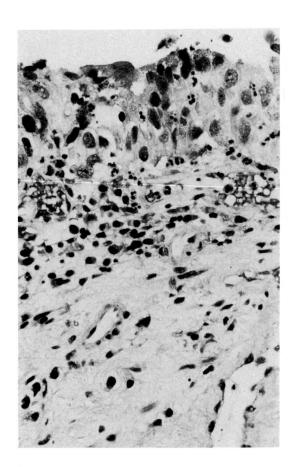

Figure 28–10. Carcinoma in situ. (Courtesy of Louis P. Dehner, M.D.)

Figure 28–11. Transitional cell papilloma. (From Mostofi, F. K., Sobin, L. H., and Torloni, H.: Histological Typing of Urinary Bladder Tumors, no. 10. International Histological Classification of Tumors. Geneva, World Health Organization, 1973.)

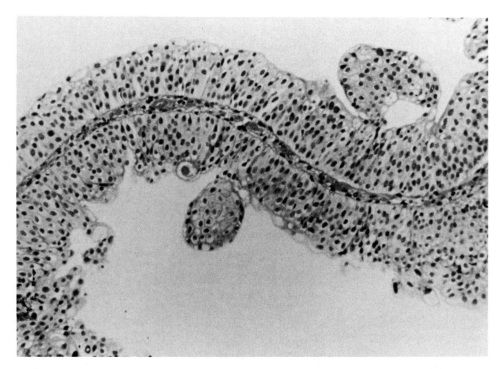

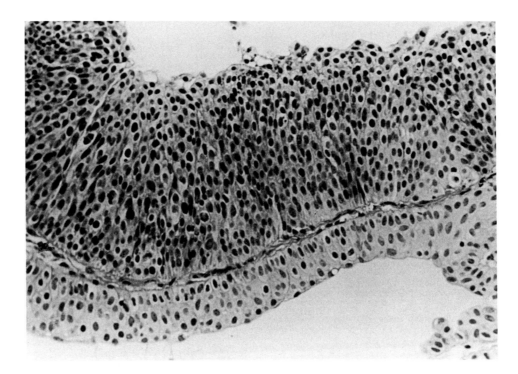

Figure 28–12. Well-differentiated transitional cell carcinoma. (From Mostofi, F. K., Sobin, L. H., and Torloni, H.: Histological Typing of Urinary Bladder Tumors, no. 10. International Histological Classification of Tumors. Geneva, World Health Organization, 1973.)

growth. Because the bladder does not have a distinct basement membrane, it is difficult to demonstrate invasion of the lamina propria. Furthermore, invagination of the normal urothelium into the submucosa as occurs with von Brunn's nests sometimes is difficult to distinguish from cancer invasion (Mostofi, 1954). Moreover, cancer invasion into the smooth muscle cells of the tunica muscularis mucosa sometimes can be mistaken for invasion into the bladder detrusor muscle (Keep et al., 1989).

Transitional cell epithelium has a great metaplastic potential; therefore, transitional cell carcinomas may contain spindle cell (Young et al., 1988), squamous cell, or adenocarcinomatous elements (Figs. 28–13 through 28–15). These elements are present in about one third of bladder cancers. Some tumors may exhibit several different elements. Transitional cell carcinomas arise most commonly in the trigone/bladder base area and on the lateral bladder walls; however, they may arise anywhere within the bladder. About 70 per cent of bladder tumors are papillary, 10 per cent are nodular, and 20 per cent are mixed.

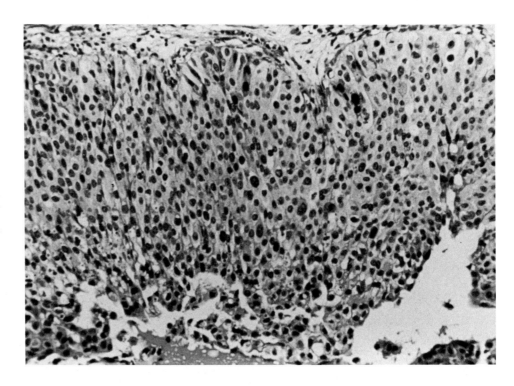

Figure 28–13. Moderately differentiated transitional cell carcinoma. (From Mostofi, F. K., Sobin, L. H., and Torloni, H.: Histological Typing of Urinary Bladder Tumors, no. 10. International Histological Classification of Tumors. Geneva, World Health Organization, 1973.)

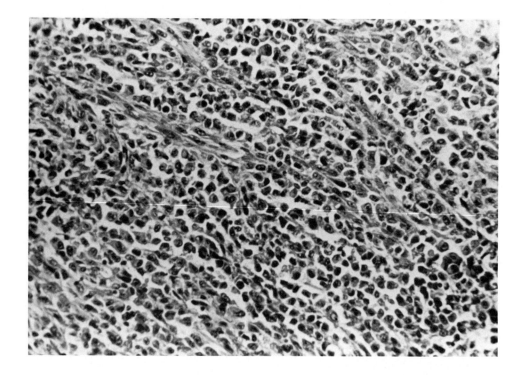

Figure 28–14. Undifferentiated transitional cell carcinoma. (From Mostofi, F. K., Sobin, L. H., and Torloni, H.: Histological Typing of Urinary Bladder Tumors, no. 10. International Histological Classification of Tumors. Geneva, World Health Organization, 1973.)

Tumor Grading

No uniformly accepted grading system for bladder cancer is defined. Most commonly used systems are based on the degree of anaplasia of the tumor cells (Broders, 1922; Koss, 1975; Mostofi et al., 1973) and group carcinomas into three grades corresponding to well-, moderately, and poorly differentiated tumors.

A strong correlation exists between tumor grade and tumor stage (Jewett and Strong, 1946), with most well-differentiated tumors being superficial and most poorly differentiated tumors being invasive. However, stage-for-stage, there is a significant correlation between tumor grade and prognosis. The correlation between tumor stage and prognosis is even stronger.

A *papilloma* (grade 0) is a papillary lesion with a thin fibrovascular core covered by normal bladder mucosa (Friedell et al., 1976) (see Fig. 28–11). *Well-differentiated* (grade 1) tumors (see Fig. 28–12) have a thin fibrovascular stalk with a thickened urothelium containing more than seven cell layers, with the cells exhibiting only slight anaplasia and pleomorphism. There also may be an increased nuclear-cytoplasmic ratio and a prominence of the nuclear membrane. The disturbance of the

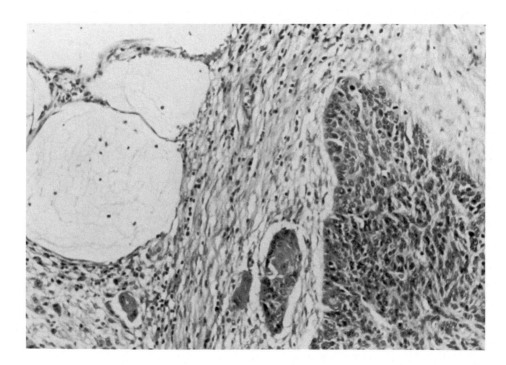

Figure 28–15. Transitional cell carcinoma with squamous and glandular metaplasia. (From Mostofi, F. K., Sobin, L. H., and Torloni, H.: Histological Typing of Urinary Bladder Tumors, no. 10. International Histological Classification of Tumors. Geneva, World Health Organization, 1973.)

base-to-surface cellular maturation is mild, and there are only rare mitotic figures. *Moderately differentiated* (grade 2) tumors (see Fig. 28–13) have a wide fibrovascular core, a greater disturbance of the base-to-surface cellular maturation, and a loss of cell polarity. The nuclear-cytoplasmic ratio is higher with nuclear pleomorphism and prominent nucleoli. Mitotic figures are more frequent. *Poorly differentiated* (grade 3) tumors (see Fig. 28–14) have cells that do not differentiate as they progress from the basement membrane to the surface. Marked nuclear pleomorphism is noted, with a high nuclear-cytoplasmic ratio. Mitotic figures may be frequent (Friedell et al., 1980).

Metaplastic Elements

It is not unusual for different tumor types to coexist in the same bladder (see Fig. 28–15); however, all epithelial tumors are believed to have a common ancestry in the transitional epithelium. The most frequent combination is a papillary transitional cell carcinoma with flat carcinoma in situ. Squamous cell carcinoma elements also are frequently seen with invasive transitional cell carcinoma. Less common is the combination of adenocarcinoma elements with invasive transitional cell carcinoma (Koss, 1975). The presence of these metaplastic elements in a transitional cell carcinoma does not change the principal classification of the tumor as a transitional cell carcinoma.

Squamous Cell Carcinoma

Etiology

Considerable variability is noted in the prevalence of squamous cell carcinoma of the bladder in different parts of the world. For example, squamous cell cancer accounts for only about 1 per cent of bladder cancers in England (Costello et al., 1984), 3 to 7 per cent in the United States (Kantor et al., 1988; Koss, 1975), but more than 75 per cent in Egypt (El-Bolkainy et al., 1981). About 80 per cent of squamous cell carcinomas in Egypt are associated with chronic infection with *S. haematobium* (Fig. 28–16). These cancers are called bilharzial bladder cancers; they occur in patients who are, on the average, 10 to 20 years younger than patients with transitional cell carcinoma. Bilharzial cancers are exophytic, nodular, fungating lesions that usually are well differentiated and have a relatively low incidence of lymph node and distant metastases. Although some investigators have speculated that the low incidence of distant metastases may be due to capillary and lymphatic fibrosis resulting from chronic schistosomal infection (Ghoneim and Awad, 1980), it is probably more related to the fact that most of these tumors are low-grade (El-Bolkainy et al., 1981).

Nonbilharzial squamous cell cancers are usually caused by chronic irritation from urinary calculi, long-term indwelling catheters, or bladder diverticula. As many as 80 per cent of paraplegics have squamous changes in the bladder, and about 5 per cent develop squamous cell carcinoma (Bejany et al., 1987; Broecher et al., 1981; Maruf et al., 1982). Cigarette smoking also has been reported to be significantly associated with an increased risk of squamous cell bladder carcinoma (Kantor et al., 1988). Male preponderance is less striking in squamous cell carcinoma (1.3:1). In general, the prognosis of squamous cell carcinoma is poor because most patients have advanced disease at the time of diagnosis.

Histology

Squamous cell carcinomas characteristically have keratinized cells that contain concentric aggregates of cells

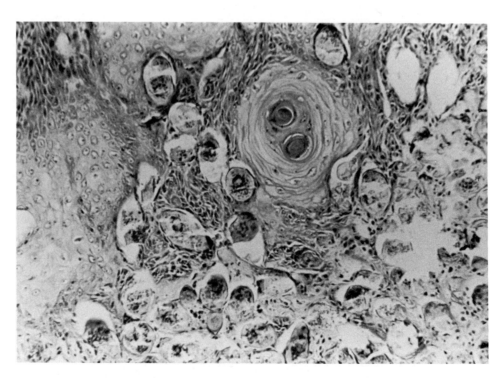

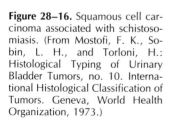
Figure 28–16. Squamous cell carcinoma associated with schistosomiasis. (From Mostofi, F. K., Sobin, L. H., and Torloni, H.: Histological Typing of Urinary Bladder Tumors, no. 10. International Histological Classification of Tumors. Geneva, World Health Organization, 1973.)

called squamous pearls (Fig. 28–17). They may show varying degrees of histologic differentiation (Koss, 1975). Squamous cell cancers shed keratinized cells into the urine that sometimes can be detected cytologically. However, cytology has been of limited usefulness in patients with this tumor. Squamous cell cancers are more frequently associated with coexistent squamous metaplasia than with carcinoma in situ.

Treatment

Squamous cell carcinoma requires aggressive surgical therapy. Transurethral resection, partial cystectomy, and radiation therapy have not been successful (Martin et al., 1989b; Newman et al., 1968). Although definitive radiation therapy with salvage cystectomy has been recommended by some (Costello et al., 1984), the best survival results have been achieved with radical cystectomy with or without planned preoperative radiation therapy (Ghoneim and Awad, 1980). The true benefit of the planned preoperative radiation therapy has not been clearly established. Chemotherapy regimens are not effective for squamous cell carcinoma (Logothetis et al., 1988; Maruf et al., 1982; Sternberg et al., 1989). Several reports suggest that stage-for-stage the prognosis of squamous cell carcinoma is comparable to that of transitional cell carcinoma (Faysal, 1981; Johnson et al., 1976; Richie et al., 1976). Active or recurrent cancer in the urethra has been reported in about half of patients with squamous cell carcinoma, suggesting that urethrectomy should be performed routinely in these patients (Bejany et al., 1987).

Adenocarcinoma

Adenocarcinoma accounts for less than 2 per cent of primary bladder cancers (Kantor et al., 1988). They are classified into three groups: (1) primary vesical, (2) urachal, and (3) metastatic. Adenocarcinomas also occur in intestinal urinary conduits, augmentations, and pouches, and with ureterosigmoidostomy (Husmann and Spence, 1990; Kalble et al., 1990; Spencer and Filmer, 1991). These are discussed in Chapters 70 and 72.

Primary Vesical Adenocarcinoma

Adenocarcinomas of the bladder arise in two common sites: (1) the bladder base area, including the trigone and the immediately adjacent lateral walls; and (2) the dome of the bladder. However, adenocarcinomas can occur anywhere in the bladder (Fig. 28–18). Adenocarcinoma is the most common type of cancer in exstrophic bladders. These tumors develop in response to chronic inflammation and irritation (Bennett et al., 1984; Nielson and Nielsen, 1983). Adenocarcinoma also has been reported with schistosomiasis (Anderstrom et al., 1983); however, it is less common than squamous cell carcinoma with schistosomiasis.

Other established risk factors have not been documented except, possibly, coffee drinking (Kantor et al., 1988). All histologic variants of enteric adenocarcinoma, including signet-ring and colloid carcinoma, may occur in the bladder. Most bladder adenocarcinomas are mucin producing (Koss, 1975). Adenocarcinomas may be papillary or solid. Signet-ring adenocarcinomas characteristically produce linitis plastica of the bladder (Blute et al., 1989; Choi et al., 1984; Sheldon et al., 1984). Most adenocarcinomas are poorly differentiated and invasive and are more commonly associated with cystitis glandularis than with carcinoma in situ. Radical cystectomy with pelvic lymphadenectomy offers the best chance for cure. Adenocarcinomas are poorly responsive to radiation therapy or cytotoxic chemotherapy (Anderstrom et al., 1983; Blute et al., 1989; Logothetis et al.,

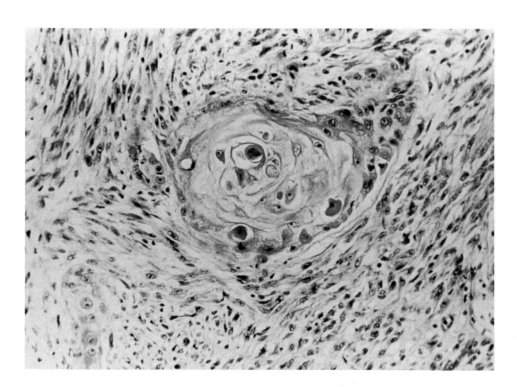

Figure 28–17. Squamous cell carcinoma. (From Mostofi, F. K., Sobin, L. H., and Torloni, H.: Histological Typing of Urinary Bladder Tumors, no. 10. International Histological Classification of Tumors. Geneva, World Health Organization, 1973.)

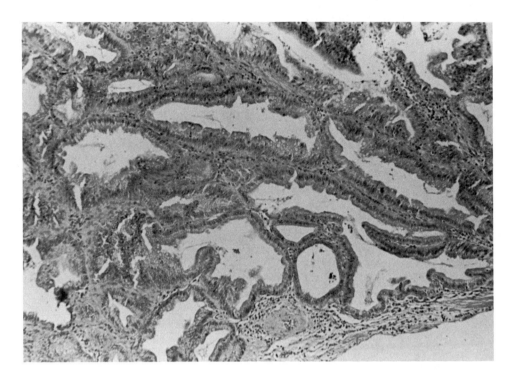

Figure 28–18. Adenocarcinoma. (From Mostofi, F. K., Sobin, L. H., and Torloni, H.: Histological Typing of Urinary Bladder Tumors, no. 10. International Histological Classification of Tumors. Geneva, World Health Organization, 1973.)

1988; Sternberg et al., 1989). The generally poor prognosis associated with adenocarcinoma is due primarily to the fact that they are diagnosed at an advanced stage. No evidence exists that, stage-for-stage, the prognosis is different from that of transitional cell carcinoma.

Urachal Carcinoma

Urachal carcinomas are extremely rare tumors that arise outside the bladder and histologically may be adenocarcinomas, transitional cell carcinomas, squamous cells carcinomas, or rarely sarcomas. Adenocarcinoma is the most common histologic type. For a tumor to be classified as urachal carcinoma, there must be a sharp demarcation between the tumor and the adjacent bladder mucosa, and the tumor must be located within the bladder wall beneath the normal urothelium (Mostofi et al., 1955). Urachal tumors invading through the urothelium and extending into the bladder may be confused with a primary vesical carcinoma (Kakizoe et al., 1983; Koss, 1975).

Urachal carcinomas may extend into the prevesical space. They may appear with a bloody or mucoid discharge from the umbilicus or produce a mucocele, occurring as a palpable mass. Many urachal tumors have stippled calcifications on radiographs (Brick et al., 1988; Narumi et al., 1988). Tumors invading the bladder lumen may produce mucus in the urine. Patients with urachal carcinomas have a worse prognosis than those with primary bladder adenocarcinomas (Mostofi et al., 1955). Tumors treated with partial cystectomy have local recurrence rates between 15 and 50 per cent (Magri, 1962). Histologically, these tumors exhibit wider and deeper infiltration of the bladder wall than expected, making partial cystectomy inadequate in a substantial proportion of cases (Kakizoe et al., 1983; Sheldon et

al., 1984). Accordingly, radical cystectomy with bilateral pelvic lymphadenectomy and en bloc excision of the urachus is the treatment of choice for all except the small, well-differentiated urachal carcinomas. Radiation therapy has not been effective in treating these tumors (Sheldon et al., 1984). Urachal carcinomas metastasize to the iliac and inguinal lymph nodes, omentum, liver, lung, and bone (Sheldon et al., 1984). As with other adenocarcinomas, urachal carcinomas are not responsive to chemotherapy. In general, the prognosis of urachal carcinoma is poor; however, Johnson and co-workers (1985) reported a 50 per cent survival rate.

Metastatic Adenocarcinoma

One of the most common forms of adenocarcinoma of the bladder is metastatic adenocarcinoma (Choi et al., 1984). The primary sites for these tumors include the rectum, stomach, endometrium, breast, prostate, and ovary (Klinger, 1951). Nevertheless, metastases to the bladder from adenocarcinoma is still a relatively rare phenomenon occurring in only 0.26 per cent of cases (Klinger, 1951). Patients with the diagnosis of adenocarcinoma of the bladder should be carefully evaluated for other primary adenocarcinomas before proceeding with definitive treatment.

ORIGIN AND PATTERNS OF DISSEMINATION

Multicentric Origin

Clinical and urinary tract mapping studies suggest that transitional cell carcinoma usually is a field change disease with tumors arising at different times and sites in the urothelium. This suggests a polyclonal etiology of bladder cancer, also supported by point mutation analysis of the p53 cancer suppressor gene on chromosome 17 (Sidransky and Vogelstein, unpublished data). However, it does not exclude the possibility that, in some cases, multiple tumors are derived from a single cell clone that has disseminated to other sites in the urinary tract by implantation or by lymphatic or vascular spread. The appearance of the same marker chromosome has been demonstrated in multiple recurrences of a bladder tumor. Also, genetically identical cells have been demonstrated in primary bladder tumor cells and cells from a metastatic site (Summers et al., 1983). Moreover, analysis with flow cytometry of normal-appearing mucosa in patients with bladder tumors has also demonstrated aneuploid stem cells, suggesting that diffuse premalignant or malignant changes may be responsible for the polychronotopicity (multiple tumors at different sites and times) of bladder cancer (Farsund et al., 1983).

Patterns of Spread

Direct Extension

Local invasion of bladder cancer can occur by three mechanisms (Jewett and Eversole, 1960). The most common is en bloc spread, occurring in about 60 per cent of tumors, characterized by cancer cells invading in a broad front directly beneath the primary mucosal lesion. Tentacular invasion, occurring in about 25 per cent of tumors, is the next most common type. Lateral spread, with tumor cells growing under normal-appearing mucosa, is observed in only about 10 per cent of tumors. Bladder cancer spreads by invading through the lamina propria into the submucosa and muscularis of the bladder wall. This process may occur either because tumor cells are not able to synthesize components of the basement membrane or because of an increased degradation of basement membrane components by enzymes produced by tumor cells (Zuk et al., 1989). In the submucosa and muscularis, tumor cells gain access to blood vessels and lymphatics through which they may metastasize to regional lymph nodes and/or distant sites. A significant correlation exists between muscle invasion and distant metastases (Jewett and Strong, 1946). Bladder cancer also may spread locally to invade adjacent organs, including the prostate, uterus, vagina, ureters, rectum, and intestine.

More than 40 per cent of men undergoing cystectomy for invasive bladder cancer have involvement of the prostate (Hardeman et al., 1988; Schellhammer et al., 1977; Wishnow and Ro, 1988). In the majority of such cases, the prostatic urethra is the site of involvement, but 6 per cent have stromal involvement without prostatic urethra involvement. Overall, about 40 per cent with prostatic involvement have invasion of the stroma (Wood et al., 1989). In such patients, there is a high incidence (80 per cent) of subsequent distant metastases. It has been suggested that patients with prostatic involvement should be treated with neoadjuvant chemotherapy (Wishnow and Ro, 1988), but the efficacy of chemotherapy in this setting has not been demonstrated.

Coexisting primary adenocarcinoma of the prostate may be present in 25 per cent of patients (Kabalin et al., 1989; Montie et al., 1989).

Tumors arising in bladder diverticula pose a special problem; they can invade directly from the mucosa into the perivesical tissues because bladder diverticula do not have a muscular wall. Often these tumors are treated with simple diverticulectomy or partial cystectomy. However, in most reported series, survival results with conservative excision are poor (Faysal and Freiha, 1981).

Metastatic Spread

About 5 per cent of patients with superficial papillary cancer and approximately 20 per cent with high-grade carcinoma in situ have vascular or lymphatic spread, presumably from invasion of tumor cells into superficial lymphatic and vascular channels just beneath the lamina propria.

LYMPHATIC SPREAD

Lymphatic metastases occur earlier and independent of hematogenous metastases in some patients. This may be evidenced in patients with lymph node metastases who are apparently cured with radical cystectomy and pelvic lymphadenectomy (Skinner and Lieskovsky, 1984). Autopsy studies have shown that about one fourth to one third of patients dying of bladder cancer do not have pelvic lymph node metastases (Babaian et al., 1980). The most common sites of metastases in bladder cancer are the pelvic lymph nodes, occurring in about 78 per cent of patients. Among these, the paravesical nodes are involved in 16 per cent, the obturator nodes in 74 per cent, and the external iliac nodes in 65 per cent. The juxtaregional common iliac lymph nodes are involved in about 20 per cent of patients (Smith and Whitmore, 1981a).

VASCULAR SPREAD

The common sites of vascular metastases from bladder cancer are liver, 38 per cent; lung, 36 per cent; bone, 27 per cent; adrenal gland, 21 per cent; and intestine, 13 per cent. Any other organ may be involved (Babaian et al., 1980).

Implantation

Bladder cancer also spreads by implantation in abdominal wounds, denuded urothelium, resected prostatic fossa, or traumatized urethra (Weldon and Soloway, 1975). Implantation occurs more commonly with high-grade tumors (van der Werf-Messing, 1984). Implantation into wound scars can be prevented by giving approximately 1000 centigray (CGy) preoperative radiation, which should be given before the performance of partial cystectomy or cystotomy for interstitial radiation therapy (van der Werf-Messing, 1969). Tumor implantation into the resected prostatic fossa is an infrequent occurrence. Some investigators have reported that bladder tumors can be safely resected at the time of transurethral resection of the prostate without conferring a significantly higher risk of tumor cell implantation into the prostatic fossa or urethra (Green and Yalowitz, 1972).

NATURAL HISTORY

Approximately 70 per cent of bladder cancers are low-grade, superficial tumors. The majority of patients develop tumor recurrences following endoscopic resection (Althausen et al., 1976; Fitzpatrick et al., 1986; Gilbert et al., 1978; Malmstrom et al., 1987). Usually, tumors that are well-differentiated and superficial at the time of initial diagnosis remain so throughout the life of the patient. Of these, about 25 per cent recur with higher-grade tumors (Gilbert et al., 1978). Most recurrences are probably new tumors arising from other areas of dysplastic urothelium, but a significant proportion may be true recurrences resulting from inadequate treatment or from tumor cell implantation (Page et al., 1978).

About 10 to 15 per cent of patients with superficial tumors subsequently develop invasive or metastatic cancer (Althausen et al., 1976; Lutzeyer et al., 1982).

Most patients (80 to 90 per cent) with invasive bladder cancer already have invasive disease at the time of initial diagnosis (Hopkins et al., 1983; Kaye and Lange, 1982). About 50 per cent of patients with muscle-invasive bladder cancer already have occult distant metastases. This limits the efficacy of local or regional forms of therapy. Most of these patients develop overt clinical evidence of distant metastases within 1 year (Babaian et al., 1980; Prout et al., 1979).

Nearly all patients with metastatic bladder cancer succumb within 2 years (Babaian et al., 1980); however, approximately 5 per cent of patients with established metastatic disease have "freak" cancers that run a more indolent clinical course, lasting 5 years or more (Marshall and McCarron, 1977). Between 10 and 35 per cent of patients with limited regional lymph node metastases survive 5 years or more without evidence of metastases following radical cystectomy and pelvic lymphadenectomy (LaPlante and Brice, 1973; Skinner and Lieskovsky, 1984; Smith and Whitmore, 1981a). It is uncertain to what extent these patients represent surgical cures of regionally metastatic bladder cancer or, simply, freak cancers. One must conclude that, at worst, patients with only limited nodal metastases have a more protracted clinical course than those with visceral or osseous metastases, and, at best, some patients with limited nodal metastases may be cured by pelvic lymphadenectomy and cystectomy. In patients with extensive nodal metastases, the prospects for cure are nil (Smith and Whitmore, 1981a). These uncertainties lead to controversy about the common policy of performing cystectomy with limited prospects for cure in patients with gross nodal metastases (approximately 10 per cent of patients coming to surgery) but not in patients with distant metastases. Many patients with incurable bladder cancer either may *not* develop severe local symptoms from the primary tumor or may have these symptoms controlled with conservative measures, such as transurethral resection or radiation therapy. It is conceivable that many such patients could retain the bladders even though they may ultimately die from metastatic bladder cancer.

Prognostic Indicators

Clinical and laboratory tests have been examined as potential means of predicting the clinical course of bladder cancer in individual patients.

Clinicopathologic Parameters in Superficial Bladder Cancer

The most clinically useful prognostic parameters for tumor recurrence and subsequent cancer progression in the patient with superficial tumors are tumor grade, depth of tumor penetration, lymphatic invasion, tumor size, urothelial dysplasia or carcinoma in situ, papillary or solid tumor configuration, multifocal tumors, frequency of tumor recurrences, and the patient's age (Fitzpatrick et al., 1986; Heney et al., 1983; Madgar et al., 1988; Wolf and Hojgaard, 1983). The most important among these are tumor grade, tumor stage, and presence of carcinoma in situ.

Tumor recurrence and progression rates are higher in patients with large (greater than 10 g) or multifocal tumors (Fitzpatrick et al., 1986), high-grade tumors (Heney et al., 1983), tumors with lamina propria invasion (Dalesio et al., 1983), those invading lymphatic spaces (Anderstrom et al., 1980), and those associated with severe urothelial dysplasia or carcinoma in situ (Althausen et al., 1976). In patients with T1, grade 3 tumors, one third exhibit cancer progression (Gilbert et al., 1978; Jakse et al., 1987).

In patients with diffuse carcinoma in situ, an important prognostic factor is the presence of irritative voiding symptoms (frequency, urgency, dysuria). For example, Riddle and co-workers (1976) reported that only one of 13 patients who were asymptomatic died of invasive bladder cancer, whereas 15 of 23 with irritative symptoms died of invasive cancer despite definitive radiation therapy or cystectomy. Another important factor is the extent of involvement with carcinoma in situ; those with only focal involvement have a more indolent course than those with diffuse involvement (Althausen et al., 1976).

Laboratory Parameters

A variety of laboratory parameters also have been evaluated for prognostic significance. Although significant correlations with tumor progression have been demonstrated, these tests have not been adopted into clinical practice to influence treatment decisions in individual patients.

THOMPSON-FRIEDENREICH (T) ANTIGEN EXPRESSION

The Thompson-Friedenreich (T) antigen is a cryptic disaccharide present on human erythrocytes, which can be exposed by neuraminidase treatment. T antigen is naturally expressed in an unmasked form on bladder cancer cells (Oda et al., 1990; Radzikowski et al., 1989). It is expressed independently of ABH blood group antigens. T antigen expression has been reported to correlate with muscle-invasive cancer and is associated with a poor prognosis (Coon et al., 1982; Javadpour, 1984). It has also been reported to be predictive of the response to treatment with BCG and interleukin-2 (Dow et al., 1989).

LECTIN-BINDING CARBOHYDRATE STRUCTURES

A decrease in lectin-binding carbohydrate structures on the surface of bladder tumor cells also has been correlated with cancer progression (Langkilde et al., 1989).

ABH BLOOD GROUP ANTIGENS

Patients with type O blood with superficial tumors have a higher incidence of high-grade tumors and cancer progression (Orihuela and Shahon, 1987).

The ABO blood group antigen system consists of carbohydrate antigens, which are carried by either glycoproteins or glycolipids on blood cells or epithelial cells. The biosynthesis of these carbohydrate antigens is presumed to be controlled by at least five different genes: ABO, Se, H, Le, and X. These genes code for specific transferase enzymes that add the respective carbohydrates to their precursors in a sequential fashion. Studies of expression of blood group antigens on bladder cancer cells suggest that, with malignant transformation, bladder cancer cells cease to express the ABH blood group antigens (Coon et al., 1982; Huben, 1984). Antigen deletion has correlated with recurrence rates and the development of invasive disease (Malmstrom et al., 1988). The best documented change has been the deletion of the A and B antigens from patients with type A and B blood, respectively, and the deletion of the H antigen from patients with type O blood (Sheinfeld et al., 1990). In general, malignant transformation appears to be associated with enhanced Lewis^x antigen expression accompanied by one or more changes in the expression of other blood group antigens (Cordon-Cardo et al., 1988). Alterations in blood group antigen expression are due to perturbations of the glycosyltransferase enzymes in the tumor cells or to the use of alternative substrates and/or competition among the transferases in the altered biosynthetic pathway (Orntoff, 1988).

ONCOFETAL PROTEIN EXPRESSION

Both carcinoembryonic antigen (Huben, 1984; Wiley et al., 1982) and human chorionic gonadotropin (Campo et al., 1989; Martin et al., 1989b) are expressed in some bladder cancers. Trophoblastic differentiation occurs in about 20 per cent of high-grade transitional cell carcinomas and is associated with poor prognosis and resistance to radiation therapy.

EPIDERMAL GROWTH FACTOR RECEPTORS

Epidermal growth factor (EGF) is a polypeptide that induces cell division in a variety of tissues. Growth factors may be important in stimulating the unrestricted growth of cancer cells. EGF receptors are similar to the *erb-b* oncogene. EGF receptors have been identified on the basal layers of normal urothelium and frequently throughout the cell layers on bladder cancer cells (Messing, 1990). Increased EGF receptors also have been found on specimens of endoscopically normal-appearing urothelium from patients with transitional cell carcinoma elsewhere in the bladder (Messing, 1990). An association has been demonstrated among EGF receptor content and tumor stage, tumor grade, and time to progression (Neal et al., 1990).

MISCELLANEOUS OTHER BIOCHEMICAL MARKERS

Other biochemical markers have been evaluated for prognostic significance in bladder cancer (Carbin et al., 1989; Carter et al., 1987; Huben, 1984; Nemoto et al., 1990; Ramaekers et al., 1985; Seymour et al., 1987; Smith et al., 1990), but definitive results are lacking.

CHROMOSOMAL ABNORMALITIES

Chromosomal abnormalities, including increased numbers of chromosomes, marker chromosomes, and chromosomes of abnormal size or position of the centromere, also have been shown to correlate with an increased risk for tumor recurrence and cancer progression (Carter et al., 1987; Falor and Ward-Skinner, 1988; Gibas and Sandberg, 1984). Tumor recurrences and cancer progression are more common among patients who have tumors with marker chromosomes and a large proportion of aneuploid tumor cell lines (Gibas and Sandberg, 1984).

Prediction of Lymph Node Metastases, Distant Metastases, and Survival

Tumor grade and depth of invasion are the most important factors in predicting the likelihood of lymph node metastases in patients with invasive bladder cancer (Kern, 1984). Nodal metastases are more common in those with anaplastic tumors and tumors with deep muscle invasion or infiltration into the perivesical fat (Kern, 1984; Prout et al., 1979). A correlation is found between lymph node metastases and the presence of distant metastases (Kern, 1984; Prout et al., 1979). However, distant metastases can occur in the absence of lymph node metastases.

Paraneoplastic Syndromes

Paraneoplastic syndromes, including hypercalcemia and leukemoid reaction, occur in patients with metastatic bladder cancer (Block and Whitmore, 1973; Michel et al., 1984) and are generally associated with a dire prognosis. These responses also have been reported in patients without metastases (Bennett et al., 1986).

Predictors of Response to Radiation Therapy

Some speculate that treatment selection might be facilitated if it were possible to identify patients with radiation-sensitive tumors. Controversial evidence suggests that papillary tumors are more responsive than solid tumors to radiation therapy (Slack and Prout, 1980), but this factor has not been confirmed in all studies (Hall and Heath, 1981; Shipley et al., 1982; Whitmore and Batata, 1985). Other studies have suggested that the presence of squamous elements and the secretion of human chorionic gonadotropin are also associated with a poor response to radiation therapy (Martin et al., 1989a, 1989b).

DIAGNOSIS

Signs and Symptoms

The most common presenting symptom of bladder cancer is painless hematuria, which occurs in about 85 per cent of patients (Varkarakis et al., 1974). The symptom complex of bladder irritability with urinary frequency, urgency, and dysuria is the second most common form of presentation and usually is associated with diffuse carcinoma in situ or invasive bladder cancer. Other signs and symptoms of bladder cancer include flank pain from ureteral obstruction, lower extremity edema, and a pelvic mass. Occasionally, patients present with symptoms of advanced disease, such as weight loss and abdominal or bone pain.

Conventional Microscopic Cytology

Malignant transitional cells can be observed on microscopic examination of the urinary sediment or bladder washings. Characteristically, tumor cells have enlarged nuclei with irregular, coarsely textured chromatin (Fig. 28–19). The limitations of microscopic cytology are due to the facts that cells from well-differentiated tumors are cytologically normal appearing and that well-differentiated cancer cells are more cohesive and are not readily shed into the urine. Therefore, microscopic cytology is more sensitive in patients with high-grade tumors. Even in patients with high-grade tumors, however, the urinary cytology may be falsely negative in 20 per cent.

False-positive cytologic findings may occur in 1 to 12 per cent of patients and are usually due to severe atypia, inflammation, or changes caused by radiation therapy or chemotherapy (Koshikawa et al., 1989). These changes are frequently observed after several months of therapy and may persist for more than 1 year after the initiation of therapy. Cytology is not a cost-effective means of screening for bladder cancer unless high-risk populations are evaluated (Gamarra and Zein, 1984).

Flow Cytometry

Flow cytometry measures the DNA content of cells; therefore, it can quantitate the aneuploid cell populations and proliferative activity (per cent S-phase cells) in a tumor. With flow cytometry, the isolated nuclei of cells stained with a DNA-binding dye flow through a small tube in which fluorescence is excited by a laser beam. DNA content is measured from fluorescent intensity. The ability to perform flow cytometry on paraffin-imbedded archival tumor tissues allows correlations to be made among flow cytometry parameters, tumor progression, and patient survival.

For diagnostic purposes, bladder wash specimens usually are required for satisfactory results (Konchuba et al., 1989). Arbitrary limits are required to define normalcy. For example, if more than 15 per cent of the cells are aneuploid, the cytologic findings are defined as being positive for cancer (Melamed, 1984).

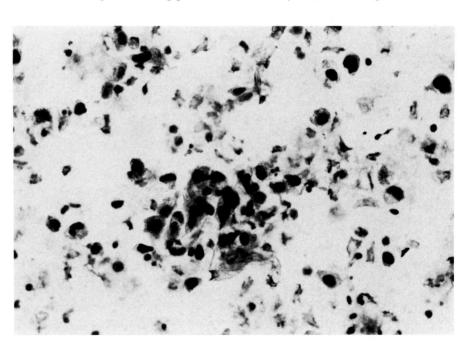

Figure 28–19. Urinary cytologic preparation showing many neoplastic cells. (Courtesy of Louis P. Dehner, M.D.)

Flow cytometry studies in bladder cancer patients have demonstrated several clinical correlations (Atallah et al., 1990; Badalament et al., 1990; Blomjous et al., 1989; Tribukait, 1987; Wijkstrom and Tribukait, 1990). Diploid tumors generally tend to be low-grade and low-stage, and patients have a favorable prognosis. Tumors with a triploid to tetraploid chromosome number have unfavorable pathologic characteristics, and patients have a poor prognosis. Patients with tumors that are tetraploid or have a greater than tetraploid chromosome number have a more favorable prognosis than triploid to tetraploid tumors but a worse prognosis than patients with diploid tumors (Tribukait, 1987; Wijkstrom and Tribukait, 1990; Winkler et al., 1989). Inflammatory cells can form a hyperdiploid cell fraction, which makes interpretation of standard flow cytometry difficult.

A correlation exists between proliferative activity, expressed as the percentage of tumor cells in the DNA synthesizing (S) phase, and tumor progression. An increased incidence of lymph node metastases occurs in patients with aneuploid tumors and in patients with tumors that have greater than 10 per cent S-phase cells. Tumors with more than one aneuploid cell population also have a higher cancer progression rate. In patients treated with radiation, the presence or persistence of triploid to tetraploid cell lines is an unfavorable prognostic indicator. In contrast, patients who have tumor cells following radiation therapy that have diploid, tetraploid, or polyploid chromosome complements have a more favorable response to radiation therapy.

Flow cytometry can measure multiple parameters simultaneously. For example, cells can be stained for DNA and cytokeratins (a marker for epithelial cells). The flow cytometer can be programmed to measure DNA content only in cells that stain positive for cytokeratins (Hijazi et al., 1989). This multiparameter approach improves the accuracy of flow cytometry because it is possible to determine not only the overall proliferative activity in a tumor but actually to measure which cells are proliferating. Current studies have exploited this type of approach and appear to demonstrate more prognostic significance than either DNA measurements alone or antigen expression measurements alone (Fradet et al., 1990). Flow cytometry also has been used to study the expression of blood group antigens and ploidy in the same tumor cells. With the technique of double labeling, changes in expression of blood group antigens during the cell cycle can be monitored (Burk and Drewinko, 1976; Vuvenoc et al., 1985).

In general, flow cytometry has not been found clinically to be more valuable than conventional cytology, although some studies have reported that it is more accurate (Denovic et al., 1982). Low-grade superficial tumors, which are usually diploid, often produce false-negative results. Aneuploidy is a common feature of high-grade tumors. Flow cytometry is especially accurate in patients with carcinoma in situ, in whom approximately 90 per cent of tumors can be correctly identified (Badalament et al., 1988; Melamed, 1984). Flow cytometry has not supplanted conventional cytology in managing bladder cancer patients. Where it is readily available, it may be an adjunct in the diagnosis of bladder

cancer, measuring the hyperdiploid cell fraction (Badalament et al., 1990). A major drawback of flow cytometry is its expense.

For predicting the likelihood of tumor progression, flow cytometry is limited because a significant proportion of bladder cancers that progress are diploid or near-diploid, and some superficial tumors that do not progress are aneuploid (Tribukait et al., 1982).

Quantitative Fluorescent Image Analysis

Quantitative fluorescent image analysis is a cytologic technique that analyzes smears on a microscope slide to quantitatively measure DNA content in the cell (Carter et al., 1987). It combines quantitative biochemical analysis and a more subjective visual evaluation of individual cells.

This technique utilizes a computer-controlled fluorescence microscope, which automatically scans and images the nucleus of each cell on a slide. The computer quantitates the amount of emitted fluorescence, which is directly proportional to the nucleic acid content, and identifies each cell that contains an abnormal amount of DNA. Thus, a cytotechnologist can focus on each abnormal cell identified in an automated analysis for morphologic evaluation. Quantitative fluorescence image analysis identifies individual cells and, thus, differs from flow cytometry, which identifies cell populations. A large number of cells are required for flow cytometry analysis, which generally requires bladder wash specimens. In contrast, quantitative fluorescence image analysis can be done with voided urine samples.

Quantitative fluorescence image analysis has been suggested as a potentially cost-effective test for screening high-risk patient groups. Specific monoclonal antibodies may serve to further increase the specificity of quantitative fluorescence image analysis for bladder cancer detection. This type of analysis also may serve as a means of monitoring treatment response. The drawback to this technique is that it requires expensive equipment. Parry and Hemstreet (1988) reported that quantitative fluorescence image analysis was more sensitive (76 versus 33 per cent) for the detection of low-grade bladder cancer than conventional cytology. It also was of comparable specificity (94 versus 96.7 per cent).

Specimen Collection

Saline bladder washings are more accurate than voided urine samples for detecting bladder cancer because the mechanical action of barbotage enhances tumor cell shedding and provides better preserved cells for examination (Trott and Edwards, 1973). In urine that has remained in the bladder for prolonged periods, cellular degeneration occurs. Therefore, first-voided morning specimens should not be sampled for cytology. Urinary tract infection, indwelling catheters, calculi, or bladder instrumentation can also produce artifactual changes in urinary cytology (Gamarra and Zein, 1984). If sheets of transitional cells are sheared off by one of these processes, the cell fragments, which can resemble papillary fragments of transitional cell carcinomas, may be mistaken for tumor fragments.

Osmotic changes from contrast media also may cause minor difficulties in interpreting cytologic preparations. Similarly, radiation therapy, intravesical chemotherapy, and intravesical BCG therapy can induce confusing abnormalities.

Some clinicians do not routinely employ urinary cytology because of its inherent inaccuracy; however, it is not unusual for a patient with a low-grade papillary tumor also to have occult high-grade carcinoma in situ either in the bladder or elsewhere in the urinary tract. In some cases, the urinary cytology may provide the only clue to the presence of carcinoma in situ.

Excretory Urography

Excretory urography is indicated in all patients with signs and symptoms suggestive of bladder cancer. Urography is not a sensitive means of detecting bladder tumors, particularly small ones. However, it is useful in screening the upper urinary tracts for associated urothelial tumors. Large bladder tumors may appear as filling defects in the bladder on the cystogram phase of the urogram (Fig. 28–20). Ureteral obstruction caused by a bladder tumor usually is a sign of a muscle-invasive cancer.

Cystoscopy

All patients suspected of having bladder cancer should have careful cystoscopy and bimanual examination. Abnormal areas should be biopsied. Random or selected site mucosal biopsy specimens also may be obtained. Retrograde pyelography also should be performed if the upper urinary tracts are not adequately visualized on the excretory urogram. If an upper urinary tract lesion is seen, a retrograde ureteropyelogram obtaining urine samples for cytologies or brush biopsies should be performed (see the section on upper tract urothelial tumors).

Resection of Bladder Tumors

The ideal method for resecting a bladder tumor is first to resect the superficial portion of the tumor, sending it to the pathologist as a separate specimen. Then, the deep portion along with some underlying bladder muscle is resected and sent as a separate specimen for histologic examination. After the tumor has been completely resected, the base of the resection site is fulgurated. This approach usually provides for complete removal of the tumor and valuable diagnostic information about the grade and depth of infiltration of the tumor. Soloway (1983) has suggested that resecting low-grade superficial tumors into the muscle layer may be unnecessary and unwise because tumor recurrence resulting from implantation would then appear to be muscle invasive, which would mandate aggressive therapy.

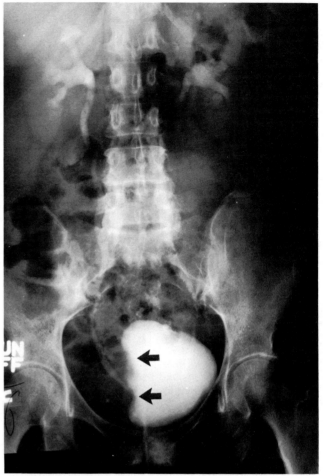

Figure 28–20. Excretory urography in bladder cancer.

It is not always necessary to perform a formal resection of superficial low-grade papillary tumors, particularly those that may be difficult to reach with a resectoscope. It is acceptable to treat these tumors with simple fulguration. The obvious disadvantage of fulguration is that it does not provide tissue for histologic documentation of tumor grade and stage. Laser therapy also has been utilized for destroying bladder tumors in this clinical setting.

It is not always necessary to attempt complete tumor resections in patients with very extensive broad-based sessile tumors, which are almost certain to require cystectomy, particularly if a tumor is located in an area that is difficult to reach with a resectoscope. Attempts at complete resection may result in bladder perforation with dissemination of tumor cells. In such cases, it may be more prudent to begin resecting at the margin of tumor and progress toward its center, resecting only enough tissue to establish the tumor grade and document the presence of muscle invasion. If this approach is taken, it is best accomplished with frozen section documentation of the adequacy of the biopsy specimens.

Tumors encroaching on the ureteral orifices should be resected without regard to the orifice. However, it is important not to fulgurate the orifice after the tumor has been resected. When the ureteral orifice is resected, a stent may be left in place for several days to prevent obstruction of the orifice by scar tissue. Some investigators have advocated passing a ureteral catheter first and then resecting around the catheter; however, the ureteral catheter may prevent adequate tumor resection.

Tumors on the lateral bladder wall may induce stimulation of the obturator nerve during resection, resulting in violent contraction of the adductor muscles of the leg. Resections of such tumors should be performed with the patient under general anesthesia with simultaneous intravenous administration of pancuronium to adequately paralyze the patient and minimize the risk of inadvertent bladder perforation associated with adductor muscle spasm.

Tumors arising in bladder diverticula should be biopsied rather than resected. Patients with tumors in a diverticulum are best treated definitively with either partial or total cystectomy. Transurethral resection should not be attempted because of the high risk of bladder perforation.

Selected Site Mucosal Biopsies

Selected site mucosal biopsies from areas adjacent to the tumor as well as from the opposite bladder wall, bladder dome, trigone, and prostatic urethra have been recommended at the time of resection of the primary tumor. They provide important prognostic information about the likelihood of tumor recurrence. About 20 to 25 per cent of patients are found to have dysplasia or carcinoma in situ (Althausen et al., 1976; Vincente-Rodriguez et al., 1987). Between 30 and 70 per cent of muscle-invasive bladder cancers are associated with carcinoma in situ. In comparison, some investigators believe that selected site mucosal biopsies are unnecessary and even potentially hazardous because they denude the urothelium and may create fertile areas for tumor cell implantation. Some believe that urinary cytology is a better indicator of the presence of concurrent carcinoma in situ (Harving et al., 1988).

Vital Staining of the Bladder

A variety of agents have been used for vital staining of the bladder mucosa as a means of detecting subclinical areas of bladder cancer. These agents include tetracycline, hematoporphyrins, acridine orange, and methylene blue. These staining methods generally are not selected because of their lack of sensitivity and specificity of staining (Benson et al., 1982; Fukui et al., 1983).

STAGING

Because tumor stage is important in determining therapy, accurate staging of bladder cancer is desirable. Nevertheless, there are considerable staging errors in bladder cancer. Understaging occurs most frequently in patients with high-grade and intermediate-stage tumors of whom approximately one third are understaged; 10 per cent are overstaged (Wijkstrom et al., 1984).

Goals of Staging

Superficial Versus Infiltrating Tumor

The first treatment decision based on tumor stage is whether the patient has a superficial or invasive tumor. If it is a superficial tumor, more elaborate staging techniques, such as bone scan, computed tomography (CT), and so forth are not indicated. Such techniques are reserved for patients with documented muscle-invasive bladder cancer.

The primary transurethral resection of the tumor is the most important test for judging the depth of penetration of the tumor. Variation occurs in the interpretation of histology sections between different pathologists in assessing the tumor grade and depth of infiltration. Part of the reason for these discrepancies is related to the smooth muscle fibers of the tunica muscularis mucosa in the lamina propria of the bladder wall, which may be confused with the detrusor muscle (Abel et al., 1988a, 1988b). In addition, bimanual physical examination provides limited information about whether there is infiltration of the bladder wall. In this regard, if the tumor is palpable on bimanual examination, it is usually infiltrating into the bladder muscle or perivesical tissues.

Localized Versus Extensive or Metastatic Tumor

The second treatment decision made on the basis of staging is to identify patients with invasive tumors who may benefit from aggressive, potentially curative therapy. For this purpose, CT scanning, ultrasonography, and magnetic resonance imaging (MRI) have been used to evaluate the local extent of bladder tumors. These staging studies may provide valuable information but are inaccurate in determining the presence or absence of microscopic muscle invasion and minimal extravesical tumor spread (Koss et al., 1981). Moreover, postoperative changes produced by the transurethral resection of the primary tumor as well as postradiation therapy or postchemotherapy fibrosis also may cause difficulties in interpreting CT, MRI, and ultrasound scans.

Staging Tests

Computed Tomography Scan

In addition to assessing the extent of the primary tumor, CT scanning also provides information about the presence of pelvic and para-aortic lymphadenopathy and the possible presence of liver or adrenal metastases (Lantz and Hattery, 1984). To accurately assess the depth of penetration, CT scanning should be done prior to transurethral resection because artifacts introduced by the resection may be confusing (Husband et al., 1989) (Fig. 28–21). Contrast-enhanced CT scanning improves the accuracy of staging (Sager et al., 1987). CT scanning is limited in accuracy because it can detect only gross extravesical tumor extension, lymph nodes that

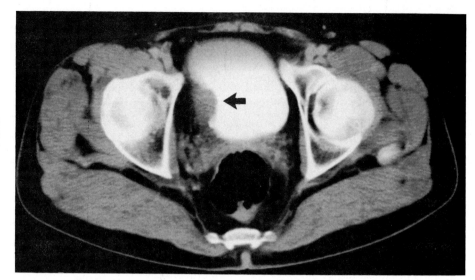

Figure 28–21. Computed tomographic scan of the pelvis showing an invasive bladder tumor infiltrating the posterior bladder wall.

are grossly enlarged, and liver metastases that are larger than 2 cm in diameter (Nurmi et al., 1988; Voges et al., 1989). Enlargement of the lymph nodes does not always indicate metastatic disease. Furthermore, hepatic lesions, such as cavernous hemangiomas, may be confused with liver metastases unless dynamic scanning is performed following injection of contrast material. CT scans fail to detect nodal metastases in up to 40 per cent of patients having them (Lantz and Hattery, 1984). Some workers have questioned the practical utility of using CT scanning for local staging of bladder cancer (Nishimura et al., 1988).

Magnetic Resonance Imaging Scan

MRI scanning is not much more helpful than CT scanning. With few exceptions (Johnson et al., 1990),

the resolution of the pelvic and abdominal anatomy with MRI has not been reported to be as good as that with CT scanning (Buy et al., 1988; Husband et al., 1989; Tavares et al., 1990; Wood et al., 1988) (Fig. 28–22). A double-surface coil may allow more accurate MRI staging of bladder cancer patients than a conventional coil MRI (Barentsz et al., 1988). With MRI, the possibility of multiplane imaging theoretically should provide better visualization of the anatomy. Soft tissue contrast may be enhanced by using paramagnetic contrast agents, such as gadolinium-diethylene–triaminepenta-acetic acid complex (Gd-DTPA) (Sohn et al., 1990). MRI spectroscopy in the future also may have the capacity to provide information about the physiologic states of different tissues, but this possibility has not yet been realized. Both CT and MRI scanning are more accurate in very advanced tumors (Vock et al., 1982).

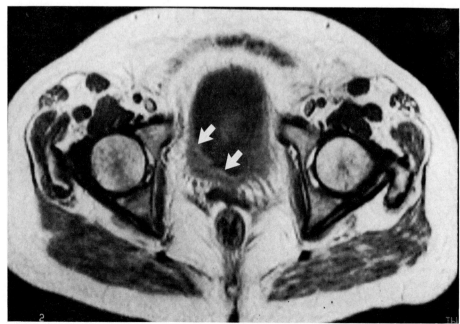

Figure 28–22. Magnetic resonance imaging scan of the pelvis demonstrating an invasive bladder cancer infiltrating the posterior bladder wall. (Courtesy of J. K. T. Lee, M.D.)

Ultrasonography

Abdominal and transurethral ultrasonography have been evaluated with limited success in the assessment of the local extent of bladder cancer, but they have not been adopted in general use (Holm et al., 1988; Lantz and Hattery, 1984; Nakamura and Nijima, 1980).

Lymphangiography

Lymphangiography can provide information about the internal architecture of the external iliac lymph nodes and, therefore, theoretically may detect metastases in nodes that are not grossly enlarged (Gibod et al., 1984; Lantz and Hattery, 1984). However, with few exceptions, pelvic lymphangiography is not superior to CT scanning in detecting regional lymph node metastases (Farah and Cerney, 1978). Lymphangiography is associated with more discomfort and morbidity than CT scanning and can identify only about 50 to 60 per cent of patients with lymph node metastases. False-negative findings are more common than false-positive findings. At most medical centers, lymphangiography has been abandoned in the routine staging of invasive bladder cancer. Both lymphangiography and CT scanning can be used in conjunction with fine-needle aspiration biopsy of pelvic lymph nodes to establish—but not to exclude—the presence of pelvic lymph node metastases (Gibod et al., 1984).

Lymphadenectomy

Pelvic lymphadenectomy is the most accurate means of staging bladder cancer patients for regional lymph node involvement. Some patients having only limited nodal metastases below the bifurcation of the common iliac arteries and without invasion of adjacent organs may be cured by pelvic lymphadenectomy (LaPlante and Brice, 1973; Skinner, 1982). The primary regions of lymphatic drainage of the bladder are the perivesical, hypogastric, obturator, external iliac, and presacral lymph nodes. The common iliac, inguinal, and para-aortic lymph nodes are juxtaregional nodes for bladder cancer.

Lymphadenectomy usually is performed in conjunction with cystectomy rather than as an independent staging procedure. Fine-needle aspiration biopsy of enlarged lymph nodes under CT guidance may be performed to document incurable lymph node metastases. In the future, laparoscopic lymphadenectomy may have a role in selected high-risk patients.

The standard staging lymphadenectomy for bladder cancer includes removal of the nodes from the iliac bifurcations to the femoral canals and from the genito-femoral nerves to the bladder pedicles. Some clinicians have routinely performed a more extensive node dissection, including nodes as high as the aortic bifurcation, whereas others have elected not to perform pelvic lymphadenectomy in patients with bladder cancer. The incidence of lymph node involvement correlates with the stage and grade of the tumor, ranging from 10 per cent in noninvasive tumors to 40 per cent in high-grade,

deeply infiltrating tumors. The potential therapeutic benefit of pelvic lymphadenectomy may be assessed as follows. Of the 10 to 40 per cent of patients with lymph node metastases who come to cystectomy, between 35 and 70 per cent have only limited metastases (one or two nodes below the iliac bifurcations), and 10 to 35 per cent of the latter patients may be cured with cystectomy and pelvic lymphadenectomy. Accordingly, the routine performance of pelvic lymphadenectomy may increase the surgical cure rate by 1 to 10 per cent. Thus, in high-risk or elderly patients, lymphadenectomy may be omitted without substantially altering the ultimate prospects for cure.

Chest Radiograph and Chest Computed Tomography Scan

A metastatic evaluation to rule out distant metastases should be performed before proceeding to pelvic lymphadenectomy. The most sensitive means of detecting pulmonary metastases is a chest CT scan; however, CT scans frequently detect small, noncalcified pulmonary lesions, most of which are granulomas. There is a direct correlation between the size of a pulmonary lesion and the likelihood of its being a metastasis. Most noncalcified lesions that are 1 cm or larger are metastases. Because standard chest films do not have sufficient resolution to demonstrate small granulomas, but rather detect only lesions larger than 1 cm in diameter, routine chest radiographs with or without tomography usually are relied upon to rule out pulmonary metastases in bladder cancer patients.

Bone and Liver-Spleen Scans

Bone and liver-spleen scans seldom reveal metastatic disease in patients with normal liver function tests, especially if the alkaline phosphatase level is normal (Berger et al., 1981; Brismar and Gustafson, 1988). CT scans are more accurate than liver-spleen scans in detecting liver metastases. Accordingly, liver-spleen scans are not a necessary part of the routine metastatic evaluation of bladder cancer patients, and bone scans are not necessary in patients who have normal alkaline phosphatase levels. A bone scan may be useful, however, as a baseline for future reference. Thus, the recommended metastatic evaluation for patients with invasive bladder cancer includes chest radiography, excretory urogram, abdominopelvic CT scan, bone scan, and liver function tests. If any of these suggest the presence of metastases, histologic confirmation should be sought by the least invasive means possible, usually fine-needle aspiration biopsy.

Staging Systems

Two main staging systems for bladder cancer are currently in use. In the United States, most urologists choose the Jewett-Strong (1946) system as modified by Marshall (1952). The other staging system was developed jointly by the International Union Against Cancer

(UICC) and the American Joint Committee on Cancer Staging (AJC) (Hermanek and Sobin, 1987).

Jewett-Strong-Marshall System

The Jewett-Strong-Marshall system categorizes noninvasive bladder cancers, including papillary noninvasive tumors and carcinoma in situ, as stage 0. In the AJC-UICC system, they are classified as Ta and Tis, respectively. Tumors that have invaded the submucosa are classified in the Jewett-Strong-Marshall system as stage A, whereas in the AJC-UICC system, they are classified as T1. Muscle-invasive tumors are classified in the Jewett-Strong-Marshall system as stage B1 and B2, depending on whether there is superficial or deep muscle invasion. These tumors are classified in the AJC-UICC system as T2 and T3a, respectively. Tumors that have invaded into the perivesical fat are classified as stage C in the Jewett-Strong-Marshall system and as T3b in the AJC-UICC system. Tumors invading the pelvic viscera or regional lymph nodes are classified as stage D1 in the Jewett-Strong-Marshall classification. The AJC-UICC system designates them as stage T4 if they invade the viscera and as N-positive if they invade the lymph nodes. In the AJC-UICC system, the regional lymph nodes for bladder cancer are considered to be the nodes of the true pelvis that lie below the bifurcation of the common iliac arteries. Laterality does not affect the N classification. N1 denotes a single positive node less than or equal to 2 cm in diameter. N2 denotes a single positive node greater than 2 cm but less than 5 cm in diameter, or multiple positive nodes less than 5 cm in diameter. N3 denotes positive nodes greater than 5 cm in diameter. The Jewett-Strong-Marshall classification considers patients having juxtaregional lymph node metastases or distant metastases as stage D2. The AJC-UICC system considers patients without distant metastases as M0 and those with distant metastases as M1. These staging systems are illustrated in Table 28–3.

MANAGEMENT OF SUPERFICIAL BLADDER CANCER (STAGES 0 AND A)

Transurethral Resection or Fulguration

Most patients with superficial bladder cancer can be adequately treated with transurethral resection or fulguration of the tumor. The overall survival rate for these patients is excellent (approximately 70 per cent 5-year survival) (Barnes et al., 1967; Nichols and Marshall, 1956). About 10 to 15 per cent of these patients ultimately require more aggressive therapy.

The incidence of subsequent muscle-invasive tumors is low in patients initially having mucosa-confined tumors but may be as high as 46 per cent in patients initially having submucosal involvement. Accordingly, patients with stage T1 tumors should be considered as having potentially aggressive tumors, particularly if they are high-grade (Abel et al., 1988a).

Table 28–3. STAGING SYSTEMS FOR BLADDER CANCER

Finding	Jewett-Strong-Marshall Stage	1987 UICC Stage
No tumor in the specimen	0	T0
Carcinoma in situ	0	Tis
Noninvasive papillary tumor	0	Ta
Submucosal invasion	A	T1
Superficial muscle invasion	B1	T2
Deep muscle invasion	B2	T3A
Invasion of perivesical fat	C	T3B
Invasion of contiguous organ	D1	T4
Regional lymph node metastases	D1	(N1–3)
Juxtaregional lymph node metastases	D2	—
Distant metastases	D2	M1

Follow-Up Cystoscopy and Urography

The traditional follow-up program recommended for patients with superficial bladder cancer includes serial cystoscopies every 3 months for 2 years, then every 6 months for 2 years, and then yearly. Either annual or biennial excretory urograms usually have been recommended. Some investigators believe that patients with low-grade tumors do not need cystoscopy as frequently (Kent et al., 1989) but rather should be followed with urinary cytology and cystoscopy less frequently. In this regard, it is advisable to obtain a postresection urinary cytology examination to ensure that complete tumor resection has been accomplished. Similarly, some investigators believe that routine monitoring of the upper urinary tracts is not necessary. Approximately 2 to 5 per cent of patients with bladder cancer subsequently develop upper tract tumors (Zincke et al., 1984). Not all of these tumors produce hematuria or positive cytologic findings (Smith et al., 1989). The mean interval to development of upper urinary tract tumors is approximately 70 months (Oldbring et al., 1989; Shinka et al., 1988; Smith et al., 1989).

Follow-up cystoscopy can be readily performed as an office procedure. The flexible cystoscope has greatly facilitated patient surveillance. A small proportion of tumors in the range of 2 mm may be overlooked when using flexible cystoscopy (Meyhoff et al., 1988), but with experience, flexible cystoscopy is nearly as accurate as rigid cystoscopy.

Adjuvant and Miscellaneous Therapies

A variety of treatments have been employed as adjuvant therapy in patients with superficial bladder cancer to prevent the recurrence and progression of the cancer. These include intravesical chemotherapy; systemic chemotherapy; intravesical immunotherapy with interferon, BCG, and other agents; photoradiation therapy; laser therapy; and vitamin therapy. Other treatments such as radiation, hyperthermia, and hydrostatic pressure have been tested but have not been adopted for general use.

Radiation Therapy for Superficial Bladder Cancer

Radiation therapy is not effective in the treatment of superficial bladder cancer. It does not prevent the occurrence of new tumors (Goffinet et al., 1975) and may be associated with considerable morbidity, particularly radiation cystitis. Interstitial radiation therapy has been used to treat superficial tumors in Europe (van der Werf-Messing, 1984). Radon seeds, [198]Au seeds, and tantalum wire have been used for interstital radiation therapy. Intracavitary radiation therapy utilizing a radium capsule in a catheter (Hewett et al., 1981) and intraoperative electron-beam therapy combined with conventional fractionated external-beam radiation therapy (Martinez and Gunderson, 1984; Matsumoto et al., 1981) are reported to be effective for superficial bladder cancer. However, experience with these treatments is limited, and they have not been widely accepted.

Cystectomy for Superficial Bladder Cancer

Total cystectomy is rarely required for patients with superficial bladder cancer except for those with symptomatic, diffuse, unresectable papillary tumors or carcinoma in situ that does not respond to intravesical therapy (Matthews et al., 1984). In appropriately selected patients, survival rates are favorable. Bracken and associates (1981a) reported that patients treated with cystectomy for stages Ta and T1 bladder cancer had survival rates comparable to those in the age-matched normal population. Preoperative radiation therapy has not been claimed to enhance survival in patients with superficial bladder cancer.

Adjuvant Intravesical Therapy

Either adjuvant intravesical chemotherapy or intravesical immunotherapy is indicated in patients who are at a high risk for tumor recurrence by virtue of having recurrent tumors, multiple tumors, high-grade tumors associated with urothelial atypia, or carcinoma in situ (Rubben et al., 1988). Thiotepa and BCG are the least expensive intravesical agents available. Doxorubicin has an intermediate cost. Mitomycin C is the most expensive. BCG currently appears to be the most effective agent for intravesical use, but the optimum strain, dose schedule, and route of administration have not been determined. Patients who fail treatment with one intravesical agent may be managed successfully with a different agent.

There is a low incidence of developing a secondary hematologic malignancy after intravesical chemotherapy with thiotepa or mitomycin (Sonneveld et al., 1990).

Triethylenethiophosphoramide (Thiotepa)

Modern intravesical chemotherapy began in the 1960s with introduction of intravesical thiotepa (Jones and Swinney, 1961). Before thiotepa, other agents used were silver nitrate, trichloroacetic acid, and podophyllin. Thiotepa is an alkylating agent that acts by cross-linking nucleic acids and proteins. Commonly administered doses are 1 mg/1ml instilled directly into the bladder and retained for 2 hours. Often, it is administered in doses of 30 mg in 30 ml of saline or 60 mg in 60 ml of saline. A frequently recommended regimen includes 6 to 8 weekly treatments followed by monthly treatments for 1 year. Thiotepa produces complete tumor remissions in approximately 35 per cent of patients and partial remissions in approximately 25 per cent (Koontz et al., 1981). Thiotepa also has been used for prophylaxis against tumor recurrence following complete resection of all visible tumor (Zincke et al., 1983). Thiotepa in doses of 30 or 60 mg given monthly following transurethral resection of a bladder tumor has been shown to reduce the tumor recurrence rate to 47 per cent at 2 years compared with a 73 per cent recurrence rate in patients not receiving prophylaxis. This benefit was observed largely in patients with grade 1 tumors (Prout et al., 1983). In this study, 16 per cent of patients receiving thiotepa prophylaxis had tumor progression, 8 per cent developed muscle-invasive disease, and 3 per cent developed distant metastases. Thiotepa is less valuable for treatment of carcinoma in situ (Koontz et al., 1981). In a prospective, randomized trial, thiotepa was shown to be less effective than BCG in the treatment of superficial bladder cancer (Brosman, 1982).

Thiotepa is readily absorbed through the urothelium because of its relatively low molecular weight (198 daltons), and it causes myelosuppression in 15 to 20 per cent of patients. White blood cell and platelet counts should be obtained before each thiotepa treatment. Some workers have advocated the administration of thiotepa immediately after tumor resection (Soloway, 1983), but there are insufficient data to determine the optimum time course of thiotepa therapy.

Etoglucid (Epodyl)

Etoglucid is available in Europe but is not available in the United States. It is an alkylating agent similar to thiotepa with a slightly higher molecular weight (262 daltons). Accordingly, it is not as readily absorbed through the urothelium and causes myelosuppression less frequently than thiotepa. It is administered in a 1 per cent solution weekly for 12 weeks and then monthly thereafter. Etoglucid causes more severe chemical cystitis than thiotepa. Complete responses occur in approximately 45 per cent of patients, and partial responses occur in approximately 35 per cent (Lamm, 1983; Robinson et al., 1977). Etoglucid was reported in a randomized trial to be more effective than transurethral resection alone or intravesical doxorubicin in preventing tumor recurrences in patients with primary bladder cancers but not in those with recurrent superficial tumors (Kurth et al., 1984). It also has been helpful in treating upper urinary tract superficial tumors (Mathiasen et al., 1988).

Mitomycin C

Mitomycin C is an antibiotic chemotherapeutic agent that acts by inhibition of DNA synthesis. It has a higher molecular weight than thiotepa or etoglucid (334 daltons) and, therefore, causes fewer problems with transurothelial absorption. Less than 1 per cent of instilled mitomycin is absorbed (van Helsdingen et al., 1988). Mitomycin C is effective as primary treatment of previously untreated bladder tumors and has been shown to be effective in patients who have failed prior treatment with thiotepa (Issell et al., 1984; Prout et al., 1982; Stricker et al., 1987). Mitomycin C is usually administered in a dose of 40 mg intravesically weekly for 8 weeks followed by monthly maintenance therapy for 1 year. Complete tumor responses occur in about 40 per cent of patients, and partial responses occur in up to another 40 per cent (Issell et al., 1984; Lamm, 1983; Prout et al., 1982). Mitomycin is reported to be more effective in the treatment of high-grade tumors (Soloway, 1984). Soloway (1984) reported that 8 per cent of complete responders, 23 per cent of partial responders, and 19 per cent of nonresponders developed muscle-invasive cancer, and 7 per cent died of metastatic bladder cancer. Similar results were reported by Hellsten and co-workers (1990). The side effects of mitomycin C include chemical cystitis (10 to 15 per cent) that may lead to bladder contraction and genital skin rashes (5 to 15 per cent).

Mitomycin C has been reported to prevent the development of invasive bladder cancer in a controversial prospective clinical trial (Huland et al., 1984). In this study, all patients had complete tumor excision and negative cytologic findings before mitomycin C treatment, thus excluding patients with multifocal disease. Moreover, 50 per cent were treated for a solitary primary tumor, and only 29 per cent had high-grade tumors. Other studies (Denovic et al., 1983; Lockhart et al., 1983) of mitomycin C prophylaxis in patients with multiple, recurrent, and high-grade tumors have not confirmed this low recurrence rate.

Doxorubicin (Adriamycin)

Doxorubicin also is an antibiotic chemotherapeutic agent. Because of its high molecular weight (580 daltons), it is minimally absorbed. A variety of dose schedules have been followed in the treatment of superficial bladder cancer. A minimal dose of 50 mg should be given for intravesical therapy. Treatment schedules have ranged from as often as three times per week to as infrequently as monthly. Complete responses occur in less than one half of patients, and partial responses occur in approximately one third. No significant differences in the response rates of patients with low-grade and high-grade tumors have been reported (Lundbeck et al., 1983, 1988).

When used for prophylaxis against tumor recurrence, doxorubicin in doses of 60 to 90 mg at intervals ranging from every 3 weeks to every 3 months has yielded mixed results. Garnick and colleagues (1984) reported a 47 per cent recurrence rate within 18 months and a 16 per cent incidence of subsequent muscle invasion. Zincke and associates (1983) reported a 31 per cent recurrence rate in patients treated with doxorubicin as compared with 30 per cent in those treated with thiotepa and 71 per cent in patients treated with placebo. Nijima and co-workers (1983) reported that doxorubicin was proportionately better than mitomycin C when given for prophylaxis against tumor recurrence. Kurth and associates (1984) reported that doxorubicin was effective in patients with recurrent tumors but was not significantly effective in reducing recurrence rates in patients with primary bladder tumors.

In the large, multi-institutional Southwest Oncology Clinical Group trial, doxorubicin was shown to be significantly less effective than intravesical BCG in the treatment of patients with carcinoma in situ and for prophylaxis against tumor recurrence (Mori et al., 1988).

The side effects of doxorubicin include chemical cystitis, which is severe in many patients and may progress to permanent bladder contracture in a small percentage (Kondas et al., 1988).

Comparison of Intravesical Chemotherapeutic Agents

All agents for intravesical chemotherapy are about equally effective (Newling, 1990). The possible exception reported is that mitomycin may be marginally superior to thiotepa in the treatment of patients with stage Ta tumors (Heney et al., 1988). The complete response rates for intravesical chemotherapeutic agents range from 33 to 57 per cent when administered for the treatment of residual papillary tumors and from 55 to 66 per cent when administered for the treatment of carcinoma in situ. When used as prophylaxis against tumor recurrence, the recurrence rates are reduced to 30 to 44 per cent compared with about 70 per cent in controls.

Combination intravesical chemotherapy with both mitomycin C and doxorubicin was no more effective than either drug alone for prophylaxis against tumor recurrence (Ferraris, 1988; Fukui et al., 1989). No conclusive evidence demonstrates that intravesical chemotherapy has a significant impact on the incidence of muscle-invasive recurrences or ultimate cancer death rates.

Systemic Chemotherapy for Superficial Bladder Cancer

Systemic chemotherapy with methotrexate (Hall and Heath, 1981), cyclophosphamide (England et al., 1981; Jenkins et al., 1988b), and cisplatin (Needles et al., 1982) has been evaluated as a means of controlling superficial bladder cancer. Although each of these agents is somewhat effective, the attendant side effects of systemic chemotherapy discourage its routine use in most patients with superficial bladder cancer. Moreover, systemic chemotherapy is not effective against carcinoma in situ.

Vitamin and Dietary Therapy

The vitamins, pyridoxine (Byar and Blackhard, 1977; Studer et al., 1984), vitamin C (Schlegel et al., 1969), and vitamin A analogues (retinoids) (Alfthan et al., 1983; Studer et al., 1984) have been given for prophylaxis against bladder cancer recurrences. They are of marginal efficacy. Retinoids cause severe dryness of mucous membranes.

Selenium also has been reported to be effective in the prevention of bladder cancer (Helzlsouer et al., 1989).

Intravesical Bacillus Calmette-Guérin Therapy

BCG is an attenuated strain of *Mycobacterium bovis* that has stimulatory effects on immune responses. BCG has been administered intravesically to treat superficial bladder cancer and has emerged as the most effective intravesical agent for this purpose (Catalona and Ratliff, 1990; Martinez-Pineiro et al., 1990). Morales and co-workers (1976) first administered BCG to humans, using the Armand Frappier strain both intravesically (120 mg in 50 ml of saline) and intradermally (5 mg with a Heaf gun) weekly for 6 weeks. Most subsequent clinical trials have verified the effectiveness of BCG therapy (reviewed by Catalona and Ratliff, 1990). BCG is commonly given in three clinical settings: (1) prophylaxis in tumor-free patients, (2) treatment of residual tumor in patients with papillary transitional cell carcinoma other than carcinoma in situ, and (3) treatment of patients with carcinoma in situ.

Several strains of BCG have been used, including the Pasteur, Armand Frappier, Tice, Connaught, Glaxo (Evans), Tokyo, Dutch (RIVM), and Moreau. All are derived from the original strain developed at the Pasteur Institute. Some doubt exists about the efficacy of the Glaxo and Dutch strains. The viability and density of BCG organisms per milligram of vaccine may vary with the strain and from lot to lot within the same strain (Cummings et al., 1989; Kelley et al., 1985). In addition to intravesical instillation, BCG has been administered with intradermal boosters and has been administered orally. All routes of administration have been reported to be effective, but it appears that intradermal immunization is unnecessary. Studies do not confirm the effectiveness of oral BCG (Lamm et al., 1990). Intralesional injections of BCG may be associated with severe anaphylactic toxic side effects (Martinez-Pineiro and Muntanola, 1977).

Prospective, randomized trials have shown that BCG is effective for prophylaxis against tumor recurrence (Brosman, 1982; Lamm et al., 1980; Pinsky et al., 1982). Lamm and co-workers (1980) reported that BCG reduced tumor recurrence rates from 42 per cent in patients treated with transurethral resection alone to 17 per cent in BCG-treated patients (mean follow-up, 15 months). BCG also is effective in the treatment of patients who have not responded to intravesical thiotepa treatment (Brosman, 1982, 1984; Netto and Lemos, 1983; Schellhammer et al., 1986).

Brosman (1982) and Netto and Lemos (1983) conducted randomized trials comparing BCG with thiotepa for prophylaxis. The recurrence rates with BCG were less than 10 per cent (mean follow-up, 18 to 21 months) as compared with 40 per cent and 43 per cent (mean follow-up, 36 to 39 months) for thiotepa. Pinsky and colleagues (1982) reported that BCG decreased the rate of progression to muscle-invasive disease from 36 per cent in control patients to 9 per cent in BCG-treated patients; however, this study included some patients who had previously had muscle-invasive tumors. Taken together, studies suggest that, using BCG for prophylaxis, the tumor recurrence rates range from 0 to 41 per cent with most being around 20 per cent, whereas patients not receiving BCG treatments (thiotepa or no treatment) had recurrence rates of 40 to 80 per cent (Brosman, 1982; Coplen et al., 1990; deKernion et al., 1985; Lamm et al., 1980; Morales and Ersil, 1979; Netto and Lemos, 1983; Shinka et al., 1989).

BCG also has been used to treat residual unresectable tumor, although BCG should not be considered as a substitute for the resection of resectable tumors (Brosman, 1984; Coplen et al., 1990; deKernion et al., 1985; Morales et al., 1981; Schellhammer et al., 1986). Overall, these series show a complete response rate of 58 per cent. In some studies, the response rates were higher in patients with low-grade tumors (Morales et al., 1981). Morales and co-workers advocated initiating BCG therapy within 10 days of tumor resection to take advantage of increased BCG adherence to the disrupted bladder mucosa. However, early administration of BCG may be associated with a greater risk of severe complications. It is prudent to wait about 2 weeks following tumor resection before starting BCG therapy.

BCG is perhaps most useful in the treatment of patients with carcinoma in situ (Coplen et al., 1990; deKernion et al., 1985; Herr et al., 1986; Lamm et al., 1982). In studies with short-term follow-up of 1 to 2 years, BCG induces a complete response rate in about 72 per cent of patients. The favorable response usually is associated with resolution of urinary irritative symptoms. Intravesical BCG in conjunction with transurethral resection of the prostate may be effective in the treatment of patients with carcinoma in situ involving the prostatic urethral mucosa (Bretton et al., 1989; Hillyard et al., 1988).

Long-term studies of BCG therapy have reported favorable responses in 50 to 89 per cent of patients. These studies suggest that patients who fail to respond to initial induction therapy may respond to more intensive regimens (Bretton et al., 1990; Coplen et al., 1990; Morales and Nickel, 1986; Sarosdy and Lamm, 1989). For example, Coplen and co-workers (1990) reported durable favorable responses after one 6-week course of intravesical BCG in only 34 per cent of patients. A second 6-week course was successful in 53 per cent of the treatment failure cases, yielding an overall tumor-free response rate of 64 per cent for patients treated for either 6 or 12 weeks. In this study, 58 per cent of patients with papillary tumors who failed to respond to the first treatment course responded to the second course, whereas only 38 per cent with carcinoma in situ who failed responded to the second course. Similarly, 16 per cent of patients who had papillary tumor at the time of failure to respond subsequently developed invasive disease, whereas 63 per cent who had carcinoma in situ at the time of failure to respond developed invasive disease. These investigators recommended a second course of BCG therapy for first-course failures. However, patients who have carcinoma in situ after the first course of BCG should be followed closely and considered for alternative therapy. Catalona and co-workers (1987) recommended alternative therapy for patients who do not respond to two courses of BCG, because the risks of developing invasive or metastatic disease in these patients exceeded the prospects for a favorable outcome with further BCG therapy.

The alternative therapy for failure of two courses of BCG depends on the type of tumor present at the time of failure. If the patient with low-grade, superficial tumor fails to respond, the other conventional conservative treatments are legitimate options. If the patient with high-grade or invasive tumor fails to respond, cystectomy should be considered.

BCG therapy has been reported to delay tumor progression, although the ultimate incidence of muscle invasion or metastatic disease has not significantly decreased (Herr et al., 1988). For example, cystectomy was required in 25 per cent of BCG-treated patients with carcinoma in situ as compared with 42 per cent of patients treated with transurethral resection alone. The median time to cystectomy was 24 months in the BCG-treated patients as compared with 8 months in patients treated with transurethral resection alone.

The value of maintenance BCG therapy is unclear; however, two prospective randomized studies have failed to demonstrate significant benefits from quarterly or monthly maintenance therapy (Badalament et al., 1987; Hudson et al., 1987). The validity of these studies has been questioned because maintenance therapy may have been given to patients treated with inadequate (6-week course) induction therapy. Further studies are required to evaluate the role of maintenance therapy.

Bladder irritability is the main side effect of BCG therapy. It can be relieved to some extent with oral oxybutynin, 5 mg three times per day, and phenazopyridine, 200 mg three times per day. The symptom complex includes dysuria (91 per cent), urinary frequency (90 per cent), hematuria (46 per cent), fever (24 per cent), malaise (18 per cent), nausea (8 per cent), chills (8 per cent), arthralgia (2 per cent), and pruritus (1 per cent). Granulomatous prostatitis also occurs commonly following BCG therapy (Oates et al., 1988)

Symptoms severe enough to require antituberculous therapy occur in up to 6 per cent of patients (Lamm et al., 1986). Systemic BCG infection has been presumed to be responsible for several deaths during treatment (Deresiewicz et al., 1990; Rawls et al., 1990). Patients having fever persisting more than 48 hours following intravesical BCG therapy and not responding to antipyretics should be treated with oral isoniazid, 300 mg/per day, plus pyridoxine, 50 mg/day. Patients with more prolonged or severe systemic symptoms should be treated with isoniazid, pyridoxine, and rifampicin, 600

mg/per day. Ethambutal, 1200 mg/per day (Steg et al., 1989), and cycloserine, 250 to 500 mg two times per day, should be added to the treatment regimen if the patient appears to be critically ill (Lamm, 1989; Sakamoto et al., 1989). Corticosteroids (40 mg prednisone daily) also have been recommended for severe reactions, but their value has not been formally tested in humans. These treatment recommendations do not correspond to the current CDC recommendations for antituberculous therapy. For both pulmonary and nonpulmonary tuberculosis, the CDC recommends a 6-month course of isoniazid plus rifampin, including pyrazinamide for the first 2 months of therapy. Pyrazinamide would not be expected to be effective against disseminated BCG infection because it is not active against *M. bovus*, the strain from which BCG is derived. The CDC has advised that streptomycin may be a better third drug than cycloserine in patients who are critically ill. In general, cycloserine is considered to be a second drug for drug-resistant or atypical myocobacterial infections. No data exist on the necessary duration of treatment for symptomatic disseminated BCG infections. It is possible that a 6-week course of treatment may suffice; however, it would seem prudent to recommend a 6-month course. A correlation exists between the intensity of BCG therapy and both its attendant toxicity and results (Brosman, 1982; Morales and Ersil, 1979). Toxicity also is related to the route of administration. Anaphylactic reactions have been reported with intralesional injections, whereas intravesical and oral administration have rarely produced severe complications. BCG may be given to patients with vesicoureteral reflux without significantly increased complications (Bohle et al., 1990). BCG should not be given to immunocompromised patients and should not be given to patients after traumatic catheterization.

Intravesical BCG therapy is believed to exert its antitumor effects through immune mechanisms (Catalona and Ratliff, 1990; Kavoussi et al., 1990). A weak correlation exists between skin test reactivity to purified protein derivative (PPD) and a favorable response to BCG therapy (Brosman, 1982; Lamm et al., 1982). BCG induces a chronic granulomatous response in the bladders of many patients (Lamm et al., 1980; Morales et al., 1976; Schellhammer et al., 1986; Torrence et al., 1988). A marginal correlation is noted between bladder granuloma formation and a favorable response to BCG therapy. These correlations are weak (Torrence et al., 1988). Some patients who have positive skin test responses and develop bladder granulomas do not respond clinically to BCG therapy. Conversely, some who have negative skin test responses and do not develop granulomas appear to have favorable responses to BCG therapy. Favorable effects of BCG have been reported to be limited to the tumors that are initially diploid and express ABH antigens or acquire these characteristics after treatment. These markers are reported to be independent of tumor grade and tumor stage (Orihuela and Shahon, 1987).

The reasons for the initial failure to respond to mild induction regimens may be related to differences in the immune competence of the hosts, differences in vaccine potency, or both (Kelley et al., 1985). It is believed that at least 10^7 organisms are required for therapy. The recommended doses for the various strains of BCG are as follows: Armand Frappier, 120 mg; Pasteur, 75 to 150 mg; Tice, 50 mg; Japanese, 40 mg; Connaught, 120 mg; and Dutch (RIVM), 120 mg. Every effort should be made to resect all tumor before initiating BCG therapy.

Intravesical Interferon

Interferons have antiproliferative and immunostimulating properties. They have been widely tested as anticancer agents in the treatment of tumors, including bladder cancer (Williams, 1988). Torti and co-workers (1988) reported that intravesical interferon as primary therapy, without concomitant surgical excision, resulted in a 25 per cent complete tumor regression rate for patients with papillary tumors, but the complete regressions were maintained in only half the patients. Interferon resulted in complete regression of carcinoma in situ in approximately one third of the patients, but also only one half of them (16 per cent) had durable responses. These durable response rates of 12 per cent for residual papillary disease and 16 per cent for carcinoma in situ are substantially lower than those that have been reported for intravesical chemotherapy or intravesical BCG therapy.

Recombinant interferon alpha-2b (IFN-α2b) has been effective in some clinical trials in the treatment of carcinoma in situ. A prospective, randomized clinical trial (Glashan, 1990) comparing low-dose (10 million units) with high-dose (100 million units) recombinant α-2b interferon weekly for 12 weeks and then monthly for 1 year in patients with carcinoma in situ revealed a 43 per cent complete response rate with the high-dose regimen and a 5 per cent response rate with the low-dose regimen. Complete responses occurred in two of nine patients who had failed to respond to prior intravesical BCG therapy. Complete responses were maintained for at least 6 months in 90 per cent of patients. Side effects were minimal. A limiting factor of high-dose interferon is its expense.

Intravesical IFN-α2b may be more effective in patients not previously treated with chemotherapy (67 per cent) than in those previously failing to respond to intravesical chemotherapy (30 per cent). Intra-arterial infusion of IFN-α2 also has been tried in patients with locally advanced bladder cancers without beneficial effects (Scheithauer et al., 1988). Further clinical studies are necessary to compare intravesical interferon with other established treatments for superficial bladder cancer.

Hematoporphyrin Derivative (Photodynamic) Phototherapy

Hematoporphyrin derivative (HpD) is a mixture of porphyrins that are preferentially concentrated in neoplastic and dysplastic tissues. With irradiation of these tissues using light of the proper wavelength (630 nm),

sensitized cells are destroyed through the release of singlet oxygen causing mitochondrial poisoning. HpD activation by white light also has been utilized to localize bladder cancer cells. HpD therapy with subsequent illumination of the bladder with a krypton-ion laser light source has shown effectiveness against superficial tumors or carcinoma in situ (greater than 90 per cent response rate) but not large or invasive tumors (Benson et al., 1982, 1983a, 1984; Hisazumi et al., 1983; Prout et al., 1987). The adverse side effects of HpD therapy include generalized cutaneous photosensitivity, which requires the patients to avoid sunlight for 6 to 8 weeks after treatment. Moreover, intense local bladder symptoms lasting 10 to 12 weeks occur in most patients, and bladder contractures can occur in up to one fifth of patients (Harty et al., 1989; Nseyo et al., 1987). It is possible that the occurrence of bladder contractures can be reduced or eliminated by reducing light exposure. HpD therapy is still considered investigational.

Laser Therapy

A variety of lasers have been employed to treat bladder tumors (Smith, 1989). Smith and Dixon (1984) used the argon laser in patients with small superficial bladder tumors and in those with carcinoma in situ. Laser energy is selectively absorbed into vascular tissues, such as tumors. The argon laser provides a 1-mm depth of penetration; therefore, it is safe but can be applied only on small tumors. The neodymium-yttrium-aluminum-garnet (Nd.YAG) laser has a 4- to 15-mm depth of penetration that can destroy larger tumors, but it is also less safe (Hofstetter et al., 1981). The Nd.YAG laser has been used in the treatment of bladder tumors with good local tumor control within the treated field (5 to 10 per cent in-field recurrence rate) (Beer et al., 1989; McPhee et al., 1988), but its proper role in the treatment of bladder cancer is unclear. Lasers also have been selected to treat the tumor bed following transurethral resection of larger tumors. It has been hypothesized that the subsequent incidence of local recurrence is less with lasers than with conventional fulguration of the tumor bed.

Laser treatment of bladder tumors also has been used in selected high-risk patients with muscle-invasive tumors who are either too ill for or refuse cystectomy. In these patients, if the tumors are not too large, the Nd.YAG laser may achieve adequate local tumor control (Beisland and Sander, 1990; McPhee et al., 1988).

Laser therapy is theoretically attractive because it can be performed through a small cystoscope utilizing local anesthesia without bleeding or obturator nerve stimulation. The main disadvantage is that limited tumor tissue is obtained for histologic examination. Laser therapy for bladder tumors has not been adopted for general use.

Hydrostatic Pressure Treatment

Hydrostatic pressure treatment was introduced by Helmstein (1972) for treating superficial bladder cancer.

With this technique, the bladder is filled with saline under pressure or a balloon is inserted in the bladder and inflated while the patient is under epidural anesthesia. The balloon pressure is maintained above the diastolic blood pressure for 5 to 7 hours. This results in necrosis of bladder tumors. A major complication of this treatment is bladder perforation. Hydrostatic pressure treatment also has been used for intractable post-radiotherapy hemorrhage (Mufti et al., 1990). This treatment has been largely abandoned.

Mucosal Denudation

Mechanical stripping of the bladder mucosa for the treatment of diffuse superficial bladder cancer has been attempted with mixed results and a high incidence of morbidity (Hansen et al., 1976).

MANAGEMENT OF INVASIVE BLADDER CANCER (STAGES B, C, AND D1)

In current years, two essentially different approaches to the treatment of muscle-invasive bladder cancer have been adopted: (1) bladder preservation and (2) bladder reconstruction (Montie, 1990). At some medical institutions, cystectomy with bladder reconstruction is performed almost exclusively, whereas at others, therapeutic efforts focus almost entirely on bladder preservation. The goal of bladder preservation is to eradicate the cancer and maintain adequate bladder function. The results of bladder salvage protocols have been reported (Rotman et al., 1990; Shipley et al., 1988; Wajsman and Klimberg, 1989). These studies often have focused only on the subgroup of patients who were able to complete the entire treatment protocol without emphasizing the fact that a patient who still has residual cancer after having undergone the initial radiation therapy and chemotherapy usually is not an ideal candidate for a cystectomy. What is known about the responses of bladder cancer to chemotherapy suggests that bladder salvage protocols are best suited for a patient with minimally invasive cancer of pure transitional cell histology. There are no adequate phase III trials comparing bladder salvage protocols with bladder reconstruction protocols.

In the bladder reconstruction approach, the initial treatment is radical cystectomy followed by urinary diversion or reconstruction, adding adjunctive chemotherapy in patients who have pathologic findings suggesting a high risk for recurrence. An advantage of this approach is that it avoids chemotherapy in patients who do not need it. The disadvantage is that chemotherapy may not be as well tolerated postoperatively.

Radical cystectomy, the most effective local therapy for patients with bladder cancer, is associated with pelvic recurrence rates of only 10 to 20 per cent as compared with recurrence rates of 50 to 70 per cent with definitive radiation therapy alone, definitive chemotherapy alone, or combinations of the two. With the development of continent urinary diversions and nerve-sparing surgery, the results of bladder reconstructive protocols appear attractive.

Currently, four different types of urinary diversions are used: (1) ileal conduit; (2) continent cutaneous diversions, such as the Kock or Indiana pouch; (3) continent orthotopic reservoirs to the urethra with ileal or ileocecal pouches, which can be done only in men; and (4) augmented rectal reservoirs, which can be done in women as well. The operative mortality of radical cystectomy has decreased from 20 to 2 per cent or less (in some series, operative mortality is less than 0.5 per cent). In comparison, mortality rates associated with chemotherapy range from 2 to 6 per cent (see Chapters 66 and 74).

Transurethral Resection for Invasive Bladder Cancer

Transurethral resection alone is inadequate therapy for most muscle-invasive bladder cancers (Nichols and Marshall, 1956). Exceptions to this rule are patients with small tumors that have only superficial muscle invasion. Barnes and co-workers (1967) reported a 40 per cent 5-year survival rate in patients with tumors that infiltrated into but not through the bladder muscle who were treated with transurethral resection alone. Current studies have confirmed these early observations. Henry and co-workers (1988) reported that 5-year survival rates in patients with stage B1 and B2 bladder tumors treated with transurethral resection alone were better than rates in those treated with preoperative radiation therapy followed by radical cystectomy, radical cystectomy alone, or definitive radiation therapy alone. In this study, however, patients treated with transurethral resections generally had smaller tumors than patients in the other groups. Herr (1987) also reported that appropriately selected patients with muscle-invasive bladder cancer had excellent survival results following transurethral resection alone.

Transurethral resection should probably be reserved for patients who have small, low-grade tumors with only superficial muscle invasion and for patients who are not medically fit for cystectomy.

Definitive Radiation Therapy with Salvage Cystectomy

Only 20 to 30 per cent of patients with invasive bladder cancer can be cured by external-beam radiation therapy alone. There appears to be no correlation between tumor grade and the responsiveness to radiation therapy (Goffinet et al., 1975; Miller and Johnson, 1973; Wallace and Bloom, 1976). These poor results may be caused in part by staging errors. Many of the patients in these radiation therapy series were staged primarily with bimanual examination (Miller and Johnson, 1973).

Of patients who have incomplete responses to radiation therapy, only 8 to 15 per cent are candidates for salvage cystectomy (Blandy et al., 1980; Goffinet et al., 1975; Goodman et al., 1981). In patients treated with salvage cystectomy, the overall 5-year survival rate is approximately 38 per cent, depending on the pathologic findings in the cystectomy specimen. If no residual tumor is found, the 5-year survival rate is approximately 70 per cent. When superficial residual tumor is present, the 5-year survival rate is 50 per cent. If deeply infiltrating cancer is present, the 5-year survival rate is only 25 per cent (Blandy et al., 1980; Crawford and Skinner, 1980; Smith and Whitmore, 1981b). The operative morbidity and mortality associated with salvage cystectomy has been reported to be only slightly higher than that associated with primary cystectomy. Definitive external-beam radiation therapy for bladder cancer includes a total tumor dose of 7000 CGy over 7 weeks (35 fractions), with 5000 CGy to the pelvis. It has not been proven that pelvic irradiation can control nodal metastases. In at least 50 per cent of patients, radiation therapy fails to control the primary tumor (Goffinet et al., 1975). In these patients, palliative cystectomy may be required for hematuria, dysuria, or intolerable urinary frequency caused by the tumor.

Representative results of radiation therapy for invasive bladder cancer include 5-year survival rates of about 35 per cent for stage A, 40 per cent for stage B1, 35 per cent for stage B2, 20 per cent for stage C, and 7 per cent for stage D (Blandy et al., 1980; Goffinet et al., 1975; Gospodarowicz et al., 1989; Greven et al., 1990; Jenkins et al., 1988a).

In the United States, there is little enthusiasm for radiation therapy as primary therapy for patients with invasive bladder cancer. In comparison, in Britain and Europe, radiation therapy continues to be the mainstay of definitive therapy; cystectomy is reserved for those who fail to respond to radiation therapy locally.

Less enthusiasm exists for the use of *postoperative* radiation therapy. Miller and Johnson (1973) reported 5-year survival rates of 41 per cent for patients with superficial tumors treated with postoperative radiation therapy, with a 23 per cent incidence of complications and a 6 per cent mortality rate. In this study, the survival rates in patients with deeply invasive tumors were dismal. This unfavorable risk-benefit ratio has discouraged the routine use of postoperative radiation therapy. Combined pre- and postoperative radiation therapy has been used with favorable survival results reported at 3 years, but long-term survival results have not been reported (Mohuiddin et al., 1981).

The theoretical advantages of radiation therapy include retaining bladder function, avoiding the need for an external appliance, and possible retention of sexual potency in men. These advantages have become less compelling with the development and popularization of the potency-sparing technique for radical cystectomy and continent urinary diversions.

Other techniques of radiation therapy for bladder cancer include combined external-beam and interstitial implantation therapy (van der Werf-Messing, 1984; van der Werf-Messing and van Putten, 1989). These techniques have an increased risk for radiation cystitis.

Clinical trials also have been initiated utilizing fast neutrons to treat bladder cancer in an attempt to improve upon the results obtained with photon radiation therapy alone. Neutrons theoretically exhibit biologic properties that may be at least threefold more effective than photons; however, the effectiveness of neutron therapy varies from tissue to tissue. Trials of neutron therapy for bladder cancer reveal that neutrons are of no greater efficacy than photons and are associated with a higher incidence of serious complications to the bowel and, in some studies, increased treatment-associated death rates (Russell et al., 1989).

Chemical Radiation Sensitizers

Misonidazole is a radiation sensitizer that has been investigated as a potential means of increasing the effectiveness of radiation therapy for bladder cancer. Early studies suggested a possible benefit; however, results have not been confirmed, and neurotoxicity has been considerable. Radiation sensitizers have not been adopted into general use in the treatment of bladder cancer (Abratt et al., 1987; Bydder et al., 1989). Misonidazole also has been recommended for integrated radiation therapy–cystectomy protocols (Ono et al., 1989).

Cis-platin and 5-fluorouracil are also considered to be potential radiation sensitizers.

Hyperthermia as an Adjunct to Radiation Therapy

Hyperthermia has been combined with radiation therapy with or without chemotherapy to achieve improved tumor responses in patients with advanced bladder cancer. This approach is based on increased susceptibility of malignant tumors to the toxic effects of hyperthermia (Hall et al., 1974; Kubota et al., 1984). Complete local responses have been reported in up to 42 per cent of patients. The toxic side effects are generally greater than those observed in patients treated with conventional radiation therapy and chemotherapy.

Complications of Radiation Therapy

Approximately 70 per cent of patients develop acute, self-limited complications during radiation therapy, including dysuria, urinary frequency, and diarrhea. Severe, persistent complications occur in less than 10 per cent of patients. One of the most troublesome complications is refractory radiation cystitis. This may require instillations of alum or formalin or require palliative cystectomy.

Intraoperative Radiation Therapy

Intraoperative radiation therapy with electron beams combined with external-beam therapy has been evaluated (Matsumoto et al., 1981; Shipley et al., 1987). With this protocol, approximately 2500 to 3000 CGy are given as a single intraoperative dose followed by 3000 to 4000 CGy as fractionated external-beam therapy. The results were favorable only in patients with superficially invasive tumors.

Integrated Preoperative Radiation Therapy and Cystectomy

The concept of planned preoperative radiation therapy followed by cystectomy was initiated by Whitmore and co-workers (1977). They proposed the following rationale: (1) well-oxygenated tumor cells are more susceptible to the effects of radiation therapy, (2) radiation therapy may sterilize peripheral microextensions of tumor as well as regional lymph node metastases, and (3) radiation therapy may preclude the metastatic potential of tumor cells disseminated at the time of cystectomy. In the early experience, 4000 CGy was delivered in 200-CGy fractions over 4 weeks; however, in 1966, they changed to a short-course dose schedule of 2000 CGy and five fractions over a 1-week period of time.

Whitmore and colleagues (1977) reported on the comparative survival of patients treated with a long-course, high-dose radiation, those treated with a short-course, low-dose radiation, and a group of patients treated with cystectomy alone at their institution between 1949 and 1959. A marginally better disease-free survival and fewer deaths were noted from tumor recurrence in patients with deeply invasive tumors treated with either course of preoperative radiation. Other clinical trials reported by Miller and Johnson (1973) and Bloom and associates (1982) that compared the results of integrated therapy with radiation therapy alone demonstrated a survival advantage for integrated therapy. In a study by Bloom and co-workers (1982), the survival differences were not statistically significant when all patients were considered, but they were significant in men younger than age 60.

Other studies examined whether integrated therapy offered a survival advantage over cystectomy alone. The Veterans Administration Cooperative Urological Research Group (Blackard et al., 1972) did not show an advantage of integrated therapy over cystectomy alone; however, they also failed to show an advantage of cystectomy over definitive radiotherapy alone. The National Cooperative Study Group (Prout, 1976) failed to demonstrate a statistically significant difference in the 5-year survival rate of patients treated with integrated therapy who completed the protocol (36 per cent) and those treated with cystectomy alone (29 per cent). Considering all patients, the 5-year survival rates were not significantly different for patients treated with preoperative radiation therapy (23 per cent) and those treated with cystectomy alone (20 per cent).

Van der Werf-Messing (1973) reported that the beneficial results of preoperative radiation were observed primarily in patients who had surgical downstaging (i.e., pathologic stage less than clinical stage). In her study, approximately two thirds of patients exhibited downstaging. A reanalysis of the National Cooperative Study (Prout, 1976) also revealed that patients with surgical downstaging (35 per cent) had more favorable survival results. In this study, the group having the highest survival rate, however, consisted of patients who did *not* receive integrated therapy and who had no residual tumor in the bladder. The National Cooperative Study has been incorrectly cited as supporting the claim that preoperative radiation therapy enhances patient survival, but the data do not support this conclusion.

Results of the National Cooperative Study (Slack and Prout, 1980) also suggested that downstaging occurred more frequently in patients who had tumors with a papillary configuration and in those without lymphatic invasion. However, subsequent studies (Hall and Heath, 1981; Shipley et al., 1982; Whitmore and Batata, 1985) failed to demonstrate a correlation between tumor histology, tumor grade, papillary configuration, and presence or absence of lymphatic invasion and tumor downstaging. Whitmore and Batata (1985) reported that downstaging occurred most frequently among patients with low-grade, low-stage tumors; tumors of transitional histology; and tumors not associated with lymph node metastases.

Whitmore (1980) reported that the results in patients treated with the short-course preoperative radiation therapy were comparable to those of patients treated with the long-course radiation therapy, although he found that downstaging was less common in patients treated with short-course therapy. He speculated that with the short course of radiation therapy, insufficient time elapsed to allow downstaging to occur.

Another purported benefit for preoperative radiation therapy was that it lowered the local tumor recurrence rate in the pelvis; however, this observation was not confirmed in other studies (Prout, 1976; Skinner and Leiskovsky, 1984). The 5-year survival results in most series of patients treated with integrated therapy are 35 to 40 per cent in patients with stage B2 and C (T3) tumors (Droller, 1982).

The validity of the concept of integrated therapy came into question in the late 1970s and early 1980s (Catalona, 1980; Mathur et al., 1981; Montie et al., 1984; Radwin, 1980; Vinnicombe and Abercrombie, 1978). The underlying assumptions of the benefits of preoperative radiation therapy, including validity of the comparison with historical controls, were questioned. The argument for decreased implantability of tumor cells based on data in patients treated with radium implantation for superficial bladder tumors may not be applicable to patients with invasive bladder cancer, because the bladder is not intentionally opened during cystectomy as it is during implantation. If, as reported, two thirds of cases are downstaged by preoperative radiation therapy and the patients have a significant survival advantage, patients as a group treated with preoperative radiation therapy should have better survival rates than patients not treated with integrated therapy; but, in fact, they do not.

Some workers suggested (Whitmore and Batata, 1985) that the apparent effects of preoperative radiation therapy on those who had surgical downstaging may not be a cause-and-effect relationship, but rather that downstaging may merely be a marker for biologically favorable tumors predetermined to do well even without radiation therapy.

Preoperative radiation therapy can cause a substantial delay in the performance of cystectomy (Prout, 1976). Theoretically, this delay might allow dissemination of the tumor to occur, whereas early cystectomy might be curative. Other potential adverse effects of preoperative radiation therapy include an increased incidence in wound infections (Prout, 1976) and bowel complications (Richie et al., 1976), especially among elderly patients receiving high-dose therapy (Whitmore and Batata, 1985).

A number of investigators have published data failing to support a survival advantage for integrated therapy (Kaplan et al., 1988; Mathur et al., 1981; Montie et al., 1984; Skinner and Leiskovsky, 1984; Vinnicombe and Abercrombie, 1978). In other series of patients treated with cystectomy alone, reported survival results were comparable to those of patients treated with integrated therapy (Mathur et al., 1981; Skinner and Leiskovsky, 1984). Skinner and Leiskovsky (1984) reported a comparison of 100 patients who received integrated therapy with 97 patients treated with cystectomy alone and found no significant survival advantage for integrated therapy. The 5-year, disease-free survival rate was 75 per cent for patients treated with cystectomy alone for stage P2 and P3a tumors, 44 per cent for patients with stage P3a and P3b tumors, and 36 per cent for patients with stage P4 tumors. No difference was observed in the tumor recurrence rate (9 per cent) in patients receiving integrated therapy and patients treated with cystectomy alone (7 per cent). Other investigators have reported similar low pelvic recurrence rates in patients not treated with preoperative radiation therapy. For example, Wishnow and Dmochowski (1988) reported a local pelvic recurrence rate of only 6 per cent with cystectomy without preoperative radiation therapy, but some of these patients also received adjuvant chemotherapy. Whitmore and Batata (1985) suggested that comparable survival results in the current cystectomy series may be due to different case selection.

In 1982, the Southwest Oncology Group initiated a randomized trial comparing 2000 rad of preoperative radiation therapy in 5 days followed by radical cystectomy with cystectomy alone in patients with invasive bladder cancer. An interim report showed no statistical difference between the two groups (Crawford et al., 1987).

In summary, critical analysis suggests that preoperative radiation therapy is not uniformly effective in patients with invasive bladder cancer. There may be a subgroup of patients with invasive tumors, who have downstaging following radiation therapy, who do better; but as a group, patients treated with integrated therapy have survival rates that are comparable to those for patients treated with cystectomy alone. Thus, the favorable response of downstaging after preoperative radiation therapy may merely identify a subset of patients with biologically favorable tumors. No convincing evidence exists that preoperative radiation therapy is responsible for the favorable prognosis. Moreover, because of the expense, delay, and potential morbidity associated with preoperative radiation therapy for bladder cancer, there is an increasing tendency to omit it prior to cystectomy in patients with invasive bladder cancer. However, marginal evidence exists, based on a randomized clinical study, suggesting that preoperative radiation may be beneficial in the treatment of patients with P3 and P4 bilharzial bladder cancer (Ghoneim and Awad, 1980). Preoperative radiation therapy also has been recommended for the patient with invasive squamous cell carcinoma of the bladder (Swanson et al., 1990).

Radiation Therapy in Bladder Salvage Protocols

A number of newer strategies attempt to preserve voiding function in patients with invasive bladder cancer. In addition to definitive transurethral resection alone and definitive radiation therapy alone, bladder salvage protocols include (1) neoadjuvant chemotherapy followed by cystectomy only when necessary and (2) neoadjuvant chemotherapy plus radiation therapy followed by cystectomy when necessary. The first approach is discussed under neoadjuvant chemotherapy. With the second approach, patients are treated with a combination chemotherapy regimen including cisplatin, vinblastine, and methotrexate (CMV) and 4000 CGy of radiation (Shipley et al., 1988). The patient is then re-evaluated, and, if there is complete evidence of tumor regression, the radiation therapy is continued for a total dose of 6480 CGy in an effort to sterilize the bladder. Patients who fail to have a complete response following 4000 CGy of radiation plus two courses of CMV are advised to undergo cystectomy. Preliminary results of this protocol have been reported (Marks et al., 1988). In this pilot study, 25 per cent of the patients had complete responses and another 19 per cent had positive cytologic findings with negative findings on biopsy. More than half the patients received the full dose of therapy, and all were alive without tumor recurrence including one with positive cytologic findings. Of the patients who failed to respond to neoadjuvant therapy, the majority are disease-free following salvage cystectomy. Overall, 84 per cent of patients are disease-free with short-term follow-up, but this approach will require larger studies with longer follow-up to evaluate its true efficacy.

In a similar study (Sauer et al., 1988), patients were treated with radiotherapy plus cisplatin. In this study, 4140 CGy was delivered to the bladder. During the 1st and 5th treatment weeks, on 5 consecutive days, patients received 25 mg per day of cisplatin. The overall complete response rate was 77 per cent, although one third of complete responders had early local recurrences or local recurrences plus distant metastases. Of the patients, 82 per cent maintained the bladder with normal function. Combination chemotherapy and radiation therapy regimens produced local objective response rates of 55 to 75 per cent. The only published randomized trial comparing standard radiation therapy alone with cisplatin plus radiation therapy did not demonstrate a survival benefit from this approach (Raghavan et al., 1989).

Numerous treatment options are available for patients with invasive bladder cancer. Further studies will be needed to determine whether it is preferable to attempt bladder salvage with chemotherapy with or without radiation therapy, resorting to cystectomy only if there is an incomplete response, or whether it is preferable to perform cystectomy and replacement intestinal cystoplasty. Moreover, the role of definitive radiation therapy with salvage cystectomy is also being reconsidered.

NEOADJUVANT CHEMOTHERAPY

Most patients with invasive bladder cancer who have tumor recurrences ultimately succumb to distant metastases. Therefore, it is believed that the therapeutic limits of regional therapy, such as radical surgery and radiation therapy, have been reached. Effective systemic therapy for occult distant metastases is needed to improve cure rates. The rationale for neoadjuvant chemotherapy is that it may not only shrink locally advanced tumor, but it also may eradicate lymph node and occult distant metastases.

The principles of neoadjuvant chemotherapy are (1) micrometastases may often be present at the time of first diagnosis, (2) micrometastases are probably best treated when the volume is minimal, (3) downstaging of bladder cancer by radiation therapy before cystectomy may increase survival benefit, (4) cisplatin may act as a radiation sensitizer, and (5) systemic chemotherapy before radiation therapy may eliminate the reduction in drug access to the tumor that occurs as result of radiation-induced vascular sclerosis (Raghavan et al., 1989, 1990).

Neoadjuvant chemotherapy has been tested largely in patients who present initially with locally advanced tumors with perivesical extension or lymph node metastases. The most promising regimen is a four-drug combination including methotrexate, vinblastine, Adriamycin (doxorubicin), and cisplatin. This regimen has been called M-VAC. Clinical studies with neoadjuvant M-VAC therapy following aggressive transurethral resection of the primary tumor and re-resection of the primary tumor site resulted in about a 50 per cent incidence of clinical complete response and about a 25 to 30 per cent incidence of pathologic complete responses (Herr, 1989; McCullough et al., 1989; Scher et al., 1988). The extent to which these responses are caused by the aggressive transurethral resection or the M-VAC chemotherapy has not been accurately quantified. The ultimate effect of neoadjuvant M-VAC therapy on long-term disease-free survival is not well documented. It also is uncertain whether patients who have clinically complete responses should be subjected to cystectomy. In this regard, there are significant errors in clinical staging in both directions following M-VAC therapy. Residual masses detectable on CT scan may contain fibrosis only in 30 to 40 per cent of instances. In comparison, approximately one third of patients who have no clinical evidence of residual tumor are found to harbor microscopic tumor if radical excision is performed. Not all studies of neoadjuvant chemotherapy are encouraging (Tannock et al., 1989), and further studies are needed to determine the clinical usefulness of neoadjuvant M-VAC therapy.

The disadvantages of neoadjuvant chemotherapy are similar to those of preoperative radiation therapy: (1) patients may experience sufficient morbidity to exclude them from the cystectomy; (2) for patients destined not to respond, the delay could allow metastases to occur; and (3) inherent inaccuracy in evaluating the response to neoadjuvant therapy may be misleading, especially in patients with clinical complete responses who then refuse cystectomy.

CYSTECTOMY

Partial Cystectomy

Partial cystectomy is a legitimate treatment option in selected patients with solitary invasive bladder cancer who cannot be managed safely with transurethral resection and who have no prior history of bladder tumor. In these patients, selected site mucosal biopsy specimens should be obtained to ensure that there is no severe atypia or carcinoma in situ elsewhere in the bladder or prostatic urethra. It is also desirable to achieve a 2-cm margin of resection around the tumor. Using these criteria, only about 10 to 15 per cent of patients with invasive bladder cancer are suitable candidates for partial cystectomy; however, the survival rates of such patients are comparable to those obtained with radical excision (Resnick and O'Connor, 1973). It may be prudent to give preoperative radiation therapy in doses of 1000 to 1200 CGy to prevent tumor cell implantation in the surgical wound. Wound implantation has been reported to occur in 10 to 20 per cent of patients from opening the bladder (Magri, 1962). Implantation can be prevented with low-dose radiation therapy (van der Werf-Messing, 1969).

If the tumor is close to a ureteral orifice, ureteral reimplantation may be required; but ureteral reimplantation generally is considered appropriate only if the tumor is cephalad or lateral to the orifice. If the tumor involves the trigone–bladder neck area, total cystectomy is usually recommended.

Pelvic lymphadenectomy is appropriate in patients undergoing partial cystectomy. Although data supporting its efficacy are lacking, at worst, knowledge of the lymph node status may influence the decision to give adjuvant chemotherapy.

Disturbingly high (70 per cent) tumor recurrence rates have been reported in patients with high-grade tumors treated with partial cystectomy (Faysal, 1981; Faysal and Freiha, 1979). Some of these patients can be salvaged with total cystectomy.

Standard Radical Cystectomy

The technique of radical cystectomy and the various forms of urinary diversion are the topics of Chapters 72 and 74 and are discussed here only briefly.

In men, the standard operation for muscle-invasive bladder cancer is radical cystoprostatectomy including pelvic lymphadenectomy (Skinner, 1982) with wide excision of the bladder and prostate along with the bladder pedicles and perivesical fat. Total urethrectomy is performed if there is tumor involvement of the prostatic urethra (Lopez-Almansa et al., 1988). In the absence of tumor involvement of the prostate, urethral recurrences occur in fewer than 5 per cent of patients. Radical cystoprostatectomy uniformly causes erectile impotence.

In women, the standard operation for invasive bladder cancer is an anterior pelvic exenteration with wide excision of the bladder and urethra in continuity with the uterus, fallopian tubes, ovaries, and anterior wall of the vagina. This operation diminishes the capacity of the vagina but does not preclude postoperative vaginal intercourse in most instances. The urethra should be removed routinely because 36 per cent of women have cancer involving the urethra (Depaepe et al., 1990).

It is important to evaluate the distal ureters, employing frozen sections to ensure that there is no evidence of residual cancer. If cancer is found, the ureters should be transected more cephalad to achieve tumor-free margins. Tumor recurrence rates are higher in patients with positive margins (Zincke et al., 1984). In rare circumstances, there may be severe atypia or carcinoma in situ involving the entire length of one or both upper urinary tracts. In these rare cases, it may not be possible to obtain tumor-free margins, and it may be necessary either to remove the entire affected renal unit or to proceed with the ureterointestinal anastomosis, despite the questionable margins. Linker and Whitmore (1975) and Johnson and co-workers (1989) reported surprisingly low tumor recurrence rates in patients with retained renal units having positive margins.

Nerve-Sparing Radical Cystoprostatectomy

A nerve-sparing modification of radical cystoprostatectomy that preserves erectile function in the majority of patients was reported by Schlegel and Walsh (1987) (Brendler et al., 1990a). It also is possible to preserve potency in patients undergoing total urethrectomy. Potency may be more readily preserved in patients in whom the urethra is left intact (Brendler et al., 1990a). Delayed urethrectomy also has been recommended to enhance the likelihood of preserving potency. With the nerve-sparing cystectomy, the vesical arteries and bladder pedicles are transected immediately adjacent to the seminal vesicles and ureters to avoid injury to the cephalad portions of the neurovascular bundles.

The advisability of performing nerve-sparing radical cystectomy has been questioned by Pritchett and co-workers (1988), who found lymph nodes in the retained bladder pedicles following nerve-sparing cystoprostatectomy in 60 per cent of patients. The clinical significance of these lymph nodes remains uncertain. The reported early results with nerve-sparing cystectomy are favorable (Brendler, 1990b).

In patients in whom it is not possible to preserve potency, sexual function usually can be restored by intracavernosal injection therapy with vasodilators or by implantation of a penile prosthesis (Boyd et al., 1989).

Urinary Diversions

A variety of urinary diversions has been used in patients undergoing cystectomy for invasive bladder cancer.

Ureterosigmoidostomy

One of the earliest forms of urinary diversion was ureterosigmoidostomy, which has been largely supplanted by other forms of diversion because of the associated adverse postoperative sequelae. Early problems with ureterosigmoidostomy were related to complications of the ureterocolonic anastomoses. Leadbetter and Clark (1955) and Goodwin and associates (1953) described antireflux techniques for the ureterocolonic anastomoses that reduced the incidence of reflux, but obstruction, urinary stone formation, electrolyte imbalance, and systemic hyperchloremic acidosis still occurred frequently. Also, colonic neoplasms occurred at the site of the ureterosigmoid anastomosis in nearly 10 per cent of patients. These adenocarcinomas are believed to be induced by the carcinogenic action of the combined fecal and urinary streams on the intestinal mucosa (Husmann and Spence, 1990). Accordingly, other forms of urinary diversion in which the urinary stream is not in continuity with the fecal stream have become more popular.

Intestinal Conduits

The time-honored urinary diversion following radical cystectomy is the ileal conduit popularized by Bricker (1950). Peristomal inflammation, parastomal hernia, stomal stenosis, urinary tract stone disease, ureteroileal anastomotic strictures, pyelonephritis, and late upper urinary tract deterioration are the principal complications of ileal conduit urinary diversion (Bracken et al., 1981b; Sullivan et al., 1980). Virtually all patients find the necessity of wearing an external collecting appliance objectionable, but most patients adjust to it with time.

In patients with radiation enteritis, a jejunal or transverse colon conduit may be selected. Jejunal conduits are infrequently chosen because of the characteristic metabolic derangement caused by losses of sodium and chloride from the jejunum. This requires careful metabolic monitoring and management with salt repletion. Colon conduits are more suitable for the performance of nonrefluxing ureterointestinal anastomoses; however, there may be an increased incidence of anastomotic strictures with tunneled nonrefluxing ureterointestinal anastomoses.

Continent Urinary Diversions

An important advance has been the development of continent urinary diversions not requiring an external collecting appliance. These techniques use bowel segments to create a reservoir that can be emptied by intermittent catheterization through a continent abdominal stoma or that can be anastomosed to the urethra to form an orthotopic neobladder. Reservoirs constructed of ileum alone (Kock pouch) (Skinner et al., 1987) or the ileocecal segment (Mainz pouch) (Thuroff et al., 1986), Indiana pouch (Rowland et al., 1987), and modifications thereof have been the most frequently utilized continent urinary diversions. These operations have a high rate of acceptance among patients (Boyd et al., 1987); however, they are technically more demanding than the ileal conduit, and the risk of complications is higher (Kock et al., 1982; Skinner et al., 1984, 1987).

The principal complications of these reservoirs include leakage of urine through the antiincontinence valves, formation of stones within the reservoirs, difficulty in catheterizing the stomas, urinary tract infections, and vesicoureteral refluxes. Continent diversions can be performed safely in previously irradiated patients, but such patients have an increased incidence of urinary leaks and postoperative diarrhea (Ahlering et al., 1988a).

One of the first efforts at neobladder formation was the Camey procedure (Lilien and Camey, 1984) in which a V-shaped loop of ileum is anastomosed on its antimesenteric border directly to the membranous urethra. Because the bowel is not detubularized with this operation, nocturnal incontinence is a significant problem, and daytime incontinence also occurs in some patients. The antireflux mechanism may fail because of the relatively high pressures generated by peristaltic contractions of the tubular ileal loop. Accordingly, the Camey procedure has been largely supplanted by detubularized ileal or ileocolonic reservoirs anastomosed to the urethra (Ghoneim et al., 1987; Kock et al., 1989; Marshall, 1988; Studer et al., 1989; Wenderoth et al., 1990). With neobladders, patients void using the Valsalva maneuver. If the neobladder has adequate capacity (500 to 800 ml) and low internal pressures, adequate emptying and satisfactory daytime and nighttime continence usually are achieved. If the neobladder is made too large, incomplete emptying can require the need for intermittent self-catheterization.

Neobladder formation cannot be performed in women with the expectation of achieving urinary continence. A valved rectal pouch modification of ureterosigmoidostomy that partially separates the fecal and urinary streams has been devised as a possible continent urinary diversion for women (Kock et al., 1988). Insufficient experience has been reported to adequately evaluate this operation.

Concerns exist about continent urinary diversions interfering with adjuvant postoperative chemotherapy in patients at high risk for tumor recurrence (Wishnow et al., 1989). In this regard, increased resorption of methotrexate has been reported in patients with urinary diversions (Fossa et al., 1990; Wishnow et al., 1989). This is even more of a problem with continent diversions in which urine is stored. Concerns also exist about cancer occurring in urinary reservoirs (Filmer and Spencer, 1990).

With any form of urinary diversion in which the urethra is left in situ, it is important to monitor the patient postoperatively with urinary cytology and urethroscopy.

Complications of Radical Cystectomy and Urinary Diversion

The complication rate for patients undergoing radical cystectomy and urinary diversion is approximately 25 to 35 per cent (Skinner et al., 1980; Sullivan et al., 1980). Among the most common complications are wound infections (10 per cent), intestinal obstruction (10 per cent), hemorrhage, and cardiopulmonary complications. Rectal injuries have been reported in approximately 4 per cent of patients. In general, if the rectal injury is small, fecal contamination is minimal, and the patient has not been irradiated, the rectum may be closed primarily, dilating the external sphincter to allow primary healing with low internal bowel pressures. In other circumstances, a temporary diverting colostomy should be strongly considered (Flechner and Spaulding, 1982). The reoperation rate following cystectomy is about 10 per cent (Wishnow et al., 1989). The mortality rate associated with radical cystectomy at most medical institutions has decreased to around 1 to 2 per cent (Bracken et al., 1981b).

MANAGEMENT OF METASTATIC DISEASE (STAGE D2)

Cytotoxic Chemotherapy

Chemotherapeutic agents that have documented activity against transitional cell carcinoma include cisplatin, methotrexate, vinblastine, and doxorubicin. When provided as single agents, these drugs induce objective tumor regression in 20 to 30 per cent of patients. Most of these responses are only partial regressions with a duration of about 6 months (Soloway, 1985; Yagoda, 1983).

Combination therapy with three or four of these drugs has been evaluated in clinical trials (Rotman et al., 1990). One of these regimens uses cisplatin, methotrexate, and vinblastine (CMV) (Harker et al., 1984). The four-drug combination, M-VAC (Sternberg et al., 1985), is believed to be the most effective regimen currently available. These combinations yield objective response rates of 57 to 70 per cent and complete responses in 30 to 50 per cent of patients. The probable reason that response rates decreased in subsequent reports is that M-VAC was administered to a wider range of patients (Sternberg et al., 1985, 1988, 1989). A 3-year experience with M-VAC in 124 patients evaluated for survival and 121 patients evaluated for response to therapy reported that only 20 per cent survived at the end of the study, with a median survival of 13 months (Sternberg et al., 1989). Although 44 patients (36 ± 9 per cent) were listed as having complete responses, in 17 of these patients, the complete response was documented by clinical criteria only. In 13 patients, the complete response required surgical resection of residual disease to be achieved. Only 14 patients had a pathologically documented complete response. Patients with only nodal metastases respond better and longer than those with more advanced disease. M-VAC was not effective against carcinoma in situ.

Among the patients with a clinical complete response, 76 per cent experienced relapse with a median response duration of 22 months. Among those who achieved a pathologic complete response, 64 per cent experienced relapse after a median response duration of 19 months. Similarly, 69 per cent of the patients who had a surgically assisted complete response experienced relapse after a median response time of 22 months. Thus, overall, two thirds of the complete responders experienced relapse before 2 years. It is likely that more relapses will occur with longer follow-up. Moreover, the M-VAC regimen was associated with substantial toxicity, the most common adverse side effects being mucositis and renal insufficiency. Myelosuppression also was common. Overall, 3 per cent of the patients died of drug-related causes. Both the mucositis and myelosuppression were ameliorated with the administration of granulocyte colony stimulating factor (Gabrilove et al., 1988).

To summarize, the patient with metastatic transitional cell carcinoma treated with M-VAC therapy has a 25 per cent chance, at best, of having a complete response to chemotherapy alone and a 33 per cent chance of having a complete response to chemotherapy with the assistance of a salvage operation. Two thirds of patients with a complete response relapse within 2 years. Thus, only 17 per cent of patients can expect to remain tumor-free 3 years from the initiation of M-VAC chemotherapy. This low durable response rate is achieved at a relatively high price in terms of toxicity to patients who require frequent hospitalizations for granulocytopenic sepsis. This therapeutic ratio leaves much to be desired. An unanswered question is to what extent the long-term survivors owe their longevity to the chemotherapy and to what extent to the biology of the tumor. Thus, although M-VAC has undisputed activity against transitional cell carcinoma, it falls short of a truly successful chemotherapeutic regimen.

Controversy exists about whether M-VAC is more effective than other methotrexate-platinum–containing regimens. For example, some investigators have found M-VAC to be no more active then single agents alone or other combinations, reporting response rates ranging from 0 to 15 per cent (Connor et al., 1989; Hillcoat et al., 1989; Tannock et al., 1989). In a prospective, randomized trial comparing M-VAC with the CISCA regimen, which uses cisplatin, cyclophosphamide, and Adriamycin (doxorubicin) (Logothetis et al., 1989), the preliminary results suggest that M-VAC may be slightly more effective. Evidence is available that M-VAC may be marginally more effective than CMV as well. Nonetheless, randomized controlled trials have failed to reveal a survival benefit for combination chemotherapy over single-agent chemotherapy, although higher objective response rates have been documented with the combined regimens (Soloway et al., 1983; Troner et al., 1987).

Attempts have been made to increase the therapeutic index of chemotherapy by giving intra-arterial infusions. In some cases, favorable response rates have been reported; however, intra-arterial chemotherapy does not appear to be effective in treating lymph node metastases. The complications of intra-arterial chemotherapy also include peripheral neuropathy and cutaneous toxicity as well as the usual renal toxicity and granulocytopenia (Eapen et al., 1989; Jacobs et al., 1989).

Logothetis and co-workers (1990) reported on a phase I trial to evaluate the use of recombinant granulocyte-macrophage colony-stimulating factor in patients with metastatic urothelial tumors who were refractory to conventional M-VAC chemotherapy. The M-VAC chemotherapy was escalated in these patients by increasing the doxorubicin dose by 50 per cent, the vinblastine dose by 30 per cent, and the cisplatin dose by 40 per

cent. Overall, 12 of 30 patients had objective responses of which seven (23 per cent) were complete responses. The duration of the complete responses was short. The hematopoietic growth factor may allow for greater likelihood of favorable responses to chemotherapy. The side effects from the growth factor included skin rash, fever, malaise, fluid retention, hypotension, chest pain, and pleuritis.

Several issues need to be resolved concerning chemotherapy for patients with advanced bladder cancer. One is whether further chemotherapy is needed in patients who have been rendered complete responders by surgical excision because there is no true salvage chemotherapy following M-VAC. Another important issue is whether further surgery is indicated in patients who achieve a complete response with chemotherapy because at least half of them harbor residual tumor. Controlled clinical trials will be required to resolve these issues.

Adjuvant Chemotherapy

Systemic chemotherapy has been employed as an adjunct to both radical cystectomy and radiation therapy. These trials have yielded conflicting results. Some studies suggest that adjuvant chemotherapy is beneficial, whereas others show little or no benefit (Soloway, 1985). With the development of newer more effective combination regimens, there is an increased impetus for the provision of chemotherapy in the adjuvant setting (Herr et al., 1983; Hill et al., 1985; Soloway, 1985).

No generally accepted prospective, randomized trials demonstrate the effectiveness of adjuvant chemotherapy. Some trials indirectly suggest a possible benefit. One trial evaluated CISCA in an adjuvant setting. It was not a prospective, randomized trial but rather a retrospective analysis of the treatment results of patients with pathologic findings suggestive of a high likelihood for tumor relapse (nodal metastases, extravesical tumor involvement, visceral invasion, or vascular or lymphatic invasion), who did or did not receive adjuvant CISCA chemotherapy. These results were compared with those of patients who did not have unfavorable pathologic findings. The high-risk patients who received adjuvant CISCA survived significantly longer than their counterparts who did not receive it, having results comparable to those of the low-risk patients. The CISCA protocol included five monthly courses of chemotherapy. Patients with only vascular or lymphatic invasion of the primary tumor were not benefited by CISCA therapy and appeared to do reasonably well whether or not they received it. Those who had pure transitional cell carcinoma and those who had transitional cell carcinoma with squamous elements with involvement of extravesical tissues, adjacent pelvic viscera, or regional lymph nodes appeared to benefit from adjuvant therapy. This study does not substitute for a controlled, randomized trial of high-risk patients, but the results indirectly suggest a potential benefit of adjuvant chemotherapy for selected high-risk patients.

In an as yet unpublished randomized clinical trial,

Donald G. Skinner and colleagues reported that adjuvant chemotherapy with cisplatin, doxorubicin, and cyclophosphamide significantly prolonged the time to progression and increased survival in patients with pure transitional cell carcinoma or transitional cell carcinoma associated with squamous and/or glandular differentiation with or without carcinoma in situ. The validity of the randomization scheme and statistical analysis of this study have been challenged by some investigators. Further review of this study is required before definitive conclusions can be drawn.

Palliative Radiation Therapy

Radiation therapy in doses of 3000 to 3500 CGy given in ten fractions often is effective in relieving pain from osseous metastases. Pain relief is usually prompt. It is advisable to utilize prophylactic radiation in minimally symptomatic metastases involving weight bearing bones, such as the spine or the femoral neck. Internal fixation may be required for the prevention or treatment of pathologic fractures.

Palliative radiation therapy in doses of 4000 to 4500 CGy may be effective in controlling local symptoms from the primary tumor, but doses of radiation in this range also can aggravate the local symptoms produced by the primary tumor (urgency, frequency, hematuria, and dysuria).

Intravesical Alum or Formalin Instillation

A 1 per cent alum solution may be effective in treating hemorrhage from radiation cystitis (Ostroff and Chenault, 1982). The solution may be instilled with continuous bladder irrigation without the need for anesthesia and is generally well tolerated. Occasionally, discontinuation may be required because of symptoms of vesical pain and irritability. Danger of possible seizures from aluminum toxicity has been reported in patients with diminished renal function (Kavoussi et al., 1986).

Formalin is a 37 per cent solution of formaldehyde gas dissolved in water. Formalin solution in concentrations of 1 to 10 per cent (0.37 to 3.7 per cent formaldehyde gas) has been given in bladder instillations to control hemorrhage from advanced bladder tumor or radiation cystitis (Brown, 1970). Formalin solution is exceedingly irritating to the bladder and, thus, requires general or regional anesthesia for intravesical instillation. Because a 10 per cent formalin solution may cause fibrosis and obstruction of the ureteral orifices, formalin instillation should begin with a 1 per cent solution and be repeated with a 4 per cent solution, if necessary. A cystogram should be performed before instillation to rule out vesicoureteral reflux. If reflux is present, Fogarty catheters should be passed up both ureters, and the patient should be tilted in the head-up position to protect the upper urinary tracts from the toxic effects of formalin (Fall and Pettersson, 1979). The formalin solution is instilled into the bladder and maintained in contact with the urothelium for about 30 minutes.

Palliative Hypogastric Artery Embolization and Palliative Cystectomy

Life-threatening hemorrhage rarely occurs from hemorrhagic cystitis or uncontrolled bladder tumors. In these instances, if fulguration, laser treatment, or intravesical alum or formalin instillations fail to control the hemorrhage, it may be necessary to perform transfemoral percutaneous hypogastric artery embolization (Carmignani et al., 1980). If hypogastric embolization or ligation fails to control the hemorrhage, palliative cystectomy may be required as a last resort.

Immunotherapy

Extensive immunologic studies have been made of bladder cancer, both in experimental animal models and in humans (Catalona et al., 1982; Droller, 1984). The most common form of immunotherapy is intravesical BCG therapy for superficial bladder cancer.

The streptococcal OK-432 vaccine has been reported to produce effects similar to those of BCG, but the data using this agent are limited (Kagawa et al., 1979). Studies with *Corynebacterium parvum* for advanced disease have not shown therapeutic effectiveness (Purves et al., 1979). Other studies suggest that interleukin-2 with or without BCG may be effective in the treatment of superficial bladder tumors (Dow et al., 1989; Huland and Huland, 1989; Pizza et al., 1984), but these results have not been confirmed. Immunotherapy with keyhole-limpet hemocyanin also has been evaluated (Flamm et al., 1990; Jurincic et al., 1988). This treatment was reported to be as effective as etoglucid (Flamm et al., 1990).

Parenteral administration of the interferon inducer poly(I:C) may reduce early tumor recurrences and provide long-term survival benefits in patients with carcinoma in situ, but these studies have not been confirmed (Herr et al., 1978; Kemeny et al., 1981).

Passive immunotherapy with immune pig lymphocytes has suggested the possibility of beneficial effects but also has not been confirmed by other studies (Symes et al., 1978). Other miscellaneous studies of immunotherapy for bladder cancer were reviewed by Droller (1984).

NONUROTHELIAL TUMORS OF THE BLADDER

Small-Cell Carcinoma

It is believed that small-cell carcinomas of the bladder are derived from neuroendocrine stem cells (Fig. 28–23). Small-cell carcinoma may be mixed with elements of transitional cell carcinoma in the same tumor. Another possible source of small-cell carcinoma is the dendritic cells in the normal urothelium. Small-cell carcinomas exhibit neuroendocrine markers, such as staining positively for neuron-specific enolase. Small-cell carcinomas are usually biologically aggressive tumors with early vascular and muscle invasion. Patients with

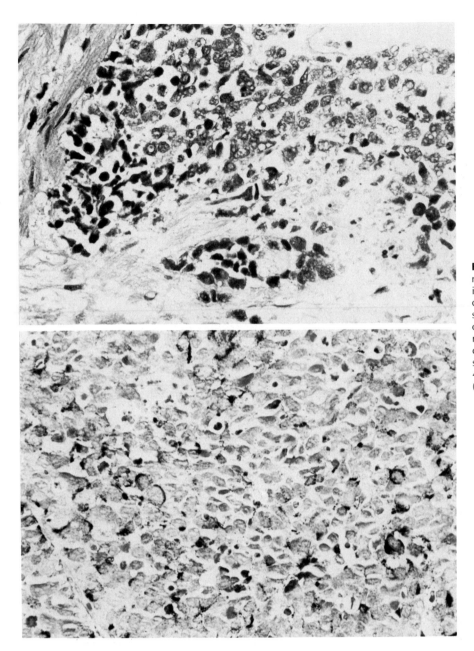

Figure 28–23. Small-cell carcinoma. Neuroendocrine carcinoma of the bladder showing infiltrating nests of small hyperchromatic cells with rounded to elliptic contours. The smaller cells with dense chromatin resemble oat cell carcinoma of the lung (top). Immunoperoxidase stained positive for neuron-specific enolase, Leu-7, and chromogranin as shown (bottom). (Hematoxylin and eosin, × 400; avidin biotin peroxidase, × 400.) (Courtesy of Louis P. Dehner, M.D.)

small-cell carcinoma should be evaluated for a primary small-cell carcinoma of the lung, which may have metastasized to the bladder (Swanson et al., 1988). Isolated reports have been made of favorable responses to chemotherapy for small-cell carcinoma (Davis et al., 1989); however, most cases are resistant to treatment with chemotherapy or radiation therapy (Mills et al., 1987).

Carcinosarcoma

Carcinosarcomas are highly malignant tumors containing both malignant mesenchymal and epithelial elements (Fig. 28–24). The mesenchymal elements are usually chondrosarcoma or osteosarcoma (Koss, 1975; Young, 1987). The epithelial elements may be transitional cell carcinoma, squamous cell carcinoma, or adenocarcinoma. These tumors are rare, usually occurring in middle-aged men. The common presenting symptom is gross, painless hematuria. The prognosis is uniformly poor despite aggressive treatment with cystoprostatectomy. For example, in one series, the 5-year survival rate was only 20 per cent (Sen et al., 1985). Carcinosarcomas are resistant to radiation therapy and chemotherapy (Schoborg et al., 1980; Uyama and Moriwaki, 1981).

Some bladder cancers exhibit a prominent spindle cell component and are sometimes referred to as sarcomatoid carcinomas. These are also aggressive tumors with a poor prognosis but should not be confused with true carcinosarcomas (Young et al., 1988). Similarly, pseudosarcomatoid inflammatory reactions may sometimes be confused with carcinosarcomas. Because of the benign nature of these lesions, it is of utmost importance to distinguish them from true carcinosarcomas.

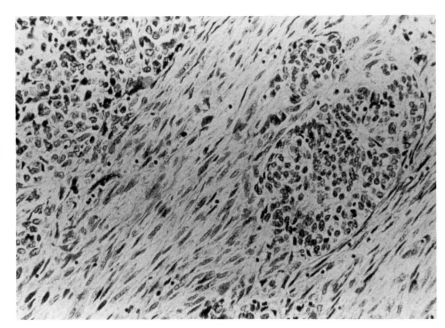

Figure 28–24. Carcinosarcoma. (From Mostofi, F. K., Sobin, L. H., and Torloni, H.: Histological Typing of Urinary Bladder Tumors, no. 10. International Histological Classification of Tumors. Geneva, World Health Organization, 1973.)

Metastatic Carcinoma

The bladder may be secondarily involved by cancers from virtually any other primary site. The most common primary sites are prostate, ovary, uterus, colon, lung, breast, and stomach as well as primary melanoma, lymphoma, and leukemia (Koss, 1975).

Nonepithelial Bladder Tumors

The three categories of nonepithelial bladder tumors are as follows: (1) primitive connective tumors, including leiomyosarcoma, rhabdomyosarcoma, chondrosarcoma, osteosarcoma, liposarcoma, and granular cell myoblastoma; (2) tumors of nonconnective tissue origin, including angiosarcoma, neurosarcoma, neurofibroma, pheochromocytoma, melanoma, and so forth; and (3) secondary nonepithelial tumors, including lymphoma, leukemia, plasmacytoma, and melanoma (Rosi et al., 1983). Approximately 1 to 5 per cent of all bladder tumors are nonepithelial in origin. The more common nonepithelial bladder tumors are reviewed in the following discussion.

Neurofibroma

A neurofibroma is a benign tumor of the nerve sheath resulting from overgrowth of the Schwann cells. Neurofibromas may occur as an inherited autosomal dominant trait of variable penetrance (Torres and Bennett, 1966). In the bladder, neurofibromas arise from the ganglia of the bladder wall and may occur as either solitary lesions or plexiform lesions. Vesical neurofibromatosis often becomes clinically manifest in childhood with symptoms of urinary tract obstruction, urinary incontinence, vesical irritability, or pelvic mass (Clark et al., 1977). Conservative management should be at-tempted unless there is severe urinary tract obstruction or unless symptoms become incapacitating. Rarely, bladder neurofibromas may undergo malignant degeneration to form neurofibrosarcomas (Clark et al., 1977).

Pheochromocytoma

Bladder pheochromocytomas account for less than 1 per cent of all bladder tumors and less than 1 per cent of all pheochromocytomas (Albores-Saavedra et al., 1969). They arise from paraganglionic cells within the bladder wall, usually in the region of the trigone (Koss, 1975). There is no sex predilection, and the peak age incidence is in the 2nd through the 4th decades. About 10 per cent of bladder pheochromocytomas are malignant and have the capacity to metastasize to the regional lymph nodes or distant sites. Malignancy is determined more by the clinical behavior than the histologic features of the tumor. Most pheochromocytomas in the bladder are metabolically active, causing paroxysmal attacks of hypertension on filling and emptying of the bladder in two thirds of patients. Hematuria develops in only about one half of patients.

On cystoscopic examination, the tumor appears as a submucosal nodule covered by intact urothelium. Histologically, the tumors are composed of nests of polyhedral cells with eosinophilic cytoplasm. Partial cystectomy is the treatment of choice for patients with pheochromocytomas. The histologic features of benign pheochromocytoma cannot be distinguished from its malignant counterpart (Koss, 1975). The regional lymph nodes also should be evaluated preoperatively with CT and gross inspection at the time of operation. If lymph node metastases are suspected, arteriography may reveal hypervascular lesions. Pelvic lymphadenectomy should be performed if lymph node metastases are present. Lifelong follow-up is required because late metastases may occur, often being heralded by return of endocrine manifestations (DeKlerk et al., 1975).

Primary Lymphoma

Primary bladder lymphoma arises in the submucosal lymphoid follicles (Koss, 1975) and is the second most common type of nonepithelial bladder tumor (Binkovitz et al., 1988). The peak age is 40 to 60 years old, and women are affected more often than men. All histologic types of malignant lymphomas occur in the bladder. Radiation therapy is the preferred treatment for localized primary bladder lymphomas. Approximately 50 per cent of patients survive 5 years with radiation therapy (Koss, 1975). With contemporary chemotherapy, the survival rate may be as high as 65 per cent.

Plasmacytoma, Granular Cell Myoblastoma, Malignant Melanoma, Choriocarcinoma, and Yolk Sac Tumor

These rare primary bladder tumors exhibit the same characteristics as their counterparts in other sites of the body and are managed in a similar fashion.

Sarcoma

Malignant connective tissue tumors containing cell types that are normally present in the bladder include angiosarcoma and leiomyosarcoma. Those that contain tissues not normally present in the bladder include rhabdomyosarcoma, liposarcoma, chondrosarcoma, and osteosarcoma. Sarcomas of the bladder account for less than 1 per cent of all malignant bladder tumors. It is believed that sarcomas arise from pluripotential mesenchymal tissues of the bladder wall.

ANGIOSARCOMA

Angiosarcomas are extremely rare tumors that arise within the bladder wall. Histologically, they contain dilated vascular channels with prominent papillary endothelial proliferation (Koss, 1975). If the tumor has not metastasized, radical cystectomy is the treatment of choice.

LEIOMYOSARCOMA

Leiomyosarcoma is the most common malignant mesenchymal tumor of the bladder occurring in adults. It is twice as common in men as in women. Grossly, it appears as a submucosal nodule or ulcerating mass. Histologically, spindle cells are arranged in parallel bundles. The presence of nuclear abnormalities distinguish a leiomyosarcoma from a benign leiomyoma. Leiomyosarcomas may sometimes be amenable to treatment with partial cystectomy, but survival results may be compromised when conservative operations are per-

formed for large or extensive tumors (Swartz et al., 1985). Total cystectomy has yielded a 5-year survival rate of 65 per cent (Tsukamoto and Lieber, 1991). Benign leiomyomas may be treated with simple enucleation or local excision (Kabalin et al., 1990; Teran and Gambrell, 1989; Vargas and Mendez, 1983).

RHABDOMYOSARCOMA

Rhabdomyosarcoma may occur at any age but is most common in young children. Embryonal rhabdomyosarcoma in children characteristically produces polypoid lesions in the base of the bladder, giving rise to the descriptive term *sarcoma botryoides*. This tumor is composed of primitive muscle cells, including the characteristic eosinophilic rhabdomyoblast containing an eccentric nucleus. Muscle fibers containing cytoplasmic cross-striations are characteristic of rhabdomyosarcomas but often may not be present. Rhabdomyosarcoma is an extremely aggressive tumor that metastasizes to lymph nodes in 20 to 40 per cent of patients; it is the sarcoma with the greatest propensity for lymph node metastases. It also spreads hematogenously to other organs of the body. Embryonal rhabdomyosarcomas in children are responsive to multimodality treatment regimens, which usually include primary chemotherapy with cyclophosphamide, actinomycin, vincristine, doxorubicin, and cisplatin followed by radiation therapy and surgical excision. In general, the current treatment philosophy is to attempt to preserve bladder function if possible by treating first with conservative excision followed by chemotherapy and radiation therapy, if necessary. Radical exenterative surgery is reserved for tumors that cannot be controlled by conservative means. Conservative approaches are of limited success in controlling the majority of rhabdomyosarcomas. Embryonal rhabdomyosarcomas are discussed in greater detail in Chapter 54.

Adult rhabdomyosarcomas include three cell types: spindle cell, alveolar cell, and giant cell. These aggressive tumors respond poorly to radiation therapy or chemotherapy, and in general, the prognosis is poor (Koss, 1975; Tsukamoto and Lieber, 1991). The rare benign counterpart of rhabdomyosarcoma, called rhabdomyoma, is treated with conservative excision alone.

The extremely rare liposarcomas, chondrosarcomas, and osteosarcomas that occur in the bladder may occur alone or with malignant epithelial elements as a carcinosarcoma. The most effective treatment for these tumors is total cystectomy, although wide segmental excision may be effective for very small localized lesions (Ahlering et al., 1988b; MacKenzie et al., 1971; Rosi et al., 1983; Wilson et al., 1979). The prognosis of patients with bladder sarcomas is generally poor regardless of treatment.

UROTHELIAL TUMORS OF THE RENAL PELVIS AND URETER

EPIDEMIOLOGY

Incidence—Age, Sex, and Race

Upper urinary tract epithelial tumors involving the renal pelvis are relatively uncommon. National incidence and mortality statistics for the United States on renal pelvis tumors are limited because they are grouped along with renal cell carcinoma (1987 Annual Cancer Statistics Review). Renal pelvis tumors account for approximately 5 to 10 per cent of all renal tumors and about 5 per cent of all urothelial tumors (Fraley, 1978). Ureteral tumors are even more uncommon, occurring with one fourth the incidence of renal pelvis tumors (Huben et al., 1988). Epidemiologic statistics are more readily available on ureteral tumors because they are classified separately.

Ureteral tumors are at least twice as common in men as in women and twice as common among whites as among blacks. The peak incidence in white men is ten cases per 100,000 per year (Tables 28–4 and 28–5) (1987 Annual Cancer Statistics). The incidence of upper urinary tract tumors is increasing, but it is unclear whether this represents a true increase in the prevalence of the disease or whether it merely represents improved detection and reporting.

Upper tract urothelial tumors rarely occur before the age of 40, the peak incidence being in the 6th and the 7th decades of life. The mean age of occurrence is 65 years (Anderstrom et al., 1989).

Association with Balkan Nephropathy

In the Balkan countries, including Bulgaria, Greece, Romania, and Yugoslavia, there is an endemic nephropathy that is associated with a high incidence of upper tract urothelial tumors (Petkovic, 1975; Radovanovic et al., 1985). In these countries, urothelial tumors account for 40 per cent of all renal cancers. Balkan nephropathy–associated transitional cell carcinoma is more commonly bilateral (10 per cent) and behaves in a more indolent fashion than the sporadic form of the disease. This syndrome has necessitated the adoption of conservative renal-sparing surgery in many patients and has provided an increased impetus to use conservative treatment of upper tract urothelial cancers in other clinical settings.

ETIOLOGY

Occupational Factors

Significantly increased risks for renal pelvic and ureteral tumors have been reported for those employed in the chemical, petrochemical, and plastics industries (relative risk = 4) and for those exposed to coal, coke (relative risk = 4), asphalt, and tar (relative risk = 5.5) (Jensen et al., 1988).

Smoking

Cigarette smoking is the major risk factor for carcinoma of the renal pelvis and ureter (Ross et al., 1989). The Copenhagen case-control study of renal pelvis and ureter cancer showed that cigarette smoking accounted for 56 per cent of upper tract tumors in Denmark (Jensen et al., 1988). In this study, there was a relative risk of 2.6 for smokers of cigarettes alone and of 3.8 for smokers of cigarettes in combination with other types of tobacco. A strong dose-effect relationship was observed; the heaviest smokers had an eightfold risk. Similarly, deep inhalation of smoke increased the risk, whereas stopping smoking or smoking of filter cigarettes decreased the risk. The increased risk of renal pelvis and ureter cancer with smoking was stronger than that of bladder tumors.

Coffee Drinking

After adjusting for smoking, there is only a slightly increased risk (relative risk = 1.3) for upper tract urothelial tumors associated with heavy coffee drinking (Ross et al., 1989).

Table 28–4. 1985 AGE-ADJUSTED PEAK URETERAL CANCER INCIDENCE RATES*: SEER PROGRAM—RACE AND SEX DIFFERENCES

	White	Black	Total
Males	10.0 (75–79†	5.6 (70–74)	9.6 (75–79)
Females	3.4 (75–79)	2.1 (80–84)	3.2 (75–79)
Total	5.9 (75–79)	3.2 (70–74)	5.7 (75–79)

*Rates are per 100,000 and are age-adjusted to the 1970 U.S. standard population.
†(Age group).
From 1987 Annual Cancer Statistics Review Including Cancer Trends: 1950–1985. Bethesda, Maryland, National Cancer Institute, pp III 34–III 42.

Table 28–5. 1985 AGE-ADJUSTED PEAK URETERAL CANCER MORTALITY RATES*: SEER PROGRAM—RACE AND SEX DIFFERENCES

	White	Black	Total
Males	2.3 (85 +)†	0.7 (75–79)	2.1 (85 +)
Females	1.5 (85 +)	0.7 (80–84)	1.4 (85 +)
Total	1.7 (85 +)	0.5 (85 +)	1.6 (85 +)

*Rates are per 100,000 and are age-adjusted to the 1970 U.S. standard population.
†(Age group).
From 1987 Annual Cancer Statistics Review Including Cancer Trends: 1950–1985. Bethesda, Maryland, National Cancer Institute, pp. IV 29–IV 37.

Analgesics

A well-documented, significant increased risk for upper tract urothelial tumors is associated with analgesic abuse (McCredie et al., 1986; Morrison, 1984). Steffens and Nagel (1988) reported that 22 per cent of patients with renal pelvis tumors and 11 per cent with ureteral tumors gave a history of phenacetin abuse. The latency period ranged from 24 to 26 years.

Long-term exposure to analgesics induces a nephropathy that is associated with up to a 70 per cent incidence of upper urinary tract transitional cell carcinoma (Johansson and Wahlqvist, 1979). In the urinary tract, analgesic abuse induces a thickening of basement membranes around subepithelial capillaries, called capillarosclerosis. This finding is pathognomonic for analgesic abuse and has been reported in 15 per cent of patients with renal pelvis and ureteral tumors (Palvio et al., 1987).

In the Copenhagen study, after adjustment for smoking and high-risk occupational exposure, the relative risk for upper tract urothelial tumors for analgesic abusers was 2.4 for men and 4.2 for women. A dose-effect relationship was observed for both phenacetin and aspirin, although based on metabolism, phenacetin is probably the most important agent (Jensen et al., 1989).

Infectious Agents

Chronic bacterial infection associated with urinary calculi and obstruction predisposes the individual to squamous cell carcinoma or, less commonly, to urothelial adenocarcinoma. Schistosomiasis involving the ureters is associated with squamous cell carcinoma of the ureter, as it is in the bladder, although to a lesser extent. A viral etiology for urothelial tumors also has been investigated, but it has not been clearly established (Fraley, 1978).

Cyclophosphamide

Cyclophosphamide has been implicated in inducing transitional cell carcinoma of the upper and lower urinary tract (Brenner and Schellhammer, 1987). This is discussed in the section on bladder cancer.

Heredity

Upper tract transitional cell carcinoma has been reported in several familial cancer syndromes (Frischer et al., 1985; Lynch et al., 1990; Orphali et al., 1986). Chromosomal abnormalities also have been described in upper tract tumors (Gibas et al., 1987; Hecht et al., 1985; Sandberg et al., 1986).

LOCATION AND DISTRIBUTION OF TUMORS

Bilateral involvement (synchronous or metachronous) occurs in 2 to 5 per cent of sporadic upper tract transitional cell carcinomas (Babaian and Johnson, 1980;

Murphy et al., 1981). Upper tract tumors occur in 2 to 4 per cent of patients with bladder cancer (Oldbring et al., 1989a) except in occupational bladder cancer, in which the incidence was reported to be as high as 13 per cent (Shinka et al., 1988). The mean interval between the bladder tumor and the upper tract tumor was reported to be 70 months with a range of 70 to 170 months (Oldbring et al., 1989a; Shinka et al., 1988). Although the performance of routine excretory urography for follow-up of the upper urinary tracts in bladder cancer patients is controversial, patients with multiple tumors, recurrent tumors, and tumors involving the ureteral orifices are appropriate candidates for upper tract monitoring.

Approximately 30 to 75 per cent of patients with upper tract urothelial tumors have bladder tumors at some point in time (Abercrombie et al, 1988; Anderstrom et al., 1989; Huben et al., 1988; Kakizoe et al., 1980). This high incidence of subsequent bladder cancer suggests the need for routine follow-up cystoscopy in patients with upper tract tumors. The explanation for the disparity between the relatively low incidence of subsequent upper tract tumors in patients with bladder cancer and the relatively high incidence of subsequent bladder tumors in patients with upper tract tumors may be related to seeding of tumor cells downstream or to the fact that the bladder mucosa has a longer exposure time to urinary carcinogens than the renal pelvis and ureter, because the former functions as a reservoir and the latter as a conduit.

Ureteral tumors are located most commonly in the lower ureter and least commonly in the upper ureter (Anderstrom et al., 1989). Babaian and Johnson (1980) reported that 73 per cent of ureteral tumors were in the distal ureters, 24 per cent in the mid-ureter, and 3 per cent in the proximal ureter.

Several investigators have reported on histologic mapping studies of upper tract urothelial tumors (Heney et al., 1981; Mahadevia et al., 1983; McCarron et al., 1982). These studies revealed associated urothelial changes ranging from hyperplasia, to dysplasia, to frank carcinoma in situ in a substantial proportion of patients. In the renal pelvis, carcinoma in situ may be patchy in distribution and extend into the collecting ducts of the kidney (Mahadevia et al., 1983), which limits the potential efficacy of conservative surgery for renal pelvis tumors. These changes are more common in association with high-grade tumors. More severe changes are associated with a greater risk for tumor recurrence in the bladder and a poorer overall prognosis.

PATHOLOGY

Transitional Cell Carcinoma

Transitional cell carcinoma accounts for more than 90 per cent of upper tract urothelial tumors. The histopathologic features are similar to those of transitional cell carcinoma of the bladder.

Squamous Cell Carcinoma

Squamous cell carcinomas account for 0.7 to 7 per cent of upper tract urinary tumors (Babian and Johnson,

1980; Blacker et al., 1985). These tumors are nearly always associated with infected staghorn calculi of long duration. Patients characteristically present with advanced disease. The response to treatment with surgery, radiation therapy, or chemotherapy is poor (Grabstald et al., 1971; Li and Cheung, 1987).

Adenocarcinoma

Adenocarcinoma of the renal pelvis is an extremely rare tumor, representing less than 1 per cent of all renal pelvis tumors. As with squamous cell carcinoma, adenocarcinoma usually is associated with calculi, long-term obstruction, and inflammation (Stein et al., 1988).

Papillary adenocarcinoma occurring in the ureter may represent the malignant counterpart of nephrogenic adenoma of the ureter (Kim et al., 1988).

Inverted Papilloma

Inverted papillomas occur in the upper urinary tracts as well as in the bladder. These tumors also have the potential to undergo malignant transformation (Stower et al., 1990).

Nonurothelial Tumors of the Upper Urinary Tracts

Rarely, sarcomas, including leiomyosarcoma (Madgar et al., 1988) and carcinosarcoma (Fleming, 1987), occur in the upper urinary tracts. These tumors behave similarly to their counterparts in the bladder. Surgical excision is the preferred treatment.

TUMOR MARKERS

No truly useful tumor markers exist for transitional cell carcinoma. Some tumors produce oncofetal protein, such as human chorionic gonadotropin or carcino-embryonic antigen (Fulks and Falace, 1985). The significance of these markers is discussed in the section on bladder cancer. Hypercalcemia also may occur in patients with advanced disease and usually portends a poor prognosis.

NATURAL HISTORY

Patterns of Spread

Transitional cell carcinoma of the upper urinary tract may spread by direct invasion into the renal parenchyma or surrounding structures, by mucosal extension (seeding), by lymphatic invasion, or by vascular invasion (Jitsukawa et al., 1985). High-grade tumors demonstrate a greater propensity to spread. Davis and co-workers (1987) reported that invasion of the renal hilar tissue by renal pelvis tumors had greater predictive value for

metastases (95 per cent) than vascular (83 per cent) or lymphatic (77 per cent) invasion.

Mucosal Invasion

Evidence exists that tumor cells seed along the mucosal surface from cephalad to caudal in the urinary tract (Johnson and Babaian, 1979). This finding is supported by clinical studies documenting a high incidence of recurrences in the ureteral stump of patients treated with nephrectomy and incomplete ureterectomy for renal pelvis tumors and by the occurrences of bladder tumors in the region of the ipsilateral ureteral orifice of patients with upper tract tumors. Johnson and Babaian (1979) reported that transitional cell carcinoma rarely develops subsequently in the upper urinary tract above the level of resection of a ureteral tumor. They could find only one such instance in the M.D. Anderson Hospital experience. However, Amar and Das (1985) reported that upper tract tumors developed in 6.4 per cent of bladder cancer patients with vesicoureteral reflux as compared with only 0.4 per cent of patients without reflux. This observation was not confirmed by Mukamel and co-workers (1985) in patients routinely treated with thiotepa instillations. An alternative explanation for the findings of Amar and Das may be that the patients with "upper tract recurrences" may have pre-existing undetected upper tract tumors that seed down to the ureteral orifice, producing bladder tumors that require resection of the ureteral orifice to completely excise them.

Lymphatic Extension

The most common sites of lymphatic extension from upper tract tumors are the para-aortic, paracaval, and pelvic lymph nodes (Batata et al., 1975), depending on the location of the primary tumor.

Hematogenous Dissemination

Venous extension into the renal veins and vena cava may occur with renal pelvis tumors as it does with renal cell carcinoma (Geiger et al., 1986; Jitsukawa et al., 1985). Surgical excision is the preferred treatment if there is no evidence of metastatic disease. The most common sites of hematogenous visceral metastases from upper tract tumors are the liver, lung, and bone (Batata et al., 1975).

Prognostic Indicators

Tumor Stage and Grade

Tumor grade and stage clinically are the most useful prognostic variables. Tumor grade and stage match in 83 per cent of patients (Huben et al., 1988). Of the two, tumor stage is the more important predictor of prognosis. Huben and colleagues (1988) reported that the median survival for low-grade tumors was 67 months; for high-grade tumors, median survival was only 14 months. Similarly, the median survival for low-stage tumors was 91 months and for high-stage tumors was 13 months.

ABH Blood Group and Thomassen-Friederich (T) Antigen Expression

ABH blood group antigen expression has been reported to be of prognostic significance in upper tract urothelial tumors, as it is in bladder cancer. However, T antigen expression was reported not to correlate with prognosis (Kagawa et al., 1985).

DNA Flow Cytometry

Flow DNA analysis correlates with the malignant potential of upper tract urothelial tumors. Oldbring and associates (1989b) reported that all grade 3 tumors and 50 per cent of grade 2 tumors were aneuploid. In a long-term follow-up study of DNA ploidy analysis by flow cytometry, Blute and co-workers (1988) found a correlation among tumor cell ploidy, grade, stage, and clinical outcome. For high-grade, high-stage tumors, ploidy provided no additional information; however, for low-grade, low-stage tumors, an aneuploid pattern identified a subgroup of patients who had significantly poorer survival rates.

DNA Synthesizing (S)-Phase Fraction

Studies measuring the S-phase fraction of renal pelvis and ureteral tumors with bromodeoxyuridine labeling revealed that all low-grade tumors have an S-phase fraction of less than 10 per cent. The average S-phase fraction for noninvasive tumors was 9.7 per cent and for invasive tumors was 20.9 per cent. The S-phase fraction also appeared to correlate with the biologic potential of the tumor (Nemoto et al., 1989).

Distribution of Tumor Stages and Grades

The distribution of tumor stages and grades differs in various published series (Anderstrom et al., 1989; Babaian and Johnson, 1980; Bloom et al., 1970; Huben et al., 1988; Zoretic and Gonzales, 1983; Zungri et al., 1990); however, the majority are low-grade, low-stage tumors.

SIGNS AND SYMPTOMS

The most common presenting symptom of upper urinary tract urothelial tumors is gross hematuria, occurring in about 75 per cent of patients (Bloom et al., 1970; Murphy et al., 1981). Hematuria throughout urination suggests bleeding from the upper urinary tracts. Vermiform clots have the same connotation.

Flank pain occurs in up to 30 per cent of patients and usually is dull because of gradual obstruction and distention of the collecting system. Acute flank pain occurs from the passage of blood clots. In some studies, 10 to 15 per cent of patients are asymptomatic, with the tumor diagnosed as an incidental finding on an imaging study obtained for other reasons. A small proportion of patients present with symptoms of advanced disease, including abdominal or flank mass, weight loss, anorexia, and bone pain.

DIAGNOSIS

Imaging Studies

Excretory Urography

Upper tract urothelial tumors usually are diagnosed as radiolucent filling defects on excretory or retrograde urography (Fein and McClennan, 1986). The differential diagnosis includes overlying bowel gas, external compression of the collecting system by a crossing vessel, blood clot, radiolucent stone, sloughed renal papilla, or fungus ball. Other less common possibilities include a fibroepithelial polyp (Blank et al., 1987), air bubble, granuloma, leukoplakia, malacoplakia, hemangioma, renal tuberculosis, cholesteatoma, and leiomyoma.

Approximately 50 to 75 per cent of patients have a filling defect (Murphy et al., 1981), which is characteristically irregular and in continuity with the wall of the collecting system (Fig. 28–25). In the kidney, the tumor may produce incomplete filling or nonfilling of a renal infundibulum or calyx. In 10 to 30 per cent of patients, the tumor causes obstruction or nonvisualization of the collecting system (Babaian and Johnson, 1980). This finding usually is associated with a greater degree of malignancy (Bloom et al., 1970).

It is important to study carefully the contralateral upper urinary tract for subtle filling defects because the

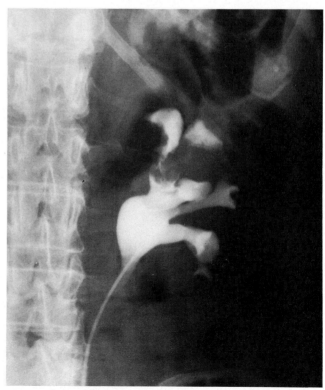

Figure 28–25. Retrograde pyelogram of renal pelvis tumor.

status of the contralateral upper tract may play an important role in treatment planning.

Retrograde Urography

Retrograde urography provides better visualization of the collecting system than excretory urography. Contrast material should be diluted by one third to one half to avoid obscuring subtle filling defects. Contrast material should be injected through a bulb tip ureteral catheter to fill the entire renal pelvis and ureter (Figs 28–26 and 28–27). Because hyperosmotic contrast material may alter the cellular detail and make cytologic studies more difficult to interpret, nonionic contrast material may be preferable for retrograde studies. Retrograde ureteropyelography is particularly helpful in patients with high-grade obstructions with poor visualization or nonvisualization on excretory urography. Ideally, retrograde ureteropyelography should be performed under fluoroscopic control to ensure adequate filling and to avoid overdistention with rupture of the renal fornices and intravasation and extravasation of contrast material. Overall, retrograde urography is accurate in establishing the diagnosis of urothelial cancer with greater than 75 per cent accuracy (Murphy et al., 1981).

After retrograde urography, a ureteral catheter should be passed into the upper urinary tract to collect urine for cytologic studies and to obtain saline barbotage specimens or to perform brush biopsy of the lesion (see following discussion).

Antegrade Pyelography

Antegrade pylography is not advisable in patients suspected of having upper tract transitional cell carcinoma because of the risk of seeding tumor cells along the needle tract. However, in exceptional clinical cir-

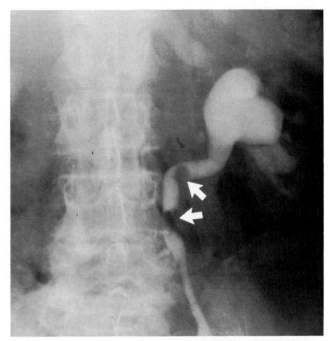

Figure 28–26. Retrograde pyelogram of upper ureteral tumor.

cumstances when the patient has a nonvisualizing kidney and it is not possible to perform a retrograde study, antegrade pyelography may be required to determine the cause of obstruction. This should be done as a procedure of last resort, however, because complete obstruction is more likely to be associated with a high-grade tumor for which the risk of tumor cell seeding is greater. In these situations, CT scanning may reveal a soft tissue mass within the collecting system and obviate the need for an antegrade study.

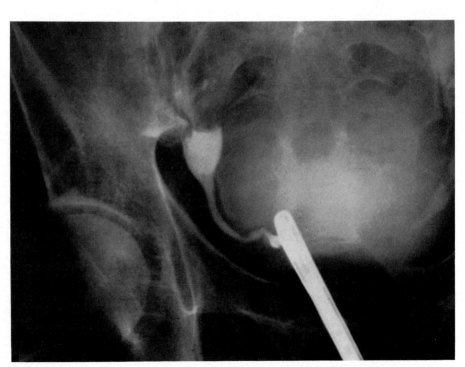

Figure 28–27. Retrograde pyelogram of lower ureteral tumor.

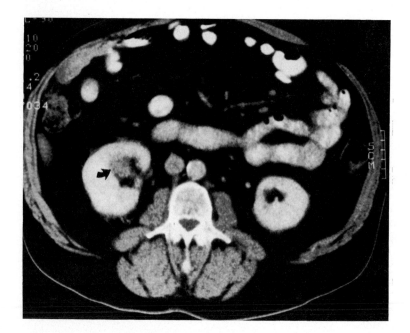

Figure 28–28. Computed tomographic scan showing a right renal pelvis tumor.

Computed Tomography

CT is useful both in the diagnosis and staging of upper tract urothelial tumors (Baghdassarian Gatewood et al., 1982; Lantz and Hattery, 1984; Milestone et al., 1990) (Figs. 28–28 and 28–29). Because CT is more sensitive than conventional radiography in visualizing minimally radiopaque substances, it can demonstrate low concentrations of contrast agents in the urine excreted by poorly functioning kidneys. Thus, CT may delineate a collecting system tumor better than excretory urography in some instances (Kenney and Stanley, 1987). In comparison, small tumors may be overlooked on CT scans, owing to volume averaging.

Uric acid stones, which are radiolucent on standard urography, are opaque on CT scans because their radiodensity is usually greater than 100 Houndsfield units (HU) (range, 80 to 250 HU) (Lantz and Hattery, 1984). Transitional cell carcinomas are recognized as a soft tissue mass with an average density of 46 HU and a range of 10 to 70 HU (Lantz and Hattery, 1984).

Ultrasonography also may be helpful in distinguishing between a urothelial tumor and a radiolucent calculus, but ultrasonography is generally of little value in the diagnosis and staging of upper tract urothelial tumors.

Large, infiltrating renal pelvis tumors may be difficult to distinguish from renal cell carcinoma. On CT, transitional cell carcinomas have a low attenuation relative to normal renal parenchyma. CT scans also can reveal necrosis and/or spontaneous hemorrhage within the tumor (Bree et al., 1990).

Magnetic Resonance Imaging

MRI has not been reported to offer any material advantage over CT scanning in the diagnosis and staging of patients with upper tract urothelial tumors (Milestone et al., 1990).

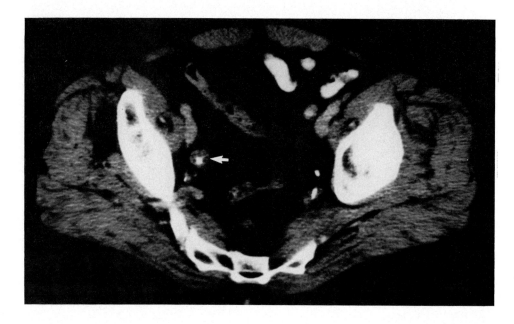

Figure 28–29. Computed tomographic scan showing mid-ureteral transitional cell carcinoma.

Cystoscopy

Because of the high incidence of associated bladder tumors in patients with upper tract transitional cell carcinoma, cystoscopy is mandatory to rule out coexistent bladder tumors. If performed at the time of bleeding, cystoscopy also may be helpful in localizing the bleeding site.

Cytopathology

A voided urine specimen for cytopathology is the most convenient, least invasive means of obtaining cells from the urinary tract for cytologic evaluation. Precautions for collecting samples for cytology are presented in the section on bladder cancer. Even under ideal circumstances, however, voided urine samples for cytopathology provide an insensitive test for establishing the diagnosis of upper tract urothelial tumors. With low-grade tumors, the cytology is read as normal in up to 80 per cent of patients (Grace et al., 1967). As with bladder tumors, there is a correlation between tumor grade and positive cytology results. Accordingly, some workers have reported that urinary cytology is of little help in diagnosing primary tumors of the renal pelvis or ureter (Nielsen and Ostri, 1988). Murphy and associates (1981) reported that cytology was accurate in 45 per cent of patients with grade 2 tumors, in 78 per cent with grade 3 tumors, and in 83 per cent with grade 4 tumors; however, many of these patients also had concomitant bladder tumors. Even if the voided cytologic finding is positive in a patient with an upper tract filling defect, one cannot be absolutely certain of the site of origin of the malignant cells.

Ureteral catheterization for collection of urine directly from the upper urinary tracts provides more accurate cytologic results (Hawtrey, 1971; Sarnacki et al., 1971), but it still is associated with substantial false-negative (22 to 35 per cent) and false-positive findings. Saline barbotage provides better cell yields because hydraulic forces release loosely adherent cells from the urothelium and improve the accuracy of cytology results.

Brush Biopsy

Gill and co-workers (1973) introduced the concept of brush biopsy to establish the diagnosis of upper tract urothelial tumors. With this technique, a fine brush mounted on the end of a guide wire is passed through a ureteral catheter into the collecting system and, under fluoroscopic guidance, is manipulated adjacent to the filling defect (Gittes, 1984). The lesion is then sampled by moving the brush back and forth within the ureteral catheter. The brush is removed through the catheter, and the sample (brushings) is sent for cytologic examination. Brush biopsies have a high positive predictive value (approaching 100 per cent) when they are read as being conclusive or suspicious for malignancy or when they show severely dysplastic cells. Brushings that show atypical cells have a positive predictive value of 75 per cent. Sheline and colleagues (1989) reported that brush biopsy has a sensitivity of 91 per cent, a specificity of 88 per cent, and an accuracy of 89 per cent. Blute and associates (1981) reported a 78 per cent overall accuracy. In general, brush biopsy is well tolerated with minimal complications; however, severe complications, including massive hemorrhage from the upper urinary tracts and ureteral perforation, have been reported (Blute et al., 1981). The risks of spreading tumor cells to areas of ureteral mucosa denuded by the manipulations associated with brush biopsy also must be borne in mind. Gittes (1984) reported that brush biopsy is not indicated in patients with radiographically obvious lesions; in those with a solitary kidney with a single, well-defined lesion; and in those with positive upper tract cytology findings, with no visible lesion or with lesions that will be approached percutaneously.

Ureteroscopy/Nephroscopy

In current years, with the development of rigid and flexible ureteroscopes, ureteroscopy has been used increasingly in establishing the diagnosis of upper tract urothelial tumors. Streem and co-workers (1986) reported that ureteropyeloscopy increased the diagnostic accuracy over the standard diagnostic regimen from 58 to 83 per cent. Similarly, Blute and colleagues (1989) reported that the diagnosis of renal pelvis tumors was made correctly in 86 per cent of renal pelvic tumors and 90 per cent of ureteral tumors by ureteropyeloscopy. The complication rate in this series was 7 per cent. The major concern about performing ureteroscopy in patients with upper tract urothelial tumors is the risk of ureteral perforation with extravasation of tumor cells, denudation of the ureteral mucosa for implantation of tumor cells, or development of complete ureteral disruption or stricture formation.

Small endoscopic biopsy forceps are available for performing biopsies through a ureteroscope. These forceps obtain very small tissue fragments that may be difficult for the pathologist to interpret. Nonetheless, the characteristic endoscopic appearance of a transitional cell carcinoma usually is sufficient to establish the correct diagnosis. Diagnostic ureteroscopy should be reserved for patients in whom the diagnosis remains in doubt after utilizing conventional diagnostic techniques and for those in whom the treatment would be influenced by the results of ureteroscopy. Diagnostic ureteropyeloscopy is discussed in greater detail in Chapter 62.

Open nephroscopy through a pyelotomy incision has been reported as a valid diagnostic technique and as a means of treating upper tract urothelial tumors (Gittes, 1984); however, tumor cell implantation in the retroperitoneum has been reported following pyeloscopy (Tomera et al., 1982).

STAGING

Staging Systems

Two staging systems are commonly used for transitional cell carcinoma of the upper urinary tract. In the

United States, most clinicians use the staging system described by Grabstald and co-workers (1971) or the modification of it described by Cummings (1980). This system is similar to the Jewett-Strong-Marshall system for bladder cancer. In the Grabstald-Cummings system, tumors confined to the mucosa are designated stage I. Tumors invading the lamina propria and involving the submucosa are called stage II. Tumors invading into the smooth muscle of the ureter, renal pelvis, or renal parenchyma are called stage III. Those that have extended through the muscle or renal capsule or that have metastasized or invaded adjacent organs are called stage IV.

The TNM staging system proposed by the AJC-UICC (Spiessl et al., 1989) categorizes upper tract tumors as follows: Tx, primary tumor cannot be assessed; T0, no evidence of primary tumor; Tis, carcinoma in situ; Ta, papillary noninvasive carcinoma; T1, tumor involving the submucosa; T2, tumor invading into smooth muscle; T3, tumor invading into the peripelvic or periureteral soft tissue or renal parenchyma; and T4, tumors that have invaded through the kidney or into adjacent organs. Regional lymph node metastases are designated N-positive. In the AJC-UICC system, the renal lymph nodes for renal pelvis and ureteral cancer are considered to be the para-aortic and paracaval nodes. Laterality does not effect the N classification. Nx denotes regional lymph nodes cannot be assessed; N0 denotes no lymph node metastases; N1 denotes a single positive node less than or equal to 2 cm in diameter; N2 denotes a single positive node greater than 2 cm, but less than 5 cm in diameter or multiple positive nodes less than 5 cm in diameter; and N3 denotes positive nodes greater than 5 cm in diameter. The AJC-UICC system considers patients without distant metastases as M0 and those with distant metastases as M1. These staging systems are shown in Table 28–6.

Metastatic Evaluation

CT scanning is helpful in determining the local extent of the primary tumor as well as in evaluating metastases. CT scanning can demonstrate extension into the renal parenchyma or periureteral soft tissue, venous involvement, lymph node involvement, or liver metastases (Lantz and Hattery, 1984). Other useful tests for the metastatic evaluation include chest radiography or CT, bone scan, and liver function tests.

In patients with compromised renal function, it is advisable to obtain a creatinine clearance value and a renal scan to determine split renal function. These results may have a bearing on whether conservative or radical surgery is performed.

TREATMENT

Current data suggest that the following generalizations are valid concerning the treatment of upper tract urothelial tumors. Patients with low-grade, low-stage tumors do well with either conservative or radical surgery. Patients with intermediate-grade tumors do better with radical surgery. Patients with high-grade, high-stage tumors do equally poorly with either conservative or radical surgery. With conservative surgery, tumor recurrence rates in the retained ipsilateral collecting system vary from 7 to 60 per cent, depending on the tumor grade. However, little evidence exists that recurrences compromise patient survival.

These generalizations are supported by an experience in which only one of 15 (7 per cent) patients with grade 1 tumors treated with conservative resections had a recurrence in the ipsilateral ureter. The 5-year survival was 88 per cent for radical surgery and 75 per cent for conservative surgery for grade 1 tumors. Of patients with grade 2 tumors, eight of 29 (28 per cent) treated with conservative resection had ipsilateral recurrences. The 2-year survival was 90 per cent for radical surgery versus 46 per cent for conservative surgery. No patient with a grade 3 or 4 tumor had an ipsilateral recurrence, probably because of short survival in all patients. Contralateral recurrences occurred in less than 2 per cent of patients (Murphy et al., 1980, 1981). These data provide the basis for the following general treatment guidelines. Most renal pelvis tumors should be treated with total nephroureterectomy. Upper and mid-ureteral tumors should be treated with segmental resection if they are solitary and low-grade and with nephroureterectomy if they are multifocal or high-grade. Distal ureteral tumors should be treated by distal ureterectomy and ureteroneocystostomy. Conservative resections are especially appropriate for solitary or functionally dominant kidneys; bilateral tumors; or small, polypoid, low-grade ureteral tumors. In the rare patient with bilateral diffuse tumors or diffuse tumors in a solitary kidney, bilateral nephrectomy with hemodialysis and, possibly, subsequent renal transplantation may be the best treatment options.

Patients with only positive cytologic findings of the upper tracts and normal radiographic findings and ureteroscopic examinations should be followed closely with excretory or retrograde urography and should *not* be treated blindly.

Nephroureterectomy

The traditional treatment for upper tract urothelial tumors is total nephroureterectomy with excision of a

Table 28–6. STAGING SYSTEMS OF UPPER TRACT UROTHELIAL TUMORS

Finding	Grabstald-Cummings Stage	1987 UICC Stage
Carcinoma in situ	I	Tis
Noninvasive papillary tumor	I	Ta
Tumor involving submucoa	II	T1
Muscle-invasive tumor	III	T2
Tumor invading renal parenchyma	III	T3
Tumor invading peripelvic or periureteral soft tissue	III	T3
Invasion of contiguous organs	IV	T4
Lymph node metastases	IV	(N1–3)
Distant metastases	IV	M1

cuff of bladder (Anderstrom et al., 1989). This is based on many studies that have demonstrated a high incidence (30 to 75 per cent) of subsequent tumor recurrence in the ureteral stump or around the ipsilateral ureteral orifice in patients treated with more conservative operations (Bloom et al., 1970; Kakizoe et al., 1980; Mullen and Kovacs, 1980). Further studies have demonstrated that conservative surgery is acceptable in selected patients (Mufti et al., 1989; Zungri et al., 1990).

Nephroureterectomy usually is performed through two incisions including a flank incision and a paramedian modified Gibson incision. This operation also can be performed through a midline incision or a single modified flank incision. Some workers have recommended endoscopic resection of the intramural ureter followed by removal of the remaining ureter in continuity with the kidney through a single flank incision. The surgical techniques of nephroureterectomy are discussed in greater detail elsewhere in this text.

Johansson and Wahlqvist (1979) recommended performing a parafascial nephroureterectomy with adrenalectomy and retroperitoneal lymphadenectomy for upper tract transitional cell carcinoma. In this series, the 5-year survival was 84 per cent with the radical operation as compared with only 51 per cent with conventional nephroureterectomy. The principal difference in prognosis was observed in patients with high-stage tumors in whom the radical operation produced a 74 per cent survival compared with a 37 per cent survival with the conservative operation. However, the patients in this series were not concurrently treated and, thus, may not have been entirely comparable. Many patients in the study had tumors associated with analgesic abuse, which also may have influenced the results. Similar results were reported by Zungri and associates (1990).

Skinner (1978) recommended routine lymphadenectomy in patients with upper tract urothelial tumors, but Babaian and Johnson (1980) suggested that there are insufficient data to justify the additional time and possible operative morbidity. The majority of reports indicate that when lymph node metastases are present, the patient has widely disseminated disease and is unlikely to benefit from regional lymphadenectomy (Heney et al., 1981). Johansson and Wahlqvist (1979) reported on two patients with lymph node metastases treated with lymphadenectomy who were alive and tumor-free 7 years later. Representative 5-year survival results reported by Batata and co-workers (1975) were stage A, 91 per cent; stage B, 43 per cent; stage C, 23 per cent; and stage D, 0 per cent.

Conservative Excision

The concept of conservative excision for upper tract urothelial tumors was first introduced by Vest (1945); however, this concept was generally ignored until the early 1970s when favorable results of conservative surgery were reported in patients with Balkan nephropathy. Most evidence suggests that for low-grade, low-stage tumors, equivalent results are achieved with conservative excision and nephroureterectomy (Anderstrom et al., 1989; Murphy et al., 1980; Zoretic and Gonzales,

1983). Zoretic and Gonzales (1983) reported on 16 patients who underwent segmental resections for ureteral tumors. The 5-year survival rate was 71 per cent with a ureteral recurrence rate of 6 per cent. Mufti and co-workers (1989) reported that the survival of patients treated with conservative resections was greater than 90 per cent. However, when urothelium was left behind after a conservative resection, there was a 22 per cent recurrence rate on the same side, noted almost exclusively in patients with multifocal tumors. Bazeed and associates (1986) reported tumor recurrences in four of nine (44 per cent) patients treated with local excision, four of whom had normal contralateral kidneys. All recurrences were reported to be successfully treated with repeat local excision.

Other series have reported tumor recurrence rates ranging from 25 to 40 per cent with segmental resection or local excision (Ghazi et al., 1979; Hatch et al., 1988; Wallace et al., 1981). The recurrence rates following conservative resection of renal pelvis tumors are higher than those following conservative resection of ureteral tumors (Mazeman, 1976; Zincke and Neves, 1984). For obvious anatomic reasons, renal pelvis tumors are more difficult to excise completely with conservative surgery than are ureteral tumors.

Partial nephrectomy also has been reported in patients with transitional cell carcinoma of the renal pelvis. Ziegelbaum and colleagues (1987) reported a 38 per cent tumor recurrence rate in patients treated with a variety of different conservative surgical procedures for upper tract urothelial tumors, and only 46 per cent of patients were tumor-free at the time of their report. These investigators recommended conservative surgery only in situations in which it is necessary to avoid renal failure.

For distal ureteral tumors, regardless of tumor grade or stage, distal ureterectomy removing a cuff of bladder with ureteral reimplantation using a psoas hitch or Boari flap, if necessary, is the preferred treatment. It is important to obtain a negative proximal ureteral margin; otherwise, a total nephroureterectomy should be performed in most instances. Using this approach, Johnson and Babaian (1979) reported a recurrence in only one of six patients.

Endoscopic Treatment of Upper Tract Urothelial Tumors

The rationale for endoscopic treatment for upper tract urothelial tumors is the same as that for endoscopic management of superficial bladder tumors. The principal differences relate to the logistic difficulties encountered in gaining access to the upper urinary tracts and in performing the manipulations necessary to treat the tumors. The other major considerations include the relative thinness of the wall of the upper urinary collecting system, which makes it more susceptible to perforation and extravasation of tumor cells. Also, the relatively smaller diameter of the upper urinary tract makes it more susceptible to obstruction by relatively minor degrees of post-treatment fibrosis.

Endoscopic treatment of upper tract urothelial tumors is also discussed in detail in Chapter 62.

Ureteroscopic Treatment

Limited data exist on the results of ureteroscopic excision, fulguration, or laser destruction of upper tract urothelial tumors. The available studies report tumor recurrence rates ranging from 15 to 45 per cent with relatively short-term follow-up (Blute et al., 1989; Huffman et al., 1985; Schmeller and Hofstetter, 1989). Huffman and co-workers (1985) recommended following such patients with ureteroscopic surveillance. The feasibility of this approach is questionable (see Chapter 62).

Little has been written about the complications of ureteroscopic management of upper tract tumors. The major complications include ureteral perforation, which occurs in less than 10 per cent of patients; tumor cell implantation on denuded urothelium; and ureteral strictures, which have been reported to occur in more than one third of patients (Schmeller and Hofstetter, 1989). Stricture formation is less with laser treatment than with electrocautery (Schmeller and Hofstetter, 1989).

Percutaneous Treatment

Data are limited about the percutaneous management of upper tract urothelial tumors (Nolan et al., 1988; Smith et al., 1987a; Tasca and Zattoni, 1990). The major concern about this form of treatment is tumor seeding along the nephrostomy tract, but insufficient information is available to assess this risk. The tumor recurrence rate within the collecting system has been reported to be as high as 45 per cent (Smith et al., 1987a). Tasca and Zattoni (1990) recommended that this approach should be restricted to patients with small, single, low-grade tumors not amenable to ureteroscopic excision.

Instillation Therapy

Anecdotal information only is available concerning instillation therapy for upper tract urothelial tumors. Smith and colleagues (1987b) reported on intravesical mitomycin C to treat distal ureteral tumors in patients with vesicoureteral reflux. DeKock and Breytenbach (1986) reported local excision and instillation of thiotepa into the upper urinary tracts with beneficial effects and no adverse side effects. BCG also has been instilled into the upper urinary tracts to treat urothelial tumors, including carcinoma in situ (Herr, 1985; Ramsey and Soloway, 1990; Smith et al., 1987a; Studer et al., 1989). BCG demonstrated efficacy in this clinical setting, but there are reports of some patients developing sepsis (Ramsey and Soloway, 1990; Studer et al., 1989).

Radiation Therapy

In patients with upper tract urothelial tumors, radiation therapy has been largely a postoperative adjuvant in those considered at high risk for local recurrence. In this clinical setting, radiation therapy has been reported to be of some benefit (Brookland and Richter, 1985); however, the numbers of patients reported were too small to permit definitive conclusions to be drawn. Radiation therapy also is effective for palliation of painful osseous metastases (see Bladder Cancer).

Angioinfarction

Angioinfarction is rarely used in the treatment of renal pelvic tumors, but it may have a role in selected patients with symptomatic primary tumors who have incurable distant metastases.

Systemic Chemotherapy

The chemotherapeutic regimens for the treatment of upper tract urothelial tumors are the same as those for the treatment of bladder cancer. Because of the rarity of these tumors, no large series have been reported. The long-term results of M-VAC chemotherapy have been disappointing with durable complete responses being reported in as few as 5 per cent of patients; as many as 41 per cent experienced neutropenic sepsis with a 2 to 3 per cent mortality (Tannock et al., 1989).

Scher and co-workers (1988) reported on patients with extravesical transitional cell carcinomas treated with M-VAC as a neoadjuvant. This study included only small numbers of patients with upper tract tumors; therefore, the results cannot be generalized. As was the case with the treatment of bladder cancer patients, M-VAC was ineffective against mixed histologic tumors and was also ineffective in preventing the development of new carcinoma in situ lesions.

Permission granted by Mosby-Year Book, Inc., Chicago, to use material from Catalona, W. J.: Adult and Pediatric Urology, 1987.

REFERENCES

Bladder Cancer

Abel, P. D., Hall, R. R., and Williams, G.: Should pT1 transitional cell cancers of the bladder still be classified as superficial? Br. J. Urol., 62:235, 1988a.

Abel, P. D., Henderson, D., Bennett, M. K., et al.: Differing interpretations by pathologists of the pT category and grade of transitional cell cancer of the bladder. Br. J. Urol., 62:339, 1988b.

Abratt, R. P., Barnes, D. R., Potin, A. R., et al.: Radical radiation and oral and intra-vesical misonidazole for bladder cancer. Int. J. Radiat. Oncol. Biol. Phys., 13:1053, 1987.

Abratt, R. P., Sealy, R., Tucker, R. D., et al.: Radical irradiation and misonidazole in the treatment of grade III and T3 bladder cancer. Int. J. Radiat. Oncol. Biol. Phys., 9:629, 1983.

Aherne, G.: Retinoblastoma associated with other primary malignant tumors. Trans. Ophthalmol. Soc. U. K., 94:938, 1974.

Ahlering, T. E., Kanellos, A., Boyd, S. D., et al.: A comparative study of perioperative complications with Kock pouch urinary diversion in highly irradiated versus nonirradiated patients. J. Urol., 139:1202, 1988a.

Ahlering, T. E., Weintraub, P., and Skinner, D. G.: Management of adult sarcomas of the bladder and prostate. J. Urol., 140:1397, 1988b.

Albores-Saavedra, J., Maldonado, M. E., Ibarra, J., et al.: Pheochromocytoma of the urinary bladder. Cancer, 23:1110, 1969.

Alfthan, O., Tarkkanen, J., Grohn, P., et al.: Tigason (etretinate) in prevention of recurrence of superficial bladder tumors: A double-blind clinical trial. Eur. Urol., 9:6, 1983.

Althausen, A. F., Prout, G. R., Jr., and Daly, J. J.: Noninvasive papillary carcinoma of the bladder associated with carcinoma in situ. J. Urol., 116:575, 1976.

Anderstrom, C., Johansson, S., and Nilsson, S.: The significance of lamina propria invasion on the prognosis of patients with bladder tumors. J. Urol., 124:23, 1980.

Anderstrom, C., Johansson, S. L., and von Schultz, L.: Primary adenocarcinoma of the urinary bladder: A clinicopathologic and prognostic study. Cancer, 52:1273, 1983.

1987 Annual Cancer Statistics Review: Including Cancer Trends: 1950–1985, NIH Publication No. 88-2789. Bethesda, Maryland, U. S. Department of Health and Human Services, National Cancer Institute.

Arce, S., Lopez, R., Almaguer, M., et al.: HLA-antigens and transitional cell carcinoma. Mater. Med. Pol., 10:98, 1978.

Atallah, A. S., Tribukait, B., El-Bedeiwy, A. -F. A., et al.: Prediction of lymph node metastases in bladder carcinoma with deoxyribonucleic acid flow cytometry. J. Urol., 144:884, 1990.

Atkin, N. B., and Fox, M. F.: 5q deletion: The sole chromosome change in a carcinoma of the bladder. Cancer Genet. Cytogenet., 46:129, 1990.

Augustine, A., Hebert, J. R., Kabat, G. C., et al.: Bladder cancer in relation to cigarette smoking. Cancer Res., 48:4405, 1988.

Babaian, R. J., Johnson, D. E., Llamas, L., et al.: Metastases from transitional cell carcinoma of the urinary bladder. Urology, 16:142, 1980.

Babu, V. R., Miles, B. J., Cerney, J. C., et al.: Chromosome 21q22 deletion: A specific chromosome change in a new bladder cancer subgroup. Cancer Genet. Cytogenet., 38:127, 1989.

Badalament, R. A., Fair, W. R., Whitmore, W. F., Jr., et al.: The relative value of cytometry and cytology in the management of bladder cancer: The Memorial Sloan-Kettering Cancer Center experience. Semin. Urol., 6:22, 1988.

Badalament, R. A., Herr, H. W., Wong, G. Y., et al.: A prospective randomized trial of maintenance versus nonmaintenance intravesical bacillus Calmette-Guérin therapy of superficial bladder cancer. J. Clin. Oncol., 5:441, 1987.

Badalament, R. A., O'Toole, R. V., Keyhani-Rofagha, S., et al.: Flow cytometric analysis of primary and metastatic bladder cancer. J. Urol., 143:912, 1990.

Barentsz, J. O., Lemmens, J. A., Ruijs, S. H., et al.: Carcinoma of the urinary bladder: MR imaging with a double surface coil. Am. J. Roentgenol., 151:107, 1988.

Barnes, R. W., Bergman, R. T., Hadley, H. T., et al.: Control of bladder tumors by endoscopic surgery. J. Urol., 97:864, 1967.

Beer, M., Jocham, D., Beer, A., et al.: Adjuvant laser treatment of bladder cancer: 8 Years' experience with the Nd-YAG laser 1064 nm. Br. J. Urol., 63:476, 1989.

Beisland, H. O., and Sander, S.: Neodymium-YAG laser irradiation of stage T2 muscle-invasive bladder cancer: Long-term results. Br. J. Urol., 65:24, 1990.

Bejany, E. C., Lockhart, J. L., and Rhamy, R. K.: Malignant vesical tumors following spinal cord injury. J. Urol., 138:1390, 1987.

Bennett, J. K., Wheatley, J. K., and Walton, K. N.: 10-Year experience with adenocarcinoma of the bladder. J. Urol., 131:262, 1984.

Bennett, J. K., Wheatley, J. K., and Walton, K. N.: Nonmetastatic bladder cancer associated with hypercalcemia, thrombocytosis and leukemoid reaction. J. Urol., 135:47, 1986.

Benson, R. C., Jr.: Endoscopic management of bladder cancer with hematoporphyrin derivative phototherapy. Urol. Clin. North Am., 11:637, 1984.

Benson, R. C., Farrow, G. M., Kinsey, J. H., et al.: Detection and localization of in situ carcinoma of the bladder with hematoporphyrin derivative. Mayo Clin. Proc., 57:548, 1982.

Benson, R. C., Jr., Kinsey, J. H., Cortese, D. A., et al.: Treatment of transitional cell carcinoma of the bladder with hematoporphyrin derivative phototherapy. J. Urol., 130:1090, 1983a.

Benson, R. C., Jr., Swanson, S. K., and Farrow, G. M.: Relationship of leukoplakia to urothelial malignancy. J. Urol., 131:507, 1984.

Benson, R. C., Jr., Tomera, K. M., and Kelalis, P. P.: Transitional cell carcinoma of the bladder in children and adolescents. J. Urol., 130:54, 1983b.

Berger, G. L., Sadlowsky, R. W., Sharp, J. R., et al.: Lack of value of routine postoperative bone and liver scans in cystectomy candidates. J. Urol., 125:637–639, 1981.

Binkovitz, L. A., Hattery, R. R., and LeRoy, A. J.: Primary lymphoma of the bladder. Urol. Radiol., 9:231, 1988.

Blackard, C. E., and Byar, D. P.: Results of a clinical trial of surgery and radiation in stages II and III carcinoma of the bladder. J. Urol., 108:875, 1972.

Blandy, J. P., England, H. R., Evans, S. J. W., et al.: T3 bladder cancer: The case for salvage cystectomy. Br. J. Urol., 52:506, 1980.

Block, N. L., and Whitmore, W. F., Jr.: Leukemoid reaction, thrombocytosis, and hypercalcemia associated with bladder cancer. J. Urol., 110:660, 1973.

Blomjous, C. E. M., Schipper, N. W., Vos, W., et al.: Comparison of quantitative and classic prognosticators in urinary bladder carcinoma: A multivariate analysis of DNA flow cytometric, nuclear morphometric and clinicopathologic features. Virchows Archiv. [A], 415:421, 1989.

Bloom, H. J. G., Hendry, W. F., Wallace, D. M., et al.: Treatment of T3 bladder cancer: Controlled trial of preoperative radiotherapy and radical cystectomy versus radical radiotherapy. Br. J. Urol., 54:136, 1982.

Blute, M. L., Engen, D. E., Travis, W. D., et al.: Primary signet ring cell adenocarcinoma of the bladder. J. Urol. 141:17, 1989.

Bohle, A., Schuller, J., Knipper, A., et al.: Bacillus Calmette-Guérin treatment and vesicorenal reflux. Eur. Urol., 17:125, 1990.

Boyd, S. D., Feinberg, S. M., Skinner, D. G., et al.: Quality of life survey of urinary diversion patients: Comparison of ileal conduits versus continent Kock ileal reservoirs. J. Urol., 138:1386, 1987.

Boyd, S. D., and Schiff, W. M.: Inflatable penile prostheses in patients undergoing cystoprostatectomy with urethrectomy. J. Urol., 141:60, 1989.

Bracken, R. B., McDonald, M. W., and Johnson, D. E.: Cystectomy for superficial bladder cancer. Urology, 28:459, 1981a.

Bracken, R. B., McDonald, M., and Johnson, D. E.: Complications of single-stage radical cystectomy and ileal conduit. Urology, 17:141, 1981b.

Brendler, C. B., Schlegel, P. N., and Walsh, P. C.: Urethrectomy with preservation of potency. J. Urol., 144:270, 1990a.

Brendler, C. B., Steinberg, G. D., Marshall, F. F., et al.: Local recurrence and survival following nerve-sparing radical cystoprostatectomy. J. Urol., 144:1137, 1990b.

Bretton, P. R., Herr, H. W., Kimmel, M., et al.: The response of patients with superficial bladder cancer to a second course of intravesical bacillus Calmette-Guérin. J. Urol., 143:710, 1990.

Bretton, P. R., Herr, H. W., Whitmore, W. F., Jr., et al.: Intravesical bacillus Calmette-Guérin therapy for in situ transitional cell carcinoma involving the prostatic urethra. J. Urol., 141:853, 1989.

Brick, S. H., Friedman, A. C., Pollack, H. M., et al.: Urachal carcinoma: CT findings. Radiology, 169:377, 1988.

Bricker, E. M.: Bladder substitution after pelvic evisceration. Surg. Clin. North Am., 30:1511, 1950.

Brismar, J., and Gustafson, T.: Bone scintigraphy in staging of bladder carcinoma. Acta Radiol., 29:251, 1988.

Broders, A. C.: Epithelioma of the genitourinary organs. Ann. Surg., 75:574, 1922.

Broecher, B. H., Klein, F. A., and Hackler, R. H.: Cancer of the bladder in spinal cord injury patients. J. Urol., 125:196, 1981.

Brosman, S. A.: Experience with bacillus Calmette-Guérin in patients with superficial bladder carcinoma. J. Urol., 128:27, 1982.

Brosman, S. A.: BCG in the management of superficial bladder cancer. Urology, 23(April suppl.):82, 1984.

Brown, R. B.: Experiences with intravesical formalin administration in advanced carcinoma of the bladder. Br. J. Urol., 42:738, 1970.

Brown, R. R., Price, J. M., Friedell, G. H., et al.: Tryptophan metabolism in patients with bladder cancer: Geographic differences. JNCI, 43:295, 1969.

Bryan, G. T.: The role of urinary tryptophan metabolites in the etiology of bladder cancer. Am. J. Clin. Nutr., 24:841, 1971.

Bryan, G. T.: The pathogenesis of experimental bladder cancer. Cancer Res., 37:2813, 1977.

Burch, J. D., Rohan, T. E., Howe, G. R., et al.: Risk of bladder cancer by source and type of tobacco exposure: A case-control study. Int. J. Cancer, 44:622, 1989.

Burk, K. H., and Drewinko, B.: Cell cycle dependency of tumor antigens. Cancer Res., 36:3535, 1976.

Buy, J. N., Moss, A. A., Guinet, C., et al.: MR staging of bladder carcinoma: Correlation with pathologic findings. Radiology, 169:695, 1988.

Byar, D., and Blackhard, C.: Comparisons of placebo, pyridoxine, and topical Thiotepa in preventing recurrence of stage I bladder cancer. Urology, 10:556, 1977.

Bydder, P. V., Burry, A. F., Gowland, S., et al.: A controlled trial of misonidazole in the curative treatment of infiltrating bladder cancer. Australas. Radiol., 33:8, 1989.

Campo, E., Algaba, R., Palacin, A., et al.: Placental proteins in high-grade urothelial neoplasms: An immunohistochemical study of human chorionic gonadotropin, human placental lactogen and pregnancy-specific beta-1-glycoprotein. Cancer, 63:2497, 1989.

Carbin, B. E., Ekman, P., Eneroth, P., et al.: Urine-TPA (tissue polypeptide antigen), flow cytometry and cytology as markers for tumor invasiveness in urinary bladder carcinoma. Urol. Res., 17:269, 1989.

Carmignani, G., Belgrano, E., Puppo, P., et al.: Transcatheter embolization of the hypogastric arteries in cases of bladder hemorrhage from advanced pelvic cancers: Follow-up in 9 cases. J. Urol., 124:196, 1980.

Carter, H. B., Amberson, J. B., Bander, N. H., et al.: Newer diagnostic techniques for bladder cancer. Urol. Clin. North Am., 14:763, 1987.

Case, R. A. M., Hosker, M. E., McDonald, D. B., et al.: Tumors of the urinary bladder in workmen engaged in the manufacture and use of certain dyestuff intermediates in the British chemical industry. Br. J. Ind. Med., 11:75, 1954.

Catalona, W. J.: Bladder carcinoma. J. Urol., 123:35, 1980.

Catalona, W. J., Hudson, M. A., Gillen, D. P., et al.: Risks and benefits of repeated courses of intravesical bacillus Calmette-Guérin therapy for superficial bladder cancer. J. Urol., 137:220, 1987.

Catalona, W. J., and Ratliff, T. L.: Bacillus Calmette-Guérin and superficial bladder cancer: Clinical experience and mechanism of action. Surg. Annu., 22:363, 1990.

Catalona, W. J., Ratliff, T. L., and McCool, R. E.: Immunology of genitourinary tumors. In Paulson, D. F. (Ed.): Genitourinary Cancer 1. Boston, Martinus Nijhoff, 1982, p. 169.

Chan, H., and Pratt, C. B.: A new familial cancer syndrome? A spectrum of malignant and benign tumors including retinoblastoma, carcinoma of the bladder and other genitourinary tumors, thyroid adenoma, and a probable case of multifocal osteosarcoma. J. Natl. Cancer Inst., 58:205, 1977.

Chapman, J. W., Connolly, J. G., and Rosenbaum, L.: Occupational bladder cancer: A case-control study. In Connolly, J. G. (Ed.): Carcinoma of the Bladder. New York, Raven Press, 1981, p. 45.

Choi, H., Lamb, S., Pintar, K., et al.: Primary signet-ring cell carcinoma of the urinary bladder. Cancer, 53:1985, 1984.

Ciccone, G., and Vineis, P.: Coffee drinking and bladder cancer. Cancer Lett., 41:45, 1988.

Clark, S. S., Marlett, M. M., Prudencio, R. F., et al.: Neurofibromatosis of the bladder in children: Case report and literature review. J. Urol., 118:654, 1977.

Clavel, J., Cordier, S., Boccon-Gibod, L., et al.: Tobacco and bladder cancer in males: Increased risk for inhalers and smokers of black tobacco. Int. J. Cancer, 44:605, 1989.

Cole, P., Hoover, R., and Friedell, G. H.: Occupation and cancer of the lower urinary tract. Cancer, 29:1250, 1972.

Connor, J. P., Olsson, C. A., Benson, M. C., et al.: Long-term follow-up in patients treated with methotrexate, vinblastine, doxorubicin, and cisplatin (M-VAC) for transitional cell carcinoma of urinary bladder: Cause for concern. Urology, 34:353, 1989.

Coon, J. S., Weinstein, R. S., and Summers, J. L.: Blood group precursor T-antigen expression in human urinary bladder carcinoma. Am. J. Clin. Pathol., 77:692, 1982.

Coplen, D. E., Marcus, M. D., Myers, J. A., et al.: Long-term follow-up of patients treated with 1 or 2, 6-week courses of intravesical bacillus Calmette-Guérin: Analysis of possible predictors of response free of tumor. J. Urol., 144:652, 1990.

Cordon-Cardo, C., Reuter, V. E., Lloyd, K. O., et al.: Blood group–related antigens in human urothelium: Enhanced expression of Le^x and Le^y determinants in urothelial carcinoma. Cancer Res., 48:4113, 1988.

Costello, A. J., Tiptaft, R. C., England, H. R., et al.: Squamous cell carcinoma of the bladder. Urology, 23:234, 1984.

Crawford, E. D., Das, S., and Smith, J. A.: Preoperative radiation therapy in the treatment of bladder cancer. Urol. Clin. North Am., 14:781, 1987.

Crawford, E. D., and Skinner, D. G.: Salvage cystectomy after irradiation failure. J. Urol., 123:32, 1980.

Cummings, J. A., Hargreave, T. B., Webb, J. M., et al.: Intravesical Evans bacille Calmette-Guérin in the treatment of carcinoma in situ. Br. J. Urol., 63:259, 1989.

Cutler, S. H., and Young, J. L., Jr. (Eds.): Third National Cancer Survey: Incidence data. NCI Monogr., 41, 1975.

Dalesio, O., Schulman, C. C., Sylvester, R., et al.: Prognostic factors in superficial bladder tumors: A study of the European Organization for Research on the Treatment of Cancer: Genitourinary Tract Cancer Cooperative Group. J. Urol., 129:730, 1983.

Davis, M. P., Murthy, M. S. N., Simon, J., et al.: Successful management of small cell carcinoma of the bladder with cisplatin and etoposide. J. Urol., 142:817, 1989.

deKernion, J. B., Huang, M., Lindner, A., et al.: The management of superficial bladder tumors and carcinoma in situ with intravesical bacille Calmette-Guérin (BCG). J. Urol., 133:598, 1985.

DeKlerk, D. P., Catalona, W. J., Nime, F. A., et al.: Malignant pheochromocytoma of the bladder: The late development of renal cell carcinoma. J. Urol., 113:864, 1975.

DeKock, M. L. S., Anderson, C. K., and Clark, P. B.: Vesical leukoplakia progressing to squamous cell carcinoma in women. Br. J. Urol., 53:316, 1981.

Del Senno, L., Maestri, I., Piva, R., et al.: Differential hypomethylation of c-myc protooncogene in bladder cancers at different stages and grades. J. Urol., 142:146, 1989.

DeMeester, L. J., Farrow, G. M., and Utz, D. C.: Inverted papillomas of the urinary bladder. Cancer, 36:505, 1975.

Denovic, M., Bovier, R., Sarkissian, J., et al.: Intravesical instillation of mitomycin C in the prophylactic treatment of recurring superficial transitional cell carcinoma of the bladder. Br. J. Urol., 55:382, 1983.

Denovic, M., Darzynkiewicz, A., Kostryrka-Claps, M. L., et al.: Flow cytometry of low stage bladder tumors. Cancer, 48:109, 1982.

Depaepe, M. E., Andre, R., and Mahadevia, P.: Urethral involvement in female patients with bladder cancer: A study of 22 cystectomy specimens. Cancer, 65:1237, 1990.

Deresiewicz, R. L., Stone, R. M., and Aster, J. C.: Fatal disseminated mycobacterial infection following intravesical bacillus Calmette-Guérin. J. Urol. 144:1331, 1990.

Dow, J. A., di Sant'Agnese, P. A., and Cockett, A. T.: Expression of blood group precursor T antigen as a prognostic marker for human bladder cancer treated by bacillus Calmette-Guérin and interleukin-2. J. Urol., 142:978, 1989.

Droller, M. J.: Bladder cancer. In Monographs in Urology. Burroughs Welcome Company, 1982, p. 131.

Droller, M. J.: Immunotherapy of genitourinary neoplasia. Urol. Clin. North Am., 11:643, 1984.

Duncan, R. E., Bennett, D. W., Evans, A. T., et al.: Radiation-induced bladder tumors. J. Urol., 118:43, 1977.

Dunn, T. L., Seymour, G. J., Gardiner, R. A., et al.: Immunocytochemical demonstration of p21^{ras} in normal and transitional cell carcinoma urothelium. J. Pathol., 156:59, 1988.

Durkee, C., and Benson, R., Jr.: Bladder cancer following administration of cyclophosphamide. Urology, 16:145, 1980.

Eapen, L., Stewart, D., Danjoux, C., et al.: Intraarterial cisplatin and concurrent radiation for locally advanced bladder cancer. J. Clin. Oncol., 7:230, 1989.

Edwards, P. D., Hurm, R. A., and Jaeschke, W. H.: Conversion of cystitis glandularis to adenocarcinoma. J. Urol., 108:56, 1972.

El-Bolkainy, M. N., Mokhtar, N. M., Ghoneim, M. A., et al.: The impact of schistosomiasis on the pathology of bladder carcinoma. Cancer, 48:2643, 1981.

England, H. R., Molland, E. A., Oliver, R. T. D., et al.: Systemic cyclophosphamide in flat carcinoma in situ of the bladder. In Oliver, R. T. D., Hendry, W. F., and Bloom, H. J. G. (Eds.): Bladder Cancer: Principles of Combination Therapy. London, Butterworths, 1981, p. 97.

Fall, M., and Pettersson, S.: Ureteral complications after intravesical formalin instillation. J. Urol., 122:160, 1979.

Falor, W. H., and Ward-Skinner, R. M.: The importance of marker chromosomes in superficial transitional cell carcinoma of the bladder: 50 Patients followed up to 17 years. J. Urol., 139:929, 1988.

Farah, R. N., and Cerney, J. C.: Lymphangiography in staging patients with carcinoma of the bladder. J. Urol., 119:40, 1978.

Farrow, G. M., Utz, D. C., and Rife, C. C.: Morphological and clinical observations of patients with early bladder cancer treated with total cystectomy. Cancer Res., 36:2495, 1976.

Farsund, T., Laerum, O. D., and Hostmark, K. J.: Ploidy disturbance of normal-appearing bladder mucosa in patients with urothelial cancer: Relationship to morphology. J. Urol., 130:1076, 1983.

Faysal, M. H.: Squamous cell carcinoma of the bladder. J. Urol., 126:598, 1981.

Faysal, M. H., and Freiha, F. S.: Evaluation of partial cystectomy for carcinoma of the bladder. Urology, 14:352, 1979.

Faysal, M. H., and Freiha, F. S.: Primary neoplasm in vesical diverticula. Br. J. Urol., 53:141, 1981.

Ferraris, V.: Doxorubicin plus mitomycin C regimen in the prophylactic treatment of superficial bladder tumors. Cancer, 62:1055, 1988.

Filmer, R. B., and Spencer, J. R.: Malignancies in bladder augmentations and intestinal conduits. J. Urol., 143:671, 1990.

Fitzpatrick, J. M., West, A. B., Butler, M. R., et al.: Superficial bladder tumors (stage pTa, grades 1 and 2): The importance of recurrence pattern following initial resection. J. Urol., 135:920, 1986.

Flamm, J., Bucher, A., Holtl, W., et al.: Recurrent superficial transitional cell carcinoma of the bladder: Adjuvant topical chemotherapy versus immunotherapy: A prospective randomized trial. J. Urol., 144:260, 1990.

Flamm, J., and Dona, S.: The significance of bladder quadrant biopsies in patients with primary superficial bladder cancer. Eur. Urol., 16:81, 1989.

Flechner, S. M., and Spaulding, J. T.: Management of rectal injury during cystectomy. Urology, 19:143, 1982.

Fossa, S. D., Heilo, A., and Bormer, O.: Unexpectedly high serum methotrexate levels in cystectomized bladder cancer patients with an ileal conduit treated with intermediate doses of the drug. J. Urol., 143:498, 1990.

Fradet, Y., Tardif, M., Bourget, L., et al.: Clinical cancer progression in urinary bladder tumors evaluated by multiparameter flow cytometry with monoclonal antibodies. Cancer Res., 30:432, 1990.

Fraley, E. E., Lange, P. H., and Hakala, T. R.: Recent studies on the immunobiology and biology of human urothelial tumors. Urol. Clin. North Am., 3:31, 1976.

Fraumeni, J. F., Jr., and Thomas, L. B.: Malignant bladder tumors in a man and his three sons. JAMA, 201:507, 1967.

Friedell, G. H., Bell, J. R., Burney, S. W., et al.: Histopathology and classification of urinary bladder carcinoma. Urol. Clin. North Am., 3:53, 1976.

Friedell, G. H., Parija, G. C., Nagy, G. K., et al.: The pathology of human bladder cancer. Cancer, 45:1823, 1980.

Friedell, G. H., Soloway, M. S., Hilgar, A. G., et al.: Summary of workshop on carcinoma in situ of the bladder. J. Urol., 136:1047, 1986.

Fujita, J., Yoshida, O., Yuasa, Y., et al.: Ha-ras activated by somatic alterations in human urinary tract tumors. Nature, 309:464, 1984.

Fukui, I., Sekine, H., Kihara, K., et al.: Intravesical combination chemotherapy with mitomycin C and doxorubicin for carcinoma in situ of the bladder. J. Urol., 141:531, 1989.

Fukui, T., Yokokawa, M., Mitani, G., et al.: In vivo staining test with methylene blue for bladder cancer. J. Urol., 130:252, 1983.

Gabrilove, J. L., Jakubowski, A., Scher, H., et al.: Effect of granulocyte colony-stimulating factor on neutropenia and associated morbidity due to chemotherapy for transitional cell carcinoma of the urothelium. N. Engl. J. Med., 318:1414, 1988.

Gamarra, M. C., and Zein, T.: Cytologic spectrum of bladder cancer. Urology, 23:23, 1984.

Garnick, M. B., Schade, D., Israel, M., et al.: Intravesical doxorubicin for prophylaxis in the management of recurrent superficial bladder carcinoma. J. Urol., 131:43, 1984.

Ghoneim, M. A., and Awad, H. K.: Results of treatment in carcinoma of the bilharzial bladder. J. Urol., 123:850, 1980.

Ghoneim, M. A., Kock, N. G., Lycke, G., et al.: An appliance-free, sphincter-controlled bladder substitute: The urethral Kock pouch. J. Urol., 138:1150, 1987.

Gibas, Z., and Sandberg, A. A.: Chromosomal rearrangements in bladder cancer. Urology, 23:3, 1984.

Gibod, L. B., Katz, M., Cochand, B., et al.: Lymphography and percutaneous fine needle node aspiration biopsy in the staging of bladder carcinoma. J. Urol., 132:24, 1984.

Gilbert, H. A., Logan, J. L., Lagan, A. R., et al.: The natural history of papillary transitional cell carcinoma of the bladder and its treatment in an unselected population on the basis of histologic grading. J. Urol., 119:486, 1978.

Glashan, R. W.: A randomized controlled study of intravesical α-2b-interferon in carcinoma in situ of the bladder. J. Urol., 144:658, 1990.

Goffinet, D. R., Schneider, M. J., Glatstein, E. J., et al.: Bladder cancer: Results of radiation therapy in 384 patients. Radiology, 117:149, 1975.

Goodman, G. B., Hislop, T. G., Elwood, J. M., et al.: Conservation of bladder function in patients with invasive bladder cancer treated by definitive irradiation and selective cystectomy. Int. J. Radiat. Oncol. Biol. Phys., 7:569, 1981.

Goodwin, W. E., Harris, A. P., Kaufman, J. J., et al.: Open, transcolonic ureterointestinal anastomosis: A new approach. Surg. Gynecol. Obstet., 97:295, 1953.

Gordon, N. S., Sinclair, R. A., and Snow, R. M.: Pelvic lipomatosis with cystitis cystica, cystitis glandularis and adenocarcinoma of the bladder: First reported case. Aust. N. Z. J. Surg., 60:229, 1990.

Gospodarowicz, M. K., Hawkins, N. V., Rawlings, G. A., et al.: Radical radiotherapy for muscle invasive transitional cell carcinoma of the bladder: Failure analysis. J. Urol., 142:1448, 1989.

Green, L. F., and Yalowitz, P. A.: The advisability of concomitant transurethral excision of vesical neoplasm and prostatic hyperplasia. J. Urol., 107:445, 1972.

Greven, K. M., Solin, L. J., and Hanks, G. E.: Prognostic factors in patients with bladder carcinoma treated with definitive irradiation. Cancer, 65:908, 1990.

Habs, M. R., and Schmahl, D.: Prevention of urinary bladder tumors in cyclophosphamide-treated rats by additional medication with uroprotectors sodium 2-mercaptoethane sulfonate (Mesna) and disodium 2,2′-dithio-bis-ethane sulfonate (Dimesna). Cancer, 51:606, 1983.

Hall, R. R., and Heath, A. B.: Radiotherapy and cystectomy for T3 bladder carcinoma. Br. J. Urol., 53:598, 1981.

Hall, R. R., Schade, R. O. K., and Swinney, J.: Effect of hyperthermia on bladder cancer. Br. Med. J., 2:593, 1974.

Hansen, R. I., Nerstrom, B., Djurhuus, J. C., et al.: Late results from mucosal denudation for urinary bladder papillomatosis. Acta Chir. Scand., 472:73, 1976.

Hardeman, S. W., Perry, A., and Soloway, M. S.: Transitional cell carcinoma of the prostate following intravesical therapy for transitional cell carcinoma of the bladder. J. Urol., 140:289, 1988.

Harge, P., Hoover, R., and Kantor, A.: Bladder cancer risks and pipes, cigars and smokeless tobacco. Cancer, 55:901, 1985.

Harker, W. G., Freiha, F. S., Shortliffe, L., et al.: Cisplatin, methotrexate, and vinblastine (CMV) for metastatic transitional cell carcinoma of the urinary tract (TCC): Chemotherapy evaluation of complete response by site. Proc. Am. Soc. Clin. Oncol., Abstract C-6773:160, 1984.

Harty, J. I., Amin, M., Wieman, T. J., et al.: Complications of whole bladder dihematoporphyrin ether photodynamic therapy. J. Urol., 141:1341, 1989.

Harving, N., Wolf, H., and Melsen, F.: Positive urinary cytology after tumor resection: An indicator for concomitant carcinoma in situ. J. Urol., 140:495, 1988.

Hellsten, S., Mansson, W., Henrikson, H., et al.: Intravesical mitomycin C for carcinoma in situ of the urinary bladder. Scand. J. Urol. Nephrol., 24:35, 1990.

Helmstein, K.: Treatment of bladder carcinoma by a hydrostatic pressure technique. Br. J. Urol., 44:434, 1972.

Helzlsouer, K. J., Comstock, G. W., and Morris, J. S.: Selenium, lycopene, alpha-tocopherol, beta-carotene, retinol, and subsequent bladder cancer. Cancer Res., 49:6144, 1989.

Heney, N. M., Ahmed, S., Flanagan, M., et al.: Superficial bladder cancer: Progression and recurrence. J. Urol., 130:1083, 1983.

Heney, N. M., Koontz, W. W., Barton, B., et al.: Intravesical thiotepa versus mitomycin C in patients with T_A, T_1 and T_{IS} transitional cell carcinoma of the bladder: A phase III prospective randomized study. J. Urol., 140:1390, 1988.

Henry, K., Miller, J., Mori, M., et al.: Comparison of transurethral resection to radical therapies for stage B bladder tumors. J. Urol., 140:964, 1988.

Hermanek, P., and Sobin, L. H. (Eds): UICC-International Union Against Cancer TNM Classification of Malignant Tumors, ed. 4. Heidelberg, Springer-Verlag, 1987, p. 135.

Herr, H. W.: Preoperative irradiation with and without chemotherapy as adjunct to radical cystectomy. Urology, 25:127, 1985.

Herr, H. W.: Conservative management of muscle-infiltrating bladder cancer: Prospective experience. J. Urol., 138:1162, 1987.

Herr, H. W.: Neoadjuvant chemotherapy for invasive bladder cancer. Semin. Surg. Oncol., 5:266, 1989.

Herr, H. W., Kemeny, N., Yagoda, A., et al.: Poly (I:C) immunotherapy in patients with papillomas or superficial carcinomas of the bladder. NCI Monogr., 49:325, 1978.

Herr, H. W., Laudone, V. P., Badalament, R. A., et al.: Bacillus Calmette-Guérin therapy alters the progression of superficial bladder cancer. J. Clin. Oncol., 6:1450, 1988.

Herr, H. W., Pinsky, C. M., Whitmore, W. F., Jr., et al.: Long-term effect of intravesical bacillus Calmette-Guérin on flat carcinoma in situ of the bladder. J. Urol., 135:265, 1986.

Herr, H. W., Yagoda, A., Batata, M., et al.: Planned preoperative cisplatin and radiation therapy for locally advanced bladder cancer. Cancer, 52:2705, 1983.

Hewett, C. B., Babiszewski, J. F., and Antunez, A. R.: Update on intracavitary radiation in the treatment of bladder tumors. J. Urol., 126:323, 1981.

Hijazi, A., Devoneck, M., Bouvier, R., et al.: Flow cytometry study of cytokeratin 18 expression according to tumor grade and deoxyribonucleic acid content in human bladder tumors. J. Urol., 141:522, 1989.

Hill, D. E., Ford, K. S., and Soloway, M. S.: Radical cystectomy and adjuvant chemotherapy. Urology, 25:151, 1985.

Hillcoat, B. L., Raghavan, D., Matthews, J., et al.: A randomized trial of cisplatin versus cisplatin plus methotrexate in advanced cancers of the urothelial tract. J. Clin. Oncol., 7:706, 1989.

Hillyard, R. W., Jr., Ladaga, L., and Schellhammer, P. F.: Superficial transitional cell carcinoma of the bladder associated with mucosal involvement of the prostatic urethra: Results of treatment with intravesical bacillus Calmette-Guérin. J. Urol., 139:290, 1988.

Hisazumi, H., Misahi, T., and Myoshi, N.: Photoradiation therapy of bladder tumors. J. Urol., 130:685, 1983.

Hoffman, D., Masuda, Y., and Wynder, E. L.: Alpha-naphthylamine and beta-naphthylamine in cigarette smoke. Nature, 221:254, 1969.

Hofstetter, A., Frank, F., Keditsch, E., et al.: Endoscopic neodymium-YAG laser application for destroying bladder tumors. Eur. Urol., 7:278, 1981.

Holm, H. H., Juul, N., Torp-Pedersen, S., et al.: Bladder tumor staging by transurethral ultrasonic scanning. Eur. Urol., 15:31, 1988.

Hoover, R., and Strasser, P. H.: Artificial sweeteners and human bladder cancer. Lancet, 1:837, 1980.

Hopkins, S. C., Ford, K. S., and Soloway, M. S.: Invasive bladder cancer: Support for screening. J. Urol., 130:61, 1983.

Hopman, A. H. N., Poddighe, P. J., Smeets, A. W. G. B., et al.: Detection of numerical chromosome aberrations in bladder cancer by in situ hybridization. Am. J. Clin. Pathol., 135:1105, 1989.

Horai, Y., Fujita, K., and Ishizaki, T.: Genetically determined N-acetylation and oxidation capacities in Japanese patients with nonoccupational urinary bladder cancer. Eur. J. Clin. Pharmacol., 37:581, 1989.

Howe, G. R., Burch, J. D., Miller, A. B., et al.: Tobacco use, occupation, coffee, various nutrients, and bladder cancer. JNCI, 64:701, 1980.

Huang, W.-L., Ro, J. Y., Griguon, D. J., et al.: Postoperative spindle cell nodule of the prostate and bladder. J. Urol., 143:824, 1990.

Huben, R. P.: Tumor markers in bladder cancer. Urology, 23:10, 1984.

Hudson, M. A., Ratliff, T. L., Gillen, D. P., et al.: Single course versus maintenance bacillus Calmette-Guérin therapy for superficial bladder tumors: A prospective randomized trial. J. Urol., 138:295, 1987.

Huland, E., and Huland, H.: Local continuous high dose interleukin-2: A new therapeutic model for the treatment of advanced bladder carcinoma. Cancer Res., 49:5469, 1989.

Huland, H., Otto, U., Droese, M., et al.: Long-term mitomycin C instillation after transurethral resection of superficial bladder carcinoma: Influence on recurrence, progression, and survival. J. Urol., 132:27–29, 1984.

Husband, J. E., Olliff, J. F., Williams, M. P., et al.: Bladder cancer: Staging with CT and MR imaging. Radiology, 173:435, 1989.

Husmann, D. A., and Spence, H. M.: Current status of tumor of the bowel following ureterosigmoidoscopy: A review. J. Urol., 144:607, 1990.

Issell, B. F., Prout, G. R., Jr., Soloway, M. S., et al.: Mitomycin C intravesical therapy in noninvasive bladder cancer after failure on thiotepa. Cancer, 53:1025, 1984.

Jacobs, S. C., Menashe, D. S., Mewissen, M. W., et al.: Intraarterial cisplatin infusion in the management of transitional cell carcinoma of the bladder. Cancer, 64:388, 1989.

Jakse, G., Loidl, W., Seeber, G., et al.: Stage T1, grade 3 transitional cell carcinoma of the bladder: An unfavorable tumor? J. Urol., 137:39, 1987.

Javadpour, N.: Multiple cell markers in bladder cancer: Principles and clinical practice. Urol. Clin. North Am., 11:609, 1984.

Jenkins, B. J., Caulfield, M. J., Fowler, C. G., et al.: Reappraisal of the role of radical radiotherapy and salvage cystectomy in the treatment of invasive (T2/T3) bladder cancer. Br. J. Urol., 62:343, 1988a.

Jenkins, B. J., England, H. R., Fowler, C. G., et al.: Chemotherapy for carcinoma in situ of the bladder. Br. J. Urol. 61:326, 1988b.

Jewett, H. J., and Eversole, S. L.: Carcinoma of the bladder: Characteristic modes of local invasion. J. Urol., 83:383, 1960.

Jewett, H. J., and Strong, G. H.: Infiltrating carcinoma of the bladder: Relation of depth of penetration of the bladder wall to incidence of local extension and metastases. J. Urol., 55:366, 1946.

Johnson, D. E., and Babaian, R. J.: Conservative surgical management for noninvasive distal ureteral carcinoma. Urology, 13:365, 1979.

Johnson, D. E., Hodge, G. B., Abdul-Karim, F. W., et al.: Urachal carcinoma. Urology, 26:218, 1985.

Johnson, D. E., Schoenwald, M. B., Ayala, A. G., et al.: Squamous cell carcinoma of the bladder. J. Urol., 115:542, 1976.

Johnson, D. E., Wishnow, K. I., and Tenney, D.: Are frozen-section examinations of ureteral margins required for all patients undergoing radical cystectomy for bladder cancer? Urology, 33:451, 1989.

Johnson, O. L., Bracken, R. B., and Ayala, A. G.: Vesical adenocarcinoma occurring in patients with pelvic lipomatosis. Urology, 15:280, 1980.

Johnson, R. J., Carrington, B. M., Jenkins, J. P., et al.: Accuracy in staging carcinoma of the bladder by magnetic resonance imaging. Clin. Radiol., 41:258, 1990.

Jones, H. C., and Swinney, J.: Thiotepa in the treatment of tumors of the bladder. Lancet, 2:615, 1961.

Jurincic, C. D., Engelmann, U., Gasch, J., et al.: Immunotherapy in human bladder cancer with keyhole limpet hemocyamin: Randomized study. J. Urol., 139:723, 1988.

Kabalin, J. N., Freiha, F. S., and Niebel, J. D.: Leiomyoma of the bladder: Report of 2 cases and demonstration of ultrasonic appearance. Urology, 35:210, 1990.

Kabalin, J. N., McNeal, J. E., Price, H. M., et al.: Unsuspected adenocarcinoma of the prostate in patients undergoing cystoprostatectomy for other causes: Incidence, histology and morphometric observations. J. Urol., 141:1091, 1989.

Kadlubar, F. F., Talaska, G., Lang, N. P., et al.: Assessment of exposure and susceptibility to aromatic amine carcinogens. IARC Sci. Publ., 1988, p. 166.

Kagawa, S., Ogura, K., Kurokawa, K., et al.: Immunological evaluation of a streptococcal preparation (OK-432) in treatment of bladder carcinoma. J. Urol., 122:467, 1979.

Kakizoe, T., Matsumoto, K., Audoh, M., et al.: Adenocarcinoma of urachus: Report of 7 cases and review of the literature. Urology, 21:360, 1983.

Kalble, T., Tricker, A. R., Friedel, P., et al.: Ureterosigmoidostomy: Long-term results, risk of carcinoma and etiological factors for carcinogenesis. J. Urol., 144:1110, 1990.

Kantor, A. F., Hartge, P., Hoover, R. N., et al.: Epidemiological characteristics of squamous cell carcinoma and adenocarcinoma of the bladder. Cancer Res., 48:3853, 1988.

Kaplan, S. A., Sawczuk, I. S., O'Toole, K., et al.: Contemporary cystectomy versus preoperative radiation therapy plus cystectomy for bladder cancer. Urology, 32:485, 1988.

Kavoussi, L. R., Brown, E. J., Ritchey, J. K., et al.: Fibronectin-mediated Calmette-Guérin bacillus attachment to murine bladder mucosa. J. Clin. Invest., 85:62, 1990.

Kavoussi, L. R., Gelstein, L. D., and Andriole, G. L.: Encephalopathy and an elevated serum aluminum level in a patient receiving intravesical alum irrigation for severe urinary hemorrhage. J. Urol., 136:665, 1986.

Kay, R., and Lattanzi, C.: Nephrogenic adenoma in children. J. Urol., 133:99, 1985.

Kaye, K. W., and Lange, P. H.: Mode of presentation of invasive bladder cancer: Reassessment of the problem. J. Urol., 128:31, 1982.

Keep, J. C., Piehl, M., Miller, A., et al.: Invasive carcinomas of the urinary bladder: Evaluation of tunica muscularis mucosae involvement. Am. J. Clin. Pathol., 91:575, 1989.

Kelley, D. R., Ratliff, T. R., Catalona, W. J., et al.: Intravesical BCG therapy for superficial bladder cancer: Effect of BCG viability on treatment results. J. Urol., 134:48, 1985.

Kemeny, N., Yagoda, A., Wang, Y., et al.: Randomized trial of standard therapy with or without poly(I:C) in patients with superficial bladder cancer. Cancer, 48:2154, 1981.

Kent, D. L., Shachter, R., Sox, H. C., Jr., et al.: Efficient scheduling of cystoscopies in monitoring for recurrent bladder cancer. Med. Decis. Making, 9:26, 1989.

Kern, W. H.: The grade and pathologic stage of bladder cancer. Cancer, 53:1185, 1984.

Kierman, M., and Gafney, E. F.: Brunn's nests and glandular metaplasia: Normal urothelial variants in the supramontanal prostatic urethra. J. Urol., 137:877, 1987.

Klinger, M. E.: Secondary tumors of the genitourinary tract. J. Urol., 65:144, 1951.

Kock, N. G., Ghoneim, M. A., Lycke, K. G., et al.: Urinary diversion to the augmented and valved rectum: Preliminary results with a novel surgical procedure. J. Urol., 140:1375, 1988.

Kock, N. G., Ghoneim, M. A., Lycke, K. G., et al.: Replacement of the bladder by the urethral Kock pouch: Functional results, urodynamics and radiological features. J. Urol., 141:1111, 1989.

Kock, N. G., Nilson, A. E., Nilsson, L. O., et al.: Urinary diversion via continent ileal reservoir: Clinical results in 12 patients. J. Urol., 128:469, 1982.

Konchuba, A. M., Schellhammer, P. F., Alexander, J. P., et al.: Flow cytometric study comparing paired bladder washing and voided urine for bladder cancer detection. Urology, 33:89, 1989.

Kondas, J., Szentgyorgyi, E., and Szoke, D.: Local adriamycin treatment for prevention of recurrence of superficial bladder tumors. Int. Urol. Nephrol., 20:611, 1988.

Koontz, W. W., and Prout, G. R., Jr., Smith W., et al.: The use of intravesical thiotepa in the management of non-invasive carcinoma of the bladder. J. Urol. 125:307, 1981.

Koshikawa, T., Leyh, H., and Schenck, U.: Difficulties in evaluating urinary specimens after local mitomycin therapy of bladder cancer. Diagn. Cytopathol., 5:117, 1989.

Koss, J. C., Arger, P. H., Coleman, B. G., et al.: CT staging of bladder carcinoma. Am. J. Roentgenol., 137:359, 1981.

Koss, L. G.: Tumors of the urinary bladder. *In* Atlas of Tumor Pathology, Second Series, Fascile 11. Washington, D. C., Armed Forces Institute of Pathology, 1975, p. 1.

Koss, L. G., Esperanza, M. T., and Robbins, M. A.: Mapping cancerous and precancerous bladder changes: A study of the urothelium in ten surgically removed bladders. JAMA, 227:281, 1974.

Kubota, Y., Shuin, T., Miura, T., et al.: Treatment of bladder cancer with a combination of hyperthermia, radiation and bleomycin. Cancer, 53:199, 1984.

Kunter, A. F., Hartge, P., Hoover, R. N., et al.: Urinary tract infection and risk of bladder cancer. Am. J. Epidemiol., 119:510, 1984.

Kunze, E., Schauer, A., and Schmitt, M.: Histology and histogenesis of two different types of inverted urothelial papillomas. Cancer, 51:348, 1983.

Kurth, K. H., Schroder, F. H., Tunn, U., et al.: Adjuvant chemotherapy of superficial transitional cell bladder carcinoma: Preliminary results of a European Organization for Research on Treatment of Cancer randomized trial comparing doxorubicin hydrochloride, ethoglucid and transurethral resection alone. J. Urol., 132:258, 1984.

Kurz, K. R., Pitts, W. R., and Vaughan, E. D., Jr.: The natural history of patients less than 40 years old with bladder tumors. J. Urol., 137:395, 1987.

Lamm, D. L.: Intravesical therapy of superficial bladder cancer. AUA Update, 2:2, 1983.

Lamm, D. L.: Editorial comment. J. Urol., 142:1074, 1989.

Lamm, D. L., DeHaven, J. I., Shriver, J., et al.: A randomized prospective comparison of oral versus intravesical and percutaneous bacillus Calmette-Guérin for superficial bladder cancer. J. Urol., 144:65, 1990.

Lamm, D. L., Stogdill, V. D., Stogdill, B. J. et al.: Complications of bacillus Calmette-Guérin immunotherapy in 1,278 patients with bladder cancer. J. Urol., 135:272, 1986.

Lamm, D. L., Thor, D. E., Harris, S. C., et al.: Bacillus Calmette-Guérin immunotherapy of superficial bladder cancer. J. Urol., 124:38, 1980.

Lamm, D. L., Thor, D. E., Stogdill, V. D., et al.: Bladder cancer immunotherapy. J. Urol., 128:931, 1982.

Langkilde, N. C., Wolff, H., and Orntoft, T. F.: Lectinohistochemistry of human bladder cancer: Loss of lectin binding structures in invasive carcinomas. APMIS, 97:367, 1989.

Lantz, E. J., and Hattery, R. R.: Diagnostic imaging of urothelial cancer. Urol. Clin. North Am., 11:576, 1984.

LaPlante, M., and Brice, M., II: The upper limits of hopeful application of radical cystectomy for vesical carcinoma: Does nodal metastasis always indicate incurability? J. Urol., 109:261, 1973.

Lazarevic, B., and Garret, R.: Inverted papilloma and papillary transitional cell carcinoma of urinary bladder. Cancer, 42:1904, 1978.

Leadbetter, W. F., and Clarke, B. G.: Five years' experience with ureteroenterostomy by combined technique. J. Urol., 73:67, 1955.

Lilien, O. M., and Camey, M.: 25-Year experience with replacement of human bladder (Camey procedure). J. Urol., 132:886, 1984.

Linker, D. G., and Whitmore, W. F., Jr.: Ureteral carcinoma in situ. J. Urol., 113:777, 1975.

Locke, J. L., Hill, D. E., and Walzer, Y.: Incidence of squamous cell carcinoma in patients with long-term catheter drainage. J. Urol. 133:1034, 1985.

Lockhart, J. L., Chaikin, L., Bondhus, M. J., et al.: Prostatic recurrences in the management of superficial bladder tumors. J. Urol., 130:256, 1983.

Logothetis, C. J., Dexeus, F. H., Chong, C., et al.: Cisplatin, cyclophosphamide and doxorubicin chemotherapy for unresectable urothelial tumors: The M. D. Anderson experience. J. Urol., 141:33, 1989.

Logothetis, C. J., Dexeus, F. H., Sella, A., et al.: Escalated therapy for refractory urothelial tumors: Methotrexate-vinblastine-doxorubicin-cisplatin plus unglycosylated recombinant human granulocyte-macrophage colony-stimulating factor. JNCI, 82:667, 1990.

Logothetis, C. J., Johnson, D. E., Chong, C., et al.: Adjuvant cyclophosphamide, doxorubicin, and cisplatin chemotherapy for bladder cancer: An update. J. Clin. Oncol., 6:1590, 1988.

Lopez-Almansa, M., Molina, Huben, R., and Huben, R. P.: Transitional cell carcinoma of the urethra in men after radical cystectomy for bladder cancer: Is prophylactic urethrectomy indicated? Br. J. Urol., 61:507, 1988.

Lower, G. M., Jr., Nilsson, T., Nelson, C. E., et al.: N-acetyltransferase phenotype and risk in urinary bladder cancer: Approaches in molecular epidemiology: Preliminary results in Sweden and Denmark. Environ. Health Perspect., 29:71, 1979.

Lucas, S. B.: Squamous cell carcinoma of the bladder and schistosomiasis. East Afr. Med. J., 59:345, 1982.

Lundbeck, R., Bruun, E., Finnerup, B., et al.: Intravesical therapy of noninvasive bladder tumors (stage Ta) with doxorubicin: Initial treatment results and the long-term course. J. Urol, 139:1212, 1988.

Lundbeck, F., Mogensen, P., and Jeppersen, N.: Intravesical therapy of noninvasive bladder tumors with doxorubicin and urokinase. J. Urol., 130:1087, 1983.

Lutzeyer, W., Rubben, H., and Dahm, H.: Prognostic parameters in superficial bladder cancer: An analysis of 315 cases. J. Urol., 127:250, 1982.

Mackenzie, A. R., Sharma, T. C., Whitmore, W. F., Jr., et al.: Nonextirpative treatment of myosarcomas of the bladder and prostate. Cancer, 28:329, 1971.

Madgar, I., Goldwasser, B., Nativ, O., et al.: Long-term follow-up of patients less than 30 years old with transitional cell carcinoma of the bladder. J. Urol., 139:933, 1988.

Magri, J.: Partial cystectomy: Review of 104 cases. Br. J. Urol., 34:74, 1962.

Malker, H. S., McLaughlin, J. K., Silverman, D. T., et al.: Occupational risks for bladder cancer among men in Sweden. Cancer Res., 47:6763, 1987.

Malmstrom, P. U., Busch, C., and Norlen, B. J.: Recurrence, progression and survival in bladder cancer: A retrospective analysis of 232 patients with greater than or equal to 5-year follow-up. Scand. J. Urol. Nephrol., 21:185, 1987.

Malmstrom, P. U., Busch, C., and Norlen, B. J., et al.: Expression of ABH blood group isoantigen as a prognostic factor in transitional cell bladder carcinoma. Scand. J. Urol. Nephrol., 22:265, 1988.

Marks, L. B., Kaufman, S. D., Prout, G. R., Jr., et al.: Invasive bladder carcinoma: Preliminary report of selective bladder conservation by transurethral surgery, upfront MCV (methotrexate, cisplatin, and vinblastine) chemotherapy and pelvic irradiation plus cisplatin. Int. J. Radiat. Oncol. Biol. Phys., 15:877, 1988.

Marshall, F. F.: Creation of an ileocolic bladder after cystectomy. J. Urol., 139:1264, 1988.

Marshall, V. F.: The relation of the preoperative estimate to the pathologic demonstration of the extent of vesical neoplasms. J. Urol., 68:714, 1952.

Marshall, V. F., and McCarron, J. P., Jr.: The curability of vesical cancer: Greater now or then? Cancer Res., 37:2753, 1977.

Martin, J. E., Jenkins, B. J., and Zuk, R. J., et al.: Clinical importance of squamous metaplasia in invasive transitional cell carcinoma of the bladder. J. Clin. Pathol., 42:250, 1989a.

Martin, J. E., Jenkins, B. J., and Zuk, R. J., et al.: Human chorionic gonadotrophin expression and histological findings as predictors of response to radiotherapy in carcinoma of the bladder. Virchows Arch. [A], 414:273, 1989b.

Martinez, A., and Gunderson, L. L.: Intraoperative radiation therapy for bladder cancer. Urol. Clin. North Am., 11:693, 1984.

Martinez-Pineiro, J. A., Jimenez Leon, J., Martinez-Pineiro, L., Jr., et al.: Bacillus Calmette-Guérin versus doxorubicin versus thiotepa: A randomized prospective study in 202 patients with superficial bladder cancer. J. Urol., 143:502, 1990.

Martinez-Pineiro, J. A., and Muntanola, P.: Nonspecific immunotherapy with BCG vaccine in bladder tumors: A preliminary report. Eur. Urol., 3:11, 1977.

Maruf, N. J., Godec C. J., Strom, R. L., et al.: Unusual therapeutic response of massive squamous cell carcinoma of the bladder to aggressive radiation and surgery. J. Urol., 128:1313, 1982.

Masters, J. R., Vesey, S. G., Mumm, C. F., et al.: C-*myc* oncoprotein levels in bladder cancer. Urol. Res., 16:341, 1988.

Mathiasen, H., Frimodt-Moller, P. C., and Nielsen, H. V.: Ureteropyeloscopic tumour treatment. Scand. J. Urol. Nephrol., 110:201, 1988.

Mathur, V. K., Krahn, H. P., and Ramse, E. R.: Total cystectomy for bladder cancer. J. Urol., 125:784, 1981.

Matsumoto, K., Kakizoe, T., Mikuriza, S., et al.: Clinical evaluation of intraoperative radiotherapy for carcinoma of the urinary bladder. Cancer, 47:509, 1981.

Matthews, P. N., Madden, M., Bidgood, K. A., et al.: The clinical pathological features of metastatic superficial papillary bladder cancer. J. Urol., 132:904, 1984.

Mayer, W. J., and McWhorter, W. P.: Black/white differences in non-treatment of bladder cancer patients and implications for survival. Am. J. Public Health, 79:772, 1989.

McCredie, M., Stewart, J. H., Ford, J. M., et al.: Phenacetin-containing analgesics and cancer of the bladder or renal pelvis in women. Br. J. Urol., 55:220, 1983.

McCullough, D. L., Cooper, R. M., Yeaman, L. D., et al.: Neoadjuvant treatment of stages T2 to bladder cancer with cis-platinum, cyclophosphamide and doxorubicin. J. Urol., 141:849, 1989.

McCullough, D. L., Lamm, D. L., McLaughlin, A. P., III, et al.: Familial transitional cell carcinoma of the bladder. J. Urol., 113:629, 1975.

McPhee, M. S., Arnfield, M. R., Tulip, J., et al.: Neodymium: YAG laser therapy for infiltrating bladder cancer. J. Urol., 140:44, 1988.

Melamed, M. R.: Flow cytometry of the urinary bladder. Urol. Clin. North Am., 11:599, 1984.

Melamed, M. R., Koss, L. G., Ricci A., et al.: Cytohistological observations on developing carcinoma of the urinary bladder in man. Cancer, 13:67, 1960.

Melicow, M. M.: Histological study of vesical urothelium intervening between gross neoplasms in total cystectomy. J. Urol., 68:261, 1952.

Messing, E. M.: Clinical implications of the expression of epidermal growth factor receptor in human transitional cell carcinoma. Cancer Res., 50:2530, 1990.

Meyers, F. J., Gumerlock, P. H., Kokoris, S. P., et al.: Human bladder and colon carcinomas contain activated *ras* p21: Specific detection of twelfth codon mutants. Cancer, 63:2177, 1989.

Meyhoff, H. H., Andersen, J. T., Klarskov, P., et al.: Flexible fiberoptic versus conventional cystourethroscopy in bladder tumor patients: A prospective study. Scand. J. Urol. Nephrol., 110:237, 1988.

Michel, F., Gattegno, B., Meyrier, A., et al.: Paraneoplastic hypercalcemia associated with bladder carcinoma: Report of 2 cases. J. Urol., 131:753, 1984.

Miller, L. S., and Johnson, D. E.: Megavoltage irradiation for bladder

cancer: Alone, postoperative or preoperative. *In* Proceedings of the Seventh National Cancer Conference. Philadelphia, J. B. Lippincott Co., 1973, p. 771.

Miller, M. E., and Cosgriff, J. M.: Acetylator phenotype in human bladder cancer. J. Urol., 130:65, 1983.

Mills, S. E., Wolfe, J. T., Weiss, M. A., et al.: Small cell undifferentiated carcinoma of the urinary bladder: A light-microscopic, immunocytochemical, and ultrastructural study of 12 cases. Am. J. Surg. Pathol., 11:606, 1987.

Mohuiddin, M., Kramer, S., Newall, J., et al.: Combined pre- and postoperative adjuvant radiotherapy for bladder cancer: Result of RTOG/Jefferson Study. Cancer, 47:2840, 1981.

Montie, J. E.: High-stage bladder cancer: Bladder preservation or reconstruction. Cleve. Clin. J. Med., 57:280, 1990.

Montie, J. E., Straffon, R. A., and Stewart, B. H.: Radical cystectomy without radiation therapy for carcinoma of the bladder. J. Urol., 131:477, 1984.

Montie, J. E., Wood, D. P., Jr., Pontes, J. E., et al.: Adenocarcinoma of the prostate in cystoprostatectomy specimens removed for bladder cancer. Cancer, 63:381, 1989.

Morales, A.: Treatment of carcinoma in situ of the bladder with BCG: A phase II trial. Cancer Immunol. Immunother., 9:69, 1980.

Morales, A., Eidinger, D., and Bruce, A. W.: Intracavitary bacillus Calmette-Guérin in the treatment of superficial bladder tumors. J. Urol., 116:180, 1976.

Morales, A., and Ersil, A.: Prophylaxis of recurrent bladder cancer with bacillus Calmette-Guérin. *In* Johnson D. E., Samuels M. L. (Eds): Cancer of the Genitourinary Tract. New York, Raven Press, 1979, p. 121.

Morales, A., and Nickel, J. C.: Immunotherapy of superficial bladder cancer with BCG. World J. Urol., 3:209, 1986.

Morales, A., Ottenhof, P., and Emerson, L.: Treatment of residual, noninfiltrating bladder cancer with bacillus Calmette-Guérin. J. Urol., 125:649, 1981.

Mori, K., Lamm, K. L., and Crawford, E. D.: A trial of bacillus Calmette-Guérin vs. adriamycin in superficial bladder cancer: A Southwest Oncology Group Study. Urol. Int., 41:254, 1988.

Morrison, A. S.: Advances in the etiology of urothelial cancer. Urol. Clin. North Am. 11:557, 1984.

Morrison, A. S. Buring, J. E., Verhock, W. G., et al.: An international study of smoking and bladder cancer. J. Urol., 131:650, 1984.

Morrison, A. S., and Cole, P.: Epidemiology of bladder cancer. Urol. Clin. North Am., 3:13, 1976.

Mostofi, F. K.: Potentialities of bladder epithelium. J. Urol., 71:705, 1954.

Mostofi, F. K., Sobin, L. H., and Torloni, H.: Histological typing of urinary bladder tumors (International Histologic Classification of Tumors, No. 10). Geneva, World Health Organization, 1973.

Mostofi, F. K., Thomson, R. V., and Dean, A. L., Jr.: Mucous adenocarcinoma of the urinary bladder. Cancer, 8:74, 1955.

Mufti, G. R., Virdi, J. S., and Singh, M.: Reappraisal of hydrostatic pressure treatment for intractable postradiotherapy vesical hemorrhage. Urology, 35:9, 1990.

Murphy, W. M., and Soloway, M. S.: Urothelial dysplasia. J. Urol., 127:849, 1982.

Nakamura, S., and Nijima, T.: Staging of bladder cancer by ultrasonography: A new technique by transurethral intravesical scanning. J. Urol., 124:341, 1980.

Narumi, Y., Sato, T., Kuriyama, K., et al.: Vesical dome tumors: Significance of extravesical extension on CT. Radiology, 169:383, 1988.

Navarre, R. J., Jr., Loening, S. A., Platz, C., et al.: Nephrogenic adenoma: A report of 9 cases and review of the literature. J. Urol., 127:775, 1982.

Neal, D. E., Bennett, N. K., Hall, R. R., et al.: Epidermal-growth factor receptors in human bladder cancer: Comparison of invasive and superficial tumors. Lancet, 1:366, 1985.

Neal, D. E., Sharples, L., Smith, K., et al.: The epidermal growth factor receptor and the prognosis of bladder cancer. Cancer, 65:1619, 1990.

Needles, B., Yagoda, A., Sogani, P., et al.: Intravenous cisplatin for superficial bladder tumor. Cancer, 50:1722, 1982.

Nemoto, R., Hattori, K., Uchida, K., et al.: Estimation of growth fraction in situ in human bladder cancer with bromodeoxyuridine labelling. Br. J. Urol., 65:27, 1990.

Netto, N. R., Jr., and Lemos, G. C.: A comparison of treatment methods for the prophylaxis of recurrent superficial bladder tumors. J. Urol., 129:33, 1983.

Newling, D.: Intravesical therapy in the management of superficial transitional cell carcinoma of the bladder: Experience of the EORTC group. Br. J. Cancer, 61:497, 1990.

Newman, D. M., Brown, J. R., Jay, A. C., et al.: Squamous cell carcinoma of the bladder. J. Urol., 100:470, 1968.

Nichols, J. A., and Marshall, V. F.: The treatment of bladder carcinoma by local excision and fulguration. Cancer, 9:559, 1956.

Nielsen, K., and Nielsen, K. K.: Adenocarcinoma in exstrophy of the bladder—the last case in Scandanavia? A case report and review of the literature. J. Urol., 130:1180, 1983.

Nijima, T., Koiso, K., Akaza, H., and The Japanese Urological Cancer Research Group for Adriamycin: Randomized clinical trial on chemoprophylaxis of recurrence in cases of superficial bladder cancer. Cancer Chemother Pharmacol, 11(Suppl.):79, 1983.

Nishimura, K., Hida, S., and Nishio, Y.: The validity of magnetic resonance imaging (MRI) in the staging of bladder cancer: Comparison with computed tomography (CT) and transurethral ultrasonography (US). Jpn. J. Clin. Oncol., 18:217, 1988.

Nseyo, U. O., Dougherty, T. J., and Sullivan, L.: Photodynamic therapy in the management of resistant lower urinary tract carcinoma. Cancer, 60:3113, 1987.

Nurmi, M., Katevuo, K., and Puntala, P.: Reliability of CT in preoperative evaluation of bladder carcinoma. Scand. J. Urol. Nephol., 22:125, 1988.

Oates, R. D., Stilmant, M. M., Freedlund, M. C., et al.: Granulomatous prostatitis following bacillus Calmette-Guérin immunotherapy of bladder cancer. J. Urol., 140:751, 1988.

Oda, H., Oda, T., Ohoka, H., et al.: Flow cytometric evaluation of Thomsen-Friedreich antigen on transitional cell cancer using monoclonal antibody. Urol. Res., 18:107, 1990.

O'Keane, J. C.: Carcinoma of the urinary bladder after treatment with cyclophosphamide. N. Engl. J. Med., 319:871, 1988.

Oldbring, J., Glifberg, I., Mikulowski, P., et al.: Carcinoma of the renal pelvis and ureter following bladder carcinoma: Frequency, risk factors and clinicopathological findings. J. Urol., 141:1311, 1989.

Ono, K., Akuta, K., Takahasi, M., et al.: Effect of misonidazole in preoperative irradiation for bladder cancer followed by total cystectomy. Radiat. Med., 7:105, 1989.

Orihuela, E., and Shahon, R. S.: Influence of blood group type on the natural history of superficial bladder cancer. J. Urol., 138:758, 1987.

Orntoff, F. F.: Activity of the human blood group ABO, Se, H, Le and X gene-encoded glycosyltransferases in normal and malignant bladder urothelium. Cancer Res., 48:4427, 1988.

Ostroff, E. B., and Chenault, O. W., Jr.: Alum irrigation for the control of massive bladder hemorrhage. J. Urol., 128:929, 1982.

Page, B. H., Levison, V. B., and Curwen, M. P.: The site of recurrence of noninfiltrating bladder tumors. Br. J. Urol., 50:237, 1978.

Parada, L. F., Tabin, C. J., Shih, C., et al.: Human EJ bladder carcinoma oncogene is homologue of Harvey sarcoma virus *ras* gene. Nature, 297:474, 1982.

Parry, W. L., and Hemstreet, G. P., III: Cancer detection by quantitative fluorescence image analysis. J. Urol., 139:270, 1988.

Patch, F. S., and Rhea, L. J.: The genesis and development of Brunn's nests and their relationship to cystitis cystica, glandularis and primary adenocarcinoma of the bladder. Can. Med. Assoc. J., 33:597, 1935.

Pedersen-Bjergaard, J., Ersboll, J., Hansen, V. L., et al.: Carcinoma of the bladder after treatment with cyclophosphamide for non-Hodgkins lymphoma. N. Engl. J. Med., 318:1028, 1988.

Pinsky, C. M., Camacho, F. J., Kerr, D., et al.: Treatment of superficial bladder cancer with intravesical BCG. In Terry, W. D., Rosenberg, S. A. (Eds.): Immunotherapy of Human Cancer. New York, Elsevier North Holland Inc., 1982, p. 309.

Piper, J. M., Tonascia J., and Metanoski, G. M.: Heavy phenacitin use and bladder cancer in women aged 20 to 49 years. N. Engl. J. Med., 313:292, 1985.

Pizza, G., Severini, G., Menniti, D., et al.: Tumour regression after intralesional injection of interleukin-2 (IL-2) in bladder cancer: Preliminary report. Int. J. Cancer, 34:359, 1984.

Pritchett, T. R., Schieff, W. M., Klatt, E., et al.: The potency-sparing radical cystectomy: Does it compromise the completeness of the cancer resection? J. Urol., 140:1400, 1988.

Prout, G. R., Jr.: The surgical management of bladder carcinoma. Urol. Clin. North Am., 3:149, 1976.

Prout, G. R., Jr., Griffin, P. O., Nocks, B. N., et al.: Intravesical therapy of low stage bladder carcinoma with mitomycin C: Comparison of results in untreated and previously treated patients. J. Urol., 127:1096, 1982.

Prout, G. R., Jr., Griffin, P. P., and Shipley, W. U.: Bladder carcinoma as a systemic disease. Cancer, 42:2532, 1979.

Prout, G. R., Jr., Koontz, W. W., Jr., Coombs, J., et al.: Long-term fate of 90 patients with superficial bladder cancer randomly assigned to receive or not to receive thiotepa. J. Urol., 130:677, 1983.

Prout, G. R., Jr., Lin, C. W., Benson, R., Jr., et al.: Photodynamic therapy with hematoporphyrin derivative in the treatment of superficial transitional-cell carcinoma of the bladder. N. Engl. J. Med., 317:1251, 1987.

Purves, E. C., Snell, M., Cope, W. A., et al.: Subcutaneous *Corynebacterium parvum* in bladder cancer. Br. J. Urol., 51:278, 1979.

Quilty, P. M., and Kerr, G. R.: Bladder cancer following low- or high-dose pelvic irradiation. Clin. Radiol., 38:583, 1987.

Radwin, H. M.: Invasive transitional cell carcinoma of the bladder: Is there a place for preoperative radiotherapy? Urol. Clin. North Am., 7:551, 1980.

Radzikowski, C. Z., Steuden, I., Wiedlocha, A., et al.: The Thomsen-Friedenreich antigen on human urothelial cell lines detectable by peanut lectin and monoclonal antibody raised against human glycophorin A. Anticancer Res., 9:103, 1989.

Raghavan, D., Shipley, W. U., Garnick, M. B., et al.: Biology in management of bladder cancer. N. Engl. J. Med., 322:1129, 1990.

Raghavan, D., Wallace, M. A., Sandeman, T., et al.: First randomized trials of pre-emptive (neoadjuvant) intravenous (IV cisplatin CDDP) for invasive transitional cell carcinoma of the bladder (TCCB) [abstract]. Proc. Am. Soc. Clin. Oncol., 8:133, 1989.

Ramaekers, F., Huysman, S. A., Moesker, O., et al.: Cytokeratin expression during neoplastic progression of human transitional cell carcinomas as detected by a monoclonal and a polyclonal antibody. Lab. Invest., 52:31, 1985.

Rawls, W. H., Lamm, D. L., Lowe, B. A., et al.: Fatal sepsis following intravesical bacillus Calmette-Guérin administration for bladder cancer. J. Urol., 144:1328, 1990.

Rehn, L.: Ueber blasentumoren bei fuchsinarbeitern. Arch. Kind. Chir., 50:588, 1895.

Renwick, A. G., Thakrar, A., Lawrie, C. A., et al.: Microbial amino acid metabolites and bladder cancer: No evidence of promoting activity in man. Hum. Toxicol., 7:267, 1988.

Resnick, M. I., and O'Connor, V. J., Jr.: Segmental resection for carcinoma of the bladder: Review of 102 patients. J. Urol., 109:1007, 1973.

Richie, J. P., Waisman, J., Skinner, D. G., et al.: Squamous cell carcinoma of the bladder: Treatment by radical cystectomy. J. Urol., 115:670, 1976.

Riddle, P. R., Chisholm, G. D., Trott, P. A., et al.: Flat carcinoma in situ of bladder. Br. J. Urol., 47:829, 1976.

Risch, H. A., Burch, J. D., Miller, A. B., et al.: Dietary factors and the incidence of cancer in the urinary bladder. Am. J. Epidemiol., 127:1179, 1988.

Ro, J. Y., Ayala, A. G., and el-Naggar, A.: Muscularis mucosa of urinary bladder: Importance for staging and treatment. Am. J. Surg. Pathol., 11:668, 1987.

Robinson, M. R. G., Sheltz, M. B., Richards, B., et al.: Intravesical epodyl in the management of bladder tumors: Combined experience of the Yorkshire Urological Cancer Research Group. J. Urol., 118:972, 1977.

Rosi, P., Selli, C., Carini, M., et al.: Myxoid liposarcoma of the bladder. J. Urol., 130:560, 1983.

Rotman, M., Aziz, H., Porrazzo, M., et al.: Treatment of advanced transitional cell carcinoma of the bladder with irradiation and concomitant 5-fluorouracil infusion. Int. J. Radiat. Oncol. Biol. Phys., 18:1131, 1990.

Rowland, R. G., Mitchell, M. E., Bihrle, P., et al.: Indiana continent urinary reservoir. J. Urol., 137:1136, 1987.

Rubben, H., Lutzeyer, W., Fischer, N., et al.: Natural history and treatment of low and high risk superficial bladder tumors. J. Urol., 139:283, 1988.

Russell, K. J., Laramore, G. E., Griffin, T. W., et al.: The fast neutron radiotherapy for treatment of carcinoma of the urinary bladder. Am. J. Clin. Oncol., 12:301, 1989.

Sager, E. M., Talle, K., Fossa, S. D., et al.: Contrast-enhanced computed tomography to show perivesical extension in bladder carcinoma. Acta Radiol., 28:307, 1987.

Sakamoto, G. D., Burden, J., and Fisher, D.: Systemic bacillus Calmette-Guérin infection after transurethral administration for superficial bladder cancer. J. Urol., 142:1073, 1989.

Santos, E., Tronick, S. R., Aaronson, S. A., et al.: T24 human bladder carcinoma oncogene is activated form of normal human homolog of BALB- and Harvey-MSV transforming genes. Nature, 298:343, 1982.

Sarosdy, M. F., and Lamm, D. L.: Long-term results of intravesical bacillus Calmette-Guérin therapy for superficial bladder cancer. J. Urol., 142:719, 1989.

Sauer, R., Schrott, K. M., Dunst, J., et al.: Preliminary results of treatment of invasive bladder carcinoma with radiotherapy and cisplatin. Int. J. Radiat. Oncol. Biol. Phys., 15:871, 1988.

Schairer, C., Harge, P., Hoover, R. N., et al.: Racial differences in bladder cancer risk: A case-control study. Am. J. Epidemiol., 128:1027, 1988.

Scheithauer, W., Theyer, G., Zechner, O., et al.: Experiences with continuous intraarterial administration of recombinant interferon alpha-2C(rIFN-alpha 2) for treatment of patients with advanced transitional cell bladder cancer. J. Biol. Regul. Homeost. Agents, 2:67, 1988.

Schellhammer, P. F., Bean, M. A., and Whitmore, W. F., Jr.: Prostatic involvement by transitional cell carcinoma: Pathogenesis, patterns and prognosis. J. Urol., 118:399, 1977.

Schellhammer, P. F., Ladago, L. E., and Fillion, M. B.: Bacillus Calmette-Guérin (BCG) for superficial transitional cell carcinoma (TCC) of the bladder. J. Urol., 135:261, 1986.

Scher, H. I., Yagoda, A., Herr, H. W., et al.: Neoadjuvant M-VAC (methotrexate, vinblastine, doxorubicin and cisplatin) effect on the primary bladder lesion. J. Urol., 139:470, 1988.

Schelegel, J. U., Pipkin, G. E., Nishimura, R., et al.: The role of ascorbic acid in the prevention of bladder tumor formation. Trans. Am. Assoc. Genitourinary Surgeons, 61:85, 1969.

Schlegel, P. N., and Walsh, P. C.: Neuroanatomical approach to radical cystoprostatectomy with preservation of sexual function. J. Urol., 138:1402, 1987.

Schoborg, T. W., Saffos, R. O., Rodriguez, A. P., et al.: Carcinosarcoma of the bladder. J. Urol., 124:724, 1980.

Schulte, P. A.: The role of genetic factors in bladder cancer. Cancer Detect. Prev., 11:379, 1988.

Schultz, R. E., Bloch, M. J., Tomaszewski, J. E., et al.: Mesonephric adenocarcinoma of the bladder. J. Urol., 132:263, 1984.

Sella, A., Dexeus, F. H., Chong, C., et al.: Radiation therapy–associated invasive bladder tumors. Urology, 33:185, 1989.

Sen, S. E., Malek, R. S., Farrow, G. M., et al.: Sarcoma and carcinosarcoma of the bladder in adults. J. Urol., 133:29, 1985.

Seymour, G. J., Walsh, M. D., Lavin, N. F., et al.: Transferrin receptor expression by human bladder transitional cell carcinomas. Urol. Res., 15:341, 1987.

Sheinfeld, J., Reuter, V. E., Melamed, M. R., et al.: Enhanced bladder cancer detection with the Lewis X antigen as a marker of neoplastic transformation. J. Urol., 143:285, 1990.

Sheldon, C. A., Clayman, R. V., Gonzalez, R., et al.: Malignant urachal lesions. J. Urol., 131:1, 1984.

Shinka, T., Hirano, A., Uekado, Y., et al.: Intravesical bacillus Calmette-Guérin treatment for superficial bladder tumors. Br. J. Urol., 63:610, 1989.

Shinka, T., Uekado, Y., Aoshi, H., et al.: Occurrence of uroepithelial tumors of the upper urinary tract after the initial diagnosis of bladder cancer. J. Urol., 140:745, 1988.

Shipley, W. U., Cummings, K. B., and Coombs, L. J.: 4,000 Rad pre-op radiation followed by prompt radical cystectomy for invasive bladder cancer: A prospective study of patient tolerance and pathologic downstaging. J. Urol., 127:48, 1982.

Shipley, W. U., Kaufman, S. D., and Prout, G. R., Jr.: Intraoperative radiation therapy in patients with bladder cancer: A review of techniques allowing improved tumor doses and providing high cure rates without loss of bladder function. Cancer, 60:1485, 1987.

Shipley, W. U., Kaufman, S. D., and Prout, G. R., Jr.: The role of radiation therapy and chemotherapy in the treatment of invasive carcinoma of the urinary bladder. Semin. Oncol., 15:390, 1988.

Silverberg, E., Boring, C. C., and Squires, T. S.: Cancer Statistics, 1990. CA, 40:9, 1990.

Silverman, D. T., Levin, L. I., Hoover, R. N., et al.: Occupational risks of bladder cancer in the United States: I. White men. JNCI, 81:1472, 1989a.

Silverman, D. T., Levin, L. I., and Hoover, R. N.: Occupational risks of bladder cancer in the United States: II. Nonwhite men. JNCI, 81:1480, 1989b.

Skinner, D. G.: Management of invasive bladder cancer: A meticulous pelvic node dissection can make a difference. J. Urol., 128:34, 1982.

Skinner, D. G., Boyd, S. D., and Lieskovsky, G.: An update on the Kock pouch for continent urinary diversion. Urol. Clin. North Am., 14:789, 1987.

Skinner, D. G., Crawford, E. D., and Kaufman, J. J.: Complications of radical cystectomy for carcinoma of the bladder. J. Urol., 123:640, 1980.

Skinner, D. G., and Lieskovsky, G.: Contemporary cystectomy with pelvic node dissection compared to preoperative radiation therapy plus cystectomy in management of invasive bladder cancer. J. Urol., 131:1069, 1984.

Skinner, D. G., Lieskovsky, G., and Boyd, S. D.: Technique of creation of a continent internal ileal reservoir (Kock pouch) for urinary diversion. Urol. Clin. North Am., 11:741, 1984.

Slack, N. H., and Prout, G. R., Jr.: The heterogeneity of invasive bladder carcinoma and different responses to treatment. J. Urol., 123:644, 1980.

Slattery, M. L., West, D. W., and Robinson, L. M.: Fluid intake and bladder cancer in Utah. Int. J. Cancer, 42:17, 1988.

Smith, H., Weaver, G., Barjenbruch, O., et al.: Routine excretory urography in follow-up of superficial transitional cell carcinoma of bladder. Urology, 34:193, 1989.

Smith, J. A., Jr.: Current concepts in laser treatment of bladder cancer. Prog. Clin. Biol. Res., 303:463, 1989.

Smith, J. A., Jr., and Dixon, J. A.: Argon laser phototherapy of superficial transitional cell carcinoma of the bladder. J. Urol., 131:655, 1984.

Smith, J. A., Jr., and Whitmore, W. F., Jr.: Regional lymph node metastases from bladder cancer. J. Urol., 126:591, 1981a.

Smith, J. A., Jr., and Whitmore, W. F., Jr.: Salvage cystectomy for bladder cancer after failure of definitive irradiation. J. Urol., 125:643, 1981b.

Smith, N. W., Strutton, G. M., Walsh, M. D., et al.: Transferrin receptor expression in primary superficial human bladder tumours identifies patients who develop recurrences. Br. J. Urol., 65:339, 1990.

Sohn, M., Neuerburg, J., Teufl, F., et al.: Gadolinium-enhanced magnetic resonance imaging in the staging of urinary bladder neoplasms. Urol. Int., 45:142, 1990.

Soloway, M. S.: The management of superficial bladder cancer. In Javadpour, N. (Ed.): Principles and Management of Urologic Cancer. Baltimore, Williams & Wilkins, 1983, p. 446.

Soloway, M. S.: Intravesical and systemic chemotherapy in the management of superficial bladder cancer. Urol. Clin. North Am., 11:623, 1984.

Soloway, M. S.: Learning to integrate systemic chemotherapy into a treatment plan for patients with advanced bladder cancer. J. Urol., 133:440, 1985.

Soloway, M. S., Einstein, A., Corder, M. P., et al.: A comparison of cisplatin and the combination of cisplatin and cyclophosphamide in advanced urothelial cancer: A National Bladder Cancer Collaborative Group A Study. Cancer, 52:767, 1983.

Sonneveld, P., Kurth, K. H., Hagemeyer, A., et al.: Secondary hematologic neoplasm after intravesical chemotherapy for superficial bladder carcinoma. Cancer, 65:23, 1990.

Sontag, J. M.: Experimental identification of genitourinary carcinogens. Urol. Clin. North Am., 7:803, 1980.

Spencer, J. R., and Filmer, R. B.: Malignancy associated with urinary tract reconstruction using enteric segments. In Lepor, H., and Lawson, R. K. (Eds.): Urologic Oncology V., Norwell, M. A, Kluwer Academic Publishers, 1991.

Stark, G. L., Feddersen, R., Lowe, B. A., et al.: Inflammatory pseudotumor (pseudosarcoma) of the bladder. J. Urol., 141:610, 1989.

Steffens, J., and Nagel, R.: Tumours of the renal pelvis and ureter: Observations in 170 patients. Br. J. Urol., 61:277, 1988.

Steg, A., Leleu, C., Debre, B., et al.: Systemic bacillus Calmette-Guérin infection "BCGitis" in patients treated by intravesical bacillus Calmette-Guérin therapy for bladder cancer. Eur. Urol., 16:161, 1989.

Steinbeck, G., Plato, N., Norell, S. E., et al.: Urothelial cancer and some industry-related chemicals: An evaluation of the epidemiologic literature. Am. J. Ind. Med., 17:371, 1990.

Sternberg, C. N., Yagoda, A., Scher, H. I., et al.: Preliminary results of M-VAC (methotrexate, vinblastine, doxorubicin and cisplatin) for transitional cell carcinoma of the urothelium. J. Urol., 133:403, 1985.

Sternberg, C. N., Yagoda, A., Scher, H. I., et al.: M-VAC (methotrexate, vinblastine, doxorubicin, and cisplatin) for advanced transitional cell carcinoma of the urothelium. J. Urol., 139:461, 1988.

Sternberg, C. N., Yagoda, A., Scher, H. I., et al.: Methotrexate, doxorubicin and cisplatin for advanced transitional cell carcinoma of the urothelium: Efficacy and patterns of response and relapse. Cancer, 64:2448, 1989.

Stricker, P. D., Grant, A. B., Hosken, B. M., et al.: Topical mitomycin C therapy for carcinoma of the bladder. J. Urol., 138:1164, 1987.

Studer, U. E., Ackermann, D., Casanova, G. A., et al.: Three years' experience with an ileal low pressure bladder substitute. Br. J. Urol., 63:43, 1989.

Studer, U. E., Biedermann, C., Chollet, D., et al.: Prevention of recurrent superficial bladder tumors by oral etretinate: Preliminary results of a randomized double-blind, multicenter trial in Switzerland. J. Urol., 131:47, 1984.

Sullivan, J. W.: Epidemiologic survey of bladder cancer in greater New Orleans. J. Urol., 128:281, 1982.

Sullivan, J. W., Grabstald, H., and Whitmore, W. F., Jr.: Complications of ureteroileal conduit with radical cystectomy: Review of 336 cases. J. Urol., 124:797, 1980.

Summers, J. L., Falor, W. H., Ward, R. M., et al.: Identical genetic profiles in primary and metastatic bladder tumors. J. Urol., 129:827, 1983.

Swanson, D. A., Liles, A., and Zagars, G. K.: Preoperative irradiation and radical cystectomy for stages T2 and T3 squamous cell carcinoma of the bladder. J. Urol., 143:37, 1990.

Swanson, T. E., Brooks, R., Pearse, H., et al.: Small cell carcinoma of the urinary bladder. Urology, 32:558, 1988.

Swartz, D. A., Johnson, D. E., Ayala, A. G., et al.: Bladder leiomyosarcoma: A review of 10 cases with 5-year follow-up. J. Urol., 133:200, 1985.

Symes, M. O., Eckert, H., Feneley R. C., et al.: Adoptive immunotherapy and radiotherapy in the treatment of urinary bladder cancer. Br. J. Urol., 50:328, 1978.

Tannock, I., Gospodarowicz, M., Connolly, J., et al.: M-VAC (methotrexate, vinblastine, doxorubicin and cisplatin) chemotherapy for transitional cell carcinoma: The Princess Margaret Hospital experience. J. Urol., 142:289, 1989.

Tavares, N. J., Demas, B. E., and Hricak, H.: MR imaging of bladder neoplasms: Correlation with pathologic staging. Urol. Radiol., 12:27, 1990.

Teran, A. Z., and Gambrell, R. D., Jr.: Leiomyoma of the bladder: Case report and review of the literature. Int. J. Fertil., 34:289, 1989.

Teulings, F. A. G., Peters, H. A., Hop, W. C. J., et al.: A new aspect of the urinary excretion of tryptophan metabolites in patients with cancer of the bladder. Int. J. Cancer, 21:140, 1978.

Thuroff, J. W., Alken, P., Riedmiller, H., et al.: The Mainz pouch (mixed augmentation, ileum and cecum) for bladder augmentation and continent diversion. J. Urol., 137:17, 1986.

Torrence, R. J., Kavoussi, L. R., Catalona, W. J., et al.: Prognostic factors in patients treated with intravesical bacillus Calmette-Guérin for superficial bladder cancer. J. Urol., 139:941, 1988.

Torres, H., and Bennett, M. J.: Neurofibromatosis of the bladder: Case report and review of the literature. J. Urol., 96:910, 1966.

Torti, F., Shortliffe, L. D., Williams, R. D., et al.: Alpha interferon and superficial bladder cancer: A Northern California Oncology Group Study. J. Clin. Oncol., 6:476, 1988.

Tribukait, B.: Flow cytometry in assessing the clinical aggressiveness of genitourinary neoplasms. World J. Urol., 5:108, 1987.

Tribukait, B., Gustafson, H., and Espositi, P. -L.: The significance of ploidy and proliferation in the clinical and biological evaluation of bladder tumors: A study of 100 untreated cases. Br. J. Urol., 54:130, 1982.

Tricker, A. R., Mostafa, M. H., Spiegelhalder, B., et al.: Urinary excretion of nitrate, nitrite and N-nitroso compounds in schistosomiasis and bilharzial bladder cancer patients. Carcinogenesis, 10:547, 1989.

Troner, M., Birch, R., Omura, G. A., et al.: Phase III comparison of cisplatin alone versus cisplatin, doxorubicin and cyclophosphamide in the treatment of bladder (urothelial) cancer: A Southeastern Cancer Study Group trial. J. Urol., 137:660, 1987.

Trott, P. A., and Edwards, L.: Comparison of bladder washings and urine cytology in the diagnosis of bladder cancer. J. Urol., 110:664, 1973.

Tsai, Y. C., Nichols, P. W., Hiti, A. L., et al.: Allelic losses of chromosomes 9, 11, and 17 in human bladder cancer. Cancer Res., 50:44, 1990.

Tsukamoto, T., and Lieber, M. M.: Sarcomas of the kidney, urinary bladder, prostate, spermatic cord paratestis and testis in adults. In Raaf, J. H. (Ed.): Management of Soft Tissue Sarcomas. Chicago, Year Book Medical Publishers, 1991.

Tuttle, T. M., Williams, G. M., and Marshall, F. F.: Evidence for cyclophosphamide-induced transitional cell carcinoma in a renal transplant patient. J. Urol., 140:1009, 1988.

Tyler, D. E.: Stratified squamous epithelium in the vesical trigone and urethra: Findings correlated with menstrual cycle and age. Am. J. Anat., 111:319, 1962.

Utz, D. C., and Farrow, G. M.: Carcinoma in situ of the urinary tract. Urol. Clin. North Am., 11:735, 1984.

Utz, D. C., Hanash, K. A., and Farrow, G. M.: The plight of the patient with carcinoma in situ of the bladder. J. Urol., 103:160, 1970.

Uyama, T., and Moriwaki, S.: Carcinosarcoma of urinary bladder. Urology, 18:191, 1981.

van der Werf-Messing, B.: Carcinoma of the bladder treated by suprapubic radium implants: The value of additional external irradiation. Eur. J. Urol., 5:277, 1969.

van der Werf-Messing, B.: Carcinoma of the bladder treated by preoperative radiation followed by cystectomy. Cancer, 32:1084, 1973.

van der Werf-Messing, B. H. P.: Carcinoma of the urinary bladder treated by interstitial radiotherapy. Urol. Clin. North Am., 11:659, 1984.

van der Werf-Messing, B. H., and van Putten, W. L.: Carcinoma of the urinary bladder category T2,3NXM0 treated by 40 Gy external irradiation followed by cesium 137 implant at reduced dose (50%). Int. J. Radiat. Oncol. Biol. Phys., 16:369, 1989.

van Helsdingen, P. J., Rikken, C. H., Sleeboom, H. P., et al.: Mitomycin C resorption following repeated intravesical instillations using different instillation times. Urol. Int., 43:42, 1988.

Vanni, R., Peretti, D., Scarpa, R. M., et al.: Cytogenetics of bladder cancer: Rearrangements of the short arm of chromosome 11. Cancer Detect. Prev., 10:401, 1987.

Vargas, A. D., and Mendez, R.: Leiomyoma of the bladder. Urology, 21:308, 1983.

Varkarakis, M. J., Gaeta, J., Moore, R. H., et al.: Superficial bladder tumor: Aspects of clinical progression. Urology, 4:414, 1974.

Vekemans, K., Vanneste, A., Van Oyen, P., et al.: Postoperative spindle cell nodule of bladder. Urology, 35:342, 1990.

Vincente-Rodriguez, J., Chechile, G., Algaba, F., et al.: Value of random endoscopic biopsy of the diagnosis of bladder carcinoma in situ. Eur. Urol., 13:150, 1987.

Vinnicombe, J., and Abercrombie, G. F.: Total cystectomy—a review. Br. J. Urol., 50:488, 1978.

Viola, M. V., Fromowitz, F., Oravez, S., et al.: Ras oncogene p21 expression is increased in premalignant lesions of high grade bladder carcinomas. J. Exp. Med., 161:1213, 1985.

Visvanathan, K. V., Pocock, R. D., and Summerhayes, I. C.: Preferential and novel activation of H-ras in human bladder. Oncogene Res., 3:77, 1988.

Vock, P., Haertel, M., Fuchs, W. A., et al.: Computed tomography in staging of carcinoma of the urinary bladder. Br. J. Urol., 54:158, 1982.

Voges, G. E., Tauschke, E., Stockle, M., et al.: Computerized tomography: An unreliable method for accurate staging of bladder tumors in patients who are candidates for radical cystectomy. J. Urol., 142:972, 1989.

Vuvenoc, M., Fontaniere, B., Blanc-Brunat, N., et al.: Simultaneous staining of nuclear DNA and blood group cell surface antigens on cells for bladder irrigation fluid. Anal. Quant. Cytol., 7:69, 1985.

Wahlqvist, L.: Chemical carcinogenesis—a review and personal observations with special reference to the role of tobacco and phenacetin in the production of urothelial tumors. *In* Pavone-Maculoso, M., et al. (Eds): Bladder Tumors and Other Topics in Urological Oncology. New York, Plenum Press, 1980, p. 47.

Wajsman, Z., and Klimberg, I. W.: Treatment alternatives for invasive bladder cancer. Semin. Surg. Oncol., 5:272, 1989.

Wallace, D. M., and Bloom, H. J. G.: The management of deeply infiltrating (T₃) bladder carcinoma: Controlled trial of radical radiotherapy and radical cystectomy (first report). Br. J. Urol., 48:587, 1976.

Wan, J., and Grosman, H. B.: Bladder carcinoma in patients age 40 years or younger. Cancer, 64:178, 1989.

Waterhouse, J., Muir, C., Shanmugartanam, K., et al.: Cancer incidence in five continents, Volume 4. Lyon, International Agency for Research on Cancer, 1982.

Weinstein, R. S., Alroy, J., Farrow, G. M., et al.: Blood group isoantigen deletion in carcinoma in situ of the urinary bladder. Cancer, 43:661, 1979.

Weinstein, R. S., Miller, A. W., III, and Pauli, B. V.: Carcinoma in situ: Comment on the pathobiology of a paradox. Urol. Clin. North Am., 7:523, 1980.

Weldon, T. E., and Soloway, M. S.: Susceptibility of urothelium to neoplastic cellular implantation. Urology, 5:824, 1975.

Wenderoth, U. K., Bachor, R., Egghart, G., et al.: The ileal neobladder: Experience and results of more than 100 consecutive cases. J. Urol., 143:492, 1990.

Whitmore, W. F., Jr.: Integrated irradiation and cystectomy for bladder cancer. Br. J. Urol., 52:1, 1980.

Whitmore, W. F., Jr., and Batata, M.: Status of integrated irradiation and cystectomy for bladder cancer. Urol. Clin. North Am. 11:681, 1985.

Whitmore, W. F., Jr., Batata, M. A., Hilaris, B. S., et al.: A comparative study of two preoperative radiation regimens with cystectomy for bladder cancer. Cancer, 40:1077, 1977.

Wick, M. R., Brown, B. A., Young, R. H., et al.: Spindle-cell proliferations of the urinary tract: An immunohistochemical study. Am. J. Surg. Pathol., 12:379, 1988.

Wiener, D. P., Koss, L. G., Sablay, B., et al.: The prevalence and significance of Brunn's nests, cystitis cystica and squamous metaplasia in normal bladders. J. Urol., 122:317, 1979.

Wijkstrom, H., Edsmyr, F., and Lundh, B.: The value of preoperative classification according to the TNM system. Eur. Urol., 10:101–106, 1984.

Wijkstrom, H., and Tribukait, B.: Deoxyribonucleic acid flow cytometry in predicting response to radical radiotherapy of bladder cancer. J. Urol., 144:646, 1990.

Wiley, E. L., Mendelsohn, G., Droller, M., et al.: Immunoperoxidase detection of carcino-embryonic antigen and blood group substances in papillary transitional cell carcinoma of the bladder. J. Urol., 128:276, 1982.

Williams, R. D.: Intravesical interferon alpha in the treatment of superficial bladder cancer. Semin. Oncol., 15:10, 1988.

Wilson, T. M., Fauver, H. E., and Weigel, J. W.: Leiomyosarcoma of urinary bladder. Urology, 13:565, 1979.

Winkler, H. Z., Nativ, O., Hosaka, Y., et al.: Nuclear deoxyribonucleic acid ploidy in squamous cell bladder cancer. J. Urol., 141:297, 1989.

Wishnow, K. I., and Dmochowski, R.: Pelvic recurrence after radical cystectomy without preoperative radiation. J. Urol., 140:42, 1988.

Wishnow, K. I., Johnson, D. E., Dmochowski, R., et al.: Ileal conduit in era of systemic chemotherapy. Urology, 33:358, 1989.

Wishnow, K. I., and Ro, J. Y.: Importance of early treatment of transitional cell carcinoma of prostate duct. Urology, 32:11, 1988.

Wolf, H.: Studies on the role of tryptophan metabolites in the genesis of bladder cancer. Acta Clin. Scand. (Suppl) 433:154, 1973.

Wolf, H., and Hojgaard, K.: Urothelial dysplasia concomitant with bladder tumors as a determinant factor for future new recurrences. Lancet, 2:134, 1983.

Wood, D. P., Montie, J. E., Pontes, J. E., et al.: The role of magnetic resonance imaging in the staging of bladder carcinoma. J. Urol., 140:741, 1988.

Wood, D. P., Montie, J. E., Pontes, J. E., et al.: Transitional cell carcinoma of the prostate in cystoprostatectomy specimens removed for bladder cancer. J. Urol., 141:346, 1989.

Yagoda, A.: Chemotherapy for advanced urothelial cancer. Semin. Urol., 1:60, 1983.

Yalla, A. V., Ivker, M., Burros, H. M., et al.: Cystitis glandularis with perivesical lipomatosis: Frequent association of two unusual proliferative conditions. Urology, 5:383, 1975.

Young, R. H.: Carcinosarcoma of the urinary bladder. Cancer, 59:1333, 1987.

Young, R. H., and Scully, R. E.: Pseudosarcomatous lesions of the urinary bladder, prostate gland, and urethra: A report of three cases and review of the literature. Arch. Pathol. Lab. Med., 111:354, 1987.

Young, R. H., Wick, M. R., and Mills, S. E.: Sarcomatoid carcinoma of the urinary bladder: A clinicopathologic analysis of 12 cases and review of the literature. Am. J. Clin. Pathol., 90:653, 1988.

Zincke, H., Garbeff, P. J., and Beahrs, J. R.: Upper urinary tract transitional cell cancer after radical cystectomy for bladder cancer. J. Urol., 131:50, 1984.

Zincke, H., Utz, D. C., Taylor, W. F., et al.: Influence of thiotepa and doxorubicin instillation at time of transurethral surgical treatment of bladder cancer on tumor recurrence: A prospective, randomized, double-blind, controlled trial. J. Urol., 129:505, 1983.

Zuk, R. J., Baithun, S. I., Martin, J. E., et al.: The immunocytochemical demonstration of basement membrane deposition in transitional cell carcinoma of the bladder. Virchows Archiv. [A], 414:447, 1989.

Urothelial Tumors of the Renal Pelvis and Ureter

Abercrombie, G. F., Eardley, I., Payne, S. R., et al.: Modified nephroureterectomy: Long-term follow-up with particular reference to subsequent bladder tumours. Br. J. Urol., 61:198, 1988.

Amar, A. D., and Das, S.: Upper urinary tract transitional cell carcinoma in patients with bladder carcinoma and associated vesicoureteral reflux. J. Urol., 133:468, 1985.

Anderstrom, C., Johansson, S. L., Pettersson, S., et al.: Carcinoma of the ureter: A clincopathologic study of 49 cases. J. Urol., 142:280, 1989.

1987 Annual Cancer Statistics Review: Including Cancer Trends: 1950–1985, NIH Publication No. 88-2789. Bethesda, Maryland, U. S. Department of Health and Human Services, National Cancer Institute.

Babaian, R. J., and Johnson, D. E.: Primary carcinoma of the ureter. J. Urol., 123:357, 1980.

Baghdassarian Gatewood, O. M., Goldman, S. M., Marshall, F. F., et al.: Computerized tomography in the diagnosis of carcinoma of the kidney. J. Urol., 127:876, 1982.

Batata, M. A., Whitmore, W. F., Jr., Milaris, B. S., et al.: Primary carcinoma of the ureter: A prognostic study. Cancer, 35:1626, 1975.

Bazeed, M. A., Scharfe, T., Becht, E., et al.: Local excision of urothelial cancer of the upper urinary tract. Eur. Urol., 12:89, 1986.

Blacker, E. J., Johnson, D. E., Abdul-Karim, F. W., et al.: Squamous cell carcinoma of renal pelvis. Urology, 25:124, 1985.

Blank, C., Lissmer, L., Kaneti, J., et al.: Fibroepithelial polyp of the renal pelvis. J. Urol., 137:962, 1987.

Bloom, N. A., Vidone, R. A., and Lytton, B.: Primary carcinoma of the ureter: A report of 102 new cases. J. Urol., 103:590, 1970.

Blute, M. L., Segura, J. W., Patterson, D. E., et al.: Impact of endourology on diagnosis and management of upper urinary tract urothelial cancer. J. Urol., 141:1298, 1989.

Blute, M. L., Tsushima, K., Farrow, G. M., et al.: Transitional cell carcinoma of the renal pelvis: Nuclear deoxyribonucleic acid ploidy studied by flow cytometry. J. Urol., 140:944, 1988.

Blute, R. D., Jr., Gittes, R. R., and Gittes, R. F.: Renal brush biopsy: Survey of indications, techniques and results. J. Urol., 126:146, 1981.

Bree, R. L., Schultz, S. R., and Hayes, R.: Large infiltrating renal transitional cell carcinomas: CT and ultrasound features. J. Comput. Assist. Tomogr., 14:381, 1990.

Brenner, D. W., and Schellhammer, P. F.: Upper tract urothelial malignancy after cyclophosphamide therapy: A case report and literature review. J. Urol., 137:1226, 1987.

Brookland, R. K., and Richter, M. P.: The postoperative irradiation of transitional cell carcinoma of the renal pelvis ureter. J. Urol., 133:952, 1985.

Cummings, K. B.: Nephroureterectomy: Rationale in the management of transitional cell carcinoma of the upper urinary tract. Urol. Clin. North Am., 7:569, 1980.

Davis, B. W., Hough, A. J., and Gardner, W. A.: Renal pelvic carcinoma: Morphological correlates of metastatic behavior. J. Urol., 137:857, 1987.

DeKock, M. L., and Breytenbach, I. H.: Local excision and topical thiotepa in the treatment of transitional cell carcinoma of the renal pelvis: A case report. J. Urol., 135:566, 1986.

Fein, A. B., and McClennan, B. L.: Solitary filling defects of the ureter. Semin. Roentgenol., 21:201, 1986.

Fleming, S.: Carcinosarcoma (mixed mesodermal tumor) of the ureter. J. Urol., 138:1234, 1987.

Fraley, E. E.: Cancer of the renal pelvis. In Skinner, D. G., and deKernion, J. B. (Eds.): Genitourinary Cancer. Philadelphia, W. B. Saunders Co., 1978, p. 134.

Frischer, Z., Waltzer, W. C., and Gonder, M. J.: Bilateral transitional cell carcinoma of the renal pelvis in the cancer family syndrome. J. Urol., 134:1197, 1985.

Fulks, R. M., and Falace, P. B.: Carcinoma of the ureter with extensive squamous differentiation and positive immunoperoxidase staining for carcinoembryonic antigen: A case report. J. Urol., 133:92, 1985.

Geiger, J., Fong, Q., and Fay, R.: Transitional cell carcinoma of renal pelvis with invasion of renal vein and thrombosis of subhepatic inferior vena cava. Urology, 28:52, 1986.

Ghazi, M. R., Morales, P. A., and Al-Askari, S.: Primary carcinoma of ureter: Report of 27 new cases. Urology, 14:18, 1979.

Gibas, Z., Griffin, C. A., and Emanuel, B. S.: Trisomy 7 and i(5p) in a transitional cell carcinoma of the ureter. Cancer Genet. Cytogenet., 25:369, 1987.

Gill, W. B., Lu, C. T., and Thomsen, S.: Retrograde brushing: A new technique for obtaining histologic and cytologic material from ureteral, renal pelvic and renal calyceal lesions. J. Urol., 109:573, 1973.

Gittes, R. F.: Retrograde brushing and nephroscopy in the diagnosis of upper-tract urothelial cancer. Urol. Clin. North Am., 11:617, 1984.

Grabstald, H., Whitmore, W. F., and Melamed, M. R.: Renal pelvic tumors. JAMA, 218:845, 1971.

Grace, D. A., Taylor, W. N., Taylor, J. N., et al.: Carcinoma of the renal pelvis: A 15-year review. J. Urol., 98:566, 1967.

Hatch, T. R., Hefty, T. R., and Barry, J. M.: Time-related recurrence rates in patients with upper tract transitional cell carcinoma. J. Urol., 140:40, 1988.

Hawtrey, C. E.: Fifty-two cases of primary ureteral carcinoma: A clinical-pathologic study. J. Urol., 105:188, 1971.

Hecht, F., Berger, C. S., and Sandberg, A. A.: Nonreciprocal chromosome translocation t(5;14) in cancers of the kidney: Adenocarcinoma of the renal parenchyma and transitional cell carcinoma of the kidney pelvis. Cancer Genet. Cytogenet., 14:197, 1985.

Heney, N. M., Nocks, B. N., Daly, J. J., et al.: Prognostic factors in carcinoma of the ureter. J. Urol., 125:632, 1981.

Herr, H. W.: Durable response of a carcinoma in situ of the renal pelvis to topical bacillus Calmette-Guérin. J. Urol., 134:531, 1985.

Huben, R. P., Mounzer, A. M., and Murphy, G. P.: Tumor grade and stage as prognostic variables in upper tract urothelial tumors. Cancer, 62:2016, 1988.

Huffman, J. L., Bagley, D. H., Lyon, E. S., et al.: Endoscopic diagnosis and treatment of upper-tract urothelial tumors: A preliminary report. Cancer, 55:1422, 1985.

Jensen, O. M., Knudsen, J. B., McLaughlin, J. K., et al.: The Copenhagen case-control study of renal pelvis and ureter cancer: Role of smoking and occupational exposures. Int. J. Cancer, 41:557, 1988.

Jensen, O. M., Knudsen, J. B., Tomasson, H., et al.: The Copenhagen case-control study of renal pelvis and ureter cancer: Role of analgesics. Int. J. Cancer, 44:965, 1989.

Jitsukawa, S., Nakamura, K., Nakayama, M., et al.: Transitional cell carcinoma of kidney extending into renal vein and inferior vena cava. Urology, 25:310, 1985.

Johansson, S., and Wahlqvist, L.: A prognostic study of urothelial renal pelvic tumors: Comparison between the prognosis of patients treated with infrafascial nephrectomy and perifascial nephroureterectomy. Cancer, 43:2525, 1979.

Johnson, D. E., and Babaian, R. J.: Conservative management for noninvasive distal ureteral carcinoma. Urology, 13:365, 1979.

Kagawa, S., Takigawa, H., Ghazizadeh, M., et al.: Immunohistological detection of T antigen and ABH blood group antigens in upper urinary tract tumours. Br. J. Urol., 57:386, 1985.

Kakizoe, T., Fujita, J., Murase, T., et al.: Transitional cell carcinoma of the bladder in patients with renal pelvic and ureteral cancer. J. Urol., 124:17, 1980.

Kenney, P. J., and Stanley, R. J.: Computed tomography of ureteral tumors. J. Comput. Assist. Tomogr., 11:102, 1987.

Kim, Y. I., Yoon, D. H., Lee, S. W., et al.: Multicentric papillary adenocarcinoma of the renal pelvis and ureter: Report of a case with ultrastructural study. Cancer, 62:2402, 1988.

Lantz, E. J., and Hattery, R. R.: Diagnostic imaging of urothelial cancer. Urol. Clin. North Am., 11:567, 1984.

Li, M. K., and Cheung, W. L.: Squamous cell carcinoma of the renal pelvis. J. Urol., 138:269, 1987.

Lynch, H. T., Ens, J. A., and Lynch, J. F.: The Lynch syndrome II and urological malignancies. J. Urol., 143:24, 1990.

Madgar, I., Goldwasser, B., Czerniak, A., et al.: Leiomyosarcoma of the ureter. Eur. Urol., 14:487, 1988.

Mahadevia, P. S., Karwa, G. L., and Koss, L. G.: Mapping of urothelium in carcinomas of the renal pelvis and ureter: A report of nine cases. Cancer, 51:890, 1983.

Mazeman, E.: Tumours of the upper urinary tract, calyces, renal pelvis and ureter. Eur. Urol., 2:120, 1976.

McCarron, J. P., Jr., Chasko, S. B., and Gray, G. F., Jr.: Systematic mapping of nephroureterectomy specimens removed for urothelial cancer: Pathological findings and clinical correlations. J. Urol., 128:243, 1982.

McCredie, M., Stewart, J. H., Carter, J. J., et al.: Phenacetin and papillary necrosis: Independent risk factors for renal pelvic cancer. Kidney Int., 30:81, 1986.

Milestone, B., Friedman, A. C., Seidmon, E. J., et al.: Staging of ureteral transitional cell carcinoma by CT and MRI. Urology, 36:346, 1990.

Morrison, A. S.: Advances in the etiology of urothelial cancer. Urol. Clin. North. Am., 11:557, 1984.

Mufti, G. R., Gove, J. R., Badenoch, D. F., et al.: Transitional cell carcinoma of the renal pelvis and ureter. Br. J. Urol., 63:135, 1989.

Mukamel, E., Nissenkorn, I., Glanz, I., et al.: Upper tract tumours in patients with vesico-ureteral reflux and recurrent bladder tumours. Eur. Urol., 11:6, 1985.

Mullen, J. B., and Kovacs, K.: Primary carcinoma of the ureteral stump: A case report and a review of the literature. J. Urol., 123:113, 1980.

Murphy, D. M., Zincke, H., and Furlow, W. L.: Primary grade 1 transitional cell carcinoma of the renal pelvis and ureter. J. Urol., 123:629, 1980.

Murphy, D. M., Zincke, H., and Furlow, W. L.: Management of high grade transitional cell cancer of the upper urinary tract. J. Urol., 135:25, 1981.

Nemoto, R., Hattori, K., Sasaki, A., et al.: Estimations of the S phase fraction in situ in transitional cell carcinoma of the renal pelvis and ureter with bromodeoxyuridine labelling. Br. J. Urol., 64:339, 1989.

Nielsen, K., and Ostri, P.: Primary tumors of the renal pelvis: Evaluation of clinical and pathological features in a consecutive series of 10 years. J. Urol., 140:19, 1988.

Nolan, R. L., Nickel, J. C., and Froud, P. J.: Percutaneous endourologic approach for transitional cell carcinoma of the renal pelvis. Urol. Radiol., 9:217, 1988.

Oldbring, J., Glifberg, I., Mikulowski, P., et al.: Carcinoma of the renal pelvis and ureter following bladder carcinoma: Frequency, risk factors and clinicopathological findings. J. Urol., 141:1311, 1989a.

Oldbring, J., Hellsten, S., Lindholm, K., et al.: Flow DNA analysis in the characterization of carcinoma of the renal pelvis and ureter. Cancer, 64:2141, 1989b.

Orphali, S. L., Shols, G. W., Hagewood, T., et al.: Familial transitional cell carcinoma of renal pelvis and upper ureter. Urology, 27:394, 1986.

Palvio, D. H., Andersen, J. C., and Falk, E.: Transitional cell tumors of the renal pelvis and ureter associated with capillarosclerosis indicating analgesic abuse. Cancer, 59:972, 1987.

Petkovic, S. D.: Epidemiology and treatment of renal pelvic and ureteral tumors. J. Urol., 114:858, 1975.

Radovanovic, Z., Krajinovic, S., Jankovic, S., et al.: Family history of cancer among cases of upper urothelial tumours in a Balkan nephropathy area. J. Cancer Res. Clin. Oncol., 110:181, 1985.

Ramsey, J. C., and Soloway, M. S.: Instillation of bacillus Calmette-

Guérin into the renal pelvis of a solitary kidney for the treatment of transitional cell carcinoma. J. Urol., 143:1220, 1990.

Ross, R. K., Paganini-Hill, A., Landolph, J., et al.: Analgesics, cigarette smoking, and other risk factors for cancer of the renal pelvis and ureter. Cancer Res., 49:1045, 1989.

Sandberg, A. A., Berger, C. S., Haddad, F. S., et al.: Chromosome change in transitional cell carcinoma of ureter. Cancer Genet. Cytogenet., 19:335, 1986.

Sarnacki, C. T., McCormack, L. J., Kiser, W. S., et al.: Urinary cytology and the clinical diagnosis of urinary tract malignancy: A clinicopathologic study of 1,400 patients. J. Urol., 106:761, 1971.

Schemeller, N. T., and Hofstetter, A. G.: Laser treatment of ureteral tumors. J. Urol., 141:840, 1989.

Scher, H. I., Yagoda, A., Herr, H. W., et al.: Neoadjuvant M-VAC (methotrexate, vinblastine, doxorubicin and cisplatin) for extravesical urinary tract tumors. J. Urol., 139:475, 1988.

Sheline, M., Amendola, M. A., Pollack, H. M., et al.: Fluoroscopically guided retrograde brush biopsy in the diagnosis of transitional cell carcinoma of the upper urinary tract: Results in 45 patients. Am. J. Roentgenol., 153:313, 1989.

Shinka, T., Uekado, Y., Aoshi, H., et al.: Occurrence of uroepithelial tumors of the upper urinary tract after the initial diagnosis of bladder cancer. J. Urol., 140:745, 1988.

Skinner, D. G.: Technique of nephroureterectomy with regional lymph node dissection. Urol. Clin. North Am., 5:253, 1978.

Smith, A. Y., Orihuela, E., and Crowley, A. R.: Percutaneous management of renal pelvic tumors: A treatment option in selected cases. J. Urol., 137:852, 1987a.

Smith, A. Y., Vitale, P. J., Lowe, B. A., et al.: Treatment of superficial papillary transitional cell carcinoma of the ureter by vesicoureteral reflux of mitomycin C. J. Urol., 138:1231, 1987b.

Spiessl, B., Beahrs, O. H., Hermanek, P., et al.: Renal pelvis and ureter. *In* Spiessl, B., Beahrs, O. H., Hermanek, P., Hutter, R. V. P., Scheibe, O., Sobin, L. H., and Wagner, G. (Eds.): UICC-TNM Atlas Illustrated Guide to the TNM/pTNM-Classification of Malignant Tumours. Berlin, Springer-Verlag, 1989, p. 260.

Steffens, J., and Nagel, R.: Tumours of the renal pelvis and ureter: Observations in 170 patients. Br. J. Urol., 61:277, 1988.

Stein, A., Sova, Y., Lurie, M., et al.: Adenocarcinoma of the renal pelvis: Report of two cases, one with simultaneous transitional cell carcinoma of the bladder. Urol. Int., 43:299, 1988.

Stower, M. J., MacIver, A. G., Gingell, J. C., et al.: Inverted papilloma of the ureter with malignant change. Br. J. Urol., 65:13, 1990.

Streem, S. B., Pontes, J. E., Novick, A. C., et al.: Ureteropyeloscopy in the evaluation of upper tract filling defects. J. Urol., 136:383, 1986.

Studer, U. E., Casanova, G., Kraft, R., et al.: Percutaneous bacillus Calmette-Guérin perfusion of the upper urinary tract for carcinoma in situ. J. Urol., 142:975, 1989.

Tannock, I., Gospodarowicz, M., Connolly, J., et al.: M-VAC (methotrexate, vinblastine, doxorubicin and cisplatin) chemotherapy for transitional cell carcinoma: The Princess Margaret Hospital experience. J. Urol., 142:28, 1989.

Tasca, A., and Zattoni, F.: The case for a percutaneous approach to transitional cell carcinoma of the renal pelvis. J. Urol., 143:902, 1990.

Tomera, K. M., Leary, F. J., and Zincke, H.: Pyeloscopy in ureteral tumors. J. Urol., 127:1088, 1982.

Vest, S. A.: Conservative surgery in certain benign tumors of the ureter. J. Urol., 53:97, 1945.

Wallace, D. M. A., Wallace, D. M., Whitfield, H. N., et al.: The late results of conservative surgery for upper tract urothelial carcinomas. Br. J. Urol., 53:537, 1981.

Ziegelbaum, M., Novick, A. C., Streem, S. B., et al.: Conservative surgery for transitional cell carcinoma of the renal pelvis. J. Urol., 138:1146, 1987.

Zincke, H., and Neves, R. J.: Feasibility of conservative surgery for transitional cell cancer of the upper urinary tract. Urol. Clin. North Am., 11:717, 1984.

Zoretic, S., and Gonzales, J.: Primary carcinoma of the ureters. Urology, 21:354, 1983.

Zungri, E., Chechile, G., Algaba, F., et al.: Treatment of transitional cell carcinoma of the ureter: Is the controversy justified? Eur. Urol., 17:276, 1990.

29
ADENOCARCINOMA OF THE PROSTATE

Thomas A. Stamey, M.D.
John E. McNeal, M. D.

It is not enough to label a tumor malignant; it is necessary to specify which characteristics, and the degree of each of them, that make it malignant.

LESLIE FOULDS, 1954

This statement, written by Leslie Foulds nearly four decades ago, is particularly appropriate for cancer of the prostate. Clinical and pathologic observations have been confounded by subjectivity of the observer, by lack of precise and consistent criteria for clinical and pathologic staging and grading, and by inconsistency in the clinical definitions and standards for measuring progression. In addition, the variable responses to endocrine therapy together with competing causes of mortality have contributed to more inconsistency in conclusions about the natural history of prostate cancer.

Although several parameters—capsule penetration, positive surgical margins, seminal vesicle invasion, and lymph node metastases—have traditionally been associated with poor prognosis, their relationship to each other has not been completely understood. It has not been appreciated that each of these parameters may occur in the absence of the others. Until the late 1980s, the failure to recognize the important differences in anatomic location between clinical stage A and stage B cancers has also led to confusion (McNeal et al., 1988c, 1988d). Lymph node metastasis and seminal vesicle invasion have long been recognized as adverse survival parameters. However, it has not been generally appreciated that 35 to 40 per cent of clinical stage TB radical prostatectomies involve extension of the cancer into the periprostatic fat along the perineural spaces in the *absence* of lymph node or seminal vesicle invasion (McNeal et al., 1990b; Villers et al., 1989). Nor has it been recognized that iatrogenic positive surgical margins are distressingly common—especially at the apex—in the absence of any other adverse histologic parameters (Stamey et al., 1990).

All things considered, it is no wonder that the natural history, diagnosis, and treatment of prostatic cancer remain highly controversial. Nevertheless, we believe that the advent of prostate-specific antigen, transrectal ultrasound biopsies, and quantitative histologic studies of radical prostatectomy specimens for clinical stage A and B disease has added a dimension to our understanding of prostate cancer that was not available in 1986. It is remarkable that so much new information has appeared in the brief years since the fifth edition of *Campbell's Urology*.

POPULATION STATISTICS

Almost all cancers that arise in the prostate are adenocarcinomas of the duct-acinar secretory epithelium. Adenocarcinoma of the prostate is the most common internal cancer of males in the United States; 122,000 newly diagnosed cases are estimated for 1991 as compared with 101,000 new cases of lung cancer in men (Boring et al., 1991). Among all races in the United States, the age-adjusted mortality rate from prostatic adenocarcinoma established for 1983 to 1984 is 22.7 deaths per 100,000 men, and the incidence is 75.3 cases per 100,000 men (Devesa et al., 1987). Prostate cancer is very uncommon before the age of 50 years, but its frequency climbs steeply with age to peak or plateau in the 9th decade for both incidence and mortality rate (Lew and Garfinkel, 1990). Although it is mainly a disease of older men, it is estimated that a death from prostate cancer represents, on average, 9.0 years of life lost (Horm and Sondik, 1989).

Many epidemiologic studies have been aimed at identifying etiologic or predisposing factors for prostate cancer; their details have been well summarized in several review articles (Carter et al., 1990a; Hutchison, 1981; Scardino, 1989; Zaridze and Boyle, 1987). No consistent evidence exists for substantial risk factors associated with diet, occupation, socioeconomic status, infectious disease history, sexual practices, body build, or hormonal factors. Because of the known androgen dependence of prostate cancer and anecdotal information that early castration is protective, differences in sex hormone status might be expected among men with prostate cancer. However, the results of several studies have been conflicting or negative, and it has been proposed that the role of androgenic hormones is only a permissive one (Carter et al., 1990a; Franks, 1973; Scardino, 1990; Wynder et al., 1971).

The differences between countries in mortality rate and incidence of clinical prostate cancer are particularly striking. The United States is near the high end of the continuum, whereas Japan is near the low end, with clinical incidence and mortality rate both less than 5 per 100,000 men (Akazaki and Stemmermann, 1973; Breslow et al., 1977; Carter et al., 1990c; Haenszel and Kurihara, 1968). However, it has been reported that the frequency of incidental finding of cancer of the prostate at autopsy is similar among countries that have widely different clinical frequencies (Breslow et al., 1977). Furthermore, Japanese immigrants to the United States and their offspring show increases in clinical incidence and mortality that approach United States values (Akazaki and Stemmermann, 1973; Haenszel and Kurihara, 1968). It has, therefore, been proposed that factors responsible for the *initiation* of prostate cancer may be similar throughout the world and that clinical differences arise from differences in unidentified environmental *promoting* factors (Carter et al., 1990c; Dhom, 1983).

Blacks in the United States have a mortality rate for prostate cancer that is two to three times the rate for whites in the same geographic area, even when it is corrected for socioeconomic status and age (Ernster et al., 1977). In contrast, in an extensive autopsy study, the frequency of incidental prostate cancer was found to be similar between the two races (Guileyardo et al., 1980). In this study and in another smaller study (McNeal et al., 1986a), the proportion of incidental cancers that were large and poorly differentiated was considerably greater in blacks than in whites. It was suggested from these data that the risk of developing histologically detectable cancer (initiation) may be similar between these two races; however, in blacks, additional factors—probably genetic—cause more rapid growth and dedifferentiation (promotion). Cancer volume and dedifferentiation have been found to correlate strongly with metastasis (McNeal et al., 1986a, 1990b).

A probable role for genetic factors in prostate cancer has also been uncovered in several studies of familial aggregation in prostate cancer cases (Fincham et al., 1990; Steinberg et al., 1990; Woolf, 1960). A two to threefold increase in risk has been reported for men having a father or brother with clinical carcinoma of the prostate, and the relative risk may exceed five if two or more first-degree relatives have had clinical prostate cancer (Steinberg et al., 1990). The increase in risk was reported to be specific for cancer in the prostate gland (Woolf, 1960).

NATURAL HISTORY

Histologic Versus Clinical Cancer

The natural history of adenocarcinoma of the prostate has been stated to be unpredictable (Catalona, 1984; Franks et al., 1958; Franks, 1973; Whitmore, 1973, 1988), although there has never been a formal study in which the predictive values of standard clinical or morphologic indices were compared with cancer in the prostate versus cancer in other organs. In fact, the results of such a study would probably not be illuminating, considering the specific nature of the prediction problem. For other cancers, generally, the certainty of a fatal outcome for the untreated disease is assumed; interest in prediction focuses on survival following attempted eradication of the cancer. Observations from the surgical resection specimen often contribute to prediction.

In comparison, for prostate cancer, it is often assumed that localized disease in most cases will probably have little or no effect on the quality or duration of life. Prediction then focuses on identifying the occasional clinically localized cancer that is likely to progress to metastatic disease (Catalona, 1984). The evidence on which to base such predictions is often limited to a small biopsy rather than the entire cancer, supplemented by clinical estimation of the extent of local disease rather than pathologic staging.

This difference in perspective has arisen because of the uniquely high prevalence of undiagnosed prostate cancer in men older than 50 years, as demonstrated at autopsy (Franks, 1954a, 1956; Scardino, 1989) or at prostatectomy for other causes (Kabalin et al., 1989b). The autopsy prevalence of prostatic adenocarcinoma is at least 15 per cent in the 6th decade and has been reported to be higher (Franks, 1954a). Autopsy prevalence of prostatic adenocarcinoma reaches 30 per cent in the 7th decade, 40 per cent in the 8th decade, and 50 per cent in the 9th decade (30 to 40 per cent overall average) (Scardino, 1989). Incidental cancer in other organs at autopsy is a relatively rare finding at any age. Hence, for the prostate, a unique dichotomy exists between the magnitude of the reservoir of malignancy in the population and the rate of emergence of clinically aggressive disease.

Using a 30 per cent overall prevalence figure, it has been calculated that only 1.05 per cent of the total population reservoir of cancer reaches clinical diagnosis in any year, and the annual mortality rate is only 0.31 per cent of the total prevalence of histologic cancer (Scardino, 1989). Because of the high autopsy prevalence and resulting clinical dichotomy, Franks proposed in 1954 that two distinct species of carcinoma occur in the prostate (Franks, 1954a, 1956). "Latent" cancer is proposed to be identical in all observable respects to the few "clinically manifest" cancers, but it is thought to be biologically incapable of ever acquiring malignant behavioral features.

Subsequently, the prognostic success of histologic

grading of adenocarcinoma of the prostate has demonstrated that the capacity for clinically aggressive behavior can, in fact, often be recognized with histologic study (Gleason, 1977). Hence, the concept of latency as originally proposed is untenable. Nevertheless, grading often has only limited predictive value for the individual patient, and this problem together with the still unexplained high prevalence of incidental (autopsy) cancer continues to be regarded by some as evidence that there are two biologically distinct species of carcinoma in the prostate (Carter et al., 1990c).

This view has been further supported by the observation that the prevalence of incidental (autopsy) cancer is also high in countries where the incidence of *clinical* cancer is much lower than in the United States. A current study compared the age-specific prevalence of autopsy cancer and clinical cancer in Japan and the United States (Carter et al., 1990c). The slopes of curves of log prevalence versus age in the two countries for both autopsy cancer and clinical cancer were interpreted in terms of the biologic concepts of *tumor progression* and *multistep carcinogenesis*. Mathematic analysis of the curves suggested that several biologic steps (presumably mutational events) were required for both the first phase—initiation of histologic (autopsy) cancer—and the second phase—progression from histologic cancer to clinical cancer.

It was concluded that, for each phase, the number of biologic (mutational) steps was the same for the two countries. For the first (initiation) phase, the probability of occurrence of these steps was similar for the United States and Japan. However, for the second phase—that is, progression to clinical cancer—the probability of occurrence of the progression steps was much lower among the Japanese. It was reasoned that those cancers that do not take the second-phase progression steps are effectively "latent," and that their identification is unpredictable by histologic or other means.

Tumor Progression

The concept of biologic tumor progression was first proposed by Foulds in 1954 (Foulds, 1954, 1958) and has become established during the last decade as an important general principle of tumor biology (Heppner, 1984; Nicolson, 1987; Weinberg, 1989; Woodruff, 1983). Evidence for its wide applicability has been found in a variety of experimental and spontaneous cancers. Progression appears to be based on an inherent genetic instability in most types of malignant cells; they spontaneously accumulate mutational events on a random basis, with a cumulative probability that is proportional to the number of cell divisions the tumor has undergone (Cohen and Ellwein, 1990; Goldie, 1987; Goldie and Coldman, 1979). Multiple steps in progression are anticipated to exist for both the premalignant and invasive phases of cancer generally (Hanahan, 1989). Progress has been made in the specific identification of these steps (Fearon and Vogelstein, 1990; Sager, 1989).

No evidence demonstrates that prostate cancer is unique in this respect. Because progression is probabilistic (Goldie, 1987), it carries an element of unpredictability for any cancer in any organ, for any cell in that cancer, and for any given mitosis of that cell. But probability is not selective, and it cannot provide a basis for discriminating two biologic races within a single type of malignancy.

It has been suggested that the dichotomy between the frequency of clinical versus histologic cancer may not be as great as initially perceived (Scardino, 1989). From the aforementioned incidence and mortality data, it was calculated that the *lifetime risk* of clinical prostate cancer in a man of age 50 in 1985 would be 9.51 per cent, whereas his lifetime prostate cancer mortality risk would be 2.89 per cent (Seidman et al., 1985). If the lifetime risk of histologic cancer (autopsy data) is taken as 42 per cent, then 7 per cent of men with histologic cancer will die of it.

Cancer Volume and Biologic Behavior

The dichotomy may be still smaller if the progression of histologic cancer to a clinically aggressive phase is a simple probabilistic function of cancer volume (McNeal, 1969; McNeal et al., 1986a; Scardino, 1989; Stamey et al., 1988). (Fig. 29–1). The hypothesis that progression is volume-related is based on the strong evidence that biologic progression in cancers generally is closely linked to cumulative cell division (Cohen and Ellwein, 1990; Goldie, 1987). Such a relationship provides the conceptual basis for a direct link between cancer volume and probability of metastasis.

The volume distribution of autopsy carcinomas is such that the (microscopic) cancers with the smallest volume are the most numerous, with an exponentially declining frequency at successive increasing volumes (McNeal et al., 1986a). This is shown in Figure 29–1 as a nearly equal frequency in *logarithmically* equivalent volume intervals. Such a volume distribution is consistent with a constant cell population doubling time for prostate cancer at all volumes, and that doubling time has been estimated to be as long as 2 years (Stamey and Kabalin, 1989). Thus, the smallest tumors, perhaps the smallest 50 per cent are, with few exceptions, predictably remote in time from aggressive behavior. Consideration of only the larger cancers (>0.3 ml) as likely to progress to metastatic potential would further increase the ratio of clinical to histologic cancer.

Much still remains unresolved about the natural history of adenocarcinoma of the prostate, but the weight of evidence indicates that the label "unpredictable" is not justified. This is particularly true when it is considered that the type of prediction usually referred to is attempted from small-sample estimates of histology and crude clinical estimates of tumor volume. Under favorable conditions—comparable to those often found in other cancers—accurate knowledge of prostate cancer volume and histologic grade can be highly predictive of biologic behavior (McNeal et al., 1990b). Prostatic adenocarcinoma is probably a single biologic entity with a very high rate of malignant transformation but a very slow and constant mass doubling time and a very slow

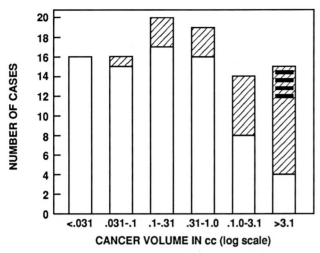

Figure 29–1. Volume distribution of prostate cancer in 100 autopsies grouped into six consecutive, logarithmically equal volume intervals. Cases with Gleason grade 4 and/or 5 elements are indicated by hatched areas. Cases with distant metastases are indicated by horizontal bars.

biologic progression rate, which is linked to cumulative cell division and, hence, to tumor volume.

PATHOLOGY

Classification of Prostate Cancers

A classification of the spectrum of malignant tumors that may be found in the prostate is outlined in Table 29–1. Adenocarcinoma comprises more than 95 per cent of all prostate cancers, and more than 90 per cent of the remainder are transitional cell carcinomas. These two, together with squamous cell carcinomas, the majority of undifferentiated carcinomas, and probably the carcinoid histologic pattern, are derived from a common precursor cell type—the embryonic urogenital sinus epithelium.

In the male, the urogenital sinus epithelium lining the prostatic urethra normally differentiates into a transitional epithelium which bears a surface layer of columnar secretory cells (Fig. 29–2), rather than the umbrella cells, which characterize the surface layer of bladder transitional epithelium (McNeal, 1988b). This specialized transitional epithelium extends for a variable distance of several millimeters into the main trunk ducts of the glandular prostate and partly or completely lines the tiny submucosal periurethral glands.

Also within the glandular parenchyma and not in continuity with the trunk ducts, microscopic foci of transitional cell metaplasia may occasionally be seen involving groups of ducts and acini, usually in response to inflammation. In the urethral lining or in any portion of the duct-acinar system, prolonged or severe inflammation may further stimulate metaplasia of an already metaplastic transitional epithelium to a squamous phenotype. Estrogenic hormone administration also readily induces the squamous phenotype, but hormone-induced squamous cells are distinctively enlarged and pale because of cytoplasmic glycogen deposition. Because these secretory and nonsecretory phenotypes can readily be interchanged in the normal epithelium, it is not surprising that transitional cell carcinoma is the second most common prostatic carcinoma, with squamous cell cancer as an occasional variant.

Transitional Cell Carcinoma

Transitional cell carcinoma in the prostate in the majority of cases is found in patients who also have bladder and/or urethral cancer, and it is usually the bladder tumor that is clinically manifest. Prostate involvement may represent direct invasion of an advanced carcinoma of the bladder (Schellhammer et al., 1977). More often, it is represented by foci of intraductal or intra-acinar prostatic transitional cell carcinomas (Fig. 29–3), which arise independently or by mucosal spread from the urethra (Mahadevia et al., 1986; Wood et al., 1989). In situ foci within the prostate have been reported in 29 per cent of cystectomies for bladder cancer (Wood et al., 1989), and they may be extensive enough to involve most of the duct-acinar system of the prostate. Invasion of intraductal transitional cell cancer into the prostate stroma is not uncommon.

Morphology of the Glandular Prostate

The prostatic acini and all ducts beyond the main trunk ducts near the urethra are lined by a single layer

Table 29–1. CLASSIFICATION OF PROSTATE CANCERS BY CELL TYPE OF ORIGIN

I. Epithelial
  A. Adenocarcinoma
    Parent epithelium: secretory lining of duct branches and acini
    Patterns (see grades): cribriform, papillary, undifferentiated, "endometrioid," and so forth
  B. Transitional cell carcinoma
    Parent epithelium
      Prostatic urethra
      Major trunk ducts in proximity to urethra
      Metaplasia (inflammatory, ischemic) in duct branches, acini
    Patterns
      Intraductal transitional cell carcinoma
      Invasive transitional cell carcinoma
      Squamous cell carcinoma
  C. Neuroendocrine carcinoma
    Parent epithelium: "serotonin cells" of duct branches, acini
    Patterns: often mixed
      Adenocarcinoma with neuroendocrine peptides
      Carcinoid tumor
      Small cell (oat cell) carcinoma
II. Stromal: rare, wide variety of types known as sarcomas
  A. Rhabdomyosarcoma: 42 per cent of sarcomas, most patients younger than 10 years
  B. Leiomyosarcoma: 26 per cent of sarcomas, most patients older than 40 years
III. Secondary
  A. Direct invasion from bladder: transitional cell carcinoma
  B. Direct invasion from colon adenocarcinoma: uncommon
  C. Metastasis: seeding from widely disseminated cancer; rare; lung, 50 per cent; melanoma, 35 per cent
  D. Lymphoma: rare

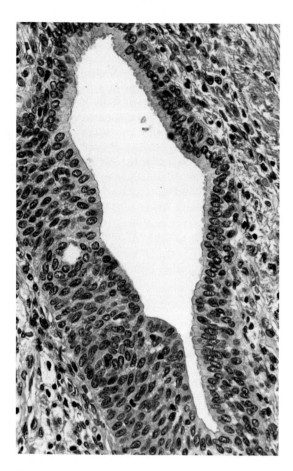

Figure 29–2. Epithelial lining of peripheral zone duct trunk near the urethra at the point of transition from urethral-type lining to more distal glandular lining *(above)*. Multilayer transitional epithelium is surmounted by a single layer of luminal secretory cells. (× 360).

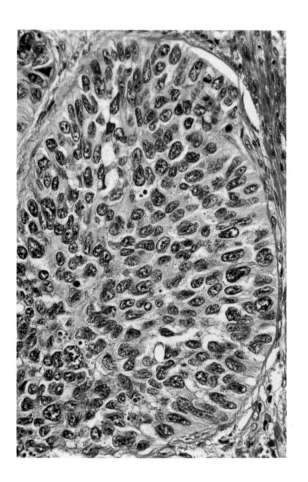

Figure 29–3. Intraductal transitional cell carcinoma in the prostate. Cells with variably enlarged, hyperchromatic, malignant nuclei resemble those in Figure 29–2, but a prominent cell disorder and no lumen are noted. Boundary with the stroma appears noninvasive, with parallel collagen bundles delineating a sharp epithelial border (× 360).

of tall columnar secretory cells, which are the parent cell type of prostatic adenocarcinoma. In the *peripheral zone*, which constitutes about 70 per cent of the normal glandular prostate, and in the normally small *transition zone* where benign prostatic hyperplasia arises, the duct-acinar architecture is simple (Fig. 29–4). The secretory cell cytoplasm is very pale to clear, with nuclei that are uniformly basal, producing a very orderly epithelial pattern (Fig. 29–5). In the *central zone*, where adenocarcinoma seldom develops, the duct-acinar architecture is complex (Fig. 29–6), and the epithelium lining larger ducts and acini appears somewhat disorderly because of cell crowding with nuclei displaced to varying levels in the cells (Fig. 29–7). The cytoplasm is somewhat less pale than in the peripheral zone (McNeal, 1988b).

In each region of the glandular prostate, the epithelium lining the ducts is secretory in appearance and is histologically identical to that of its acini (McNeal, 1988b) (see Figs. 29–4 and 29–6). In both ducts and acini of all zones, cytoplasmic pallor is due to the presence of numerous small, clear vacuoles, which are well visualized only by electron microscopy. All secretory cells of ducts and acini of all regions have a cytoplasm that stains with uniform intensity using immunohistochemical techniques for prostate-specific antigen (PSA) (see Fig. 29–4) and prostatic acid phosphatase (PAP). The keratin composition of intermediate filaments is also apparently the same between ducts and acini of all zones. Because the ducts and acini are of similar size in any zone, they cannot be distinguished microscopically, except in fortuitous planes of section that view the duct-acinar system in profile (see Figs. 29–4 and 29–6).

It has been suggested that in the prostate, ducts and acini have identical biologic roles; they are secretory reservoirs for the storage and intermittent expulsion of small volumes of secretion (McNeal, 1988b). The absence of biologic or morphologic distinction between ducts and acini makes it unlikely that there are morphologically or biologically different "ductal" and "acinar" carcinomas in the prostate.

In other organs, such as the pancreas, that are specialized for continuous and high-volume secretion, morphologic distinction between ducts and acini is readily apparent in the normal tissue and consistently reflected in their neoplasms. The term "ductal" is probably also inappropriate to describe transitional cell carcinoma in the prostate. Only a small portion of the prostatic duct system is normally lined by transitional epithelium (McNeal, 1988b). Furthermore, the possibility that a given cancer may have originated with transitional cell metaplasia in an acinus can never be discounted.

Unusual Adenocarcinomas

The *prostatic utricle* is lined by a secretory epithelium that is histologically identical to that of the ducts and acini of the peripheral zone or transition zone. The epithelial cells show strong, diffuse cytoplasmic staining with immunohistochemical techniques for PSA and PAP. Therefore, it is evident that, in the adult, this embryonic müllerian vestige has undergone prostatic differentiation, and any carcinomas that might arise here would expectedly be prostatic.

Previously, the term "endometrioid carcinoma" was applied to prostatic adenocarcinomas that showed prominent growth into the urethral lumen near the verumontanum and that histologically often showed ribbons or papillations of tall columnar cells (Melicow and Pachter, 1967; Melicow and Tannenbaum, 1971). Such tumors have subsequently been shown to be positive for PSA and PAP; they appear to represent simply invasive or intraductal growth toward the urethra of prostatic adenocarcinomas, which are usually of fairly large size (Epstein and Woodruff, 1986).

Very uncommonly, moderately differentiated carcinomas appear in the prostate, which show a pure histologic pattern that is indistinguishable from that of carcinoid tumor of the lung or intestine (Azumi et al., 1984). Also uncommon are undifferentiated cancers with all of the histologic features of pulmonary small cell or "oat cell" carcinoma (Schron et al., 1984). Typically, both of these histologic patterns are composed of cells that are negative for PSA and PAP but are positive for serotonin and other "neuroendocrine" markers, such as calcitonin and neuron-specific enolase.

The characteristic dense core secretory granules of neuroendocrine cells are often found in the cells of these tumors by electron microscopy (di Sant'Agnese and de Mesy Jensen, 1984). The parent benign cell of carcinoid and small cell tumors is represented in the normal prostate by individual scattered small cells, often with dendritic morphology, which are tucked between columnar secretory cells toward their basal aspect and seldom reach the lumen of the duct or acinus. These cells are too inconspicuous to identify reliably with routine stains but consistently are serotonin positive with immunohistochemical staining and often contain calcitonin or other neuropeptides.

It was initially proposed that these cells and their tumors, whether in the prostate or other organs, represent direct descendents of embryonic migratory neural crest epithelium. However, it has since been shown that, in at least some organs, cells that are functionally and morphologically neuroendocrine embryologically may simply represent an alternative pattern of differentiation for the normal epithelial cell type of that organ (di Sant'Agnese and de Mesy Jensen, 1987). In the prostate, this appears to be the case because occasionally carcinomas develop that, in part or entirely, show mixtures of adeno- and neuroendocrine differentiation in their morphology, their immunohistochemical staining patterns, or both.

Basal Cell Layer in Carcinoma

It would therefore appear that, in the prostate, malignant tumors rarely arise from any cells other than those that are found lining normal ducts and acini. Even among these populations, there is one cell type—the basal cell—which appears to rarely undergo malignant transformation. These are inconspicuous cells, which

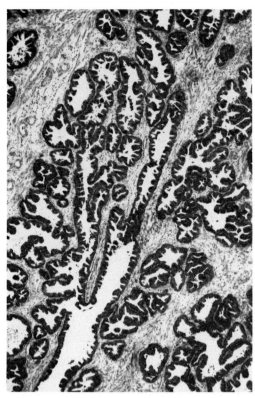

Figure 29–4. Peripheral zone subsidiary duct with branches and acini. Architectural pattern is simple, with small oval acini. Tissue is treated with immunohistochemical stain for prostate-specific antigen (PSA), which produces uniform black color throughout the cytoplasm of all the ductal and acinar cells (× 90).

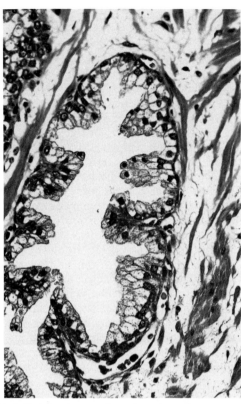

Figure 29–5. Peripheral zone acinus of simple oval contour set in loose fibromuscular stroma and lined by pale columnar cells with uniform basal nuclei (× 360). (From McNeal, J. E.: Am. J. Surg. Pathol., 12:619, 1988b).

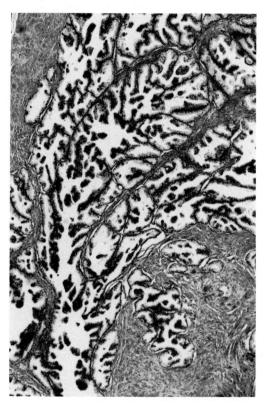

Figure 29–6. Central zone subsidiary duct with branches and acini. Architectural pattern is complex—acini are polygonal and closely spaced with intraluminal ridges. Stroma is denser than the peripheral zone (× 90). (From McNeal, J. E.: Am. J. Surg. Pathol., 12:619, 1988b).

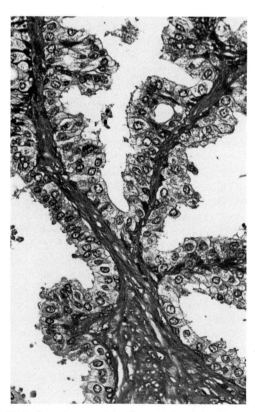

Figure 29–7. Central zone acini with somewhat darker, more crowded epithelium and larger more randomly placed nuclei than peripheral zone (× 360). (From McNeal, J. E.: Am. J. Surg. Pathol., 12:619, 1988b).

form an extremely thin and perhaps discontinuous layer between the columnar secretory cells, to whose deep surface they are attached, and the basement membrane, whose production is their only known function. It is definite that they are not myoepithelial cells, as are the similar-appearing cells of the breast ducts (Mao and Angrist, 1966). They have been proposed to contain the stem cell population, which renews the secretory epithelium, but this is still debated. In routine preparations, they are recognized only as naked, slit-like, dark nuclei scattered randomly and with extremely variable density in the narrow potential space between the secretory cells and the fibromuscular stroma (Cleary et al., 1983). They are distinguished immunohistochemically by absent PSA and PAP staining and by expression of keratin intermediate filaments 5 and 14, whereas the secretory cells express mainly keratins 8 and 18 (Brawer et al., 1985).

Invasive adenocarcinomas of the prostate are never seen to form a basal cell layer, even an incomplete one. In the best differentiated carcinomas, the malignant cells are in direct contact with the stroma, and yet they consistently express secretory cell keratins (8 and 18) rather than basal cell keratins. The malignant phenotype is therefore explicitly secretory, but a more subtle role for basal cells in malignant transformation has not been ruled out.

Adenocarcinoma: Anatomic Site of Origin

HISTORICAL PERSPECTIVE. Within most visceral organs, except the gastrointestinal tract, the relative predilection of the epithelium of different regions for malignant transformation has not been an issue of major interest. For the prostate, it has been a focus of controversy for 80 years.

In 1912, Lowsley first proposed that, in this small organ whose histologic composition was then thought to be homogeneous, there could be great differences in cancer prevalence between regions that were only millimeters apart. He stated that adenocarcinoma originated selectively in the posterior lobe, a region that was defined precisely by his studies of the patterns of clustering of duct buds in the development of the embryonic prostate. He described a posterior cluster, which budded from the posterior urethral wall distal to the verumontanum and reached the rectal surface as a narrow, vertical midline strip directly posterior to the ejaculatory ducts, expanding only slightly laterally. It was a relatively small region compared with the adjacent lateral lobes, which composed the bulk of the glandular prostate.

Two major problems are associated with this concept. First, Lowsley's investigations were confined to fetuses, and no concurrent studies of adults were published to confirm his claim of regional predisposition to cancer. Second, no one has ever established the presence of anatomic landmarks in the normal adult prostate that define a posterior lobe. The idea was nevertheless popular for many years, and different studies reported quite different territorial boundaries for a posterior lobe, within which all or most carcinomas were said to occur.

Acceptance of Lowsley's concept was never universal, and several studies over the years, which mapped the exact locations of small cancers found at autopsy, showed no correspondence of tumor distribution to Lowsley's posterior lobe (Blennerhassett and Vickery, 1966; Gaynor, 1938; Karube, 1961; McNeal, 1969). Franks (1954b) proposed to resolve this confusion with his findings that there were no anatomic landmarks to define *any* lobes within the adult prostate; the only anatomic boundary of biologic significance was between a large "outer gland," which was uniformly susceptible to carcinoma, and a small "inner gland" near the urethra, which was susceptible to benign prostatic hyperplasia (BPH) but not cancer. The inner prostate was reported to be composed of submucosal glands and smaller mucosal glands. Their boundary with the outer prostate was shown diagrammatically, but exact landmarks within the prostate for this fundamental partitioning were not explicitly defined.

The view of Franks has prevailed in Great Britain. Unfortunately, in the United States, the characteristic lateral masses and midline dorsal mass of BPH within the inner prostate have been mislabeled as "lobes," implying erroneously that they are to be found in normal anatomy. Because the "lateral lobes" and "middle lobe" are precisely defined in this misconception, the entire outer prostate as described by Franks is, by default, labeled as "posterior lobe." Following this transformation, Franks and Lowsley are forced into semantic agreement on the site of cancer origin, although their concepts are quite incompatible.

ANATOMIC BOUNDARIES IN THE ADULT PROSTATE IN RELATION TO CARCINOMA. Anatomic landmarks that more precisely define Franks' inner prostate have subsequently been delineated (McNeal, 1978, 1988b). Two subregions, designated as the *transition zone* and the *periurethral glands*, have been identified. Both compartments are related exclusively to the proximal segment of the prostatic urethra—that 50 per cent of its length between the bladder neck and the base (proximal extent) of the verumontanum.

All of the major ducts of the prostate enter the urethra in its distal segment (50 per cent), and the proximal segment is completely sheathed by the *preprostatic sphincter*, a continuous sleeve of smooth muscle fibers that would preclude the passage of major ducts (Figs. 29–8 and 29–9) (McNeal, 1978). The posterior wall of the entire proximal segment of the prostatic urethra is abruptly angled anteriorly about 35 degrees relative to the urethra below the base of the verumontanum. The separation of this proximal urethral segment from the main glandular prostate is made possible by the absence of any major duct origins, and the resulting space accommodates the periurethral stroma and surrounding preprostatic sphincter.

The periurethral stroma contains scattered tiny periurethral glands, whose number and points of origin along the proximal urethral segment are variable. They remain confined within the periurethral stroma and branch proximally toward the bladder neck. The periurethral glands and stroma are often involved in BPH, but generally to a minor degree.

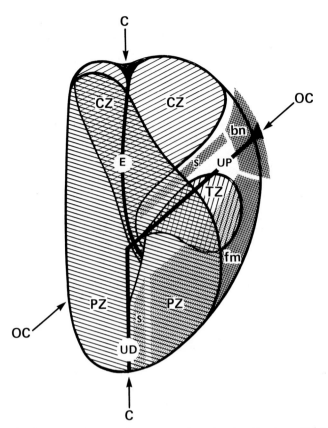

Figure 29–8. Diagram of prostate and urethra in side view. Distal prostatic urethral segment (UD), proximal urethral segment (UP), and ejaculatory ducts (E) in relation to sagittally cut anteromedial nonglandular tissues. (Bladder neck, bn; anterior fibromuscular stroma, fm; preprostatic sphincter, s; distal striated sphincter, s.) These structures are shown in relation to a three-dimensional representation of the glandular prostate. (Central zone, CZ; peripheral zone, PZ; transitional zone, TZ.) Oblique coronal plane (OC) of Figure 29–9 and coronal plane (C) of Figure 29–10 are indicated by arrows. (From McNeal, J. E.: Am. J. Surg. Pathol., 12:619, 1988b.)

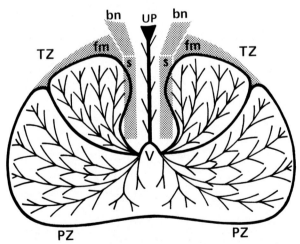

Figure 29–9. Oblique coronal section diagram of prostate showing location of peripheral zone (PZ) and transition zone (TZ) in relation to proximal urethral segment (UP), verumontanum (V), preprostatic sphincter (s), bladder neck (bn), and periurethral region with periurethral glands. Branching pattern of prostatic ducts is indicated. Medial transition zone ducts penetrate into sphincter. (From McNeal, J. E.: Am. J. Surg. Pathol., 12:619, 1988b.)

The transition zone in a normal young adult is represented by two small lobes of glandular tissue, whose ducts leave the urethra immediately below the distal border of the preprostatic sphincter and branch proximally along its external aspect toward the bladder (see Fig. 29–9). These ducts are situated lateral to the sphincter and extend ventrally to a variable degree. The lateral hyperplastic masses, which usually form the greater portion of BPH tissue, originate here, especially medially, where the transition zone ducts penetrate between the fibers of the preprostatic sphincter (McNeal, 1978).

Thus, this "inner prostate" is not only medial (periurethral) but also anterior, constituting the anterior aspect of the glandular prostate just below the bladder neck and bulging toward the prostate apex to a degree that is proportional to the magnitude of BPH. Transverse section maps through the prostate made many years ago to diagram the locations of small autopsy cancers show a density of cancer foci in this anteromedial region, which is comparable to that found elsewhere (Blennerhassett and Vickery, 1966; Gaynor, 1938; Karube, 1961). Several studies have emphasized the occurrence of anteromedial cancer (Christensen et al., 1990; Epstein et al., 1988; McNeal et al., 1988c) or transition zone cancer (McNeal et al., 1988d), its presence in the region of the prostate afflicted by BPH, and the fact that it is usually recognized clinically as incidental cancer in transurethral resection for BPH (stage TA) (Christensen et al., 1990; Epstein et al., 1988; McNeal et al., 1988c, 1988d; Price et al., 1990).

The majority of adenocarcinomas, however, originate outside the transition zone boundary in Franks' outer prostate. In the outer gland, there are two distinct duct systems, which define two histologically and biologically different regions (Fig. 29–10) (McNeal, 1968, 1988b). The peripheral zone—roughly 70 per cent of the volume of the young adult prostate—arises from ducts that mainly extend laterally from the urethra along its entire distal segment. These duct origins form a continuous line with those of the proximal urethral segment, and the architecture and epithelial morphology of peripheral zone and transition zone are the same (see Figs. 29–4, 29–5, and 29–11).

A separate set of ducts arises on the convexity of the verumontanum in proximity to the ejaculatory duct orifices; these ducts branch directly proximally, giving rise to a wedge of glandular tissue where the base coincides with almost the entire base of the prostate. This tissue is the central zone—roughly 25 per cent of the normal glandular prostate. Its glandular tissue is architecturally and cytologically distinctive, as was first described by Gil-Vernet in 1953 (see Figs. 29–6 and 29–7). Its cells are biologically unique; they secrete pepsinogen II (Reese et al., 1986) and tissue plasminogen activator (Reese et al., 1988), which are not found elsewhere in the prostate. The boundary lines of the peripheral zone with both the transition zone and the central zone are usually clearly visible in the normal prostate and are further accentuated by differences in stromal composition among the three zones (see Figs. 29–5, 29–7, and 29–11) (McNeal, 1978, 1988b; McNeal et al., 1988d).

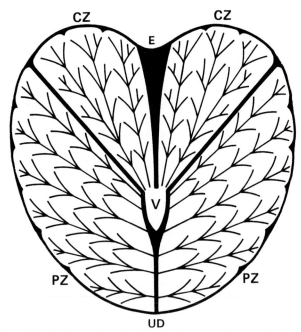

Figure 29–10. Coronal section diagram of prostate showing location of central zone (CZ) and peripheral zone (PZ) in relation to distal urethral segment (UD), verumontanum (V), and ejaculatory ducts (E). Branching pattern of prostatic ducts is indicated. Subsidiary ducts provide uniform density of acini along the entire main duct course. (From McNeal, J. E.: Am. J. Surg. Pathol., 12:619, 1988b.)

The central zone gives rise to only 5 to 10 per cent of all adenocarcinomas (McNeal, 1968, 1969; McNeal et al., 1988d) although it contains as much as 40 per cent of the total prostate epithelium because of its very high epithelial-to-stromal ratio. Hence, small cancers are uncommon at the prostate base. For the remainder of Franks' outer prostate and the inner gland (transition zone) as well, the susceptibility to carcinoma is best regarded as uniform to a very rough approximation.

More than half of all cancers arise in the peripheral zone, which is normally the largest region and the one most accessible to rectal palpation of cancer. However, in the anterolateral "wings" of the peripheral zone—as in the transition zone—only relatively large tumors would be expected to be palpable. Because of the tremendously variable contribution of BPH to transition zone mass, the susceptibility of the transition zone to carcinoma is not easily determined, but certainly more than 20 per cent of adenocarcinomas occur there. The proposal made at one time, that BPH increases susceptibility to carcinoma, was subsequently disputed; such a tendency is not clearly evident in radical prostatectomy specimens.

Composite maps showing the exact distribution of small cancers sometimes show a shallow gradient of increasing frequency in progression from urethra to capsule. This gradient is paralleled by a similar gradient in the density of secretory glandular tissue. The gradient is not steep enough to support the proposal that cancer origin is selectively subcapsular. In studies in which that observation was made, care was not taken to limit evaluation to cancers of microscopic size (Byar et al., 1972). The peripheral zone is seldom more than 1.5 cm in thickness measured from the capsule surface. Even

by the time they reach a relatively small diameter of 1 cm, most cancers would, therefore, expectedly have grown to a partly subcapsular location. Any evaluation of the relative location of cancer origins that includes cancers of grossly visible size would necessarily be inaccurate.

Adenocarcinoma: Precursor Changes

HISTORICAL PERSPECTIVE. Attention was first directed to the mode of origin of prostatic adenocarcinoma in the early studies of Moore (1935) more than 50 years ago. Moore noted that atrophy with aging was an early event in the prostate, seen commonly in small foci by the 5th decade. He often found invasive carcinoma in association with atrophy and concluded that atrophy was a premalignant lesion.

Franks (1954c) subsequently expanded on this concept with more detailed histologic description, including a classification of prostatic atrophy into several different categories. "Sclerotic atrophy" was noted to be focal and accompanied by marked gland shrinkage and distortion with periglandular fibrosis (Fig. 29–12). In "postatrophic hyperplasia," cell enlargement and close packing of small glands were superimposed on the

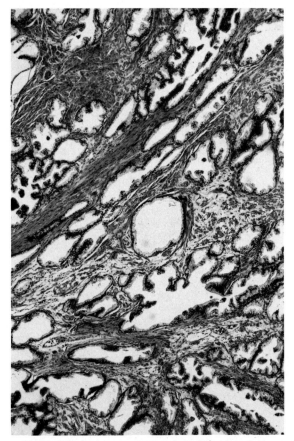

Figure 29–11. Histologic appearance of the boundary between the peripheral zone (lower right) and the transition zone (upper left) in a normal prostate from a young man. Coarse-fibered transition zone stroma is further compacted into a narrow band at the boundary, with the abrupt appearance of a loose peripheral zone stroma below the boundary. Glandular tissue is similar in both zones (× 90). (From McNeal, J. E.: Am. J. Surg. Pathol., 12:619, 1988b.)

original sclerotic atrophy, and a close histologic similarity of this change to moderately differentiated invasive carcinoma was demonstrated and presented as evidence of biologic association. The relationship of this lesion to cancer was subsequently disputed.

Evidence has been presented that focal atrophy is a consequence of inflammation (McNeal, 1968, 1988b). Focal inflammation of unknown cause is common in the prostate, and postinflammatory atrophy is seen even in the 3rd decade. Atrophy with aging is diffuse and is uncommon until after the age at which carcinoma becomes common.

During the last 20 years, interest in the nature of premalignant changes in the prostate has progressively increased. A number of different histologic patterns have been proposed to be associated with cancer origin (Andrews, 1949; Brawn, 1982; Kastendieck et al., 1976; Kovi et al., 1988; McNeal, 1965; McNeal and Bostwick, 1986; Quinn et al., 1990). All of the lesions reported have been proliferative in type, and no further evidence has arisen linking malignancy to atrophy in the prostate. Several investigators have thought that their evidence, limited to morphologic similarity and frequency of association with invasive carcinoma, did not warrant definite conclusions on the biologic significance of the lesion described.

The histologic description of a premalignant phase is best established for carcinomas of hollow organs and body surfaces, where a suspect lesion can be identified grossly and followed over time until the emergence of invasive cancer. In solid organs, such as the prostate, sequential blind biopsies can never provide such a reliable and convenient approach for tracing the behavior of a suspect lesion.

CATEGORIES OF PRECURSOR LESION. Two general categories of proliferative lesions have been described in association with prostatic adenocarcinoma (Brawn, 1982; Gleason, 1985; Kastendieck et al., 1976; McNeal, 1965). One of these categories is represented by the proliferation of new architectural units, similar to those seen in glandular BPH nodules. It is referred to as "atypical adenomatous hyperplasia" or "adenosis" (Brawn, 1982) and is mainly distinguished from BPH by details of architectural pattern. Often, the gland units are very small and closely packed and have a monotonously uniform, round-to-oval contour. The cells of these acinar units are tall columnar cells with normally pale cytoplasm and only inconstant nuclear enlargement and atypia. In other foci, glands may be quite variable in size, usually with bizarre contours in the larger glands. Despite the variety of architectural patterns included in this diagnosis of adenosis, histologic criteria are not clearly defined.

The second type of proliferative lesion thought to be premalignant is characterized by proliferation of cells within pre-existing duct-acinar units (Andrews, 1949; Kastendieck et al., 1976; Kovi et al., 1988; McNeal, 1965; McNeal and Bostwick, 1986; Quinn et al., 1990). Cytologic atypia, which is usually absent in adenosis, is invariably present here. Although some new architecture is occasionally described, and proliferation of cells to fill pre-existing ducts is included by some investigators, cytologic atypia with abnormal nuclei is probably a more consistently important feature than actual increase in cell numbers or cell crowding.

Essentially the same lesion has been rediscovered by a number of investigators over the last two decades. Descriptions differ in their completeness; the relative emphasis on atypia versus proliferation; and the inclusion by some of a variety of architectural abnormalities, which others have classed with adenosis. The earliest precise description of this type of lesion was provided by Andrews in 1949. In 1965, more specific diagnostic criteria were proposed, and the lesion defined was demonstrated in direct transition to invasive carcinoma (McNeal, 1965). At present, these relatively stringent diagnostic criteria have been further refined and are generally accepted (Quinn et al., 1990). The lesion is referred to as "duct-acinar dysplasia" (McNeal, 1988a; Quinn et al., 1990) or "prostatic intra-epithelial neoplasia," and it appears to be the best candidate for a biologic precursor to the majority of prostatic adenocarcinomas.

FEATURES OF PROSTATIC DUCT-ACINAR DYSPLASIA (PROSTATIC INTRAEPITHELIAL NEOPLASIA). Dysplastic foci are found in roughly 40 per cent of prostates from men older than 50 years without adenocarcinoma and in 80 per cent of prostates from men with adenocarcinoma (McNeal and Bostwick, 1986; Oyasu et al., 1986; Quinn et al., 1990). Dysplasia is most often a sharply delimited, small focal lesion, with a darkly stained thickened epithelium that sets it off clearly from the surrounding normal glands (Fig. 29–13). In prostates without cancer, foci larger than 4 mm are uncommon, but they are often seen in prostates with cancer, especially in tissue immediately adjacent to the invasive tumor. Multifocality is common, and foci tend to be more numerous in glands with cancer.

Nuclear enlargement, cell crowding or pseudostratification, and alterations of cytoplasmic staining are cytologic changes that are usually seen in dysplasia. They are also occasional features of a variety of nonspecific atypias, which are very common in the prostate. Dysplasia is most specifically characterized by increased variation in nuclear size (anisokaryosis) and usually by increased variation in contour, which may be a more subtle abnormality. Almost equally significant is some degree of disorder in cell-cell relationships, evidenced by variable nuclear spacing, inconstant distance of nuclei from the cell base, and partial loss of polarity (Fig. 29–14). In more severe degrees of dysplasia (grade II), these abnormalities are usually accentuated and typically accompanied by hyperchromasia with occasional prominent nucleoli and darkening of the cytoplasm (McNeal and Bostwick, 1986). The addition to the aforementioned features of very large, prominent nucleoli in most nuclei identifies grade III dysplasia. This most severe degree of dysplasia is not often found in prostates without cancer. Its identification as an isolated lesion on needle biopsy suggests a need for further biopsy to rule out concurrent invasive cancer (McNeal and Bostwick, 1986, Quinn et al., 1990).

The aforementioned histologic features appear to represent a one-dimensional continuum of increasing severity. They are thought also to represent a temporal continuum of deviation from normal toward the emer-

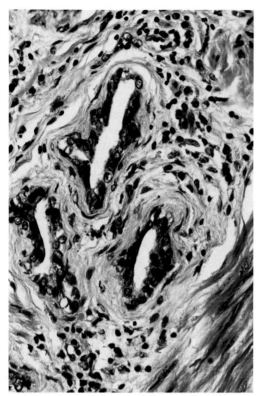

Figure 29–12. Postinflammatory atrophy is characterized by shrunken glands with a periglandular pale scar displacing the darker muscle bundles *(lower* and *upper right).* Epithelial cytoplasm is scant with variably prominent nuclei. A few residual, tiny dark inflammatory cell nuclei are present (× 360). (From McNeal, J. E.: Am. J. Surg. Pathol., 12:619, 1988b.)

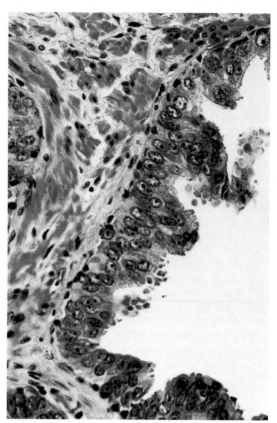

Figure 29–13. Duct-acinar dysplasia with markedly thickened epithelium compared with Figure 29–5. Crowding and multilayering of enlarged nuclei with prominent nucleoli are noted. The dysplastic cell cytoplasm is dark, and the basal cell layer is visible (× 360).

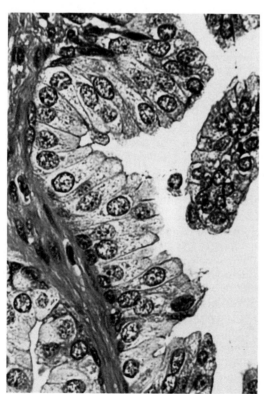

Figure 29–14. Dysplastic epithelium demonstrating variable nuclear enlargement with irregular contour and disordered spacing. Hyperchromasia is prominent, but there is not much evidence of crowding, multilayering, or dark cytoplasm (× 720).

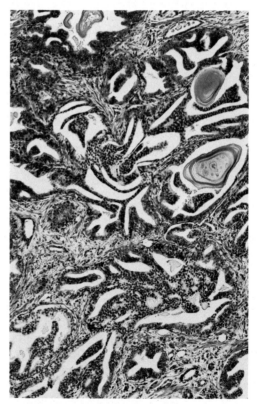

Figure 29–15. Development of intraductal carcinoma from dysplasia. Branching duct above shows transluminal trabeculae. Note the corpora amylacea. Branching duct below shows evolution of cribriform pattern from trabeculae (× 70).

gence of invasive carcinoma, which has been demonstrated at its point of origin from grade III and grade II dysplasia (Bostwick and Brawer, 1987; McNeal et al., 1991; Quinn et al., 1990).

Nuclear crowding, sometimes to the point of distinct multilayering of nuclei, is a common and visually striking accompaniment of dysplasia. When severe, it produces tufts or pseudopapillations of densely crowded nuclei, with an intrusion into the gland lumen that creates a markedly scalloped epithelial border. Occasionally, in foci of grade III dysplasia, markedly elongated pseudopapillations fuse to completely bridge the lumen, producing a network of trabeculations across the lumen or a cribriform pattern (Fig. 29–15). This pattern, referred to as *cribriform intraductal carcinoma,* appears to reflect a further stage of progression beyond dysplasia. Its presence correlates even more strongly with the presence of concurrent invasive cancer, and the associated tumors are usually large, with areas that are poorly differentiated (McNeal et al., 1986b).

The biologic features of dysplasia and their relation to those of invasive carcinoma have yet to be thoroughly studied. Preliminary evidence using immunohistochemical staining for cytoplasmic markers of differentiation (PSA, PAP) shows consistently reduced intensity of staining in dysplasia, with progression to frequent complete absence of staining in grade III dysplasia (McNeal et al., 1988a). Studies of carbohydrate moieties in cell membrane proteins have also described characteristic abnormalities in dysplasia (McNeal et al., 1988b; Perlman and Epstein, 1990).

The basal cell layer, which probably provides the most reliable morphologic distinction between invasive and noninvasive epithelium, is often focally absent in the lining of the ducts and acini of dysplastic foci (Bostwick and Brawer, 1987), suggesting a transition phase to invasive cancer (McNeal et al., 1991). A lesion that appears almost identical to dysplasia has been induced in rats by long-term high-dose androgen-estrogen treatment (Leav et al., 1988) and has been found to occur spontaneously in a strain of rats that is susceptible to prostatic adenocarcinoma (Isaacs, 1984).

The identification of an animal model for dysplasia may contribute to a better understanding of its early biologic features and the nature of its relationship to invasive cancer.

Adenocarcinoma: Histologic Features

The smallest prostatic adenocarcinomas that are histologically detectable are almost invariably at least moderately well-differentiated tumors (Catalona, 1984; McNeal, 1969; McNeal et al., 1986a; Scardino, 1989). In unselected autopsy populations, in which perhaps 70 per cent of tumors are less than 1 ml in volume, these smallest tumors are the most numerous group (see Fig. 29–1) (McNeal, 1969; McNeal et al., 1986a). In contrast, roughly 80 per cent of clinically detected carcinomas are larger than 1 ml (Scardino, 1989). The biologic relationship between autopsy cancers and clinical cancers has been debated, but there is so far no strong evidence

that any factor other than the passage of time distinguishes them. Approximately half of patients with clinical prostate cancer have additional unsuspected carcinomas. Among those patients who have two cancers (one unsuspected), about half also have a third tumor, and about half of those with three tumors also have a fourth tumor (Villers et al., 1991).

Importantly, the volume distribution of these additional incidental carcinomas is practically the same as that of incidental autopsy cancers. Hence, in a patient whose clinical cancer is larger than 1 ml, the presence of multiple tumors will usually not represent a very great increment in total (sum) cancer volume. Only an occasional patient will have two apparently separate cancers, each larger than 1 ml. The clinical designations of "diffuse" or "multifocal" to describe the distribution of clinically evident tumor in the prostate are seldom justified by precise quantitative analysis of the surgical specimen.

The diversity of histologic patterns commonly seen among different tumors and even within different areas of a single carcinoma in the prostate may be greater than that which is typical of cancer in any other organ. Because histologic diversity is rare in the smallest prostate cancer and progressively more common in tumors larger than 1 ml, it has been suggested that these additional histologic patterns, especially those which are less well differentiated, develop within the tumor through morphologic evolution (tumor progression) with the passage of time and increasing tumor volume (McNeal et al., 1986a). This hypothesis has been contested, and the issue is not settled.

Cytologic Features

The majority of prostatic carcinomas, across a broad range of architectural differentiation, have relatively abundant cytoplasm with some features of glandular secretory epithelial differentiation. Hence, cytoplasmic differentiation is not generally a useful feature for distinguishing between grades of prostate cancer, in contrast to its value for squamous carcinoma and other malignancies.

More refined methods for immunohistochemical demonstration of PSA and PAP as cytoplasmic differentiation markers show general distinctions between architecturally well-differentiated, moderately differentiated, and poorly differentiated tumors. Higher grade carcinomas tend to show a predominance of areas that are faintly stained or unstained (Epstein and Eggleston, 1984). However, in better differentiated cancers, intensity of staining often appears to be randomly variable within various areas having similar histologic appearance. The significance of any given staining level may not be reliably interpreted at present.

The cell cytoplasm in most areas of invasive carcinoma, like that of severe dysplasia, is dark because of the loss of the numerous small, clear vacuoles, which fill the cytoplasm in normal epithelium. However, there are "clear cell carcinomas" (McNeal et al., 1988c, 1988d, 1990b) in which most or all areas of the tumor retain the clear to pale, diffusely vacuolated cytoplasm

(Fig. 29–16). Most often, such tumors are also well differentiated architecturally, and the best differentiated subset of these has been designated by Gleason (1977) as grades 1 and 2, which are said to have the best prognosis for the patient of all prostate cancers. Cancers showing a preponderance of grade 1 and/or grade 2 areas are almost exclusively of transition zone origin (McNeal, 1988b; McNeal et al., 1988c, 1990b).

Nuclear Features

Nuclear enlargement of variable degree is a nearly universal feature of prostatic adenocarcinoma although it may be seen in only some of the nuclei in the best differentiated cancers, such as Gleason grades 1 and 2 (Gleason, 1985). Hyperchromasia and enlarged prominent nucleoli invariably accompany nuclear enlargement.

The nuclear features of prostate cancer have been subjected to detailed quantitative analysis using computerized planimetry, with calculation of a number of morphologic indices. "Nuclear roundness" (Diamond et al., 1982a, 1982b; Epstein et al., 1984; Mohler et al., 1988a, 1988b), a morphometric index, has been reported to be strongly correlated to patient prognosis. It attaches a numerical value to the degree of deviation of the nuclear perimeter from that of a perfect circle. The usefulness of nuclear roundness and other indices for grading and estimating patient prognosis from specimens obtained by needle biopsy or transurethral resection (TUR) may be limited because of the great frequency of significant nuclear distortion in such specimens (Mohler et al., 1988a). The performance of nuclear morphometry by computer is time-consuming, and the indices have never been translated into criteria that can be visually estimated. It is likely that such indices cannot be reliably estimated without computer planimetry.

Currently, no conceptual basis exists for understanding the nuclear shape changes and hyperchromasia that characterize prostatic carcinoma and many other malignancies. These features cannot be related to differentiation as can cytoplasmic and architectural features. They are probably not related to ploidy because we are unable to distinguish between the nuclei of diploid versus aneuploid cancers microscopically.

Although, in general, aneuploidy is a common and distinctive change in the nuclei of malignant tumors, its biologic determinants are obscure, and its relationship to natural history is somewhat different for each type of cancer. The development of aneuploidy in cancers of the prostate is clearly related to tumor progression (Frankfurt et al., 1985; Jones et al., 1990; Lee et al., 1988b; Lundberg et al., 1987; Stephenson et al., 1987; Winkler et al., 1988) as it is in many other cancers, but its practical value for estimating prognosis in this malignancy must be determined empirically. The relationship between ploidy and natural history varies among types of cancer; generalization is not possible.

For the prostate, evidence has been presented that aneuploidy is usually not among the changes that coincide with the inception of invasive tumor or its early growth; it is uncommon in cancers smaller than 4 ml in volume (Jones et al., 1990). Aneuploidy is progressively more common with increasing clinical stage and with volume greater than 4 ml, but various studies have shown that up to one third of prostatic carcinomas remain diploid, even at high stages or grades (Frankfurt et al., 1985; Jones et al., 1990; Winkler et al., 1988). Lymph node metastases tend to show a higher frequency of aneuploidy than primary tumors, but as many as 42 per cent of lymph node samples may be diploid (Stephenson et al., 1987). Aneuploidy in nodal deposits has been reported to correlate with more rapid progression of metastatic disease (Stephenson et al., 1987).

Among carcinomas without distant metastasis, aneuploidy does not distinguish a clear-cut class of more aggressive tumors. Along with grade, volume, and local extension, it is among the factors related to the occurrence of nodal or distant metastasis. Its prognostic importance relative to these other variables and the extent to which it behaves as an independent determinant is not yet clear. It has been reported that half of cancers show heterogeneity of ploidy between different samples of the same cancer (Lundberg et al., 1987) and that 60 per cent of diploid prostate cancers have aneuploid metastatic deposits (Babiarz et al., 1991). It is therefore probable that ploidy is not sufficiently uniform throughout a given cancer to circumvent the problems of sampling error in small biopsy samples.

The presence of extremely large, prominent, densely stained nucleoli is a striking feature of many prostatic adenocarcinomas. A threshold nucleolar size is likely, which is rarely exceeded by benign prostatic cells (Gleason, 1985; Kelemen et al., 1990; Myers et al., 1982). This factor has been subjected to quantitation, and the visual impression is confirmed by mathematic analysis. A computer-generated scale devised for grading has been shown to have value in predicting individual patient prognosis (Tannenbaum et al., 1982). However, it is doubtful whether this system can be used without computer analysis.

Evaluation of nucleolar size by eye is of great importance in distinguishing between very well differentiated carcinoma and the great variety of common atypias in the prostate, which do not at present have reliable diagnostic criteria (Gleason, 1985) (Fig. 29–17). When at least occasional large, prominent nucleoli are not demonstrable, the diagnosis of carcinoma should not be made.

Architectural Features

The unique histologic diversity expressed by prostatic adenocarcinoma is mainly a function of its great variety of architectural patterns. These patterns are ordered into a linear scale of progressive dedifferentiation, the challenge being to group the many patterns into a manageable number of categories with objective criteria. A number of different architectural grading systems have been devised (Brawn, 1982; Gaeta et al., 1980; Gleason, 1977; Harada et al., 1977; Mostofi, 1975; Utz and Farrow, 1969). Their prognostic success is largely based on a circumstance of nature—that the behavior of an individual prostate cancer is reflected with unusual

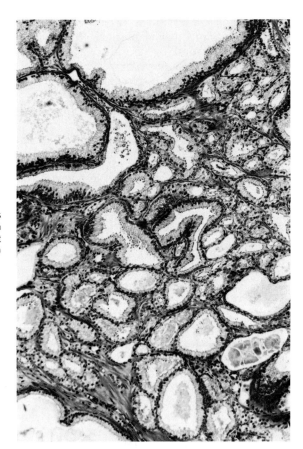

Figure 29–16. Clear-cell transition zone carcinoma, Gleason grade 1-2. Pale cells with uniform basal nuclei mimic normal epithelium. Little appearance of invasion is evident. Variable gland size and contour, which are shown here, are often not present (× 90). (From McNeal, J. E., et al.: Am. J. Surg. Pathol., 12:897, 1988.)

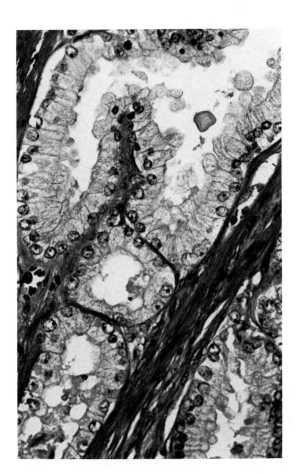

Figure 29–17. Clear-cell transition zone carcinoma demonstrating the orderly appearance of cells and nuclei. Gland borders do not appear invasive, but basal cells are absent. Nucleoli of very large size are diagnostic of carcinoma (× 360).

fidelity in its morphologic appearance compared with the situation for other malignancies.

This architectural diversity also creates a complication in grading, in that multiple distinct architectural patterns are often found within different areas of the same tumor, especially in carcinomas larger than 1 ml. Different grading systems have varied in their efforts to cope with the presence of different histologic patterns in the same biopsy sample. A potential problem is that there may be histologic patterns in any tumor that contribute to the behavior of that tumor but which by chance were not sampled in the biopsy specimen (Epstein and Steinberg, 1990; Lange and Narayan, 1983). This problem leads to inevitable inaccuracy in estimating prognosis from biopsy specimens.

Grading systems based on nuclear features would have a practical advantage if these cytologic features remain relatively constant throughout different areas of a given cancer, circumventing the sampling problem inherent in architectural grading. This possibility has yet to be substantiated (Catalona, 1984). Furthermore, the problem of nuclear distortion in biopsy sampling is considerable, and no solution has been proposed. A few grading systems have included nuclear features together with architectural features (Gaeta et al., 1980) and have the advantage of allowing estimation by eye rather than by computer planimetry. Unquestionably, degree of nuclear deviation from normal correlates with loss of differentiation by architectural criteria; however, it is possible that both measure nearly the same thing, and therefore nuclear features might be largely redundant in estimating the patient's prognosis.

GLEASON GRADING SYSTEM. The grading system in most general use is the Gleason system, based purely on architectural criteria (Gleason, 1977). Its value for clinical prediction has been established in a series with a greater number of patient-years of follow-up than that for any other system. Criteria for assigning grade are clearly defined and relatively reproducible.

The diversity of histologic patterns in biopsy samples is handled by assigning a "primary" grade to that pattern occupying the greatest area of the specimen and a "secondary" grade to the pattern occupying the second largest area. Additional patterns of smaller areas and any patterns occupying less than 5 per cent of the total cancer area are ignored. Primary and secondary grades, which are the same number in tumors of pure pattern, are added to give a "score" or "sum." Because there are five grades, the score or sum comprises nine intervals from 2 to 10.

The five grades were referred to in original publications as "histologic patterns" to conform to a nomenclature system established as part of the data analysis in the original series of 2911 patients. This nomenclature has been awkward to apply in practice, and the term "grade" has increased in general usage (Partin et al., 1989) because the procedure involved is the same as that for assigning histologic grade to cancers of other organs. The Gleason system has been given the sanction of two consensus conferences as the preferred system for current use (Gardner et al., 1988; Murphy and Whitmore, 1979), pending the establishment of scientifically verified improvements.

As with grading systems generally, in the Gleason system there is not the same *number of patients* in each grade (or grade sum) category, and there are not equivalent *differences in prognosis* between all adjacent categories, as shown in Figure 29–18. This arrangement reduces the maximum potential information of the grading process in general, and makes some grading decisions more important than others. From Figure 29–18, and with the knowledge that any grade score is usually the sum of identical or adjacent grades, it can be concluded that the distinction between grade 3 or better versus grade 4 or worse makes the greatest prognostic impact on the greatest number of patients. This distinction is superficially a distinction between well-differentiated carcinoma and poorly differentiated carcinoma.

Grade 3 or better (grades 1, 2) carcinomas, with one notable exception, share the general architectural pattern of independent glands, each lined by a single row of epithelial cells, which completely encloses a lumen and, in turn, is completely enclosed by stroma. Except for the absence of basal cells, the preceding general pattern is similarly true of benign glands. The malignant glands of grade 1 to 3 cancer, however, show loss of the orderly branching pattern of benign prostatic ducts and acini; malignant glandular units tend to be random in their size, contour, and spacing (Figs. 29–19 and 29–20). This pattern deviation is important in the diagnosis of well-differentiated carcinoma, but its recognition requires experience in the recognition of the normal pattern. A further appearance of invasiveness is often conveyed by blurring of the normally sharp epithelial-stromal interface.

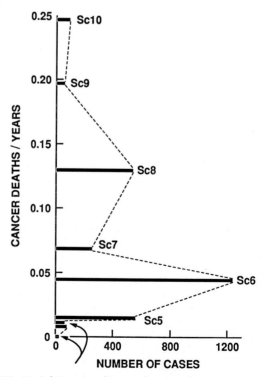

Figure 29–18. Relative mortality as a function of score (primary grade plus secondary grade) in Gleason's series of 2911 cases. Length of horizonatal bar for each score shows the number of patients in that category. Double-headed arrow indicates score 2, score 3, and score 4.

Variation in individual expression of the aforementioned abnormalities can create cancers of a variety of superficially different appearances, which are all grade 3. If gland spacing is close and uniform and invasiveness is equivocal or slight, the cancer may be grade 1 or 2. However, this diagnosis can be made only if cell cytoplasm is clear rather than dark, which further increases the resemblance to normal tissue. In very small samples of grade 1 or 2, distinction from benign tissue may be impossible architecturally without resort to the cytologic criterion of very large nucleoli (Gleason, 1985).

A dramatic exception to these rules for identifying well-differentiated cancer is a Gleason cribriform variant of grade 3 carcinoma. This pattern consists of multiple small masses of cells, each of which is perforated by multiple lumens. Here, lumens are surrounded by more than a single cell row, and several lumens share a group of epithelial cells without stromal partitioning. These features are identical to those of a common histologic pattern of grade 4 carcinoma, but they are distinguished by the fact that the cell masses are small and discrete, with sharp boundaries, as opposed to the large invasive sheets of grade 4. The cell masses often have the size and contour of large ducts, and this pattern, in fact, almost always represents intraductal carcinoma. This pattern has already been described in this chapter as an evolutionary pattern of dysplasia produced by cell proliferation within ducts and acini (see Fig. 29–15). Cribriform grade 3 cancer was not recognized by Gleason as intraductal; statistically, it is usually associated with relatively large cancers having grade 4 areas (McNeal et al., 1986b).

The Gleason grade 4 histologic pattern shows greater diversity of histologic appearances than any other grade. All grade 4 variants have in common the *absence* of "complete" gland formation as defined for grade 3. Four general variants can be described, but the distinctions between them are not always sharp.

A *cribriform* pattern has been identified, and its histologic appearance has just been outlined for intraductal cancer. However, in grade 4, either there are circumscribed cribriform masses, which are much larger than ducts, or there are large, more diffuse sheets with ragged, invasive-appearing borders (Fig. 29–21).

Alternatively, there is a *fused gland* pattern. It bears close resemblance to a grade 3 pattern in which narrow tubular glands with small, well-defined lumens run closely parallel to each other and are separated by extremely thin stromal septa. In this grade 4 variant, however, the septa are incomplete, and the adjacent glands have a common epithelial lining over much of the field (Fig. 29–22).

Another variant is characterized by *cell nests* with absent lumens. Superficially, the large, featureless sheets in this variant suggest grade 5, but narrow septa partly subdivide the sheet into small packets, often of fairly uniform size. Within the packets, the cells have abundant cytoplasm, and nuclei are often arranged in rows or around central foci that have failed to generate lumens.

Lastly, *cell cords* are seen in some grade 4 cancer areas, mimicking tiny tubular glands, which are widely separated by stroma and exist as individual tubules. However, lumens are only sporadically differentiated, and the intervening parts of the tubules are solid cords, often only a single cell in width (Fig. 29–22).

Grade 5 carcinoma often has a pattern similar to that last described, distinguished only by the near absence of any true lumens in cell cords and, sometimes, by fields that are much more cellular and may show breakup of tubules into individual cells or cell groups (Fig. 29–23). Usually, cytoplasm is distinctively scant in this grade. *Comedocarcinoma* is a visually distinct variant of grade 5 carcinoma. It represents intraductal cancer with little evidence of cribriform patterning and with central cores of total cell necrosis (Fig. 29–24). This is the only situation in which necrotic cell fields are seen in prostatic adenocarcinoma. Statistics show this noninvasive pattern to be associated with extremely poor patient prognosis, which is similar to that of frankly invasive grade 5 cancer.

GRADE, VOLUME, AND PROGNOSIS. Conceptually, the Gleason and other architectural grading systems trace a continuum of dedifferentiation, as defined by the loss of capacity of newly formed malignant cells to form glands that mimic those of the benign epithelium. That morphology mirrors biology in this regard, except perhaps for Gleason grades 1 and 2, is demonstrated in the survival data from Gleason's series (see Fig. 29–18) and subsequent experience correlating grade with lymph node metastases (Kramer et al., 1980).

It has been the general experience, however, that the biopsy grade of a tumor has often not been an accurate predictor of clinical course *for the individual patient* (Sagalowsky et al., 1982; Whitmore, 1988, 1990). The proliferation of new grading systems has partly represented a response to this limitation in the Gleason system, but it is not yet established that any other system is clearly better. Limitations on the predictive value of grading may to a great extent be inherent based on two considerations. First, cancer of the prostate expresses an unusually great diversity of histologic patterns, even within the same tumor, and yet the usual biopsy specimen represents a relatively tiny sample in most cases. There may not be any grading parameters that are constant throughout a tumor and therefore avoid significant sampling problems.

Second, loss of differentiation may reflect a set of biologic factors whose sum does not represent the dominant biologic determinant of cancer behavior. In the original study by Gleason (1977), the addition of clinical staging information to grade produced additional predictive value, suggesting that additional independent variables might be measured. Subsequently, several studies have indicated that cancer volume, which is an important factor among those involved in clinical staging, correlates strongly with grade and with tumor behavior as measured by distant metastases or lymph node metastases (Partin et al., 1989; Sharkey et al., 1984; Zincke and Utz, 1984).

In a series of radical prostatectomies for adenocarcinoma, knowledge of quantitated cancer volume and whole tumor Gleason grade together provided an extremely accurate prediction of lymph node metastasis

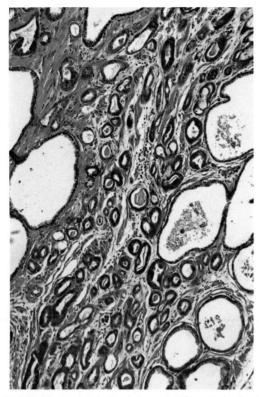

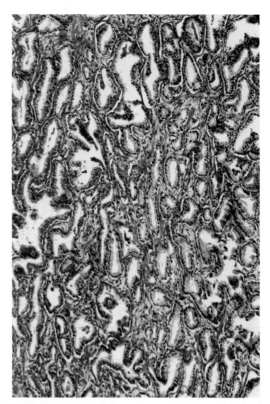

Figure 29–19. Gleason grade 3 carcinoma. Malignant glands of moderately variable size and contour are lined by a single epithelial layer. Each is completely surrounded by stroma. Gland spacing is quite variable. An indefinite, invasive border with benign tissue at right and left is noted (× 90).

Figure 29–20. Gleason grade 3 carcinoma. Malignant glands of widely variable contour and size are each lined by a single epithelial layer and completely surrounded by stroma. Glands are closely spaced. Variability of gland spacing is not as great as usually seen (× 90).

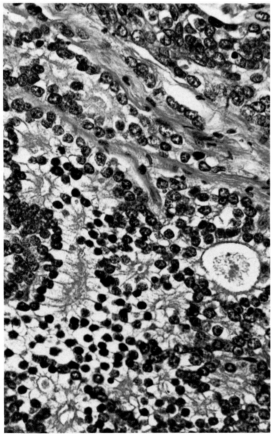

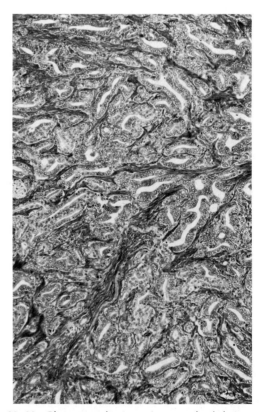

Figure 29–21. Gleason grade 4 carcinoma—cribriform pattern. Individual gland lumens are lined by a usually single epithelial layer but are not separated by stroma. Invasive border *(upper right)* is important to distinguish from intraductal carcinoma (× 360).

Figure 29–22. Gleason grade 4 carcinoma—gland fusion pattern. Closely packed, well-formed glands are lined by a single epithelial layer. They often appear independent, but in many areas they share a common lining epithelium (× 90).

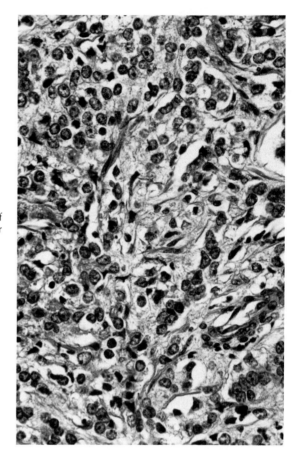

Figure 29–23. Gleason grade 5 carcinoma—invasive pattern. Featureless sheets of cells invade randomly. Cell cytoplasm is scant, and no evidence exists of glandular differentiation (× 360).

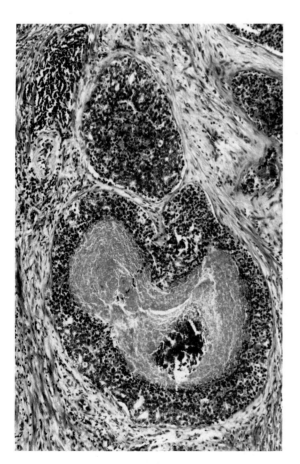

Figure 29–24. Gleason grade 5 carcinoma—intraductal comedocarcinoma pattern. Two ducts show noninvasive stromal border and are filled with malignant cells. They superficially resemble transitional cell carcinoma seen in Figure 29–2. A few remaining tiny cribriform lumens help to identify this tissue as glandular. Large area of luminal granular necrosis in larger duct is an essential criterion for comedocarcinoma. Dark focus within necrotic area is calcification (× 90).

(Fig. 29–25) (McNeal et al., 1990b). The significance of high grade was different at different volumes.

Although these data are preliminary, they suggest that cancer volume and level of dedifferentiation together reflect accurately a set of biologic determinants that are dominant in the production of at least one type of distant spread. In addition, there is strong evidence that lymph node metastasis predicts distant metastasis (Gervasi et al., 1989; Zincke and Utz, 1984). As a corollary conclusion, inaccuracy in clinical estimation of volume and grade rather than unpredictable biologic behavior are the main determinants of inadequate prediction for the individual patient.

Adenocarcinoma: Growth and Local Spread

Throughout a broad range of volumes and including the smallest tumors, the physical configuration of prostatic adenocarcinomas typically deviates markedly from that of a sphere or cube. The boundaries of any tumor often appear to be random, presumably determined by its invasiveness and the direction of local tissue planes. However, as cancers increase in volume, certain patterns to their contours reflect the interaction of tumor invasiveness with constraining anatomic boundaries in the prostate; the features of these interactions also partly determine capsule penetration and seminal vesicle invasion (McNeal et al., 1988d).

TRANSITION ZONE BOUNDARY—STAGE TA VERSUS STAGE TB. The boundary between the peripheral zone and transition zone appears to represent a partial barrier to invasion for most cancers (see Fig. 29–11) (McNeal et al., 1988d). At volumes less than 4 ml, most cancers that reach this boundary from either side grow along it, conforming to it rather than invading outside their zone of origin. Even at larger tumor volumes, disruption of the transition zone boundary is not universal (Fig. 29–26), and a partially intact boundary may precisely delineate part of the anterior margin of some peripheral zone carcinomas as large as 12 ml.

This compartmentalization tends to constrain many peripheral zone carcinomas to a somewhat crescentic outline in transverse section. Inhibition of anterior invasion may also result in earlier spread toward and along the capsular surface, thus possibly increasing the likelihood of detection by rectal examination (Fig. 29–27). Conversely, transition zone cancers tend to have a globular contour, similar to that of the masses of BPH tissue that they often displace. This restricted local spread tends to confine them to the tissues near to the proximal segment of the prostatic urethra and relatively remote from the rectal surface of the gland. Hence, transition zone cancers are usually detected incidentally at TUR for BPH and are seldom palpable rectally until larger than 4 ml in volume (Christensen et al., 1990; McNeal et al., 1988c).

Clinical stage A carcinoma, strictly defined by detection incidentally at TUR or enucleation of BPH nodules, is nearly equivalent to transition zone cancer because both these surgical procedures seldom sample tissue outside the transition zone (Price et al., 1990). However, a small minority of peripheral zone carcinomas disregard the transition zone boundary and grow close enough to the urethra to be sampled at TUR. Although they tend to be relatively large tumors, the amount of malignant tissue resected is likely to be small because most of

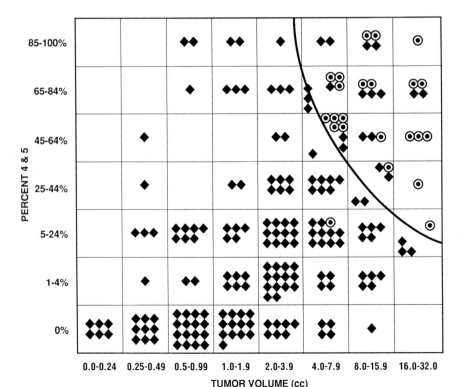

Figure 29–25. Log cancer volume (eight consecutive ranges) versus per cent of Gleason histologic grade 4–5 cancer (consecutive ranges) for 209 prostatic carcinomas. Grade-volume coordinates for each cancer without lymph node metastases are indicated by a diamond. Grade-volume coordinates for each cancer having lymph node metastases are indicated by a circle with a central dot. Those sets of coordinates that correspond to 3.2 ml of Gleason histologic grade 4–5 cancer (cancer volume × per cent of grade 4–5) are joined by a curved line. There are 38 data points (cases) with more than 3.2 ml Gleason histologic grade 4–5 cancer and 171 cases with less than 3.2 ml, grade 4–5 cancer. (McNeal, J. E., et al.: Cancer, 66:1225, 1990.)

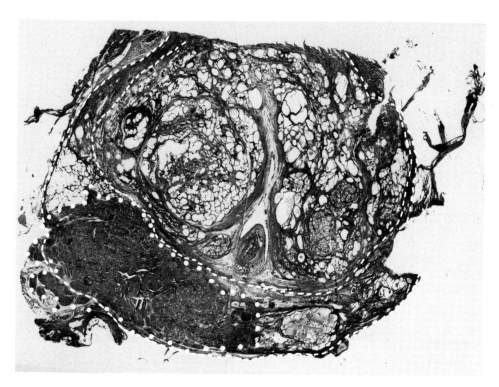

Figure 29-26. Transverse section through the mid-prostate with large benign hyperplasia nodules in the transition zone. The transition zone boundary and prostate capsule are marked by a broken white line. Large carcinoma in the left peripheral zone is molded to the contour of the transition zone boundary along the anterior surface. Invasion of the prostate capsule is noted at the lower left on the lateral aspect of the rectal surface. No invasion of the transition zone boundary has occurred. (From McNeal, J. E., et al.: Am. J. Surg. Pathol., 12:897, 1988.)

these carcinomas have a broad base against the capsule surface and a narrow apex near the urethra.

Except for the occasional non–transition zone tumor, stage A carcinomas are often smaller than the average stage B carcinoma because histologic detection, unlike clinical palpation, has no volume threshold. Stage A carcinomas have a relatively low frequency of capsule penetration compared with stage B tumors (Christensen et al., 1990; McNeal et al., 1988c, 1988d), and they seldom show seminal vesicle invasion. The seminal ves-

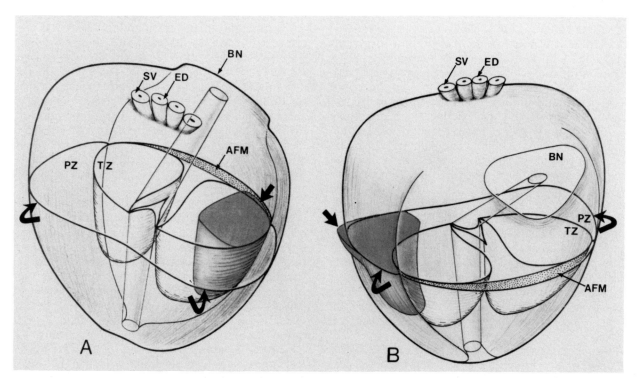

Figure 29-27. Transparent three-dimensional images of prostate showing the two zones of cancer origin. A representative cancer in each zone is related to a transverse section through the mid-prostate *(curved arrows)*. *A*, Transition zone cancer on left is viewed from the rectal surface and base. Cancer conforms to the TZ boundary but invades anteriorly, into fibromuscular stroma *(arrow)*. *B*, Nontransition zone cancer on right is viewed from the anterior surface. Cancer conforms to the TZ boundary but invades posterolaterally through the capsule *(arrow)* in the region where nerve penetration of capsule is common. (TZ, transition zone; PZ, peripheral zone; AFM, anterior fibromuscular stroma; B, bladder neck; ED, ejaculatory duct; SV, seminal vesicle.) (From McNeal, J. E., et al.: Am. J. Surg. Pathol., 14:240, 1990.)

icles and most of the prostatic capsule lie beyond the confines of the transition zone boundary. These factors of size and location undoubtedly contribute to the better prognosis ascribed to patients with stage A tumors. Whether transition zone cancers are biologically less malignant than non–transition zone cancers of comparable grade and volume is not clear and has been disputed (Christensen et al., 1990; McNeal et al., 1988d).

CAPSULE PENETRATION. Capsule penetration is a very common phenomenon in non–transition zone carcinomas, and both its frequency and extent show strong correlation with clinical prognosis and with other measures of aggressive behavior (McNeal et al., 1990b). In some earlier studies, ambiguity existed concerning the anatomy of the capsule and definition of penetration. The prostate capsule is variable in thickness and in its proportion and distribution of smooth muscle versus collagenous tissue. Its only constant landmark is its external smooth surface, often covered by loose, fibrofatty tissue. At its inner aspect, it blends with prostatic glandular tissue without any line of demarcation (Ayala et al., 1989; McNeal et al., 1990b).

Fortunately, the weight of evidence now indicates that only complete penetration through the prostate capsule with perforation of its external surface correlates with prognosis or other measures of aggressive behavior (Byar et al., 1972; McNeal et al., 1986a; 1990b; Stamey et al., 1988). Interestingly, even complete capsule penetration, if it is limited to a small area—roughly 0.5 cm^2 of the prostate surface or less—appears to have no adverse prognostic significance. In contrast, the thickness or bulk of the area of extracapsular growth beyond the prostate surface is not usually an important variable because capsule penetration areas are almost always less than 2 mm in thickness, except for very large cancers (>12 ml in volume) with extensive extraprostatic spread.

Greater than 0.5 cm^2 (equivalent to 1 cm measured length) penetration of the prostate capsule by carcinoma is relatively rare in tumors less than 4 ml in volume (Fig. 29–28). Both frequency and extent of penetration increase rapidly above 4 ml, and almost all cancers greater than 12 ml in volume show extensive invasion through the capsule even though 50 per cent of these large cancers show less than 5 per cent invasion of the seminal vesicles and apparently have no detectably positive pelvic lymph nodes at surgical staging. A very similar volume dependency is characteristic of the frequency of lymph node metastases and of the frequency and proportion of poorly differentiated (grades 4 and 5) areas in the cancer. The close interrelationship of these variables makes it difficult at present to assign a definite independent clinical significance to capsule invasion in prostate cancer, except as a cause of positive surgical margins.

Most penetration of the capsule by prostate cancer is *facilitated spread* represented by extension of cancer through the capsule along conduits provided by the perineural spaces (Villers et al., 1989). Long ago, perineural spaces were thought to be the lymphatic channels, which provided cancers with access to the nodes and general circulation. When they were discovered not to

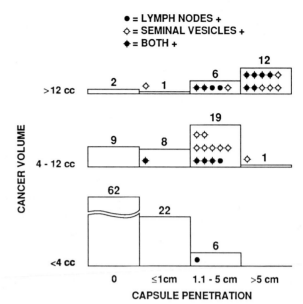

Figure 29–28. Relationships of the extent of capsule penetration (cm) and cancer volume (cc) to each other and to the presence of lymph node metastases (filled circle) and seminal vesicle invasion (open circle) in 148 nontransition zone cancers. For each of three volume categories, the extent of capsule penetration is divided into four consecutive ranges. The number of cases in each range is represented by the height of the appropriate box and that number is also printed at the top of each box. Within the box that represents the number of cases in each volume and capsule penetration category, those individual cases in which seminal vesicle invasion or lymph node metastases occurred are each represented by a symbol according to the key shown. (From McNeal, J. E., et al.: Am. J. Surg. Pathol., 14:240, 1990.)

be lymphatics (Shanthaveerappa and Bourne, 1966), and perineural spread was found in nearly 100 per cent of prostate cancers (Rodin et al., 1967), no other possible role in the spread of carcinoma was considered. However, it now appears that most prostate cancers may inherently not have sufficient destructive capability for direct invasion through the prostate capsule unless aided by perineural transport. This observation is particularly significant because the success of surgical treatment for prostate cancer conceptually relies on the effectiveness of a capsule barrier, which is often less than a millimeter thick, overlying areas of carcinoma (Epstein, 1990).

The importance of perineural space invasion through the capsule is evident in the striking regional localization of capsule penetration to the areas of the superior and inferior nerve pedicles, where the nerve fibers cluster as they penetrate the capsule on their way to the neurovascular bundle (Color Figure 1). The larger superior pedicle is draped over the posterolateral aspect of the prostate base and receives many nerve branches, which extend superiorly through the capsule obliquely relative to the capsule surface. This oblique nerve course toward the prostate base is responsible for the fact that many carcinomas show capsule penetration mainly toward the superior aspect of the intraprostatic tumor, the portion that is nearest to the prostate base.

The inferior nerve pedicle is much smaller and receives nerve branches from a small posterolateral apical area. Nerve branches penetrate the capsule directly

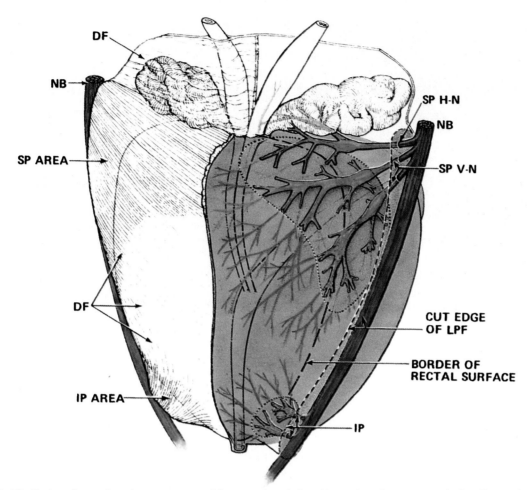

Color Figure 1. Distribution of nerve branches to prostate—right posterolateral view. Nerves from the neurovascular bundle (NB) branch to supply the prostate in the large superior pedicle (SP) at the prostate base and the small inferior pedicle (IP) at the prostate apex. Branches leave lateral pelvic fascia to travel in the Denonvilliers fascia (DF), which has been cut away from the right half of the prostate. Nerve branches from the superior horizontal subdivision (H-N) cross base to the midline. Large vertical subdivision (V-N) fans out extensively over the prostate surface as far distally as mid-prostate. Branches continue their course within the prostate after penetrating the capsule inside the large nerve penetration area *(dotted line)*. Small inferior pedicle has limited ramification and nerve penetration area *(dotted line)*. (From Villers, A., et al.: J. Urol., 142:763, 1989.)

rather than obliquely. Because of the small cross-sectional area of the average prostate apex, relatively fewer cancer origins would be expected there. However, in the volume range of clinically detected cancers, roughly 80 per cent of tumors show extension of at least some portion of the tumor within 8 mm of the apical extremity of the prostate. Thus, most carcinomas are at risk for capsule penetration along apical nerve branches.

Transition zone carcinomas also often grow close to the apex. Because the transition zone boundary is less definite at the apex, and because the distance to the posterior capsule is reduced, these normally anterior tumors may have access to the inferior nerve pedicle. In addition, they may show anterolateral capsule penetration, which is conversely seldom found in non–transition zone cancers. However, above the apex, transition zone carcinomas can only reach the nerve branches of the superior pedicle by penetrating the zone boundary and traversing a relatively broad expanse of peripheral zone tissue, which they rarely do until very large. Overall, capsule penetration is only about half as frequent in transition zone carcinomas and tends to be of lesser extent.

SEMINAL VESICLE INVASION. Seminal vesicle invasion has traditionally been regarded as an index of poor prognosis (Jewett et al., 1972). However, its close association with cancer volume and capsule penetration makes it difficult to be sure that it has an independent prognostic role (Fig. 29–29) (Villers et al., 1990). Furthermore, the type of invasion associated with poor prognosis in early descriptions was characterized by extensive replacement of the seminal vesicle and surrounding tissues by cancer (Jewett et al., 1972). Today, we associate this degree of involvement mainly with cancers larger than 12 ml, having extensive capsule penetration and lymph node metastases (Villers et al., 1990). It is likely that lesser degrees of seminal vesicle invasion in smaller cancers with better prognosis were often overlooked in earlier studies because prostates were not studied systematically.

Seminal vesicle invasion almost always results from direct spread of tumor into the ejaculatory duct wall inside the prostate and near the prostate base (Villers et al., 1990). Hence, the seminal vesicles are first invaded medially near their junction with the prostate base; only fairly large cancers commonly show more

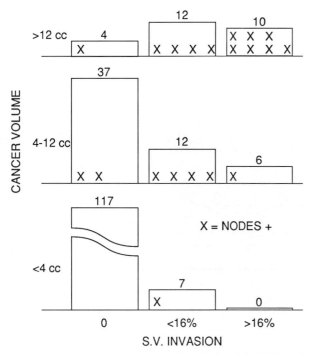

Figure 29–29. Frequency and extent of seminal vesicle (SV) invasion (0, less than 16 per cent, and greater than 16 per cent) found in each cancer volume range (less than 4 cc, 4 to 12 cc, and greater than 12 cc). The number of cases in each category of cancer volume and seminal vesicle invasion is indicated by the relative height of each column and the number above it. Each case with lymph node metastases is indicated by an X in the appropriate column. (From Villers, A., et al.: J. Urol., 142:763, 1989.)

than 1-cm extension along the length of the seminal vesicle. With less than systematic study, the frequency of invasion found could vary considerably with the location of the section taken.

With more systematic sectioning of seminal vesicles, it seems likely that the significance attached to this type of extraprostatic spread would be considerably modified in any given case by the features of the intraprostatic tumor. Cancers arising near the base tend to invade the seminal vesicles while still small and well differentiated. Apical carcinomas and transition zone cancers generally cannot even reach the basal prostate surface until large and poorly differentiated. When cancer volume and grade are known, seminal vesicle status may have little additional prognostic value.

CLASSIFICATION FOR CLINICAL STAGING

The need for a uniform clinical staging system to classify patients who present with prostate cancer is obvious. The staging system devised by the Organ Systems Coordinating Center (OSCC) of the National Cancer Institute was published in 1988 by Whitmore. It is based on the TNM system and is especially useful for the T categorization (digital rectal examination), avoiding the inconsistencies of the Union Internationale Contre le Cancer (UICC) and American Joint Commit-

tee on Cancer (AJCC) systems. An editorial by Catalona and Whitmore (1989) discusses the history of and the controversies surrounding the AJC-UICC classifications.

The Organ Systems Classification of the Whitmore Committee is shown in Table 29–2. To show the versatility of this attractive system, we have added in italics the proper place and suggested designations for cancers detected by transrectal ultrasound, by PSA, or by palpation of normal feeling asymmetric or non-nodular, abnormally firm prostates.

TA—Digitally Unrecognizable Cancer

The Whitmore system in Table 29–2 essentially is based on prior American criteria, but it uses the UICC (TNM) broad designations. However, many prostate cancers are detected using transrectal ultrasound, an elevated serum level of PSA, or an asymmetric but normal-feeling prostate without any induration on rectal examination. Where do these cancers fit into the T-category definition? No separate status has been proposed for these new situations, and because these prostates feel normal to digital palpation, there is a current tendency in the literature to place them in a stage A category. This is a serious mistake, which promises to lead to increasing confusion in the interpretation of data. In the past, stage TA has been limited to cancer detected by TUR or enucleation, which 90 per cent of the time is equivalent pathologically to transition zone cancer (McNeal et al., 1988c, 1988d). Impalpable cancers discovered by transrectal ultrasound (TRUS), PSA levels, or normal-feeling asymmetry on digital rectal examination (DRE) are almost all peripheral or central zone cancers, which are different morphologically from stage TA, transitional zone cancers. Because, in the OSCC classification, TA *is* digitally unrecognizable neoplasm, proved histologically, it is reasonable to add three subgroups within the TAX category: TAX-TRUS, TAX-PSA, and TAX-Asym.

Observe that the TA1 and TA2 classification in the OSCC system in Table 29–2 indicates that any high-grade cancer in the TUR chips (or in an enucleated specimen) automatically classifies the tumor as TA2, even when less than 5 per cent of the total surgical specimen is involved with cancer. In terms of clinical progression, this important observation on high-grade cancer has been confirmed by almost all investigators, but there has been confusion as to which score in the Gleason grading system constitutes a "high-grade" cancer.

Some investigators have used a Gleason score (range 2 to 10) of 5 or less (Cantrell et al., 1981), whereas others have used a score of 7 or less (Epstein et al., 1986) to characterize the absence of high-grade cancer. Of the five Gleason grades—remembering that the heterogeneity of prostate cancer led Gleason to exclude any grade that constituted less than 5 per cent of the cancer in the biopsy or TUR prostate (TURP) chips— the high-grade cancer in the Gleason grading system should be grade 4 or grade 5 for purposes of classifying any cancer as clinical stage TA2 rather than TA1. This

Table 29–2. ORGAN SYSTEMS COORDINATING CENTER CLASSIFICATION FOR CLINICAL STAGING OF PROSTATE CANCER

Primary Tumor (T)

TX	Anatomic relationships indefinable (e.g., prior total prostatectomy)
TA	Digitally unrecognizable cancer (confirmed histologically and substaged if traditional TUR cancer)
TA1	≤5% of total surgical specimen and of low to medium grade
TA2	>5% of specimen, any grade, or ≤5% of specimen with any high grade
TAX	TA, but not A1 or A2
TAX-TRUS	*Detected by ultrasound, confirmed by biopsy*
TAX-PSA	*Detected by PSA, testing confirmed by biopsy*
TAX-Asym	*Detected by DRE as a normal feeling but asymmetric prostate*
TB	Digitally palpated cancer, organ-confined
TB1	≤½ of one lobe, regardless of location
TB2	>½ of one lobe but not >1 lobe
TB3	>1 lobe or bilaterally palpable cancer
TBX	Palpable, organ-confined cancer, not otherwise characterized
TBX-asym	*Abnormally firm (non-nodular)*
TBX-sym	*Abnormally firm (non-nodular)*
TBC*	Palpable cancer extending beyond prostate capsule
TC1	Extension beyond margin unilaterally (may include seminal vesicle)
TC2	Extension bilaterally (may include seminal vesicle)
TC3	Extension into bladder, rectum, levator muscles, or pelvic side walls

Lymph Node Status (N)

N0 (C and/or H)	No regional lymph node metastases, clinically (C) and/or histologically (H)
N1 (H)	Microscopic regional lymph node metastasis, proved histologically
N2 (C and/or H)	Gross regional lymph node metastases
N3 (C and/or H)	Extraregional lymph node metastases
NX	Minimal requirements have not been met

Distant Metastasis (M)†

M0	No evidence of metastases
M1	Elevated acid phosphatase only (three consecutive elevations)
M2 (V and/or B)	Visceral (V) and/or bone (B) metastases
MX	Minimal requirements not met

*TBC, in addition to the TC categories, requires TB specification of the extent of the intracapsular cancer.
†Excludes lymph nodes.
Abbreviations: TUR, transurethral resection; TRUS, transrectal ultrasound; PSA, prostate-specific antigen; DRE, digital rectal examination.

is so not only because Gleason grade 4 and grade 5 cancers are usually larger than Gleason grades 3, 2, and 1 cancers (McNeal et al., 1986a, 1990a), but also because the finding of positive lymph nodes is strongly correlated with the absolute volume of grade 4 and/or grade 5 cancer (McNeal et al., 1990a). In more than 400 radical prostatectomies, we have never seen positive lymph nodes in the patient whose cancer was composed exclusively of Gleason grades 1 to 3, and metastases are rarely (0.5 per cent) found with less than 3 ml of grade 4/5 tumor.

We believe that the Gleason score for a clinical stage A cancer to be classified as a TA1 must be 6 or less. Almost all of these cancers will be 2 + 1, 2 + 2, 3 + 2, or

3 + 3, which is the most common of all grades in the scoring system. If Gleason grade 4 cancer is present, the score will be at least 7 (3 + 4, 4 + 4), and the patient should be classified as a TA2 even though 5 per cent or less of the chips contain cancer. Scores such as 4 + 1 or 4 + 2, where there is an apparent skip in the Gleason grades, are extremely rare and usually indicate a serious sampling error. In our analysis of residual cancer in 22 TA1 and 22 TA2 cancers (Voges et al., 1991), any patient who had any grade 4 cancer in the TURP chips had at least 1.7 ml of residual cancer in the radical prostatectomy specimen—a volume that surely warrants radical prostectomy in patients with an anticipated life expectancy of 15 years or more.

TB—Digitally Palpable, Organ-Confined Cancer

The TB category in Table 29–2 is a substantial improvement over the classification most commonly utilized in the United States. Generally, TB1 has been defined as either a nodule less than 2 cm in diameter (Middleton and Smith, 1982) or something less than complete involvement of one lobe (Catalona and Stein, 1982). TB2 refers to any cancer greater than these two different B1 definitions of unilobar disease. Catalona's B1 classification does not distinguish the important small nodule in the Whitmore classification (TB1), and neither his nor Middleton's B2 categories distinguish between unilobar and bilobar involvement—a distinction that can be practically important in performing TRUS and in making decisions relating to unilateral or bilateral nerve-sparing radical prostatectomies. Even more confusing is the practice of designating a unilobar palpable B1 cancer as a B2 on the basis of a contralateral positive needle biopsy (Catalona and Stein, 1982). Also, note in Table 29–2 that we have added TBX–asymetrically firm and TBX–symetrically firm in italics to distinguish non-nodular, abnormally firm prostates, which we have shown to carry a 36 per cent positive biopsy rate (Hodge et al., 1989a).

One advantage to adopting the OSCC classification—which clearly attempts to relate the DRE to increasing palpable cancer volume—is that 80 per cent of TB1 nodules in the Stanford series of radical prostatectomies were less than 4 ml, which makes the DRE a reasonably accurate voluming tool for TB1 nodules (Stamey et al., 1988). Once, however, the nodule occupies more than one half of one lobe (TB2), identical-feeling prostates can range from 2 to 40 ml in cancer volume. Indeed, in these larger palpable tumors (TB2 and TB3), we believe that there is more volume information obtained by the Yang PSA (Y-PSA) than by the DRE (Stamey and Kabalin, 1989).

Whitmore's OSCC Committee further noted: "For purposes of prospective studies, preparation of a two-dimensional diagram indicating the *estimated actual size* in centimeters and shape of the prostate, and the size, shape, location, and degree of induration (first degree or equivocal, //// one crosshatch; second degree or moderate, ❋ two crosshatches; third degree or stony hard, ❋ three crosshatches) of the tumor is recommended. The diagram should include a transverse sectional view(s), at a specified level(s) of the prostate, to characterize any asymmetry of the rectal surface of the gland. The diagram provides information regarding estimated absolute and relative (to the prostate) two-dimensional tumor size and location that supplements the specific T categorization and is intended to indicate the perceived actual size, shape, and induration of the prostate and the tumor. As imaging techniques permitting objective measurements of prostatic size and/or tumor size evolve and are utilized, they will serve to supplement the prostatic diagram."

TBC—Palpable Cancer Thought to Extend Beyond Capsule

Primary tumor stage TBC is fairly straightforward as shown in Table 29–2. Note that the TC categories also require a TB indication of the extent of palpable cancer within the prostate. This makes sense because a relatively small tumor may occasionally have palpable extension beyond the capsule. It must be remembered, however, that penetration of small or moderate size cancers into the periprostatic fat occurs frequently to a microscopic extent. This is virtually never detected on DRE or with any imaging modality and cannot play any role in clinical staging.

N—Lymph Node Status

Lymph node status category (N) as shown in Table 29–2 is very useful.

M—Distant Metastases; Question of M1 (DO) Disease

No classification can accurately forecast future developments, but Whitmore's Committee sought to assure a minimal common denominator in staging that, *with the exception of M1 disease* (see Table 29–2), they appear to have achieved. The M1 category, although not stated, surely applies only to serum *enzymatic* elevations of acid phosphatase and not to radioimmunoassays of PAP. Even this clarification and limitation to enzymatic serum acid phosphatase is clouded by the issue of precisely what constitutes an "elevation"—1 per cent, 5 per cent, or 20 per cent. Because substrates vary from one enzymatic assay to the other, are they all equally sensitive in detecting M1 disease? Serum enzymatic assays for acid phosphatase are also very unstable, requiring special handling immediately after drawing the blood serum, a procedure that has been rarely observed.

In addition to these real issues surrounding the interpretation of an "elevated" enzymatic acid phosphatase,

it is very probable that PSA is so elevated in these cases that the same information may be available from PSA determinations. In fact, Babaian and associates (1991a) reported on 37 of 440 cases with prostate cancer who had an "elevation" of the Roy enzymatic serum PAP; the mean PSA (Hybritech) was 138 ng/ml, range 9.2 to 946 ng/ml. These important issues relating to enzymatic serum acid phosphatase—the so-called DO stage introduced by Whitesel and co-workers (1984)—should be clarified by carefully designed studies before the urologist can accept that an elevation indicates distant metastases in clinical stage TA and TB disease. It is unlikely that the classification of the M1 category in Table 29–2 will stand the test of time, and it should probably be dropped.

Systems of Classification for Pathologic Staging (p)

Currently, no generally accepted classification for pathologic staging has been developed, which is based on standardized systematic evaluations of the surgical specimen, and which tabulates separately those features that may independently affect prognosis. Because the Stanford series of radical prostatectomies represent the largest number of closely sectioned and quantitatively measured specimens ever studied, it is useful to consider the results of 312 of these radical prostatectomies for clinical stage TB prostate cancer (Fig. 29–30).

Of particular note is the discordance between different types of prostatic spread. Ten per cent of patients had microscopic lymph node metastases undetected by frozen section at the time of surgical staging, most of whom, but not all, had seminal vesicle invasion; 15 per cent had seminal vesicle invasion in the absence of lymph node metastases; 35 per cent had capsular penetration into the periprostatic fat without lymph node metastases or seminal vesicle invasion; and 40 per cent were organ confined, including absence of any positive surgical margins. These data are based on 3-mm step sections throughout the prostate with special sections through the apex and base of the prostate to assess apical margins, invasion of Denonvilliers' fascia, and invasion of the seminal vesicles.

The UICC "p" category system shown in Table 29–3 is an example of inadequate histopathologic categories for the primary tumor. Note that pT3 groups penetration through the capsule with seminal vesicle invasion; because a much larger volume of cancer is required for seminal vesicle invasion than for capsular penetration, this category is morphologically incorrect. The pT1 (focal) cancer category does not indicate the upper limits of what constitutes a "focus." Is a single 1-ml or 2-ml cancer a focal cancer? The pT2 category describes a "diffuse" carcinoma. Unilobar or bilobar? If pT2 includes extension *to* the capsule, and pT3 through the capsule, into which category does the common cancer with extension *into* the capsule but not into the periprostatic fat fit? Where do cases of positive surgical margins fit in the histologic classification in Table 29–3?

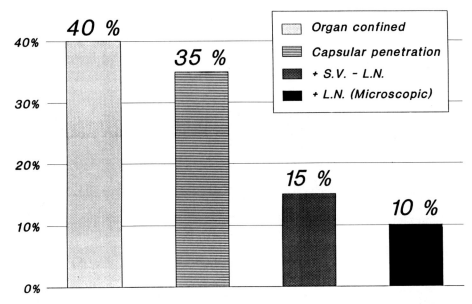

Figure 29–30. A total of 312 clinical stage TB cancers from radical prostatectomy specimens were examined histologically by the Stanford technique. Of the pelvic lymph nodes, 10 per cent thought to be free of cancer at surgical staging were later found to contain microscopic deposits of metastatic cancer. Of the seminal vesicles, 15 per cent were invaded by cancer in patients who did not have positive lymph nodes. Capsular penetration refers to those cancers that had penetrated through the capsule into the periprostatic fat. Only 40 per cent of cases were completely confined within the prostate, including those with invasion into but not through the capsule.

All proposed pathologic staging systems have failed to state as a first principle the minimum number and planes of histologic sections that must be examined to form a basis for distinguishing between these various categories. For example, the average weight of more than 400 radical prostatectomies for clinical stage B cancer at Stanford is about 44 g. In the cephalocaudal direction on the rectal surface, these prostates measure about 4 cm on average (range 2.4 to 6.5 cm). The pathologist who examines these average prostates with four 1-cm cross-sections will report organ-confined cancer five times more often than the pathologist who examines the prostate at 2-mm intervals.

Clearly, a need exists for agreement on a histopathologic classification that recognizes positive surgical margins, reasonable differences in increasing cancer volume and grade, degree of capsular penetration into the periprostatic fat, extent of seminal vesicle invasion, and presence of cancer in Denonvilliers' fascia. These histologic determinants of potential biologic behavior will be of little use unless the method of sectioning and examining the prostate is standardized. Until there is agreement on this important issue, investigators should report in detail their own techniques of examining the surgical specimens and accept the fact that a comparison

of published data from different institutions will have very limited value.

Clinical Stage at Initial Presentation with Prostate Cancer

Several reports describe the frequency with which patients present with specific clinical stages of prostate cancer (Murphy et al., 1982; Veterans Administration Cooperative Urological Research Group, 1967a). Given the lack of uniformity in standards for clinical classification, the subjectivity of the rectal examination, the varying quality and often falsely positive radionuclide bone scans, the current impact of PSA and TRUS in diagnosing impalpable cancer in the peripheral and central zones of the prostate, and the introduction of mass screening programs, these reports are not very useful for the 1990s.

However, the results of an excellent population-based study are available. Johannson and associates (1989) accrued 654 new cases of prostate cancer in a population-based study from a restricted geographic area in Sweden. All patients had bone scans, chest radiography, and intravenous urograms. As seen in Table 29–4, 24 per cent had metastatic disease at presentation (M+), 17 per cent were in clinical stage TA, only 5 per cent had a small palpable TB nodule (TB1), 25 per cent had

Table 29–3. POSTSURGICAL HISTOPATHOLOGIC CLASSIFICATION FOR THE PRIMARY TUMOR

pT	Primary tumor
pTis	Preinvasive carcinoma (carcinoma in situ)
pT0	No evidence of tumor found on histologic examination of specimen
pT1	Focal (single or multiple) carcinoma
pT2	Diffuse carcinoma with or without extension to capsule
pT3	Carcinoma with invasion beyond the capsule and/or invasion of seminal vesicles
pT4	Tumor with invasion of adjacent organs
pTX	Extent of tumor invasion cannot be assessed

Adapted from Spiessl, B., Hermanek, P., Scheibe, O., and Wagner, G.: Prostate. *In* TNM Atlas: Illustrated Guide to the Classification of Malignant Tumours, Ed. 2. New York, Springer-Verlag, 1982, p. 180.

Table 29–4. CLINICAL STAGE OF PROSTATE CANCER ON INITIAL PRESENTATION*

Bone metastases by bone scan (M2)	24%
Stage A (TA1 and TA2)	17%
Small, palpable B nodule (TB1)	5%
Larger, palpable B nodules (TB2 and TB3)	25%
Stage C (TBC)	28%
Total	99%

*Data compiled from 654 new cases of prostate cancer. All patients had bone scan, chest radiograph, and intravenous urogram.

Adapted from Johansson, J. E., et al.: Natural history of localised prostate cancer: A population-based study in 223 untreated patients. Lancet, 1:799, 1989.

larger TB nodules (TB2 and TB3), and 28 per cent were clinical stage TC on DRE (TBC).

Because only 40 per cent of palpable TB nodules will be confined within the prostate capsule at the time of radical prostatectomy (see Fig. 29–30), and most of these are made up of TB1 nodules, the magnitude of the problem of curing prostate cancer by radical prostatectomy is readily apparent. Indeed, these dismal statistics constitute the main reason for early detection programs in the population at large.

About 30 per cent of patients with apparently localized disease on DRE (TA and TB) have pelvic lymph node metastases (Donohue et al., 1982; Gervasi et al., 1989; Smith et al., 1983). Almost all of these metastases occur in clinical stages TA2, TB2, and TB3. Fifty per cent of patients with stage TC prostate cancer will have positive lymph nodes (Donohue et al., 1982; Zincke et al., 1986).

TUMOR MARKERS

To find a serum marker that would determine the presence and extent of malignant disease, gauge its progression over time, and verify the success or failure of therapy has been an important goal of research on cancer in every organ. Prostatic carcinoma was the first malignancy for which such biochemical evaluation became possible with tests for serum acid phosphatase (Gutman and Gutman, 1938). Many biochemical tests for other cancers have since been developed, but in 1991, PSA is the most unique marker in cancer biology. It is the first and only organ-specific cancer marker with the possible exception of thyroglobulin.

Prostatic Acid Phosphatase

Three years after the Gutmans (1938) showed that serum enzymatic acid phosphatase titers were elevated in 11 of 15 patients with metastatic prostate cancer, Huggins and Hodges (1941) demonstrated its unique role as a measure of response to bilateral orchiectomy or estrogen administration.

For the ensuing 4 decades, serum enzymatic acid phosphatase was the standard marker for prostate cancer until Foti, Herschman, and Cooper (1975) introduced an immunologically specific radioimmunoassay for human PAP. From the comprehensive tables in the review of PAP by John Heller (1987), serum enzymatic assays utilizing a variety of substrates were elevated in 12 per cent of patients with clinical stage A disease, in 15 to 20 per cent with stage B disease, in 29 to 38 per cent with stage C disease, and in 60 to 82 per cent with metastatic bone disease in those studies reporting at least 25 patients in each category. In contrast, investigators employing radioimmunoassays (RIA-PAP) reported elevations in 12 to 33 per cent, 16 to 78 per cent, 16 to 71 per cent, and 63 to 92 per cent, respectively, for the same clinical stages.

Interpretation of the usefulness of serum enzymatic assays in the literature is complicated by the different substrates employed for enzymatic hydrolysis, the lack of specificity of phosphatase enzymes, the instability at room temperature (requiring immediate icing after venopuncture or stabilization with an acid citrate buffer), the biologic variability within a 24-hour period, and the repeated failure of many investigators to precisely define what is meant by an abnormal elevation. (See Heller, 1987, for precise references.) Sodium thymolphthalein monophosphate (Roy et al., 1971) is widely thought to be the best of the enzymatic assays, but this conclusion is not supported by inspection of Heller's (1987) tables in terms of per cent elevations at different clinical stages of cancer.

Because acid phosphatases occur in many other organs and tissues besides the prostate, it is not surprising that gastric, pancreatic, lung, and breast cancer can all elevate serum enzymatic acid phosphatases (Heller, 1987). Rectal carcinoid tumors, leukemia, multiple myeloma, and even Paget's disease can also cause elevations of the enzymatic phosphatase. BPH causes elevations of RIA-PAP in 14 per cent of patients, primarily in those with greater than 40 g of benign hyperplasia (Stamey et al., 1987). Prostates with large amounts of BPH can cause elevation in serum enzymatic acid phosphatase.

Bone marrow acid phosphatase has no value in staging prostate cancer (Belville et al., 1981; Schellhammer et al., 1982).

It has not been shown that measuring the l-tartrate inhibitable fraction of serum acid phosphatase ("prostate" acid phosphatase) has any value over measuring total serum acid phosphatase (Heller, 1987).

Because of the instability of serum acid phosphatase levels as well as the inconvenience of expressing the results in international units (the amount of substrate converted per minute per unit volume of serum), RIAs—with their ability to measure precise quantities in nanograms per milliliter of relatively immunologically unique PAP—have virtually replaced all enzymatic assays in the United States in 1991. Two observations are important. First, whether these RIA-PAP assays are monoclonal or polyclonal, they are not completely immunologically specific for PAP. If they were, serum levels would not remain in the normal range after cystoprostatectomy or radical prostatectomy for organ-confined cancer. Second, and of much more importance, although RIA-PAP assays are several times more sensitive and reproducible than enzymatic assays, they are almost never as sensitive as PSA levels at any given clinical stage.

Figure 29–31 compares an RIA-PSA with an RIA-PAP in 230 untreated patients with prostate cancer (Stamey and Kabalin, 1989). Both assays are polyclonal, double-antibody, competitive-binding RIAs. Similar results have been reported by Schellhammer and colleagues (1991) in 143 untreated patients and by Robles and associates (1988) in 1383 patients. Ahmann and Schifman (1987) reported that PSA levels were superior to RIA-PAP and enzymatic acid phosphatase levels (Roy method) in 80 patients with metastatic cancer; Rock et al. (1987) have made similar comparisons with all three assays. These data indicate that an RIA-PAP, in the presence of an RIA-PSA, adds no unique infor-

Figure 29–31. Relationship of prostate-specific antigen (PSA) (Yang Pros-Check) and prostate acid phosphatase (PAP) concentrations to clinical cancer stage TA1 to D2 cancers in 230 patients. The mean values of PSA and PAP (ng/ml) are shown above each standard error (SE) bar for each stage. The range of serum PSA for normal individuals, 0 to 2.5 ng/ml, is indicated by the lighter shaded area; that for PAP, 0 to 2.1 ml/ml, by the darker shaded area. The number of patients (n) in each clinical stage is shown at the bottom of the figure. D1 is microscopic pelvic lymph node metastases; D2 is metastases to bone or viscera. Both PSA and PAP are radioimmunoassays. (Modified from Stamey, T. A., and Kabalin, J. N.: J. Urol., 141:1070, 1989.)

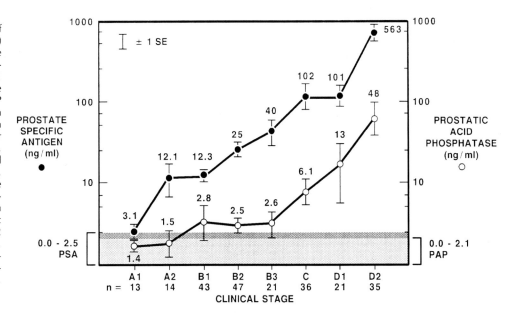

mation. Thus, physicians should rely exclusively on RIA-PSA and save their patients the expense of a simultaneous RIA-PAP.

The question of whether an elevated serum enzymatic acid phosphatase level always indicates metastatic cancer was considered earlier in this chapter in the discussion of the so-called DO disease in relation to Whitmore's OSCC M1 classification in Table 29–2.

Prostate-Specific Antigen

PSA is a unique enzyme. A glycoprotein, produced only by prostate epithelial cells, it hydrolyzes (lyses) the coagulum of the ejaculate (Lee et al., 1989; Lilja and Lourell, 1985). Its function is clearly related to male fertility and, probably for this reason, it is highly conserved in evolution. PSA has a molecular weight of about 30,000, contains 240 amino acids with 7 per cent carbohydrates, and has extensive homology with proteases of the kallikrein family (Watt et al., 1986). It occurs in seminal plasma in milligram quantities. Various investigators recognized this prominent protein in semen: Hara and co-workers (1971) called it gammaseminoprotein; Li and Beling (1973), semen E1 antigen; and Sensabaugh (1978), p30.

Sensabaugh, a biochemist, and the first to characterize this remarkable protein, was seeking a better marker than PAP in the forensic analysis of sexual assault evidence (Graves et al., 1985). In 1990, Sensabaugh and Blake published in detail their two-column technique for purifying PSA from seminal plasma. In this article, and in an accompanying article by Graves and associates (1990a), the identity of seminal plasma protein p30 with PSA is firmly established. In 1979, Wang and his colleagues at Roswell Park, seeking a better marker for prostate cancer, isolated PSA from prostatic tissue using immunodiffusion techniques and showed that it did not cross-react with other tissues. The three-dimensional antigenic domain of PSA has been characterized (Chu

et al., 1989), and its kallikrein-like gene sequence of 6 kilobases has been identified (Riegman et al., 1989; Schedlich et al., 1987). (See Sensabaugh and Blake, 1990, for a discussion of the kallikrein gene family.)

Several publications from Roswell Park between 1980 and 1986 confirmed that PSA was organ-specific, that serum elevations of PSA occurred in both prostate cancer and BPH, and that PSA was an important prognostic marker for monitoring patients with prostate cancer. (See Oesterling, 1991, for a review of all related references.)

Prostate-Specific Antigen Level and Volume of Intracapsular Cancer

Our interest in PSA began in early 1985 when Dr. Norman Yang suggested to us that his PSA assay might be proportional to the volume of prostate cancer. We had determined the cancer volumes on our first 25 radical prostatectomies in 1984 and had stored the preprostatectomy sera at −70°C. The PSA values on these sera were indeed proportional to the volume of *intracapsular* cancer and, after radical prostatectomy, PSA levels fell to 0 (<0.3 g/ml) (half-life 2.2 ± 0.8 days) (Stamey et al., 1987). In contrast, PAP (enzymatic or immunologic) remained at normal levels after radical prostatectomy, failing to reflect the removal of substantial volumes of prostate cancer.

The relationship of serum PSA level to volume of intracapsular prostate cancer, as seen in Figure 29–32, is unique among tumor markers (Stamey et al., 1987, 1989c). As shown in Table 29–5, this proportionality among our patients at Stanford with clinical stage TA and TB disease is not dependent on the presence of extracapsular penetration, seminal vesicle invasion, or lymph node metastases; the PSA level rises at an overall average rate of 3.5 ng/ml per gram of intracapsular cancer regardless of extracapsular penetration, probably indicating that the volume of extracapsular cancer in clinical stages TA and TB is not significant when com-

CANCER VOLUME vs. PSA

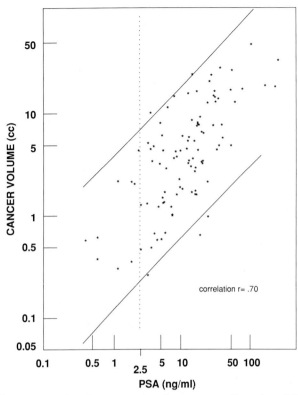

Figure 29–32. Bivariate scatterplot of prostate-specific antigen (PSA) (Yang Pros-Check) against cancer volume for 102 patients, with the axes on a logarithmic scale. Correlation is between the log PSA and the log cancer volume. The 95-per cent prediction limits for the prediction of cancer volume from a given value of PSA for a new patient are read from the appropriate points on the upper and lower solid lines. The vertical dotted line indicates the upper limit PSA for "normal" men (2.5 ng/ml). (From Stamey, T. A., et al.: J. Urol., 141:1076, 1989.)

pared with the volume of intracapsular cancer. We also observed that BPH, in prostates without cancer elevated serum levels of PSA by only 0.3 ng/ml per gram of BPH (Stamey et al., 1987), a number that has been confirmed in both England and France (Perrin et al., 1991). Carter and co-workers (1991) have shown that the change in PSA levels over time in 17 men ultimately proved to have prostate cancer (4.2 ± 0.8 to 14 ± 3.6 ng/ml, Hybritech assay) was much steeper than the rise in PSA levels in 20 men ultimately proven to have BPH (3.0 ± 0.4 to 3.4 ± 0.4 ng/ml).

Because serum PSA level is proportional to intracapsular cancer volume, and because prostate cancer pro-

gression (including cancer penetration into the periprostatic fat, the seminal vesicles, and the pelvic lymph nodes) is also proportional to intraprostatic cancer volume (McNeal et al., 1986a; Stamey et al., 1988), it follows that preoperative serum PSA levels should be very useful in predicting pathologic stage after radical prostatectomy. Several investigators, however, utilizing different assays than the Yang polyclonal assay and different histologic techniques in examining the prostate, have not found preoperative serum PSA level to be very helpful as a predictor of pathologic stage. (See review by Oesterling, 1991.) However, as noted in our original report of 78 patients undergoing radical prostatectomy (Stamey et al., 1987), and as shown by the results from 301 patients (Fig. 29–33), we believe that preoperative serum PSA level by the Yang assay is very helpful in assessing the likelihood of adverse pathologic findings.

The three most unfavorable parameters shown in Figure 29–33 are the presence of microscopic, undetectable pelvic lymph node metastases at surgical staging; the presence of a cancer volume greater than 12 ml within the prostate; and the presence of seminal vesicle invasion, especially when extensive (Villers et al., 1990). Thirteen per cent of all our radical prostatectomies (n = 408) for clinical stage A and B disease have histologic cancer volumes greater than 12 ml. None of these 54 patients, including 25 who had neither lymph node metastases nor more than 5 per cent of the seminal vesicles invaded, have maintained an undetectable postoperative PSA level 4 years after radical prostatectomy. Thus, we believe that cancer volumes greater than 12 ml are incurable by radical prostatectomy alone.

Observe in Figure 29–33 that the difference between having a preoperative Yang serum PSA level of less than 10 ng/ml compared with having one greater than 50 ng/ml represents a difference of 0 per cent versus 45 per cent for microscopic lymph node metastases, of less than 1 per cent versus 64 per cent for cancer volumes greater than 12 ml within the prostate, of 5 per cent versus 73 per cent for seminal vesicle invasion, of 11 per cent versus 55 per cent for invasion into the periprostatic fat extending for more than 0.5 cm² along the side of the capsule, and of 27 per cent versus 91 per cent for having a Gleason score of 7 to 10 when the entire cancer is examined. Note that the percentages of these adverse pathologic findings for the Yang categories of PSA levels between 10 to 20 ng/ml and 20 to 50 ng/ml show a progressive increase. The mean PSA levels for all cancers in the four subgroups of PSA levels in Figure 29–33 are 5, 15, 30, and 97 ng/ml.

Prostate-Specific Antigen Level and Volume of Extracapsular Cancer

PSA, as might be expected, is also proportional to the volume of untreated extracapsular cancer in clinical stages C, D1, and D2 disease (Stamey et al., 1987; Stamey and Kabalin, 1989) when compared with the earlier clinical stages (see Fig. 29–31). The clinical staging system used at Stanford for the categories shown in Figure 29–31 is illustrated in Figure 29–34 and is similar to the one adopted by Whitmore's OSCC Com-

Table 29–5. PSA PER GRAM OF PROSTATE CANCER IN 102 RADICAL PROSTATECTOMIES

	Organ-Confined (n = 66)	+LN, +SV, CP > 1 cm (n = 36)
Mean PSA level (ng/ml)	10.9	44.6
Mean cancer volume (cm³)	3.1	12.6
Ratio of PSA level to cancer volume (ng/ml/g)	3.5	3.5

Abbreviations: PSA, prostate-specific antigen; LN, lymph nodes; SV, seminal vesicles; CP, capsular penetration into periprostatic fat.

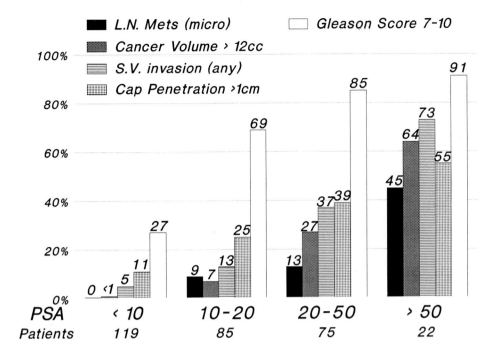

Figure 29–33. Serum prostate-specific antigen (PSA) (Yang Pros-Check) was collected on an ambulatory basis before prostate manipulation in 301 patients undergoing radical prostatectomies for clinical stage TA and TB prostate cancer. Although all five adverse pathologic parameters rise with increasing PSA, the differences between a PSA of <10 ng/ml and >50 ng/ml are very useful clinically.

mittee, which was discussed previously and presented in Table 29–2. These data show an increasing serum PSA level from the earliest clinical stages to metastatic bone disease; PSA averaged 563 ng/ml in 35 untreated patients with bone metastases. Other investigators have also confirmed the rising PSA level with increasing clinical stage (Chan et al., 1987; Hudson et al., 1989).

Although it is true that there is a variable and somewhat less intense immunohistochemical staining of malignant cells with PSA as loss of differentiation occurs with increasing Gleason grades of prostate cancer, there is also an increase in tumor volume, offsetting any net decrease in PSA production per cancer cell. Under these circumstances, it is not surprising that the PSA level continues to rise in the serum in reasonable proportion to increasing tumor burden in the untreated patient. Only 2 per cent of 419 patients with stage D2 disease with no prior hormonal therapy had a normal PSA level in the prospective study reported by Smith and associates (1991). The unique use and limitation of PSA levels in clinical stage A disease are discussed in the final sections of this chapter, which deal with the treatment of patients with each clinical stage of prostate cancer.

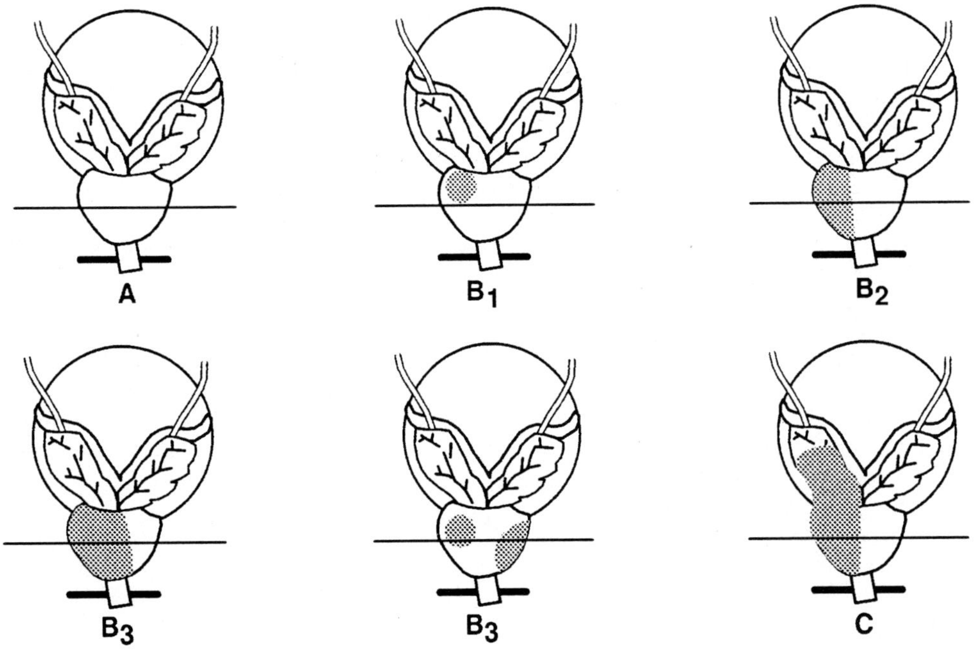

Figure 29–34. Palpable findings on digital rectal examination for clinical stages TA, TB, and TC (see Table 29–2 for further detail). (Modified from Stamey, T. A., and Kabalin, J. N.: J. Urol., 141:1070, 1989.)

A

B₁

B₂

B₃

B₃

C

Value of Prostate-Specific Antigen Level in Monitoring Therapy for Prostate Cancer

Although the PSA level is of most use in estimating the tumor burden in patients with untreated prostate cancer, it is also helpful in monitoring patients after radical prostatectomy, radiation therapy, and hormonal therapy. If we ever develop effective cytotoxic chemotherapeutic agents for prostate cancer, PSA levels will probably serve as the primary marker of therapeutic success or failure.

RADICAL PROSTATECTOMY. We observed in 1987 that any patient who had a detectable PSA level 3 weeks or more after radical prostatectomy had residual cancer (Stamey et al., 1987). With the Yang polyclonal assay, any value below 0.3 ng/ml is statistically similar to 0.0 ng/ml. As reviewed by Oesterling (1991), the Hybritech cutoff for a significant detectable PSA level indicative of residual disease was 0.4, 0.5, 0.6, and 0.6 ng/ml at four university centers, all of whom have a major interest in prostate cancer and use this assay exclusively. Kleinschmidt and associates (1991) measured PSA by the Hybritech assay in 50 patients after cystoprostatectomy for bladder cancer; the mean PSA was 0.21 ± 0.16 ng/ml, with a range of 0.1 to 0.6 ng/ml. They concluded that based on a 95 per cent confidence interval, the minimum level of PSA detected by the Hybritech assay is 0.5 ng/ml. They also observed that PSA was 98 per cent organ specific, whereas an RIA-PAP was only 17 per cent organ specific.

Following serum PSA level at frequent intervals after radical prostatectomy allows much earlier assessment of therapeutic efficacy than the historical alternative of waiting months or years for the positive bone scan. It also creates the possibility of initiating adjunctive therapy (radiation therapy, hormonal therapy, or it is hoped someday chemotherapy) when the tumor burden is extremely small. As might be expected, the worse the pathologic stage at the time of radical prostatectomy, the sooner the PSA level becomes detectable. (See Oesterling for review, 1991.)

In our Stanford series, only 1.4 per cent (2/139) of organ-confined cancers developed a detectable PSA level on follow-up compared with 20 per cent (10/51) of patients who had less than 0.5 cm^2 of capsular penetration into the periprostatic fat in the absence of seminal vesicle invasion or lymph node metastases. Seven of these ten patients, however, had positive margins compared with only six positive margins in the 41 patients who still have an undetectable PSA level, strongly suggesting that positive margins may be more important than minimal extracapsular penetration (Eigner et al., 1991).

This example emphasizes how PSA can indicate the need for early changes in therapeutic approaches to prostate cancer, in this instance, the critical importance of avoiding positive margins. It also emphasizes the need for consistent, systematic histopathologic sectioning of the prostate at closely spaced intervals.

Paulson and Frazier (1991) performed 189 radical prostatectomies in 3½ years, dividing them into organ-confined (94), specimen-confined (54), and prostates with positive margins (41). By conventional criteria of surgical failure, such as serum enzymatic acid phosphatase elevation, local palpable recurrence, or recurrence on imaging study, 2 of 94, 3 of 54, and 5 of 41 failed within the short follow-up period. Using PSA level greater than 0.5 ng/ml (Hybritech) as a criterion, however, 16 of 94, 24 of 54, and 29 of 41 failed.

Lightner and co-workers (1990) performed random needle biopsies of the urethrovesical anastomotic area in postradical prostatectomy patients with PSA levels greater than 0.4 ng/ml by the Hybritech assay who were otherwise without evidence of disease, including a nondiagnostic DRE. Forty-two per cent had positive biopsy findings despite a nondiagnostic rectal examination. These investigators had no positive biopsies in 30 patients with undetectable PSA levels.

RADIATION THERAPY

"Definitive" Radiation of the Prostate and Pelvis. Of 183 patients treated with radiation therapy, 11 per cent had an undetectable PSA level at a mean follow-up of 5 years (Stamey et al., 1989a). We observed a decrease in serum PSA levels in 82 per cent of patients during the first year of radiation; serum PSA levels in 52 per cent rose in the second year after completion of therapy (Stamey et al., 1989a). Schellhammer and colleagues (1991) found an undetectable PSA level (≤ 0.5 ng/ml) by the Hybritech method in 30 of 212 patients (7 per cent) followed 3 years or more after radiation therapy. In our experience, a progressive rise in serum PSA levels after completion of radiation therapy is always indicative of radiation failure. The clinician should also recognize that metastatic bone disease can occur at very low levels of PSA after pelvic radiation—even as low as 8 ng/ml by the Yang assay, levels that are incompatible with metastases in the untreated patient (563 ± 104 ng/ml) (Stamey and Kabalin, 1989; Stamey et al., 1989a).

Kabalin and co-workers (1989a) performed systematic, TRUS-guided biopsies of the prostate in 27 consecutive patients who completed definitive radiation therapy for at least 18 months or more (mean 5.2 years). Many of these patients had normal or impalpable prostates as well as low or even undetectable serum levels of PSA. A total of 93 per cent (25/27) had histologically identified prostate cancer, including 16 of 18 (89 per cent) with localized clinical stage TA and TB disease prior to radiation therapy. An increase in the Gleason grade of the prostate cancer, when compared with the preradiation biopsy, was not uncommon. We concluded that there is an unacceptably high local failure rate to radiation therapy, which cannot be appreciated by DRE, serum acid phosphatase, or a PSA level that is in the normal or low normal range.

Irradiation Post–Radical Prostatectomy. We reported the first six patients to receive adjunctive pelvic radiation therapy when the only evidence of persistent prostate cancer was a biochemical abnormality, i.e., PSA (Stamey et al., 1987). With greater experience, we have learned that, although serum PSA will fall to undetectable levels after radiation in about 60 per cent of patients, this encouraging response has not proven to be durable in most cases (Table 29–6). This finding includes not only those patients whose PSA never returns to undetectable levels after radical prostatectomy, in whom only one of 12 patients (stage D1, 31 months follow-up) has had a durable undetectable PSA level after radiation, but also those whose PSA levels fell to 0 ng/ml after prostatectomy (less than 0.3 ng/ml by the Yang assay) and in whom months or years later, PSA levels became detectable.

As seen in Table 29–6, we are more optimistic about adjunctive radiation when the only adverse pathologic finding is capsular penetration into the periprostatic fat or positive surgical margin (Link et al., 1991). All of the patients described in Table 29–6 had a detectable and rising PSA level at the time of radiation therapy. Whether immediate radiation based on pathologic stage, without waiting for PSA levels to become detectable, would produce better adjunctive radiation results is unknown. Because some patients with seminal vesicle invasion and others with capsular penetration into the periprostatic fat will be cured by radical prostatectomy alone, and because the significance of minutely positive surgical margins is uncertain, proceeding to radiation therapy without awaiting a detectable and rising PSA level carries some risk of unnecessary treatment.

Lange and associates (1990) have reported somewhat similar results for radiation therapy after radical prostatectomy in those patients who have a detectable PSA level. However, our series was prospective, and we radiated at low levels of PSA, usually between 1 and 2 ng/ml by the Yang assay. To potentially cure, at the most, six of 25 patients, when the pelvic tumor residual is so small that it cannot be palpated or imaged, argues strongly that prostate cancer is resistant to 7000 rads of external beam therapy.

ENDOCRINE THERAPY. Both Kuriyama and colleagues (1981) and Killian and colleagues (1985) recognized the usefulness of PSA levels in monitoring patients with advanced prostatic cancer. In general, the level of serum PSA was inversely proportional to survival time as well as the likelihood of cancer remission, but the relationship between pre- and post-hormonal PSA was not explored as a measure of favorable prognosis.

We reported on 11 consecutive patients with untreated D2 metastatic disease in whom the PSA level fell from a preoperative mean of 1088 ng/ml to 74 ng/ml (a 95 per cent mean decrease) within 6 months of initiating hormonal therapy (Stamey et al., 1989b). In three of the 11 (27 per cent), PSA fell to undetectable levels and remained in that range at 6 months and beyond. Seven of the remaining eight patients whose PSA did not fall to undetectable levels at 6 months died within 18 months of initiating hormonal therapy; their PSA response was characterized by a dramatic early fall in PSA, followed by a steady increase well before the 6-month end point.

These data suggested that an early fall to near undetectable or undetectable levels of PSA that is maintained for at least 6 months can be predictive of a long-term response to hormonal therapy. Conversely, a dramatic fall to even normal levels that is not maintained at 6 months is predictive of a short-term response to antiandrogen therapy. Siddall and associates (1986), using goserelin acetate in monthly injections in 65 patients, were the first to observe the importance of the 6-month PSA assessment in achieving a prolonged clinical response. Miller and co-workers (1991) have reported similar observations, although many of their patients with stage D2 disease had been treated with nonhormonal therapies, and the investigators required only that PSA fall to normal levels (less than 4 ng/ml, Hybritech).

Arai and associates (1990) reported on 44 patients whose initial PSA level was greater than 10 ng/ml. They utilized an enzyme competitive binding assay with a minimal detectable PSA value of 1.5 ng/ml. Despite this disturbingly high minimal detectable level, the patients whose PSA levels decreased 80 per cent or more within 1 month of initiating hormonal therapy survived significantly longer free of disease progression ($P < .001$).

Ercole and colleagues (1987) determined PSA and PAP (RIA) retrospectively in 49 patients with stage D2 disease before and during endocrine therapy. PSA and PAP levels fell in 31 patients who had a favorable response but rose in 18 patients with an unfavorable response. The failure to observe a temporary fall in PSA levels in patients with an unfavorable response probably reflects the limitations of available sera in the early period after initiating antiandrogen treatment. An initial fall in PSA levels is almost universal on initiation of hormonal therapy. Smith and co-workers (1991) reported that 98 per cent of 411 patients with stage D2

Table 29–6. PELVIC RADIATION THERAPY FOLLOWING RADICAL PROSTATECTOMY BASED SOLELY ON A DETECTABLE PSA LEVEL

Worst Pathologic Stage	Total Number of Patients	Number of Patients			Follow-up (months)*
		PSA Level Was Never <0.3 ng/ml Before XRT	PSA Level Fell to <0.3 ng/ml After XRT	Last PSA Level Was Still <0.3 ng/ml	
D1	8	7	4	1 (13%)	31
C_{sv}	8†	3	4†	2 (25%)	19, 50†
C_m	6	2	5	2 (33%)	24, 30
C_{cp}	3	0	2	1 (33%)	30

*Follow-up in months since initiation of radiation therapy for patients whose last PSA level was less than 0.3 ng/ml.
†A patient with only 1 per cent involvement of his seminal vesicle but who also had a positive surgical margin.
Abbreviations: D1, pelvic lymph node metastasis; C_{sv}, seminal vesicle involvement; C_m, positive surgical margin; C_{cp}, capsule penetration with negative margin; PSA, prostate-specific antigen; XRT, x-ray therapy.
Adapted from Link, P., et al: Adjuvant radiation therapy in patients with detectable prostatic specific antigen following radical prostatectomy. J. Urol., 145:532, 1991.

disease who had received no prior hormonal therapy had a decrease in PSA levels with a median decrease of 97.7 per cent after 3 months of therapy.

Our practice is to obtain a PSA level before starting endocrine therapy, and at 1 month, 3 months, and 6 months after bilateral orchiectomy or leuprolide hormonal therapy. The intervening values are used to determine whether to add flutamide if PSA reverses its downward trend (see section in this chapter on hormonal therapy).

Although PSA is undoubtedly androgen-dependent, evidence has been presented that the fall in PSA levels may be independent of cell inhibition or death. (See Oesterling, 1991, for review.) Because clinical experience is now overwhelming, with few exceptions (perhaps 5 per cent), that PSA level reflects the clinical course of hormonally treated patients with stage D2 disease, these experimental observations with nude mice and immortal prostate cancer cell lines are probably inappropriate to the clinical situation.

Clinical Precautions for Use of Prostate-Specific Antigen as a Tumor Marker

Serum PSA level shows no evidence for a circadian-type pattern from 8 A.M. to 8 P.M. (Dejter et al., 1988), perhaps explaining why we found excellent reproducibility on two consecutive serum samples, 6 weeks apart, in 31 ambulatory patients with newly diagnosed prostate cancer who had had no intervening treatment or prostate examinations (Stamey et al., 1987).

Although Maatman found no daily fluctuations beyond the error of the laboratory assay when the PSA level was measured every 4 hours in eight men admitted to the hospital with clinical stage D2 prostate cancer (Maatman, 1989), the ambulatory PSA level falls 18 ± 11 per cent when prostate cancer patients are admitted to the hospital overnight (Stamey et al., 1987). Thus, interpretation of serum PSA levels should be based on outpatient, ambulatory assays with full knowledge of whether the patient's prostate has been treated by TURP, radical prostatectomy, radiation therapy, or hormones, because any type of therapy to the prostate changes the meaning of PSA levels (Stamey and Kabalin, 1989; Stamey et al., 1989a–c).

Moreover, acute bacterial prostatitis with chills, fever, and bacteriuria elevates serum PSA levels dramatically in our experience, often requiring several months to return to baseline values. Nonbacterial prostatitis—even with purulent expressed prostatic secretion—causes neither an elevation in PSA levels nor a detectable change in TRUS of the prostate.

Although there is some controversy over whether DRE elevates serum levels of PSA (see Oesterling, 1991, for review), it is irrational to massage a prostate that contains PSA at a concentration of 1 to 2 million ng/ml of prostatic fluid in a serologic environment that averages 1.1 ± 0.7 ng/ml (Yang assay) and then draw a blood serum. Using the Yang assay, we found nearly a twofold increase in serum PSA levels after rectal examination, and a fourfold increase when cystoscopic examination was combined with palpation of the prostate against the cystoscope. A 53 to 57 fold increase in serum PSA levels was measured after needle biopsy or TUR of the prostate (Stamey et al., 1987). That most of this increase was caused by creating communications between normal prostatic glands and the venous system, as opposed to communications with cancerous glands, was suggested by very small increases in serum PSA levels when large amounts of high-grade cancer were biopsied or resected.

Because these biopsies across normal glands can potentially increase serum PSA to extraordinary levels (several hundred nanograms per milliliter), the physician should wait at least 4 weeks for PSA to reach baseline levels after biopsy, just as it is necessary to wait this long in patients after radical prostatectomy who have very high preoperative serum levels of PSA. Yuan and Catalona (1991) observed that 27 (30 per cent) of 89 men failed to return to prebiopsy levels by 2 weeks after systematic needle biopsies. Oesterling and Bergstralh (1991) carefully studied 27 patients after TRUS-guided biopsies or TURP. All had returned to baseline serum levels of PSA by 4 weeks. Thus, both these investigations are in agreement that any PSA collected within 4 weeks of prostate biopsy or TURP should not be used to estimate tumor burden or pathologic stage. Because the rise in serum PSA levels after prostatic examination is minimal compared with biopsy or TURP, 1 week will suffice for any elevation secondary to DRE for PSA to return to baseline levels.

The two most common commercial assays for PSA available in the United States are the polyclonal Yang Pro-Check PSA and the monoclonal Hybritech Tandem-R PSA (see Oesterling, 1991, for review). Both assays are approved by the Food and Drug Administration (FDA). Major differences between the two assays include the problem of restricted monoclonal recognition of antigenic epitopes versus polyclonal recognition of multiple epitopes, which probably accounts for the greater sensitivity of the Yang assay to prostatic manipulation; differences caused by standards in female sera versus 1 per cent bovine serum albumin; potential problems with the "hook" effect, which occurs at lower concentrations with the monoclonal assay as compared with the polyclonal assay (Graves et al., 1990b); and substantial differences in the definition of normal ranges, which occur in opposite direction to what the differences in standards should dictate. The decision of Hybritech to substitute horse serum albumen for female serum in their assay substantially complicates the meaning of past observations.

In general, the Yang polyclonal assay gives values 1.4 to 1.9 times higher than the Hybritech monoclonal assay (Graves et al., 1990b). Others have obtained similar differences (Chan et al., 1987; Hortin et al., 1988); but all of these observations were made before horse serum albumen was substituted for female serum in the Hybritech assay. When we purified PSA to serve as an independent standard employing the technique of Sensabaugh and Blake (1990), we found the Yang assay standards to be equivalent to the independent standard; however, the assigned values for the Hybritech assay were very low, perhaps secondary to the binding of PSA to serum proteins in the female sera diluent (Graves et al., 1990b). Because of these observations, we urged the adoption of an international standard.

Based on these data, a panel of immunologists at the FDA on December 6, 1990, formally recommended to the Centers for Disease Control (CDC) and the National Research Council of the World Health Organization that an international standard be adopted. The adoption of such a standard would have great advantages to practicing urologists, because many different commercial laboratories use either the Hybritech or the Yang assay. Adoption of an international standard would substantially diminish the differences between various assays, especially the Hybritech and the Yang.

Until such a time when international standards are established, and the definition of normal controls is agreed upon and their values determined, the real meaning of PSA values determined by different assays can only be judged against clinical studies that utilize the specific assay. Unfortunately, for the scientific and clinical community, interinstitutional comparisons when different assays are employed will be relatively meaningless. The need for a better definition of normal controls is emphasized by the report that 51 (21 per cent) of 241 men in a screening program who had evidence of BPH on rectal examination or ultrasound had a normal PSA level by the Hybritech assay of less than 4 ng/ml (Hudson et al., 1991).

Prostate-Specific Antigen as a Kallikrein-Like Serine Protease

PSA possesses chymotrypsin-like activity and is bound to α_1-antichymotrypsin and α_2-macroglobulin (Christensson et al., 1990). However, the proportion of the PSA-α_1-antichymotrypsin complex is higher in patients with prostate cancer than in those with BPH, which could improve the clinical sensitivity for cancer (Stenman et al., 1991). PSA is known to lyse high molecular weight seminal vesicle proteins (Lee et al., 1990; Lilja and Lourell, 1985). Many questions remain about its protease activity. Are there other substrates than those in seminal vesicle fluid? What prevents PSA from acting on prostate-derived proteins? Is PSA active in the normal blood clotting cascade? Could PSA account for the disseminated intravascular coagulation (DIC) syndrome in patients with metastatic prostate cancer?

The availability of purified PSA was limited at one time and it was extremely expensive. Sensabaugh and Blake (1990) have published their simple two-column technique for purifying p30 from seminal plasma. In a companion article (Graves et al., 1990a), we have shown that PSA and p30 have identical purification profiles, and we have developed a rapid and continuous technique for purifying PSA in large quantities, which should make PSA readily accessible for some much needed physiologic studies. Lastly, these publications establish that PSA, p30, and gamma-seminoprotein are all one and the same protein.

Prostate-Specific Antigen as a First-Line Detection Test

Because DRE and TRUS involve subjective interpretations, and because a blood test is more acceptable to patients, interest has developed in the use of PSA level as a primary, initial screening test. This interest has been enhanced by the general observation that an abnormal PSA level is just as sensitive as an abnormal DRE for detecting prostate cancer. For example, in 2648 urologic outpatients followed by Cooner (1991), 288 cancers were diagnosed using an abnormal DRE (10.9 per cent), whereas 306 cancers were diagnosed using an abnormal PSA level (11.6 per cent) using the Hybritech assay ($\geq$4.1 ng/ml).

However, as reviewed in the next section, Diagnosis of Prostate Cancer, inclusion of patients with a PSA level between 4.1 and 10 ng/ml imposes a huge financial burden as well as an unconscionable number of biopsies (6.1) and ultrasounds (18.2) for every cancer detected in urologically referred patients with normal-feeling prostates. True screening studies on unselected patients with normal-feeling prostates will require an even greater number of ultrasounds and unnecessary biopsies in the intermediate range of PSA levels (4.1 to 10 ng/ml, Hybritech). Despite these obvious limitations, Catalona and co-workers (1990) have been advocates of this approach. The role of PSA levels in primary screening is currently debated; some are strong advocates of its use (Catalona et al., 1990 and 1991), others are critics (Cooner et al., 1990; Scardino, 1989).

Because of the National Prostate Cancer Awareness Week, considerable direct information is now available on the frequency distribution of PSA levels in these "screening" populations for which all patients are selected solely by their response to news bureau advertisements (Table 29–7). In terms of the Hybritech assay, about 85 to 90 per cent of men 50 years or older will have a PSA level less than or equal to 4 ng/ml; 8 to 12 per cent will have a PSA level between 4.1 and 10 ng/ml; and 3 per cent or less will have a PSA level greater than 10 ng/ml (Boxer, 1991; Brawer et al., 1991; Hudson et al., 1991—this study included men older than 40 years).

Table 29–7. DISTRIBUTION OF PROSTATE-SPECIFIC ANTIGEN LEVELS IN "SCREENING" VERSUS UROLOGICALLY REFERRED PATIENTS IN MEN 50 YEARS OR OLDER

Number of Patients	Prostate-Specific Antigen(ng/ml)*		
	$0 \leq 4$	$4.1–10$	>10
Urologic† (n = 2648)	65%	20%	15%
"Screening"‡ (n = 2659)	85–90%	8–12%	$\leq$3%

*Hybritech assay; Yang equivalents: 0–$\leq$7.3, 7.4–18.4, >18.4 ng/ml.
†Cooner, W. H.: Prostate-specific antigen, digital rectal examination, and transrectal ultrasonic examination of the prostate in prostate cancer detection. Monogr. Urol., 12:3, 1991. Thirty-three per cent had an abnormal digital rectal examination.
‡Stanford series, 478; Brawer, 1240; Boxer, 700; Hudson, 241. Seventeen per cent had an abnormal digital examination.

We screened 478 men at Stanford University during the National Prostate Cancer Awareness Week in 1990. Eighty-nine per cent (427/478) had a Yang PSA level of ≤7.3 ng/ml (Hybritech, ≤4 ng/ml); 9 per cent (43/478) had a Yang PSA level of 7.4 to 18.4 ng/ml (Hybritech, 4.1 to 10 ng/ml); and 2 per cent (8/478) had a Yang PSA level of >18.4 ng/ml. This distribution, as seen in Table 29–7, is substantially different from that found by Cooner (1991) in 2648 patients. Only 65 per cent had a PSA level of ≤4.0 ng/ml, 20 per cent had a PSA level of 4.1 to 10 ng/ml, and 15 per cent had a PSA level of >10 ng/ml (Hybritech). Moreover, in our screening study at Stanford University, we found only 17 per cent with an abnormal DRE (Hudson and associates, 1991, found 17.3 per cent) compared with Cooner's finding of 33 per cent with abnormal DRE (Table 29–7).

This trend among "screening" populations toward a smaller elevation of serum PSA levels and half as many positive DRE examinations (Table 29–7) suggests that using these modalities in the urologist's office will be more cost-effective in detecting cancer than using them for screening the general population. However, the distribution of PSA levels in the two groups in Table 29–7 clearly indicates that smaller cancers will be detected by PSA screening in the community.

Babaian and colleagues (1991) have reported the distribution of PSA levels in relation to prostate volume determined by TRUS in 331 men without clinical or biopsy evidence of prostate cancer on sequential step-section TRUS analysis. Some 81 per cent had a PSA level of ≤4 ng/ml, 15.7 per cent had a PSA level of 4.1 to 10 ng/ml, and 3.2 per cent had a PSA level of >10 ng/ml by the Hybritech assay. The association between serum PSA level and gland volume was highly significant in these patients without clinical evidence of prostate cancer ($P < .00005$). This study reminds us that BPH causes significant elevation of PSA levels (>4 ng/ml) in nearly 20 per cent of all men without cancer, which markedly degrades the efficiency of PSA levels alone as a screening tool for cancer, except at PSA levels of >10 ng/ml (18.4 ng/ml by the Yang assay).

Men who present with acute urinary retention from BPH tend to have higher serum PSA levels than those who present for elective surgery (Armitage et al., 1988).

DIAGNOSIS OF PROSTATE CANCER

Digital Rectal Examination and Finger-Guided Biopsies

We have relied on DRE and digitally guided biopsies for diagnosis of prostate cancer for many decades, a combination that has a detection rate in population studies as high as 1.7 per cent when a high index of suspicion is used for abnormalities found on DRE of the prostate (Chodak et al., 1989). Most investigators have reported lower detection rates of 0.8 to 1.4 per cent. (See Scardino, 1989, for review.)

Transrectal Ultrasound-Guided Biopsies in Screening Studies

The advent of TRUS, especially TRUS-guided biopsies of hypoechoic areas, as opposed to "blind" finger-guided biopsies, has clearly increased the detection rate of prostate cancer in screening (advertising through local news bureaus) populations. The detection rate was 2.6 per cent in one study of 784 men (Lee et al., 1988a), and it was 2.3 per cent in 2427 men, aged 55 to 70 years old, who were similarly screened by the National Prostate Cancer Detection Project (Mettlin, 1990).

As seen in Table 29–8, of the 56 cancers detected in the Mettlin report, DRE would have missed 32 per cent of the tumors if TRUS had not been performed, and TRUS would have missed 14.3 per cent of the tumors if DRE had not been done. Thus, although DRE appears to have missed half of the cancers, this finding is misleading because, in another 25 cancers (44.6 per cent as shown in Table 29–8), TRUS and DRE both detected the tumor. Hence, if all DRE suspicious examinations are submitted to TRUS, the final detection rate is 59 per cent for DRE and 77 per cent for TRUS, a much smaller difference, but still an important one. Thus, there are clearly some impalpable cancers in the peripheral zone that cannot be detected by DRE but that can be proved by ultrasound biopsy of hypoechoic areas in the peripheral or central zones. Note in Table 29–8 that five cancers were detected by multiple biopsies taken because of elevated PSA levels in cases for which neither TRUS nor DRE were diagnostic.

The conclusions from this important study are as follows: (1) In a screening study, some cancers are palpable but cannot be seen on TRUS because they are isoechoic; hence, TRUS should never be performed without being preceded by a carefully executed rectal examination. (2) If every patient is studied with TRUS, some impalpable cancers will be detected (18/56 or 32 per cent in the Mettlin report) but at the substantial expense of many biopsies. (3) PSA testing appears to play a major role because an additional five (8.9 per cent) cancers were found in patients in whom neither

Table 29–8. METHOD OF DETECTING 56 CANCERS (2.3%) IN 2427 MEN SCREENED FOR PROSTATE CANCER

Method	No. of Cancers (n = 56)	Cancer Detected (%)
PSA alone	5/56	8.9
DRE alone	8/56	14.3
TRUS alone	18/56	32.1
DRE or TRUS*	25/56	44.6
Total by DRE	33/56	59
Total by TRUS	43/56	77

*These 25 cancers were palpated and seen on TRUS.
Abbreviations: PSA, prostate-specific antigen; DRE, digital rectal examination; TRUS, transrectal ultrasound.
Adapted from Mettlin, C.: Preliminary findings from the American Cancer Society National Prostate Cancer Detection Project. Presented at the 5th International Symposium on Transrectal Ultrasound in the Diagnosis and Management of Prostate Cancer. Chicago, IL, September 14, 1990, pp. 84–85.

an abnormal DRE nor a hypoechoic area on TRUS was found. (4) Twice as many patients underwent biopsy for a suspicious ultrasound (330 men or 13.6 per cent of the population) as underwent biopsy because of a suspicious DRE (153 men or 6.3 per cent). This significant difference in number of patients undergoing biopsy to detect the cancers in each group further blurs the statistical advantage of TRUS over DRE when all DRE-positive patients are submitted to a TRUS-guided biopsy.

Repeat Screening of the Same Population at Yearly Intervals

Lee (1990) screened 394 men as a subset of the Mettlin study shown in Table 29–8, detecting cancer in 2.5 per cent. The second year, 228 returned for repeat examination; cancer was found in an additional 2.6 per cent. The third year, 176 returned, and another 1.1 per cent were found to have cancer. These 18 cancers among the 394 men originally in the study represent a cumulative detection rate of 4.6 per cent when a group of men are repeatedly screened for 3 consecutive years with DRE and TRUS. None of Lee's subset were diagnosed by PSA level alone.

DRE, PSA Testing, and TRUS in a Urologic Practice

Cooner and associates (1990) have published studies utilizing DRE, PSA testing, and TRUS in 1807 men between 50 and 89 years old who were referred to their urologic practice. In this classic study, *all* patients were included regardless of their symptoms or findings on DRE (Cooner et al., 1990). This study is unique because two urologists had to agree as to whether the DRE was abnormal or normal (BPH was considered normal); all patients had an ambulatory serum PSA level taken prior to prostate manipulation; and all ultrasounds were performed by one person (Cooner), both an expert ultrasonographer and urologist.

Cooner has expanded the number of patients from 1807 to 2648 (Cooner, 1991)—a 47 per cent expansion—without significantly changing overall percentages, an impressive accomplishment considering the subjectivity of both DRE and TRUS. The results for these 2648 patients are presented in Tables 29–9 through 29–11. Cooner has used the Hybritech assay, dividing the DRE data into those patients with PSA levels of ≤4 ng/ml, 4.1 to 10 ng/ml, and >10 ng/ml. The Yang assay equivalents are approximately ≤7.3 ng/ml, 7.4 to 18.4 ng/ml, and >18.4 ng/ml (Graves et al., 1990b).

In the 2648 patients in Cooner's early detection program, the overall cancer detection rate was 14.5 per cent (383/2648), a huge increase over the maximum detection rate by DRE alone with finger-guided biopsies. However, the detection rate was six times higher in those with an abnormal DRE, 32 per cent (288/896), compared with those with a normal DRE, 5.4 per cent (95/1752). As seen in Table 29–9, when these 288 patients with abnormal DRE were divided into three levels of PSA, the 10.3 per cent cancer detection rate

Table 29–9. CANCER DETECTION RATE RELATED TO LEVELS OF SERUM PSA AND DRE IN 2648 PATIENTS

PSA (ng/ml)*	No. of Cancers/No. of Patients	
	DRE +	DRE −
≤ 4.0	$\frac{46}{446}$ = 10.3%	$\frac{31}{1265}$ = 2.5%
4.1–10.0	$\frac{74}{194}$ = 38.1%	$\frac{19}{343}$ = 5.5%
<10.0	$\frac{168}{256}$ = 65.6%	$\frac{45}{144}$ = 31.3%
Total	$\frac{288}{896}$ = 32%	$\frac{95}{1752}$ = 5.4%

*Hybritech assay.
Abbreviations: PSA, prostate-specific antigen; DRE, digital rectal examination. Adapted from Cooner, W. H.: Prostate-specific antigen, digital rectal examination, and transrectal ultrasonic examination of the prostate in prostate cancer detection. Monogr. Urol., 12:3, 1991.

in those with a PSA level of ≤4 ng/ml progressively rose to 65.6 per cent when the PSA level was >10 ng/ml as measured by the Hybritech assay (18.4 ng/ml by the Yang assay).

Note in Table 29–10, however, that the number of patients undergoing biopsy ranged from 67 per cent to 99 per cent. This table also reflects the number of hypoechoic areas found in those patients with abnormal-feeling prostates because only biopsies of hypoechoic areas were done. In our institution, we would have performed biopsies on 100 per cent of these patients because of the possibility of isoechoic cancers, which are reported to occur in as many as 32 per cent of patients with significant tumors, although this percentage includes stage A cancers (Shinohara et al., 1989). Cooner performed biopsies of these DRE-positive, isoechoic ultrasound areas too; however, he excluded them from the data analysis to be consistent in the biopsy of hypoechoic lesions on TRUS. Note in Table 29–10 that, for every cancer detected in a DRE-positive patient with a PSA level of ≤4 ng/ml, 9.7 patients received sonograms and 6.5 underwent biopsy.

Table 29–10. NUMBER OF BIOPSIES PERFORMED RELATED TO LEVELS OF SERUM PSA AND DRE IN 2648 PATIENTS

PSA (ng/ml)*	No. of Biopsies/No. of Patients	
	DRE +	DRE −
≤ 4.0	$\frac{300}{446}$ = 67.3%	$\frac{265}{1265}$ = 21.0%
4.1–10.0	$\frac{177}{194}$ = 91.2%	$\frac{116}{343}$ = 33.8%
<10.0	$\frac{255}{256}$ = 99.6%	$\frac{123}{144}$ = 85.4%
Total	$\frac{732}{896}$ = 82%	$\frac{504}{1752}$ = 29%

*Hybritech assay.
Abbreviations: PSA, prostate-specific antigen; DRE, digital rectal examination. Adapted from Cooner, W. H.: Prostate-specific antigen, digital rectal examination, and transrectal ultrasonic examination of the prostate in prostate cancer detection. Monogr. Urol., 12:3, 1991.

It can be argued that all abnormalities of the prostate on DRE, BPH excluded, should be evaluated by biopsy under TRUS guidance, although patients with a PSA level or ≤4 ng/ml will not often have cancer. For example, in our Stanford studies, a true TB nodule, as shown in Figure 29–34, carried a positive biopsy rate of 76 per cent. Abnormally firm prostates, when associated with a hypoechoic area in the peripheral or central zones, had a positive biopsy rate of 36 per cent (Hodge et al., 1989a). To abnormally firm areas (TBX in Table 29–2), we can now add a 30 per cent positive biopsy rate in asymmetric prostates in which one palpably soft lobe projects more posteriorly toward the rectum (TAX-Asym in Table 29–2). These positive biopsy rates are clearly cost-effective in any early detection program. It is highly likely that the 288 cancers Cooner found by the biopsies of hypoechoic areas in the peripheral or central zones would have been detected by our technique of six systematic biopsies (Hodge et al., 1989b), even if the ultrasonographer was far less experienced in TRUS technology.

In any early detection or screening program, more patients will have normal-feeling, symmetric prostates (including BPH) than abnormal prostates on DRE, as confirmed by Cooner's classic series in which two thirds of all patients examined had normal-feeling prostates (see Table 29–9). Thus, it is these 1752 patients, 5.4 per cent of whom had a hypoechoic area and cancer on biopsy, that deserve our greatest attention. Note in Tables 29–9 through 29–11 that, at PSA levels of 4 ng/ml or less by Hybritech assay, the cancer detection rate was only 2.5 per cent; 21 per cent of these 1265 patients needed a biopsy; 8.5 patients had a biopsy for every cancer detected; and 41 patients had ultrasounds for every cancer detected. Moreover, most of the cancers detected in this PSA range were in men over 65 years old.

In comparison, when the PSA level was >10 ng/ml by Hybritech assay, 31 per cent had cancer, almost all patients (85 per cent) underwent biopsy, only 2.7 patients underwent biopsy for every cancer detected, and only three patients had ultrasounds for every tumor discovered.

Dr. Cooner's work has delineated important conclusions about how we should employ these diagnostic modalities. For men with a normal DRE and a PSA level equal to or less than 4 ng/ml (Hybritech), we should proceed no further. For men with a PSA level greater than 10 ng/ml, we should immediately proceed to TRUS and biopsy, to which we would add systematic biopsies. These data represent a major contribution to the early detection of prostate cancer.

Dilemma of a Normal DRE and a Hybritech PSA Level of 4.1 to 10 ng/ml

What remains undefined from Cooner's study, however, is what to do with the intermediate PSA group (4.1 to 10 ng/ml), who have a normal DRE. Is a 5.5 per cent cancer detection rate (Table 29–9) cost-effective when, because of the nonspecificity of hypoechoic areas, 34 per cent of all patients in this category must undergo biopsy (Table 29–10)? Because only one in six patients undergoing biopsy will have cancer in this PSA range, and 18 ultrasounds will need to be performed for each cancer detected (Table 29–11), it is at least a legitimate question as to whether the nation can afford it.

Because of the annual Prostate Cancer Awareness Week sponsored by the American Urological Association and Schering Corporation, some good approximations are now available for the level of PSA in men older than 50 years in the community who answer news bureau advertisements for free DRE and PSA testing. The frequency distribution of PSA levels in Cooner's urologically referred patients is contrasted with that for a similar number of patients screened at four different centers in Table 29–7. As expected, the screened population does not have as high levels of PSA as urologically referred patients.

Another problem with investigating this group of patients is that, after we have detected cancer in one of six patients who undergo biopsy, and in one of 18 for whom we perform TRUS, we cannot tell the other 17 patients, including the five with negative biopsy results—after all this effort—that they do not have a significant cancer in the transition zone BPH area, where roughly 25 per cent of all prostate cancers arise. TRUS like DRE, with rare exceptions, cannot detect cancer in the BPH zone.

McLeary (1990) noted that, at Ann Arbor, they have detected only 12 cancers in the transition zone area out of 6437 TRUS examinations (one per 536 ultrasounds). To detect even these 12 cancers, they biopsied the transition zone area in 112 patients. These numbers make it perfectly clear that TRUS is not a technique for the detection of anteromedially located BPH cancers. To be sure, if the PSA level is very elevated and systematic biopsies in the peripheral and transition zones produce negative results, then random sampling of the transition zone may be indicated to disclose cancer.

Nonspecificity of Hypoechoic Areas

It is important to recognize from the data in Tables 29–9 and 29–10 the nonspecificity of hypoechoic areas in the peripheral and central zones of the prostate. If DRE was positive, 2.5 patients with hypoechoic areas needed biopsy for every cancer detected (732/288); if DRE was negative, 5.3 hypoechoic areas needed biopsy

Table 29–11. NUMBER OF SONOGRAMS AND BIOPSIES OF HYPOECHOIC AREAS NEEDED TO DETECT 1 CANCER (2648 PATIENTS)

PSA (ng/ml)*	No. of Sonograms Needed		No. of Biopsies Needed	
	DRE+	DRE−	DRE+	DRE−
≤4.0	9.7	40.8	6.5	8.5
4.1–10.0	2.6	18.2	2.4	6.1
>10.0	1.5	3.2	1.5	2.7

*Hybritech assay.
Abbreviations: PSA, prostate-specific antigen; DRE, digital rectal examination.
Adapted from Cooner, W. H.: Prostate-specific antigen, digital rectal examination, and transrectal ultrasonic examination of the prostate in prostate cancer detection. Monogr. Urol., 12:3, 1991.

for every cancer discovered (504/95). Overall, regardless of DRE findings, 3.2 patients must undergo biopsy because of hypoechoic areas for every patient proved to have cancer (1236/383).

What are the pathologic findings of these noncancerous, hypoechoic areas in the peripheral and central zones? McLeary and Lee reported their findings from 954 biopsies (14.8 per cent) in 6437 patients (McLeary, 1990). Of the 954 biopsies of hypoechoic areas, 35 per cent contained cancer and 6 per cent contained dysplasia. However, whereas 12 per cent showed some inflammation, 18 per cent were histologically normal, 19 per cent showed hyperplasia, and 10 per cent contained some atrophy. These last three categories, which fit within a general category of histologic "normality," constituted 47 per cent of all hypoechoic areas biopsied—a number that clearly emphasizes the nonspecificity of hypoechoic findings in the peripheral and central zones.

Six Systematic Biopsies Versus Directed Hypoechoic Biopsies

Because hypoechoic lesions in the peripheral and central zones of the prostate are not specific for cancer, and because the average prostate extends for only 4 cm in the cephalocaudal direction, we recommended six systematic biopsy specimens taken under TRUS guidance as the best way to diagnose prostate cancer. We take three 15-mm cores equally spaced between apex and base in the mid-parasagittal plane of each lobe and process all six biopsies separately (Hodge et al., 1989b). TRUS allows precise placement of the 15-mm core biopsy so that the full thickness of the peripheral zone, which seldom exceeds 10 mm in the mid-parasagittal plane, is within the biopsy core. Because the distal (deepest) part of the needle core will sample the acini and tubules of the transition zone, it is useful to mark with ink the distal end of the biopsy core before placing it in formalin so that cancer arising from transition zone tissue can be identified.

Systematic biopsies offer substantial additional information as to (1) extent (volume) of the cancer, (2) estimate of the overall Gleason grade of the whole tumor, and (3) location of the cancer at the apex or bladder neck, which may be helpful in avoiding positive surgical margins. In addition, systematic biopsies represent the only technique currently available to detect isoechoic cancers, which are said to represent as many as 21 per cent of palpable stage B cancers (Shinohara et al., 1989). They are also the only way to judge the isoechoic spread of unilobar palpable TB1 and TB2 cancers (see Fig. 29–34) into the contralateral, normal-feeling lobe (Hodge et al., 1989b). Moreover, it is well known that the more differentiated cancers (Gleason grades 3 or less) tend to be less hypoechoic to isoechoic (see Chapter 8). Because these are the more favorable cancers for potential cure, systematic biopsies are often required to detect them in the peripheral or central zone.

Most ultrasonographers take three or four routine biopsies of any hypoechoic area; thus, obtaining six

spatially separated biopsies entails minimal additional effort as the price of obtaining substantial additional, and sometimes unique, information. As we have also emphasized, measuring the actual millimeters of cancer in each core biopsy is a powerful voluming tool (Hodge et al., 1989b).

The only criticism of systematic biopsies is the possibility of detecting microscopically small—and, therefore, insignificant—foci of cancer (Cooner et al., 1989; Cooner, 1991; Scardino, 1989). We described techniques in our original publication to minimize this possibility (Hodge et al., 1989b). Indeed, the finding of hypoechoic lesions is so nonspecific for cancer that even directed biopsies at hypoechoic areas are clearly at risk of also detecting insignificant cancers. Because 47 per cent of all directed biopsies at hypoechoic areas show histologically normal prostate tissue, a 15-mm long biopsy can just as easily hit an insignificant cancer as can systematic, spatially oriented biopsies. This is especially possible in TRUS biopsies in DRE-negative patients who have a Hybritech PSA level between 4.1 and 10 ng/ml. In this large group of patients, only one of six hypoechoic directed biopsies are positive for cancer (see Table 29–11).

We have sought objective evidence on this question by looking at the volume distribution of cancer in 408 consecutive radical prostatectomies as well as in a subset of 124 patients who had systematic biopsies. As seen in Table 29–12, in only nine of 408 radical prostatectomies (2 per cent) was the cancer <0.2 ml (largest cancer in each prostate if multiple). Observe that only 9 per cent (37/408) were <0.5 ml. This distribution is no different in the subset of 124 patients undergoing radical prostatectomies who had systematic biopsies. Among these 124 patients, ten had normal or normal-feeling prostates. The volumes of the cancers (largest cancer in each prostate) ranged from 0.35 to 7 ml. In fact, the 0.35-ml cancer was accompanied by a secondary cancer of 0.32 ml. The remaining nine cancers ranged from 0.89 to 7 ml. These numbers do not suggest that we are detecting too many insignificant cancers by this highly useful technique.

Two other investigators have employed systematic biopsies extensively. Vallancien in Paris performed biopsies on 100 consecutive men with normal or normal-feeling BPH prostates (Vallancien et al., 1991a). Fourteen were found to have cancer, seven of whom were younger than 70 years of age. Table 29–13 compares the per cent positive biopsies in Cooner's (Cooner et al., 1990) and Vallancien's (Vallancien et al., 1991a) patients of the same age, stratified according to PSA levels. In the PSA range of >4 ng/ml, the systematic

Table 29–12. VOLUME DISTRIBUTION IN RADICAL PROSTATECTOMIES

	Volume (ml)				
	0–<0.2	0–<0.5	0–<4	4–12	>12
Total (n = 408)	9 (2%)	37 (9%)	240 (59%)	114 (28%)	54 (13%)
Systematic biopsies (n = 124)	4 (3%)	9 (7%)	81 (65%)	32 (26%)	11 (9%)

Table 29–13. DIRECTED VERSUS SYSTEMATIC BIOPSY IN MEN YOUNGER THAN 70 YEARS OF AGE WITH NORMAL-FEELING PROSTATES

PSA (ng/ml)*	Directed		Systematic	
	% Bx +	No. of Patients	% Bx +	No. of Patients
≤4.0	1.5	10/659	0.0	0/44
4.1–10.0	6.4	8/124	16.0	2/12
>10.0	19.0	8/42	33.0	5/15
>4.0	9.6	16/166	26.0	7/27

*Hybritech assay.

Abbreviations: PSA, prostate-specific antigen; bx, biopsy.

Adapted from Cooner, W. H., et al.: Prostate cancer detection in a clinical urological practice by ultrasonography, digital rectal examination and prostate-specific antigen. J. Urol., 143:1146, 1990 and Vallancien, G., et al.: Systematic prostatic biopsies in 100 men with no suspicion of cancer on digital rectal examination. J. Urol., 146:1308, 1991a.

positive biopsy rate was more than twice that of Cooner's directed biopsies at hypoechoic areas. In the series of Vallancien and colleagues, all seven patients younger than 70 years of age had radical prostatectomies with pathologic calculated cancer volumes of 2.2 to 11.2 ml. Apparently, five of these seven highly significant cancers were not seen as hypoechoic areas on TRUS.

Huland and Hammerer in West Berlin have performed the largest number of systematic biopsies reported to date (n = 419) and have shared their data with us (Table 29–14). Their DRE classification of normal (including normal BPH), abnormally firm, and palpable nodules (TA and TB) is similar to the classification we used when biopsies were taken of only hypoechoic lesions (Hodge et al., 1989a). The similarities between these two studies—our standard biopsies of hypoechoic lesions and Huland and Hammerer's systematic biopsies—are striking.

In the DRE-negative, abnormally firm, and nodular prostates, their cancer detection rate was 12 per cent, 32 per cent, and 71 per cent, respectively, compared with our 5 per cent, 36 per cent, and 79 per cent. Whereas Huland and Hammerer's cancer detection rate for patients with normal DRE was twice ours (and Cooner's as shown in Table 29–9), their finding of 12 per cent is close to that of Vallancien at 10 per cent for

Table 29–14. CANCER DETECTION RATES FROM SIX SYSTEMATIC BIOPSIES IN 419 MEN

Digital Rectal Examination	Prostate-Specific Antigen*		
	0–3.99 ng/ml (n = 162)	4–10 ng/ml (n = 84)	>10 ng/ml (n = 173)
Negative† (n = 59)	3% (1/35)	13% (2/15)	44% (4/9)
Abnormally firm (n = 192)	6% (4/63)	32% (12/38)	52% (47/91)
TB or TC (n = 168)	42% (27/64)	74% (23/31)	96% (70/73)
Total	20% (32/162)	44% (37/84)	70% (121/173)

*Hybritech assay.

†Negative digital rectal examination includes normal-feeling benign prostatic hyperplasia.

Data from H. Huland and P. Hammerer, 1991.

seven cancers in 71 patients. All seven cancers were known to be of substantial volume. The progressive rise in cancer detection rates with increasing PSA levels in all three categories in Table 29–14 also argues strongly that systematic biopsies are detecting biologically significant cancer.

We conclude that systematic biopsies, an important and informative technique for obtaining maximum histologic and clinically useful information on prostate cancer, are probably no more likely to detect insignificant, microscopic cancers than biopsy of nonspecific hypoechoic areas on TRUS. Systematic biopsies are far more likely to detect significant *isoechoic* cancers, which can be missed by relying on nonspecific, subjective hypoechoic areas. Indeed, the report from Scardino's group that 10 (20 per cent) of 51 cases undergoing biopsy by both TRUS and digital guidance were positive by digital biopsy and negative by ultrasound guidance is a strong argument for systematic biopsies (Shabsigh et al., 1989).

Systematic biopsies are especially advantageous in normal or normal-feeling prostates, for which the positive biopsy rate is more than twice that of hypoechoic-directed biopsies (Tables 29–13 and 29–14). Equally useful, however, is the spatial information obtained in relation to potentially positive surgical margins. Better representation of the true Gleason grade of the whole cancer is an obvious advantage of six evenly spaced biopsies.

Aspiration Biopsies

Aspiration biopsies are now less popular because of the Swedish Biopty instrument, which produces an 18-gauge needle core 15 mm in length and which, for most patients, is less painful than aspiration biopsy. Most pathologists believe that the Gleason grading system and its architectural classification cannot be utilized in cytologic grading. Grade 3 dysplasia cannot be readily distinguished from invasive cancer because the nucleoli, nuclei, and cells have essentially the same appearance. Aspiration also has the disadvantage of yielding no volumetric information; therefore, measuring the millimeters of cancer in solid-core biopsies is a powerful tool. Before the advent of TRUS-guided biopsy, aspiration had the advantage of covering a greater internal area of the prostate by moving the needle through a larger area of the prostate. Overall, although we believe fine needle aspiration of the prostate is not nearly as useful as six systematic Biopty needle cores, a balanced presentation on some of the advantages and disadvantages of aspiration biopsies has been published by Stilmant and colleagues (1989).

Cystoscopy and Intravenous Urograms

Unless the patient has microscopic hematuria, there is no need for either of these examinations in the evaluation of patients with clinical stage A or B prostate cancer.

Computed Tomography and Magnetic Resonance Imaging

Probably 50 per cent of the new patients seen at Stanford for clinical stage A and B disease with the diagnosis of prostate cancer arrive with the results of a computed tomographic (CT) scan, magnetic resonance imaging (MRI), or sometimes both. Like RIA-PAP, these examinations are useless, exceedingly expensive, and create an unnecessary cost to the health care system. The physician who orders a CT scan or MRI for clinical stage TA or TB carcinoma understands little about the biology of prostate cancer at this stage of the disease and the limitations of these imaging modalities at the microscopic level. If the biopsy cores are loaded with undifferentiated cancer and the PSA level is greater than 100 ng/ml by the Yang assay, there may be some reason to seek the presence of large retroperitoneal lymph nodes, which might be aspirated to save surgical exploration. In such an instance, CT serves as well as MRI, but the sensitivity of detecting positive lymph nodes is so low with both of these imaging modalities as to make them almost useless.

Most CT and MRI scans are actually ordered with the mistaken idea that they will identify either intra- or extra-prostatic cancer and, thus, add useful information. Capsular penetration into the periprostatic fat and into the seminal vesicles is a microscopic phenomenon (McNeal et al., 1990b) that is far from the resolving power of even MRI (Rifkin et al., 1990) unless exceedingly gross disease is present, which should be detectable on rectal examination or indicated by the level of serum PSA. TRUS, when combined with systematic biopsies, yields much better information than can ever be obtained with MRI or CT. Even so, TRUS is also a very insensitive imaging modality for detecting periprostatic or seminal vesicle invasion at the microscopic level (Rifkin et al., 1990). Terris and associates (1990) have reported the TRUS findings in 300 patients whose seminal vesicles were examined histologically.

Cystoscopy, intravenous urograms, CT, MRI, and RIA-PAP should almost never be obtained in the evaluation of clinical stage A and B prostate cancer. Even in the case of clinical stage C disease of any size, CT and MRI add little to what an inexpensive ultrasound of the kidneys can do in assessing obstructive disease.

Bone Scans

Bone scans are useful, but PSA testing has greatly restricted their need. Oesterling (1991) has argued convincingly that any radical prostatectomy candidate with a Hybritech serum PSA level ≤20 essentially has no chance of demonstrating bone metastases. In postradical prostatectomy patients, Terris and co-workers (1991a) have shown that as long as PSA remains undetectable, there is no need to obtain a bone scan. Lange and his associates (Lightner et al., 1988) have presented an abstract with the same conclusion. Rare exceptions may occur.

TREATMENT OF PROSTATE CANCER

General Considerations

The treatment of prostate cancer is largely determined by the volume and grade of the tumor at the time of therapy. With a cancer volume of 1.5 ml, perineural space invasion into the periprostatic fat is not uncommon; with 3 ml, invasion of the seminal vesicle can occur in clinical stage B cancer but not in stage A cancers; and with 3.2 ml of Gleason grade 4 or 5 cancer, microscopic lymph node invasion is common (see Fig. 29–25) (McNeal et al., 1986a, 1990a; Stamey et al., 1988).

Because escape of prostate cancer into the periprostatic fat and seminal vesicles and lymph node invasion are microscopic, there is no imaging modality capable of signaling early spread into these areas. CT and MRI are particularly insensitive to the spread of cancer until the invasion is gross and more readily discerned by other methods, such as PSA testing and DRE. Seminal vesicle invasion can be measured by direct biopsy under TRUS guidance (Hodge et al., 1989a; Vallancien et al., 1991b), but with this single exception, TRUS and MRI are equally poor as early staging modalities for prostate cancer (Rifkin et al., 1990).

When treatment is by radical prostatectomy, the presence of positive surgical margins, often iatrogenic, interposes further serious restrictions on the outcome of therapy, which may have little to do with the otherwise natural history of prostate cancer in the absence of positive margins.

Natural History

In addition to these confounding variables of measuring early local spread by clinically inadequate imaging modalities, and the importance of the surgeon avoiding iatrogenically positive surgical margins, another critical issue is a prolonged natural history of prostate cancer in the absence of interventional therapy, especially in the early clinical stages.

Utilizing serial PSA determinations in 43 untreated patients with prostate cancers, we reported that over two thirds of all clinical stage A and B cancers were doubling at rates exceeding 4 years (Schmid et al., 1991; Stamey and Kabalin, 1989). These measurements are in keeping with the prolonged natural history of palpable clinical stage B prostate cancers described by Whitmore and co-workers (1991). Whitmore followed 29 clinical stage B1 cancers for a median of 10.3 years. Whereas all of these cancers progressed in their palpable size, and 69 per cent of the patients received "expectant" treatment (nine had ^{125}I seed implantation, two received hormones, and nine had a TURP), the actuarial 15-year survival was 67 ± 12 per cent (standard error, SE). Only three patients died of prostatic cancer during this period of follow-up, and only four died of other causes; six of the 29 developed metastases.

George (1988), Johansson and associates (1989), and Adolfsson and Carstensen (1991) have presented somewhat similar data in terms of the high rate of local progression but a low rate of metastases, although the follow-up in these three studies is relatively short—5 to 7 years, 5 years, and 8 years, respectively—accounting in part for the relatively few deaths from prostate cancer. In the report by Adolfsson and Carstensen (1991) on 61 patients younger than 70 years of age with clinical stage TB nodules, the cumulative 5- and 10-year probabilities for tumor progression to stage C disease, for developing metastases, and for dying of prostate cancer were 49 per cent and 72 per cent, 8 per cent and 23 per cent, and 2 per cent and 8 per cent, respectively. As in the Whitmore series, a number of these patients received endocrine and radiation therapy, and three were even subjected to radical prostatectomy. Nevertheless, Whitmore's long-term study of 29 "expectantly" treated clinical stage B1 cancers, 80 per cent of which will be less than 4 ml in volume, serves to emphasize the steady but slow progression of early palpable prostate cancer.

The finding that local progression occurs long before identifiable distant metastases indicates the importance for the clinician and patient of giving proper consideration to the competing causes of death in this age group. It is fair to state that assessing the life expectancy of patients with prostate cancer prior to treatment is far more important than for any other genitourinary malignancy. If the patient does not have an estimated 10- to 15-year life expectancy, neither radical prostatectomy nor irradiation therapy should be considered unless there are unusual mitigating circumstances. As discussed further on, these patients are probably well served by simple expectant therapy with TURP for obstruction or hormonal therapy, singly or combined.

Contrary to the findings in these highly selected series of expectantly treated patients are those in the two large series of patients treated by Bagshaw (1988) and Lerner and co-workers (1991). Bagshaw observed a 35 per cent 15-year actuarial risk of prostate cancer death in patients whose tumors were judged to be limited to the prostate and a 65 per cent risk if extracapsular disease was present. In the studies by Lerner, the 10-year risk of prostate cancer death was 30 ± 7 per cent in patients with clinically localized disease. Why are these cancer-specific death rates so much higher in radiation-treated patients than in the more expectantly managed patients just discussed? Although the answer is not entirely clear, Lerner and colleagues (1991) have provided an excellent discussion of this topic.

Prostate cancer is thought to be less malignant in men older than 70 than in men younger than 60 years of age, but there is little objective data to support this concept (Adami et al., 1986). To prove this hypothesis would require detecting cancers of equivalent volumes and grades among the age groups under comparison, which would be very difficult to do.

Dilemma of a 40 Per Cent Histologic Incidence and Only an 8 Per Cent Lifetime Probability of Being Diagnosed with Prostate Cancer

Applying the Surveillance, Epidemiology and End Results (SEER) data from the National Cancer Institute

for the probability of men in the United States to be diagnosed with prostate cancer at 5-year age intervals, and applying United States mortality rates from insurance companies for the probability of surviving to the start of these 5-year intervals, it is possible to calculate what the lifetime probability is for a man to be diagnosed with prostate cancer. Seidman and co-workers (1985) calculated this probability to be 9.5 per cent with a lifetime risk of dying of prostate cancer at 2.9 per cent. Dr. Alice Whittemore, Chief of Epidemiology at Stanford University School of Medicine, independently calculated the lifetime probability of being diagnosed with prostate cancer and found it to be 8.8 per cent in 1989. If we take the last figure and reduce it by 0.8 per cent to withdraw those patients in the SEER data who were diagnosed with clinical stage A1 or A2 cancers and whose tumors are too small to be of any consequence (about 9 per cent of the 8.8 per cent), we have a lifetime probability risk of 8 per cent for a man to be diagnosed with clinical stage A1, A2, B1 to B3, C, D1, or D2 cancer. This 8 per cent figure is also in agreement with case control studies of spouses of men known to have prostate cancer (Steinberg et al., 1990). However, because at least 40 per cent of men older than 50 years of age in the United States have histologic evidence of prostate cancer, how do we know whom to treat if four of five men with histologic cancer do not need therapy?

One answer is to take an unselected series of human prostates from men who are not known to have cancer and determine the volume of the largest cancer. If the series is large enough and the cancers are evenly distributed throughout all volumes, the 8 per cent largest cancers should represent the 8 per cent of men who were destined to have prostate cancers large enough to be diagnosed during their lifetimes, if the prostates had not been removed.

We have determined the volume of cancer in 139 consecutive patients followed by F. S. Freiha at Stanford, none of whom were known to have prostate cancer, and all of whom were having cystoprostatectomy for bladder cancer (Stamey et al., 1991). As seen in Figure 29–35, 55 of the 139 prostates were cancerous (40 per cent). Cancers equal to or greater than 0.5 ml in volume represent 7.9 per cent of the 139 prostates. Unfortunately, 0.2-ml cancers, which are both palpable on DRE and readily visible in the peripheral or central zones on TRUS (Stamey, 1989), represent 12.2 per cent of the population—far in excess of the 8 per cent of men who will have tumors large enough to be diagnosed in their lifetime. In comparison, cancers greater than 1.0 ml in volume represent only 4.3 per cent of the 139 patients, only one half of the 8 per cent who will develop a cancer large enough to be detected in the SEER surveillance system.

We conclude from this information that cancers of volume 0.5 ml or greater are appropriate for therapy, and those less than 0.5 ml need not be treated.

Regional Lymph Node Metastases

Johansson and associates (1989) did not know the lymph node status of their patients (see Table 29–4),

VOLUME DISTRIBUTION OF 55 UNSUSPECTED LARGEST PROSTATE CANCERS IN 139 CYSTOPROSTECTOMIES

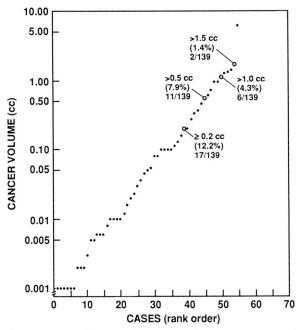

Figure 29–35. In 139 patients undergoing cystoprostatectomies for bladder cancer, none was known to have prostate cancer. On digital rectal examination (DRE), 137 had normal-feeling prostates. The two abnormal prostate glands on DRE did not contain cancer in the area of the palpable abnormality. The volume of the largest cancer in each prostate is presented on a logarithmic scale. The number and percentage of cancers ≥0.2 cc, 0.5 cc, 1.0 cc, and 1.5 cc are indicated along the plot. Cancer volumes of 0.5 cc or larger (7.9 per cent) correspond most closely to the 8-per cent probability of these men developing prostate cancer (see text), if the bladder tumors had not required removal of the prostates. (From Stamey, T. A., et al.: National Conference on Prostate Cancer, American Cancer Society. Cancer, 1992.)

but it is well known that nearly 30 per cent of stage TA and TB patients will have at least microscopic metastases to the pelvic lymph nodes (Donohue et al., 1982; Gervasi et al., 1989; Smith et al., 1983). Most of these metastases occur in patients with either clinical stage TA2 or palpable TB2 to TB3 disease. For example, in 34 of 417 patients undergoing radical prostatectomy at Stanford who had microscopic, undetectable positive pelvic lymph nodes at staging, only four cases had a palpable TB1 nodule. Sixteen were in stage TB2, eight were in stage TB3, two were suspected of being in early stage TC, two were in stage TA2, and two had large, benign-feeling prostates with high serum levels of PSA. Fifty per cent of all patients with clinical stage C disease are known to have positive lymph nodes (Donohue et al., 1982; Zincke et al., 1986).

Even a single microscopic metastatic focus in only one of multiple pelvic lymph nodes is a hallmark of prostate cancer that is incurable by any currently available modality of treatment; 70 per cent of these patients will die of prostate cancer rather than an unrelated cause (see Scardino, 1989, for review). However, because of the long natural history of prostate cancer, many of these patients will do well for 10 years.

Scardino's group (Gervasi et al., 1989) reported a cancer specific mortality rate at 10 years of 57 per cent using a combination of radioactive gold seed implantation and external beam irradiation. From the group of 146 surgically staged and then irradiated patients that we previously reported (Freiha and Bagshaw, 1984), we followed up on all 62 patients who had metastasis to their pelvic lymph nodes and whose positive lymph node bearing area was included in the radiation field—not a single patient was cured of cancer. Most died of carcinoma, and the few who are still alive have progressive tumor. Smith and associates (1984) have presented similar data.

Possible Role of Transurethral Resection in the Dissemination of Prostate Cancer

McGowan (1980) and Hanks and colleagues (1983) suggested that TURP disseminates prostate cancer cells, influencing both survival and time to progression, especially in TC1 to TC3 tumors (see Table 29–2). However, when greater efforts were made to compare patients with similar cancer stages and grades, little evidence was found to support these reputed adverse effects from TURP (Forman et al., 1986; Kuban et al., 1985; Meacham et al., 1989; Paulson and Cox, 1987).

Radiation Therapy

External Beam Irradiation

Dr. Malcolm Bagshaw and associates reported their 30-year radiation experience with 900 patients at Stanford in 1988, precisely outlining the clinical staging system they used to classify their radiation results. If these results are referenced to the clinical staging system used in Table 29–2 and Figure 29–34, this report shows that the actuarial 15-year survival rate for irradiation treatment of TB1 cancer occupying less than half of one lobe is almost as good as that for radical prostatectomy (about 48 per cent) for this earliest of all palpable stages of prostate cancer. However, if the induration or nodule occupies more than half of one lobe, or extends bilaterally (clinical stages TB2 and TB3 in Figure 29–34), the 15-year actuarial survival falls to 23 per cent (Fig. 29–36). Because Whitmore reports an actuarial survival for "expectantly" treated B1 nodules of 67 ± 12 per cent (SE), it is a reasonable assumption that these excellent results on radiation for TB1 nodules are the result of the natural history of the cancer. That a patient with any palpable cancer larger than a TB1 nodule has only a 23 per cent survival rate 15 years after radiation is of substantial concern.

Freiha and Bagshaw (1984) reported that 61 per cent of patients undergoing finger-guided, perineal biopsies 18 months or more following completion of radiotherapy had biopsy samples positive for cancer, and that these distinguished patients at a higher risk for development of metastases. Kabalin and co-workers (1989a), employing systematic, TRUS-guided needle biopsies of 27 consecutive patients who presented at a mean of 5.2 years

STAGE B PROSTATIC CANCER - (Node Status Unknown)

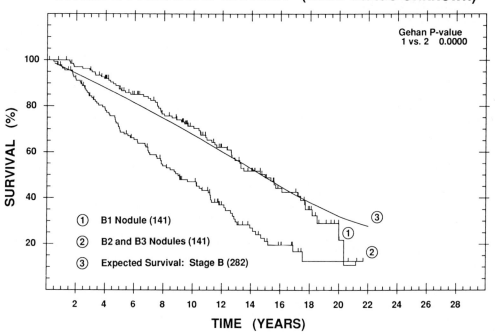

Figure 29–36. Actuarial survival curves (Kaplan and Meier) for 141 clinical stage TB1 nodules and 141 TB2 and TB3 nodules (combined) radiated at Stanford University School of Medicine. Curve 3 represents the expected survival of age-matched males for these 282 patients with clinical stage TB cancer. Observe that the 15-year acturial survival for TB2 and TB3 patients is 23 per cent. The bone status and serum prostate-specific antigen (PSA) at the time of follow-up is unknown. (Modified from Bagshaw, M. A., et al.: NCI Monographs, 7:47, 1988.)

after external beam radiation therapy, found that 93 per cent were positive for cancer, including 20 of 22 with normal postirradiation DREs. These positive biopsy findings occurred at all levels of serum PSA, including 83 per cent of patients with levels <10 ng/ml (Yang assay). These two studies emphasize an extraordinarily high failure rate of external beam radiation therapy to sterilize the local cancer.

Indeed, survival rates for 101 patients with TA, TB, and TC (NOMO) prostate cancers treated conservatively with TURP or simple retropubic enucleation appear to be as good as those for historical controls (Moskovitz et al., 1987).

Combined Gold Seed Implantation and External Beam Radiotherapy

Scardino and Wheeler (1988) have compared the actuarial 5-, 10-, and 15-year survival rates for combined radiotherapy to survival rates for external beam results alone. For all clinical stage TA2 and TB patients, the actuarial survival rates at 5, 10, and 15 years for combined therapy are 86 per cent, 59 per cent, and 28 per cent, compared with 81 per cent, 60 per cent, and 34 per cent for external beam therapy. For clinical stage TC patients, combined gold seed implantation plus external beam radiotherapy was associated with actuarial survival rates of 74 per cent, 34 per cent, and 17 per cent at 5, 10, and 15 years, compared with external beam therapy results at Stanford of 61 per cent, 35 per cent, and 17 per cent.

Retropubic Interstitial Implantation of Iodine 125 Seeds

Although ^{125}I interstitial seed implantation was begun at Sloan-Kettering Memorial Hospital in New York in

1970, and a minimal follow-up of 5 years for the first 100 patients was published by Whitmore (1980), only later have 10-year follow-ups been published (Whitmore and Hilaris, 1989). At 10 years, 40 per cent of TB1 and 70 per cent of TB2 tumors had progressed. This form of radiation therapy has no serious advocates at the present time.

One of the limitations of all forms of brachytherapy has been the nonhomogeneous distribution of the interstitial seed implants despite the best of efforts. Holm was an early advocate of ultrasound-guided, perineal implantation techniques to achieve a better distribution of the seeds with less morbidity (Carter et al., 1989). Although there are clear technical advantages to this approach, it is highly likely that this will prove to be one more form of inadequate radiation therapy. Palladium implants are thought by most clinicians to offer no advantages over other available isotopes.

A few radiation treatment centers are combining 5000 rads of external beam therapy with subsequent retropubically guided iridium 192 implantation using perineal template removable implants (Brindle et al., 1989). At Stanford, this procedure is combined with interstitial hyperthermia by microwave activation of the implants.

Irradiation Therapy for Local Control in Clinical Stage TC and D1(N+) Disease

What is the role of radiotherapy in achieving local control in large cancers, both N+ and N0? Surya and Provet (1989) reviewed the manifestations and treatment of advanced prostate cancer. In general, there are only two clinical consequences of prostate cancer: local growth and metastatic disease. Is irradiation an effective way to control morbidity from local growth of prostate cancer?

Gibbons and associates (1979) reported excellent local control in 209 patients with clinical stage TC cancer treated with external beam radiation therapy; they remain advocates of this approach today (personal communication). Holzman and colleagues (1989), however, reported local tumor recurrence in 53 per cent of their patients who also experienced serious morbidity. Other investigators have reported no differences in local progression when radiated patients are compared with non-radiated controls (Smith et al., 1984; Steinberg et al., 1990). Paulson and co-workers (1984) reported no difference in the time to first evidence of distant metastases in patients randomly assigned to external beam irradiation and those expectantly treated with delayed hormonal therapy at the time of metastases.

One serious problem of irradiation for stage TC or D1 cancer is the 33 per cent rate of urinary incontinence following a TURP for progressive urinary obstruction months or years after completion of irradiation (Green et al., 1990). This unexpected complication has been experienced on several occasions at Stanford. The prostatic chips removed at TUR nearly always show 100 per cent involvement with Gleason grade 5 cancer. Even though the resection is carefully limited to the area proximal to the midverumontanum, the resulting incontinence is severe and presumably derives from a combination of irradiation to and invasion of the sphincter combined with resection of vesical neck and preprostatic sphincter mechanisms. We now avoid TUR in these patients if at all possible. We prefer early hormonal therapy or simple vesical neck incisions rather than risk postirradiation urinary incontinence.

Thus, the urologist does have a viable and simpler alternative than irradiation to treat incurable prostate cancer in a manner that controls the local disease. The judicious use of TURP without irradiation, plus early hormonal therapy when it seems indicated, may be as good for local control of the disease as radiotherapy. Further randomized studies would help with this dilemma. As is discussed in the section on hormonal therapy, early hormone therapy is preferable to delayed treatment.

Significance of Postirradiation Positive Biopsies

Whereas Cox and Kline (1983) did not believe that biopsy of the prostate after irradiation was predictive of subsequent survival, further reports by Freiha and Bagshaw (1984), Schellhammer and associates (1987), and Scardino and Wheeler (1988) all show clearly that the presence of positive biopsy findings 18 months or more after irradiation therapy strongly correlates with biologically active disease and treatment failure. A rising or elevated PSA level 1 year or longer after radiotherapy is also indicative of irradiation failure (Kabalin et al., 1989a; Stamey et al., 1989a).

Salvage Prostatectomy After Radiation Failure

If a patient has a life expectancy of 10 to 15 years at the time radiation failure is detected, the possibility of salvage radical prostatectomy may be considered. However, the seminal vesicles should be negative for cancer as determined by TRUS-guided biopsy. In addition, the serum level of PSA must not be too elevated, and bone scan findings should be negative. If a CT scan of the pelvis and abdomen shows no visible lymph nodes, we reluctantly offer the patient a salvage radical prostatectomy. In a small series of 20 patients at Stanford, one third are completely dry, one third have stress urinary incontinence at the end of the day, and one third are very incontinent. Patients who are dry are usually those who had 7000 rads of irradiation without a prior staging lymphadenectomy. Of these patients, 50 per cent have an undetectable PSA level with a follow-up of 6 months to 6 years.

At the 1990 meeting of the American College of Surgeons in San Francisco, Scardino presented his results on 30 patients, 77 per cent of whom had prior pelvic lymph node dissection and 70 per cent of whom had retropubic interstitial seed implantations. Fifty-four per cent were continent (0 to 1 pad per day), and 53 per cent had no recurrence with an undetectable PSA level at a mean follow-up of 32 months (range 2 to 70 months).

The decision to perform salvage prostatectomy is difficult because of the possibility that early hormone therapy might offer equivalent survival advantage with a potentially better quality of life.

Radical Prostatectomy

The nerve-sparing retropubic radical prostatectomy developed by Walsh and associates (Walsh and Donker, 1982; Walsh et al., 1983) and the recognition of an unsuspected and extraordinarily high failure rate of 7000 rads to sterilize local prostate cancer (Freiha and Bagshaw, 1984; Kabalin et al., 1989a) have greatly increased the number of radical prostatectomies performed in the United States for clinically localized stage A and B cancer.

Significance of Capsular Penetration

From careful histopathologic studies at Stanford, however, we now recognize, as shown in Figure 29–30, that only 40 per cent of clinical stage TB prostate cancers thought to be localized on DRE are actually confined to the prostate (McNeal et al., 1986a, 1990b; Stamey et al., 1988). The 10 per cent of patients with microscopic lymph node metastases are clearly incurable, as are 75 per cent of those with seminal vesicle invasion when post–radical prostatectomy PSA level is chosen as a measure of cure (Stein et al., 1992). However, it is likely that many of the 35 per cent of patients with clinical stage TB prostate cancers who have some capsular penetration into the periprostatic fat can be cured by radical prostatectomy, provided that the neurovascular nerve bundle is not separated from the prostate capsule.

Based on our histologic information that capsular penetration into the periprostatic fat most commonly occurs precisely in the area of the neurovascular bundle, we argued that the nerve-sparing radical prostatectomy could potentially compromise the chance for a surgical cure in 27 per cent of clinical stage B1 nodules and in 88 per cent of stage B2 and B3 nodules (Stamey et al., 1988). Bigg and co-workers (1990) reported an alarmingly high incidence of positive surgical margins in nerve-sparing radical prostatectomies of clinical stage TB2 and TB3 cancers (tumor >2 cm on DRE or bilateral, histologically proven tumor by the investigators' definition).

In a report on 250 patients undergoing nerve-sparing radical prostatectomy, 68 patients had capsular penetration (27 per cent) and, surprisingly, *all* but one of these had positive surgical margins (Catalona and Bigg, 1990). We examined 98 cases from 335 patients with clinical stage TB cancer who underwent radical prostatectomy and who had cancer penetration into the periprostatic fat but no seminal vesicle invasion or lymph node metastases. Only 33 per cent (32/98) of our cases with capsular penetration were associated with positive surgical margins. We are unable to explain this discrepancy between the significance of capsular penetration and positive surgical margins in Catalona's series and the Stanford series, but our data support our contention that positive margins can be avoided in two thirds of all patients with capsular penetration if the proper surgical procedure is performed in patients without seminal vesicle or pelvic lymph node invasion.

Significance of Positive Surgical Margins

Eggleston and Walsh (1985) initially reported only a 7 per cent overall incidence of positive surgical margins in their first 100 radical prostatectomies. Catalona and Bigg (1990) reported a 30 to 33 per cent incidence of positive surgical margins even in patients with no seminal vesicle invasion or pelvic lymph node metastases who were operated on for clinical stage TA and TB disease. Stamey and associates (1990) reported a 23 per cent positive margin rate in 136 clinical stage B radical prostatectomies with cancer volumes <12 ml. In the last study, positive margins for the first time were divided into those associated with capsular penetration of the cancer and those caused by inadvertent surgical incisions through the capsule into cancer within the prostate; surgical recommendations were made on how to avoid many of these positive margins (see 1990 video from Schering Corporation on the Stanford radical retropubic prostatectomy).

Organ-Confined Versus Non–organ-Confined Cancers in Clinical Stage TA and TB Disease

Because clinical stage TA and TB disease are spatially different tumors (see earlier discussion), it is interesting to note that, although 65 per cent of 49 stage A transition zone cancers were organ confined (see Fig. 29–37) compared with 40 per cent of clinical stage B peripheral zone cancers (see Fig. 29–38), the volume distribution between organ-confined and non–organ-confined can-

cers was extraordinarily similar for stage A and B disease. This similarity of volume distribution, especially in the non–organ-confined groups, argues strongly for the fact that clinical stage A and B cancers are not biologically different malignancies as thought by Christensen and colleagues (1990). We should not forget the survival data of Barnes and co-workers (1976), who could not distinguish TA from TB cancers.

ESCAPE OF NON–ORGAN-CONFINED CANCERS FROM THE PROSTATE. From our analysis of 243 radical prostatectomies, we concluded that 50 per cent of all prostate cancers escape the boundaries of the prostate by following the perineural spaces into the periprostatic fat; 23 per cent follow the ejaculatory ducts into the seminal vesicles (peripheral or central zone cancers only, not transition zone tumors); 21 per cent invade Denonvilliers' fascia, especially in the "midprostate" area; 2 to 4 per cent invade by direct tumor extension laterally; and the remaining 4 to 5 per cent invade the bladder neck or membranous urethra (Villers et al., 1989, 1990). Anatomic knowledge of the precise areas where prostate cancer escapes from the prostate should improve the results from radical retropubic prostatectomy, especially in those patients with extraprostatic extension who do not have lymph node metastases (Stamey et al., 1990).

Cancer Location in Relation to Digital Rectal Examination and Transurethral Resection

In terms of radical prostatectomy, it is worth noting that 94 per cent of clinically palpable stage B tumors are located in the peripheral or central zones of the prostate. Of the remaining 6 per cent, 3 per cent were large transition zone cancers (2.5 to 26 ml in volume) palpable on DRE, and 3 per cent were palpable BPH nodules in which cancer was diagnosed fortuitously in the transition zone (Villers et al., 1990). Of all clinical stage A cancers detected at the time of TURP, about 9 per cent will represent impalpable peripheral zone cancers invading the transition zone, where they are partially removed by the resectoscope.

Role of Volume and Grade in Determining Prognosis After Radical Prostatectomy

Although the extent of cancer penetration into the periprostatic fat, the per cent Gleason grade 4 and 5 of the whole cancer, and the extent of seminal vesicle invasion all increase with increasing cancer volume, volume and cancer grade are the two most important variables (McNeal et al., 1986a, 1990a; Stamey et al., 1988). The heterogeneity of the cancer grade in the Gleason grading system makes it difficult to employ grade as a biologic marker unless the biopsy is representative of the whole tumor, perhaps from systematic biopsies.

As seen in Table 29–15, and recalling that any grade in the Gleason system must occupy at least 5 per cent

Table 29–15. GLEASON GRADE DISTRIBUTION BY VOLUME IN 408 RADICAL PROSTATECTOMIES

	Volume (ml)			
	0–<0.5 (n = 37)	0–<4 (n = 240)	4–12 (n = 114)	>12 (n = 54)
No. with ≥5% Gleason grade 4 + 5	9 (24%)	95 (40%)	93 (82%)	51 (94%)
No. with ≥50% Gleason grade 4 + 5	3 (8%)	36 (15%)	45 (39%)	26 (48%)

of the cancer in the biopsy, even cancers <4 ml in volume can have 5 per cent or more of Gleason grade 4+5 in as many as 40 per cent of cases, and 15 per cent of these cancers will have 50 per cent or more of Gleason grade 4+5 in the whole cancer. Hence, the presence of some Gleason grade 4+5 cancer in these pre–radical prostatectomy biopsies is not a useful marker of volume.

Table 29–15 also indicates that the percentage of Gleason grade 4+5 cancer, whether ≥5 per cent or ≥50 per cent, will not distinguish cancer volumes of 4 to 12 ml from those >12 ml. Thus, we are left with cancer volume as our most important clinical index, because we know that patients with cancers <4 ml fall into an excellent prognostic group, whereas there is no cure for stage TB cancers >12 ml (Stamey et al., 1990), even in the absence of seminal vesicle invasion and positive pelvic lymph nodes.

To be sure, PSA levels after radical prostatectomy in cancers >12 ml, which unfortunately represents 13 per cent of all our clinical stage TA and TB disease (see Table 29–12), can remain undetectable for as long as 3 or 4 years before becoming detectable and starting to rise. Of our 54 radical prostatectomies with cancer volumes >12 ml (see Table 29–12), 14 (26 per cent) have an undetectable PSA level; however, seven have been followed for less than 12 months, 12 for less than 24 months, and one each at 25 and 34 months.

Because we do well with cancers <4 ml in volume and probably should not operate on cancers >12 ml in volume until we have effective chemotherapeutic agents, we believe that a combination of DRE, PSA testing, six systematic biopsies with spatial separation of each core, and measurement of the millimeters of cancer in each biopsy will allow a reasonable and easy distinction between ≤4 ml and ≥12 ml of cancer. But how well do we do in recognizing cancer volumes between 4 and 12 ml? We are not sure, and this area deserves substantial research.

In general, 80 per cent of B1 nodules will be less than 4 ml in volume, and almost all are curable by radical prostatectomy if positive surgical margins are not created. We all know that TB2 and TB3 nodules represent larger cancers and therefore carry a progressively greater risk of surgically positive margins (especially if nerve-sparing operations are done), seminal vesicle invasion, and lymph node metastases. Jewett's survival rate for stage TB cancers larger than the smallest palpable nodule (a little larger than the TB1 nodule classified in Table 29–2 and shown in Figure 29–34), was only 18

per cent alive without disease at 15 years (Jewett, 1975). These statistics are, of course, true survivals (not actuarials) and represent an era prior to 1951.

A series at Johns Hopkins, Baltimore, from 1951 to 1963 reported a similar 15-year survival of 25 per cent, free of disease, in these larger TB2 and TB3 cancers, and a 51 per cent survival rate for patients with the smaller TB1 tumors (Elder et al., 1982; Jewett, 1980). Gibbons and associates (1989) reported similar results.

These series all involve perineal prostatectomies, and Bagshaw's 15-year actuarial survival rate of 23 per cent for approximately similar sized TB2 and TB3 nodules in Figure 29–36 is about the same as that for 7000 rads of external beam radiotherapy (Bagshaw et al., 1988). In comparison, Bagshaw's data are actuarial rather than crude survivals, and it is not known whether the patients are free of disease or not. The combination of 5000 rads of external beam therapy and gold seed implantation shows similar survival rates to Bagshaw's data (Scardino and Wheeler, 1988). Whether a more radical retropubic prostatectomy can improve on these dismal 15-year results on larger clinical stage B2 to B3 cancers remains to be seen (Stamey et al., 1990).

Optimum surgical extirpation for clinical stage TB cancer then depends on reliably estimating the volume and grade of intracapsular cancer because the smaller volumes are likely to be organ-confined (Figs. 29–37 and 29–38). Urologists now have at their disposal at least three tools that were unavailable to Jewett and Gibbons when their classic series were accumulating. The preoperative level of serum PSA is the most important advance. Systematic biopsies, spatially separated, with quantitation (mm) of the cancer in each 15-mm core and improved utilization of Gleason grade 4+5, are the second most important advance (Hodge et al., 1989b; McNeal et al., 1990a). The third advance is measurement of the volume of hypoechoic cancer on TRUS (Shinohara et al., 1989). The latter measurement, however, is the least useful because, like DRE, it grossly underestimates the volume of cancer in the prostate (Terris et al., 1991b). DRE as an estimate of volume for clinical stage TB disease is helpful only for stage TB1 disease, as illustrated in Figure 29–34, for which 80 per cent of all such palpable cancers will be less than 4 ml in volume.

In addition to these critical preoperative estimates of intracapsular volume and grade, there are no reliable preoperative staging techniques to detect the 35 per cent of patients who have microscopic capsular penetration into the periprostatic fat or the 10 per cent of patients who have microscopic pelvic lymph node metastases observed in Figure 29–30. The 15 per cent of patients with microscopic seminal vesicle invasion can probably be detected by TRUS-guided biopsies (Hodge et al., 1989a; Vallancien et al., 1991b), but it must be remembered that the *degree* (extent) of seminal vesicle invasion may be important prognostically (Villers et al., 1990).

As repeatedly emphasized in this chapter, MRI and CT scans are not useful for clinical stage TA and TB cancers. TRUS is no better than MRI (Rifkin et al., 1990) for detection of microscopic extracapsular prostate cancer. However, ultrasound has a real advantage in

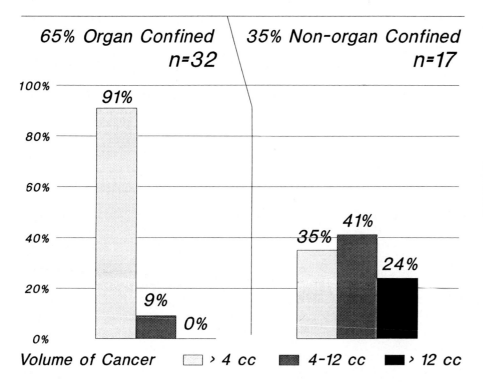

Figure 29–37. Volume distribution of 49 transition zone cancers (clinical stage TA) for both organ-confined (65 per cent) and non-organ–confined (35 per cent) cancers. (Compare with Figure 29–38.)

TRUS-guided biopsies and can readily distinguish microscopic invasion of the seminal vesicles (Vallancien et al., 1991b). For all the emphasis on "downstaging" of prostate cancer by hormonal therapy prior to radical prostatectomy, the only potential for true downstaging that could possibly be proved preoperatively would be invasion of the seminal vesicle. Disappearance of preoperatively proven seminal vesicle invasion would be highly unlikely in the radical prostatectomy specimen.

Radical Prostatectomy for Clinical Stage A Disease

Decisions as to cancer volume and grade are relatively simple in clinical stage B cancers, for which the peripheral and central zones can be palpated as well as subjected to systematic biopsy and ultrasound. Clinical stage TA cancer, which we regard as nearly equivalent to transition zone cancer, is much more complicated and

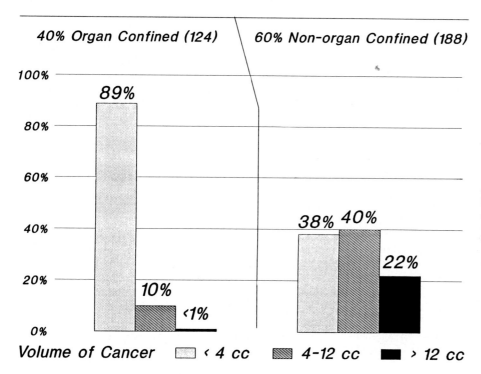

Figure 29–38. Volume distribution of 312 peripheral and central zone cancers (clinical stage TB) for both organ-confined (40 per cent) and non-organ–confined (60 per cent) cancers. Note the equivalent distribution by volume in both organ-confined and non-organ–confined cancers in clinical stage TA (see Fig. 29–37) and TB tumors.

uncertain. Because TUR can remove most of the BPH tissue from the transition zone, and retropubic or suprapubic enucleation can remove virtually all of the BPH, the very operation that discovered the cancer can theoretically remove it all or at least reduce the tumor to an insignificant residual volume. Indeed, the reason clinical stage TA cancer is so difficult to treat is precisely because it is so difficult to estimate the residual volume of cancer in comparison to clinical stage TB disease.

Much has been learned from morphometric examinations of prostates removed for clinical stage TA disease (see earlier discussions on growth and local spread of prostate cancer). Stage TA cancers tend to be much smaller than stage TB tumors, demonstrate much less capsular penetration, tend to have an architectural pattern of clear cell Gleason grade 1 and 2 cancer, and rarely invade the seminal vesicles because the transition zone is separated from the central zone, which contains the ejaculatory ducts along which peripheral zone cancer courses to invade the seminal vesicles.

Despite these favorable morphologic considerations, some untreated clinical stage TA cancers progress locally, metastasize to the pelvic lymph nodes, and then later metastasize to the bones. Because patients older than 70 years often make up a significant portion of clinical stage TA patients, mortality from intercurrent disease is usually so high that survival is an inadequate measure for statistical analysis. Accordingly, most observers have studied time to progressive disease, utilizing both local progression and distant metastases.

GLEASON GRADE IN STAGE TA. Because a majority of stage TA cancers were recognized decades ago to be low-grade, and because patients with high-grade cancers were not thought to be good candidates for radical prostatectomy (see Jewett), most patients with stage TA cancer were left untreated after diagnosis. For this reason, there are several excellent studies on the natural history of progression in clinical stage TA cancers. Cantrell and co-workers (1981) and Epstein and co-workers (1986), using <5 per cent and ≥5 per cent cancer involvement of the resected specimen as the distinction between stage TA1 and TA2 disease, reported 2 per cent progression for stage TA1 cancer at 4 years and 16 to 25 per cent progression at an average of 10 years (Epstein et al., 1988). For stage TA2 cancer, 32 per cent had progressed at 4 years. Extent (<5 per cent or ≥5 per cent) and grade of disease were strong predictors of progression.

All observers realized that "high-grade" cancer in stage TA disease carries a poor prognosis. Within the Gleason grading system, however, confusion exists as to what constitutes high-grade cancer on biopsy. Because the Gleason score must be used for biopsies, and because the presence of 3.2 ml of grade 4 cancer is strongly correlated with metastases to pelvic lymph nodes (McNeal et al., 1990b), it is rational to insist that stage TA1 cancers include only scores of 2 to 6, and that the presence of any Gleason score of 7 to 10 in resections for which <5 per cent of the chips contain cancer should automatically place that TA1 cancer into a TA2 category. Employing this rationale in our analysis of residual cancer volume in 44 radical prostatectomy specimens

for stage TA1 and TA2 disease (Voges et al., 1991), the presence of any Gleason grade 4 cancer (even a small piece of one chip) in patients with less than 5 per cent cancer was associated with a residual cancer of at least 1.7 ml in the radical prostatectomy specimen.

PROGRESSION IN CLINICAL STAGE TA IS PROPORTIONAL TO CANCER VOLUME AND GRADE. Lowe and Listrom (1988) reported on 232 patients with clinical stage TA cancers, also using the criteria of <5 per cent or ≥5 per cent tumor in the resected specimen. Only 9 per cent (21 patients) presented with Gleason scores of 7 or greater, and 62 per cent (144) had <5 per cent of the chips involved with cancer; 34 per cent (79) had less than 1 per cent of the surgical specimen involved. Overall, only 6 per cent died of cancer, 10 per cent died of intercurrent disease with documented tumor progression, and 10 per cent were alive with progressive disease. Thus, only 26 per cent overall had clinical detection of progressive disease.

Increasing grade and volume of the resected tumor were highly and significantly related to progression. Median time to progression by actuarial analysis for untreated stage TA1 cancer was 17.5 years, but for TA2 it was 4.75 years. Tumor volume in the TUR specimen significantly affected the probability of progression. Only 5 of 79 (6 per cent) progressed with <1 per cent cancer in the TUR chips, 8 of 65 (12 per cent) with 1 to 5 per cent involvement, and 47 of 89 (53 per cent) with ≥5 per cent cancer. The Gleason score similarly influenced the percentage of patients with recurrence: 7, 27, 38, and 57 per cent progressed with Gleason sums of 2 to 3, 4, 5 to 6, and 7 to 9, in that order.

So consistently were volume and grade related to progression, that highly useful probability tables were constructed for disease progression at 5 and 10 years based on 5-year age intervals at the time of diagnosis. Urologists should refer to these tables as part of the rationale of which patients with clinical stage TA disease should be treated. Nowhere in the urologic literature can one find better evidence that prostate cancer is indeed a predictable disease and that this predictability is directly related to cancer volume and grade.

PREDICTION OF RESIDUAL CANCER IN CLINICAL STAGE TA. Although these studies on natural history of untreated stage TA disease are impressive, our ability to decide—even with excellent probability tables—who should be treated on the basis of stage TA1 to TA2 categories of <5 per cent or ≥5 per cent tumor involvement of the resected specimen is limited. Because not everyone progresses, and because a few are even cured of cancer by TUR, how do we know who has significant residual cancer when stage TA tumor is discovered? Although there is little question about the desirability of treatment in high-grade (score of 7 or greater) stage TA2 disease, how do we recognize those patients with stage TA1 or TA2 cancers who will progress with Gleason scores of 2 to 6?

We have emphasized throughout this chapter that volume and grade are critically important to the progression of prostate cancer. How well does the TA1 and TA2 classification predict a significant residual volume of cancer in the radical prostatectomy specimen? Not very well according to our studies at Stanford University (Voges et al., 1991) and the studies of Scardino's group at Baylor University (Greene et al., 1991).

For example, among our 44 radical prostatectomies for stage TA cancer (22 TA1, 22 TA2), eight patients (4 TA1, 4 TA2) had either no residual cancer at all (2 TA2) or no single cancer as large as 0.2 ml in the radical prostatectomy specimen. Thus, 18 per cent of 44 TA1 and TA2 cancers had a needless radical prostatectomy if a significant tumor is defined as one with at least a 0.2-ml cancer (Scardino, 1989). However, Figure 29–35, from our radical cystoprostatectomy data, suggests that, for a cancer to become clinically significant, at least a tumor of 0.5 ml or greater must be present. Table 29–16 shows that an additional six radical prostatectomies (four TA1, two TA2) were unnecessary because the residual volume was <0.5 ml, thereby making 32 per cent of this series unlikely to have shown significant clinical progression.

Note in Table 29–16 that this analysis of the largest residual cancer (regardless of location) shows that only in the largest volume range did the TA2 category predict an excess of larger residual tumors in comparison to the TA1 category. In our studies and Scardino's studies, there is no comfort that this TA1–TA2 separation allows the urologist to avoid unnecessary surgery in almost one third of patients with clinical stage TA disease who have a radical prostatectomy.

Currently, there is no way to identify the subset of patients who have had complete or nearly complete resection of cancer. It is also possible that progression of clinical stage TA cancer is related to the total original volume of cancer in the transition zone and not to the residual volume after TUR, a possibility that would be more in keeping with our observations on histologic progression of clinical stage TB cancers. For example, 86 per cent of our radical prostatectomy specimens for clinical stage TA show residual cancer in contact with the border of the TUR defect (Voges et al., 1991). This portion of the residual cancer could represent the most invasive part of the original tumor, and it certainly would be closer to the lateral capsule. Under these circumstances, its malignant potential might be better estimated by its original, total cancer volume (TUR chips plus residual TUR cancer). These biologic considerations deserve further investigation.

SERUM PSA LEVEL IN CLINICAL STAGE TA.
In addition to the presence of Gleason grade 4 cancer

in the resected tissue as a predictor of substantial residual cancer volume (>1.7 ml), we found that the level of serum PSA at least 4 weeks after TURP was predictive of substantial residual cancer volume (Voges et al., 1991). In our study using the Yang assay, 19 of 20 patients with a PSA level >2.5 ng/ml had >0.9 ml of cancer, whereas seven of eight patients with a Yang PSA level of <1.0 ng/ml had a residual volume of <0.4 ml. Twelve of 44 patients (27 per cent) had a serum PSA level between 1 and 2.5 ng/ml, which was associated with both significant as well as insignificant cancers.

Employing the Hybritech assay, Carter and associates (1990b) found that their stage TA1 patients with a PSA level ≤1 ng/ml had a residual cancer volume of 0.5 ml and that their stage TA1 and TA2 patients combined with a PSA level >10 ng/ml had cancer volumes >0.5 ml. However, because 51 per cent of their patients had PSA levels between 1 and 10 ng/ml (Yang equivalent of 1.5 to 18.4 ng/ml) with cancer volumes both less than and greater than 0.5 ml, the Hybritech assay does not appear nearly as sensitive as the Yang assay in predicting residual cancer volume before radical prostatectomy in clinical stage TA disease.

IMPALPABLE PERIPHERAL ZONE CANCER IN STAGE TA. We found that eight of 44 (18 per cent) prostates with stage TA disease had a peripheral zone cancer that was larger than the original transition zone cancer found at TURP (Voges et al., 1991). Because six of these eight cancers were >0.5 ml in volume, it is important to be aware of these impalpable peripheral zone cancers, both in follow-up with regular DRE and in TRUS evaluation for significant residual tumors. Greene and colleagues (1991) have presented similar concerns.

ESTIMATING RESIDUAL VOLUME AND GRADE IN STAGE TA BEFORE RADICAL PROSTATECTOMY. Because the TA1 and TA2 categories are not very helpful in predicting significant residual cancer for the individual patient, what can the urologist do to avoid unnecessary radical prostatectomies in one third of patients with clinical stage TA cancers?

First, the urologist must make a careful search for Gleason grade 4 cancers in the TURP chips. Second, if the Yang assay is >2.5 ng/ml 1 month or longer after the TUR, the patient probably has at least 0.9 ml of residual tumor. Third, the urologist needs to remember that 18 per cent of patients will have larger, impalpable cancer in the peripheral zone, which should be assessed by careful DRE and systematic biopsies of the peripheral zone. Fourth, our positive biopsy rate is 28 per cent in clinical stage TA patients who have our routine six systematic biopsies; however, when we include two additional anteriorly directed biopsies along the proximal urethral defect, our rate increases to 47 per cent; if we include microscopic foci of 3 mm or less, the positive biopsy rates are 52 and 68 per cent, respectively (Terris et al., 1991c). We have not biopsied through the urethral lumen to obtain tissue directly anterior to the urethra, where we know some patients have residual cancer (McNeal et al., 1988c). Fifth and lastly, when all these biopsy findings are negative, and the Yang PSA level is <2.5 ng/ml, we follow the patient with serial

Table 29–16. LARGEST RESIDUAL CANCER AFTER RADICAL PROSTATECTOMY FOR CLINICAL STAGE TA DISEASE

Residual Cancer Volume (ml)	A1	A2
0.0	0	2
0.001–0.190	4	2
0.20–0.49	4	2
0.50–0.99	6	3
≥1.0	8	13
Total	22	22

Adapted from Voges, G. E., et al.: The predictive significance of substaging stage A prostate cancer (A1 vs. A2) for volume and grade of total cancer in the prostate. J. Urol., 1991. In press.

PSA level determination every 6 months and then repeat the eight biopsies in 2 years.

Zhang and associates (1991) recalled 52 patients (mean age 68) with clinical stage TA1 cancer who had been conservatively followed for a mean of 5.8 years (1 to 14 years). Eight patients (15 per cent) had abnormal findings on digital examination; ten had elevated PSA levels by Hybritech assay (4.6 to 14.6 ng/ml), and 29 had abnormal findings on TRUS. Random biopsies were done in all 52 patients. Moderately to poorly differentiated cancers were found in five patients (10 per cent), two of whom had TB cancers. All five were treated including three who had radical prostatectomy for what proved to be organ-confined cancer. Three patients had normal DRE with "focal" cancer and were not treated. The investigators believed that TRUS should be an integral part of the follow-up for stage TA1 cancer.

Agatstein and co-workers (1987) recommended fine needle aspiration of all patients undergoing a TURP for BPH. They detected 17 cancers in 98 aspirates. Apparently, all 17 proved to have stage A2 cancer at TURP, and no stage TA1 cancers were detected. Our data and that of the Baylor group on reconstructed stage TA radical prostatectomies would suggest that some clinical stage TA1 cancers with closely similar volumes to clinical stage TA2 cancers should have been detected in these aspirates (see Table 29–16).

We believe that this practice of aspirating BPH before TURP, if acted on by radical prostatectomy without TURP, will surely lead to unnecessary procedures. The best way to detect unsuspected cancer in patients with BPH is to do a TURP, except in unusual circumstances for which the serum level of PSA is extraordinarily elevated.

Radical Prostatectomy for Clinical Stage TC and D1 Disease

Flocks and associates reported in 1973 and 1975 some astonishing 10- and 15-year disease-free survivals for clinical stage C disease treated by injecting 2 ml of gold 198 into the bladder, the "urogenital diaphragm," and the ligated ends of the vas (Table 29–17). Schroeder and Belt (1975) and Scott and Boyd (1969) reported substantial series with 15-year survival rates of 20 per cent obtained by combining hormonal therapy with radical prostatectomy. Most patients in these two series

had very small stage TC cancers or even large stage TB cancers, and many were selected on the basis of preoperative estrogen sensitivity. The Mayo Clinic has reported a large series of patients who underwent radical prostatectomies for stage C disease, half of whom had adjuvant therapy, mostly hormonal (Zincke et al., 1986).

The increase in practice of radical retropubic prostatectomy has created the following dilemmas: (1) what to do when the lymph nodes are found unexpectedly to be positive at surgical staging—that is, clinical stage D1 disease, TA(N+), TB(N+), or TC(N+), and (2) what to do for the 10 per cent of patients in whom the results of surgical examination of the pelvic lymph nodes are initially negative but later, with more extensive and permanent histologic sectioning, are found to be positive. The clinical dilemma is whether to proceed with radical prostatectomy as the best means of achieving local control (Steinberg et al., 1990), to combine radical prostatectomy with immediate hormonal therapy (Myers et al., 1983; Zincke, 1989), to combine radical prostatectomy with delayed hormonal therapy (deKernion et al., 1990), or to leave the prostate in situ and treat with radiation or hormonal therapy.

No clear answer can be given in response to this array of questions. In the preceding discussion of radiation therapy, we pointed out the disadvantages of radiation for large stage TB and TC cancers. Probably no difference occurs in progression rates—local or distant—between radiation and hormonal therapy. In the Steinberg report, for example, there was no difference in local progression in clinical stage D1 disease between those patients expectantly treated (without surgery) and those treated with radiation (Steinberg et al., 1990).

In 1991, there is a definite tendency toward removing these prostates for local control, recognizing that the surgery is not curative. Without question, the impotent patient with obstructive urinary symptoms is better treated with a noncurative radical prostatectomy in the presence of unexpected D1 disease of microscopic volume (discovered by frozen section rather than gross inspection). Moreover, the role of DNA ploidy in potential selection of cases remains highly controversial (deKernion et al., 1990; Zincke, 1989). We need to remember that 40 per cent of clinical stage TB patients had diploid pelvic lymph node metastases (Stephenson et al., 1987). These options will require a decade of research to learn what is best for the patient.

Table 29–17. RADICAL PROSTATECTOMY FOR CLINICAL STAGE C DISEASE

Source	No. of Patients	Lymph Node Status	Stage	Additional Therapy	10-Year Survival (%)	15-Year Survival (%)
Flocks (1973) (1975)	69	+	C	[198]Au interstitial radiation plus lymphadenectomy	67*	28*
	32	–	C		12	12
Schroeder and Belt (1975)	213†	?	C	Estrogen	36‡	20‡
Scott and Boyd (1969)	33 at 10 years, 31 at 15 years	?	C	Estrogen-responsive tumors, low-grade	51	20
Zincke, Utz, and Taylor (1986)	101	49 negative 52 positive	C	47, None; 48, hormone; 6, radiation	60‡	—

*Cancer-free.
†Twenty-nine per cent >71 years of age at time of radical prostatectomy. Pathologic stage C; many may have been clinical stage B.
‡Actuarial survival rates, not actual survivors at 10 and 15 years.

Complications of Radical Prostatectomy

Igel and colleagues (1987) reported on 692 consecutive radical retropubic prostatectomies from the Mayo Clinic. Perioperative or early operative mortality was 0.6 per cent, pulmonary emboli occurred in 2.7 per cent, and severe to total urinary incontinence was present in 5 per cent. Walsh (1988) noted that preoperative autologous donation has reduced the need for homologous transfusion to 2 per cent of patients; pulmonary emboli occurred in 0.3 per cent. In 450 radical prostatectomies at Stanford in the past 5 years, there have been no perioperative or early postoperative deaths. We believe that autologous transfusion, the use of Allen stirrups and leg pumps, ambulation the night of surgery, and early discharge by the 5th or 6th postoperative day have all contributed to minimal operative morbidity.

With direct anastomosis of the bladder mucosa to the urethral mucosa, avoiding the Vest-type sutures, anastomotic strictures should occur in less than 10 per cent of patients. Most of these strictures will require, at the most, two to three urethral dilatations with smooth van Buren sounds.

Rectal injury can occur distal to the apex of the prostate during dissection of Denonvilliers' fascia from the underlying longitudinal muscle of the rectum (2 per cent in our series). We have closed all of these injuries in two layers with copious irrigation and never had to resort to a diverting colostomy. Small asymptomatic lymphoceles are probably common after the routine pelvic lymphadenectomy, but rarely will patients (less than 1 per cent) require temporary, percutaneous drainage.

Erectile impotency occurs in 90 per cent of patients after radical prostatectomy, although Finkel and Taylor (1981) found that 43 per cent of patients had erectile potency after perineal prostatectomy. Although several investigators report high rates of successful sexual intercourse after the Walsh nerve-sparing radical prostatectomy, we believe that the definition of a single sexual event in the past 12 months—without any description of the *quality* of that event—is an inadequate assessment of sexual postoperative functioning. Except for the very young, we believe only a few patients in fact find the quality of their sexual life to be equivalent to that before surgery.

Fortunately, because orgasmic function is invariably maintained even when all the periprostatic fascias with their enclosed neurovascular bundles are excised with the prostate, there are numerous ways to provide satisfactory erectile function for the impotent patient. Moreover, the wait for spontaneous return of the erectile function can be much longer than 12 months, and as Bahnson and Catalona have reported (1988), there are frequently other factors than injury to the neurovascular bundles responsible for postoperative impotence. Indeed, we offer all patients at 3 months postoperatively the option of mechanical erection devices, like the ErecAid or intracavernous injection therapy.

Hormonal Therapy

Our Stanford data show that only 40 per cent of 312 clinical stage TB cancers and 65 per cent of 49 clinical stage TA cancers were confined to the prostate at radical prostatectomy (see Figs. 29–37 and 29–38). Although many patients with only capsular penetration will be cured by radical prostatectomy, these numbers essentially mean that approximately 75 per cent of all new patients who present with prostate cancer (see Table 29–4) will ultimately require some form of therapy other than radical prostatectomy. Given the information that all forms of radiation therapy now appear essentially incapable of sterilizing prostate cancer confined to the pelvis (Kabalin et al., 1989a; Link et al., 1991; Scardino and Wheeler, 1988; Whitmore and Hilaris, 1989), and recognizing that we currently have no effective chemotherapeutic agent, hormonal therapy will be required for most patients diagnosed with prostate cancer unless there are significant improvements in early detection.

Three significant clinical issues must be addressed. First, should hormonal therapy be started immediately upon recognition of an incurable stage of prostate cancer or can it be delayed as long as the patient remains asymptomatic? Second, should hormonal therapy be combined with some other form of therapy that is inadequate by itself, such as radiotherapy or radical prostatectomy, for most non–organ-confined disease? Third, which form of hormonal therapy should be used?

In the presence of untreated metastatic bone disease confirmed by bone scans, hormonal therapy produces improvement in 60 to 80 per cent of men; however, hormonally resistant progression appears during the first 12 months of therapy in 35 to 40 per cent of these patients (Sogani and Fair, 1987). From the National Cancer Institute (NCI) randomized study, half of the patients who received leuprolide and flutamide were dead by 3 years, but patients with less extensive metastatic disease lived for at least 5 years (Crawford et al., 1989). It is known that 5 to 15 per cent of patients receiving hormonal therapy for metastatic disease live 10 years; whereas retrospective analysis of these patients has failed to discern the causes of such long-term survival (Reiner et al., 1979), it is possible that clinical estimates of tumor burden in past years were too crude to recognize those patients with very minimal metastatic cancer.

Ishikawa and associates (1989) observed the influence of serum testosterone levels on survival—free of progression—in patients with metastatic disease. Chodak and co-workers (1991), in a randomized clinical trial of orchiectomy versus goserelin acetate implants, reported that survival was strongly influenced by four independent prognostic factors: bone pain ($P = .0001$), serum testosterone level ($P = .0048$), serum alkaline phosphatase level ($P = .0056$), and performance status ($P = .0084$). Combinations of these factors were able to predict differences in 2-year survival rates of 84 per cent versus 8 per cent. As noted by the investigators, stratification of these variables among patients in clinical trials could be important.

Cohen and colleagues (1990) have demonstrated a significant correlation between survival and the absence of neuroendocrine cells in the prostates of patients with metastatic cancer. All patients died within 4 years if they tested positive for neuron-specific enolase, whereas 90 per cent of those who tested neuroendocrine negative were alive 6 years after diagnosis. This information suggests that neuroendocrine cells may be important in the final, progressive, androgen-resistant phase of metastatic prostate cancer. In a related study, elevated serum chromogranin-A levels have been identified in 48 per cent of patients with advanced stage D2 cancer (Kadmon et al., 1991).

Early or Delayed Hormonal Therapy

Most of us have waited until very late into the later clinical stages of prostate cancer before starting hormonal therapy, especially if the patient was asymptomatic. This philosophy of delayed hormonal therapy was largely based on findings from Study I of the Veterans Administration Cooperative Urological Research Group (VACURG). When patients were randomized between immediate hormonal therapy and placebo therapy with later hormonal treatment once they became symptomatic, there was no difference in average survival rates (VACURG, 1967b). Indeed, the VACURG group recommended that therapy ". . . be withheld until the patient's symptoms were so severe as to require relief," a recommendation that many of us have followed assiduously.

Sarosdy (1990), however, has analyzed the VACURG Study I in great detail, withdrawing the 26 to 40 per cent of cardiovascular deaths in patients treated with estrogen and calculating the cancer-specific deaths. These recalculations show that those patients who received immediate estrogen therapy did better than those who were initially treated with placebo and later given estrogens when needed (3 per cent cancer deaths in the estrogen therapy group versus 8.4 per cent in the placebo group, P = .008). More importantly, Sarosdy points out that the VACURG studies were never designed to determine the effectiveness of early versus delayed hormonal therapy, and that the conclusion was inappropriate in view of modern-day designs for large-scale clinical trials.

Evidence from current studies suggests that early hormonal therapy may increase patient survival in comparison to delayed hormonal therapy, even though a definitive randomized study to test this possibility has not been reported. Byar and Corle (1988) observed that, in the VACURG Study II, patients who received 1 mg per day of diethylstilbestrol (DES) beginning at diagnosis experienced an increased overall survival in clinical stages TC and D2 disease when compared with patients who received placebo (delayed hormonal therapy). The significance of this advantage to early hormonal therapy, however, may be somewhat lessened by the fact that only 44 per cent of the placebo-treated patients were later given delayed hormonal therapy. Kozlowski and

associates (1991) have reviewed the literature in favor of early hormone therapy; they provide an excellent discussion of a risk-benefit analysis that strongly supports early hormone therapy.

In the 1989 NCI study by Crawford and colleagues, leuprolide—an analogue of gonadatropin-releasing hormone—was coupled with either placebo or flutamide, a nonsteroidal antiandrogen that competitively inhibits the binding of androgens to the cell nucleus (Simard et al., 1986). They found an increased median length of survival of 28.3 months versus 35.6 months for the flutamide combination (P = .035). In an update of a subgroup of 82 patients whose metastatic disease was limited to the axial skeleton and/or pelvis and who had a good performance status, the 41 patients who received leuprolide plus placebo had a median survival of 41.5 months, whereas the 41 men receiving leuprolide plus flutamide have not yet reached median survival at 60 months (personal communication, 1991, Joanne Swanson, Schering Corporation). Thus, it appears that combination therapy—combined androgen deprivation—is clearly superior to leuprolide alone in prolonging life. Of equal importance, however, is that early hormonal therapy for less extensive disease appears to prolong life in both arms of the study: 41.5 versus 28 months for patients treated with leuprolide and placebo, and 60 versus 35 months for patients treated with leuprolide plus flutamide.

The ideal way to study early versus delayed hormonal therapy is to use immediate or deferred orchiectomy for similar clinical stages of advanced disease. The Medical Research Council in England has been conducting such a study since 1985 (Kirk, 1987). As of November, 1990, 750 patients have been recruited to this study, but another 1000 are needed for effective randomization in the different clinical stages (Kirk, D., personal communication, November, 1990). One interesting subset of 270 patients with advanced local disease but NXMO (see Table 29–2) received orchiectomy, radiotherapy, or both. Orchiectomy was as effective as radiotherapy in achieving local control and, not surprisingly, more effective in delaying time to metastases. Van Aubel and co-workers (1985) reported similar results in 30 patients treated for stage D1 prostate cancer by orchiectomy alone. These investigators observed a median interval to distal progression of greater than 45 months.

Immediate or Delayed Hormonal Therapy in Stage D1 Cancer of the Prostate

Myers and associates (1983), Zincke and associates (1986, 1989), Kramolowsky (1988), and deKernion and associates (1990) all show significant differences in favor of early hormonal therapy as opposed to delayed therapy in patients with radical prostatectomies who are found to have metastatic cancers in their pelvic lymph nodes. Despite these very suggestive studies that immediate hormonal therapy lengthens survival, none of them were randomized, the numbers are relatively small, the choice of treatment was made by individual physicians, and the Kaplan-Myer projections were used to predict survival before half the patients were dead (i.e., reached median survival). Although the references here relate to D1 disease, for which there is the most information, especially for those patients thought to have clinical stage TB2 or TB3 disease prior to radical prostatectomy, the identical choice of early versus delayed therapy applies equally to the 28 per cent of patients who present with clinical stage C disease (Table 29–4). To our knowledge, data are unavailable on the effectiveness of combining radiotherapy with hormonal treatment.

Forms of Hormonal Therapy

DIETHYLSTILBESTROL. The VACURG studies clearly established the high cardiovascular risk of 5 mg per day of DES. Studies of treatment with 3 mg per day of DES versus treatment with orchiectomy (Glashan and Robinson, 1981; Henriksson and Edhag, 1986) and leuprolide (Leuprolide Study Group, 1984) established the significant number of side effects and cardiovascular complications associated with 3 mg per day of DES (7 per cent in the Leuprolide Study Group). The dosage of 1 mg per day of DES, however, is as effective as 5 mg per day in delaying progression of stage TC to D2 disease (Byar, 1973; Byar and Corle, 1988). Although incomplete suppression of serum testosterone has been reported with DES at a dosage of 1 mg per day (Kent et al., 1973; Shearer et al., 1973), the completed European Organization on Research and Treatment of Cancer (EORTC) Protocol 30805 in which patients were randomized to 1 mg DES daily versus bilateral orchiectomy has shown no differences in survival or cardiovascular thromboembolic events (Robinson, 1987; Robinson, M.R.G., personal communication, April, 1991). These data suggest the need for randomized studies for combined androgen deprivation in which flutamide and 1 mg/day of DES is compared with flutamide and leuprolide or flutamide and bilateral orchiectomy. While awaiting the outcome of these studies, it is clear that combined androgen deprivation with DES and flutamide is a viable alternative to both flutamide and leuprolide as well as flutamide and orchiectomy.

BILATERAL ORCHIECTOMY. Bilateral orchiectomy has been the gold standard for hormonal therapy since the report by Huggins and associates in 1941. With the recognition of unexpected severe cardiovascular toxicity from 5 mg of DES daily in the VACURG studies, bilateral orchiectomy has been an attractive and important alternative to DES therapy. It is the least expensive long-term therapy when compared with current non-DES alternatives in the United States—luteinizing hormone–releasing hormone (LHRH) agonist and the nonsteroidal antiandrogen, flutamide.

However, unlike LHRH, DES, and flutamide, bilateral orchiectomy is not reversible; its main disadvantages are psychologic trauma, generally permanent loss of libido, and erectile impotence. It does have the advantage of complete therapeutic compliance, and it rapidly removes 95 per cent of the most powerful circulating androgen, testosterone. Orchiectomy can be performed safely and quickly with minimal morbidity on an outpatient basis. Indeed, in the impotent patient, bilateral orchiectomy is the ideal form of therapy. If psychologic resistance is expected, a subcapsular orchiectomy or even artificial testicular implant placement can be performed at the time of orchiectomy.

LHRH AGONISTS. Based on Schally's Nobel Prize–winning isolation and subsequent synthesis of native LHRH, which causes an initial testosterone release (termed the flare period) followed by a fall in testosterone to castrate levels (Schally et al., 1976), treatment with an LHRH analogue (leuprolide) at 1 mg subcutaneously per day was compared with treatment with 3 mg of DES per day (Leuprolide Study Group, 1984). Time to progression and actuarial survival rates at 1 year were the same. Impotence and hot flashes were the principal side effects of leuprolide, but cardiovascular complications and gynecomastia were much less than in the DES-treated group. Because LHRH agonists have no effect on adrenal androgen production, LHRH therapy can probably be considered equivalent to 3 mg per day of DES or to bilateral orchiectomy and probably equivalent to 1 mg/day of DES (Robinson, 1987; Robinson, M.R.G., personal communication, April, 1991).

The initial "flare" from the temporary release of testosterone can cause bone pain in the 1st week of therapy (7.7 per cent in the leuprolide-only arm of Crawford and co-workers, 1989 during the first week of therapy and 7 per cent in the Leuprolide Study Group, 1984). A potential for spinal cord injury exists if vertebral metastases are present. Therefore, LHRH agonists should be avoided in any patient with metastatic cancer who has the slightest suggestion of neurologic symptoms. The flare reaction can be greatly blunted by starting flutamide simultaneously with LHRH agonists (Kuhn et al., 1989; Crawford et al., 1989; Lubrie et al., 1987a). It can also be avoided by 1 day of therapy with ketoconazole (Trachtenberg and Point, 1983).

All LHRH analogues appear clinically equivalent; goserelin acetate—an LHRH agonist implanted subcutaneously every 28 days—has been shown to be equivalent to bilateral orchiectomy in suppressing testosterone, in time to disease progression, and in survival rates (Peeling, 1989). Leuprolide is now available in a monthly depot injection of 7.5 mg, and goserelin acetate is available as a 3.6-mg implant for monthly subcutaneous injections using a 16-gauge needle.

ANTIANDROGENS. DES, orchiectomy and LHRH agonists eliminate or markedly suppress androgen production by the testes, which accounts for about 95 per cent of circulating testosterone. However, the weakly androgenic steroids from the adrenal cortex, dehydroepiandrosterone and androstenedione, which are present in the serum in significant concentrations (Coffey, 1986), are converted into strong androgens in peripheral tissues, including the prostate (see Labrie et al., 1987b for review).

True antiandrogens, especially the active metabolite of the nonsteroidal agent flutamide (flutamide-OH), are important because they act as competitive inhibitors for dihydrotestosterone (DHT) and testosterone (T) receptor proteins, which act on specific DNA sites in the nucleus of the prostate cell. Labrie and colleagues (1982) were the first to use flutamide and LHRH agonist in the treatment of metastatic prostate cancer in an effort to block the effects of the adrenal androgens. Their later observations on the competitive affinities of flutamide-OH, DHT, and T for the receptor proteins in cytosol from human prostate cancers (and other androgen sensitive animal tissues) are important (Simard et al., 1986). The relative affinities of DHT, T, and flutamide-OH clearly show that high concentrations of flutamide are required in order to prevent the access of androgens to the receptor. Thus, the weak affinity of flutamide for the DHT and T receptor proteins is a strong argument to always block testicular androgens by medical or surgical castration when using flutamide. Indeed, the observations that about one third of patients respond to flutamide after failure of medical or surgical castration (Fossà et al., 1990; Labrie et al., 1988), whereas almost no one responds to castration after failure of flutamide as initial monotherapy (Sogani et al., 1984) suggests that flutamide *alone* encourages more androgen resistance than castration alone.

Labrie has consistently presented strong arguments that flutamide should always be given in conjunction with medical or surgical castration. His calculations based on known affinities of DHT and flutamide-OH and their respective intraprostatic concentrations indicate that flutamide administered alone leaves 40 per cent of DHT free to bind to the androgen receptor in prostatic tissue. When flutamide is combined with castration, however, only 5 per cent of DHT is available to the androgen receptor (Labrie et al., 1987b; Labrie et al., 1988).

Steroidal antiandrogens, such as cyproterone acetate and megestrol acetate, compete with dihydrotestosterone for cytosolic receptor sites as flutamide does. They also have strong progestational activity, which inhibits LH release and can produce castrate levels of testosterone. The gradual increase in levels of serum testosterone that occurs with chronic administration of cyproterone acetate can be prevented with 0.1 mg of DES daily. Loss of libido and erectile impotency are disadvantages to therapy with the steroidal antiandrogens. Cyproterone acetate is widely prescribed in Europe and Canada. The Urological Group of the EORTC randomized trials (protocol 30761), however, have not shown cyproterone acetate to be as effective as DES in retarding the progression of prostate cancer. Indeed, in EORTC protocol 30805, 1 mg per day of DES was as effective as cyproterone acetate *plus* bilateral orchiectomy (Robinson, 1987; Robinson, M.R.B., personal communication, April, 1991).

Ketoconazole impairs the production of androgen by inhibiting the enzymes of gonadal and adrenal corticosteroid synthesis (Sonino, 1987). Castrate levels of androgens occur within 4 to 8 hours of a 400-mg oral dose (Trachtenberg and Point, 1983). It is primarily helpful when there is a need for a rapid androgen response such as occurs in impending spinal cord compression. Both Trump and co-workers (1989) and Gerber and Chodak (1990) described excellent responses in a small subset of patients who failed orchiectomy or leuprolide mono-

therapy. Liver failure can be an important complication of ketoconazole therapy.

COMBINATION THERAPY. Total androgen suppression with flutamide in combination with medical (LHRH agonist) or surgical castration was reported by Labrie and co-workers (1982, 1985). Their dramatic results, at least in comparison to historical controls, were viewed with some skepticism and led to several large-scale randomized trials. In the best randomized double-blind study, sponsored by the NCI, Crawford and associates (1989) studied 603 patients within 15 months from 93 contributing institutions. All men received leuprolide in combination with placebo or flutamide. Those who received leuprolide and flutamide had a longer progression-free survival (16.5 versus 13.9 months; P = .039) and an increase in the median length of survival (35.6 versus 28.3 months; P = .05).

In an update of a subset of patients with metastatic disease limited to the axial skeleton and/or pelvis who had a good performance status, the median survival for 41 patients who received leuprolide plus placebo was 41.5 months, whereas the 41 patients who received leuprolide and flutamide had not reached median survival at 60 months (personal communication, Joanne Swanson, Schering Corporation, 1991). These data will probably translate into an extra 2 years of life for this subset of patients with less metastatic disease who are treated with flutamide plus primary gonadal suppression (leuprolide or orchiectomy).

In a Canadian study giving a different nonsteroidal antiandrogen, Anandron (nilutamide), 203 patients were randomly assigned to either castration plus placebo or castration plus anandron (Canadian Anandron Study Group, 1990). Median survival of the placebo arm was 19 months versus 26 months for the anandron arm (P = .048). A similar double-blind, placebo-controlled multicenter study, involving 457 untreated patients with metastatic disease, has been reported by the International Anandron Study Group (Janknegt, et al., 1991). Statistically significant differences were found in favor of orchiectomy plus Anandron in complete or partial response (P = <0.001) and cancer-related survival (P = 0.046) versus patients treated with orchiectomy alone.

Smith and colleagues (1991) reported that 98 per cent of 411 prospectively treated stage D2 patients had a decrease in PSA levels with a median decrease of 97.7 per cent 3 months after randomization to leuprolide plus placebo or leuprolide plus nilutamide (another nonsteroidal antiandrogen). PSA level normalized in 76 per cent of those treated with nilutamide plus leuprolide compared with 52 per cent of those treated with placebo plus leuprolide (P = <.0001).

Bilateral orchiectomy was compared with goserelin acetate implants (3.6 mg) and flutamide in a randomized EORTC study of 327 patients (EORTC 30853 Study, Keuppens et al., 1990). A substantial benefit occurred in the flutamide group in delaying the time to first progression (P = 0.004). Because orchiectomy is presumably equivalent to goserelin, the delay in time to progression is due to the addition of flutamide. Although these investigators reported no differences in time to death, median survival had not occurred (only one third had died in each group). Even if median survival had been reached, this study and the Danish study (DAPROCA 86), with which it was combined (Iversen et al., 1990), cannot possibly draw conclusions on survival. The flutamide patients were withdrawn from the study at the time of progression, and obviously the orchiectomy group continued original treatment. These last two studies (Iversen et al., 1990; Keuppens et al., 1990) emphasize the importance of properly designed studies from the start, especially in terms of survival.

One of the reasons the NCI trial of leuprolide with and without flutamide (Crawford et al., 1989) was so successful is that the goal of 600 patients was accomplished in an astonishingly short time of 15 months and that the investigators waited until half the patients in each arm had died before reporting results. In some of the studies reviewed, although not all, median survival had not been reached, which allows actuarial predictions to be "loaded up front" with earlier recruits and prevents valid assessments of true survival. In general, trials with complete androgen blockade have shown a greater number of positive objective responses, a greater delay in time to progression, or an increased survival. Taken together, the European data notwithstanding, these studies strongly suggest an advantage to flutamide plus ablation of testicular androgens.

In conclusion, the NCI trials clearly suggest that there is some merit to the Labrie hypothesis (1982, 1985) and that flutamide was a powerful addition to leuprolide in prolonging life when given early in metastatic disease. What is not known is whether flutamide combined with 1 mg per day of DES is as effective as flutamide combined with orchiectomy or LHRH agonists.

Chemotherapy

Effective chemotherapeutic agents are urgently needed for prostate cancer. In view of the 3-year doubling time for most cancers (Schmid et al., 1991), cell cycle–nonspecific agents will be required rather than those that rely on DNA replication for cell killing. Effective chemotherapeutic agents could greatly increase the indications for radical prostatectomy when provided as adjunctive therapy. The M.D. Anderson group at Houston combined hormonal therapy with cytotoxic chemotherapy (Johnson et al., 1989).

Unfortunately, there are no effective chemotherapeutic drugs for prostate cancer. Those that have been tried show short responses without any significant survival advantage (Eisenberger, 1988; Gibbons, 1987). At Stanford, doxorubicin is administered intravenously for pain palliation in the terminally ill patient at a dosage of 20 mg/m² once a week, on an outpatient basis (Torti et al., 1983). Cardiac toxicity is a serious limitation. DES diphosphate at a dosage of 1 g per day given intravenously for 5 days is widely thought to provide repeated relief for a few months, regardless of prior therapy (Ferro, 1991). Estramustine phosphate sodium (Emcyt) is probably no better than DES. Suramin was initially reported with some enthusiasm despite substantial toxicity (Linehan et al., 1990). In vitro tissue cultures with human prostatic epithelial cells in our laboratory, however, have shown suramin to be cytostatic rather than cytocidal (Peehl et al., 1991). Unfortunately, it is also highly toxic.

Local radiation therapy is most useful for pain control. In general, 3000 rads is given for chest (rib) pain, 4000 rads for vertebral pain or impending collapse of a vertebra, and 5000 rads for hip or long bone pain. Strontium 89 is reported to be effective for bone pain (Robinson et al., 1990).

In some patients with the pain of terminal disease, intrathecal narcotics and epidural or subcutaneous narcotic pumps are helpful.

REFERENCES

Adami, H. -O., Norlén, B. J., Malker, B., and Meirik, O.: Long-term survival in prostatic carcinoma, with special reference to age as a prognostic factor. Scand. J. Urol. Nephrol., 20:197, 1986.

Adolfsson, J., and Carstensen, J.: Natural course of clinically localized prostate adenocarcinoma in men less than 70 years old. J. Urol., 146:96, 1991.

Agatstein, E. A., Hernandez, F. J., Layfield, L. J., Smith, R. B., and deKernion, J. B.: Use of fine needle aspiration for detection of stage A prostatic carcinoma before transurethral resection of the prostate: A clinical trial. J. Urol., 138:551, 1987.

Ahmann, F. R., and Schifman, R. B.: Prospective comparison between serum monoclonal prostate specific antigen and acid phosphatase measurements in metastatic prostatic cancer. J. Urol., 137:431, 1987.

Akazaki, K., and Stemmermann, G. N.: Comparative study of latent carcinoma of the prostate among Japanese in Japan and Hawaii. JNCI, 50:1137, 1973.

Andrews, G. S.: Latent carcinoma of the prostate. J. Clin. Pathol., 2:197, 1949.

Arai, Y., Yoshiki, T., and Yoshida, O.: Prognostic significance of prostate specific antigen in endocrine treatment for prostatic cancer. J. Urol., 144:1415, 1990.

Armitage, T. G., Cooper, E. H., Newling, D. W. W., Robinson, M. R. G., and Appleyard, I.: The value of the measurement of serum prostate specific antigen in patients with benign prostatic hyperplasia and untreated prostate cancer. Br. J. Urol., 62:584, 1988.

Ayala, A. G., Ro, J. Y., Babaian, R., Tronosco, P., and Grignon, D. J.: The prostatic capsule: Does it exist? Its importance in the staging and treatment of prostatic carcinoma. Am. J. Surg. Pathol., 13:21, 1989.

Azumi, N., Shibuya, H., and Ishikura, M.: Primary prostatic carcinoid tumor with intracytoplasmic prostatic acid phosphatase and prostate-specific antigen. Am. J. Surg. Pathol., 8:545, 1984.

Babaian, R. J., Evans, R. B., Miyashita, H., and Ramirez, E. I.: The distribution of PSA in a normal population: Relationship to gland volume and age. J. Urol., 145:381A, 1991. (Abstract no. 675.)

Babaian, J. R., Camps, J. L., Frangos, D. N., Ramirez, B. S., Tenney, D. M., Hassell, J. S., and Fritsche, H. A.: Monoclonal PSA in untreated prostate cancer. Cancer, 67:2200, 1991.

Babiarz, B., Peters-Gee, J. M., Crissman, J. D., Cerny, J. C., and Miles, B. J.: DNA quantitation in prostatic adenocarcinoma: A comparison between primary tumor and lymph node metastasis. J. Urol., 145:215A, 1991. (Abstract, no. 11.)

Bagshaw, M. A.: Radiation therapy for cancer of the prostate. In Skinner, D. G., and Lieskovsky, G. (Eds.): Diagnosis and Management of Genitourinary Cancer. Philadelphia, W. B. Saunders Co., 1988, pp. 425–445.

Bagshaw, M. A., Cox, R. S., and Ray, G. R.: Status of radiation treatment of prostate cancer at Stanford University. NCI Monogr., 7:47, 1988.

Bahnson, R. H., and Catalona, W. J.: Papaverine testing of impotent patients following nerve-sparing radical prostatectomy. J. Urol., 139:773, 1988.

Barnes, R., Hirst, A., and Rosenquist, R.: Early carcinoma of the prostate: Comparison of stages A and B. J. Urol., 115:404, 1976.

Belville, W. D., Mahan, D. E., Sepulveda, R. A., Bruce, A. W., and Miller, C.: Bone marrow acid phosphatase by radioimmunoassay: 3 Years of experience. J. Urol., 125:809, 1981.

Bigg, S. W., Kavoussi, L. R., and Catalona, W. J.: Role of nerve-sparing radical prostatectomy for clinical stage B2 prostate cancer. J. Urol., 144:1420, 1990.

Blennerhassett, J. B., and Vickery, A. L., Jr.: Carcinoma of the prostate gland. Cancer, 19:980, 1966.

Boring, C. C., Squires, T. S., and Tong, T.: Cancer statistics, 1991. CA, 41:19, 1991.

Bostwick, D. G., and Brawer, M. K.: Prostatic intra-epithelial neoplasia and early invasion in prostate cancer. Cancer, 59:788, 1987.

Boxer, R. J.: Prostate cancer screening using prostate specific antigen in a community hospital. J. Urol., 1991. In press.

Brawer, M. K., Chetner, M. P., Beatie, J., and Lange, P. H.: Prostate specific antigen and early detection of prostatic carcinoma. J. Urol., 145:382A, 1991. (Abstract, no. 677.)

Brawer, M. K., Peehl, D. M., Stamey, T. A., and Bostwick, D. G.: Keratin immunoreactivity in the benign and neoplastic human prostate. Cancer Res., 45:3663, 1985.

Brawn, P. N.: Adenosis of the prostate: A dysplastic lesion that can be confused with prostate adenocarcinoma. Cancer, 49:826, 1982.

Brawn, P. N., Ayala, A. G., Von Eschenbach, A. C., Hussey, D. H., and Johnson, D. E.: Histologic grading study of prostate adenocarcinoma: The development of a new system and comparison with other methods—a preliminary study. Cancer, 49:525, 1982.

Breslow, N., Chan, C. W., Dhom, G., Drury, R. A. B., Franks, L. M., Gellei, B., Lee, Y. S., Lundberg, S., Sparke, B., Sternby, N. H., and Tulinius, H.: Latent carcinoma of prostate at autopsy in seven areas. Int. J. Cancer, 20:680, 1977.

Brindle, J. S., Martinez, A., Schray, M., Edmundson, G., Benson, R. C., Zincke, H., Diokno, A., and Gonzalez, J.: Pelvic lymphadenectomy and transperineal interstitial implantation of IR 192 combined with external beam radiotherapy for bulky stage C prostatic carcinoma. Int. J. Radiat. Oncol. Biol. Phys., 17:1063, 1989.

Byar, D. P.: The Veterans Administration Cooperative Urological Research Group's studies of cancer of the prostate. Cancer, 32:1126, 1973.

Byar, D. P., and Corle, D. K.: Hormone therapy for prostate cancer: Results of the Veterans Administration Cooperative Urological Research Group studies. NCI Monogr., 7:165, 1988.

Byar, D. P., Mostofi, F. K., and the Veterans Administration Cooperative Urological Research Group: Carcinoma of the prostate: Prognostic evaluation of certain pathologic features in 208 radical prostatectomies. Cancer, 30:5, 1972.

Canadian Anandron Study Group: Total androgen ablation in the treatment of metastatic prostatic cancer. Semin. Urol., 8:159, 1990.

Cantrell, B. B., DeKlerk, D. P., Eggleston, J. C., Boitnott, J. K., and Walsh, P. C.: Pathological factors that influence prognosis in stage A prostatic cancer: The influence of extent versus grade. J. Urol., 125:516, 1981.

Carter, B. S., Carter, H. B., and Isaacs, J. T.: Epidemiologic evidence regarding predisposing factors to prostate cancer. Prostate, 16:187, 1990a.

Carter, H. B., Andres, R., Metter, E. J., Fozard, J. L., Chan, D. W., and Walsh, P. C.: Early detection of prostate cancer using serial PSA measurements. J. Urol., 145:382A, 1991. (Abstract, no. 679.)

Carter, H. B., Partin, A. W., Epstein, J. I., Chan, D. W., and Walsh, P. C.: The relationship of prostate specific antigen levels and residual tumor volume in stage A prostate cancer. J. Urol., 144:1167, 1990b.

Carter, H. B., Piantadosi, S., and Isaacs, J. T.: Clinical evidence for and implications of the multistep development of prostate cancer. J. Urol., 143:742, 1990c.

Carter, S. St. C., Trop-Pedersen, S. G., and Holm, H. H.: Ultrasound-guided implantation techniques in treatment of prostate cancer. Urol. Clin. North Am., 16:751, 1989.

Catalona, W. J.: Prostate Cancer. New York, Grune & Stratton, 1984.

Catalona, W. J., and Bigg, S. W.: Nerve-sparing radical prostatectomy: Evaluation of results after 250 patients. J. Urol., 143:538, 1990.

Catalona, W. J., Smith, D. S., Ratliff, T. L., Dodds, K. M., Coplen, D. E., Yuan, J. J. J., Petros, J. A., and Andriole, G. L.: Measurement of prostate specific antigen in serum as a screening test for prostate cancer. N. Engl. J. Med., 324:1156, 1991.

Catalona, W. J., Ratliff, T. L., and Yuan, J. J. J.: Serum prostate specific antigen as a first-line screening test for prostate cancer. J. Urol., 143:313A, 1990. (Abstract no. 499.)

Catalona, W. J., and Stein, A. J.: Staging errors in clinically localized prostatic cancer. J. Urol., 127:452, 1982.

Catalona, W. J., and Whitmore, W. F., Jr.: New staging systems for prostate cancer [Editorial]. J. Urol., 142:1302, 1989.

Chan, D. W., Bruzek, D. J., Oesterling, J. E., Rock, R. C., and Walsh, P. C.: Prostate-specific antigen as a marker for prostatic cancer: Monoclonal and a polyclonal immunoassay compared. Clin. Chem., 33:1916, 1987.

Chodak, G. W., Keller, P., and Schoenberg, H. W.: Assessment of screening for prostate cancer using the digital rectal examination. J. Urol., 141:1136, 1989.

Chodak, G. W., Vogelzang, N. J., Caplan, R. J., Soloway, M., and Smith, J. A.: Independent prognostic factors in patients with metastatic (stage D2) prostate cancer. JAMA, 265:618, 1991.

Christensen, W. N., Partin, A. W., Walsh, P. C., and Epstein, J. I.: Pathologic findings in clinical stage A2 prostate cancer. Cancer, 65:1021, 1990.

Christensson, A., Laurell, C.-B., and Lilja, H.: Enzymatic activity of PSA and its reactions with extracellular serine proteinase inhibitors. Eur. J. Biochem., 194:755, 1990.

Chu, T. M., Kawinski, E., Hibi, N., Croghan, G., Wiley, J., Killian, C. S., and Corral, D.: Prostate-specific antigenic domain of human prostate-specific antigen identified with monoclonal antibodies. J. Urol., 141:152, 1989.

Cleary, K. R., Choy, H. Y., and Ayala, A. G.: Basal cell hyperplasia of the prostate. Am. J. Clin. Pathol., 80:850, 1983.

Coffey, D.: Endocrine control of normal and abnormal growth of the prostate. In Rajfer, J., (Ed.): Urologic Endocrinology. Philadelphia, W. B. Saunders Co., 1986, p. 170.

Cohen, R. J., Glezerson, G., Haffejee, Z., and Afrika, D.: Prostatic carcinoma: Histological and immunohistological factors affecting prognosis. Br. J. Urol., 66:405, 1990.

Cohen, S. M., and Ellwein, L. B.: Cell proliferation in carcinogenesis. Science, 249:1007, 1990.

Cooner, W. H.: Prostate-specific antigen, digital rectal examination, and transrectal ultrasonic examination of the prostate in prostate cancer detection. Monogr. Urol., 12:3, 1991.

Cooner, W. H., Mosley, B. R., Rutherford, C. L., Jr., Beard, J. H., Pond, H. S., Terry, W. J., Igel, T. C., and Kidd, D. D.: Prostate cancer detection in a clinical urological practice by ultrasonography, digital rectal examination and prostate specific antigen. J. Urol., 143:1146, 1990.

Cox, J. D., and Kline, R. W.: Do prostatic biopsies 12 months or more after external irradiation for adenocarcinoma, stage III, predict long-term survival? Int. J. Radiat. Oncol. Biol. Phys., 9:299, 1983.

Crawford, E. D., Eisenberger, M. A., McLeod, D. G., Spaulding, J. T., Benson, R., Dorr, F. A., Blumenstein, B. A., Davis, M. S., and Goodman, P. J.: A controlled trial of leuprolide with and without flutamide in prostatic carcinoma. N. Engl. J. Med., 321:419, 1989.

Dejter, S. W., Jr., Martin, J. S., McPherson, R. A., and Lynch, J. H.: Daily variability in human serum prostate-specific antigen and prostatic acid phosphatase: A comparative evaluation. Urology, 32:288, 1988.

deKernion, J. B., Neuwirth, H., Stein, A., Dorey, F., Stenzl, A., Hannah, J., and Blyth, B.: Prognosis of patients with stage D1 prostate carcinoma following radical prostatectomy with and without early endocrine therapy. J. Urol., 144:700, 1990.

Devesa, S. S., Silverman, D. T., Young, J. L., Pollock, E. S., Brown, C. C., Horn, J. W., Percy, C. L., Myers, M. H., McKay, F. W., and Fraumeni, J. F., Jr.: Cancer incidence and mortality trends among whites in the United States, 1947–84. JNCI, 79:701, 1987.

Dhom, G.: Epidemiologic aspects of latent and clinically manifest carcinoma of the prostate. J. Cancer Res. Clin. Oncol., 106:210, 1983.

Diamond, D. A., Berry, S. J., Jewett, H. J., Eggleston, J. C., and Coffey, D. S.: A new method to assess metastatic potential of human prostate cancer: Relative nuclear roundness. J. Urol., 128:729, 1982a.

Diamond, D. A., Berry, S. J., Umbricht, C., Jewett, H. J., and Coffey, D. S.: Computerized image analysis of nuclear shape as a prognostic factor for prostatic cancer. Prostate, 3:321, 1982b.

di Sant'Agnese, P. A., and de Mesy Jensen, K. L.: Endocrine-paracrine cells of the prostate and prostatic urethra: An ultrastructural study. Hum. Pathol., 15:1034, 1984.

di Sant'Agnese, P. A., and de Mesy Jensen, K. L.: Neuroendocrine differentiation in prostatic carcinoma. Hum. Pathol., 18:849, 1987.

Donohue, R. E., Mani, J. H., Whitesel, J. A., Mohr, S., Scanavino, D., Augspurger, R. R., Biber, R. J., Fauver, H. E., Wettlaufer, J. N., and Pfister, R. R.: Pelvic lymph node dissection: Guide to patient management in clinically locally confined adenocarcinoma of prostate. Urology, 20:559, 1982.

Eggleston, J. C., and Walsh, P. C.: Radical prostatectomy with preservation of sexual function: Pathological findings in the first 100 cases. J. Urol., 134:1146, 1985.

Eigner, E. B., McNeal, J. E., and Stamey, T. A.: Prognosis in pathologically localized carcinoma of the prostate. J. Urol., 1991. Submitted for publication.

Eisenberger, M. A.: Chemotherapy for prostate carcinoma. NCI Monogr., 7:151–163, 1988.

Elder, J. S., Jewett, H. J., and Walsh, P. C.: Radical perineal prostatectomy for clinical stage B2 carcinoma of the prostate. J. Urol., 127:704, 1982.

El-Shirbiny, A., Bhargava, A., Beckley, S., Fitzpatrick, J., and Murphy, G. P.: Comparison of immunologic and enzymatic assay of prostatic acid phosphatase for follow-up and assessment of clinical status of stage D prostate cancer. J. Surg. Oncol., 26:256, 1984.

Epstein, J. I.: Evaluation of radical prostatectomy capsular margins of resection. Am. J. Surg. Pathol., 14:626, 1990.

Epstein, J. I., Berry, S. J., and Eggleston, J. C.: Nuclear roundness factor: A predictor of progression in untreated stage A2 prostate cancer. Cancer, 54:1666, 1984.

Epstein, J. I., and Eggleston, J. C.: Immunohistochemical localization of prostate-specific acid phosphatase and prostate-specific antigen in stage A2 adenocarcinoma of the prostate: Prognostic implications. Hum. Pathol., 15:853, 1984.

Epstein, J. I., Oesterling, J. E., and Walsh, P. C.: The volume and anatomical location of residual tumor in radical prostatectomy specimens removed for stage A1 prostate cancer. J. Urol., 139:975, 1988.

Epstein, J. I., Paull, G., Eggleston, J. C., and Walsh, P. C.: Prognosis of untreated stage A1 prostatic carcinoma: A study of 94 cases with extended follow-up. J. Urol., 136:837, 1986.

Epstein, J. I., and Steinberg, G. D.: The significance of low-grade prostate cancer on needle biopsy. Cancer, 66:1927, 1990.

Epstein, J. I., and Woodruff, J. M.: Adenocarcinoma of the prostate with endometrioid features. Cancer, 57:111, 1986.

Ercole, C. J., Lange, P. H., Mathisen, M., Chiou, R. K., Reddy, P. K., and Vessella, R. L.: Prostate specific antigen and prostatic acid phosphatase in the monitoring and staging of patients with prostatic cancer. J. Urol., 138:1181, 1987.

Ernster, V. L., Winkelstein, W., Jr., Selvin, S., Brown, S. M., Sacks, S. T., Austin, D. F., Mandel, S. A., and Bertolli, T. A.: Race, socioeconomic status, and prostate cancer. Cancer Treat. Rep., 61:187, 1977.

Fearon, E. R., and Vogelstein, B.: A genetic model for colorectal tumorigenesis. Cell, 61:759, 1990.

Ferro, M. A.: Use of intravenous stilbestrol diphosphate in patients with prostatic carcinoma refractory to conventional hormonal manipulation. Urol. Clin. North Am., 18:139, 1991.

Fincham, S. M., Hill, G. B., Hanson, J., and Wijayasinghe, C.: Epidemiology of prostatic cancer: A case-control study. Prostate, 17:189, 1990.

Finkel, A. L., and Taylor, S. P.: Sexual potency after radical prostatectomy. J. Urol., 125:350, 1981.

Fleishner, N., Zadra, J. A., and Bruce, A. W.: Comparison of two assays of prostate specific antigen with clinical correlation. J. Urol., 141:183A, 1989. (Abstract no. 53.)

Flocks, R. H.: The treatment of stage C prostatic cancer with special reference to combined surgical and radiation therapy. J. Urol., 109:461, 1973.

Flocks, R. H., O'Donoghue, E. P. N., Milleman, L. A., and Culp, D. A.: Surgery of prostatic carcinoma. Cancer, 36(Suppl.):705, 1975.

Forman, J. D., Order, S. E., Zinreich, E. S., Lee, D. -J., Wharam, M. D., and Mellits, E. D.: The correlation of pretreatment transurethral resection of prostatic cancer with tumor dissemination and disease-free survival: A univariate and multivariate analysis. Cancer, 58:1770, 1986.

Fosså, S. D., Hosbach, G., and Paus, E.: Flutamide in hormone-resistant prostate cancer. J. Urol., 144:1411, 1990.

Foti, A. G., Herschman, H., and Cooper, J. F.: A solid-phase radioimmunoassay for human prostatic acid phosphatase. Cancer Res., 35:2446, 1975.

Foulds, L.: The experimental study of tumor progression: A review. Cancer Res., 14:327, 1954.

Foulds, L.: The natural history of cancer. J. Chronic Dis., 8:2, 1958.

Frankfurt, O. S., Chin, J. L., Englander, L. S., Greco, W. R., Pontes, J. E., and Rustum, Y. M.: Relationship between DNA ploidy, glandular differentiation, and tumor spread in human prostate cancer. Cancer Res., 45:1418, 1985.

Franks, L. M.: Latent carcinoma of the prostate. J. Pathol. Bacteriol., 68:603, 1954a.

Franks, L. M.: Benign nodular hyperplasia of the prostate: A review. Ann. R. Coll. Surg. Engl., XIV:92, 1954b.

Franks, L. M.: Atrophy and hyperplasia in the prostate proper. J. Pathol. Bacteriol., 68:617, 1954c.

Franks, L. M.: Latency and progression in tumours: The natural history of prostatic cancer. Lancet, 2:1037, 1956.

Franks, L. M.: Etiology, epidemiology, and pathology of prostate cancer. Cancer, 32:1092, 1973.

Franks, L. M., Fergusson, J. D., and Murnaghan, G. F.: An assessment of factors influencing survival in prostatic cancer: The absence of reliable prognostic features. Br. J. Cancer, 12:321, 1958.

Freiha, F. S., and Bagshaw, M. A.: Carcinoma of the prostate: Results of post-irradiation biopsy. Prostate, 5:19, 1984.

Gaeta, J. F., Asirwatham, J. E., Miller, G., and Murphy G. P.: Histologic grading of primary prostatic cancer: A new approach to an old problem. J. Urol., 123:689, 1980.

Gardner, W. A., Jr., Coffey, D., Kam, J. P., Chiarodo, A., Epstein, J., McNeal, J. E., and Miller, G.: A uniform histopathologic grading system for prostate cancer. Hum. Pathol., 19:119, 1988.

Gaynor, E. P.: Zur frage des prostatakrebses. Virchows Arch. f. Path. Anat., 301:602, 1938.

George, N. J. R.: Natural history of localised prostatic cancer managed by conservative therapy alone. Lancet, 1:494, 1988.

Gerber, G. S., and Chodak, G. W.: Prostate specific antigen for assessing response to ketoconazole and prednisone in patients with hormone refractory metastatic prostate cancer. J. Urol., 144:1177, 1990.

Gervasi, L. A., Mata, J., Easley, J. D., Wilbanks, J. H., Seale-Hawkins, C., Carlton, C. E., and Scardino, P. T.: Prognostic significance of lymph nodal metastases in prostate cancer. J. Urol., 142:332, 1989.

Gibbons, R. P.: Prostate cancer: Chemotherapy. Cancer, 60:586, 1987.

Gibbons, R. P., Correa, R. J., Brannen, G. E., and Weissman, R. M.: Total prostatectomy for clinically localized prostatic cancer: Long-term results. J. Urol., 141:564, 1989.

Gibbons, R. P., Mason, J. T., and Correa, R. J.: Carcinoma of the prostate: Local control with external beam radiation therapy. J. Urol., 121:310, 1979.

Gil-Vernet, S.: In Biologia et Pathologia de la Prostata. Madrid, Paz-Montalvo, 1953.

Glashan, R. W., and Robinson, M. R. G.: Cardiovascular complications in the treatment of prostatic cancer. Br. J. Urol., 53:624, 1981.

Gleason, D. F.: Histologic grading and staging of prostatic carcinoma. In Tannenbaum, M. (Ed.): Urologic Pathology: The Prostate. Philadelphia, Lea & Febiger, 1977, pp. 171–197.

Gleason, D. F.: Atypical hyperplasia, benign hyperplasia and well differentiated adenocarcinoma of the prostate. Am. J. Surg. Pathol., 9(Suppl 1):53, 1985.

Goldie, J. H.: Scientific basis for adjuvant and primary (neoadjuvant) chemotherapy. Semin. Oncol., 14:1, 1987.

Goldie, J. H., and Coldman, A. J.: A mathematic model for relating the drug sensitivity of tumors to their spontaneous mutation rate. Cancer Treat. Rep., 63:1727, 1979.

Graves, H. C. B., Kamarei, M., and Stamey, T. A.: Identity of prostate specific antigen and the semen protein p30 purified by a rapid chromatography technique. J. Urol., 144:1510, 1990a.

Graves, H. C. B., Sensabaugh, G. F., and Blake, R. T.: Postcoital detection of male-specific semen protein: Application to the investigation of rape. N. Engl. J. Med., 312:338, 1985.

Graves, H. C. B., Wehner, N., and Stamey, T. A.: Comparison of a polyclonal and monoclonal immunoassay for PSA: Need for an international antigen standard. J. Urol., 144:1516, 1990b.

Green, N., Treible, D., and Wallack, H.: Prostate cancer: Post-irradiation incontinence. J. Urol., 144:307, 1990.

Greene, D. R., Egawa, S., Neerhut, G., Flanagan, W., Wheeler, T. M., and Scardino, P. T.: The distribution of residual cancer in radical prostatectomy specimens in stage A prostate cancer. J. Urol., 145:324, 1991.

Guileyardo, J. M., Johnson, W. D., Welsh, R. A., Akazaki, K., and Correa, P.: Prevalence of latent prostate carcinoma in two U.S. populations. JNCI, 65:311, 1980.

Gutman, A. G., and Gutman, E. B.: "Acid" phosphatase occurring in the serum of patients with metastasizing carcinoma of prostate gland. J. Clin. Invest., 17:473, 1938.

Haenszel, W., and Kurihara, M.: Studies of Japanese migrants: I. Mortality from cancer and other diseases among Japanese in the United States. JNCI, 40:43, 1968.

Hanahan, D.: Transgenic mice as probes into complex systems. Science, 246:1265, 1989.

Hanks, G. E., Leibel, S., and Kramer, S.: The dissemination of cancer by transurethral resection of locally advanced prostate cancer. J. Urol., 129:309, 1983.

Hara, M., Inorre, T., and Fukuyama, T.: Some physico-chemical characteristics of gamma-seminoprotein, an antigenic component specific for human seminal plasma. Jpn. J. Legal Med., 25:322, 1971.

Harada, M., Mostofi, F. K., Corle, D. K., Byar, D. P., and Trump, B. F.: Preliminary studies of histologic prognosis in cancer of the prostate. Cancer Treat. Rep., 61:223, 1977.

Heller, J. E.: Prostatic acid phosphatase: Its current clinical status. J. Urol., 137:1091, 1987.

Henriksson, P., and Edhag, O.: Orchidectomy versus oestrogen for prostatic cancer: Cardiovascular effect. Br. Med. J., 293:413, 1986.

Heppner, G. H.: Tumor heterogeneity. Cancer Res., 44:2259, 1984.

Hodge, K. K., McNeal, J. E., and Stamey, T. A.: Ultrasound guided transrectal core biopsies of the palpably abnormal prostate. J. Urol., 142:66, 1989a.

Hodge, K. K., McNeal, J. E., Terris, M. K., and Stamey, T. A.: Random systematic versus directed ultrasound guided transrectal core biopsies of the prostate. J. Urol., 142:71, 1989b.

Holzman, M., Seale-Hawkins, C., and Scardino, P. T.: The frequency and morbidity of local tumor recurrence after definitive radiotherapy for stage C prostate cancer. J. Urol., 141:347A, 1989. (Abstract no. 709.)

Horm, J. W., and Sondik, E. J.: Person-years of life lost due to cancer in the United States, 1970 and 1984. Am. J. Public Health, 79:1490, 1989.

Hortin, G. L., Bahnson, R. R., Daft, M., Chan, K. M., Catalona, W. J., and Ladenson, J. H.: Differences in values obtained with 2 assays of prostate specific antigen. J. Urol., 139:762, 1988.

Hudson, M. A., Bahnson, R. R., and Catalona, W. J.: Clinical use of prostate specific antigen in patients with prostate cancer. J. Urol., 142:1011, 1989.

Hudson, M. A., Migliore, P., Weinberg, A., Hedrick, T., Wargo, M., and Scardino, P. T.: Use of digital rectal exam, transrectal ultrasonography and serum PSA in prostate cancer screening. J. Urol., 145:381A, 1991. (Abstract, no. 676.)

Huggins, C., and Hodges, C. V.: Studies on prostatic cancer: Effect of castration, of estrogen and of androgen injection on serum phosphatases in metastatic carcinoma of the prostate. Cancer Res., 1:293, 1941.

Huggins, C., Stevens, R. E., and Hodges, C. V.: Studies on prostatic cancer: II. The effects of castration on advanced carcinoma of the prostate gland. Arch. Surg., 43:209, 1941.

Hutchinson, G. B.: Incidence and etiology of prostate cancer. Urology, 17(Suppl.):4, 1981.

Igel, T. C., Barrett, D. M., Segura, J. W., Benson, R. C., Jr., and Rife, C. C.: Perioperative and postoperative complications from bilateral pelvic lymphadenectomy and radical retropubic prostatectomy. J. Urol., 137:1189, 1987.

Isaacs, J. T.: The aging ACI/Seg versus Copenhagen male rat as a model system for the study of prostatic carcinogenesis. Cancer Res., 44:5785, 1984.

Ishikawa, S., Soloway, M. S., Van Der Zwaag, R., and Todd, B.: Prognostic factors in survival free of progression after androgen

deprivation therapy for treatment of prostate cancer. J. Urol., 241:1139, 1989.

Iversen, P., Suciu, S., Sylvester, R., Christensen, I., and Denis, L.: Zoladex and flutamide versus orchiectomy in the treatment of advanced prostatic cancer: A combined analysis of two European Studies, EORTC 30853 and DAPROCA 86. Cancer, 66:1067, 1990.

Janknegt, R. A.—International Anandron Study Group: Efficacy and tolerance of a total androgen blockade with Anandron and orchiectomy: A double-blind placebo-controlled multicenter study. J. Urol., 145:425A, 1991. (Abstract, no. 852.)

Jewett, H. J.: The present status of radical prostatectomy for stages A and B prostatic cancer. Urol. Clin. North Am., 2:105, 1975.

Jewett, H. J.: Radical perineal prostatectomy for palpable, clinically localized, non-obstructive cancer: Experience at the Johns Hopkins Hospital 1909–1963. J. Urol., 124:492, 1980.

Jewett, H. J., Eggleston, J. C., and Yawn, D. H.: Radical prostatectomy in the management of carcinoma of the prostate: Probable causes of some therapeutic failures. J. Urol., 107:1034, 1972.

Johansson, J. E., Adami, M. D., Andersson, S. O., Bergstrom, R., Krusemo, U. B., and Kraaz, W.: Natural history of localised prostate cancer: A population-based study in 223 untreated patients. Lancet, 1:799, 1989.

Johnson, D. E., Logothetis, C. J., and von Eschenback, A. C.: Systemic Therapy for Genitourinary Cancers. Chicago, Year Book Medical Publishers, 1989.

Jones, E. C., McNeal, J., Bruchovsky, N., and deJong, G.: DNA content in prostatic adenocarcinoma. Cancer, 66:752, 1990.

Kabalin, J. N., Hodge, K. K., McNeal, J. E., Freiha, F. S., and Stamey, T. A.: Identification of residual cancer in the prostate following radiation therapy: Role of transrectal ultrasound guided biopsy and prostate specific antigen. J. Urol., 142:326, 1989a.

Kabalin, J. N., McNeal, J. E., Price, H. M., Freiha, F. S., and Stamey, T. A.: Unsuspected adenocarcinoma of the prostate in patients undergoing cystoprostatectomy for other causes: Incidence, histology and morphometric observations. J. Urol., 141:1091, 1989b.

Kadmon, D., Thompson, T. C., Lynch, G. R., and Scardino, P. T.: Elevated serum chromogranin-A levels in patients with advanced prostate cancer. J. Urol., 145:215A, 1991. (Abstract no. 10.)

Karube, K.: Study of latent carcinoma of the prostate in the Japanese based on necropsy material. Tohoku J. Exp. Med., 74:265, 1961.

Kastendieck, H., Altenähr, E., Hüsselmann, H., and Bressel, M.: Carcinoma and dysplastic lesions of the prostate. Z. Krebsforsch, 88:33, 1976.

Kelemen, P. R., Buschmann, R. J., and Weisz-Carrington, P.: Nucleolar prominence as a diagnostic variable in prostatic carcinoma. Cancer, 65:1017, 1990.

Kent, J. R., Bischoff, A. J., Arduino, L. J., Mellinger, G. T., Byar, D. P., Hill, M., and Kozbur, X.: Estrogen dosage and suppression of testosterone levels in patients with prostatic carcinoma. J. Urol., 109:858, 1973.

Keuppens, F., Denis, L., Smith, P., Carvalho, A. P., Newling, D., Bond, A., Sylvester, R., DePauw, M., Vermeylen, K., Ongena, P., and the EORTC GU Group: Zoladex and flutamide versus bilateral orchiectomy. A randomized Phase III EORTC 30853 Study. Cancer, 66:1045–1057, 1990.

Killian, C. S., Yang, N., Enrich, L. J., Vargas, F. P., Kuriyama, M., Wang, M. C., Slack, N. H., Papsidero, L. D., Murphy, G. P., Chu, T. M., and Investigators of the National Prostatic Cancer Project: Prognostic importance of prostate-specific antigen for monitoring patients with stages B2 to D1 prostate cancer. Cancer Res., 45:886, 1985.

Kirk, D.: Trials and tribulations in prostate cancer. Br. J. Urol., 59:375, 1987.

Kleinschmidt, K., Gottfried, H.-W., Riska, P., Miller, K., Wenderoth, U. K., and Hautmann, R.: Organ specificity of PSA and PAP. Impact on detection of residual tumor following radical prostatectomy. J. Urol., 145:383A, 1991. (Abstract no. 684.)

Kovi, J., Mostofi, F. K., Heshmat, M. Y., and Enterline, J. P.: Large acinar atypical hyperplasia and carcinoma of the prostate. Cancer, 61:555, 1988.

Kozlowski, J. M., Ellis, W. J., and Grayhack, J. T.: Advanced prostatic carcinoma: Early versus late endocrine therapy. Urol. Clin. North Am., 18:15, 1991.

Kramer, S. A., Spahr, J., Brendler, C. B., Glenn, J. F., and Paulson, D. F.: Experience with Gleason's histopathologic grading in prostatic cancer. J. Urol., 124:223, 1980.

Kramolowsky, E. V.: The value of testosterone deprivation in stage D1 carcinoma of the prostate. J. Urol., 139:1242, 1988.

Kuban, D. A., el-Mahdi, A. M., Schellhammer, P. F., and Babb, T. J.: The effect of transurethral prostatic resection on the incidence of osseous prostatic metastasis. Cancer, 56:961, 1985.

Kuhn, J. -M., Billebaud, T., Navratil, H., Moulonguet, A., Fiet, J., Grise, P., Louis, J. -F., Costa, P., Husson, J. -M., Dahan, R., Bertagna, C., and Edelstein, R.: Prevention of the transient adverse effects of a gonadotropin-releasing hormone analogue (buserelin) in metastatic prostatic carcinoma by administration of an antiandrogen (nilutamide). N. Engl. J. Med., 321:413–418, 1989.

Kuriyama, M., Wang, M. C., Lee, C. L., Killian, C. S., Papsidero, L. D., Inaji, H., Loor, R. M., Lin, M. F., Nishiura, T., Slack, N. H., Murphy, G. P., and Chu, T. M.: Use of human prostate-specific antigen in monitoring prostate cancer. Cancer Res., 41:3874, 1981.

Labrie, F., Dupont, A., and Belanger, A.: Complete androgen blockade for the treatment of prostate cancer. *In* DeVita, V. T., Jr., Hellman, S., and Rosenberg, S. A. (Eds.): Important Advances in Oncology. Philadelphia, J. B. Lippincott Co., 1985, p. 193.

Labrie, F., Dupont, A., Belanger, A., Cusan, L., Lacourclere, Y., Monfette, G., Laberge, J. G., Edmond, J. P., Fazekas, A. T. A., Raynaud, J. P., and Husson, J. M.: New hormonal therapy in prostatic cancer: Combined treatment with an LHRH agonist and an anti-androgen. Clin. Invest. Med., 5:267, 1982.

Labrie, F., Dupont, A., Belanger, A., and Lachance, R.: Flutamide eliminates the risk of disease flare in prostatic cancer patients treated with a luteinizing hormone-releasing hormone agonist. J. Urol., 138:804–806, 1987a.

Labrie, F., Dupont, A., Giguere, M., Borsanyi, J. -P., Lacourciere, Y., Monfette, G., Emond, J., and Bergeron, N.: Benefits of combination therapy with flutamide in patients relapsing after castration. Br. J. Urol., 61:341–346, 1988.

Labrie, F., Luthy, I., Veilleux, R., Simard, J., Belanger, A., and Dupont, A.: New concepts on the androgen sensitivity of prostate cancer. *In* Murphy, G. P., Khoury, S., Küss, R., Chatelain, C., and Denis, L. (Eds.): Proceedings of Second International Symposium on Prostate Cancer. Prostate Cancer, Part A: Research, Endocrine Treatment, and Histopathology. New York, Alan R. Liss, Inc., 1987b, pp. 145–172.

Lange, P. H., Lightner, D. J., Medini, E., Reddy, P. K., and Vessella, R. L.: The effect of radiation therapy after radical prostatectomy in patients with elevated prostate specific antigen levels. J. Urol., 144:927, 1990.

Lange, P. H., and Narayan, P.: Understaging and undergrading of prostate cancer. Urology, 21:113, 1983.

Leav, I., Ho, S., Ofner, P., Merk, F. B., Kwan, P. W., and Damassa, D.: Biochemical alterations in sex hormone-induced hyperplasia and dysplasia of the dorsolateral prostates of Noble rats. JNCI, 80:1045, 1988.

Lee, C., Keefer, M., Zhao, Z. W., Kroes, R., Berg, L., Liu, X., and Sensibar, J.: Demonstration of the role of prostate-specific antigen in semen liquefaction by two-dimensional electrophoresis. J. Androl., 10:432, 1989.

Lee, F.: Prostate cancer: Preliminary results of an early detection program. Presented at the 5th International Symposium on Transrectal Ultrasound in the Diagnosis and Management of Prostate Cancer. Chicago, IL, September 14, 1990, pp. 86–91.

Lee, F., Littrup, P. J., Torp-Pedersen, S. T., Mettlin, C., McHugh, T. A., Gray, J. M., Kamasaka, G. H., and McLeary, R. D.: Prostate cancer: Comparison of transrectal US and digital rectal examination for screening. Radiology, 168:389, 1988a.

Lee, S. E., Currin, S. M., Paulson, D. F., and Walther, P. J.: Flow cytometric determination of ploidy in prostatic adenocarcinoma: A comparison with seminal vesicle involvement and histopathological grading as a predictor of clinical recurrence. J. Urol., 140:769, 1988b.

Lerner, S. P., Seale-Hawkins, C., Carlton, C. E., Jr., and Scardino, P. T.: The risk of dying of prostate cancer in patients with clinically localized disease. J. Urol., 1991. In press.

Leuprolide Study Group: Leuprolide versus diethylstilbestrol for metastatic prostate cancer. N. Engl. J. Med., 311:1281, 1984.

Lew, E. A., and Garfinkel, L.: Mortality at ages 75 and older in the Cancer Prevention Study (CPSI). CA, 40:210, 1990.

Li, T. S., and Beling, C. G.: Isolation and characterization of two specific antigens of human seminal plasma. Fertil. Steril., 24:2134, 1973.

Lightner, D. J., Lange, P. H., Ercole, C. J., Unger, K., Sauees, J. B., Mathiasen, M. L., and Vessella, R. L.: Serum prostate specific antigen (PSA) and the utility of isotopic bone scans (BoS) in the monitoring of patients with carcinoma of the prostate (CaP) [Abstract 461]. Proc. Am. Soc. Clin. Oncol., 7:120, 1988.

Lightner, D. J., Lange, P. H., Reddy, P. K., and Moore, L.: Prostate specific antigen and local recurrence after radical prostatectomy. J. Urol., 144:921, 1990.

Lilja, H., and Lourell, C. B.: The predominant protein in human seminal coagulate. Scand. J. Clin. Lab. Invest., 45:635, 1985.

Linehan, W. M., LaRocca, R., Stein, Cy., Walther, M., Cooper, M., Weiss, G., Choyke, P., Cassidy, J., Uhrich, M., and Myers, C. E.: Use of suramin in treatment of patients with advanced prostate carcinoma. J. Urol., 143:221A, 1990. (Abstract no. 131.)

Link, P., Freiha, F. S., and Stamey, T. A.: Adjuvant radiation therapy in patients with detectable prostatic specific antigen following radical prostatectomy. J. Urol., 145:532, 1991.

Lowe, B. A., and Listrom, M. B.: Incidental carcinoma of the prostate: An analysis of the predictors of progression. J. Urol., 140:1340, 1988.

Lowsley, O. S.: The development of the human prostate gland with reference to the development of other structures at the neck of the urinary bladder. Am. J. Anat., 13:299, 1912.

Lundberg, S., Carstensen, J., and Rundquist, I.: DNA flow cytometry and histopathological grading of paraffin-embedded prostate biopsy specimens in a survival study. Cancer Res., 47:1973, 1987.

Maatman, T. J.: The role of prostate specific antigen as a tumor marker in men with advanced adenocarcinoma of the prostate. J. Urol., 141:1378, 1989.

Mahadevia, P. S., Koss, L. G., and Tar, I. J.: Prostatic involvement in bladder cancer: Prostate mapping in 20 cystoprostatectomy specimens. Cancer, 58:2096, 1986.

Mao, P., and Angrist, A.: The fine structure of the basal cell of the human prostate. Lab. Invest., 15:1768, 1966.

McGowan, D. G.: The adverse influence of prior transurethral resection on prognosis in carcinoma of prostate treated by radiation therapy. Int. J. Radiat. Oncol. Biol. Phys., 6:1121, 1980.

McLeary, R. D.: Biopsy techniques, strategic and systematic. Presented at the 5th International Symposium on Transrectal Ultrasound in the Diagnosis and Management of Prostate Cancer. Chicago, IL, September 14, 1990, pp. 7–17.

McNeal, J. E.: Morphogenesis of prostatic carcinoma. Cancer, 18:1659, 1965.

McNeal, J. E.: Regional morphology and pathology of the prostate. Am. J. Clin. Pathol., 49:347, 1968.

McNeal, J. E.: Origin and development of carcinoma in the prostate. Cancer, 23:24, 1969.

McNeal, J. E.: Origin and evolution of benign prostatic enlargement. Invest. Urol., 15:340, 1978.

McNeal, J. E.: Significance of duct-acinar dysplasia in prostatic carcinogenesis. Prostate, 13:91, 1988a.

McNeal, J. E.: Normal histology of the prostate. Am. J. Surg. Pathol., 12:619, 1988b.

McNeal, J. E., Alroy, J., Leav, I., Redwine, E. A., Freiha, F. S., and Stamey, T. A.: Immunohistochemical evidence for impaired cell differentiation in the premalignant phase of prostate carcinogenesis. Am. J. Clin. Pathol., 90:23, 1988a.

McNeal, J. E., and Bostwick, D. G.: Intraductal dysplasia: A premalignant lesion of the prostate. Hum. Pathol., 17:64, 1986.

McNeal, J. E., Bostwick, D. G., Kindrachuk, R. A., Redwine, E. A., Freiha, F. S., and Stamey, T. A.: Patterns of progression in prostate cancer. Lancet, 1:60, 1986a.

McNeal, J. E., Leav, I., Alroy, J., and Skutelsky, E.: Differential lectin staining of central and peripheral zones of the prostate and alterations in dysplasia. Am. J. Clin. Pathol., 89:41, 1988b.

McNeal, J. E., Price, H. M., Redwine, E. A., Freiha, F. S., and Stamey, T. A.: Stage A versus stage B adenocarcinoma of the prostate: Morphological comparison and biological significance. J. Urol., 139:61, 1988c.

McNeal, J. E., Redwine, E. A., Freiha, F. S., and Stamey, T. A.: Zonal distribution of prostatic adenocarcinoma. Am. J. Surg. Pathol., 12:897, 1988d.

McNeal, J. E., Reese, J. H., Redwine, E. A., Freiha, F. S., and Stamey, T. A.: Cribriform adenocarcinoma of the prostate. Cancer, 58:1714, 1986b.

McNeal, J. E., Villers, A. A., Redwine, E. A., Freiha, F. S., and

Stamey, T. A.: Capsular penetration in prostate cancer: Significance for natural history and treatment. Am. J. Surg. Pathol., 14:240, 1990a.

McNeal, J. E., Villers, A. A., Redwine, E. A., Freiha, F. S., and Stamey, T. A.: Histologic differentiation, cancer volume, and pelvic lymph node metastasis in adenocarcinoma of the prostate. Cancer, 66:1225, 1990b.

McNeal, J. E., Villers, S., Redwine, E. A., Freiha, F. S., and Stamey, T. A.: Microcarcinoma in the prostate: Its association with duct-acinar dysplasia. Hum. Pathol., 1991. In press.

Meacham, R. B., Scardino, P. T., Hoffman, G. S., Easley, J. D., Wilbanks, J. H., and Carlton, C. E., Jr.: The risk of distant metastases after transurethral resection of the prostate versus needle biopsy in patients with localized prostate cancer. J. Urol., 142:320, 1989.

Melicow, M. M., and Pachter, M. R.: Endometrial carcinoma of prostatic utricle (uterus masculinus). Cancer, 20:1715, 1967.

Melicow, M. M., and Tannenbaum, M.: Endometrial carcinoma of uterus masculinus (prostatic utricle): Report of 6 cases. J. Urol., 106:892, 1971.

Mettlin, C.: Preliminary findings from the American Cancer Society National Prostate Cancer Detection Project. Presented at the 5th International Symposium on Transrectal Ultrasound in the Diagnosis and Management of Prostate Cancer. Chicago, IL, September 14, 1990, pp. 84–85.

Middleton, R. G., and Smith, J. A., Jr.: Radical prostatectomy for stage B2 prostatic cancer. J. Urol., 127:702, 1982.

Miller, J. I., Ahmann, F. R., Drach, G. W., and Bottaccini, M. R.: Serum PSA levels predict duration of remission and survival post hormone therapy of metastatic prostate cancer. J. Urol., 145:384A, 1991. (Abstract no. 688.)

Mohler, J. L., Partin, A. W., Epstein, J. I., Lohr, W. D., and Coffey, D. S.: Nuclear roundness factor measurement for assessment of prognosis of patients with prostatic carcinoma: II. Standardization of methodology for histologic sections. J. Urol., 139:1085, 1988a.

Mohler, A. L., Partin, A. W., Lohr, W. D., and Coffey, D. S.: Nuclear roundness factor measurement for assessment of prognosis of patients with prostatic carcinoma: I. Testing of a digitization system. J. Urol., 139:1080, 1988b.

Moore, R. A.: The morphology of small prostatic carcinoma. J. Urol., 33:224, 1935.

Moskovitz, B., Nitecki, S., and Levin, D. R.: Cancer of the prostate: Is there a need for aggressive treatment? Urol. Int., 42:49, 1987.

Mostofi, F. K.: Grading of prostatic carcinoma. Cancer Chemother Rep. (Part 1), 59:111, 1975.

Mostofi, F. K.: Problems of grading carcinoma of prostate. Semin. Oncol., 3:161, 1976.

Murphy, G. P., Natarajan, N., Pontes, J. E., Schmitz, R. L., Smart, C. R., Schmidt, J. D., and Mettlin, C.: The national survey of prostate cancer in the United States by the American College of Surgeons. J. Urol., 127:928, 1982.

Murphy, G. P., and Whitmore, W. F., Jr.: A report of the workshops on the current status of the histologic grading of prostate cancer. Cancer, 44:1490, 1979.

Myers, R. P., Neves, R. J., Farrow, G. M., and Utz, D. C.: Nucleolar grading of prostatic adenocarcinoma: Light microscopic correlation with disease progression. Prostate, 3:423, 1982.

Myers, R. P., Zincke, H., Fleming, T. R., Farrow, G. M., Furlow, W. L., and Utz, D. C.: Hormonal treatment at time of radical retropubic prostatectomy for stage D1 prostate cancer. J. Urol., 130:99, 1983.

Nicolson, G. L.: Tumor cell instability, diversification, and progression to the metastatic phenotype: From oncogene to oncofetal expression. Cancer Res., 47:1473, 1987.

Oesterling, J. E.: Prostate-specific antigen: A critical assessment of the most useful tumor marker for adenocarcinoma of the prostate. J. Urol., 145:907, 1991.

Oesterling, J. E., and Bergstralh, E. J.: Prostate-specific antigen (PSA) following prostate bipopsy (Bx) and transurethral resection of the prostate (TURP): Length of time necessary to achieve a stable value. J. Urol., 145:251A, 1991. (Abstract no. 154.)

Oyasu, R., Bahnson, R. R., Nowels, K., and Garnett, J. E.: Cytological atypia in the prostate gland: Frequency, distribution and possible relevance to carcinoma. J. Urol., 135:959, 1986.

Partin, A. W., Epstein, J. I., Cho, K. R., Gittelsohn, A. M., and

Walsh, P. C.: Morphometric measurement of tumor volume and per cent of gland involvement as predictors of pathological stage in clinical stage B prostate cancer. J. Urol., 141:341, 1989.

Paulson, D. F., and Cox, E. B.: Does transurethral resection of the prostate promote metastatic disease? J. Urol., 138:90, 1987.

Paulson, D. F., and Frazier, H. A.: Is PSA of clinical importance in evaluating outcome after radical surgery? J. Urol., 145:383A, 1991. (Abstract, no. 683.)

Paulson, D. F., Hodge, G. B., Jr., Hinshaw, W., and the Uro-Oncology Research Group: Radiation therapy versus delayed androgen deprivation for stage C carcinoma of the prostate. J. Urol., 1341:901, 1984.

Peehl, D. M., Wong, S. T., and Stamey, T. A.: Cytostatic effects of suramin on prostate cancer cells cultured from primary tumors. J. Urol., 145:624–630, 1991.

Peeling, W. B.: Phase III studies to compare goserelin (Zoladex) with orchiectomy and with diethylstilbestrol in treatment of prostatic carcinoma. Urology, 33(Suppl.):45, 1989.

Perlman, E. J., and Epstein, J. I.: Blood group antigen expression in dysplasia and adenocarcinoma of the prostate. Am. J. Surg. Pathol., 14:810, 1990.

Perrin, P., François, O., Maquet, J. H., Bringeon, G., Duteil, P., and Devonec, M.: Circulating prostate-specific antigen in benign hypertrophy and localized cancer of the prostate: Can PSA be considered as a screening examination for localized cancer? Progrès en Urologie, 2:(April), 1991.

Price, H., McNeal, J. E., and Stamey, T. A.: Evolving patterns of tissue composition in benign prostatic hyperplasia as a function of specimen size. Hum. Pathol., 21:578, 1990.

Quinn, B. D., Cho, K. R., and Epstein, J. I.: Relationship of severe dysplasia to stage B adenocarcinoma of the prostate. Cancer, 65:2328, 1990.

Reddy, P. K., and Lange, P. H.: Stirrups to minimize complications of prolonged dorsal lithotomy positioning. J. Urol., 139:326, 1988.

Reese, J. H., McNeal, J. E., Redwine, E. A., Samloff, I. M., and Stamey, T. A.: Differential distribution of pepsinogen II between the zones of the human prostate and the seminal vesicle. J. Urol., 136:1148, 1986.

Reese, J. H., McNeal, J. E., Redwine, E. A., Stamey, T. A., and Freiha, F. S.: Tissue plasminogen activator as a marker for functional zones within the human prostate gland. Prostate, 12:47, 1988.

Reiner, W. G., Scott, W. W., Eggleston, J. C., and Walsh, O. C.: Long-term survival after hormonal therapy for stage D prostatic cancer. J. Urol., 122:183, 1979.

Riegman, P. H. J., Vlietstra, R. J., van der Korpert, J. A. G. M., Romijn, J. C., and Trapman, J.: Characterization of the prostate-specific antigen gene: A novel human Kallikrein-like gene. Biochem. Biophys. Res. Commun., 159:95, 1989.

Rifkin, M. D., Zerhouni, E. A., Gasonis, C. A., Quint, L. E., Paushter, D. M., Epstein, J. I., Hamper, U., Walsh, P. C., and McNeil, B. J.: Comparison of magnetic resonance imaging and ultrasonography in staging early prostate cancer: Results of a multi-institutional cooperative trial. N. Engl. J. Med., 323:621, 1990.

Robey, E. L., Schellhammer, P. F., Wright, G. L., Jr., and El-Mahdi, A. M.: Cancer serum index and prostatic acid phosphatase for detection of progressive prostatic cancer. J. Urol., 134:787, 1985.

Robinson, M. R. G.: Complete androgen blockade: the EORTC experience comparing orchidectomy versus orchidectomy plus cyproterone acetate versus low-dose stilbestrol in the treatment of metastatic carcinoma of the prostate. In Murphy, G. P., Khoury, S., Küss, R., Chatelain, C., and Denis, L. (Eds.): Proceedings of Second International Symposium on Prostate Cancer. Prostate Cancer, Part A: Research, Endocrine Treatment, and Histopathology. New York, Alan R. Liss, Inc., 1987, pp. 383–390.

Robinson, R. G., Mebust, W. K., Davis, B. E., Weigel, J. W., and Baxter, K. G.: Treatment of metastatic prostate carcinoma in bone with strontium-89. J. Urol., 143:222A, 1990. (Abstract no. 133.)

Robles, J. M., Morell, A. R., Redorta, J. P., de Torres Mateos, J. A., and Roselló, A. S.: Clinical behavior of prostatic specific antigen and prostatic acid phosphatase: a comparative study. Eur. Urol., 14:360–366, 1988.

Rock, R. C., Chan, D. W., Bruzek, D., Waldron, C., Oesterling, J., and Walsh, P.: Evaluation of a monoclonal immunoradiometric assay for prostate-specific antigen. Clin. Chem., 33:2257–2261, 1987.

Rodin, A. E., Larson, D. L., and Roberts, D. K.: Nature of the perineural space invaded by prostatic carcinoma. Cancer, 20:1772, 1967.

Roy, A. V., Brower, M. E., and Hayden, J. E.: Sodium thymolphthalein monophosphate: A new acid phosphatase substrate with greater specificity for the prostatic enzyme in serum. Clin. Chem., 17:1093, 1971.

Sagalowsky, A. I., Milam, H., Reveley, L. R., and Silva, F. G.: Prediction of lymphatic metastases by Gleason histologic grading in prostatic cancer. J. Urol., 128:951, 1982.

Sager, R.: Tumor suppressor genes: The puzzle and the promise. Science, 246:1406, 1989.

Sarosdy, M. F.: Do we have a rational treatment plan for stage D-1 carcinoma of the prostate? World J. Urol., 8:27, 1990.

Scardino, P. T.: Early detection of prostate cancer. Urol. Clin. North Am., 16:635, 1989.

Scardino, P. T., and Wheeler, T. M.: Local control of prostate cancer with radiotherapy: Frequency and prognostic significance of positive results of postirradiation prostate biopsy. NCI Monogr., 7:95, 1988.

Schally, A. V., Kastin, A. J., and Coy, D. H.: LH-releasing hormone and its analogues: Recent basic and clinical investigations. Int. J. Fertil., 1:1, 1976.

Schedlich, L. J., Bennetts, B. H., and Morris, B. J.: Primary structure of a human glandular kallikrein gene. DNA, 6:429, 1987.

Schellhammer, P. F., Bean, M. A., and Whitmore, W. F., Jr.: Prostatic involvement by transitional cell carcinoma: Pathogenesis, patterns and prognosis. J. Urol., 118:399, 1977.

Schellhammer, P. F., El-Mahdi, A. M., Higgins, E. M., Schultheiss, T. E., Ladaga, L. E., and Babb, T. J.: Prostate biopsy after definitive treatment by interstitial ^{125}Iodine implant or external beam radiation therapy. J. Urol., 137:897, 1987.

Schellhammer, P. F., Schlossberg, S. M., El-Mahdi, A. M., Wright G. L., and Brassil, D. N.: PSA levels after definitive irradiation for carcinoma of the prostate. J. Urol., 1991. In press.

Schellhammer, P. F., Warden, S. S., Wright, G. L., and Sieg, S.: Bone marrow acid phosphatase by counter-immune electrophoresis: Pre-treatment and post-treatment correlations. J. Urol., 127:66, 1982.

Schmid, H. -P., McNeal, J. E., and Stamey, T. A.: Observations on the doubling time of prostate cancer as measured by serial PSA in untreated patients with prostate cancer. N. Engl. J. Med., 1991. Submitted for publication.

Schroeder, F. H., and Belt, E.: Carcinoma of the prostate: A study of 213 patients with stage C tumors treated by total perineal prostatectomy. J. Urol., 114:257, 1975.

Schron, D. S., Gipson, T., and Mendelsohn, G.: The histogenesis of small cell carcinoma of the prostate. Cancer, 53:2478, 1984.

Scott, W. W., and Boyd, H. L.: Combined hormone control therapy and radical prostatectomy in the treatment of selected cases of advanced carcinoma of the prostate—a retrospective study based upon 25 years of experience. J. Urol., 101:86, 1969.

Seidman, H., Mushinski, M. H., Gelb, S. K., and Silverberg, E.: Probabilities of eventually developing or dying of cancer—United States, 1985. CA, 35:36, 1985.

Sensabaugh, G. F.: Isolation and characterization of a semen-specific protein from human seminal plasma: A potential new marker for semen identification. J. Forensic Sci., 23:106, 1978.

Sensabaugh, G. F., and Blake, E. T.: Seminal plasma protein p30: Simplified purification and evidence for identity with prostate specific antigen. J. Urol., 144:1523, 1990.

Shabsigh, R., Carter, S. Stc., Egawa, S., Wright, C. D., Carlton, C. E., Jr., and Scardino, P. T.: Transrectal ultrasound and/or digital guided biopsy of the prostate. J. Urol., 141:282A, 1989. (Abstract no. 449.)

Shanthaveerappa, T. R., and Bourne, G. H.: Perineural epithelium: A new concept of its role in the integrity of the peripheral nervous system. Science, 154:1464, 1966.

Sharkey, F. E., Dusenbery, D. M., Moyer, J. E., and Barry, J. D.: Correlation between stage and grade in prostatic adenocarcinoma: A morphometric study. J. Urol., 132:602, 1984.

Shearer, R. J., Hendry, W. F., Sommerville, I. F., and Fergusson, J. D.: Plasma testosterone: An accurate monitor of hormone treatment in prostatic cancer. Br. J. Urol., 45:668, 1973.

Shinohara, K., Wheeler, T., and Scardino, P. T.: The appearance of prostate cancer on transrectal ultrasonography: Correlation of imaging and pathological examinations. J. Urol., 142:76, 1989.

Siddall, J. K., Hetherington, J. W., Cooper, E. H., Newling, D. W. W., Robinson, M. R. G., Richards, B., and Denis, L.: Biochemical monitoring of carcinoma of prostate treated with an LH-RH analogue (Zoladex). Br. J. Urol., 58:676–682, 1986.

Simard, J., Luthy, I., Guay, J., Bélanger, A., and Labrie, F.: Characteristics of interaction of the antiandrogen flutamide with the androgen receptor in various target tissues. Mol. Cell Endocrinol., 44:261–270, 1986.

Smith, J. A., Jr., Crawford, E. D., Lange, P. H., Lynch, D. F., Al-Juburi, A., Bracken, R. B., Wise, H. A., Heyden, N., and Bertagna, C.: PSA correlation with response and survival in advanced carcinoma of the prostate. J. Urol., 145:354A, 1991. (Abstract no. 685.)

Smith, J. A., Jr., Haynes, T. H., and Middleton, R. G.: Impact of external irradiation on local symptoms and survival free of disease in patients with pelvic lymph node metastasis from adenocarcinoma of the prostate. J. Urol., 131:705, 1984.

Smith, J. A., Jr., Seaman, J. P., Gleidman, J. B., and Middleton, R. G.: Pelvic lymph node metastasis from prostatic cancer: Influence of tumor grade and stage in 452 consecutive patients. J. Urol., 130:290, 1983.

Sogani, P. C., and Fair, W. R.: Treatment of advanced prostatic cancer. Urol. Clin. North A., 14:353, 1987.

Sogani, P. C., Vagaiwala, M. R., and Whitmore, W. F.: Experience with flutamide in patients with advanced prostatic cancer without prior endocrine therapy. Cancer, 54:744, 1984.

Sonino, N.: The use of ketoconazole as an inhibitor of steroid production. N. Engl. J. Med., 317:812, 1987.

Spiessl, B., Hermanek, P., Scheibe, O., and Wagner, G.: Prostate. In TNM Atlas: Illustrated Guide to the Classification of Malignant Tumours, Ed. 2. New York, Springer-Verlag, 1982, p. 180.

Spigelman, S. S., McNeal, J. E., Freiha, F. S., and Stamey, T. A.: Rectal examination in volume determination of carcinoma of the prostate: Clinical and anatomical correlations. J. Urol., 136:1228, 1986.

Stamey, T. A.: Prostate cancer: Some basic clinical and morphometric observations. Monogr. Urol., 10:79, 1989.

Stamey, T. A., Freiha, F. S., McNeal, J. E., Redwine, E. A., Whittemore, A. S., and Schmid, H. -P.: Relationship of clinical significance for treatment to tumor volume in prostate cancer. J. Urol., 1991. National Conference on Prostate Cancer, American Cancer Society. Cancer, 1992.

Stamey, T. A., and Kabalin, J. N.: Prostate specific antigen in the diagnosis and treatment of adenocarcinoma of the prostate: I. Untreated patients. J. Urol., 141:1070, 1989.

Stamey, T. A., Kabalin, J. N., and Ferrari, M.: Prostate-specific antigen in the diagnosis and treatment of adenocarcinoma of the prostate: III. Radiation treated patients. J. Urol., 141:1084, 1989a.

Stamey, T. A., Kabalin, J. N., Ferrari, M., and Yang, N.: Prostate specific antigen in the diagnosis and treatment of adenocarcinoma of the prostate: IV. Anti-androgen treated patients. J. Urol., 241:1088, 1989b.

Stamey, T. A., Kabalin, J. N., McNeal, J. E., Johnston, I. M., Freiha, F., Redwine, E. A., and Yang, N.: Prostate specific antigen in the diagnosis and treatment of adenocarcinoma of the prostate: II. Radical prostatectomy treated patients. J. Urol., 141:1076, 1989c.

Stamey, T. A., McNeal, J. E., Freiha, F. S., and Redwine, E.: Morphometric and clinical studies on 68 consecutive radical prostatectomies. J. Urol., 139:1235, 1988.

Stamey, T. A., Villers, A. A., McNeal, J. E., Link, P. C., and Freiha, F. S.: Positive surgical margins at radical prostatectomy: Importance of the apical dissection. J. Urol., 143:1166, 1990.

Stamey, T. A., Yang, N., Hay, A. R., McNeal, J. E., Freiha, F. S., and Redwine, E.: Prostate-specific antigen as a serum marker for adenocarcinoma of the prostate. N. Engl. J. Med., 317:909, 1987.

Stein, A., deKernion, J. B., Smith, R. B., Dorey, F., and Patel, H.: Post radical prostatectomy PSA levels in patients with organ confined and locally extensive prostate cancer. J. Urol. (Special Editorial Supplement), March, 1992.

Steinberg, G. D., Carter, B. S., Beaty, T. H., Childs, B., and Walsh, P. C.: Family history and the risk of prostate cancer. Prostate, 17:337, 1990.

Steinberg, G. D., Epstein, J. I., Piantodosi, S., and Walsh, P. C.: Management of stage D1 adenocarcinoma of the prostate: The Johns Hopkins Experience 1974 to 1987. J. Urol., 144:1425, 1990.

Stenman, U. -H., Leinonen, J., Alfthan, H., Rannikko, S., Tuhkanen, K., and Alfthan, O.: A complex between prostate-specific antigen and α_1-antichymotrypsin is the major form of prostate-specific antigen in serum of patients with prostatic cancer: assay of the complex improves clinical sensitivity for cancer. Cancer Res., 51:222–226, 1991.

Stephenson, R. A., James B. C., Gay, H., Fair, W. R., Whitmore, W. F., Jr., and Melamed, M. R.: Flow cytometry of prostate cancer: Relationship of DNA content to survival. Cancer Res., 47:2504, 1987.

Stilmant, M. M., Freedlund, M. C., de las Morenas, A., Shepard, R. L., Oates, R. D., and Siroky, M. B.: Expanded role for fine needle aspiration of the prostate: A study of 335 specimens. Cancer, 63:583, 1989.

Surya, B. V., and Provet, J. A.: Manifestations of advanced prostate cancer: Prognosis and treatment. J. Urol., 142:921, 1989.

Tannenbaum, M., Tannenbaum, S., DeSanctis, P. N., and Olsson, C. A.: Prognostic significance of nucleolar surface area in prostate cancer. Urology, 19:546, 1982.

Terris, M. K., Klonecke, A. S., McDougall, I. R., and Stamey, T. A.: Utilization of bone scans in conjunction with prostate specific antigen levels in the surveillance for recurrence of adenocarcinoma after radical prostatectomy. J. Nucl. Med., 32:1713, 1991a.

Terris, M. K., McNeal, J. E., and Stamey, T. A.: Invasion of the seminal vesicles by prostatic cancer: Detection with transrectal sonography. AJR, 155:811, 1990.

Terris, M. K., McNeal, J. E., and Stamey, T. A.: Estimation of prostate cancer volume by transrectal ultrasound imaging. J. Urol., 1991b. In press.

Terris, M. K., McNeal, J. E., and Stamey, T. A.: Transrectal ultrasound and ultrasound guided prostate biopsies in the detection of residual carcinoma in clinical stage A carcinoma of the prostate. J. Urol., 1991c. Submitted for publication.

Torti, F. M., Aston, D., Lum, B. L., Kohler, M., Williams, R. D., Spaulding, J. T., Shortliffe, L., and Freiha, F. S.: Weekly doxorubicin in endocrine refractory carcinoma of the prostate. J. Clin. Oncol., 1:477, 1983.

Trachtenberg, J., and Point, A.: Ketoconazole: A novel and rapid treatment for advanced prostate cancer. J. Urol., 130:152, 1983.

Trump, D. L., Havlin, K. H., Messing, E. M., Cummings, K. B., Lange, P. H., and Jordan, V. C.: High-dose ketoconazole in advanced hormone-refractory prostate cancer: Endocrinologic and clinical effects. J. Clin. Oncol., 7:1093, 1989.

Utz, D. C., and Farrow, G. M.: Pathologic differentiation and prognosis of prostatic carcinoma. JAMA, 209:1701, 1969.

Vallancien, G., Prapotnich, D., Veillon, B., Brisset, J. M., and Andre-Bougaran, J.: Systematic prostatic biopsies in 100 men with no suspicion of cancer on digital rectal examination. J. Urol., 146:1308, 1991a.

Vallancien, G., Prapotnich, D., Veillon, B., Brisset, J. M., and Andre-Bougaran, J.: Seminal vesicle biopsies in the preoperative staging of prostatic cancer. Eur. Urol., 19:343, 1991b.

van Aubel, O. G., Hoekstra, W. J., and Schröder, F. H.: Early orchiectomy for patients with stage D1 prostatic carcinoma. J. Urol., 134:292, 1985.

Veterans Administration Cooperative Urological Research Group: Treatment and survival of patients with cancer of the prostate. Surg. Gynecol. Obstet., 124:1011, 1967a.

Veterans Administration Cooperative Urological Research Group: Carcinoma of the prostate: Treatment comparisons. J. Urol., 98:516, 1967b.

Villers, A., McNeal, J. E., Redwine, E. A., Freiha, F. S., and Stamey, T. A.: The role of perineural space invasion in the local spread of prostatic adenocarcinoma. J. Urol., 142:763, 1989.

Villers, A., McNeal, J. E., Redwine, E. A., Freiha, F. S., and Stamey, T. A.: Pathogenesis and biological significance of seminal vesicle invasion in prostatic adenocarcinoma. J. Urol., 143:1183, 1990.

Villers, A., McNeal, J. E., Freiha, F. S., and Stamey, T. A.: Multiple cancers in the prostate: morphologic features of clinically recognized vs. incidental tumors. Cancer (Submitted).

Voges, G. E., McNeal, J. E., Redwine, E. A., Freiha, F. S., and Stamey, T. A.: The predictive significance of substaging stage A prostate cancer (A1 vs. A2) for volume and grade of total cancer in the prostate. J. Urol., 1991. In press.

Walsh, P. C.: Radical retropubic prostatectomy with reduced morbidity: An anatomic approach. NCI Monogr., 7:133, 1988.

Walsh, P. C., and Donker, P. J.: Impotence following radical prostatectomy: Insight into etiology and prevention. J. Urol., 128:492, 1982.

Walsh, P. C., Lepor, H., and Eggleston, J. C.: Radical prostatectomy with preservation of sexual function: Anatomical and pathological considerations. The Prostate, 4:473, 1983.

Wang, M. C., Valenzuela, L. A., Murphy, G. P., and Chu, T. M.: Purification of a human prostate specific antigen. Invest. Urol., 17:159, 1979.

Watt, K. W. K., Lee, P. J., M'Timkulu, T., Chan, W. P., and Loor, R.: Human prostate-specific antigen: Structural and functional similarity with serine proteases. Proc. Natl. Acad. Sci. USA, 83:3166, 1986.

Weinberg, R. A.: Oncogenes, antioncogenes, and the molecular bases of multistep carcinogenesis. Cancer Res., 49:3713, 1989.

Whitesel, J. A., Donohue, R. E., Mani, J. H., Mohr, S., Scanavino, D. J., Angspurger, R. R., Biber, R. J., Fauver, H. E., Wettlaufer, J. N., and Pfister, R. R.: Acid phosphatase: Its influence on the management of carcinoma of the prostate. J. Urol., 131:70, 1984.

Whitmore, W. F., Jr.: The natural history of prostatic cancer. Cancer, 32:1104, 1973.

Whitmore, W. F., Jr.: Interstitial radiation therapy for carcinoma of the prostate. Prostate, 1:157, 1980.

Whitmore, W. F., Jr.: Overview: Historical and contemporary. NCI Monogr., 7:7, 1988.

Whitmore, W. F., Jr.: Locoregional prostatic cancer: Advances in management. Cancer, 65:667, 1990.

Whitmore, W. F., Jr., Catalona, W. J., Grayhack, J. T., Hanks, G., Peters, P. C., Shipley, W. U., and Walsh, P. C.: Organ systems program staging classification for prostate cancer. In Coffey, D. S., Resnick, M. I., Dorr, F. A., and Karr, J. P. (Eds.): A Multidisciplinary Analysis of Controversies in the Management of Prostate Cancer. New York, Plenum Press, 1988, p. 295.

Whitmore, W. F., Jr., and Hilaris, B.: Treatment of localized prostate cancer by interstitial 125-I. In Karr, J. P., and Yamanaka, H. (Eds.): Prostate Cancer: The Second Tokyo Symposium. New York, Elsevier Science Publishing Co., 1989, p. 344.

Whitmore, W. J., Jr., Warner, J. A., and Thompson, I. M., Jr.: Expectant management of localized prostatic cancer. Cancer, 67:1091, 1991.

Winkler, H. Z., Rainwater, L. M., Myers, R. P., Farrow, G. M., Therneau, T. M., Zincke, H., and Lieber, M. M.: Stage D1 prostatic adenocarcinoma: Significance of nuclear DNA ploidy patterns studied by flow cytometry. Mayo Clin. Proc., 63:103, 1988.

Wood, D. P., Jr., Montie, J. E., Pontes, J. E., Medendorp, S. V., and Levin, H. S.: Transitional cell carcinoma of the prostate in cystoprostatectomy specimens removed for bladder cancer. J. Urol., 141:346, 1989.

Woodruff, M. F. A.: Cellular heterogeneity in tumours. Br. J. Cancer, 47:589, 1983.

Woolf, C. M.: An investigation of the familial aspects of carcinoma of the prostate. Cancer, 13:739, 1960.

Wynder, E. L., Mabuchi, K., and Whitmore, W. F., Jr.: Epidemiology of cancer of the prostate. Cancer, 28:344, 1971.

Yuan, J. J. J., and Catalona, W. J.: Effects of digital rectal examination, prostate massage, transrectal ultrasonography and needle biopsy of the prostate on serum prostate specific antigen levels. J. Urol., 145:213A, 1991. (Abstract no. 2.)

Zaridze, D. G., and Boyle, P.: Cancer of the prostate: Epidemiology and aetiology. Br. J. Urol., 59:493, 1987.

Zhang, G. K., Wasserman, M. F., Kapoor, D. A., Smiley, D. G., and Reddy, P. K.: Early detection of local progressive disease from stage A1 prostate cancer (CAP) by transrectal ultrasonography (TRUS). J. Urol., 145:215A, 1991. (Abstract no. 9.)

Zincke, H.: Extended experience with surgical treatment of stage D1 adenocarcinoma of prostate. Urology, 33(Suppl.):27, 1989.

Zincke, H., Farrow, G. M., Myers, R. P., Benson, R. C., Furlow, W. L., and Utz, D. C.: Relationship between grade and stage of adenocarcinoma of the prostate and regional pelvic lymph node metastases. J. Urol., 128:498, 1982.

Zincke, H., and Utz, D. C.: Observations on surgical management of carcinoma of the prostate with limited nodal metastases. Urology, 24:137, 1984.

Zincke, H., Utz, D. C., and Taylor, W. F.: Bilateral pelvic lymphadenectomy and radical prostatectomy for clinical stage C prostatic cancer: Role of adjuvant treatment for residual cancer and in disease progression. J. Urol., 135:1199, 1986.

30
NEOPLASMS OF THE TESTIS

Jerome P. Richie, M.D.

Testicular cancer, although relatively rare, represents the most common malignancy in men in the 15- to 35-year-old age group and evokes widespread interest for several reasons. Testicular cancer has become one of the most curable solid neoplasms and serves as a paradigm for the multimodal treatment of malignancies. The dramatic improvement in survival resulting from the combination of effective diagnostic techniques, improved tumor markers, effective multidrug chemotherapeutic regimens, and modifications of surgical technique has led to a diminution in patient mortality from greater than 50 per cent before 1970 to less than 10 per cent in 1990. With the availability of effective treatment even for patients with advanced disease, attention has been turned to reduction of morbidity by altering protocols in selected subsets of patients. These changes in treatment philosophy are based on the knowledge of effective backup should alternative methods of treatment fail.

Testicular cancer is one of the few neoplasms associated with accurate serum markers—human beta-subunit chorionic gonadotropin (β-hCG) and alpha-fetoprotein (AFP). These accurate tumor markers allow careful follow-up with intervention earlier in the course of disease. Additional characteristics of testicular tumors that favor successful therapeutic manipulation include origin from germ cells, which are generally sensitive to both radiation therapy and a wide variety of chemotherapeutic agents; capacity for differentiation into histologically more benign counterparts; rapid rate of growth; predictable and systematic pattern of spread; and occurrence in young individuals without comorbid disease who may tolerate multimodal treatment. Nonetheless, it is of interest that, in patients whose tumors arise outside the testicle (extragonadal germ cell tumors), the prognosis with similar treatment is approximately half that expected in patients whose tumors are of primary germ cell origin.

The burgeoning field of molecular biology holds promise for the identification of intracellular changes that alter the kinetics of growth of normal testicular cells. Whereas in the 1980s cell surface antigens and morphologic characteristics could be evaluated, the potential for better understanding and possible elucidation of the etiology of testicular cancer may well be achieved in the not-too-distant future.

CLASSIFICATION

Histology

The testis is covered by a series of tunics that are acquired during descent from the genital ridge in the retroperitoneum through the inguinal canal into the scrotum. These tunics include the tunica vaginalis, the internal spermatic fascia, the cremasteric fascia, the external spermatic fascia, and the scrotum with skin and dartos tunic. The testicular tubules, arranged in a series of lobules, have a dense fascial covering called the tunica albuginea. On its posterior surface, the tunica albuginea is invaginated into the body of the testis to form the mediastinum testis. The mediastinum sends septa into the testis, dividing it into lobules. The upper pole of the testis has a vestigial remnant, the appendix testis. On the posterior surface of the testis, the adnexal structures are the epididymis, vas deferens, and spermatic cord.

The normal testis is composed of seminiferous tubules arranged in 200 to 350 lobules, which converge at the mediastinum testis where they connect with 12 to 20 efferent ducts that drain into the globus major of the epididymis. The tubuli recti coalesce in the mediastinum to form the rete testis, which merges into the efferent ductules that traverse in the testis to enter the globus major of the epididymis.

The seminiferous tubules contain two cell populations, the supporting, or Sertoli cells, and the spermatogenic cells, called spermatogonia. The supporting Sertoli cells line the basement membrane of the tubules and envelop the germ cells as they pass through various stages of spermatogenesis. The stroma between the seminiferous tubules is connective tissue in which the interstitial cells of Leydig are arranged in clusters. These cells are the androgen-producing cells, which are essential for spermatogenesis to occur. The majority of primary neoplasms of the testis arise from germinal elements, accounting for 90 to 95 per cent of all testicular neoplasms. The nongerminal elements, accounting for roughly 5 per cent of all primary testicular neoplasms, include neoplasms arising from gonadal stroma, mesenchymal structures, and ducts in addition to other miscellaneous lesions. Metastatic tumors to the testis are distinctly uncommon, although involvement by neoplasms of the reticuloendothelial system may occur.

The blood supply to the testis is derived from the site of origin near the genital ridge. The internal spermatic arteries arise from the aorta below the renal arteries and course through the spermatic cord directly to the testis. The artery to the vas deferens anastomoses with the internal spermatic artery. Venous drainage from the testis starts at the pampiniform plexus of the spermatic cord. This plexus, at the internal ring, joins to form the spermatic vein and drains into the vena cava on the right and into the left renal vein on the left. Lymphatics tend to follow the cord to the area of the lumbar lymphatics around the area of the great vessels.

The appendages of the testis and epididymis are embryologic remnants. The appendix testis, a remnant of the müllerian duct, represents the only müllerian remnant in the area of the testis. The remaining appendages include the appendix epididymis and paradidymis, which arise from the mesonephric or wolffian duct. The appendix epididymis is attached to the globus major of the epididymis. The paradidymis is attached at the junction of the epididymis and vas deferens. The appendix testis is found in 90 per cent of autopsy cases; the appendix epididymis is present in roughly 33 per cent of patients.

Histologic classifications, grading systems, and staging evaluations have traditionally provided a major clinical basis for therapeutic decisions (Table 30–1). Morphologic descriptions provide standardized means of identifying a given tumor and, in conjunction with past clinical experience, of estimating its potential for local growth, distant metastases, or both. Clinical and surgical staging indicates the extent to which a given tumor's potential has been realized at the time of evaluation. Although histologic and staging systems play important roles in treatment selection, grading schema have not been uniformly employed. At least six major attempts have been made since 1940 to classify germinal tumors with a clinical basis that will be meaningful for therapeutic decisions. A major distinction between British and American systems is the fact that British pathologists refer to all nonseminomatous germ cell tumors as malignant teratomas of one cell type or another, whereas American pathologists generally prefer the term embryonal carcinoma for the more undifferentiated form of teratoma. Nonetheless, these classifications can be correlated (Table 30–2).

Freidman and Moore (1946) provided one of the first generally accepted histologic classifications; this system, later modified by Dixon and Moore (1952) and Mostofi (1973), has become the North American standard classification. Teilum (1959) suggested the incorporation of the endodermal sinus tumor (infantile embryonal type) in the germ cell category (Pierce, 1975). Mostofi and Price (1973) subdivided teratomas into mature and immature varieties and coined the term "polyembryoma."

Table 30–1. HISTOLOGIC CLASSIFICATION

I. Primary neoplasms
  A. Germinal neoplasms (demonstrating one or more of the following components)
    1. Seminoma
      a. Classic (typical) seminoma
      b. Anaplastic seminoma
      c. Spermatocytic seminoma
    2. Embryonal carcinoma
    3. Teratoma (with or without malignant transformation)
      a. Mature
      b. Immature
    4. Choriocarcinoma
    5. Yolk sac tumor (endodermal sinus tumor, embryonal adenocarcinoma of the prepubertal testis)
  B. Nongerminal neoplasms
    1. Specialized gonadal stromal neoplasms
      a. Leydig cell tumor
      b. Other gonadal stromal tumors
    2. Gonadoblastoma
    3. Miscellaneous neoplasms
      a. Adenocarcinoma of the rete testis
      b. Mesenchymal neoplasms
      c. Carcinoid
      d. Adrenal rest "tumor"
II. Secondary neoplasms
  A. Reticuloendothelial neoplasms
  B. Metastases
III. Paratesticular neoplasms
  A. Adenomatoid
  B. Cystadenoma of epididymis
  C. Mesenchymal neoplasms
  D. Mesothelioma
  E. Metastases

The British Testicular Tumour Panel (Pugh and Cameron, 1976) formalized the English version of testicular tumor nomenclature. The World Health Organization (Mostofi and Sobin, 1977) modified the earlier system of Mostofi and Price (1973) by including the term "yolk sac" and by subdividing the embryonal carcinoma with teratoma category. The commonly used histologic classifications are summarized and compared in Tables 30–1 and 30–2.

Carcinoma In Situ

The early detection of preneoplastic change could improve survival for patients with many types of tumors, including testicular cancer. Controversy exists, however, concerning the premalignant alteration of intratubular germ cell neoplasia with the development of frank malignancy. One of the investigators of intratubular germ cell neoplasia has been Skakkebaek and associates. In several articles, they described the occurrence of intratubular germ cells that are atypical in nature when seen on the testicular biopsy samples from infertile men (Skakkebaek, 1972). In one series, four of six patients with intratubular germ cell neoplasia developed "invasive tumor" between 1 and 5 years after initial biopsy (Skakkebaek, 1978). One problem, however, is that "invasive" as defined by this methodology involves invasion of the basement membrane. This finding differs from the standard germ cell tumor that is seen in a patient with a palpable mass within the testis.

Table 30–2. GERM CELL NOMENCLATURE

Friedman and Moore (1946)	Mostofi and Price (1973)	Pugh (British, 1976)	Mostofi and Sobin (1977)
Seminoma	Seminoma ("typical")	Seminoma	Seminoma
	Spermatocytic	Spermatocytic	Spermatocytic
	Anaplastic	—	—
Teratoma	Teratoma	Teratoma, differentiated (TD)	Teratoma
	Mature		Mature
	Immature		Immature
	With malignant transformation		With malignant transformation
Teratocarcinoma	Embryonal carcinoma with teratoma	Malignant teratoma, intermediate (MTI)	Embryonal carcinoma and teratoma
Embryonal carcinoma	Embryonal carcinoma (adult type)	Malignant teratoma, undifferentiated (MTU)	Embryonal carcinoma (adult type)
	Polyembryoma		
Chorioepithelioma	Choriocarcinoma with or without embryonal carcinoma and/or teratoma	Malignant teratoma, trophoblastic (MTT)	Choriocarcinoma with or without embryonal carcinoma and/or teratoma
—	Embryonal carcinoma (juvenile type)	Yolk sac tumor	Yolk sac tumor (endodermal sinus tumor)

Precancerous changes have been observed as well in the adjacent, apparently uninvolved areas of the testis in patients with germinal tumors (Skakkebaek, 1975). These findings raise the difficult question of how to deal with the opposite gonad, particularly because there is a known tendency for a patient to develop a contralateral tumor in approximately 1 per cent of cases.

The rate of intratubular germ cell neoplasia is well defined and described. How should one deal with this finding and in what percentage of patients will clinically apparent testicular tumors develop? These questions remain unanswered.

Experimental Models

Teratocarcinomas contain primitive malignant cells, embryonal carcinoma cells, and various tissues that are partially or fully differentiated, including cartilage, bone, muscle, and respiratory and transitional epithelium. This admixture of tissues suggests the capability of differentiation or dedifferentiation. In fact, murine embryonal carcinoma cells, when placed in a mouse blastocyst, may differentiate in an orderly fashion and participate in the creation of a normal mouse. These studies emphasize the effect of the environment on the development of the malignant or normal cell. In the embryonal carcinoma cell, both neoplasia and embryogenesis come together. This feature has allowed the embryonal carcinoma cell and the blastocyst to serve as models for tumor-host interactions.

Teratoma or teratocarcinoma rarely develops spontaneously in mice. However, with careful inbreeding of strains with low frequency, strains such as the 129-TERSv have been obtained in which up to 30 per cent of male offspring have spontaneous congenital testicular teratocarcinoma. Stevens (1967) developed and successfully manipulated a testicular teratoma line in a strain of the 129 mouse. The tumors are first visible as embryonic cell clusters within the seminiferous tubules as early as day 14 of fetal development. Unfortunately, this murine model has been of limited value because the tumors can rarely be sustained by serial transplantation in the new hosts. In this model, more primitive-appearing embryonal cells occasionally persisted and, if these were implanted within the peritoneal cavity, yolk sac tumors and "embryoid bodies" were produced.

In the 129-TERSv strain mice, Stevens also found microscopic teratomas in the genital ridges. By transplantation of the genital ridge of appropriate strains of fetal mice into the testes of syngeneic adult mice, teratomas and teratocarcinomas can be developed. The Stevens model is effective in producing teratocarcinomas between the 12th and 16th day of development with an approximately 80 per cent rate of tumor production (Stevens, 1968). The grafts, however, fail if ridge transplantation is attempted to other sites outside the scrotum. Also, some strains of mice that are susceptible to embryo-derived tumors do not form tumors when genital ridges are transplanted. For example, the strain A/He—with a very low rate of incidence of spontaneous tumors—will allow genital ridge transplantation at a success rate of about 80 per cent. In other strains with no germ cells in the genital ridge, however, transplantation fails to produce tumors. Thus, the importance of genetic predisposition as well as environmental factors and timing sequences in oncogenesis is apparent.

Damjanov and Solter (1976) observed that transplantation of very early stage (day 1 to 7) mouse embryos from some strains (C2H, A, CBA) to extrauterine sites resulted in the production of rapidly growing teratocarcinomas. These teratocarcinomas could be retransplanted in vivo or cultivated in vitro. After the 8th day of gestation, however, transplantation resulted in the production of teratoma only. The teratomas were composed of mature somatic elements with slow growth rates, and they were not transplantable. These experiments provide evidence favoring the concept of the misplaced embryo as the origin of germinal tumors.

Primordial germ cells, early embryos, and embryonal carcinoma cells share similar characteristics, including the following: (1) pluripotency, (2) ultrastructural appearance, (3) alkaline phosphatase content, (4) formation of embryoid bodies, and (5) surface antigens. During the process of differentiation, these features become altered. Artz and Jacob (1974) noted that some cell surface antigens remain unchanged, whereas others, notably histocompatibility antigens, do not make their appearance until primitive elements have matured into adult forms.

GERM CELL NEOPLASM

Epidemiology

Incidence

Approximately 5500 new cases related to testicular cancer are reported in the United States annually (Silverberg, 1990). Estimates indicate that for American white males the lifetime probability of developing testicular cancer is approximately 0.2 per cent, or one in 500 (Zdeb, 1977). The average annual age-adjusted incidence rate of testicular cancer for American males from 1969 to 1971 was 3.7 per 100,000—nearly twice the rate of 2.0 per 100,000 from 1937 to 1939. The average rate among American black males is 0.9 per 100,000; this rate has remained unchanged for the last 40 years.

Similar trends have been noted in Denmark, where the age-adjusted incidence rose from 3.4 to 6.4 per 100,000 between 1945 and 1970 (Clemmesen, 1974). Data compiled by Muir and Nectoux (1979) indicate considerable variability in the worldwide incidence of adult germ cell tumors. The average annual rate (age-adjusted) is highest in Scandinavia (Denmark, Norway), Switzerland, Germany, and New Zealand; intermediate in the United States and Great Britain; and low in Africa and Asia. In data collected by Clemmesen (1974) the age-adjusted rate rose from 3.2 to 6.7 per 100,000 in Copenhagen between 1943 and 1967. Prevalence rates in Copenhagen were double those of rural Denmark during the same period.

Age

Peak incidences of testicular tumors occur in late adolescence to early adulthood (20 to 40 years), in late adulthood (over 60 years), and in infancy (0 to 10 years). Overall, the highest incidence is noted in young adults, making these neoplasms the most common solid tumor in men between 20 and 34 years of age and the second most common solid tumor in men between 35 and 40 years of age in the United States and Great Britain. Seminoma is rare in those younger than the age of 10 and above the age of 60, but it is the most common histologic type overall with a peak incidence between the ages of 35 and 39 years. Spermatocytic seminoma (approximately 10 per cent of seminomas) occurs most often in patients over the age of 50 years. Embryonal carcinoma and teratocarcinoma occur predominantly between the ages of 25 and 35 years. Choriocarcinoma (1 to 2 per cent of germ cell tumors) occurs more often in the 20- to 30-year age group. Yolk sac tumors are the predominant lesions of infancy and childhood, but they are frequently found in combination with other germ cell elements in young adults. Histologically benign, pure teratoma occurs most often in the pediatric age group but frequently appears in combination with other germ cell elements in adults. Malignant testicular lymphomas are predominantly tumors of men over 50 years of age.

Racial Factors

Variable incidence rates are noted for different ethnic groups within a given geographic region. The incidence of testicular tumors in the American black is approximately one third of that in the American white but 10 times that in the African black. In Israel, Jews have at least an eightfold higher incidence of testicular tumors in comparison with non-Jews. In Hawaii, the incidence among Filipino/Japanese sectors is approximately one tenth of that for the Chinese/white/native Hawaiian populations.

Graham and Gibson (1972) presented data indicating a higher incidence among professional men. Mack and Henderson (1980) noted higher incidence rates in upper and middle socioeconomic classes of whites in Los Angeles County. Although similar trends have been noted in American blacks (Ross et al., 1979), the rate is still less than one third of that for whites of comparable social status.

Genetic Factors

Although a relatively higher incidence of testicular tumors has been reported in twins, brothers, and family members, the evidence for a predominant genetic influence is not overwhelming (Johnson, 1976). In nearly 7000 sets of twins from the Danish Twin Registry, Harvald and Hauge (1963) found no higher incidence of cancer in twins than was expected in the general population. Muller (1962) reported that there was a familial history of malignant disease in approximately 16 per cent of cases. The 2 to 3 per cent incidence of bilateral tumors may suggest the potential importance of genetic (or congenital) factors.

Laterality and Bilaterality

Testicular neoplasms appear to be slightly more common in the right testis than in the left, similar to the slightly greater incidence of right-sided cryptorchidism. Approximately 2 to 3 per cent of testicular tumors are bilateral, occurring either simultaneously or successively. If secondary testicular tumors are excluded, the incidence of bilateral tumors is between 1 and 2.8 per cent of all cases of germinal neoplasms (Sokal et al., 1980). Similar rather than different histology in the two testes predominates with bilateral tumors. Bach and co-workers (1983) tabulated the histology in 337 cases of bilateral testicular tumors. Bilateral seminoma was the most common histologic type (48 per cent); bilateral similar nonseminomas were found in 15 per cent; germinal tumors with different histology were found in 15 per cent; and nongerminal tumors with similar histology were found in 22 per cent. A history of cryptorchidism (uni- or bilateral) in nearly half of these men is consistent with observations that bilateral dysgenesis occurs frequently in cases of unilateral maldescent (Sohval, 1956). Long-term surveillance of patients with a history of cryptorchidism or previous orchiectomy for a germ cell tumor is mandatory.

Frequency of Histologic Types

Germinal tumors constitute between 90 and 95 per cent of all primary testicular malignancies. Variability in the reported frequency of histologic types may reflect true differences in the incidence of such tumors. It is possible, however, that such variations merely reflect demographic differences, variance of histologic interpretations, or other unquantified selection factors. The overall incidence rates have been tabulated as follows: seminoma, 40 per cent; embryonal carcinoma, 20 to 25 per cent; teratocarcinoma, 25 to 30 per cent; teratoma, 5 to 10 per cent; and pure choriocarcinoma, 1 per cent. When combined histologic patterns (more than one histologic pattern) are considered as a separate entity, the frequency approximates the following: seminoma, 30 per cent; embryonal carcinoma, 30 per cent; teratoma, 10 per cent; teratocarcinoma, 25 per cent; choriocarcinoma, 1 per cent; and combined patterns (e.g., seminoma plus embryonal carcinoma, embryonal carcinoma plus choriocarcinoma), 15 per cent (Mostofi, 1973).

Etiology

Experimental and clinical evidence supports the importance of congenital factors in the etiology of germ cell tumors. During development, the primordial germ cell may be altered by environmental factors, resulting in disturbed differentiation. The germ cell is conceivably detained from normal development by cryptorchidism, gonadal dysgenesis, hereditary predisposition, chemical carcinogens, trauma, or orchitis. The teratocarcinoma tumor model (Stevens, 1968) suggests the crucial influence of temporal relationships on normal versus abnormal differentiation.

Congenital Causes

CRYPTORCHIDISM. LeComete (1851) is credited with the initial observation that testicular maldescent and tumor formation are interrelated. Pooled data from several large series indicate that approximately 7 to 10 per cent of patients with testicular tumors have prior histories of cryptorchidism (Whitaker, 1970). Mostofi (1973) lists five possible, but unquantified, factors that may play a causative role in the cryptorchid/malignant testis: abnormal germ cell morphology, elevated temperature, interference with blood supply, endocrine dysfunction, and gonadal dysgenesis.

The exact incidence of cryptorchidism is unknown because much of the relevant information on testicular maldescent includes data on patients with retractile testes. From accumulated series, Scorer and Farrington (1971) estimated that approximately 4.3 per cent of neonates, 0.8 per cent of infants and children, and 0.7 per cent of adult males over the age of 18 years (army selectees) harbor a truly cryptorchid testis. In reviewing more than 7000 cases of testicular tumor, Gilbert and Hamilton (1940) found a history of cryptorchidism in 840 men (12 per cent). Based on the observed incidence of cryptorchidism in military inductees (0.23 per cent, roughly 1 in 500), they calculated the estimated risk of tumorigenesis in a man with a history of maldescent to be 48 times that of a man with normally descended testes. Later epidemiologic studies have reported the relative risk of testicular cancer in patients with cryptorchidism to be much lower, that is, three to 14 times the normal expected incidence (Farrer et al., 1985; Henderson et al., 1979; Schottenfeld et al., 1980).

Between 5 and 10 per cent of patients with histories of cryptorchidism develop malignancy in the contralateral, normally descended gonad. This observation is consistent with the findings of Berthelsen and associates (1982). They have provided biopsy data in 250 patients with testicular cancer relative to the contralateral testis. Carcinoma in situ (CIS) was found in 13 (5.2 per cent), representing one third of patients with atrophy of the remaining testis and one fifth of patients with a history of cryptorchidism. Two of the patients (10 per cent) with contralateral CIS subsequently developed a second testis cancer. Campbell (1942) noted that roughly 25 per cent of patients with bilateral cryptorchidism and history of testis cancer were subject to the risk of a second germ cell tumor.

Campbell (1942) indicated that nearly half of patients with malignancy associated with cryptorchidism have impalpable abdominal testes. Although the anatomic position (inguinal versus abdominal) may play a role in determining the degree of gonadal damage (and the risk of subsequent tumor formation), the relative influence upon the cryptorchid testis may depend largely on the observer (Gilbert and Hamilton, 1940).

Ultrastructural abnormalities of the spermatogonia and Sertoli cells are readily apparent in the cryptorchid testis by the age of 3 years. Cellular degeneration is followed by progressive fibrosis, destruction of the basement membrane, and deposition of myelin and lipids (Mengel et al., 1982). Considerations of these histologic changes and other social factors have favored the practice of early orchiopexy. Such a philosophy, however, has not completely prevented tumor formation in the testis (Batata et al., 1982; Martin, 1979).

Acquired Causes

TRAUMA. Although trauma is considered a contributing factor in zinc- or copper-induced fowl teratomas, there is little to suggest a cause-and-effect relationship in humans (Carleton et al., 1953). Most investigators conclude that trauma to the enlarged testis is an event that prompts medical evaluation rather than being a causative factor.

HORMONES. Sex hormone fluctuations may contribute to the development of testicular tumors in experimental animals and humans. The administration of estrogen to pregnant mice may cause maldescent and dysgenesis of the testis in the offspring (Nomura and Kanzak, 1977). Similar findings have been noted in the male offspring of women exposed to diethylstilbestrol

(Cosgrove et al., 1977) or oral contraceptives (Rothman and Louik, 1978). Exogenous estrogen administration has also been linked to the induction of Leydig cell tumors. Epidemiologic studies found relative risk rates ranging from 2.8 to 5.3 per cent for testicular tumor in the male progeny of diethylstilbestrol-treated mothers (Henderson et al., 1983; Schottenfeld et al., 1980).

ATROPHY. Nonspecific or mumps-associated atrophy of the testis has been suggested as a potential causative factor in testicular cancer. Gilbert (1944) collected 80 cases of testicular tumor occurring in patients with a history of nonspecific atrophy and 24 additional cases related to a previous history of mumps orchitis among 5500 cases of testicular tumors. Although a causative role for atrophy remains speculative, it is tempting to invoke local hormonal imbalance as a possible cause for malignant transformation.

Pathogenesis and Natural History

Local growth characteristics and patterns of spread have been well defined by the clinical observation of patients with germinal testicular tumors. Following malignant transformation, intratubular CIS extends beyond the basement membrane and may eventually replace most of the testicular parenchyma. Local involvement of the epididymis or spermatic cord is hindered by the tunica albuginea, and seemingly, as a consequence, lymphatic or hematogenous spread may occur first. Approximately half of patients with nonseminomatous tumors present with disseminated disease (Bosl et al., 1981). Involvement of the epididymis or cord may lead to pelvic and inguinal lymph node metastasis, whereas tumors confined to the testis proper are usually spread to retroperitoneal nodes. Hematogenous spread to lung, bone, or liver is occasioned either directly by vascular invasion or indirectly by previously established lymphatic metastasis, by way of the thoracic duct and subclavian veins or other lymphaticovenous communications. The natural history of germinal testis tumors has been the subject of numerous treatises and appears sufficiently well defined to permit the following generalizations (Whitmore, 1968):

1. Complete spontaneous regressions are rare.
2. All germinal testis tumors in adults should be regarded as malignant. Although the infantile teratoma may be regarded as "benign," teratoma of the adult testis may be associated with vascular invasion microscopically and a definite mortality risk in patients treated with orchiectomy alone (as high as 29 per cent, according to Mostofi and Price, 1973). Clinical experience has shown that retroperitoneal teratoma in the adult, whether resulting from maturation of embryonal carcinoma or from regression of the embryonal carcinoma component of a teratocarcinoma (spontaneous or induced), may be accompanied by unrelenting local growth and ultimate fatality (Hong et al., 1977).
3. The tunica albuginea is a natural barrier to expansile local growth. Extension through this dense membrane occurs at the testicular mediastinum, where the blood vessels, lymphatics, nerves, and efferent tubules exit the testis proper. Local involvement of the epididymis or spermatic cord occurs in 10 to 15 per cent of cases and increases the risk of lymphatic or bloodborne metastasis.
4. Lymphatic metastasis is common to all forms of germinal testis tumors, although pure choriocarcinoma almost uniformly disseminates by means of vascular invasion as well. The spermatic cord contains four to eight lymphatic channels that traverse the inguinal canal and retroperitoneal space. As the spermatic vessels cross ventral to the ureter, these lymphatics fan out medially and drain into the retroperitoneal lymph node chain. The primary drainage of the right testis is usually located within the group of lymph nodes in the interaortocaval region at the level of the second vertebral body; the first echelon of nodes draining the left testis is located in the para-aortic region in the compartment bounded by the left ureter, the left renal vein, the aorta, and the origin of the inferior mesenteric artery. Subsequent cephalad drainage is to the cisterna chyli, thoracic duct, and supraclavicular nodes (usually left), but retrograde spread may occur to common iliac, external iliac, and inguinal lymph nodes.

Although the thoracic duct–subclavian vein juncture is the major site of communication, other lymphaticovenous communications may be occasioned by massive retroperitoneal lymph node deposits. Furthermore, it has been demonstrated by spermatic lymphangiography that testicular lymphatics can rarely communicate directly with the thoracic duct, bypassing the retroperitoneal nodes. Lymphatics of the epididymis drain into the external iliac chain, affording locally extensive testicular tumors access to pelvic lymph nodes. Inguinal node metastasis may result from scrotal involvement by the primary tumor, prior inguinal or scrotal surgery, or retrograde lymphatic spread secondary to massive retroperitoneal lymph node deposits.

5. Extranodal distant metastasis results from either direct vascular invasion or tumor emboli from lymphatic metastasis by means of major thoracoabdominal channels or minor lymphaticovenous communications. Most, but not all, bloodborne metastasis occurs following lymph node involvement. This finding is of obvious practical importance in treatment and prognosis. Despite surgical excision of negative retroperitoneal lymph nodes, the failure rate with distant metastasis is approximately 5 per cent (Whitmore, 1973). In programs reserving further treatment following inguinal orchiectomy for clinical stage A nonseminoma patients, approximately 30 per cent will fail—most with retroperitoneal lymph node metastasis (80 per cent of failures) and the remainder with extralymphatic distant metastasis (20 per cent of failures) independent of retroperitoneal deposits (Duchesne et al., 1990). Primary and secondary deposits of nongerminal tumors frequently vary histologically. Pure seminomas, however, rarely metastasize as another form of germinal tumor; nonseminomas rarely metastasize as pure seminomas unless the primary lesion has combined histology containing seminomatous elements (Ray et al., 1979). Although the clinical incidence of nonseminomatous metastasis from an apparently pure seminoma is less than 10 per cent,

30 to 45 per cent of patients who die from apparently pure seminoma harbor nonseminomatous metastases (Bredael et al., 1982).

With the exception of seminoma, the growth rate among germ cell tumors tends to be high. Doubling times calculated on the basis of serial chest radiographs usually range from 10 to 30 days. Alterations in the production of tumor marker substances (β-hCG, AFP, lactate dehydrogenase) are in keeping with rapid metabolic activity and growth. The anticipated rapid demise of patients who fail to respond to treatment has been confirmed by clinical observation. Approximately 85 per cent of patients who die from germ cell tumors do so within 2 years, and the majority of the remainder die within 3 years. Because of a sometimes indolent course, seminoma may recur from 2 to 10 years following apparently successful initial management.

Because of the short natural history of germinal tumors, it has become customary to regard 2-year survival as an endpoint for judging the effectiveness of therapy. With the evolution of multimodal therapy, "surviving" patients may not be actually "cured" of their neoplasm, and a disease-free interval of 5 years may be a more appropriate assessment of curability. Longer follow-up after chemotherapy is mandatory, however, because relapse has been noted up to 10 years after treatment.

Clinical Manifestations

In general, survival in patients with germ cell tumors is related to the stage at presentation and, therefore, the amount of tumor burden as well as the effectiveness of subsequent treatment. Those patients who present with advanced disease (stage III) generally have a much poorer prognosis than do those with disease confined to the testis or those with regional nodal involvement only. Delay in diagnosis of 1 to 2 months or more is not uncommon in these patients. Delay in diagnosis seems to be related directly to patient factors, such as ignorance, denial, and fear, as well as physician factors, such as misdiagnosis.

Almost half of patients will present with metastatic disease (Bosl et al., 1981). The need clearly exists for patient education through programs such as advocation of testicular self-examination. Only through these widespread public health techniques will the knowledge of testicular tumors be promulgated so that diagnosis can be achieved earlier. Physician-related causes still remain major factors in delay of treatment, emphasizing the need for continuing physician education. It is of interest that denial is such a strong force in a patient with testicular tumor. Some present with masses as large as grapefruits within the scrotal contents.

Signs and Symptoms

The usual presentation of a testicular tumor is a nodule or painless swelling of one gonad. This finding may be noted incidentally by the patient or by his sexual partner. The classic description is that of a lump, swelling, or hardness of the testis. Approximately 30 to 40 per cent of patients may complain of a dull ache or a heavy sensation in the lower abdomen, anal area, or scrotum. In approximately 10 per cent of patients, acute pain will be the presenting symptom. Occasionally, patients with a previously small atrophic testis will note enlargement. On rare occasions, infertility may be the presenting complaint (Skakkebaek, 1972). Acute onset of pain is rare unless there is associated epididymitis or bleeding within the tumor.

In approximately 10 per cent of patients, the presenting manifestations may be due to metastases, including a neck mass (supraclavicular lymph node metastasis); respiratory symptoms, such as cough or dyspnea (pulmonary metastasis); gastrointestinal disturbances, such as anorexia, nausea, vomiting, or hemorrhage (retro-duodenal metastasis); lumbar back pain (bulky retroperitoneal disease involving the psoas muscle or nerve roots); bone pain (skeletal metastasis); central and peripheral nervous system manifestations (cerebral, spinal cord, or peripheral root involvement); and unilateral or bilateral lower extremity swelling (iliac or caval venous obstruction or thrombosis).

Gynecomastia, seen in about 5 per cent of patients with testicular germ cell tumors, may be regarded as a systemic endocrine manifestation of these neoplasms. The breast is a target organ for the action of both androgen and estrogen. In normal men, the breast fails to enlarge because there is a quantitative predominance of androgen production over estrogen secretion. Gynecomastia occurs in men with excessive estrogen secretion or deficient androgen production. In men with malignant testicular neoplasms, either one of these two mechanisms may be operative.

Excessive estrogen production occurs in patients with gonadotropin-producing neoplasms, most commonly choriocarcinomas, and also less frequently in patients with embryonal carcinomas, teratocarcinomas, and seminomas. The cause of increased estrogen production in these patients may be twofold: (1) the testis is stimulated by excessive amounts of hCG and more estrogen than androgen is produced, and (2) the trophoblastic tumors synthesize and secrete estradiol (Walsh, 1977). Furthermore, in men with a history of cryptorchidism or following orchiectomy, androgen deficiency may be a contributing factor.

Physical Examination

Physical examination of the testis is performed by bimanual examination of the scrotal contents, beginning with the normal contralateral testis. This examination provides a baseline and allows the examiner to appreciate the relative size, contour, and consistency of the normal testis as well as of the suspected gonad. Physical examination of the testis is performed by careful palpation of the testis between the thumb and first two fingers of the examining hand. The normal testis is homogenous in consistency, freely movable, and separable from the epididymis. Any firm, hard, or fixed area within the substance of the tunica albuginea should be considered suspicious until proved otherwise. Further appreciation of the suspected tumor should be directed toward possible involvement of the cord, scrotal invest- ments, or skin. In general, seminoma tends to expand within the testis as a painless, rubbery enlargement. Embryonal carcinoma or teratocarcinoma may produce an irregular rather than discrete mass, although this distinction is not always appreciated.

Testicular tumors tend to remain ovoid, being limited by the tough investing tunica albuginea. In 10 to 15 per cent of patients, spread to the epididymis or cord may occur. A hydrocele may be present and may increase the difficulty in appreciation of a testicular neoplasm. Ultrasonography of the scrotum is a rapid and reliable technique to exclude hydrocele or epididymitis and should be utilized in patients if there is any suspicion of testicular tumor.

Physical examination should include palpation of the abdomen for evidence of nodal disease or visceral in- volvement. Routine assessment of the supraclavicular lymph nodes may reveal adenopathy in patients with advanced disease. Examination of the chest may disclose gynecomastia or the presence of respiratory tract in- volvement.

Rarely, patients present with advanced disease with- out a recognizable primary tumor in the testis. Some of these primary tumors may be extragonadal germ cell tumors, with the patient having an inherently worse prognosis. Others, however, may represent a small primary testicular tumor with large extragonadal metas- tasis. Palpation of the testes is important to exclude primary germ cell tumor in origin. In patients with a diagnosis of "extragonadal" germ cell tumor, ultrasound of the testis is mandatory to be certain one is not dealing with a primary germ cell tumor.

Differential Diagnosis

The differential diagnosis of a testicular mass includes testicular torsion, epididymitis, and epididymo-orchitis. Less common problems include hydrocele, hernia, he- matoma, spermatocele, or syphilitic gumma. In any patient with a solid, firm, intratesticular mass, testicular cancer must be the considered diagnosis until proved otherwise. In patients in whom the diagnosis is unclear, or in whom a hydrocele precludes adequate examina- tion, ultrasonography of the scrotal contents should be employed as an important second step. Ultrasonography of the scrotum is basically an extension of the physical examination. Any hypoechoic area within the tunica albuginea is markedly suspicious for testicular cancer. With the advent of scrotal ultrasonography and its general availability, the delay in diagnosis resulting from confusion with epididymitis should be markedly re- duced.

Imaging Studies

Immersion and high-resolution ultrasonography may aid in the clinical evaluation of scrotal masses (Friedrich et al., 1981; Richie et al., 1982). Intrascrotal fluid collections are no barrier to the examination of the underlying testicular parenchyma by ultrasonography. In patients with palpably normal genitalia and evidence of extragonadal germ cell malignancy, sonography has been reported to be successful in identifying occult testicular neoplasms (Glazer et al., 1982).

Clinical Staging of Germ Cell Neoplasm

Once the diagnosis of the germ cell neoplasm has been established by radical orchiectomy, clinical staging is necessary to define further treatment modalities. Stag- ing evaluations should take into account the pathologic examination of the primary specimen, the history and physical findings, and a variety of other diagnostic modalities. Clinical staging attempts to define the extent of disease at the time of diagnosis as well as during the course of treatment and at subsequent follow-up evalu- ation. The accuracy of clinical assessment is imperative if the physician is to be able to make a logical decision as to therapy. The importance of clinical staging cannot be overemphasized; this knowledge allows the orderly decision of appropriate treatment as well as reasonable expectations for prognosis. With the advent of alterna- tive treatment protocols for patients with clinical low- stage testicular cancer, the impact of staging and its accuracy is ever more critical.

Sites of Metastases

In order for staging to be effective and complete, familiarity with the likely routes of spread and usual sites for metastasis from primary germ cell tumors is necessary. The majority of testicular cancers spread through the lymphatics in an orderly fashion, although vascular dissemination can occur early in some tumors. The primary lymphatic drainage from the right testicle is to the interaortal caval lymph nodes, primarily, and subsequently to precaval, preaortic, and paracaval lymph nodes. Once the interaortal caval nodes are involved, there tends to be spread to the left para-aortic area, more commonly from the right to left side. Sub- sequent drainage can occur to the left common iliac and left external iliac nodes, once extensive involvement occurs in the left para-aortic region. The primary drain- age of the left testis is to the left para-aortic nodes just below the level of the left renal vein and, subsequently, to preaortic nodes.

Cross-metastases occur more commonly in patients with right-sided tumors because of the lymphatic drain- age from right to left. Iliac lymph nodes may be involved primarily when the tumor has invaded the epididymis or spermatic cord, and secondarily when para-aortic disease is present. Inguinal metastases may occur when the tunica albuginea has been invaded or when previous surgery, such as inguinal herniorrhaphy or orchiopexy, has altered the normal lymphatic flow. Although the suprahilar area was thought to be involved commonly in patients with more extensive retroperitoneal nodal cases, in actuality, the lymphatics tend to follow the aorta below the crus of the diaphragm into the retrocrural space. Landing sites for minimal, moderate, or extensive disease have been determined and reported by Donohue and associates (1982).

Distant spread of testicular cancer occurs most commonly to the pulmonary region, with intraparenchymal pulmonary involvement. Subsequent spread may be noted to liver, viscera, brain, or bone (Johnson et al., 1976). In general, bony metastases are encountered rather late in the course of disease. Central nervous system metastases may be understaged.

Staging Systems

The predictable mode of metastasis in patients with germ cell tumors, along with technologic advances in imaging and biochemical marker assays, has improved the accuracy of initial clinical evaluations, although they are far from perfect. A variety of clinical staging systems have been advocated during the past 40 years or more. For testicular tumors, the system proposed by Boden and Gibb in 1951 has been the mainstay of clinical staging. This ABC system has been refined by Skinner (1976) with subclassification of regional nodal involvement into B1, B2, and B3. Refinement in staging and treatment has led to the development of many substages with different prognostic and therapeutic import. More commonly used clinical staging systems are shown in Table 30–3. These clinical staging systems are based on noninvasive diagnostic techniques. Pathologic staging systems, based on retroperitoneal lymph node dissection, are detailed in Table 30–4. Confusion exists because of differences among these clinical and pathologic staging systems, making interinstitutional comparisons sometimes difficult.

Findings noted at orchiectomy, predominantly histologic findings in the primary tumor, plus physical examination, radiologic procedures, and laboratory studies are essential in assessing clinical stage of disease. Radiologic procedures can include chest radiograph, intravenous urography, lymphangiography, computed tomographic (CT) scan, or magnetic resonance imaging scan. Laboratory studies include tumor markers, β-hCG, and AFP, and a multiple screening analysis (SMA). Metastases may be assessed not only clinically but also by surgical methods. Some investigators have advocated routine supraclavicular lymph node biopsy for the staging of patients with testicular tumors (Fowler et al., 1979). The relative lack of yield of subclinical metastases along with the potential morbidity of this procedure contraindicate routine supraclavicular node biopsy in a patient without a palpable supraclavicular mass (Lynch and Richie, 1980).

Staging classifications should aid in the determination of (1) the decision for proper therapy; (2) the evaluation of treatment results; and (3) the capability of comparing results of therapy from a variety of institutions, both regionally and internationally. Staging systems should be utilized in tumors with similar biologic characteristics; thus, a clinical staging system for seminoma has been developed as well as one for nonseminomatous germ cell tumors. Although numerous staging classifications are currently employed, the majority are a modification or extension of the one originally proposed by Boden and Gibb in 1951. These investigators separated extent of disease into three stages: stage I, tumor limited to the testis with no evidence of spread through the capsule or to the spermatic cord; stage II, clinical or radiologic evidence of tumor extension beyond the testicle, but contained within the regional lymph nodes; and stage III, disseminated disease above the diaphragm, or visceral disease. A variety of systems have been developed related to differences in treatment among various med-

Table 30–3. CLINICAL STAGING SYSTEMS

Boden/Gibb Stage	MSKCC	Royal Marsden Hospital	M.D. Anderson Hospital	American Joint Committee
A (I) Tumor confined to testis	A	I	I	TX Unknown status T0 No evidence of primary T1 Confined to testis T2 Beyond tunica T3 Invasion of rete testis or epididymis T4a Invasion of cord T4b Invasion of scrotum
B (II) Spread to regional nodes	B1 <5 cm B2 >5 cm B3 >10 cm ("bulky")	IIA <2 cm IIB >2, <5 cm IIC >5 cm	IIA Negative lymphangiogram (LAG)/positive nodes IIB Positive LAG/positive nodes	
C (III) Spread beyond retroperitoneal nodes	C3	III Supraclavicular nodal (SCN) or mediastinal involvement IV Extralymphatic metastasis		

Table 30–4. PATHOLOGIC STAGING SYSTEMS

Skinner	Walter Reed	TNM
A	I	N0
Confined to testis		
B		
Spread to retroperitoneum		
B1	IA	N1,
< 6 Positive nodes, no node >2		N2A
cm, no extranodal extension		
B2	IIB	N2B
> 6 Positive nodes, any node >2		
cm		
B3	IIC	N3
Massive retroperitoneal disease		
C	III	M+
Metastatic		

ical centers, differences in methods to assess the extent of disease, and differences in the needs among various treating specialties responsible for these patients. A convenient dividing point for staging systems is cases of seminomas and of nonseminomatous tumors. Patients with pure seminomas are usually staged by clinical means. Staging may employ surgical techniques in patients with nonseminomatous tumors.

Findings at Orchiectomy

Radical or inguinal orchiectomy, with early clamping of the spermatic cord at the deep inguinal ring, effectively removes a primary tumor and allows staging in patients with testicular cancer. The orchiectomy specimen should be processed carefully to ensure that all elements within the tumor are recognized and that the histologic diagnosis is reasonably accurate. Of equal import is determination of the local extent of tumor. The pathologist should record whether the tumor is confined within the body of the testis (stage T1), extends beyond the tunica albuginea (stage T2), involves the rete testis or epididymis (stage T3), or invades either the spermatic cord (stage T4a) or scrotal wall (stage T4b). The histologic report should also determine whether lymphatic or vascular invasion is seen within the tumor mass as well as the percentage of subtypes of tumors present.

The extent of staging is in part determined by decisions for therapy; for example, if surveillance protocols are to be considered, every effort should be made to exclude patients with any evidence of retroperitoneal disease. If retroperitoneal lymphadenectomy is likely to be elected as the primary treatment for low-stage, nonseminomatous tumors, efforts should be directed toward delineation of regional nodal versus distant metastases.

Imaging Studies

Chest Radiograph

Posteroanterior and lateral chest radiographs should be the initial radiographic procedure performed. These radiographs provide the minimal assessment of the lung parenchyma and mediastinal structures. Whole lung tomography is not obtained routinely at the Brigham and Women's Hospital and the Dana Farber Cancer Institute, Boston. In a review of 120 studies performed, whole lung tomography altered the therapeutic decision in only four of 120 patients (Jochelson et al., 1984).

Chest CT scans provide more sensitive evaluations of the thorax and may increase the detection of pulmonary metastases. Chest CT, however, will delineate lesions as small as 2 mm in size. Approximately 70 per cent of these small lesions will turn out to be benign processes. Thus, if CT scanning is used, a critical high index of suspicion should be present, with recognition that small lesions may in fact be benign and not related to the primary testicular cancer.

Computerized Tomography

Abdominal CT scans have been recommended as being the most effective means to identify retroperitoneal lymph node involvement. CT scanning has replaced intravenous urography and pedal lymphangiography as the procedure of choice for evaluation of the retroperitoneum. Pedal lymphangiography has an error rate of roughly 25 per cent false negatives and 10 per cent false positives. Given the overall inaccuracy of lymphangiography, coupled with its invasive nature, lymphangiography is no longer needed for staging purposes. CT has largely supplanted intravenous pyelography in visualization of the kidneys and course of the ureters and is much more sensitive in the detection of extensive retroperitoneal disease. Abdominal CT scans, especially with third- and fourth-generation scanners, can identify small lymph node deposits less than 2 cm in diameter in the upper para-aortic regions. CT scanning provides a generally accurate three-dimensional estimate of tumor size and identifies involvement of soft tissue structures and regional viscera. In addition, CT gives a view of the retrocrural space in the para-aortic region above the crus of the diaphragm, an important site of metastasis. CT scanning, however, is not sufficiently accurate to distinguish fibrosis, teratoma, or malignancy by size criteria alone (Stomper et al., 1985).

Tumor Markers

Germinal testis tumors are among a select group of neoplasms identified as producing the so-called marker proteins that are relatively specific and readily measurable in minute quantities with highly sensitive radioimmunoassay (RIA) technology. Applied to the study of body fluids and tissue sections, these biochemical markers theoretically may be capable of detecting small tumor burdens (10^5 cells) that are not distinguished by currently available imaging techniques (Bagshawe and Searle, 1977). The study of biochemical marker substances, particularly AFP and β-hCG, is clinically useful in the diagnosis, staging, and monitoring of treatment responses in patients with germ cell neoplasms and may be useful as a prognostic index. Germ cell tumor markers belong to two main classes: (1) oncofetal substances associated with embryonic development (AFP and β-hCG) and (2) certain cellular enzymes, such as lactic acid dehydrogenase (LDH) and placental alkaline phosphatase (PLAP).

The production by germ cell tumors of oncofetal substances provides evidence that oncogenesis and ontogenesis are closely related. AFP is a dominant serum protein of the early embryo, and hCG is a secretory product of the placenta. During normal maturation of the fetus, both products fall to barely detectable levels soon after birth. The production of AFP and hCG by trophoblastic and syncytiotrophoblastic cells, respectively, within germ cell neoplasms implies the re-expression of repressed genes (presumably lost during differentiation) or malignant transformation of a pluripotential cell that has retained the ability to differentiate into cells capable of producing oncofetal proteins (Abelev, 1974; Uriel, 1979).

Alpha-Fetoprotein

AFP is a single-chain glycoprotein (molecular weight approximately 70,000) first demonstrated by Bergstrand and Czar (1954) in normal human fetal serum. In the fetus, AFP is a major serum-binding protein produced by the fetal yolk sac, liver, and gastrointestinal tract. The highest concentrations noted during the 12th to 14th weeks of gestation gradually decline so that 1 year following birth, AFP is detectable only at low levels (<40 ng/ml). In 1963, Abelev and colleagues detected AFP in embryos of mice and in the sera of mice with chemically induced liver tumors. Further investigation led to the discovery of elevated levels in humans with hepatomas and testis tumors. The metabolic half-life of AFP in humans is between 5 and 7 days, a fact that is useful in evaluating treatment response.

After the first 6 weeks of postnatal life, an elevated AFP level may be detected in association with a number of malignancies (testis, liver, pancreas, stomach, lung), normal pregnancy, benign liver disease, ataxia telangiectasia, and tyrosinemia. In endodermal sinus (or yolk sac) tumors, immunofluorescent methods indicate that the epithelial lining of the cysts and tubules is the site of the synthesis of AFP (Teilum et al., 1975). AFP may be produced by pure embryonal carcinoma, teratocarcinoma, yolk sac tumor, or combined tumors but not by pure choriocarcinoma or pure seminoma (Javadpour, 1980a, 1980b). These observations indicate that yolk sac elements are not always recognizable by conventional light microscopy in individuals with elevated serum AFP levels due to germ cell tumors. Binding studies with lectins have shown that AFP produced in the fetal liver has a different molecular structure from that produced in yolk sac tumors, a characteristic that may discriminate benign from malignant liver disease (Ruoslahti et al., 1978).

Human Chorionic Gonadotropin

This glycoprotein (molecular weight 38,000) is composed of alpha and beta polypeptide chains and is normally produced by trophoblastic tissue. Pituitary hormones (luteinizing hormone, follicle-stimulating hormone, thyroid-stimulating hormone) possess alpha subunits closely resembling that of hCG. The beta subunit of hCG is structurally and antigenically distinct from that of the pituitary hormones and allows the production of specific antibodies against the purified β-hCG subunit in RIA techniques (Vaitukaitis, 1979).

During pregnancy, hCG is secreted by the placenta for the maintenance of the corpus luteum. Zondek (1930) was the first to demonstrate that hCG is detectable in the sera of some patients with germ cell tumors. An elevated hCG level may also be demonstrated in those with various other malignancies (liver, pancreas, stomach, lung, breast, kidney, bladder) and perhaps in marijuana smokers. In germ cell tumors, syncytiotrophoblastic cells have been found responsible for the production of hCG. Some of the RIA techniques for β-hCG variously cross-react with luteinizing hormone (LH), and accordingly, caution should be exercised with the patient whose LH value may be physiologically elevated (e.g., postcastration).

The serum half-life of hCG is between 24 and 36 hours, but the individual subunits are cleared much more rapidly (20 minutes for the alpha subunit and 45 minutes for the beta subunit). All patients with choriocarcinoma and 40 to 60 per cent of patients with embryonal carcinoma are expected to have elevated serum levels of β-hCG. Approximately 5 to 10 per cent of patients with "pure" seminomas have detectable levels of β-hCG (usually below the level of 500 ng/ml), apparently produced by the syncytiotrophoblast-like giant cells occurring in some seminomas.

Clinical Applications of AFP and β-hCG

Among patients with nonseminomatous testis tumors, approximately 50 to 70 per cent have elevated levels of AFP and approximately 40 to 60 per cent have elevated levels of β-hCG when sensitive RIA techniques are employed. If both markers are measured simultaneously, approximately 90 per cent of patients will have elevations of one or both marker substances (Barzell and Whitmore, 1979; Fraley et al., 1979; Javadpour, 1980a). These values are derived from patient populations having clinical stages I, II, and III tumors. In patients with clinical stage I tumors only, the incidence of positive markers is lower.

Clinical Staging Accuracy

The overall sensitivity of any test or marker will vary with the amount of tumor burden. Determinations of AFP and β-hCG, in concert with other staging modalities, have helped reduce the understaging error in germ cell tumors to a level of 10 to 15 per cent. Expressed another way, approximately 10 to 15 per cent of patients with nonseminomatous germ cell tumors can be expected to have normal marker levels even at advanced stages of disease. Although large numbers of patients with clinical stage I nonseminoma have not had markers drawn before orchiectomy, data from the University of

Minnesota suggest that roughly two thirds will have elevated levels of AFP, β-hCG, or both (Lange and Raghavan, 1983). Up to 90 per cent of such patients are expected to produce marker substances in the presence of advanced disease.

Following orchiectomy, persistent elevation of one or both markers suggests residual tumor, and although a rapid normalization of previously elevated markers conceivably represents elimination of tumor, this is not categorically the case. In patients with disease clinically confined to the testis (clinical stage I), approximately 30 per cent will develop metastatic disease while under surveillance despite negative tumor markers immediately following inguinal orchiectomy. Similarly, a persistent marker elevation following a technically satisfactory retroperitoneal lymph node dissection indicates the presence of residual disease (stage III), whereas normal values do not categorically exclude the possibility of future recurrence.

Monitoring Therapeutic Response

The rate of tumor marker decline relative to expected marker half-life following treatment has been proposed as a prognostic index. Patients whose values decline according to negative half-lives following treatment appear more likely to be disease-free than those whose marker decline is slower or those whose markers never return to normal levels (Lange and Raghavan, 1983). Serial determinations of AFP and β-hCG levels closely reflect the effectiveness of therapy in patients with testicular tumors. The rate of marker decline following treatment (surgery, irradiation, chemotherapy) is proportional to the decrease in tumor burden and viability. Following apparently successful treatment, serologic relapse may precede clinical detection by an appreciable but unquantified interval. Alternative therapy may be initiated when minimal tumor burden is thereby perceived.

Following treatment of metastatic disease with irradiation, systemic drugs, or surgery, persistent marker elevation indicates an incomplete response. Because of a therapeutic lag following irradiation or chemotherapy, definition of the "expected" rate of decline and subsequent normalization of markers remains somewhat uncertain; no clear endpoint of tumor destruction can be identified. Such an endpoint has been precisely defined for surgery, in that serum markers should fall immediately according to half-life, if such a procedure eradicates the tumor. Nevertheless, marker determinations do act as guidelines following primary chemotherapy or irradiation. Clinical experience has shown that if a patient with advanced disease fails to achieve normalization of tumor markers following aggressive combination chemotherapy, attempts at surgical excision almost uniformly fail. Normalization of marker levels after treatment cannot be equated with the absence of residual disease. Between 20 and 30 per cent of patients receiving combined systemic chemotherapy for bulky metastatic disease, and subsequently subjected to retroperitoneal lymph node dissection, will have viable tumor confirmed histologically despite normal preoperative tumor marker levels. Similarly, failure to achieve normal levels of AFP and β-hCG following definitive irradiation indicates persistent tumor.

Histologic Diagnosis

Classification of germ cell neoplasms according to morphologic appearance is invaluable in treatment selection. The broad distinction between seminomas and nonseminomas has been particularly important in determining management strategies for retroperitoneal lymph node metastasis. In that germ cell tumors arise from pluripotential cells, a variety of elements may inhabit a given primary tumor or its secondary metastatic sites. Ray and co-workers (1979) noted that in the majority of patients (71 of 75, or 95 per cent), a primary tumor containing embryonal carcinoma and seminoma metastasized as pure embryonal carcinoma or combined with other elements but rarely metastasized as pure seminoma (two of 75, or 3 per cent). Heterogeneity among germ cell neoplasms is an expected consequence of their pluripotential origin. Biochemical marker "probes" can provide a means of delineating tumor heterogeneity, which may be of assistance in treatment selection.

Relative to seminoma, the detection of an elevated AFP level strongly suggests the presence of a nonseminomatous element. Step sections of the primary tumor may further define the source of the marker abnormality. Metastatic disease accompanied by an elevated serum AFP level from a pure seminoma indicates a nonseminomatous element, and treatment plans should be restructured accordingly. Parenthetically, 30 to 45 per cent of patients dying with seminoma are found to have elements of nonseminomatous histology at autopsy. It is generally accepted that between 5 and 10 per cent of patients with "pure" seminoma will have mild elevation of β-hCG level because of the presence of syncytiotrophoblastic giant cell forms. If step sections of the primary tumor fail to disclose nonseminomatous elements, conventional therapy is justified. If the β-hCG normalizes after orchiectomy, the patient should be treated as having pure seminoma. Current clinical evidence has indicated that β-hCG levels as high as 500 ng/ml may be found in association with a pure seminoma, although such an occurrence is rare.

Prognostic Value

Heterogeneity within nonseminomatous tumors is indicated by differences in growth rate, metastatic potential, and response to therapy and survival. The identification of factors associated with a poor prognosis or high risk provides a basis for altering therapeutic guidelines. Analyses concerning the prognostic implications of elevated marker values are conflicting. The degree of AFP or β-hCG elevation does appear directly proportional to the amount of tumor burden (stage and number of metastatic sites). The importance attached to the elevation of one tumor marker or another is not readily appreciated unless all potential variables are subjected to multivariate analysis. In studying interrelationships among tumor histology, tumor markers, tumor burden, and number of metastatic sites, Bosl and associates (1983) identified elevation of β-hCG and/or LDH levels and number of metastatic sites as the most important prognostic factors in determining survival in patients with germ cell tumors. Elevation of either tumor marker associated with multiple sites of metastasis implies a high risk of treatment failure despite aggressive multi-drug chemotherapy regimens.

Lactic Acid Dehydrogenase

LDH is a ubiquitous cellular enzyme (molecular weight 134,000) with particularly high levels detectable in smooth, cardiac, and skeletal muscles; liver; kidney; and brain. Elevation of serum LDH levels or one of its isoenzymes (LDH I–IV) has been reported useful in monitoring the treatment of germ cell tumors. Because of its low specificity (high false-positive rate), serum LDH levels must be correlated with other clinical findings in making therapeutic decisions.

In evaluating experience with serum LDH as a tumor marker for nonseminomatous germ cell tumors, Boyle and Samuels (1977) reported a direct relationship between tumor burden and LDH levels. Increased LDH values were noted in seven of 92 (8 per cent) patients with stage I disease, 15 of 42 (32 per cent) with stage II disease, and 57 of 70 (81 per cent) with stage III disease. Recurrence rates in patients with stage I and II disease were higher in those with elevated pretreatment LDH values—15 of 22 (77 per cent)—than in those with normal levels—42 of 112 (40 per cent). The first fraction (LDH-I) as determined by agar gel electrophoresis was responsible for LDH elevation in 25 of 29 patients studied. Skinner and Scardino (1980) found that an elevated LDH level may be the sole biochemical abnormality in as many as 10 per cent of patients with persistent or recurrent nonseminomatous tumors. Serum LDH may be even more helpful as a marker substance in the surveillance of patients with advanced seminomas. In reviewing their experience in patients with advanced "pure" seminomas, Stanton and colleagues (1983) found elevation of LDH levels in 21 of 26 patients (81 per cent). LDH seems to be most helpful as a marker for "bulk" tissue.

Placental Alkaline Phosphatase and Gamma-Glutamyl Transpeptidase

PLAP is a fetal isoenzyme structurally different from adult alkaline phosphatase. Small studies with enzyme-linked immunoabsorbent assays indicate that as many as 40 per cent of patients with advanced disease have elevated levels of PLAP (Javadpour, 1983). Gamma-glutamyl transpeptidase (GGT) is a hepatocellular enzyme frequently elevated in benign or neoplastic diseases of the liver. Its presence has been documented in humans in the placenta, normal testis, and seminal fluid, and in sacrococcygeal teratocarcinoma and testicular seminoma (Krishnaswamy et al., 1977). Javadpour (1983) found that one third of patients with active seminomas had elevated levels of GGT. Although the individual sensitivity of PLAP and GGT testing is low,

simultaneous determinations revealed elevation of one or both in 25 of 30 patients (80 per cent) considered to have active disease.

Treatment of Germ Cell Neoplasm

Principal treatment strategies for patients with germ cell tumor of the testis have evolved from conceptions of tumor natural history, clinical staging (assessment of the extent of disease), and effectiveness of treatment (alteration of natural history). Analysis of the tumor histology and of the frequency and pattern of spread indicates some predictable features of germ cell neoplasms. Pathologic stage is a function of disease progression, and clinical staging is an application of the methods available for assessment of pathologic stage. Selection of treatment alternatives is dependent on the relative advantages and disadvantages of different regimens. Multimodal therapy has been largely credited with treatment successes, but the current accuracy of clinical staging, the ability to recognize failure early, and the high probability of successful treatment of such failures have prompted investigations aimed at reducing the therapeutic burden.

Each of the major treatment alternatives—surgery, irradiation, and chemotherapy—has a particular but imperfectly defined role in the management of testicular tumors. As a means of establishing local control, inguinal or "radical" orchiectomy is clearly preferred. Such a procedure provides histologic diagnosis and local staging information (P category); controls the neoplasm locally with virtually 100 per cent effectiveness, the rare exception usually being attributable to iatrogenic influence; results in the cure of the patient with tumor confined to the testis; and is accomplished with minimal morbidity and virtually no mortality. Surgical excision of a retained spermatic cord remnant or of the "contaminated" scrotum is recommended following scrotal violation or tumor spillage, although additional irradiation of groin and ipsilateral hemiscrotum will suffice when pure seminoma is diagnosed. Because more than half of patients with testicular tumors present with metastatic disease, further treatment following orchiectomy is usual.

Clinical staging in addition to treatment of the retroperitoneal lymph nodes is a logical next step if no evidence of disease is detected in supradiaphragmatic or extralymphatic sites. It is now generally acknowledged that the majority of patients with large retroperitoneal metastatic deposits are best managed by chemotherapy initially.

Histologic diagnosis is a major factor in the natural history of testicular neoplasms. Between 65 and 85 per cent of all seminomas are clinically confined to the testis, whereas 60 to 70 per cent of nonseminomas appear with recognizable metastatic disease. Both the relatively low rate of spread and radiosensitivity have made radiation therapy the most widely accepted form of treatment for seminomas following inguinal orchiectomy. Radiation therapy, principally in Europe, and surgical excision, in

North America, have been employed in the management of regional lymph node metastasis from nonseminomas.

SEMINOMA

Seminoma is the most common histologic testis tumor in adults and accounts for approximately 60 to 65 per cent of all germ cell tumors of the testis. The established treatment for low-stage seminoma has been inguinal orchiectomy followed by therapeutic or adjuvant radiation therapy (Fig. 30–1). This regimen represents a highly effective method of treating low-stage disease with minimal morbidity. With the advent of multidrug chemotherapy for cure of patients with more disseminated disease, the overall cure rate for all stages exceeds 90 per cent.

Seminoma is very sensitive to radiation therapy and usually occurs at an early stage. Approximately 75 per cent of patients with seminomas will present with stage I disease, and in this group, greater than 90 per cent survival should routinely be anticipated. Postorchiectomy external beam radiation therapy to the retroperitoneal lymph nodes achieves very high cure rates for these patients.

The optimum treatment of patients who present with distant metastases or bulk retroperitoneal disease is chemotherapy initially. The role of salvage chemotherapy, surgical removal, or radiation therapy in clinical situations for which there are persistent radiographic masses remains controversial. Controversy exists about the treatment of bulk stage II disease as well.

Autopsy studies in patients dying with seminoma reveal that liver and lung involvement is common and is seen in approximately 75 per cent of patients. Bone and brain metastases are observed in 50 and 25 per cent of patients, respectively. Of major import is the fact that roughly one third of patients with histologically pure seminoma of the testes who ultimately die of the disease are found to harbor nonseminomatous elements in metastatic sites (Bredael et al., 1982).

Because seminoma occurs in a young population, and because surgical extirpation, radiation therapy, and multidrug chemotherapy all have salient benefits, treatment should be aimed not only at consideration of cure, but also at attempted maintenance of fertility and avoidance of potential harmful long-term sequelae. Although the role of irradiation therapy is unquestioned in patients with low-stage disease, it has become apparent that survival in patients with nonseminomatous germ cell tumors now parallels or exceeds that of patients with seminoma when compared stage for stage, especially for patients with advanced stage disease. Analyses of treatment failures have exposed a number of controversial issues in the management of patients with seminomatous tumors. An obligation exists to explore integrated therapeutic regimens in patients with more advanced disease and to attempt to reduce treatment burden in others.

Staging

Staging evaluation by physical examination, radiographic studies, and biochemical marker determinations indicates that approximately 75 per cent of seminomas are confined to the testis at the time of clinical presentation. Between 10 and 15 per cent will harbor metastatic disease in regional retroperitoneal lymph nodes, and no more than 5 to 10 per cent will have advanced to juxtaregional lymph node or visceral metastases. Data on the incidence of retroperitoneal lymph node involvement in clinical stage I seminoma are sparse but suggest that roughly 15 per cent of patients with negative findings in the history, physical examination, and intravenous pyelogram (IVP) have nodal metastasis documented by retroperitoneal lymphadenectomy (Whitmore, 1968). Because of the recognized effectiveness of radiation therapy, improved staging methods, and favorable natural history, few advocate lymph node dissection in patients with stage I seminoma.

Following inguinal orchiectomy, determination of serum tumor markers may provide additional clinicopathologic information relative to treatment selection for patients with "pure" seminomas. Although no ideal tumor marker exists for seminoma, determination of AFP and β-hCG levels supplements the histologic characterization of all germ cell tumors. An elevated AFP level virtually excludes a diagnosis of pure seminoma in that step sectioning of the primary tumor or histologic examination of secondary deposits almost uniformly discloses nonseminomatous elements. An elevated β-hCG level occurs in 5 to 10 per cent of pure seminomas, although levels over 1000 ng/ml have not been reported (Javadpour et al., 1978). Syncytiotrophoblastic giant cell elements responsible for the production of β-hCG have been detected by immunoperoxidase techniques. A specific predictive value of an elevated β-hCG level has not been noted; however, patients in whom the β-hCG level does not normalize should generally be treated as if they have nonseminomatous elements.

After radical orchiectomy, clinical evaluation for possible extragonadal metastatic disease should include postorchiectomy testing for serum tumor markers, chest radiograph, and retroperitoneal CT scan. In the past, bipedal lymphangiography was recommended for pa-

Therapy of Patients with Seminoma

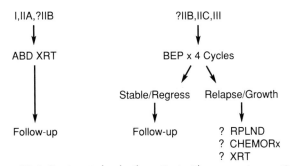

Figure 30–1. Treatment plan for the patient with pure seminoma. (BEP, bleomycin, etoposide, and cisplatin; ABD XRT, abdominal radiation therapy; RPLND, retroperitoneal lymph node dissection; CHEMORx, chemotherapy; XRT, radiation therapy.)

tients with pure seminoma. This recommendation was based on suggested treatment to one portal higher than that at which lymphatic involvement occurred. Thus, if the lymphangiogram results were positive, patients were treated with supplemental mediastinal and supraclavicular nodal radiation. With the advent of effective chemotherapy for salvage, radiation therapy above the diaphragm should be avoided. Therefore, the need for lymphangiography has diminished substantially. Some medical centers, however, still advocate routine lymphangiography for patients with seminoma to increase the amount of radiation therapy to the retroperitoneum.

The system of Boden and Gibb (1951) has been modified through the years as clinical staging procedures have become more precise and better correlated with treatment results. For the most part, extent of disease has been defined by three clinical stages: stage I, tumor confined to the testis ± epididymis and/or spermatic cord; stage II, metastasis present in retroperitoneal lymph nodes only; and stage III, spread beyond retroperitoneal lymph nodes. Currently, most workers subdivide stage II into stage IIA (nonbulky retroperitoneal deposits) and stage IIB (palpable or radiographically bulky, >10 cm diameter, retroperitoneal disease). Others distinguish between supradiaphragmatic lymph node metastasis (stage III) and visceral involvement (stage IV). A comparison among various common staging systems is shown in Table 30–5.

Histology

Three subtypes of pure seminomas have been described: "classic," anaplastic, and spermatocytic. The histologic and biochemical properties, natural history, and response to therapy of these subtypes have been characterized.

Several histopathologic characteristics of the primary tumor have been evaluated with regard to prognostic features as well as predictive value for likelihood of metastatic involvement (Hoeltl et al., 1987). Unfortunately, however, no significant predictors have been identified that will reliably detail the likelihood of metastatic involvement. Because most patients are treated with retroperitoneal irradiation, and surgical confirmation is not obtained, a small difference with these risk factors would not be identified.

Typical Seminoma

Typical or classic seminoma accounts for 82 to 85 per cent of all seminomas, occurring most commonly in the

4th decade but not uncommonly in the 5th and 6th decades. Seminoma rarely, if ever, occurs in the infant or adolescent but may occur in the patient over the age of 60 years. Histologically, it is composed of islands or sheets of relatively large cells with clear cytoplasm and densely staining nuclei. Syncytiotrophoblastic elements occur in 10 to 15 per cent, and lymphocytic infiltration occurs in approximately 20 per cent. The incidence of syncytiotrophoblastic elements corresponds to the frequency of β-hCG production. The slower growth rate of seminomas may be inferred from the observation that treatment failures may become evident 2 to 10 years following apparently adequate irradiation of metastatic sites.

Anaplastic Seminoma

Anaplastic seminoma accounts for between 5 and 10 per cent of all seminomas and has an age distribution similar to that of the typical subtype. Despite its rarity, discrimination of the anaplastic seminoma is noteworthy because up to 30 per cent of patients dying with seminoma have an anaplastic morphology. A number of features suggest that the anaplastic seminoma is a more aggressive and potentially more lethal variant of the typical seminoma. These characteristics include the following: (1) a greater mitotic activity, (2) a higher rate of local invasion, (3) an increased rate of metastatic spread, and (4) a higher rate of tumor marker production (β-hCG).

Histologically, anaplastic seminoma is typified by increased mitotic activity (three or more mitoses per high-power field), nuclear pleomorphism, and cellular anaplasia (Mostofi, 1973). Morphologically, histiocytic lymphoma and embryonal carcinoma may closely resemble anaplastic seminoma. Relative to the rate of metastasis, Percarpio and colleagues (1979) noted in a series of 77 patients with anaplastic seminoma that 19 (25 per cent) had clinical evidence of stage II disease. Shulman and co-workers (1983) reported a similar incidence of metastatic disease (29 per cent), a relatively high rate of extragonadal extension (46 per cent), and an unexpectedly high rate (36 per cent) of elevated β-hCG in 14 patients with anaplastic seminoma.

The less favorable results of treatment for patients with anaplastic seminoma may merely reflect a greater metastatic potential; there is no difference from classic seminoma when patients are treated appropriately and compared stage for stage. Analyses of treatment results indicate that inguinal orchiectomy plus radiation therapy

Table 30–5. COMPARISON OF CLINICAL STAGING SYSTEMS IN SEMINOMA

Clinical Extent of Disease	Walter Reed (Maier and Sulak, 1973)	M.D. Anderson (Doornbos et al., 1975)	Royal Marsden (Peckham et al., 1982)	UCLA (Crawford et al., 1983)
Testis/cord	IA (IIB-IA but positive RPLND)	I	I	I
Retroperitoneal nodes	II	IIA <10 cm	IIa <2 cm IIb 2–5 cm	IIA <2 cm IIB 2–10 cm
Nodes above diaphragm	III	III	III	III
Viscera	III	III	IV	III

Abbreviations: RPLND, retroperitoneal lymph node dissection.

is equally effective in controlling anaplastic and classic seminoma.

Spermatocytic Seminoma

This lesion is composed of cells varying in size with deeply pigmented cytoplasm and rounded nuclei containing characteristic filamentous chromatin. The cells closely resemble different phases of maturing spermatogonia. Spermatocytic seminoma accounts for 2 to 12 per cent of all seminomas, and nearly half occur in men over the age of 50 years. Bilateral tumors have been reported, but no cases have occurred in conjunction with cryptorchidism. The association of spermatocytic seminoma with other nonseminomatous tumors is rare.

The metastatic potential of spermatocytic seminoma is extremely low, and prognosis is accordingly favorable. Reviews by Thackray and Crane (1976) and Weitzner (1979) document no cases of metastatic disease. When histologic and staging evaluations have confirmed the diagnosis and the fact that disease is limited to the testis, treatment beyond inguinal orchiectomy appears unwarranted.

Treatment

The natural history and radiosensitivity of seminoma favor megavoltage irradiation in relatively modest amounts as the treatment of choice in the majority of patients following inguinal orchiectomy. Because the staging error may be 15 to 25 per cent for stage I seminoma, any treatment (or lack of it) should produce a cure in 75 per cent of patients, or better. The overall effectiveness of radiation therapy is confirmed, however, in that 2500 to 3500 cGy delivered over a 3-week period to the periaortic and ipsilateral inguinopelvic lymph nodes results in 5-year survival rates of 90 to 95 per cent. In stage II disease, 5-year survival rates of roughly 80 per cent are anticipated following therapeutic retroperitoneal irradiation with or without additional treatment of the mediastinum. Deposits in supradiaphragmatic nodes or distant sites and bulky abdominal disease respond less favorably to primary radiation therapy, which by itself yields survival rates as low as 20 to 30 per cent. Evidence indicates that seminoma is exquisitely sensitive to various chemotherapy regimens, particularly platinum-based ones, with response rates of 60 to 100 per cent being reported.

Stages I and IIA

In stage I and low-volume stage II seminoma, irradiation of para-aortic and inguinopelvic lymphatics is delivered through anterior and posterior parallel opposing fields. The retroperitoneal lymph node groups included in radiation treatment fields are the ipsilateral external iliac, the bilateral common iliac, the paracaval, and the para-aortic nodes superiorly, including coverage of the cisterna chyli. CT scanning is useful in planning and simulation of treatment fields. The exact field depends on characteristics of the individual patient as well as the equipment. The para-aortic field is bounded superiorly by the origin of the thoracic duct and includes the anterior surface of the 11th or 10th thoracic vertebra, anteriorly to the internal inguinal ring and inguinal excision, laterally to include the ipsilateral renal hilum, and more generously on the left side than on the right. The contralateral para-aortic nodes are treated on an individual basis. The pelvic segment stretches from the 4th lumbar vertebra to the inguinal ligament and includes the orchiectomy scar. In a patient with retained spermatic cord remnant or contaminated scrotum, the field may be widened considerably.

In patients with histories of herniorrhaphy or prior orchiopexy, with potential alteration in lymphatic drainage, the inferior portion of the field should include the contralateral inguinal region as well. The contralateral testis should be shielded.

Fields are treated with conventional fractionation of 150 cGy per day, 5 days per week, including both anterior and posterior fields treated on a daily basis. Elective supradiaphragmatic irradiation for patients with stage I neoplasm is not recommended. Prophylactic treatment of the mediastinum or supraclavicular area is not indicated.

Treatment Results

STAGE I

Patients with stage I seminoma treated with postorchiectomy radiation enjoy outstanding 5-year survival rates approximating 95 per cent. Five-year disease-free survival rates roughly equate with cure in that late relapses with death are exceedingly rare beyond that time. Results for disease-free survival in patients with postorchiectomy radiation therapy for clinical stages I and II seminoma are presented in Table 30–6. Routine survival rates above 95 per cent are to be expected in patients with clinical stage I seminoma. This survival rate does not seem altered by the addition of prophylactic mediastinal irradiation. In fact, prophylactic mediastinal irradiation has been discontinued in the majority of institutions (Thomas et al., 1982). With the advent of effective chemotherapy against disseminated disease, mediastinal or supradiaphragmatic irradiation could potentially compromise the patient's ability to receive effective therapy (Loehrer et al., 1987).

STAGE II

Patients with clinical stage II seminoma treated with postorchiectomy radiation therapy have 5-year survival rates of approximately 80 per cent with a range of 70 to 92 per cent (see Table 30–6). This subset of patients creates increasing controversy in the decision for radiation therapy versus combination chemotherapy as primary treatment. Treatment results are reported depending on the staging system utilized. Some medical centers designate stage IIA as less than 10 cm in diameter and stage IIB as greater than 10 cm in diameter. Others employ different definitions for bulk retroperitoneal disease. Certainly, patients with less than 5-cm masses have a reasonably good 5-year survival with radiation

Table 30–6. RADIATION THERAPY IN CLINICAL STAGES I AND II SEMINOMA (DISEASE-FREE SURVIVAL)

Source	Stage I		Stage II		
	No. of Patients	*Survival (%)*	*No. of Patients*	*Survival (%)*	*Years of Follow-Up (A/C)*
Maier and Sulak (1973)	284	97	34	91	5 (A)
Earle and co-workers (1973)	71	100	27	85	5 (A)
Peckham and McElwain (1974)	78	98	27	93	4 (A)
Doornbos and co-workers (1975)	79	94	48	77	3 (C)
Blandy (1976)	98	93	35	71	5 (A)
van der Werf-Messing (1976)	91	100	67	85	5 (A)
Batata and co-workers (1979)	227	88	53	62	5 (C)
Dosoretz and co-workers (1981)	135	97	18	92	5 (A)
Thomas and co-workers (1982)	338	94	86	74	5 (A)

Abbreviations: A, actuarial survival; C, crude survival.

therapy alone. Patients with stage IIA disease have survival rates above 90 per cent, which statistically does not differ from patients with stage I disease. For patients with stage IIB disease treated by extended radiation therapy alone, approximately one third of patients will develop metastatic disease outside the treated fields. In a study from the Royal Marsden Hospital in London, 10 per cent of patients with stage IIA disease, defined as less than 2-cm retroperitoneal metastases, relapsed; 18 per cent of patients with less than 5-cm nodes relapsed, but 38 per cent of patients with greater than 5-cm nodes relapsed (Peckham et al., 1981).

ADVANCED SEMINOMA

The overall disease-free survival in patients with stage IIB or greater disease treated with abdominal irradiation is only approximately 50 per cent. Radiation was the treatment of choice for patients with advanced seminoma prior to the advent of platinum-based combination chemotherapy (Table 30–7). Patients had experienced relapse with equal frequency in the abdomen or in distant sites, regardless of whether prophylactic mediastinal or supraclavicular irradiation was used. Patients who had experienced relapse might be salvaged with radiation therapy, although the response rate was poor.

Prior to the 1970s, alkylating agents were used against metastatic seminoma. The combination of *cis*-platinum, vinblastine, and bleomycin has been found to be effective against disseminated testicular seminomas as well as nonseminomatous tumors. More than 90 per cent of

patients who present with stage III disease will achieve a complete response to chemotherapy alone, and approximately 90 per cent of these responders remain disease-free during follow-up evaluations to 4 years (Table 30–8).

Response rates seem to be somewhat better when *cis*-platinum–based chemotherapy is given as the primary treatment with no prior radiation, but reasonable results can be obtained for relapse after initial irradiation. Extensive prior irradiation can produce an impact on the amount of chemotherapy received as well as the response rate. Thus, response rates seem to be higher in patients treated with chemotherapy than in those treated with primary radiation alone. One difficulty in a patient with advanced seminoma treated with *cis*-platinum combination chemotherapy is the lack of complete resolution of masses on CT scan. Controversy exists about the need for further treatment as opposed to observation. Attempts to remove bulk residual disease after chemotherapy for seminoma are fraught with difficulty. Because seminoma involves the retroperitoneum as a fibrotic process similar to retroperitoneal fibrosis, clean retroperitoneal dissection is rarely achieved. In most patients explored after chemotherapy, only residual necrosis or fibrosis is found. However, in a study involving a review of patients at Sloan-Kettering Memorial Hospital, New York, with bulky stage II or III seminoma for which the residual mass was 3 cm or greater, residual viable tumor was found in approximately 50 per cent of patients (Motzer et al., 1987).

Irradiation and chemotherapy are both highly effec-

Table 30–7. RADIATION THERAPY IN CLINICAL STAGES IIB AND III SEMINOMA (DISEASE-FREE SURVIVAL)

Source	Stage IIB		Stage III	
	No. of Patients	Survival (%)	No. of Patients	Survival (%)
Maier and Sulak (1973)	—	—	18	17
Doornbos and co-workers (1975)	22	61	14	21
Blandy (1976)	—	—	17	12
van der Werf-Messing (1976)	21	75	30	43
Smith (1978)	7	29	14	14
Batata and co-workers (1979)	—	—	24	42
Dosoretz and co-workers (1981)	7	43	9	44
Thomas and co-workers (1982)	46	48	20	32
Green and co-workers (1983)	18	94*	—	—

*Five of 18 patients lost to follow-up in <2 years.

Table 30–8. PRIMARY CHEMOTHERAPY FOR ADVANCED SEMINOMA

Source	Regimen	No. of Patients	Prior Irradiation No. (%)	Follow-Up CR + PR	NED	Mo
Einhorn and Williams (1980a)	PVB (A)	19	13 (68)	12 + 7	11 (58)	19
Vugrin and co-workers (1981b)	DDP + Cy	9	6 (67)	5 + 4	7 (78)	19
Morse and co-workers (1983)*	VAB-VI	22	8 (38)	9 + 10	17 (77)	17
Wajsman and co-workers (1983)	DDP + VBPr/ VP-16	12	4 (33)	12	12 (100)	—
Crawford and co-workers (1983)†	VAC	16	1 (7)	15	15 (94)	48

*Both series contain patients with extragonadal primary tumors and patients who received additional surgery ± radiation therapy.
†Fifteen of 16 patients received radiation therapy following chemotherapy.
Abbreviations: CR, complete response; PR, partial response; NED, no evidence of disease; PVB(A), *cis*-platinum, vinblastine, bleomycin, adriamycin; DDP, *cis*-platinum; Cy, cyclophosphamide; VAB, vinblastine-actinomycin D-bleomycin; VBPr, vinblastine, bleomycin, prednisone; VAC, vincristine, actinomycin, cyclophosphamide.

tive against pure seminoma. Natural history of seminoma generally favors a minimal therapeutic burden, which justifies radiation therapy after orchiectomy in the majority of patients (see Fig. 30–1). In patients with bulk or advanced disease, however, initial treatment should be platinum-based chemotherapy with surgery or radiation therapy reserved for those patients in whom treatment failed. Because of the effectiveness of chemotherapy, surveillance has been advocated by certain medical centers (Duchesne et al., 1990; Oliver et al., 1990).

Patients with advanced seminomas seem to have a chemosensitive tumor with potential cure with chemotherapy that is comparable to that observed for patients with nonseminomatous germ cell tumors. More than 85 per cent of patients have achieved continuous disease-free status with *cis*-platinum combination chemotherapy. Therefore, multidrug, *cis*-platinum–based chemotherapy should be given initially in patients with advanced seminoma, and no further treatment should be given in patients with radiographically complete responses. With residual mass, close and careful observation is favored as opposed to consolidation with radiation therapy or surgical excision (Fossa et al., 1987). Although surveillance can be considered following orchiectomy for stage I seminoma, the excellent results with minimal morbidity and toxicity from low-dose, retroperitoneal irradiation make this the treatment of choice.

NONSEMINOMA

Tumors designated as "nonseminoma" include those that are histologically composed of embryonal carcinoma, teratoma, choriocarcinoma, and yolk sac elements, alone or in various combinations. Tumors containing both seminomatous and nonseminomatous elements are generally regarded as nonseminomas, a consideration that may have practical bearing upon treatment selection. Aside from morphologic differences, distinctions between seminoma and nonseminoma are made relative to natural behavior, clinical staging, and treatment strategies.

Natural History

Clinical evidence is strong that nonseminomas follow a potentially less favorable natural history than do pure seminomas. Depending to some degree on referral patterns and staging criteria, 50 to 70 per cent of patients with nonseminomas, but only 20 to 30 per cent of those with seminomas, will present with metastatic disease at the time of diagnosis. The first echelon of spread for all germ cell tumors is most commonly the retroperitoneal lymph nodes. Evidence for this generalization stems from postmortem and clinical experiences. Autopsy studies indicate that roughly three quarters of patients dying with germ cell tumors have a concomitant or prior history of retroperitoneal nodal and parenchymal metastases, despite therapeutic retroperitoneal irradiation or lymphadenectomy. After retroperitoneal lymph nodes, lung is the next most common site of spread for metastases. This observation is evident from autopsy studies and from the follow-up of patients after lymph node dissection, in that lung metastasis represents the most frequently recognized site of treatment failure regardless of lymph node status. Next in frequency of spread are liver, brain, bone, and kidney, although almost any site may be involved.

Clinical Staging

The natural history and frequency of disease dissemination favor the accurate clinical staging of nonseminomatous tumors. The rapid development of precise imaging techniques and tumor-indexing substances frequently produced by nonseminomas also foster staging accuracy. The principal differences between staging systems for seminomas and nonseminomas relate to the roles of surgical lymph node sampling and serum tumor markers.

Histology

Embryonal carcinoma is generally discovered as a small, rounded but irregular mass invading the tunica vaginalis and not infrequently involving contiguous cord structures. The cut surface reveals a variegated, grayish white, fleshy tumor, often with areas of necrosis or hemorrhage and a poorly defined capsule. The typical histologic appearance is that of distinctly malignant epithelioid cells arranged in glands or tubules. The cell borders are usually indistinct, the cytoplasm pale or vacuolated, and the nuclei rounded with coarse chromatin and one or more large nucleoli. Pleomorphism, mitotic figures, and giant cells are features common to these highly malignant tumors.

Pure choriocarcinoma may occur as a palpable nodule, with size depending on the extent of local hemorrhage. Patients with pure choriocarcinoma may present with evidence of advanced distant metastasis and what seems a paradoxically small intratesticular lesion that may not distort the normal testicular size or shape. Central hemorrhage with viable grayish white tumor at the periphery may be seen on the cut surface if the lesion can be demonstrated grossly.

Microscopically, two distinct and appropriately oriented cell types must be demonstrated to satisfy the histologic diagnosis of choriocarcinoma—syncytiotrophoblasts and cytotrophoblasts. The syncytiotrophoblasts may be large multinucleated cells containing abundant, often vacuolated, eosinophilic cytoplasm and large, hyperchromatic, irregular nuclei. Less commonly, the syncytial elements may be spindle-shaped and contain one large, dark-staining nucleus. The cytotrophoblasts are closely packed, intermediate-sized, uniform cells with a distinct cell border, clear cytoplasm, and a single vesicular nucleus.

Teratoma contains more than one germ cell layer in various stages of maturation and differentiation. "Mature" elements resemble benign structures derived from normal ectoderm, entoderm, and mesoderm. "Immature" teratoma consists of undifferentiated primitive tissues from each of the three germ cell layers. Grossly, the tumors are usually large, lobulated, and nonhomogeneous in consistency. The cut surface may reveal variably sized cysts containing gelatinous, mucinous, or hyalinized material interspersed with islands of solid tissue, often containing cartilage or bone. Histologically, the cysts may be lined by squamous, cuboidal, columnar, or transitional epithelium. The solid component may contain any combination of cartilage; bone; intestinal, pancreatic, or liver tissue; smooth or skeletal muscle; and neural or connective tissue elements. On rare occasions, malignant changes may be recognized in such differentiated tissues, justifying the designation "malignant teratoma."

Yolk sac tumor is the most common testis tumor of infants and children. In adults, it occurs most frequently in combination with other histologic types and is presumably responsible for the production of AFP. The terms endodermal sinus tumor, infantile testis adenocarcinoma, juvenile embryonal carcinoma, and orchioblastoma are used synonymously. In its pure form, the lesion has a homogeneous yellowish, mucinous appearance. Microscopically, the tumor is composed of epithelioid cells that form glandular and ductal structures arranged in columns, papillary projections, or solid islands within a primitive mesenchymal stroma. The individual epithelial tumor cells may be columnar, cuboidal, or flat, with poorly defined cell borders and vacuolated cytoplasm containing glycogen and fat. The large, irregularly shaped nuclei contain one or more prominent nucleoli and variable amounts of chromatin. Embryoid bodies, a common finding in yolk sac tumors, resemble 1- to 2-week-old embryos. These ovoid structures, commonly measuring less than 1 mm in diameter, consist of a cavity surrounded by loose mesenchyme containing syncytiotrophoblasts and cytotrophoblasts.

In classifying over 6000 testis tumors, Mostofi (1973) found that in roughly 40 per cent, more than one histologic pattern was identified. Because of its frequent occurrence (24 per cent of testis tumors), the combination of teratoma and embryonal carcinoma, termed "teratocarcinoma," is usually classified as a specific entity. Teratocarcinomas are frequently large and frequently disseminated. Metastatic deposits associated with teratomas usually contain embryonal carcinoma (80 per cent) and, less frequently, teratoma or choriocarcinoma. The bisected tumor exhibits cysts, typical of teratoma, within the solid, sometimes hemorrhagic stroma containing embryonal elements.

The pluripotential nature of germ cell tumors, and in particular nonseminomatous tumors, is evident from the varied histologic patterns of metastasis, over half of which display different morphologies in primary versus metastatic sites, although pure choriocarcinoma invariably spreads unaltered. Whereas postmortem studies document that 30 to 45 per cent of patients dying with seminoma harbor nonseminomatous metastases, the converse is rarely documented.

Treatment—Stage I

Removal of the testis by means of an inguinal approach, the so-called radical orchiectomy, remains the definitive procedure for pathologic diagnosis as well as local treatment of testicular neoplasms. Morbidity is minimal and mortality should be virtually zero while allowing 100 per cent local control. Transscrotal biopsy is to be condemned. The inguinal approach permits early control of the vascular and lymphatic supply as well as en bloc removal of the testis with all its tunics.

In patients with nonseminomatous germ cell tumors, following inguinal orchiectomy, the accuracy of clinical staging is critical as a determinant for further treatment selection. Because of the inexactitude of clinical staging, retroperitoneal lymphadenectomy remains the mainstay of surgical therapy in patients with nonseminomatous germ cell tumors (Table 30–9). These tumors generally spread to the retroperitoneal lymph nodes before further dissemination, and the primary landing sites are well identified. After spread to the retroperitoneum, the next most common site of metastasis is to the lungs, where metastases can be identified early with plain radiographs. Furthermore, these tumors often produce β-hCG or AFP, both of which are measurable in the serum at nanogram levels.

Historical Perspectives

Anatomic studies at the turn of the century by Most (1898) and Cuneo (1901) as well as later work by

Table 30–9. TWO- TO FIVE-YEAR SURVIVAL AFTER ORCHIECTOMY AND RPLND IN PATHOLOGIC STAGE I NSGCTT

Source	NED No.	NED %	Years of Follow-Up
Whitmore (1970)	50/58	86	5
Walsh and co-workers (1971)	24/25	96	3
Bradfield and co-workers (1973)	28/40	70	3
Staubitz and co-workers (1974)	42/45	93	3
Johnson and co-workers (1976)	65/72	90	5
Skinner (1976)*	39/43	91	2
Donohue and co-workers (1978)	27/30	90	3
Fraley and co-workers (1979)	28/28	100	2
Bredael and co-workers (1983)†	126/138	91	3
Total	429/479	Average 90	

*Adjuvant actinomycin D.
†Thirty patients received adjuvant chemotherapy.
Abbreviations: RPLND, retroperitoneal lymph node dissection; NSGCTT, non-seminomatous germ cell testicular tumor; NED, no evidence of disease.

Jamieson and Dobson (1910) and Rouviere (1938) demonstrated the lymphatic drainage of the testis. The primary echelon of drainage for right-sided tumors is the interaortal caval nodes and for left-sided tumors, left para-aortic and preaortic nodes. Some crossover exists, especially from right to left. These anatomic studies provided the basis for regional control after establishing local control by orchiectomy.

The first site of metastasis in patients with nonseminomatous tumors is generally the retroperitoneal lymph nodes (90 per cent). In approximately 10 per cent of patients, the first site of metastasis will be outside the borders of a standard retroperitoneal lymph node dissection. Thorough excision of the retroperitoneal lymph nodes remains the epitome or gold standard of staging. Although noninvasive staging techniques are somewhat accurate, 20 to 25 per cent of patients with clinical stage I disease are understaged by all available modalities of nonsurgical staging. The cure rate for patients with pathologically confirmed stage I disease is roughly 95 per cent with surgery alone. The 5 to 10 per cent of patients who may experience relapse following negative findings on retroperitoneal lymph node dissection for stage I disease have a high cure rate with salvage chemotherapy.

The 5 to 10 per cent of patients who experience relapse will generally do so within the first 2 years after diagnosis. Thus, careful follow-up is necessary for the first 2 years, generally with monthly chest radiographs and tumor markers for the 1st year and every other month for the 2nd year. Because relapse beyond 2 years is rare, these patients can be followed annually for the next several years. Patients who experience relapse generally do so in the lungs, suggesting hematogenous spread that preceded lymphatic dissemination. Recurrences in the retroperitoneum have been recognized rarely in patients who previously had negative lymph node dissection findings.

Retroperitoneal lymph node dissection was established as a primary therapy for nonseminomatous germ cell tumors by Lewis in 1948. Kimbrough and Cook (1953) fostered inguinal orchiectomy plus retroperitoneal lymphadenectomy as the preferred local regional treatment for patients with testis tumors. In Europe, conversely, radiation therapy was used as a primary means for sterilizing nodal deposits. Lewis reported a 46 per cent 5-year survival among 28 patients treated with lymphadenectomy and/or radiation therapy after orchiectomy.

A variety of surgical approaches have been advocated for retroperitoneal lymphadenectomy. Cooper and associates popularized the transthoracic approach in 1950. Staubitz and co-workers (1974) and Whitmore (1979) practiced the transabdominal approach. The question of bilateral suprahilar dissection was raised by Donohue and associates (1982). This issue led to important mapping studies for the distribution of retroperitoneal lymph node metastases in patients with minimal, moderate, or advanced retroperitoneal disease. This work has allowed tailoring of the surgical procedure to the amount of retroperitoneal adenopathy that is present.

Retroperitoneal lymph node dissection, by way of a transabdominal or thoracoabdominal approach, is a generally well tolerated, 3- to 4-hour procedure with negligible mortality and minimal morbidity. The mortality rate is less than 1 per cent. Morbidity ranges from 5 to 25 per cent and is usually related to atelectasis, pneumonitis, ileus, lymphocele, or pancreatitis.

Fertility After Retroperitoneal Lymph Node Dissection

Semen quality as an indicator of potential fertility has been studied by many investigators before, during, and after various treatments for testicular cancer. Approximately 50 to 60 per cent of males are reportedly subfertile at the time of diagnosis of a nonseminotamous germ cell tumor. Controversy exists as to whether spermatogenesis is impaired prior to the clinical manifestation of testicular cancer or whether semen quality is impaired as a result of diagnosis and/or initial therapy. Nonetheless, in a large proportion of patients, spermatogenesis impairment may be reversible.

EMISSION AND EJACULATION. Before 1980, a high incidence of infertility was noted following retroperitoneal lymph node dissection in patients with testicular cancer. This infertility was largely due to either failure of seminal emission or retrograde ejaculation secondary to damage to the sympathetic nerve fibers involved in ejaculation.

Early descriptions of retroperitoneal lymphadectomy included a complete bilateral dissection from above the renal hilar area bilaterally, encompassing both ureters down to where each ureter crossed the common iliac artery. Retroperitoneal tissue was removed both anterior to and posterior to the great vessels to completely remove all node-bearing tissue. Thorough removal of all lymphatic tissue was considered essential because of the lack of effective alternative therapies. Indeed, retroperitoneal lymph node dissection using the aforementioned template has been curative in patients with minimal nodal involvement, even without the use of adjunctive chemotherapy.

With the development of effective combination *cis*-platinum–based chemotherapy, testicular cancer has become one of the most curable of all genitourinary tumors. As survival rates have improved, the long-term effects of infertility resulting from retroperitoneal lymph node dissection have assumed greater import. A major impetus for close observation or surveillance therapy has been the long-term effect of ejaculatory compromise and infertility in patients with low-stage testicular cancer.

MODIFIED RETROPERITONEAL LYMPH NODE DISSECTION. In the early 1980s, Narayan and associates (1982) published an important article concerning ejaculation after extended retroperitoneal lymph node dissection. This article showed that modification of surgical boundaries could allow return of ejaculation in approximately half of patients with low-stage testicular cancer following retroperitoneal lymph node dissection. Even with more extensive dissections for stage BII or BIII retroperitoneal involvement, ejaculatory capability returned in approximately one third of patients.

Richie (1990) reported a prospective study of modified lymph node dissection in 85 patients with clinical stage I nonseminomatous germ cell tumor of the testis. The dissection is bilateral above the level of the inferior mesenteric artery but unilateral below the inferior mesenteric artery. The technique involves a thoracoabdominal approach through the ipsilateral side with mobilization of the peritoneal envelope completely. Once the peritoneum is peeled from the posterior rectus fascia, an incision is made in the peritoneum and palpation is carried out to be certain there is no bulk disease or more extensive disease, which would preclude retroperitoneal rather than transperitoneal lymphadenectomy. By peeling the peritoneal envelope and remaining in a retroperitoneal fashion, along with preservation of the inferior mesenteric artery, injury to the nerves controlling ejaculation on the contralateral side of the aorta and great vessels below the inferior mesenteric artery is avoided (Figs. 30–2 and 30–3).

Thus, for a right-sided tumor, the dissection would encompass the renal hilar area bilaterally to the level of the left ureter or gonadal vein. On the left side, dissection is carried down to the level of the inferior mesenteric artery, then across to the right side and down the right side of the aorta, encompassing the right common iliac artery. All node-bearing tissue in the interaortic caval area is removed, and the posterior margin is the anterior spinous ligament. Both sympathetic chains are preserved. On the right side, the dissection is carried along the right renal hilar area to the level of the right ureter and down to where the ureter crosses the common iliac artery. The ipsilateral spermatic vessels are removed to the level of the deep inguinal ring and the previously ligated stump of the cord (Fig. 30–2).

For left-sided dissection, a similar dissection is performed with the exception of the right lateral margin (Fig. 30–3). Because nodal spread tends to occur from

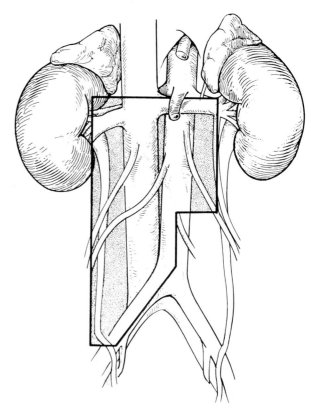

Figure 30–2. Modified right-sided retroperitoneal lymph node dissection template. The dissection is complete above the level of the inferior mesenteric artery but limited to the unilateral/ipsilateral side below the level of the inferior mesenteric artery.

right to left, dissection is only carried to the lateral margin of the inferior vena cava rather than all the way over to the right ureter. This dissection is bilateral above the inferior mesenteric artery and unilateral below the inferior mesenteric artery.

The final pathology report of the 85 patients who underwent modified retroperitoneal lymph node dissection noted stage A disease in 64 patients and stage BI disease in 21 patients. Patients have been followed from 12 to 84 months with a median of 38 months. Seven patients have experienced relapse, all with pulmonary metastases. All patients have been salvaged with chemotherapy and remain free of disease. No retroperitoneal recurrences have been noted other than one retrocrural recurrence.

With respect to preservation of ejaculatory function, 75 of 85 patients have reported spontaneous return of antegrade ejaculation, usually within 1 month postoperatively. An additional five patients have regained antegrade ejaculation with imipramine (Tofranil). Thus, 80 of 85 patients (94 per cent) have recovered antegrade ejaculation, either spontaneously or with medication. Five patients continue to have retrograde ejaculation, as documented by sperm in the urine following ejaculation. Sperm counts have been obtained in 65 patients. The counts range from a low of 2×10^6/ml to a high of 120×10^6/ml. Volume has ranged from 0.5 to 4.5 ml. Most patients report that post–node dissection ejaculate volume is approximately one half that of pre–node

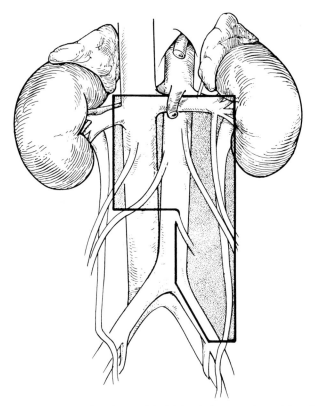

Figure 30–3. Template for modified left-sided retroperitoneal lymph node dissection. The right-sided border is near the right margin of the inferior vena cava.

dissection ejaculate volume. Thus far, there have been 11 pregnancies reported by this group of patients in their partners.

The template or boundary method of retroperitoneal lymph node dissection has significant advantages. By application of this technique, a complete bilateral dissection can be performed in the area most likely to be involved with retroperitoneal nodal disease, yet modification in a less likely area can spare some of the ejaculatory consequences. This type of procedure is universally transferable to surgeons with some experience in performance of retroperitoneal lymph node dissection and requires no additional new skills or techniques of identification. The aforementioned techniques represent a therapeutically and diagnostically sound method for the treatment of patients with pathologic stage A and stage BI disease, with preservation of ejaculation in more than 90 per cent of patients.

Several medical centers have described modifications of retroperitoneal lymph node dissections with a variety of techniques to preserve ejaculation. Donohue and associates (1990) reported modifications with preservation of ejaculation in two thirds of patients with right-sided tumors and one third of those with left-sided tumors. Pizzocaro (1985) reported on unilateral retroperitoneal lymph node dissection with excellent preservation of ejaculation. Ninety per cent of patients with stage A and stage BI testicular cancer had preservation of ejaculation, whereas only 23 per cent of patients with stage BII testicular cancer had preservation of ejaculation (Pizzocaro, 1985).

Attempts have been made to identify individual retroperitoneal sympathetic nerves responsible for antegrade ejaculation. Jewett and Torbey (1988) described early experience with nerve-sparing techniques with excellent return of ejaculation. Likewise, Donohue and associates (1990) have performed a similar procedure with excellent return of ejaculation in short-term follow-up. These techniques involve removal of node-bearing tissue from around the postganglionic fibers. The techniques are somewhat more time-consuming and may require a steeper learning curve as well. Thus far, recurrence rates with these modified techniques are not different from those with standard techniques.

Radiation Therapy

Megavoltage irradiation has been available since the 1950s and in common use since the 1960s, by which time retroperitoneal lymph node dissection (RPLND) had already become established, especially in the United States. Radiation therapy of the retroperitoneum in patients with clinical stage I nonseminomatous germ cell testicular tumor (NSGCTT) remains accepted practice in many treatment centers outside North America. The main objections to retroperitoneal lymph node irradiation have been the inaccuracy of clinical staging of the retroperitoneal lymph nodes; the resultant lack of survival data that could be reasonably compared with surgical data; and the concern that, in the event of postirradiation relapse, the prior irradiation might preclude adequate chemotherapy or surgical excision. Modern staging techniques have reduced the falsely negative staging error in clinical stage I disease to approximately 20 per cent. In patients with clinical stage I disease subjected to RPLND, 10 to 15 per cent will harbor undetected nodal metastasis, and another 5 to 10 per cent will experience relapse following surgery, almost always in extranodal sites.

The tumoricidal dose for NSGCTT ranges between 4000 and 5000 cGy, far in excess of that required to sterilize seminoma. A dose of 4000 to 4500 cGy delivered in 4 to 5 weeks to the para-aortic and ipsilateral pelvic lymph nodes is the recommended radiation standard in clinical stage I NSGCTT. The long-term complications of para-aortic irradiation include radiation enteritis, bowel obstruction, and bone marrow suppression, with a reported frequency of between 5 and 10 per cent. Secondary malignancy has been reported following abdominal radiation therapy for Hodgkin's disease, but such reports following treatment for testis tumors are anecdotal.

The overall success rate of radiation therapy in the treatment of clinical stage I NSGCTT in terms of 5-year survival is between 80 and 95 per cent when chemotherapy is used to treat relapses (Table 30–10). Relapse rates following radiation therapy for clinical stage I disease are as high as 24 per cent (14/59), with 3 per cent within the irradiated volume and 21 per cent outside (Raghavan et al., 1982).

Surveillance

If staging modalities were sufficiently accurate to identify patients whose disease is truly confined to the

Table 30–10. SURVIVAL AFTER ORCHIECTOMY AND RADIOTHERAPY FOR CLINICAL STAGES I AND II NSGCTT (2–5 YEARS)

Source	Stage I		Stage II		Total	
Battermann and co-workers (1973)	24/30	(80%)	6/19	(32%)	30/49	(61%)
Tyrrell and Peckham (1976)	73/88	(84%)	14/29	(48%)	87/117	(74%)
van der Werf-Messing (1976)*	26/29	(90%)	16/35	(46%)	42/64	(66%)
Maier and Mittemeyer (1977)	25/29	(86%)	9/11	(82%)	34/40	(85%)
Peckham and co-workers (1981)†	37/39	(95%)	17/21	(81%)	54/60	(90%)
Blandy and co-workers (1983)	125/162	(77%)	—		125/162	(77%)
Total	310/377	(82%)	62/115	(54%)	372/492	(76%)

*Extrapolated from actuarial tables.
†Includes patients treated successfully for relapse and patients in stage II treated primarily with preirradiation chemotherapy.
Abbreviation: NSGCTT, nonseminomatous germ cell testicular tumor.

testis, orchiectomy alone should yield survival results equal to therapeutic strategies that incorporate treatment of the regional lymph nodes. With the inaccuracies of staging, however, RPLND remains the only modality that can accurately delineate pathologic stage I from pathologic stage II testicular cancer. Clinical understaging approximates 25 per cent even in the best of series. Nonetheless, approximately 70 per cent of patients who undergo RPLND are found to have pathologic stage I disease and, therefore, receive no therapeutic benefit from the operation. Additionally, 5 to 10 per cent of patients will relapse outside of the field of the retroperitoneal node dissection.

With the advent of effective chemotherapy, coupled with concerns about the need for RPLND in all patients with clinical stage I testicular cancer as well as the complications of loss of ejaculation and infertility, postorchiectomy observation or surveillance has a certain appeal. Several large surveillance programs have been undertaken throughout the world. In several of the largest series, detailed in Table 30–11, the relapse rate is approximately 30 per cent. Unfortunately, the death rate in those patients who relapse has been 7 per cent, or 1.8 per cent of the entire series. Even with monitoring, 80 per cent of relapses are noted at more advanced stages compared with those patients who undergo RPLND and who tend to experience relapse with pulmonary metastases at a lower stage of advanced disease (Rowland et al., 1982). Considering that the majority of these patients have very favorable factors in order to enter a surveillance protocol, death rates should be exceedingly rare in this subset of patients.

As more experience is generated, patient selection should identify those individuals at low risk for metastases in whom close observation could be elected. These patients require meticulous evaluation before entering a well-designed and well-managed surveillance protocol. Staging should be carried out compulsively in selected patients with no evidence of suspicious nodes or pulmonary masses.

Several series have evaluated prognostic factors associated with relapse (Dunphy et al., 1988; Fung et al., 1988). Patients with a significant percentage of embryonal carcinoma in the primary tumor are thought to be at high risk of relapse. The local T stage or extent of involvement of the tumor is also an important prognostic factor. Patients with invasion of the epididymis or tunica albuginea (T2 or greater) have a higher rate

of relapse. Lastly and most importantly, the presence of vascular or lymphatic invasion is significantly associated with relapse.

In patients in whom surveillance therapy is elected, this should be considered an active form of treatment with careful follow-up being mandatory. Physical examination, chest radiographs, and tumor marker levels are performed monthly for the 1st year, every 2 months for the 2nd year, and every 3 to 6 months thereafter. Because of the difficulty with assessment of the retroperitoneum, CT scan should be performed approximately every 2 to 3 months for the first 2 years and at least every 6 months thereafter. Surveillance is necessary for a minimum of 5 years and possibly 10 years following orchiectomy.

Treatment—Stage II (Spread to Retroperitoneal Lymph Nodes)

Surgical Treatment

The potential advantages of RPLND in the treatment of testis cancer stem from the fact that retroperitoneal deposits are usually the first and frequently the sole evidence of extragonadal spread. Such therapy is capable of eradicating resectable disease in over half of patients with stage II tumors. Analysis of different surgical experiences reveals that several uncontrolled variables exist. These variables include the clinical staging accuracy, the extent and quality of node dissection, the criteria of surgical resectability, the pathologic examination of surgical specimens, and the use of adjuvant or "salvage" (for recurrent disease) chemotherapy.

A variety of surgical approaches to retroperitoneal lymphadenectomy have been explored. Thoracoabdominal and midline transperitoneal exposures are common today. The usual distribution of nodal metastasis, as determined by anatomic studies, surgical exploration, and lymphangiography, extends from the superior border of the renal vessels around the aorta and vena cava to either ureter laterally and along the common iliac vessels to just beyond their bifurcations. The extent of lymph node dissection is individualized from the following considerations: (1) serum tumor marker levels after orchiectomy, (2) lymphangiographic or abdominal CT scan interpretations, and (3) findings at laparotomy. Positive markers following orchiectomy or positive

Table 30–11. SURVEILLANCE STUDIES IN PATIENTS WITH CLINICAL STAGE I NONSEMINOMATOUS GERM CELL TUMOR

Series	No. of Patients	No. Relapsed (%)	No. Dead
Read and co-workers (1983)	45	11 (24)	0
Johnson and co-workers (1984)	36	12 (33)	2
Pizzocaro and co-workers (1986)	85	23 (27)	1
Freedman and co-workers (1987)	259	70 (27)	3
Gelderman and co-workers (1987)	54	11 (20)	0
Rørth and co-workers (1987)	79	24 (30)	2
Raghavan and co-workers (1988)	46	13 (8)	2
Sogani and co-workers (1988)	45	10 (22)	2
Thompson and co-workers (1988)	36	12 (33)	2
Total	680	179 (26)	12 (7%)

radiographic studies indicate the need for a complete bilateral lymphadenectomy.

Clinical experience has shown that surgical exploration alone is more than 90 per cent accurate in assessing the presence or absence of lymph node metastasis. When suspicious-looking lymph nodes are encountered at laparotomy, a complete bilateral lymphadenectomy is recommended. Suprarenal nodal metastasis occurs infrequently in the absence of advanced infrarenal disease. Routine suprahilar lymph node dissection in the absence of palpable metastasis in this region has not demonstrably improved local control rates. When serum markers, CT scan, and laparotomy findings are collectively negative, a modified bilateral dissection may be performed.

Since it was popularized by Lewis (1948), RPLND has been used with varying success to treat regional metastasis from testis cancer. RPLND is certainly capable of controlling regional node metastasis in selected patients. The majority of surgical series furnish little information relating the frequency of relapse and curability to the size, number, site, or histology of the nodal metastasis. Surgicopathologic correlation according to criteria in Table 30–12 may provide some relevant data.

Chemotherapy

The high relapse and unresectability rates in patients with bulky retroperitoneal disease, coupled with the demonstrated effectiveness of multidrug regimens in treating disseminated cancer, prompted the choice of chemotherapy as initial therapy for those with advanced nodal or pulmonary metastases during the mid-1970s (Fig. 30–4). Almost simultaneously, advances in clinical

staging identified patients who might benefit from such a strategy. Because chemotherapy was so effective in treating disseminated disease, it appeared prudent to redefine the role of surgery following primary chemotherapy. This question was approached by systematically administering combination-drug therapy and subjecting patients to surgical excision of residual disease, if such were judged feasible. The results from different institutions using varying drug combinations and techniques of lymphadenectomy indicated that chemotherapy is capable of sterilizing bulky disease, with resultant tumor necrosis and fibrosis, in roughly one third of cases. Another 20 per cent, however, harbored residual malignant elements and the remainder, teratoma. Survival was excellent in patients with necrotic tumor or fibrosis and in those with teratoma or completely resected viable cancer. Complete resection was rarely feasible in patients with persistently elevated serum markers following chemotherapy. Negative results of tests for post-treatment serum markers did not exclude the possible existence of a histologically viable cancer.

The recognition of teratoma within surgically excised

Table 30–12. PATHOLOGIC STAGING OF NONSEMINOMATOUS GERM CELL TUMORS

Stage	Description of Retroperitoneal Nodes
I (A)	Negative
II (B)	Positive
N1	Microscopic involvement
N2	Nodes grossly involved
A (B1)	< 5 Nodes involved with none >2 cm diameter
B (B2)	> 5 Nodes involved and/or nodes >2 cm diameter
N3	Extranodal extension (gross or microscopic), resectable
N4 (B3)	Incompletely resected/unresectable disease

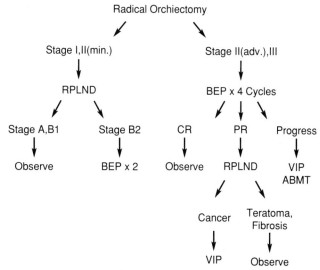

Figure 30–4. Treatment algorithm for patients with nonseminomatous germ cell testicular tumors (NSGCT). (RPLND, retroperitoneal lymph node dissection; BEP, bleomycin, etoposide, and cisplatin; VIP, vinblastine, ifosfamide, and cisplatin; ABMT, autologous bone marrow transplantation; CR, complete response; PR, partial response.)

residual masses following combination chemotherapy for advanced disease was noted in the late 1970s (Hong et al., 1977; Merrin et al., 1975). The surgical removal of benign "mature" or "immature" teratoma should be accomplished for five reasons: (1) preoperative studies cannot rule out the possibility of residual malignancy; (2) pathologic examination may not detect small malignant foci within an apparently benign mass; (3) expansion of benign solid and cystic teratomatous elements may compromise vital organ function; (4) teratoma may exist as or degenerate into a malignant sarcomatous form; and (5) chemotherapy and radiation therapy are ineffective against benign or malignant teratoma.

Roughly one third of patients with advanced NSGCTT who have normal levels of serum tumor markers following preoperative cytoreductive chemotherapy have a malignant component within the excised residual tissues (Einhorn et al., 1981a; Vugrin et al., 1981b). Although pathologic techniques vary, it is unlikely that step sectioning is routine in the assessment of all resected material, implying that a malignant element may be overlooked because of sampling error. Logothetis and associates (1982) described the "growing teratoma syndrome" after observing the enlargement of teratomatous deposits during or following chemotherapy. Whereas the early recognition and resection of teratoma have been accompanied by an excellent prognosis, untreated disease may possess a lethal potential due to the continued local growth or the putative subsequent malignant transformation of histologically benign components. These considerations, together with the inability to distinguish between teratoma and carcinoma and the uncertain natural history of untreated teratoma, warrant surgical resection of residual masses following chemocytoreduction. Although irradiation may have favorable effects in such a setting, relevant pathologic data are wanting.

Surgical excision of residual nodal tissue or extranodal masses following treatment with multidrug chemotherapy is recommended. If chemotherapy is given initially for pulmonary metastasis alone (when pretreatment studies fail to demonstrate significant retroperitoneal disease), and there is no serologic or radiographic evidence of neoplasm after therapy, surveillance without RPLND may be undertaken but with an apparently substantial risk.

Radiation Therapy

An alternative approach to patients with clinical stage I NSGCTT is lymph node irradiation. This approach had been fairly routine outside of the United States before the development of effective chemotherapy and routine abdominal CT scan, but it was abandoned in most institutions because of a lack of evidence that prophylactic irradiation was effective. No randomized prospective study had been successfully completed comparing radiotherapy with any other modality when this approach was largely abandoned. However, it fell into disuse along with the development of effective chemotherapy.

The efficacy of lymph node irradiation still remains in

question, although one randomized study that has reached maturity now exists. Between 1980 and 1984, 153 patients with clinical stage I NSGCTTs were randomized after orchiectomy to either prophylactic x-ray therapy (XRT) or observation. With a minimal follow-up of 5 years, 23 of 85 (27 per cent) patients experienced relapse with 14 of the 23 (61 per cent) relapsing primarily in the retroperitoneum. Only 11 of 68 (16 per cent) patients treated with XRT experience relapse, with 0 of 11 (0 per cent) in the retroperitoneum. All patients in both groups who experienced relapse were salvaged with chemotherapy with the exception of one patient in the XRT-treated group.

This data would suggest that XRT can be an effective modality for low-stage NSGCTT, and the failure to demonstrate its efficacy previously may be due to a high proportion of understaged patients in historical controls not evaluated by CT scanning. If, however, "prophylactic" XRT is effective, it would appear that less than 50 per cent of those patients with retroperitoneal disease truly benefit from this therapy. Similar to RPLND, prophylactic XRT likely eradicates disease in the retroperitoneum; however, coexistent disease exists outside of the retroperitoneum in a large proportion of these patients. Unlike RPLND, XRT gives no information regarding the need for adjuvant chemotherapy. Furthermore, many patients are treated unnecessarily (although the morbidity is low) and, for those patients who have a relapse, there is potentially a greater likelihood of morbid consequences from chemotherapy.

The evolution of effective multidrug regimens has changed the attitudes of both radiation and surgical oncologists. Many radiotherapists now recommend chemotherapy as initial treatment for (1) nodal metastasis clinically judged larger than 2 cm in diameter, (2) supradiaphragmatic node involvement, and (3) extralymphatic spread. Supplementary irradiation is delivered to initially large nodal deposits, with surgical excision being reserved for selected patients with residual masses (Peckham et al., 1981). The main drawback of such an approach is that, if relapse occurs following radiation therapy for small-volume disease or following an integrated scheme, the effectiveness of chemotherapy may be undermined by cumulative myelosuppression. Furthermore, surgical treatment of focally persistent disease may be complicated by prior irradiation.

Treatment—Stage III

Before the 1970s, advanced stages of testicular cancer were treated with chemotherapy, albeit with modest response rates. Li and colleagues (1960) described the so-called triple therapy, consisting of chlorambucil, methotrexate, and actinomycin D, for patients with disseminated testicular cancer. They reported a 50 per cent objective response rate and a 5 to 10 per cent complete response rate with chemotherapy based predominantly on actinomycin D. Subsequently, MacKenzie (1966) reviewed the Memorial Sloan-Kettering Cancer Center experience in 154 patients with disseminated nonseminomatous germ cell tumor and concluded that actinomycin D was the most effective and active agent, either alone or in combination with the aforementioned agents.

During the 1960s, additional agents, such as mithramycin, vinblastine, and bleomycin, were also shown to be active in this disease (Kennedy, 1970). Samuels and Howe (1970) were among the first to recognize the utility of vinblastine in the treatment of patients with disseminated testicular cancer. They reported four complete responses in 21 patients with advanced disease employing this regimen. In 1972, investigators at Sloan-Kettering Memorial Hospital utilized the combination of vinblastine, actinomycin D, and bleomycin (VAB-I) with partial remission in 19 per cent and complete response in 19 per cent (Wittes et al., 1976). With all the previously mentioned regimens, response rate was generally on the order of 10 to 15 per cent with at least a 50 per cent relapse rate.

The concept of a combination of vinblastine with bleomycin was initially described by Samuels and associates (1975). Although intermittent therapy was utilized initially, these investigators switched to continuous infusion of bleomycin in combination with vinblastine in 1973 (Samuels et al., 1976). This so-called VB-III regimen of continuous infusion resulted in overall response rates in the 60 per cent range.

Cis-platinum, arguably the single most active agent in the treatment of testicular cancer, was identified initially in studies of agents that inhibit bacterial replication (Rosenberg et al., 1965). Nephrotoxicity and ototoxicity were potential problems, although doses of 20 mg/m^2 could be given with adequate hydration.

VAB Protocols

Beginning in 1972, the Memorial Sloan-Kettering Cancer Center (MSKCC) group began using combination chemotherapy with vinblastine, actinomycin D, and bleomycin, resulting in 19 per cent complete response (CR) and 19 per cent partial response (PR) rates (Wittes et al., 1976). From 1974 to 1975, cis-platinum was added to continuous infusion bleomycin (VAB-II) (Cheng et al., 1978). These investigators reported a 50 per cent CR rate and a 34 per cent PR rate; 12 patients (24 per cent) remained alive and disease-free. A number of patients were subjected to second-look surgical procedures following VAB-II chemotherapy.

The 50 per cent relapse rate in patients who had achieved CR with VAB-II led to the inauguration of the VAB-III regimen from 1975 through 1976. Modifications in the protocol with the addition of cyclophosphamide to the induction phase and adriamycin to the maintenance schedule resulted in a 61 per cent overall CR rate, but the durable CR rate was only 44 per cent (Cvitkovic et al., 1978). VAB-III involved two major inductions spaced approximately 6 months apart. In September 1976, additional modifications resulted in the VAB-IV combination, associated with a CR rate of 80 per cent; 24 of 48 patients (50 per cent) remained disease-free (Cvitkovic et al., 1978). In 1977, patients with poor prognostic features, such as bulky retroperitoneal metastases, liver, brain, or multiple sites of involvement, and high elevations of serum tumor markers, underwent a more intensive VAB-V regimen. The CR rate, however, was only 47 per cent, and toxicity was quite severe. This regimen was abandoned in 1978.

The VAB-VI regimen was initiated in 1979 and accrued 166 patients by 1982. This VAB-VI regimen was a major departure from prior VAB programs. Cis-platinum was given monthly for three courses at a dose of 120 mg/m^2, along with vinblastine, 4 mg/m^2; cyclophosphamide, 600 mg/m^2; actinomycin, 1 mg/m^2; and bleomycin, 30 units. This regimen was repeated every 4 weeks for three cycles with bleomycin held on the third cycle. The interval between inductions was shortened, and chlorambucil was omitted. Maintenance therapy was compared with no maintenance therapy in a randomized study. Complete response rate was 57 per cent. Overall relapse was 12 per cent (Bosl et al., 1986).

PVB Studies

One of the major contributors to the development of combination chemotherapy for patients with disseminated testicular cancer has been the group at Indiana University. Beginning in 1974, cis-platinum was added to the standard two-drug regimen of vinblastine and bleomycin (Einhorn and Donohue, 1977). Originally, this regimen consisted of cis-platinum, 20 mg/m^2, every 3 weeks; vinblastine, 0.2 mg/kg, on day 1 and 2 every 3 weeks; and bleomycin, 30 units intravenous (IV) push. This cycle was repeated four times. Saline hydration was used to prevent nephrotoxicity. In their early trial, CR was achieved in 70 per cent, and virtually 100 per cent objective response rate was noted.

Because of toxicity with high-dose vinblastine, specifically causing myalgias, neuropathy, and ileus, a second randomized prospective trial was introduced to study the standard platinum, vinblastine, and bleomycin (PVB) regimen with a lower total dose of vinblastine (0.3 mg/kg). Maintenance vinblastine was used for 2 years after achievement of response. In this trial, there was no significant difference in efficacy with the lower vinblastine dosage with or without the addition of adriamycin (Einhorn and Williams, 1980b). Thus, the lower dose of vinblastine, 0.3 mg/kg, was shown to be equally effective with long-term, durable response rates.

Beginning in 1978, a third-generation study was performed in a randomized prospective fashion, comparing four cycles of PVB chemotherapy with or without maintenance vinblastine. This study confirmed the fact that cure rates could be achieved with four cycles of chemotherapy without the need for maintenance (Einhorn et al., 1981b). Overall, 80 per cent of patients in this study were alive and disease-free with follow-up greater than 5 years.

Etoposide (VP-16) has single-agent activity in patients with testicular cancer. Because of the toxicity, especially neuromuscular toxicity, with vinblastine, VP-16 was studied in a randomized prospective trial under the auspices of the Southeastern Cancer Study Group (Williams et al., 1987a). In this multi-institutional trial, 121 patients were treated with PVB with a 61 per cent CR rate. A total of 123 patients were treated with bleomycin, platinum, and VP-16 with a 60 per cent CR rate. Including patients rendered disease-free after resection of teratoma, 74 per cent were disease-free in the PVB group versus 83 per cent in the platinum, bleomycin, VP-16 group. Toxicity was similar in both arms. Thus, bleomycin, etoposide, platinum (BEP) would seem to be a superior combination chemotherapy and has become the standard for patients with disseminated germ cell tumor.

Randomized studies have compared three cycles with four cycles of BEP. The response rate is equivalent in both groups. Thus, for patients without adverse risk factors (vide infra), three cycles of BEP chemotherapy should suffice.

Adjuvant Chemotherapy

Surgical excision has been the standard treatment for patients with clinical stage I or low stage II nonseminomatous germ cell tumors. At issue is whether adjuvant chemotherapy is necessary in patients with disease in the retroperitoneum that has been resected completely. In patients with pathologic stage II nonseminomatous germ cell tumors, controversy exists concerning the role of adjunctive chemotherapy. The 2-year disease-free survival rate for such patients is 60 to 80 per cent, indicating that 20 to 40 per cent of these cases will recur, usually in the lungs. These patients can be salvaged with three or four cycles of combination chemotherapy.

A national intergroup study published by Williams and associates (1987b) reported a 48 per cent relapse rate for patients with any positive nodes who were observed following retroperitoneal lymphadenectomy. This relapse rate was compared with a 2 per cent relapse rate in patients who received two cycles of adjuvant chemotherapy, either VAB-VI or PVB, postoperatively. This study included all patients with positive retroperitoneal lymph nodes dissected, from stage N1 to N3. No difference was found in relapse rate among patients with nodal stages—40 per cent for stage N1, 53 per cent for stage N2a, and 60 per cent for stage N2b.

In a review of 39 patients who underwent RPLND at the Brigham and Women's Hospital for pathologic stage BI disease, with less than six positive nodes and no node greater than 2 cm, only three of 39 patients have had relapse with a median follow-up of 3.5 years (Richie and Kantoff, 1991). Thus, for patients with minimal retroperitoneal disease, resected completely, careful follow-up is recommended. For patients with more extensive disease, adjuvant chemotherapy with two cycles can be initiated relatively shortly after RPLND. The other alternative is careful follow-up with three or four cycles of chemotherapy at the time of relapse. Two cycles of cis-platinum–based adjuvant chemotherapy will almost always prevent relapse.

Salvage Chemotherapy

Cis-platinum combination chemotherapy will effect cure rates in approximately 70 per cent of patients with disseminated germ cell tumors. In patients in whom serum markers have normalized after four cycles of chemotherapy, residual masses should be resected surgically. The operative procedures for surgical resection are more extensive and are discussed in a separate chapter. Surgeons should be aware of potential bleomycin-related complications, especially with pulmonary fibrosis. Barneveld and colleagues (1987) reported eight of 93 patients with evidence of bleomycin pneumonitis, one of whom died from bleomycin toxicity. Bleomycin toxicity can be minimized by careful monitoring intra- and postoperatively, reduction in the forced inspiratory oxygen (less than 0.25), and restriction of free water intraoperatively and immediately postoperatively.

In patients who have residual cancer that has been resected after chemotherapy, or more commonly in patients who do not respond to the traditional courses of induction therapy, salvage therapy with different agents is available and should be considered (see Fig. 30–4). In patients who show evidence of progression during cis-platinum combination chemotherapy, salvage chemotherapy with cis-platinum should not be administered. In patients who progress after having received cis-platinum, cis-platinum may still be useful and should be considered in salvage regimens.

Ifosfamide is an active agent in patients with testicular cancer with a 22 per cent single-agent response rate (Wheeler et al., 1986). Ifosfamide in combination with vinblastine and cis-platinum (VIP regimen) has achieved an approximate 30 per cent disease-free status in patients who have failed initial chemotherapy regimens (Lauer et al., 1987). In patients who receive ifosfamide, mesna should be used before starting ifosfamide to prevent the complication of hemorrhagic cystitis. In patients who initially receive vinblastine, etoposide should be used in the VIP regimen. In patients who initially receive etoposide, vinblastine should be used.

Third-line chemotherapy for patients who have failed first- and second-line therapy includes autologous bone marrow transplantation with high-dose chemotherapy regimens. Carboplatin, an agent with activity similar to cisplatin, has myelosuppression as its dose-limiting toxicity. Therefore, carboplatin can be given in lieu of cisplatin in patients who are undergoing autologous bone marrow transplantation.

Management of High-Risk Testicular Cancer Patients

Patients with stage C nonseminomatous testicular cancer can be subdivided into patients who will respond to standard chemotherapy and patients who will require more aggressive chemotherapy. The Indiana University staging system detailed in Table 30–13 has proved to be a workable model with therapeutic advantages. Patients with minimal or moderate disease did well with standard chemotherapy, with response rates in the 91 to 95 per cent category (Birch et al., 1986). Patients with advanced disease, however, had only a 53 per cent therapeutic response. Therefore, more aggressive chemotherapy should be utilized in patients with advanced extent disease according to this category.

Table 30–13. INDIANA UNIVERSITY STAGING SYSTEM FOR DISSEMINATED TESTICULAR CANCER

Minimal Extent

1	Elevated markers only
2	Cervical nodes (± nonpalpable retroperitoneal nodes)
3	Unresectable nonpalpable retroperitoneal disease
4	Fewer than five pulmonary metastases per lung field AND largest <2 cm (± nonpalpable retroperitoneal nodes)

Moderate Extent

1	Palpable abdominal mass only (no supradiaphragmatic disease)
2	Moderate pulmonary metastases: 5–10 metastases per lung field and largest <3 cm OR solitary pulmonary metastasis of any size >2 cm (± nonpalpable retroperitoneal disease)

Advanced Extent

1	Advanced pulmonary metastases: primary mediastinal nonseminomatous germ cell tumor OR > 10 pulmonary metastases per lung field OR multiple pulmonary metastases
2	Palpable abdominal mass plus supradiaphragmatic disease
3	Liver, bone, or central nervous system metastases

EXTRAGONADAL TUMORS

Primary tumors of extragonadal origin are rare, with fewer than 1000 cases described in the literature. Distinction between a primary extragonadal germ cell tumor (EGT) and metastatic disease from an undetected testis primary tumor may be difficult but has obviously important clinical implications. Surgical and autopsy series have confirmed the absence of a "burned-out" testicular primary lesion in a number of cases, laying to rest some of the skepticism surrounding the diagnosis of EGT in the past (Luna and Valenzuela-Tamariz, 1976). Testicular ultrasonography has emerged as a sensitive technique for the detection of tiny neoplasms a few millimeters in size within the clinically "normal" testis. Although the exact incidence of EGTs is unknown, clinical data suggest that roughly 3 to 5 per cent of all germ cell tumors are of extragonadal origin.

The most common sites of origin are, in decreasing order of frequency, the mediastinum, retroperitoneum, sacrococcygeal region, and pineal gland, although many unusual sources have also been reported. Two schools of thought exist as to the origin of these neoplasms: (1) displacement of primitive germ cells during early embryonic migration from the yolk sac entoderm and (2) persistence of pluripotential cells in sequestered primitive rests during early somatic development. The theory of misplaced germ cells holds that during ontogeny, migration through the retroperitoneum is misdirected cephalad to the mediastinum and pineal gland or caudad to the sacrococcygeal region, rather than to the genital ridges. The alternative hypothesis maintains that primitive pluripotential cells may be dislocated during early embryogenesis (blastema or morula phase). A germ cell rest in the third brachial cleft, for example, could result in a mediastinal tumor, which, interestingly, often resembles a thymoma histologically.

Males are predominantly affected, although a female predominance has been noted with sacrococcygeal lesions. With the exception of sacrococcygeal tumors in the newborn, these tumors generally lack encapsulation, unlike their testicular counterparts, and tend to invade or envelop contiguous structures. The majority of adults with EGTs present with advanced local disease and distant metastases. These tumors most commonly spread to regional lymph nodes, lung, liver, and bone. Histologically, all germ cell types are represented, with pure seminoma accounting for roughly half the tumors in the mediastinum and retroperitoneum. In general, sacrococcygeal tumors of the newborn and young adult are functionally and histologically benign, whereas tumors discovered during infancy prove malignant in about half the cases.

EGTs may reach a large size with no or relatively few symptoms. Diagnosis of mediastinal EGT is most commonly established during the third decade, with or without signs and symptoms of chest pain, cough, or dyspnea. Patients with primary retroperitoneal tumors may present with abdominal or back pain, other vague constitutional symptoms, palpable mass, or vascular obstruction. Sacrococcygeal tumors are most often diagnosed in the neonate (1 in 40,000 births) and less frequently in infants or adults, with findings of palpable mass, skin discoloration or hairy nevus, or bowel or urinary obstruction. Tumors of the pineal gland occur in children and young adults, producing symptoms of increased intracranial pressure (headache, visual impairment), oculomotor dysfunction (diplopia, ptosis), hearing loss, hypopituitarism (abnormal menses), and hypothalamic disturbances (diabetes insipidus).

Complete local excision of mediastinal or retroperitoneal tumors is rarely feasible because of frequent local extension and high rates of metastatic disease. In reviewing 30 cases of primary mediastinal tumors, Martini and colleagues (1974) found only four of 30 patients who presented with no metastasis. Three of these four had pure seminoma. In the ten patients with pure seminoma, only four were long-term survivors following surgery or radiotherapy. Of 20 patients with elements of embryonal carcinoma, only one was alive at 20 months following surgery, radiotherapy, and chemotherapy.

Sterchi and Cordell (1975) reviewed the cases of 108 patients with mediastinal seminoma, finding a 5-year survival rate of 58 per cent following primary radiation therapy or surgery. The MSKCC experience involving 21 cases of extragonadal seminoma with primary cisplatin-based chemotherapy was reviewed; only one patient died of metastatic disease, with the remainder disease-free at 19+ to 46+ months' follow-up. Patients with primary retroperitoneal seminoma appear equally responsive to intensive chemotherapy regimens (Stanton et al., 1983). In contrast, patients with nonseminomatous EGT have done poorly despite surgery, radiotherapy, and chemotherapy (Recondo and Libshitz, 1978; Reynolds et al., 1979). Disappointingly, only two of 18 patients treated at MSKCC with successive VAB protocols have achieved CR. Although Garnick and co-workers (1983) reported similar results, those of Hainsworth and co-workers (1982), using the PVB regimen, were superior. The reason for this apparent discrepancy remains unclear.

Wide local excision is the treatment of choice for sacrococcygeal tumors, in that the majority are benign. Limited experience renders uncertain the advisability of adjunctive irradiation or chemotherapy for malignant tumors. Radical excisions for pineal tumors have been disappointing from the standpoints of local control and operative morbidity. Such procedures have been largely abandoned in favor of primary radiation therapy, although a cerebrospinal fluid shunt may be required (Cole, 1971).

OTHER TESTIS NEOPLASMS

Under the designation "other testis neoplasms" are included a heterogeneous group of tumors of relatively infrequent occurrence. Together, they constitute between 5 and 10 per cent of all testis tumors.

Sex Cord-Mesenchyme Tumors (Gonadal Stromal Tumors, Sex Cord-Stromal Tumors)

Both semantic and histogenetic uncertainties have contributed to the continuing difficulties in the classification of such lesions. Distinguishing between hyperplasia and benign and malignant tumors has added to the problems of classification. Teilum (1946, 1971) was principally responsible for calling attention to this group of tumors and for emphasizing the comparative pathology of the analogous ovarian and testicular neoplasms. The cell type, architecture, and degree of differentiation of these tumors may closely duplicate the supporting tissues in the gonads of either sex. In the testis, the microscopic appearance may be that of an undifferentiated gonadal stroma, a Sertoli cell tumor in germ cell–free seminiferous tubules, or a Leydig cell tumor. More rarely, tumors that are apparently composed of granulosa cells or theca cells occur.

Interstitial Cell Lesions (Leydig Cell Tumors)

Various degrees of apparent focal or diffuse interstitial cell hyperplasia may be noted with a variety of conditions associated with seminiferous tubule atrophy. To what extent these represent absolute or relative increases in interstitial cells may be difficult to assess. Interstitial cell tumors, the most common of the sex cord-mesenchyme lesions, make up between 1 and 3 per cent of all testis tumors. Although the majority have been reported in men between the ages of 20 and 60 years, approximately one fourth have been reported before puberty.

The etiology of Leydig cell tumors is unknown. In contrast to germ cell tumors, there appears to be no association with cryptorchidism. The experimental production of Leydig cell tumors in mice following long-term estrogen administration or intrasplenic testicular autografting is consistent with a hormonal basis.

The lesions are generally small, yellow to brown, well-circumscribed, and rarely exhibit hemorrhage or necrosis. Microscopically, the tumors consist of relatively uniform, polyhedral, closely packed cells with round and slightly eccentric nuclei and eosinophilic granular cytoplasm with lipoid vacuoles, brownish pigmentation, and occasional characteristic inclusions known as Reinke crystals. Pleomorphism with large and bizarre cell forms may occur, and mitotic figures may or may not be identified. None of these features appears to be consistently related to malignant potential. Furthermore, limited observations suggest that ultrastructural features will not categorically distinguish between normal and neoplastic Leydig cells, whether benign or malignant.

Approximately 10 per cent of interstitial cell tumors are malignant, but there are no consistently reliable histologic criteria for making this judgment. Large size, extensive necrosis, gross or microscopic evidence of infiltration, invasion of blood vessels, and excessive mitotic activity are all features that suggest the possibility of malignancy, but metastasis is generally regarded as the only reliable criterion of malignancy. Like other testis tumors, malignant lesions may involve retroperitoneal lymph nodes, lung, and bone. Of importance is the observation that malignancy is nonexistent in the prepubertal age group.

CLINICAL PRESENTATION. In the prepubertal cases (average age 5 years), presenting manifestations are usually those of isosexual precocity with prominent external genitalia, mature masculine voice, and pubic hair growth. Hormonal assays in such patients have been few and generally incomplete or have been carried out by antiquated techniques. An increased testosterone production is usually demonstrable, and urinary 17-ketosteroid output may or may not be elevated. Virilizing types of congenital adrenocortical hyperplasia may also produce the endocrine signs and symptoms of interstitial cell tumors; differential tests must be carried out to clarify the diagnosis. Such tests include estimation of urinary 17-hydroxy- and 17-ketosteroid levels as well as plasma cortisol levels before and after corticotropin (ACTH) stimulation and dexamethasone suppression.

Because interstitial cell carcinomas have been shown to possess 21-hydroxylase activity and to be capable of forming cortisol and hydroxylating steroids at the 11-beta position, it is clear that interstitial cell tumors may possess some of the same functional activities as adrenocortical tissue. The similar embryologic origin of interstitial cells and adrenocortical cells and the occurrence of adrenal rests in the testis complicate interpretation. The paradox of the tumor's arising in the interstitial cells of a prepubertal testis and behaving metabolically like its adult counterpart, in conjunction with cells in the normal prepubertal testis containing enzymes capable of producing testosterone, explains the occurrence of spermatogenesis in the seminiferous tubules more remote from the tumor.

In adults, the majority of reported cases have shown manifestations of endocrine imbalance, although some do not. The endocrinologic manifestations may precede the palpable testis mass, which is the most common presenting feature. In the remaining adult cases, symptoms of a feminizing nature, such as impotence, decreased libido, and gynecomastia, may occur. The slow progression of these neoplasms is suggested by the long duration of gynecomastia, which may precede recognition of the testicular mass. In contrast to the situation with adult germ cell tumors, the duration of gynecomastia with adult interstitial cell tumors has ranged from 6 months to 10 years and averages more than 3 years. Elevation of urinary and plasma estrogen values in association with this tumor is relatively common.

Lockhart and associates (1976) reported a nonfunctioning interstitial cell tumor of the testis of a malignant type in which there was neither clinical nor chemical manifestation of endocrinopathy. Hormonal disturbance, therefore, is not an essential feature. In cases in which a testicular swelling was not clinically apparent, Gabrilove and colleagues (1975) performed selective venous catheterization and measurement of the testicular venous effluent to assess gynecomastia of obscure etiology. Measurement of AFP and β-hCG may be helpful in differential diagnosis. Occasionally, magnetic resonance imaging will detect a small nonpalpable Leydig cell tumor not seen by ultrasonography (Kaufman et al., 1990). Other considerations in the differential diagnosis include feminizing adrenocortical disorders, Klinefelter's syndrome, and other feminizing testicular disorders.

TREATMENT. Radical inguinal orchiectomy is the initial procedure of choice. With documentation of Leydig cell tumor, endocrinologic studies and further clinical staging evaluations are indicated. In the event of histopathologic suspicion of malignancy, lymphangiogram, CT scan, or ultrasound (alone or in combination) of the retroperitoneum is indicated to seek retroperitoneal adenopathy. As with germ cell tumors of the adult testis, spread to the lung, liver, or supradiaphragmatic lymph nodes is possible. The potential production of hormones by metastatic tumor invites exploration of these substances as markers for metastatic disease, but data are lacking. Urinary estrogens, androgens, corticoids, and pregnanediol have each demonstrated abnormalities on the basis of the metabolic activity of different interstitial cell tumors.

RPLND has been recommended as routine in patients whose interstitial cell tumors appear histologically or biochemically malignant. Total experience with any form of therapy, however, is limited by the small number of patients who have been treated, although the existing data suggest the relative radioresistance of this tumor. *Ortho-para*-DDD has been used with evidence of benefit in some patients (Azer and Braumstein, 1981). A variety of chemotherapeutic agents, including *cis*-platinum, vinblastine, bleomycin, cyclophosphamide, doxorubicin, and vincristine, have been employed in various combination regimens without convincing benefit, but experience is very limited. Evidence of estrogen receptors in various mouse Leydig cell tumor lines provides an experimental basis for trials of endocrine therapy (Sato et al., 1978). In addition, inhibition of mitochondrial protein synthesis with concomitant arrest of in vivo

growth of solid Leydig cell tumors in rats by oxytetracycline has been reported (van der Bogert et al., 1983).

The prognosis for Leydig cell tumors is good because of their generally benign nature. The persistence of virilizing and feminizing features following orchiectomy is not necessarily an indication of malignancy because these changes are to some extent irreversible. As might be anticipated from the characterization of malignancy, i.e., metastasis, the average survival time from surgery for patients with a malignant Leydig cell tumor is approximately 3 years.

Sertoli Cell Tumors (Androblastoma, Gonadal Stromal Tumor, Sertoli Cell–Mesenchyme Tumor)

Nodules of immature seminiferous tubules with lumina lined by undifferentiated cells are found not infrequently in cryptorchid testes and in roughly one fourth of patients with testicular feminization. Such lesions were formerly considered tubular adenomas, but it seems probable that they are not neoplastic, and malignant change appears not to have been reported.

True Sertoli cell–mesenchyme tumors constitute less than 1 per cent of all testicular tumors and may occur in any age group, including infancy. Although rare in humans, they are the most common testicular tumor in dogs. The majority of Sertoli cell tumors are benign, but approximately 10 per cent have proved malignant on the basis of the currently accepted criterion of malignancy—the demonstration of metastasis. As with Leydig cell tumors, definitive histologic criteria of malignancy remain to be established.

The etiology of these tumors has not been determined. The majority have arisen in apparently normal intrascrotal testes, although occurrence in maldescended or cryptorchid testes has been reported.

Grossly, these tumors vary in size from 1 cm to more than 20 cm in diameter. The cut surface is usually graywhite to creamy yellow, with a uniform consistency interrupted by cystic change that becomes increasingly evident with increasing tumor size. The benign lesions are usually well-circumscribed, whereas the malignant lesions tend to be larger and less demarcated. Invasion of paratesticular structures may occur and is suggestive of malignancy.

The precise origin of these tumors remains somewhat uncertain, although derivation from the primitive gonadal mesenchyme is suspected. A diversity of microscopic appearances is evident not only among tumors but also among different areas within the same tumor. The essential diagnostic features include epithelial elements resembling Sertoli cells and varying amounts of stroma. The amount and organization of these two components have led to various attempts to subclassify the tumors.

The epithelial element, on the one hand, may be arranged in tubules with or without lumina and lined by radially arranged cells in one or multiple layers. On the other hand, the epithelial cells may form columns or sheets of trabeculae growing between stromal elements. The stromal elements may be scant, or the tumor may be largely composed of stroma resembling a fibroma but containing strands of epithelial cells. Secretory material forming Call-Exner–like bodies is occasionally seen within tubules, and the morphologic appearance resembles that of granulosa cell tumors. Furthermore, the stromal elements may be sufficiently well differentiated to be recognizable as Leydig cells. The enormous potential for variation both in stromal and epithelial components and in degrees of differentiation accounts for the wide range of morphologic appearances described for these lesions and contributes to the difficulty in their classification.

Although large size, poor tumor demarcation, invasion of adjacent structures, blood vessel and lymphatic invasion, and increased mitotic activity are all suggestive of a malignant potential, as with Leydig cell tumors, the designation of malignancy can be made with certainty only in the presence of metastasis.

The presenting signs and symptoms are those of testicular mass with or without pain and with or without gynecomastia. Although the lesions have been reported in all age groups, approximately one third of the recorded patients have been 12 years of age or less. About one third of the patients have had gynecomastia. Gynecomastia in the presence of a testis tumor in the prepubertal age group is an important finding in differential diagnosis, because feminization in boys with Leydig cell tumors is always superimposed on virilism.

Studies of the endocrinologic activity of these tumors have been uncommon. Gynecomastia is presumably a consequence of estrogen production, but whether or not the Sertoli cells or the stromal elements are responsible for estrogen production remains to some extent uncertain. Gabrilove and colleagues (1980) reported an elevated plasma testosterone value in association with some virilizing features in a young patient with Sertoli cell tumor.

Radical orchiectomy is the initial procedure of choice and will, of course, be curative in the 90 per cent of cases that are benign. In the small proportion of patients in whom malignancy has been demonstrated by the presence of metastasis, retroperitoneal lymph node involvement has been common, and RPLND has been performed with apparent therapeutic success (Rosvoll and Woodard, 1968). The course of the disease, even in patients with metastasis, may be protracted compared with that of patients with metastatic germ cell tumors. Lung and bone metastases may occur and warrant the inclusion of chest films and bone scans in the staging evaluation. The value of radiation therapy and chemotherapy in the management of patients with this disease is uncertain. Although hormone production is a potential marker for follow-up in patients with apparently malignant tumors, clinical evidence on this point is lacking.

Gonadoblastoma (Tumors of Dysgenetic Gonads, Mixed Germ Cell Tumor, Gonadocytoma)

These rare tumors, occurring almost exclusively in patients with some form of gonadal dysgenesis, constitute approximately 0.5 per cent of all testis neoplasms. They occur in all age groups from infancy to beyond 70 years, although the majority are in individuals under 30 years of age.

Grossly, the lesions may be unilateral or bilateral and may vary in size from microscopic to greater than 20 cm in diameter. Aggressive growth may replace and obscure the nature of the gonad from which the tumor arose, and lesions weighing more than 1000 g have been reported. The tumors generally are round, with a smooth and slightly lobulated surface, and vary in consistency from soft and fleshy to firm or hard. Calcified areas are frequent and probably reflect the extensive spontaneous retrogressive changes common with these lesions. The cut surface is grayish white to yellow but may vary considerably, depending on the histologic makeup of the tumor.

Although gonadoblastomas are currently regarded as neoplasms, the possibility that they represent hamartomas or nodular hyperplasia in response to pituitary gonadotrophins has been suggested. First clearly described by Scully (1953), the tumors consist of three elements—Sertoli cells, interstitial tissue, and germ cells—the proportions of which show considerable variation. In about half such tumors, germ cell overgrowth, with the evolution of what is readily recognized as seminoma, or germ cell elements with histologic features of embryonal carcinoma, teratoma, choriocarcinoma, or yolk sac tumor may occur. Throughout the tubules, characteristic Call-Exner bodies may be identified, consisting of periodic acid–Schiff (PAS)-positive material similar to that seen in the basement membrane of the tubules.

The clinical manifestations in patients with this tumor are the consequence of three factors: (1) the usual concurrence of gonadal dysgenesis with resultant abnormalities in the external genitalia and gonads; (2) the presence of germ cells with malignant potential; and (3) the endocrine function of the gonadal stromal components of the tumor, usually with the production of androgen. Although interstitial cells may not be evident by light microscopy, a steroidogenic potential of the tumor may exist. Furthermore, demonstration of Leydig cells in the tumor does not necessarily dictate virilism, either because the resultant steroids may be biologically inactive or because the end organs may be defective. The usual appearance is that of solid tubules of varying size containing germ cells in close association with Sertoli cells and of mature interstitial cells evident between the tubules.

The germ cells of gonadoblastoma are similar to those of seminoma, and if germ cell proliferation occurs, it may progress from an in situ stage to invasive germinoma (seminoma), referred to as gonadoblastoma with germinoma (seminoma).

Approximately four fifths of patients with gonadoblastomas are phenotypic females, usually presenting with primary amenorrhea and sometimes with lower abdominal masses. The remainder are phenotypic males, almost always presenting with cryptorchidism, hypospadias, and some female internal genitalia. However, gonadoblastoma has been described in an anatomically normal male (Talerman, 1972). In the phenotypic females, the breasts are small, the internal genitalia are hypoplastic, and the gonads are usually of the streak type. The test result for sex chromatin is negative, and the chromosome analysis usually shows XY, XO, or XO/XY patterns. Virilization in the phenotypic female usually manifests as hypertrophy of the clitoris. In the phenotypic male, gynecomastia may occasionally be present, and there is often hypospadias, some female internal genitalia, and dysgenetic testes usually located in the abdomen or inguinal region. The test result for sex chromatin is negative, and the chromosome pattern is XY or XO/XY.

In general, 90 per cent of patients with gonadal dysgenesis and gonadoblastoma have chromatin-negative findings and more than half have an XY karyotype, with the remainder demonstrating mosaicism. The external sex organs of patients with gonadoblastomas show a wide range of appearances ranging from normal to completely ambiguous. The secondary sex organs usually consist of a hypoplastic uterus and two normal or slightly hypoplastic fallopian tubes. Male internal sex organs, such as epididymis, vas deferens, and prostate, are found sometimes in phenotypic virilized females and always in phenotypic male pseudohermaphrodites.

Radical orchiectomy is the first step in therapy, and the high incidence of bilaterality (50 per cent) argues for contralateral gonadectomy when gonadal dysgenesis is present. The prognosis is excellent for the patient with gonadoblastoma or gonadoblastoma with germinoma. In the presence of seminoma or other germ cell types, clinical staging employing the techniques used for the staging of germ cell tumors of the adult testis may be indicated, although experience is too limited to justify categoric recommendations. As with germ cell tumors of the adult testis, therapy may logically be based on tumor histology and the results of clinical staging.

Neoplasms of Mesenchymal Origin

A variety of neoplasms derived from mesenchymal elements may arise on the tunica albuginea or, more rarely, within the testis. Included are benign fibroma, angioma, neurofibroma, and leiomyoma. Occurring as painless masses, they are of concern chiefly because of the possibility of a malignant tumor. Differential diagnosis includes abnormalities of the testicular appendages, fibrous pseudotumors, adenomatoid tumors, and non-neoplastic cystic lesions. Varying from minute, "shot-like" lesions on the surface of the testis to masses of several centimeters in diameter, the reported lesions have been variously treated by local excision or orchiectomy.

Malignant mesothelioma may arise from any site on the mesothelial membrane—pleura, peritoneum, pericardium, or tunica vaginalis. Fewer than 20 cases involving the tunica vaginalis have been reported. The lesion occurs in patients from 21 to 78 years of age, and the usual presentation is with a hydrocele. Radical orchiectomy is indicated for local control, but local recurrence and abdominal and pulmonary metastases may ensue. Limited experience suggests that surgery

and irradiation may be of some value in controlling intra-abdominal metastasis. The value of chemotherapy remains to be defined, although doxorubicin appears active.

Miscellaneous Primary Non–Germ Cell Tumors

The testis may be the primary site of a number of tumors of unrelated histogenesis and varied pathologic type, including the following.

Epidermoid Cyst

Representing an estimated 1 per cent of testis tumors (Shah et al., 1981), approximately half occur in the 3rd decade, and most of the remainder occur between the 2nd and 4th decades. Grossly, these lesions appear as round, sharply circumscribed, firm, and encapsulated intratesticular nodules. The cut surface reveals a grayish-white to yellowish, cheesy, amorphous mass. Microscopically, the wall is composed of dense fibrous tissue lined by stratified squamous keratinized epithelium, desquamations from which, with degeneration and microcalcification, make up the amorphous interior.

Although the histogenesis remains uncertain, a common thesis is that the tumor represents a monolayer teratoma. Such a histogenesis is circumstantially supported by the age and racial incidences of such tumors and by the occasional association with cryptorchidism. This histogenesis, in turn, supports radical orchiectomy as the usual treatment, because the possibility of other germ cell elements in association with such lesions can be excluded only by careful microscopic examination. Nevertheless, the clinical behavior of these tumors has been consistently benign; apparently, no instance of associated, clinically unrecognized but microscopically confirmed germ cell tumor has been reported.

Rare instances of bilaterality have been reported (as with germ cell tumors) (Forrest and Whitmore, 1984). Testicular ultrasonography may demonstrate a well-circumscribed lesion with a solid central core and may aid in the distinction from a germ cell tumor. Although most have been managed by radical orchiectomy, local excision in a small number of patients appears to have been equally successful. The weakness in the last approach stems from uncertainty in clinical diagnosis and the potential risks of spillage of a germ cell tumor.

Adenocarcinoma of the Rete Testis

These rare but highly malignant tumors occur uniformly in adults over a wide age range (20 to 80 years). Jacobellis and associates (1981) reported the 19th case. The usual clinical presentation is a painless scrotal mass, commonly with an associated hydrocele. Pathologic evaluation reveals a multicystic papillary adenocarcinoma composed of small cuboidal cells with elongated nuclei and scanty cytoplasm, presumably arising from the rete tubules of the testicular mediastinum. Despite radical orchiectomy, half of the patients die within 1 year from the time of diagnosis. Metastasis has occurred in inguinal and retroperitoneal lymph nodes, lungs, bone, and liver. The observation that retroperitoneal deposits may represent the sole site of metastasis supports the rationale of retroperitoneal lymphadenectomy in the absence of distant metastasis. Irradiation and chemotherapy with methotrexate, 5-fluorouracil, actinomycin D, or cyclophosphamide in the treatment of metastasis have been of limited, if any, benefit.

Adrenal Rest Tumors

The association of bilateral testis tumors with congenital adrenal hyperplasia and the remission of both endocrine manifestations and tumors following appropriate corticoid treatment call attention to these unusual lesions. Whether they represent neoplasms or hyperplasia and whether they derive from "normal" adrenal rests or from abnormal interstitial cells remain uncertain in some cases. Kirkland and co-workers (1977) suggested that LH may contribute to the growth of these tumors because (1) high serum levels of LH may be observed in association with incomplete suppression of adrenal steroid secretion, and (2) there is evidence of gonadotrophin secretion with testicular tumors in some patients with congenital adrenal hyperplasia (CAH).

Nevertheless, these tumors are primarily dependent on ACTH for growth and steroid secretion. The most likely circumstance is that they may arise from the adrenal cortical rests that may occur normally in the testis but that are abnormally stimulated in the syndrome of CAH. Recognition of CAH and appropriate medical treatment may obviate surgical treatment of the testis "tumors."

Adenomatoid Tumors (Angiomatoid Tumors of the Endothelium, Adenofibroma, Mesothelioma, Lymphangioma, Adenofibromyoma, Adenoma)

These lesions are characteristically small benign tumors peculiar to the genital tract of males and females. They consist of a fibrous stroma in which disoriented spaces of epithelial cells occur, resembling endothelium, epithelium, or mesothelium. Histogenesis remains debatable. Although the lesion occurs primarily in the epididymis in the male, occasional instances of tumor confined to the testis have been reported.

Carcinoid

Carcinoid is uncommon outside the gastrointestinal tract. Nearly 150 cases of carcinoid in the ovary have been recorded as well as 23 cases in the testis, 17 of which were primary and six metastatic (Talerman et al., 1978). On gross pathologic examination, the tumors have been circumscribed and limited to the testis, with diameters ranging up to 8 cm. Microscopically, the tumors are composed of islands, nests, or discrete masses of round, oval, or polygonal cells separated by fibrous strands and exhibiting a solid acinar structure. Although most of the reported cases have been pure carcinoids, a few have arisen in association with teratoma. In primary ovarian carcinoids, the majority have arisen in association with teratoma.

The histogenesis of these tumors remains uncertain, but one-sided development of a teratoma or origin from argentaffin or enterochromaffin cells within the gonad are the alternatives. A slow, progressive, painless testicular enlargement is the most frequent presentation. Although minimal symptoms suggestive of carcinoid syndrome were noted in one patient, estimations of serum serotonin and 5-hydroxyindoleacetic acid have not been performed preoperatively. Treatment has been inguinal orchiectomy, which apparently has been curative in patients with primary testicular carcinoid. In contrast, patients with metastatic carcinoid to the testis have a poor prognosis.

Secondary Tumors of the Testis

Lymphoma

Testicular involvement by lymphoma may be a manifestation of primary extranodal disease, an initial manifestation of clinically occult nodal disease, or a later manifestation of disseminated nodal lymphoma. Accounting for about 5 per cent of all testis tumors, these lesions constitute the most common secondary neoplasms of the testis and the most frequent of all testis tumors in patients over 50 years of age. The median age of occurrence is approximately 60 years. Primary lymphoma of the testis may occur in children; eight cases in patients ranging from 2 to 12 years of age having been reviewed by Weitzner and Gropp (1976).

Grossly, the testis is diffusely enlarged, usually to a diameter of 4 to 5 cm or more, bulging with a granular gray to light tan to pink solid tumor. Foci of hemorrhage and necrosis may be evident, and there may be gross extension to the epididymis or cord. Microscopically, all varieties of reticuloendothelial neoplasms, including Hodgkin's disease, have been described in the testis. However, the majority are diffuse. Of these, most are histiocytic (74 per cent), according to the Rappaport classification, or large noncleaved (70 per cent), according to the Lukes and Collins classification. Diffuse replacement of the normal architecture is the rule, with focal sparing of the seminiferous tubules.

Malignant lymphoma confined to the testis at the time of clinical onset of disease is rare compared with the frequency with which the gonadal mass represents the initial clinical manifestation of occult or apparent nodal disease. However, when lymph node disease is limited to the regional nodes, it is possible that the neoplasm arose in the gonad and metastasized to the regional nodes. The pattern of dissemination of testicular lymphomas is similar to that of testicular germ cell tumors. In autopsy cases, a pattern of pulmonary nodules not contiguous to the mediastinum or hilum strongly suggests a propensity of testicular lymphomas to spread by the hematogenous route, consistent with the observation of vascular invasion not infrequently seen in patients with testicular lymphoma.

A poor prognosis may be anticipated when there is evidence of generalized disease within a year after diagnosis. As with lymphomas elsewhere, patients with poorly differentiated lymphocytic types tend to survive longer than those with the histiocytic type. Disease-free survivals of 60 months or longer in patients with testicular lymphoma treated by orchiectomy alone provide strong circumstantial evidence that a true primary testicular lymphoma occurs occasionally. However, even patients whose disease seems to be limited to the gonads after clinical and surgical staging may still have a short survival time. In comparison, patients who have no clinical evidence of systemic spread 1 year after therapy have a high probability of cure. Whether the long-term survival following orchiectomy alone is a reflection of a cured primary testicular tumor, spontaneous regression, or prolonged remission of a generalized disease remains debatable.

A common clinical presentation is a painless enlargement of the testis, although about one fourth of the patients have generalized constitutional symptoms, including weight loss, weakness, and anorexia. Bilateral tumors occur in almost half the patients, simultaneously in roughly 10 per cent, and metachronously in the remainder.

Investigation may include a complete blood count, peripheral smears, bone marrow studies, chest radiograph, bone scan, CT scan or IVP, lymphogram, and liver and spleen scans. Apparently, a high probability of generalized disease exists if para-aortic nodes are involved, indicating the importance of retroperitoneal staging. Although radical orchiectomy provides the diagnosis and initial treatment, once the diagnosis of lymphoma has been established, referral to a medical oncologist is advisable for staging evaluation and decisions regarding further treatment.

Survival is poor in patients with bilateral disease and in patients presenting with lymphoma at other sites and later experiencing a testicular relapse. However, among patients with disease apparently confined to the testis, Turner and colleagues (1981) reported eight of 14 to be alive and well for 7 to 87 months (mean 2.5 years).

Leukemic Infiltration of the Testis

The testicle appears to be a prime initial site of relapse in male children with acute lymphocytic leukemia. Stoffel and co-workers (1975) reported an 8 per cent incidence of extramedullary involvement of the testis in children with acute leukemia, the majority of patients being in complete remission at the time of testicular enlargement. The interval from testicular involvement to death ranges from 5 to 27 months, with a median of 9 months. Kuo and associates (1976) reported seven children who developed testicular swelling during bone marrow remission in whom needle biopsy confirmed leukemic infiltration.

The leukemic infiltration is mainly in the interstitial spaces, with destruction of the tubules by infiltration in advanced cases. Enlargement is bilateral in 50 per cent of cases and is commonly associated with scrotal discoloration. Testicular irradiation with doses of 1200 CGy over 6 to 8 days is clinically successful in local control. Because of the frequency of bilateral involvement microscopically, bilateral irradiation seems advisable, even with apparent unilateral involvement. Almost all patients can be expected to develop subsequent marrow relapse, despite control of testicular involvement by irradiation, unless effective systemic chemotherapy is given.

Biopsy is essential to the diagnosis, orchiectomy is probably unwarranted, and treatment of choice is testicular irradiation with 2000 CGy in ten fractions plus reinstitution of adjunctive chemotherapy. Reinduction therapy is needed in children who experience relapse in the testis while on chemotherapy. The prognosis of male children who undergo such a bout of testicular infiltration is guarded.

Metastatic Tumors

Approximately 200 cases of metastatic carcinoma to the testis have been reported. In the majority, it is discovered incidentally at autopsy in cases of widespread metastatic disease. In rare circumstances, a metastatic focus in the testis may be the presenting feature of an occult neoplasm or the first evidence of a recurrent, previously diagnosed, and treated neoplasm.

The usual pathologic feature of secondary testicular cancers is the microscopic demonstration of neoplastic cells in the interstitium, with relative sparing of the tubules. The route of dissemination to the testis may be hematogenous or lymphatic or by direct invasion from contiguous masses. Renal adenocarcinoma may involve the testis by way of spermatic vessels. Rarely, dropped metastasis from a diffuse intra-abdominal malignancy can involve the cord and testis through a patent processus vaginalis. Retrograde extension through the vas deferens presumably may be a source as well.

The common primary sources in decreasing order of frequency are prostate, lung, gastrointestinal tract, melanoma, and kidney. A relatively high incidence of prostatic lesions reflects in part the frequency of carcinoma of the prostate and the use of orchiectomy in its treatment. Metastatic tumors to the testis occur later in life, usually in the 6th or 7th decade, in contrast to primary testicular tumors. Metastasis has been bilateral in a small proportion of cases. Approximately 2.5 per cent of lymphomas are found in the testis in metastatic fashion.

TUMORS OF TESTICULAR ADNEXA

Epithelial Tumors

Epithelial tumors of the testicular adnexal structures are rare, even though the epididymis and paratesticular tissues may be involved by extensions from primary germinal cell testicular tumors. With the exception of cystadenomas of the epididymis, the majority of tumors involving the testicular adnexal structures are of mesenchymal origin.

Adenomatoid Tumors

Adenomatoid tumors are the most common tumors of the paratesticular tissues, accounting for approximately 30 per cent of all paratesticular tumors. In the male they are located in a restricted anatomic distribution of the epididymis, testicular tunics, and rarely the spermatic cord. In the female they have been described in the uterus, fallopian tubes, and rarely the ovary. In men, the majority of these tumors arise in or adjacent to the lower or upper pole of the epididymis, with a slightly higher incidence in the lower pole.

Clinical Features

The majority of these tumors occur in individuals in the 3rd or 4th decade of life, but cases have been seen in patients ranging from 20 to 80 years of age. Clinically, an adenomatoid tumor occurs as a small, solid, asymptomatic mass, which is generally found on routine examination. These rounded, discrete masses lie anywhere in the epididymis and may be embedded in the testicular tunics. An occasional patient will present with mild pain or discomfort in association with the nodule. Most of these tumors have been present for several years without obvious change in size. These tumors uniformly behave in a benign fashion.

Histology

On gross examination, the tumors are small, ranging from 0.5 to 5 cm in diameter. The tumors are usually attached to the testicular tunics. On sectioning, the tumors appear uniformly white, yellow, or tan with a fibrous appearance.

On microscopic examination, there are two different elements: epithelial-like cells and fibrous stroma. The epithelial-like cells are usually arranged in a framework of poorly delineated spaces, sometimes with flattened or cuboidal cells.

A fairly common feature of adenomatoid tumors is the presence of vacuoles within the epithelial cells (Mostofi and Price, 1973). The vacuoles may range from minute to large and may, in fact, replace most of the cytoplasm of the cell. The nuclei show marked uniformity in size and chromatin distribution. Nuclei are generally round or oval and centrally placed with a single nucleolus present. The cytoplasm is acidophilic and finely granular. The stroma ranges from loose tissue to dense, collagenized tissue with occasional hyalinization. Variations in the amount of stroma are common.

The origin of this tumor is unknown. Some pathologists have considered this to be a reaction to injury or inflammation. Jackson in 1958 as well as other investigators have suggested that adenomatoid tumor may be of mesothelial origin, predominantly on the basis of histology. Occasional misclassification of adenomatoid tumors has been reported as mesothelioma. Others have

suggested that adenomatoid tumors are of endothelial origin and may represent a specialized hemangioma or lymphangioma. Ultrastructural findings by Marcus and Lynn (1970) failed to confirm any similarities to hemangioma. These investigators found morphologic similarity to pleural mesotheliomas.

These tumors behave in a benign fashion, and there has never been a documented case of metastases. Cellular atypia and local invasion have been observed occasionally. Nonetheless, the long history of these tumors and the absence of distant metastases suggest a benign nature. Treatment, therefore, is surgical excision (Soderstrom and Leidberg, 1966).

Mesothelioma

Paratesticular mesothelioma is more common in older age groups but may be encountered in any age group, including children. Usually, the tumor occurs as a firm, painless scrotal mass in association with a hydrocele. Gradual enlargement of the hydrocele or sometimes the mass itself is observed in approximately 50 per cent of patients. Most of these patients are treated by orchiectomy.

On gross examination, there is a poorly demarcated lesion, whitish or yellowish, with intermittent firm and shaggy and friable areas. Microscopically, there is a background of papillary and solid structures against densely fibrous fibroconnective tissue. The complex structure has papillary processes combined with solid sheets of cells. Tumor cells tend to have a generous amount of cytoplasm and poorly defined cytoplasmic borders. Nuclei are often vesicular with a single small nucleolus. Mitotic activity is usually absent. Calcifications may be seen scattered throughout these neoplastic structures. Solid mesotheliomas may have small or rather extensive areas of spindle-shaped cells resembling sarcomas. This feature, although devoid of clinical significance, may lead to an erroneous diagnosis of soft tissue sarcoma. Psammoma bodies are sometimes found within papillary areas within the tumor.

Approximately 15 per cent of testicular mesotheliomas have been documented to result in metastatic involvement of inguinal lymph nodes or abdominal structures (Kasdon, 1969). The pure papillary tumors nearly always prove benign. Those of a more complex structure, however, may recur and may develop multiple recurrences or even metastases.

Clinical management should consist of adequate surgical excision with follow-up examination and local biopsy if a metastatic focus is suspected (Hollands et al., 1982). Antman and associates (1984) reported a patient in whom conservative management failed. Limited experience with chemotherapy and radiation therapy has been utilized in these rare tumors without any conclusions. Staging can include CT scans of the chest and abdomen and, rarely, laparotomy if there is a clinical suspicion of recurrent disease.

Cystadenoma

Cystadenoma of the epididymis corresponds to benign epithelial hyperplasia. Sherrick described the first case in 1956, and about 20 cases have been the subjects of subsequent reports. Approximately one third of the cases are bilateral and may be seen as part of von Hippel-Lindau disease. The tumor occurs most often in young adults and produces either minimal local discomfort or no symptoms. When seen in the elderly individual, it is frequently an incidental finding at the time of orchiectomy.

On gross examination, the lesion is partially cystic, ranging from 1.5 to 5 cm in diameter. The cut section may be multicystic, well-encapsulated, or circumscribed. The wall is studded by one or several nodules of epithelial cells arranged in small glands and papillary structures. Many of the glands are lined by columnar and ciliated cells, many of which display a vacuolated or clear cytoplasm. Staining shows abundant glycogen as well as stainable lipids in the clear cells. This pattern is similar to that of renal cell carcinoma, and distinction from metastases of renal cell carcinoma may be difficult.

Paratesticular Tumors

Occasionally, purely testicular mesenchymal tumors (one-sided teratomas) are reported (Davis, 1962). For the most part, the overwhelming majority of mesenchymal tumors in this area arise from paratesticular structures, although sometimes it may be difficult to determine whether the primary origin was the spermatic cord, the epididymis, or the tunica vaginalis.

Most investigators agree that rhabdomyosarcoma, in its juvenile form, accounts for approximately 40 per cent of all paratesticular tumors, benign and malignant. Leiomyosarcoma appears to be the second most common lesion in this area, followed by occasional occurrences of fibrosarcoma, liposarcoma, and undifferentiated mesenchymal tumors, which complete the spectrum of this group. Cooperative study groups have described some of their results with these tumors as well. One is dependent on this sort of accrual of data, because the rarity of the tumor makes certain conclusions on therapy still tentative. In one report (Kingston et al., 1983), four boys with primary paratesticular tumors were described. Late relapses, defined as recurrence or tumor persistence 2 years after diagnosis and treatment, have now been reported. This finding should be kept in mind for follow-up evaluation of such tumors.

Rhabdomyosarcoma

Paratesticular rhabdomyosarcoma occurs predominantly in children and adolescents and, with some exceptions, is most commonly seen during the first 2 decades of life. Clinically, this tumor usually appears as a large intrascrotal mass that compresses the testis and the epididymis, sometimes reaching the external inguinal ring. The location varies somewhat, depending on the exact point of origin. On gross inspection, it can appear circumscribed; however, on microscopic examination, it often extends well beyond the margin seen by the naked eye. The cut surface is solid, grayish-white, and firm, and is rarely hemorrhagic. Some patches of necrosis can

be noted, especially around the central portion of the lesion.

The microscopic features of paratesticular rhabdomyosarcoma are largely characterized by pronounced variation from case to case and even within the same tumor. Most of them show more than one pattern of the spectrum, ranging from totally undifferentiated mesenchymal elements to the distinctive features of skeletal muscle fibers. A characteristic finding is a combination of various patterns containing an admixture of cellular elements, accurately described by Patton and Horn (1962).

Some paratesticular rhabdomyosarcomas are partially or predominantly arranged in an "alveolar" fashion identical with the distinctive pattern frequently seen in other locations. This pattern was first designated as "alveolar rhabdomyosarcoma" by Riopelle and Theriault (1956) and is currently accepted as a variant of embryonal rhabdomyosarcoma.

Riehle and Venkatachalam (1982) make the point that has often been made about other sarcomas, namely, that electron microscopic diagnosis assisted more frequently in sorting out aberrations, variance, and, particularly, identification of the sarcoma in question. Electron microscopy has been successfully used to identify the cytoplasmic myofilaments and Z bands in a paratesticular rhabdomyosarcoma.

Testicular and Paratesticular Tumor Management

The primary testicular or paratesticular tumor should be removed by inguinal orchiectomy with high ligation of the cord. The primary lymphatic drainage of the testis and the cord courses through lymphatics parallel to the testicular vessels; these lymphatics intercommunicate with para-aortic nodes at the level of the renal vessels. The lower para-aortic and iliac nodes serve as a route of lymphatic spread when the primary spermatic lymphatics have become occluded by fibrosis or tumor (Burrington, 1969). Several papers discussing these tumors have recommended routine RPLND (Ghavimi et al., 1973; Johnson, 1975). The fact that rhabdomyosarcoma is the most common malignant spermatic cord tumor has been reaffirmed. The 5-year survival rate using multimodal treatment approximates 75 per cent. Current adjuvant therapy is reviewed in the following discussion.

RADIOTHERAPY. Cobalt-60 teletherapy can be delivered in a total tumor dose of 4000 to 6000 CGy over a period of 5 to 8 weeks through ports extending well beyond the known confines of the tumor. Dose and port size are determined by the primary site and extent of the tumor and by the age of the patient. Radiotherapy can be used for local tumors, even when the tumor is generalized.

CHEMOTHERAPY. Chemotherapy with vincristine (1.5 mg/m^2), cyclophosphamide (300 mg/m^2), and dactinomycin (0.4 mg/m^2) is utilized. A report by Ghavimi and co-workers (1973) described 29 children younger than 15 years of age with embryonal rhabdomyosarcoma who were treated according to a multidisciplinary protocol, which consisted of surgical removal of the tumor, if possible, followed by chemotherapy, and by radiation therapy in patients with gross or microscopic residual disease. Radiation therapy was given in a dose in the 4500- to 7000-rad range. Additional new trials of chemotherapy consisted of cycles of sequential administration of dactinomycin, doxorubicin (Adriamycin), vincristine, and cyclophosphamide, with obligatory periods of rest. The drug therapy was continued for 2 years. In addition, at the present time, early phase II trials are also employing a method of IV administration of methyl-CCNU (Semustine) that appears promising.

Tumor stage and site are now considered important prognostic indicators. Grosfeld and associates (1983) stated that chemotherapy improves survival in patients with stage I (91 per cent) and stage II tumors (86 per cent) and may shrink bulky stage III tumors, allowing less radical procedures in certain selective sites, particularly the urinary tract. It is still true, however, that survival is poor in stage III disease, with 35 per cent survival, and dismal in stage IV disease, with 5.2 per cent survival despite combined therapy. Relapses are generally fatal despite attempts at second-look resection, altered chemotherapy, and radiation (Grosfeld et al., 1983).

Leiomyosarcoma

Smooth muscle tumors of the spermatic cord and epididymis are rare, and their exact incidence is difficult to determine for the following reasons: first, because the clinical and histologic differences between benign smooth muscle tumors and malignant ones are very slight; and second, because some adenomatoid tumors are erroneously classified as leiomyomas, especially those that exhibit a significant component of smooth muscle (Wilson, 1949). Most cases of benign and malignant smooth muscle tumors described in the literature are in patients between the 5th and 8th decades of life. Of extratesticular tumors occurring within the scrotum, 90 per cent are found in the spermatic cord. Of the latter, 30 per cent are malignant, and 70 per cent are benign. Of the malignant variety, the majority are mesenchymal sarcomas, e.g., fibrosarcoma, myxosarcoma, liposarcoma, rhabdomyosarcoma, and leiomyosarcoma. More than 25 cases have been reported of leiomyosarcoma of the spermatic cord. Local invasion of the adjacent tissues was found in five of the 13 cases in which this detail was described. The first recurrence was usually local, in the scrotum or at the distal spermatic stump. This feature was described in six cases.

Distant spread has been hematogenous in a large number of cases, i.e., in tumors of humerus, liver, ileum, and lung. Autopsies were not done in many cases, however, and the clinical finding of abdominally palpable masses probably represented metastatic disease in the para-aortic lymph nodes. The ratio of the number of cases in which hematogenous spread was known to have occurred to the number with known lymphatic spread is 6:2. These facts, at least, support the opinion of Strong (1942) and of others who believe that the spread is as frequently hematogenous as lymphatic. The

importance of electron microscopy in the documentation of these particular tumors, as contrasted to light microscopy, has been emphasized (Gaffney et al., 1984).

The philosophy and planning of treatment have been greatly affected by the mode of spread. It is agreed that all cases of tumor of the spermatic cord should be explored, and the growth should be removed. If it is benign, simple excision is all that is necessary. The standard therapy for leiomyosarcoma has been radical orchiectomy in which a high ligation of the cord is carried out. Because of the high incidence of hematogenous spread, the surgeon should carry out early clamping of the cord to prevent escape of tumor cells.

Electron microscopy is extremely helpful in the differentiation of the type of testicular sacrcoma. Although, at present, management may not be radically changed, depending on the histologic description, there are differences as to the extent of dissection of the nodes. In young persons, the complications of node dissection have been minimal, although these obviously have to be considered in adults as well (Waters et al., 1982). Particularly important for young individuals is a discussion with the parents concerning obvious difficulties with fertility in the future. This aspect has been addressed but chiefly in adult patients (Lipshultz, 1982). The additional use of tumor markers must be further explored in these entities, and experience at the present time is limited in comparison with what might be called adult testis tumors (Vugrin et al., 1982).

Miscellaneous Mesenchymal Tumors of the Spermatic Cord

Isolated cases of other mesenchymal tumors of the spermatic cord, including liposarcoma, lipoma, fibrosarcoma, and myxochondrosarcoma, have been recorded. Liposarcoma is probably the most significant one in this group because of its greater frequency. Samellas (1964), in his review of 112 tumors of the spermatic cord, added one case of his own to three cases already reported. Gowing and Morgan (1964) found two cases in their review of paratesticular tumors of connective tissue.

On histologic examination, liposarcomas of the spermatic cord and of the scrotal area show essentially the same features as those described in other soft tissue sites, although most of the recorded cases just mentioned were predominantly characterized as well differentiated. The Armed Forces Institute of Pathology collected 14 paratesticular liposarcomas, which also appear to show this tendency to be well-differentiated. In most cases, these lesions appear as discrete nodular masses, sometimes attaining a large size, frequently located near the spermatic cord, and entirely separate from the testicle.

On histologic examination, mesenchymal tumors of the spermatic cord are characterized by the presence of a rather uniform pattern of interwoven bundles of long spindle-shaped cells with blunt-ended nuclei and with cytoplasmic myofibrils extending along their longitudinal axis. Leiomyoma is separated from leiomyosarcoma on the basis of occasional or absent mitotic figures and because of its uniform cellular arrangement. Approximately 70 per cent of those tumors considered malignant on initial histologic examination either recur or metastasize (or both), regardless of their location.

Malignant neoplasms arising within the spermatic cord are uncommon, with 161 cases reported in the literature by 1969 (Arlen et al., 1969). Sporadic cases have continued to appear, but the cumulative number remains relatively small. Although Banlowsky and Shultz (1970) have described 19 histologic types of sarcoma originating from the spermatic cord and the tunics, none was classified as neurofibrosarcoma. Johnson and associates (1975) have described such a case.

REFERENCES

Abelev, G. I.: Alpha-fetoprotein as a marker of embryo-specific differentiation in normal and tumor tissue. Transplant. Rev., 20:3, 1974.

Abelev, G. I., Perova, S. D., Kramkova, N. I., Postnikova, Z. A., and Irlin, I. S.: Production of embryonal alpha I globulin by transplantable mouse hepatomas. Transplantation, 1:174, 1963.

Antman, K., Cohen, S., Dimitrov, N. V., Green, M., and Mussia, F.: Malignant mesothelioma of the tunica vaginalis testis. J. Clin. Oncol., 2:447, 1984.

Arlen, M., Grabstald, H., and Whitmore, W. F., Jr.: Malignant tumors of the spermatic cord. Cancer, 23:525, 1969.

Artz, K., and Jacob, R.: Absence of serologically detectable H2 on primitive teratocarcinoma cells in culture. Transplantation, 17:632, 1974.

Azer, P. C., and Braumstein, G. D.: Malignant Leydig cell tumor. Cancer, 47:1251, 1981.

Bach, D. W., Weissbech, L., and Hartlapp, J. H.: Bilateral testicular tumors. J. Oncol., 129:989, 1983.

Bagshawe, K. D., and Searle, F.: Tumour markers. In Marks, C. N., and Hales, C. N. (Eds.): Essays in Medical Biochemistry, Vol. 3. London, Biochemical Society, 1977, pp. 25–74.

Banowsky, L. H., and Shultz, G. N.: Sarcoma of the spermatic cord and tunics: Review of the literature, case report and discussion of the role of retroperitoneal lymph node dissection. J. Urol., 103:628, 1970.

Barneveld, P. W., Sleijfer, D. T., VanderMark, T. W., et al.: Natural course of bleomycin-induced pneumonitis. Am. Rev. Respir. Dis., 135:48, 1987.

Barzell, W. E., and Whitmore, W. F., Jr.: Clinical significance of biological markers: Memorial Hospital experience. Semin. Oncol., 6:48, 1979.

Batata, M. A., Chu, F. C. H., Hilaris, B. S., Unal, A., Whitmore, W. F., Jr., Grabstald, H., and Golbey, R. B.: Radiation therapy role in testicular germinomas. Adv. Med. Oncol., 6:279, 1979.

Batata, M. A., Chu, F. C. H., Hilaris, B. S., Whitmore, W. F., Jr., and Golbey, R. B.: Testicular cancer in cryptorchids. Cancer, 49:1023, 1982.

Battermann, J. J., Delemarre, J. F. M., Hart, A. A. M., et al.: Testicular tumors: A retrospective study. Arch. Chir. Neerl., 25:457, 1973.

Bergstrand, C. G., and Czar, B.: Demonstration of new protein from carcinoma of the colon. J. Urol., 72:712, 1954.

Berthelsen, J. G., Skakkebaek, N. E., Sorensen, B. C., and Mogensen, P.: Screening for carcinoma in situ of the contralateral testis in patients with germinal testicular cancer. Br. Med. J., 285:1683, 1982.

Birch, R., Williams, S. D., Cohn, A., et al.: Prognostic factors for a favorable outcome in disseminated germ cell tumors. J. Clin. Oncol., 4:400, 1986.

Blandy, J. P.: Urology, Vol. 2. Oxford, Blackwell Scientific Publications, 1976, p. 1203.

Blandy, J. P., Oliver, R. T. D., and Hope-Stone, H. F.: A British approach to the management of patients with testicular tumors. Testes Tumors, 7:207, 1983.

Boden, G., and Gibb, R.: Radiotherapy and testicular neoplasms. Lancet, 2:1195, 1951.

Bosl, G. J., Geller, N. L., Cirrincione, C., et al.: Multivariate analysis of prognostic variables in patients with metastatic testicular cancer. Cancer Res., 43:3404, 1983.

Bosl, G. J., Gluckman, R., Geller, N. L., et al.: VAB-VI: An effective chemotherapy regimen for patients with germ cell tumors. J. Clin. Oncol., 4:1493, 1986.

Bosl, G. J., Vogelzang, N. J., Goldman, A., Fraley, E. E., Lange, P. H., Levitt, S. H., and Kennedy, B. J.: Impact of delay in diagnosis on clinical stage of testicular cancer. Lancet, 2:970, 1981.

Boyle, L. E., and Samuels, M. L.: Serum LDH activity and isoenzyme patterns in nonseminomatous germinal (NSG) testis tumors. Proc. Am. Soc. Clin. Oncol., 18:278, 1977.

Bradfield, J. S., Hagen, R. O., and Ytredal, D. O.: Carcinoma of the testis: An analysis of 104 cases with germinal tumors of the testis other than seminoma. Cancer, 31:633, 1973.

Bredael, J. J., Vugrin, D., and Whitmore, W. F., Jr.: Autopsy findings in 154 patients with germ cell tumors of the testis. Cancer, 50:548, 1982.

Bredael, J. J., Vugrin, D., and Whitmore, W. F., Jr.: Recurrences in surgical stage I nonseminomatous germ cell tumors of the testis. J. Urol., 130:476, 1983.

Burrington, J. D.: Rhabdomyosarcoma of the paratesticular tissues in children. Report of eight cases. J. Pediatr. Surg., 4:503, 1969.

Campbell, H. E.: Incidence of malignant growth of the undescended testicle. Arch. Surg., 44:353, 1942.

Carleton, R. L., Freidman, N. B., and Bomge, E. J.: Experimental teratomas of the testis. Cancer, 6:464, 1953.

Cheng, E., Cvitkovic, E., Wittes, R. E., and Golbey, R. B.: Germ cell tumors: VAB II in metastatic testicular cancer. Cancer, 42:1262, 1978.

Clemmesen, J.: Statistical studies in malignant neoplasms. Microbiol. Scand. (Suppl.), 247:1, 1974.

Cole, H.: Tumours in the region of the pineal. Clin. Radiol., 22:110, 1971.

Cooper, J. F., Leadbetter, W. F., and Chute, R.: The thoracoabdominal approach for retroperitoneal gland dissection: Its application to testis tumors. Surg. Gynecol. Obstet., 90:46, 1950.

Cosgrove, M. D., Benton, B., and Henderson, B. E.: Male genitourinary abnormalities and maternal diethylstilbestrol. J. Urol., 117:220, 1977.

Crawford, E. D., Smith, R. B., and deKernion, J. B.: Treatment of advanced seminoma with preradiation therapy. J. Urol., 19:75, 1983.

Cuneo, B.: Note sur les lymphatiques du testicle. Bull. Soc. Anat. (Paris), 76:105, 1901.

Cvitkovic, E., Wittes, R., Golbey, R., et al.: Primary combination chemotherapy for metastatic or unresectable germ cell tumors. Proc. Am. Assoc. Cancer Res., 19:174, 1978.

Damjanov, I., and Solter, D.: Animal model: Embryo-derived teratomas and teratocarcinomas in mice. Am. J. Pathol., 83:241, 1976.

Davis, A. E., Jr.: Rhabdomyosarcoma of the testicle. J. Urol., 87:148, 1962.

Dixon, F. J., and Moore, R. A.: Tumors of the Male Sex Organs, Fascicle 32. Washington, DC, Armed Forces Institute of Pathology, 1952, pp. 48–103.

Donohue, J. P., Foster, R. S., Rowland, R. G., Bihrle, R., Jones, J., and Geier, G.: Nerve-sparing retroperitoneal lymphadenectomy with preservation of ejaculation. J. Urol., 144(2 Pt 1):287, discussion 291, 1990.

Donohue, J. P., Zachary, J. M., and Maynard, B. R.: Distribution of nodal metastases in nonseminomatous testis cancer. J. Urol., 128:315, 1982.

Doornbos, J. F., Hussey, D. H., and Johnson, D. E.: Radiotherapy for pure seminoma of the testis. Radiology, 116:401, 1975.

Dosoretz, D. E., Shipley, W. U., Blitzer, P. H., Gilbert, S., Prat, J., Parkhurst, E., and Wang, C. C.: Megavoltage irradiation for pure testicular seminoma: Results and patterns of failure. Cancer, 48:2184, 1981.

Duchesne, G. M., Horwich, A., Dearnaley, D. P., et al.: Orchidectomy alone for Stage I seminoma of the testis. Cancer, 65:1115, 1990.

Dunphy, C. H., Ayala, A. G., Swanson, D. A., et al.: Clinical stage I nonseminomatous and mixed germ cell tumors of the testis. A clinicopathologic study of 93 patients on a surveillance protocol after orchiectomy alone. Cancer, 62:1202, 1988.

Earle, J. D., Bagshaw, M. A., and Kaplan, H. S.: Supervoltage radiation therapy of the testicular tumors. Am. J. Roentgenol., 117:653, 1973.

Einhorn, L. H., and Donohue, J. P.: *Cis*-diaminedichloroplatinum, vinblastine, and bleomycin combination chemotherapy in disseminated testicular cancer. Ann. Intern. Med., 87:293, 1977.

Einhorn, L. H., and Williams, S. D.: Chemotherapy of disseminated testicular cancer. Cancer, 46:1339, 1980a.

Einhorn, L. H., and Williams, S. D.: Chemotherapy of disseminated seminoma. Cancer Clin. Trials, 3:307, 1980b.

Einhorn, L. H., Williams, S. D., Mandebaum, I., and Donohue, J. P.: Surgical resection in disseminated testicular cancer following chemotherapeutic cytoreduction. Cancer, 48:904, 1981a.

Einhorn, L. H., Williams, S. D., Troner, M., et al.: The role of maintenance therapy in disseminated testicular cancer. N. Engl. J. Med., 305:727, 1981b.

Farrer, J. H., Walker, A. H., and Rajfer, J.: Management of the postpubertal cryptorchid testis: A statistical review. J. Urol., 134:1071, 1985.

Forrest, J. B., and Whitmore, W. F., Jr.: Bilateral synchronous epidermoid cysts. World J. Urol., 2:76, 1984.

Fossa, S., Borge, L., Aass, N., et al.: The treatment of advanced metastatic seminoma: Experience in 55 cases. J. Clin. Oncol., 5:1071, 1987.

Fowler, J. E., Jr., McLeod, D. G., and Stutzman, R. E.: Critical appraisal of routine supraclavicular lymph node biopsy in staging of testicular tumors. Urology, 14:230, 1979.

Fraley, E. E., Lange, P. H., and Kennedy, B. J.: Germ-cell testicular cancer in adults. N. Engl. J. Med., 301:1370, 1420, 1979.

Freedman, L. S., Jones, W. G., Peckham, M. J., et al.: Histopathology in the prediction of relapse of patients with stage I testicular teratoma treated by orchidectomy alone. Lancet, 2:294, 1987.

Freidman, N. B., and Moore, R. A.: Tumors of the testis: A report on 922 cases. Milit. Surg., 99:57, 1946.

Friedrich, M., Claussen, C. D., and Felix, R.: Immersion ultrasound of testicular pathology. Radiography, 141:235, 1981.

Fung, C. Y., Kalish, L. A., Brodsky, G. L., Richie, J. P., and Garnick, M. B.: Stage I nonseminomatous germ cell testicular tumor: Prediction of metastatic potential by primary histopathology. J. Clin. Oncol., 6:1467, 1988.

Gabrilove, J. L., Freiberg, E. K., Leiter, E., and Nicolis, G. L.: Feminizing and non-feminizing Sertoli cell tumors. J. Urol., 124:757, 1980.

Gabrilove, J. L., Nicolis, G. L., Mitty, H. A., and Sohval, A. R.: Feminizing interstitial cell tumor of the testis: Personal observations and a review of the literature. Cancer, 35:1184, 1975.

Gaffney, E. F., Harte, P. J., and Browne, H. J.: Paratesticular leiomyosarcoma: An ultrastructural study. J. Urol., 133:133, 1984.

Garnick, M. B., Canellos, G. P., and Richie, J. P.: The treatment and surgical staging of testicular and primary extragonadal germ cell cancer. JAMA, 250:1733, 1983.

Gelderman, W. A. H., Koops, H. S., Sleijfer, D. F., et al.: Orchidectomy alone in stage I nonseminomatous testicular germ cell tumor. Cancer, 59:578, 1987.

Ghavimi, F., Exelby, P. R., D'Angio, G. J., Whitmore, W. F., Jr., Lieberman, P. H., Lewis, J. L., Jr., Miké, V., and Murphy, M. L.: Proceedings: Combination therapy of urogenital embryonal rhabdomyosarcoma in children. Cancer, 32:1178, 1973.

Gilbert, J. B.: Tumors of the testis following mumps orchitis: Case report and review of 24 cases. J. Urol., 51:296, 1944.

Gilbert, J. B., and Hamilton, J. B.: Studies in malignant testis tumors; incidence and nature of tumors in ectopic testis. Surg. Gynecol. Obstet., 71:731, 1940.

Glazer, H. S., Lee, J. K. T., Melson, G. L., and McClennan, B. C.: Sonographic detection of occult testicular neoplasms. Am. J. Radiol., 138:67, 1982.

Gowing, N. F., and Morgan, A. D.: Paratesticular tumors of connective tissue and muscle. Br. J. Urol., 36(Suppl):78, 1964.

Graham, S., and Gibson, R.: Social epidemiology of cancer of the testis. Cancer, 29:1324, 1972.

Green, N., Broth, E., George, F. W., Kaplan, R., Lombardo, L., Skaist, L., Weinstein, E., and Petrovich, Z.: Radiation therapy in bulky seminoma. Urology, 21:467, 1983.

Grosfeld, J. L., Weber, T. R., Weetman, R. M., and Baener, R. L.: Rhabdomyosarcoma in childhood: Analysis of survival in 98 cases. J. Pediatr. Surg., 18:141, 1983.

Hainsworth, J. D., Einhorn, L. H., Williams, S. D., Stewart, M., and

Greco, F. A.: Advanced extragonadal germ cell tumors: Successful treatment with combination chemotherapy. Ann. Intern. Med., 97:7, 1982.

Harvald, B., and Hauge, M.: Heredity of cancer elucidated by a study of unselected twins. JAMA, 186:749, 1963.

Henderson, B. E., Benton, B., Jing, J., Hu, M. C., and Pike, M. C.: Risk factors for cancer of the testis in young men. J. Cancer, 3:598, 1979.

Henderson, B. E., Ross, R. K., Pike, M. C., and Depue, R. H.: Epidemiology of testis cancer. *In* Skinner, D. G. (Ed.): Urological Cancer. New York, Grune & Stratton, 1983, pp. 237–250.

Hoeltl, W., Kosak, D., Paunt, J., et al.: Testicular cancer: Prognostic implications of vascular invasion. J. Urol., 137:683, 1987.

Hollands, M. J., Dottori, V., and Nash, A. G.: Malignant mesothelioma of the tunica vaginalis testis. Eur. Urol., 8:121, 1982.

Hong, W. K., Wittes, R. E., Hajdu, S. T., Cvitkovic, E., Whitmore, W. F., Jr., and Gobley, R. B.: The evolution of mature teratoma from malignant testicular tumors. Cancer, 40:2987, 1977.

Jackson, J. R.: The histogenesis of the "adenomatoid" tumor of the genital tract. Cancer, 11:337, 1958

Jacobellis, U., Ricco, R., and Ruotolo, G.: Adenocarcinoma of the rete testis 21 years after orchiopexy: Case report and review of the literature. J. Urol., 125:429, 1981.

Jamieson, J. K., and Dobson, J. F.: The lymphatics of the testicle. Lancet, 1:493, 1910.

Javadpour, N.: The role of biologic tumour markers in testicular cancer. Cancer, 45:1755, 1980a.

Javadpour, N.: Significance of elevated serum alpha-fetoproteins (AFP) in seminoma. Cancer, 45:2166, 1980b.

Javadpour, N.: Multiple biochemical tumour markers in testicular cancer. Cancer, 52:887, 1983.

Javadpour, N., McIntire, K. R., and Waldmann, T. A.: Human chorionic gonadotropin (hCG) and alpha-fetoprotein (AFP) in sera and tumor cells of patients with testicular seminoma. Cancer, 42:2768, 1978.

Jewett, M. A. S., and Torbey, C.: Nerve-sparing techniques in retroperitoneal lymphadenectomy in patients with low-stage testicular cancer. Semin. Urol., 6:233, 1988.

Jochelson, M., Garnick, M. B., Balikian, J., and Richie, J. P.: The efficacy of routine whole lung tomography in germ cell tumors. Cancer, 54:1007, 1984.

Johnson, D. E.: Epidemiology of testicular tumors. *In* Johnson, D. E. (Ed.): Testicular Tumors, Ed. 2. Flushing, NY, Medical Examination Publishing Co., 1976, pp. 37–46.

Johnson, D. E., Appelt, G., Samuels, M. C., and Luna, M.: Metastases from testicular carcinoma. Urology, 8:234, 1976.

Johnson, D. E., Kaesler, K. E., Mackay, B. M., and Ayala, A. G.: Neurofibrosarcoma of the spermatic cord. Urology, 5:680, 1975.

Johnson, D. E., Lo, R. K., von Eschenbach, A. C., et al.: Surveillance alone for patients with clinical stage I non-seminomatous germ cell tumors of the testis: Preliminary results. J. Urol., 131:491, 1984.

Johnson, D. G.: Trends in surgery for childhood rhabdomyosarcoma. Cancer, 35:916, 1975.

Kasdon, E. J.: Malignant mesothelioma of the tunica vaginalis propria testis. Report of two cases. Cancer, 23:1144, 1969.

Kaufman, E., Akiya, F., Foucar, E., Gambort, F., and Cartwright, K. C.: Virilization due to Leydig cell tumor diagnosis by magnetic resonance imaging: Case management report. Clin. Pediatr., 29:414, 1990.

Kennedy, B. J.: Mithramycin therapy in advanced testicular neoplasms. Cancer, 26:755, 1970.

Kimbrough, J. C., and Cook, F. E., Jr.: Carcinoma of the testis. JAMA, 153:1436, 1953.

Kingston, J. E., McElwain, T. J., and Malpas, J. S.: Childhood rhabdomyosarcoma: Experience of the Children's Solid Tumor Group. Br. J. Cancer, 48:195, 1983.

Kirkland, R. T., Kirkland, J. L., Keenan, B. S., Bongiovanni, A. M., Rosenberg, H. S., and Clayton, G. W.: Bilateral testicular tumors in congenital adrenal hyperplasia. J. Clin. Endocrinol. Metab., 44:367, 1977.

Krishnaswamy, P. R., Tate, S., and Meister, A.: Gamma-glutamyl transpeptidase of human seminal fluid. Life Sci., 20:681, 1977.

Kuo, T. T., Tschang, T. P., and Chu, J. Y.: Testicular relapse in childhood acute lymphocytic leukemia during bone marrow remission. Cancer, 38:6204, 1976.

Lange, P. H., and Raghavan, D.: Clinical application of tumor markers in testicular cancer. *In* Donohue, J. P. (Ed.): Testis Tumor. Baltimore, Williams & Wilkins, 1983, pp. 111–130.

Lauer, R. L., Roth, B., Loehrer, P. J., et al.: *Cis*-platinum plus ifosfamide plus either VP-16 or vinblastine as third-line therapy for metastatic testicular cancer. Proc. Am. Soc. Clin. Oncol., 6:99, 1987.

LeComete (1851): Quoted by Grove, J. S.: The cryptorchid problem. J. Urol., 71:735, 1954.

Lewis, L. G.: Testis tumor: Report on 250 cases. J. Urol., 59:763, 1948.

Li, M. C., Whitmore, W. F., Jr., Golbey, R., and Grabstald, H.: Effects of combined drug therapy on metastatic cancer of the testis. JAMA, 174:1291, 1960.

Lipshutz, L. I.: Management of infertility following treatment for testicular carcinoma. Cancer Bull., 34:31, 1982.

Lockhart, J. L., Dalton, D. L., Vollmer, R. T., and Glenn, J. F.: Nonfunctioning interstitial cell carcinoma of the testis. Urology, 8:392, 1976.

Loehrer, P. J., Birch, R., Williams, S. D., et al.: Chemotherapy of metastatic seminoma: The Southeastern Cancer Study Group Experience. J. Clin. Oncol., 5:1212, 1987.

Logothetis, C. J., Samuels, M. C., Trindade, A., and Johnson, D. E.: The growing teratoma syndrome. Cancer, 50:1629, 1982.

Luna, M. A., and Valenzuela-Tamariz, J.: Germ cell tumors of the mediastinum: Post-mortem findings. Am. J. Clin. Pathol., 65:450, 1976.

Lynch, D. F., and Richie, J. P.: Supraclavicular node biopsy in staging testis tumors. J. Urol., 123:39, 1980.

Mack, T. M., and Henderson, B. E.: Cancer Registries for Special and General Uses. In US-USSR monograph, NIH publ. no. 80-2044, 1980, pp. 57–61.

MacKenzie, A. R.: The chemotherapy of metastatic seminoma. J. Urol., 96:790, 1966.

Maier, J. G., and Mittemeyer, B. T.: Carcinoma of the testis. Cancer, 39:981, 1977.

Maier, J. G., and Sulak, M. H.: Radiation therapy in malignant testis tumors: Part I. Seminoma. Cancer, 32:1212, 1973.

Marcus, J. B., and Lynn, J. A.: Ultrastructural comparison of an adenomatoid tumor, lymphangioma, hemangioma and mesothelioma. Cancer, 25:171, 1970.

Martin, D. C.: Germinal cell tumors of the testis after orchiopexy. J. Urol., 121:42, 1979.

Martini, N., Golbey, R. B., Hajdu, S. I., Whitmore, W. F., Jr., and Beattie, E. J.: Primary mediastinal germ cell tumors. Cancer, 33:763, 1974.

Mengel, W., Wronecki, K., Schroeder, J., and Zimmermann, F. A.: Histopathology of the cryptorchid testis. Urol. Clin. North Am., 9:331, 1982.

Merrin, C., Baumastner, G., and Wajsman, Z.: Benign transformation of testicular carcinoma by chemotherapy. Lancet, 1:43, 1975.

Morse, M. J., Herr, H. W., Sogani, P. C., Bosl, G. J., and Whitmore, W. F., Jr.: Surgical exploration of metastatic seminoma following VAB-6 chemotherapy [Abstract C-559]. Proc. Am. Soc. Clin. Oncol., 2:143, 1983.

Most, H.: Über maligne loden geschwulste und ihre metastatasin. Arch. Pathol. Anat., 54:73, 1898.

Mostofi, F. K.: Testicular tumors: Epidemiologic, etiologic and pathologic features. Cancer, 32:1186, 1973.

Mostofi, F. K., and Price, E. B.: Tumors of the male genital system. *In* Atlas of Tumor Pathology, Second Series, Fascicle 8. Washington, DC, Armed Forces Institute of Pathology, 1973.

Mostofi, F. K., and Sobin, L. H.: International Histological Classification of Tumors of Testes (No. 16). Geneva, World Health Organization, 1977.

Motzer, R., Bosl, G., Heelen, R., et al.: Residual mass: An indication for surgery in patients with advanced seminoma following systemic chemotherapy. J. Clin. Oncol., 5:1064, 1987.

Muir, C. S., and Nectoux, J.: NCI Monogr., 53:157, 1979.

Muller, K.: Cancer Testis [Thesis]. Copenhagen, Munksgaard, 1962.

Narayan, P., Lange, P. H., and Fraley, E. E.: Ejaculation and fertility after extended retroperitoneal lymph node dissection for testicular cancer. J. Urol., 127:685, 1982.

Nomura, T., and Kanzak, T.: Induction of urogenital anomalies and some tumor in the progeny of mice receiving diethylstilbestrol during pregnancy. Cancer Res., 37:1099, 1977.

Oliver, R. T., Lore, S., and Ong, J.: Alternatives to radiotherapy in the management of seminoma. Br. J. Urol., 65:61, 1990.

Patton, R. B., and Horn, R. C., Jr.: Rhabdomyosarcoma: Clinical and pathological features and comparison with human fetal and embryonal skeletal muscle. Surgery, 52:572, 1962.

Peckham, M. J.: Testicular tumours, investigation and staging; General aspects and staging classifications. *In* Peckham, M. J. (Ed.): The Management of Testicular Tumours. Chicago, Year Book Medical Publishers, 1982, pp. 89–101.

Peckham, M. J., Barrett, A., McElwain, T. J., Hendry, W. F., and Raghavan, D.: Nonseminoma germ cell tumours (malignant teratoma) of the testis: Results of treatment and an analysis of prognostic factors. Br. J. Urol., 53:162, 1981.

Peckham, M. J., and McElwain, T. J.: Radiotherapy of testicular tumors. Proc. R. Soc. Med., 67:300, 1974.

Percarpio, B., Clements, J. C., McLeod, D. G., Sorgen, S. D., and Cardinale, F. S.: Anaplastic seminoma: An analysis of 77 patients. Cancer, 43:2510, 1979.

Pierce, G. B.: Teratocarcinoma: Introduction and perspectives. *In* Sherman, M. I., and Solter, D. (Eds.): Teratomas and Differentiation. New York, Academic Press, 1975, pp. 3–12.

Pizzocaro, G., Salveoni, R., and Zanoni, F.: Unilateral lymphadenectomy in intraoperative stage I nonseminomatous germinal testicular cancer. J. Urol., 134:485, 1985

Pizzocaro, G., Zanoni, F., Milani, A., et al.: Orchiectomy alone in clinical stage I nonseminomatous testis cancer: A critical appraisal. J. Clin. Oncol., 4:35, 1986.

Pugh, R. C. B., and Cameron, K.: Teratoma. *In* Pugh, R. C. B. (Ed.): Pathology of the Testis. Oxford, Blackwell Scientific Publications, 1976, pp. 199–244.

Raghavan, D., Colls, B., Levi, J., et al.: Surveillance for stage I non-seminomatous germ cell tumours of the testis: The optimal protocol has not yet been defined. Br. J. Urol., 61:522, 1988.

Raghavan, D., Peckham, M. J., Heyderman, E., Tobias, J. S., and Austin, D. E.: Prognostic factors in clinical stage I non-seminomatous germ-cell tumours of the testis. Br. J. Cancer, 45:167, 1982.

Ray, B., Hajou, S. I., and Whitmore, W. F., Jr.: Distribution of retroperitoneal lymph node metastases in testicular germinal tumors. Cancer, 33:30, 1979.

Read, G., Johnson, R. J., Wilkinson, P. M., et al.: Prospective study on follow-up alone in stage I teratoma of the testis. Br. Med. J., 287:1503, 1983.

Recondo, J., and Libshitz, H. I.: Mediastinal extragonadal germ cell tumors. Urology, 11:369, 1978.

Reynolds, T. F., Tagoda, A., Vugrin, D., and Golbey, R. B.: Chemotherapy of mediastinal germ cell tumors. Semin. Oncol., 6:113, 1979.

Richie, J. P.: Modified retroperitoneal lymphadenectomy for clinical stage I testicular cancer. J. Urol., 144:1160, 1990.

Richie, J. P., Birnholz, J., and Garnick, M. B.: Ultrasonography as a diagnostic adjunct for the evaluation of masses in the scrotum. Surg. Gynecol. Obstet., 154:695, 1982.

Richie, J. P., and Kantoff, P.: Is adjuvant chemotherapy necessary for patients with stage B$_1$ testicular cancer? J. Clin. Oncol., 1991. In press.

Riehle, R. A., and Venkatachalam, H.: Electron microscopy in diagnosis of adult paratesticular rhabdomyosarcoma. Urology, 19:658, 1982.

Riopelle, J. L., and Theriault, J. P.: Sur une forme meconnue de sarcoma des parties molles: Le rhabdomyosarcome alvéolaire. Ann. Anat. Pathol. (Paris), 1:88, 1956.

Rorth, M., von der Maase, H., Nielsen, E. S., et al.: Orchidectomy alone versus orchidectomy plus radiotherapy in stage I non-seminomatous testicular cancer: A randomized study by the Danish Carcinoma Study Group. Int. J. Androl., 10:255, 1987.

Rosenberg, B., VanCamp, L., and Krigas, T.: Inhibition of cell division in *E. coli* by electrolysis products from a platinum electrode. Nature, 205:678, 1965.

Ross, R. K., McCurtis, J. W., Henderson, B. F., et al.: Descriptive epidemiology of testicular and prostatic cancer in Los Angeles. Br. J. Cancer, 39:284, 1979.

Rosvoll, R. V., and Woodard, J. R.: Malignant Sertoli cell tumor of the testis. Cancer, 22:8, 1968.

Rothman, K. J., and Louik, C.: Oral contraceptives and birth defects. N. Engl. J. Med., 299:522, 1978.

Rouviere, H.: Anatomy of the Human Lymphatic System (translated by M. J. Tobias). Ann Arbor, MI, Edwards Bros., 1938.

Rowland, R. G., Weisman, D., Williams, S., Einhorn, L., and

Donohue, J. P.: Accuracy of preoperative staging in Stage A and B non-seminomatous germ cell testis tumors. J. Urol., 127:718, 1982.

Ruoslahti, E., Engvall, E., Pakkala, A., and Seppala, M.: Developmental changes in carbohydrate moiety of human alpha-fetoprotein. Int. J. Cancer, 22:515, 1978.

Samellas, W.: Malignant neoplasms of spermatic cord. Liposarcoma. N.Y. State J. Med., 64:1213, 1964.

Samuels, M. L., and Howe, C. D.: Vinblastine and the management of testicular cancer. Cancer, 25:1009, 1970.

Samuels, M. L., Johnson, D. E., and Holoye, P. Y.: Continuous intravenous bleomycin therapy with vinblastine in stage III testicular neoplasia. Cancer Chemother. Rep., 59:563, 1975.

Samuels, M. L., Lanzotti, V. J., Holoye, P. Y., et al.: Combination chemotherapy and germinal cell tumors. Cancer Treat. Rev., 3:185, 1976.

Sato, B., Huseby, R. A., and Samuels, L. T.: Characterization of estrogen receptors in various mouse Leydig cell tumor lines. Cancer Res., 38:2842, 1978.

Schottenfeld, D., Warshauer, M. E., Sherlock, S., Zauber, A. G., Leder, M., and Payne, R.: The epidemiology of testicular cancer in young adults. Am. J. Epidemiol., 112:232, 1980.

Scorer, C. C., and Farrington, G. H.: Congenital Deformities of the Testis and Epididymis, Chap. 2. New York, Appleton-Century-Crofts, 1971.

Scully, R. E.: Gonadoblastoma: A gonadal tumor related to the dysgerminoma (seminoma) and capable of sex-hormone production. Cancer, 6:455, 1953.

Shah, K. H., Maxted, W. C., and Chun, B.: Epidermoid cysts of the testis. Cancer, 47:577, 1981.

Sherrick, J. C.: Papillary cystadenoma of the epididymis. Cancer, 9:403, 1956.

Shulman, Y., Ware, S., Al-Askari, S., and Morales, P.: Anaplastic seminoma. Urology, 21:379, 1983.

Silverberg, E.: Cancer statistics. Cancer, 40:9, 1990.

Skakkebaek, N. E.: Possible carcinoma in situ of the testis. Lancet, 2:516, 1972.

Skakkebaek, N. E.: Atypical germ cells in the adjacent "normal" tissue of testicular tumors. Acta Pathol. Microbiol. Scand., 83:127, 1975.

Skakkebaek, N. E.: Carcinoma in situ of the testis: Frequency in relationship to invasive germ cell tumors in infertile men. Histopathology, 2:157, 1978.

Skinner, D. G.: Nonseminomatous testis tumors: A plan of management based on 96 patients to improve survival in all stages by combined therapeutic modalities. J. Urol., 115:65, 1976.

Skinner, D. G., Melamud, A., and Lieskovsky, G.: Complications of thoracoabdominal retroperitoneal lymph node dissection. J. Urol., 127:1107, 1982.

Skinner, D. G., and Scardino, P. T.: Relevance of biochemical tumor markers and lymphadenectomy in management of nonseminomatous testis tumors: Current perspective. J. Urol., 123:378, 1980.

Smith, R. B.: Management of testicular seminoma. In Skinner, D. G., and deKernion, J. B. (Eds.): Genitourinary Cancer. Philadelphia, W. B. Saunders Co., 1978, pp. 460–469.

Soderstrom, J., and Leidberg, C. F.: Malignant "adenomatoid" tumour of the epididymis. Acta Pathol. Microbiol. Scand., 67:165, 1966.

Sogani, P. C., Whitmore, W. F., Jr., Herr, H. W., et al.: Long-term experience with orchiectomy alone in treatment of clinical stage I non-seminomatous germ cell tumour of the testis. J. Urol., 133:246A, 1988.

Sohval, A. R.: Testicular dysgenesis in relation to neoplasm of the testicle. J. Urol., 75:285, 1956.

Sokal, M., Peckham, M. J., and Hendry, W. F.: Bilateral germ cell tumours of the testis. Br. J. Urol., 5:158, 1980.

Stanton, G. F., Bosl, G. J., Vugrin, D., Whitmore, W. F., Jr., Myers, W. P. L. M., and Golbey, R. B.: Treatment of patients with advanced seminoma with cyclophosphamide, bleomycin, actinomycin D, vinblastine and cis-platin (VAB-6) [Abstract C-551]. Proc. Am. Soc. Clin. Oncol., 2:1, 1983.

Staubitz, W. J., Early, K. S., Magoss, I. V., and Murphy, G. P.: Surgical management of testis tumors. J. Urol., 111:205, 1974.

Sterchi, M., and Cordell, A. R.: Seminoma of the anterior mediastinum. Ann. Thorac. Surg., 19:371, 1975.

Stevens, L. C.: Origin of testicular teratomas from primordial germ cells in mice. JNCI, 38:549, 1967.

Stevens, L. C.: The development of teratomas from intratesticular grafts of tubal mouse eggs. J. Embryol. Exp. Morphol., 20:329, 1968.

Stoffel, T. J., Nesbit, M. E., and Levitt, S. H.: Extramedullary involvement of the testis in childhood leukemia. Cancer, 35:1203, 1975.

Stomper, P. C., Jochelson, M. S., Garnick, M. B., and Richie, J. P.: Residual abdominal masses following chemotherapy for nonseminomatous testicular cancer: Correlation of CT and histology. AJR, 145:743, 1985.

Strong, G. H.: Lipomyxoma of the spermatic cord: Case report and review of literature. J. Urol., 48:527, 1942.

Talerman, A.: A distinctive gonadal neoplasm related to gonadoblastoma. Cancer, 30:1219, 1972.

Talerman, A., Gramata, S., Miranda, S., and Okagaka, T.: Primary carcinoid tumor of the testis. Cancer, 42:2696, 1978.

Teilum, G.: Arrhenoblastoma-androblastoma: Homologous ovarian and testicular tumors. Acta Pathol. Microbiol. Scand., 23:252, 1946.

Teilum, G.: Endodermal sinus tumors of ovary and testis: Comparative morphogenesis of so-called mesonephroma ovarie (Schiller) and extraembryonic structure of rat placenta. Cancer, 12:1092, 1959.

Teilum, G.: Special Tumors of Ovary and Testis and Related Extragonadal Lesions. Philadelphia, J. B. Lippincott Co., 1971.

Teilum, G., Albrechtson, R., and Norgaard-Pederson, B.: The histogenetic embryologic basis for reappearance of alpha-fetoprotein in endodermal sinus tumors (yolk sac tumors) and teratoma. Acta Pathol. Microbiol. Scand., 83:80, 1975.

Thackray, A. C., and Crane, W. A. J.: Seminoma. In Pugh, R. C. B. (Ed.): Pathology of the Testis. Oxford, Blackwell Scientific Publications, 1976.

Thomas, G. M., Rider, W. D., Dembo, A. J., et al.: Seminoma of the testis: Results of treatment and patterns of failure after radiation therapy. Int. J. Radiat. Oncol. Biol. Phys., 8:165, 1982.

Thompson, P. I., Nixon, J., and Harvey, V. J.: Disease relapse in patients with stage I non-seminomatous germ cell tumor of the testis on active surveillance. J. Clin. Oncol., 6:1597, 1988.

Turner, R. R., Colby, T. V., and MacKintosh, F. R.: Testicular lymphomas. Cancer, 48:2095, 1981.

Tyrrell, C. J., and Peckham, M. J.: The response of lymph node metastasis of testicular teratoma to radiation therapy. Br. J. Urol., 48:363, 1976.

Uriel, J.: Retrodifferentiation and the fetal patterns of gene expression in cancer. Adv. Cancer Res., 29:127, 1979.

Vaitukaitis, J. L.: Human chorionic gonadotropin: A hormone secreted for many reasons. N. Engl. J. Med., 301:324, 1979.

van der Bogert, C., Dontje, B. H. J., and Kroon, A. M.: Arrest in in vivo growth of a solid Leydig cell tumor by prolonged inhibition of mitochondrial protein synthesis. Cancer Res., 43:2247, 1983.

van der Werf-Messing, B.: Radiotherapeutic treatment of testicular tumors. Int. J. Radiat. Oncol. Biol. Phys., 1:235, 1976.

Vugrin, D., Cvitkovic, E., Whitmore, W. F., Jr., Cheng, E., and Golbey, R. B.: VAB-4 combination chemotherapy in the treatment of metastatic testis tumors. Cancer, 47:833, 1981a.

Vugrin, D., Whitmore, W. F., Jr., and Batata, M.: Chemotherapy of disseminated seminoma with combination of cis-diamminedichloroplatinum (II) and cyclophosphamide. Cancer Clin. Trials, 4:42, 1981b.

Vugrin, D., Whitmore, W. F., Jr., Nisselbaum, J., and Watson, R. C.: Correlation of serum tumor markers and lymphangiography with degrees of nodal involvement in surgical Stage II testis cancer. J. Urol., 127:683, 1982.

Wajsman, Z., Beckley, S. A., and Pontes, J. E.: Changing concepts in the treatment of advanced seminomatous tumors. J. Urol., 129:303, 1983.

Walsh, P. C.: The endocrinology of testicular tumors. In Grundmann, E., and Vahlensieck, W. (Eds.): Recent Results in Cancer Research, Vol. 60. Berlin, Springer-Verlag, 1977, p. 196.

Walsh, P. C., Kaufman, J. J., Coulson, W. F., and Goodwin, W. E.: Retroperitoneal lymphadenectomy for testicular tumors. JAMA, 217:309, 1971.

Waters, W. B., Garnick, M. B., and Richie, J. P.: Complications of retroperitoneal lymphadenectomy in the management of nonseminomatous tumors of the testis. Surg. Gynecol. Obstet., 154:501, 1982.

Weitzner, S.: Spermatocytic seminoma. Urology, 6:74, 1979.

Weitzner, S., and Gropp, A.: A primary reticulum cell sarcoma of the testis in a 12-year-old. Cancer, 37:935, 1976.

Wheeler, B. M., Loehrer, P. J., Williams, S. D., and Einhorn, L. H.: Ifosfamide and refractory germ cell tumors. J. Clin. Oncol., 4:28, 1986.

Whitaker, R. H.: Management of the undescended testis. Br. J. Hosp. Med., 4:25, 1970.

Whitmore, W. F., Jr.: The treatment of germinal tumors of the testis. *In* Proceedings of the Sixth National Cancer Conference. Philadelphia, J. B. Lippincott Co., 1968, pp. 347–355.

Whitmore, W. F., Jr.: Germinal tumors of the testis. *In* Proceedings of the Sixth National Cancer Conference. Philadelphia, J. B. Lippincott Co., 1970, pp. 219–221.

Whitmore, W. F., Jr.: Germinal tumors of the testis. *In* Proceedings of the Seventh National Cancer Conference. Philadelphia, J. B. Lippincott Co., 1973, pp. 485–499.

Whitmore, W. F., Jr.: Surgical treatment of adult germinal testis tumors. Semin. Oncol., 6:55, 1979.

Williams, S. D., Birch, R., Einhorn, L. H., et al.: Treatment of disseminated germ cell tumors with cis-platinum, bleomycin and either vinblastine or etoposide. N. Engl. J. Med., 316:1435, 1987a.

Williams, S. D., Stablain, D. M., Einhorn, L. H., et al.: Immediate adjuvant chemotherapy versus observation with treatment at relapse in pathologic stage II testicular cancer. N. Engl. J. Med., 317:1433, 1987b.

Wilson, W. W.: Adenomatoid leiomyoma of the epididymis. Br. J. Surg., 37:240, 1949.

Wittes, R. E., Yagoda, A., Silvay, O., Magill, G. B., Whitmore, W. F., Jr., Krakoff, I. H., and Golbey, R. B.: Chemotherapy of germ cell tumors of the testis. Cancer, 37:637, 1976.

Zdeb, M. S.: The probability of developing cancer. Am. J. Epidemiol., 106:6, 1977.

Zondek, B.: Versuch einer biologischen (Hormonalen) diagnostik beim malignen hodentumor. Chirurg, 2:1072, 1930.

31
TUMORS OF THE PENIS

Paul F. Schellhammer, M.D.
Gerald H. Jordan, M.D.
Steven M. Schlossberg, M.D.

Coverage of the subject of abnormal penile growths must include discussion of both benign and malignant tumors. Some penile lesions are strictly benign, and some are premalignant or at least possess the potential for malignancy. A description of these lesions serves to establish their anatomic, etiologic, and histologic relationship to squamous cell carcinoma of the penis, which is the most common malignant lesion of the penis. Malignancies of different histology also occur and are described in this chapter.

BENIGN NONCUTANEOUS LESIONS

Congenital inclusion cysts have been reported to occur in the penoscrotal raphe (Cole and Helwig, 1976). Acquired inclusion cysts subsequent to trauma or circumcision are more common. Retention cysts arise from the sebaceous glands located on the mucosal surface of the prepuce and on the skin of the shaft (Fig. 31–1). Retention cysts may also occur in the parameatal area as a result of urethral gland obstruction (Shiraki, 1975). Sebaceous glands are not found on the glans penis.

Benign tumors of the supporting structures include angiomas, fibromas, neuromas, lipomas, and myomas. (These are discussed in the differential diagnosis of sarcomas of the penis.) Angiomas are usually superficial. They appear as punctate reddish macules or papules that occur most frequently on the coronal aspect of the glans and resemble the small angiokeratomas found on the scrotum.

Penile masses and deformities, or pseudotumors, may be secondary to self-administered injections or foreign body implants (Nitidandhaprabhas, 1975). Testosterone in oil (Zalar et al., 1969) and other common oils (Engelman et al., 1974) have been placed on or injected into the penis, producing a destructive lipogranuloma-tous process that may grossly mimic carcinoma. Endogenous lipoid degeneration may at times produce a similar inflammatory response (Smetana and Bernhard, 1950).

Occasionally, phlebitis (Grossman et al., 1965), lymphangitis (Ball and Pickett, 1975; Nickel and Plumb, 1962), or angiitis (Rubenstein and Wolff, 1964) may produce subcutaneous penile nodules or cords.

When a diagnosis is in question, all benign lesions are best treated with local excision and careful histologic examination to rule out malignancy.

BENIGN CUTANEOUS LESIONS

Cutaneous nevi occurring on the skin of the penis must be distinguished from malignant melanoma by biopsy (vide infra) (Fig. 31–2). Penile melanosis describes hyperpigmentation of the basal layer of the epidermis without cellular hyperplasia or atypia (Revuz and Clerici, 1989).

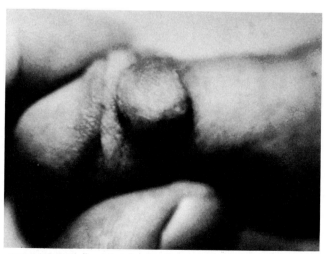

Figure 31–1. Epithelial inclusion cyst of the skin of the shaft just proximal to the coronal sulcus. It was removed by enucleation.

We wish to acknowledge Dr. H. Grabstald who directed our efforts in the previous two editions and L. Neilson for manuscript preparation.

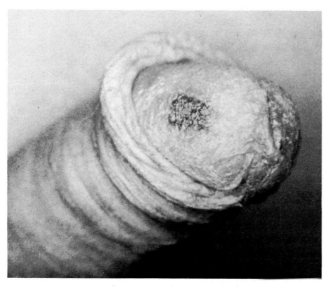

Figure 31–2. Blue nevus of the glans penis. (Courtesy of Dr. Peter Scardino.)

Hirsute papillomas, pearly penile papules, or coronal papillae are common and normal findings on the glans penis and are more frequent in uncircumcised males. They occur in about 15 per cent of postpubertal males (Neinstein and Goldenring, 1984). These lesions consist of linear, curved, or irregular rows of conical or globular excrescences that are arranged along the coronal sulcus and vary in color from white to yellow to red. They are considered acral angiofibromas. When larger than usual, they may be confused with small condylomata acuminata. Treatment is rarely necessary, but when indicated, the CO_2 laser has been described as a successful modality (Magid and Garden, 1989). No association with infection or malignancy is reported (Tannenbaum and Becker, 1965).

The entire range of rashes and ulcers secondary to initiation, allergy, or infection must be considered in the differential diagnosis of the cutaneous lesion.

PREMALIGNANT CUTANEOUS LESIONS

Although the true incidence of progression of any one of these entities to squamous cell carcinoma is unknown, all have been associated with this cancer. In one series, 42 per cent of patients with squamous cell cancer had a history of pre-existing penile lesions (Bouchot et al., 1989).

Cutaneous Horns

The cutaneous horn rarely occurs on the penis. This lesion is characterized by an overgrowth and a cornification of the epithelium, forming a solid protuberance (Fig. 31–3). On microscopic examination, extreme hyperkeratosis, dyskeratosis, and acanthosis are observed. This process usually develops over a pre-existing skin

condition (e.g., wart, nevus, area of trauma, and malignant change) and may enlarge quite rapidly. Treatment consists of surgical excision to include a margin of normal tissue around the base of the lesion. A penile horn may recur and subsequent biopsy findings may prove malignant, whereas initial biopsy findings were benign (Fields et al., 1987). Because this growth may evolve into a carcinoma or may be stimulated by an underlying carcinoma, careful histologic study of the base and close follow-up of the scar are necessary (Hassan et al., 1967; Pressman et al., 1962).

Balanitis Xerotica Obliterans

The most frequent manifestation of balanitis xerotica obliterans is a white patch on the prepuce or on the glans that extends to and around the urethral meatus and occasionally into the fossa navicularis. The meatus itself may appear white, indurated, and edematous (see Fig. 31–3). The lesions may be multiple, involving a large portion of the glans and the prepuce, and may assume a mosaic appearance. Glandular erosions, fissures, and meatal stenosis may occur. Symptoms consist of pain, discharge, pruritus, local penile discomfort, painful erections, and urinary obstruction (Bainbridge et al., 1971).

The lesion occurs in both circumcised and uncircumcised males, but it is more frequent in the latter (Bainbridge et al., 1971). It is most common in middle-aged men but has been reported in children (McKay et al., 1975). The histologic characteristics of the lesion are similar to those of lichen sclerosus et atrophicus found on other cutaneous surfaces (Laymon and Freeman, 1944). The character of the lesion is confirmed by

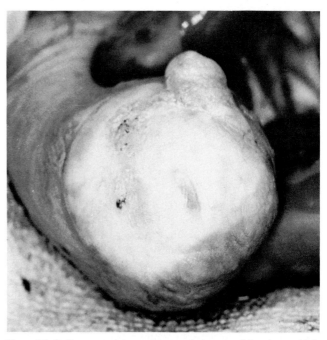

Figure 31–3. Cutaneous horn and mucosal changes of the glans, which histologically demonstrated carcinoma in situ (erythroplasia of Queyrat/Bowen's disease) and balanitis xerotica obliterans of the perimeatal area.

biopsy, which shows an atrophic epidermis with loss of rete pegs, an homogenization of the collagen on the upper third of the dermis, and a zone of lymphocytic and histocytic infiltration.

Treatment is directed at relief of meatal stenosis by meatotomy, urethral dilatation, or local application of topical steroids (Poynter and Levy, 1967). Well-localized lesions on the glans may be treated with a corticosteroid injection (Poynter and Levy, 1967). Surgical excision has also been employed (Rheinschild and Olsen, 1970). Because there are rare reports of malignant degeneration (Jamieson et al., 1986; Laymon and Freeman, 1944; Rheinschild and Olsen, 1970), the lesions require periodic examination and follow-up biopsy if a change in clinical appearance occurs.

Leukoplakia

Leukoplakia is a descriptive term that implies a sharply defined, white, cutaneous plaque, which may be hypertrophic or atrophic. It may be associated with a number of entities. The lesion may be associated with local irritative symptoms. Histologic examination is necessary to determine the presence of malignancy. On histologic examination, hyperkeratosis, parakeratosis, and hypertrophy of the rete pegs with dermal edema and lymphocytic infiltration are seen. Treatment is aimed at elimination of the sources of chronic irritation. Circumcision is warranted in the uncircumcised patient. Both surgical excision and radiation have been employed in the treatment of leukoplakia. Because leukoplakia may coexist with or may antecede the occurrence of carcinoma (Hanash et al., 1970; Reece and Koontz, 1975), close follow-up of the excision scar and periodic biopsy of lesions that have not been completely excised are necessary to detect early evidence of malignant degeneration.

VIRAL-RELATED DERMATOLOGIC LESIONS

A number of penile lesions are related by virtue of an increasing body of information supporting a common viral etiology. The offending virus is the human papillomavirus (HPV).

Condyloma Acuminatum

Condylomata acuminata are typically soft, friable, reddish, cyanotic, papillary lesions, which are also termed "venereal warts" or "genital warts." They have a predilection for the moist, glabrous areas of the body and the mucocutaneous surfaces of the genital and perineal areas. Condylomata may occur singularly on a narrow pedicle or in a grape-like cluster on a sessile, broad base. Condylomata acuminata rarely occur before puberty (Copulsky et al., 1975; Redman and Meacham, 1973).

In the male, condylomata occur most commonly on

the prepuce, the penile shaft, and the glans. The lesions, single or multiple, are apt to recur in the same area or different areas after treatment. Careful inspection may reveal intrameatal lesions, and approximately 5 per cent of patients with condylomata acuminata will demonstrate urethral involvement, which may extend as far proximally as the prostatic urethra (Culp et al., 1944). Bladder involvement, although rare, has been reported, and adequate treatment presents a formidable task (Bissada et al., 1974; Kleiman and Lancaster, 1962).

Condylomata acuminata, on histologic study, appear as an undulating outer layer of keratinized tissue covering papillary fronds that are supported by connective tissue stroma. The epithelial pegs consist of well-ordered rows of squamous cells. A dermal lymphocytic infiltrate is normally present. Caution must be exercised in the interpretation of microscopic abnormalities of condylomata acuminata in the patient who has received treatment with podophyllin. This agent, which affects cell division, can induce histologic changes consistent with carcinoma (King and Sullivan, 1947). Therefore, preliminary biopsy for definitive histologic identification of lesions that appear to be condylomata acuminata, but that are large or atypical, is advisable before podophyllin therapy.

A dramatic increase has occurred in both the knowledge and interest in genital condyloma. The terms, "genital condyloma," "venereal warts," "genital warts," and "genital HPV infection," all refer to a sexually transmitted disease caused by HPV. This interest in HPV infection has occurred for three reasons. First, although it is not a reportable sexually transmitted disease, a current estimate puts the number of new cases of HPV infection at 500,000 to 1 million annually. Prevalence figures are unknown (Stone, 1989). Second, HPV infection is the main etiologic agent in cervical cancer and dysplasia (Lancaster et al., 1986). Third, a significant number of male partners of women with cervical condyloma will have lesions not seen by simple inspection (Sedlacek et al., 1986).

On histologic analysis, the classic finding of a koilocyte (a cell characterized by an empty cavity surrounding an atypical nucleus) is pathognomonic for HPV infection (Schneider, 1989). DNA hybridization techniques have been used to identify infection. This approach is mainly employed as a research tool, but it raises the question of how to treat patients with biopsy results that show viral DNA without the pathologic change typical of viral infection (Carpiniello et al., 1990; Schultz et al., 1990). With the aid of DNA analysis, more than 40 different HPV subtypes have been found. Viral types 6, 11, and 42 to 44 tend to be associated with gross condyloma and low-grade dysplasia. Types 16, 18, 31, 33, 35, and 39 have a higher malignant association (Smotkin, 1989). Different treatment plans have been proposed based on DNA typing (Carpiniello et al., 1990).

If no obvious lesions are seen in a patient referred for diagnosis, a 5 per cent acetic acid soak of the penis for 3 to 5 minutes followed by inspection with magnification identifies subclinical disease (Ferenczy, 1990). Careful inspection of the genitalia, the urethral meatus, and, at times, the entire urethra should be performed. Some urologists utilize a small nasal speculum, whereas others utilize urethroscopy. Any patient with condyloma at the meatus should have a complete urethroscopy (Barrasso et al., 1987; Culp et al., 1944). Because the clinical findings of aceto-white lesions are often nonspecific, it is mandatory that a biopsy of the suspicious lesion be performed before establishing the diagnosis of HPV infection (Krebs, 1989a and b).

A variety of different options exist for the treatment of genital condyloma. Since the reported success in 1944 of podophyllin in the treatment of condylomata acuminata among army recruits (Culp et al., 1944), this agent has been commonly used to eradicate the lesion. Care must be taken to supervise therapy carefully, because normal skin is also disrupted by podophyllin (King and Sullivan, 1947). A 0.5 per cent podophyllotoxin solution has been safely and effectively used in a self-application regimen (Edwards et al., 1988). Trichloroacetic acid applied topically for 3 weeks has provided successful therapy (Ferenczy, 1990). Circumcision is advisable to remove preputial lesions, to gain exposure for treatment, and to permit patient and physician to watch for recurrences. Fulguration and local excision of large, bulky lesions may be advisable to expedite treatment and to avoid large areas of maceration and secondary infection.

Patients with extensive disease will benefit from laser therapy. Both the CO_2 and neodymium-yttrium-aluminum-garnet (Nd:YAG) lasers have been selected to treat genital condyloma. Multifocal, small lesions seen with acetic acid staining and magnification are ideally treated with the CO_2 laser mounted on an operating microscope (Carpiniello et al., 1987). The Nd:YAG laser is an excellent tool for larger lesions on the penis and external genitalia (Bahmer et al., 1984; Stein, 1986). Properly applied laser therapy of the superficial to mid layers of the dermis usually provides an excellent cosmetic result with good eradication of disease.

Intraurethral condyloma can be extremely difficult to treat. Small lesions within the fossa navicularis can be eradicated with the CO_2 laser, with or without a meatotomy (Rosemberg et al., 1982). More proximal urethral lesions are better treated through a cystoscope with the Nd:YAG laser. In addition, a pediatric resectoscope is often helpful in debulking extensive lesions. Every effort should be made to employ minimal electrocautery, which will decrease the potential for developing urethral stricture. Either as a primary or an adjuvant therapy, 5-fluorouracil cream is extremely useful for intraurethral condyloma (Bissada et al., 1974; Boxer and Skinner, 1977; Dretler and Klein, 1975). Care must be taken to protect the scrotal skin from contact with the cream, which can be quite irritating. A scrotal support or zinc oxide cream may be helpful.

Interferon therapy has also been used in the treatment of condyloma (Geffen et al., 1984). A randomized study has shown that intralesional interferon-α 2b, injected three times a week for 3 weeks, has activity against condyloma (Eron et al., 1986). Although these results are encouraging, interferon has thus far been reserved for the treatment of extensive or resistant lesions (Ferenczy, 1990; Krebs, 1989a and b).

Currently, controversy centers on the best method of treatment, whether DNA typing is necessary in all patients, what extent of treatment is necessary in the male, and whether total eradication of HPV infection is truly possible. Initial enthusiasm for extensive and aggressive treatment in the male appeared mainly in the gynecologic literature (Krebs and Schneider, 1987; Levine et al., 1984; Sand et al., 1986; Sedlacek et al., 1986). The incidence of asymptomatic infection in the male partners of women with cervical condyloma or neoplasia varied from 53 to 90 per cent.

As urologists began to evaluate the success rate of laser treatment, recurrence rates varied from 13 per cent (Stein, 1986) to 66 per cent (Carpiniello et al., 1987). In addition, adjuvant 5-fluorouracil did not improve the success rate (Carpiniello et al., 1988). The difference in results may attest to the extent of follow-up and to the various viral subtypes present initially. Recurrences and reinfection may also originate from subclinical intraurethral disease. A treatment protocol has been proposed based on the extent of the initial disease (Carpiniello et al., 1990).

HPV infection is extremely common and potentially carcinogenic. Condyloma have been associated with squamous cell carcinoma of the penis (Beggs and Spratt, 1961; Dawson et al., 1965; Rhatigan et al., 1972). Malignant transformation of condyloma to squamous cell carcinoma has been reported (Boxer and Skinner, 1977; Coetzee, 1977; Pereira-Bringel and de Andrade Arruda, 1982). Condylomata acuminata located in the perianal areas and the oral cavity have undergone malignant degeneration (Siegel, 1962). An increased incidence of penile intraepithelial neoplasia has been found in the male partners of women with cervical intraepithelial neoplasia (Barrasso et al., 1987). HPV infection has been implicated in the development of bowenoid papulosis, a variant of carcinoma in situ (vide infra). The role that HPV plays in the development of condylomatous lesions and their transformation to malignant lesions may be of significant importance, but this area awaits further epidemiologic and molecular study.

Bowenoid Papulosis

Carcinoma in situ of the penis is well recognized since its description many years ago. A new condition, bowenoid papulosis, has been described, which has a similar histologic appearance but a benign clinical course (Kopf and Bart, 1977; Wade et al., 1978).

Bowenoid papulosis occurs as multiple papules, which are often pigmented. These lesions are seen most commonly on the penile skin in the male and vulva in the female and have a peak incidence during the 2nd and 3rd decades of life. Lesions range in size from 0.2 cm to 3 cm in diameter. Smaller lesions will often coalesce into larger ones, explaining the variation in size (Patterson et al., 1986). Pigmented lesions are usually seen on the penile skin, whereas glanular lesions tend to be flat papules (Gross et al., 1985). Clinically, a benign diagnosis is usually made, stressing the importance of biopsy for verification of the malignant process (Peters and Perry, 1981).

Histologically, these lesions meet all the criteria for

carcinoma in situ (Gross et al., 1985; Patterson et al., 1986; Peters and Perry, 1981; Wade et al., 1978). Different growth patterns identified histologically correlate with flat, endophytic and exophytic clinical appearances (Gross et al., 1985). Specific histologic studies seeking a viral etiology have demonstrated intranuclear HPV (Zelickson and Prawer, 1980). A subsequent study extracted total DNA content from 12 biopsy specimens. DNA sequences closely related to HPV 16 were found in all of the samples (Gross et al., 1985).

Bowenoid papulosis has been treated with all the modalities used for external genital lesions. Therapies have included electrodesiccation, cryotherapy, laser, and 5-fluorouracil cream. In general, these treatments have been successful. We treated one 31-year-old man with recurrent disease who experienced failure of conservative therapy with excision of the penile skin and skin grafting. In an analogous situation, vulvectomy has been performed in the female.

In summary, bowenoid papulosis represents a variant of carcinoma in situ of the external genitalia that occurs in younger patients. HPV has been found in these lesions and may have a causative role. To date, progression to an invasive lesion has not been reported.

Kaposi's Sarcoma

Kaposi's sarcoma, first described in 1972 by the dermatologist Moretz Kaposi (1982), is a disease of the reticuloendothelial system, which appears as a cutaneous neovascular tumor. Kaposi's sarcoma occurs as an elevated, painful, bleeding papule or ulcer with bluish discoloration. On histologic examination, the tumor is vasoformative with endothelial proliferation and spindle cell formation.

Initially, Kaposi's sarcoma occurred only rarely in Europe and North America. The condition was characterized by a slowly progressive tumor affecting the lower extremities of older men, usually of Italian or Eastern European Jewish ancestry. The neoplasm is also reported in other distinct populations, namely, young black African men and patients receiving immunosuppressive therapy. Kaposi's sarcoma has been closely associated with patients with acquired immunodeficiency syndrome (AIDS), and in these patients, it is a much more virulent malignancy.

Kaposi's sarcoma is now subcategorized as follows: (1) classic Kaposi's sarcoma, which occurs in a patient without known immunodeficiency and has an indolent and a rarely fatal course; (2) immunosuppressive treatment–related Kaposi's sarcoma, which occurs in a patient receiving immunosuppressive treatment for organ transplantation or other indications and which is often reversed with dose modification of immunosuppressive agents; (3) African Kaposi's sarcoma, which occurs in young males and even prepubescent children and which can be indolent or aggressive in nature; and (4) epidemic Kaposi's sarcoma, which occurs in a patient with AIDS.

The classic and immunosuppressive categories are considered nonepidemic. Nonepidemic Kaposi's sarcoma restricted to involvement of the penis should be aggressively treated because it is rarely associated with diffuse organ involvement. Localized surgical excision or small-field external beam or electron beam radiation has proved effective. With wider areas of involvement, partial penectomy is indicated. In the immunosuppressed patient, Kaposi's sarcoma will frequently regress with discontinuation of the immunosuppressive therapy. If this regression does not occur, local excision or external beam radiation should be considered. Systemic treatment for multisystem involvement with Kaposi's sarcoma has employed interferon and cytotoxic therapy (National Cancer Institute Position Statement, 1990).

The underlying immune deficiency associated with AIDS predisposes the host to Kaposi's sarcoma. The first case of AIDS epidemic Kaposi's sarcoma was reported in 1981 (Friedman, 1981), and the first case involving the penis was reported in 1986 (Seftel et al., 1986). Since that time, Kaposi's sarcoma of the penis has become a relatively common lesion in the patient with AIDS. Kaposi's sarcoma involves the penis more in the homosexual male population than in other patients with AIDS. In the first 1000 cases of AIDS reported by the Centers for Disease Control, the incidence of penile Kaposi's sarcoma was 44 per cent in homosexual and bisexual male patients compared with only 16 per cent in intravenous drug abusers with AIDS and 0 per cent in hemophilic patients with AIDS (Bayne and Wise, 1988; Jaffe et al., 1983).

In many patients with AIDS, Kaposi's sarcoma appears as the presenting sign of disease. However, Kaposi's sarcoma of the penis is rarely the first area of involvement and is usually associated with other systemic lesions. The treatment of the sarcoma itself is, therefore, directed toward palliation (Lowe et al., 1989). Particular problems arise when the sarcoma involves the glans penis or corpus spongiosum, causing urethral obstruction.

A number of options exist, with the simplest being the creation of a cutaneous urethrostomy proximal to the lesion. With such distal urethral involvement, the urethrostomy created at the penoscrotal junction allows for voiding in the erect position. In some patients with exceptionally large lesions involving the distal penis or with diffuse involvement of the penis extending to the pendulous portion of the penile urethra, a partial penectomy or total penectomy with creation of a perineal urethrostomy is an option.

Other than surgical excision and urethrostomy, the Nd:YAG laser has been used in some instances for lesions of the glans penis and fossa navicularis to alleviate urethral obstruction (Wishnow and Johnson, 1988). Additionally, partial responses with radiotherapy delivered by either external beam techniques or intraurethral luminal techniques have been noted.

BUSCHKE-LÖWENSTEIN TUMOR (VERRUCOUS CARCINOMA, GIANT CONDYLOMA ACUMINATUM)

The characteristics of the Buschke-Löwenstein tumor were recognized by Buschke and Löwenstein in 1925, and later by Löwenstein in 1939 in the United States. A histologically identical lesion termed "verrucous carcinoma" was described as occurring in the oral cavity (Ackerman, 1948). Whereas verrucous carcinomas of nonpenile sites do metastasize, metastasis from Buschke-Löwenstein tumors is extremely rare. Because of its large size and its resemblance to condyloma acuminatum, the term "giant condyloma" has also been used to identify this lesion. Frequently, it is grossly indistinguishable from squamous cell carcinoma. It may originally occur as a small, localized papillary growth, which over a period of time develops into a large, necrotic, exophytic lesion that may cover and destroy much of the penis. Urethral erosion and fistulization occur. This progressive growth, associated with discharge, odor, and bleeding, prompts the patient to seek medical attention.

The true incidence of the Buschke-Löwenstein tumor is unknown. It is undoubtedly higher than reported, because many of these tumors are labeled as low-grade squamous cell carcinoma of the penis. Retrospective analyses of series of penile carcinomas have revealed a number of verrucous cancers or giant condylomata included under the category of low-grade squamous cell carcinomas (Davies, 1965; Hanash et al., 1970).

As in the case of condyloma acuminatum, the etiology may be viral (Dawson et al., 1965; Ubben et al., 1979). HPV 6 and 11 have been identified in these tumors (Boshart and zur Hausen, 1986). The Buschke-Löwenstein tumor differs from condyloma acuminatum in that the latter, no matter how large, remains superficial, sparing adjacent tissue. The Buschke-Löwenstein tumor, however, displaces, penetrates, and destroys adjacent structures by compression. Apart from this unrestrained local growth, it shows no signs of malignancy on histologic examination. On microscopic examination, the tumor forms a luxuriant mass composed of broad, rounded rete pegs, which often extends far into the underlying tissue. The pegs are composed of well-differentiated squamous cells that show no cellular anaplasia. These epithelial pegs are characteristically surrounded by a dense band of acute and chronic inflammatory cells.

Lymph node metastases are rare with verrucous carcinoma (Ackerman, 1948; Davies, 1965), and their presence probably reflects malignant degeneration in the primary lesion. Malignant alterations are known to evolve in verrucous carcinoma of the larynx, the oral cavity, and the female genital area (Davies, 1965; Dawson et al., 1965). Anecdotal cases of malignant degeneration have been reported in association with carcinoma of the penis (Youngberg et al., 1983).

Excisional biopsy or multiple deep biopsies are necessary to distinguish the lesion from true penile carcinoma. Once the diagnosis has been established, treatment consists of excision, sparing as much of the penis as possible. Large lesions, however, may require total amputation. Because of the high frequency of recurrence after surgery, close follow-up is required. Treatment with podophyllin has proved unsuccessful, probably because of its inability to penetrate the thick layer of stratum corneum that is characteristic of the tumor. Topical administration of 5-fluorouracil has also been reported to be unsuccessful (Bruns et al., 1975).

At present, topical chemotherapy has no place in the treatment of any large, exophytic penile cancer. Bleomycin has been suggested as a primary or adjunctive mode of therapy for verrucous carcinoma (Misma and Matunalea, 1972). Radiation therapy is not advised. It is ineffective and has been associated with rapid malignant changes when directed at verrucous carcinoma in other locations (Kraus and Perez-Mesa, 1966; Lepow and Leffler, 1960; Proffitt et al., 1970).

SQUAMOUS CELL CARCINOMA

Carcinoma In Situ (Erythroplasia of Queyrat, Bowen's Disease)

Carcinoma in situ of the penis is appropriately discussed here. This lesion has not routinely been identified as carcinoma of the penis. Urologists and dermatologists refer to this lesion as erythroplasia of Queyrat or Bowen's disease. This nomenclature has served to separate carcinoma in situ from the mainstream of the thinking and reporting of penile carcinoma. However, the epidemiology and natural history of this lesion parallel that of early carcinoma of the penis, and carcinoma in situ can precede and progress to invasive carcinoma.

The erythroplasia described originally by Queyrat in 1911 consists of a red, velvety, well-marginated lesion found on the glans penis and, less frequently, on the prepuce (Fig. 31–4) (Aragona et al., 1985) invarably in the uncircumcised male. It occasionally is superficially ulcerative and is associated with discharge and pain.

On histologic examination, the normal mucosa is replaced by atypical hyperplastic cells characterized by disorientation, vacuolation, multiple hyperchromatic nuclei, and mitotic figures at all levels. The epithelial rete extends into the submucosa and appears elongated, broadened, and bulbous. The submucosa shows capillary proliferation and ectasia with a surrounding inflammatory infiltrate, usually rich in plasma cells. These microscopic features distinguish it from chronic localized balanitis, which it may grossly resemble. HPV has been identified in carcinoma in situ (Pfister and Haneke, 1984).

Intraepithelial neoplasm of the skin associated with a high occurrence of subsequent internal malignancy was described as a distinct entity by Bowen in 1912. When Bowen's disease occurs on the penis, it is called erythroplasia of Queyrat, and the two conditions are similar on histologic examination (Graham and Helwig, 1973). They are both characterized by the noninvasive epithelial cellular changes of carcinoma in situ. Visceral malignancy is not associated with erythroplasia of Queyrat and, although traditionally Bowen's disease was believed to be a marker for internal malignancy, case-control studies have not confirmed this association (Epstein, 1960). Therefore, penile carcinoma in situ does not warrant a specific search for internal malignancy.

Treatment requires proper identification of malignancy. Therefore, biopsies should be multiple and of adequate depth to detect invasion. When lesions are

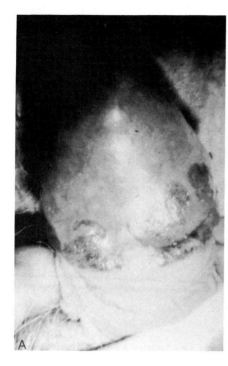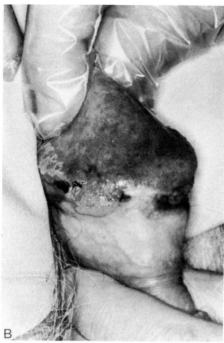

Figure 31–4. Erythroplasia of Queyrat's disease characterized by superficial erythematous lesions on the glans penis and coronal sulcus.

small and noninvasive, local excision that spares penile anatomic structure and function is adequate. If a lesion is preputial, circumcision will suffice. Fulguration is occasionally successful but often is associated with recurrences. Radiation therapy has been successful in eradicating the lesion, and appropriately delivered and planned radiation results in minimal morbidity (Grabstald and Kelley, 1980; Kelley et al., 1974).

Topical 5-fluorouracil has been administered with good success and few complications (Goette, 1974; Graham and Helwig, 1973; Hueser and Pugh, 1969; Lewis and Bendl, 1971). Five per cent 5-fluorouracil base cream causes denudation and dissolution of areas involved with malignant and premalignant changes while preserving normal skin. Cosmetic results are excellent. Recurrences are treated simply with repeated application. Systemic absorption of 5-fluorouracil is minimal (Dillaha et al., 1965). Isolated reports about CO_2 laser therapy (Rosemberg and Fuller, 1980), liquid nitrogen cryosurgery (Madej and Meyza, 1982; Mortimer et al., 1983; Sonnex et al., 1982), and Nd:YAG laser (Landthaler et al., 1986) have described both excellent control of disease and cosmetic outcome.

Invasive Carcinoma

Incidence

Penile carcinoma constitutes less than 1 per cent of all malignancies among the United States' male population—an incidence of 1 to 2 cases per 100,000 per annum. It is most commonly diagnosed during the 6th and 7th decades of life; in two studies, the mean age was 58 years (Gursel et al., 1973) and 55 years (Derrick et al., 1973). It is not rare, however, among males in the 4th and 5th decades of life. Of patients in one large series, 22 per cent were younger than 40 years of age

(Dean, 1935). Carcinoma of the penis has been reported in children (Kini, 1944; Narasimharao et al., 1985).

No identifiable racial predisposition has been encountered in some series (Beggs and Spratt, 1961); others have found an increased incidence in the black population (Johnson et al., 1973). Rather than showing genetic predilection, the proportionally greater frequency among blacks may be a reflection of the greater number of uncircumcised black males (Schrek and Lenowitz, 1947).

Etiology

The incidence of carcinoma of the penis varies markedly with the hygienic standards and the cultural and religious practices of different countries. Circumcision has been well established as a prophylactic measure that virtually eliminates the occurrence of penile carcinoma. Development of penile carcinoma among the uncircumcised has been attributed to the chronic irritative effects of smegma, a by-product of bacterial action on desquamated cells that are retained within the preputial sac. This chronic irritation and exposure are accentuated by the presence of phimosis, which most large series report to occur in 25 to 75 per cent of patients presenting with carcinoma of the penis.

Although definite evidence that smegma is a carcinogen is lacking (Reddy and Baruah, 1963), it nevertheless must be suspect (Plaut and Kohn-Speyer, 1947; Pratt-Thomas et al., 1956). Carcinoma of the scrotum has been clearly identified as being associated with chemical irritants that act as carcinogens (e.g., coal, dust, tar, paraffin); however, a relationship between carcinoma of the penis and these chemicals does not exist, although its exposure must be identical to that of the scrotum.

Carcinoma of the penis is almost unknown among the Jewish population, among whom neonatal circumcision is customary. When it does occur, the rarity warrants comment (Licklider, 1961). In the United States, where neonatal circumcision is frequent, penile carcinoma composes less than 1 per cent of malignancies in the male. This figure is in marked contrast to the incidence of carcinoma of the penis among the uncircumcised African tribes (Dodge, 1965) and the uncircumcised Asian population, among whom it composes 10 to 20 per cent of all malignancies in the male. In Paraquay, penile carcinoma is the most common genitourinary malignancy (Lynch and Krush, 1969). In India, carcinoma of the penis is extremely rare among the neonatally circumcised Jewish population. It is somewhat more frequent among Muslims who practice prepubertal circumcision and it is quite common among the uncircumcised Christian and Hindu population (Paymaster and Gangadharan, 1967).

Data from most large series reveal that the tumor, although rarely developing in the neonatally circumcised, is more frequent when circumcision is delayed until puberty (Frew et al., 1967; Gursel et al., 1973; Johnson et al., 1973). Adult circumcision offers little or no protection against the future appearance of penile carcinoma (Thomas and Small, 1963). Some period of exposure to smegma, however brief, may account for the decreased effectiveness of pubertal circumcision and the negligible protective effect of adult circumcision.

Routine neonatal circumcision is periodically decried as a form of aesthetic and sexual mutilation (Morgan, 1965; Preston, 1970). The American Academy of Pediatrics Task Force on Circumcision reported as follows: The 1971 edition of Standards and Recommendations of Hospital Care of Newborn Infants by the Committee on the Fetus and Newborn of the American Academy of Pediatrics (AAP) stated that "there are no valid medical indications for circumcision in the neonatal period." In 1975, an ad hoc task force of the same committee reviewed this statement and concluded that "there is no absolute medical indication for routine circumcision of the newborn." The 1975 recommendation was reiterated in 1983 by both the AAP and the American College of Obstetrics and Gynecology in the jointly published *Guidelines to Perinatal Care* (Schoen et al., 1989).

Since the 1975 report, new evidence has suggested possible medical benefits from newborn circumcision. Data now suggest that the incidence of urinary tract infection in male infants may be reduced when this procedure is performed during the newborn period. Additional information has been published concerning the relationship of circumcision to sexually transmitted diseases and, in turn, the relationship of viral sexually transmitted diseases to cancer of the penis and cervix. In 1988, the Task Force (Schoen et al., 1989) revised its assessment as follows: "Newborn circumcision has potential medical benefits and advantages as well as disadvantages and risks. When circumcision is being considered, the benefits and risks should be explained to the parents and informed consent obtained."

It is reasonable to consider that circumcision may not be as important in countries in which good hygiene is practical and soap and water are readily available. However, argument against circumcision must take into account the fact that penile carcinoma represents the only neoplasm for which there exists a predictable and simple means of prophylaxis that spares the organ at risk (Dagher et al., 1973) and must also now consider the findings of the task force regarding infection.

Although a history of trauma often predates the appearance of carcinoma of the penis, it is thought that this finding is coincidental rather than causal (Hanash et al., 1970). However, the development of carcinoma in the scarred penile shaft skin after mutilating circumcision has been reported as a distinct entity (Fig. 31–5) (Bissada et al., 1986). No consistent etiologic relationship of penile carcinoma to venereal disease (syphilis, granuloma inguinale, and chancroid) has been found, and any association of these diseases with penile carcinoma is probably coincidental (Schrek and Lenowitz, 1947).

An etiologic factor of current interest is viral infection. The association of penile carcinoma and cervical carcinoma has related both to herpesvirus infection. A threefold to eightfold increase in the incidence of cervical carcinoma among the sexual partners of patients with penile carcinomas has been documented in several series (Goldberg et al., 1979). However, this relationship has not been confirmed by others (Redd et al., 1977). Penile carcinoma has also been associated with sexually transmitted HPV. A study from Brazil found HPV 18 DNA sequences in seven of 18 cases (Villa and Lopes, 1986).

Although the state of immune suppression among the renal transplant population is associated with a marked increase in squamous cell malignancies, only one case of penile cancer in a transplant recipient has been reported (Previte et al., 1979).

Natural History

Carcinoma of the penis usually begins with a small lesion, which gradually extends to involve the entire glans, shaft, and corpora. The lesion may be papillary and exophytic or flat and ulcerative; if untreated, penile autoamputation may eventually occur. The rates of growth of the papillary and ulcerative lesions are quite similar, but the flat ulcerative tumor has a tendency to earlier nodal metastasis and is associated with poorer 5-year survival rates (Dean, 1935; Marcial et al., 1962). Lesions larger than 5 cm (Beggs and Spratt, 1961) and those extending to cover 75 per cent of the shaft (Staubitz et al., 1955) are also associated with an increased incidence of metastases and a decreased survival rate. However, a consistent relationship of lesion size to the presence of metastasis and to decreased survival has been questioned (Ekstrom and Edsmyr, 1958; Puras et al., 1978).

Buck's fascia acts as a temporary natural barrier, protecting the corporal bodies from invasion of neoplasm. Penetration of Buck's fascia and the tunica albuginea permits invasion of the vascular corpora and establishes the potential for vascular dissemination. Urethral and bladder involvement is rare (Riveros and Gorostiaga, 1962; Thomas and Small, 1963).

Metastases to the regional femoral and iliac nodes represent the earliest route of dissemination from penile

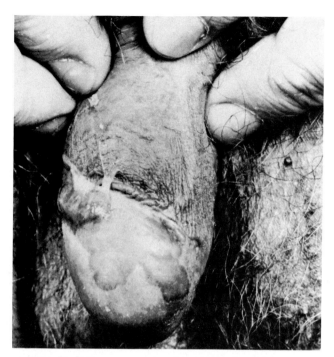

Figure 31–5. Cancer appearing along dorsal circumcision scar.

carcinoma. A detailed description of lymphatic drainage of the penis is found elsewhere in this text. Briefly, the lymphatics of the prepuce form a connecting network that joins with lymphatics from the skin of the shaft. These tributaries drain into the superficial inguinal nodes (the nodes above the fascia lata). The lymphatics of the glans join the lymphatics draining the corporal bodies, and they form a collar of connecting channels at the base of the penis that drain by way of the superficial nodes, hence, to the deep inguinal nodes (the nodes beneath the fascia lata) and, from there, to the pelvic nodes (external iliac, internal iliac, and obturator). Penile lymphangiogram studies demonstrate a consistent pattern of drainage that proceeds from superficial inguinal to deep inguinal to pelvic node sites without evidence of skip drainage (Cabanas, 1977). Multiple cross-communications exist throughout all levels of drainage, so that penile lymphatic drainage is bilateral to both inguinal areas.

Metastatic enlargement of the regional nodes eventually leads to skin necrosis, chronic infection, and death from inanition, sepsis, or hemorrhage secondary to erosion into the femoral vessels. Clinically detectable distant metastatic lesions to the lung, liver, bone, or brain are uncommon and are reported as occurring in 1 to 10 per cent of large series (Beggs and Spratt, 1961; Derrick et al., 1973; Johnson et al., 1973; Kossow et al., 1973; Puras et al., 1978; Riveros and Gorostiaga, 1962; Staubitz et al., 1955). Such metastases usually occur late in the course of the disease after the local lesion has been treated. Distant metastases in the absence of regional node metastases are unusual.

Carcinoma of the penis is characterized by a relentless progressive course, causing death for the majority of untreated patients within 2 years (Beggs and Spratt, 1961; Derrick et al., 1973; Skinner et al., 1972). Rarely, long-term survival will occur, even with advanced local disease and regional node metastases (Beggs and Spratt, 1961; Furlong and Uhle, 1953). No report of spontaneous remission of carcinoma of the penis is known. About 5 to 15 per cent of patients have been reported to subsequently develop a second primary neoplasm (Beggs and Spratt, 1961; Buddington et al., 1963; Gursel et al., 1973). One analysis reported secondary carcinoma in 17 per cent of patients (Hubbell et al., 1988).

Modes of Presentation

Signs

Almost without exception, the penile lesion itself calls attention to the possibility of carcinoma. It may appear as an area of induration or erythema, a small bump, a pimple, a warty growth, or a more luxuriant, exophytic lesion. Alternatively, it may appear as a shallow-based, nonhealing erosion or a deeply excavating ulcer with elevated or rolled-in margins (Fig. 31–6). Phimosis may obscure a lesion and thus result in a prolonged period of neglect. Eventually, erosions through the prepuce, a foul preputial odor, and discharge with or without bleeding call attention to disease (Fig. 31–7).

Penile carcinoma is most frequent on the glans, the coronal sulcus, and the prepuce. It is less commonly found on the shaft or at the meatus. A possible explanation is that the shaft and the meatus—unlike the glans, coronal sulcus, and inner surface of the prepuce—are not constantly exposed to smegma and other irritants contained within the preputial sac.

Occasionally a mass, an ulceration, a necrosis, a suppuration, and a hemorrhage in the inguinal area resulting from nodal metastases present before a lesion concealed in the phimotic preputial sac (Fig. 31–8).

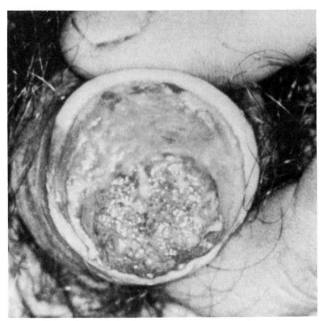

Figure 31–6. Ulcerating invasive lesion of the glans penis obscuring meatus. Foreskin has been retracted.

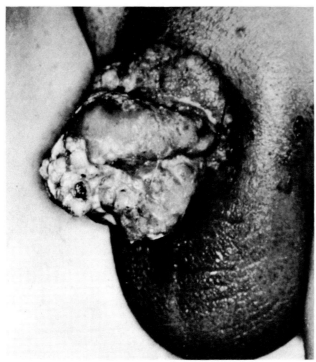

Figure 31–7. Ulcerating lesion perforating phimotic prepuce, associated with extensive purulence and secondary infection.

Local corporal involvement rarely progresses to the stage at which urinary retention and urinary fistula are among the presenting signs, but these symptoms associated with autoamputation of the penis may occur (Fig. 31–9).

Symptoms

Pain does not develop in proportion to the extent of the local destructive process and usually is not a presenting complaint. Weakness, weight loss, fatigue, and systemic malaise occur secondary to chronic suppuration. Occasionally, significant blood loss from the penile lesion or the nodal lesion, or both, occurs. Presenting symptoms referable to distant metastases are rare because local and regional nodal disease are characteristically far advanced before distant metastases are detectable.

Diagnosis

Delay

The time from the initiation of signs and symptoms to the time of the patient's presentation to a physician is usually long, considering the rather advanced condition of the lesions. From 15 to 50 per cent of patients have been reported to delay medical care for more than 1 year (Buddington et al., 1963; Dean, 1935; Furlong and Uhle, 1953; Gursel et al., 1973; Hardner et al., 1972). Patients with carcinoma of the penis, more than patients with other types of carcinoma, delay seeking medical attention (Lynch and Krush, 1969). Explana-

tions are multiple, namely, personal neglect, embarrassment, guilt, fear, and ignorance. No reason appears justified, however, because the penis is an organ that is handled and observed on a daily basis.

Of even greater concern are the estimates of the length of delay by the physician in initiating appropriate therapy (Lynch and Krush, 1969). According to some studies (Ekstrom and Edsmyr, 1958; Johnson et al., 1973), the difference in survival rates between patients who present early and those who present later is negligible. However, decreased survival rates associated with longer delay have been noted by others (Hardner et al., 1972). It appears logical that patients would have achieved better survival rates if they had been treated earlier.

Examination

At clinical presentation, the majority of lesions are confined to the penis (Derrick et al., 1973; Johnson et al., 1973; Skinner et al., 1972). The penile lesion is assessed with regard to its size, location, fixation, and involvement of the corporal bodies. Inspection of the base of the penis and scrotum is necessary to rule out extension into these areas. Rectal and bimanual examination provide information regarding perineal body invasion or the presence of a pelvic mass. Careful bilateral palpation of the inguinal area for adenopathy is of extreme importance.

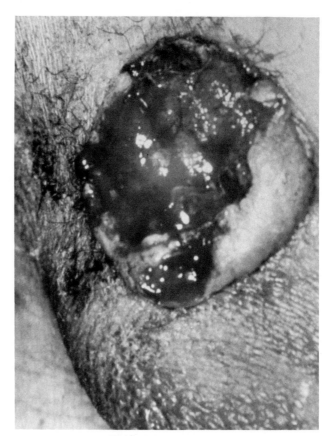

Figure 31–8. Ulcerating inguinal nodal metastasis from carcinoma of the penis.

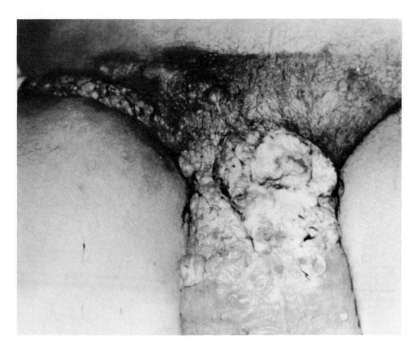

Figure 31–9. Extensive invasive carcinoma of the penis with autoamputation of the glans and shaft. Extensive inguinal nodal metastasis shows ulceration and secondary infection. Multiple satellite lesions involve the scrotal skin.

Biopsy

Identifying carcinoma of the penis and depth of invasion by microscope study of a biopsy specimen is mandatory before initiation of therapy. Biopsy may be a separate procedure from amputation. Frequently, a dorsal slit is necessary to gain adequate exposure of the lesion for appropriate biopsy. No harmful effects regarding tumor dissemination secondary to biopsy are recognized. Biopsy with confirmation of tumor by frozen section while the patient is still anesthetized, and immediate surgical excision with partial or total amputation (with full prior informed consent from the patient) would constitute an alternative means of diagnosis and simultaneous treatment.

Histology

The majority of tumors of the penis are squamous cell carcinomas demonstrating keratinization, epithelial pearl formation, and various degrees of mitotic activity. The normal rete pegs are disrupted. Invasive lesions penetrate the basement membrane and surrounding structures.

Grading

Most malignancies of the penis are low grade (Murrell and Williams, 1965; Staubitz et al., 1955). Lack of correlation between grade and survival has been noted by a number of investigators (Beggs and Spratt, 1961; Edwards and Sawyers, 1968; Hardner et al., 1972; Johnson et al., 1973; Kuruvilla et al., 1971; Staubitz et al., 1955). In contrast, other series have reported reduced survival rates among patients with anaplastic neoplasms (Ekstrom and Edsmyr, 1958, Frew et al., 1967; Hanash et al., 1970; Marcial et al., 1962; Puras et al., 1978). One review emphasized the association of high-grade disease with regional nodal metastases

(Fraley et al., 1989). Patterns of growth have occasionally been a prognostic aid (Frew et al., 1967). A relationship between the degree of plasma cell, lymphocytic, or eosinophilic infiltrate and survival has not been found (Kuruvilla et al., 1971).

The loss of cell surface blood group antigens has been associated with invasion and metastases (Prasad and Veliath, 1986). The determination of DNA ploidy using archival pathology material has been related to the prognosis in a number of urogenital and nonurogenital malignancies. Aneuploidy may predict disease of greater biologic potential for growth and metastases. Ploidy analysis of squamous cell carcinoma of the penis is limited to a small number of patients and thus far has not provided significant prognostic information (Hoofnagle et al., 1990; McConnell, J. D., personal communication, 1990).

The strongest prognostic indicator for survival is the presence or absence of nodal metastasis (Tables 31–1 and 31–2).

Laboratory Studies

Laboratory evaluation findings in patients with penile carcinoma are usually normal. Anemia, leukocytosis, and hypoalbuminemia may be present in patients with chronic illness, malnutrition, and extensive suppuration at the area of the primary and inguinal metastatic sites. Azotemia may occur secondary to urethral or ureteral obstruction. Hypercalcemia in the absence of detectable osseous metastasis associated with penile carcinoma has been noted (Anderson and Glenn, 1965; Rudd et al., 1972).

In a review from Memorial Sloan-Kettering Cancer Center (Sklaroff and Yagoda, 1982), 17 of 81 patients (20.9 per cent) with penile carcinoma were hypercalcemic; 16 of 17 patients (94 per cent) with clinical inguinal metastases were hypercalcemic. Hypercalcemia seems to be largely a function of the bulk of the disease.

Table 31–1. CARCINOMA OF THE PENIS—PROGNOSTIC INDICATORS FOR SURVIVAL

Series	Number of Patients	Clinical and Pathologic Characteristics of Inguinal Adenopathy			5-Year Survival Rates (%)	
		Per Cent with Palpable Nodes	Per Cent Clinically False-Positive (Nodes Palpable, Histologic Findings Negative)	Per Cent Clinically False-Negative (Nodes Not Palpable, Histologic Findings Positive)	Inguinal Nodes Negative on Histologic or Repeated Physical Examination	Inguinal Nodes Resected and Positive on Histologic Examination of Adenectomy Specimen
Ekstrom and Edsmyr 1958	229	33	48	—	80[a]	42
Beggs and Spratt 1961	88	35	36	20	72.5	45
Thomas and Small 1963	190	—	64	20	—	26
Edwards and Sawyers 1968	77	—	—	0	68	25
Hanash and co-workers, 1970	169	—	58[b]	2[b]	77[c]	
Kuruvilla and co-workers, 1971	153	39	63	10	69	33
Hardner and co-workers, 1972	100	42	41[b]	16[b]	—	—
Gursel and co-workers, 1973	64	53	60[b]	—	58	—
Skinner and co-workers, 1972	34	29	40	—	75 / 87[d]	20 / 50[d]
DeKernion and co-workers, 1973	48	54	38[b]	—	84[e]	55[e]
Derrick and co-workers, 1973	87	29	52	—	53 / 76[d]	22 / 55[d]
Johnson and co-workers, 1973	153	—	—	—	64.4	21.8
Kossow and co-workers, 1973	100	51	49	25	—	—
Puras and co-workers, 1978	576	82	47	38[b]	89	67[g] / 29[h]
Cabanas, 1977	80	96	65	100	90	70[i] / 50[j] / 20[k]
Fossa and co-workers, 1987	79	—	—	13	90	80[l] / 20[m]
Srinivas and co-workers, 1987	199	63	14[u]	18	74	82[n] / 54[o] / 40[p] / 12[q]
McDougal and co-workers, 1986	65	—	—	66	100	83[r] / 66[s] / 38[t]

[a]Majority of patients received prophylactic or preoperative radiotherapy to inguinal area.
[b]Histologic classification based on node biopsy, not node dissection.
[c]Corrected 5-year survival; i.e., patients dying before 5 years without evidence of disease are excluded.
[d]Patients dying free of cancer before 5 years are considered surgical cures.
[e]Three-year survival.
[f]Omitted.
[g]Positive findings in inguinofemoral nodes.
[h]Positive findings in inguinofemoral and pelvic nodes.
[i]Single inguinal node with positive findings.
[j]More than one inguinal node with positive findings.
[k]Three-year survival with positive findings in inguinal and pelvic nodes.
[l]N1–2.
[m]N3.
[n]One node positive.
[o]One to six nodes positive.
[p]Greater than six nodes positive.
[q]Bilateral nodes positive.
[r]Adjunctive adenectomy.
[s]Immediate therapeutic adenectomy.
[t]Delayed therapeutic adenectomy.
[u]After antibiotic therapy.

It is often associated with inguinal metastases and may resolve with surgical removal of the inguinal nodes (Block et al., 1973). Parahormone-like substances may be produced by the tumor and metastases (Malakoff and Schmidt, 1975). Medical treatment includes saline hydration and administration of diuretics, steroids, calcitonin, and mithramycin (Linderman and Papper, 1975).

Radiologic Studies

Metastases to lung, bone, and brain are rarely identified on radiographic examination or scanning. Intravenous pyelography usually demonstrates normal findings unless there is massive retroperitoneal adenopathy. The role of lymphangiography is not well established because certain difficulties are inherent in the study.

Table 31–2. FIVE-YEAR SURVIVAL RELATED TO EXTENT OF NODAL METASTASIS

Series	Number of Patients	Number of Positive Nodes	
		≤2	>2
Fraley and co-workers, 1989	31	15/17 (88%)	1/14 (7%)
Johnson and Lo, 1984a	22	6/7 (85%)*	2/15 (13%)
Srinivas and co-workers, 1987	119	5/6 (82%)	7/34 (20%)
			9/16 (54%)†
Fossa and co-workers, 1987	18	11/12 (88%)‡	2/6 (33%)§

*Approximate.
†A subset with one to six positive nodes.
‡N1–2.
§N3.

The filling of external iliac nodes might be suboptimal because of the inflammatory or metastatic obstruction in the superficial and deep inguinal systems, and distinction between inflammatory and metastatic nodal changes is difficult in the inguinal area. However, lymphangiography has been utilized to direct fine needle aspiration assessment of nodes and would seem to be most helpful in identification of nodal abnormalities in the common iliac and para-aortic nodes.

In patients with high-grade or invasive histology, inguinal adenopathy, or abnormalities on bimanual examination, computed tomography of the abdomen and pelvis can identify pelvic and para-aortic adenopathy. Positive identification of tumor in these nodes by needle aspiration cytology or biopsy contraindicates surgery alone and identifies patients for investigational studies, combining chemotherapy with surgery (see discussion of chemotherapy).

Staging

Accurate assessment of the extent of the primary lesion and identification of regional and distant metastatic disease are necessary in directing appropriate initial therapy and assessing end results. However, clinical evaluation for the presence of inguinal metastases is subject to significant inaccuracy. Furthermore, no universally accepted staging system for penile carcinoma exists (Baker and Watson, 1975).

The most commonly employed classification was suggested by Jackson (Table 31–3) (Jackson, 1966). The cross-comparison of results among different series is often quite impossible. Specifically, the characteristics of the initial primary lesion—whether it is confined to the epidermis, superficially or deeply invasive, small, large, limited to the glans or involving other structures—are not stated. Also, the characteristics of nodal metastases—whether they are solitary or multiple, unilateral or bilateral, superficial inguinal, deep inguinal, pelvic, or any combination of these—are not stated.

The Jackson staging system for penile carcinoma is a clinical one. However, histopathology of the primary lesion provides important prognostic features, including grade and extent of invasion, which, in turn, direct treatment decisions. Therefore, a description of the lesion should supplement stage designation. The tumor, node, and metastasis (TNM) staging system (Table 31–4 and Fig. 31–10) most precisely describes depth of invasion. Table 31–5 lists the diagnostic criteria for TNM designations.

Stage distribution at clinical presentation varies with the geographic origin of the series. For example, a less than 5 per cent incidence of stage IV penile carcinoma was found in a series from Dallas (Ewalt and McConnell, 1990) compared with a 35 per cent incidence of stage IV in a series from India (Kaushal and Sharma, 1987).

Differential Diagnosis

A number of penile lesions must be considered in the differential diagnosis of penile carcinoma. They include some of the lesions previously discussed, namely, condyloma acuminatum, Buschke-Löwenstein tumor, and a number of inflammatory lesions, such as chancre, chancroid, herpes, lymphopathia venereum, granuloma inguinale, and tuberculosis. These diseases can be identified by appropriate skin tests, tissue studies, serologic examinations, cultures, or specialized staining techniques.

TREATMENT OF THE PRIMARY NEOPLASM

Amputation by partial or total penectomy has been the gold standard of therapy. The low incidence of distant metastatic disease, the significant morbidity that can result from untreated local disease, and the success of long-term palliation and survival even with advanced local disease, support aggressive local therapy whenever possible. The disfigurement that occurs with amputation has directed efforts toward organ-sparing techniques employing partial excision or Mohs surgery and nonsurgical techniques employing x-ray, laser, or cryodestruc-

Table 31–3. CLASSIFICATION FOR CARCINOMA OF THE PENIS

Stage I (A)	Tumors confined to glans, prepuce, or both
Stage II (B)	Tumors extending onto shaft of penis
Stage III (C)	Tumors with inguinal metastasis that are operable
Stage IV (D)	Tumors involving adjacent structures; tumors associated with inoperable inguinal metastasis or distant metastasis

Adapted from Jackson, S. M.: The treatment of carcinoma of the penis. Br. J. Surg., 53:33, 1966. By permission of the publisher, Butterworth-Heinemann Ltd.

Table 31–4. TNM CLASSIFICATION OF
PENILE CARCINOMA

Primary Tumor (T)
TX   Primary tumor cannot be assessed
T0   No evidence of primary tumor
Tis Carcinoma in situ
       Ta Noninvasive verrucous carcinoma
T1   Tumor invades subepithelial connective tissue
T2   Tumor invades corpus spongiosum or cavernosum
T3   Tumor invades urethra or prostate
T4   Tumor invades other adjacent structures

Regional Lymph Nodes (N)
NX   Regional lymph nodes cannot be assessed
N0   No regional lymph node metastasis
N1   Metastasis in a single, superficial, inguinal lymph node
N2   Metastasis in multiple or bilateral superficial inguinal lymph
       nodes
N3   Metastasis in deep inguinal or pelvic lymph node(s),
       unilateral or bilateral

Distant Metastases (M)
MX   Presence of distant metastasis cannot be assessed
M0   No distant metastases
M1   Distant metastases

Adapted from Union Internationale Contre le Cancer (UICC): TNM Atlas: Illustrated Guide to the TNM/pTNM-Classification of Malignant Tumours, Ed. 3. New York, Springer-Verlag, 1989, pp 237–244 and American Joint Committee on Cancer: from Manual Staging for Cancer, Ed. 3. Philadelphia, J. B. Lippincott Co., 1988, pp 189–191.

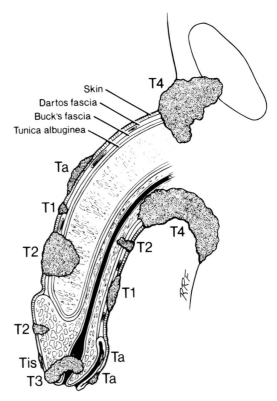

Figure 31–10. Because treatment decisions for inguinal node dissections are currently based on the characteristics of the primary lesion (see Treatment of Inguinal Nodes), a careful assessment of the *depth of invasion* of the primary is required. The diagram illustrates the importance of depth of invasion in assigning tumor (T) stage.

tion. The necessary goal of any of these treatment modalities is complete destruction of the primary tumor.

Conventional Surgical Treatment

In certain selected cases of small lesions involving only the prepuce, complete tumor excision with tumor-free margins may be accomplished by circumcision (Ekstrom and Edsmyr, 1958). Circumcision alone, however, is frequently followed by tumor recurrence (Gursel et al., 1973; Hardner et al., 1972; Marcial et al., 1962). Two series documented postcircumcision recurrence rates of 50 per cent (Narayana et al., 1982) and 32 per cent (McDougal et al., 1986).

For lesions involving the glans and the distal shaft, even when they are apparently superficial, partial amputation with a 2-cm margin proximal to the tumor is necessary to minimize local recurrence. Frozen section of the proximal margin is recommended for microscopic confirmation of a tumor-free margin of resection. Following this guideline, recurrent tumor at the line of resection is rare, even with deep corporal invasion, because tumor spread is by embolic metastases and not by lymphatic permeation (deKernion et al., 1973; Ekstrom and Edsmyr, 1958; Hardner et al., 1972).

One series reported no local recurrences with total amputation and a 6 per cent local recurrence rate after partial amputation (McDougal et al., 1986). In contrast, local wedge excision has been associated with recurrence rates that approach 50 per cent (Jensen, 1977). Adequate partial amputation in the absence of inguinal metastases can produce a 5-year survival rate of 70 to 80 per cent (see Table 31–1). The residual penile stump is usually servicable for upright micturition and sexual function.

If the proximal penile shaft is involved by malignancy to the extent that resection will leave a close margin and a stump that prohibits upright voiding and satisfactory sexual function, total penectomy is performed to ensure an adequate margin and to allow more convenient micturition in a sitting position by way of perineal urethrostomy (Fig. 31–11). For the rare lesion of the skin of the penile shaft that involves epidermis only, removal of the skin and subcutaneous tissue may be adequate (Fig. 31–12A and B) (Grabstald, 1970). In more advanced tumors with local extension to scrotum

Table 31–5. MINIMAL DIAGNOSTIC CRITERIA FOR CARCINOMA OF THE PENIS

Primary Tumor (T)
Clinical examination
Incisional-excisional biopsy of lesion and histologic examination for grade and depth of invasion

Regional and Juxtaregional Lymph Nodes (N)
Clinical examination
CT scan
Superficial inguinal node dissection for high-grade or invasive histology
Lymphangiography and aspiration cytology (optional)

Distant Metastases(M)
Clinical examination
Chest radiograph, CT scan
MRI, bone scan (optional)
Biochemical determinations (liver functions, calcium)

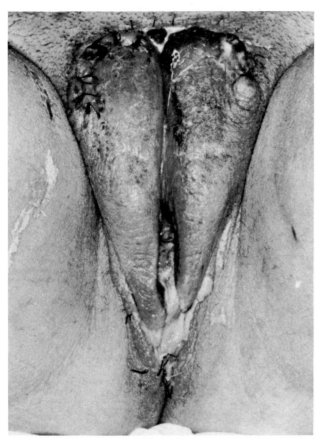

Figure 31–11. Appearance after total penectomy and partial scrotectomy and formation of perineal urethrostomy.

or pubis (stage T4), or with fixed inguinal nodes (N3), hemipelvectomy or hemicorporectomy with combination chemotherapy merits consideration in well-selected individuals (Fig. 31–13) (Block et al., 1973).

Mohs Micrographic Surgery

Mohs micrographic surgery (MMS) is a method of surgically removing skin cancer by excising tissue in thin layers. MMS includes color coding of excised specimens with tissue dyes, accurate orientation of excised tissue through construction of tissue maps, and microscopic examination of the horizonal frozen sections. The technique, first introduced in 1941 by Dr. Frederic Mohs, was described as microscopically controlled chemosurgery. The term "chemosurgery" has been replaced with a more descriptive term, "Mohs micrographic surgery."

MMS is a much more time-consuming modality than many of the traditional tissue-sparing techniques. The American College of Mohs Micrographic Surgery frowns on the use of additional personnel for the examination of these carefully prepared sections. They state that "the precise accuracy of MMS can be maintained only if the Mohs micrographic surgeon is responsible for all of the steps in the process. Variations from the technique or extra steps involving additional personnel may introduce errors which reduce the cure rate" (Cottel et al., 1988).

The capability of MMS to trace out silent tumorous "extensions" with a cure rate equivalent to the more radical surgical techniques, while at the same time allowing the maximum preservation of normal, uninvolved tissue, makes it an attractive modality for the treatment of some carcinomas of the penis. In the Mohs series and other series, MMS seems to be ideally suited for small, distally located carcinomas (Brown et al., 1987; Mohs et al., 1985). Mohs reported a 100 per cent cure rate in the lesions he treated that were less than 1 cm in diameter but only a 50 per cent cure rate in lesions that were greater than 3 cm.

After MMS, the areas of excision are allowed to heal by secondary intention, and meatal stenosis can be a complication. Meatal stenosis is treated by standard techniques with island flaps to reconstruct the meatus and/or a Y-V advancement technique to relieve the stenosis. In the majority of patients treated with MMS, patients have adequate functional shaft length. However, the glans penis is misshapen or totally absent (Fig. 31–14). These patients may seek reconstructive surgery, which oftentimes is difficult to perform.

Often, the appearance of the distal shaft of the penis can be improved by recreating a coronal margin. This can be accomplished by placing a split-thickness skin graft into a small circumcising groove, thus providing a pigmented line mimicking the coronal margin. A further cosmetic effort is achieved by tubing and burying the split-thickness graft, which can provide a tissue contour variance along with a pigmentation difference. It is difficult to recreate the bulky shape of the normal glans penis. The ventral fascial flap with a skin island, described by Jordan (1987) for reconstruction of the fossa navicularis, has been employed in a limited number of patients to provide bulk on the distal end of the penis (Figs. 31–15, 31–16, 31–17, and 31–18).

Like most methods to control local tumor, MMS does not represent a panacea. However, for small lesions and in select patients, MMS seems to provide cure rates at least equal to the results of partial penectomy, while leaving the patient with less long-term functional and cosmetic disability. The reconstructive surgeon is often faced with a delicate dilemma in patients who have had MMS for larger lesions. These patients have essentially undergone partial penectomy, and it is difficult to achieve a satisfactory result with lesser reconstructive techniques. In comparison, the more aggressive techniques of total phallic construction often do not provide an acceptable option.

Laser Surgery

Laser therapy has been employed to treat stage Tis, Ta, T1, and some T2 penile cancer. Potential advantages of laser therapy in penile cancer are destruction of the lesion with preservation of normal structure and function. However, several disadvantages exist, which are especially apparent when laser therapy is used to treat larger lesions. Depth of laser destruction may be difficult to determine, and histologic documentation of depth of malignant penetration may not be available. Therefore, it is imperative to adequately stage the tumor with deep

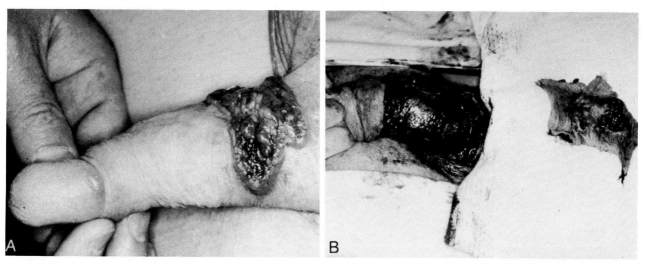

Figure 31–12. *A*, Erosive but superficial lesion of the skin of the proximal shaft was treated by sleeve resection of the skin and preservation of the penis. *B*, Postresection appearance together with excised lesion and surrounding skin.

biopsies before applying laser therapy. In the properly selected patient, laser therapy offers a very viable treatment option.

Treatment of Tis tumors (Bowen's disease, erythro-

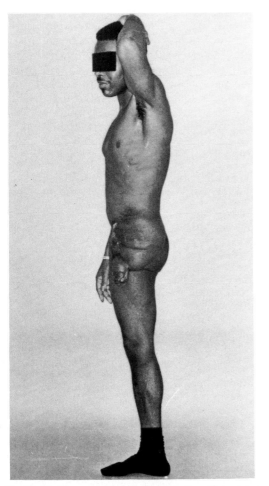

Figure 31–13. Hemicorporectomy in young male with invasive penile carcinoma with inguinal nodal metastasis but without evidence of positive juxtaregional nodes or distant metastasis.

plasia of Queyrat, Bowenoid papulosis) can be achieved with any of the common surgical lasers. Several reports have documented the ability of the CO_2 laser to treat these lesions (Bandieramonte et al., 1987; Rosemberg and Fuller, 1980). Because these lesions are superficial, often multifocal, and require precise treatment, the CO_2 laser and operating microscope are the ideal approach. In addition, 5 per cent acetic acid staining may be helpful in determining the full extent of the lesion. The Nd:YAG laser has also been used successfully in the treatment of stage Tis tumors (Malloy et al., 1988).

Treatment of T1 and T2 tumors has not been as uniformly successful. Several different techniques have been used applying both the CO_2 and Nd:YAG lasers. The most aggressive use of the CO_2 laser has been reported by Bandiermonte and co-workers (1987, 1988). Total resection of the surface of the glans penis was carried out for T1 tumor. By using a very short pulse with a high peak power at the base of the lesion and around the meatus, precise excision providing a specimen for pathologic examination can be achieved.

Despite magnification, positive surgical margins have been noted, however, and a 15 per cent recurrence rate has been reported (Bandieramonte et al., 1988). The Nd:YAG laser has received more widespread attention either as primary therapy or as an adjunct to excision. Utilization of the focusing handpiece and iced saline irrigation, six of nine patients with T1 tumors were tumor-free with a mean follow-up of 26 months. Tumor was not completely destroyed in two patients with stage T2 disease (Malloy et al., 1988). Laser excision with the aid of a sapphire tip, followed by laser coagulation of the base in stage T1 and T2 tumors, was associated with an 81 per cent success rate at a mean follow-up of 17 months (Boon, 1988).

Another approach, described by Rothenberger (1986), applies a penile tourniquet to create a bloodless field, scalpel excision of gross tumor, and Nd:YAG radiation of the base of the tumor. With a mean observation period of 5 years, no local recurrences were seen in 11 stage T1 and 6 stage T2 tumors so treated (Roth-

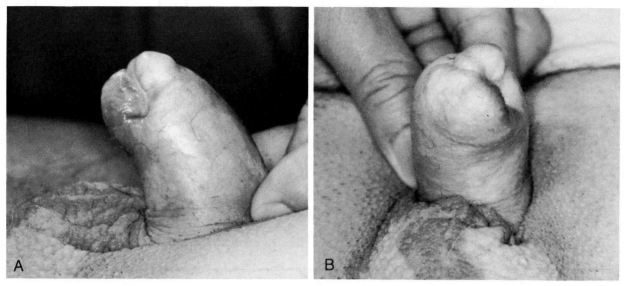

Figure 31–14. *A* and *B,* The classic deformity of the glans and distal shaft following Mohs micrographic surgery is illustrated. Note the small and deformed glans with the near totally absent coronal margin. Additionally, observe the appearance of the stenotic urethral meatus.

enberger, 1986). The largest series using Nd:YAG laser destruction for stage Tis, T1, T2, and some T3 tumors reported an actuarial survival at 5 years of 89 per cent for node-negative and 25 per cent for node-positive patients. Local recurrence was seen in only two of 28 patients with invasive tumor followed for 5 years (Kriegmair et al., 1990). This study supports an earlier series with Nd:YAG laser, which also reported excellent control of the primary lesion at 2- to 3-year follow-up (Hofstetter and Frank, 1983).

In conclusion, laser therapy can effectively be employed in carcinoma of the penis. Carcinoma in situ is eradicated safely with either the CO_2 or Nd:YAG laser. Treatment of T1 and T2 tumors may be successfully accomplished with laser surgery alone. Whether partial excision with subsequent laser coagulation will provide better results awaits further experience with various techniques. Comparable results to partial penectomy can be achieved in properly staged and treated patients. Because some patients treated with laser therapy may develop local recurrence, close follow-up is mandatory to determine whether repeat laser treatment or amputation excision will be necessary (Boon, 1988).

Radiation Therapy

The sole advantage of initial radiation therapy over initial surgery rests on the preservation of penile ana-

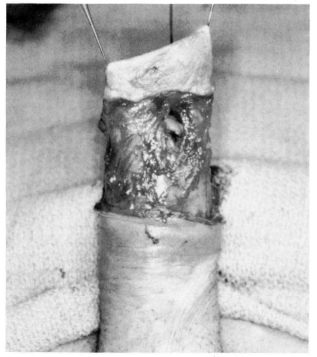

Figure 31–15. A transverse ventral skin island is elevated on a dartos fascia pedicle. The fascial pedicle is buttonholed, allowing transposition of the flap to the dorsum of the penis.

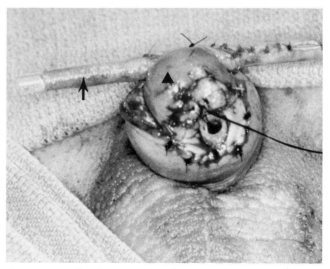

Figure 31–16. The placement of a tubed skin graft *(arrow)* for coronoplasty is illustrated. Note the transverse skin island *(dart)* transposed to the dorsum of the shaft of the penis.

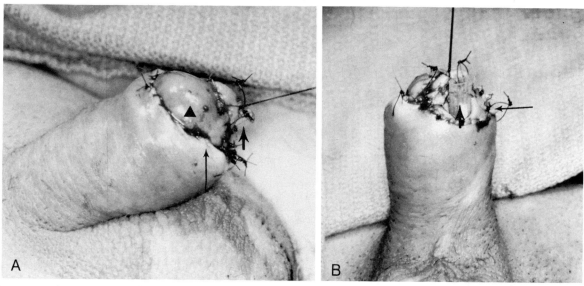

Figure 31–17. *A and B,* Appearance of the immediate postoperative result with the stenting urethral catheter *(short arrow)* and buried stenting tube *(long arrow)* for the first stage coronoplasty. The transverse ventral skin island that has been transposed to the dorsum of the penis provides bulk and dorsal "glans" *(arrowhead).*

tomic structure and function—a consideration that is especially important among young patients. However, this is an end result that can now be achieved with the advances in Mohs, laser, and reconstructive techniques as already described. Surgical amputation must follow if radiation therapy fails. Partial penectomy, although anatomically deforming, does not necessarily preclude upright micturition and satisfactory sexual function. Among elderly patients, preservation of an aesthetic anatomic structure and sexual function are often of secondary importance.

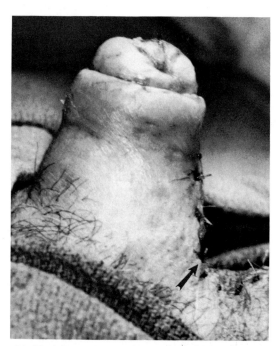

Figure 31–18. A later postoperative result illustrating the appearance of the coronal margin with the improved bulk of the glans penis. Not infrequently, the patient so treated requires a release of the penoscrotal tethering. This has been accomplished *(arrow).*

Objections to radiation therapy in the treatment of primary lesions rest on a number of observations. First, squamous cell carcinoma is characteristically radioresistant, and the doses of radiation (i.e., 6000 rads) (Kelley et al., 1974) necessary to sterilize deeply infiltrating penile tumors frequently result in urethral fistula, stenosis, and stricture, with or without penile necrosis, pain, and edema. These complications may require secondary penectomy (Duncan and Jackson, 1972).

Second, infection, so frequently associated with penile carcinoma, markedly decreases the effect of radiation therapy on the neoplasm and increases the incidence of damage to the radiosensitive penile tissue (low therapeutic index) (Murrell and Williams, 1965).

Third, the lengthy treatment schedule of 3 to 6 weeks, followed by several months of morbidity after the termination of treatment, represents a formidable burden for the elderly—a group for whom partial penectomy, in contrast, represents a relatively direct and expeditious procedure.

Lastly, it is well accepted that, if radiation therapy is to equal the success rate of initial surgical treatment, radiation failures (i.e., those cases without complete resolution of the treated lesion at 3 to 6 months after therapy or those with evidence of recurrences) must be promptly treated with penectomy in order not to jeopardize survival. Therefore, careful long-term follow-up of the patient to detect recurrence is mandatory. In one series seven (63 per cent) of 11 recurrences were detected after 2 years, and two (18 per cent) of 11 recurrences were detected after 5 years (Mazeron et al., 1984). Such follow-up may be a difficult task among a group of patients who have already demonstrated unreliability and neglect in seeking prompt attention for the original primary lesion. Furthermore, distinguishing postradiation ulcer, scar, and fibrosis from possible recurrent carcinoma represents a diagnostic problem often requiring repeated biopsy.

Radiation therapy does warrant consideration in a

select group of patients: (1) young individuals presenting with small (2 to 3 cm), superficial, exophytic, noninvasive lesions on the glans or coronal sulcus (radiation may also be considered after a course of topical 5-fluorouracil cream has failed in the treatment of carcinoma in situ); (2) patients refusing surgery as an initial form of therapy; and (3) patients with inoperable or distant metastases who require local therapy to the primary tumor but who express desire to retain the penis. Before radiation therapy, circumcision (or, at the very least, a dorsal slit) is necessary to expose the lesion, to allow resolution of surface infection, and to prevent moist maceration and preputial edema.

Evaluation of the overall success of radiation in the treatment of primary lesions of carcinoma of the penis is made difficult by the lack of uniformity of radiation treatment within single series and between different series. Time schedules of treatment, total radiation exposure, and the type of delivery system used—such as external beam therapy (Jackson, 1966), radium mold (Jackson, 1966), electron beam (Kelley et al., 1974), and interstitial implants (Pierquin et al., 1971)—vary considerably (Mazeron et al., 1984).

Radiation therapy to select, small, superficial lesions is quite successful. A 90 per cent rate of control of the primary tumor among 20 patients treated with megavoltage radiation has been reported (Duncan and Jackson, 1972). However, the dosages employed (5000 to 5700 rads over 3 weeks) produced a significant number of complications, namely, penile necrosis in 10 per cent of patients and urethral stricture in 30 per cent.

The most successful series employing radiation therapy is that reported by Memorial Sloan-Kettering Cancer Center (Kelley et al., 1974). Applying electron beam therapy, a 100 per cent success rate in controlling lesions in ten carefully selected patients was achieved clinically and confirmed histologically by negative biopsy findings of the lesion. A 5- to 10-year update on this series reported that nine patients were tumor-free. In one patient, carcinoma developed at another penile site, suggesting a new primary tumor. Nine patients retained sexual function. The most common complication was urethral stricture in four patients (Grabstald and Kelley, 1980). A series from the M.D. Anderson Hospital and Tumor Institute also reports good control of smaller lesions without significant morbidity (Haile and Delclos, 1980), and similar success with well-selected cases has been reported by other centers (Daly et al., 1982; Mazeron et al., 1984; Raynal et al., 1977; Salaverria et al., 1979).

When radiation therapy is employed as the initial treatment for penile carcinoma, control of the primary lesions occurs with much less frequency than when surgery is primarily employed (Table 31–6). A patient's prognosis is not altered if surgery is promptly performed when radiation fails to control the carcinoma (Murrell and Williams, 1965). Jackson (1966), however, did show that nodal metastases develop more frequently during or after a course of radiation therapy than after surgery; this finding suggests the potential for metastases to occur during or following a course of unsuccessful radiation therapy.

In summary, small, superficial tumors will respond well to radiotherapy, and with careful planning, complications can be minimized. The treatment of larger, invasive malignancies is less successful, may be associated with severe local complications, and theoretically may provide an interval during which metastatic dissemination may occur. Other untoward effects of radiation include testicular damage and secondary neoplasia (Lederman, 1953). In the case of a sexually active young patient with an invasive lesion, surgical amputation followed by penile reconstruction (vide infra) rather than primary radiation therapy should be considered.

TREATMENT OF INGUINAL NODES

The prognosis for patients with carcinoma of the penis is markedly worsened by the presence of inguinal metastases. This factor affects the prognosis more than tumor grade, gross appearance, or morphologic and microscopic patterns of the tumor. Nodal metastases are more frequently associated with high-grade or invasive histology.

Surgical Treatment

Controversial issues concerning the treatment of regional lymph nodes center on the timing and extent of surgery and involve the following questions: (1) Should lymphadenectomy be performed for a patient with palpable inguinal lymphadenopathy that is persistent after treatment of the primary penile lesion and a course of antibiotics in order to allow for subsidence of nodal enlargement secondary to inflammation? (2) Should lymphadenectomy be performed on a prophylactic or adjunctive basis in a patient with clinically negative inguinal examination findings? (3) Should adenectomy be performed bilaterally if only unilateral nodes are palpable, or should node dissections be limited to the side of palpable adenopathy? (4) Should lymphadenectomy be extended to the pelvic lymph nodes, unilaterally or bilaterally, or should it be restricted to the inguinal lymph node area?

The rarity of penile carcinoma will make it impossible to conduct adequate prospective randomized trials to resolve these controversies surrounding the treatment of regional nodes. Based on historic and retrospective data accumulated from the literature, these questions are discussed individually as follows. Although guidelines can be developed from retrospective analysis, treatment must often be individualized according to the dictates of a particular case.

Should lymphadenectomy be performed in the presence of clinically palpable inguinal nodes after appropriate treatment of the primary lesion and subsidence of inflammation? This question can be answered in the affirmative. The recommendation for inguinal node dissection for patients having positive nodes at presentation is well substantiated. Evidence to support this statement is based on the following findings: Patients with penile carcinomas and inguinal metastases who do not undergo treatment rarely survive 2 years and almost never survive

Table 31–6. SURGERY REQUIRED AFTER RADIATION THERAPY FOR CARCINOMA OF THE PENIS

Series	Number of Patients	Amputation for Recurrent or Persistent Disease, or Both (%)*	Other Surgery (%)	Total (%)
Lederman, 1953	48	35	—	35
Murrell and Wiliams, 1965	92	48	—	48
Jackson, 1966	58	51	—	51
Knudsen and Brennhovd, 1967	145	62	6†	68
Almgard and Edsmyr, 1973	33	52	18‡	70
Engelstad, 1948	64	45§	8†	53
Raynal and co-workers, 1977	45	22	8†	30
Salaverria and co-workers, 1979	13	23	—	23
Haile and Delclos, 1980	20	10	10†	20
Daly and co-workers, 1982	22	5	10†	15
Sagerman and co-workers, 1984	15	40	—	40
Mazeron and co-workers, 1984	50	20	10	30
Fossa and co-workers, 1987	11	33	—	33

*Difference from 100 per cent indicates cure from radiation alone.
†Penectomy for radiation complications.
‡Local excision or electrocoagulation of recurrent neoplasm.
§Includes seven radiation therapy failures not having further surgery.

5 years. No spontaneous regression of penile carcinoma has been reported. However, 20 to 50 per cent of patients with clinically palpable adenopathy and histologically proven inguinal node metastases who are treated by inguinal lymphadenectomy achieve a 5-year disease-free survival (see Table 31–1). When extent of nodal disease has been identified, patients with limited nodal involvement fare even better.

A series from Memorial Sloan-Kettering Cancer Center (MSKCC) reported an 82 per cent 5-year survival after adenectomy for patients with a single positive node (Srinivas et al., 1987). A series from the Norwegian Radium Hospital (Fossa et al., 1987) reported an 88 per cent 5-year survival after adenectomy for patients with minimal nodal metastases. Other series have reported that survivors routinely have two or less positive nodes (see Table 31–2) (Beggs and Spratt, 1961; Fraley et al., 1989; Johnson and Lo, 1984a).

Palpable adenopathy at initial presentation does not inevitably indicate the presence of tumor. A false-positive rate of up to 50 per cent related to node enlargement caused by inflammation has been reported (see Table 31–1). However, the persistence of adenopathy after treatment of the primary tumor and a course of antibiotics or the appearance of adenopathy during follow-up is much more likely because of metastasis than inflammatory reaction. In the Memorial Sloan-Kettering Cancer Center series reported by Srinivas and associates (1987), 66 of 76 patients (86 per cent) with palpable adenopathy after 6 weeks of antibiotic therapy had pathologically positive nodes.

Should complete *inguinal lymphadenectomy be routinely performed in patients with clinically negative groin examination findings the time of presentation of the primary lesion?* This question invites the greatest amount of controversy. As stated, the cure rate with inguinal adenectomy when nodes are positive for malignancy may be as high as 80 per cent. A cure rate of this magnitude with surgery in the face of regional nodal metastases parallels the urologist's experience with testicular carcinoma, in which surgical monotherapy results

in cure in a significant number of node-positive patients. In contrast, for other common genitourinary malignancies—bladder, prostate, and renal—surgical cure is unusual in the presence of nodal metastases. Why then is there any discussion concerning the wisdom of node dissection for treatment of a tumor when the potential for cure is substantial, especially in view of the fact that node dissections are frequently advocated in the treatment of urologic malignancies when evidence of their efficacy is marginal at best?

The problem arises from the significant morbidity of inguinal node dissection in contrast to the limited morbidity of retroperitoneal and pelvic lymphadenectomy. Early complications of phlebitis, pulmonary embolism, wound infection, flap necrosis, and late complications of lymphedema can occur with disconcerting frequency after inguinal adenectomy (Fig. 31–19) (Fraley et al., 1989; Johnson and Lo, 1984b; McDougal et al., 1986; Skinner et al., 1972). However, postoperative complications have been lessened in the last decade by improved pre- and postoperative care; advances in surgical technique; preservation of the dermis, Scarpa's fascia, and the saphenous vein; and modification of the extent of node dissection (Catalona, 1988). Furthermore, it has been suggested that the performance of a node dissection in the setting of microscopic disease may be less likely to cause complications than node dissection in the setting of bulky nodal metastasis (Fraley et al., 1989).

Mortality after lymphadenectomy was reported only in association with surgery done simultaneously with amputation of the primary tumor and was related to sepsis. Mortality was not reported when adenectomy was delayed several weeks after amputation (Ekstrom and Edsmyr, 1958). An operative mortality of 3.3 per cent was reported in an early series (Beggs and Spratt, 1961). Johnson and Lo (1984b) reported a surgical mortality of 0 per cent. Postoperative mortality should be much less than 1 per cent.

The admonition of Hippocrates—"Primum non nocere" ("First, do no harm")—deserves serious consideration and represents a significant issue in developing

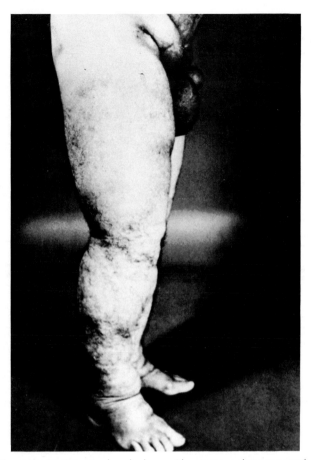

Figure 31–19. Extensive lymphedema with cutaneous changes secondary to recurrent lymphangitis and phlebitis.

the role of prophylactic or adjunctive adenectomy in the absence of palpable adenopathy. The incidence of metastases to the inguinal nodes has been reported in 2 to 25 per cent of patients presenting with penile carcinomas who have clinically negative inguinal examination findings (see Table 31–1). A very large series reported a 38 per cent false-negative rate (Puras et al., 1978), on the basis of impalpable microinvolvement of the nodes or changes in the inguinal area, such as postsurgical induration, scar, or obesity, that make accurate examination impossible.

The incidence of metastases to clinically normal nodes is based on information derived from both complete node dissections and limited lymph node biopsies. Because some patients will subsequently develop positive nodes after initial limited dissections or selected biopsy findings were negative, and because the detection of metastases on pathologically submitted material is dependent on the number of sections per node examined—that is, how hard the pathologist looks for tumor—the incidence rates for false-negative clinical examinations represent the minimum. These patients with clinically negative but histologically positive nodes are at risk for death from penile cancer. A review calculated that 17 per cent of patients who presented initially with negative nodes died of disease (Catalona, 1980).

The curative benefit of lymphadenectomy in the presence of grossly palpable nodes involved with tumor has been established; therefore, it is logical to presume that a lymphadenectomy performed in the setting of microscopic nodal disease would confer an even greater survival advantage. However, reports from the Ellis Fischel State Cancer Hospital (Columbia, Missouri) showed no apparent reduction in 5-year survival rates among those patients with negative nodes initially who were carefully followed and later, upon clinical appearance of adenopathy, had node dissection (Lesser and Schwarz, 1955). The 5-year survival rate in this group paralleled that of patients presenting with metastatic adenopathy initially who were treated with node dissection (Baker et al., 1976). This expectant treatment philosophy was also supported by Frew and colleagues (1967). However, with this protocol, adenectomy is being undertaken in the presence of grossly palpable tumor. This observation does not exclude the possibility that adenectomy for clinically imperceptible, that is, microscopic disease, might yield better results. However, it is difficult to justify a broad recommendation for lymph node dissection to patients with negative clinical inguinal examination results for whom the procedure will not be therapeutic in approximately 75 per cent.

Unfortunately, most series have not separately analyzed postlymphadenectomy survival of patients with clinically palpable nodes that are positive for neoplasm on histologic examination compared with survival of patients with clinically negative nodes that are positive for neoplasm on histologic examination. Three analyses compared 5-year survival free of disease between patients who had either immediate adjunctive or delayed therapeutic lymphadenectomy.

McDougal and co-workers (1986) reported a series of 23 patients with invasive primary lesions and nonpalpable nodes; nine were treated with immediate adjunctive lymph node dissection (six were node-positive), and 14 were treated with surveillance and delayed lymph node dissection. The 5-year survival in the node-positive immediate adjunctive lymphadenectomy group was 88 per cent (5/6); in the surveillance group, the 5-year survival was 38 per cent. However, only one patient in the surveillance group had lymph node dissection; presumptively, the others had either progressed to inoperable local disease status or had progressed to distant disease before clinical manifestation of adenopathy (emphasizing the role of careful, frequent follow-up and the difficulty of enforcing it). A third subset of patients in this series manifested adenopathy at presentation and had immediate therapeutic lymph node dissection with ten of 15 (66 per cent) surviving 5 years (McDougal et al., 1986).

The best results, therefore, were from *immediate* adjunctive lymph node dissection (88 per cent); the next best results were from immediate therapeutic lymph node dissection (66 per cent); and the worst results (38 per cent) were from surveillance and delayed lymph node dissection when nodes became palpable. The interval of opportunity for cure appears to have been lost with this last group. Fraley reported that immediate adjunctive lymphadenectomy resulted in a survival free of disease at 5 years in six of nine (66 per cent) node-positive patients compared with one of 12 (8 per cent) patients who had been followed and treated by delayed lymphadenectomy (Fraley et al., 1989). Whereas only two of six of the immediate lymphadenectomy group had more than two positive nodes (these two patients died of cancer), all of the patients treated by delayed lymphadenectomy had three or more positive nodes.

A series from the M.D. Anderson Hospital compared 5-year disease-free survival for 14 patients with early adjunctive lymphadenectomy for clinically impalpable but histologic node-positive disease with that for eight patients who were followed and submitted to later lymphadenectomy when clinical nodal enlargement appeared (Johnson and Lo, 1984a). The primary tumors were a similar stage. The 5-year disease-free survival was 57 per cent for early adenectomy compared with 13 per cent for delayed adenectomy. The number of involved nodes in the first group (median = 2) was half of that in the second group (median = 4), and no patient with more than two positive nodes survived more than 5 years.

Also supporting early lymphadenectomy are the following studies. A series from Puerto Rico (Puras et al., 1978) identified surgical removal of the primary tumor followed within 1 month by routine lymphadenectomy as the treatment protocol associated with the highest 5-year survival rate. A series from Uraguay (Cabanas, 1977) reported improved survival by employing early node biopsy, which, if findings are positive, is followed by prompt complete node dissection. Information from several series supports better survival with resection of low-volume nodal disease. Adjunctive or early lymphadenectomy gives greater assurance that surgical intervention will occur when tumor volume is small (see Table 31–2) (Fossa et al., 1987; Fraley et al., 1989; Johnson and Lo, 1984; Srinivas et al., 1987).

It is important to identify indicators that predict for increased risk of nodal involvement so as to be able to select patients who are most likely to harbor subclinical metastasis.

Primary tumor stage assessment* is of paramount importance (deKernion et al., 1973; McDougal et al., 1986). Lesions that invade through the basement membrane of the penile integument are more likely to be associated with nodal metastases, and proposals have been made for ilioinguinal node dissection in medically suited patients with clinically negative nodes, whose primary lesion is invasive (Catalona, 1980; deKernion et al., 1973; McDougal et al., 1986).

Grade can provide information about the likelihood of nodal metastasis (Fraley et al., 1989). Fraley's study of tumor grade and relationship to nodal metastasis showed a higher correlation than do most other series; one of 19 patients with well-differentiated tumor, five of 19 patients with moderately differentiated tumor, and all 16 patients with poorly differentiated tumor developed nodal metastases.

Sentinel node biopsy, node dissection superficial to

*Several series have identified patients with stage II penile cancer at high risk because of *invasive* histology. However, the Jackson staging system is a clinical system. Jackson described stage II disease only as "tumor involving the penile shaft" to distinguish shaft lesions from glans lesions (stage I) and made no reference to invasion (see Tables 31–3 and 31–4).

fascia lata, and aspiration cytology are staging procedures less extensive than complete inguinal lymphadenectomy that can provide useful information. The concept of sentinel node biopsy as described by Cabanas is predicated on detailed penile lymphangiographic studies that have demonstrated consistent drainage of the penile lymphatics into a sentinel node or group of nodes located superomedial to the junction of the saphenous and femoral veins in the area of the superficial epigastric vein (Cabanas, 1977). In this series, when this sentinel node was negative for tumor, metastases to other ilionguinal lymph nodes did not occur. Metastases to this node indicated the need for a complete superficial and deep inguinal dissection.

The accuracy of sentinel node histology to identify inguinal metastasis has been questioned by a number of reports (deKernion et al., 1973; Perinetti et al., 1980; Wespes et al., 1986). Because nodal metastasis became palpable within 1 year of a negative sentinel node biopsy in some patients in these series, a false-negative biopsy result must be presumed. In one large series, five of 82 (6 per cent) sentinel node–negative groins in five of 41 patients (12 per cent) with negative sentinel node biopsy subsequently developed inguinal metastasis (Fossa et al., 1987). In Cabanas' series, three of 31 patients with negative sentinel nodes did not survive; this finding may indicate a false-negative rate for identifying metastasis of 10 per cent (Cabanas, 1977). McDougal and associates (1986) reported a 50 per cent false-negative rate with inguinal node biopsy.

Superficial inguinal node dissection has been proposed for the patient without palpable adenopathy. Superficial node dissection involves removal of those nodes superficial to the fascia lata (Figs. 31–20, 31–21, and 31–22). Total lymphadenectomy—that is, removal also of those nodes deep to the fascia lata contained within the femoral triangle—is performed if the superficial nodes are positive (deKernion et al., 1973).

The advantage of the superficial dissection is that it provides more information than does biopsy of a single node, it avoids the possibility of misidentifying the sentinel node, and it is associated with minimal morbidity. The incidence, if any, of positive inguinal nodes deep to the fascia lata in the absence of positive superficial inguinal nodes is not readily available. Although corporal lymphatics have been presumed to occasionally drain directly to the deep inguinal nodes, clinical evidence supports the superficial nodes as the first echelon of metastasis and an accurate marker for deep and more proximal node involvement. Also, penile lymphatic studies show no evidence, by lymphangiography, of direct pelvic node drainage (Riveros et al., 1967).

The experience with aspiration cytology is limited, and most information is derived from a single large series (Scappini et al., 1986). The procedure requires pedal and/or penile lymphangiography for node localization, followed by aspiration under fluoroscopic or computed tomography scan guidance. Multiple nodes must be sampled (e.g., 170 node chains in 29 patients in this series). Of the 20 patients who had lymphadenectomy for histologic confirmation, there was complete agreement between aspiration cytology and histologic results. However, two of nine patients whose cytology

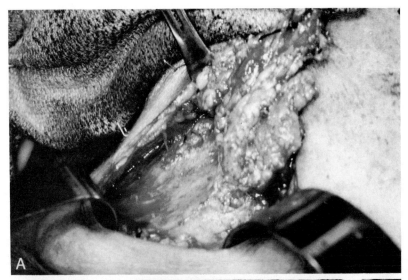

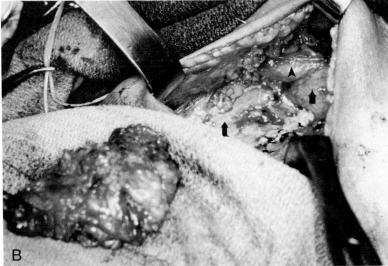

Figure 31–20. *A*, Reflection of superficial node packet from fascia lata with dissection proceeding cephalad to inguinal ligament. *B*, Superficial inguinal node packet removed exposing fascia lata *(curved arrow)* external oblique fascia *(solid arrow)* and spermatic cord *(dart)*. The saphenous vein has been suture ligated at its junction with the common femoral vein.

was negative subsequently died of metastatic disease (a presumptive 20 per cent false-negative result). This finding and the procedural difficulty with lymphangiography and multiple samplings make aspiration less practical than sentinel biopsy and superficial node dissection. However, direct aspiration of palpable nodes, if positive, can provide immediate information with which to advise patients regarding further treatment.

Should inguinal lymphadenectomy be bilateral rather than unilateral for patients presenting with unilateral adenopathy at initial presentation of the primary tumor? The answer to this question is yes. The anatomic crossover of lymphatics of the penis is well established, and bilateral drainage is, therefore, the rule. Bilateral lymphadenectomy is recommended in patients presenting with unilateral palpable adenopathy in conjunction with the primary lesion. The contralateral node dissection may be limited to the area superficial to the fascia lata if no histologic evidence of positive superficial inguinal nodes is found. Clinical support for a bilateral procedure is based on the finding of contralateral metastases in greater than 50 per cent of patients so treated, even if the contralateral nodal region appears negative to clinical palpation (Ekstrom and Edsmyr, 1958).

Should bilateral inguinal lymphadenectomy be performed in patients who present with unilateral adenopathy sometime after the initial presentation in treatment of the primary tumor? The answer to this question would logically appear to be affirmative based on the data provided in the preceding paragraph. However, it is generally believed that a bilateral node dissection in this setting is not necessary. This recommendation of unilateral rather than bilateral node dissection with delayed unilateral adenopathy is supported by the elapsed disease-free observation on the normal side.

If one assumes that nodal metastases will enlarge at the same rate, the clinical palpation of metastases, if present in both groins, should appear at approximately the same time. The absence of clinical adenopathy on one side dictates a higher probability of freedom from disease on that side (Ekstrom and Edsmyr, 1958). However, this situation should occur much less frequently than in the past because of identification of high-risk patients for immediate bilateral lymphadenectomy. The low-risk patients with superficial, well-differentiated lesions who are selected for expectant treatment will probably have a less than 10 per cent incidence of nodal metastases after treatment of the primary tumor (de-

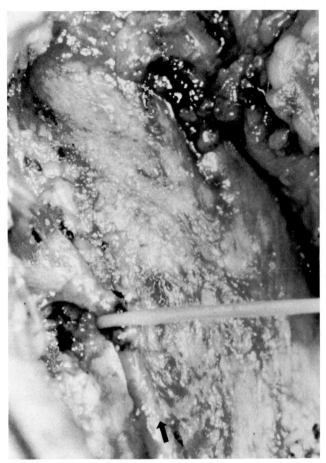

Figure 31–21. Alternatively, the vein may be preserved *(arrow)*.

Kernion et al., 1973; Hardner et al., 1972; McDougal et al., 1986).

Should pelvic lymphadenectomy be performed in patients with positive inguinal metastases? Therapeutic gain of extending nodal dissection to include the iliac nodes is undetermined. Information is limited regarding the frequency of pelvic node metastases in the setting of positive or negative inguinal nodes. Histologic evaluation of pelvic nodes has demonstrated metastatic spread in two of four patients having staging laparotomy (Uehling, 1973). Iliac nodes have been found to be positive for tumor metastases in five of 13 patients (35 per cent) at autopsy (Gursel et al., 1973), in 15 of 45 patients (30 per cent) (Riveros and Gorostiaga, 1962), in nine of 30 patients (29 per cent) with positive inguinal nodes (Puras et al., 1978), and in 11 of 73 (15 per cent) of patients with positive inguinal nodes (Srinivas et al., 1987).

Puras and co-workers (1978) found no evidence of positive iliac nodes among 40 patients having ilioinguinal node dissection and negative inguinal nodes. Srinivas and associates (1987) related extent of inguinal metastases to iliac metastases. Only one of 16 (6 per cent) patients with less than six positive inguinal nodes had iliac metastasis, whereas ten of 27 (37 per cent) patients with greater than six positive inguinal nodes had iliac node metastases. Srinivas and colleagues (1987) reported no instance of positive pelvic nodes in the absence of positive inguinal nodes.

Survival of patients with positive iliac nodes is limited. Of 11 patients in the Srinivas series, none survived to 3 years, and most died within 7 months. For this reason, specific recommendations against pelvic node dissection have appeared (Hanash et al., 1970). Until more information is available, a definitive statement about the advisability of pelvic node dissection is not possible. However, because involvement of pelvic nodes on microscopic examination may occur with some frequency, because survival with positive pelvic nodes has been documented (Cabanas, 1977; deKernion et al., 1973; Puras et al., 1980) (see Table 31–1), and because duration of survival has been lengthened after iliac node dissection (Hardner et al., 1972), the procedure is reasonable for the young male, who is a good surgical risk.

Information specifying the location of positive nodes found at dissection (femoral, iliac, bilateral, unilateral) and the number of nodes involved with tumor or histologic examination is generally unavailable. A larger body of data relating the pattern and extent of nodal metastases to patient survival will aid in accurately defining the natural history of node-positive penile carcinoma and identifying indications for extent of lymphadenectomy.

On the basis of available information, several options for treatment of inguinal nodes are proposed. As previously mentioned, because staging systems are imprecise, a description of the location, extent of invasion, and histologic grade of a lesion is required.

Stage Tis, Ta, T1, N0M0 (I, II)

This stage describes lesions that involve only the glans mucosa or shaft skin and that are totally exophytic and superficial. These penile neoplasms, in the absence of palpable adenopathy, are very unlikely (less than 10 per cent) to involve nodal metastases (deKernion et al., 1973; McDougal et al., 1986) and, therefore, may be followed with periodic examination of the inguinal area after treatment of the primary tumor. The appearance of unilateral adenopathy provides indications for unilateral inguinal node dissection with added pelvic node dissection as determined by the histology of the inguinal nodes and the patient's medical status.

A contralateral superficial inguinal node dissection is also a consideration. If a contralateral dissection is not performed and adenopathy later presents on the opposite side, a superficial and deep node dissection should be undertaken. Because most inguinal metastases occur within a 2- to 3-year period following initial therapy (Beggs and Spratt, 1961; Derrick et al., 1973; Johnson et al., 1973), this period of risk must be closely supervised with examinations at 2- to 3-month intervals.

The patient should be taught careful self-examination of the inguinal areas for early detection of metastases. Delayed appearance of inguinal metastases may occur; therefore, the patient should never be dismissed from close physical examination. Such a program requires close cooperation of the patient—a formidable responsibility in a group of patients who historically have demonstrated a lack of reliability by presenting rather late in the course of the original penile lesion.

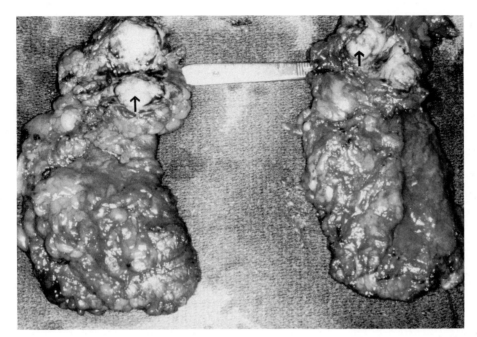

Figure 31–22. Bilateral superficial node packet with single, bisected positive node (arrow) on each side.

In the past, approximately 20 per cent of stage I patients were expected to develop inguinal metastases (Whitmore, 1970). However, this group included patients with stage I invasive glans lesions who would now be selected for immediate nodal evaluation. Immediate assessment of the inguinal nodes by bilateral superficial inguinal node dissection is another option for superficial penile lesions of this description, especially in the young patient.

Stage T2, T3, N0M0 (I, II)

These lesions, although limited to the glans or shaft, demonstrate invasion of Buck's fascia, tunica albuginea, and corporal bodies. The incidence of nodal metastases increases significantly in the presence of a tumor that invades the corporal tissue. Nodes were positive in 17 of 25 (68 per cent) invasive penile carcinomas (de-Kernion et al., 1973) and in six of nine (66 per cent) invasive tumors in the absence of palpable adenopathy (McDougal et al., 1986). Therefore, immediate bilateral adjunctive node dissection is indicated. The decision whether to limit dissection to these nodes superficial to the fascia lata, if all such nodes are negative on frozen section, or to perform both a superficial and deep node dissection, employing the limited boundary technique (to maximize staging accuracy and therapeutic value and to minimize morbidity) described by Catalona (1988) should be based on personal preference. Either option appears reasonable.

Stage Tis, Ta, T1–3, N1–3, M0 (III)

Patients with penile carcinoma and palpable adenopathy require control of the primary tumor, followed by a reevaluation of the inguinal nodes 2 to 6 weeks after infection is controlled and inflammatory adenopathy has resolved. This reevaluation serves not only to permit more accurate assessment of the cause of adenopathy

(inflammatory versus neoplastic) but also markedly reduces the potential operative morbidity secondary to sepsis.

If bilateral adenopathy persists, bilateral radical inguinal node dissections are recommended. If adenopathy is unilateral, metastases necessitating complete inguinal node dissection are anticipated in approximately 50 per cent of the clinically normal contralateral groins. A superficial node dissection only, if histology is negative, may be considered for the normal contralateral groin, or a deep node dissection with limited boundaries may be used. If adenopathy resolves with antibiotic therapy, then the decision for adjunctive lymphadenectomy is based on primary tumor stage as discussed in the preceding sections.

Stage Any T, Any N, M1; T4; Inoperable N (IV)

This category includes patients with distant metastases, inguinal adenopathy that is inoperable because of invasion and fixation, and extensive adjacent organ invasion. Treatment is often limited to palliative chemotherapy or radiotherapy, but aggressive combined modality therapy with chemotherapy and surgery—especially for the young patient—is warranted. In selected patients with fixed nodes but no distant metastases, neoadjuvant chemotherapy (vide infra) followed by inguinal and pelvic adenectomy with consideration of hemicorporectomy or hemipelvectomy is an option. Prior staging laparotomy is necessary to exclude abdominal visceral disease or high common iliac or para-aortic nodal metastasis.

Radiation Therapy

Assessment of the treatment of the inguinal area by irradiation is hampered by the uncertainty arising from the inaccuracy of clinical staging and the frequent lack of histologic confirmation of nodal metastases. Objections to the treatment of inguinal node metastases are that inguinal areas tolerate radiation poorly and are subject to skin maceration and ulceration. Infectious adenopathy will reduce the effectiveness of radiation therapy and magnify complications. The perilymphatic fat that frequently surrounds nodes may act as a protective barrier to the effective radiation treatment of intranodal metastatic deposits (Harlin, 1952). Information concerning the use of radiation therapy as a primary mode of treatment for penile carcinoma comes primarily from European countries.

The adjunctive or therapeutic use of radiation in treatment is controversial. Even if metastases are documented by node biopsy, the efficacy of subsequent radiation is impossible to judge because all tumor may have been removed by the biopsy. In one series, 70 per cent of nodal metastases involved a solitary node, and 5-year survival in this group was 70 per cent (Cabanas, 1977). Radiotherapy for inguinal metastases documented by histologic examination has been compared with surgery for the node-positive groin. A 50 per cent 5-year survival rate was observed among the surgically treated group, and a 25 per cent 5-year survival rate was observed among the irradiated group (Staubitz et al., 1955). Other series report that radiation to the inguinal areas has not proved therapeutically effective (Jensen, 1977; Murrell and Williams, 1965).

Several Scandinavian centers have delivered radiation therapy to inguinal nodes as well as to primary tumor in all cases of penile carcinoma; surgical adenectomy followed if palpable nodes persisted or appeared subsequently (Ekstrom and Edsmyr, 1958; Engelstad, 1948).

In a series of 130 patients initially having clinically impalpable nodes, 18 subsequently developed palpable nodal disease requiring lymphadenectomy, and another 11 patients had metastases but no surgery. Therefore, 29 of 130 (22 per cent) of men who received prophylactic groin irradiation subsequently developed inguinal metastases (Ekstrom and Edsmyr, 1958).

Murrell and Williams (1965) found that three of 11 patients (25 per cent) who received radiation therapy to the inguinal area without initially palpable nodes subsequently developed inguinal metastases. These percentages closely approximate the incidence of subclinical metastases that are encountered if node dissection is performed when the clinical examination is normal (see Table 31–1), and they suggest that radiation therapy did not alter the course of disease. Furthermore, the clinical evaluation of the groin following radiation therapy is difficult, and the complications encountered with groin dissection after radiation can be significant.

Lastly, the 5-year survival rate for patients with prophylactically irradiated groins followed as necessary by lymphadenectomy differs little from that for patients having surgery alone. Although a large, randomized, controlled study might definitely answer the question of efficacy of radiation therapy for inguinal metastases, both microscopic and macroscopic, it is unlikely that such a study could be realized. Present information identifies surgical therapy for inguinal metastasis as superior to radiation therapy.

Radiation therapy may be considered in patients presenting with inoperable fixed and ulcerative inguinal lymph nodes. Occasionally, radiation to these areas is well tolerated, may result in significant palliation, and may postpone local complications for prolonged periods (Furlong and Uhle, 1953; Staubitz et al., 1955; Vaeth et al., 1970).

In summary, radiation therapy to the inguinal area is not as effective therapeutically as lymph node dissection, but it may be useful if surgery cannot be performed. Furthermore, palliation can, at times, be achieved for inoperable nodes. Our policy has been not to combine preoperative radiation therapy with inguinal lymphadenectomy, but others have advocated the combination (Ekstrom and Edsmyr, 1958; Engelstad, 1948).

Chemotherapy

Reports from Japan (Ichikawa et al., 1969) have described a substantial and reproducible response of penile and scrotal carcinoma to treatment with bleomycin. Ichikawa and colleagues (1969) reported excellent response in six previously untreated patients with carcinoma of the penis. Reports from Uganda (Kyalwazi and Bhana, 1973) describe complete or partial regression in the majority of treated patients. A review of 67 patients from the world literature who could be evaluated revealed a 73 per cent response rate to bleomycin (Blum et al., 1973). However, these promising results have not been confirmed in a study from MSKCC, where 14 patients with advanced disease were treated with bleomycin. Only one complete and two partial responses were noted (Ahmed et al., 1984).

Cis-platinum and methotrexate, also tested at MSKCC, have shown more activity than bleomycin. *Cis*-platinum produced objective response in three of nine patients (Sklaroff and Yagoda, 1979). A later study using 70 or 120 mg/m^2 of *cis*-platinum every 3 weeks reported responses in three of 12 patients in spite of prior chemotherapy and irradiation therapy (Ahmed et al., 1984). However, a Cooperative Southwest Oncology Group study evaluated 26 patients treated with *cis*-platinum therapy and found only a 15 per cent partial response rate of minimal duration (1 to 3 months) (Gagliano et al., 1989).

Methotrexate given in high doses with folinic acid rescue produced a complete remission in one of three patients, and low-dose methotrexate produced partial remission in two of five patients treated (Sklaroff and Yagoda, 1980). Methotrexate has been demonstrated to be effective in other reports (Garnick et al., 1979; Mills, 1972). Methotrexate and bleomycin or bleomycin alone in combination with irradiation have achieved significant responses in single case reports (Abratt, 1984; Edsmyr et al., 1985).

Chemotherapy in the neoadjuvant and adjuvant setting was employed at the Milan National Tumor Institute (Pizzocaro and Piva, 1988). A protocol of 12 weekly courses of vincristine, bleomycin, and methotrexate was administered to 12 patients after adenectomy as adjuvant therapy and to five patients before node dissection as neoadjuvant therapy. The patients treated with adjuvant chemotherapy were at high risk, i.e., nine showed extranodal tumor growth, five had pelvic nodal involvement, and five had bilateral metastasis. At a follow-up ranging between 18 and 102 months, only one case had recurred.

The same regimen was employed as neoadjuvant therapy for five patients with large nodal tumor metastases (nodes ranged from 6 to 11 cm in size). Three achieved a partial response, were successfully resected, and continued without disease at 20 to 72 months. In another neoadjuvant study, four patients with stage III disease treated with two cycles of cisplatin (100 mg/m²) and continuous infusion of 5-fluorouracil (1.0 g daily times 5 days) showed objective regression of nodal disease. Two patients had no persistent tumor in the lymphadenectomy specimen, and none of the four have recurred at 6 to 40 months after lymphadenectomy (Fisher et al., 1990).

The rarity of penile carcinoma in the United States will make it difficult to accumulate sufficient numbers of patients to adequately test agents in phase II or III trials. This information will need to come from trials in South America and Asia. Such information will be of significant value in identifying agents to be given as (1) neoadjuvant therapy in patients with stage III disease, (2) adjuvant therapy when pathologic node evaluation reveals extensive inguinal metastasis or pelvic metastasis that predicts for diminished survival (Fraley et al., 1989; Johnson and Lo, 1984a; Srinivas et al., 1987), and (3) palliative therapy in patients with locally inoperable tumors or distant metastases.

RECONSTRUCTION FOLLOWING PENECTOMY AND EMASCULATION

Partial Penectomy

The patient who has undergone partial penectomy has the option of penile reconstruction. Free flap reconstruction of the penis with a radial forearm flap would, in most centers, be considered the modality of choice (Chang and Hwang, 1984; Devine et al., 1987; Gilbert et al., 1987, 1988). Modifications of the radial forearm flap (Biemer, 1988; Farrow et al., 1989) have enhanced its versatility. In addition, the upper lateral arm flap has proved to be of value in reconstruction of the penis. This flap is a source of thin, relatively nonhirsute epithelium with a dependable blood supply and dependable cutaneous innervation.

Because these free flaps have dependable innervation, which can be elevated with the flap, they provide phallic reconstructive covering with erogenous sensibility. This erogenous sensibility serves a purpose beyond sexual gratification. Sensation must be present before a prosthesis is placed. The patient with a partial penectomy can undergo the reconstruction and placement of a prosthesis with good success. The proximal corporal bodies serve well to seat the prosthesis; the distal corpora are constructed with a vascular graft material, usually Gore-Tex, which allows for tissue ingrowth and stability.

Partial penectomy for penile carcinoma should not be avoided based on strictly cosmetic criteria because modern penile reconstructive surgery can provide excellent cosmetic results and allow resumption of sexual activity.

Total Penectomy

Phallic reconstruction following loss of the penis provides genitourinary surgery with one of its greatest challenges. The anatomy and physiology of the erectile corpora cavernosa are unique and are not reproduced by the transfer of any other human tissues. The earlier attempts at phallic construction/reconstruction consisted of the "tube within a tube" concept, utilizing a tubed flap of abdominal skin for the urethra enclosed within another covering flap of abdominal skin. The "phallus" was transferred to the area of the penis by sequential steps of delay. Such reconstructions were often unsuccessful because of the multiple procedures involved. Additionally, the phallus lacked sensation and had suboptimal aesthetic appearance.

Arterialized flaps (superficial groin flap) and myocutaneous flaps (gracilis, rectus femoris, and rectus abdominis) have been tried with moderate success in phallic reconstruction. Although these local flaps ostensibly diminished the number of reconstructive stages, they too were insensate and tended to atrophy.

Newer concepts in microsurgical reconstruction have produced improvements in the function and appearance of the neophallus. Ideally, phallic reconstruction should address the following requirements: (1) one-stage microsurgical procedure, (2) creation of a competent urethra to achieve normal voiding, (3) restoration of a phallus that has both tactile and erogenous sensibility, (4) enough bulk to allow implantation of a prosthetic stiffener for vaginal penetration, and (5) aesthetic acceptance by the patient.

In an attempt to meet these five reconstructive criteria, we first embarked on a technique employing microneurovascular transfers (see Chapter 83). These advances in free tissue transfer have been employed to help accomplish the criteria described for successful phallic reconstruction.

Following total penectomy, successful reconstruction of a phallus with microvascular transfer is technically straightforward. Prosthetic placement, however, is more difficult in that total reconstruction of the corporal body is a necessity. Gore-Tex has served well at this center for "corporal" reconstruction. The Gore-Tex corpora allows for tissue ingrowth, thus limiting migration of prosthetic elements. Additionally, the Gore-Tex sleeves can be anchored in the perineum to the ischial tuberosities, thus stabilizing the devices posteriorly. This stabilization allows for better rigidity and limits migration of the prosthetic elements. In that the Gore-Tex is placed to allow for tissue ingrowth and anchoring only, the ultrathin Gore-Tex grafts serve well and limit the amount of foreign body placed.

With collaboration of the urologist and the plastic surgeon, the reconstruction of a neophallus is becoming more of a reality. Experience with microneurovascular tissue transfers has demonstrated that a successful one-stage phallic reconstruction is now possible.

Inguinal Reconstruction Following Node Dissection

Changes in the technique and the incisions employed have limited the complications seen previously with lymph node dissection. Previously, flaps were elevated on the dermal and subdermal blood supply, and tissue loss was a frequent occurrence. The realization that skin lymphatics are not involved in the metastatic process permits dissection deep to Scarpa's fascia, which lessens the incidence of skin flap loss. The transposition of the sartorius muscle over the vessels has minimized the incidence of vascular erosion and thrombosis. Nonetheless, wound problems do occur, and certain patients require the excision of a wide area of skin because of the mass of metastatic tumor contained in the superficial groin nodes.

The majority of wound problems are secondary to the loss of skin at the edge of the wound. These skin problems arise because the blood supply to the skin of the lower leg is, for the most part, musculocutaneous in distribution (McCraw and Dibbell, 1977; McCraw et al., 1977). With the elevation of flaps as cuticular entities, the deep perforator vessels are divided and, hence, the flaps are left to survive as random flaps. In some instances, flap elevation exceeds the cutaneous vascular territory.

The superior aspect of the wound represents a "tidal zone" between cuticular vascular territories and musculocutaneous vascular territories (Brown et al., 1975; Cormack and Lamberty, 1985; Hester et al., 1984). The superior aspect of the wound may be placed below the cutaneous vascular territory, and the results are flap ischemia and necrosis (Fig. 31–23). Likewise, the inferior aspect of the wound is clearly in a musculocutaneous vascular area and, with elevation, becomes a random flap, which may again exceed the abilities of the dorsal plexus to provide vascularity.

In most instances, only a small amount of superficial skin is lost. These small areas of skin loss can be simply covered with split-thickness skin grafting. However, with deeper skin loss or with the excision of a large cuticular area with the specimen, more substantial tissue transfer is required. A number of local flaps are available for transposition into these tissue defects. The gracilis musculocutaneous unit is totally expendable and transposed without difficulty into a groin defect (Orticochea, 1972a, 1972b).

For situations requiring larger flaps, the tensor fasciae latae musculofascial cutaneous system represents an excellent tissue transfer unit (Nahai et al., 1979; Nahai, 1980). The tensor fasciae latae is simply transposed to the groin, and its large size and bulk make it an ideal choice for coverage of large defects.

The inferiorly based rectus abdominis musculocutaneous flap also represents an excellent transfer unit for groin defects (Taylor et al., 1984). The contralateral inferior rectus abdominis muscle flap can be transposed across the infrapubic space to the opposite groin without difficulty if the ipsilateral flap is not usable.

Muscle, fascial, or musculocutaneous fascial cutaneous units described previously are invariably sufficient for coverage of the femoral vessels. However, if unavailable, pedicle omental flaps represent a valuable option (Arnold et al., 1983). The rich arterial supply of this flap has been proved to cause neovascularization in the host site. The abundance of lymphatics in the flap helps in the control of infection and reabsorption of extracellular fluid (Bunkis and Walton, 1990; Hoffman and Trengove-Jones, 1990; McCraw and Arnold, 1986; Samson, 1990; Taylor et al., 1990; Trier, 1990).

NONSQUAMOUS MALIGNANCY

Melanoma and basal cell carcinoma rarely occur on the penis, presumably because the organ's skin is protected from sun exposure. Malignancies arising from the supporting structures of the penis are also quite rare and include any combination of tumors of smooth or striated muscle or of fibrous, fatty, or vascular tissue. Information regarding appropriate treatment of these malignancies is derived from the review of single case reports and small series.

Basal Cell Carcinoma

The rarity of basal cell carcinoma of the penis contrasts with the frequency of this lesion on other cutaneous surfaces. Less than 15 cases have been well documented (Goldminz et al., 1989). Treatment is by local excision, which is virtually always curative (Goldminz et al., 1989; Hall et al., 1968). No cases of metastasis or local recurrence after local excision have been reported.

Melanoma

Fewer than 60 cases of melanoma of the penis have been reported. Of 1200 melanomas treated at MSKCC, only two were of penile origin (Das Gupta and Grabstald, 1965). At the M. D. Anderson Cancer Treatment Center, less than 1 per cent of all primary penile carcinomas were malignant melanomas (Johnson and Ayala, 1973).

Melanoma appears as a blue-black to reddish-brown, pigmented papule, plaque, or ulceration on the glans penis; less frequently, it is found on the prepuce. Definitive diagnosis is accomplished by histologic examination of biopsy specimens, which reveals atypical junctional

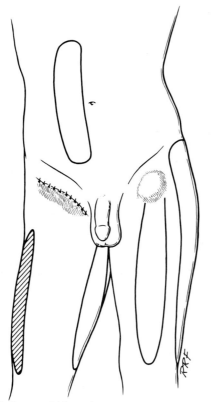

Figure 31–23. Flaps useful in groin coverage.

On the left, the tensor fasciae latae musculocutaneous transfer unit is outlined on the lateral part of the leg. The biceps femoris musculocutaneous transfer unit is illustrated on the anterior thigh.

On the right, the vastus lateralis muscle flap is illustrated on the lateral leg. The vastus can be included with the tensor fasciae latae unit, thus making the cutaneous tip more reliable. The gracilis musculocutaneous unit is illustrated medially. On the abdomen is illustrated the vertical rectus abdominis muscle flap. This flap can be transposed to the ipsilateral or the contralateral groin.

On the right groin is illustrated the tidal zone of skin loss following lymph node dissection; on the left groin is illustrated a bulky tumor, which may require en bloc skin removal with the node dissection.

cell activity with displacement of pigmented cells into the dermis.

Prognostic characteristics that have been found significant for melanoma in other sites, such as depth of invasion and thickness of the tumor, have unfortunately not been applied to penile lesions. When this information is available, local excision might be possible in select cases (Martin et al., 1988). Distant metastatic spread has been found in 60 per cent of patients studied (Abeshouse, 1958; Johnson et al., 1973). Hematogenous metastases occur by means of the vascular structures of the corporal bodies; lymphatic spread to the regional ilioinguinal nodes occurs by lymphatic permeation.

Surgery is the primary mode of treatment with radiotherapy and chemotherapy being of only adjunctive or palliative benefit. For stage I melanoma (localized lesion without metastases) and stage II melanoma (metastases confined to one regional area), adequate excision of the primary tumor by partial or total penile amputation together with en bloc bilateral ilioinguinal node dissection offers the greatest prospect for cure (Bracken and Diokno, 1974; Johnson et al., 1973; Manivel and Fraley,

1988). However, the prognosis for the patient with this neoplasm is poor, with few reported 5-year survivors (Reid, 1957; Wheelock and Clark, 1943) because of the frequency of metastases occurring beyond the confines of surgical resection.

Sarcomas

Primary mesenchymal tumors of the penis are very rare. A thorough review of 46 such tumors from the Armed Forces Institute of Pathology revealed an equal number of benign and malignant lesions (Dehner and Smith, 1970). The patients ranged in age from newborn to the 8th decade of life. The presenting signs and symptoms of subcutaneous mass, penile pain and enlargement, priapism, and urinary obstruction were the same for both benign and malignant lesions. A sarcoma has been reported to "masquerade" as a Peyronie's plaque (Moore et al., 1975).

Malignant lesions were found more frequently on the proximal shaft; benign lesions were more often located distally. The most common malignant lesions were those of vascular origin (hemangioendothelioma), followed in frequency by those of neural, myogenic, and fibrous origin (Ashley and Edwards, 1957). Single case reports of sarcomatous lesions have been published, e.g., malignant fibrous histiocytoma (Parsons and Fox, 1988), angiosarcoma (Rasbridge and Parry, 1989), and epithelioid sarcoma (Leviav et al., 1988).

Sarcomas have been classified as superficial when they arise from the integumentary supporting structures and as deep when they arise from the corporal body supporting structures (Pratt and Ross, 1969). Wide local surface excision and partial penile amputation for the superficial tumors have been suggested and used successfully in isolated case reports (Dalkin and Zaontz, 1989; Pak et al., 1986). Total penile amputation has been reserved for tumors of deep corporal origin. However, local recurrences are characteristic of sarcomas (Dehner and Smith, 1970). To avoid local recurrences, a total amputation, even for superficial malignancies of any cell type, should be considered.

Regional metastases are rare; therefore, unless adenopathy is palpable, node dissections are not recommended (Hutcheson et al., 1969). Distant metastases have also been unusual (Dehner and Smith, 1970), and this fact encourages aggressive local treatment in anticipation of cure. Radiation therapy and chemotherapy have not been used extensively enough to comment upon their efficacy.

Paget's Disease

Paget's disease of the penis is extremely rare. Less than 15 cases have been reported (Mitsudo et al., 1981). It appears grossly as an erythematous, eczematoid, well-demarcated area that cannot be clinically distinguished from erythroplasia of Queyrat, Bowen's disease, or, therefore, carcinoma in situ of the penis. Clinical presentation includes local discomfort, pruritus, and occasionally, a serosanguineous discharge. On microscopic examination, identification is clearly made by the presence of large, round or oval, clear-staining hydropic cells with hypochromatic nuclei, i.e., "Paget cells."

Paget's disease may often herald a deeply seated carcinoma with Paget cells moving through ducts or lymphatics to the epidermal surface. In the penis, a sweat gland carcinoma (Mitsudo et al., 1981) or peri-urethral gland adenocarcinoma (Jenkins, 1989) may be the primary neoplasm. Complete local surgical excision of the skin and subcutaneous tissue is the recommended form of therapy. If inguinal adenopathy is present, radical node dissection is advised (Hagan et al., 1975). Careful observation for recurrence at the margins is necessary.

Lymphoreticular Malignancy

Primary lymphoreticular malignancy rarely occurs on the penis (Dehner and Smith, 1970). Leukemia may infiltrate the corpora, resulting in priapism (Pochedly et al., 1974). When lymphomatous infiltration of the penis is diagnosed, a thorough search for systemic disease is necessary. If the penile lesion is indeed a primary tumor, treatment with systemic chemotherapy may be used. It is the most effective therapy for local disease, for potential occult deposits that may exist elsewhere, and for preservation of form and function (Marks et al., 1988). Local low-dose irradiation has also been reported as successful (Stewart et al., 1985).

Kaposi's sarcoma, usually a cutaneous manifestation of a generalized lymphoreticular disorder, may produce genital lesions and now is most frequently associated with AIDS (vide supra).

Metastasis

Metastatic lesions to the penis are unusual. Approximately 200 cases have been reported in the literature. Their infrequency is somewhat puzzling when one considers the rich blood and lymphatic supply to the organ and its proximity to the bladder, the prostate, and the rectum—areas frequently involved with neoplasm. It is from these three organs that the majority of metastatic penile lesions originate (Abeshouse, 1958). Renal and respiratory neoplasms have also metastasized to the penis. The most likely routes of spread are by direct extension, retrograde venous and lymphatic transport, and arterial embolism.

The most frequent sign of penile metastases is priapism; penile swelling, nodularity, and ulceration have also been reported (Abeshouse and Abeshouse, 1961; McCrea and Tobias, 1958; Weitzner, 1971). Urinary obstruction and hematuria may occur. The most common histologic feature of penile invasion by metastatic lesions is the replacement of one or both corpora cavernosa, a ready explanation for the frequent finding of priapism. Solitary cutaneous, preputial, and glanular deposits are less common.

The differential diagnosis includes idiopathic pria-pism; venereal or other infectious ulcerations; tuberculosis; Peyronie's plaque; and primary, benign, or malignant tumors.

Penile metastases represent an advanced form of virulent disease and usually appear rather rapidly after recognition and treatment of the primary lesion (Abeshouse and Abeshouse, 1961; Hayes and Young, 1967; Mukamel et al., 1987). On rare occasions, a long period may elapse between the treatment of the primary lesion and the appearance of penile metastases (Abeshouse and Abeshouse, 1961), or the penile lesion may occur as the initial and only site of metastases.

Because of the association of a penile metastatic lesion with advanced disease, survival after its presentation is limited, and the majority of patients die within 1 year (Mukamel et al., 1987; Robey and Schellhammer, 1984). Successful treatment may occasionally be possible in the case of solitary nodules or localized distal penile involvement if complete excision by partial amputation succeeds in removing the entire area of malignant infiltration (Spaulding and Whitmore, 1978). The prospect for surgical cure is minimal if proximal corporal invasion is present. Penectomy is occasionally indicated after failure of other modalities to palliate intractable pain (Mukamel et al., 1987). Pain can also be managed by dorsal nerve section (Hill and Khalid, 1988). Treatment with radiation therapy has been generally unsuccessful, and chemotherapy has not been employed in a sufficient number of cases to warrant definitive recommendations.

REFERENCES

Abeshouse, B. S.: Primary and secondary melanoma of the genito-urinary tract. South. Med. J., 51:994, 1958.

Abeshouse, B. S., and Abeshouse, G. A.: Metastatic tumors of the penis: A review of the literature and a report of two cases. J. Urol., 86:99, 1961.

Abratt, R. P.: The treatment of bilateral ulcerated lymph node metastases from carcinoma of the penis. Cancer, 54:1720–1722, 1984.

Ackerman, L. V.: Verrucous carcinoma of the oral cavity. Surgery, 23:670, 1948.

Ahmed, T., Sklaroff, R., and Yagoda, A.: Sequential trials of methotrexate, cisplatin and bleomycin for penile cancer. J. Urol., 132:465, 1984.

Almgard, L. E., and Edsmyr, F.: Radiotherapy in treatment of patients with carcinoma of the penis. Scand. J. Urol. Nephrol., 7:1, 1973.

Anderson, E. E., and Glenn, J. F.: Penile malignancy and hypercalcemia. JAMA, 192:128, 1965.

Aragona, F., Serretta, V., Marconi, A., Spinelli, C., and Arganini, M.: Queyrat's erythroplasia of the prepuce: A case-report. Acta Chir. Belg., 85:303, 1985.

Arnold, P. G., Witzke, D. J., Irons, G. B., and Woods, J. E.: Use of omental transposition flaps for soft-tissue reconstruction. Ann. Plast. Surg., 11:508, 1983.

Ashley, D. J. B., and Edwards, E. C.: Sarcoma of the penis: Leiomyosarcoma of the penis: Report of a case with a review of the literature of sarcoma of the penis. Br. J. Surg., 43:170, 1957.

Bahmer, F. A., and Tang, D. E., and Payeur-Kirsch, M.: Treatment of large condylomata of the penis with the neodymium-YAG-laser. Acta Derm. Venereol. (Stockh.), 64:361–363, 1984.

Bainbridge, D. R., Whitaker, R. H., and Shepheard, B. G. F.: Balanitis xerotica obliterans and urinary obstruction. Br. J. Urol., 43:487, 1971.

Baker, B. H., Spratt, J. S., Perez-Mesa, C., et al.: Carcinoma of the penis. J. Urol., 116:458, 1976.

Baker, B. H., and Watson, F. R.: Staging carcinoma of the penis. J. Surg. Oncol., 7:243, 1975.

Ball, T. P., and Pickett, J. D.: Traumatic lymphangitis of penis. Urology, 6:594, 1975.

Bandieramonte, G., Lepera, P., Marchesini, R., Andreola, S., and Pizzocaro, G.: Laser microsurgery of superficial lesions of the penis. J. Urol., 138:315, 1987.

Bandieramonte, G., Santoro, O., Boracchi, P., Piva, L., Pizzocaro, G., and DePalo, G.: Total resection of glans penis surface by CO_2 laser microsurgery. Acta Oncol., 27:575, 1988.

Barrasso, R., De Brux, J., Croissant, O., and Orth, G.: High prevalence of papillomavirus-associated penile intraepithelial neoplasia in sexual partners of women with cervical intraepithelial neoplasia. N. Engl. J. Med., 317:916, 1987.

Bayne, D., and Wise, G. J.: Kaposi sarcoma of the penis and genitalia: A disease of our times. Urology, 31:22, 1988.

Beggs, J. H., and Spratt, J. S.: Epidermoid carcinoma of the penis. J. Urol., 91:166, 1961.

Biemer, E.: Penile construction by the radial arm flap. Clin. Plast. Surg., 15:425, 1988.

Bissada, N. K., Cole, A. T., and Fried, F. A.: Extensive condylomas acuminata of the entire male urethra and the bladder. J. Urol., 112:201, 1974.

Bissada, N. K., Morcos, R. R., and El-Senoussi, M.: Post-circumcision carcinoma of the penis. I. Clinical aspects. J. Urol., 135:283, 1986.

Block, N. L., Rosen, P., and Whitmore, W. F.: Hemipelvectomy for advanced penile cancer. J. Urol., 110:703, 1973.

Blum, R. H., Carter, S. K., and Agre, K.: A clinical review of bleomycin—a new antineoplastic agent. Cancer, 31:903, 1973.

Boon, T. A.: Sapphire probe laser surgery for localized carcinoma of the penis. Eur. J. Surg. Oncol., 14:193, 1988.

Boshart, M., and zur Hausen, H.: Human papillomaviruses (HPV) in Buschke-Lowenstein tumors: Physical state of the DNA and identification of a tandem duplication in the non-coding region of a HPV 6-subtype. J. Virol., 58:963, 1986.

Bouchot, O., Auvigne, J., Peuvrel, P., Glemain, P., and Buzelin, J. M.: Management of regional lymph nodes in carcinoma of the penis. Eur. Urol., 16:410, 1989.

Bowen, J.: Precancerous dermatoses: A review of two cases of chronic atypical epithelial proliferation. J. Cutan. Dis., 30:241, 1912.

Boxer, R. J., and Skinner, D. G.: Condylomata acuminata and squamous cell carcinoma. Urology, 9:72, 1977.

Bracken, R. B., and Diokno, A. C.: Melanoma of the penis and the urethra: 2 Case reports and review of the literature. J. Urol., 111:198, 1974.

Brown, M. D., Zachary, C. B., Grekin, R. C., and Swanson, N. A.: Penile tumors: Their management by Mohs micrographic surgery. J. Dermatol. Surg. Oncol., 13:1163, 1987.

Brown, R. G., Vasconez, L. O., and Jurkiewicz, M. J.: Transverse abdominal flaps and the deep epigastric arcade. Plast. Reconstr. Surg., 55:416, 1975.

Bruns, T. N. C., Lauvetz, R. J., Kerr, E. S., and Ross, G.: Buschke-Lowenstein giant condylomas: Pitfalls in management. Urology, 5:773, 1975.

Buddington, W. T., Kickham, C. J. E., and Smith, W. E.: An assessment of malignant disease of the penis. J. Urol., 89:442, 1963.

Bunkis, J., and Walton, R. L.: The rectus abdominis flap for groin defects, Chap. 327. In: Strauch, B., Vasconez, L. O., and Hall-Findlay, E. J. (Eds.): Grabb's Encyclopedia of Flaps, Vol. III. Boston, Little, Brown & Co., 1990, pp. 1410–1415.

Buschke, A., and Löwenstein, L.: Uber carcinomahnliche condylomata acuminata des penis. Klin. Wochenschr., 4:1726, 1925.

Cabanas, R.: An approach to the treatment of penile carcinoma. Cancer, 39:456, 1977.

Carpiniello, V. L., Malloy, T. R., Sedlacek, T. V., and Zderic, S. A.: Results of carbon dioxide laser therapy and topical 5-fluorouracil treatment for subclinical condyloma found by magnified penile surface scanning. J. Urol., 140:53, 1988.

Carpiniello, V. L., Schoenberg, M., and Malloy, T. R.: Long-term followup of subclinical human papillomavirus infection treated with the carbon dioxide laser and intraurethral 5-fluorouracil: A treatment protocol. J. Urol., 143:726, 1990.

Carpiniello, V. L., Zderic, S. A., Malloy, T. R., and Sedlacek, T. V.: Carbon dioxide laser therapy of subclinical condyloma found by magnified penile surface scanning. Urology, 24:608, 1987.

Catalona, W. J.: Role of lymphadenectomy in carcinoma of the penis. Urol. Clin. North Am., 7:785, 1980.

Catalona, W. J.: Modified inguinal lymphadenectomy for carcinoma of the penis with preservation of saphenous veins: Technique and preliminary results. J. Urol., 140:306, 1988.

Chang, T. S., and Hwang, W. Y.: Forearm flap in one-stage reconstruction of the penis. Plast. Reconstr. Surg., 74:251, 1984.

Coetzee, T.: Condyloma acuminatum. S. Afr. J. Surg., 15:75, 1977.

Cole, L. A., and Helwig, E. B.: Mucoid cysts of the penile skin. J. Urol., 115:397, 1976.

Copulsky, J., Whitehead, E. D., and Orkin, L. A.: Condyloma acuminata in a three-year-old boy. Urology, 5:372, 1975.

Cormack, G. C., and Lamberty, B. G. H.: The blood supply of thigh skin. Plast. Reconstr. Surg., 75:342, 1985.

Cottel, W. J., et al.: Essentials of Mohs micrographic surgery. J. Dermatol. Surg. Oncol., 14:11, 1988.

Culp, O. S., Magid, M. A., and Kaplan, I. W.: Podophyllin treatment of condylomata acuminata. J. Urol., 51:655, 1944.

Dagher, R., Selzer, M. L., and Lapides, J.: Carcinoma of the penis and the anti-circumcision crusade. J. Urol., 110:79, 1973.

Dalkin, B., and Zaontz, M. R.: Rhabdomyosarcoma of the penis in children. J. Urol., 141:908, 1989.

Daly, N. J., Douchez, J., and Combes, P. F.: Treatment of carcinoma of the penis by iridium 192 wire implant. Int. J. Radiat. Oncol. Biol. Phys., 8:1239, 1982.

Das Gupta, T., and Grabstald, H.: Melanoma of the genitourinary tract. J. Urol., 93:607, 1965.

Davies, S. W.: Giant condyloma acuminata: Incidence among cases diagnosed as carcinoma of the penis. J. Clin. Pathol., 18:142, 1965.

Dawson, D. F., Duckworth, J. K., Bernhardt, H., and Young, J. M.: Giant condyloma and verrucous carcinoma of the genital area. Arch. Pathol., 79:225, 1965.

Dean, A. L.: Epithelioma of the penis. J. Urol., 33:252, 1935.

Dehner, L. P., and Smith, B. H.: Soft tissue tumors of the penis. Cancer, 25:1431, 1970.

deKernion, J. B., Tynbery, P., Persky, L., and Fegen, J. P.: Carcinoma of the penis. Cancer, 32:1256, 1973.

Derrick, F. C., Lynch, K. M., Kretkowski, R. C., and Yarbrough, W. J.: Epidermoid carcinoma of the penis: Computer analysis of 87 cases. J. Urol., 110:303, 1973.

Devine, P. D., Winslow, B. H., Jordan, G. H., Horton, C. E., and Gilbert, D. A.: Reconstructive phallic surgery. In Libertino, J. A. (Ed.): Pediatric and Adult Reconstructive Urologic Surgery, Ed. 2. Baltimore, Williams & Wilkins, 1987, p. 552.

Dillaha, C. J., Jansen, T., Honeycutt, W. M., and Holt, G. A.: Further studies with topical 5-fluorouracil. Arch. Dermatol., 92:410, 1965.

Dodge, O. G.: Carcinoma of the penis in East Africans. Br. J. Urol., 37:223, 1965.

Dretler, S. P., and Klein, L. A.: The eradication of intraurethral condyloma acuminata with 5-fluorouracil cream. J. Urol., 113:195, 1975.

Duncan, W., and Jackson, S. M.: The treatment of early cancer of the penis with megavoltage x-rays. Clin. Radiol., 23:246, 1972.

Edsmyr, F., Andersson, L., and Esposti, P.: Combined bleomycin and radiation therapy in carcinoma of the penis. Cancer, 56:1257, 1985.

Edwards, A., Atma-Ram, A., and Thin, R. N.: Podophyllotoxin 0.5% v podophyllin 20% to treat penile warts. Genitourin. Med., 64:263–265, 1988.

Edwards, R. H., and Sawyers, J. L.: The management of carcinoma of the penis. South. Med. J., 61:843, 1968.

Ekstrom, T., and Edsmyr, F.: Cancer of the penis: A clinical study of 229 cases. Acta Chir. Scand., 115:25, 1958.

Engelman, E. R., Herr, H. W., and Ravera, J.: Lipogranulomatosis of external genitalis. Urology, 3:358, 1974.

Engelstad, R. B.: Treatment of cancer of the penis at the Norwegian Radium Hospital. Am. J. Roentgenol., 60:801, 1948.

Epstein, E.: Association of Bowen's disease with visceral cancer. Arch. Dermatol., 82:349, 1960.

Eron, L. J., Judson, F., Tucker, S., Prawer, S., Mills, J., Murphy, K., Hickey, M., Rogers, M., Flannigan, S., Hien, N., Katz, H. I., Goldman, S., Gottlieb, A., Adams, K., Burton, P., Tanner, D., Taylor, E., and Peets, E.: Interferon therapy for condylomata acuminata. N. Engl. J. Med., 315:1059, 1986.

Ewalt, D. H., and McConnell, J. D.: Penile neoplasms—30 year experience 1958–1988 [Abstract 651]. J. Urol., 143:351A, 1990.

Farrow, G. A., Boyd, J. B., and Semple, J. L.: Total reconstruction of the penis employing the "cricket bat flap" single stage forearm free graft [Abstract 77]. J. Urol., 141:52A, 1989.

Ferenczy, A.: Strategies to eradicate genital HPV infection in men. Contemp. Urol., 2:19, 1990.

Fields, T., Drylie, D., and Wilson, J.: Malignant evolution of penile horn. Urology, 30:65–66, 1987.

Fisher, H. A. G., Barada, J. H., Horton, J., and VonRoemeling, R.: Neoadjuvant therapy with Cisplatin and 5-Fluorouracil for stage III squamous cell carcinoma of the penis [Abstract 653]. J. Urol., 143:352A, 1990.

Fossa, S. D., Hall, K. S., Johannessen, M. B., Urnes, T., and Kaalhus, O.: Carcinoma of the penis: Experience at the Norwegian Radium Hospital 1974–1985. Eur. Urol., 13:372, 1987.

Fraley, E. E., Zhang, G., Manivel, C., and Niehans, G. A.: The role of ilioinguinal lymphadenectomy and significance of histological differentiation in treatment of carcinoma of the penis. J. Urol., 142:1478–1482, 1989.

Frew, I. D. O., Jefferies, J. D., and Swiney, J.: Carcinoma of the penis. Br. J. Urol., 39:398, 1967.

Friedman, K. A. E.: Disseminated Kaposi's sarcoma syndrome in young homosexual men. J. Am. Acad. Dermatol., 5:468, 1981.

Furlong, J. H., and Uhle, C. A. W.: Cancer of penis: A report of eighty-eight cases. J. Urol., 60:550, 1953.

Gagliano, R. G., Blumenstein, B. A., Crawford, E. D., Stephens, R. L., Coltman, C. A., Jr., and Costanzi, J. J.: Cis-diamminedichloroplatinum in the treatment of advanced epidermoid carcinoma of the penis: A Southwest Oncology Group. J. Urol., 141:66, 1989.

Garnick, M. B., Skarin, A. T., and Steele, G. D.: Metastatic carcinoma of the penis: Complete remission after high-dose methotrexate chemotherapy. J. Urol., 122:265–266, 1979.

Geffen, J. R., Klein, R. J., and Friedman-Kien, A. E.: Intralesional administration of large doses of human leukocyte interferon for the treatment of condylomata acuminata. J. Infect. Dis., 150:612–615, 1984.

Gilbert, D. A., Horton, C. E., Terzis, J. K., Devine, C. J., Jr., Winslow, B. H., and Devine, P. C.: New concepts in phallic reconstruction. Ann. Plast. Surg., 18:128, 1987.

Gilbert, D. A., Williams, M. W., Horton, C. E., Terzis, J. K., Winslow, B. H., Gilbert, D. M., and Devine, C. J., Jr.: Phallic reinnervation via the pudendal nerve. J. Urol., 140:295, 1988.

Goette, D. K.: Erythroplasia of Queyrat. Arch. Dermatol., 110:271, 1974.

Goldberg, H. M., Pell-Ilderton, R., Daw, E., and Saleh, N.: Concurrent squamous cell carcinoma of the cervix and penis in a married couple. Br. J. Obstet. Gynecol., 86:585, 1979.

Goldminz, D., Scott, G., and Klaus, S.: Penile basal cell carcinoma: Report of a case and review of the literature. J. Am. Acad. Dermatol., 20:1094, 1989.

Grabstald, H.: Carcinoma of the penis involving skin of base. J. Urol., 104:438, 1970.

Grabstald, H., and Kelley, C. D.: Radiation therapy of penile cancer. Urology, 15:575, 1980.

Graham, J. H., and Helwig, E. B.: Erythroplasia of Queyrat. Cancer, 32:1396, 1973.

Gross, G., Hagedorn, M., Ikenberg, H., Rufli, T., Dahlet, C., Grosshans, E., and Gissmann, L.: Bowenoid papulosis: Presence of human papillomavirus (HPV) structural antigens and of HPV 16–related DNA sequences. Arch. Dermatol., 121:858, 1985.

Grossman, L. A., Kaplan, H. J., Grossman, M., and Ownby, F. D.: Thrombosis of the penis: Interesting facet of thromboangitis obliterans. JAMA, 192:329, 1965.

Gursel, E. O., Georgountzos, C., Uson, A. C., Melicow, M. M., and Veenema, R. J.: Penile cancer. Urology, 1:569, 1973.

Hagan, K. W., Braren, V., Viner, N. A., Page, D. L., and Rhamy, R. K.: Extramammary Paget's disease in the scrotal and inguinal areas. J. Urol., 114:154, 1975.

Haile, K., and Delclos, L.: The place of radiation therapy in the treatment of carcinoma of the distal end of the penis. Cancer, 45:1980, 1980.

Hall, T. C., Britt, D. B., and Woodhead, D. M.: Basal cell carcinoma of the penis. J. Urol., 99:314, 1968.

Hanash, K. A., Furlow, W. L., Utz, D. C., and Harrison, E. G.: Carcinoma of the penis: A clinicopathologic study. J. Urol., 104:291, 1970.

Hardner, G. J., Bhanalaph, T., Murphy, G. P., Albert, D. J., and Moore, R. H.: Carcinoma of the penis: Analysis of therapy in 100 consecutive cases. J. Urol., 108:428, 1972.

Harlin, J. C.: Carcinoma of the penis. J. Urol., 67:326, 1952.

Hassan, A. A., Orteza, A. M., and Milam, D. F.: Penile horn: Review of literature with 3 case reports. J. Urol., 97:315, 1967.

Hayes, W. T., and Young, J. M.: Metastatic carcinoma of the penis. J. Chronic Dis., 20:891, 1967.

Hester, T. R., Jr., Nahai, F., Beegle, P. E., and Bostwick, J., III: Blood supply of the abdomen revisited, with emphasis on the superficial inferior epigastric artery. Plast. Reconstr. Surg., 74:657, 1984.

Hill, J. T., and Khalid, M. A.: Point of technique—penile denervation. Br. J. Urol., 61:167, 1988.

Hoffman, W. Y., and Trengove-Jones, G.: The rectus femoris flap, Chap. 326. In Strauch, B., Vasconez, L. O., and Hall-Findlay, E. J. (Eds.): Grabb's Encyclopedia of Flaps, Vol. III. Boston, Little, Brown & Co., 1990, pp. 1408–1409.

Hofstetter, A., and Frank, F.: Laser use in urology. In Dixon, J. A. (Ed.): Surgical Application of Lasers. Chicago, Year Book Medical Publishers, 1983, pp. 146–162.

Hoofnagle, R. F., Mahin, E. J., Lamm, D. L., and Kandzari, S. J.: Deoxyribonucleic acid flow cytometry of squamous cell carcinoma of the penis [Abstract 654]. J. Urol., 143:352A, 1990.

Hubbell, C. R., Rabin, V. R., and Mora, R. G.: Cancer of the skin with blacks: V. A review of 175 black patients with squamous cell carcinoma of the penis. J. Am. Acad. Dermatol., 18:292–298, 1988.

Hueser, J. N., and Pugh, R. P.: Erythroplasia of Queyrat treated with topical 5-fluorouracil. J. Urol., 102:595, 1969.

Hutcheson, J. B., Wittaker, W. W., and Fronstin, M. H.: Leiomyosarcoma of the penis: Case report and review of literature. J. Urol., 101:874, 1969.

Ichikawa, T., Nakano, I., and Hirokawa, I.: Bleomycin treatment of the tumors of penis and scrotum. J. Urol., 102:699, 1969.

Jackson, S. M.: The treatment of carcinoma of the penis. Br. J. Surg., 53:33, 1966.

Jaffe, H. W., Bregman, D. J., and Selik, R. M.: Acquired immunodeficiency syndrome in the United States: The first one thousand cases. J. Infect. Dis., 148:339, 1983.

Jamieson, N. V., Bullock, K. N., and Barker, T. H. W.: Adenosquamous carcinoma of the penis associated with balanitis xerotica obliterans. Br. J. Urol., 58:730–731, 1986.

Jenkins, I. L.: Extra-mammary Paget's disease of the penis. Br. J. Urol., 63:103, 1989.

Jensen, M. S.: Cancer of the penis in Denmark 1942 to 1962 (511 cases). Dan. Med. Bull., 24:66, 1977.

Johnson, D. E., and Ayala, A. G.: Primary melanoma of penis. Urology, 2:174, 1973.

Johnson, D. E., Fuerst, D. E., and Ayala, A. G.: Carcinoma of the penis: Experience in 153 cases. Urology, 1:404, 1973.

Johnson, D. E., and Lo, R. K.: Management of regional lymph nodes in penile carcinoma: Five-year results following therapeutic groin dissections. Urology, 24:308–311, 1984a.

Johnson, D. E., and Lo, R. K.: Complications of groin dissection in penile carcinoma: Experience with 101 lymphadenectomies. Urology, 24:312, 1984b.

Jordan, G. H.: Reconstruction of the fossa navicularis. J. Urol., 138:102, 1987.

Kaposi, M.: Idiopathic multiple pigmented sarcoma of the skin [Reprinted from Arch. Dermatol. Syphil., 4:265, 1892]. Cancer, 32:342, 1982.

Kaushal, V., and Sharma, S. C.: Carcinoma of the penis: A 12-year review. Acta Oncol., 26:413–417, 1987.

Kelley, C. D., Arthur, K., Rogoff, E., and Grabstald, H.: Radiation therapy of penile cancer. Urology, 4:571, 1974.

King, L. S., and Sullivan, M.: Effects of podophyllin and of colchicine on normal skin, on condyloma acuminatum and on verruca vulgaris. Arch. Pathol., 43:374, 1947.

Kini, M. G.: Cancer of the penis in a child, aged two years. Indian Med. Gaz., 79:66, 1944.

Kleiman, H., and Lancaster, Y.: Condyloma acuminata of the bladder. J. Urol., 88:52, 1962.

Knudsen, O. S., and Brennhovd, I. O.: Radiotherapy in the treatment of the primary tumor in penile cancer. Acta Chir. Scand., 133:69, 1967.

Kopf, A. W., and Bart, R. S.: Tumor conference number 11: Multiple bowenoid papulosis of the penis: A new entity? J. Dermatol. Surg. Oncol., 3:265, 1977.

Kossow, J. H., Hotchkiss, R. S., and Morales, P. A.: Carcinoma of penis treated surgically: Analysis of 100 cases. Urology, 2:169, 1973.

Kraus, F. T., and Perez-Mesa, C.: Verrucous carcinoma: Clinical and pathologic study of 105 cases involving oral cavity, larynx, and genitalia. Cancer, 19:26, 1966.

Krebs, H. B.: Genital HPV infections. Clin. Obstet. Gynecol., 32:180, 1989a.

Krebs, H. B.: Management strategies. Clin. Obstet. Gynecol., 32:200, 1989b.

Krebs, H. B., and Schneider, V.: Human papillomavirus–associated lesions of the penis: Colposcopy, cytology, and histology. Obstet. Gynecol., 70:299, 1987.

Kriegmair, M., Rothenberger, K. H., Spitzenpfeil, E., Schmeller, N. T., and Hofstetter, A. G.: Neodymium-YAG-laser treatment for carcinoma of the penis [Abstract 650]. J. Urol., 143:351A, 1990.

Kuruvilla, J. T., Garlick, F. H., and Mammen, K. E.: Results of surgical treatment of carcinoma of the penis. Aust. N. Z. J. Surg., 41;157, 1971.

Kyalwazi, S. K., and Bhana, D.: Bleomycin in penile carcinoma. East Afr. Med. J., 50:331, 1973.

Lancaster, W. D., Castellano, C., Santos, C., Delgado, G., Kurman, R. J., and Jenson, A. B.: Human papillomavirus deoxyribonucleic acid in cervical carcinoma from primary and metastatic sites. Am. J. Obstet. Gynecol., 154:115, 1986.

Landthaler, M., Haina, D., Brunner, R., et al.: Laser therapy of Bowenoid papulosis and Bowen's disease. J. Dermatol. Surg. Oncol., 12:1253, 1986.

Laymon, C. W., and Freeman, C.: Relationship of balanitis xerotica obliterans to lichen sclerosus et atrophicus. Arch. Dermatol. Syph., 49:57, 1944.

Lederman, M.: Radiotherapy of cancer of the penis. Br. J. Urol., 25:224, 1953.

Lepow, H., and Leffler, N.: Giant condylomata acuminata (Buschke-Lowenstein tumor): Report of two cases. J. Urol., 83:853, 1960.

Lesser, J. H., and Schwarz, H., II: External genital carcinoma: Results of treatment at Ellis Fischel State Cancer Hospital. Cancer, 8:1021, 1955.

Leviav, A., Devine, P. C., Schellhammer, P. F., and Horton, C. E.: Epithelioid sarcoma of the penis. Clin. Plast. Surg., 15:489, 1988.

Levine, R. U., Crum, C. P., Herman, E., Silvers, D., Ferenczy, A., and Richart, R. M.: Cervical papillomavirus infection and intraepithelial neoplasia: A study of male sexual partners. Obstet. Gynecol., 64:16, 1984.

Lewis, R. J., and Bendl, B. J.: Erythroplasia of Queyrat: Report of a patient successfully treated with topical 5-fluorouracil. Can. Med. Assoc. J., 104:148, 1971.

Licklider, S.: Jewish penile carcinoma. J. Urol., 86, 98, 1961.

Linderman, R. D., and Papper, S.: Therapy of fluid and electrolyte disorders. Ann. Intern. Med., 82:64, 1975.

Lowe, F. C., Lattimer, G., and Metroka, C. E.: Kaposi's sarcoma of the penis in patients with acquired immunodeficiency syndrome. J. Urol., 142:1475, 1989.

Löwenstein, L. W.: Carcinoma-like condylomata acuminata of the penis. Med. Clin. North Am., 5:789, 1939.

Lynch, H. T., and Krush, A. J.: Delay factors in detection of cancer of the penis. Nebr. State Med. J., 54:360, 1969.

Madej, G., and Meyza, J.: Cryosurgery of penile carcinoma. Oncology, 39:350, 1982.

Magid, M., and Garden, J. M.: Pearly penile papules: Treatment with the carbon dioxide laser. J. Dermatol. Surg. Oncol., 15:552–554, 1989.

Malakoff, A. F., and Schmidt, J. D.: Metastatic carcinoma of penis complicated by hypercalcemia. Urology, 5:519, 1975.

Malloy, T. R., Wein, A. J., and Carpiniello, V. L.: Carcinoma of the penis treated with neodymium YAG laser. Urology, 31:26, 1988.

Manivel, J. C., and Fraley, E. E.: Malignant melanoma of the penis and male urethra: 4 Case reports and literature review. J. Urol., 139:813, 1988.

Marcial, V. A., Figueroa-Colon, J., Marcial-Rojas, R. A., and Colon, J. E.: Carcinoma of the penis. Radiology, 79:209, 1962.

Marks, D., Crosthwaite, A., Varigos, G., Ellis, D., and Morstyn, G.: Therapy of primary diffuse large cell lymphoma of the penis with preservation of function. J. Urol., 139:1057, 1988.

Martin, R. W., III, Russell, R. C., Trautmann, V. F., and Klingler, W. G.: Conservative excision of penile melanoma. Ann. Plast. Surg., 20:266–269, 1988.

Mazeron, J. J., Langlois, D., Lobo, P. A., Huart, J. A., Calitchi, E., Lusinchi, A., Raynal, M., Le Bourgeois, J. P., Abbou, C. C., and Piequin, B.: Interstitial radiation therapy for carcinoma of the penis using iridium 192 wires: The Henri Mondor experience (1970–1979). Int. J. Radiat. Oncol. Biol. Phys., 10:1891, 1984.

McConnell, J. D.: Personal communication, 1990.

McCraw, J. B., and Arnold, P. G.: McCraw and Arnold's Atlas of Muscle and Musculocutaneous Flaps. Norfolk, Hampton Press Publishing, 1986, pp. 265–294 (vertical rectus), 423–443 (tensor fascia lata), 445–461 (rectus femoris), 463–482 (vastus lateralis).

McCraw, J. B., and Dibbell, D. G.: Experimental definition of independent myocutaneous vascular territories. Plast. Reconstr. Surg., 60:212, 1977.

McCraw, J. B., Dibbell, D. G., and Carraway, J. H.: Clinical definition of independent myocutaneous vascular territories. Plast. Reconstr. Surg., 60:341, 1977.

McCrea, L. W., and Tobias, G. L.: Metastatic disease of the penis. J. Urol., 80:489, 1958.

McDougal, W. S., Kirchner, F. K., Jr., Edwards, R. H., and Killion, L. T.: Treatment of carcinoma of the penis: The case of primary lymphadenectomy. J. Urol., 136:38, 1986.

McKay, D. L., Fuqua, F., and Weinberg, A. G.: Balanitis xerotica obliterans in children. J. Urol., 114:773, 1975.

Mills, E. E. D.: Intermittent intravenous methotrexate in the treatment of advanced epidermoid carcinoma. S. Afr. Med. J., 46:398, 1972.

Misma, Y., and Matunalea, M.: Effect of bleomycin on benign and malignant cutaneous tumors. Acta Derm. Venereol. (Stockh.), 52:211, 1972.

Mitsudo, S., Nakanishi, I., and Koss, L. G.: Paget's disease of the penis and adjacent skin. Arch. Pathol. Lab. Med., 105:518, 1981.

Mohs, F. E.: Chemosurgery: A microscopically controlled method of cancer excision. Arch. Surg., 42:279, 1941.

Mohs, F. E., Snow, S. N., Messing, E. M., and Kuglitsch, M. E.: Microscopically controlled surgery in the treatment of carcinoma of the penis. J. Urol., 133:961, 1985.

Moore, S. W., Wheeler, J. E., and Hefter, L. G.: Epithelioid sarcoma masquerading as Peyronie's disease. Cancer, 35:1706, 1975.

Morgan, W. K. C.: The rape of the phallus. JAMA, 193:223, 1965.

Mortimer, P. S., Sonnex, T. S., and Dawber, R. P. R.: Cryotherapy for multicentric pigmented Bowen's disease. Clin. Exp. Dermatol., 8:319, 1983.

Mukamel, E., Farrer, J., Smith, R. B., and deKernion, J. B.: Metastatic carcinoma of penis: When is total penectomy indicated? Urology, 24:15, 1987.

Murrell, D. S., and Williams, J. L.: Radiotherapy in the treatment of carcinoma of the penis. Br. J. Urol., 37:211, 1965.

Nahai, F.: The tensor fascia lata flap. Clin. Plast. Surg., 7:51, 1980.

Nahai, F., Hill, H. L., and Hester, T. R.: Experiences with the tensor fascia lata flap. Plast. Reconstr. Surg., 63:788, 1979.

Narasimharao, K. L., Chatterjee, H., and Veliath, A. J.: Penile carcinoma in the first decade of life. Br. J. Urol., 57:358, 1985.

Narayana, A. S., Olney, L. E., Loening, S. A., Weimar, G. W., and Culp, D. A.: Carcinoma of the penis: Analysis of 219 cases. Cancer, 49:2185, 1982.

National Cancer Institute (NCI) Position Statement: Kaposi's sarcoma. *In* PDQ, Physician Data Query (Database). Bethesda, MD, August 21, 1990, pp. 1–11.

Neinstein, L. S., and Goldenring, J.: Pink pearly papules: An epidemiologic study. J. Pediatr., 105:594, 1984.

Nickel, W. R., and Plumb, R. T.: Nonvenereal sclerosing lymphangitis of penis. Arch. Dermatol., 86:761, 1962.

Nitidandhaprabhas, P.: Artificial penile nodules: Case reports from Thailand. Br. J. Urol., 47:463, 1975.

Orticochea, M.: Musculo-cutaneous flap method: Immediate and heroic substitute for the method of delay. Br. J. Plast. Surg., 25:106, 1972a.

Orticochea, M.: New method of total reconstruction of the penis. Br. J. Plast. Surg., 25:347, 1972b.

Pak, K., Sakaguchi, N., Takayama, H., and Tomoyoshi, T.: Rhabdomyosarcoma of the penis. J. Urol., 136:438, 1986.

Parsons, M. A., and Fox, M.: Malignant fibrous histiocytoma of the penis. Eur. Urol., 14:75, 1988.

Patterson, J. W., Kao, G. F., Graham, J. H., and Helwig, E. B.: Bowenoid papulosis: A clinicopathologic study with ultrastructural observations. Cancer, 57:823, 1986.

Paymaster, J. C., and Gangadharan, P.: Cancer of the penis in India. J. Urol., 97:110, 1967.

Pereira-Bringel, P. J., and de Andrade Arruda, R.: 5-Fluorouracil cream 5% in the treatment of intraurethral condylomata acuminata. Br. J. Urol., 54:295, 1982.

Perinetti, E. P., Crane, D. C., and Catalona, W. J.: Unreliability of sentinel lymph node biopsy for staging penile carcinoma. J. Urol., 124:734, 1980.

Peters, B. S., and Perry, H. O.: Bowenoid papules of the penis. J. Urol., 126:482, 1981.

Pfister, H., and Haneke, E.: Demonstration of human papilloma virus type 2 DNA in Bowen's disease. Arch. Dermatol. Res., 276:123, 1984.

Pierquin, B., Chassagne, D., and Cox, J. D.: Toward consistent local control of certain malignant tumors. Radiology, 99:661, 1971.

Pizzocaro, G., and Piva, L.: Adjuvant and neoadjuvant vincristine, bleomycin, and methotrexate for inguinal metastases from squamous cell carcinoma of the penis [Fasc. 6b]. Acta Oncol., 27:823–824, 1988.

Plaut, A., and Kohn-Speyer, A. C.: The carcinogenic action of smegma. Science, 195:391, 1947.

Pochedly, C., Mehta, A., and Feingold, E.: Priapism with hyperacute stem-cell leukemia. N.Y. State J. Med., 75:540, 1974.

Poynter, J. H., and Levy, J.: Balanitis xerotica obliterans: Effective treatment with topical and sublesional steroids. Br. J. Urol., 39:420, 1967.

Prasad, K. R., and Veliath, A. J.: Cell surface blood group antigens in carcinoma of the penis. Appl. Pathol., 4:192, 1986.

Pratt, R. M., and Ross, R. T. A.: Leiomyosarcoma of the penis. Br. J. Surg., 56:870, 1969.

Pratt-Thomas, H. R., Heins, H. C., Latham, E., Dennis, E. J., and McIver, F. A.: The carcinogenic effect of human smegma: An experimental study. Cancer, 9:671, 1956.

Pressman, D., Rolnick, D., and Turbow, B.: Penile horn. Am. J. Surg., 104:640, 1962.

Preston, E. N.: Whither the foreskin? A consideration of routine neonatal circumcision. JAMA, 213:1853, 1970.

Previte, S. R., Karian, S., Cho, S. I., and Austen, G., Jr.: Penile carcinoma in renal transplant recipient. Urology, 13:298, 1979.

Proffitt, S. D., Spooner, T. R., and Kosek, J. C.: Origin of undifferentiated neoplasm from verrucous epidermal carcinoma of oral cavity following irradiation. Cancer, 26:389, 1970.

Puras, A., Fortuno, R., Gonzalez-Flores, B., and Sotolongo, A.: Staging lymphadenectomy in the treatment of carcinoma of the penis. Proc. Kimbrough Urol. Semin., 14:15, 1980.

Puras, A., Gonzalez-Flores, B., et al.: Treatment of carcinoma of the penis. Proc. Kimbrough Urol. Semin., 12:143, 1978.

Queyrat, L.: Erythroplasie du gland. Soc. Franc. Dermatol. Syphilol., 22:378, 1911.

Rasbridge, S. A., and Parry, J. R. W.: Angiosarcoma of the penis. Br. J. Urol., 63:440, 1989.

Raynal, M., Chassagne, D., Baillet, F., and Pierquin, B.: Endocuritherapy of penis cancer. Recent Results Cancer Res., 60:135, 1977.

Redd, C. R. R. M., et al.: A study of 80 patients with penile carcinoma combined with cervical biopsy study of their wives. Int. Surg., 62:549, 1977.

Reddy, D. G., and Baruah, I. K. S. M.: Carcinogenic action of human smegma. Arch. Pathol., 75:414, 1963.

Redman, J. F., and Meacham, K. R.: Condyloma acuminata of the urethral meatus in children. J. Pediatr. Surg., 8:939, 1973.

Reece, R. W., and Koontz, W. W., Jr.: Leukoplakia of the urinary tract: A review. J. Urol., 114:165, 1975.

Reid, J. D.: Melanosarcoma of the penis. Cancer, 10:359, 1957.

Revuz, J., and Clerici, T.: Penile melanosis. J. Am. Acad. Dermatol., 20:567–570, 1989.

Rhatigan, R. M., Jimenez, S., and Chopskie, E. J.: Condyloma acuminatum and carcinoma of the penis. South. Med. J., 65:423, 1972.

Rheinschild, G. W., and Olsen, B. S.: Balanitis xerotica obliterans. J. Urol., 104:860, 1970.

Riveros, M., Garcia, R., and Cabanas, R.: Lymphadenography of the dorsal lymphatics of the penis. Cancer, 20:2026, 1967.

Riveros, M., and Gorostiaga, R.: Cancer of the penis. Arch. Surg., 85:377, 1962.

Robey, E. L., and Schellhammer, P. F.: Four cases of metastases to the penis and a review of the literature. J. Urol., 132:992, 1984.

Rosemberg, S. K., and Fuller, T. A.: Carbon dioxide rapid super-pulsed laser treatment of erythroplasia of Queyrat. Urology, 16:181, 1980.

Rosemberg, S. K., Jacobs, H., and Fuller, T.: Some guidelines in the treatment of urethral condylomata with carbon dioxide laser. J. Urol., 127:906, 1982.

Rothenberger, K. H.: Value of the neodymium-YAG laser in the therapy of penile carcinoma. Eur. Urol., 12:34, 1986.

Rubenstein, M., and Wolff, S. M.: Penile nodules as a major manifestation of subacute angitis. Arch. Intern. Med., 114:449, 1964.

Rudd, F. V., Rott, R. K., Skoglund, R. W., and Ansell, J. S.: Tumor-induced hypercalcemia. J. Urol., 107:986, 1972.

Sagerman, R. H., Yu, W. S., Chung, C. T., and Puranki, A.: External beam irradiation of cancer of the penis. Radiology, 152:183, 1984.

Salaverria, J. C., Hope-Stone, H. F., Paris, A. M. I., Molland, E. A., and Blandy, J. P.: Conservative treatment of carcinoma of the penis. Br. J. Urol., 51:32, 1979.

Samson, R. H.: Omental flap for coverage of exposed groin vessels, Chap. 325. In Strauch, B., Vasconez, L. O., and Hall-Findlay, E. J. (Eds.): Grabb's Encyclopedia of Flaps, Vol. III. Boston, Little, Brown & Co., 1990, pp. 1404–1407.

Sand, P. K., Bowen, L. W., Blischke, S. O., and Ostergard, D. R.: Evaluation of male consorts of women with genital human papilloma virus infection. Obstet. Gynecol., 68:679, 1986.

Scappini, P., Piscioli, F., Pusiol, T., Hofstetter, A., Rothenberger, K., and Luciani, L.: Penile cancer: Aspiration biopsy cystology for staging. Cancer, 58:1526–1533, 1986.

Schneider, V.: Microscopic diagnosis of HPV infection. Clin. Obstet. Gynecol., 32:148, 1989.

Schoen, E. J., Anderson, G., Bohon, C., Hinman, F., Jr., Poland, R. L., and Wakeman, E. M.: Task force on circumcision, report of the task force on circumcision. Pediatrics, 84:388, 1989.

Schrek, R., and Lenowitz, H.: Etiologic factors in carcinoma of penis. Cancer Res., 7:180, 1947.

Schultz, R. E., Miller, J. W., MacDonald, G. R., Auman, J. R., Peterson, N. R., Ward, B. E., and Crum, C. P.: Clinical and molecular evaluation of acetowhite genital lesions in men. J. Urol., 143:920, 1990.

Sedlacek, T. V., Cunnane, M., and Carpiniello, V.: Colposcopy in the diagnosis of penile condyloma. Am. J. Obstet. Gynecol., 154:494, 1986.

Seftel, A. D., Sadick, N. S., and Waldbaum, R. S.: Kaposi's sarcoma of the penis in a patient with the acquired immune deficiency syndrome. J. Urol., 136:673, 1986.

Shiraki, I. W.: Parameatal cysts of the glans penis: A report of nine cases. J. Urol., 114:544, 1975.

Siegel, A.: Malignant transformation of condyloma acuminatum. Am. J. Surg., 103:613, 1962.

Skinner, D. G., Leadbetter, W. F., and Kelley, S. B.: The surgical management of squamous cell carcinoma of the penis. J. Urol., 107:273, 1972.

Sklaroff, R. B., and Yagoda, A.: Cis-diamminedichloride platinum II (DDP) in the treatment of penile carcinoma. Cancer, 44:1563, 1979.

Sklaroff, R. B., and Yagoda, A.: Methotrexate in the treatment of penile carcinoma. Cancer, 45:214, 1980.

Sklaroff, R. B., and Yagoda, A.: Penile cancer: Natural history and therapy. In Chemotherapy and Urological Malignancy. New York, Springer-Verlag, 1982, pp. 98–105.

Smetana, H. F., and Bernhard, W.: Sclerosing lipogranuloma. Arch. Pathol., 50:296, 1950.

Smotkin, D.: Virology of human papillomavirus. Clin. Obstet. Gynecol., 32:117, 1989.

Sonnex, T. S., Ralfs, I. G., Plaza de Lanza, M., and Dawber, R. P. R.: Treatment of erythroplasia of Queyrat with liquid nitrogen cryosurgery. Br. J. Dermatol., 106:581, 1982.

Spaulding, J. T., and Whitmore, W. F., Jr.: Extended total excision of prostatic adenocarcinoma. J. Urol., 120:188, 1978.

Srinivas, V., Morse, M. J., Herr, H. W., Sogani, P. C., and Whitmore, W. F., Jr.: Penile cancer: Relation of extent of nodal metastasis to survival. J. Urol., 137:880–882, 1987.

Staubitz, W. J., Melbourne, H. L., and Oberkircher, O. J.: Carcinoma of the penis. Cancer, 8:371, 1955.

Stein, B. S.: Laser treatment of condylomata acuminata. J. Urol., 136:593, 1986.

Stewart, A. L., Grieve, R. J., and Banerjee, S. S.: Primary lymphoma of the penis. Eur. J. Surg. Oncol., 11:179, 1985.

Stone, K. M.: Epidemiologic aspects of genital HPV infection. Clin. Obstet. Gynecol., 32:112, 1989.

Tannenbaum, M. H., and Becker, S. W.: Papillae of the corona of the glans penis. J. Urol., 93:391, 1965.

Taylor, G. I., Corlett, R. J., and Boyd, J. B.: The versatile deep inferior epigastric (inferior rectus abdominis) flap. Br. J. Plast. Surg., 37:330, 1984.

Taylor, G. I., Corlett, R. J., and Boyd, J. B.: The deep inferior epigastric artery island rectus musculocutaneous flap, Chap. 328. *In* Strauch, B., Vasconez, L. O., and Hall-Findlay, E. J. (Eds.): Grabb's Encyclopedia of Flaps, Vol. III. Boston, Little, Brown & Co., 1990, pp. 1416–1420.

Thomas, J. A., and Small, C. S.: Carcinoma of the penis in southern India. J. Urol., 160:520, 1963.

Trier, W. C.: Local skin flaps, Chap. 321. *In* Strauch, B., Vasconez, L. O., and Hall-Findlay, E. J. (Eds.): Grabb's Encyclopedia of Flaps, Vol. III. Boston, Little, Brown & Co., 1990, pp. 1393–1395.

Ubben, K., Kryzek, R., and Ostrow, R.: Human papilloma virus DNA detected in two verrucous carcinomas. J. Invest. Dermatol., 22:195–210, 1979.

Uehling, D. T.: Staging laparotomy for carcinoma of penis. J. Urol., 110:213, 1973.

Vaeth, J. M., Green, J. P., and Lowry, R. O.: Radiation therapy of carcinoma of the penis. Am. J. Roentgenol. Radiat. Ther. Nucl. Med., 108:130, 1970.

Villa, L. L., and Lopes, A.: Human papillomavirus DNA sequences in penile carcinomas in Brazil. Int. J. Cancer, 37:853, 1986.

Wade, T. R., Kopf, A. W., and Ackerman, A. B.: Bowenoid papulosis of the penis. Cancer, 42:1890, 1978.

Weitzner, S.: Secondary carcinoma in the penis: Report of three cases and literature review. Am. Surg., 37:563, 1971.

Wespes, E., Simon, J., and Schulman, C. C.: Cabanas' approach: Is sentinel node biopsy reliable for staging of penile carcinoma? Urology, 28:278, 1986.

Wheelock, M. C., and Clark, P. J.: Sarcoma of penis. J. Urol., 49:478, 1943.

Whitmore, W. F.: Tumors of the penis, urethra, scrotum, and testes. *In* Campbell, M. F., and Harrison, H. H. (Eds.): Urology, Ed. 3. Philadelphia, W. B. Saunders Co., 1970, pp. 1190–1229.

Wishnow, K. I., and Johnson, D. E.: Effective outpatient treatment of Kaposi's sarcoma of the urethral meatus using the neodymium:YAG laser. Lasers Surg. Med., 8:428, 1988.

Youngberg, G. A., Thornthwaite, J. T., and Inoshita, T.: Cytologically malignant squamous-cell carcinoma arising in a verrucous carcinoma of the penis. J. Dermatol. Surg. Oncol., 9:474, 1983.

Zalar, J. A., Knode, R. E., and Mir, J. A.: Lipogranuloma of the penis. J. Urol., 102:75, 1969.

Zelickson, A. S., and Prawer, S. E.: Bowenoid papulosis of the penis: Demonstration of intranuclear viral-like particles. Am. J. Dermatopathol., 2:305, 1980.

X
EMBRYOLOGY AND ANOMALIES OF THE GENITOURINARY TRACT

32
NORMAL DEVELOPMENT OF THE URINARY TRACT

Max Maizels, M.D.

"Most pediatric patients who require urologic surgery have an underlying congenital anomaly. It follows that urologists, especially pediatric urologists, require a basic understanding of embryology, not only of the urinary organs but also of the cloacal derivatives. . . . Pediatric urologists should understand normal embryology so that they can better understand malformation syndromes that involve the urogenital system" (Stephens, 1982).

This chapter presents concepts of normal embryonic and fetal development of the urinary tract and of selected pathologic developments. As there are few embryos with uropathies to study, grasping the embryology is difficult because one is expected to use schematic drawings to infer the appearances of embryonic tissues. Herein, a "realistic" view of normal development is presented using mostly photographs.

". . . The urinary organs, basically, may be maldeveloped owing to genetic defects or to environment. However, the etiology of the majority of malformations is not known (Stephens, 1982)." Few theories regarding the mechanisms of pathologic development have been tested, yet many theories have become accepted. Although it is plausible that urologic malformations arise from aberrations of normal development, this logic may be incorrect. Some conditions are difficult to explain as an anomaly of normal development (Currarino and Weisbruch, 1989). Unscientific speculation, inaccurate description, and apparently logical mistakes have led to notions about abnormal development that are not necessarily accurate (Hamilton and Mossman, 1976).

The periods of development are presented by gestational age. When necessary, gestational age was derived from crown rump length cited in the literature by interpolation using data from FitzGerald (1978) (Table 32–1). A time table of development in humans is also presented (Table 32–2).

MORPHOGENESIS OF THE GERM LAYERS

PERIOD OF THE ZYGOTE (CONCEPTION TO 1ST WEEK). Development begins after a sperm fertilizes an ovum. The combined cell, a zygote, begins its development by division, cleavage, into about 30 smaller cells, blastomeres. The blastomeres arrange themselves as a hollow sphere, the blastula, which is about the same size as the parent zygote (Fig. 32–1A). Darkly colored cells form an inner cell mass that will give rise to the tissues of the embryo.

PERIOD OF THE LAMINAR EMBRYO (2ND TO 3RD WEEK). During the 2nd week, the inner cell mass flattens. A separate sheet of cells, the endoderm, appears on the undersurface of the inner cell mass. The cells that appose the endoderm compose the ectoderm. The lamination of the inner cell mass into an endoderm and an ectoderm marks the blastoderm. A cleft appears above the ectoderm and enlarges as the yolk sac (Fig. 32–1B). During the 3rd week, cell migration between the ectoderm and endoderm streaks the previously smooth surface of the blastoderm (Fig. 32–1C, D). These cells develop into mesoderm. At the region of the caudal end of the primitive streak, the endoderm

Table 32–1. CROWN-RUMP LENGTH RELATED TO GESTATIONAL AGE

Age (weeks)	Length (mm)
4	5
5	8
6	12
8	23
12	56
16	110
20	160
24	200
28	240
32	280
36	310
40	350

After FitzGerald, M. J. T. (Ed.): Abdominal and pelvic organs. In Human Embryology. New York, Harper & Row, 1978.

1301

Table 32–2. TIME TABLE OF THE DEVELOPMENT OF THE HUMAN URINARY SYSTEM

Days after Ovulation	Developmental Event
	Period of the Embryo
18	Cloacal membrane at caudal end of primitive streak (Fig. 32–1)
20	Para-axial mesoderm and lateral plate mesoderm (Figs. 32–3 and 32–4); tail end of embryo folds to create cloaca
22	Intermediate mesoderm; pronephric duct present (Fig. 32–4)
24	Nephrotomes of the pronephros disappear Mesonephric ducts and tubules appear (Fig. 32–4)
26	Caudal portions of the wolffian ducts end blindly short of the cloaca
28	Wolffian duct has fused to the cloaca; ureteral buds appear (Figs. 32–5 and 32–6); septation of cloaca begins (Figs. 32–21, 32–23, 32–24)
32	Common excretory ducts dilate and extend into the cloaca (Fig. 32–29); metanephric mesenchyme caps the ureteral buds (Figs. 32–5, 32–6, 32–8, 32–10)
33	Ureteral buds have extended and appear as primitive pelves (Fig. 32–6)
37	Metanephrol are reniform (Fig. 32–7); ureteral bud ampullae divide into cranial and caudal poles (Fig. 32–6); elongate growth of ureter (Fig. 32–14); Chawalla's membrane (Fig. 32–15)
41	Müllerian ducts appear (Figs. 32–38 and 32–42); cloaca partitioning (Fig. 32–21); genital tubercle prominent (Figs. 32–20 and 32–22); lumen of ureter is discrete
44	Urogenital sinus separate from rectum (Fig. 32–21); wolffian ducts and ureters drain separately into the urogenital sinus (Figs. 32–27, 32–28, 32–29)
	Indifferent Stage of Embryo Begins
48	First nephrons appear (Fig. 32–8); collecting tubules appear; urogenital membrane ruptures
51	Kidneys in lumbar region (Fig. 32–11); orifices of ureters cranial to those of the wolffian ducts; müllerian ducts descend adjacent to the mesonephric ducts (Figs. 32–27, 32–28, 32–38)
52	Glomeruli appear in the kidney
54	Müllerian ducts are fused behind the urogenital sinus; Müller's tubercle distinct (Fig. 32–27); testis distinguishable
	Period of the Fetus Begins
8 weeks	1° and 2° urethral grooves (Fig. 32–22C)
9 weeks	First likelihood of renal function
	Indifferent Stage of Embryo Ends
10 weeks	Genital ducts of opposite sex degenerate (Fig. 32–41), bladder muscularization
12 weeks	External genitalia become distinctive for sex; male penile urethra forming; feminization of female begins (Fig. 32–37) Urogenital union (Fig. 32–39); apex of bladder separates from allantoic diverticulum; prostate appears (Fig. 32–35); Cowper's glands (Fig. 32–36) and Skene's glands appear
13 weeks	Bladder becomes muscularized
14 weeks	Ureter begins to attain submucosal course in bladder
16 weeks	Mesonephros involuted; glandar urethra forms (Fig. 32–33); sinus vagina (Fig. 32–44)
18 weeks	Ureteropelvic junction apparent (Fig. 32–39)
20–40 weeks	Further growth and development complete the urogenital organs including, among others, testis descent after 26 weeks (Fig. 32–40); differentiation of myometrium (Fig. 32–45)

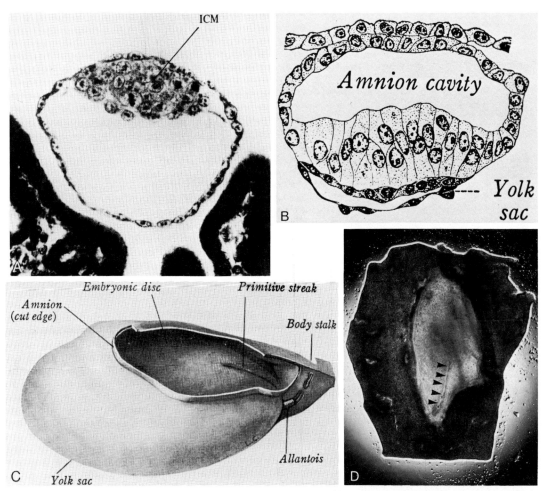

Figure 32–1. Morphogenesis of the germ layers. *A,* Blastocyst consists of cells arranged as a sphere. Some cells aggregate as the inner cell mass (ICM) (blastocyst of bat). (From Austin, C. R., and Short, R. V.: Reproduction in Mammals, Book 2. Embryonic and Fetal Development. 2nd ed. Cambridge, Cambridge University Press, 1973.) *B,* The inner cell mass laminates into endoderm and ectoderm. Clefts above and below the cell layers develop into the amnion cavity and yolk sac, respectively (monkey). (From Arey, L. B.: Developmental Anatomy. Philadelphia, W. B. Saunders Co., 1974.) Cell migration between the endoderm and ectoderm streaks the smooth blastoderm. These migrating cells develop into mesoderm. *C,* Primitive streak of the human. (From Arey, L. B.: Developmental Anatomy. Philadelphia, W. B. Saunders Co., 1974.) *D,* Primitive streak (*arrowheads*) is located in the center of the clear blastoderm (wet mount of the chick embryo viewed by transillumination).

remains apposed to the ectoderm without intervening mesoderm. The layers remain apposed in this area during later stages of development as the cloacal membrane (see Development of the Cloaca). Thereby, there are three germ layers.

PERIOD OF THE SOMITE EMBRYO (3RD TO 6TH WEEK). The primordial germ cells are visible in somite embryos (Fig. 32–2).

During the period of the embryo (to 8 weeks of development), the germ layers form the organs of the body; during the period of the fetus (9 weeks to term), development involves maturation of the formed organs.

OVERVIEW OF NORMAL DEVELOPMENT OF THE URINARY SYSTEM

The definitive urinary system results from complex interactions of embryonic mesoderm with itself and with endoderm. This development is commonly viewed to repeat that of lower vertebrates: the pronephros persists in adult cyclostomes (lampreys); the mesonephros is the functional kidney of most anamniotes (fish); and the metanephros is the definitive kidney of most amniotes (birds and mammals). These phases are repeated in humans. The pronephros is the first urinary tissue to appear; next, the mesonephros; and, finally, the metanephros.

Pronephros

During the 4th week of development, condensed mesoderm adjacent to the midline segments into blocklike units, somites (Fig. 32–3). The pronephros appears in the cervical region of the ten-somite embryo between the 2nd and 6th somites (Hamilton and Mossman, 1976). Cells, presumably derived from the intermediate mesoderm, cluster and differentiate into pronephric tubules. The tubules do not function. It is believed that the duct of the pronephric tubule continues caudally as the mesonephric duct (Fig. 32–4*A*). Soon, the pronephros is not apparent.

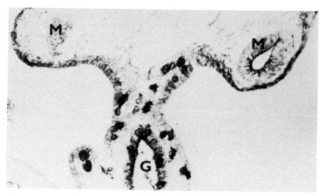

Figure 32–2. Germ cells. Migration of primordial germ cells, which are darkly stained by reaction with alkaline phosphatase, is evident in somite embryos (26 to 44 days). Alkaline phosphatase is lost from the endodermal cells of the allantois and gut but not from the primordial germ cells (28-day-old human embryo). (G, gut; M, mesonephric vesicle; × 37). (From Jirasek, J. E.: Birth Defects. Original Article Series, Vol. 2, no. 2:13, 1977. The National Foundation.)

Elongate growth of ducts pervades development of the genitourinary tract as shown by descent of the pronephric, mesonephric, and müllerian ducts toward the cloaca and ascent of the ureter toward the lumbar retroperitoneum. Mechanisms for elongate growth have been studied in the pronephric duct of the axolotl. The pronephric duct elongates by rearrangement of the cells

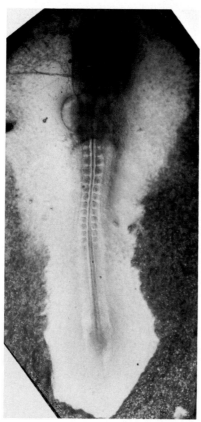

Figure 32–3. Somite stage of development. Mesenchyme condenses as block-like structures, the somites. A row of somites flanks each side of the midline (wet mount of chick embryo).

at the tip of the duct. Here, the duct's diameter is narrower than elsewhere, and the cells actively migrate. Poole and Steinberg (1982) concluded that a craniocaudal gradient of adhesion established by the mesoderm guides the migration of the adjacent duct cells. Philopodia mediate the cell contact. The distribution of cell surface alkaline phosphatase activity is consistent with this enzyme being involved in guiding the descent of the pronephric duct (Zackson and Steinberg, 1988).

Mesonephros

The mesonephric (wolffian) duct descends from the level of the cervical somites to reach the caudal region of the embryo by elongate growth of the terminus of the duct. The duct is adjacent to mesoderm intermediate between the somites and the coelom (primitive peritoneum) (Fig. 32–4B). After the duct and mesoderm appose, mesonephric tubules appear. The nephrons of the mesonephros are induced by the advancing ampulla of the mesonephric duct analogous to the induction of nephrons of the kidney during period 3 of ureteral bud development (see Development of the Ureteral Bud). The mesenchyme condenses, the renal s-shaped vesicles form, the tubules connect to the mesonephric duct, and the tubules segment into glomerulus, proximal tubule, distal tubule, and collecting duct. During its descent, the mesonephric duct induces about 40 pairs of tubules (Potter, 1972). By 28 days, the mesonephric duct has descended to contact the urogenital sinus, and it later drains into the sinus. By 37 days, the mesonephroi are fully developed; they appear as paired retroperitoneal organs, which are close to the midline and bulge into the peritoneum (Fig. 32–5). After 10 weeks of development, the caudal mesonephric nephrons degenerate (Felix, 1912a). The cranial nephrons persist and become incorporated into the genital duct system (see Development of the Ducts of the Genitalia).

The human mesonephros is believed to function. Dilatation of the allantois and bulging, followed by rupture of the cloacal membrane, are interpreted as resulting from the hydrostatic pressure generated from secretion of mesonephric urine (Muecke, 1979). Convolution of tubules and appearance of glomeruli are also interpreted as evidence of function. Because the mesonephroi of several mammals can excrete marker dyes (e.g., phenol red) (Hamilton and Mossman, 1976), it is believed that the human mesonephros can clear the plasma of unwanted metabolites.

Kidney

DEVELOPMENT OF THE URETERAL BUD. After the mesonephric duct drains into the urogenital sinus, the ureteral bud appears. The bud originates as a diverticulum from the posteromedial aspect of the mesonephric duct at the point where the terminus of the duct bends to enter the cloaca (Fig. 32–6A). Potter (1972) has offered the most cohesive view of the later development of the ureteral bud. Based on microdissections

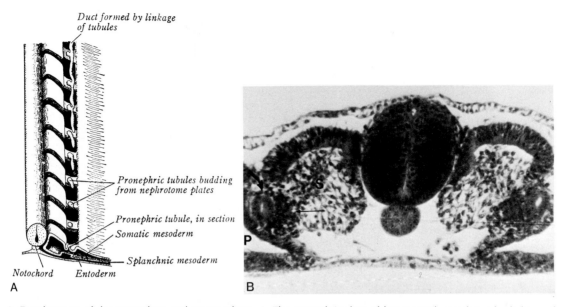

Figure 32–4. Development of the pronephros and mesonephros. *A,* The pronephric duct of lower vertebrates forms by linkage of pronephric tubules. In humans, the pronephric duct probably continues caudally as the mesonephric duct (From Arey, L. B.: Developmental Anatomy. Philadelphia, W. B. Saunders Co., 1974.) *B,* The mesonephric duct (*curved arrow*) apposes mesoderm (*straight arrow*) intermediate between the somite (S) and the coelom (P). Mesonephric tubules appear after the inductive interaction between the duct and mesoderm (chick embryo). (From Maizels, M., and Stephens, F. D.: The induction of urologic malformations: Understanding the relationship of renal ectopia and congenital scoliosis. Invest. Urol., 17:209, 1979.)

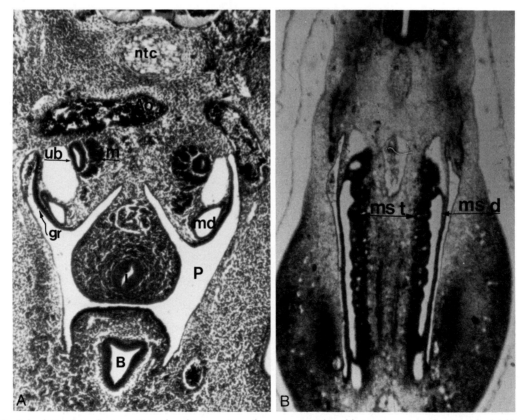

Figure 32–5. Spatial relationship of retroperitoneal and intraperitoneal organs. *A,* Kidney blastema consists of ureteral bud (ub) and its apposed mesenchyme (m). The mesonephric duct (md) is between the renal blastema and gonadal ridge (GR). Note the thickened epithelium. Bladder (B) is an epithelial tube (transverse section of chick embryo) (i, intestine; Ao, aorta; ntc, notochord; P, peritoneum). *B,* Mesonephric tubules (Ms) extend longitudinally along retroperitoneum and drain into mesonephric duct (MsD) (coronal section of chick embryo).

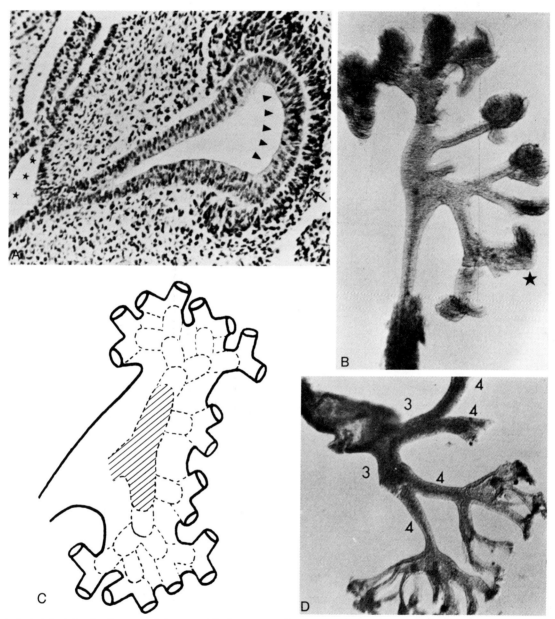

Figure 32–6. Period 1 of the development of the ureteral bud. *A,* Ureteral bud (*arrowheads*) arises as a diverticulum from the mesonephric duct (*asterisks*). Metanephric mesenchyme (*black arrow*) surrounds the ampulla of the ureteral bud (28-day-old embryo) (see Fig. 32–4A).

B, The ampullae branch dichotomously. The branches then dilate to establish the primitive pelvis and calyces (8-week-old human embryo) (*asterisk,* see *D*).

C, Schematic of *B* to show how dichotomous branchings (*dashed lines*) of the primitive ureteral bud (*hatches*) dilate to create the renal pelvis (*solid outline*).

D, Rapid branchings of the ampullae create a bush-like appearance. The base of the bush becomes a bulbous chamber, a calyx (10-week-old human fetus; numbers refer to generations of ampullary divisions).

E, Schematic of *D* to show development of a calyx. Rapid division of an ampulla (*solid black*) produces multiple short branches of the ureteral bud (*hatches* and *stippling*). The resultant bulbous chamber is the primitive calyx.

F, Development of a papilla. With secretion of urine and growth of nephrons, the renal tissue flattens the contour of the calyx (*left*) and then intrudes into the lumen of the calyx as the renal papilla (*right*). (From Potter, E. L.: Normal and Abnormal Development of the Kidney. Chicago, Year Book Medical Publishers, 1972.)

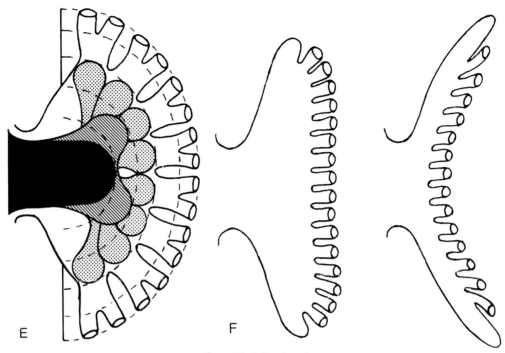

E   F

Figure 32–6 *Continued*

of human embryonic kidneys at various stages of development, the ureteral bud appears to develop further over four periods.

The pattern of nephrogenesis depends on whether the ureteral bud branches symmetrically or not. Branches that are symmetric show similar activities. During period 1, the branchings are symmetric—each one leads to form the pelvis and calyces; during periods 1 and 2, the branchings are symmetric—each one induces tubules. Conversely, branches that are asymmetric show different activities. During period 3, the branchings are asymmetric—one branch of the bud induces tubules, the other simply extends towards the cortex.

PERIOD 1 (5TH TO 14TH WEEK). The initial four to six dichotomous branchings of the ampullae mold the renal pelvis. The metanephrogenic mesenchyme proliferates to appose all of the new ampullae of the new ureteral bud branches. The initial branching establishes the inferior and superior poles of the future kidney. Branching near the poles of the kidney occurs faster than branching near the midsection. Because of this asynchrony, by 7 weeks there are about six generations of ampullae at the poles of the kidney and only four generations of ampullae at the midsection of the kidney. The asynchronous branching helps maintain the reniform shape of the kidney (Hamilton and Mossman, 1976) (Fig. 32–7).

This primitive network of ureteral bud branches dilates and creates the appearance of the pelvis and calyces (Figs. 32–6*B*, *C*). Because the dilatation is not uniform, the appearance of the pelvis and calyces in the newborn may be varied.

The subsequent three to five generations of branchings contribute to the calyces. The branchings occur so rapidly that the many branches appear to arise from a common stem that initially resembles a bulbous chamber (Figs. 32–6*D*, *E*). With later growth, the renal parenchyma projects into this chamber as a conical papilla.

This projection converts the bulbous chamber into the cup-like shape of the definitive calyx (Fig. 32–6*F*). The branchings that occur after 7 weeks are the first to induce nephrons (Fig. 32–8). The bud branching is symmetric. Each branch leads to nephron formation (see the subsequent discussion of nephrogenesis).

Figure 32–7. Time lapse, motion picture prints showing lobular development of mouse kidney in vitro. Branching of the ureteral bud yields lobular renal architecture. (From Saxen, L., Toivonen, S., Vainio, T., and Korhonen, D.: Z. Naturforsch., 20b:340, 1965.)

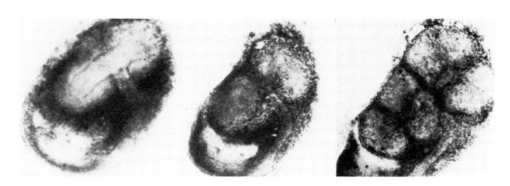

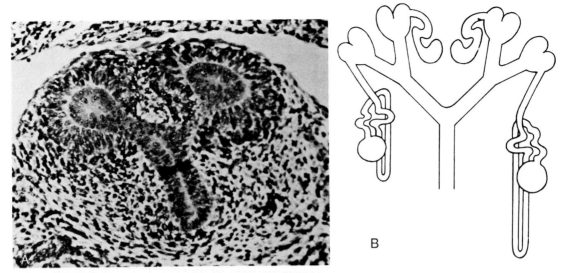

Figure 32–8. Induction of nephrons during period 1 of development of the ureteral bud. *A*, Ampullae branch dichotomously. Each branch remains capped by condensed mesenchyme. *B*, Each branch induces a nephron from its cap of undifferentiated metanephric mesenchyme (schematic). (From Potter, E. L.: Normal and Abnormal Development of the Kidney. Chicago, Year Book Medical Publishers, 1972.)

The next five to seven generations of branchings of the ampulla of the ureteral bud create the collecting ducts. During this interval, the bud branches progressively more slowly. Therefore, as the ampullae extend toward the periphery of the kidney, the collecting ducts laid down close to the calyces are short and wide; the collecting ducts laid down close to the periphery are long and slender.

PERIOD 2 (15TH TO 22ND WEEK). During this period, the ampullae divide infrequently and a family of nephrons is induced by a single ampulla. Interstitial growth of the collecting ducts causes the ampullae to extend centrifugally toward the surface of the kidney. As each ampulla extends, a family of about four (range of two to eight) nephrons is laid down seriatim as "arcades" or tiers of nephrons (Fig. 32–9). The site where the collecting ducts begin centrifugal growth is the corticomedullary junction. The central zone, the medulla, contains the mass of collecting ducts; the peripheral zone, the cortex, contains the nephrons that are attached to collecting ducts. The collecting ducts in the cortex are straight (without branches).

PERIOD 3 (22ND TO 32ND WEEK). As the ampulla grows, it extends farther toward the cortex of the kidney. As the ampulla migrates, it induces about four to six nephrons in series (see Fig. 32–9). This period of development creates nephrons in which the glomeruli lie in the outer half of the cortex. About 75 per cent of the kidney's glomeruli are induced during periods 2 and 3 of development.

PERIOD 4 (32ND TO 36TH WEEK TO ADULTHOOD). The ureteral bud ampullae cease to induce new nephrons and are no longer apparent. During this period the collecting ducts elongate, the proximal tubules convolute, and the loops of Henle penetrate deeper into the medulla. A typical collecting duct drains about 9 to 11 nephrons. Nephron induction by a branching ureteral bud causes the kidney surface to appear lobular at birth (see Fig. 32–7).

Proliferation and branching of the ureteral bud are likely affected by local environmental factors. Mellins

(1984) theorized that variations in bud growth and branching could lead to uropathies of the kidney and ureter, such as a bifid or an extrarenal pelvis and the anomalous appearance of the collecting system of a pelvic kidney. Or, as another example, Middleton and Pfister (1974) theorized that if after the pelvis and calyces are established further branchings of the ureteral bud fail to induce nephrons, perhaps the branches coalesce and appear in later life as a calyceal diverticulum.

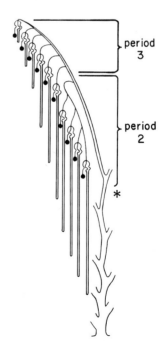

Figure 32–9. Periods 2 and 3 of the development of the ureteral bud. During period 2, as the ampullae migrate toward the cortex, a family of about four nephrons is induced seriatim as "arcades" or tiers by each ampulla. During period 3, a series of about five nephrons are induced, which attach directly to the collecting duct. (*Asterisk* marks site of corticomedullary junction.) (After Potter, E. L.: Normal and Abnormal Development of the Kidney. Chicago, Year Book Medical Publishers, 1972.)

Molecular Biology of Nephrogenesis

Molecular biologic research has probed normal development mostly in embryonic rodent or avian tissues, which grow in vitro or as grafts on a vascular membrane. Unless otherwise cited, the information presented here largely derives from a review by Saxen (1987). Tubulogenesis involves the following steps: initially, induction of unspecialized mesenchyme; then, proliferation of mesenchyme; next, alteration of distribution of cytoskeletal and extracellular matrix proteins that precedes the morphogenesis of the mesenchyme. The mesenchyme now appears as tubules. These steps are followed by segmentation and, finally, vascularization of the nephron.

INDUCTION OF THE NEPHRON. Nephrons are always induced by the interactions between an ampulla of the ureteral bud and its adjacent metanephrogenic mesenchyme. These interactions occur during period 1 when the ampullae branch dichotomously, during period 2 when the ampullae establish tiers of nephrons, and during period 3 when the ampullae advance centrifugally.

Close cell contacts are important to induction. Grobstein (1956) showed the metanephrogenic blastema will not differentiate into tubules if the metanephrogenic mesenchyme does not closely contact the ureteral bud or another inductor tissue. Cell processes from the ureteral bud will reach out even across the pores of a filter in vitro to the metanephrogenic mesenchyme to initiate induction (Lehtonen et al., 1975). If the tissues are separated to prevent close contact, the ureteral bud does not branch, and the metanephrogenic blastema does not differentiate.

Furthermore, the basement membrane of the ureteral bud epithelium is discontinuous only where induction occurs, at the tips of the ampullae. This discontinuity permits close cell contact with the metanephrogenic mesenchyme (Saxen, 1987). This observation through electron microscopy is further supported by the results of immunohistochemical experiments (see Altered Cytoskeletal Proteins and Extracellular Matrix Constituents).

Inductive tissue interactions—one cell population significantly alters the behavior of an adjacent cell population—are common in organ development. They commonly involve an epithelium and its mesenchyme. (See also the discussions of the development of the prostate, uterus, and vagina and the regression of the müllerian duct.) However, inductive interactions during tubulogenesis are unique, as the renal mesenchyme converts into an epithelium and attains a basement membrane.

Tissues other than the ureteral bud can induce the metanephrogenic blastema to differentiate into tubules (Unsworth and Grobstein, 1970). For example, nervous tissue, especially thoracic spinal cord, can also induce nephrons across a filter (Sariola et al., 1989). The neurons within the tissue are the cells responsible for induction. Nervous tissue, treated by immunologic cell lysis to be comprised of only glial and undifferentiated cells, does not induce tubules. In comparison, nervous tissue that contains neurons does induce tubules. A miscellany of other tissues shows cell processes that penetrate the filter but do not induce tubules. It is unlikely that neurons themselves are involved in nephrogenesis in vivo, but cells expressing neurofilaments are noted around the wolffian duct. In the mouse, neurons are noted in the medullae and septa between renal lobules after tubules have already formed.

The only tissue capable of differentiating into renal tubules is the metanephrogenic blastema. The blastema will differentiate into a nephron in vitro, suggesting that early epithelial mesenchymal induction alone is responsible for nephrogenesis (Avner et al., 1983). Other factors such as hormones or urine production are not required.

PROLIFERATION. Proliferation of the induced metanephrogenic mesenchymal cells apparently involves two mechanisms. First, persistent direct contact with an inductor tissue (ureteral bud in vivo or spinal cord in vitro) stimulates the metanephrogenic mesenchyme to proliferate. The proliferation is probably mediated by a mitogen. After induction, a burst of DNA synthesis, as an uptake of radiolabeled thymidine, is observed, and cell division follows. Second, after the period of inductive contact, the mesenchymal cells may continue to differentiate without requiring direct contact with an inductor. However, the mesenchyme is now responsive to growth factors within the embryo. Transferrin, a chelator of iron that is synthesized in the liver and likely is involved with transmembrane iron transport, appears to stimulate mitosis of the metanephrogenic mesenchyme. The now increased number of cells aggregate, and the renal rudiment grows. Furthermore, the larger number of cells promotes morphogenesis, as the mass of cells can now express a new phenotype (tubular epithelium).

ALTERED CYTOSKELETAL PROTEINS AND EXTRACELLULAR MATRIX CONSTITUENTS. It appears that components of extracellular matrix may participate to initiate morphogenesis of nephrons. Using immunohistologic techniques, it was shown that connective tissue antigens (e.g., collagens and fibronectin), which are present prior to induction, are lost during induction (Ekblom et al., 1986). The collagens are lost at the ampullae of the ureteral bud, and fibronectin is lost from the mesenchyme. Fibronectin disappears perhaps because either the newly formed cells are not able to elaborate the glycoprotein or the proteolytic enzymes in the interstitium degrade it. As fibronectin has been shown to promote cell "mobility," the absence of this product could be responsible for condensation of mesenchyme. Reduced cell mobility leads to increased cell density. Or, it may be that the loss of extracellular matrix permits closer cell apposition, restricts cell mobility, and thereby the cells aggregate. Laminin, which appears intensely after induction, may further encourage aggregation of the cells (Saxen, 1987).

The importance of extracellular matrix materials is further strengthened by the finding of syndecan in the blastema. This is a cell surface proteoglycan, which binds to interstitial collagens and fibronectin. The distribution of syndecan correlates temporally with renal differentiation, namely, syndecan first appears intensely in the metanephrogenic mesenchyme adjacent to the ureteral bud. The shift in distribution of interstitial glycoprotein as described follows the appearance of syndecan. Syndecan is still present in the differentiating epithelium and is gradually lost as the nephron matures. Syndecan appears specific to tubule induction because the proteoglycan is not expressed when metanephrogenic mesenchyme is cultured with tissues that do not show induction (i.e., liver). Mixed-species grafting experiments show that syndecan is elaborated by the renal mesenchyme and not from the inductor tissue. As syndecan is a "new" molecule, which appears after induction and is lost after nephrogenesis is advanced, it may become a marker to study induction in the kidney.

Other proteins with "adhesive" properties, such as a neural cell adhesion molecule (N-CAM) and uvomorulin, may help maintain the initial cell adhesion. For example, in mouse renal blastema, the metanephrogenic mesenchyme shows N-CAMs before induction. After induction, the N-CAMs are lost, and a new CAM, uvomorulin, is expressed. It appears that N-CAMs are important adhesives for predetermined, but as yet uninduced, nephrogenic mesenchyme. The N-CAMs are not expressed as a consequence of induction (Klein et al., 1988).

The inductive signal appears to spread away from the ureteral bud ampullae via migration of "induced" metanephrogenic mesenchyme. Spread of the signal would bring the yet uninduced mesenchymal cells, which are deep in the renal blastema, into contact with the "inductor" (Saxen, 1987).

Just as changes in the distribution of constituents of the extracellular matrix are noted with induction, the distribution of constituents of the cytoskeleton also varies. One such change involves vimentin filaments. These filaments are present in uninduced mesenchyme. Induction of mesenchyme is associated with loss of the filaments. The filaments remain only in undifferentiated mesenchyme between new renal tubules.

MORPHOGENESIS. The primitive tubule is the nephric vesicle and appears from the aggregated metanephrogenic cells. Then, a discontinuous basement membrane lines the vesicle. Next, the induced mesenchymal cells condense, and the nuclei polarize to a basal position to form an epithelium. It appears the transition of the mesenchyme to epithelium is also associated with synthesis of large-size proteoglycans (Lash, 1983). The cells laminate into a comma-shaped, double-layered structure; then, swell as a vesicle; and, finally, connect with the collecting tubule. The tubules then elongate and coil.

In the mouse, genes in which expression is linked to collagen type IV production (α_1 and α_2) become active during the period of nephrogenesis when this collagen is incorporated into basement membrane formation. The genes then become quiescent after the period of nephrogenesis (Sawczuk, 1988).

The two phases of induction, change in the extracellular matrix and morphogenesis of the tubules, show different metabolic characteristics. Inhibitors of DNA, RNA, or protein synthesis impair the morphogenesis of tubules when they are applied to the metanephrogenic blastema during induction but not when they are applied later, as during tubulogenesis (Ekblom, 1981).

SEGMENTATION. Immunohistochemical studies can identify the glomerular podocytes, the brush border of proximal tubules, and the Tamm-Horsfall protein of the distal tubules. These studies show that the segmentation of the nephron is sequential and follows the order of glomerulus, proximal tubule, and then distal tubule. The cells that participate in creating the visceral layer of Bowman's capsule flatten, and angiogenic cells invade to create vascular tufts (see Vascularization of the Nephron). Potter (1972) counted 822,300 glomeruli in the kidney of a 40-weeks-old fetus. Glomerular counting of whole fetal kidneys of rats shows an initial phase involving a burst of glomerular differentiation, followed by a second phase of elaboration of tubular development on the basis of tubular length (Okada and Morikawa, 1988). Glomerular counting in the rabbit also shows a burst of new glomerular development during the early part of gestation (McVary and Maizels, 1989).

Perhaps abnormal tubular segmentation accounts for renal tubular dysgenesis—an autosomal recessive condition characterized by a kidney that contains collecting ducts and glomeruli but tubules are not apparent (Swinford, 1989.)

VASCULARIZATION OF THE NEPHRON. After the nephric vesicle appears, the primitive Bowman's capsule segments from the renal tubule. Mesenchymal cells migrate into the cleft of the vesicle. These cells differentiate into endothelial cells. Primitive capillaries later form and then contain mature erythrocytes, presumably derived from the general circulation.

The endothelial cells do not derive from the renal blastema. When mouse metanephric blastema is grafted on the CAM of quail eggs, the glomerular capillaries show the nuclear marker of quail cells, whereas the glomerular podocytes show a mouse origin.

Perhaps the alteration in cellular constituents, as described, promotes vascularization of the nephron, namely, the degradation of collagens and fibronectin makes "split products." These products show angiogenic activity. The nearby mesenchyme may thereby differentiate to vascularize the Bowman's capsule.

Other grafting experiments have demonstrated that the glomerular basement membrane is formed from constituents of both the glomerular epithelium and endothelial cells. The origin of the mesangial cells is unknown. From immunologic studies, it appears that the mesangial cells, similar to the glomerular endothelium, do not derive from the renal blastema. Also, explants of murine renal blastema develop Bowman's capsules but do not show capillary endothelium or mesangial cells (Avner et al., 1983).

MORPHOGENESIS OF RENAL DYSPLASIA

The morphogenesis of renal dysplasia is examined, using experiments that test the knowledge of normal renal development.

Importance of Metanephrogenic Mesenchyme

Metanephrogenic cells are required for normal nephrogenesis. The absence of these cells leads to dysplasia experimentally (Maizels and Simpson, 1983). Chick renal blastemas, which are depleted of condensed metanephrogenic mesenchyme by tissue culture, develop further as "primitive ducts" consistent with those seen in human renal dysplasia (Fig. 32–10).

Sariola and co-workers (1988) showed that when the mesenchyme does not remain condensed against the ureteral bud, abnormal morphogenesis results. Application of an antibody against the ganglioside G_{D3}, which is on the cell surface of the metanephrogenic mesenchyme, caused both reduced branching of the ureteral bud and tubule epithelium formation during in vitro nephrogenesis of the embryonic kidney (Sariola et al., 1988). Perhaps the antibody blocks development by affecting cell-cell interactions between the epithelium and mesenchyme.

Importance of the Extracellular Environment

SIMPLE MOLECULES. Support for the view that renal dysplasia may follow an abnormal interaction between the ureteral bud and metanephrogenic mesenchyme comes from observing the effects of altered potassium concentration. In vitro differentiation of young renal rudiments (after 7 weeks' gestation) appears to require high local concentrations of potassium (Crocker, 1973). Abnormal ureteral bud branching and nephrogenesis follow in vitro exposure of human renal rudiments to low potassium concentration. There are fewer ureteral bud branches, ampullae, and nephrons. These effects were not seen when older rudiments were similarly cultured. Bud branchings that contribute to formation of the pelviocalyceal system were not affected.

MATRIX. We found that perturbing the normal shifts in the distribution of major glycoprotein (fibronectin and laminin) constituents of the interstitium causes an impact on later renal development (Spencer and Maizels, 1987). The glutamine analogue, 6-diazo-5-oxo-L-norleucine (DON), inhibits the synthesis of glycosoaminoglycans and glycoproteins and inhibits in vitro tubulogenesis in a dose-dependent manner. The effect is specific when DON is applied to the tissues during the induction period. When explants are treated with similar inhibitors and CAM is grafted to observe their further in vivo development, the specimens show primitive ducts (Spencer and Maizels, 1987).

The importance of the extracellular matrix to development is seen in other experiments. When DON is injected locally into the posterolateral body wall, avoiding the peritoneal cavity, of chick embryos during the induction period of the renal tubules, the kidneys that develop 1 week following injection show a halving of the surface area of the tubules compared with controls.

Dysplasia did not appear, but the paucity of nephrons resembles hypoplasia (Howe et al., 1989). This view is further underscored by the conclusions of Lelongt and co-workers (1988) who examined the effect of perturbing proteoglycan synthesis in murine renal development. In vitro, the treated kidney showed loose mesenchyme, reduced ureteric bud branching, and fewer nephrons. The importance of laminin in development was investigated similarly in the murine lung. Antilaminin inhibited in vitro branching of the bronchial tree; branches were dilated; and a dose-dependent, lower rate of growth than controls was observed (Schuger et al., 1990).

Ekbloom (1986) concluded that carbohydrates are associated with the actual induction process. Saxen (1987) suggests that the molecules critical to induction, perhaps glycoproteins and/or carbohydrates, lie at the interface between the ureteral bud ampulla and metanephrogenic mesenchyme.

Obstructed Urine Drainage May Not Be of Primary Importance

Clinical observations led to inferences that obstruction of urine drainage may cause renal dysplasia (Bernstein, 1971), but the validity of these inferences has not been well supported by experimental data. Obstruction by suture ligation of the ureter of normal renal blastemas of the chick embryo (Berman and Maizels, 1982) or of mammalian fetuses (Fetterman et al., 1974; Javadpour et al., 1974; Tanaglio, 1972) leads to hydronephrosis not to dysplasia. However, abnormal blastemas (e.g., ureteral buds denuded of condensed metanephrogenic mesenchyme) that are obstructed develop dysplasia more often than abnormal blastemas that develop without ligation of the ureter (Maizels et al., 1983).

Clinical Renal Dysplasia

ABNORMAL URETERAL BUD AND METANEPHROGENIC MESENCHYME INTERACTIONS. On the one hand, when the ureters of duplex kidneys drain onto the trigone, their associated renal units are normally formed. On the other hand, when the ureters of duplex kidneys drain outside the trigone (e.g., urethra and bladder diverticulum), their associated renal units likely are poorly formed (hypoplasia or dysplasia). Ureters that drain outside the trigone are presumed to have originated from ureteral buds that are defective, perhaps because they were abnormally positioned on the wolffian duct. Malpositioned buds may interact poorly with the metanephrogenic mesenchyme, and hypodysplasia may thereby follow (Stephens, 1983).

The notion that obstruction is not required to cause renal dysplasia is further supported by the observations of Kirillova and associates (1982). Microdissection of a human embryo (8 weeks' gestation) showed that the right kidney appeared as a cyst. The ureter was twisted within its mesenchymal coat (see Development of the Ureter), but it was not obstructed or discontinuous.

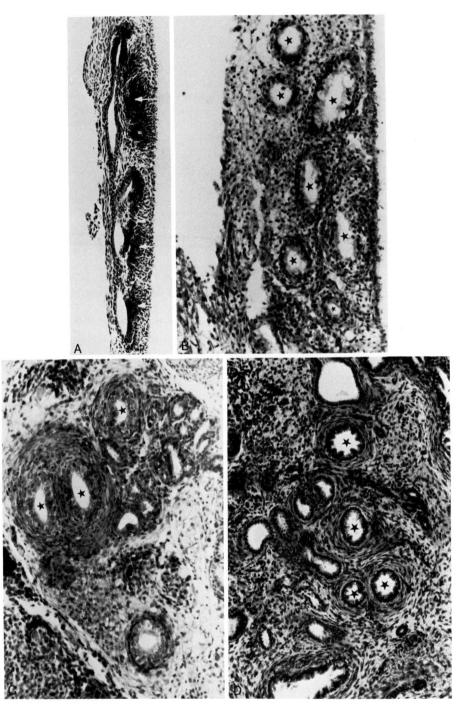

Figure 32–10. Induction of primitive ducts.

A, Longitudinal section of renal blastema microdissected from chick embryo after 8 days of incubation. Visible are segmental branches of the ureteral bud (*asterisks*) and condensed metanephrogenic mesenchyme (*arrow*).

B, Renal blastema microdissected from chick embryo and then cultured in vitro. Ureteral bud branches (*asterisks*) are numerous, but the metanephrogenic mesenchyme is no longer condensed or apparent. Renal tubules do not develop in vitro.

C, Renal blastema microdissected from chick embryo; then cultured in vitro to provide branched ureteral buds without condensed metanephrogenic mesenchyme; and, finally, further cultured in ovo, as a graft develops into tissue composed primarily of primitive ducts (*asterisks*). The ducts are lined by tall epithelium and are surrounded by whorled mesenchymal cells.

D, Nephrectomy specimen in newborn with prune belly syndrome. Primitive ducts (*asterisks*) typical of renal dysplasia are surrounded by whorled fibromuscular cells and resemble those induced in the chick embryos. (From Maizels, M., and Simpson, S. B., Jr.: Primitive ducts of renal dysplasia induced by culturing ureteral buds denuded of condensed renal mesenchyme. Science, 219:509, 1983. Copyright 1983 by the AAAS.)

Histologic sections showed that the "cyst" was actually the dilated upper ureter that came to resemble a giant pelvis. Collecting tubules drained into the cyst. Metanephrogenic mesenchyme and tubulogenesis were reduced. These observations were interpreted as being consistent with the specimen being the embryonic progenitor of a unilateral multicystic kidney. It was speculated that an inherent reduction in branching of the ureteral bud was responsible. Coalescence of the ureteral bud branches, which were destined to become calyces, led to cyst formation. The paucity of bud ampulla led to only sparse nephrogenesis.

GENETICS. It is likely that genetic problems are interwoven with unilateral/bilateral renal agenesis, especially as associated with müllerian anomalies as seen in Mayer-Rokitansky-Küster syndrome. The genetics may be characterized as a single autosomal dominant gene with variable expression (Pavanello et al., 1988). Furthermore, almost all cases of females with bilateral renal agenesis associated with the Potter syndrome have the Mayer-Rokitansky-Küster syndrome (Pavanello et al., 1988). The importance of genetic makeup in ureteral abnormalities is emphasized by noting that single ureter vaginal ectopia is likely 15 times more common in Japanese than in whites. Furthermore, in Japanese the kidney develops more normally than in whites where dysplasia is routine (Gotoh et al., 1983). (See Development of the Ducts of the Genitalia [Female].)

In summary, it is plausible that dysplasia results from an abnormal interaction between inherently defective metanephrogenic mesenchyme and ureteral bud ampullae. The mesenchyme does not become specialized enough to elaborate tubules and differentiates only into the fibromuscular collar of the primitive duct. Perhaps this mesenchyme may also differentiate heterotopically into cartilage or bone marrow as is seen clinically. In fact, hemopoiesis, granulopoiesis, and chondrogenesis have also been observed in embryonic renal tissue in amphibians, mice, and birds (Saxen, 1987). The development of dysplasia may be accentuated by coexisting renal obstruction (e.g., ureteropelvic junction obstruction and ureterocele).

As an additional possibility, it could be that renal dysplasia begins in the setting of a normal renal blastema that is then harmed, perhaps by an adverse environment (e.g., ischemia and toxins). Dysplasia may be induced reliably in the chick model, but no model simulates the multicystic kidney.

ASCENT OF THE KIDNEY

The renal blastema originates at the level of the upper sacral segments. The final position of the kidney at the level of the upper lumbar vertebrae is attributed to the ascent of the renal blastema. Some mechanisms that lead to normal renal ascent are presented subsequently.

Anatomic studies show that normal ascent of the renal rudiment from the level of the sacral segments of the human embryo to the level of the lumbar segments of the newborn seems to occur by four mechanisms: (1) caudal growth of the spine; (2) elongate growth of the ureter; (3) molding of the renal parenchyma; and (4) fixation of the kidney to the retroperitoneum, which follows elongate spine growth (Fig. 32–11) (Boyden, 1932; Gruenwald, 1943).

The contribution of elongate growth of the spine to renal ascent above the umbilical arteries (mechanism 4) was examined experimentally (Maizels and Stephens, 1979). The caudal spine of the developing chick embryo was deformed mechanically to perturb elongate spine growth. In the surviving chicks, induced scoliosis was statistically associated with incomplete ascent of the kidneys up the retroperitoneum, namely, renal ectopia.

The dependence of renal ascent on elongate growth of the spine may be similar to the passive ascent of the spinal cord. For example, the caudal portion of the spinal cord, the conus medullaris, "ascends" from the coccygeal level in the newborn to the lumbar level in the adult because the spine grows faster longitudinally than the spinal cord.

In addition to scaling the retroperitoneum, the kidney also rotates medially on its polar axis, causing the pelvis to face the spine. Kidneys ectopic within the bony pelvis are often not reniform. This abnormal shape may be the persistence of the normal molding of the renal parenchyma during its failed attempt to hurdle the umbilical artery (mechanism 3).

Congenital crossed renal ectopia, as seen on an intravenous pyelogram (IVP), can be distinguished from acquired cross lateral displacement by imaging the kid-

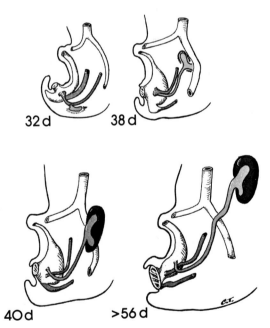

Figure 32–11. Schematic of renal ascent in the human embryo. The ureteral bud has originated from the mesonephric duct and actively elongates to reach the umbilical arteries. By 38 days, the umbilical artery tilts the upper pole of the kidney ventrally. At 40 days, the renal parenchyma elongates and then by 44 days the kidney rounds itself to elevate the lower pole of the kidney above the umbilical artery. After 56 days, the kidney fixes to the tissues of the retroperitoneum. Axial growth of the spine elevates the kidney to its final position. (From Maizels, M.: An Investigation of Urologic Malformations: Experimental Elucidation of Renal Ectopia. Masters Thesis, Evanston, IL, Northwestern University, 1978.)

neys with a cross-table, lateral view on a renogram. The kidney that becomes displaced across the midline will be anterior to the great vessels, whereas a kidney that shows congenital crossed ectopia will be aligned with the native kidney posterior to the great vessels (de Jonge et al., 1988).

APPEARANCE OF THE FETAL KIDNEY BY ULTRASOUND

As the fetal kidney advances during gestation, it more often resembles its postnatal ultrasonographic appearance, probably because fat is progressively deposited in the pararenal space and renal sinus (Tables 32–3 and 32–4) (Bowie et al., 1983).

Normative postnatal polar kidney size in children born from 26 weeks' gestation to term was described by de Vries and Levene (Fig. 32–12). The ratio of polar kidney to fetal crown rump length was about 0.78, irrespective of gestational age; the right and left kidneys were of similar length (de Vries and Levene, 1983). The medulla is evident by 27 weeks' gestation (Jeanty et al., 1982.)

DEVELOPMENT OF THE RENAL ARTERIES

Three groups of branches of the dorsal aorta appear early in development. They course ventrally to the intestine, laterally to the intermediate mesoderm, and dorsolaterally to the body wall and spine. The lateral branches are well developed only in the areas of the mesonephroi. Endothelial branchings continue to originate from the aorta until the aorta has developed a mesodermal coat (tunica media). The branchings create two to three arteries at each segmental level between the mesonephric arteries and the dorsolateral segmental arteries. The arterial branches anastomose as a plexus (see Fig. 32–12A, B). This plexus anastomoses with renal vessels at more cranial segmental levels, as the kidneys ascend the retroperitoneum. Portions of the plexus contribute to the adult pattern of the renal arteries.

Local mechanical forces may determine which portions of the plexus involute. For example, in species that have large mesonephroi, the segmental vessels may

Table 32–4. BLADDER CAPACITY AND VOIDED VOLUMES DURING GESTATION

Gestational Age (weeks)	Bladder Capacity (ml)	Urine Output (nl/hr)
20	(Evident)	—
32	10	12
Term	40	26

From Campbell, S., Wladimiroff, J. W., and Dewhurst, C. J.: J. Obstet. Gynaecol. [Br. Commonw.], 80:680, 1973.

be pulled ventrally to obliterate the periaortic plexus; in species that have acute curvature of the caudal trunk, the segmental vessels may be pulled dorsally to obliterate the periaortic plexus. Because human embryos do not have large mesonephroi or acute curvature of the caudal trunk, the portions of the periaortic plexus that persist may be variable, and thereby the renal vasculature may also be variable (Fig. 32–13C) (Bremer, 1915).

Persistence of the embryonic caudal vasculature may tether the rotation of the kidney during lumbar ascent. Nonrotated kidneys with aberrant arterial supply then develop (Nathan and Glezer, 1984).

FUNCTION OF THE FETAL KIDNEY

The first renal tubules are induced after 7 weeks. Correlations of morphology with renal function of animal embryos have led to projections that the tubules of the human fetus probably function after about 9 weeks of development (Gersh, 1937). The tubules secrete dyes in vitro by 14 weeks (Cameron and Chambers, 1983). Also, by the 14th week of gestation, the loop of Henle is functional, and tubular reabsorption occurs (Smith and Robillard, 1989).

In the laboratory, the exteriorized fetus model permits one to measure normal rates of glomerular and tubular clearance; blood flow; and tubular resorption of electrolytes, water, and solutes (Alexander and Nixon, 1961). Such measurements have not yet been applied clinically. The low glomerular filtration rate (GFR) in fetal life

Table 32–3. SONOGRAPHIC IDENTIFICATION OF THE FETAL KIDNEY DURING GESTATION

Gestational Age (weeks)	Sonographic Appearances			
	Identify (%)	Reniform Outline	Echogenic Outline	Central Complex of Renal Sinus
<12	10	+	–	–
12–24	80	+ +	+	+
24–36	100	+ +	+ +	+ +

Ratio of kidney circumference/abnormal circumference is normally constant during pregnancy at .27 to .3.
From Grannum, P., Bracken, M., Silverman, R., and Hobbins, J. C.: Am. J. Obstet. Gynecol., 136:249, 1980.

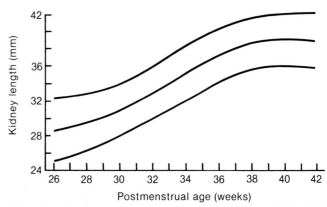

Figure 32–12. Smoothed cross-sectional growth chart of the fetal kidney. (Redrawn from de Vries, L., and Levene, M. I.: Measurement of renal size in preterm and term infants by real-time ultrasound. Arch. Dis. Child., 58:145, 1983.)

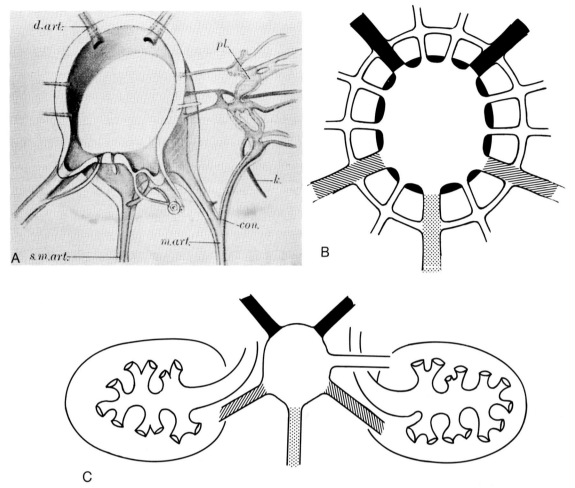

Figure 32–13. Development of renal arteries. *A,* Ventral (s.m. art.); dorsolateral (d. art.); and lateral (m. art.) groups of branches appear at each segmental level of the aorta. A capillary vascular plexus (pl.) exists laterally and supplies the kidney. The lateral plexus connects to the mesonephric artery (m. art.) by a thick-walled vessel (con.) and to the aorta by three slender vessels of endothelium only (reconstruction of cat embryo at second lumbar segment). The left side of the drawing is incomplete. (After Bremer, J. L.: Am. J. Anat., 18:179, 1915.) *B,* Schematic of *A. C,* The lateral vascular plexus may be the framework for the variability of the renal arteries. If the plexus involutes, there will be a single renal artery (*left*). If the plexus persists, there may be double or multiple renal arteries (*right*).

likely relates to the kidneys receiving a smaller per cent of the cardiac output (3 per cent in utero compared with 17 per cent in newborns), high renal vascular resistance, and low filtration fraction. The rise in GFR during gestation likely relates to an increase in kidney mass rather than to an improved function of the tissues (Smith and Robillard, 1989).

The GFR appears to correlate with gestational age between 27 weeks' gestation and term. The GFR increase in the weeks following birth likely relates to the recruitment of superficial cortical nephrons, which thereby enhances glomerular perfusion.

DEVELOPMENT OF THE URETER

Embryonic

After 28 days of development, the ureteral bud originates from the mesonephric duct as an evagination. Previously, the primitive ureter had been thought to ascend the pelvis as simple elongation of a hollow tube.

However, Ruano-Gil and co-workers (1975) presented new data on the early development of the ureter. They studied human embryos and showed the patency of the ureter changes during development.

Between 28 and 35 days of development, the entire length of the ureter is patent. Perhaps because the cloaca is still imperforate at this stage, mesonephric urine fills the ureter, raises the intraluminal pressure, and maintains this patency.

Between 37 and 40 days of development, the lumen of the ureter is not apparent histologically except perhaps at the midportion. Perhaps rapid elongate growth of the ureter obliterates the lumen.

After this period, the lumen extends cranially and caudally from the midportion of the ureter, and after 40 days the entire length of the ureter is again apparent (Fig. 32–14). These observations may help to understand why congenital strictures of the ureter are most common at the ureteropelvic or ureterovesical junctions. As the ureter lumens at these two sites are the last to become patent again, they may be more likely to remain narrow as strictures. A similar mechanism may account for

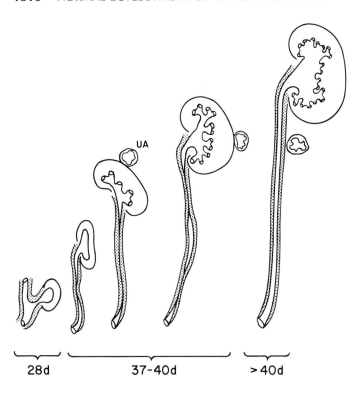

Figure 32–14. Early development of the ureter. At 28 days, the ureteral bud appears from the mesonephric duct. Between 37 and 40 days, the lumen of the ureter is first progressively lost, beginning at its midportion. Then, the lumen of the ureter becomes apparent again, beginning at its midportion. After 40 days, the lumen of the ureter is apparent throughout its length (UA, umbilical artery).

instances of subglottic stenosis of the larynx (O'Rahilly and Tucker, 1973). Alcaraz and colleagues (1989) identified a membrane between the lumen of the primitive ureter and the chamber of the urogenital sinus (37 days' gestation). The membrane, probably reflective of Chawalla's membrane, is initially one cell layer and then thickens (39 days' gestation) (Fig. 32–15). Persistence of this membrane may cause an impact on obstructive uropathy of the lower ureter.

Fetal

By 8 weeks of development, the ureter is a patent tube without muscle that has elongated pari passu, with ascent of the kidney in the retroperitoneum. Muscularization of the ureter is described in Table 32–5 and Figs. 32–16 and 32–17. After 10 weeks, the epithelium of the ureter is two layers thick. By 14 weeks, there is transitional epithelium. At 18 weeks, the ureter shows intrin-

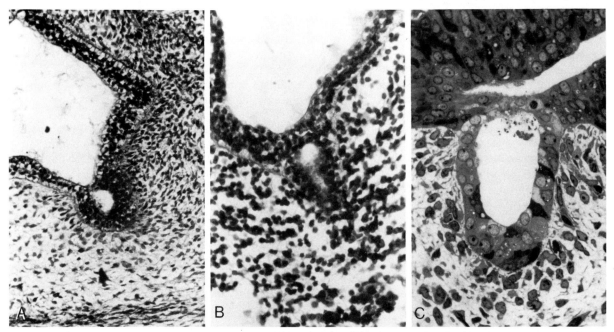

Figure 32–15. Chwalla's membrane in human and rat. The membrane marks the ureterovesical junction in humans (A, × 400; B, × 640; about 42 days' gestation) and resembles that (C) in the rat embryo (× 500; 27 days' gestation). (From Alcaraz, A., Vinaixa, F., Tejedo-Mateu, A., et al.: Acta Urol. Esp., 13:318, 1989.)

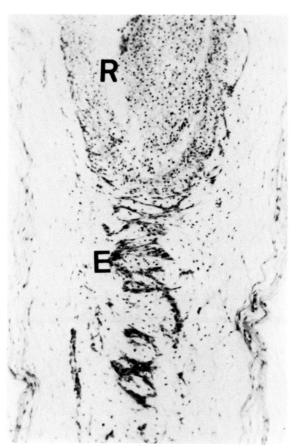

Figure 32–16. Upper ureter of human fetus (17 weeks' gestation). Early muscle bundles (E) course spirally (R, lumen of ureter). (From Matsuno, T., Tokunaka, S., and Koyanagi, T.: J. Urol., 132:148, 1984.)

sic narrowings at the UPJ, pelvic brim, and ureterovesical junction, and complementary intrinsic dilatations at the spindles of the ureter. The fetal ureter may elongate more than the kidney ascends. The ureter may absorb the excess length by becoming tortuous or folding its wall as pleats—the "fetal folds" of Ostling (1942) (Fig. 32–18).

The first secretion and drainage of renal urine (9 weeks' gestation) precede muscularization of the upper ureter (12 weeks' gestation) (see Table 32–5) (Matsuno et al., 1984). Urine flow in the ureter may mechanically stimulate myogenesis (see discussion of the development of the bladder).

The elastic fibers in the human fetal ureter were examined by Escala and co-workers (1989). After 12 weeks' gestation, the elastic fiber architecture does not change. In the adventitia, where the fibers appear first, the elastic fibers are longitudinally orientated; in the muscular layer, the fibers are randomly orientated; and in the submucosa, the fibers radiate from the basement membrane (see Fig. 32–17). During later development, the fibers in each layer increase according to the ratio of 5:1:2, respectively. It is plausible that asynchrony between urine formation and elastic deposition contributes to dilatations of the pelvis/ureter during development.

Postnatal

The infant grows taller faster than the ureter elongates. Thereby, the ureter may straighten and unfold (Ostling, 1942). These fetal pleats are not ordinarily obstructive. However, a pleat that intrudes into the lumen of the ureter and becomes fixed by adventitia of the ureter may obstruct urine drainage as a valve (Fig. 32–19) (Maizels and Stephens, 1980).

DEVELOPMENT OF THE CLOACA

During the period of the laminar embryo, the cloacal membrane is in the caudal region where ectoderm directly apposes endoderm. Growth of mesenchyme near the cloacal membrane lifts the tail end of the embryo off the blastoderm. This lifting folds the tail end and creates a chamber, the cloaca, the dilated terminus of the hindgut. The cloaca is lined with endoderm. Further growth of the tail fold flexes the tail end farther, and the cloacal membrane becomes positioned on the ventrum of the embryo. Continued growth of mesenchyme lateral to the cloacal membrane elevates the ectoderm as labioscrotal swellings. Growth of mesen-

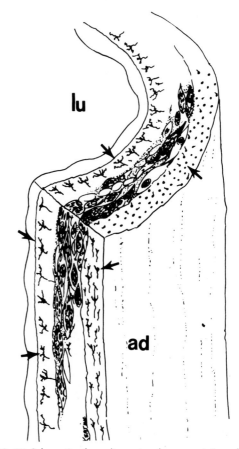

Figure 32–17. Schematic, three-dimensional representation of the elastic fiber orientation of a longitudinal and transverse section of a human fetal ureter (12 weeks' gestation) (lu, ureter lumen; ad, adventitia). (From Escala, J. M., Keating, M. A., and Boyd, G.: J. Urol., 141:969, 1989.)

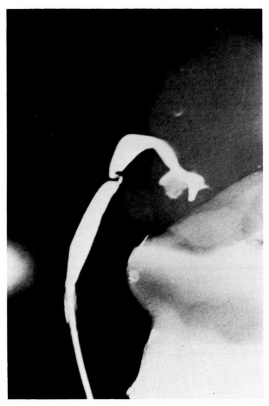

Figure 32–18. Pleats of the ureter. Retrograde pyelogram of a newborn kidney and ureter specimen shows the wall of the ureter folds and pleats of the lumen of the ureter. The pleats probably do not usually obstruct urine drainage.

chyme cranial to the cloacal membrane elevates the ectoderm as the genital tubercle—the primordium of the phallus (Fig. 32–20). When the mesoderm extends further cranially, the infraumbilical body wall becomes prominent.

The classic view holds that septation of the cloaca begins at about 28 days (Stephens, 1983). The urorectal

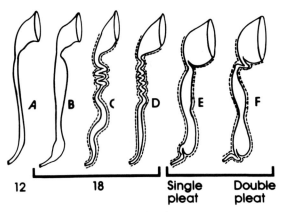

Figure 32–19. Possible embryogenesis of valves of the ureter. *A,* By 12 weeks of gestation, the caliber of the lumen of the ureter is uniform. *B,* At 18 weeks, pelvic and abdominal spindles of the ureter appear. If elongate growth of the ureter occurs faster than that of trunk, the ureter may become tortuous (*C*) or acquire pleats (*D*). *E* and *F,* Pleats are normally not obstructive but may persist as valves. (From Maizels, M., and Stephens, F. D.: Valves of the ureter as a cause of primary obstruction of the ureter: Anatomic, embryologic and clinical aspects. J. Urol., 123:742, 1980.)

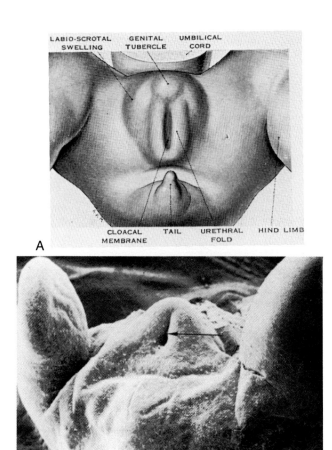

Figure 32–20. *A,* External appearance of the cloaca at about 7 weeks. Growth of the mesenchyme at the caudal end of the embryo lifts the embryo off the blastoderm and creates the tail fold. Further growth and migration of the mesenchyme around the cloacal membrane creates the genital tubercle and the labioscrotal swellings. (From Hamilton, W. J., and Mossman, H. W.: Human Embryology Prenatal Development of Form and Function. New York, The Macmillan Press Ltd., 1976.) *B,* Scanning electron micrograph of the genital tubercle of the same stage as in *A.* The urethral folds flank the urethral groove (*arrow*). (See also Fig. 32–22*A* and *C.*) (Rowsell, A. R., and Morgan, B. D. G.: Br. J. Plast. Surg., 40:201, 1987.)

septum, Tourneux's fold, extends in the coronal plane toward the cloacal membrane. At the same time, Rathke's plicae appear as two tissue folds from the lateral aspects of the hindgut. These plicae meet each other in the midline, and by 7 weeks' gestation the cloaca is divided. The rectum and primitive urogenital sinus are separate (Figs. 32–21, 32–24, and 32–26*C*). The portion of the primitive urogenital sinus cranial to the mesonephric ducts is the vesicourethral canal, and that caudal to the mesonephric ducts is the urogenital sinus (Fig. 32–22) (Hamilton and Mossman, 1976). Shortly, the müllerian ducts form Müller's tubercle on the posterior wall of the vesicourethral canal (see Fig. 32–28). The confluence of the urorectal septum with the cloacal membrane marks the perineal body.

A new twist on development of the cloaca was offered by van der Putte (1986). He studied embryos from pigs with hereditary anorectal malformations. Natural mark-

Table 32–5. TIME TABLE OF MUSCULAR DEVELOPMENT OF THE HUMAN URINARY TRACT

Gestational Age (weeks)	Prostate	Urethra	Bladder	Ureter	Pelvis
6	←——————————————————————— No muscle ———————————————————————→				
7	←——————————— No muscle ———————————→		Muscle in dome and extends caudally	←——————— No muscle ———————→	
8		Mesenchyme condenses as rare muscle U-shaped distribution of muscle	Muscle diffuse in bladder	Ureter drains into the bladder	Dilated chamber
11			←——————————————————— No muscle ———————————————————→		
12		Striated muscle laying outside of and adjacent to smooth muscle cells	Muscle bundles appear	Muscle in upper ureter; superficial ureteral sheath at UVJ	Muscle appears
16	Prostate epithelial buds grow into mesenchyme (Figs. 32–34 and 32–35)	Striated muscle encircles urethra at urogenital diaphragm (muscle is smaller than pelvic floor striated muscle) Enhancement of smooth muscle cell		Upper ureter muscle appears as bundles that have a spiral course	
17			Muscle layering is almost complete and advanced beyond that of trigone	Muscle at intramural ureter immature with muscle bundles Spiral muscle more prominent in ureter (Fig. 32–16). Longitudinal muscle orientation in intravesical ureter and attached to deep periureteral sheath. Waldeyer's sheath separates superficial and deep periurethral sheath.	
21			Bulky middle circular muscle layer	Spiral muscle layer Superficial periureteral sheath at UVJ is well developed	
40	←——————————————————————— Muscularization complete ———————————————————————→				

Adapted from Matsuno, T., Tokunaka, S., and Koyanagi, T.: J. Urol., 132:148, 1984.

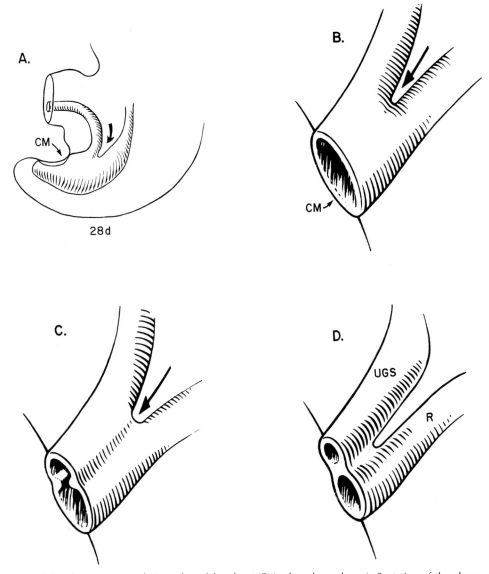

Figure 32–21. Septation of the cloaca. A, Lateral view of caudal embryo (CM, cloacal membrane). Septation of the cloaca occurs in a coronal plane as Tourneux's fold (B) extends to the cloacal membrane from above, and (C) as Rathke's plicae extend toward each other from the sides. D, Septation establishes the primitive urogenital sinus (UGS) and rectum (R). (From Stephens, F. D., and Smith, E. D.: Anorectal Malformations in Children. Chicago, Year Book Medical Publishers, 1971.)

ers of the pig cloaca were used (e.g., specific epithelia identify regions of the cloaca, an epithelial tag marks the dorsal cloacal wall, and smooth muscle and epithelia are topographically related) to track normal and anomalous development. Rather than viewing the fusion of the folds of Rathke and Tourneax to produce the septation of the cloaca, the septation is observed as a shift of the dorsal cloaca toward the cloacal membrane, which "carries" the urorectal septum caudally (Fig. 32–23). High imperforate anus may relate to excessive mesenchyme in the dorsal part of the cloacal membrane; the membrane does not rupture owing to no anorectal orifice; and a rectal fistula is forced to the urinary tract (see Figs. 32–24 and 32–25).

Figure 32–22. Development of the urogenital sinus. A, By 9 weeks of development, the urogenital sinus consists of a narrow pelvic part near the bladder and an expanded phallic part near the urogenital membrane (anterior portion of cloacal membrane). (From Arey, L. B.: Developmental Anatomy. Philadelphia, W. B. Saunders Co., 1974.) B, Transverse section through phallic part of urogenital sinus (plane BB seen in A). The endodermal cells lining the phallic portion of the cloacal membrane (urogenital membrane, *asterisk*) thicken and then degenerate to create the secondary urethral groove. The secondary urethral groove remains as the vestibule in the female and closes as the penile urethra in the male. (From Hamilton, W. J., and Mossman, H. W.: Human Embryology Prenatal Development of Form and Function. New York, The Macmillan Press Ltd., 1976.) C, Transillumination of the phallus of a 9-week-old human fetus viewed from below (2, labioscrotal fold; 3, phallus; 4, urethral groove continuous with urogenital sinus; 5, urethral fold). (From England, M. A.: Color Atlas of Life Before Birth. Chicago, Year Book Medical Publishers, 1983.)

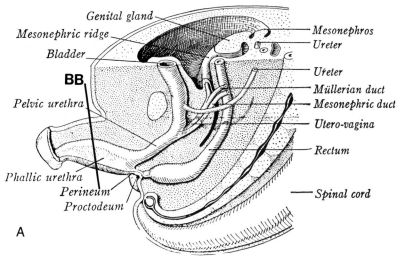

A

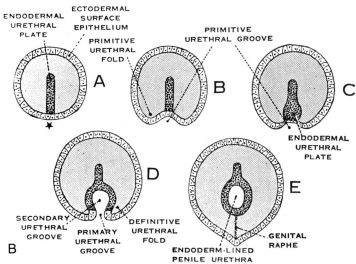

B

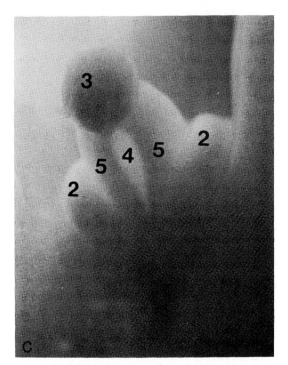

C

Figure 32–22 *See legend on opposite page*

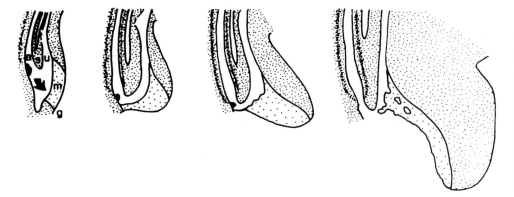

Figure 32–23. Successive stages shown semidiagrammatically in the development of the pig cloaca (11-, 13-, 17-, 25-mm embryos). The epithelial tag (black spot) marks the junction of the gut and dorsal cloacal wall. The tag and dorsal cloaca descend to the cloacal membrane (m) giving the appearance of primary descent of the urorectal septum (s). The membrane ruptures without contacting the septum. (a, anus; u, urethra.) (From van der Putte, S. C. J.: J. Pediatr. Surg., 21:434, 1986.)

Figure 32–24. Normal development of the human cloaca. *A,* At about 6 weeks of development, the cloaca (c) is bounded by the genital tubercle (t), urorectal septum (s), postanal swelling (p), and cloacal membrane (m) (midsagittal section, × 120) (cf. 17-mm pig embryo in Fig. 32–23). *B,* At about 7 weeks of development, the cloacal membrane is not evident, and the anorectal and urogenital sinuses show separate openings (midsagittal section, × 30) (cf. 25-mm pig embryo in Fig. 32–23). (From van der Putte, S. C. J.: J. Pediatr. Surg., 21:434, 1986.)

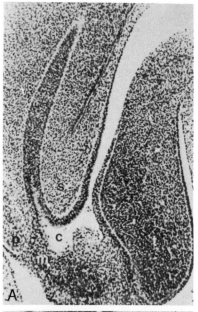

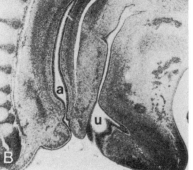

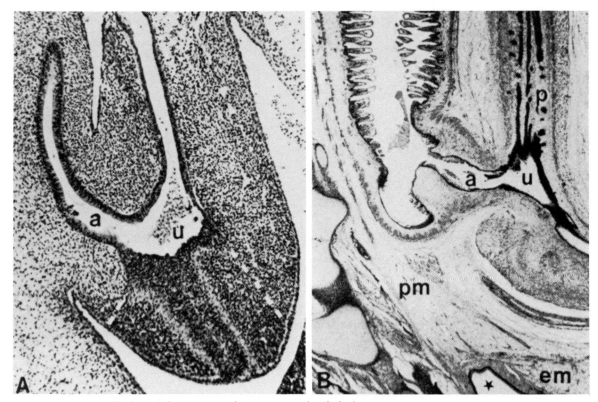

Figure 32–25. Development of high imperforate anus in the pig compared with the human.

A, Anorectal agenesis in a pig (stage is equivalent to before 6 weeks of development in the human) shows persistent communication between the anorectal (a) and urogenital (u) part of the cloaca. Tracking of tissues (see text) leads to the impression that in this condition excessive mesenchyme in the dorsal portion of the cloacal membrane may interfere with descent of the dorsal cloaca, and only a single urogenital orifice appears (sagittal section, × 80).

B, Anorectal agenesis in a human at about 19 weeks of development. Anal sinus (a) communicates with urethra (u) distal to the prostate (p). The puborectal (pm) and external sphincter muscles (em) have developed at their normal sites (× 20). (From van der Putte, S. C. J.: J. Pediatr. Surg., 21:434, 1986.)

Such views of normal development may permit predictions that anomalous interactions between the descending urorectal septum and the cloaca would result in specific anomalous developments of the bladder (distention consequent to absent urethral orifice) and rectum (distention consequent to imperforate anus), and in anomalous müllerian duct and external genitalia development (Escobar et al., 1987).

DEVELOPMENT OF THE TRIGONE AND BLADDER

Trigone

Understanding the development of the trigone is based predominantly on reconstructions of embryos that are examined histologically and on inferences from clinical studies of the bladders of children.

After the mesonephric ducts drain into the urogenital sinus, the epithelium of the urogenital sinus (endoderm) fuses with that of the mesonephric duct (mesoderm). At this time, the ureteral bud evaginates from the mesonephric duct (see Development of the Ureter). By 33 days of gestation, the segment of the mesonephric duct beyond the ureteral bud dilates as the common excretory

duct—the precursor of the hemitrigone (Alcaraz et al., 1989). The right and left common excretory ducts are absorbed into the urogenital sinus (Hamilton and Mossman, 1976). The mesenchyme of the right and left common excretory ducts is believed to migrate toward the midline, because the endodermal mucosa of the bladder does not persist in the midsection of the trigone (Hamilton and Mossman, 1976). The epithelia of the ducts fuse toward the midline as a triangular area—the primitive trigone. The terminus of the ureter enters the bladder directly by day 37 (Alcaraz et al., 1989). The mesonephric duct orifices grow caudally and flank the paramesonephric ducts at the level of the urogenital sinus—the site of the future verumontanum (Figs. 32–27 and 32–28).

The mechanism of absorption of the primitive ureter into the trigone is based on inferences derived from clinical observations of the trigone in newborns with duplex kidneys (Fig. 32–29). As the common excretory duct is absorbed into the urogenital sinus, the orifice of the duct is believed to move caudally and the orifice of the ureter cranially. Continued growth of the epithelium and mesoderm of the absorbed common excretory ducts separates the ureteral orifices laterally and establishes the framework of the primitive trigone. The ureteral orifice that drains the upper pole of the kidney rotates

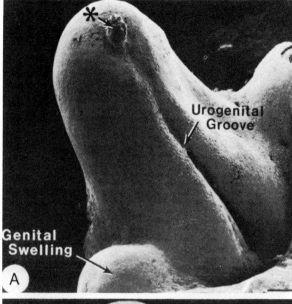

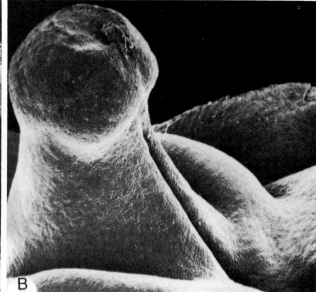

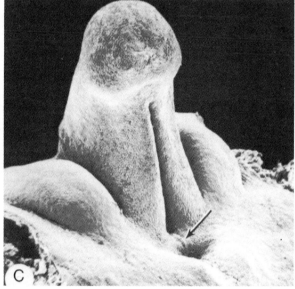

Figure 32–26. Indifferent stage of external genitalia. Ventrum of genital tubercle (8-week-old human embryo) viewed in a scanning electron micrograph. *A,* The urethral groove is between the paired urethral folds. The labioscrotal (genital) swellings are present. An epithelial tag is at the tip of the tubercle (*asterisk*). *B,* Slightly later, the urethral groove is deeper and the genital swellings more prominent. *C,* Still later, the perineal body (*arrow*) is between the urethral groove and the proctodeal depression (see Fig. 32–22A and C). (From Waterman, R. E.: Human embryo and fetus. *In* Hafez, E. S. E., and Kenemans, P. (Eds.): Atlas of Human Reproduction. Hinghman, MA, Kluwer Boston, Inc., 1982.)

clockwise, as viewed from outside the bladder, so that the orifice lies caudal and medial to the orifice of the lower pole ureter. Weigert and later Meyer recognized the regularity of this relationship, which has come to be known as the Weigert-Meyer rule. Similarly, when the orifices of the ureters of duplex kidneys are adjacent to each other on the trigone, they are situated next to each other such that the orifice of the upper pole ureter is medial to the orifice of the lower pole ureter (Stephens, 1958).

Following this logic, several concepts are plausible. Perhaps the laterally ectopic ureter had originated from a ureteral bud that was abnormally low on the wolffian duct and came to drain farther laterally on the trigone than usual. Vesicoureteral reflux would result. In caudal ectopy of the ureteral orifice, the ureteral bud may have originated abnormally high on the wolffian duct and come to drain on the bladder neck (Mackie and Stephens, 1979) or retained its connection with the wolffian duct (persistent mesonephric duct) (Stephens, 1983).

Triplicate ureters do not conform regularly to the Weigert-Meyer rule (Stephens, 1983). Inverted Y duplication of the ureter also does not readily conform to these embryologic notions (Ecke and Klatte, 1989).

The separate development of the trigone and bladder accounts for the contiguity of the muscle of the ureter with the muscle laminae of the trigone and not with the detrusor. This separate development may account for the different pharmacologic responses of the musculature of the bladder neck and trigone from those of the detrusor.

Vesicoureteral Reflux In Utero

The period when the ureter attains the oblique submucosal course of the newborn bladder is uncertain but likely occurs after 14 weeks (Felix, 1912b). Booth and co-workers (1975) reported the incidence of reflux is 3.6 per cent at about 25 weeks' gestation on cystograms

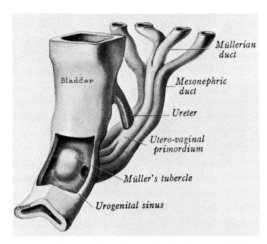

Figure 32–27. Diagrammatic view of the development of the ducts of the genitalia (cf. Fig. 32–28). The paramesonephric ducts descend toward the pelvis medial to the mesonephric ducts. After the mesonephric ducts are absorbed into the trigone, they migrate medially and caudally, flanking the paramesonephric ducts. The termini of these four ducts are at the site of the verumontanum in the male and the cervix in the female (From Arey after Broman. Arey, L. B.: Developmental Anatomy, 7th ed. Philadelphia, W. B. Saunders Co., 1974.)

obtained accidentally during in utero fetal paracentesis for erythroblastosis. From historical series, the incidence of reflux is 1.2 per cent on cystograms in normal premature and term infants. This reduced incidence in older infants is consistent with the notion of spontaneous resolution of reflux (Booth et al., 1975).

Bladder

By 10 weeks' gestation the bladder is a cylindric tube lined by connective tissue (Fig. 32–21A) (Lowsley, 1912). The wall of the bladder over the trigone is twice as thick as elsewhere. The apex of the vesicoallantoic canal tapers as the urachus. The urachus is contiguous with the allantoic duct, but the allantois probably does not contribute to the formation of the urachus or bladder (Arey, 1974; Felix, 1912c). By 12 weeks, the segment of the bladder contiguous with the allantoic diverticulum involutes. This segment is between the apex of the bladder and the umbilicus. It becomes a thick tube and then a fibrous cord—the median umbilical ligament (Moore, 1977).

By 13 weeks, mesenchyme surrounding the bladder develops into circular, interlacing, and longitudinal strands of smooth muscle. The muscle fibers of the ureters are contiguous with those of the trigone. Muscularization is more abundant at the bladder base, especially at the upper limit of the trigone, than elsewhere. Rapid muscularization causes the wall of the trigone to now become five times thicker than elsewhere. The bladder lumen narrows at the internal vesical sphincter.

By 16 weeks, the entire bladder has discrete inner and outer longitudinal layers and a middle circular layer. Fascicles from the longitudinal layer interlace with the circular layer (Stephens, 1958). According to Wood-

Jones (1901), the outer longitudinal layer is a complete muscle coat that "originates" from the puboprostatic ligament and sweeps up to the bladder apex and down the posterior wall to "insert" into the upper aspect of prostate in boys or anterior wall of the vagina in girls. The middle circular layer at 20 weeks' gestation is

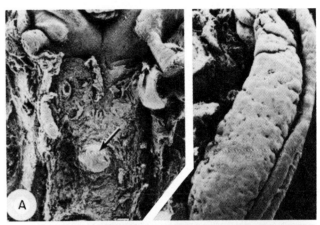

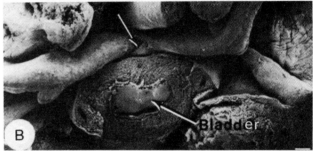

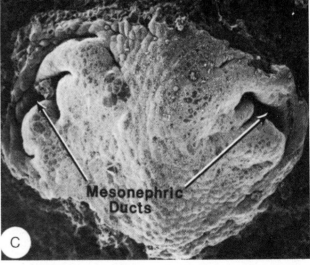

Figure 32–28. Human embryo (8 weeks old) showing the relationships of the genital ducts and bladder. A, The müllerian and mesonephric ducts lie adjacent to each other; a pair of such ducts from each side come toward each other in the midline (*arrow*) behind the bladder. Umbilical arteries are seen on each side of the bladder. The colon is behind the arrow. B, After removal of the bladder, the müllerian tubercle is seen (*arrow*) on the posterior wall of the bladder remnant. C, At higher magnification, the fused müllerian ducts cause the region to bulge between the ostia of both mesonephric ducts. (From Waterman, R. E.: Human embryo and fetus. *In* Hafez, E. S. E., and Kenemans, P. (Eds.): Atlas of Human Reproduction. Hinghman, MA, Kluwer Boston, Inc., 1982.)

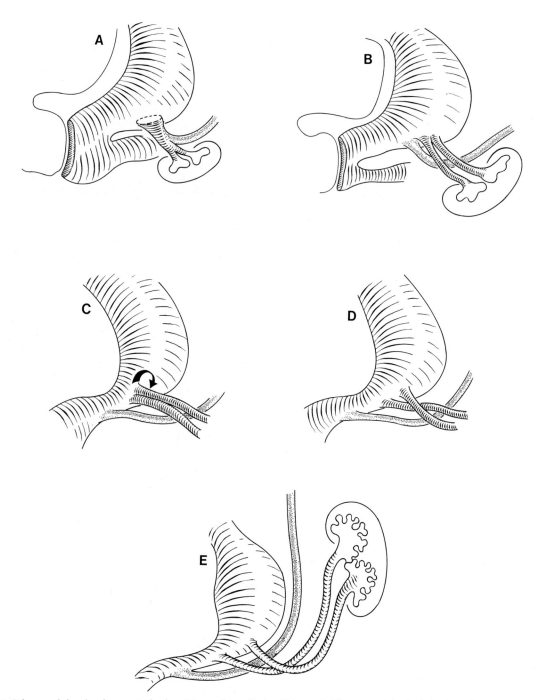

Figure 32–29. Schema of the development of a hemitrigone for a duplex kidney. *A,* The ureteral buds drain into the common excretory duct (*shaded*). *B,* The buds and duct are absorbed into the urogenital sinus such that the orifice of the mesonephric duct is caudal and medial to that of the ureteral orifice. *C to E,* Continued absorption of the ureters into the trigone is associated with the clockwise rotation of the ureter draining the upper pole around the ureter draining the lower pole.

comprised of fine muscle bundles, which are comparable to those at the bladder neck sphincter. For the internal sphincter the circular layer at the bladder neck heaps up, especially posteriorly, and the muscle fibers are fine closely packed fibers. The sphincteric muscle is quite thick at 20 weeks.

By term, the muscle bundles of the circular layer of the bladder are more coarse than those of the sphincter. The inner longitudinal layer is complete on the anterior bladder wall but, posteriorly, it is evident only in the region of the trigone where it extends distally to become contiguous with the longitudinal layer in the urethra. Development to term results in further increase in the size of the muscles of the detrusor, trigone, and sphincter (Fig. 32–30).

The mechanics of bladder distention may stimulate bladder muscularization. Continence of bladder urine may be possible at about 16 weeks, when the urethral sphincter muscle encircles the urethra. This is prior to completion of the muscular framework of the trigone (21 weeks). Normal cycles of bladder expansion (storage of urine) and emptying may aid normal trigone development. "Fetal bladder dysfunction" could thereby lead to anomalous development of the trigone and uretero-vesical junction (reflux, obstruction, ureterocele) (Matsuno, 1984).

As imaged by ultrasonography the fetal bladder varies in size, emptying about 16 ml every 90 minutes near term (Wladimiroff and Campbell, 1974). Bladder volume shows circadian rhythm with a trough between 6:00 P.M. and 6:00 A.M. (Kogan and Iwamoto, 1989). Because fetal imaging to check for urine in the bladder relies on a change in bladder volume, in instances when bilateral renal agenesis is suspected, the bladder should not be examined during this time interval because the bladder volume may not change for up to 3 hours in the normal fetus. However, other workers have not shown such a circadian rhythm (Wladimiroff and Campbell, 1974).

The rate of fetal urine production is linearly related to gestational age (30 to 40 weeks), with mean values of 9.6 and 27.3 ml/hour, respectively (Wladimiroff and Campbell, 1974). The fetal sheep bladder during the later part of gestation shows spontaneous contractions after induced diuresis. It is responsive to parasympathomimetic (bethanecol) and parasympathoplegic (atropine) drugs and beta-sympathomimetic (ritodrine) and parasympathoplegic (propranolol) drugs. These responses might help in understanding the causes of neonatal bladder dysfunction (incomplete bladder emptying) (Kogan and Iwamoto, 1989).

Developmental interactions between the bladder epithelium and mesenchyme are similar to those in the kidney, uterus, and vagina.

DEVELOPMENT OF THE UROGENITAL SINUS

Indifferent Stage

By 6 weeks of development, the urogenital sinus is apparent. The portion of the sinus near the bladder is narrow—the pelvic urethra. The portion near the urogenital membrane is expanded—the phallic urethra. The genitalia are sexually indifferent until about 10 weeks of development (see Figs. 32–20, 32–22, and 32–26).

During the 5th week, a plate of endodermal cells thickens the inner portion of the urogenital membrane. This plate extends distally toward the genital tubercle. The tip of the tubercle shows an epithelial tag, which is transient. Mesenchyme grows along the lateral margins of the phallic portion of the urogenital sinus to raise the overlying ectoderm and create the primitive urethral groove (see Fig. 32–26). In the 7th week after the urogenital membrane disintegrates (FitzGerald, 1978), the phallic part of the urogenital sinus is seen as a trough lined by endoderm. The endodermal cells thicken to become the urethral plate. By 8 weeks, the superficial cells of the endodermal plate disintegrate. This cell death establishes the superficial, primary, and deep, secondary, urethral grooves (see Figs. 32–22B, C and Fig. 32–26). The mesenchyme on either side of the urethral plate proliferates to form urethral folds, which eclipse the urethral groove. The folds do not reach the genital tubercle. From these events the secondary urethral groove is lined by endoderm and is limited by the 2-degree urethral fold; the primary urethral groove is lined by ectoderm and is limited by the 1-degree urethral fold.

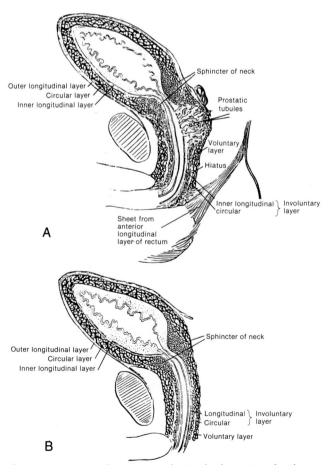

Figure 32–30. Semidiagrammatic longitudinal section of a human bladder and adjacent urethra (9 months' gestation). *A,* Male. *B,* Female. (From Wood-Jones, F.: J. Anat. Physiol., 36:51(2), 1901–02.)

In normal male development, the penis is straight when the phallic urethra is formed. In normal female development, the clitoris shows ventral curvature, perhaps because as there is no underlying urethra, there is no ventral support. In the male, if hypospadias develops, the deficient phallic urethra may permit the ventral curvature to remain as chordee; whereas in the female, if an accessory phallic urethra develops, the ventral curvature may straighten the clitoris and make it prominent (Bellinger and Duckett, 1982).

Thus, the genitalia at the close of the indifferent stage show characteristic features. The genital tubercle is prominent and is flanked laterally by labioscrotal swellings. The ventrum of the tubercle shows the superficial and deep urethral grooves. The paired müllerian ducts have reached the urogenital sinus (Waterman, 1982) and have fused in the midline as the müllerian tubercle. The tubercle protrudes but does not open into the posterior wall of the urogenital sinus. After 10 weeks, the external genitalia of the male and female develop differently.

Urogenital Sinus in the Male

PENIS. By the 10th week, the external genitalia of a boy masculinize. The genital tubercle elongates into a cylindric phallus. Mesenchyme in the tubercle condenses as the primitive cavernous tissue. At about 12 weeks, an oblique groove appears at the corona of the glans. This groove demarcates the glans from the shaft of the phallus. The organ is now a penis. A ridge of skin (primitive foreskin) proximal to the groove accentuates the coronal margin. The glans ventrum becomes excavated (analogous to excavation of the endodermal urethral plate) to form the fossa navicularis (Fig. 32–31). The fossa remains filled with desquamated cells. At about 14 weeks' gestation, the penis is bigger; however, the skin on the penile shaft is disproportionately excessive, especially on the dorsum where it folds on itself ". . . as if it were developing at a much more rapid rate of growth than the differentiating mesoderm into cavernous tissue . . . and appears as if flowing over the dorsum of the glans" (Hunter, 1935).

URETHRA

Penile Urethra. The phallic portion of the urogenital sinus develops into the bulbar and penile urethra. The endodermal edges of the secondary urethral groove fuse to tubularize the penile urethra in the 12th week (see Fig. 32–32 and Fig. 32–22B). The ectodermal edges of the groove fuse as the median raphe. The penis appears straight (Fig. 32–32). The scrotal swellings round, mi-

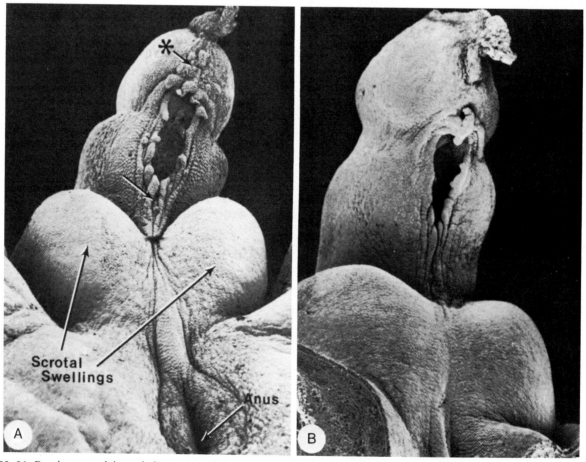

Figure 32–31. Development of the male human genitalia (10 weeks old). Scanning electron micrograph of the ventrum of the genitalia. *A,* The urethral folds are fusing to form the penile urethra. The paired scrotal swellings are converging toward each other. The asterisk marks the urethral plate. The fossa will come to be filled with squames, and the process of fusion of the urethral folds will continue on the glans to complete the glandular urethra during the 4th month. *B,* The urethral folds have fused further to form the penile urethra. The fusion is complete by the end of the 12th week. A sulcus separates the glans from the shaft of the phallus. (From Waterman, R. E.: Human embryo and fetus. *In* Hafez, E. S. E., and Kenemans, P. (Eds.): Atlas of Human Reproduction. Hinghman, MA, Kluwer Boston, Inc., 1982.)

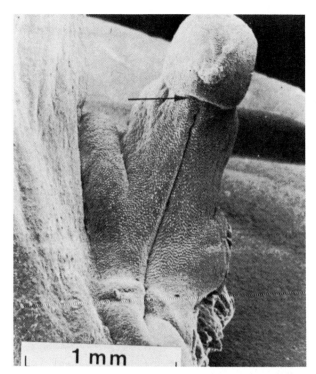

Figure 32–32. Development of male human genitalia (penis) (12 weeks old). The coronal sulcus (*arrow*) separates the glans from the shaft of the penis. The urethral folds have met in the middle on the ventrum of the shaft. An epithelial tag just above the arrow on the glans likely is the site of excavation. (From Rowsell, A. K., and Morgan, B. D. G.: Br. J. Plast. Surg., 40:201, 1987.)

grate caudally, and fuse to form the scrotum at the base of the penis. By term, the urethra shows an outer circular and an inner longitudinal layer, both of which are contiguous with their respective layers of bladder.

Glandar Urethra. During the 16th week the glandar urethra appears (Waterman, 1982). Debate regarding the mechanisms involved in formation of the glandar urethra has involved whether there is ventral fusion of urethral folds or primary excavation of the glans. From review of the archival histologic material of Hunter (1935) and scanning electron microscopic images of Rowsell and Morgan (1987), it is likely that both mechanisms are involved.

The glans and foreskin likely develop in three steps. First, the fossa navicularis lumen originates from the canalization of a cord of epithelial cells that had grown in from the tip of the glans (Rowsell and Morgan, 1987). The desquamated cells that cover the glans become a thick layer, and after 20 weeks the desquamated cells fill the fossa navicularis. Second, the urethral folds now at the level of the glans corona extend ventrally to fuse in the midline. This ventral fusion of the folds extends distally to make the floor of the glandar urethra. Ventral fusion of the glandar urethral folds "traps" the squames, which now appear to "plug" the glandar urethra. The urethral meatus is now at its definitive glandar position. Third, the foreskin grows ventrally until it completely encircles the glans. The preputial and urethral folds fuse on the ventrum of the glans as the frenulum (Fig. 32–33).

It is plausible that the many anatomic variants of distal shaft hypospadias stem from combinations of anomalous development of these three mechanisms. For example, cases in which the glandar urethral folds did not fuse, but in which the preputial folds did fuse would appear as hypospadias with a complete foreskin (Hatch et al., 1989). Alternatively, absent fusion of the glandar urethral folds, along with failure of glans canalization, would lead to the globular configuration of the glans in some cases of hypospadias.

PREPUCE. Separation of the prepuce from the glans was studied by Diebert (1933) using histologic sections of human material (3 months' gestation to 6 months old). Separation begins by 6 months' gestation and involves keratinization of the apposed preputial and glandar epithelia. Keratinization begins at opposite sites, the glans corona and distal margin of the prepuce, which extend toward each other. Keratinization leads to

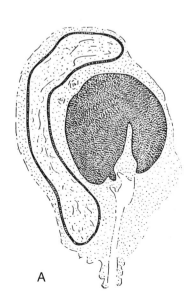
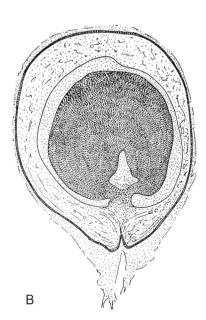

Figure 32–33. Glans penis of the human fetus. *A*, At about 16 weeks' gestation, urethral folds extend ventrally. They will later meet and fuse in the midline. This pattern of fusion traps a plug of squames. *B*, After 20 weeks' gestation, the glandular urethra is complete, and the frenulum marks the site where the preputial and urethral folds fused. (From Hunter, R. H.: J. Anat., 70:68, 1935.)

A   B

"pearl" formation. Cavitation of the pearl creates a lumen. When several longitudinally arranged pearls coalesce, the foreskin is separable from the glans. After birth, larger newborns show more preputial glandar separation than smaller ones. Separation should be sufficient by 10 days old to allow mechanical retraction without likelihood of tearing the epithelia. At surgery for circumcision or hypospadias repair, the degree of pearl formation is quite variable. When excess preputial skin still remains after circumcision, it may adhere to the underlying glans. Perhaps this occurs in the child in whom pearl formation is deficient and the artificial separation by circumcision was premature. In other children who experience balanitis from infected smegma, perhaps pearl formation is excessive and chemical irritation, bacterial superinfection, or both follow.

PROSTATE. The pelvic part of the urogenital sinus develops into the lower portion of the prostatic urethra and the membranous urethra (Hamilton and Mossman, 1976). Prostatic differentiation in the human embryo begins in the mesenchyme of the prostatic part of the urethra. Mesenchymal cells under the basal lamina develop into fibroblasts by the 8th week of development. Testicular Leydig's cells are differentiated at this time (Kellokumpu-Lehtinen and Pelliniemi, 1988).

By the 10th week, epithelial outgrowths from the prostatic segment of the urethra grow and branch out into the surrounding mesenchyme. By 12 weeks, five groups of tubules form the lobes of the prostate (Lowsley, 1912): Group 1, the middle lobe is made up of about ten branching tubules that originate on the floor of the urethra between the bladder and the orifices of the ejaculatory ducts. The middle lobe is rarely absent. Groups 2 and 3, the lateral lobes originate from about 35 tubules on the lateral walls of the urethra. Group 4, the posterior lobe originates from the floor of the urethra distal to the openings of the ejaculatory ducts. The tubules of the posterior lobe grow back behind the lateral lobes from which they are separated by a fibrotic capsule. As the tubules grow out, they "push" the circular musculature and "scatter" the fibers. These scattered fibers of circular urethral muscle become the prostate capsule (Wood-Jones, 1901) (Figs. 32–34 and 32–30). Group 5, the anterior lobe is prominent until 16 weeks of development and then involutes to become an insignificant structure by 22 weeks (Fig. 32–35) (Lowsley, 1912).

Lumens appear in the epithelial buds at the period of maximal testosterone secretion (10 weeks) and contain acid phosphatase. Androgens accelerate the differentiation of a secretory epithelium in vitro after the mesenchyme has begun to differentiate in vivo (Kellokumpu-Lehtinen and Pelliniemi, 1988). The epithelia of the nearby wolffian/müllerian ducts do not appear to contribute to the prostate as the urethra does. All three duct systems (urethra, wolffian, and müllerian) contribute to the epithelium of the seminal colliculus. The epithelial cells in the luminal part of the region are columnar, whereas those in the outer part of the prostatic urethra are cuboidal (Kellokumpu-Lehtinen and Pelliniemi, 1988). Cuhna (1984) showed by tissue recombinant experiments that depending on the androgen

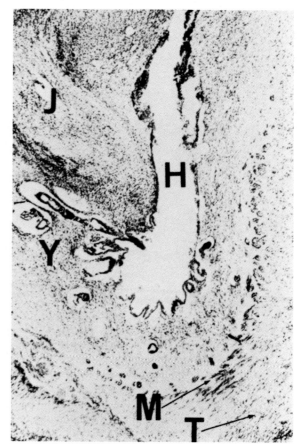

Figure 32–34. Posterior urethra of human fetus at 16 weeks' gestation (sagittal orientation). Prostate buds (Y); striated muscle around the urethra (T), which bounds an inner layer of circular smooth muscle (M); and ejaculatory duct (J) are apparent. (H, lumen of urethra.) (From Matsuno, T., Tokunaka, S., and Koyanagi, T.: J. Urol., 132:148, 1984.)

level, mesenchyme but not epithelium of the urogenital sinus induced specific epithelial morphogenesis. During embryonic and neonatal periods, mesenchyme alone exhibits androgen receptor activity. Androgens can accelerate the differentiation of human urethral epithelial cells into secretory prostatic cells in vitro (Kellokumpu-Lehtinen and Pelliniemi, 1988).

The external urethral sphincter is a cylindric layer of circular fibers, which extend between the lower prostatic and membranous portions of the urethra. The sphincter is aided by a broad sheet of muscle fibers, which originates from the anterior surface of the rectum and inserts at the junction of the membranous and bulbar urethra (see Fig. 32–30).

COWPER'S GLANDS. Cowper's glands are present by 12 weeks of development. They originate as endodermal buds of the urogenital sinus. The buds penetrate the surrounding compact mesenchyme of the corpus spongiosum. The buds enlarge as racemose glands at the level of the membranous urethra and remain as small glands at the level of the bulbar urethra. After 18 weeks, a glandular epithelium appears (Fig. 32–36).

The urogenital sinus epithelium and genital tubercle can convert the testosterone produced by the testis to a more potent androgen, dihydrotestosterone (George et

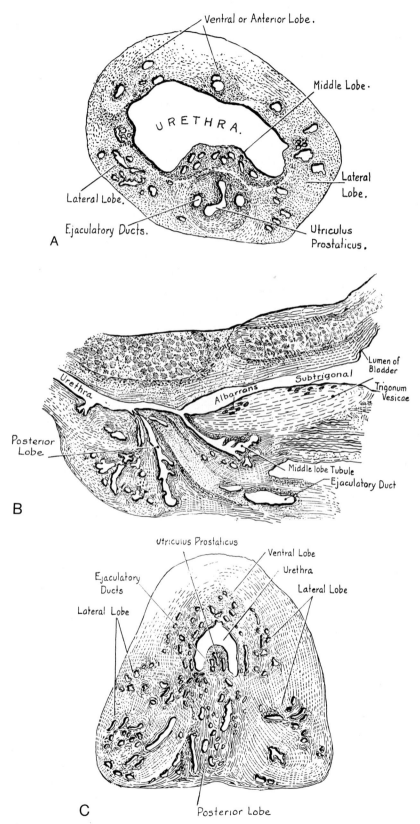

Figure 32–35. Development of the prostate. *A,* At 4 months (transverse section). *B,* At 5 months (longitudinal section). *C,* At 7½ months (transverse section). (From Lowsley, O. S.: Am. J. Anat., 13:299, 1912. Reprinted by permission of Wiley-Liss, a division of John Wiley and Sons, Inc.)

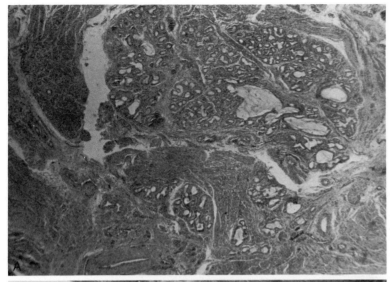

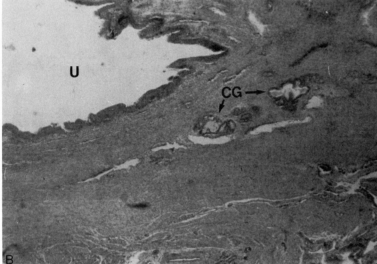

Figure 32–36. Cowper's gland consists of (*A*) glands with racemose drainage at the level of the membranous urethra and (*B*) as small glands (C) near the bulbar urethra (U) (histologic section of stillborn fetus.) (Courtesy of F. D. Stephens.)

al., 1988). Dihydrotestosterone mediates the differentiation of the derivatives of the urogenital sinus, namely, the prostate, from the pelvic portion of the urogenital sinus (Cunha, 1972; Kellokumpu-Lehtinen and Pelliniemi, 1988), and the external genitalia, from the phallic portion of the urogenital sinus (Süteri and Wilson, 1974). Testosterone mediates the differentiation of the derivatives of the wolffian duct, namely, the seminal vesicle, epididymis, and vas deferens.

This different responsiveness of target organ to androgen helps in the understanding of why in cases in which the external genitalia cannot convert testosterone to dihydrotestosterone (reductase is needed but is deficient) the external genitalia do not masculinize, whereas the internal genitalia in the same cases do masculinize (reductase not needed) (George et al., 1988).

Urogenital Sinus in the Female

URETHRA. The pelvic part of the urogenital sinus develops into the lower portion of the definitive urethra and vagina (Hamilton and Mossman, 1976). Epithelial tubules originate from the primitive urethra after about 11 weeks (Stephens, 1983) to become the paraurethral glands of Skene (Hamilton and Mossman, 1976). These glands are the female homologues of the prostate. Mesenchymal differentiation in the female urethra is less prominent than in the analogous segment in the male (Kellokumpu-Lehtinen and Pelliniemi, 1988).

EXTERNAL GENITALIA. Absence of androgen or androgen insensitivity permits feminization of the external genitalia from 12 to 28 weeks' gestation (Fig. 32–37).

HYMEN AND VAGINAL INTROITUS. The embryogenesis of the hymen is important clinically. Examination of many thousands of female newborns without major anomalies of the urogenital tract shows the hymen is uniformly present (Jenny, 1987; Mor and Merlob, 1988). This is in distinction to those with urogenital anomalies (atresia, duplication), in whom hymenal absence is observed.

Variations in the normal skin distribution in the introitus should be considered during the examination

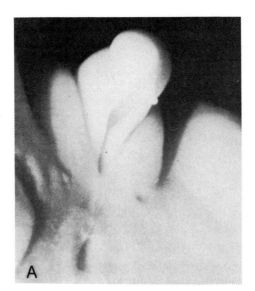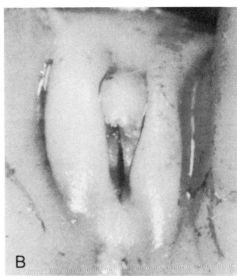

Figure 32–37. Feminization of the external genitalia. *A,* Feminization beginning in a human fetus at about 12 weeks' gestation. The phallus bends ventrally, the labioscrotal swellings remain separate, and the urethral folds do not fuse. *B,* By about 18 weeks' gestation, the labia and clitoris are apparent. The hymen is present. (From Jirasek, J. E.: Birth Defects. Original Article Series, 2:13, 1977. The National Foundation.)

of girls for sexual abuse. Failure of midline fusion of skin across the posterior fourchette may leave this area covered only by mucosa, which is comparable to that of the hymen. This mucosa would extend to the anus. As the mucosa resembles that of the normal hymen, this appearance of the external genitalia is a congenital anomaly rather than a result of sexual abuse (Adams and Horton, 1989). Estrogen effect may be responsible for edema and hypertrophy of hymenal tissues that appear as hymenal bands or tags. The bands should involute by a few weeks after birth as the estrogen effects wane (Muecke, 1979).

VESTIBULE. The phallic portion of the urogenital sinus remains a vestibule because the urethral plate does not extend as far to the genital tubercle as in the male (Fig. 32–22*A*). The urethra and vagina open into the vestibule (see Fig. 32–37). The labial swellings grow posterior to the vestibule and meet to form the posterior commissure. The swellings also grow lateral to the vestibule to form the labia majora. Urethral folds that flank the urogenital sinus develop into the labia minora (Hamilton and Mossman, 1976). The phallic part of the urogenital sinus (the undersurface of the elongated genital tubercle) contains the urethral grooves, which remain open and thereby contribute to the vaginal vestibule (Bellinger and Duckett, 1982). After the 9th week of development, Bartholin's glands begin as evaginations of the vestibule endoderm and then grow into the labia majora (Stephens, 1983). These glands are the homologues of Cowper's glands in the male. This development is complete by 12 weeks (Waterman, 1982).

Hormonal factors, such as androgen exposure (most commonly congenital adrenal hyperplasia), may lead the urethral folds to fuse. The union of the folds in utero is recognized as posterior labial fusion in the newborn. The time period when the folds are exposed to androgen may influence the outcome. If the exposure is before 12 to 14 weeks' gestation, posterior fusion and clitoromegaly result, whereas exposure after this period results only in clitoromegaly (Klein et al., 1989). A familial form of posterior labial fusion characterized by autoso-

mal dominant inheritance has been described. Knowledge of the embryology helps distinguish between posterior labial fusion (a union of the urethral folds in utero) and labial adhesion (an agglutination of the labia minora as a consequence of inflammation). Labial fusion is congenital, does not show a midline raphe, and does not recur after operative correction. In contrast, labial adhesion is rare in the newborn, shows a midline raphe that is a result of labial inflammation, and may recur after surgical correction (Klein et al., 1989).

DEVELOPMENT OF THE DUCTS OF THE GENITALIA

Indifferent Stage

The genital ducts appear during the 5th to 6th week. As they remain structurally the same for genetic males and females, the appearance of the ducts begins the indifferent stage of sexual development until the 10th week.

The müllerian ducts appear during the 6th week of gestation. Each duct originates as a funnel-shaped invagination of the coelomic epithelium (peritoneum) near each side of the developing diaphragm (Fig. 32–38). The müllerian duct is also referred to as the paramesonephric duct, because it descends to the pelvis adjacent to the basement membrane on the lateral aspect of the mesonephric duct (Gruenwald, 1941). The lower segment of the müllerian duct crosses anterior to the mesonephric duct. At about the 8th week of gestation, the medial segments of the müllerian ducts at the level of the bladder fuse to form the uterovaginal primordium (müllerian vagina) (see Figs. 32–27 and 32–28). This primordium in the female later merges with an expansion of the urogenital sinus (sinus vagina) to make the vagina contiguous (see Female) (see Figs. 32–43*A* and 32–44). The uterovaginal primordium elevates but does not penetrate the dorsal wall of the pelvic portion of the urogenital sinus as the müllerian tubercle (see Fig.

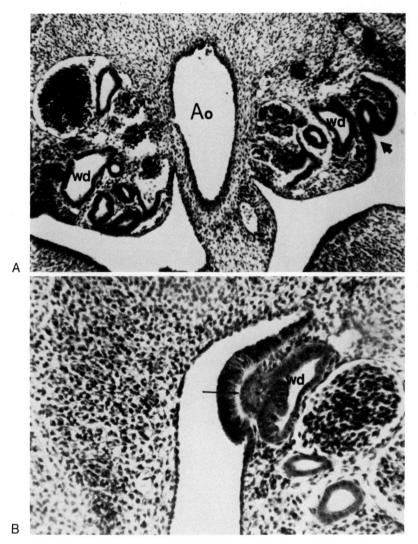

Figure 32–38. Early formation of the müllerian ducts. *A,* The ducts begin as an invagination of the "peritoneum" (*arrow*) near the developing diaphragm (Ao, aorta). *B,* They descend as a solid core (*arrow*) toward the pelvis alongside the mesonephric duct (wd) (chick embryo). (From Maizels, M., and Stephens, F. D.: The induction of urologic malformations: Understanding the relationship of renal ectopia and congenital scoliosis. Invest. Urol., 17:209, 1979.)

32–28). This tubercle lies between and cranial to the mesonephric duct orifices. During the indifferent stage the mesonephroi begin to degenerate.

Between 4 and 8 weeks, the thoracic portions of the mesonephroi degenerate, but formation of new tubules caudally maintains the bulk of the organ in the lumbar region (Felix, 1912d). Of the remaining tubules, the upper 5 to 12 tubules compose the epigenitalis and a similar number of tubules at the lower portion compose the paragenitalis. The glomeruli of the epigenitalis degenerate, but their connections to the collecting ducts of the mesonephric duct remain. The ends of the collecting ducts become surrounded by the indifferent gonad. By 8 weeks' gestation, enzymes necessary for androgen synthesis are present in the human fetal testis. The male gonad differentiates into a testis. The female gonad differentiates into an ovary later during midgestation.

Male

UROGENITAL UNION. After 12 weeks, urogenital union, the fusion of testicular and mesonephric ducts,

begins. The rete tubules in the testis connect to the epigenitalis of the mesonephros (Wood-Jones, 1901). These epigenital ducts now become the efferent ducts (Felix, 1912e, f), and the mesonephric duct becomes the vas deferens. During the 4th month, the efferent ducts adjacent to the testis remain straight, whereas those adjacent to the vas deferens coil. The upper portion of the vas deferens also coils and becomes the epididymis, whereas the lower portion near the müllerian tubercle dilates fourfold to become an ampulla (Felix, 1912g). The lower portion of the vas deferens develops concentric layers of mesenchyme by about 12 weeks, but muscle fibers are not seen until 28 weeks (Felix, 1912g). After 12 weeks, a septum divides the ampulla of the distal portion of the vas deferens into the ejaculatory duct and seminal vesicle (Fig. 32–39) (Felix, 1912g).

The remaining mesonephric tubules become vestigial. Epigenital tubules that do not participate in urogenital union remain as the appendix of the epididymis. The paradidymis comprises the lower group of the lumbar mesonephric tubules (paragenitalis). The paragenitalis degenerates, but tubules between the head of the epididymis and the testis may remain as the organ of Giraldés.

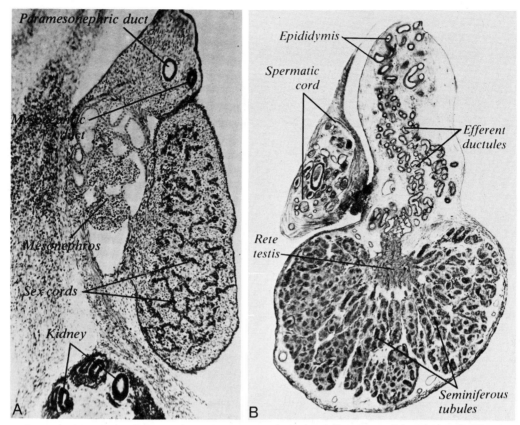

Figure 32–39. Development of the testis and urogenital union. A, By 8 weeks, the medullary sex cords have begun to differentiate. The glomeruli of the epigenitalis degenerate, and the collecting tubules will later drain the tubules of the testis. B, By 20 weeks, the rete tubules of the testis drain into the coiled efferent ducts. (From FitzGerald, M. J. T.: Human Embryology. New York, Harper & Row, 1978.)

The development of the vas may help in understanding how an atretic ureter may drain into a seminal vesicle cyst. It is plausible that a ureteral bud failed to separate from the common excretory duct and "vas." The ureter might eventually communicate with the ipsilateral seminal vesicle to appear as a seminal vesicle cyst (Oyen et al., 1988). As the renal blastema is likely abnormal, kidney development would be abortive.

The clinical findings in bilateral agenesis of the vas deferens support these ideas concerning embryology (Fonzo et al., 1983). As the vasa are absent so are the seminal vesicles. Thereby, the ejaculate volume is low, acid, and devoid of fructose and coagulable proteins. As the ureteral bud is not likely formed, renal agenesis may be seen but is not uniform, perhaps because the wolffian duct had become atretic after the ureteral bud formed. Because the body and tail of the epididymis are commonly absent, there may have been a mesonephric abnormality. The head of the epididymis is present and likely derives from the gonadal ridge.

ANATOMY OF TESTIS DESCENT. Heyns (1987) studied the anatomy of the gubernaculum and testis through dissection of 178 human male fetuses. At the stage of the intra-abdominal testis, the epididymis and lower pole of the testis are attached to the gubernaculum—a cylinder of jelly-like tissue that resembles Wharton's jelly in the umbilical cord. The gubernaculum is covered by peritoneum except posteriorly where it is adjacent to the mediastinum of the testis (Fig. 32–40).

The caudal end of the gubernaculum enters the internal inguinal ring. The inguinal canal is short with the internal and external rings almost on top of each other.

Heyns observed the following:

1. Before 23 weeks' gestation, the gubernaculum is above the external ring.
2. The gubernaculum begins to swell, as monitored by wet weight. The swelling peaks at about 28 weeks.
3. The gubernaculum bulges through the external ring and does not have scrotal extensions (see Fig. 32–40).
4. The testis, epididymis, and gubernaculum move through the inguinal canal as a unit.
5. The gubernaculum becomes smaller and fibrous. By comparison, the wet weight of Wharton's jelly of the umbilicus does not change during this period.

Heyns concluded that there are three anatomic phases of testis descent:

1. In the embryo, internal descent of the testis toward the internal ring is caused by differential growth of the lumbar vertebral column and pelvis.
2. Quick passage of the testis through the inguinal canal is mediated by gubernacular swelling.
3. The testis descends from the external ring into the scrotum after 26 weeks' gestation. During prenatal ultrasound examination, 60 per cent of males show testis descent by 30 weeks, and 93 per cent after 32 weeks (Birnholz, 1983).

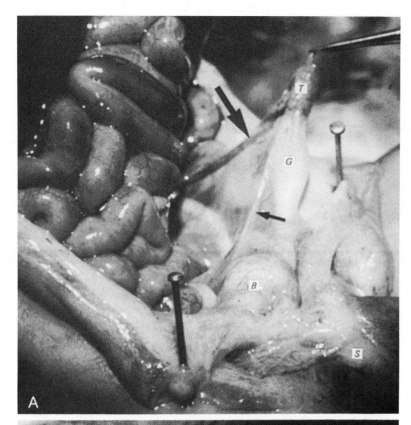

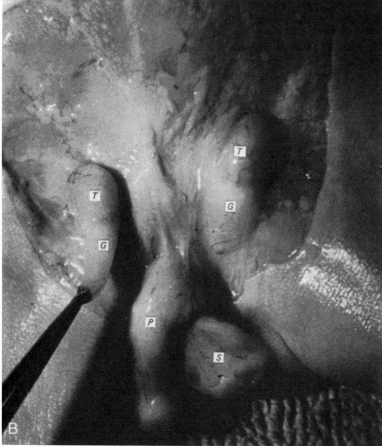

Figure 32–40. Anatomy of testis descent in the human fetus. *A,* At 22 weeks' gestation, testicular vessels (*large arrow*), vas deferens (*small arrow*), and gubernaculum (G) are enveloped in a fold of peritoneum (mesorchium). *B,* At 25 weeks' gestation, the skin over the lower anterior abdominal wall and scrotum have been removed. The gubernaculum does not show distal attachments. No extensions to the crural or scrotal area are evident. (T, testis; B, bladder; S, scrotum; P, penis.) (From Heyns, C. F.: J. Anat., 153:93, 1987.)

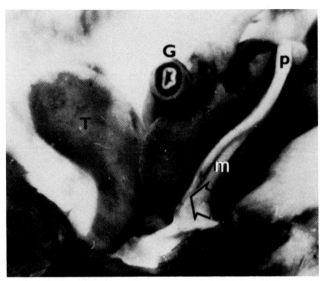

Figure 32–41. Regression of the paramesonephric duct begins at the caudal (*arrow*) and cranial (not shown) ends of the duct. This is an oblique view of the abdomen of a 2-month-old human fetus; and both testes are shown. (T, testis; p, paramesonephric ducts; G, gut.) (From Jirasek, J. E.: The National Foundation. Original Article Series, 15:13, 1977.)

MÜLLERIAN DUCTS. The müllerian ducts degenerate when exposed to müllerian inhibiting substance (MIS), which is produced by Sertoli's cells after 8 weeks of development. The degeneration occurs mostly in a craniocaudal direction. In the laboratory, the cranial portion of the duct is more sensitive to the effect of MIS than the caudal portion of the duct. (Donahoe et al., 1977). Clinically, however, regression extends both caudally and cranially (Fig. 32–41) (Jirasek, 1977). The cranial end of the degenerating müllerian duct may persist as the appendix of the testis (cf. appendix of epididymis) (Fig. 32–42).

By 16 weeks, the caudal end of the müllerian duct is degenerated to the level of the ejaculatory ducts (Deibert, 1933). The müllerian vagina does not form, and testosterone inhibits formation of the sinus vagina (see Fig. 32–44 and Development of the Ducts of the Genitalia. In the Female) (Bok and Drews, 1983). At this level, the müllerian ducts are fused as the uterovaginal primordium. This primordium persists as the prostatic utricle (see Fig. 32–35). The utricle becomes quite large and a dense layer of stroma surrounds it. The utricle opens into the urogenital sinus in the midline adjacent to the orifices of the ejaculatory ducts (Fig. 32–28C) (Deibert, 1933).

By 22 weeks, the utricle and ejaculatory ducts expand under the floor of the urethra and elevate the wall of the urethra to create the verumontanum (Deibert, 1933). The verumontanum causes the lumen of the prostatic urethra to appear semilunar (Fig. 32–35C). Later, the utricle contracts to become only a small structure on the tip of the verumontanum.

By 30 weeks, the seminal vesicles have grown back behind the base of the bladder, and the ejaculatory ducts are surrounded by thick musculature.

MOLECULAR BIOLOGY OF MÜLLERIAN DUCT REGRESSION. The biologic mechanisms whereby MIS causes regression of the müllerian ducts are becoming better understood (Donahoe et al., 1977; Josso, 1973). MIS is a polypeptide that is produced by fetal Sertoli cells. The steroids testosterone, medroxyprogesterone, and progesterone augment the effect of MIS in vitro (Ikawa, 1982). This augmentation is believed to be mediated by the binding of the steroids to the receptors of the mesenchyme that surround the müllerian duct. After local absorption of the substance, the mesenchyme may then alter the extracellular matrix by increased hyaluronidase activity or fibronectin lysis. These alterations may facilitate breakdown of the müllerian duct basement membrane (Ikawa et al., 1982; Trelstad et al., 1982). MIS can also act as a hormone (Donahoe et al., 1976). In the rat, only 24 hours of exposure of the müllerian duct to MIS is needed to degenerate the duct (Donahoe et al., 1977). The gene for MIS is mapped to the short arm of chromosome 19 (Cohen-Haguenaur et al., 1987).

The syndrome of hernia uteri inguinale results from a lack of MIS at the end of the indifferent stage of development. The müllerian duct structures (uterus,

Figure 32–42. Development of müllerian and wolffian ducts. Excisional biopsy of ducts draining a streak gonad in a child with intersex. Müllerian duct (md) elaborates to resemble an oviduct, and wolffian duct (wd) has coiled as a rudimentary epididymis. In normal development, the müllerian duct would involute to become the appendix testis.

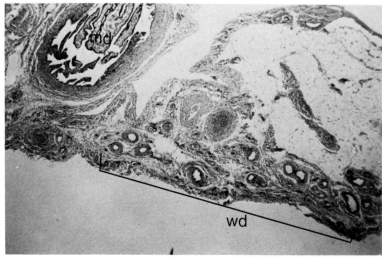
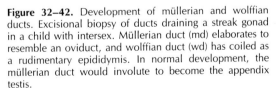

fallopian tube) persist. This syndrome appears in a genotypically and phenotypically normal boy who has cryptorchidism and hernia. Müllerian structures are found inside the hernia sac. The condition is genetically heterologous and may involve an X-linked or an autosomal recessive transmission pattern (Naguib et al., 1989). This syndrome has been described in women who present with inguinal hernias that contain an ovary, fallopian tube, and unicornous uterus but is not shown to be related to an aberration of the normal MIS expression (Elliott et al., 1989).

Androgen binding is noted in the developing male rat in the tissue primordia of the glans, the corpora, the urethral epithelium and its mesenchyme, and the prepuce (Murakami, 1987). The female shows much weaker binding in these sites. The cells that are especially labeled are mesenchymal, suggesting that, as in the prostate, the mesenchymal cells are the targets whereby androgens mediate morphogenesis. Insensitivity to testosterone may explain why in males with the testicular feminization syndrome and diminished androgen receptor activity (Chuna et al., 1984), the distal vagina (sinus vagina formation requires absence of androgen activity) persists, whereas the proximal vagina (müllerian vagina involution is dependent on MIS) does not (Bok and Drews, 1983). Also in this syndrome the prostate, a derivative of the urogenital sinus and thereby dependent on androgen is absent.

Ultrasound examination is accurate in determining the gender of the fetus by visualizing the genitalia (70 per cent of cases at 15 weeks' gestation and 90 per cent of cases after 20 weeks' gestation) (Birnholz, 1983).

Female

UTERUS AND VAGINA. After about 9 weeks' gestation, the septum between the fused müllerian ducts is absent. The mesonephric ducts degenerate around the 10th week. By the 11th week, the vaginal plate lined by squamous epithelium is seen. The uterovaginal primordium remains Y-shaped until the 12th week (FitzGerald, 1978). The cranial unfused portion of the müllerian ducts becomes the oviducts; the caudal fused portion becomes the uterus and cervix. The bicornuate uterus becomes a single chamber by upward expansion of the fused müllerian ducts as the fundus (FitzGerald, 1978). By the end of the 13th week, cervical glands develop. By the 14th week, the caudal vagina increases markedly in size. During the 15th week, the solid epithelial anlage of the anterior and posterior vaginal fornices appear (Cunha et al., 1988). The solid epithelial tip of the fused müllerian ducts (müllerian vagina) contact the dorsal wall of the urogenital sinus. Sinovaginal expansions or "bulbs" derive from the caudal end of the wolffian ducts, as they extend into the urogenital sinus (Figs. 32–43A and 32–44). These bulbs link the müllerian vagina with the sinus vagina. The meeting of the sinus vagina and müllerian vagina forms a contiguous lumen at about 24 weeks (Waterman, 1982).

Absence of testosterone allows feminine development by permitting the müllerian and dilated caudal wolffian ducts to fuse and thereby form the sinus portion of the vagina (Bok and Drews, 1983). Testosterone appears to inhibit this fusion because it leads the dilated segments of the wolffian ducts to become surrounded by dense mesenchyme. Male differentiation then follows (see Fig. 32–44) (Bok and Drews, 1983).

In the human fetus, the histologic development of the uterus shows undifferentiated mesenchyme at 12 weeks' gestation. At 14 weeks, there is an inner and outer layer of mesenchyme around the müllerian epithelium. The mesenchymal differentiation to smooth muscle is evident at 18 weeks, as judged by ultrastructure. Further differentiation of these two layers shows that by 31 weeks, the outer layer of the uterine wall is a myometrium and the inner layer of the wall is endometrial stroma (Fig. 32–45) (Konoishi et al., 1984).

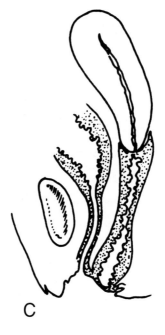

Figure 32–43. Diagram of the normal descent of the vaginal orifice between 12 weeks (A) and 16 weeks (C) of development. (From Bargy, F., Laude, F., Barbet, J. P., and Houette, A.: Surg. Radiol. Anat., 11:103, 1989.)

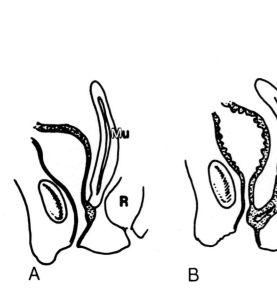

A   B   C

XX day 19

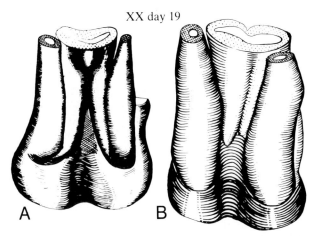

Figure 32–44. Development of the lower vagina. *A,* Mouse embryo genital tracts cultured without exogenous testosterone show female development. The müllerian ducts fuse with the adjacent wolffian ducts to form the sinovaginal bulbs. This fusion permits the link of the müllerian ducts with the urogenital sinus. *B,* Exogenous testosterone prevents fusion, and male development follows. (From Bok, G., and Drews, U.: J. Embryol. Exp. Morphol., 73:275, 1983. Company of Biologists, Ltd.)

The dual origin of the vagina (lower one third from urogenital sinus and upper two thirds from fused müllerian ducts) is further supported by noting that the septum in midvaginal atresia is lined on its superior portion with columnar epithelium consistent with müllerian duct origin and is lined on its inferior portion with squamous epithelium consistent with urogenital sinus origin (Toaff, 1984). Segmental absence of muscle differentiation in the ampullary part of the fallopian tubes has been reported (Tuluson, 1984).

The pathoembryogenesis of a vaginal ectopic ureter in a female may be analogous to that of a seminal vesicle cyst in a male (see preceding discussion). It is plausible that a ureteral bud failed to separate from the common excretory duct. The ureter maintained contact with the mesonephric duct and thereby became associated with the descending müllerian ducts (see Development of the Ducts of the Genitalia. Indifferent Stage). As the mesonephric duct normally degenerates, the ureter would come to drain adjacent to the müllerian ducts, clinically, most commonly near the lateral margin of the fornix of the cervix or hymen (Currarino, 1982). Occlusion of one limb of a duplicated müllerian system is associated with ipsilateral renal anomalies (agenesis or ipsilateral ureter opening into the occluded müllerian duct) (Gilsanz et al., 1982).

Incomplete fusion of the müllerian ducts likely results in the variety of patterns of duplication anomalies of the uterus and vagina (Gilsanz and Cleveland, 1982). The duplication may be the only anomaly or may occur in conjunction with renal, bladder, or cloacal exstrophy. In cloacal exstrophy, descensus of the urorectal septum is poor. Gilsanz and Cleveland's view is that poor descensus leads to failure of the normal fusion of the müllerian ducts and hence the high incidence of vaginal/ uterine duplication in cloacal exstrophy. This is distinct from bladder exstrophy, in which it may be viewed that the abdominal wall mesoderm fails to cover the anterior

abdomen because of an expansive cloacal membrane, perhaps extending to the umbilicus, or because the membrane ruptured prematurely but after müllerian fusion occurred. Hence, in bladder exstrophy as the müllerian ducts form and fuse normally, vaginal and uterine duplications are less common (90 per cent and 10 per cent, respectively).

Transverse vaginal septa should be divided to avoid dystocia in later years. For example, a fetus with a breech presentation could straddle the septum and delay delivery (Carey and Steinberg, 1989).

MOLECULAR BIOLOGY OF UTERINE AND VAGINAL DEVELOPMENT. The müllerian ducts develop in a feminine manner spontaneously unless they are inhibited by MIS. The mesonephric duct degenerates, but remnants may remain as Gartner's duct. The duct lies along the margin of the oviduct and uterus and opens adjacent to the cervix.

Morphogenesis of the vaginal epithelium involves an epithelial mesenchymal interaction. The epithelium takes on the phenotype determined by the stroma it is cultured with, but there is leeway in the expression of this interaction. For example, a combination of vaginal epithelial mesenchyme with uterine stroma leads to a uterine epithelial differentiation, and alternatively uterine epithelium with vaginal stroma leads to a vaginal epithelial differentiation (Cunha et al., 1988).

In the mouse, uterine epithelium appears to play an

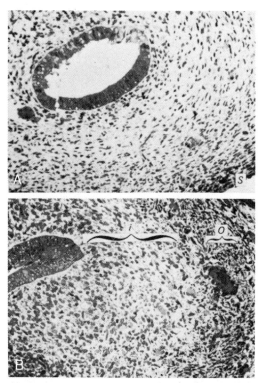

Figure 32–45. Development of the uterus in the human. *A,* By 12 weeks' gestation, the müllerian epithelium is surrounded by loose mesenchyme. *B,* At 14 weeks' gestation, the mesenchyme has arranged itself into an outer (o) and inner (i) layer. Further differentiation into endometrium and myometrium is complete by 31 weeks of development. (From Konishi, I., Fujii, S., Okamura, H., and Mori, T.: J. Anat., 139:239, 1984.)

important role in differentiation of its mesenchyme into muscle, analogous to that of the ureteral bud and its associated mesenchyme (Cunha et al., 1989). This differentiation does not appear to depend on estrogens. Bartol and co-workers (1988) studied the morphogenesis of the endometrium in sheep with respect to glycosoaminoglycan components of the extracellular matrix. The tissues were intensely stained (components stable and thereby accumulate) when morphogenetic events were not active, and they were weakly stained (components actively synthesized but then degraded and thereby do not accumulate) when morphogenetic events were active.

These components were present at the epitheliomesenchymal interface from just after fusion of the paired paramesonephric ducts during the 2nd quarter of gestation. They were present again in ewes from birth to 2 weeks. Ablation experiments show that the development of the endometrial glands is not altered by the absence of the ovary up to 2 weeks old, and this finding is consistent with the data of Bigsby and Cuhna (1986). These show that proliferation of uterine epithelium in the mouse is independent of gonads and adrenals and of steroids. The proliferation is likely an expression of the constitutive nature of the epithelial cells. However, exogenous estrogen administered during this interval caused permanent abnormalities. Excess progesterone does not appear to influence development of müllerian derivative (Cunha et al., 1988). Perhaps insults encountered during critical periods of uterine development may later contribute to pathologic conditions of the formed uterus.

GENETICS OF UROPATHIES

It is likely that a genetic basis exists for urologic birth defects, as there are many reports of sibling and familial uropathology (Dwoskin et al., 1986). Most defects are not of a recognized chromosomal abnormality, but specific HLA loci are seen in familial UPJO and ureteral reflux (Mackintosh et al., 1989).

The familial nature of urologic malformations in fetal bilateral renal agenesis/dysgenesis was studied by Roodhooft and co-workers (1984). In affected individuals, 12 per cent of family members had asymptomatic renal malformations. The mothers tended to be more often affected than the fathers. This tendency was also seen in sibs of index patients who had the same mother but different fathers (Moore et al., 1987). In one of ten children's karyotype, there was a 45,X,47,XXX mosaicism. However, when compared with controls, only those affected by renal agenesis had relatives with other renal anomalies that were more frequent than those in the general population.

Trisomy 7 has been associated with agenesis. The rate of occurrence of malformations among siblings of index patients was .04, which is 250 times greater than the prevalence rate of .016 in the general population. Parents should be so counseled regarding future pregnancies. If an immediate relative of an index patient is similarly affected, sonography of the extended family members could be done. Some of these conditions may be the result of the expression of a single gene that shows an autosomal dominant pattern of inheritance (Biedel et al., 1984). This screening may identify such an autosomal dominant pattern of inheritance and so aid genetic counseling (Moore et al., 1987). Screening could also involve a maternal fetal ultrasound after 14 weeks' gestation to check for oligohydramnios. Oligohydramnios is marked in all fetuses with bilateral agenesis at this stage, because of the absence of urine that normally contributes to amniotic fluid volume. However, the risk of false-positive diagnosis needs to be more clearly known before the role of such ultrasound is established (Moore et al., 1987).

The familial nature of renal anomalies when index children have renal agenesis/dysgenesis in association with an obstructive uropathy was examined by Moore and colleagues (1987). The families exhibited a low risk of recurrence of agenesis/dysgenesis, but they are at increased risk for structural urinary anomalies (renal ectopia and UPJO).

REFERENCES

Abramovich, D. R., Garden, A., Jandial, L., and Page, K. R.: Fetal swallowing and voiding in relation to hydramnios. Obstet. Gynecol., 54:15, 1979.

Adams, J. A., and Horton, M.: Is it sexual abuse? Confusion caused by a congenital anomaly of the genitalia. Clin. Pediatr., 28:146, 1989.

Alcaraz, A., Vinaixa, F., Tejedo-Mateu, A., Fores, M., Gotzens, V., Talbot-Wright, R., Alvarez-Vijande, R., and Carretero, P.: [Congenital obstructive disease of the ureter]. Acta Urol. Esp., 13:318, 1989.

Alexander, D. P., and Nixon, D. A.: The fetal kidney. Br. Med. Bull., 17:112, 1961.

Arey, L. B.: Developmental Anatomy, 7th ed. Philadelphia, W. B. Saunders Co., 1974.

Avner, E. D., Villee, D. B., Schneeberger, E. E., and Grupe, W. E.: An organ culture model for the study of metanephric development. J. Urol., 129:660, 1983.

Bargy, F., Laude, F., Barbet, J. P., and Houette, A.: The anatomy of intersexuality. Surg. Radiol. Anat., 11:103, 1989.

Bartol, F. F., Wiley, A. A., and Goodlett, D. R.: Ovine uterine morphogenesis: Histochemical aspects of endometrial development in the fetus and neonate. J. Anim. Sci., 66:1303, 1988.

Bellinger, M. F., and Duckett, J. W.: Accessory phallic urethra in the female patient. J. Urol., 127:1159, 1982.

Berman, D. J., and Maizels, M.: The role of urinary obstruction in the genesis of renal dysplasia: A model in the chick embryo. J. Urol., 128:1091, 1982.

Bernstein, J.: The morphogenesis of renal parenchymal maldevelopment (renal dysplasia). Pediatr. Clin. North Am., 18:395, 1971.

Biedel, C. W., Pagon, R. A., and Zapata, J. O.: Müllerian anomalies and renal agenesis: Autosomal dominant urogenital adysplasia. J. Pediatr., 104:861, 1984.

Bigsby, R. M., and Cunha, G. R.: Estrogen stimulation of DNA synthesis in epithelium lacking estrogen receptors. Endocrinology, 119:390, 1986.

Birnholz, J. C.: Determination of fetal sex. N. Engl. J. Med., 309:942, 1983.

Bok, G., and Drews, U.: The role of the wolffian ducts in the formation of the sinus vagina: An organ culture study. J. Embryol. Exp. Morph., 73:275, 1983.

Booth, E. J., Bell, T. E., McLain, C., and Evans, A. T.: Fetal vesicoureteral reflux. J. Urol., 113:258, 1975.

Bowie, J. D., Rosenberg, E. R., Andreotti, R. F., and Fields, S. I.: The changing sonographic appearance of fetal kidneys during pregnancy. J. Ultrasound Med., 2:505, 1983.

Boyden, E. A.: Congenital absence of the kidney. An interpretation based on a 10-mm human embryo exhibiting unilateral renal agenesis. Anat. Rec., 52:325, 1932.

Bremer, J. L.: The origin of the renal artery in mammals and its anomalies. Am. J. Anat., 18:179, 1915.

Cameron, G., and Chambers, R.: Direct evidence of function in kidney of an early human fetus. Am. J. Physiol., 123:482, 1983.

Campbell, S., Wladimiroff, J. W., and Dewhurst, C. J.: The antenatal measurement of fetal urine production. J. Obstet. Gynaecol. [Br. Commonw.], 80:680, 1973.

Carey, M. P., and Steinberg, L. H.: Vaginal dystocia in a patient with a double uterus and a longitudinal vaginal septum. Aust. N. Z. J. Obstet. Gynaecol., 29:74, 1989.

Chamberlanin, P. F., Manning, F. A., Morrison, I., and Lange, I. R.: Circadian rhythm in bladder volumes in the term human fetus. Obstet. Gynecol., 64:657, 1984.

Cohen-Haguenaur, O., Picard, J. V., Mattei, M. G., Serero, S., Nguyen, V. C., de Tand, M. F., Guerrier, D., Hors-Cayla, M. C., Josso, N., and Frezal, J.: Mapping of the gene for anti-müllerian hormone to the short arm of human chromosome 19. Cytogenet. Cell Genet., 44:2, 1987.

Crocker, J. F.: Human embryonic kidneys in organ culture: Abnormalities of development induced by decreased potassium. Science, 21:1178, 1973.

Cunha, G. R.: Epithelio-mesenchymal interactions in primordial gland structures which become responsive to androgen stimulation. Anat. Rec., 172:179, 1972.

Cunha, G. R., Taguchi, O., Sugimura, Y., Lawrence, W. D., Mahmood, F., and Robboy, S. J.: Absence of teratogenic effects of progesterone on the developing genital tract of the human female fetus. Hum. Pathol., 19:777, 1988.

Cunha, G. R.: Androgenic effects upon prostatic epithelium are mediated via trophic influences from stroma. Prog. Clin. Biol. Res., 145:81, 1984.

Cunha, G. R., Taguchi, O., Sugimura, Y., Lawrence, W. D., Mahmood, F., and Robboy, S. J.: Absence of teratogenic effects of progesterone on the developing genital tract of the human fetus. Hum. Pathol., 19:777, 1988.

Cunha, G. R., Young, P., and Brody, J. R.: Role of uterine epithelium in the development of myometrial smooth muscle cells. Biol. Reprod., 40:861, 1989.

Currarino, G.: Single vaginal ectopic ureter and Gartner's duct cyst with ipsilateral renal hypoplasia and dysplasia (or agenesis). J. Urol., 128:988, 1982.

Currarino, G., and Weisbruch, G. J.: Transverse fusion of the renal pelvis and single ureter. Urol. Radiol., 11:88, 1989.

Deibert, G. A.: The separation of the prepuce in the human penis. Anat. Rec., 57:387, 1933.

de Jonge, M. K., Van Nouhys, J. M., and Tjabbes, D.: How to differentiate between ectopia and displacement in patient with crossed kidney. Urology, 31:450, 1988.

de Vries, L., and Levene, M. I.: Measurement of renal size in preterm and term infants by real-time ultrasound. Arch. Dis. Child., 58:145, 1983.

Donahoe, P. K., Ito, Y., and Hendren, W. H., III: A graded organ culture assay for detecting of müllerian inhibiting substance. J. Surg. Res., 23:141, 1977.

Donahoe, P. K., Ito, Y., Marfatia, S., and Hendren, W. H., III: The production of müllerian inhibiting substance by the fetal, neonatal and adult rat. Biol. Reprod., 15:329, 1976.

Dwoskin, J. Y., Noe, H. N., Gonzalez, E. T., Jr., Firlit, C. F., Chaviano, A. H., and Lebowitz, R. L.: Sibling uropathology. Dialog. Pediatr. Urol., 9:6, June, 1986.

Ecke, M., and Klatte, D.: Inverted Y-ureteral duplication with an uterine ectopy as caused of ureteric enuresis. Urol. Int., 44:116, 1989.

Ekblom, P.: Determination and differentiation of the nephron. Med. Biol., 59:139, 1981.

Ekblom, P., Vestweber, D., and Kemler, R.: Cell-matrix interactions and cell adhesion during development. Annu. Rev. Cell Biol., 2:27, 1986.

Elliott, D. C., Beam, T. E., and Danapoli, T. S.: Hernia uterus inguinale associated with unicornuate uterus. Arch. Surg., 124:872, 1989.

Escala, J. M., Keating, M. A., Boyd, G., Pierce, A., Hutton, J. L., and Lister, J.: Development of elastic fibres in the upper urinary tract. J. Urol., 141:969, 1989.

Escobar, L. F., Weaver, D. D., Bixler, D., Hodes, M. E., and Mitchell, M.: Urorectal septum malformation sequence. Report of six cases and embryological analysis. Am. J. Dis. Child., 141:1021, 1987.

Felix, W.: The development of the urinogenital organs. In Keibel, F. and Mall, F. P. (Eds.): Manual of Human Embryology. Philadelphia, J. B. Lippincott Co., 1912. [Vol. II, Chapt. XIX., a. 866; b. 880; c. 752; d. 815; e. 829; f. 830; g. 938.]

Fetterman, G. H., Ravitch, M. M., and Sherman, F. F.: Cystic changes in fetal kidneys following ureteral ligation. Kidney Int., 5:111, 1974.

FitzGerald, M. J. T. (Ed.): Abdominal and pelvic organs. In Human Embryology. New York, Harper & Row, 1978, p. 106.

Fonzo, D., Manenti, M., Varengo, M., Quadri, R., Frea, B., Tizzani, A., and Carone, R.: Andrological and hormonal findings in subjects with ductus deferens agenesis. Andrologia, 15:614, 1983.

Friedland, G. W., and De Vries, P.: Renal ectopia and fusion—embryologic basis. Urology, 5:698, 1975.

George, F. W., Peterson, K. G., Frankel, P. A., and Wilson, J. D.: The androgen receptor in the fetal epididymis is similar to that in the mature rabbit. Proc. Soc. Exp. Biol. Med., 188:500, 1988.

Gersh, I.: The correlation of structure and function in the developing mesonephros and metanephros. Contrib. Embryol., 26:35, 1937.

Gilsanz, V., and Cleveland, R. H.: Duplication of the müllerian ducts and genitourinary malformations. Part I. The value of excretory urography. Radiology, 144:793, 1982.

Gilsanz, V., Cleveland, R. H., and Reid, B. S.: Duplication of the müllerian ducts and genitourinary malformations. Part II. Analysis of malformations. Radiology, 144:797, 1982.

Gotoh, T., Morita, H., Tokunaka, S., Koyanagi, T., and Tsuji, I.: Single ectopic ureter. J. Urol., 129:271, 1983.

Grannum, P., Bracken, M., Silverman, R., and Hobbins, J. C.: Assessment of fetal kidney size in normal gestation by comparison of ratio of kidney circumference to abdominal circumference. Am. J. Obstet. Gynecol., 136:249, 1980.

Grobstein, C.: Trans-filter induction of tubules in mouse metanephrogenic mesenchyme. Exp. Cell Res., 10:424, 1956.

Gruenwald, P.: The relation of the growing müllerian duct to the wolffian duct and its importance for the genesis of malformations. Anat. Rec., 81:1, 1941.

Gruenwald, P.: The normal changes in the position of the embryonic kidney. Anat. Rec., 85:163, 1943.

Hamilton, W. J., and Mossman, H. W. (Eds.): Determination, differentiation, the organizer mechanism, abnormal development, and twinning. In Human Embryology Prenatal Development of Form and Function. New York, Macmillan Press Ltd., 1976, p. 201.

Hamilton, W. J., and Mossman, H. W. (Eds.): The urogenital system. In Human Embryology Prenatal Development of Form and Function. New York, Macmillan Press Ltd., 1976, p. 377.

Hatch, D. A., Maizels, M., Zaontz, M. R., and Firlit, C. F.: Hypospadias hidden by a complete prepuce. Surg. Gynecol. Obstet., 169:233, 1989.

Heyns, C. F.: The gubernaculum during testicular descent in the human fetus. J. Anat., 153:93, 1987.

Howe, S. C., Cromie, W. J., and Kay, N. W.: Development of an in vitro model for the disruption of extracellular matrix components in the study of congenital renal parenchymal dysmorphism. J. Urol., 142:612, 1989.

Hunter, R. H.: Notes on development of prepuce. J. Anat., 70:68, 1935.

Ikawa, H., Hutson, J. M., Budzik, G. P., MacLaughlin, D. T., and Donahoe, P. K.: Steroid enhancement of müllerian duct regression. J. Pediatr. Surg., 17:453, 1982.

Javadpour, N., Graziano, A. B., and Terril, R.: Experimental induction of patent allantoic duct by intrauterine bladder outlet obstruction. J. Surg. Res., 17:341, 1974.

Jeanty, P., Dramaix-Wilmet, M., Elkhazen, N., Hubinont, C., and van Regemorter, N.: Measurements of fetal kidney growth on ultrasound. Radiology, 144:159, 1982.

Jenny, C., Kuhns, M. L. D., and Arakawa, F.: Hymens in newborn female infants. Pediatrics, 80:399, 1987.

Jirasek, J. E.: Morphogenesis of the genital system in the human. Birth Defects. The National Foundation. Original Article Series, 15:13, 1977.

Josso, N.: In vitro synthesis of müllerian inhibiting hormone by seminiferous tubules isolated from the calf fetal testis. Endocrinology, 93:829, 1973.

Kellokumpu-Lehtinen, P., and Pelliniemi, L. J.: Hormonal regulation of differentiation of human fetal prostate and Leydig cells in utero. Folia Histochem. Cytobiol., 26:113, 1988.

Kirillova, I. A., Kulazhenko, V. P., Kulazhenko, L. G., and Novikova, I. V.: Cystic kidney in an 8-week human embryo. Acta Anat., 114:68, 1982.

Klein, G., Langegger, M., Goridis, C., and Ekblom, P.: Neural cell adhesion molecules during embryonic induction and development of the kidney. Development, 102:749, 1988.

Klein, V. R., Willman, S. P., and Carr, B. R.: Familial posterior labial fusion. Obstet. Gynecol., 73(Part 3):500, 1989.

Kogan, B., and Iwamoto, H.: Lower urinary tract function in the sheep fetus: Studies of autonomic control and pharmacologic responses of the fetal bladder. J. Urol., 141:1019, 1989.

Konishi, I., Fujii, S., Okamura, H., and Mori, T.: Development of smooth muscle in the human fetal uterus: an ultrastructural study. J. Anat., 139:239, 1984.

Langman, J.: Medical Embryology, 2nd ed. Baltimore, Williams & Wilkins Co., 1969, p. 301.

Lash, J. W., Saxen, L., and Ekblom, P.: Biosynthesis of proteoglycans in organ cultures of developing kidney mesenchyme. Exp. Cell Res., 147:85, 1983.

Lehtonen, E., Wartiovaara, J., Nordling, S., and Saxen, L.: Demonstration of cytoplasmic processes in millipore filters permitting kidney tubule induction. J. Embryol. Exp. Morph., 33:187, 1975.

Lelongt, B., Makino, H., Dalecki, T. M., and Kanwar, Y. S.: Role of proteoglycans in renal development. Dev. Biol., 128:256, 1988.

Liu, K. W., and Fitzgerald, R. J.: An unusual case of complete urethral duplication in a female child. Aust. N. Z. J. Surg., 58:587, 1988.

Lowsley, O. S.: The development of the human prostate gland with reference to the development of other structures at the neck of the urinary bladder. Am. J. Anat., 13:299, 1912.

Mackie, G. G., and Stephens, F. D.: Duplex kidneys: A correlation of renal dysplasia with position of the ureteral orifice. J. Urol., 114:274, 1979.

Mackintosh, P., Almarhoos, G., and Heath, D. A.: HLA linkage with familial vesicoureteral reflux and familial pelviureteric junction obstruction. Tissue Antigens, 34:185, 1989.

Maizels, M., and Simpson, S. B., Jr.: Primitive ducts of renal dysplasia induced by culturing ureteral buds denuded of condensed renal mesenchyme. Science, 219:509, 1983.

Maizels, M., Simpson, S. B., Jr., and Firlit, C. F.: Simulation of human renal dysplasia in a chick embryo model. Abstract #765. American Urological Association, Las Vegas, 1983.

Maizels, M., and Stephens, F. D.: The induction of urologic malformations: Understanding the relationship of renal ectopia and congenital scoliosis. Invest. Urol., 17:209, 1979.

Maizels, M., and Stephens, F. D.: Valves of the ureter as a cause of primary obstruction of the ureter: Anatomic, embryologic and clinical aspects. J. Urol., 123:742, 1980.

Matsuno, T., Tokunaka, S., and Koyanagi, T.: Muscular development in the urinary tract. J. Urol., 132:148, 1984.

McVary, K. T., and Maizels, M.: Urinary obstruction reduces glomerulogenesis in the developing kidney: A model in the rabbit. J. Urol., 142:646, 1989.

Mellins, H. Z.: Cystic dilatations of the upper urinary tract: A radiologist's developmental model. Radiology, 145:291, 1984.

Middleton, A. W., Jr., and Pfister, R. C.: Stone-containing pyelocaliceal diverticulum: Embryogenic, anatomic, radiologic and clinical characteristics. J. Urol., 111:2, 1974.

Moore, D., Tudehope, D., Lewis, B., and Masel, J.: Familial renal abnormalities associated with the oligohydramnios tetrad secondary to renal agenesis and dysgenesis. Aust. Paediatr. J., 23:137, 1987.

Moore, K. L.: The Developing Human, 2nd ed. Philadelphia, W. B. Saunders Co., 1977.

Mor, N., and Merlob, P.: Congenital absence of the hymen only a rumor? (Letter.) Pediatrics, 82:679, 1988.

Mor, N., Merlob, P., and Reisner, S. H.: Tags and bands of the female external genitalia in the newborn infant. Clin. Pediatr., 22:122, 1983.

Muecke, E. C.: The embryology of the urinary system. In Campbell's Urology, 4th ed. Philadelphia, W. B. Saunders Co., 1979, p. 1286.

Murakami, R.: Autoradiographic studies of the localization of androgen-binding cells in the genital tubercles of fetal rats. J. Anat., 151:209, 1987.

Naguib, K. K., Teebi, A. S., Farag, T. I., al-Awadi, S. A., el-Khalifa, M. Y., and el-Sayed, M.: Familial uterine hernia syndrome: report of an Arab family with four affected males. Am. J. Med. Genet., 33:180, 1989.

Nathan, H., and Glezer, I.: Right and left accessory renal arteries arising from a common trunk associated with unrotated kidneys. J. Urol., 132:7, 1984.

Okada, T., and Morikawa, Y.: Histometry of the developing kidney in fetal rats. Nippon Juigaku Zasshi, 50:269, 1988.

O'Rahilly, R., and Tucker, J. A.: The early development of the larynx in staged human embryos. Part 1. Embryos of the first five weeks. Ann. Oto. Rhino. Laryngol., Supp. 7, Vol. 82, 1973.

Ostling, K.: The genesis of hydronephrosis: Particularly with regard to the changes at the ureteropelvic junction. Acta Chir. Scand., [Supp.] 86:72, 1942.

Oyen, R., Gielen, J., van Poppel, H., and Baert, L.: Seminal vesicle cyst and ipsilateral renal agenesis. Case report. Eur. J. Radiol., 8:122, 1988.

Pavanello, R. de C., Eigier, A., and Otto, P. A.: Relationship between Mayer-Rokitansky-Küster (MRK) anomaly and hereditary renal adysplasia (HRA). Am. J. Med. Genet., 29:845, 1988.

Poole, T. J., and Steinberg, M. S.: Evidence of the guidance of pronephric duct migration by a craniocaudally traveling adhesion gradient. Devel. Biol., 92:144, 1982.

Potter, E. L.: Normal and Abnormal Development of the Kidney. Chicago, Year Book Medical Publishers, 1972.

Roodhooft, A. M., Birnholz, J. C., and Holmes, L. B.: Familial nature of congenital absence and severe dysgenesis of both kidneys. N. Engl. J. Med., 310:1341, 1984.

Rowsell, A. R., and Morgan, B. D. G.: Hypospadias and the embryogenesis of the penile urethra. Br. J. Plast. Surg., 40:201, 1987.

Ruano-Gil, D., Coca-Payeras, A., and Tejedo-Mateu, A.: Obstruction and normal recanalization of the ureter in the human embryo: Its relation to congenital ureteric obstruction. Eur. Urol., 1:293, 1975.

Sariola, H., Aufderheide, E., Bernhard, H., Henke-Fahle, S, Dippold, W., and Ekbolm, P.: Antibodies to cell surface ganglioside GD3 perturb inductive epithelial-mesenchymal interactions. Cell, 54:235, 1988.

Sariola, H., Ekblom, P., and Henke-Fahle, S.: Embryonic neurons as in vitro inducers of differentiation of nephrogenic mesenchyme. Dev. Biol., 132:271, 1989.

Sawczuk, I. S., Olsson, C. A., Buttyan, R., Nguyen-Huu, M. C., Zimmerman, K. A., Alt, F. W., Zaker, Z., Wolgemuth, D., and Reitelman C.: Gene expression in renal growth and regrowth. J. Urol., 140:1145, 1988.

Saxen, L.: Organogenesis of the kidney. In Barlow, P. W., Green, P. B., and Wylie, C. C. (Eds.): Development and Cell Biology Series. Cambridge, Cambridge University Press, 1987.

Saxen, L., Toivonen, S., Vainio, T., and Korhonen, P.: Untersuchungen uber die Tubulogenese der Niere. III. Die Analyse der Fruhentwicklung mit der Zeitraffermethode. Z. Naturforsch., 20b:340, 1965.

Schuger, L., O'Shea, S., Rheinheimer, J., and Varani, J.: Laminin in lung development: Effects of anti-laminin antibody in murine lung morphogenesis. Dev. Biol., 137:26, 1990.

Siiteri, P. K., and Wilson, J. D.: Testosterone formation and metabolism during male sexual differentiation in the human embryo. J. Clin. Endocrin. Metab., 38:113, 1974.

Smith, F. G., and Robillard, J. E.: Pathophysiology of fetal renal disease. Semin. Perinatol., 13:305, 1989.

Spencer, J., and Maizels, M.: Inhibition of protein glycosylation causes renal dysplasia in the chick embryo. J. Urol., 138:984, 1987.

Stephens, F. D.: Anatomical vagaries of double ureters. Aust. N. Z. J. Surg., 28:27, 1958.

Stephens, F. D.: Embryopathy of malformations. J. Urol. [Guest editorial.], 127:13, 1982.

Stephens, F. D.: Congenital Malformations of the Urinary Tract. New York, Praeger Publishers, 1983.

Stonestreet, B. S., Hansen, N. B., Laptook, A. R., and Oh, W.: Glucocorticoid accelerates renal function maturation in fetal lambs. Early Hum. Dev., 8:331, 1983.

Swinford, A. E., Bernstein, J., and Toriello, H. V.: Renal tubular dysgenesis: Delayed onset of oligohydramnios. Am. J. Med. Gent., 32:127, 1989.

Tanagho, E. A.: Surgically induced partial ureteral obstruction in the fetal lamb. III. Ureteral obstruction. Invest. Urol., 10:35, 1972.

Toaff, M. E.: Origin of the epithelium of atretic hemivaginas. Am. J. Obstet Gynecol. (Letter.), 149:237, 1984.

Trelstad, R. L., Hayashi, K., et al.: The epithelial mesenchymal interface of the male müllerian duct: Basement membrane integrity and ductal regression. Dev. Biol., 92:27, 1982.

Tuluson, A. H.: Complete absence of the muscular layer of the ampullary part of the fallopian tubes. Arch. Gynecol., 234:279, 1984.

Unsworth, B., and Grobstein, C.: Induction of kidney tubules in mouse metanephrogenic mesenchyme by various embryonic mesenchymal tissues. Dev. Biol., 21:547, 1970.

Vainio, S., Lehtonen, E., Jalkanen, M., Bernfield, M., and Saxen, L.: Epithelial mesenchymal interactions regulate the stage-specific expression of a cell surface proteoglycan, syndecan, in the developing kidney. Dev. Biol., 134:382, 1989.

van der Putte, S. C. J.: Normal and abnormal development of the anorectum. J. Pediatr. Surg., 21:434, 1986.

Waterman, R. E.: Human embryo and fetus. *In* Hafez, E. S. E., and Kenemans, P. (Eds.): Atlas of Human Reproduction. Hingham, MA, Kluwer Boston, Inc., 1982.

Wladimiroff, J. W., and Campbell, S.: Fetal urine production rates in normal and complicated pregnancy. Lancet, 1(849):151, 1974.

Wood-Jones, F.: The musculature of the bladder and urethra. Anatomical Society, Great Britain and Ireland. J. Anat. Physiol., 36:51(2), 1901–2.

Zackson, S. L., and Steinberg, M. S.: A molecular marker for cell guidance information in the axolotl embryo. Dev. Biology, 127:435, 1988.

33
RENAL FUNCTION IN THE FETUS AND NEONATE

Robert L. Chevalier, M.D.
James Mandell, M.D.

The development of renal function in the fetus and neonate can be viewed as a continuing evolution of interdependent morphologic and physiologic stages. During gestation, the functional changes are determined by increases in nephron number, growth, and maturation, whereas hemostasis of the fetus is maintained predominantly by the placenta. At birth, the kidney must suddenly assume this previously maternal role. The kidney's response to this demand is governed to a great extent by its anatomic development (gestational age at delivery), and thus important functional differences are seen in the premature and term neonate.

In this chapter, we review the anatomic stages and functional aspects of fetal renal development and postnatal functional development and the evaluation of postnatal renal function and hormonal control of renal function during development.

ANATOMIC STAGES OF FETAL RENAL DEVELOPMENT

The major morphogenic stages of the human kidney appear quite early in development and, except for the last one, are transitory (Fig. 33–1) (Potter, 1972). The pronephros appears at 3 weeks, never progresses beyond a rudimentary stage, and involutes by 5 weeks. The mesonephros is seen at 5 weeks of gestation, appears to have transitory function, and degenerates by 11 to 12 weeks. Its major role in renal development is related to the fact that its ductal system gives rise to the ureteric bud. The last is critical for development of the metanephric or definitive kidney. The metanephros begins its inductive phase after 5 weeks of gestation, and in the human nephrogenesis is completed by 34 to 36 weeks.

Original studies by Dr. Chevalier were supported by an Established Investigatorship of the American Heart Association and by NIH grants AM25727, HL40209, and DK40558.

In the developing metanephric kidney, there is a centrifugal pattern of nephrogenesis and maturation with the outer cortical nephrons being the last to complete development.

FUNCTIONAL FETAL RENAL DEVELOPMENT

Information regarding the functional development of the metanephric kidney is gained primarily through animal studies. One must be careful in extrapolating such data from species in which there is dissimilarity of structural maturation at comparable gestational ages. Urine production in the human kidney is known to begin around 10 to 12 weeks. Salt and water hemostasis, however, is primarily handled by the placenta throughout gestation.

Fetal renal blood flow remains at a relatively low stable rate in utero. The ratio of renal blood flow to cardiac output at 20 weeks is 0.03 compared with the postnatal ratio of 0.2 to 0.3 (Rudolph and Heyman, 1976). This diminished renal blood flow is probably related to several different factors. The number of vascular channels is low early in gestation, and arteriolar resistance in these channels is increased (Ichikawa et al., 1979; Robillard et al., 1987). Studies in animals have demonstrated roles for renal innervation and for the renin-angiotensin system as chronic modulators of this effect (Robillard et al., 1987). These findings are discussed in greater detail subsequently.

Glomerular filtration rate (GFR) in the fetus is theoretically equal to the single nephron GFR times the number of functioning glomeruli. This value is difficult to determine, however, because GFR is much higher in juxtamedullary compared with subcortical glomeruli (Spitzer et al., 1974). Glomerular filtration rate parallels renal mass and correlates with gestational age, because

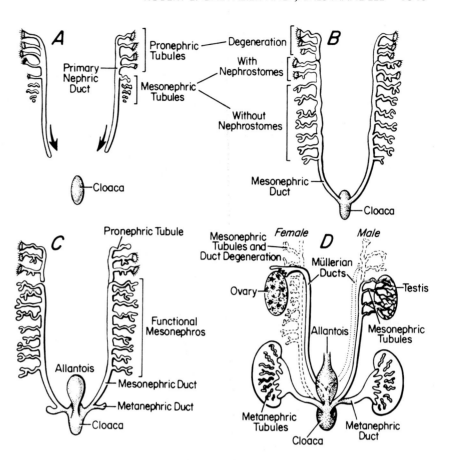

Figure 33–1. Relations of pronephros, mesonephros, and metanephros at various stages of development. To simplify, the tubules have been drawn as if they had been pulled out to the side of the ducts. The first rudimentary pronephros (A) is elaborated as a group of tubules emptying on either side into the primary nephric ducts, which extend caudad to discharge ultimately into the cloaca. A little later in development a second group of tubules arises more caudal in position than the pronephric tubule. These are mesonephric tubules (A). In their growth, they extend toward the primary nephric ducts and soon open into them (B).

The plan, as shown in C, represents approximately the conditions attained by the human embryo toward the end of the 4th week. In D are depicted the conditions after sexual differentiation has taken place: female left side: male right side. The müllerian ducts (shown in D) arise in human embryos during the 8th week, in close association with the mesonephric ducts. The müllerian ducts are the primordial tubes from which the oviducts, uterus, and vagina of the female are formed. Note that although both mesonephric and müllerian ducts appear in all young embryos, the müllerian ducts become vestigial in the male and the mesonephric ducts become vestigial in the female. (From Patten, B. M.: Human Embryology, 3rd ed. New York, McGraw-Hill, 1968.)

nephrogenesis continues from 10 to 12 weeks of gestation until 34 weeks (Smith and Robillard, 1989).

Fractional excretion of sodium (FE_{NA}) shows a negative correlation with gestational age. The fetus produces hypotonic or isotonic urine with high sodium content and in large volumes. Potassium excretion similarly increases with gestation, which may be related to a rise in fetal plasma aldosterone concentration. A maturational increase in glucose transport of the fetal kidneys also occurs. Other tubular functions, such as bicarbonate reabsorption and acid production, are low in the fetus. They are, however, responsive to parathyroid excretion, intravascular volume, and acid infusion.

POSTNATAL FUNCTIONAL DEVELOPMENT

At birth, several dramatic events occur that alter renal function. The kidney's response to the changing milieu and its attempt at regaining homeostasis are heavily influenced by the gestational age at delivery.

Renal blood flow increases sharply at birth, with a 5- to 18-fold rise in different animal studies (Aperia and Herin, 1975; Gruskin et al., 1970). This finding reflects several factors: a redistribution of flow from the inner to outer cortex (Aperia et al., 1977a) and a drop in renal vascular resistance, associated with increased intrarenal prostaglandins (Gruskin et al., 1970).

GFR doubles during the 1st week in term infants (Guignard et al., 1975). Because of the dependence of

GFR on gestational age, for infants born before 34 weeks, GFR rises slowly. After reaching a postconceptional age of 34 weeks, a rapid rise is observed. Factors responsible for this rapid rise include diminished renal vascular resistance (Gruskin et al., 1970) and greater perfusion pressure, glomerular permeability, and filtration surface (John et al., 1981). In experimental animals, the increase in surface area for filtration accounts for most of the maturation increase in GFR (Spitzer et al., 1974). Serum creatinine levels, which reflect maternal levels at birth, also decrease by 50 per cent in the 1st week of life in term or near-term infants. The GFR continues to rise, reaching adult levels by 2 years of age (Rubin et al., 1949).

In the neonate, tubular function changes in association with the rise in GFR. A blunted response to sodium loading remains, however, owing to the inability of the distal tubule to appropriately decrease its fractional excretion of sodium (Kim and Mandell, 1988). This effect is probably related to the high circulating renin and aldosterone levels and to a diminished renal response to atrial natriuretic peptide (see discussion further on). Conversely, premature infants, less than 35 weeks' gestation, subject to sodium deprivation may develop hyponatremia because of tubular immaturity and sodium wasting (Engelke et al., 1978; Roy et al., 1976). Thus, sodium supplementation is frequently required in premature infants.

In terms of concentrating ability, the neonatal kidney can dilute fairly well (25 to 35 mOsm/L) but has limited concentrating capacity (600 to 700 mOsm/L) (Hansen and Smith, 1953). Concentrating capacity is even more restricted in the premature infant (500 mOsm/L). The factors responsible for this include anatomic immaturity of the renal medulla, decreased medullary concentration of sodium chloride and urea, and diminished responsiveness of the collecting ducts to antidiuretic hormone (Schlondorff et al., 1978; Stanier, 1972).

Acid-base regulation in the neonate is characterized by a reduced threshold for bicarbonate reabsorption (Svenningsen, 1974). Bicarbonate reabsorption is gradually raised with increasing GFR. An inability to respond to an acid load eventually improves by 4 to 6 weeks postnatally. This inability is accentuated in the premature infant who tends to be slightly acidotic in comparison to the adult.

Glucose transport matures with the rising GFR in the neonate. This effect is more readily observed in the premature infant, because fractional excretion of glucose is higher before 34 weeks of gestation (Arant, 1978).

Calcium-phosphate metabolism also changes shortly after birth. Parathyroid hormone (PTH) is suppressed at birth, and serum calcium concentration falls. This secondarily causes an increase in PTH release. Initially, tubular reabsorption of phosphate is high in the premature infant and remains so until regular feedings commence at term (Arant, 1978).

EVALUATION OF POSTNATAL RENAL FUNCTION

Glomerular Function

Measurement of the GFR in the infant is problematic for a number of reasons. The first difficulty is obtaining an accurately timed urine collection in the incontinent patient without bladder catheterization. The second is the inherent inaccuracy in measurement of the most readily available index of GFR, plasma creatinine concentration, because precision of the assay in most clinical laboratories is $\pm$ 0.3 mg/dl. Thus, calculated GFR in the infant can be overestimated or underestimated by 100 per cent under the best circumstances of sample collections. The third is the rapidly changing GFR with normal growth: GFR factored for adult surface area (1.73 m²) increases several fold during the first 2 months of life (Fig. 33–2). Moreover, GFR increases with postconceptional age from 34 to 40 weeks' gestation (Fig. 33–3). Within the first 2 days of life, plasma creatinine reflects maternal levels and may not reflect GFR of the infant. By 7 days in term infants, plasma creatinine concentration is normally less than 1 mg/dl, whereas in preterm infants, the concentration can remain as high as 1.5 mg/dl for the 1st month of life (Trompeter et al., 1983). In view of these considerations, it is important to obtain serial values of serum creatinine. A progressive increase in the neonatal period suggests renal insufficiency regardless of gestational age.

Long-term monitoring of GFR in children with urologic abnormalities should account for increasing muscle mass that results in increasing serum creatinine concentration with age. A simple and reliable estimate of creatinine clearance (C_{cr}) can be derived from the serum

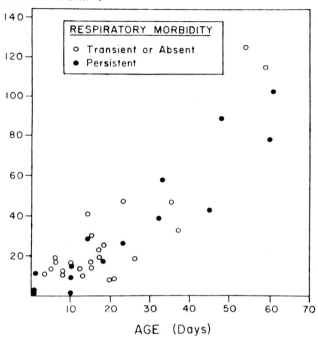

CREATININE CLEARANCE
(ml/min/1.73 M²)

Figure 33–2. Creatinine clearance in relation to postnatal age during the first 60 days of life for preterm infants (birth weight mean of 1380 g: gestational age mean of 31 weeks). During the first 10 days of life, creatinine clearance was lower (7.5 ml/min/1.73 m²) in infants with persistent respiratory dysfunction than in those without respiratory dysfunction (14.7 ml/min/1.73 m²) (P < .05). Beyond the 11th day, no difference was noted between groups. (From Ross, B., Cowett, R. M., and Oh, W.: Renal functions of low birth weight infants during the first two month of life. Pediatr., Res., 11:1162, 1977.)

creatinine concentration (P_{cr}) and the patient's height, using the following empiric formula developed by Schwartz and co-workers (1987):

$$C_{cr} = k \times L/P_{cr}$$

where C_{cr} = creatinine concentration (ml/min/1.73 m²), k = a constant (0.33 for preterm, 0.45 for full-term infants), and L = body length (cm). Although C_{cr} is constant at 80 to 140 ml/min/1.73 m² after 2 years of age, the marked increase during the first 2 years of life should be taken into account when interpreting values for young infants.

A more accurate determination of GFR can be obtained by creatinine clearance based on a 24-hour urine collection. As with the estimated C_{cr} described here, the value should be corrected for adult surface area by multiplying by 1.73 and dividing by the patient's surface area [S.A.]. This last value is derived from a nomogram (Cole, 1984). Thus,

C_{cr} (ml/min/1.73 m²) =
     "uncorrected" C_{cr} (ml/min) $\times$ 1.73/S.A.

Expression of all pediatric C_{cr} in this fashion should reduce confusion and ambiguity in comparing the result with expected normal ranges (see Figs. 33–2 and 33–3).

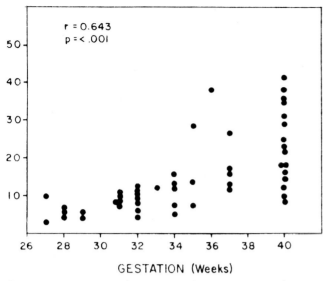

CREATININE CLEARANCE
(ml/min/1.73 M²)

Figure 33–3. Creatinine clearance in relation to gestational age in clinically well infants studied from 24 to 40 hours after birth. (From Siegel, S. R., and Oh, W.: Renal function as a marker of human fetal maturation. Acta Paediatr. Scand., 65:481, 1976.)

Accuracy of the calculated C_{cr} depends on adequacy of the timed urine collection.

For more precise measurement of GFR, and to determine the relative contribution of each kidney to total GFR, a radiolabeled tracer that is cleared solely by glomerular filtration can be infused intravenously. Plasma concentration of the isotope can then be measured sequentially with concurrent scintigraphy. An agent frequently used for this purpose is ^{99m}Tc-diethylenetriaminepenta-acetic acid (Tc-DTPA). Although precision of measurement of Tc-DTPA is greater than that of creatinine and urine collection is not required, adequate venous access and patient cooperation during scintigraphy are necessary. The latter may limit the usefulness of the technique in infants and younger children. As with C_{cr}, measurement of GFR by Tc-DTPA clearance should be corrected for adult surface area as previously described.

Tubular Function

SODIUM EXCRETION. In the fetus and neonate, external sodium balance is positive as a consequence of sodium accretion necessary for rapid growth. In older infants and children, however, urinary sodium excretion is generally equivalent to sodium intake as long as a steady state exists. The 24-hour urine sodium excretion, therefore, reflects the quantity of sodium ingested over the previous day and is normally 1 to 3 mEq/kg/day. Patients with obligatory renal sodium losses ("salt wasting") must increase sodium intake to compensate for these ongoing losses. A diagnosis of salt wasting nephropathy must be made while the patient is maintained on a restricted sodium intake (<1 mEq/kg/day) for 3 to 5 days. To prevent dangerous volume depletion or hyponatremia, the patient's blood pressure, weight, urine output, and serum sodium concentration should be closely monitored during the study.

The 24-hour urine sodium excretion can also be helpful in monitoring compliance of the patient on a restricted sodium intake (for example, one with hypertension, nephrogenic diabetes insipidus, or nephrotic syndrome). The parents of a patient with sodium excretion greater than 3 mEq/kg/day may be counseled to improve the diet.

Of even greater clinical utility, the fraction of filtered sodium appearing in the urine (FE_{NA}) can be used to isolate the tubular from the glomerular contribution to sodium excretion. This information may be employed to distinguish "prerenal" causes of oliguria from "renal parenchymal" or "postrenal" causes. A timed urine collection is not necessary, because sodium and creatinine concentrations can be measured in a random urine sample (U_{NA}, U_{cr}) and concurrent plasma sample (P_{NA}, P_{cr}):

$$FE_{NA} = 100\% \ (U_{NA} \times P_{cr})/(P_{NA} \times U_{cr})$$

In the oliguric neonate (urine flow less than 1 ml/kg/hour), FE_{NA} less than 2.5 per cent suggests a prerenal condition (Mathew et al., 1980). In the older infant or child, a value below 1 per cent is consistent with prerenal oliguria. Similar criteria can be utilized to differentiate causes of hyponatremia: FE_{NA} is increased in renal sodium wasting, adrenal insufficiency, and the syndrome of inappropriate antidiuretic hormone secretion (SIADH). In each case, the urine sample must be obtained, by bladder catheterization if necessary, before administration of any drugs that affect urine sodium excretion, such as diuretics.

URINARY ACIDIFICATION. Although renal insufficiency can interfere with urinary acidification, retention of organic acids due to decreased GFR results in an increase in unmeasured anions. In renal tubular acidosis (RTA), this "anion gap" is in the normal range (5 to 15 mEq/L) and is defined as follows:

$$\text{Anion gap} = Na^+_s - [Cl^-_s + HCO_3^-{}_s]$$

where Na^+_s = serum sodium concentration, Cl^-_s = serum chloride concentration, and $HCO_3^-{}_s$ = serum bicarbonate (or total CO_2) concentration in mEq/L.

A classification of RTA has been developed, based on the nephron segment affected and the transport defect involved. Thus, RTA can result from a defective distal tubular acidification (type I), a decreased threshold for proximal tubular bicarbonate reabsorption (type II), a combined proximal and distal abnormality (type III), or a distal defect involving impaired potassium secretion (type IV). During the first 3 weeks of life, the threshold for bicarbonate reabsorption can be as low as 14.5 mEq/L in the normal infant (Brown et al., 1978). This value should not be regarded as RTA, as treatment with alkali has been shown not to alter growth and development (Brown et al., 1978). Congenital hydronephrosis can result in type I or type IV RTA in the infant or child (Hutcheon et al., 1976; Rodriguez-Soriano et al., 1983). Appropriate evaluation and treatment are important to prevent the sequelae of RTA. These include growth retardation, osteodystrophy, nephrocalcinosis or nephrolithiasis, and polyuria.

The approach to the infant or child with suspected RTA is shown diagrammatically in Figure 33–4. The presence of metabolic acidosis in the infant can be difficult to ascertain on the basis of serum total CO_2, because problems in obtaining the sample (venous access, small sample volume) can result in spuriously low values. It is therefore important to obtain the sample from a vein with good blood flow and to transfer it expeditiously to the laboratory in a capped syringe on ice, as with arterial blood for blood gas analysis. Accurate measurement of urine pH is also crucial to the diagnosis, and a urine sample should be obtained at the time of the blood sample from a freshly voided or bagged specimen. The urine should be withdrawn into a syringe, the air should be expressed, and the sample should be transferred immediately to the laboratory for measurement by pH meter. Dipsticks are not sufficiently accurate. A urine pH below 5.5 in the presence of a total CO_2 below normal for the patient's age suggests gastrointestinal bicarbonate loss or a defect in proximal tubular bicarbonate reabsorption with intact distal acidification (type II). Inappropriately high urine pH is consistent with distal or type I RTA. Elevated serum potassium concentration in the presence of normal renal function suggests type IV RTA.

Because of the difficulty in infants when pursuing bicarbonate infusion to rule out type II, or acid infusion to rule out type I, alternative approaches have been developed to define the type of RTA. The simplest is to initiate alkali therapy with sodium bicarbonate or sodium citrate (Shohl's solution or Bicitra) at a dosage of 3 mEq/kg/day divided in four daily doses. The aim is to increase serum total CO_2 to the normal range (generally >20 mEq/L) and to raise urine pH above 7.8. Patients with type II RTA or infants with type I may require much greater doses of alkali (10 or more mEq/kg/day) to maintain a normal plasma total CO_2 concentration and to allow a normal growth rate. The fractional excretion of bicarbonate can then be calculated from random paired blood and urine samples as for FE_{NA} (see previous discussion). In contrast to types I and IV, in which the fractional bicarbonate excretion is less than 15 per cent, the value in type II is greater than 15 per cent because of the reduced threshold for bicarbonate reabsorption (Chan, 1983). An alternative means to distinguish type II from other forms of RTA is to measure blood and urine CO_2 partial pressure (PCO_2) after correction of acidosis with alkali therapy. In patients with type II, the difference between urine and blood PCO_2 is greater than 20 mm Hg, whereas in those with type I, the difference is less than 15 mm Hg (Donckerwolke et al., 1983). Another option to identify a patient with a distal tubular acidification defect (types I or IV) is to calculate the urinary anion gap:

$$\text{Urinary anion gap (mEq/L)} = Na^+ + K^+ - Cl^-$$

Normal patients and those with intact distal urinary acidification have negative urinary anion gaps; those with types I or IV RTA have positive gaps (Batlle et al., 1988). However, for infants under 3 weeks of age, the urinary anion gap is not a reliable index of urinary ammonium excretion (Sulyok and Guignard, 1990).

Although the aforementioned studies should permit separation of type II from types I and IV, the last two forms are usually distinguishable, prior to treatment with alkali, by the presence of hyperkalemia in type IV but not type I. In addition, infusion of furosemide, 1 mg/kg, should result in acidification of urine in patients with type IV but not in those with type I (Stine et al., 1985).

Although a number of causes of RTA in children are known (Chan, 1983), congenital obstructive nephropathy (Hutcheon et al., 1976; Rodriguez-Soriano et al., 1983) and Fanconi's syndrome should always be considered (see subsequent discussion). Tests for serum electrolytes, calcium, phosphorus, parathyroid hormone, and thyroid function data should be obtained. A urinalysis should be performed to screen for glucosuria. In addition, the urine amino acid pattern may reveal diffuse aminoaciduria. A 24-hour urine collection should be obtained for calculation of creatinine clearance, protein excretion, calcium excretion, and tubular reabsorption of phosphorus. Sonographic examination of the urinary tract should be performed not only to identify hydronephrosis but also to reveal nephrocalcinosis or nephrolithiasis that can develop in children with type I RTA.

As previously described, most infants and children with RTA respond well to alkali therapy (sodium bicarbonate or Shohl's solution). Some patients with type IV, however, may have persistent hyperkalemia despite correction of acidosis, which can be managed by admin-

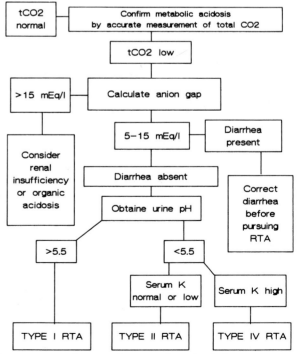

Figure 33–4. Evaluation of suspected renal tubular acidosis in the infant. (See text for details.)

istration of chlorothiazide, 10 to 20 mg/kg/day, or polystyrene sodium sulfonate (Kayexalate), 1 g/kg/day. Patients receiving diuretics need to be monitored closely for development of volume contraction, which can actually reduce potassium excretion. Infants receiving Kayexalate may undergo volume expansion from exchange of sodium for potassium and may develop bowel obstruction from inspissated resin in the intestinal tract. As long as adequate GFR is maintained, most children with RTA due to urologic abnormalities will need indefinite treatment to ensure normal growth and to prevent complications, such as nephrocalcinosis. The dose of alkali may need to be adjusted every 3 to 6 months in the rapidly growing infant.

URINARY CONCENTRATION. Most disorders of urinary concentration in infants and children are due to renal maldevelopment (renal dysplasia and obstructive nephropathy), interstitial nephritis (pyelonephritis), or renal insufficiency. Additional causes include renal tubular acidosis, sickle cell nephropathy, and medullary cystic disease. These generally result in a mild to moderate impairment in concentration, such that the urine specific gravity is greater than 1.005. Evaluation should include serum electrolytes, blood urea nitrogen (BUN), and creatinine levels; urinalysis and urine culture; renal ultrasonography; and, possibly, voiding cystourethrogram. Infants with diabetes insipidus usually have urine specific gravity consistently less than 1.005.

No physiologic definition of polyuria exists, and screening of urinary concentrating ability in a child may be initiated based on parental concern over excessive voiding frequency. Measurement of urine output and interpretation of thirst in the infant are problematic. For these reasons, the infant with unexplained dehydration or hypernatremia should be screened for a urine concentrating defect.

A urine specific gravity greater than 1.020 generally rules out a serious abnormality of urinary concentration. In the younger infant, overnight fluid restriction can result in dangerous volume depletion and hypernatremia. Such a patient should undergo a formal water deprivation test in the hospital. This test should begin with fluid restriction starting in the morning, with close monitoring of body weight and vital signs until loss of 3 per cent body weight or until urine osmolality exceeds 600 mOsm in neonates and 800 mOsm in older infants and children. If tachycardia or hypotension develops at any time, the test should be terminated.

In a patient failing to produce concentrated urine during water deprivation, fluid should be restricted on a separate day, and 1-deamino-(8-D-arginine)-vasopressin (DDAVP, 10 μg for infants or 20 μg for children) is instilled into the nostrils. Urine osmolality should be measured at 2-hour intervals for 4 to 6 hours. Renal response to DDAVP should be considered normal if the urine osmolality exceeds 600 mOsm for neonates or 800 mOsm for older infants and children. Such patients should be evaluated for central diabetes insipidus by an endocrinologist.

CALCIUM EXCRETION. Urinary calcium excretion in the neonate is most simply assessed by determination of the calcium/creatinine ratio in a random urine sample. In contrast to the older child, in whom a ratio exceeding 0.2 should be considered abnormal (Moore et al., 1978), the ratio in the infant receiving breast milk can rise to 0.4 in the term neonate and to 0.8 in the preterm neonate (Karlen et al., 1985). The most common etiology of hypercalciuria in a neonate is administration of calciuric drugs, such as furosemide and glucocorticoids, particularly in the management of bronchopulmonary dysplasia. Such a patient may be at risk for development of nephrocalcinosis or nephrolithiasis (Jacinto et al., 1988). Although it may not be feasible to discontinue glucocorticoids, substitution of chlorothiazide for furosemide may reduce urinary calcium excretion.

PHOSPHORUS, GLUCOSE, AND AMINO ACID EXCRETION. Because serum phosphorus concentration is higher in the neonate than in the older infant or child, any neonate with serum phosphorus below 4 mg/dl should be evaluated for renal phosphorus wasting. This evaluation can be accomplished in the neonate by measurement of phosphate and creatinine concentrations in urine (U_{cr}, UPO_4) and plasma (P_{cr}, PPO_4) and by calculation of the fractional tubular reabsorption of phosphorus (TRP) as follows:

$$TRP = 100\% \, [1 - (UPO_4 \times P_{cr})/(PPO_4 \times U_{cr})]$$

After the 1st week of life in the neonate, the TRP should be greater than 95 per cent in term infants and greater than 75 per cent in preterm infants (Karlen et al., 1985). Values below these ranges suggest a proximal tubular disorder or hyperparathyroidism.

In preterm infants, the threshold for tubular glucose reabsorption is lower than in the term infant or older child. The most common cause of glucosuria in hospitalized infants is intravenous infusion of dextrose at rates exceeding the tubular reabsorptive threshold.

Similar to glucose handling, the proximal tubule of the neonate is limited in its ability to reabsorb amino acids when compared with the older infant. This limitation results in a generalized aminoaciduria that is normal during the neonatal period. Thus, in evaluation of aminoaciduria, it is important to compare results with those of age-matched normal infants (Brodehl, 1978).

HORMONAL CONTROL OF RENAL FUNCTION DURING DEVELOPMENT

RENIN-ANGIOTENSIN SYSTEM. Fetal and neonatal renal function is significantly modulated by a number of circulating hormones. The best studied is the renin-angiotensin system (RAS). Inasmuch as angiotensin II receptors have been identified in the fetal rat by the 10th day of gestation (term = 21 days) (Jones et al., 1989), and renin appears in the mesonephric and renal arteries by the 15th day (Richoux et al., 1987), a role for the RAS has been postulated in the process of angiogenesis. In the human fetus, renin is present in the transient mesonephros and can be identified as early as the 8th week of gestation in the metanephros (Celio et al., 1985). By the 19th day of gestation in the rat, renin messenger (m) RNA (demonstrated by in situ hybridization histochemistry) as well as the renin protein (demonstrated by immunocytochemistry) is distributed along arcuate and interlobular arteries (Gomez et al., 1986; Gomez et al., 1989). However, in the early postnatal period, renin becomes localized to the juxtaglomerular apparatus, which persists to adulthood (Gomez et al., 1986). In addition to these developmental changes in distribution of renin, there is an eightfold decrease in the renal renin mRNA content during early development in the rat (Gomez et al., 1988a). These developmental changes are not irreversible: inhibition of angiotensin II formation by chronic intake of enalapril in the adult rat caused a redistribution of renin upstream along afferent arterioles and an increase in renal renin mRNA content, reminiscent of the fetal pattern (Gomez et al., 1988b; Gomez et al., 1990). In view of these findings, it is possible that as a result of normal maturation, the sensitivity of the renal vasculature to angiotensin II increases, with secondary inhibition of renin gene expression.

Although plasma renin activity (PRA) remains low during fetal life (Pernollet et al., 1979), a marked increase occurs in the perinatal period in most mammalian species, including humans (Fiselier et al., 1984; Osborn et al., 1980; Siegel et al., 1980; Wallace et al., 1980). The mechanism underlying this increase in PRA, which is triggered by vaginal delivery (Jelinek et al., 1986), may relate to a rise in prostaglandin synthesis (Joppich et al., 1982) or sympathetic nervous activity (Vincent et al., 1980). However, studies in piglets failed to support the increased sympathetic nervous activity (Osborn et al., 1980). It is likely that contraction of the extracellular space resulting from physiologic postnatal natriuresis contributes to the perinatal increase in PRA (Aperia et al., 1977b).

In addition to developmental changes in renin synthesis, the adrenal response to angiotensin increases during fetal and early postnatal life. In the fetal lamb, furosemide infusion does not increase either PRA or plasma aldosterone concentration (Siegel et al., 1980). In late gestation, however, PRA increases without a mineralocorticoid response, whereas in the neonate both PRA and aldosterone concentration increase after furosemide infusion (Siegel et al., 1980). Maturation of the mineralocorticoid response can also be demonstrated by angiotensin II infusion, which results in greater plasma aldosterone concentrations in adult than in fetal sheep (Robillard et al., 1983). The physiologic significance of these events may rest in the response to hemorrhage, which causes a greater increase in PRA, plasma angiotensin II, and aldosterone in late compared with early gestation in the ovine fetus (Robillard et al., 1982). Because blood pressure was maintained during moderate hemorrhage in late but not in earlier gestation (Robillard et al., 1982), the RAS may play a critical role in modulation of hemodynamics in the perinatal period.

ATRIAL NATRIURETIC PEPTIDE. Atrial natriuretic peptide (ANP) is a newly discovered peptide secreted by cardiac myocytes. It possesses a number of systemic hemodynamic and renal effects, including increases in GFR, natriuresis, diuresis, and vascular permeability, inhibition of renin and aldosterone release and vasorelaxation (Goetz, 1988). Circulating ANP

binds to specific receptors coupled to particulate guanylate cyclase, resulting in formation of cyclic gyanosine monophosphate (GMP), a putative second messenger responsible for the physiologic effects of ANP (Inagami, 1989). In addition, ANP binds to an even greater number of receptors not coupled to guanylate cyclase. Classified as "clearance" receptors, these are believed to contribute to the regulation of plasma ANP levels by removal of ANP from the circulation (Inagami, 1989). The precise role of ANP in regulation of sodium and fluid homeostasis remains unclear at present. However, evidence has accumulated to suggest that ANP plays a role in the physiologic adaptation of the fetus and neonate to its changing environment.

ANP is present in the fetal rat heart shortly after completion of organogenesis (Dolan et al., 1987; Toshimori et al., 1987). ANP mRNA first appears in the ventricles before becoming localized to the atria in the perinatal period (Wei et al., 1987). Compared with the mother, plasma ANP concentration is significantly higher in the fetus (Castro et al., 1988; Yamaji et al., 1988). Because metabolic clearance of ANP by the fetus exceeds that of the adult (Ervin et al., 1988), release of ANP from fetal cardiac myocytes must be far greater than in adults.

A number of stimuli have been shown to increase fetal plasma ANP levels. Acute volume expansion in the ovine fetus (Ross et al., 1987) and intrauterine blood transfusion in the human fetus (Robillard et al., 1988) raise plasma ANP concentration. Induction of atrial tachycardia in the fetal lamb results in hydrops and an elevation in plasma ANP concentration (Nimrod et al., 1988). Fetal hypoxia has also been shown to result in contraction of circulating volume as well as an increase in ANP levels (Cheung et al., 1988). By increasing vascular permeability, ANP may therefore contribute to regulation of blood volume in these aforementioned pathologic states.

Atrial ANP content decreases in the perinatal period, with a subsequent rise during the first 15 days of postnatal life in the rat (Dolan et al., 1989). This pattern is the opposite of that observed for plasma ANP concentration, which is elevated in the first several days of life and decreases with maturation (Kikuchi et al., 1988; Weil et al., 1986). It is likely that reduction in atrial ANP during the perinatal period results from a greater release into the circulation. In preterm infants, plasma ANP levels are initially even higher than those in fullterm infants, and the ensuing postnatal decline in levels is correlated with decreasing atrial size and decreasing body weight (Bierd et al., 1990). It is therefore likely that ANP plays a role in physiologic postnatal natriuresis and diuresis. Following the initial postnatal diuresis, however, the neonate enters a state of positive sodium balance necessary for rapid somatic growth.

The renal effects of infused ANP are reduced in the fetus compared with the adult (Brace et al., 1989; Hargrave et al., 1989). The natriuretic effect of ANP in the neonate is also reduced (Braunlich, 1987; Chevalier, 1988). Systemic clearance of ANP is increased compared with that of the adult (Chevalier, 1988). Moreover, compared with the adult, the neonatal renal natriuretic and diuretic response to acute volume expansion is attenuated (Schoeneman, 1980). In addition, the increment in plasma ANP concentration following acute saline volume expansion is less in preweaned than in postweaned rats or goats (Chevalier et al., 1990; Olsson et al., 1989). It is possible that rather than reflecting functional immaturity, the cardiac release, systemic clearance, and renal response to ANP in the neonate reflects an adaptation to the requirement for sodium conservation during this period.

VASOPRESSIN. Similar to the adult, fetal and newborn sheep have been shown to respond to both osmolar and nonosmolar stimuli for release of arginine vasopressin (AVP) (Leake et al., 1979; Robillard et al., 1979). Despite circulating levels of AVP that can be significantly higher than those in the adult (Pohjavuori et al., 1980), the fetal collecting duct appears to be less sensitive to AVP than the adult (Robillard et al., 1980). This finding may be due to a reduced density of AVP receptors, which increase during early development (Rajerison et al., 1982). In addition, the tubular effects of vasopressin may be antagonized by increased prostanoid synthesis in early development (Melendez et al., 1990).

In the postnatal period, when the collecting ducts develop full responsiveness to AVP, excessive or inappropriate AVP secretion due to birth asphyxia, intracerebral hemorrhage, or respiratory distress syndrome can result in severe hyponatremia (Kaplan and Feigin, 1978; Moylan et al., 1978; Stern et al., 1979). Conversely, infants born with nephrogenic diabetes insipidus do not respond to circulating AVP and may develop life-threatening hypernatremia.

FUNCTIONAL RESPONSE OF DEVELOPING KIDNEYS TO MALFORMATION OR INJURY

REDUCED FUNCTIONING RENAL MASS. A reduction in the number of functioning nephrons in early development is most often the result of a congenital malformation or a perinatal vascular accident, such as a renal embolus or renal vein thrombosis. Whereas loss of functioning renal mass in the postnatal period results in compensatory renal growth, the response of the fetus is less certain. Uninephrectomy in the fetal rat does not appear to result in hypertrophy of the remaining kidney (Goss and Walker, 1971; Rollason, 1969), whereas removal of a kidney in the ovine fetus may enhance growth of the single kidney (Moore et al., 1979). These short-term experimental studies are technically difficult to perform and to provide adequate controls. An infant with a single functioning kidney due to unilateral multicystic dysplasia (Laufer and Griscom, 1971) or to unilateral renal agenesis (Dinkel et al., 1988) does not have renomegaly at birth. This suggests that compensatory renal hypertrophy does not play a significant role in fetal life, possibly the result of placental clearance of putative renotropins.

Perhaps not surprising in view of the rapid growth of the normal kidney in the early postnatal period, compensatory renal growth in the neonate greatly exceeds that in the adult (Dicker and Shirley, 1973; Hayslett,

1979; Shirley, 1976). Whereas compensatory increase in renal mass in the adult is largely due to cellular hypertrophy, hyperplasia is also stimulated in the uninephrectomized weanling rat (Karp et al., 1971; Phillips and Leong, 1967). Neonatal glomerular hypertrophy results also from increased glomerular basement membrane surface area and proliferation of mesangial matrix (Olivetti et al., 1980). As in the adult, the majority of the compensatory increase in renal mass in the neonate is due to an increase in tubular volume (Hayslett et al., 1968; Horster et al., 1971).

Previously, compensatory renal growth in the uninephrectomized neonatal rat was thought to involve an increase in nephrogenesis of the remaining kidney (Bonvalet et al., 1972). This was subsequently disproved by careful serial morphologic studies (Kaufman et al., 1975; Larsson et al., 1980). In the guinea pig, approximately 20 per cent of glomeruli are underperfused during the first several weeks of life and cannot be identified by uptake of colloidal carbon (India ink) injected in vivo (Chevalier, 1982a). Following uninephrectomy at birth, however, these glomeruli are "recruited" within the 1st 3 weeks of life, resulting in an earlier increase in the number of perfused glomeruli per kidney (Chevalier, 1982a). The prior confusion regarding apparent compensatory nephrogenesis in animals subjected to uninephrectomy during early development is, therefore, likely due to incorrectly describing newly perfused glomeruli as newly formed glomeruli.

As with the enhanced increase in compensatory renal growth observed in the neonate with reduced renal mass, the functional adaptation by remaining nephrons is greater in early development than in the adult. In dogs subjected to 75 per cent renal ablation at birth, GFR increased markedly such that at 6 weeks of age, it was not different from that of sham-operated litter mates (Aschinberg et al., 1978). However, dogs undergoing renal ablation at 8 weeks of age had a GFR 6 weeks later that was less than 50 per cent that of sham-operated controls (Aschinberg et al., 1978). Reduced renal mass in the neonatal guinea pig or rat results in acceleration of the normal "centrifugal" functional nephron maturation, such that the compensatory increase in single nephron GFR is greater in superficial than in deep nephrons (Chevalier, 1982b; Ikoma et al., 1990). These studies indicate that functional as well as morphologic correlates of compensatory renal growth are augmented in early postnatal development compared with the adult.

Because glomerular hyperfiltration and glomerular hypertrophy have been implicated in the progression of most forms of renal insufficiency (Brenner et al., 1982; Fogo and Ichikawa, 1989), the neonate with reduced renal mass is theoretically at greater risk than the adult for long-term renal dysfunction. In this regard, reduced renal mass causes greater proteinuria and glomerular sclerosis in the immature than in the mature animal (Celsi et al., 1987; Ikoma et al., 1990; Okuda et al., 1987).

Likewise, congenital unilateral renal agenesis in humans has been associated with focal glomerular sclerosis and progression to renal insufficiency in adulthood (Bhathena et al., 1985; Kiprov et al., 1982; Wikstad et al., 1988). However, this increased risk has not been confirmed (Fotino, 1989). The critical question is, what is the number of functioning nephrons below which progression is inevitable? In oligomeganphronia, a form of renal hypoplasia in which the number of nephrons is reduced to less than 50 per cent, glomeruli develop marked hypertrophy and sclerosis leading to renal failure in later childhood (Bhathena et al., 1985; Elema, 1976). These considerations underscore the importance of attempting to maximize functional renal mass in the neonate or infant with renal impairment of any etiology.

CONGENITAL URINARY TRACT OBSTRUCTION. The response of the developing kidney to ureteral obstruction differs from that of the adult. Complete unilateral ureteral obstruction (UUO) during mid gestation in the fetal sheep results in dysplastic development of the ipsilateral kidney (Beck, 1971). When subjected to UUO later in gestation, however, dysplastic changes do not develop (Glick et al., 1983). In the infant, ureteral atresia in early gestation results in irreversible multicystic dysplasia of the ipsilateral kidney (Griscom et al., 1975). Ureteropelvic junction obstruction presumably develops later in gestation and causes less severe functional renal impairment, which may be minimized by early release of obstruction postnatally (King et al., 1984). These studies illustrate the critical importance of the timing of urinary tract obstruction with respect to renal development and the greater susceptibility to injury of the fetal kidney.

Even in the early postnatal period, the maturing kidney appears to be more susceptible to injury resulting from UUO than the adult kidney. As in uninephrectomy (see previous discussion), partial UUO in the neonatal guinea pig results in a greater adaptive increase in GFR of the intact opposite kidney than UUO in older animals (Taki et al., 1983). However, despite lower intraureteral hydrostatic pressure in neonatal than adult guinea pigs (Chevalier, 1984a), the decrement in GFR due to ipsilateral UUO is more severe in younger than older animals (Taki et al., 1983), and renal growth of kidneys with partial UUO since birth is arrested by 3 weeks of age (Chevalier et al., 1988).

Morphologically, the neonatal guinea pig with ipsilateral partial UUO develops contraction of glomerular volume, glomerular sclerosis, and tubular atrophy (Chevalier et al., 1987). Most importantly, growth arrest could not be prevented and function is not restored by release of obstruction after 10 days even though intraureteral pressure is normalized (Chevalier et al., 1988). In contrast, release of obstruction after a similar period in the adult animal does not cause renal atrophy and allows restoration of a normal glomerular perfusion pattern and renal blood flow (Chevalier et al., 1987).

As with UUO in the adult, chronic partial UUO in the neonatal guinea pig results in a marked increase in vascular resistance of the ipsilateral kidney. Whereas normal renal development in the guinea pig is characterized by a progressive increase in renal blood flow and recruitment of perfused glomeruli (Chevalier, 1982a; Chevalier and Kaiser 1983b), these events are prevented by ipsilateral UUO at birth (Chevalier et al., 1987; Chevalier and Gomez, 1989). Normal renal growth and hemodynamic maturation can be restored, however, by removal of the intact opposite kidney at the time of

ureteral obstruction (Chevalier and Kaiser, 1984). This finding suggests that growth factors regulated by total functional renal mass can modulate the response of the developing kidney to ipsilateral UUO.

The greater hemodynamic impairment of the neonatal kidney subjected to UUO may relate to the greater renal vascular resistance of the immature kidney and activity of the RAS (see previous discussion). Renin content of the neonatal guinea pig kidney with ipsilateral UUO is increased compared with sham-operated controls, and release of obstruction returns renin content to normal levels (Chevalier and Gomez, 1989). Inhibition of endogenous angiotensin II formation by long-term administration of enalapril to neonatal guinea pigs with UUO restores the normal maturational rise in renal blood flow, the number of perfused glomeruli, and the increase in glomerular volume of the ipsilateral kidney (Chevalier et al., 1987; Chevalier and Peach, 1985). Although administration of enalapril does not restore the renal blood flow of the neonatal guinea pig kidney after release of 5 or 10 days of ipsilateral UUO, enalapril reduces renal vascular resistance of the intact opposite kidney by 40 per cent after release of contralateral UUO (Chevalier and Gomez, 1989). Moreover, the vasoconstrictor response of the intact kidney to exogenous angiotensin II is increased, following release of contralateral UUO (Chevalier and Gomez, 1989). These studies indicate a dynamic functional balance between the two kidneys, which appears to be mediated or modulated by the intrarenal RAS.

As previously discussed, the intrarenal distribution of renin changes dramatically during development. In the fetus and early postnatal period, microvascular renin extends along interlobular and afferent arterioles, becoming localized to the juxtaglomerular region by the 20th postnatal day in the rat (Gomez et al., 1986).

In 4-week-old rats subjected to complete UUO during the 1st 2 days of life, renal renin content is increased in the obstructed kidney and immunoreactive renin extends along the afferent arteriole (El Dahr et al., 1990b). Thus, UUO from birth results in persistence of the fetal or early neonatal pattern even after the time of weaning (21 days). Furthermore, the proportion of juxtaglomerular apparatuses with renin gene expression (identified by in situ hybridization histochemistry) is increased in the obstructed kidney of 4-week-old rats (El Dahr et al., 1990b). In adult rats, however, 4 weeks of UUO did not alter the juxtaglomerular localization of renin (El Dahr et al., 1990a). Moreover, rather than an increase in renin gene expression of the obstructed kidney, UUO in the adult resulted in a decreased proportion of juxtaglomerular apparatuses containing identifiable renin mRNA in the intact opposite kidney (El Dahr et al., 1990a). These studies indicate that even at the level of renin gene expression, the renal response to UUO is age-dependent, with the neonate manifesting a greater activity of the RAS.

As with the functional studies of the RAS previously described in the neonatal guinea pig, UUO in the neonatal rat influences the intact opposite kidney. Similar to the obstructed kidney, renin is redistributed along the afferent arteriole of the hypertrophied intact kidney 4 weeks after contralateral UUO at birth, although renal renin content and renin mRNA are not increased (El Dahr et al., 1990b). This finding suggests that the immunoreactive renin along the afferent arterioles of the intact kidney represents inactive renin (prorenin), which may have been synthesized earlier in development or taken up from the circulation. The changes in distribution of intrarenal renin of the intact kidney are not due to hypertrophy alone, as uninephrectomy at birth results in a similar degree of hypertrophy without changes in microvascular renin distribution (El Dahr et al., 1990b). To determine whether renal nerves mediate or modulate renin gene expression during UUO, as well as the renin distribution of the intact kidney, neonatal rats with UUO have been subjected to denervation study (El Dahr et al., 1991). This practice prevents the increase in renin mRNA of the obstructed kidney as well as the redistribution of renin in the intact opposite kidney (El Dahr et al., 1991). The unifying pattern that emerges from the evidence to date therefore implicates the intrarenal RAS in the response of both obstructed and intact opposite kidneys of the neonate with UUO. Future attempts to preserve renal function of the infant with obstructive nephropathy should take into account the delicate balance between the two kidneys, which appears to involve the renal sympathetic innervation.

PERINATAL ISCHEMIA AND HYPOXIA. Renal dysfunction in the fetus and neonate is often the result of circulatory disturbances in the perinatal period. In response to hemorrhage or hypoxia, renal vascular resistance in the ovine fetus is increased while GFR is maintained, suggesting predominant efferent arteriolar vasoconstriction (Gomez et al., 1984; Robillard et al., 1981). This may be mediated at least in part by angiotensin (Robillard et al., 1982). Catecholamine release may be more important in mediating renal vascular resistance in early fetal life, whereas vasopressin appears to play a greater role in the more mature ovine fetus (Gomez et al., 1984).

In the neonatal lamb, hypoxia increases plasma renin activity, aldosterone, and vasopressin (Weismann and Clarke, 1981). Although GFR is reduced during hypoxia, the effect does not change during the 1st month of life (Weismann and Clarke, 1981). The preterm infant, however, may have renal responses to ischemia and hypoxia that are more similar to the fetus than the neonate.

One of the homeostatic mechanisms for preservation of renal perfusion in the presence of hypotension is autoregulation of renal blood flow. Compared with adult rats, young rats manifest autoregulation of renal blood flow at lower perfusion pressures, commensurate with the lower mean arterial pressure during early development (Chevalier and Kaiser, 1983). Interestingly, whereas adult rats with prior uninephrectomy maintain autoregulation (albeit at higher levels of renal blood flow), uninephrectomy at birth impairs autoregulation in young rats (Chevalier and Kaiser, 1983). These observations raise the possibility that following reduction in functioning renal mass, the neonatal kidney may be at greater risk for renal ischemia in the presence of superimposed hypotension. Following temporary complete occlusion of the renal artery, however, mortality has been shown to be greater in adult than young rats

(Kunes et al., 1978). Although this study suggests that the neonatal kidney may be more resistant than the adult kidney to certain insults, perinatal circulatory disorders can result in a variety of persistent glomerular and tubular functional abnormalities (Dauber et al., 1976; Stark and Geiger, 1990).

TOXIC NEPHROPATHY. Neonates are increasingly exposed to a variety of potentially nephrotoxic agents. Fortunately, the developing kidney appears to be more resistant than the adult to a number of toxic agents. Sodium dichromate and uranyl nitrate, both experimental models of toxic acute renal failure, cause less renal injury in young than in adult animals (Appenroth and Braunlich, 1988; Pelayo et al., 1983). More relevant clinically, renal concentrations of aminoglycosides (Lelievre-Pegorier et al., 1985; Marre et al., 1980; Provoost et al., 1985) and cis-platin (Jongejan et al., 1986) are lower in young than adult animals receiving high doses. This effect may be due to the normally reduced perfusion of superficial cortical nephrons in the developing kidney, such that these nephrons receive a lower dose of toxin. Another possibility is the proportionately greater renal mass compared with body weight in early development.

Few studies have addressed the potential long-term impact of toxic renal injury, however. Following uninephrectomy for Wilms' tumor, for example, irradiation and chemotherapy cause greater impairment of compensatory renal growth in younger than older infants and children (Luttenegger et al., 1975; Mitus et al., 1969).

REFERENCES

Aperia, A., and Herin P.: Development of glomerular perfusion rate and nephron filtration rate in rats 17–60 days old. Am. J. Physiol., 228:1319, 1975.

Aperia, A., Broberger, O., and Herin P.: Renal hemodynamics in the perinatal period: A study in lambs. Acta Physiol. Scand., 99:261, 1977a.

Aperia, A., Broberger, O., Herin, P., et al.: Sodium excretion in relation to sodium intake and aldosterone excretion in newborn pre-term and full-term infants. Acta Paediatr. Scand., 68:813, 1977b.

Appenroth, D., and Braunlich, H.: Age-dependent differences in sodium dichromate nephrotoxicity in rats. Exp. Pathol., 33:179, 1988.

Arant, B. S., Jr.: Developmental patterns of renal functional maturation compared in the human neonate. J. Pediatr., 92:705, 1978.

Aschinberg, L. C., Koskimies, O., Bernstein, J., et al.: The influence of age on the response to renal parenchymal loss. Yale J. Biol. Med., 51:341, 1978.

Batlle, D. C., Hizon, M. H., Cohen, E., et al.: The use of the urinary anion gap in the diagnosis of hyperchloremic metabolic acidosis. N. Engl. J. Med., 318:594, 1988.

Beck, A. D.: The effect of intra-uterine urinary obstruction upon the development of the fetal kidney. J. Urol., 105:784, 1971.

Bhathena, D. B., Julian, B. A., McMorrow, R. G., et al.: Focal sclerosis of hypertrophied glomeruli in solitary functioning kidneys of humans. Am. J. Kidney Dis., 5:226, 1985.

Bierd, T. M., Kattwinkel, J., Chevalier, R. L., et al.: The interrelationship of atrial natriuretic peptide, atrial volume, and renal function in premature infants. J. Pediatr., 116:753, 1990.

Bonvalet, J. P., Champion, M., Wanstok, F., et al.: Compensatory renal hypertrophy in young rats: increase in the number of nephrons. Kidney Int., 1:391, 1972.

Brace, R. A., Bayer, L. A., and Cheung, C. Y.: Fetal cardiovascular, endocrine, and fluid responses to atrial natriuretic factor infusion. Am. J. Physiol., 257:R580, 1989.

Braunlich, H., and Solomon, S.: Renal effects of atrial natriuretic factor in the rats of different ages. Physiol. Bohemoslov., 36:119, 1987.

Brenner, B. M., Meyer, T. W., and Hostetter, T. H.: Dietary protein intake and the progressive nature of kidney disease: The role of hemodynamically mediated glomerular injury in the pathogenesis of progressive glomerular sclerosis in aging, renal ablation, and intrinsic renal disease. N. Engl. J. Med., 307:652, 1982.

Brodehl, J.: Renal hyperaminoaciduria. *In* Edelmann, C. M., Jr. (Ed.): Pediatric Kidney Disease. Boston, Little, Brown, 1978, p. 1047.

Brown, E. R., Stark, A., and Sosenko, I.: Bronchopulmonary dysplasia: Possible relationships to pulmonary edema. J. Pediatr., 92:982, 1978.

Castro, L. C., Law, R. W., Ross, M. G., et al.: Atrial natriuretic peptide in the sheep. J. Dev. Physiol., 10:235, 1988.

Celio, M. R., Groscurth, P., and Imagami, T.: Onotogeny of renin immunoreactive cells in the human kidney. Anat. Embryol., 173:149, 1985.

Celsi, G., Bohman, S-O., and Aperia, A.: Development of focal glomerulosclerosis after unilateral nephrectomy in infant rats. Pediatr. Nephrol., 1:290, 1987.

Chan, J. C. M.: Renal tubular acidosis. J. Pediatr., 102:327, 1983.

Cheung, C. Y., and Brace, R. A.: Fetal hypoxia elevates plasma atrial natriuretic factor concentration. Am. J. Obstet. Gynecol., 159:1263, 1988.

Chevalier, R. L.: Glomerular number and perfusion during normal and compensatory renal growth in the guinea pig. Pediatr. Res., 16:436, 1982a.

Chevalier, R. L.: Functional adaptation to reduced renal mass in early development. Am. J. Physiol., 242:F190, 1982b.

Chevalier, R. L.: Hemodynamic adaptation to reduced renal mass in early postnatal development. Pediatr. Res., 17:620, 1983.

Chevalier, R. L.: Chronic partial ureteral obstruction in the neonatal guinea pig. II. Pressure gradients affecting glomerular filtration rate. Pediatr. Res. 18:1271, 1984.

Chevalier, R. L., and Gomez, R. A.: Response of the renin-angiotensin system to relief of neonatal ureteral obstruction. Am. J. Physiol., 255:F1070, 1989.

Chevalier, R. L., Gomez, R. A., Carey, R. M., Peach, M. J., and Linden, J. M.: Renal effects of atrial natriuretic peptide infusion in young and adult rats. Pediatr. Res., 24:333, 1988.

Chevalier, R. L., Gomez, R. A., and Jones, C. A.: Developmental determinants of recovery after relief of partial ureteral obstruction. Kidney Int., 33:775, 1988.

Chevalier, R. L., and Kaiser, D. L.: Autoregulation of renal blood flow in the rat: effects of growth and uninephrectomy. Am. J. Physiol., 244:F483, 1983.

Chevalier, R. L., and Kaiser, D. L.: Chronic partial ureteral obstruction in the neonatal guinea pig. I. Influence of uninephrectomy on growth and hemodynamics. Pediatr. Res., 18:1266, 1984.

Chevalier, R. L., and Peach, M. J.: Hemodyamic effects of enalapril on neonatal chronic partial ureteral obstruction. Kidney Int., 28:891, 1985.

Chevalier, R. L., Sturgill, B. C., Jones, C. E., et al.: Morphologic correlates of renal growth arrest in neonatal partial ureteral obstruction. Pediatr. Res. 21:338, 1987.

Chevalier, R. L., Thornhill, B. A., Peach, M. J., et al.: Hematocrit modulates the response of ANP to volume expansion in the immature rat. Am. J. Physiol., 258:R729, 1990.

Cole, C. H.: The Harriet Lane Handbook, 10th ed. Chicago, Year Book Medical Publishers, 1984.

Dauber, I. M., Krauss, A. N., Symchych, P. S., et al.: Renal failure following perinatal anoxia. J. Pediatr., 88:851, 1976.

Dicker, S. E., and Shirley, D. G.: Compensatory renal growth after unilateral nephrectomy in the newborn rat. J. Physiol., 228:193, 1973.

Dinkel, E., Britscho, J., Dittrich, M., et al.: Renal growth in patients nephrectomized for Wilms' tumor as compared to renal agenesis. Eur. J. Pediatr., 147:54, 1988.

Dolan, L. M., and Dobrozsi, D. J.: Atrial natriuretic polypeptide in the fetal rat: ontogeny and characterization. Pediatr. Res., 22:115, 1987.

Dolan, L. M., Young, C. A., Khoury, J. C., et al.: Atrial natriuretic factor during the perinatal period: Equal depletion in both atria. Pediatr. Res., 25:339, 1989.

Donckerwolke, R. A., Valk, C., and van-Wijngaargen-Peterman, M. J.: The diagnostic value of the urine to blood carbon dioxide tension gradient for the assessment of distal tubular hydrogen secretion in pediatric patients with renal tubular disorders. Clin. Nephrol., 19:254, 1983.

El Dahr, S., Gomez, R. A., Khare, G., et al.: Expression of renin and its mRNA in the adult rat kidney with chronic ureteral obstruction. Am. J. Kidney Dis., 15:575, 1990a.

El Dahr, S., Gomez, R. A., Gray, M. S., et al.: In situ localization of renin and its mRNA in neonatal ureteral obstruction. Am. J. Physiol., 258:F854, 1990b.

El Dahr, S., Gomez, R. A., Gray, M. S., et al.: Renal nerves modulate renin gene expression in the developing rat kidney with ureteral obstruction. J. Clin. Invest., 87:800, 1991.

Elema, J. D.: Is one kidney sufficient? Kidney Int., 9:308, 1976.

Engelke, S. C., Shah, R. L., Vasan, U., et al.: Sodium balance in very low birth weight infants. J. Pediatr., 93:837, 1978.

Ervin, M. G., Ross, M. G., Castro, R., et al.: Ovine fetal and adult atrial natriuretic factor metabolism. Am. J. Physiol., 254:R40, 1988.

Fiselier, T., Monnens, L., and van Munster, P., et al.: The renin angiotensin aldosterone system in infancy and childhood in basal conditions and after stimulation. Eur. J. Pediatr., 143:18, 1984.

Fogo, A., and Ichikawa, I.: Evidence for the central role of glomerular growth promoters in the development of sclerosis. Semin. Nephrol., 9:329, 1989.

Fotino, S.: The solitary kidney: A model of chronic hyperfiltration in humans. Am. J. Kidney Dis., 13:88, 1989.

Glick, P. L., Harrison, M. R., Noall, R. A., et al.: Correction of congenital hydronephrosis in utero. III. Early mid-trimester ureteral obstruction produces renal dysplasia. J. Pediatr. Surg., 18:681, 1983.

Goetz, K. L.: Physiology and pathophysiology of atrial peptides. Am. J. Physiol., 254:E1, 1988.

Gomez, R. A., Chevalier, R. L., Everett, A. D., et al.: Recruitment of renin gene-expressing cells in adult rat kidneys. Am. J. Physiol., 259:F660, 1990.

Gomez, R. A., Chevalier, R. L., Sturgill, B. C., et al.: Maturation of the intrarenal renin distribution in Wistar-Kyoto rats. J. Hypertens., 4 (Suppl 5):S31, 1986.

Gomez, R. A., Lynch, K. R., Chevalier, R. L., et al.: Renin and angiotensinogen gene expression in the maturing rat kidney. Am. J. Physiol., 254:F582, 1988a.

Gomez, R. A., Lynch, K. R., Chevalier, R. L., et al.: Renin and angiotensinogen gene expression and intrarenal renin distribution during ACE inhibition. Am. J. Physiol., 254:F900, 1988b.

Gomez, R. A., Lynch, K. R., Sturgill, B. C., et al.: Distribution of renin mRNA and its protein in the developing kidney. Am. J. Physiol., 257:F850, 1989.

Gomez, R. A., Meernik, J. G., Kuehl, W. D., et al.: Developmental aspects of the renal response to hemorrhage during fetal life. Pediatr. Res., 18:40, 1984.

Goss, R. J., and Walker, M. J.: Compensatory renal hypertrophy in fetal rats. J. Urol., 106:360, 1971.

Griscom, N. T., Vawter, G. P., and Fellers, F. X.: Pelvoinfundibular atresia: the usual form of multicystic kidney: 44 unilateral and two bilateral cases. Semin. Roentgenol., 10:125, 1975.

Gruskin, A. B., Edelmann, C. M., Jr., and Yuan, S.: Maturational changes in renal blood flow in piglets. Pediatr. Res., 4:7, 1970.

Guignard, J. P., Torrado, A., DaCunha, O., et al.: Glomerular filtration rate in the first three weeks of life. J. Pediatr., 87:268, 1975.

Hansen, J. P. L., and Smith, C. A.: Effects of withholding fluid in the immediate postnatal period. Pediatrics, 12:99, 1953.

Hargrave, B. Y., Iwamoto, H. S., and Rudolph, A. M.: Renal and cardiovascular effects of atrial natriuretic peptide in fetal sheep. Pediatr. Res., 26:1, 1989.

Hayslett, J. P.: Functional adaptation to reduction in renal mass. Physiol. Rev., 59:137, 1979.

Hayslett, J. P., Kashgarian, M., and Epstein, F. H.: Functional correlates of compensatory renal hypertrophy. J. Clin. Invest., 47:774, 1968.

Horster, M., Kemler, B. J., and Valtin, H.: Intracortical distribution of number and volume of glomeruli during postnatal maturation in the dog. J. Clin. Invest., 50:796, 1971.

Hutcheon, R. A., Shibuya, M., Leumann, E., et al.: Distal renal tubular acidosis in children with chronic hydronephrosis. J. Pediatr., 89:372, 1976.

Ichikawa, I., Maddox, D. A., and Brenner, B. M.: Maturational development of glomerular ultrafiltration in the rat. Am. J. Physiol., 236:F465, 1979.

Ikoma, M., Yoshioka, T., Ichikawa, I., et al.: Mechanism of the unique susceptibility of deep cortical glomeruli of maturing kidneys to severe focal glomerular sclerosis. Pediatr. Res., 28:270, 1990.

Inagami, T.: Atrial natriuretic factor. J. Biol. Chem., 264:3043, 1989.

Jacinto, J. S., Modanlou, H. D., and Crade, M.: Renal calcification incidence in very low birth weight infants. Pediatrics, 81:31, 1988.

Jelinek, J., Hackenthal, R., Hilgenfeldt, U., et al.: The renin-angiotensin system in the perinatal period in rats. J. Devel. Physiol., 8:33, 1986.

John, E., Goldsmith, D. I., and Spitzer, A.: Quantitative changes in the canine glomerular vasculature during development: Physiologic implications. Kidney Int., 20:223, 1981.

Jones, C., Millan, M. A., Naftolin, F., et al.: Characterization of angiotensin II receptors in the rat fetus. Peptides, 10:459, 1989.

Jongejan, H. T. M., Provoost, A. P., Wolff, E. D., et al.: Nephrotoxicity of cis-platin comparing young and adult rats. Pediatr. Res., 20:9, 1986.

Joppich, R., and Hauser, I.: Urinary prostacyclin and thromboxane A2 metabolites in preterm and full-term infants in relation to plasma renin activity and blood pressure. Biol. Neonate, 42:179, 1982.

Kaplan, S. L., and Feigin, R. D.: Inappropriate secretion of antidiuretic hormone complicating neonatal hypoxic ischemic encephalopathy. J. Pediatr., 92:431, 1978.

Karlen, J., Aperia, A., and Zetterstrom, R.: Renal excretion of calcium and phosphate in preterm and term infants. J. Pediatr., 106:814, 1985.

Karp, R., Brasel, J. A., and Winick, M.: Compensatory kidney growth after uninephrectomy in adult and infant rats. Am. J. Dis. Child., 121:186, 1971.

Kaufman, J. M., Hardy, R., and Hayslett, J. P.: Age-dependent characteristics of compensatory renal growth. Kidney Int., 8:21, 1975.

Kikuchi, K., Shiomi, M., Horie, K., et al.: Plasma atrial natriuretic polypeptide concentration in healthy children from birth to adolescence. Acta Paediatr. Scand., 77:380, 1988.

Kim, M. S., and Mandell, J.: Renal function in the fetus and neonate. In King, L. R., Jr. (Ed.): Urologic Surgery in Neonates and Young Infants. Philadelphia, W. B. Saunders Co., 1988, p. 41.

King, L. R., Coughlin, P. W. F., Bloch, E. C., et al.: The case for immediate pyeloplasty in the neonate with ureteropelvic junction obstruction. J. Urol., 132:725, 1984.

Kiprov, D. D., Colvin, R. B., and McCluskey, R. T.: Focal and segmental glomerulosclerosis and proteinuria associated with unilateral renal agenesis. Lab. Invest., 46:275, 1982.

Kunes, J., Capek, K., Stejskal, J., et al.: Age-dependent difference of kidney response to temporary ischaemia in the rat. Clin. Sci., 55:365, 1978.

Larsson, L., Aperia, A., and Wilton, P.: Effect of normal development on compensatory renal growth. Kidney Int., 18:29, 1980.

Laufer, I., and Griscom, N. T.: Compensatory renal hypertrophy: absence in utero and development in early life. Am. J. Roentgenol. Radium Ther. Nucl. Med., 113:464, 1971.

Leake, R. D., Weitzman, R. E., Weinberg, J. A., et al.: Control of vasopressin secretion in the newborn lamb. Pediatr. Res., 13:257, 1979.

Lelievre-Pegorier, M., Sakly, R., Meulemans, A., et al.: Kinetics of gentamicin in plasma of nonpregnant, pregnant, and fetal guinea pigs and its distribution in fetal tissues. Antimicrob. Agents Chemother., 28:565, 1985.

Luttenegger, T. J., Gooding, C. A., and Fickenscher, L. G.: Compensatory renal hypertrophy after treatment for Wilms' tumor. Am. J. Roentgenol. Radium Ther. Nucl. Med., 125:348, 1975.

Marre, R., Tarara, N., Louton, T., et al.: Age-dependent nephrotoxicity and the pharmacokinetics of gentamicin in rats. Eur. J. Pediatr., 133:25, 1980.

Mathew, O. P., Jones, A. S., James, E., et al.: Neonatal renal failure: Usefulness of diagnostic indices. Pediatrics, 65:57, 1980.

Melendez, E., Reyes, J. L., Escalante, B. A., et al.: Development of the receptors to prostaglandin E2 in the rat kidney and neonatal renal functions. Dev. Pharmacol. Ther., 14:125, 1990.

Mitus, A., Tefft, M., and Fellers, F. X.: Long-term follow-up of renal functions of 108 children who underwent nephrectomy for malignant disease. Pediatrics, 44:912, 1969.

Moore, E. S., Coe, F. L., McMann, B. J., et al.: Idiopathic hypercalciuria in children: Prevalence and metabolic characteristics. J. Pediatr., 92:906, 1978.

Moore, E. S., deLeon, L. B., Weiss, L. S., et al.: Compensatory renal hypertrophy in fetal lambs. Pediatr. Res., 13:1125, 1979.

Moylan, F. M. B., Herin, J. T., Ktishnamoorthy, K.: Inappropriate antidiuretic hormone secretion in premature infants with cerebral injury. Am. J. Dis. Child., 132:399, 1978.

Nimrod, C., Keane, P., Harder, J., et al.: Atrial natriuretic peptide production in association with nonimmune fetal hydrops. Am. J. Obstet. Gynecol., 159:625, 1988.

Okuda, S., Motomura, K., Sanai, T., et al.: Influence of age on deterioration of the remnant kidney in uninephrectomized rats. Clin. Sci., 72:571, 1987.

Olivetti, G., Anversa, P., Melissari, M., et al.: Morphometry of the renal corpuscle during postnatal growth and compensatory hypertrophy. Kidney Int., 17:438, 1980.

Olsson, K., Dahlborn, K., and Karlberg, B. E.: Temporary lack of ANP response to intravenous saline loads in goat kids. Acta Physiol. Scand., 135:591, 1989.

Osborn, J. L., Hook, J. B., and Baile, M. D.: Regulation of plasma renin in deleloping piglets. Dev. Pharmacol. Ther., 1:217, 1980.

Patten, B. M.: Human Embryology, 3rd ed. New York, McGraw-Hill, 1968.

Pelayo, J. C., Andrews, P. M., Coffey, A. K., et al.: The influence of age on acute renal toxicity of uranylnitrate in the dog. Pediatr. Res., 17:985, 1983.

Pernollet, M. G., Devynck, M. A., MacDonald, G. J., et al.: Plasma renin activity and adrenal angiotensin II receptors in fetal newborn, adult and pregnant rabbits. Biol. Neonate, 36:119, 1979.

Phillips, T. L., and Leong, G. F.: Kidney cell proliferation after unilateral nephrectomy as related to age. Cancer Res., 27:286, 1967.

Pohjavuori, M., and Fyhrquist, F.: Hemodynamic significance of vasopressin in the newborn infant. J. Pediatr., 97:462, 1980.

Potter, E. L.: Normal and Abnormal Development of the Kidney. Chicago, Year Book, 1972.

Provoost, A. P., Adejuyigbe, O., Wolff, E. D.: Nephrotoxicity of aminoglycosides in young and adult rats. Pediatr. Res., 19:1191, 1985.

Rajerison, R. M., Butten, D., and Jard, S.: Ontogenic development of kidney and liver vasopressin receptors. In Spitzer, A. (Ed.): The Kidney During Development: Morphology and Function. New York, Masson Publishing, 1982, p. 249.

Richoux, J. P., Amsaguine, S., Grignon, G., et al.: Earliest renin containing cell differentiation during ontogenesis in the rat. Histochemistry, 88:41, 1987.

Robillard, J. E., Gomez, R. A., Meernik, J. G., et al.: Role of angiotensin II on the adrenal and vascular responses to hemorrhage during development in the fetal lambs. Circ. Res., 50:645, 1982.

Robillard, J. E., Nakamura, K. T., Wilkin, M. K., et al.: Ontogeny of renal hemodynamic response to renal nerve stimulation in sheep. Am. J. Physiol., 252:F605, 1987.

Robillard, J. E., and Weiner, C.: Atrial natriuretic factor in the human fetus: Effect of volume expansion. J. Pediatr., 113:552, 1988.

Robillard, J. E., and Weitzman, R. E.: Developmental aspects of the fetal response to exogenous arginine vasopressin. Am. J. Physiol., 238:F407, 1980.

Robillard, J. E., Weitzman, R. E., Burmeister, L., et al.: Developmental aspects of the renal response to hypoxemia in the lamb fetus. Circ. Res., 48:128, 1981.

Robillard, J. E., Weitzman, R. E., Fisher, D. A., et al.: The dynamics of vasopressin release and blood volume regulation during fetal hemorrhage in the lamb fetus. Pediatr. Res., 13:606, 1979.

Robillard, J. E., Weismann, D. N., Gomez, R. A., et al.: Renal and adrenal responses to converting-enzyme inhibition in fetal and newborn life. Am. J. Physiol., 244:R249, 1983.

Rodriguez-Soriano, J., Vallo, A., and Oliveros, R.: Transient pseudohypoaldosteronism secondary to obstructive uropathy in infancy. J. Pediatr., 103:375, 1983.

Rollason, H. D.: Mitotic activity in the fetal rat kidney following maternal and fetal nephrectomy. In Nowinski, W. W., and Goss, R. J. (Eds.): Compensatory Renal Hypertrophy. New York, Academic Press, 1969, p. 61.

Ross, B., Cowett, R. M., and Oh, W.: Renal functions of low birth weight infants during the first two months of life. Pediatr. Res., 11:1162, 1977.

Ross, M. G., Ervin, M. G., Lam, R. W., et al.: Plasma atrial natriuretic peptide response to volume expansion in the ovine fetus. J. Pediatr., 157:1292, 1987.

Roy, R. N., Chance, G. W., Radde, I. C., et al.: Late hyponatremia in very low birth weight infants (<1.3 kilograms). Pediatr. Res., 10:526, 1976.

Rubin, M. I., Bruck, E., and Rapaport, M.: Maturation of renal function in childhood: clearance studies. J. Clin. Invest., 28:1144, 1949.

Rudolph, A. M., and Heyman, M.: Circulatory changes during growth in the fetal lamb. Circ. Res., 26:289, 1976.

Schlondorff, D., Weber, H., Trizna, W., et al.: Vasopressin responsiveness of renal adenylate cyclase in newborn rats and rabbits. Am. J. Physiol., 234:F16, 1978.

Schoeneman, M. J., Spitzer, A.: The effect of intravascular volume expansion on proximal tubular reabsorption during development. Proc. Soc. Exp. Biol. Med., 165:319, 1980.

Schwartz, G. J., Brion, L. P., and Spitzer, A.: The use of plasma creatinine concentration for estimating glomerular filtration rate in infants, children, and adolescents. Pediatr. Clin. North Am., 34:571, 1987.

Shirley, D. G.: Developmental and compensatory renal growth in the guinea pig. Biol. Neonate, 30:169, 1976.

Siegel, S. R., and Fisher, D. A.: Ontogeny of the renin-angiotensin-aldosterone system in the fetal and newborn lamb. Pediatr. Res., 14:99, 1980.

Siegel, S. R., and Oh, W.: Renal function as a marker of human fetal maturation. Acta Paediatr. Scand., 65:481, 1976.

Smith, F. G., and Robillard, J. E.: Pathophysiology of fetal renal disease. Semin. Perinatol., 13:305, 1989.

Spitzer, A., and Brandis, M.: Functional and morphologic maturation of the superficial nephrons: Relationship to toal kidney function. J. Clin. Invest., 53:279, 1974.

Stanier, M. W.: Development of intra-renal solute gradients in foetal and postnatal life. Pfluegers Arch., 336:263, 1972.

Stark, H., Geiger, R.: Renal tubular dysfunction following vascular accidents of the kidneys in the newborn period. J. Pediatr., 83:933, 1990.

Stern, P., LaRochette, F. T., Jr., and Little, G. A.: Role of vasopressin in water imbalance in the sick newborn. Kidney Int., 16:956, 1979.

Stine, K. C., and Linshaw, M. A.: Use of furosemide in the evaluation of renal tubular acidosis. J. Pediatr., 107:559, 1985.

Sulyok, E., and Guignard, J. P.: Relationship of urinary anion gap to urinary ammonium excretion in the neonate. Biol. Neonate, 57:98, 1990.

Svenningsen, N. W.: Renal acid-base titration studies in infants with and without metabolic acidosis in the postnatal period. Pediatr. Res., 8:659, 1974.

Taki, M., Goldsmith, D. I., and Spitzer, A.: Impact of age on effects of ureteral obstruction on renal function. Kidney Int., 24:602, 1983.

Toshimori, H., Toshimori, K., Oura, C., et al.: Immunohistochemical study of atrial natriuretic polypeptides in the embryonic, fetal and neonatal rat heart. Cell Tiss. Res., 248:627, 1987.

Trompeter, R. A., Al-Dahhan, J., Haycock, G. B., et al.: Normal values for plasma creatinine concentration related to maturity in normal term and preterm infants. Int. J. Pediatr. Nephrol., 4:145, 1983.

Vincent, M., Dessary, Y., Annat, G., et al.: Plasma renin activity, aldosterone and dopamine-B-hydroxylase activity as a function of age in normal children. Pediatr. Res., 14:894, 1980.

Wallace, K. B., Hook, J. B., and Bailie, M. D.: Postnatal development of the rcnin-angiotensin system in rats. Am. J. Physiol., 238:R432, 1980.

Wei, Y., Rodi, C. P., Day, M. L., et al.: Developmental changes in the rat atriopeptin hormonal system. J. Clin. Invest., 79:1325, 1987.

Weil, J., Bidlingmaier, F., Dohlemann, C., et al.: Comparison of plasma atrial natriuretic peptide levels in healthy children from birth to adolescence and in children with cardiac diseases. Pediatr. Res., 20:1328, 1986.

Weismann, D. N., and Clarke, W. R.: Postnatal age-related renal responses to hypoxemia in lambs. Circ. Res., 49:1332, 1981.

Wikstad, I., Celsi, G., Larsson, L., et al.: Kidney function in adults born with unilateral renal agenesis or nephrectomized in childhood. Pediatr. Nephrol., 2:177, 1988.

Yamaji, T., Hirai, N., Ishibashi, M., et al.: Atrial natriuretic peptide in umbilical cord blood: Evidence for a circulation hormone in human fetus. J. Clin. Endocrinol. Metab., 63:1414, 1988.

34
ANOMALIES OF THE UPPER URINARY TRACT

Stuart B. Bauer, M.D.
Alan D. Perlmutter, M.D.
Alan B. Retik, M.D.

Congenital anomalies of the upper urinary tract comprise a diversity of abnormalities, ranging from complete absence to aberrant location, orientation, and shape of the kidney as well as aberrant collecting system and blood supply. This wide range of anomalies results from a multiplicity of factors that interact to influence renal development in a sequential and an orderly manner. Abnormal maturation or inappropriate timing of these processes at critical points in development can produce any number of deviations in the development of the kidney and ureter.

The embryology of the urinary tract is described in Chapter 32. The reader is encouraged to review this material in order to appreciate the complexity of renal and ureteral development and the factors involved in the formation of an abnormality.

The classification of renal and ureteral anomalies used in this chapter is based on structure rather than function. The chapter is divided into four parts, including anomalies of the kidney, the collecting system, the ureteropelvic junction, and the ureter.

ANOMALIES OF THE KIDNEY

Anomalies of the kidney may be classified as follows:

I. Anomalies of number
  A. Agenesis
    1. Bilateral
    2. Unilateral
  B. Supernumerary kidney
II. Anomalies of volume and structure
  A. Hypoplasia
  B. Multicystic kidney
  C. Polycystic kidney
    1. Infantile
    2. Adult
  D. Other cystic disease
  E. Medullary sponge kidney
  F. Medullary cystic disease
III. Anomalies of ascent
  A. Simple ectopia
  B. Cephalad ectopia
  C. Thoracic kidney

IV. Anomalies of form and fusion
  A. Crossed ectopia with and without fusion
    1. Unilateral fused kidney (inferior ectopia)
    2. Sigmoid or S-shaped kidney
    3. Lump kidney
    4. L-shaped kidney
    5. Disc kidney
    6. Unilateral fused kidney (superior ectopia)
  B. Horseshoe kidney
V. Anomalies of rotation
  A. Incomplete
  B. Excessive
  C. Reverse
VI. Anomalies of renal vasculature
  A. Aberrant, accessory, or multiple vessels
  B. Renal artery aneurysms
  C. Arteriovenous fistula

ANOMALIES OF NUMBER

Agenesis

Bilateral Agenesis

Of all the anomalies of the upper urinary tract, bilateral renal agenesis has the most profound effect on the individual. Fortunately, it occurs infrequently when compared with other renal abnormalities. Although bilateral renal agenesis was first recognized in 1671 by Wolfstrigel, it was not until Potter's eloquent and extensive description of the constellation of associated defects that the full extent of the syndrome could be appreciated and recognized (Potter, 1946a and b, 1952). Subsequently, many investigators have attempted to understand all the facets of this syndrome and to explain them by employing one unifying etiology (Fitch and Lachance, 1972). But there is no unanimity regarding this topic, and controversy still exists concerning the exact mechanism of formation.

INCIDENCE. The anomaly is quite rare, only slightly more than 475 cases having been cited in the literature. Potter (1965) estimated that bilateral renal agenesis occurs once in 4800 births, but in British Columbia the incidence is once in 10,000 births (Wilson and Baird, 1985). Davidson and Ross (1954) noted a 0.28-per cent incidence in autopsies of infants and children. As with most anomalies, there is significant male predominance (nearly 75 per cent). Neither maternal age and disease nor a specific complication of pregnancy appears to influence its development (Davidson and Ross, 1954). The anomaly has been observed in several sets of siblings (Rizza and Downing, 1971; Dicker et al., 1984) and even in monozygotic twins (Thomas and Smith, 1974). Interestingly, in two pairs of monozygotic twins, one sibling of each pair was anephric, whereas the other had normal kidneys (Kohler, 1972; Mauer et al., 1974). An autosomal recessive inheritance pattern may exist (Dicker et al., 1984). If there is a genetic predisposition to this syndrome, it must have a low level of penetrance, although when siblings and parents of an index child with bilateral renal agenesis were screened, 4.5 per cent had unilateral renal agenesis (Roodhooft, et al., 1984), and 3.5 per cent had bilateral renal agenesis (McPherson et al., 1987).

EMBRYOLOGY. Complete differentiation of the metanephric blastema into adult renal parenchyma requires the presence and orderly branching of a ureteral bud. These occur normally between the 5th and 7th weeks of gestation, after the ureteral bud arises from the mesonephric or wolffian duct. It is theorized that induction of ureteral branching into major and minor calyces depends on the presence of normal metanephric blastema (Davidson and Ross, 1954). The absence of a nephrogenic ridge on the dorsolateral aspect of the coelomic cavity or the failure of a ureteral bud to develop from the wolffian duct will lead to agenesis of the kidney. The absence of both kidneys, therefore, requires a common factor causing renal or ureteral maldevelopment on both sides of the midline.

It is impossible to say which factor is most important.

Certainly no kidney can form in the absence of a metanephric blastema, but the presence of a ureteral bud and orderly branching are also necessary for the renal anlage to attain its potential. In an extensive autopsy analysis, Ashley and Mostofi (1960) found many clues to the multifactorial nature of this developmental process and shed some light on the causes of bilateral renal agenesis. Most anephric children in their series had at least a blind-ending ureteral bud of variable length. Thus, the embryologic insult in some cases was thought to affect the ureteral bud just as or soon after it arose from the mesonephric duct. Even with complete ureteral atresia, structures of wolffian duct origin (vas deferens, seminal vesicle, and epididymis) were usually present and normally formed, suggesting that the injury occurred at about the time the ureteral bud formed (the 5th or 6th week of gestation). When the ureter was absent, a rudimentary kidney was discovered in only a few instances, supporting the concept of the interdependency of the two processes. Conversely, in some instances, the ureter was normal in appearance up to the level of the ureteropelvic junction, where it ended abruptly. In those cases, no recognizable renal parenchyma could be identified. In a small number of autopsies, the gonads were absent as well, indicating an abnormality or insult that occurred prior to the 5th week, involving the entire urogenital ridge (Carpentier and Potter, 1959). Although the nephric and genital portions of the urogenital ridge are closely approximated on the dorsal aspect of the coelomic cavity, an extensive lesion affecting this area is necessary to produce such a condition in the developing fetus. Thus, several etiologies can be implicated for the absence of the kidneys.

DESCRIPTION. The kidneys are completely absent on gross inspection of the entire retroperitoneum. Occasionally, there might be a small mass of mesenchymal tissue, which is poorly organized and contains primitive glomerular elements. Tiny vascular branches from the aorta may be seen penetrating into this structure, but no identifiable major renal artery is present (Ashley and Mostofi, 1960) (Fig. 34–1).

Besides the absence of functioning kidneys, each ureter may be either wholly or partially absent. Complete ureteral atresia is observed in slightly more than 50 per cent of affected individuals (Ashley and Mostofi, 1960). The trigone, if developed, is poorly formed, owing to failure of mesonephric duct structures to be incorporated into the base of the bladder. The bladder, when present (about 50 per cent of cases), is usually hypoplastic from the lack of stimulation by fetal urine production. Alternatively, it has been postulated that ureteral bud and wolffian duct structures migrating into the ventral cloacal region are needed to initiate bladder development; their absence and not the *lack* of urine is the cause (Katz and Chatten, 1974; Levin, 1952).

ASSOCIATED ANOMALIES. Other findings in this syndrome have been extensively described by Dr. Potter, following an exhaustive investigation of these unfortunate infants. The infants have low birth weights, ranging from 1000 to 2500 g. At birth, oligohydramnios (absent or minimal amniotic fluid) is present. In addition, the characteristic facial appearance and deformity

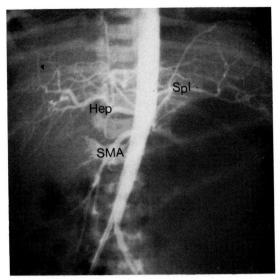

Figure 34–1. Aortogram via an umbilical artery catheter in a newborn with Potter's facies outlines major branches of the aorta but fails to demonstrate either renal artery or kidney.

of the extremities sets these children apart from normal newborns. The infants generally look prematurely senile and have ". . . a prominent fold of skin that begins over each eye, swings down in a semi-circle over the inner canthus and extends onto the cheek" (Potter, 1946a and b). It is Dr. Potter's contention that this facial feature is a sine qua non of non-functioning renal parenchyma. He even suggests that its absence confirms the presence of kidneys (Fig. 34–2A). In addition to this finding, the nose is blunted, and a prominent depression between the lower lip and chin is evident. The ears appear to be somewhat low set, drawn forward, and are often pressed against the side of the head, making the lobes seem unusually broad and exceedingly large (Fig. 34–2B). The ear canals are not displaced downward, but the appearance of the ear lobes gives that impression. The legs are often bowed and the feet clubbed, with excessive flexion at the hip and knee joints. Occasionally, the lower extremities are completely fused as well (sirenomelia) (Bain et al., 1960).

The skin can be excessively dry and appears too loose for the body. This may be secondary to severe dehydration or loss of subcutaneous fat. The hands are relatively large and claw-like.

It is thought that these characteristic facial abnormalities and limb features are caused by the effects of oligohydramnios rather than by multiple organ system defects (Fitch and Lachance, 1972; Thomas and Smith, 1974). Compression of the fetus against the internal uterine walls without the cushioning effect from amniotic fluid could explain all the findings of this syndrome.

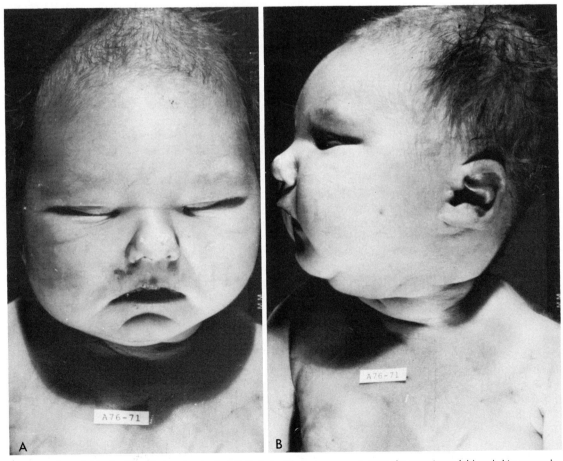

Figure 34–2. An anephric child who lived 2 days has typical Potter's facial appearance. A, Note the prominent fold and skin crease beneath each eye, blunted nose, and depression between lower lip and chin. B, The ears give an impression of being low-set because lobes are broad and drawn forward, but actually the ear canals are located normally.

Normally, urine produced by the developing kidney is the major source of amniotic fluid, constituting greater than 90 per cent by the 3rd trimester (Thomas and Smith, 1974); but, the skin, gastrointestinal tract, and central nervous system also contribute small amounts, particularly before urine production begins at 14 weeks. Thus, the absence of kidneys reduces severely the amount of amniotic fluid produced during the later stages of pregnancy.

Pulmonary hypoplasia and a bell-shaped chest are common. Originally, these findings were thought to be secondary to uterine wall compression of the thoracic cage as a result of the oligohydramniotic state (Bain and Scott, 1960). Subsequently, it was believed that the amniotic fluid itself was responsible for pulmonary development (Fitch and Lachance, 1972). However, this theory was discounted when it was discovered that there is a significant reduction in the number of airway generations as well as in acini formation (Hislop et al., 1979). Pulmonary airway divisioning occurs between the 12th and 16th weeks of gestation (Reid, 1977). A reduction in the number of divisions implies an interference with this process before the 16th week of gestation. The contribution from the kidneys to the amniotic fluid volume before that time is small, if any. Therefore, the oligohydramnios seen in cases of bilateral renal agenesis is a later finding in pregnancy, occurring long after the structural groundwork of the lung has been laid out. Hislop suggests that the anephric fetus fails to produce proline, which is needed for collagen formation in the bronchiolar tree. The kidney is the primary source of proline (Clemmons, 1977). Thus, pulmonary hypoplasia may result from absence of renal parenchyma and not from diminished amniotic fluid. In support of this hypothesis is the finding of normal lungs in two babies with prolonged leakage of amniotic fluid, beginning at a time when one would have expected pulmonary hypoplasia if the amniotic fluid alone were responsible for the defect (Perlman et al., 1976).

In the male, penile development is usually normal but a few cases of penile agenesis have occurred. Hyposadias is rare, but its occurrence is not related to the presence or absence of testes. In 43 per cent of the cases, however, the testes are undescended (Carpentier and Potter, 1959). They did not find any infants without testes, but Ashley and Mostofi (1960) noted testicular agenesis in 10 per cent. The vas deferens is normal in most cases. The presence of vasa implies that whatever caused the renal agenesis influenced the ureteral bud only after it formed or that the insult affected just the nephrogenic ridge.

Although this syndrome occurs uncommonly in females, they have a relatively high incidence of genitourinary anomalies (Carpentier and Potter, 1959). The ovaries are frequently hypoplastic or absent. The uterus is usually either rudimentary or bicornuate; occasionally, it is absent entirely, as in sirenomelia. The vagina is either a short blind pouch or completely absent.

The adrenal glands are rarely malpositioned or absent (Davidson and Ross, 1954), but anomalies of other organ systems are not unusual. The legs are frequently abnormal, with clubbed or even fused feet producing sirenomelia. A lumbar meningocele with or without the Arnold-Chiari malformation is not infrequently observed (Ashley and Mostofi, 1960; Davidson and Ross, 1954). Other malformations include abnormalities of the cardiovascular and gastrointestinal systems, which are present in up to 50 per cent of these infants.

DIAGNOSIS. The characteristic Potter facies and the presence of oligohydramnios are pathognomonic and should alert one to this severe urinary malformation. Amnion nodosum—small white keratinized nodules found on the surface of the amniotic sac—may also suggest this anomaly (Bain et al., 1960; Thompson, 1960). Of newborns, 90 per cent void during the first day of life (Clarke, 1977; Sherry and Kramer, 1955). Failure to urinate in the first 24 hours is not uncommon and should not arouse one's suspicion. Anuria after the first 24 hours without distention of the bladder should suggest renal agenesis (Williams, 1974). However, most infants who are born alive suffer from severe respiratory distress within the first 24 hours of life. When this becomes the focus of attention the anuria may be unnoticed, with the renal anomaly being thought of only secondarily.

When the association is made, excretory urography may be attempted but is generally fruitless. Renal ultrasonography is probably the simplest way to identify the kidneys and bladder in order to confirm the presence or absence of urine within these structures. If abdominal ultrasonography is inconclusive, a renal scan can be performed. The absence of uptake of the radionuclide in the renal fossa above background activity will confirm the diagnosis of bilateral renal agenesis. Umbilical artery catheterization and an aortogram can be undertaken if other modalities are unavailable or not diagnostic. These procedures will define the absent renal arteries and kidneys.

As maternal ultrasonic screening becomes more pervasive, these unfortunate babies are being diagnosed in the 2nd and 3rd trimesters when severe oligohydramnios is noted and no kidney tissue is detected. Termination of the pregnancy has been considered when the clinician is certain of the diagnosis (Rayburn and Laferla, 1986).

PROGNOSIS. Nearly 40 per cent of these affected infants are stillborn. Most of the children born alive do not survive beyond the first 24 to 48 hours because of the respiratory distress associated with pulmonary hypoplasia. Those infants who do not succumb at this time generally remain alive for variable periods, depending on the rate at which renal failure develops. The longest surviving child lived 39 days (Davidson and Ross, 1954).

Unilateral Renal Agenesis

Complete absence of one kidney occurs more commonly than does bilateral renal agenesis. In general, there are no signs (as with bilateral renal agenesis) that suggest an absent kidney (Campbell, 1928). The diagnosis is usually not suspected and remains undetected, unless careful examination of the external and internal genitalia reveals an abnormality that is associated with renal agenesis or an imaging study done for other reasons reveals only one kidney.

INCIDENCE. The clinically silent nature of this anomaly precludes a completely accurate account of its incidence. Most autopsy series, however, suggest that unilateral agenesis occurs once in 1100 births (Doroshow and Abeshouse, 1961). In a survey of excretory urograms performed at the Mayo Clinic, the clinical incidence approaches 1 in 1500 (Longo and Thompson, 1962), but Wilson and Baird (1985) noted a 1 in 5000 occurrence in British Columbia. Ultrasonic screening of 280,000 schoolchildren in Taipei [Taiwan] revealed an incidence of unilateral agenesis to be 1 in 1200 (Shieh et al., 1990).

The higher incidence of bilateral renal agenesis noted in males is not nearly as striking in the unilateral condition, but males still predominate in a ratio of 1.8:1 (Doroshow and Abeshouse, 1961). This finding is not surprising, considering the timing of embryologic events. Wolffian duct differentiation occurs earlier in the male than does müllerian duct development in the female, occurring closer to the time of ureteral bud formation. Thus, it is postulated that the ureteral bud is influenced more by abnormalities of the wolffian duct than by those of the müllerian duct.

Absence of one kidney occurs somewhat more frequently on the left side. A familial tendency has been noted. Siblings within a single family and even monozygotic twins have been reported (Kohn and Borns, 1973; Uchida et al., 1990). In a study of several families, McPherson and co-workers (1987) noted a familial pattern of inheritance and concluded that an autosomal dominant transmission with a 50- to 90-per cent penetrance exists in this study group. This inheritance pattern has been confirmed by others who evaluated families with more than one affected individual (Biedel et al., 1984; Roodhooft et al., 1984).

EMBRYOLOGY. The embryologic basis for unilateral renal agenesis does not differ significantly from that described for the bilateral type. The fault lies most probably with the ureteral bud. Complete absence of a bud or aborted ureteral development prevents maturation of the metanephric blastema into adult kidney tissue.

It is unlikely that the metanephros is responsible because the ipsilateral gonad derived from adjacent mesenchymal tissue is rarely absent, malpositioned, or non-functioning (Ashley and Mostofi, 1960). The high incidence of absent or malformed proximal mesonephric duct structures in the male and müllerian duct structures in the female strengthens the argument that the embryologic insult affects the ureteral bud primarily early in its development and even influences its precursor, the mesonephric duct. The abnormality most likely occurs no later than the 4th or 5th week of gestation, when the ureteral bud forms and the mesonephric or wolffian duct in the male begins to develop into the seminal vesicle, prostate, and vas deferens. The müllerian duct in the female at this time starts its medial migration, crossing over the degenerating wolffian duct (6th week) on its way to differentiating into the fallopian tube, uterine horn and body, and proximal vagina (Woolf and Allen, 1953; Yoder and Pfister, 1976).

Magee and associates (1979) proposed an embryologic classification based on the timing of the faulty differentiation (Fig. 34–3). If the insult occurs before the 4th week (type I), non-differentiation of the nephrogenic ridge with retardation of the mesonephric and müllerian components results, leading to complete unilateral agenesis of genitourinary structures. The individual has a solitary kidney and a unicornous uterus. In type II anomalies, the defect occurs early in the 4th week of gestation, affecting both the mesonephric and ureteral buds. The maldeveloped mesonephric duct prevents crossover of the müllerian duct and subsequent fusion. As a consequence, didelphia with obstruction of the ipsilateral horn and the vagina is produced. If the insult occurs after the 4th week (type III), the mesonephric and müllerian ducts develop normally; only the ureteral bud and metonephric blastema are affected. Normal genital architecture is present despite the absence of one kidney.

ASSOCIATED ANOMALIES. The ipsilateral ureter is completely absent in slightly more than half the patients (Ashley and Mostofi, 1960; Collins, 1932; Fortune, 1927). Many of the remaining individuals have only a partially developed ureter. In no instance is the ureter totally normal. Partial ureteral development is

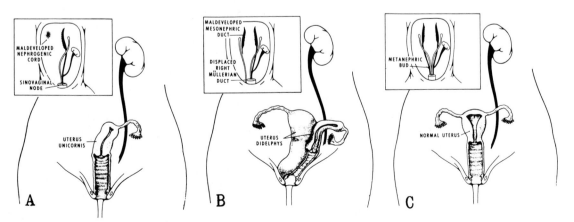

Figure 34–3. A proposed categorization of genital and renal anomalies in females. (From Magee, M.: J. Urol., 121:265, 1979.)

associated with either complete luminal atresia or patency of a variable degree. A hemitrigone in association with complete ureteral agenesis or an asymmetric trigone in the presence of a partially developed ureter is recognizable at cystoscopy. Segmental ureteral atresia on one side has been associated with contralateral ureteral or renal ectopia (Limkakeng and Retik, 1972). Except for ectopia or malrotation, anomalies of the contralateral kidney are very infrequently encountered (Longo and Thompson, 1952).

Ipsilateral adrenal agenesis is rarely encountered with unilateral agenesis, noted in less than 10 per cent of autopsy reports (Ashley and Mostofi, 1960; Collins, 1932; Fortune, 1927) and in 17 per cent of affected individuals evaluated by computed tomography (CT) (Kenney et al., 1985). These findings are not surprising in view of the different embryologic derivations of the adrenal cortex and medulla, which arise separately from the metanephros.

Genital anomalies, in comparison, are much more frequently observed. Despite the predominance of males with unilateral renal agenesis, a greater number of reproductive organ abnormalities seem to occur in females, amounting to at least 25 to 50 per cent as compared with 10 to 15 per cent in males. Although a genital anomaly is less difficult to detect in the female, which may account for the difference in incidence between the two sexes, a more plausible explanation may be related to the difference in timing and interaction of the male and female genital ducts with the developing mesonephric duct and ureteral bud. The incidence of a genital organ malformation for both sexes varies from 20 to 40 per cent (Doroshow and Abeshouse, 1961; Smith and Orkin, 1945; Thompson and Lynn, 1966).

Regardless of the sex, the gonad is usually normal. But structures derived from the müllerian or wolffian duct are most often anomalous. In the male, the testis and globus major, which contains the efferent ductules and arises from mesonephric tubules, are invariably present; all structures proximal to that point, which develop from the mesonephric duct (globus minor, vas deferens, seminal vesicle, ampulla, ejaculatory duct), are frequently absent, with an incidence approaching 50 per cent (Charny and Gillenwater, 1965; Collins, 1932; Ochsner et al., 1972; Radasch, 1908). In a further survey and review of the literature of adult males with absence of the vas deferens (Donohue and Fauver, 1989), 79 per cent were found to have an absent kidney on the ipsilateral side. Left-sided lesions predominated in a ratio of 3.5:1. Occasionally, the mesonephric duct structures may be rudimentary or ectopic rather than absent (Holt and Peterson, 1974). Seminal vesicle cyst is but one example (Beeby, 1974; Furtado, 1973). Six cases were noted among 119 boys (5 per cent) found to have unilateral agenesis during ultrasonic screening of schoolchildren (Shieh et al., 1990). Rarely has ipsilateral cryptorchidism been noted.

In the female, a variety of anomalies may result from incomplete or altered müllerian development caused by mesonephric duct maldevelopment. Approximately one third of women with renal agenesis have an abnormality of the internal genitalia (Thompson and Lynn, 1966).

Conversely, 43 per cent of women with genital anomalies have unilateral agenesis (Semmens, 1962). Most common of these is a true unicornous uterus with complete absence of the ipsilateral horn and fallopian tube or a bicornuate uterus with rudimentary development of the horn on the affected side. The fimbriated end of the fallopian tube, however, is usually fully formed and corresponds in its development to the globus major in the male (Shumacker, 1938).

Partial or complete midline fusion of the müllerian ducts may result in a double (didelphic) or septate uterus with either a single or duplicated cervix (Fortune, 1927; Radasch, 1908). Complete duplication or separation of the vagina, proximal vaginal atresia associated with a small introital dimple, and even complete absence of the vagina have been reported (D'Alberton et al., 1981; Woolf and Allen, 1953). Obstruction of one side of a duplicated system is not uncommon, and unilateral hematocolpos or hydrocolpos associated with a pelvic mass or pain, or both, has been described in the pubertal girl (Gilliland and Dick, 1976; Vinstein and Franken, 1972; Weiss and Dykhuizen, 1967; Wiersma et al., 1976; Yoder and Pfister, 1976) (Fig. 34–4). In rare instances, this anomalous condition has been mistaken for a large or infected Gartner's duct cyst. Sometimes, a true Gartner's duct cyst has been found in a prepubertal girl in association with an ectopic ureter that is blind-ending at its proximal end or one that is connected to a rudimentary kidney (Currarino, 1982). Six per cent of girls with

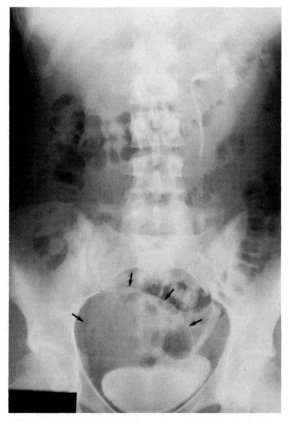

Figure 34–4. A 16-year-old girl with a solitary left kidney had abdominal pain and a pelvic mass that proved to be an obstructed duplicate vagina with hematocolpos.

unilateral agenesis had a Gartner's cyst on mass screening of schoolchildren (Shieh et al., 1990).

Radiologic investigation of the upper urinary tract in individuals with anomalies of the internal genitalia often will lead to the discovery of an absent kidney on the affected side (Bryan et al., 1949; Phelan et al., 1953). In fact, because unilateral agenesis is so frequently associated with anomalies of the internal female genitalia, the clinician should evaluate the entire genitourinary system in any girl with any of the aforementioned abnormalities.

In addition, anomalies of other organ systems are found frequently in affected individuals. The more common sites involve the cardiovascular (30 per cent), gastrointestinal (25 per cent), and musculoskeletal (14 per cent) systems (Emanuel et al., 1974) (Fig. 34–5). The anomalies include septal and valvular cardiac defects; imperforate anus and anal or esophageal strictures or atresia; and vertebral or phalangeal abnormalities (Jancu et al., 1976). Several syndromes are associated with unilateral renal agenesis—Turner's syndrome, Poland's syndrome (Mace et al., 1972), and dysmorphogenesis (Say and Gerald, 1968). Thirty per cent of children with the VATER syndrome (V = vertebral; A = imperforate anus; TE = tracheoesophageal atresia; R = renal) have renal agenesis (Barry and Auldist, 1974). Thus, a comprehensive review of all organ systems should be undertaken when more than one anomaly is discovered. In a small number of children the constellation of defects is incompatible with life and gestational or neonatal death ensues.

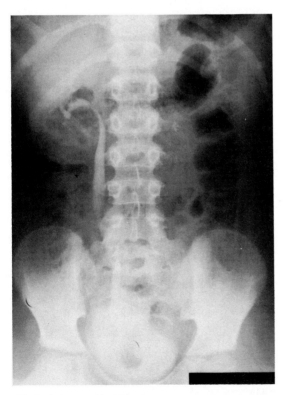

Figure 34–5. A 4-year-old girl had an excretory urogram because of imperforate anus and duplicate vagina. Note absence of left kidney and medial placement of the splenic flexure. At cystoscopy, a hemitrigone was noted.

DIAGNOSIS. In general, no specific symptoms herald an absent kidney. Most reports are composed of surveys from autopsy series. The contralateral kidney does not appear to be more prone to disease because it is solitary unless the absent kidney is really secondary to a multicystic dysplastic organ that went unrecognized at birth. In this case, there may be a mild ureteropelvic junction obstruction in the remaining functioning kidney.

The diagnosis, however, should be suspected during a physical examination when the vas deferens or body and tail of the epididymis are missing, or when an absent septate or hypoplastic vagina is associated with a unicornous or bicornuate uterus (Bryan et al., 1949). Radiologically, an absent left kidney can be surmised when a plain film of the abdomen demonstrates the gas pattern of the splenic flexure of the colon having a medial position, because the colon now occupies the area normally reserved for the left kidney (Mascatello and Lebowitz, 1976) (Fig. 34–5). When this characteristic gas pattern is present, it is a very reliable sign. A similar finding showing the hepatic flexure positioned in the right renal fossa suggests congenital absence of the right kidney (Curtis et al., 1977). The diagnosis of agenesis usually can be confirmed by renal ultrasonography and excretory urography, which will reveal an absent kidney and nephrogram, respectively, on that side and compensatory hypertrophy of the contralateral kidney (Cope and Trickey, 1982; Hynes and Watkin, 1970). However, a multicystic kidney can be mistaken for true agenesis in anyone over 1 year of age because the cysts involute as the fluid gets absorbed during the first several months of life. The colonic gas pattern will not occupy a closer position to the midline if a multicystic kidney was present during gestation. This provides an excellent clue to the diagnosis when no kidney can be detected by ultrasonography later in life.

Failure of one kidney to "light up" during the total body image phase of a radionuclide technetium scan is compatible with the diagnosis of an absent kidney, but this may not be infallible. Radionuclide imaging of the kidney using an isotope that traces renal blood flow will clearly differentiate unilateral renal agenesis from other conditions in which the renal function may be severely impaired. Isotope scanning and ultrasonography have largely replaced arteriography in defining agenesis. Fluoroscopic monitoring of the renal fossa at the end of a cardiac catheterization or renal ultrasonography at the end of an echocardiograph has demonstrated an absent kidney on occasion.

Cystoscopy, if performed, usually reveals an asymmetric trigone or hemitrigone, suggesting either partial or complete ureteral atresia and renal agenesis. Cystoscopy has been relegated to a minor diagnostic tool since the development of other, more sophisticated noninvasive radiographic studies (Kroovand, 1985).

PROGNOSIS. No clear-cut evidence exists that a patient with a solitary kidney has an increased susceptibility to other diseases. Most reviews dealing with this subject were conducted in the preantibiotic era, and they report a high incidence of "pyelitis," nephrolithiasis, ureterolithiasis, tuberculosis, and glomerulonephritis. The increased ability to prevent infection and its sequelae has reduced the incidence of morbidity and mortality among patients with a solitary kidney. In Ashley and Mostofi's series (1960), only 15 per cent of the patients died as a result of renal disease, the nature of which in almost every case would have been bilateral had two kidneys been present initially. Renal trauma resulted in death in 5 per cent. Some patients in this instance might have lived had there been two kidneys. Because the source of the autopsy material included many military personnel, the potential risk of injury was accentuated, however. Unilateral renal agenesis with an otherwise normal contralateral kidney is not incompatible with longevity and does not predispose the patient with the remaining contralateral kidney to greater than normal risks (Dees, 1960; Gutierrez, 1933). One should be prudent, however, in advising individuals to participate in contact sports or strenuous physical exertion.

Rugui et al. (1986) found an increased occurrence of hypertension and hyperuricemia and decreased renal function but no proteinuria in a small group of patients with congenital absence of one kidney. Only one patient had a renal biopsy. The specimen showed focal glomerular sclerosis, similar to what has been found in the remaining kidney in patients with the hyperfiltration syndrome noted after unilateral nephrectomy. Thus, these investigators concluded that unilateral renal agenesis may carry the same potential factor. Focal glomerulosclerosis has been confirmed in six other individuals with unilateral renal agenesis (Nomura and Osawa, 1990).

Supernumerary Kidney

Parenchymal development is controlled, in part, by as yet an unidentified substance that acts to limit the amount of functioning renal tissue. It is, therefore, interesting to find that nature has created, albeit rarely, a condition in which the individual has three separate kidneys and an excessive amount of functioning renal parenchyma. In such instances, the two main kidneys are usually normal and equal in size whereas the third is small. The supernumerary kidney is truly an accessory organ with its own collecting system, blood supply, and distinct encapsulated parenchymal mass. It may be totally separate from the normal kidney on the same side or connected to it by loose areolar tissue (Geisinger, 1937). The ipsilateral ureters may be bifid or completely duplicated. The condition is not analogous to a single kidney with ureteral duplication in which each collecting system drains portions of one parenchymatous mass surrounded by a single capsule.

INCIDENCE. The true incidence of this anomaly cannot be calculated because of its very infrequent occurrence. Approximately 75 cases have been reported since it was first described in 1656; it represents a very rare anomaly of the urinary system (Sasidharan, et al., 1976; McPherson, 1987). It affects males and females equally. A higher predilection for the left side has been noted (N'Guessan and Stephens, 1983). Campbell (1970) recorded one case involving bilateral supernu-

merary kidneys, an anomaly that has been observed even in other animals—cow and pig.

EMBRYOLOGY. The sequence of interdependent events involved in ureteral bud formation and metanephric blastema development, which is required for the maturation of the normal kidney, probably also allows for the occurrence of a supernumerary kidney. It is postulated that a deviation involving both of these processes must take place to create the anomaly. A second ureteral outpouching off the wolffian duct or a branching from the initial ureteral bud appears as a necessary first step. Next, the nephrogenic anlage may divide into two metanephric tails, which separate entirely when induced to differentiate by the separate or bifid ureteral buds (N'Guessan and Stephens, 1983). The twin metanephroi develop only when the bifid or separate ureteral buds enter them. N'Guessan and Stephens do not accept that this condition is the result of widely divergent bifid or separate ureteral buds. Geisinger (1937) proposed that the separate kidneys may have been caused either by fragmentation of a single metanephros or by linear infarction producing separate viable fragments that develop only when a second ureteral bud is present.

DESCRIPTION. The supernumerary kidney is a distinct parenchymatous mass that may be either completely separate or only loosely attached to the major kidney on the ipsilateral side. In general, it is located somewhat caudad to the dominant kidney, which is in its correct position in the renal fossa. Occasionally, the supernumerary kidney lies either posterior or craniad to the main kidney, or it may even be a midline structure anterior to the great vessels and loosely attached to each of the other two kidneys (Fig. 34–6).

The supernumerary kidney is reniform in shape but smaller than the main ipsilateral organ. In about a third of cases, the kidney or its collecting system is abnormal.

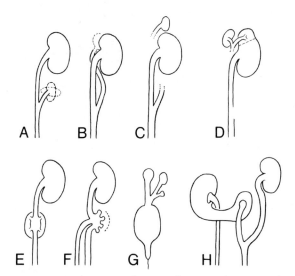

Figure 34–6. Various patterns of urinary drainage when ureters form a common stem. All kidney positions are relative only and are depicted on the left side for ease of interpretation. Dashed lines indicate that detail was not defined. (From N'Guessan, G., and Stephens, F. D.: J. Urol., 130:649, 1983.)

In almost half the reported cases the collecting system is severely dilated with the parenchyma thinned, indicative of an obstructed ureter.

The ureteral interrelationships on the side of the supernumerary kidney are quite variable (Kretschmer, 1929). Convergence of the ipsilateral distal ureters to form a common stem and a single ureteral orifice occurs in 50 per cent of the cases (Exley and Hotchkiss, 1944; N'Guessan and Stephens, 1983). Two completely independent ureters, each with its own entrance into the bladder is seen in the other 50 per cent of cases. The Weigert-Meyer principle, however, usually is obeyed, but in 10 per cent the caudal kidney has a ureter that does not follow the rule and enters the trigone below the ipsilateral ureter (Tada et al., 1981) (Fig. 34–7). Rarely, the supernumerary kidney has a completely ectopic ureter opening into the vagina or introitus (Carlson, 1950; Rubin, 1948). Individual case reports have described calyceal communications between the supernumerary and dominant kidney or fusion of the dominant kidney's ureter with the pelvis of the supernumerary kidney to create a single distal ureter (Kretschmer, 1929), which then enters the bladder (see Fig. 34–6). The vascular supply to the supernumerary kidney is, as one might expect, very anomalous, depending on its position in relation to the major ipsilateral kidney. Although some investigators believe that the blood supply to the individual parenchymal masses should be separate as well in order to consider this a true supernumerary kidney (Kaneoya et al., 1989), we do not believe that this is a necessary criteria.

ASSOCIATED ANOMALIES. Usually the ipsilateral and contralateral kidneys are normal. Except for an occasional ectopic orifice from the ureter draining the supernumerary kidney, no genitourinary abnormalities are present in any consistent pattern. Few of the case reports describe anomalies of other organ systems.

SYMPTOMS. Although this anomaly is obviously present at birth, it is rarely discovered in childhood. It may not produce symptoms until early adulthood. The average age at diagnosis in all reported cases was 36 years. Pain, fever, hypertension, and a palpable abdominal mass are the usual presenting complaints. Urinary infection, obstruction, or both are the major conditions that lead to an evaluation. Ureteral ectopia from the supernumerary kidney may produce urinary incontinence, but this is extremely rare because of the hypoplastic nature of the involved renal element (Hoffman and McMillan, 1948; Shan, 1942).

A palpable abdominal mass secondary to development of a carcinoma in the supernumerary kidney has been noted in two patients. In 25 per cent of all reported cases, however, the supernumerary kidney remains completely asymptomatic and is discovered only at autopsy (Carlson, 1950).

DIAGNOSIS. When the supernumerary kidney is normal and not symptomatic, it is usually diagnosed when excretory urography or abdominal ultrasonography is performed for other reasons. The kidney may be inferior and distant enough from the ipsilateral kidney so that it does not disturb the latter's architecture. If it is in close proximity, its mere presence may displace the major kidney or its ureter very slightly.

When the supernumerary organ is hydronephrotic, it may distort the normal ipsilateral kidney and ureter. If the collecting system is bifid, the dominant kidney is usually involved in the same disease process. When the ureters are separate, the ipsilateral kidney may show the effects of an affected supernumerary kidney. Voiding cystourethrography, ultrasonography, and even retrograde pyelography may be needed to help delineate the pathologic process. Cystoscopy will reveal one or two ureteral orifices on the ipsilateral side, depending on whether or not the ureters are completely duplicated and, if so, to what extent ureteral ectopia exists in or outside the bladder. Occasionally, a supernumerary kidney may not be accurately diagnosed until the time of surgery or may be noted at autopsy.

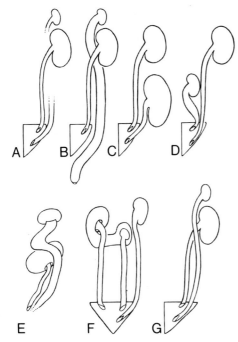

Figure 34–7. Various patterns of urinary drainage of supernumerary and ipsilateral kidneys when ureters are completely separated. All kidney positions are relative only and are depicted on the left side for ease of interpretation. Dashed lines indicate that detail was not defined. (From N'Guessan, G., and Stephens, F. D.: J. Urol., 130:649, 1983.)

ANOMALIES OF VOLUME AND STRUCTURE

These anomalies, as outlined at the beginning of this section, are discussed elsewhere in this text.

ANOMALIES OF ASCENT

Simple Renal Ectopia

When the mature kidney fails to reach its normal location in the "renal" fossa, the condition is known as renal ectopia. The term is derived from the Greek *ek* (out) and *topos* (place) and, literally, this means out of place. It is to be differentiated from renal ptosis, in which the kidney initially is located in its proper place and has normal vascularity but moves downward in relation to body position. The ectopic kidney, on the other hand, has never resided in the appropriate location.

An ectopic kidney can be found in one of the following positions: pelvic, iliac, abdominal, thoracic, and contralateral or crossed. Only the ipsilateral retroperitoneal location of the ectopic kidney is discussed here. Thoracic kidney and crossed renal ectopia with and without fusion is dealt with subsequently.

INCIDENCE. Renal ectopia has been known to exist since it was described by 16th century anatomists, but it did not achieve clinical interest until the mid-19th century. In modern times, with greater emphasis on diagnostic acumen and uroradiologic visualization including prenatal imaging, this condition has been noted with increasing frequency.

The actual incidence among autopsy series varies from 1 in 500 (Campbell, 1930) to 1 in 1200 (Anson and Riba, 1939; Bell, 1946; Stevens, 1937; Thompson and Pace, 1937), but the average occurrence is about 1 in 900 (Abeshouse and Bhisitkul, 1959). With increasing clinical detection, the incidence among hospitalized patients has approached the autopsy rate (Abeshouse and Bhisitkul, 1959). In autopsy studies no significant difference is noted in incidence between the sexes. Clinically, renal ectopia is more readily recognized in females because they undergo uroradiologic evaluations more frequently than males as a result of the higher rate of urinary infections and associated genital anomalies (Thompson and Pace, 1937).

The left side is favored slightly over the right. Pelvic ectopia has been estimated to occur once in 2100 to once in 3000 autopsies (Stevens, 1937). A solitary ectopic kidney occurs once in 22,000 autopsies (Delson, 1975; Hawes, 1950; Stevens, 1937). As of 1973, 165 cases of solitary pelvic kidney have been recorded (Downs et al., 1973). Bilateral ectopic kidneys have been observed even more rarely and are reported in only 10 per cent of patients with renal ectopia (Malek et al., 1971).

EMBRYOLOGY. The ureteral bud first arises from the wolffian duct at the end of the 4th week of gestation. It then grows craniad toward the urogenital ridge and acquires a cap of metanephric blastema by the end of the 5th week. At this point, the nephrogenic tissue is opposite the upper sacral somites.

As elongation and straightening of the caudal end of the embryo commence, the developing reniform mass migrates on its own, is forcibly extruded from the true pelvis, or appears to move as the tail uncurls and differential growth between the body and tail of the embryo occurs. Whatever the mechanism or driving force for renal ascent, it is during this migration that the upper ureteral bud matures into a normal collecting system and medial rotation of the renal pelvis takes place. This process of migration and rotation is completed by the end of the 8th week of gestation. Factors that may prevent the orderly movement of kidneys include the following: ureteral bud maldevelopment

(Campbell, 1930); defective metanephric tissue that by itself fails to induce ascent (Ward et al., 1965); genetic abnormalities; and maternal illnesses or teratogenic causes, because genital anomalies are common (Malek et al., 1971). A vascular barrier that prevents upward migration secondary to persistence of the fetal blood supply has also been postulated (Baggenstoss, 1951), but the existence of this "early" renal blood supply does not appear to affect the kidney's ultimate position. More probably it is the end result, not the cause, of renal ectopia.

DESCRIPTION. The classification of ectopia is based on the position of the kidney within the retroperitoneum: the *pelvic* kidney is opposite the sacrum and below the aortic bifurcation; the *lumbar* kidney rests near the sacral promontory in the iliac fossa and anterior to the iliac vessels; and the *abdominal* kidney is so named when it is above the iliac crest and adjacent to the second lumbar vertebra (Fig. 34–8). The ectopic kidney may be found in any one of these locations with just about equal frequency (Dretler et al., 1971).

The kidney is generally smaller and may not conform to the usual reniform shape, owing to the presence of fetal lobulations. The renal pelvis is usually anterior instead of medial to the parenchyma because there is an aborted attempt at rotation of the kidney. The axis of the kidney is slightly medial or vertical, but it may be tilted by as much as 90 degrees laterally, so that it lies in a true horizontal plane (Fig. 34–9).

The ureter is usually an appropriate length for the position of the kidney but it might be slightly tortuous. It is generally not redundant, unlike a ptotic kidney in which the ureter has achieved its full length before the kidney drops (Fig. 34–10). The ureter usually enters the bladder on the ipsilateral side with its orifice in the normal location. Therefore, cystoscopy does not distinguish renal ectopia from a normal kidney. The arterial and venous network is predictable only by the fact that

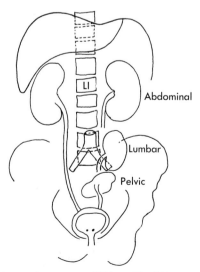

Figure 34–8. Incomplete ascent of kidney: The kidney may halt at any level of the ascent from the pelvis. (From Gray, S. W., and Skandalakis, J. E.: Embryology for Surgeons. Philadelphia, W. B. Saunders Co., 1972.)

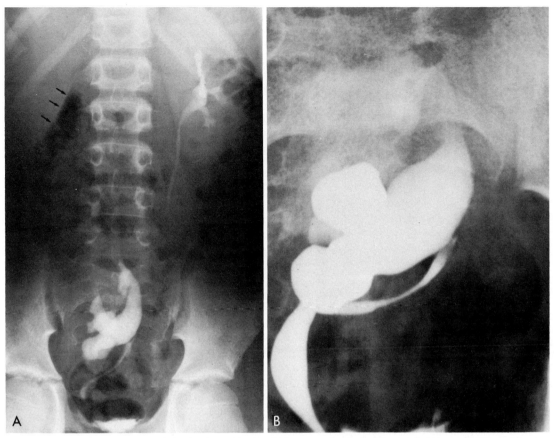

Figure 34–9. Evaluation for one urinary tract infection in a 13-year-old boy reveals: *A,* A right pelvic kidney. Position of the hepatic flexure suggests failure of renal ascent. *B,* Voiding cystourethrography reveals vesicoureteral reflux.

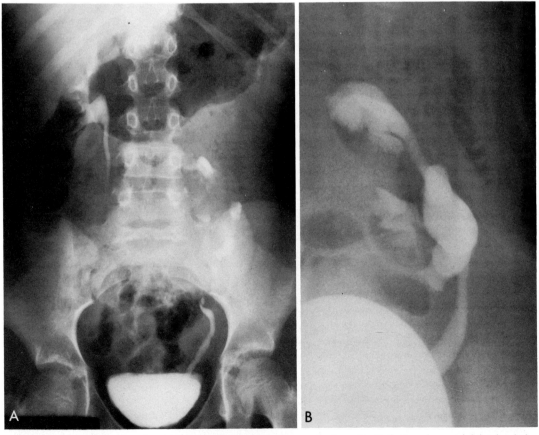

Figure 34–10. *A,* Excretory urography in a 9-year-old girl investigated for recurrent urinary tract infection shows a left lumbar kidney. *B,* Voiding cystourethrography demonstrates reflux to the ectopic kidney. At cystoscopy, the ureteral orifice was located at the bladder neck.

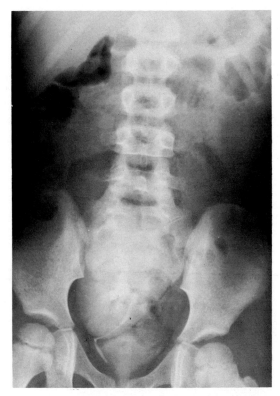

Figure 34–11. A 6-year-old boy with mild infundibular pulmonic stenosis underwent cardiac catheterization. A late abdominal film reveals a solitary pelvic kidney. At cystoscopy, a hemitrigone with an absent left ureteral orifice was discovered.

it is anomalous; its vascular pattern is dependent on the ultimate resting place of the kidney (Anson and Riba, 1939). One or two main renal arteries may arise from the distal aorta or the aortic bifurcation with one or more aberrant arteries coming off the common or external iliac or even the inferior mesenteric artery. The kidney may be supplied entirely by multiple anomalous branches, none of which arises from the aorta. In no instance has the main renal artery arisen from that level of the aorta, which would be its proper origin for a normally positioned kidney.

ASSOCIATED ANOMALIES. Although the contralateral kidney is usually normal, it is often associated with a number of congenital defects. Malek et al. (1971) and Thompson and Pace (1937) found the incidence of contralateral agenesis to be rather high, suggesting that a teratogenic factor affecting both ureteral buds and metanephric blastemas may be responsible for the two anomalies (Fig. 34–11). Bilateral ectopia is seen in a very small number of patients (Fig. 34–12).

The most striking feature is the association of genital anomalies in the patient with ectopia. The incidence varies from 15 per cent (Thompson and Pace, 1937) to 45 per cent (Downs et al., 1973), depending on how carefully the patient is evaluated. Of females, 20 to 66 per cent have one or more of the following abnormalities of the reproductive organs: bicornuate or unicornous uterus with atresia of one horn (McCrea, 1942); rudimentary or absent uterus and proximal or distal vagina (D'Alberton et al., 1981; Tabisky and Bhisitkul, 1965); and duplication of the vagina. In males, 10 to 20 per cent have a recognizable associated genital defect—undescended testes, duplication of the urethra, and hypospadias are the most common (Thompson and Pace, 1937).

Rarely, the adrenal gland is absent or abnormally positioned. A small number of patients (21 per cent) have anomalies of other organ systems (Downs et al., 1973). Most of these involve the skeletal or cardiac systems.

DIAGNOSIS. With the increasing use of radiography, ultrasonography, and radionuclide scanning to visualize the urinary tract, the incidence of fortuitous discovery of an asymptomatic ectopic kidney is also increasing. The steady rise in reported cases in recent years attests to this fact.

Most ectopic kidneys are clinically asymptomatic. A vague abdominal symptom of frank ureteral colic secondary to an obstructing stone is still the most frequent symptom leading to discovery of the misplaced kidney. The abnormal position of the kidney results in a pattern of direct and referred pain that is generally atypical for colic and may be misdiagnosed as acute appendicitis or

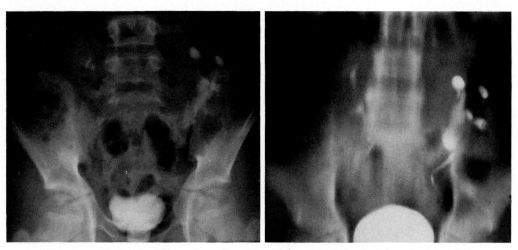

Figure 34–12. A palpable abdominal mass in an 8-year-old girl proved to be bilateral pelvic kidneys.

as pelvic organ disease in the female. It is rare to find symptoms of compression from organs adjacent to the ectopic kidney. Renal ectopia may also appear initially with a urinary infection or a palpable abdominal mass.

Malposition of the colon may be a clue to the ectopic position of a lumbar or pelvic kidney (as discussed in Agenesis). The diagnosis is made when the excretory urogram fails to reveal the kidney in its proper location. The fact that many of these kidneys overlie the bony pelvis obscuring the collecting system can lead to a misdiagnosis with failure to recognize the true position of the kidney.

Nephrotomography during an excretory urogram, when the diagnosis is suspected early enough; ultrasonography; radionuclide scanning; or retrograde pyelography usually satisfies the diagnostician. Cystoscopy alone is rarely useful because the trigone and ureteral orifices are invariably normal, unless the ureteral orifice is also ectopic which is a rare event. Arteriography may be helpful in delineating the renal vascular supply in anticipation of surgery on the ectopic kidney. This is especially important in cases of solitary ectopia.

PROGNOSIS. The ectopic kidney is no more susceptible to disease than the normally positioned kidney except for the development of hydronephrosis or urinary calculus formation. This occurrence is due, in part, to the anteriorly placed pelvis and malrotated kidney, which may lead to impaired drainage of urine from a high ureteropelvic junction or an anomalous vasculature that partially blocks one of the major calyces or the upper ureter. In addition, there is an increased exposure to injury from blunt abdominal trauma because the kidney is low lying and unprotected by the rib cage, which normally surrounds it.

Renovascular hypertension secondary to an anomalous blood supply has been reported, but a higher than normal incidence is yet unproved. Anderson and Harrison (1965), in a review of pregnant women with renal ectopia, could find no increased occurrence of difficult deliveries or maternal or fetal complications related to the ectopic kidney (Anderson and Harrison, 1965; Delson, 1975). Dystocia from a pelvic kidney is a very rare finding, but when it does occur, early recognition is mandatory and cesarean section is indicated. Although two cases of cancer within an ectopic kidney have been reported, there does not appear to be any increased risk of malignant change. No deaths have been directly attributable to the ectopic kidney but in at least five instances a solitary ectopic kidney has been mistakenly removed, with disastrous results, because the kidney was thought to represent a pelvic malignancy (Downs et al., 1973). This should not happen today with the multiplicity of imaging techniques to accurately diagnose the condition.

Cephalad Ectopia

The mature kidney may be positioned more craniad than normal in a patient who has had a history of omphalocele (Pinckney et al., 1978). When the liver herniates into the omphalocele sac with the intestines, the kidneys continue to ascend until they are stopped by the diaphragm. In all reported cases, both kidneys were affected and were immediately beneath the diaphragm at the level of the tenth thoracic vertebra (Fig. 34–13). The ureters are excessively long but otherwise normal. Angiograms in these patients demonstrate that the origin of the renal artery is more cephalad than normal, but no other abnormality of the vascular network is present. Patients with this anomaly usually have no symptoms referable to the malposition, and urinary drainage is not impaired.

Thoracic Kidney

A very rare form of renal ectopia exists when the kidney is positioned considerably higher than normal. Intrathoracic ectopia denotes either a partial or a complete protrusion of the kidney above the level of the diaphragm into the posterior mediastinum. Less than 5 per cent of all patients with renal ectopia have an intrathoracic kidney (Campbell, 1930). This condition is to be differentiated from a congenital or traumatic diaphragmatic hernia, in which other abdominal organs as well as the kidney have advanced into the chest cavity.

INCIDENCE. Prior to 1940, all reports of this condition were noted as a part of autopsy series (DeCastro

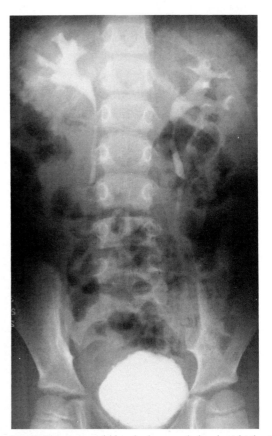

Figure 34–13. This 6-year-old boy had an omphalocele at birth. At the time, the liver was noted to be in the sac. An excretory urogram following a urinary tract infection revealed the kidneys more cephalad than usual and opposite T10.

and Shumacher, 1969). Since 1940, however, at least 92 cases have been collected in the literature; four of these have involved bilateral kidneys (Berlin et al., 1957; Hertz and Shahin, 1969; Lundius, 1975; N'Guessan and Stephens, 1984; Liddell et al., 1989). There appears to be a slight left-sided predominance of 1.5:1, and the sex ratio favors males 3:1 (Lozano and Rodriguez, 1975). This entity has been discovered in all age groups, from a neonate (Shapira et al., 1965) to a 75-year-old man evaluated for prostatic hypertrophy (Burke et al., 1967).

EMBRYOLOGY. The kidney reaches its adult location by the end of the 8th week of gestation. At this time, the diaphragmatic leaflets are formed as the pleuroperitoneal membrane separates the pleural cavity from the peritoneal cavity. Mesenchymal tissues associated with this membrane eventually form the muscular component of the diaphragm. It is uncertain whether the delayed closure of the diaphragmatic anlage allows for protracted renal ascent above the level of the future diaphragm, or whether the kidney overshoots its usual position because of accelerated ascent prior to normal diaphragmatic closure (Burke et al., 1967; N'Guessan and Stephens, 1984; Spillane and Prather, 1952). Renal angiography has demonstrated a normal site of origin for the renal artery from the aorta supplying the thoracic kidney (Lundius, 1975); however, a more cranial origin than normal has been encountered (Franciskovic and Martincic, 1959).

DESCRIPTION. The kidney is situated in the posterior mediastinum and generally has completed the normal rotation process (Fig. 34–14). Except for location, the renal contour and collecting system are normal. The kidney usually lies in the posterolateral aspect of the diaphragm in the foramen of Bochdalek. The diaphragm at this point thins out, and a flimsy membrane surrounds the protruding portion of kidney. Thus, the kidney is not within the pleural space, and there is no pneumothorax (N'Guessan and Stephens, 1984). The lower lobe of the adjacent lung may be hypoplastic secondary to compression by the kidney mass. The renal vasculature and the ureter enter and exit from the pleural cavity through the foramen of Bochdalek.

ASSOCIATED ANOMALIES. The ureter is elongated to accommodate the excessive distance to the bladder, but it never enters ectopically into the bladder or other pelvic sites. The adrenal gland has been mentioned in only two reports; in one it accompanied the kidney into the chest (Barloon and Goodwin, 1957), and in the other it did not (Paul et al., 1960). However, N'Guessan and Stephens (1984) analyzed ten cases and found that the adrenal gland is below the kidney in its normal location in the majority of patients. When this condition occurs unilaterally the contralateral kidney is usually normal. No consistent anomalies have been described in other organ systems; however, one child did have trisomy-18 (Shapira et al., 1965) and another patient had multiple pulmonary and cardiac anomalies, in addition to the thoracic kidney (Fusonie and Molnar, 1966).

SYMPTOMS. The majority of individuals with this

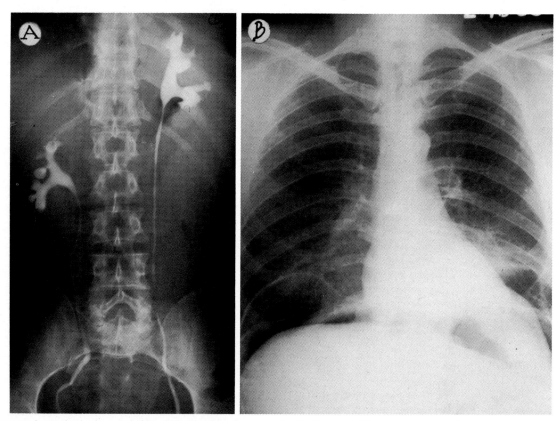

Figure 34–14. Radiograph of a thoracic kidney. The left kidney lies above the diaphragm. *A,* Diagnostic urogram. *B,* Diagnostic pneumoperitoneum. (From Hill, J. E., and Bunts, R. C.: J. Urol., 5:98, 1960.)

anomaly have remained asymptomatic. Pulmonary symptoms are exceedingly rare and even more infrequent are urinary ones. Most cases are discovered on routine chest radiographs or at the time of thoracotomy for a suspected mediastinal tumor (DeNoronha et al., 1974).

DIAGNOSIS. The diagnosis is most commonly made following a routine chest radiograph in which the affected hemidiaphragm is elevated slightly. A smooth rounded mass is seen, extending into the chest near the midline on an anteroposterior film and along the posterior aspect of the diaphragmatic leaflet on a lateral view. Excretory urography or renal scintilligraphy (Williams et al., 1983) usually suffices to clarify the diagnosis. In some instances, retrograde pyelography may be needed. Rarely, when arteriography has been employed to delineate a cardiac or pulmonary anomaly, it has revealed the presence of a thoracic kidney at the same time (Fusonie and Molnar, 1966).

PROGNOSIS. Neither autopsy series nor clinical reports suggest that a thoracic kidney results in serious urinary or pulmonary complications. Because the majority of such patients are discovered fortuitously and have no specific symptoms referable to the misplaced kidney, no treatment is necessary once the diagnosis has been confirmed.

ANOMALIES OF FORM AND FUSION

Crossed Ectopia With and Without Fusion

When a kidney is located on the side opposite from which its ureter inserts into the bladder, the condition is known as crossed ectopia. Of crossed ectopic kidneys, 90 per cent are fused to their ipsilateral mate. Except for the horseshoe anomaly, they account for the majority of fusion defects. The various renal fusion anomalies associated with ectopia are discussed in this section, whereas horseshoe kidney, the most common form of renal fusion, is presented separately.

Fusion anomalies of the kidney were first logically categorized by Wilmer (1938), but McDonald and McClellan (1957) refined and expanded this classification to include crossed ectopia with fusion; crossed ectopia without fusion; solitary crossed ectopia; and bilaterally crossed ectopia (Fig. 34–15). The fusion anomalies have been designated as (1) unilateral fused kidney with inferior ectopia; (2) sigmoid or S-shaped; (3) lump or cake; (4) L-shaped or tandem; (5) disc, shield, or doughnut; and (6) unilateral fused kidneys with superior ectopia (Fig. 34–16). Although this classification has little clinical significance, it does lend some order to an understanding of the embryology of renal ascent and rotation.

Incidence

The first reported case of crossed ectopia was described by Pamarolus in 1654. Abeshouse and Bhisitkul, in 1959, conducted the last significant review of the subject and collected exactly 500 cases of crossed ectopia with and without fusion. Subsequently, numerous case reports have been published.

A total of 62 patients with crossed ectopia without fusion have been reported (Diaz, 1953; Winram and Ward-McQuaid, 1959). This number represents approximately 10 per cent of all crossed ectopic kidneys (Lee, 1949). The anomaly occurs more commonly in males in a ratio of 2:1, and left-to-right ectopia is seen three times more frequently than right-to-left (Lee, 1949).

Solitary crossed ectopia has been reported in 27 patients (Miles et al., 1985), and males predominate in a ratio of 2:1. Generally, the crossed ectopia involves migration of the left kidney to the right side with absence of the right kidney, rather than the reverse (Kakei et al., 1976). Bilateral crossed renal ectopia has been described in five patients (Abeshouse and Bhisitkul, 1959; McDonald and McClelland, 1957) and is considered the rarest form.

Abeshouse and Bhisitkul (1959) compiled 443 reports of crossed ectopia with fusion and estimated its occurrence at one in 1000. This figure varies with the type of fusion anomaly; the unilaterally fused kidney with inferior ectopia is the most common variety, whereas fusion

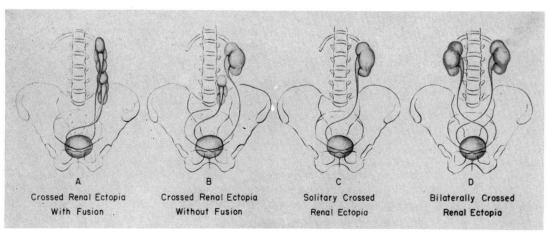

A
Crossed Renal Ectopia
With Fusion

B
Crossed Renal Ectopia
Without Fusion

C
Solitary Crossed
Renal Ectopia

D
Bilaterally Crossed
Renal Ectopia

Figure 34–15. Four types of crossed renal ectopia.

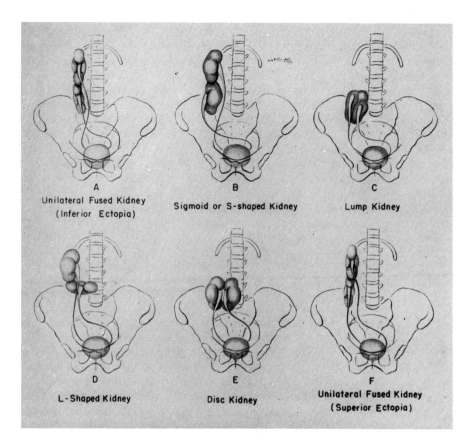

A
Unilateral Fused Kidney
(Inferior Ectopia)

B
Sigmoid or S-shaped Kidney

C
Lump Kidney

D
L-Shaped Kidney

E
Disc Kidney

F
Unilateral Fused Kidney
(Superior Ectopia)

Figure 34–16. Six forms of crossed renal ectopia with fusion.

with superior ectopia is the least common. The autopsy incidence has been calculated at one in 2000 (Baggenstoss, 1951). Crossed ectopia with fusion has been discovered in newborns (Bauer, 1977) but also has been reported in a 70-year-old man undergoing urologic evaluation for benign prostatic hypertrophy. There is a slight male predominance (3:2), and a left-to-right crossover occurs somewhat more frequently than right-to-left.

Embryology

The ureteral bud enters the metanephric blastema while the latter is situated adjacent to the anlage of the lumbosacral spine. During the next 4 weeks, the developing kidney comes to lie at the level of the L1–L3 vertebrae. Because the factor responsible for the change in kidney position during gestation is still undetermined, the reasons for crossed ectopia are similarly uncertain. Wilmer in 1938 suggested that crossover occurs as a result of pressure from abnormally placed umbilical arteries that prevent cephalad migration of the renal unit, which then follows the path of least resistance to the opposite side.

Potter (1952) and Alexander and co-workers (1950) theorized that crossed ectopia is strictly a ureteral phenomenon, with the developing ureteral bud wandering to the opposite side and inducing differentiation of the contralateral nephrogenic anlage. Ashley and Mostofi (1960) deduced that strong but undetermined forces are responsible for renal ascent and that these forces attract one or both kidneys to their final place on the opposite side of the midline.

Cook and Stephens (1977) postulated that crossover is the result of malalignment and abnormal rotation of the caudal end of the developing fetus, with the distal curled end of the vertebral column being displaced to one side or the other. This effect results either in the cloaca and wolffian duct structures lying to one side of the vertebral column, allowing one ureter to cross the midline and enter the opposite nephrogenic blastema, or in the kidney and ureter being transplanted to the opposite side of the midline during "normal" renal ascent (Hertz et al., 1977; Maizels and Stephens, 1979).

Kelalis and co-workers (1973) implicated teratogenic factors because they noted an increased incidence of associated genitourinary and other organ system anomalies. Finally, genetic influences may play a role because similar anomalies have occurred within a single family (Greenberg and Nelsen, 1971; Hildreth and Cass, 1978).

Fusion of the metanephric masses may occur when the renal anlage is still in the true pelvis prior to or at the start of cephalad migration, or it may occur during the later stages of ascent. The extent of fusion is determined by the proximity of the developing renal anlage to one another. Following fusion, advancement of the kidneys toward their normal location is impeded by midline retroperitoneal structures—the aortic bifurcation, the inferior mesenteric artery, and the base of the small bowel mesentery (Joly, 1940).

Description

Fusion of a crossed ectopic kidney is related to the time when it comes in contact with its mate. The crossed kidney usually lies caudad to its normal counterpart on that side. It is likely that migration of each kidney begins simultaneously, but ascent of the ectopic renal unit probably lags behind because of crossover time. Thus, it is the superior pole of the ectopic kidney that generally joins with the inferior aspect of the normal kidney. Ascent continues until either the uncrossed kidney reaches its normal location or one of the retroperitoneal structures prevents further migration of the fused mass. The final shape of the fused kidneys depends on the time and extent of fusion and the degree of renal rotation that has occurred. No further rotation is likely once the two kidneys have joined (Fig. 34–17). Therefore, the position of each renal pelvis may provide a clue as to the chronology of the congenital defect. An anteriorly placed pelvis suggests early fusion, whereas a medially positioned renal pelvis indicates that fusion probably occurred after rotation was completed.

Of crossed ectopic kidneys, 90 per cent are fused with their mate. When they are not fused, the uncrossed kidney generally resides in its normal dorsolumbar location and is orientated properly. The ectopic kidney is inferior and either in a diagonal or horizontal position with an anteriorly placed renal pelvis. The two kidneys in this situation are usually separated by a variable but definite distance, and each is surrounded by its own capsule of Gerota's fascia. In every case of crossed ectopia without fusion, the ureter from the normal kidney enters the bladder on the same side, whereas that of the ectopic kidney crosses the midline at the

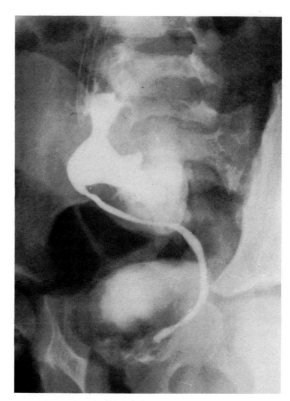

Figure 34–18. A solitary crossed pelvic kidney was found in a 7-year-old girl with recurrent urinary infection and abdominal pain. Voiding cystogram reveals vesicoureteral reflux with pyelotubular backflow.

pelvic brim and enters the bladder on the contralateral side.

In cases of solitary crossed ectopia, the kidney is usually located in the opposite renal fossa at the level of L1–L3 and is orientated normally, having completed rotation on its vertical axis (Alexander et al., 1950; Purpon, 1963). When the kidney remains in the pelvis or ascends only to the lower lumbar region, it may assume a horizontal line with an anteriorly placed pelvis because it has failed to rotate fully (Tabrisky and Bhisitkul, 1965) (Fig. 34–18). Here too, the ureter crosses the midline and enters the bladder on the opposite side. The contralateral ureter, if present, is often rudimentary (Caine, 1956). The patient with bilateral crossed ectopia may have perfectly normal-appearing kidneys and renal pelves; however, the ureters cross the midline at the level of the lower lumbar vertebrae (Abeshouse and Bhisitkul, 1959).

INFERIOR ECTOPIA. Of all unilaterally fused kidneys, two thirds involve inferior ectopia. The upper pole of the crossed kidney is attached to the inferior aspect of the normally positioned mate (Fig. 34–19). Both renal pelves are anterior; thus, fusion probably occurs relatively early.

SIGMOID OR S-SHAPED KIDNEY. The sigmoid or S-shaped kidney is the second most common anomaly of fusion. The crossed kidney is again inferior, with the two kidneys fused at their adjacent poles. Fusion of the two kidneys occurs relatively late, after complete rotation on the vertical axis has taken place. Thus, each renal pelvis is oriented correctly and faces in opposite

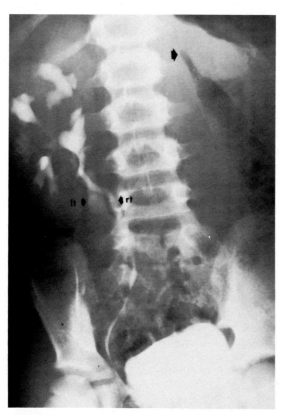

Figure 34–17. An 8-year-old boy with a left-to-right crossed, fused ectopia, in which the two kidneys lie abreast of one another. Splenic flexure lies in empty right renal fossa.

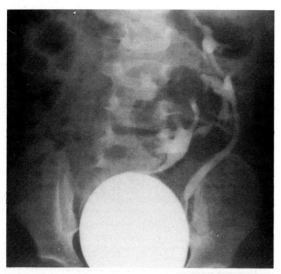

Figure 34–19. Urologic investigation in a 3-year-old girl with facial clefting syndrome and hypertelorism revealed a unilateral fused kidney with inferior ectopia. Voiding cystourethrography demonstrates bilateral reflux into each collecting system. At cystoscopy, both ureteral orifices were lateral and the trigone was poorly formed.

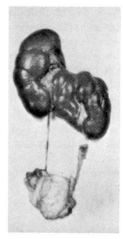

Figure 34–21. Renal fusion. L-kidney in a 1-year-old child in whom a considerable portion of the left renal segment lies across the lower lumbar spine. On each side the pelvic outlet faces anteriorly. (From Campbell, M. F.: *In* Campbell, M. F., and Harrison, J. H. (Eds.): Urology, Vol. 2, 3rd ed. Philadelphia, W. B. Saunders Co., 1970.)

directions from one another. The lower convex border of one kidney is directly opposite to the outer border of its counterpart, and there is an S-shaped appearance to the entire renal outline. The ureter from the normal kidney crosses downward anterior to the outer border of the inferior kidney, and the ectopic kidney's ureter crosses the midline before entering the bladder.

LUMP KIDNEY. The lump or cake kidney is a relatively rare form of fusion (Fig. 34–20). Extensive joining has taken place over a wide margin of maturing renal anlage. The total kidney mass is irregular and lobulated. Generally, ascent progresses only as far as the sacral promontory, but in many instances the kidney remains within the true pelvis. Both renal pelves are anterior and drain separate areas of parenchyma. The ureters do not cross.

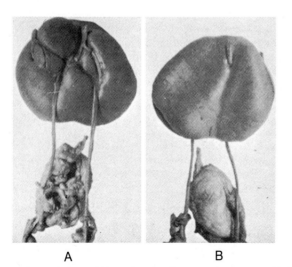

A   B

Figure 34–20. *A*, Lump kidney showing the unusual anatomy with the anterior blood supply coming from above and the ureters leaving from below. *B*, Posterior view of *A*, with the blood supply entering from above and a deep grooving of the parenchyma indicating where the kidney pressed against the spine. (Courtesy of Dr. H. S. Altman.)

L-SHAPED KIDNEY. The L-shaped or tandem kidney occurs when the crossed kidney assumes a transverse position at the time of its attachment to the inferior pole of the normal kidney (Fig. 34–21). The crossed kidney lies in the midline or in the contralateral paramedian space anterior of the L-4 vertebra (Fig. 34–22). Rotation about the long axis of the kidney may produce either an inverted or a reversed pelvic position. The ureter from each kidney enters the bladder on its respective side.

DISC KIDNEY. Disc, shield, doughnut, or pancake kidneys, as labeled by various investigators, are kidneys that have joined at the medial borders of each pole to produce a doughnut-shaped or ring-shaped mass. When more extensive fusion occurs along the entire medial aspect of each kidney, a disc or shield shape is created. The lateral aspect of each kidney retains its normal contour. Thus, this type of fusion differs from the lump or cake kidney in that the reniform shape is better preserved, because there is a somewhat less extensive degree of fusion. The pelves are anteriorly placed, and the ureters remain uncrossed. Each collecting system drains its respective half of the kidney and does not communicate with the opposite side (Fig. 34–23).

SUPERIOR ECTOPIC KIDNEY. The least common variety of renal fusion is the crossed ectopic kidney that lies superior to the normal kidney. The lower pole of the crossed kidney is fused to the upper pole of the normal kidney. Each renal unit retains its fetal orientation with both pelves lying anteriorly, suggesting that fusion occurred very early.

The vascular supply to each kidney is variable. The crossed ectopic kidney is supplied by one or more branches from the aorta or common iliac artery (Rubinstein et al., 1976). The normal kidney frequently has an anomalous blood supply, with multiple renal arteries originating from various levels along the aorta. In one rare instance, Rubinstein discovered that one renal artery had crossed the midline to supply the tandem

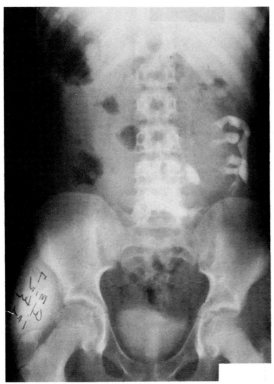

Figure 34–22. An excretory urogram in a 13-year-old child with abdominal pain reveals a tandem or L-shaped crossed ectopia.

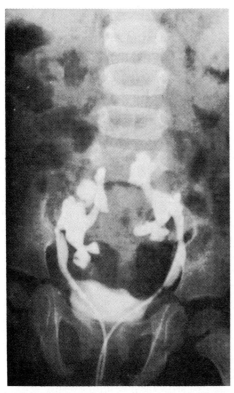

Figure 34–23. Pelvic fused kidney in a 2-year-old girl examined because of the low abdominal mass thought to be an ovarian cyst. (From Campbell, M. F.: In Campbell, M. F., and Harrison, J. H. (Eds.): Urology, Vol. 2, 3rd ed. Philadelphia, W. B. Saunders Co., 1970.)

ectopic kidney. The solitary crossed ectopic kidney has been found to receive its blood supply generally from that side of the aorta or iliac artery on which it is positioned (Tanenbaum et al., 1970).

Associated Anomalies

In all the fusion anomalies the ureter from each kidney is usually not ectopic. Except for solitary crossed ectopia, in which there may be a hemitrigone or a poorly developed trigone with the rudimentary or absent ureter on the side of the ectopic kidney, most patients with crossed ectopia have normal trigones with no indication that an anomaly of the upper urinary tract is present (Magri, 1961; Tanenbaum et al., 1970; Yates-Bell and Packham, 1972). An ectopic ureteral orifice from the crossed renal unit has been observed about 3 per cent of the time (Abeshouse and Bhisitkul, 1959; Hendren et al., 1976; Magri, 1961). Occasionally, the ureter from the uncrossed renal segment of a fusion anomaly may have an ectopic orifice (Hendren et al., 1976). In one instance, Malek and Utz (1970) discovered an ectopic ureterocele associated with an uncrossed kidney. Vesicoureteral reflux was noted frequently into the collecting system of the ectopic kidney (Kelalis et al., 1973) (see Figs. 34–18 and 34–19). Currarino and Weisbruch (1989) collected ten cases of midline renal fusion in which a single ureter divided into two pelves that stretched across the midline to drain one respective half of the total parenchymatous mass. In four of the ten cases, a second ureter was present that drained a separate duplex system on either the right or the left side. Most of the affected individuals had imperforate anus and/or abnormal vertebrae.

Most orthotopic units are normal. If an abnormality exists, it usually involves the ectopic kidney and consists of cystic dysplasia, ureteropelvic junction obstruction, and carcinoma (Abeshouse and Bhisitkul, 1959; Caldamone and Rabinowitz, 1981; Gerber et al., 1980; Macksood and James, 1983; Nussbaum et al., 1987).

The highest incidence of associated anomalies occurs in children with solitary renal ectopia and involves both the skeletal system and genital organs (Miles et al., 1985). This occurrence seems to be related more to renal agenesis than to the ectopic anomaly per se. Of patients with solitary crossed renal ectopia, 50 per cent have a skeletal anomaly and 40 per cent have a genital abnormality. The most common is either cryptorchidism or absence of the vas deferens in the male, or vaginal atresia or a unilateral uterine abnormality in the female (Kakei et al., 1976; Yates-Bell and Packham, 1972). Imperforate anus has also been observed in 20 per cent of the patients with solitary crossed ectopia.

In general, the occurrence of an associated anomaly in crossed renal ectopia, excluding solitary crossed ectopia, is low. The most frequent are imperforate anus (4 per cent), orthopedic anomalies (4 per cent), skeletal abnormalities, and septal cardiovascular defects.

Symptoms

Most individuals with crossed ectopic anomalies have no symptoms. The defects are often discovered incidentally at autopsy, during routine perinatal ultrasound screening, or following bone scanning. If manifestations do occur, common signs and symptoms usually develop in the 3rd or 4th decades of life and include vague lower abdominal pain, pyuria, hematuria, and urinary tract infection. Hydronephrosis and renal calculi have been discovered in conjunction with some of these symptoms. The abnormal kidney position and the anomalous blood supply may impede urinary drainage from the renal collecting system, thus creating a predisposition in the patient to urinary tract infection and calculus formation.

In one third of these patients, an asymptomatic abdominal mass may be the presenting sign (Abeshouse and Bhisitkul, 1959; Nussbaum et al., 1987). In a few individuals, hypertension has led to the discovery of an ectopic fusion anomaly (Abeshouse and Bhisitkul, 1959), and in one case this was attributable to a vascular lesion in one of the anomalous vessels (Mininberg et al., 1971).

Diagnosis

In the past, the usual method of detection had been excretory urography, but ultrasonography and radionuclide scanning for unrelated reasons have been discovering more asymptomatic cases. Nephrotomography can be used when necessary to define further the renal outlines (Dretler et al., 1971). Cystoscopy and retrograde pyelography are useful in mapping out the collecting system and pattern of drainage. Renal angiography may be a requirement prior to extensive surgery on the ectopic or normal kidney, because the blood supply to the kidneys is usually very anomalous.

Prognosis

Most individuals with crossed renal ectopia have normal longevity and prognosis. However, some patients with an obstructive-appearing collecting system are at risk for developing urinary tract infection or renal calculus or both (Kron and Meranze, 1949). Boatman and co-workers (1972) noted that one third of their symptomatic patients required a pyelolithotomy for an obstructing stone. Stubbs and Resnick (1977) reported a struvite staghorn calculus in a patient with crossed renal ectopia. Urinary infection in association with either vesicoureteral reflux or hydronephrosis has been implicated in the formation of these calculi.

Horseshoe Kidney

The horseshoe kidney is probably the most common of all renal fusion anomalies. It should not be confused with asymmetric or off-center fused kidneys, which may give the impression of being horseshoe-shaped. The anomaly consists of two distinct renal masses lying vertically on either side of the midline connected at their respective lower poles by a parenchymatous or fibrous isthmus that crosses the midplane of the body. It was first recognized during an autopsy by DeCarpi in 1521, but Botallo in 1564 provided the first extensive description and illustration of a horseshoe kidney (Benjamin and Schullian, 1950). In 1820, Morgagni described the first diseased horseshoe kidney. Since then, more has been written about this condition than about any other renal anomaly. Almost every renal disease has been described in the horseshoe kidney.

INCIDENCE. Horseshoe kidney occurs in 0.25 per cent of the population, or about one in 400 (Bell, 1946; Campbell, 1970; Dees, 1941; Glenn, 1959; Nation, 1945). As in other fusion anomalies, it is found more commonly in males by a 2 to 1 margin. The abnormality has been discovered clinically in all age groups ranging from fetal life to 80 years, but in autopsy series it is more prevalent in children (Segura et al., 1972). This early age prevalence is related to the high incidence of multiple congenital anomalies associated with the horseshoe kidney, some of which are incompatible with long-term survival.

Horseshoe kidneys have been reported in identical twins (Bridge, 1960) and among several siblings within the same family (David, 1974). From the rarity of these reports and the relative frequency of the anomaly, it is doubtful that these observations represent a particular genetic predisposition, but they might be the result of a genetic expression with a low degree of penetrance (Leiter, 1972).

EMBRYOLOGY. The abnormality occurs between the 4th and 6th week of gestation, after the ureteral bud has entered the renal blastema. In view of the ultimate spatial configuration of the horseshoe kidney, the entrance of the ureteral bud had to have taken place before rotation and considerably before renal ascent ensued. Boyden (1931) described a 6-week-old embryo with a horseshoe kidney, the youngest fetus ever discovered with this anomaly. He postulated that at the 14-mm stage (4½ weeks), the developing metanephric masses lie close to one another; any disturbance in this relationship might result in joining at their inferior poles. A slight alteration in the position of the umbilical or common iliac artery could change the orientation of the migrating kidneys, thus leading to contact and fusion (Fig. 34–24). It has been postulated that an abnormality in the formation of the tail of the embryo or another pelvic organ could account for the fusion process (Cook and Stephens, 1977).

Whatever the actual mechanism responsible for horseshoe kidney formation, the fusion process occurs before the kidneys have rotated on their long axes. In its mature form, the pelves and ureters of the horseshoe kidney are usually anteriorly placed, crossing ventrally to the isthmus (Fig. 34–25). Very rarely, the pelves are anteromedial, suggesting that fusion occurred somewhat later, after some rotation had taken place. In addition, migration is usually incomplete, with the kidneys lying lower than normal. It is presumed that the inferior mesenteric artery prevents full ascent by obstructing the movement of the isthmus.

DESCRIPTION. Several variations are noted in the basic shape of the horseshoe kidney (Fig. 34–26). In 95 per cent of patients, the kidneys join at the lower pole; in a small number, however, the isthmus connects both upper poles instead (Love and Wasserman, 1975).

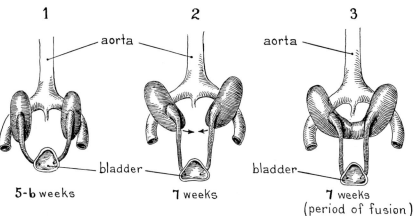

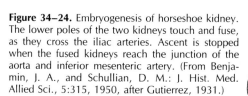

Figure 34–24. Embryogenesis of horseshoe kidney. The lower poles of the two kidneys touch and fuse, as they cross the iliac arteries. Ascent is stopped when the fused kidneys reach the junction of the aorta and inferior mesenteric artery. (From Benjamin, J. A., and Schullian, D. M.: J. Hist. Med. Allied Sci., 5:315, 1950, after Gutierrez, 1931.)

Generally, the isthmus is bulky and consists of parenchymatous tissue with its own blood supply (Glenn, 1959; Love and Wasserman, 1975). Occasionally, it is just a flimsy midline structure made up of fibrous tissue

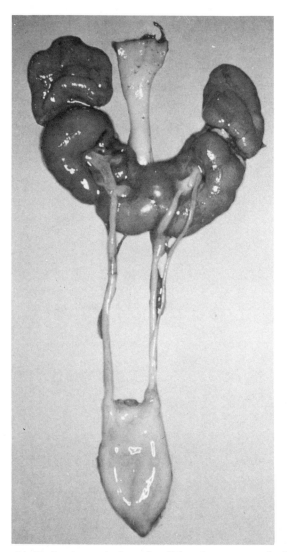

Figure 34–25. Specimen of a horseshoe kidney in a neonate who had multiple anomalies, including congenital heart disease. Note the thick parenchymatous isthmus.

that tends to draw the renal masses close together. It is located adjacent to the L-3 or L-4 vertebra, just below the junction of the inferior mesenteric artery with the aorta. As a result, the paired kidneys tend to be somewhat lower than normal in the retroperitoneum. In some instances, the anomalous kidneys are very low, anterior to the sacral promontory or even in the true pelvis behind the bladder (Campbell, 1970). In general, the isthmus lies anterior to the aorta and vena cava, but it is not unusual for it to pass between the inferior vena cava and the aorta or even behind both great vessels (Dajani, 1966; Jarmin, 1938; Meek and Wadsworth, 1940).

The calyces, normal in number, are atypical in orientation. Because the kidney fails to rotate, the calyces point posteriorly, and the axis of each pelvis remains in the vertical or obliquely lateral plane on a line drawn from lower to upper poles. The lowermost calyces extend caudally or even medially to drain the isthmus and may overlie the vertebral column.

The ureter may insert high on the renal pelvis and lie laterally, probably as the result of incomplete renal rotation. It courses downward and has a characteristic bend as it crosses over and anterior to the isthmus—a deviation that is proportionate to the thickness of the midline structure. Despite upper ureteral angulation, the lower ureter usually enters the bladder normally and rarely is ectopic.

The blood supply to the horseshoe kidney can be quite variable (Fig. 34–27). In 30 per cent of cases, it consists of one renal artery to each kidney (Glenn, 1959), but it may be atypical with duplicate or even triplicate renal arteries supplying one or both kidneys. The blood supply to the isthmus and lower poles is also very variable. The isthmus and adjacent parenchymal masses may receive a branch from each main renal artery, or they may have their own arterial supply from the aorta, originating either above or below the level of the isthmus. Not infrequently, this area may be supplied by branches from the inferior mesenteric, common or external iliac, or sacral arteries (Boatman et al., 1971; Kolln et al., 1972). Three cases of retrocaval ureter and isthmus have been reported (Eidelman et al., 1978; Heffernan et al., 1978).

ASSOCIATED ANOMALIES. The horseshoe kidney, even though it produces no symptoms, is frequently

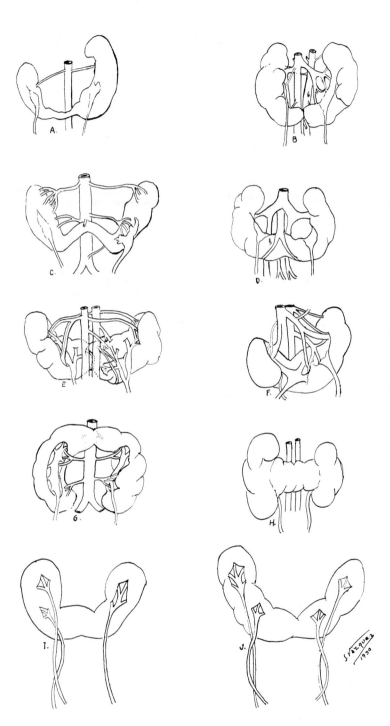

Figure 34–26. Variations in the horseshoe kidney and the number of their ureters. (From Benjamin, J. A., and Schullian, D. M.: J. Hist. Med. Allied Sci., 5:315, 1950, after Gutierrez, 1931.)

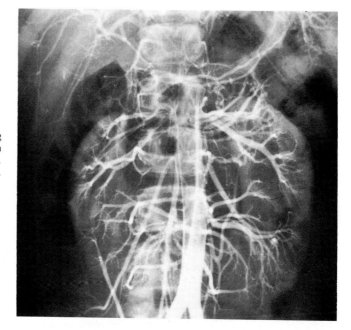

Figure 34–27. Arteriogram in a patient with a horseshoe kidney showing multiplicity of arteries supplying kidney arising from aorta and common iliac arteries. (From Kelalis, P. P.: *In* Kelalis, P. P., and King, L. R. (Eds.): Clinical Pediatric Urology. Philadelphia, W. B. Saunders Co., 1976.)

found in association with other congenital anomalies. Boatman and co-workers (1972) discovered that nearly one third of the 96 patients they studied had at least one other abnormality. Many newborns and infants with multiple congenital anomalies have a horseshoe kidney. Judging from autopsy reports, the incidence of other anomalies is certainly greater in those who die at birth or early infancy than in those who reach adulthood (Zondek and Zondek, 1964). This finding implies that horseshoe kidneys may occur more often in patients with another serious congenital anomaly. The organ systems most commonly involved include the skeletal; cardiovascular, primarily ventriculoseptal defects (Voisin et al., 1988); and central nervous systems. Horseshoe kidney is found in 3 per cent of children with neural tube defects (Whitaker and Hunt, 1987). Anorectal malformations are frequently encountered in these patients. Horseshoe kidney may also be seen in 20 per cent of patients with trisomy 18 and as many as 60 per cent of females with Turner's syndrome (Lippe et al., 1988; Smith, 1970).

Boatman and colleagues (1972) also discovered an increased occurrence of other genitourinary anomalies in patients with horseshoe kidney. Hypospadias and undescended testes each occurred in 4 per cent of males, and bicornuate uterus or septate vagina or both were noted in 7 per cent of females.

Duplication of the ureter occurs in 10 per cent of these patients (Boatman et al., 1972; Zondek and Zondek, 1964). In some cases, this finding has been associated with an ectopic ureterocele. Vesicoureteral reflux has been noted in more than half the individuals (Pitts and Muecke, 1975; Segura et al., 1972). Cystic disease, including multicystic dysplasia (Novak et al., 1977) and adult polycystic kidney disease, has been reported in horseshoe kidney (Campbell, 1970; Correa and Paton, 1976; Gutierrez, 1934; Pitts and Muecke, 1975).

SYMPTOMS. Nearly one third of all patients with horseshoe kidney remain asymptomatic (Glenn, 1959;

Kolln et al., 1972). In most instances, it is an incidental finding at autopsy (Pitts and Muecke, 1975). When symptoms are present, however, they are related to hydronephrosis, infection, or calculus formation. The most common symptom that reflects these conditions is vague abdominal pain that may radiate to the lower lumbar region. Gastrointestinal complaints may be reported as well. The so-called Rovsing sign—abdominal pain, nausea, and vomiting on hyperextension of the spine—has been infrequently observed. Signs and symptoms of urinary tract infection occur in 30 per cent of patients, and calculi have been noted in 20 to 80 per cent (Evans and Resnick, 1981; Glenn, 1959; Kolln et al., 1972; Pitts and Muecke, 1975; Sharma and Bapna, 1986). About 5 to 10 per cent of horseshoe kidneys are detected following palpation of an abdominal mass (Glenn, 1959; Kolln et al., 1972).

Ureteropelvic junction obstruction causing significant hydronephrosis occurs in as many as one third of individuals (Whitehouse, 1975; Das and Amar, 1984) (Fig. 34–28). The high insertion of the ureter into the renal pelvis, its abnormal course anterior to the isthmus, and the anomalous blood supply to the kidney may individually or collectively contribute to this obstruction.

DIAGNOSIS. Except for the possibility of a palpable midline abdominal mass (Grandone et al., 1985), the horseshoe kidney does not by itself produce symptoms. The clinical features from a diseased kidney, however, are often vague and nonspecific. The anomalies, therefore, may not be suspected until a renal ultrasound or an excretory urogram is obtained. The classic radiologic features are then recognized and a diagnosis is readily made (Fig. 34–29). Findings that suggest a horseshoe kidney singly or collectively include the following: kidneys that are somewhat low lying and close to the vertebral column; vertical or outward axis, so that a line drawn through the midplane of each kidney bisects the midline inferiorly; continuation of the outer border of the lower pole of each kidney toward and across the

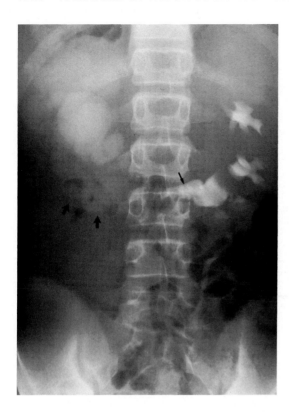

Figure 34–28. An excretory urogram in a 14-year-old boy with gross, painless hematuria following minor trauma revealed a horseshoe kidney with a right-sided ureteropelvic junction obstruction. Arrows identify the lower pole of each kidney. The left ureter can be seen crossing over the isthmus.

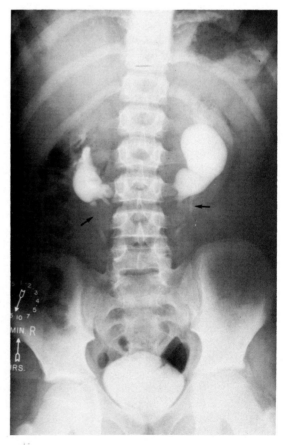

Figure 34–29. Excretory urogram in an 11-year-old boy evaluated for nocturnal incontinence reveals a horseshoe kidney. Note vertical renal axis and medial orientation of the collecting system. The ureters *(arrows)* are laterally displaced and bow over the isthmus.

midline; characteristic orientation of the collecting system, which is directly posterior to each renal pelvis, with the lowermost calyx pointing caudally or even medially; and high insertion of the ureter into the pelvis and the anteriorly displaced upper ureter that appears to drape over a midline mass. However, obstruction from either a calculus or a ureteropelvic junction stricture may obscure the radiologic picture (Christoffersen and Iversen, 1976; Love and Wasserman, 1975). Other studies, such as retrograde pyelography or computed tomography, may be necessary to confirm the diagnosis.

PROGNOSIS. Although Smith and Orkin (1945) believed that horseshoe kidneys are almost always associated with disease, subsequent investigators have not found this to be so. Glenn (1959) followed patients with horseshoe kidneys for an average of 10 years after discovery and found that nearly 60 per cent remained symptom-free. Only 13 per cent had persistent urinary infection or pain, and 17 per cent developed recurrent calculi. Operations to remove these stones or relieve obstructions were necessary in only 25 per cent. In this series, no patients benefited from division of the isthmus for relief of pain; this idea has now been largely repudiated (Glenn, 1959; Pitts and Muecke, 1975).

Many patients with horseshoe kidney have other congenital anomalies, some of which are incompatible with life beyond the neonatal period or early infancy. Excluding that group, survival is not reduced merely by the presence of this anomaly. Often a horseshoe kidney is found incidentally, and it is rarely a cause of death (Boatman et al., 1972; Dajani, 1966).

Many disease processes have been described with a horseshoe kidney but this only reflects the relative frequency of the congenital defect. In one study, 111 cases of renal carcinoma within a horseshoe kidney were reported (Buntley, 1976); more than half of these cancers were hypernephromas. However, renal pelvic tumors and Wilms' tumor each account for 25 per cent of the total. Except for renal pelvic tumors, a surprisingly high number of these cancers appear to have arisen in the isthmus (Blackard and Mellinger, 1968).

It has been suggested that the increased occurrence of chronic infection, obstruction, and stone formation may be instrumental in producing a higher than expected incidence of renal pelvic tumors in this group (Castor and Green, 1975; Shoup et al., 1962). Wilms' tumor, which is also commonly seen, frequently originates in the isthmus as well (Beck and Hlivko, 1960), often creating a very bizarre radiologic picture (Walker, 1977). The incidence of tumors within horseshoe kidneys seems to be increasing when compared with the incidence of tumors in the general population (Dische and Johnston, 1979). Survival is related to the pathology and stage of the tumor at diagnosis and not to the renal anomaly (Murphy and Zincke, 1982).

Because it is located above the pelvic inlet, a horseshoe kidney should not adversely affect pregnancy or delivery (Bell, 1946). The development of renal failure associated with adult polycystic kidney disease is not any greater in the presence of a horseshoe kidney (Correa and Paton, 1976).

The last Transplantation Registry report failed to reveal any patient with a horseshoe kidney receiving a renal transplant (Advisory Committee to the Human Transplant Registry, 1975). Since then, however, several individuals have successfully undergone transplantation (Garg, 1990).

ANOMALIES OF ROTATION

The adult kidney, as it assumes its final location in the "renal" fossa, orients itself so that the calyces point laterally and the pelvis faces medially. When this alignment is not exact, the condition is known as malrotation. Most often, this inappropriate orientation is found in conjunction with another renal anomaly, such as ectopia with or without fusion or horseshoe kidney. This discussion centers on malrotation as an isolated renal entity. It must be differentiated from other conditions that mimic it as the result of extraneous forces, such as an abnormal retroperitoneal mass.

Incidence

The true incidence of this developmental anomaly cannot be accurately calculated because minor degrees of malrotation are never reported and generally do not cause much concern. Campbell (1963) found renal malrotation once in 939 autopsies, and Smith and Orkin (1945) noted one case in 390 admissions. It is frequently observed in patients with Turner's syndrome (Gray and Skandalakis, 1972). Males are affected twice as often as females. There does not appear to be any predilection for one side or the other. In other animals, e.g., reptiles and birds, the "malrotated kidney" is actually properly oriented.

Embryology

It is thought that medial rotation of the collecting system occurs simultaneously with renal migration. Thus, the kidney starts to turn during the 6th week just when it is leaving the true pelvis and completes this process, having rotated 90 degrees toward the midline, by the time that ascent is completed at the end of the 9th week of gestation.

It has been postulated that rotation is actually the result of unequal branching of successive orders of the ureteral tree, with two branches extending ventrally and one dorsally during each generation or division (Felix, 1912). Each ureteral branch then induces differentiation of the metanephrogenic tissue surrounding it to encase it as a cap. More parenchyma develops ventrally than dorsally, and the pelvis seems to rotate medially. Weyrauch (1939) accepted this theory of renal rotation as the result of excessive ventral branching versus dorsal branching of the ureteral tree and concluded that the fault of malrotation lies entirely with the ureter. A late-appearing ureteral bud may insert into an atypical portion of the renal blastema leading to a lessened propensity for the developing nephric tissue to shift. Late appearance of the ureteral bud is almost always associated with an aberrant origin from the wolffian duct, translating into ureteral ectopia at the level of the lower urinary tract. Mackie and colleagues (1975) did not describe any malrotation anomalies in their study of renal ectopia, however. The renal blood supply does not appear to be a cause or a limiting factor in malrotation but rather follows the course of renal hyporotation, hyper-rotation, or reverse rotation.

Description

The kidney and renal pelvis normally rotate 90 degrees ventromedially during ascent. Weyrauch (1939), in an exhaustive and detailed study, outlined the various abnormal phases of medial and reverse rotation, and labeled each according to the position of the renal pelvis (Fig. 34–30).

VENTRAL POSITION. The pelvis is ventral and in the same anteroposterior plane as the calyces, which point dorsally, because they have undergone no rotation at all. This position is the most common form of malrotation. Very rarely, this ventral position may represent excessive medial rotation, in which a complete 360-degree turn has occurred. In one such presumed case reported by Weyrauch (1939), the vasculature had rotated with the kidney and passed around dorsally and laterally to it before entering the anteriorly placed hilus.

VENTROMEDIAL POSITION. The pelvis faces ventromedially because of an incompletely rotated kidney. Excursion probably stops during the 7th week of gestation, when the kidney and pelvis normally reach this position. The calyces thus point dorsolaterally.

DORSAL POSITION. Renal excursion of 180 degrees occurs to produce this position. Thus, the pelvis is dorsal to the parenchyma, and the vessels pass behind the kidney to reach the hilum. This is the rarest form of malrotation.

LATERAL POSITION. When the kidney and pelvis rotate more than 180 degrees but less than 360 degrees, or when reverse rotation of up to 180 degrees takes place, the pelvis faces laterally and the kidney parenchyma resides medially. The renal vascular supply provides the only clue to the actual direction of excursion. Vessels that course ventral to the kidney to enter a laterally or dorsolaterally placed hilum suggest reverse rotation, whereas a path dorsal to the kidney implies excessive ventral rotation. Both types of anomalous turning have been cited in Weyrauch's series (1939).

In cases of isolated malrotation, certain other characteristic features may be present. The kidney shape may be discoid, elongated, oval, or triangular, with flattened anterior and posterior surfaces. Fetal lobulations are invariably present and accentuated beyond normal limits. A dense amount of fibrous tissue encases the hilar area, possibly even distorting and fixing the pelvis. The ureteropelvic junction may be distorted as well. The upper ureter initially courses laterally, and it too may be encased in this fibrous matting. The pelvis is elongated and narrow, and calyces, especially the superior calyx, may be stretched. The blood supply, as previously described, may vary widely, depending on the direction and degree of rotation. The vasculature may consist of a single vessel with or without multiple additional branches entering the parenchyma along the course of the renal artery. In addition, there may be a polar vessel in conjunction with the main renal artery. The vascular orientation around the kidney provides the only clue to the type and extent of renal rotation, i.e., whether medial or lateral rotation has occurred.

Symptoms

Rotation anomalies per se do not produce any specific symptoms. The excessive amount of fibrous tissue encasing the pelvis, ureteropelvic junction, and upper ureter, however, may lead to a relative or actual obstruction of the upper collecting system. Vascular compression from an accessory artery may contribute to impaired drainage. Dull aching flank pain may be experienced during periods of increased urine production. Hydronephrosis is the most frequent cause of these symptoms. Hematuria, which occurs occasionally within a hydronephrotic collecting system from jostling of sidewalls, may be noted as well. Infection and calculus formation, each with its attendant symptoms, may also develop secondary to poor urinary drainage.

Diagnosis

The diagnosis may be surmised when a renal calculus is detected in an abnormal location, but confirmation should be obtained from a renal ultrasound, an excretory urogram, or a retrograde pyelogram (Fig. 34–31). The study should reveal the abnormal orientation of the renal pelvis and calyces, a flattened and elongated pelvis, a stretched superior calyx with blunting of the remaining

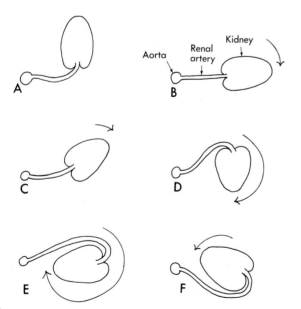

Figure 34–30. Rotation of the kidney during its ascent from the pelvis. The left kidney with its renal artery and the aorta are viewed in transverse section to show normal and abnormal rotation during its ascent to the adult site. *A*, Primitive embryonic position, hilus faces ventrad (anterior). *B*, Normal adult position, hilus faces mediad. *C*, Incomplete rotation. *D*, Hyper-rotation, hilus faces dorsad (posterior). *E*, Hyper-rotation, hilus faces laterad. *F*, Reverse rotation, hilus faces laterad. (From Gray, S. W., and Skandalakis, J. E.: Embryology for Surgeons. Philadelphia, W. B. Saunders Co., 1972.)

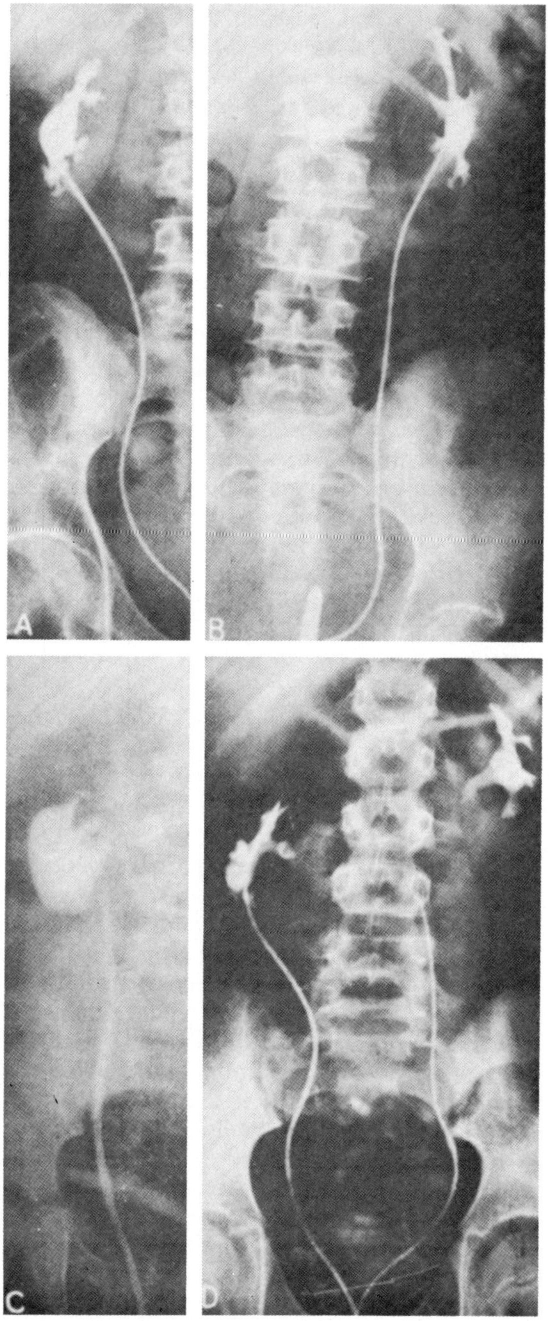

Figure 34–31. Congenital renal malrotation. *A,* Complete, the pelvis faces median. *B,* Pelvis faces posteriorly. *C,* Complete renal rotation in a 20-month-old girl with abnormally high insertion of the ureter into the pelvis. *D,* Diminutive malrotated pelvis in a 5-year-old girl. Urinary infection was the indication for urologic examination in cases *A* to *D.* (From Campbell, M. F.: *In* Campbell, M. F., and Harrison, J. H.: Urology, Vol. 2, 3rd ed. Philadelphia, W. B. Saunders Co., 1970.)

calyces, and a laterally displaced upper third of the ureter. Bilateral malrotation is not uncommon and may lead to the diagnosis of horseshoe kidney. However, careful inspection for an isthmus and observation of the lower pole renal outline should help to distinguish the two entities.

Prognosis

No abnormality of function of the kidney has been detected secondary to the malrotation. This anomaly is therefore compatible with normal longevity. Hydrone-phrosis resulting from impaired urinary drainage may lead to infection and calculus formation with their se-quelae.

ANOMALIES OF RENAL VASCULATURE

Aberrant, Accessory, or Multiple Vessels

Knowledge of the anatomy of the renal blood supply is important to every urologic surgeon, and fortunately this subject lends itself to simple investigation. Anatomists were keenly interested in renal vascular patterns before the turn of the century, but the advent of aortography in the 1940s and 1950s spearheaded a systematic clinical approach to this topic. Most of the classic work was performed by investigators in the middle to late 1950s and early 1960s (Anson and Kurth,

1955; Anson and Daseler, 1961; Geyer and Poutasse, 1962; Graves, 1954, 1956; Merklin and Michele, 1958).

The kidney is divided into various segments, each supplied by a single "end"-arterial branch that generally courses from one main renal artery. "Multiple renal arteries" is the correct term to describe any kidney supplied by more than one vessel. The term "anomalous vessels" or "aberrant vessels" should be reserved for those arteries that originate from vessels other than the aorta or main renal artery. The term "accessory vessels" denotes two or more arterial branches supplying the same renal segment.

INCIDENCE. It is observed that 71 (Merklin and Michele, 1958) to 85 per cent (Geyer and Poutasse, 1962) of kidneys have one artery that supplies the entire renal parenchyma. A slightly higher percentage of right-sided kidneys (87 per cent) have a single renal artery compared with left-sided kidneys (Geyer and Poutasse, 1962). This figure does not seem to be influenced significantly by either sex or race. True aberrant vessels are rare except in patients with renal ectopia, with or without fusion, and in individuals with a horseshoe kidney.

EMBRYOLOGY. The renal arterial tree is derived from three groups of primitive vascular channels that coalesce to form the mature vascular pattern for all retroperitoneal structures. The cranial group consists of two pairs of arteries dorsal to the suprarenal gland that shift dorsally to form the phrenic artery. The middle group is made up of three pairs of vessels that pass through the suprarenal area. They retain the same lateral position and become the adrenal artery. The caudal group has four pairs of arteries that cross ventral to the suprarenal area and become the main renal artery. Sometimes they are joined by the most inferior pair from the middle group (Guggemos, 1962). It is believed that during renal migration this network of vessels selectively degenerates, and the remaining adjacent arteries assume a progressively more important function. By a process of elimination, one primitive renal arterial pair eventually becomes the dominant vessel, the completed process being dependent on the final position of the kidney (Graves, 1956). Polar arteries or multiple renal arteries to the normally positioned kidney represent a failure of complete degeneration of all primitive vascular channels. The multiple vessel pattern that has been described for renal ectopia should be considered as an arrested embryonic state for that particular renal position (Gray and Skandalakis, 1972).

DESCRIPTION. On the basis of vascular supply, the renal parenchyma is divided into five segments—apical, upper, middle, lower, and posterior (Fig. 34–32). The main renal artery divides initially into an anterior and a posterior branch. The anterior branch almost always supplies the upper, middle, and lower segments of the kidney. The posterior branch invariably nourishes the posterior segment. The vessel to the apical segment has the greatest variation in origin as noted, arising from (a) the anterior division (43 per cent), (b) the junction of the anterior and posterior divisions (23 per cent), (c) the main stem renal artery or aorta (23 per cent), or (d) the posterior division of the main renal artery (10 per

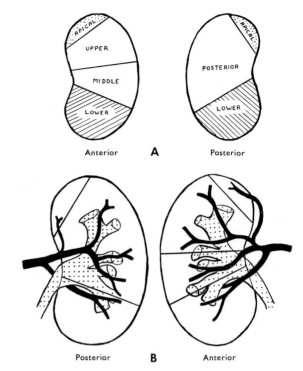

Figure 34–32. Usual pattern of arteries to the kidney. *A*, The five vascular lobes of Graves. *B*, Relationships of renal artery branch and renal pelvis to the five lobes. (From Graves, F. T.: Br. J. Surg., 42:132, 1954. By permission of the publisher, Butterworth-Heinemann Ltd.)

cent) (Graves, 1954). Rarely, the upper segment is supplied from a branch totally separate from the main renal artery (Merklin and Michele, 1958).

The lower renal segment, however, is often fed by an accessory vessel. This vessel is usually the most proximal branch when it arises from the main renal artery or its anterior division (Graves, 1954). However, it may originate directly from the aorta near the main renal artery, or it may be aberrant, arising from the gonadal vessel. A summary of findings from Merklin and Michele (1958), who analyzed reports of almost 11,000 kidneys, is depicted in Table 34–1. The relationship of the main renal artery and its proximal branches to the renal vein can be seen in Figure 34–33.

SYMPTOMS. The symptoms attributable to renal vascular anomalies are those that might result from inadequate urinary drainage. Multiple, aberrant, or accessory vessels may constrict an infundibulum (Fig. 34–34A), a major calyx, or a ureteropelvic junction (Fig. 34–35). Pain, hematuria secondary to hydronephrosis, or signs and symptoms of urinary tract infection or calculus formation may result.

DIAGNOSIS. Excretory urography may suggest multiple renal vessels or an aberrant artery when (a) a filling defect in the pelvis is consistent with an anomalous vascular pattern; (b) hydronephrosis is noted along with a sharp cutoff in the superior infundibulum (Fig. 34–34B) (Fraley, 1966, 1969); (c) ureteropelvic junction obstruction is seen in association with an angulated ureter near the renal pelvis and a kidney whose pole-to-pole axis is more vertical than normal; or (d) differences are noted in the timing and concentration of one

Table 34–1. VARIATIONS IN THE ARTERIAL SUPPLY TO THE KIDNEY*

	Condition	Per Cent
	1 Hilar artery	71.1
	1 Hilar artery and 1 upper pole branch	12.6
	2 Hilar arteries	10.8
	1 Hilar artery and 1 upper pole aortic artery	6.2
	1 Hilar artery and 1 lower pole aortic artery	6.9
	1 Hilar artery and 1 lower pole branch	3.1
	3 Hilar arteries	1.7
	2 Hilar arteries, one with upper pole branch	2.7
	Other variations	—

*From Gray, S. W., and Skandalakis, J. E. (Eds.): Embryology for Surgeons. Philadelphia, W. B. Saunders Co., 1972.

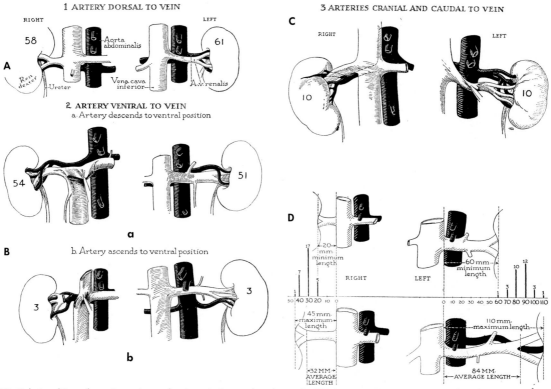

Figure 34–33. Relationships of renal arteries and veins. *A,* Artery dorsal to vein (47.6 per cent). *B,* Artery ventral to vein (*B a,* 42 per cent; *B b,* 2.4 per cent). *C,* Artery cranial and caudal to vein (8.0 per cent). *D,* Maximum, minimum, and average lengths of the renal pedicle in 30 successive specimens. (From Anson, B. J., and Daseler, E. H.: Surg. Gynecol. Obstet., 112:439, 1961. By permission of Surgery, Gynecology, and Obstetrics.)

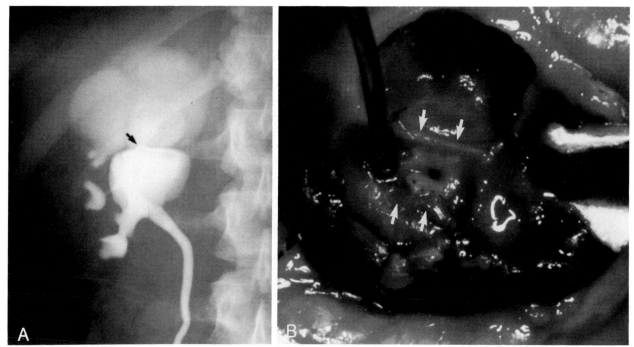

Figure 34–34. *A,* A 14-year-old girl with right flank pain underwent an excretory urogram, and this retrograde pyelogram revealed dilated upper calyces and a narrow upper infundibulum *(arrow)*. *B,* At surgery, the infundibular channel was found sandwiched between two segmental arteries *(arrows)*.

renal segment or in the entire kidney when compared with the opposite side, especially when hypertension is present.

PROGNOSIS. None of these variations in the vascular tree increase the kidney's susceptibility to disease. Hydronephrosis secondary to a vascular anomaly is indeed a very rare finding, especially when one considers the relative frequency of all renal vascular aberrations. Hypertension is no more frequent in the patient with multiple renal arteries than in the one with a single renal vessel (Geyer and Poutasse, 1962). Nathan (1958) did

report the development of orthostatic proteinuria in seven patients with a lower pole renal artery that wrapped around and compressed the main renal vein. He thought there might have been a causal relationship but did not prove it.

Renal Artery Aneurysm

Aneurysmal dilation was the first disease process of the renal artery to be recognized (Poutasse, 1957); it

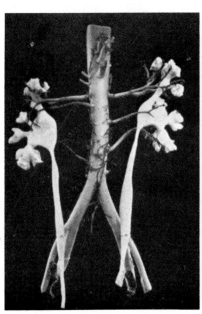
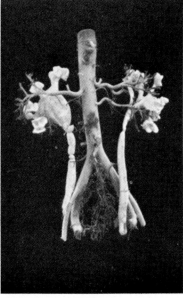

Figure 34–35. Accessory renal vessels demonstrated by celluloid corrosion preparation.

A, In a full-term fetus. The renal pelves and ureters are shown in relationship to the main arterial distribution. On each side there are two accessory renal vessels above and one below, the lower one on the left being in proximity to the ureterovesical junction.

B, In an 8-month-old fetus. The kidney on the right had one renal artery but the organ on the left had an accessory branch to the lower renal pole. Yet, the location of the lower accessory vessel on the left does not suggest that it might cause ureteral obstruction. On the right, there are early hydronephrosis, secondary kinking, and narrowing at the ureterovesical junction. (Courtesy of Dr. Duncan Morison.)

A   B

was considered a rare occurrence until selective renal angiography came into vogue. Since then, the overall incidence has been calculated to be between 0.1 and 0.3 per cent. Abeshouse (1951), in a comprehensive review, classified renal artery aneurysms as follows: saccular, fusiform, dissecting, and arteriovenous. The saccular aneurysm, a localized outpouching that communicates with the arterial lumen by a narrow or wide opening, is the most common type, accounting for 93 per cent of all aneurysms (Hageman et al., 1978; McKeil et al., 1966; Stanley et al., 1975; Zinman and Libertino, 1982). When the aneurysm is located at the bifurcation of the main renal artery and its anterior and posterior divisions or at one of the more distal branchings, it is considered to be congenital in origin and is called the fusiform type (Poutasse, 1957). The presence of similar aneurysms at branching points in the vasculature of other organ systems attests to this possible origin (Lorentz et al., 1984). Acquired aneurysms may be located anywhere and result from inflammatory, traumatic, or degenerative factors. A localized defect in the internal elastic tissue and the media allows the vessel to dilate at that point. It is a true aneurysm because its walls are composed of most of the layers that compose the normal artery (Poutasse, 1957). The outpouchings may vary in size from 1 to 2 cm up to 10 cm (Garritano, 1957).

Most renal artery aneurysms are silent, especially those in children. Some produce symptoms at a later age in relation to their size because of a tendency for them to enlarge with time. Pain, hematuria (microscopic and macroscopic), and hypertension secondary to compression of adjacent parenchyma or to altered blood flow within the vascular tree can occur (Glass and Uson, 1967). The hypertension is renin-mediated, secondary to relative parenchymal ischemia (Lorentz et al., 1984).

The diagnosis may be suspected when a pulsatile mass is palpated in the region of the renal hilum or when a bruit is heard on abdominal auscultation. A wreath-like calcification in the area of the renal artery or its branches (30 per cent) is highly suggestive (Silvis et al., 1956). Selective renal angiography (Cerney et al., 1968) or digital subtraction angiography is needed to confirm the diagnosis.

Many asymptomatic renal artery aneurysms come to light following the discovery and work-up of hypertension. Some 50 per cent are diagnosed when a renal arteriogram is performed for other reasons (Zinman and Libertino, 1982). Generally, excision is recommended if (a) the hypertension cannot be easily controlled; (b) an incomplete ring-like calcification is present; (c) the aneurysm is larger than 2.5 cm (Poutasse, 1975); (d) the patient is female and likely to become pregnant; (e) the aneurysm increases in size on serial angiograms; or (f) an arteriovenous fistula is present. The likelihood of spontaneous rupture (about 10 per cent) with its dire consequences, dictates attentive treatment in the foregoing situations.

Renal Arteriovenous Fistula

Although rare, renal arteriovenous fistulas have been discovered with increasing frequency since they were first described by Varela in 1928. Two types exist, congenital and acquired (Maldonado et al., 1964), with the latter secondary to trauma, inflammation, renal surgery, or postpercutaneous needle biopsy accounting for the increased incidence. Only the congenital variant is discussed here.

Less than 25 per cent of all arteriovenous fistulas are of the congenital type. They are identifiable by their cirsoid configuration and multiple communications between the main or segmental renal arteries and the venous channels (Cho and Stanley, 1978; Crummy et al., 1965). Although they are considered congenital because similar arteriovenous malformations can be found elsewhere in the body, they rarely appear clinically before the 3rd or 4th decade. Females are affected three times as often as males, and the right kidney is involved slightly more than the left (Cho and Stanley, 1978). The lesion is generally located in the upper pole (45 per cent of cases), but it may be found in the midportion (30 per cent) or lower pole (25 per cent) of the kidney (Yazaki et al., 1976). A total of 91 cases have been reported (Takaha et al., 1980) when the last review was conducted.

The exact cause remains an enigma, but the condition is thought to be present at birth or the result of a congenital aneurysm that erodes into an adjacent vein and slowly enlarges (Thomason et al., 1972). The pathophysiology involved in the shunting of blood, which bypasses the renal parenchyma and rapidly joins the venous circulation and returns to the heart, results in a varied clinical picture. The myriad of symptoms are based on the size of the arteriovenous malformation and the length of time it has existed (Messing et al., 1976).

The hemodynamic derangement produces a loud bruit in 75 per cent of cases. Diminished perfusion of renal parenchyma distal to the fistulous site leads to relative ischemia and renin-mediated hypertension (40 to 50 per cent) (McAlhany et al., 1971). The increased venous return and high cardiac output with concomitant diminution in peripheral resistance may result in left ventricular hypertrophy and eventually in high-output cardiac failure (50 per cent) (Maldonado et al., 1964). In addition, the arteriovenous fistula usually is located close to the collecting system. As a result, macroscopic and microscopic hematuria may occur in more than 75 per cent of affected individuals (Cho and Stanley, 1978; Messing et al., 1976). Although flank or abdominal pain may be present, a mass is rarely felt (10 per cent).

Excretory urography may reveal diminished or absent function in either one segment or the entire portion of the involved kidney (DeSai and DeSautels, 1973), an irregular filling defect in the renal pelvis or calyces secondary to either clot or encroachment by the fistula, and calyceal distortion or obstruction distal to the site of the lesion (Gunterbert, 1968). Despite these specific radiographic features, an abnormality may be noted in only 50 per cent of excretory urograms. Selective renal arteriography or digital subtraction angiography is the most definitive method for diagnosing the lesion. A cirsoid appearance with multiple small tortuous channels, a prompt venous filling, and an enlarged renal and possibly a gonadal vein are pathognomonic for a renal arteriovenous fistula (DeSai and DeSautels, 1973).

The symptomatic nature of this lesion, which causes progressive alterations in the cardiovascular system, often dictates surgical intervention. The congenital variant rarely behaves like its acquired counterpart, which may disappear spontaneously after several months. Nephrectomy, partial nephrectomy, vascular ligation (Boijsen and Kohler, 1962), selective embolization (Bookstein and Goldstein, 1973), and balloon catheter occlusion (Bentson and Crandalls, 1972) have been employed to obliterate the fistula.

ANOMALIES OF THE COLLECTING SYSTEM

Anomalies of the collecting system may be classified as follows:

I. Calyx and infundibulum
  A. Calyceal diverticulum
  B. Hydrocalycosis
  C. Megacalycosis
  D. Unipapillary kidney
  E. Extrarenal calyces
  Г. Anomalous calyx (pseudotumor of the kidney)
  G. Infundibulopelvic dysgenesis
II. Pelvis
  A. Extrarenal pelvis
  B. Bifid pelvis

CALYX AND INFUNDIBULUM

Calyceal Diverticulum

A calyceal diverticulum is a cystic cavity lined by transitional epithelium, encased within the renal substance, and situated peripheral to a minor calyx to which it is connected by a narrow channel. This abnormality, first described by Rayer in 1841, may be multiple, with the upper calyx being most frequently affected.

An incidence of 4.5 per 1000 excretory urograms has been reported (Timmons et al., 1975). A similar incidence has been noted in both children and adults, with no predilection for either size or sex.

Congenital and acquired factors have been suggested to explain the formation of calyceal diverticula. The similarity in incidence in children and adults is consistent with an embryologic etiology (Abeshouse, 1950; Devine et al., 1969; Mathieson, 1953; Middleton and Pfister, 1974). At the 5-mm stage of the embryo, some of the ureteral branches of the third and fourth generation, which ordinarily degenerate, may persist as isolated branches, resulting in the formation of a calyceal diverticulum (Lister and Singh, 1973).

A localized cortical abscess draining into a calyx has also been postulated as an etiologic factor. Other proposed causes include obstruction secondary to stone formation or infection within a calyx, renal injury, achalasia, and spasm or dysfunction of one of the supposed sphincters surrounding a minor calyx. Small diverticula are usually asymptomatic and are found incidentally at excretory urography. Distention of a diverticulum with urine trapped within it sometimes causes pain. Infection, milk of calcium (crystallization of calcium salts without actual stone formation) (Patriquin et al., 1985), and true stone formation are complications of stasis or obstruction that can produce symptoms (Lister and Singh, 1973; Siegel and McAlister, 1979). Hematuria, pain, and urinary infection may be seen in the presence of stones. In the Mayo Clinic series (Timmons et al., 1975), 39 per cent of patients with calyceal diverticula had calculi.

The diagnosis is made using excretory urography. Delayed films are helpful in demonstrating pooling of contrast material in the diverticulum. Retrograde pyelography (Fig. 34–36) and computed tomography with contrast and magnetic resonance imaging are sometimes useful in making the diagnosis and defining the precise anatomy. Milk of calcium appears as a crescent-shaped density on excretory urography, which changes as the patient assumes different positions. Ultrasonography characteristically demonstrates a layering effect between clear fluid above and echo-dense debris without shadowing below, within the diverticulum (Patriquin et al., 1985). In fact, ultrasonography may be more definitive because it is less difficult to image the milk of calcium within the diverticulum as the patient changes positions.

In general, patients who are asymptomatic do not require treatment. Persistent pain, resistant urinary infections, hematuria, and milk of calcium or true calculus formation are indications for surgery (Siegel and McAlister, 1979). If feasible, partial nephrectomy is the treatment of choice.

Hydrocalycosis

Hydrocalycosis is a very rare cystic dilation of a major calyx with a demonstrable connection to the renal pelvis—it is lined by transitional epithelium. The dilatation may be caused by a congenital or acquired intrinsic obstruction, such as a parapelvic cyst (Fig. 34–37).

Dilation of the upper calyx due to obstruction of the upper infundibulum by vessels or stenosis has been described (see Fig. 34–34) (Fraley, 1966; Johnston and Sandomirsky, 1972). Cicatrization of an infundibulum may result from infection or trauma. Conversely, hydrocalycosis has been reported to occur without an obvious cause (Williams and Mininberg, 1968). It has been postulated that achalasia of a ring of muscle at the entrance of the infundibulum into the renal pelvis causes

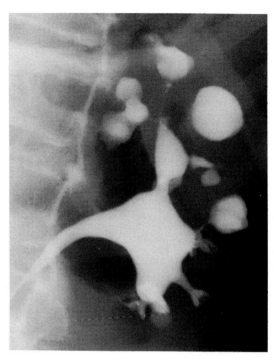

Figure 34–36. A 13-year-old girl with hematuria had a retrograde pyelogram demonstrating multiple calyceal diverticula.

a functional obstruction (Moore, 1950; Williams and Mininberg, 1968).

Mild upper calyceal dilation due to partial infundibular obstruction is relatively common but usually asymptomatic. The most frequent presenting symptom is upper abdominal or flank pain. A mass may be palpated on occasion. Stasis can lead to hematuria or urinary infection or both.

Hydrocalycosis must be differentiated from multiple dilated calyces secondary to ureteral obstruction, calyceal clubbing as a result of recurrent pyelonephritis or medullary necrosis, renal tuberculosis, large calyceal diverticulum, and megacalycosis. These entities can be distinguished by a combination of excretory urography, findings at surgery, histopathology of removed tissue, and findings of bacteriology.

Hydrocalycosis due to vascular obstruction is usually treated by dismembered infundibulopyelostomy, thus changing the relationship of the infundibulum to the vessel. When the cystic dilatation is due to an intrinsic stenosis of the infundibulum, an intubated infundibulotomy or partial nephrectomy is performed. Percutaneous treatment of these narrowed areas has also been successful and is probably the approach of choice today. Although clinical improvement is apparent in most instances, the radiologic appearance often is not altered significantly.

Megacalycosis

Megacalycosis is best defined as nonobstructive enlargement of calyces due to malformation of the renal papillae (Fig. 34–38). It was first described by Puigvert in 1963. The calyces are generally dilated and malformed and may be increased in number. The renal pelvis is neither dilated nor is its wall thickened. The ureteropelvic junction is normally funneled without evidence of

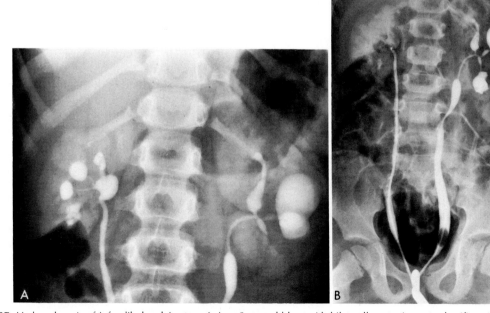

Figure 34–37. Hydrocalycosis of infundibulopelvic stenosis in a 3-year-old boy with bilaterally ectopic ureteral orifices (at the vesical neck) and other congenital anomalies, who presented with urinary infection. Reflux was not demonstrable, and the patient has remained uninfected on suppressive treatment. There has been no urographic change for 5 years. *A*, Long-term excretory urogram. Right infundibular and left infundibulopelvic stenosis. *B*, Retrograde ureteropyelogram (bilateral). Mildly dilated left ureter. Note diffuse tubular backflow on right. (From Malek, R. S.: *In* Kelalis, P. P., and King, L. R. (Eds.): Clinical Pediatric Urology, Philadelphia, W. B. Saunders Co., 1976.)

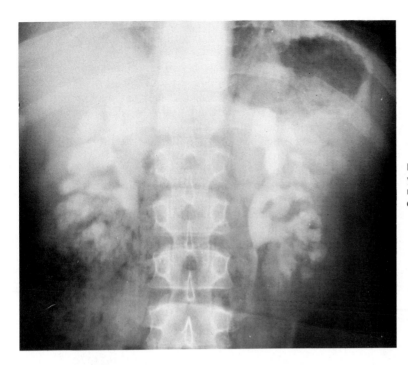

Figure 34–38. Bilateral megacalyces discovered in an 11-year-old boy with abdominal pain and hematuria. He had no history of urinary infection, and voiding cystography did not demonstrate vesicoureteral reflux.

obstruction. The cortical tissue around the abnormal calyx is normal in thickness and shows no signs of scarring or chronic inflammation. The medulla, however, is underdeveloped, assuming a falciform crescent appearance instead of its normal pyramidal shape. The collecting tubules are not dilated but are definitely shorter than normal, and they are oriented transversely rather than vertically from the corticomedullary junction (Puigvert, 1963). A mild disorder of maximum concentrating ability has been reported (Gittes and Talner, 1972), but acid excretion is normal after an acid load (Vela Navarrete and Garcia Robledo, 1983). Other functions of the kidney—glomerular filtration, renal plasma flow, and isotope uptake—are not altered (Gittes, 1984).

Megacalycosis is most likely congenital in origin. It occurs predominantly in males in a ratio of 6:1 and has been found only in whites. Bilateral disease has been seen almost exclusively in males, whereas segmental unilateral involvement is seen only in females. This suggests that an X-linked partially recessive gene with reduced penetrance in females is the causative factor (Gittes, 1984). Except for one report of two similarly affected brothers, the entity has not been thought to be familial (Briner and Thiel, 1988).

It has been theorized by Puigvert (1964) and endorsed by Johnston and Sandomirsky (1972), that there is transient delay in the recanalization of the upper ureter after the branches of the ureteral bud hook up with the metanephric blastema. This delay produces a short-lived episode of obstruction when the embryonic glomeruli start producing urine. The fetal calyces may dilate and then retain an obstructed appearance despite the lack of evidence of obstruction in postnatal life (Gittes and Talner, 1972). The increased number of calyces frequently seen in this condition may be an aborted response by the branching ureteral bud to the obstruction.

Primary hypoplasia of juxtamedullary glomeruli has been suggested as an etiology by Galian and colleagues (1970), which explains the reason for the lack of concentrating ability. This theory has not been corroborated by others, however.

The abnormality is noticed in children, usually when radiographs are obtained following a urinary tract infection or as part of an evaluation when other congenital anomalies are present. Adults frequently present with hematuria secondary to renal calculi, which leads to excretory urographic investigation.

The calyces are dilated and usually increased in number, but the infundibula and pelvis may not be enlarged. Although the ureteropelvic junction does not appear obstructed, there may be segmental dilation of the distal third of the ureter (Kozakewich and Lebowitz, 1974). Megacalycosis associated with an ipsilateral segmental megaureter has been described in 12 children (Mandell et al., 1987). This occurs mostly in males, with a left-sided predominance, who have normal caliber ureters interposed between the two abnormalities (Fig. 34–39). This anatomic picture has been mistaken, but not frequently, for congenital ureteropelvic or ureterovesical junction obstruction, with surgery being performed to correct the suspected defect. Postoperatively, the calyceal pattern remains unchanged.

Diuretic renography reveals a normal pattern for the uptake and washout of the isotope, whereas a Whitaker test fails to generate high pressures in the collecting system. Thus, an obstructive picture cannot be proved. Long-term follow-up of patients with this anomaly does not reveal any progression of the anatomic derangement or functional impairment of the kidney (Gittes, 1984).

Unipapillary Kidney

The unipapillary kidney is an exceptionally rare anomaly in humans. Only six cases have been reported (Harrison et al., 1976; Morimoto et al., 1979; Neal and

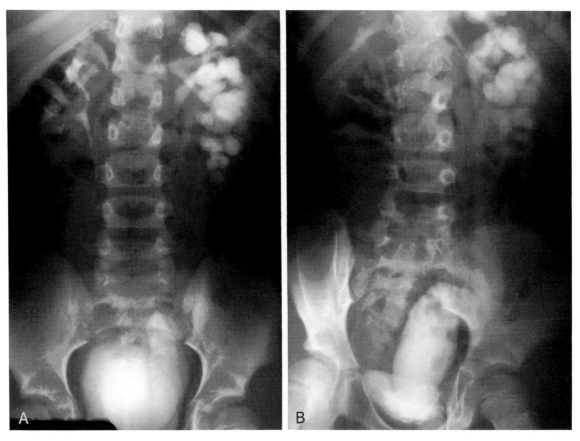

Figure 34–39. An 8-year-old boy with urinary infection was found to have left-sided megacalycosis and a distal megaureter *(A and B).* Note the normal caliber upper ureter. A voiding cystogram revealed no reflux, and a diuretic renogram did not demonstrate any obstruction.

Murphy, 1960; Sakatoku and Kitayama, 1964; Topper-cer, 1980). This anomaly is present not uncommonly in monkeys, rabbits, dogs, marsupials, insectivores, and monotremes. The etiology is thought to be a failure of progressive branching after the first three to five generations of the ureteral bud, which creates the pelvis (Potter, cited by Harrison et al., 1976). The solitary calyx drains a ridge-like papilla. Nephrons attach to fewer collecting tubules, which then drain directly into the pelvis.

The kidney is smaller than normal but usually is in its correct location. The arterial tree, although sparse, has a normal configuration. The opposite kidney is frequently absent. Genital anomalies are often present. The condition is frequently asymptomatic, being discovered fortuitously in most instances.

Extrarenal Calyces

Extrarenal calyces is an uncommon congenital anomaly in which the major calyces as well as the renal pelvis are outside the parenchyma of the kidney (Fig. 34–40). This entity was originally reviewed by Eisendrath in 1925 and then more extensively by Malament and associates in 1961. The kidney is usually discoid, with the pelvis and the major and minor calyces located outside the renal parenchyma. The renal vessels have an anomalous distribution into the kidney usually at the circum-ferential edge of the flat widened hilus. Malament considered this condition to result from abnormal nephrogenic anlage or a too early and rapidly developing ureteral bud.

Extrarenal calyces usually do not produce symptoms, although failure to drain normally may lead to stasis, infection, and calculi. Sometimes, the calyces are blunted, mimicking the radiographic changes usually seen with pyelonephritis and obstruction. This condition should be distinguished from these other entities. Surgery is reserved for those patients in whom infection or obstruction is demonstrated.

Anomalous Calyx (Pseudotumor of the Kidney)

A number of normal variants of the pyelocalyceal system in the kidney have been described. One such entity appears as a localized mass, usually situated between the infundibula of the upper and middle calyceal groups, and is called a hypertrophied column of Bertin (Fig. 34–41). The column may be sufficiently large to compress and deform the adjacent pelvis and calyces, suggesting a mass on the excretory urogram—the so-called pseudotumor. The individual calyces, however, are normally shaped and developed.

It is important to differentiate this calyceal anomaly from true disease of the calyx and from a parenchymal

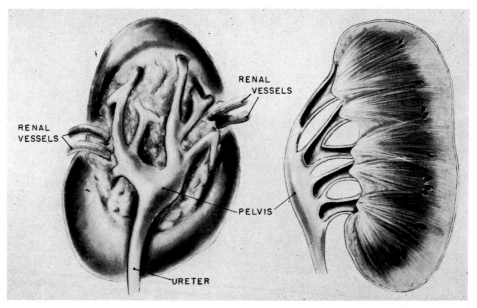

Figure 34–40. Extrarenal calyces. These represent delayed rather than insufficient ureteral growth. (From Malament, M., et al., Am. J. Roentgenol., 86:823, 1961.)

tumor. A renal scan will show normal uptake of the radioisotope in this area (Parker et al., 1976), whereas a renal ultrasound will show a normal echogenic pattern of parenchyma to the area in question.

Infundibulopelvic Dysgenesis

Infundibulopelvic stenosis most likely forms a link between cystic dysplasia of the kidney and the grossly hydronephrotic organ (Kelalis and Malek, 1981; Uhlenhuth et al., 1990). This condition includes a variety

of roentgenographically dysmorphic kidneys with varying degrees of infundibular or infundibulopelvic stenosis that may be associated with renal dysplasia (Fig. 34–42). Although not called infundibulopelvic dysgenesis, the first case involving the entire pelvis and all the infundibula of both kidneys was reported by Boyce and Whitehurst in 1976. Rayer had described a focal form of the disease in 1841, and several reports noting narrowing of one or two infundibula appeared between 1949 and 1976 (Uhlenhuth et al., 1990). These reports tried to link the focal form to cystic dysplasia secondary to obstruction, in which multicystic kidney disease is the

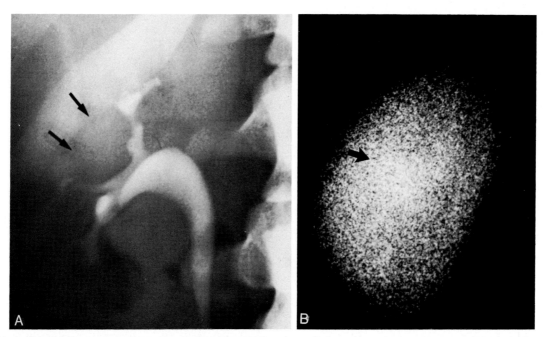

Figure 34–41. *A,* This child has a mass effect with splaying of the middle calyces. *B,* A renal scan demonstrates normal uptake in the area *(arrow),* suggesting the "pseudotumor" is really a hypertrophied column of Bertin.

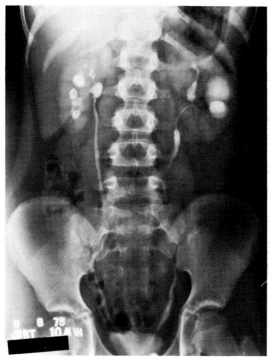

Figure 34–42. Excretory urogram in an 18-year-old male with one urinary tract infection shows severe stenosis of the infundibula and left ureteropelvic junction and a milder form of infundibulopelvic dysgenesis in the right kidney. Vesicoureteral reflux was absent on voiding cystourethrography. (Courtesy of Dr. Panos Kelalis.)

severest form in the spectrum. Uhlenhuth and co-workers (1990) believe that this phenomenon is the result of extensive dysgenesis of the pyelocalyceal system but with preservation of renal function.

Infundibulopelvic stenosis is usually bilateral and is commonly associated with vesicoureteral reflux, suggesting an abnormality of the entire ureteral bud (Kelalis and Malek, 1981). The patient usually presents with urinary infection or flank pain. Sometimes, an asymptomatic child with multiple anomalies is evaluated and found to have this condition. Despite extensively dysmorphic kidneys, the function is either normal or only slightly affected (Kelalis and Malek, 1981).

PELVIS

Extrarenal Pelvis

An extrarenal pelvis is of clinical importance only when drainage is impaired. This condition is sometimes associated with a variety of kidney abnormalities, including malposition and malrotation, that predispose the patient to urinary stasis, infection, and calculous disease.

Bifid Pelvis

Approximately 10 per cent of normal renal pelves are bifid, the pelvis dividing first at or just within its entrance to the kidney to form two major calyces. Bifid pelvis should be considered a variant of normal. No increased incidence of disease has been reported in patients with this entity. When further division of the renal pelvis occurs, triplication of the pelvis may result but is extremely rare.

ANOMALIES OF THE URETEROPELVIC JUNCTION

Anomalies of the ureteropelvic junction may be classified as follows:

I. Ureteropelvic junction obstruction
   A. Intrinsic
   B. Extrinsic
   C. Secondary

URETEROPELVIC JUNCTION OBSTRUCTION

Hydronephrosis due to congenital ureteropelvic junction obstruction is one of the more common anomalies seen in childhood. It is defined as an impediment to urinary flow from the renal pelvis into the ureter. Inefficient drainage of urine at this point leads to progressive dilation of the collecting system and a further diminution in the efficiency of pelvic emptying (Whitaker, 1975; Koff et al., 1986; Koff, 1990). Initially,

the muscle of the renal pelvis hypertrophies, and glomerular filtration diminishes to accommodate the obstructive process. Eventually, when the limit of kidney compromise is reached, destruction of renal parenchyma and impairment of function ensue.

Only primary congenital ureteropelvic junction obstruction is considered in this chapter. Other conditions that delay proximal urinary drainage and secondarily affect the ureteropelvic junction are discussed elsewhere is this text.

Incidence

Ureteropelvic junction obstruction is seen in all pediatric age groups. At one time, about 25 per cent of cases were discovered within the first year of life (Fig. 34–43) (Williams and Kenawi, 1976). Today, with the widespread use of ultrasonographic imaging of fetuses, nearly all cases are being discovered and diagnosed in the perinatal period (Brown et al., 1987). In fact,

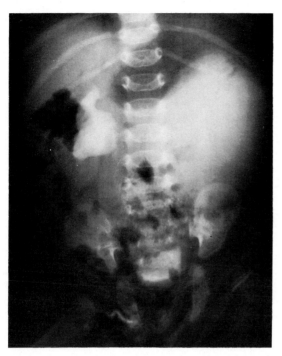

Figure 34–43. Palpation of a smooth, soft abdominal mass that transilluminated in a 3-year-old boy led to this excretory urogram, which at 6 hours reveals a ureteropelvic junction obstruction with severe hydronephrosis. An intrinsic narrowing at the ureteropelvic junction was found at surgery.

ureteropelvic junction obstruction is *the* most common cause of dilation of the collecting system in the fetal kidney, accounting for 80 per cent of all dilations of the collecting system and far exceeding the incidence of multicystic dysplastic kidneys (Colodny et al., 1980; Brown et al., 1987). Relatively few cases are detected beyond puberty and into adulthood, but those that are, are due to an aberrant vessel to the lower pole parenchyma crossing over the ureteropelvic junction area (Lowe and Marshall, 1984). The obstruction occurs more commonly in males (Johnston et al., 1977; Kelalis et al., 1971; Williams and Karlaftis, 1966), especially in the newborn period, when the ratio exceeds 2:1 (Johnston et al., 1977; Robson et al., 1976; Williams and Kenawi, 1976). Left-sided lesions predominate. In the neonate more than two thirds occur on the left side. Bilateral ureteropelvic junction obstruction is present in 10 to 40 per cent of cases (Fig. 34–44) (Johnston et al., 1977; Lebowitz and Griscom, 1977; Nixon, 1953; Robson et al., 1976; Uson et al., 1968; Williams and Kenawi, 1976). Bilaterality is more commonly found in the newborn or the infant less than 6 months of age (Perlmutter et al., 1980; Snyder et al., 1980). Unilateral and bilateral ureteropelvic junction obstructions affecting members of more than one generation have been reported in several families (Cohen et al., 1978). A dominant autosomal pattern of inheritance with variable penetrance has been suggested but not proven.

Etiology

The exact etiology of ureteropelvic junction obstruction remains an enigma despite investigations along embryologic (Allen, 1973; Osathanondh and Potter, 1963; Ruano-Gil et al., 1975), anatomic (Johnston, 1969; Nixon, 1953), functional (Whitaker, 1975), and histologic (Hanna et al., 1976; Murnaghan, 1958; Notley, 1968) lines. Hydronephrosis is most often due to a narrowing at the ureteropelvic junction (Allen, 1973; Lebowitz and Griscom, 1977). A localized area of developmental arrest, produced by fetal vessels compressing the ureter, has been suggested by Allen (1973) and Osathanondh and Potter (1963). Ruano-Gil and colleagues showed that the embryonic ureter goes through a solid phase with subsequent recanalization. Failure of complete canalization of the upper end of the ureter may be the cause of ureteropelvic junction obstruction.

INTRINSIC. An intrinsic lesion within the ureteropelvic wall may sometimes be the basis of obstruction even in the absence of a gross anatomic cause. Murnaghan (1958) demonstrated an interruption in the development of the circular musculature of the ureteropelvic junction. Whitaker (1975) incorporated these findings and theorized that the renal pelvis cannot effectively create a bolus of fluid at its junction with the ureter when it is not funnel-shaped. During an episode of diuresis, the pelvis distends more and loses its already poorly funneled appearance, so that emptying is further impeded (Whitaker, 1975). Notley (1968) and Hanna and associates (1976) learned from electron microscopic studies of the ureteropelvic junction that the muscle cell orientation is normal, but there is an excessive amount of collagen fibers and ground substance between and around the muscle cells. As a result, muscle fibers are widely separated, and their points of connection, or nexus, are attenuated. Many cells are actually atrophic. These findings are thought to be responsible for a functional discontinuity of the ureteropelvic muscular contractions that result in inefficient emptying and apparent ureteropelvic junction obstruction. Koff and associates (1986) showed in experimentally induced obstructions in dogs that the resistance to flow is fixed and pressure-dependent when an intrinsic obstruction exists, whereas in cases of intrinsic and extrinsic obstruction the exit flow is not related linearly to the intrapelvic pressure. In fact, with increasing pressure during a period of diuresis the exit flow might plateau or even diminish, accentuating the obstruction even more (Koff, 1990).

Less common causes of intrinsic ureteropelvic junction obstruction include valvular mucosal folds (Maizels and Stephens, 1980), persistent fetal convolutions (Leiter, 1979), and upper ureteral polyps (Colgan et al., 1973; Gup, 1975; Thorup et al., 1981; Williams and Kenawi, 1976; Williams et al., 1980).

Congenital folds are a variant of ureteral valves and are common findings in the upper ureter of fetuses after the 4th month of development. These folds may persist until the newborn period (Fig. 34–45). They are mucosal infoldings with an axial offshoot of adventitia that does not flatten when the ureter is distended or stretched (Fig. 34–46). The exterior surface of the ureter has a smooth appearance because of the adventitial bridges (Johnston, 1969). The epithelial folds are secondary to differing growth rates of the ureter and the body of the

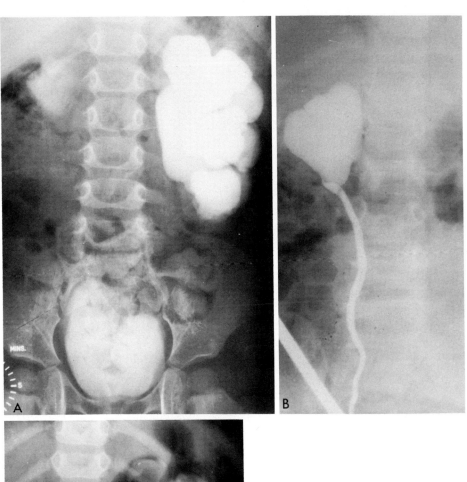

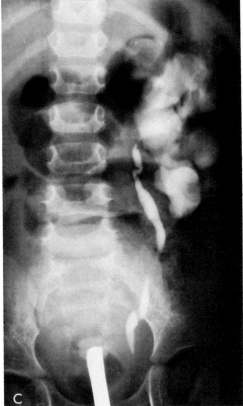

Figure 34–44. *A*, An excretory urogram in a 2-year-old girl with recurrent urinary tract infection demonstrates bilateral ureteropelvic junction obstruction. *B* and *C*, Bilateral retrograde pyelograms confirm the diagnosis.

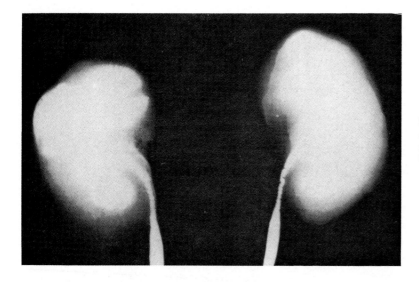

Figure 34–45. Congenital mucosal folds are outlined on a retrograde injection of this specimen taken from an 8-month-old gestational age stillborn fetus. The convolutions do not distend during the injection.

child, with excessive ureteral length occurring early in gestation. This provides a "length reserve" for the ureter, which traverses a shorter distance in the newborn than in the adult (Östling, 1942). Other workers believed that congenital folds may represent a phenomenon similar to the persistence of Chwalla's membrane in the lower ureter, which may subsequently produce a ureteral valve (Mering, et al., 1972). Östling thought that folds were a precursor of actual ureteropelvic junction obstruction because they are frequently discovered in babies who have contralateral ureteropelvic obstructions. Ordinarily, folds are not obstructive and disappear with linear growth (Leiter, 1979). They are rarely seen in the older child or the adult. Exaggerated or persistent fetal folds containing muscle, or high insertion of a valvular

leaflet at the ureteropelvic junction, however, might indeed become obstructive (Maizels and Stephens, 1980). This type of obstruction sometimes can be relieved by dissecting the folds and eliminating the kinking (Johnston, 1969); but, more commonly the ureteral portion containing the valve needs to be excised. Severe vesicoureteral reflux can produce kinking and angulation of the ureter that resembles this picture of fetal folds and may well represent a return to the fetal state. Obstruction at the ureteropelvic junction secondary to severe reflux can be a consequence of this condition.

EXTRINSIC. The most common cause of extrinsic ureteropelvic obstruction is an aberrant, accessory, or early branching vessel to the lower pole of the kidney. These vessels pass anteriorly to the ureteropelvic junc-

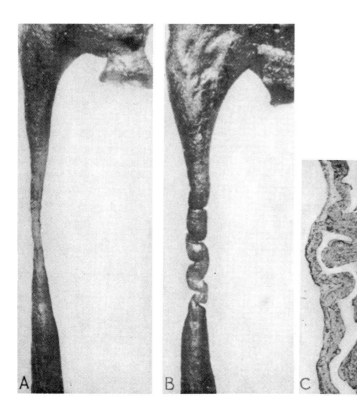

Figure 34–46. Embryologic considerations in the genesis of ureteral fold, kinks, and strictures.

A, Cast of the ureter and the renal pelvis in a newborn. There is physiologic narrowing of the upper ureter below, which is the normal main spindle of the ureter. No ureteral folds are present.

B, Cast of the ureter and the renal pelvis in the newborn. The ureteral folds proceed alternately from the opposite sides.

C, Ureteral kinks that appear as muscular folds with axial offshoots of the loose adventitia. (Courtesy of Dr. Karl Östling.) (From Campbell, M. F.: In Campbell, M. F., and Harrison, J. H. (Eds.): Urology, Vol. 2, 3rd ed. Philadelphia, W. B. Saunders Co., 1970.)

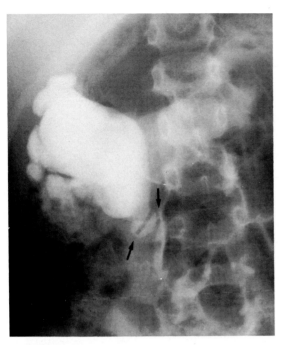

Figure 34–47. A 7-year-old boy with a right ureteropelvic junction obstruction. A retrograde study demonstrates a double kink at the upper end of the ureter. At surgery, the ureter was draped over a vessel to the lower pole.

tion or upper ureter and have been suggested as a cause of obstruction. Nixon (1953) reported that 25 of 78 cases of ureteropelvic obstruction were secondary to vascular compression (Fig. 34–47). The incidence in other series

has varied from 15 to 52 per cent and was found to be the major cause of obstruction in adults (Lowe and Marshall, 1984; Ericsson et al., 1961; Johnston et al., 1977; Stephens, 1982; Williams and Kenawi, 1976). This association has been questioned, however. It is believed by a number of observers that the vessel may well exacerbate a pre-existing intrinsic lesion, because freeing the involved vessel does not always appear to relieve the obstruction. However, there is no doubt that a certain number of ureteropelvic obstructions are vascular in origin. Stephens (1982) has theorized that when an aberrant or accessory renal artery to the lower pole of the kidney is present and the ureter courses behind it, the ureter may angulate at two places—the ureteropelvic junction and the point at which it drapes over the vessel as the pelvis fills and bulges anteriorly. The angulated ureter at the ureteropelvic junction becomes fixed to the pelvis by an array of fascial adhesions. As the ureter arches over the vessel, its lumen is compressed by kinking (Fig. 34–48). Thus, a two-point obstruction is created (Johnston, 1969; Nixon, 1953). Freeing the ureter of its adhesions and lifting it off the vessel allows for the free flow of urine in most cases. Stephens (1982) found no evidence of fibrosis or stricture at these points when this maneuver was performed in his series of patients. In addition, he noted that the lumen had a generous caliber in these so-affected individuals; however, he suggested that with time these areas may become ischemic, fibrotic, and finally stenotic.

SECONDARY. Ureteropelvic obstruction may also be due to severe vesicoureteral reflux, which coexists in 10 per cent of cases. The ureter elongates and develops

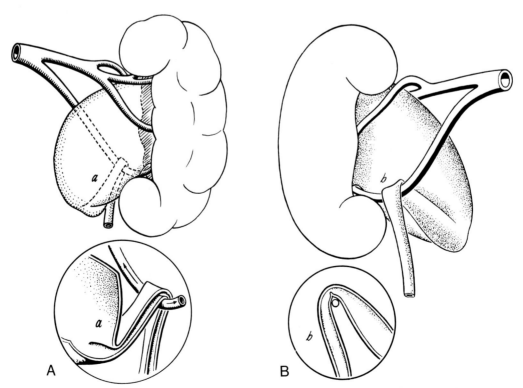

Figure 34–48. The renal pelvis protrudes anteriorly between the middle and lower vessels, angulating the ureteropelvic junction and hooking the ureter over the vessel. A and B are anterior and posterior views, respectively, with insets showing flattening and obstructive mechanisms at the ureteropelvic junction and upper ureter. (From Stephens, F. D.: J. Urol., 128:984, 1982.)

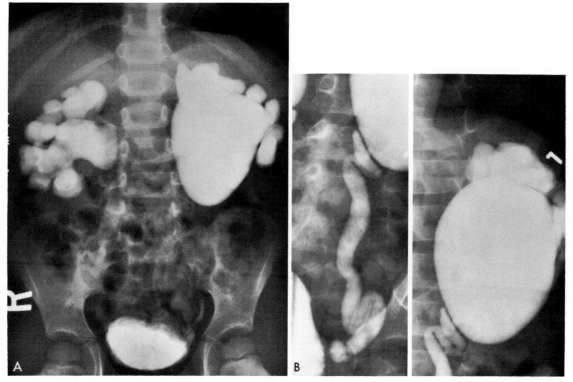

Figure 34–49. A 4-year-old boy with recurrent abdominal pain and episodic low-grade fever had *(A)* an excretory urogram that reveals bilateral ureteropelvic junction obstruction. *B,* A preoperative voiding cystogram demonstrates severe bilateral vesicoureteral reflux with a markedly redundant and kinked left upper ureter producing a secondary ureteropelvic junction obstruction. The milder right-sided obstruction was relieved following correction of the reflux.

a tortuous course in response to the obstructive element of reflux and the ureteropelvic junction area, being a point of fixation, may develop a kink in this area and obstruct secondarily (Fig. 34–49) (Lebowitz and Blickman, 1983). An obstruction may also develop secondary to lower urinary tract obstruction for the same reason (Hutch et al., 1962; Shopfner, 1966).

Associated Anomalies

The incidence of associated congenital anomalies, especially contralateral renal malformations, is high. Another urologic abnormality may be found in almost 50 per cent of affected babies (Lebowitz and Griscom, 1977; Robson et al., 1976; Uson et al., 1968). Ureteropelvic junction obstruction is the most common anomaly encountered in the opposite kidney; it occurs in 10 to 40 per cent of cases (Fig. 34–50). Renal dysplasia and multicystic kidney disease are the next most frequently observed contralateral lesions (Williams and Karlaftis, 1966). In addition, unilateral renal agenesis has been noted in almost 5 per cent of children (Johnston et al., 1977; Robson et al., 1976; Williams and Kenawi, 1976). Ureteropelvic junction obstruction may also occur in the upper or the lower half, usually the lower, of a duplicated collecting system (Amar, 1976; Joseph et al., 1989) (Fig. 34–51) or of a horseshoe or ectopic kidney.

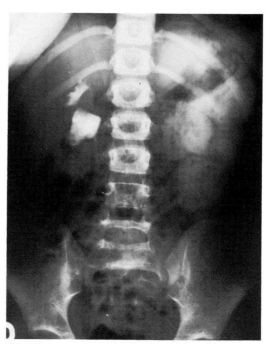

Figure 34–50. An excretory urogram in a 5-year-old girl demonstrates a high-grade obstruction on the left, presumably at the ureteropelvic junction, with a suggestion of a minor ureteropelvic junction obstruction on the right.

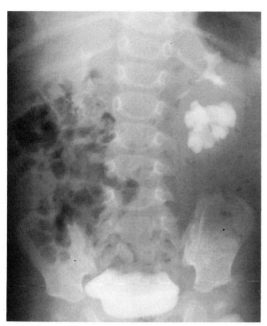

Figure 34–51. This 1-year-old boy with a duplication on the left has an obstruction at the ureteropelvic junction of the lower pole collecting system.

Minor degrees of vesicoureteral reflux have been noted in as many as 40 per cent of affected children (Lebowitz and Blickman, 1983; Juskiewenski et al., 1983; Williams and Kenawi, 1976). Generally, this degree of reflux does not contribute to the upper urinary tract obstruction, subsides spontaneously, and is thought to result possibly from the presence of urinary tract infection. However, more severe grades of reflux may have a profound effect on the ureteropelvic junction area as noted earlier. Anomalies of other organ systems are frequently observed and have no consistent pattern of obstruction. Ureteropelvic junction obstruction was observed in 21 per cent of children with the VATER complex (Uehling et al., 1983).

Symptoms

Ureteropelvic junction obstruction in the neonate or infant used to be discovered as an asymptomatic mass that was palpated on routine physical examination (Johnston et al., 1977; Robson et al., 1976; Williams and Karlaftis, 1966). Nearly 50 per cent of cases were discovered in this manner in the era before ultrasound but that has changed dramatically in the past several years (Brown et al., 1987). It is being diagnosed with increasing frequency prenatally as maternal ultrasonography has gained wide popularity (Fig. 34–52) (Fourcroy et al., 1983). Occasionally, failure to thrive, feeding difficulties, sepsis secondary to urinary tract infection, or pain and hematuria from a calculus in the kidney as a result of stasis have led the pediatrician to suspect the diagnosis and obtain a renal ultrasound or excretory urogram. Urinary tract infection is the presenting sign in 30 per cent of affected children beyond the neonatal period (Snyder et al., 1980). In the older child, intermittent flank or upper abdominal pain, sometimes associated with vomiting, is a prominent symptom (Kelalis et al., 1971; Williams and Kenawi, 1976). Hematuria, which is seen in 25 per cent of the children (Fig. 34–53), may occur following minor abdominal trauma (Kelalis et al., 1971; Williams and Kenawi, 1976). The hematuria is most probably due to rupture of mucosal vessels in the dilated collecting system (Kelalis et al., 1971).

In the young adult, episodic flank pain, especially during diuresis, is a common manifestation. Hypertension has also been noted as a presenting sign of ureteropelvic junction obstruction in both adults and children (Grossman et al., 1981; Johnston et al., 1977; Munoz et al., 1977; Squitieri et al., 1974). The pathophysiology is thought to be due to functional ischemia with reduced renal blood flow, as a result of the enlarged collecting system, producing renin-mediated hypertension (Belman et al., 1968).

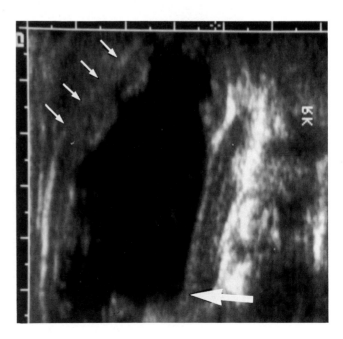

Figure 34–52. A newborn female with a prenatal diagnosis of hydronephrosis underwent confirmatory studies with this postnatal ultrasound. The ureteropelvic junction area is narrow (*single arrow,* lower right) and the parenchyma is thinned (*row of arrows,* upper left). Note the very dilated calyces.

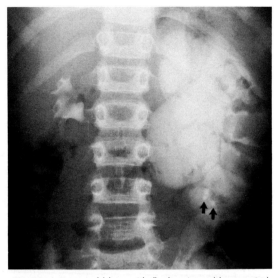

Figure 34–53. A 7-year-old boy with flank pain and hematuria has an obvious ureteropelvic junction obstruction on the left and several stones *(arrows)* in the lowermost calyx, the result of stasis of urine.

Diagnosis

Whenever the diagnosis of hydronephrosis is suspected in a prenatal examination, it must be confirmed by a postnatal examination, preferably performed after the 1st week of life (Grignon et al., 1986). The fetal and neonatal kidney may sometimes mistakenly produce a picture suggesting hydronephrosis on ultrasonography because the pyramids and medullary areas are sonolucent in the immature kidney. The diagnosis may be confirmed by radioisotope scanning in the newborn period and by excretory urography in the somewhat older child. Often, older children with abdominal complaints have a complete gastrointestinal work-up that proves to be normal. The urinary tract is then evaluated as an afterthought.

The excretory urogram reveals a distended renal pelvis and calyces, with an abrupt cutoff at the ureteropelvic junction. It is important to obtain delayed films in order to determine that a hydroureter is not present as well (Lebowitz and Griscom, 1977; Snyder et al., 1980). Severe partial obstruction may be present even when the ureter can be visualized beyond the ureteropelvic junction. The appearance of calyceal crescents is the result of dilated collecting ducts that have become oriented transversely; it is a reliable sign of upper urinary tract obstruction with remarkably recoverable renal function (Fig. 34–54). A retrograde pyelogram performed at the time of surgical correction often helps to delineate the limits of the narrowed area and the anatomy of the entire but especially the upper ureter. Many surgeons believe this radiograph is not needed in most cases, but all agree if it is to be performed, it should be done immediately prior to surgical correction. In the neonatal male, this diagnostic test is not always feasible because of the constraints of urethral size preventing an instrument of adequate caliber to be passed into the bladder.

If the obstruction is equivocal, it is worthwhile to obtain a diuretic renogram. The rate of uptake of the isotope delineates the degree of function, and the washout curve following the administration of furosemide determines the severity of the obstruction (Krueger et

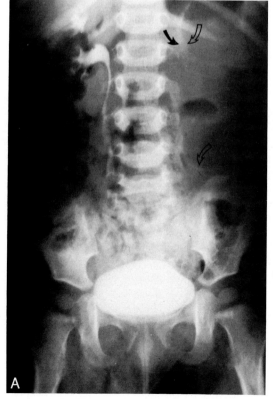

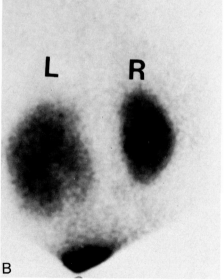

Figure 34–54. *A,* An excretory urogram in a 13-month-old boy with a severe left ureteropelvic junction obstruction. The study shows poor excretion, but several calyceal crescents *(arrows)* are noted. *B,* Despite a poor visualization on excretory urography, a renal scan reveals that the left kidney supplies 35 per cent of the total renal function.

al., 1980; O'Reilly et al., 1979). Kass and colleagues (1985) and Kass and Fink-Bennett (1990) have devised a reliable protocol for assessing obstruction with diuretic renography. Sometimes a patient has intermittent obstruction, which is precipitated only by a diuresis. The individual may have a normal excretory urogram when asymptomatic, but an obstructed one during an episode of pain (Malek, 1983) (Fig. 34–55). To help define these less clear-cut conditions, a fluoroscopic pressure-flow study can be performed by injecting contrast medium through a percutaneously placed nephrostomy tube and recording intrapelvic pressures during the constant infusion (Krueger et al., 1980; Whitaker, 1973). Alternatively, a furosemide-induced diuresis during an excretory urogram or renal scan (Koff, 1982) can be done to determine the efficiency of pelvic emptying (Segura et al., 1974). The diuresis created during the test may also produce flank pain if the patient has given a history of it (Nesbit, 1956). The intermittent nature of the signs and symptoms in these patients is usually associated with a vessel crossing the ureteropelvic junction, causing the obstruction.

It is imperative to obtain a voiding cystourethrogram on every patient with ureteropelvic junction obstruction to rule out the possibility of obstruction secondary to vesicoureteral reflux (Lebowitz and Blickman, 1983; Whitaker, 1976).

Prognosis

As more kidneys with ureteropelvic junction obstructions are being detected in the perinatal period, a debate has raged regarding timing of surgical correction. Early in the 1980s, prenatal decompression was thought to be mandatory if salvageable renal function was hoped for (Manning, 1987). This proved to be unnecessarily aggressive treatment, and now it is universally accepted that early intervention is warranted only in cases of bilateral progressive obstruction associated with increasing oligohydramnios, and even then prenatal treatment is controversial (Mandell et al., 1990).

Several investigators have shown that early but not immediate postnatal intervention is safe, reliable, and effective in allowing the affected kidney to regain a considerable portion of its potentially recoverable renal function (Bernstein et al., 1988; Dowling et al., 1988; Dejter et al., 1988; Perlmutter et al., 1980; King et al., 1984; Roth and Gonzales, 1983). In comparison, Ransley (1990) has shown little deterioration in renal function in children with moderate obstruction followed nonoperatively for 5 to 7 years. These children, however, are undergoing pyeloplasty at an older age because of the secondary effects of obstruction (calculus disease, pain, and urinary infection).

When the diagnosis is not made until later in childhood or in early adulthood, severe chronic obstruction may lead to progressive loss of renal function. With severe stasis and repeated infection, stone formation sometimes occurs. Renin-mediated hypertension secondary to obstruction may also develop.

Even in older individuals most obstructed kidneys can be salvaged by pyeloplasty. A quantitative renal scan using Tc-99m dimercaptosuccinic acid (DMSA) that determines individual renal function is sometimes helpful in deciding whether to do a nephrectomy or pyeloplasty, especially when the excretory urogram reveals a kidney with poor concentrating ability. Most affected kidneys provide at least one third of overall renal function, and these should be saved. Even poorly functioning kidneys will show some improvement after surgery (Belis et al., 1982; Parker et al., 1981). Only rarely will such kidneys have less than 10 per cent of overall renal function at presentation, and these should probably be removed. The techniques of surgical correction are discussed elsewhere in this text.

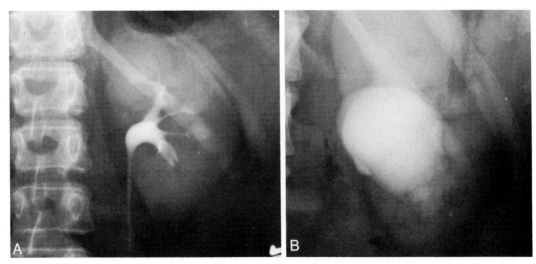

Figure 34–55. *A* and *B,* A 16-year-old boy with intermittent flank pain has a normal collecting system when asymptomatic but severe obstruction when symptomatic.

ANOMALIES OF THE URETER

Anomalies of the ureter may be classified as follows:

I. Anomalies of number
  A. Agenesis
  B. Duplications
      1. Blind-ending duplication
      2. Inverted Y duplication
  C. Triplication and supernumerary ureters
II. Anomalies of structure
  A. Atresia and hypoplasia
      1. Distal ureteral atresia
  B. Megaureter
      1. Reflux
      2. Obstructed
      3. Nonreflux-nonobstructed
      4. Megaureter in prune belly syndrome
      5. Dysplastic
  C. Ureteral stenosis and stricture
  D. Ureteral valves
  E. Spiral twists and folds of the ureter
  F. Ureteral diverticula
  G. Congenital high insertion of the ureter
III. Anomalies of termination
  A. Vesicoureteral reflux
  B. Ectopic ureter
  C. Ureterocele
      1. Simple
      2. Ectopic
IV. Anomalies of position
  A. Vascular anomalies
      1. Accessory renal vessels
      2. Preureteral vena cava
      3. Preureteral iliac artery (retroiliac ureter)
      4. Ovarian vein syndrome
      5. Distal ureteral vascular obstructions
  B. Herniation of the ureter

EMBRYOLOGY

Before the individual conditions are considered in detail, the disordered embryogenesis common to many ureteral anomalies is reviewed. Normal embryology of the kidney and ureter is presented in Chapter 32. The stages of normal embryogenesis are well documented, and there are widely accepted explanations and theories for some of the more common primary ureteral anomalies as well. In a review article, Tanagho (1976) correlated and synthesized these into a unified hypothesis for the development of lower ureteral anomalies. These concepts are used as the basis of the following summary.

Briefly, the ureteral bud normally develops from the mesonephric duct at its "elbow," where the duct swings ventrally and medially to join the cloaca. The segment of mesonephric duct between the ureteral bud and the future urogenital sinus is termed the *combined nephric duct* or the *common excretory duct*. Tanagho also calls it the trigone precursor, as it will become absorbed

progressively into the developing sinus (vesicourethral canal) and contributes mesenchyme to the muscularization of the trigone and underlying detrusor of that area. As the common excretory duct is absorbed into the urogenital sinus, the ureteral bud and mesonephric duct acquire separate openings, with the ureteral bud initially located medial and distal to the mesonephric duct. The two orifices migrate in opposing directions, rotating as they do so. The ureteral orifice migrates cephalad and laterally with the developing vesicourethral canal, and the mesonephric duct crosses over the ureter as it moves medially and caudally. Muscularization of the bladder begins after the orifices are well separated, resulting in a distinct hiatus for each duct.

Variations in the site of origin of the ureteral bud on the mesonephric duct and supernumerary budding explain a variety of ureterorenal anomalies. The anomalous budding, cephalic or caudal, is associated with varying hypoplasia or dysplasia, or both, of the affected renal segment, related in general to the degree of dislocation (Mackie and Stephens, 1975; Schwartz et al., 1981). This hypothesis of embryogenesis will now be applied to vesicoureteral reflux, ureteral duplication, and ectopic ureter.

Vesicoureteral Reflux (Fig. 34–56). In primary reflux the ureteral bud arises more caudally than normally from the mesonephric duct, resulting in a short common excretory duct. Absorption of the short duct is completed early, giving the now separated ureteral duct a longer period to migrate cranially and laterally before completing its movement. As a result, the separation between the ureter and the mesonephric duct is greater than normal and there is a large trigone with superior and lateral ureteral orifices. Because the common duct was short, its mesenchymal contribution to the muscular development of the trigone is decreased. Thus, the trigone is not only large but also poorly muscularized. Because there has been less time for the common mesenchyme to accumulate around the developing ureteral bud, the intramural ureter will also be deficient in musculature.

The ultimate result is a large, poorly muscularized trigone with a poorly fixated, laterally positioned ureteral orifice and decreased musculature of the terminal ureter. Because of the poor attachments of the ureter, the orifice is patulous or gaping and has a deficient submucosal tunnel. The variations encountered clinically in severe vesicoureteral reflux and in altered ureterotrigonal anatomy can be related directly to the degree of dislocation of the ureteral bud toward the urogenital sinus. Additional considerations regarding developmental anatomy in vesicoureteral reflux are found in Chapter 44.

Complete Ureteral Duplication (Double Ureters) (Fig. 34–57). The commonly accepted explanation of duplication is that an additional ureteral bud arises from the mesonephric duct. The bud closest to the urogenital

1402

PRIMARY REFLUX

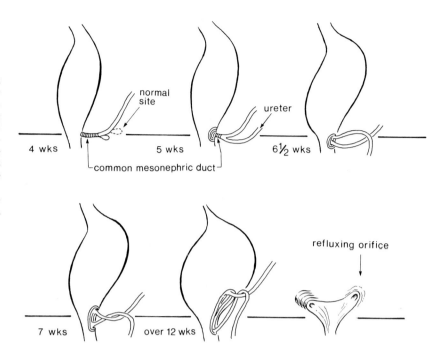

Figure 34–56. Simplified diagram of the changing position of the ureter and mesonephric duct in the development of primary reflux. In Figures 34–56 through 34–59, the caudomedial looping of the distal mesonephric duct against the urogenital sinus, which contributes to its absorption, is omitted to simplify structural relationships. The close position of the ureteral bud to the urogenital sinus results in early absorption into the sinus and more time for cranial and lateral migration of the orifice. (See text.) (Redrawn from Tanagho, E. A.: Embryologic basis for the lower ureteral anomalies: A hypothesis. Urology, 7:451, 1976.)

sinus becomes the lower pole ureter. This bud is absorbed first. The second, higher bud migrates with the mesonephric duct, rotating with it medially and then caudally before it is attached adjacent but distal to the lower pole orifice at the otherwise normal trigonal location following the Weigert-Meyer law. For addi-

tional discussion of the relationship of the ureteral orifices in duplication, see the discussion in this chapter, Duplications of the Ureter.

An alternative theory of the genesis of complete duplication is that of immediate fission of a single (junctional) bud. Just as a bud dividing during its early

URETER DUPLICATION

normal development

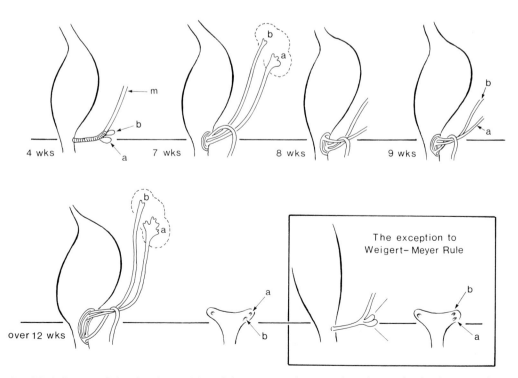

Figure 34–57. Simplified diagram of the changing position of the ureters and mesonephric duct in the development of complete duplication. (Redrawn from Tanagho, E. A.: Embryologic basis for lower ureteral anomalies: A hypothesis. Urology, 7:451, 1976.)

growth results in a bifid ureter, a junctional bud dividing immediately could result in complete duplication, for the common base would ultimately be absorbed into the urogenital sinus after absorption of the common excretory duct is completed. Stephens (1958, 1963) proposes this explanation to account for rarely encountered exceptions of the Weigert-Meyer law (see Fig. 34–61). The attachment of the two orifices to the urogenital sinus occurs somewhat later in this circumstance, providing less time for full rotation of the two ureters (see Duplications of the Ureter in this chapter).

The terms *orthotopic*, referring to the lower pole ureteral orifice, and *ectopic* or *accessory*, referring to the upper pole ureteral orifice, have been in common use despite the fact that at times either or both orifices may occupy a dislocated position. For this reason and to avoid ambiguity, the Committee on Terminology, Nomenclature and Classification of the Section on Urology, American Academy of Pediatrics, has proposed an alternative terminology (Glassberg et al., 1984). The following terms are used throughout this chapter: The kidney with two pyelocalyceal systems is a *duplex kidney*. A *bifid system* relates to two pelves joining at the ureteropelvic junction *(bifid pelvis)* or two ureters joining above the bladder *(bifid ureter)*. Two ureters associated with complete duplication are *double ureters*. The ureter draining the upper pole of a duplex kidney is the *upper pole ureter*, and its orifice is the *upper pole orifice*. Similarly, the lower pole pelvis is drained by the *lower pole ureter*, and its orifice is the *lower pole orifice*.

An *ectopic ureter* is one draining to a site on the proximal lip of the bladder neck or beyond, whether associated with a duplex or a single system. *Lateral ectopia* of a ureteral orifice is one lateral to the normal position. Caudal or medial ectopia of an orifice is one situated at the proximal lip of the bladder neck or beyond. The terminology for ureterocele is also simplified. *Intravesical ureterocele* is located entirely within the bladder. It is usually associated with a single system, uncommonly with an upper pole of a completely duplicated system and, rarely, with a lower pole ureter. *Ectopic ureterocele* has some portion of its structure situated at the bladder neck or in the urethra. Its orifice, however, may be within the bladder, bladder neck, or urethra. Most ectopic ureteroceles are associated with complete duplication, rarely with a single system.

A number of anomalies of ureteral termination associated with double ureters can result from various alterations in the sites of origin of the two ureteral buds. Clinically, reflux via the lower pole orifice into the lower pelvis is the most common anomaly. Here, the first ureteral bud originates too close to the urogenital sinus, and the second or upper pole bud arises from a normal location at the elbow of the mesonephric duct. As a result, the lower pole orifice will be high and lateral, allowing reflux to occur, and the upper pole orifice will terminate more normally on the trigone.

Other combinations can be explained by the same hypothesis. As an example, Figure 34–58 shows the origin of the refluxing lower pole orifice in combination with an ectopic orifice to the bladder neck. In this instance, the two ureteral ducts originate well apart on the mesonephric duct, one caudally and one cranially, and they become widely separated by rotation and migration before muscularization begins, with the result that separate hiatuses form in the bladder musculature.

It is not uncommon to encounter symmetric parenchymal thinning of the lower pole segment of a dupli-

URETER DUPLICATION

reflux and ectopy

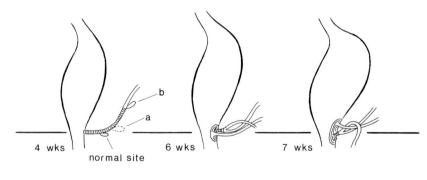

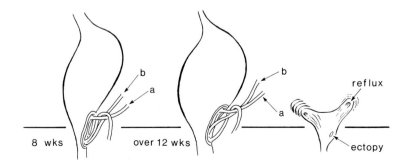

Figure 34–58. Simplified diagram of the changing position of the ureters and mesonephric duct in the development of reflux and ectopia in complete duplication. High origin of the second ureteral bud results in migration with the mesonephric duct before delayed absorption in the ectopic position into the urogenital sinus. (See text.) (Redrawn from Tanagho, E. A.: Embryologic basis for lower ureteral anomalies: A hypothesis. Urology, 7:451, 1976.)

cated ureter in the presence of severe reflux to that unit, and diffuse narrowing is more consistent with segmental primary hypoplasia than scarring. Mackie and associates (1975) and Mackie and Stephens (1975) have related this finding to an abnormality of segmental renal development, specifically to the portion of the nephrogenic ridge encountered by the ureteral bud. A normally positioned bud will strike the normal central portion of the ridge, and a normal kidney will result. A bud caudally or cranially misplaced may strike the poorer lower or upper end zones of nephrogenic ridge, resulting in variable degrees of hypoplasia and dysplasia of the induced renal segment. Schwartz and colleagues (1981) graded hypoplasia and compared this with degrees of lateral or caudal ectopy of the associated ureteric orifice. Despite considerable overlap, the degree of hypodysplasia generally correlates with the degree of orifice ectopia.

Ectopic Ureter (Fig. 34–59). Ectopic termination of a single system or of the accessory ureter in a duplex system can be explained by a high (cranial) origin of the involved ureteral bud from the mesonephric duct. As a result, the ureter migrates for a longer period and for a greater distance while attached to the mesonephric duct before the long common segment is completely absorbed and the ureter separates from it. There is little or no time for migration and ascent of the ureter. In the most extreme case, there is no separation, and in the male the ureter remains attached to the mesonephric duct, i.e., to the ejaculatory duct or to the seminal vesicle, which develops at 13 weeks as a diverticulum from the mesonephric duct (Arey, 1974).

In both sexes, the ectopic ureter can insert along an ectopic pathway (Stephens, 1963) onto the trigone,

bladder neck, or urethra. In both sexes, failure of the ureter to separate from the mesonephric duct results in drainage via the genital tract. In the male, urine drains into mesonephric duct-derived structures and never beyond the normal opening of the future ejaculatory duct, proximal to the external urinary sphincter. In the female, however, urine drains through the genital tract into paramesonephrically (müllerian duct) derived structures—uterus, cervix, and vagina—causing incontinence (Fig. 34–60).

In the female, the mesonephric duct degenerates except for a vestigial remnant, the duct of the epoöphoron, which to a varying degree remains in the medial and distal portion as Gartner's duct. In its full extent, Gartner's duct lies within the muscular wall of the genital tract, extending from the level of the internal cervical os along the lateral or anterolateral vaginal wall to the hymen. Distention of Gartner's duct with urine causes it to rupture through the thin tissue plane between the duct and the developing genital tract, establishing an extraurinary tract for drainage (Ellerker, 1958; Gray and Skandalakis, 1972; Meyer, 1946). The terminal portion of an incontinent ectopic ureter, therefore, might actually include a segment of the common excretory duct, although this is unproved (Ellerker, 1958).

In a patient with a bilateral single-system ectopia into the urethra (a rare lesion), the bladder is small and poorly formed, and the bladder neck is ill defined or nonexistent. Because the mesenchyme from the common excretory duct intended for the muscularization of the trigone and bladder neck region is displaced bilaterally along with the ectopic ureter, these normal structures fail to develop. Embryologic development specific

SINGLE ECTOPIC URETER

Figure 34–59. Simplified diagram of the changing position of the ureter and mesonephric duct in the development of a single ectopic ureter. High origin of the ureteral bud results in migration with the mesonephric duct before delayed absorption in the ectopic position into the urogenital sinus. In bilateral single ectopy, the bladder is small and the bladder neck poorly developed or nonexistent. (See text.) (Redrawn from Tanagho, E. A.: Embryologic basis for lower ureteral anomalies: A hypothesis. Urology, 7:451, 1976.)

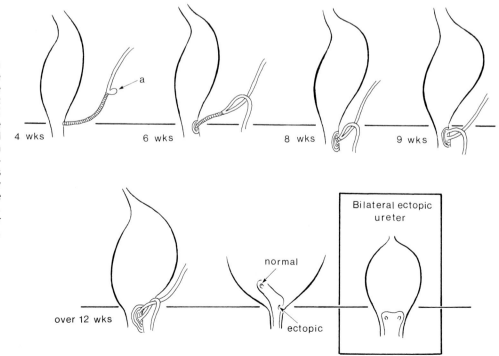

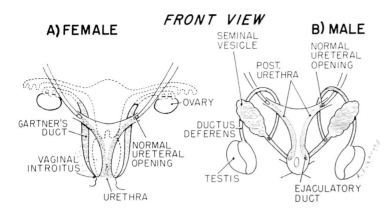

Figure 34–60. Ectopic ureteral orifices in male and female. Stippled and shaded areas indicate sites at which such openings may occur. (From Uson, A. C., and Donovan, J. T.: Am. J. Dis. Child., 98:152, 1959. Copyright 1959, American Medical Association.)

to ureterocele is considered in a further section of this chapter.

ANOMALIES OF NUMBER

Ureteral Agenesis

Bilateral ureteral agenesis can occur, along with bilateral renal agenesis, in monsters with multiple anomalies. Because it is incompatible with life, the condition is a medical curiosity only.

Unilateral ureteral agenesis should in theory indicate complete failure of ureteral bud development and be accompanied by ipsilateral renal agenesis. The hemitrigone will be totally absent because no mesonephric duct or ureteral bud anlage has been absorbed into the urogenital sinus. If some degree of ipsilateral trigonal development is evident, ureteral hypoplasia or atresia may be present (see Atresia and Hypoplasia in this chapter).

Clinically apparent unilateral ureteral agenesis when the hemitrigone is totally absent is not incompatible but actually consistent with the probability of a single-system ectopic ureter on the affected side. The subject of ureteral ectopia is presented in a subsequent section.

Duplications of the Ureter

A duplicated ureter usually drains a duplex kidney (double-collecting system) or, rarely, a normal supernumerary kidney. Ureteral duplications may be classified as *bifid ureter* (partial duplication) or *double ureters* (complete duplication). In complete duplication, a second orifice enters the bladder, urethra, or other structure. Table 34–2 summarizes the gradations in ureteral and renal duplications, excluding ectopia and ureterocele. Duplication is the most common ureteral anomaly, and in many situations it is an incidental finding causing no functional disturbance. However, there is a higher than expected incidence of duplication in cases of urinary infection, and it may be associated with upper urinary tract stasis, obstruction, or reflux. Among the manifestations of double ureters are ectopic insertion of the upper pole ureter and ectopic ureterocele.

INCIDENCE. The reported incidence of ureteral duplication varies widely among different series, depending in part on whether the survey was based on autopsy or clinical data and on the composition of patient material, and on whether or not bifid pelves were separately recorded. As it is generally recognized that clinical series usually contain a disproportionate number of duplication anomalies, unselected autopsy data are more accurate in predicting the true incidence. At least two large autopsy series have provided data not too dissimilar regarding partial and complete ureteral duplication (Campbell, 1970; Nation, 1944) (Table 34–3). Nation (1944) reviewed 230 cases of duplication; 121 of these were clinical. He identified 109 cases in approximately 16,000 autopsies, an incidence of 1 in 147 or 0.68 per cent. Campbell's personal series of 51,880 autopsies in adults, infants, and children included 342 ureteral duplications, an incidence of one in 152 or 0.65 per cent. There were 281 duplications in the 32,834 adults, an incidence of one in 117, or 0.85 per cent, but only 61 of the 19,046 children had this abnormality, one in 312 or 0.32 per cent. Because the anomaly should be found with equal frequency in unselected autopsies on adults or children, Campbell concluded that some of the duplications in children had been overlooked. Combining Nation's autopsy series and Campbell's adult series, the projected incidence of duplication is one in 125 or 0.8 per cent.

Despite a wealth of information about sex differences in the incidence of duplication in clinical series (the anomaly is identified in females at least two times more frequently), there are no reliable data on sex differences in unselected series. Campbell's autopsy data do not document such a difference. Of Nation's 109 autopsy cases, 56 were female and 53 male. However only 40 per cent of the 16,000 autopsies were done in women. Calculating a correction for this difference, one could project a female to male ratio of 1.6 to 1, or 62 per cent. These statistics, however, may not be reliable in view of the small number of cases recorded.

Clinical and autopsy data are in substantial agreement about other aspects of duplication, however (see Table 34–3). Unilateral duplication occurs about six times more often than bilateral, with the right and left sides being involved about equally. Excluding bifid pelvis, there does not appear to be a difference in the literature

Table 34–2. GRADATIONS IN URETERAL AND KIDNEY DUPLICATIONS

Temporal Relationships	Spatial Relationships

Abortive duplication of ureter (early)

Bifid ureter (Incomplete duplication of ureter) (late)

Double ureters (Complete duplication of ureter) (early)

Inverted Y ureter ← Rejoined tips of ureteric buds

Ureteral diverticulum ← Blindly ending branch

Bifid pelvis ← Narrow divergence of ureteric buds

Double pelvis ← Medium divergence of ureteric buds

Supernumerary kidney ← Wide divergence of ureteric buds

From Gray, S. W., and Skandalakis, J. E. (Eds.): Embryology for Surgeons. Philadelphia, W. B. Saunders Co., 1972.

in the incidence of bifid ureter versus double ureters. A small percentage of individuals with bilateral duplications have a mixed condition, i.e., bifid ureter on one side and double ureters on the other.

GENETICS. Evidence exists that duplication may be genetically determined by an autosomal dominant trait with incomplete penetrance (Cohen and Berant, 1976). In parents and siblings of probands with duplication, the incidence of duplication increases from the predicted one in 125 to one in eight (Whitaker and Danks, 1966) or one in nine (Atwell et al., 1974). Two reports of geographic foci suggest environmental factors can also play a role (Barnes and McGeorge, 1989; Phillips et al., 1987).

POSITION OF ORIFICES. In *double ureters* the two orifices are characteristically inverted in relation to the collecting systems they drain. The orifice to the lower pole ureter occupies the more cranial and lateral position and that of the upper pole ureter has a caudal and medial position. This relationship is so consistent that it

has been termed the Weigert-Meyer law, which is based on the original description of Weigert (1877) as modifed by Meyer (1946). When the two orifices are not immediately adjacent, the orifice from the upper pole can be found anywhere along a predictable pathway, which Stephens (1958, 1963) has called the ectopic pathway (Fig. 34–61).

Rare exceptions to the Weigert-Meyer law have been observed, in which the upper pole orifice is cranial, although still medial, to the orthotopic orifice. Stephens collected four examples from the literature and added seven more. The pattern of rotation of the ectopic orifice around the orthotopic orifice in this situation is also shown in Figure 34–61. Stephens studied the positional relationship between the lower portions of the ureters and noted that it too varies according to the terminal position of the upper pole orifice. With the rare cranially placed upper pole orifice, the ureter lies anterior to the lower pole ureter, the ureters being uncrossed. With a medial orifice, the upper pole ureter lies medially; and

Table 34–3. URETERAL DUPLICATION: CLINICAL, RADIOGRAPHIC, AND AUTOPSY STUDIES

Author, Year	Data Base		No. Duplications	Female	Male	Unilateral	Bilateral	Complete	Partial	Unilateral Complete/Partial	Bilateral Complete/Partial	Bilateral Mixed
Archangelski, 1926	110	R A	619 3 (2.7%)			502 (80%)	117 (20%)					
Colosimo, 1938	1500	X	50 (3.3%)	(68%)								
Nation, 1944	16000	A C	109 (0.68%) 121 230 total	* (63%) 88 (73%)	* 33	177 (77%)	53 (23%)	102 (44%)	118 (51%)	78 (44%)/99 (56%)	35 (45%)/19 (36%)	10 (4.3%)
Nordmark, 1948	4744	X	138 (2.8%)			119 (86%)	19 (14%)	70 (51%)	65 (47%)	59/60	11/5	3 (2.1%)
Payne, 1959	5000	C X	141 83	87 (62%)	54	120 (85%)	21 (15%)	45	78 + 18 bifid pelvis			
Johnston, 1961		C A	73 9 82 total	57 (70%)	25			63 (77%)	19 (33%)			
Kaplan and Elkin, 1968	(partial dupls. only)	X	51	33 (65%)	18	43 (84%)	8 (16%)					
Campbell, 1970	51880 (19046 child) (32834 adult)	A	342 (0.65%) 61 (0.32%) 281 (0.85%)			293 (85%)	53 (15%)	101 (30%)			4	"one in five cases"
Timothy et al., 1971		C	46	39 (85%)	7			24 (52%)	16 (35%)	13/15	11/1	6 (13%)
Privett et al., 1976	5196 (1716 child) (3480 adult) (2896 male) (2300 female)	X	91 (1.8%)	63 (66%)	32	79 (85%)	16 (15%)	33 (29%) (but 21 not known)	57 (52%)			

A = Autopsy.
C = Clinical.
R = Review.
X = X-ray.
* = See text.

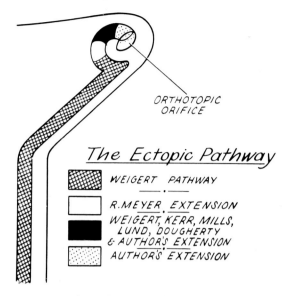

ORTHOTOPIC
ORIFICE

The Ectopic Pathway

WEIGERT PATHWAY

R.MEYER EXTENSION

WEIGERT, KERR, MILLS,
LUND, DOUGHERTY
& AUTHOR'S EXTENSION

AUTHOR'S EXTENSION

Figure 34–61. "Author's extension" refers to Stephens' observations. (Stephens, F. D.: Aust. N. Z. J. Surg., 28:28, 1958.)

with a caudally placed orifice, it spirals in an anterior-to-medial direction around the lower pole ureter as it descends, terminating posterior to the lower pole orifice. Ahmed and Pope (1986) documented a case of uncrossed complete ureteral duplication and reflux into the upper pole, which fits this pattern.

An embryonic hypothesis to explain the exception to the Weigert-Meyer law was proposed by Stephens (1958) and is based on the premise that an upper pole orifice located craniomedially arises from a junctional ureteral bud—one that bifurcated immediately—rather than from a second bud. This hypothesis is presented in detail elsewhere, and the embryology is diagrammed in Figure 34–57.

ASSOCIATED FINDINGS. The distribution of the renal mass drained by each ureter in duplication varies somewhat. About one third of the renal parenchyma is served by the upper collecting system, on the average. In a detailed radiographic review, Privett and associates (1976) reported a number of observations about duplication. The mean total number of calyces for single-system kidneys was 9.4, and for duplex units it was 11.3, with a mean of 3.7 calyces in the upper and 7.6 in the lower collecting systems. These investigators also observed that 97 per cent of the single-system kidneys in their series were radiographically normal, whereas 29 per cent of the duplex units had scarring, dilatation, or both. Reflux also was more common in the duplex units in patients who had voiding cystograms. Two of 17 nonduplex units refluxed (12 per cent) compared with 13 of 31 duplex units (42 per cent).

Hydronephrosis of the lower pole segment is not infrequent and is generally associated with severe reflux into that unit. However, primary ureteropelvic junction obstruction can involve the lower pelvis (Christoffersen and Iversen, 1976; Dahl, 1975; Johnston, 1961; Privett et al., 1976).

Other anomalies are encountered with increased frequency. In Nation's (1944) series, 27 (12 per cent) had other urinary tract anomalies, with just over half of

these being on the same side. The anomalies included renal hypoplasia and aplasia (today probably termed dysplasia) and various ureteral anomalies, among them ectopic insertion of the upper pole ureter in four cases (3 per cent of the complete duplications). Coexisting urologic anomalies were encountered in 129 of Campbell's (1970) series of 342 duplications. Nonurologic anomalies were found in 63 cases. These were not recorded in detail, but most of the urologic anomalies were, as in Nation's series, a variety of ipsilateral renal and ureteral lesions; 22 were anomalies of the contralateral kidney. The nonurologic lesions mainly involved the gastrointestinal tract plus a few cardiopulmonary lesions. Both these series, however, were autopsy series. Rarely, the pelvocalyceal systems communicate, presumably from late fusion of the ureteral buds during pelvocalyceal expansion (Beer and Mencher, 1938; Braasch, 1912).

The increased incidence of duplications in investigations of childhood urinary infections is well established. Campbell (1970) reported a personal series of 1102 children with pyuria, 307 of whom proved to have ureteropelvic anomalies. Of these, 82 (27 per cent) were duplications or 7.5 per cent of the total group. Kretschmer (1937) reviewed 101 cases of hydronephrosis in infancy and childhood and noted 24 renoureteral anomalies, over half of which were duplications.

Based on three cases of duplication with some form of ureteral ectopy, coexistent renal dysplasia, and nodular renal blastema, Cromie and colleagues (1980) raised the possibility that this pattern of findings might be more than a coincidental association, accounting for an increased risk of neoplasm (Pendergrass, 1976). This concept deserves further investigation.

Bifid ureter is often clinically unimportant, but stasis and pyelonephritis do occur. When the Y junction is extravesical, free to-and-fro peristalsis of urine from one collecting system to the other may appear, with preferential retrograde waves passing into slightly dilated limbs instead of down the common stem. This results in stasis that is more marked when the Y junction is more distal, when the bifid limbs are wide, or when the Y junction is large. Increased urinary reprocessing from vesicoureteral reflux may enhance this phenomenon, and loin pain can result. About one quarter of the patients studied with nuclear renography by O'Reilly and co-workers (1984) had significant urodynamic abnormalities. Treatment by ureteroneocystostomy is effective when the junction is sufficiently close to the vesical wall that resection of the common sheath or common stem will permit placement of both orifices within the bladder. Reimplantation of the common stem may be effective when vesicoureteral reflux is severe and the Y junction is higher up. In the absence of reflux, ureteropyelostomy or pyelopyelostomy with resection of one ureteral limb, preferably the upper limb, down to the Y junction, is effective in eliminating regurgitation of urine (Kaplan and Elkin, 1968; Lenaghan, 1962).

Blind-Ending Duplication of the Ureter

Rarely, a ureteral duplication does not drain a renal segment, hence, the term blind-ending. Less than 70 of these have been reported, although they occur considerably less infrequently than the published data indicate. Most blind-ending ureteral duplications involve one limb of a bifid system; even more unusual is one involving a complete duplication (Szokoly et al., 1974; Jablonski et al., 1978). Although the Y junction in the bifid type may be at any level, most are found in the mid- or distal ureter. Blind-ending segments are diagnosed three times more frequently in women than in men and twice as often on the right side (Albers et al., 1971; Schultz, 1967). The condition has been reported in twins (Bergman et al., 1977) and in sisters (Aragona et al., 1987).

Many of these blind segments cause no problems. Symptomatic patients mostly complain of vague abdominal or chronic flank pain, sometimes complicated by infection or calculi, or both (Marshall and McLoughlin, 1978). The majority of cases are not diagnosed until the third or fourth decade of life.

As the blind segment does not always fill on excretory urography, retrograde pyelography may be required for diagnosis (Fig. 34–62). At times, however, urinary stasis from disordered peristalsis (ureteroureteral reflux) may be demonstrated (Lenaghan, 1962), with secondary dilatation of the branch. This may be the cause of the pain (van Helsdingen, 1975). As the lesion is more common in women and on the right side, the propensity for dilation of the right urinary tract with pregnancy might explain the relatively late age at onset of symptoms.

EMBRYOLOGY. The embryogenesis of blind-ending ureteral duplication is similar to that for duplications in general. It is postulated that the affected ureteral bud is abortive and fails to make contact with the metanephros. Histologically, the blind segment contains all normal ureteral layers. Anatomically, the blind end tends to have a bulbous dilatation. Most of these blind segments are not surrounded by any abortive renal tissue, but in a few segments there is a fibrous stalk (ureteral atresia), extending into a dysplastic renal segment. The blind limb may vary from a short stump of a few centimeters to one extending all the way into the renal fossa.

The area of union between the two limbs is invested in a common sheath that may be attenuated proximally. The blind segment and the adjacent normal ureter share a common blood supply (Albers et al., 1968; Peterson et al., 1975). When the surgery is necessary, excision of the blind segment is indicated. Because the ensheathment is less dense at the upper or proximal end, the dissection should start there. Care should be taken to denude only the blind segment and not to enter the normal ureter. Some investigators suggest leaving a short stump at the junction with the common stem (Peterson et al., 1975; Rao, 1975).

Diverticula of the ureter have also been described. Controversy in the literature exists about the distinction between some diverticula and blind-ending duplications. In most cases, it may simply be a matter of terminology. For example, Campbell (1936) described a case of a finger-like extension from the lower ureter that he called a ureteral diverticulum, but he ascribed it developmentally to an abortive duplication. Similarly, Youngen and Persky (1965) labeled as a diverticulum a tubular, finger-like appendage from the pelvis but also ascribed its

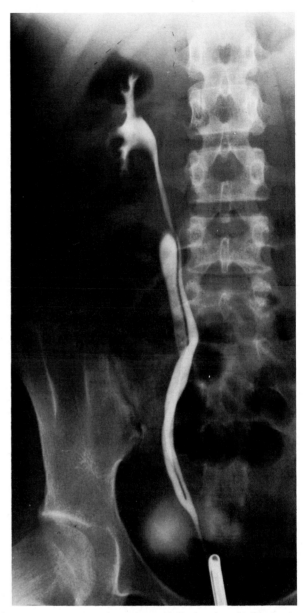

Figure 34–62. Retrograde pyelogram. Blind-ending duplication in an 18-year-old girl noted in evaluation of transitory hematuria. Only the distal portion of this blind-ending duplication has been visualized on intravenous pyelogram.

origin to an abortive budding. Rank and co-workers (1960) and Gray and Skandalakis (1972) agree that congenital ureteral diverticula have the same embryogenesis as blind duplications. Gray and Skandalakis specifically note that a diverticulum from the mid- or distal ureter originates as a blind ureteral duplication, whereas a diverticulum from the ureteropelvic area represents a primitive calyx that has failed to meet nephrogenic mesenchyme. Sarajlic and colleagues (1989) believe that all these lesions should be described as congenital diverticula.

For some investigators, the distinction between a diverticulum and blind-ending ureter is one of morphology—the typical blind-ending ureteral segment of a Y ureter joining the normal ureter at an acute angle and extending upward parallel to the normal ureter. It is at least twice as long as it is wide (Culp, 1947). A congenital diverticulum, in comparison, has a ballooned appearance. Histologically, both are similar, and both arise from disordered ureteral budding. Additional descriptions of ureteral diverticula are presented in a subsequent section.

Inverted Y Ureteral Duplication

This is the rarest of the anomalies of ureteral branching. It consists of two ureteral limbs distally that fuse proximally to become a single channel draining the kidney. This condition is more common in females. One of the distal ureteral limbs not uncommonly ends in an ectopic ureter or ureterocele (Beasley and Kelly, 1986; Harrison and Williams, 1986; Ecke and Klatte, 1989; Klauber and Reid, 1972; Mosli et al., 1986). In several cases, one distal segment was atretic (Britt et al., 1972; Suzuki et al., 1977). In one case of bilateral inverted Y duplication in a 12-year-old girl, there was an atretic distal limb on each side, each with a calculus (Suzuki et al., 1977).

The embryology of inverted Y ureteral duplication is ascribed to two separate ureteral buds whose tips coalesce and fuse into a single duct before joining the metanephros. The frequently ectopic position of one limb is caused by widely separated buds on the mesonephric duct, with the second bud relatively cephalad. To explain the distal atresia of the ectopic limb in their case, Britt and associates (1972) offered two possibilities. One is failure of Chwalle's membrane to rupture. The second, also postulated by Hawthorne (1936), is atresia of the wolffian duct—a normal regression in the female—prior to absorption of the too cephalad second ureteral bud into the urogenital sinus distally. Bingham (1986) reported a woman with a single right ureter that divided into two segments and then rejoined, showing the features of a bifid ureter distally and an inverted Y proximally. He postulated a split of the ureteral bud after beginning migration, which then refused before entering the metanephros.

Treatment is directed toward any problems resulting from an ectopic limb, generally resection of the accessory channel.

Ureteral Triplication and Supernumerary Ureters

Just as two buds from the mesonephric duct or premature fission of a single bud can explain double and bifid ureters, so the presence of three buds from the mesonephric duct or two with early fission of one of them can explain rarely encountered complete and partial triplications (Marc et al., 1977). Most investigators use the classification of Smith (1946). He classified four varieties of triplicate ureter:

1. Complete triplication—three ureters from the kidney with three draining orifices to the bladder, urethra, or elsewhere.

2. Incomplete triplication—a bifid ureter plus a single ureter, with three ureters from the kidney and two orifices draining below.

3. Trifid ureter—all three ureters unite and drain through a single orifice. This appears to be the most common form encountered.

4. Two ureters from the kidney, one becoming an inverse Y bifurcation, resulting in three draining orifices below.

In one apparently unique case, Fairchild and associates (1979) reported a typical bifid system with a third, lateral ureter that appeared to communicate with the lower pole calyx.

Triplication has been reported with renal fusion anomalies (Golomb and Ehrlich, 1989; Pode et al., 1983). Patients with triplication also may, of course, present with symptoms and signs of reflux or obstruction, ureterocele (Arap et al., 1982; Finkel et al., 1983; Juskiewenski et al., 1987; Rodo Salas et al., 1986), or ectopia, as in duplication anomalies. Treatment is based on the same principles as those for duplication anomalies (see Chapter 45).

ANOMALIES OF STRUCTURE

Atresia and Hypoplasia

Atresia and hypoplasia of the ureter are both caused by varying degrees of failure of ureteral bud development. The trigone on the same side may appear normal or hypoplastic and have a tiny dimple for an orifice (total atresia). A fibrous stalk may represent the ureter, or there may be a hypoplastic or normal ureteral segment of varying length that terminates blindly or in an atretic segment (fibrous stalk) capped by some form of an anomalous dysplastic renal remnant. In ureteropelvic atresia with a multicystic kidney, the fibrous segment may contain a minute lumen (Mackie, 1977).

In a study of the morphology of instrinsic ureteral lesions in infants and children derived from both autopsy and clinical sources, Cussen (1971) noted five of 147 dilated ureters that had atretic segments below the dilated areas. The lumen and its epithelium were absent for a distance of 0.5 to 5 cm, and the ureter was replaced by a fibrous strand, sometimes surrounded by a peripheral band of smooth muscle. Distal to the lesion, the morphology of the ureter was normal in every case.

When atresia involves the ureteropelvic area only, a multicystic dysplastic kidney caps the atretic segment (see Chapter 35). Ureteral atresia of longer lengths or lower positions will alter the prognosis. In 29 cases of congenital multicystic dysplastic kidneys, De Klerk and colleagues (1977) noted that 13 of 14 infants with isolated ureteropelvic atresia had no contralateral renal anomalies, the one exception being a simple cyst. In contrast, six of 15 infants with a lower level or long segment ureteral atresia with or without associated pelvic atresia had contralateral renal anomalies, generally multicystic dysplasia or hydronephrosis. Only seven of the 15 survived 1 year.

Ureteral hypoplasia involving the entire ureter is a part of the spectrum of ureteral atresia. Hydronephrosis was associated in three cases reported by Allen and Husmann (1989) with significant renal dysplasia and minimal function. The ureter itself may not be reconstructible.

Segmental atretic lesions involving the ureter, regardless of the associated renal anomaly, are apparently related to defective development of the ureteral bud.

Blind-ending single ureters per se that are associated with segmental ureteral atresia should cause no symptoms and generally require no treatment. Treatment should be directed toward any contralateral disease. In some institutions, patients who have palpable but otherwise asymptomatic multicystic kidneys with ureteropelvic atresia are being followed nonoperatively without any difficulty, at least on short-term basis (Vinocur et al., 1988).

Distal Ureteral Atresia

The term distal ureteral atresia is preferred to blind-ending ureter, which has been used as a synonym for atresia of the proximal ureter (Campbell, 1970) but also can be used to describe atresia at the distal end. Here, the ureter has developed proximally and blindly ends distally, at an orthotopic or ectopic position relative to the bladder base. Maldevelopment occurs early in the formation of the ureter. If it occurs after the onset of urinary secretion, a greatly dilated cystic or tubular segment of ureter and nonfunctioning kidney may be present. The surgical importance lies in the differential diagnosis of a cystic mass, often detected antenatally and palpable postnatally. The mass may be of spectacular size and may displace other viscera. Cystography,

ultrasonography, and renal scan are aids to diagnosis. At times, gastrointestinal contrast studies will be helpful. Surgical exploration may be the ultimate diagnostic test as well as definitive therapy. With ectopic termination, a duplicated segment may be involved, and ipsilateral lower pole may be obstructed from the mass (Gordon and Reed, 1962; Kornblum and Ritter, 1939; Slater, 1957; Uson et al., 1972).

Megaureters

The term megaureter simply means a large ureter. Caulk (1923) first described a condition he called megalourecter in a young woman with a disporportionately dilated ureter almost to the ureterovesical junction and a near-normal pyelocalyceal system. Most typically, a megaureter of this type has minimal or no tortuosity and is not associated with a demonstrable anatomic obstruction, although because the ureter appears to be obstructed at its lower end, it has given rise to terms such as ureteral achalasia (Creevy, 1970), primary obstructive megaureter (Williams and Hulme-Moir, 1970), aperistaltic distal ureteral segment, and functionally obstructed megaureter. Disagreements about terminology and differences in interpretation of morphologic observations have caused confusion in the literature. However, studies of ureteral structure and ultrastructure help in our understanding of the manifestations and pathophysiology of megaureter.

Gradually the term megaureter has acquired a wide usage so that it now includes a variety of secondary as well as primary lesions, despite the opinion of some that it should be limited to the functionally obstructed condition. A review of the subject of megaureter, including

Table 34–4. A PROPOSED CLASSIFICATION

	Megaureter (Wide) Examples				
Reflux Megaureter		**Obstructed megaureter**		**Nonreflux-nonobstructed megaureter**	
Primary	Secondary	Primary	Secondary	Primary	Secondary
Primary reflux megaureter †Prune-belly	Urethral obstruction Neuropathic bladder	Intrinsic obstruction: -stenosis -adynamic segment	Urethral obstruction Neuropathic bladder Extrinsic obstruction: -retroperitoneal tumor	‡Nonreflux-nonobstructed megaureter	Polyuria Infection / Remaining wide after relief of distal obstruction

E X A M P L E S

Adapted from Report of Working Party to Establish an International Nomenclature for the Large Ureter. *In* Bergsma, D., and Duckett, J. W. (Eds.): Urinary system malformations in children. Birth Defects: Original Article Series, *13*, No. 5. New York, Alan R. Liss for The National Foundation—March of Dimes, 1977.

†Some conditions (e.g., prune-belly, ureteroceles, ectopic ureters) may appear under several other columns.

‡As proved not to be obstructed.

Note: An occasional megaureter may show reflux and apparent obstruction.

a classification developed at the International Pediatric Urologic Seminar in 1976 (Smith, 1977), has provided the practicing urologist with a workable classification (Table 34–4). Examples of the various kinds of megaureters as listed are not intended to be complete. The remainder of this section describes mainly the various forms of primary megaureter as outlined in Table 34–4.

Table 34–5 summarizes a review by Stephens (1974) of the changes of muscular hyperplasia and hypertrophy in various forms of megaureter, compared with the normal. The data were derived from studies by Cussen (1967a, b, 1971), who used a graph-and-grid technique to quantitate numbers of muscle cells and their size per unit area.

Reflux Megaureter

Reflux megaureter can be a manifestation of primary reflux or of secondary elevated intravesical pressure. No site of obstruction exists in primary reflux megaureter in contrast to primary obstructed megaureter, although its cystographic appearance resembles the intravenous pyelogram (IVP) of the latter. The degree of muscular hypertrophy and hyperplasia is less (see Table 34–5). Additional descriptions of reflux megaureter can be found in Chapter 44.

Obstructed Megaureter

The primary form of obstructed megaureter is associated most commonly with a distal adynamic segment (the functionally obstructed megaureter), but infrequently it is linked with a demonstrable anatomic obstruction (stenosis). The typical radiographic appearance is that of a dilated upper ureter without appreciable tortuosity that becomes progressively widened distally. The most distal portion has a marked fusiform or bulbous dilatation, which abruptly changes into a short, undilated ureteral segment, 0.5 to 4 cm in length, which enters the bladder (Pfister et al., 1971; Williams and Hulme-Moir, 1970).

Despite the ureteral dilatation, the calyces generally are normally cupped, and the pelvis is normal or somewhat plump. Renal function usually remains near normal, and radiographic visualization is good.

Fluoroscopic study shows disturbed peristalsis, with failure of at least the more distal portion of the dilated segment to coapt, during contraction, behind the bolus of contrast material. This causes much of the bolus to be regurgitated into the upper ureter after reaching the bottom of the dilated segment, simulating or inducing reverse peristalsis, and only a small portion passes through the undilated segment into the bladder. The result is a churning or "yo-yo" effect (Pfister et al., 1971). However, retrograde catheterization of the undilated segment generally is unimpeded and fails to confirm any anatomic obstruction, although in a minority of cases some narrowing is present (Williams and Hulme-Moir, 1970). If untreated, the condition can at times progress, with development of advancing hydronephrosis and increasing ureteral dilatation and tortuosity (Williams and Hulme-Moir, 1970). Occasionally, reflux to a varying degree will occur into a primary obstructed megaureter (Blickman and Lebowitz, 1984). In this situation, the orifice is variably anomalous, consistent with reflux.

Primary obstructed megaureter occurs 3.5 to 5 times more often in males. It is two to three times more common on the left side, and is bilateral in 15 to 25 per cent of patients. In a few cases, there is contralateral agenesis or dysplasia (Johnston, 1967; Pfister et al., 1971; Williams and Hulme-Moir, 1970). Rarely, megaureter coexists with ureteropelvic junction obstruction (McGrath et al., 1987; Waltzer, 1983). Familial megaureter has been described in a mother and her adult daughter and is exceedingly rare (Tatu and Brennan, 1981).

PATHOLOGY. A number of histologic findings in the undilated segment and the adjacent portion of the dilated ureter have been described by different investigators. Some specimens appear normal by light microscopy, whereas in others the musculature of the proximal end of the undilated segment may be disorganized, abnormal, or absent. An excessive amount of circular fibers has been described (Murnaghan, 1957; Tanagho et al., 1970). The ureteral musculature is normally organized in a felt-like network of opposing helixes except for the mainly longitudinal pattern of the intramural segment. In some megaureters, the undilated distal segment has an excessively tight helix, which results in a predominantly circular orientation (Hanna et al., 1976b; McLaughlin et al., 1973).

In many cases, the area of abrupt transition between the dilated and normal-size ureter shows faulty muscular development, with a segment partially or completely deficient in muscle. The muscle that is found is maloriented. An excessive amount of collagen tends to occur within the undilated segment of ureter and in its adventitia as well (Gregoir and Debled, 1969; MacKinnon et al., 1970).

Regardless of whether or not light microscopic studies show obvious pathology, ultrastructure studies have

Table 34–5. MUSCLE HYPERTROPHY AND HYPERPLASIA IN LARGE URETERS

Disorder	No. Ureters	Hypertrophy (Cell Size)	Hyperplasia (Cell Density)
Obstruction			
intrinsic ureteral	129	2 to 3 times normal	3 to 5 times normal
urethral	72	3 to 5 times normal	5 to 50 times normal
Reflux		slight; normal range	slight; 1 to 3 times normal
Idiopathic megaureter	18	slight; normal range	none

From Stephens, F. D.: Idiopathic dilations of the urinary tract. J. Urol., 112:819, 1974.

consistently revealed an increase in collagen between the muscle bundles of the obstructing segment and between the individual muscle cells (Hanna et al., 1976b; Notley, 1972). The adjacent muscle cells in the most distal portion of the dilated segment are abnormal ("sick") as well (Hanna et al., 1976b). Hanna and his associates noted a progressive improvement in muscle cell morphology extending more proximally up the dilated portion of the megaureter; muscular hypertrophy and hyperplasia are quite marked (see Table 34–5) (Cussen, 1971; Hanna et al., 1976b). In the absence of an anatomic stenosis, obstruction may be due to failure of peristaltic transmission through the distal ureteral segment. Although various workers have blamed this on a preponderance of circular fibers, increased collagen, or focal muscle absence, the common mechanism appears to be attenuation or frank disruption of muscular continuity, either grossly or at the cellular level; this separates nexus and thus prevents spread of the action potential (Hanna et al., 1976b).

Hofmann and colleagues (1984) reported increased acetylcholinesterase activity in the juxtavesical segment of obstructed megaureters adjacent to the narrow segment. Hertle and Nawrath (1985) observed an altered (tonic) response to norepinephrine in isolated strips of obstructed megaureter as opposed to increased phasic activity of normal ureters. They ascribed this response to an increased fraction of intracellularly stored calcium in megaureters.

Tokunaka and Koyanagi, with various other associates, have published a series of articles involving light and electron microscopic studies in nonrefluxing megaureter, further defining the pathogenesis of the condition (Tokunaka et al., 1980, 1982, 1984; Tokunaka and Koyanagi, 1982). They identified two groups of nonrefluxing megaureters: a larger group (group 1), with relatively normal histopathology of the dilated segment and abnormalities limited to the intravesical segment; and a smaller group (group 2), with abnormalities involving the dilated portion of the ureter. In group 1, the abnormal findings of the intravesical ureter included deranged muscle bundle orientation and increased connective tissue. A generously developed ("bulky") periureteral sheath appeared to contribute to obstruction, especially with bladder filling. The kidneys of these megaureters were normal or showed hydronephrosis without dysmorphism. In group 2, the length of the distal narrowed segment was variable, in some cases extending extravesically. Histology was normal. The dilated portion of the ureter, in contrast, was abnormal with a marked reduction of muscle cells, which were small and widely separated in a collagen matrix. Muscle bundles were absent, nexus were attenuated, and no thick myofilaments were present. Extending ultrastructure observations to a variety of congenital disorders, this group reported muscle dysplasia in the dilated portion of the ureter in different kinds of megaureters: eight of 34 nonrefluxing megaureters, one of 22 refluxing megaureters, and four of 23 single system and four of nine duplex ectopic ureters. Extensive dysplasia of the entire ureter was associated with severe renal dysplasia or hypoplasia. For single and duplex ureteroceles, in all but one case, muscle dysplasia was limited to the ureterocele dome (present in 17 of 19 cases) and spared the involved ureter.

In the secondarily obstructed megaureter from posterior urethral valves, muscular hypertrophy and hyperplasia tend to be more marked than in intrinsic obstruction (see Table 34–5). In either case, the hypertrophy and hyperplasia are a response to an increased workload and appear in utero.

The favorable results often achieved with corrective surgery of obstructed megaureter in infancy may be related to the greater number of mesenchymal cells still present at that age that can continue to differentiate into muscle postoperatively. Chronic or recurrent infection may damage the muscle cells of the megaureter, altering the expected histologic findings and interfering with muscle cell function (Hanna et al., 1977).

Nonreflux-Nonobstructed Megaureter (Idiopathic Megaureter)

The primary form is quite uncommon and appears to be a developmental variant wherein the ureteral bud widens excessively during its differentiation, resulting in a large caliber ureter. The ureteral enlargement can be segmental (Mandell et al., 1986). Characteristically, a normal-appearing pyelocalyceal system drains into a wide ureter without evidence of anatomic or functional obstruction. Uncommonly, megacalycosis is associated (Gittes and Talner, 1972; Mandell et al., 1986; Von Neiderhausern and Tuchschmid, 1971). Intraluminal pressures remain in the normal range during physiologic flow rates and during perfusion studies (Hanna and Edwards, 1972; Whitaker, 1973). Muscular hypertrophy is negligible, and there is no hyperplasia (see Table 34–5) (Cussen, 1971).

Megaureter in Prune-Belly Syndrome

The dilated ureter in this condition has features that make it relatively unique. It is most often nonobstructed. Reflux is usually but not invariably present. A diffuse and variable abnormality of the ureteral musculature consists of a marked decrease in muscle bundles. Patchy areas may be noted, in which fibrous tissue has replaced muscle. The individual muscle bundles are surrounded by increased amounts of collagen. The individual muscle cells are also abnormal—there is a developmental myopathy, with ultrastructural studies showing attenuation of myofilaments (Hanna et al., 1977; Palmar and Tesluk, 1974; Williams and Burkholder, 1967) (see also Chapter 48).

Dysplastic Megaureter

This condition possibly belongs in a category of miscellaneous primary or acquired lesions. Hanna and associates (1977) studied two such ureters associated with dysplastic renal segments by light and electron microscopy. In addition to a marked unit reduction in muscle cells, an increase in inflammatory cells and collagen was seen. The individual muscle cells were severely abnormal, with marked atrophy and various degenerative changes. These investigators could not determine whether the findings were related to underdevelopment or to deterioration from repeated infections.

Tokunaka and colleagues (1984) studied muscle dysplasia, also using light and electron microscopy, in nonreflux and reflux megaureters, ureteroceles, and ectopic ureters from single and double systems. They defined ureteral muscle dysplasia as small, smooth muscle cells widely separated with connective tissue (collagen), attenuated nexus, and a lack of thick myosin filaments. They found muscle dysplasia in each category of megaureter studied, although the incidence varied by category. They noted, like Hanna, that extensive dysplasia involving the length of the ureter was associated with a high incidence of renal dysmorphism. Huang (1987) reported 21 cases of giant megaureter with muscular disorganization or dysplastic and variable renal hypodysplasia or relatively mild hydronephrosis for the degree of ureteral enlargement.

The management of megaureter and additional details of evaluation are presented elsewhere in this text.

Ureteral Stenosis and Stricture

Congenital anatomic narrowing or narrowing of the ureteral lumen as detected by calibration is referred to as congenital ureteral stenosis and congenital ureteral stricture, but developmentally the term "stricture" should refer only to obstructions involving a histologic lesion in the ureter. Cussen (1971), in his series of 147 ureteral lesions, noted 81 (55 per cent) with ureteral stenosis. His histologic studies of the stenotic zone revealed normal transitional epithelium, a diminished population of otherwise normal-appearing smooth muscle cells, and no increase in fibrous tissue in the wall of the stenotic zone. Ultrastructure studies were not done.

The cause of congenital ureteral stenosis is not certain, but ultrastructure studies such as those of Notley (1972) and Hanna and associates (1976 and 1977) may provide the answer. Developmentally, simple narrowing probably results from a disturbance in embryogenesis around the 11th to 12th week, with disturbed development of the mesenchyme contributing to the ureteral musculature (Allen, 1977). A spectrum of histologic abnormalities, with or without demonstrable anatomic narrowing, may occur at the zone of obstruction (Hanna et al., 1976b). The reader is referred to the previous discussion of megaureter for a description of the reported ultrastructure abnormalities.

Three areas of the ureter are particularly liable to ureteral stenosis. They are, in order of decreasing frequency, the distal ureter just above the ureterovesical junction, the ureteropelvic junction, and, rarely, the midureter at the pelvic brim (Allen, 1970; Campbell, 1952). More than one area of segmental stenosis may be present in the same ureter with a widened length of ureter between the segments, suggesting a developmental defect that affects the entire ureteral bud.

The clinical manifestations and treatment of ureteral stenoses and strictures involving the ureteropelvic junction are included in the section in this chapter on ureteropelvic junction obstruction and elsewhere in this text.

Ureteral Valves

Ureteral valves are uncommon causes of ureteral obstruction consisting of transverse folds of redundant mucosa that contain smooth muscle (Wall and Wachter, 1952). These are single annular or diaphragmatic lesions with a pinpoint opening (Figs. 34–63 and 34–64). The ureter is dilated above the obstruction and normal below it. As determined in a review of 40 congenital ureteral valves, ureteral valves are distributed throughout the length of the ureter, although least commonly in the middle third or at the pelviureteral junction (Dajani et al., 1982).

Transverse, nonobstructing mucosal folds are present in 5 per cent of ureters in newborns and gradually disappear with growth (Wall and Wachter, 1952). They may be one of the normal findings described by Östling (1942) and Kirks and associates (1978). Cussen (1971, 1977) has identified what he terms ureteral valves in 46 of 328 abnormal ureters from infants and children at surgery or at autopsy. Unlike the diaphragmatic valves described previously, these are cusps demonstrated by perfusing the upper ureter with fixative, dilating the lumen, flattening the mucosa, and accentuating the valves. In a patient with valvular obstruction, Cussen noted that the long axis of the distal ureter was eccentric relative to the long axis of the dilated proximal segment, with the fold being an eccentric cusp (Fig. 34–65). He also noted that these flaps could be found in the presence of a normal or stenotic distal ureter. In Cussen's series of 328 intrinsic ureteral lesions, he reported 24 primary valves with no distal obstruction, i.e., the ureteral valves were considered the cause of the obstruction. A total of 19 valves were reported to be in association with a more distal obstruction, these valves thought to be either primary or secondary.

Others have observed ureteral obstructions from eccentric cusps, believed to be distinct from secondary folds and kinks associated with ureteral dilation and elongation (Gosalbez et al., 1983; Maizels and Stephens, 1980). The cusp need not contain smooth muscle (Gosalbez et al., 1983; Reinberg et al., 1987). However, Williams (1977) believed that eccentric obstructing valves may be more infrequent than Cussen reported. Many of the apparent valves may be artifacts of distention because the dilated ureter at its junction with the undilated segment assumes a kinked and eccentric position from elongation and pull of the surrounding adventitia.

In summary, diaphragmatic annular valves are a rare, although definite, form of ureteral obstruction. Eccentric, cusp-like flaps or folds can be obstructing but can also be secondary to the elongation and tortuosity that occurs with ureteral distention at the site of an underlying anatomic or functional obstruction.

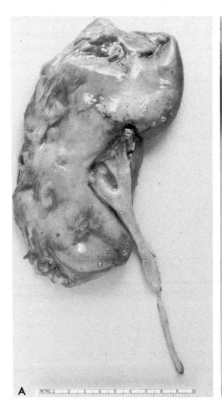
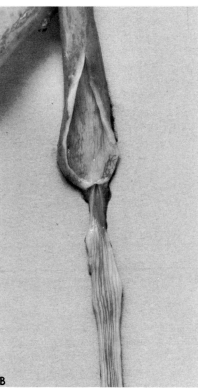

Figure 34–63. Congenital ureteral valve. *A,* Extended view. *B,* Long section showing greatly dilated ureter above the valve and normal size below. (From Simon, H. B., et al.: J. Urol., 74:336, 1955.)

Spiral Twists and Folds of the Ureter

Campbell (1970) observed this anomaly only twice in 12,080 autopsies in children (Fig. 34–66). He ascribed it to failure of the ureter to rotate with the kidney. This explanation may be simplistic, as the illustration shows more than one twist. Obstruction and hydronephrosis may result from spiral twists. The condition may arise from one of a number of possible persistent manifestations of normal fetal upper ureteral development, as described by Östling (1942) (see Figs. 34–46 and 34–66). These manifestations include ureteral mucosal redundancy (see Ureteral Valves) and apparent folds and convolutions that may have a spiral appearance. Radiographic evidence of such findings is often present in the excretory urograms of otherwise normal newborns. However, most of these folds will gradually disappear

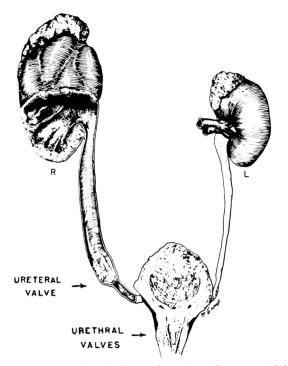

Figure 34–64. Complete diaphragm obstructing right ureter, with hydroureter and hydronephrosis above. (From Roberts, R. R.: J. Urol., 76:62, 1956.)

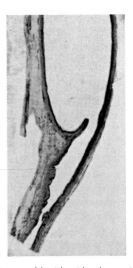

Figure 34–65. A 12-year-old girl with obstructing distal congenital ureteral valve in an ectopic, duplicated ureter. (Courtesy of Dr. Laurence R. Wharton.)

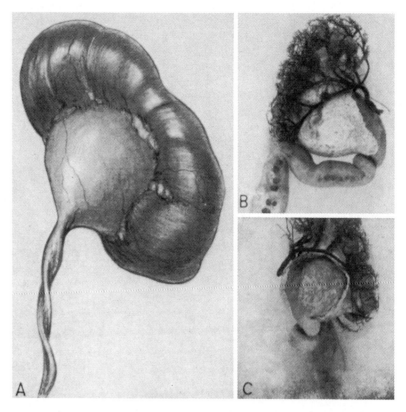

Figure 34–66. Torsion (spiral twists) of the ureter. *A,* Observed in an infant at autopsy. There is secondary hydronephrosis. Ureteral twists of the ureter of late fetal life; corrosion specimens. *B,* Anterior view. *C,* Lateral view from pelvic aspect. (Courtesy of Dr. Karl Östling.)

with normal growth of the infant. Occasionally, ureteral convolutions that are enclosed by investing fascia persist as a form of ureteropelvic obstruction (Gross, 1953) (see Ureteropelvic Junction Obstruction).

Persistent fetal folds are described in a previous paragraph. An isolated single fold or "kink" demonstrated radiographically with otherwise normal upper tracts may be acquired, nonobstructing, and reversible, and represents acute or intermittent elongation of the ureter with distal obstruction or reflux. Campbell (1970) believed that isolated primary obstructing congenital kinks could occur as an uncommon disorder, but the example he presented did not demonstrate convincing obstruction. Nevertheless, this sort of deformity is often one manifestation of ureteropelvic junction obstruction in association with ensheathment by dense fibrous bands (Gross, 1953).

Ureteral Diverticula

Diverticula of the ureter have been classified by Gray and Skandalakis (1972) into three categories: (1) abortive ureteral duplications (blind-ending bifid ureters) (see Blind-Ending Duplication of the Ureter); (2) true congenital diverticula containing all tissue layers of the normal ureter; and (3) acquired diverticula representing mucosal herniations. Congenital diverticula are very uncommon and have been reported as arising from the distal ureter above the ureterovesical junction, midureter, and ureteropelvic junction (Culp, 1947; McGraw and Culp, 1952; Richardson, 1942). These can become very large, and secondary hydronephrosis can ensue.

The patient may present with abdominal pain or renal colic and palpable cystic mass. McGraw and Culp's patient, a 64-year old woman, had a cystic lesion at surgery extending from under the right costal margin to the pelvic brim.

A typical congenital diverticulum in a 20-year old man is shown in Figure 34–67. Even small diverticula may be symptomatic. Sharma and co-workers (1980) reported two cases—a man with repeated infections and a girl with intermittent colic. Fluoroscopy in the second patient demonstrated stasis and peristaltic dysfunction with to-and-fro ("yo-yo") ureter to diverticulum reflux. She was cured by diverticulectomy.

As discussed in the previous section on blind-ending duplications, congenital diverticula below the level of the ureteropelvic junction arise from premature cleavage of the ureteral bud with abortive development of the accessory limb. Those from the ureteropelvic junction region arise from primitive calyceal formation that similarly failed to encounter metanephric tissue (Gray and Skandalakis, 1972).

Single acquired diverticula may be associated with strictures or calculi or may follow trauma (Culp, 1947). Multiple diverticula, small in size (under 5 mm), have been ascribed to the effect of chronic infection (Holly and Sumcad, 1957; Rank and Mellinger, 1960). However, Norman and Dubowy (1966) reported two cases of multiple diverticula that were demonstrable on retrograde pyelography but not on high-dose pyelography even with compression. Hansen and Frost (1978) reported a third case demonstrated by retrograde ureteropyelography. Such lesions, demonstrable only by unphysiologic pressures, may be congenital variants with

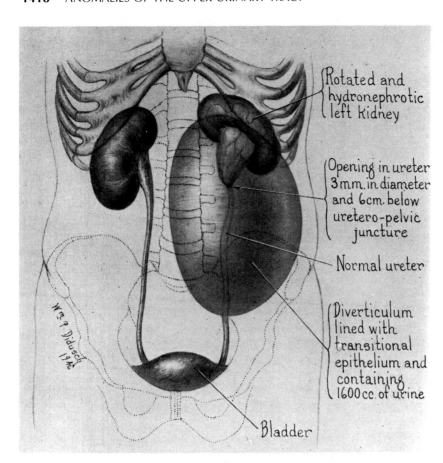

Figure 34–67. Congenital diverticulum of left ureter containing 1600 ml of urine. The kidney was hydronephrotic. (From Culp, O. S.: J. Urol., 58:309, 1947.)

weaknesses of the ureteral wall rather than acquired conditions (Hensen and Frost, 1978). However, the published reports do not contain histologic observations to support either hypothesis.

Large diverticula can generally be removed without sacrificing the kidney unless it is irreversibly involved in a dense inflammatory process.

Congenital High Insertion of the Ureter

This rare malformation may drain an otherwise normal and unobstructed kidney (Fig. 34–68). Most high insertions, however, are encountered with ureteropelvic junction obstruction, as discussed previously in this chapter.

ANOMALIES OF TERMINATION

Vesicoureteral Reflux

Primary congenital vesicoureteral reflux is classified as a disorder of ureteral termination in which the orifice is too high and lateral and is loosely attached to the angle of a poorly developed trigone. The embryologic origin is described in the first part of this chapter. In summary, the ureteral bud is thought to originate more caudally than normal from the mesonephric duct, placing it too close to the future bladder. Thus, it separates prematurely from the mesonephric duct when the normally short common segment is absorbed into the developing bladder. Because it has more time to migrate, the orifice finally comes to rest in a high and lateral position, resulting in a large and poorly developed trigone. The mesenchymal precursors of the trigonal and ureteral musculature are deficient as well, thereby contributing to the defect (Ambrose and Nicolson, 1962; Stephens and Lenaghan, 1962; Tanagho, 1965). As the degree of caudal displacement of the ureteral bud varies, the range of severity of the ureterovesical incompetence varies with it.

Vesicoureteral reflux is relatively common in total ureteral duplication (Privett et al., 1976) and most frequently involves the lower pole ureter, the so-called orthotopic orifice. The upper pole ureter is less likely to reflux. Even when it inserts close to the orthotopic lower pole orifice, its migratory pathway almost always places it more distally, so that its intravesical segment is longer (see Fig. 34–57). However, it too can reflux, generally to a lesser degree, when both buds have originated more caudally than normal so that the two orifices both terminate too high and lateral. Primary reflux into the upper pole segment may also occur, often alone, when its orifice into the distal trigone or bladder neck is ectopic, entering through a separate muscular hiatus (Ambrose and Nicolson, 1964; Tanagho, 1976).

Refer to Chapter 44 for a full presentation of vesicoureteral reflux and an extensive bibliography.

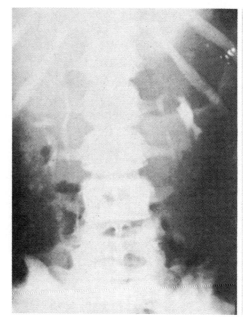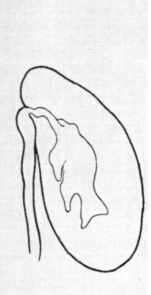

Figure 34–68. A 4-year-old girl with high ureteropelvic insertion and no obstruction.

Ectopic Ureter

An ectopic ureter is one that does not open at the normal location at the angle of the trigone. Although a refluxing ureteral orifice might be considered to belong in this category because of its tendency to have a more cranial and lateral position (called by some "lateral ectopia"), the term ectopic ureter by convention refers to any ureter in which the ultimate termination is determined by a delay in, or lack of, separation from the mesonephric duct. This is the converse of reflux, which results from early separation of the ureteral bud from the mesonephric duct. Of all ectopic ureters, 80 per cent are associated with a duplicated system, and most of these occur in females (Schulman, 1976). The embryology of ectopic ureter is detailed in that part of this chapter.

Anatomy

The ectopic ureteral orifice may open into the urinary or genital tract (see Fig. 34–60), following an ectopic pathway (see Fig. 34–61) (Stephens, 1958, 1963). When located anywhere along the trigone to the level of the vesical neck, it is unlikely to cause symptoms and is rarely of clinical concern. Openings from the vesical neck distally can cause clinical symptoms from obstruction; reflux; and, in the female, incontinence.

Stephens (1963) divided the female urethra into an upper urethral internal sphincter zone and a lower urethral external sphincter zone. An orifice in the internal sphincter region is apt to be obstructed, but the patient will be continent. An orifice in the distal urethra will have a lesser obstruction, but the patient will be incontinent.

Openings also occur in the vestibule and vagina, and rarely, in the cervix or uterus. These openings result from rupture of Gartner's duct into the developing ureterovaginal canal at some point along their common wall. The vestibular opening is the most common form and represents the terminal extent of Gartner's duct. It is likely that the terminal portion of the mesonephric duct (commonly excretory duct) fails to regress totally in some cases, although proof is not conclusive (Ellerker, 1958). Abeshouse (1943) found several reports of a ureter opening into a dilated Gartner's duct and, in one case, into a dilated vaginal (Gartner's) cyst. Termination of an ectopic ureter into a Gartner's cyst is the least common manifestation of ureteral ectopy and has been described with a single-system vaginal ectopic ureter. The associated kidney is small and dysplastic or absent (Currarino, 1982). The cyst may be closed or may communicate with the vagina, bladder, bladder neck, or urethra (Kjaeldgaard and Fianau, 1982). In one patient with a bifid system, there was sufficient renal function that treatment included ureteroneocystostomy (Kjaeldgaard et al., 1981).

Three cases of an ectopic ureter entering an apparent urethral diverticulum have been reported, the latter probably representing the terminal mesonephric duct. Two of these were in infant girls who had a small outpouching below the bladder neck (Vanhouette, 1970). Vanhouette was unable to find any true congenital urethral diverticula in young girls and emphasized that this radiographic finding should indicate an ectopic ureter. The third case was a 26-year old woman with lifelong incontinence (Wilmarth, 1948). The "diverticulum" was large but eccentric, opening at the side of the ectopic ureter, which suggests its congenital origin.

Other reports suggest that single unilateral vaginal ectopic ureter is less rare than previously believed and is not uncommon in Japan (Weiss et al., 1984). Rarely, hydrocolpos (urocolpos) and a single vaginal ectopic ureter occur in combination with a vaginal atresia (transverse vaginal septum), the latter representing arrested development of the vaginal plate (Feldman and Ross, 1980). Another rare variant is a vesicoureterovaginal communication in which the ectopic ureter has a connection with both bladder and vagina (Kondo et al., 1982). In one girl treated by nephrectomy at age 3 years for a single ectopic system, recurrent incontinence occurred 5 years later from spontaneous vesicovaginal fistula through the stump of the ectopic ureter, suggesting rupture of a thin hypoplastic membrane (Koyanagi et al., 1977).

Cases of ectopic ureter opening at the vestibule or distal urethra without incontinence have been described. In some, incontinence never developed, and the lesion was discovered during investigation of urinary infection or flank pain. In others, incontinence did not appear until adolescence or after pregnancy. In all these cases, the ectopic ureter presumably passed through some portion of the external urethral sphincter musculature, allowing ureteral drainage only during voiding. It is likely that the changes of puberty or of childbirth caused attenuation of this muscular support in some patients, allowing late-onset incontinence (Childlow and Utz, 1970; Davis, 1930; DeWeerd and Litin, 1958; Honke, 1946; Koyanagi et al., 1980; Moore, 1952; Ogawa et al., 1976; Wesson, 1934; Verbaeys et al., 1980).

In the male, ectopic ureters are found at any level of the ectopic pathway into the prostatic urethra at the level of the verumontanum proximal to the external urinary sphincter. Incontinence is not a symptom. The ectopic ureter can also drain into the genital tract through the seminal vesicle, vas deferens, or ejaculatory duct. The ipsilateral mesonephric derivatives may also be maldeveloped; seminal vesical cysts have been reported as well as one case of agenesis of the corresponding testis (Das and Amar, 1980; Deilmann and Moormann, 1978). Two cases are described of a single-system ectopic ureter terminating in the epididymis (Jona et al., 1979; Ostermayer and Frei, 1981) plus a third with a direct connection of the ectopic ureter to the lower pole calyx (Brown et al., 1988).

In a few instances, the ectopic ureter has drained into the utriculus, which is of paramesonephric (müllerian) duct origin. As the mesonephric and paramesonephric ducts lie closely applied in a common mesenchyme at their early attachment to the cloaca, it is likely that a communication develops between them in this situation (Ellerker, 1958) from shifting or fusion of the bud with the paramesonephric duct (Abeshouse, 1943). Based on the termination of the ectopic ureter described earlier, Das and Amar (1981) have classified it as follows: Type I—urogenital sinus ectopia, in which the ureter terminates in the posterior urethra, and type II—mesonephric duct ectopia, in which the ureter terminates in a mesonephric derivative.

An unusual variant of a persistent common excretory duct involves an ectopic vas deferens opening into the ureter, with a common duct terminating on the trigone in a relatively normal location. This common duct has been termed a persisting mesonephric duct, the terminal portion of which resembles the ureter rather than the vas (Schwarz and Stephens, 1978). In one 7-year-old boy, the orifice was entirely normal, with no reflux (Alfert and Gillenwater, 1972). In two infants, vesicoureteral reflux was present (Borger and Belman, 1975). All three patients had other anomalies. In another

example, a 13-year-old boy with bilateral ectopic vasa had a large, poorly emptying, hypotonic bladder with a megatrigone and bilateral reflux but no other anomalies (Redman and Sulieman, 1976).

Gibbons and colleagues (1978) reviewed 11 cases with 13 ectopic vasal insertions; ureteral ectopia was encountered in one third of the cases, and vesicoureteral reflux in nine of the 13 renal units. In five instances, the vas terminated in the bladder. Strictly speaking, these cases of ectopic vasa do not necessarily involve ectopic ureters, but the embryologic features, which are similar to those for ectopic insertion of the ureter into the seminal tract, justify inclusion here. Although the embryology of the ectopic vas is not fully understood, the common excretory duct appears to have failed to absorb completely but did not migrate distally, apparently behaving instead like a ureteral duct in its migration and development.

Ureteral openings into the rectum are extremely rare. Leef and Leader (1962) noted three instances in the literature and described an adult with a single-system ectopic ureter into the rectum plus a 2-cm blind-ending ureteral stump into the ipsilateral trigone. Uson and Schulman (1972) provided long-term follow-up data on an infant reported earlier with bilateral duplication—ectopic orifice into the rectum on one side and ectopic ureterocele on the other.

Occasionally, ureters terminate blindly in a site ectopic from the trigonal region. These appear clinically as tubular or rounded cystic masses draining a dysplastic, nonfunctioning kidney. Conversely, the upper end of an ectopic ureter may end blindly, representing an abortive ectopic ureteral bud (Gray and Skandalakis, 1972; Varney and Ford, 1954).

Incidence

The true incidence of ectopic ureter is uncertain, as many cause no symptoms. Campbell (1970) noted ten examples in 19,046 autopsies in children (1 in 1900) but thought that some had been overlooked. Of all ectopic orifices, 80 per cent are associated with a duplicated collecting system. In females, more than 80 per cent are duplicated, whereas in males the majority of ectopic ureters drain single systems (Schulman, 1976). This is particularly true when ectopic ureteroceles are excluded from consideration.

Ectopic ureter appears more commonly in females—clinically, from 2 to 12 times more frequently—with the lesser frequency probably reflecting the incidence more accurately (Burford et al., 1949; Eisendrath, 1938; Lowsley and Kerwin, 1956; Mills, 1939). Ellerker (1958) noted 366 females and 128 males in his review of 494 ectopic ureters, including autopsies, for female-to-male ratio of 2.9:1. Between 7.5 and 17 per cent of ectopic ureters appear bilaterally (Eisendrath, 1938; Ellerker, 1958). A small percentage involve a solitary kidney. With unilateral ectopic ureter, a contralateral ureteral duplication is not uncommon.

The distribution of ectopic ureters by location is itemized in Table 34–6. In the male, the posterior urethra is the most common site of ectopic ureter.

Table 34–6. LOCATION OF 494 ECTOPIC URETERS (INCLUDING AUTOPSIES)

	Number	Per Cent
128 Males		
Posterior urethra	60	47
Prostatic utricle	13	10
Seminal vesicle	42	33
Ejaculatory duct	7	5
Vas deferens	6	5
366 Females		
Urethra	129	35
Vestibule	124	34
Vagina	90	25
Cervix or uterus	18	5
Gartner's duct	3	<1
Urethral diverticulum	2	<1

From Ellerker, A. G.: Br. J. Surg., 45:344, 1958. By permission of the publisher, Butterworth-Heinemann Ltd.

Drainage into the genital tract involves the seminal vesicle three times more often than the ejaculatory duct and vas deferens combined (Ellerker, 1958; Lucius, 1963; Riba et al., 1946). In the female, the urethra and vestibule are the most common sites. The age at diagnosis ranges widely, with many examples not detected during life (Ellerker, 1958).

Associated Anomalies

The earlier reports failed to provide adequate descriptions of the upper tracts, but later reports emphasize that the degree of ectopia is related directly to the degree of renal maldevelopment—the more remote the ureteral opening, the greater the degree of renal maldevelopment (Schulman, 1976). With duplicated systems this means hypoplasia or dysplasia of the upper pole segment. In ten cases of ectopic ureter that drained a single system and opened into the male seminal tracts, the kidney was not visualized radiographically in all (Rognon et al., 1973). Of 16 single renal ducts drained by an ectopic ureter, renal dysplasia was present in seven (Prewitt and Lebowitz, 1976). The anomalous single kidney may be ectopic as well. The ectopic ureter itself is also abnormal, usually to a greater degree in the single than in the duplicated system. Usually the ureter is variably dilated, and drainage is impaired (Williams and Royle, 1969). Muscle cells may show severe alterations on ultrastructure studies. Whether these changes are developmental or acquired is not yet known (Hanna et al., 1977).

Symptoms

In males an ectopic ureter may remain undiagnosed unless symptoms of ureteral obstruction or infection appear. Although urinary incontinence should not be a complaint, urgency and frequency can be a response to the trickle of urine into the posterior urethra (Ellerker, 1958; Williams, 1954). Incontinence in males, in fact, may be a feature of the uncommon circumstance of bilateral single ectopic ureters, for reasons to be discussed later in this section.

When the ectopic ureter drains into the seminal tract it often does not become symptomatic until the onset of sexual activity. In addition to dysuria and frequency, symptoms and signs may include prostatitis, seminal vesiculitis and epididymis, painful defecation, constipation, pelvic pain, epididymal swelling, bloody or painful ejaculation, and a palpable painful cystic mass on rectal palpation (Brannan and Henry, 1973; Schnitzer, 1965). At cystoscopic evaluation, a hemitrigone will be present with a single system, and the posterolateral floor of the bladder may be displaced or elevated by a cystic mass behind it. The intravesical bulge of the dilated ureter can resemble an ectopic ureterocele (Cumes et al., 1981).

In affected females, about half present with urinary incontinence. The diagnosis may be suspected after toilet training, if not before. Typically, normal cyclic bladder function will be evident despite constant dampness or wetness.

When the offending renal unit is small and poorly functioning, identification may be difficult by ultrasonography. With any functioning parenchyma, however, nuclear scanning should demonstrate the renal tissue. At times, angiography has defined a tiny, dysplastic, duplicated segment (Kittredge and Levin, 1973). Diagnostic approaches and treatment are detailed in Chapter 45.

Treatment and Prognosis

Prognosis is generally good for the ectopic ureter in a duplicated system. Partial nephrectomy and ureterectomy, ureteroneocystostomy, or pyelopyelostomy with distal ureterectomy is the usual choice of therapy.

Single Ectopic Ureters—Additional Features

In reports from countries with mostly white populations, single-system ectopic ureters constitute 20 per cent of all ectopic ureters and most occur in males. In Japan, by contrast, 70 per cent of all ectopic ureters are single system, mostly noted in females with vaginal drainage (Gotoh et al., 1983). Single-system ectopic ureters present some differences from those involving double ureters. When bilateral, they also present more problems. Prewitt and Lebowitz (1976) reported that of 16 patients, seven had other anomalies—congenital heart disease in three and high imperforate anus in four. The high incidence of ipsilateral renal hypoplasia and dysplasia had been described earlier. Poor function or nonfunction of these anomalous and often ectopically located kidneys and a tiny blood supply make their detection difficult at times (Gibbons and Duckett, 1978; Schulman, 1976, 1978; Scott, 1981).

With a unilateral single-system ectopic ureter, the ipsilateral hemitrigone fails to develop, and one side of the bladder neck is incompletely developed. Nevertheless, with unilateral ectopia, the hemitrigone and bladder neck are generally adequate for urinary control provided that, in the female, the ectopic ureter is above the continence zone of the urethra (Mogg, 1974).

With bilateral single ectopic ureter into the urethra, the bladder fails to develop properly (see Fig. 34–59). The trigone is absent, and the bladder is generally small because it never contains more urine than is regurgitated from the urethra. Continuous incontinence is usual, although not inevitable. Even males tend to dribble, although they are generally able to retain enough volume to void as well. Boys appear to have a lesser degree of bladder underdevelopment. The bladder neck region is not clearly defined; the vesical outflow is widely funneled and shortened, resembling the condition in epispadias. In extreme cases, the bladder fails to develop at all, and the ureters enter the vestibule, a condition often incompatible with life because of severe renal insufficiency or other anomalies. The presence of varying associated anal, rectal, and genital anomalies suggests a field defect occurring in early embryogenesis (Kesavan et al., 1977). Most of these patients are females (Koyanagi et al., 1977; Mogg, 1974; Noseworthy and Persky, 1982; Sorenson and Middleton, 1983; Williams and Lightwood, 1972). Survival is possible for some in these extreme cases; however, rehabilitation may require intestinal diversion (Glenn, 1959) or bladder substitution.

In their review of bilateral single ectopic ureters, Williams and Lightwood (1972) added ten cases, seven girls and three boys, to 23 previously reported cases. The girls generally had more severe renal deformities and a lesser degree of bladder development. The results of surgical reconstruction, namely, ureteral reimplantation and construction of a vesical neck, were disappointing, especially for the girls. Only three of the seven gained adequate control. One of these underwent diversion later for upper tract dilatation, and three of the four patients who experienced failure also underwent diversion. These workers pointed out that success or failure of the reconstruction was related to the severity of the underlying condition. Ritchey and colleagues (1988) reported an experience similar to that of Williams and Lightwood.

Ureterocele

Ureterocele is a cystic dilation of the intravesical submucosal ureter. The size may vary from a small bulge of 1 or 2 cm in diameter to a lesion that almost fills the bladder. The appearance is that of a thin-walled, often translucent mass. The outer surface is vesical epithelium and the inner is ureteral epithelium. Between them is a thin layer of patchy muscle and collagen. Ureterocele may involve either a single collecting system or the ureter to the upper pole of a duplicated system. The opening for either may be intravesical in location or ectopic and at the bladder neck or more distal.

Classification and Anatomy

A number of classifications of varying complexity have appeared through the years, but a simple one in common use is that of Ericsson (1954). He divided ureterocele into two groups: simple and ectopic. Henceforth, simple ureterocele is described as intravesical ureterocele.

Intravesical ureterocele is entirely contained within the urinary bladder. It may arise from a single or occasionally supernumerary ureter that always ends in a normal or near normal bladder location. Intravesical ureteroceles, when associated with a single system, tend to be small.

Ectopic ureterocele extends into the bladder neck or urethra. The orifice terminates ectopically. As with ectopic ureters generally, most involve the upper pole of a double ureter. A single system is uncommon. Three reports describe the rare finding of a ureterocele involving the lower pole ureter of a double system. In two cases, the upper segment was normal (Ahmed, 1981; Arap et al., 1983; Lima and Cavalcanti, 1981). Ectopic ureteroceles tend to be much larger than intravesical ureteroceles.

Intravesical ureteroceles have also been termed *adult ureteroceles* because they resemble the small lesions of the adult that typically involve a single system. The ureter proximal to the ureterocele is variably dilated, to a lesser degree than the ureterocele itself. However, with the largest ectopic ureteroceles, immense dilatation and tortuosity of the ureter may occur.

Although Ericsson's classification of ureterocele has wide clinical applicability, Stephens' (1963) classification is useful for a more detailed understanding of the pathologic anatomy. He defined three major types—stenotic, sphincteric, and sphincterostenotic.

The *stenotic ureterocele* has a narrowed orifice located on the dome of a rounded intravesical mass and is usually located in a normal or near-normal intravesical location, i.e., the equivalent of Ericsson's "simple" ureterocele. The degree of stenosis may vary. When slight, the size of the ureterocele varies with peristalsis, and when extreme, the ureterocele remains tense and urine dribbles from the orifice between periodic, needle-like jets. Histologically, the wall of a stenotic ureterocele contains a surprising amount of muscle, although it is less dense than that in the ureteral wall above. Its orientation tends to be longitudinal.

The *sphincteric ureterocele* is a form of ectopic ureterocele in which the orifice is within the internal sphincter (bladder neck or proximal urethra). The orifice may be normal or even generous in size, the ureterocele being obstructed by the sphincter-like action of the vesical outlet, emptying only during voiding when the bladder neck opens. At times, there is reflux during voiding through this large proximal urethral orifice. Histologically, the sphincteric and the sphincterostenotic ureterocele contain variable muscle bundles, which are considerably less dense than those in the normal distal ureter but are oriented in a more random or helical pattern than the mainly longitudinal bundles of the normal intravesical ureter (Stephens, 1963; Tanagho, 1976).

The *sphincterostenotic ureterocele* is another variant of ectopic ureterocele in which the orifice is tiny as well as ectopic. This form of ureterocele achieves a large size, often almost filling the bladder. It is continuously distended and may extend into the vesical outlet, obstructing it to a varying degree. Prolapse of a large ureterocele through the urethra onto the perineum may occasionally occur (Diard et al., 1981; Eklöf et al., 1978; Fenelon and Alton, 1981; Klauber and Crawford, 1980; Orr and Glanton, 1953).

In addition to these three forms of ureterocele, there is an uncommon variant of ectopic ureterocele, the so-called cecoureterocele. Upward migration of the developing ectopic ureteral orifice leaves a tongue of more distal ureter underneath the urethral mucosa. The underlying urethral musculature may be attenuated or deficient, resulting in urinary incontinence (Gomez and Stephens, 1983). The orifice in a cecoureterocele is proximal to the bladder neck (Stephens, 1968).

Rarely, a ureterocele may end blindly if regression of the mesonephric duct has involved the termination of the ectopic ureter as well (Ericsson, 1954; Stephens, 1968) and may be found without associated renal tissue, presumably from disappearance of renal tissue during embryogenesis (Passerini-Glazel et al., 1986).

Ureteroceles are not inevitably associated with a dilated upper tract. Bauer and Retik (1978) described five children with a small, dysplastic renal unit and an undilated ureter in association with the ectopic ureterocele. Share and Lebowitz (1989) reported eight with ectopic ureteroceles and double ureters, all of whom had nonfunction of the involved renal segment. The ureter and calyces above the ureterocele were diminutive in each case. Some intact ureteroceles also reflux (Borden and Martinez, 1977; Leong et al., 1980).

Large ectopic ureteroceles can obstruct the lower pole ipsilateral ureter or even the contralateral side as well as the bladder neck. The lower pole ipsilateral ureter at times refluxes. On occasion, dilation of the lower pole segment is due to an intrinsic rather than an extrinsic obstruction (Androulakakis et al., 1981). As is true for ectopic ureters generally, the renal segment associated with an ectopic ureterocele tends to be abnormal and is often poorly functioning or nonfunctioning. Hypoplasia, dysplasia, and hydronephrotic atrophy are frequently present, as is superimposed pyelonephritis (Perrin et al., 1974; Williams and Woodard, 1964). The generally smaller sized intravesical ureterocele associated with a single system as encountered in adults often causes a relatively mild degree of obstruction. When diagnosed in children, however, it can be associated with a severe degree of hydronephrosis and hydroureter. Snyder and Johnston (1978) noted nonfunction of the involved kidney in five of 20 intravesical ureteroceles.

Sen and Ahmed (1988) reported 15 single-system ureteroceles, with an equal sex ratio. Single-system ureteroceles constituted 25 per cent of their series of ureteroceles; 20 per cent were bilateral. Unfortunately, they did not distinguish between intravesical and ectopic ureteroceles.

All of these forms of ureterocele and their clinical import are illustrated and described in detail in Chapter 45.

Incidence

Incidence has varied in different reports. Campbell (1951) noted an autopsy incidence in children of one in 4000. Uson and associates (1961) observed six in 3200 pediatric autopsies or one in 500. Undoubtedly, some small ureteroceles at autopsy are not recognized because they have collapsed. The clinical incidence varies also. In one series, ureterocele occurred in one in 100 pediatric urologic admissions (Uson et al., 1961) and in from one in 5000 to one in 12,000 general pediatric admissions (Malek et al., 1972). Ureterocele is three to four times more frequent in girls. It is more common on the left side. Between 10 and 15 per cent are bilateral (Bruézière et al., 1979; Campbell, 1951; Gross, 1953; Malek et al., 1972; Mandell et al., 1980).

Familial occurrence of ureterocele has been described. Two siblings had simple ureteroceles (Abrams et al., 1980); fraternal twins had ectopic ureteroceles (Ayalon et al., 1979); a mother and daughter had ectopic ureteroceles, and all their first-degree relatives had ureteral duplication to some extent (Babcock et al., 1977). Two brothers with ureterocele had concurrent agenesis of the corpus callosum (Lachiewicz et al., 1985).

In most pediatric series, ectopic ureteroceles are more common than intravesical ones. They composed 14 of 20 in Ericsson's (1954) series and 21 of 30 in Stephens' (1963) series, most of these involving duplicated systems. In a series of 93 ureteroceles, 34 were intravesical—24 of these being single systems. Fifty-nine were ectopic, with double ureters (Bruézière et al., 1979). Ectopic single systems are uncommon. None of Ericsson's series had this anomaly, but in his review of the literature he found two single systems in 14 ectopic ureteroceles. Similarly, Williams and Royle (1969) found three single systems in 15 ectopic ureteroceles. Malek and associates (1972) had two in 14; there are other sporadic reports (Prewitt and Lebowitz, 1976).

Single-system ectopic ureterocele is more common in males and appears to have a high likelihood of other anomalies. Two reports have been made of crossed renal ectopia involving the ureterocele (Farkas et al., 1978; Fishman and Borden, 1982). Johnson and Perlmutter (1980) reported seven children with single-system ectopic ureteroceles, and six were boys. Five had a nonfunctioning hypodysplastic kidney; four had major cardiac anomalies. Three boys had abdominal testes—two with bilateral nonunion to the vas. Eklöf and colleagues (1987) in a review of 35 ectopic ureteroceles in males, reported nine single systems without other associated anomalies.

Embryology

The details of the embryology of ureterocele are incompletely understood. Most investigators have ascribed the formation of intravesical ureterocele to delayed rupture of Chwalle's membrane (Chwalle, 1927)—

an occluding, two-layered epithelial membrane normally present in the 15-mm embryo and located between the developing ureter and the urogenital sinus—when the ureter has established its separate attachment to the sinus. This membrane then bulges and the adjacent primitive ureter expands, presumably from early metanephric secretion, before the membrane disappears by the 35-mm stage (Gyllensten, 1949). Delayed opening of the membrane results in further dilatation of the terminal ureteral segment and stenosis of the orifice.

The explanation for ectopic ureterocele includes delayed separation of the ureteral bud from the mesonephric duct because of its too cranial origin, which allows more time for the occurrence of ampullary terminal ureteral dilatation (Tanagho, 1976). When the ectopic orifice is in the proximal urethral or bladder neck region, there may be no intrinsic stenosis. Developmental expansion of the vesicourethral canal may also involve the developing ectopic orifice, causing it to enlarge. Obstruction of the ureterocele in this instance occurs because of sphincteric action from the vesical neck region. This mechanism explains the tendency for these ureteroceles to empty somewhat during voiding or, alternatively, for vesicoureteral reflux during voiding (Stephens, 1963 and 1968).

These explanations do not account for the fact that not all ectopic ureters are associated with ureterocele formation.

An intrinsic alteration in ureteral bud development with excessive expansion of the developing terminal ureter and altered development of the musculature of the developing intravesical ureter in the ectopic ureterocele segment may explain the difference (Stephens, 1963). Stephens compared the intravesical ureteral musculature of ectopic ureteroceles with the ectopic ureters that had a long intravesical course and orifices terminating in the internal sphincter zone. The intravesical portion of the ectopic ureter was well muscularized, and the fibers were not limited to the longitudinal orientation typical of a normal ureter. The ectopic ureterocele, in contrast, had a variable deficiency of musculature. The muscle fibers included bundles oriented in both circular and longitudinal axes. The relatively muscular-deficient distal ureter expanded more than the better muscularized, more proximal ureter.

Tokunaka and associates (1981) studied muscle structure, by light and electron microscopy, of several ureteroceles, both intravesical and ectopic. They noted a paucity of muscle bundles in the dome of the ureterocele in contrast to well-developed bundles in the proximal ureter. Muscle cells were smaller in the ureterocele than in the proximal ureter. Thick myofibrils were absent in the muscle of the ureterocele. They concluded that these findings indicated a segmental embryonic arrest of the most distal ureter, which plays a role in ureterocele formation.

Stephens did note that some ectopic ureters were deficient in musculature. However, these ureters terminated more distally, below the internal sphincter zone. He believed that when the ureteral orifice was in this location the ultimate size of the ectopic ureter was less predictable, as it was related more to alterations of

ureteral bud development than to muscular endowment (Stephens, 1963). In contrast to ectopic ureteroceles, ectopic ureters may enter the lower urinary tract through a hiatus separate from that for the orthotopic ureter, as the mesenchyme of the developing trigone accumulates between the widely separated ureteral buds (Tanagho, 1976). This accumulation would tend to keep the terminal ectopic ureter from expanding excessively, even if poorly muscularized.

In summary, embryonic obstruction; delayed absorption of the developing ureter into the urogenital sinus; and altered ureteral bud differentiation, consisting of arrested muscular development of the most caudal ureter associated with excessive caudal widening, have all been proposed as factors in ureterocele formation.

ANOMALIES OF POSITION

Vascular Anomalies Involving the Ureter

A variety of vascular lesions can cause ureteral obstruction. In these, the vascular system rather than the urinary system is generally anomalous. With the exception of accessory renal blood vessels, all of these lesions are relatively uncommon, although all have clinical relevance.

Accessory Renal Blood Vessels

Accessory or aberrant vessels to the lower pole of the kidney can cross ventral to the ureteropelvic junction, causing obstruction. These are described previously in this chapter and elsewhere in this text.

Preureteral Vena Cava

ANATOMY. This anomaly is commonly known to the urologist as *circumcaval ureter* or *retrocaval ureter*, terms that are anatomically descriptive but misleading in regard to development. Of the two terms, circumcaval ureter is preferred, because rarely a ureter may lie behind (dorsal to) the vena cava for some portion of its lumbar course without encircling the cava, and this form of retrocaval ureter appears to be developmentally different (Dreyfuss, 1959; Lerman et al., 1956; Peisojovich and Lutz, 1969). In the case of Dreyfuss (1959), there was also a small branch vein between the vena cava and right iliopsoas muscle, over which (cephalad to it) the ureter coursed to enter the retrocaval area. The term "preureteral vena cava" emphasizes that the circumcaval ureter results from altered vascular, rather than ureteral, development.

This disorder involves the right ureter, which typically deviates medially behind (dorsal to) the inferior vena cava, winding about and crossing in front of it from a medial to a lateral direction, to resume a normal course distally, to the bladder. The renal pelvis and upper ureter are typically elongated and dilated in a J- or "fishhook"-shape before passing behind the vena cava (Fig. 34–69). However, the collecting system is not inevitably obstructed. Bateson and Atkinson (1969), Crosse and associates (1975), and Kenawi and Williams (1976) have classified circumcaval ureters into two clinical types: the more common type I has hydronephrosis and a typically obstructed pattern demonstrating some degree of fishhook-shaped deformity of the ureter to the level of the obstruction, and type II has a lesser degree of or absent hydronephrosis. Here the upper ureter is not kinked but passes behind the vena cava at a higher level, the renal pelvis and upper ureter lying nearly horizontal before encircling the vena cava in a smooth curve. In type I, the obstruction appears to occur at the edge of the iliopsoas muscle, at which point the ureter deviates cephalad before passing behind the vena cava. In type II, the obstruction, when present, appears to be at the lateral wall of the vena cava as the ureter is compressed against the perivertebral tissues.

EMBRYOLOGY. The definitive inferior vena cava develops on the right side from a plexus of fetal veins (Fig. 34–70). Initially, the venous retroperitoneal pathways consist of symmetrically placed vessels, both ventral and dorsal. The posterior cardinal and supracardinal veins lie dorsally, and the subcardinals lie ventrally. These channels, with their anastomoses, form a collar on each side through which the ascending kidneys pass. Normally, the left supracardinal veins and the lumbar portion of the right posterior cardinal vein atrophy. The subcardinals become the internal spermatic veins. The definitive right-sided inferior vena cava forms from the right supracardinal vein. If the subcardinal vein in the lumbar portion fails to atrophy and becomes the primary right-sided vein, the ureter is trapped dorsal to it.

When the definitive vena cava forms normally and the ventral portion of the primitive ring also persists, a double right vena cava is formed because of the persistence of both the right subcardinal vein dorsally and the right subcardinal vein ventrally. This double vena cava traps the right ureter between its limbs (Fig. 34–71) (Gruenwald and Surks, 1943; Sasai et al., 1986).

Although bilateral and left-sided venae cavae can occur (Clements et al., 1978; Mayo et al., 1983), a bilateral circumcaval ureter has been reported only once, in an acardiac monster (Gladstone, 1905), and a left circumcaval ureter has been described in a case of situs inversus (Brooks, 1962). In cases of bilateral venae cavae associated with a circumcaval ureter, the circumcaval ureter has been reported only on the right side, denoting that the right vena cava developed abnormally from a persistent subcardinal vein, whereas the left vena cava developed from the left supracardinal vein but otherwise normally (Pick and Anson, 1940).

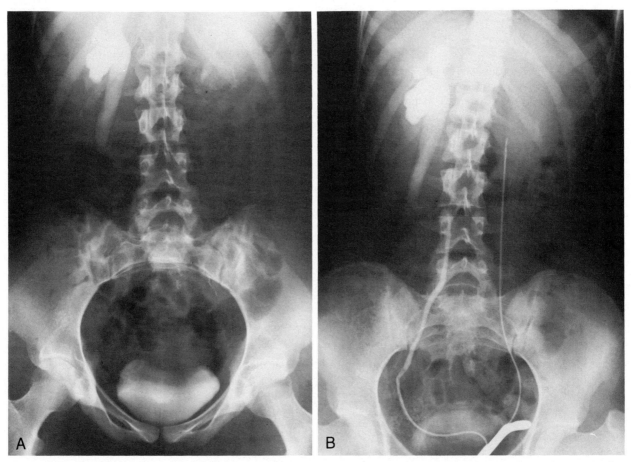

Figure 34–69. Circumcaval ureter in a 20-year-old woman with intermittent flank pain. *A,* Intravenous pyelogram. *B,* Retrograde ureteropyelogram.

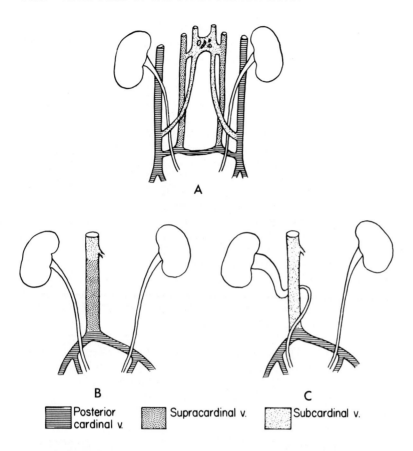

Figure 34–70. Diagrammatic representation depicting (A) fetal venous ring, (B) normal vena cava, and (C) preureteric vena cava. (Redrawn from Hollinshead, W. H.: Anatomy for Surgeons, Vol. 2, New York, Hoeber Medical Division of Harper and Row, 1956.)

INCIDENCE. The incidence of preureteral vena cava is about one in 1500 cadavers (Heslin and Mamonas, 1951) and is three to four times more common in male than in female cadavers. Gray and Skandalakis (1972) consider this frequency too high because of the preponderance of male autopsies performed. Clinically preureteral vena cava occurs 2.8 times more frequently in males, Kenawi and Williams (1976), in reviewing the literature, recorded 114 males and 41 females, with seven not known. The symptoms of preureteral vena cava are those of obstruction. Although the lesion is congenital, most patients do not present until the 3rd or 4th decade of life (Kenawi and Williams, 1976).

OTHER ANOMALIES. Several instances of horseshoe kidney have been reported (Cendron and Reis, 1972; Cukier et al., 1969; Eidelman et al., 1978; Heffernan et al., 1978; Kumeda et al., 1982; Taguchi et al., 1986). Contralateral anomalies include a variety of left renal anomalies, such as agenesis, hydronephrosis, malrotation, and hypoplasia (Kenawi and Williams, 1976). There has been one case of left hydronephrosis with ensheathing of both ureters by a single fibrous membrane below the level of the venous anomaly (Salem and Luck, 1976). An obstructing branch of the right spermatic vein has mimicked circumcaval ureteral obstruction (Psihramis, 1987), as has an anomalous tendon of the iliopsoas muscle (Guarise et al., 1989).

DIAGNOSIS. Excretory urography often fails to visualize the portion of the ureter beyond the J hook (i.e.,

extending behind the vena cava), but retrograde ureteropyelography will demonstrate an S curve to the point of obstruction (see Fig. 34–69), with the retrocaval segment lying at the level of L-3 or L-4 (Kenawi and Williams, 1976). Ultrasound (Murphy et al., 1987; Schaffer et al., 1985) and computed tomography (CT) or magnetic resonance imaging (MRI) also have been useful in defining the vascular malformation. When necessary, CT may be the procedure of choice to confirm the diagnosis and avoid retrograde ureteropyelogram (Hattori et al., 1986; Kellman et al., 1988; Lautin et al., 1988; Murphy et al., 1987; Sasai et al., 1986). Treatment of the obstruction is detailed in Chapter 68. Briefly, surgical correction involves ureteral division, with relocation and ureteroureteral or ureteropelvic reanastomosis, generally with excision or bypass of the retrocaval segment, which can be aperistaltic.

Preureteral Iliac Artery (Retroiliac Ureter)

A ureter coursing behind the common iliac artery is rare (Corbus et al., 1960; Dees, 1940; Hanna, 1972; Iuchtman et al., 1980; Seitzman and Patton, 1960; Radhkrishnan et al., 1980). Either side can be involved; in two cases, it was bilateral (Hanna, 1972; Radhkrishnan et al., 1980). Obstruction occurs at the level of L-5 or S-1 as the ureter is compressed behind the artery. Coexisting anomalies are common (Nguyen et al., 1989).

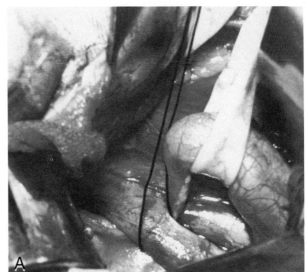

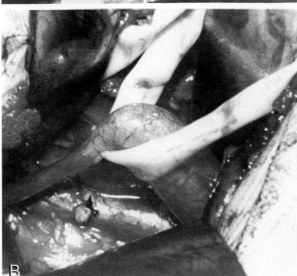

Figure 34–71. A 4-year-old boy with right ureteral obstruction from double right vena cava. Site of obstruction is apparent distally, as the ureter lies between the ventral and dorsal limbs of the double cava. Before (A) and after (B) division of ventral limb.

Gray and Skandalakis (1972) believe that the condition is vascular in origin. Normally the primitive ventral root of the umbilical artery is replaced by development of a more dorsal branch between the aorta and the distal umbilical artery. Persistence of the ventral root as the dorsal root fails to form will trap the ureter dorsally (Fig. 34–72). Dees (1940) also considered the possibility that aberrant upward migration of the kidney in the case he reported might have placed it dorsal to the iliac artery, which was redundant.

Ureteral or mesonephric duct ectopia is often present. In Dees' case there was evidence, although not definite proof, that the ureteral orifice was ectopic in the vesical neck, supporting the concept of anomalous renoureteral development. The case of Seitzman and Patton (1960) involved an ectopic ureter emptying, along with the ipsilateral vas deferens, via a persistent common mesonephric duct into the proximal posterior urethra. The case of Radhkrishnan and colleagues (1980) with bilateral retroiliac ureters also involved bilateral ectopic

termination of the vasa deferentia into the ureters. Iuchtman and associates (1980) described ectopic vaginal termination of the involved ureter, with urometrocolpos from an imperforate hymen.

Taibah and co-workers (1987) reported the unusual finding of left ureteral obstruction from a retrointernal iliac artery ureter in an otherwise normal young woman.

Vascular Obstruction of the Distal Ureter

Obstruction of the distal ureter from uterine, umbilical, obturator, and hypogastric vessels close to the bladder has been described (Campbell, 1933, 1936, 1970; Greene et al., 1954; Hyams, 1929; Scultety and Varga, 1975; Young and Kiser, 1965). However, it is not always clear that vascular impressions upon a dilated ureter are the cause of the obstruction. At times these findings may be an artifact, as when a dilated ureter from an

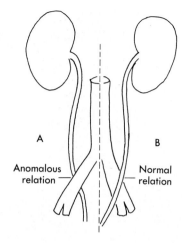

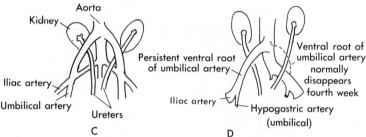

Figure 34–72. Preureteral iliac artery (postarterial ureter).
A, Anomalous relationship of ureter and artery.
B, Normal relationship of ureter and artery.
C, Relationships of ureter and iliac and umbilical arteries in the embryo.
D, Development of normal iliac channel on the right, anomalous iliac channel (persistence of proximal umbilical artery) on the left. (From Gray, S. W., and Skandalakis, J. E.: Embryology for Surgeons. Philadelphia, W. B. Saunders Co., 1972.)

intrinsic obstruction is secondarily compressed against the adjacent vessel (Campbell, 1970). Judging from the paucity of contemporary reports describing this lesion, it is likely that primary terminal ureteral obstruction by vascular lesions is a rare occurrence.

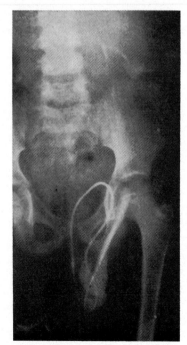

Figure 34–73. A 9-year-old boy with herniation of the left ureter into the scrotum. No hernial sac is present. Obstructed system was treated by ureteral resection and reanastomosis. (Courtesy of Dr. Hugh J. Jewett.)

Herniation of the Ureter

This is another extremely rare condition. Dourmashkin (1937) searched the literature and tabulated a series of inguinal, scrotal, and femoral herniations of the ureter. Most of these were paraperitoneal, i.e., a loop of herniated ureter extended alongside a peritoneal hernial sac. Only a minority were extraperitoneal, i.e., no hernial sac was present. In paraperitoneal ureteral hernias, the ureteral loop is always medial to the peritoneal sac. Of six scrotal hernias, four did not have peritoneal sacs. When the ureter extended into the scrotum, it was more likely to be dilated, causing upper tract obstruction.

Watson (1948) collected 102 cases of inguinal or femoral hernias involving the ureter. Jewett and Harris (1953) described a case of left ureteral hernia into the scrotum in a 9-year-old boy with left hydronephrosis (Fig. 34–73). This hernia was of the extraperitoneal type: a mesentery-like blood source supplied two loops of ureter within the scrotum that were adherent to the cord structures. Powell and Kapila (1985) reported a unique case of a 1-week-old male with bilateral megaureters presenting as left inguinal hernias. The loop of the dilated left ureter was lateral, in the inguinal canal, to an incomplete hernial sac.

Dourmashkin (1937) believed that herniation of the ureter could be acquired or congenital, the acquired form being a "sliding hernia" and the congenital form being present since birth. In the latter form, he proposed that the loop of ureter had been drawn down with the descent of the testis, and the developing ureter had adhered to migrating vas.

Internal hernias of the ureter are even more exceptional. Reports have been made of sciatic hernia containing ureter—one was diagnosed using CT in an elderly woman (Beck et al., 1952; Lindblom, 1947; Oyen et al., 1987)—and of herniation between the psoas muscle and iliac vessels (Page, 1955).

REFERENCES

Bilateral Agenesis

Ashley, D. J. B., and Mostofi, F. K.: Renal agenesis and dysgenesis. J. Urol., 83:211, 1960.

Bain, A. D., and Scott, J. S.: Renal agenesis and severe urinary tract dysplasia: A review of 50 cases, with particular reference to associated anomalies. Br. Med. J., 1:841, 1960.

Bain, A. D., Beath, M. M., and Flint, W. F.: Sirenomelia and monomelia with renal agenesis in amnion nodosom. Arch. Dis. Child., 35:250, 1960.

Carpentier, P. J., and Potter, E. L.: Nuclear sex and genital malformation in 48 cases of renal agenesis with special reference to nonspecific female pseudohermaphroditism. Am. J. Obstet. Gynecol., 78:235, 1959.

Clark, D. A.: Times of first void and first stool in 500 newborns. Pediatrics, 60:457, 1977.

Clemmons, J. J. W.: Embryonic renal injury: a possible factor in fetal malnutrition. Pediatr. Res., 11:404, 1977.

Davidson, W. M., and Ross, G. I. M.: Bilateral absence of the kidneys and related congenital anomalies. J. Pathol. Bacteriol. 68:459, 1954.

Dicker, D., Samuel, N., Feldberg, D., and Goldman, J. A.: The antenatal diagnosis of Potter syndrome—a lethal and not so rare malformation. Eur. J. Obstet. Gynecol. Reprod. Biol., 18:17, 1984.

Fitch, N., and Lachance, R. C.: The pathogenesis of Potter's syndrome of renal agenesis. Can. Med. Assoc. J., 107:653, 1972.

Hislop, A., Hey, E., and Reid, L.: The lungs in congenital bilateral renal agenesis and dysplasia. Arch. Dis. Child., 54:32, 1979.

Katz, S. H., and Chatten, J.: The urethra in bilateral renal agenesis. Arch. Pathol., 97:269, 1974.

Kohler, H. G.: An unusual case of sirenomelia. Teratology, 6:659, 1972.

Levin, H.: Bilateral renal agenesis. J. Urol., 67:86, 1952.

Mauer, S. M., Dobrin, R. S., and Vernier, R. L.: Unilateral and bilateral renal agenesis in monoamniotic twins. J. Pediatr., 84:236, 1974.

McPherson, E., Carey, J., Kramer, A., Hall, J. G., Pauli, R. M., et al.: Dominantly inherited renal adysplasia. Am. J. Med. Genet., 26:863, 1987.

Perlman, M., Williams, J., and Hirsh, M.: Neonatal pulmonary hypoplasia after prolonged leakage of amniotic fluid. Arch. Dis. Child., 51:349, 1976.

Potter, E. L.: Bilateral renal agenesis. J. Pediatr., 29:68, 1946a.

Potter, E. L.: Facial characteristics in infants with bilateral renal agenesis. Am. J. Obstet. Gynecol., 51:885, 1946b.

Potter, E. L.: Pathology of the Fetus and the Newborn. Chicago, Year Book Medical Publishers, 1952.

Potter, E. L.: Bilateral absence of ureters and kidneys. A report of 50 cases. Obstet. Gynecol., 25:3, 1965.

Rayburn, W. F., and Laferla, J. J.: Mid-gestational abortion for medical or genetic indications. Clin. Obstet. Gynecol., 13:71, 1986.

Reid, L.: The lung: its growth and remodeling in health and disease. Am. J. Roentgenol., 129:777, 1977.

Rizza, J. M., and Downing, S. E.: Bilateral renal agenesis in two female siblings. Am. J. Dis. Child., 121:60, 1971.

Roodhooft, A. M., Birnholz, J. C., and Holmes, L. D.: Familial nature of congenital absence and severe dysgenesis of both kidneys. N. Engl. J. Med., 310:1341, 1984.

Selby, G. W., and Parmelee, A. H., Jr.: Bilateral renal agenesis and oligohydramnios. J. Pediatr., 48:70, 1976.

Sherry, S. N., and Kramer, I.: The time of passage of first stool and first urine by the newborn infant. J. Pediatr., 46:158, 1955.

Sirtori, M., Ghidini, A., Romero, R., and Hobbins, J. C.: Prenatal diagnosis of sirenomelia. J. Ultrasound Med., 8:83, 1989.

Thomas, I. T., and Smith, D. W.: Oligohydramnios, cause of the nonrenal features of Potter's syndrome, including pulmonary hypoplasia. J. Pediatr., 84:811, 1974.

Thompson, V. M.: Amnion nodosum. J. Obstet. Gynaecol. Br. Commonw., 67:611, 1960.

Williams, D. I.: Personal communication, 1974.

Wilson, R. D., and Baird, P. A.: Renal agenesis in British Columbia. Am. J. Med. Genet., 21:153, 1985.

Wolf, E. L., Berdon, W. E., Baker, D. H., Wigger, H. J., and Blanc, W. A.: Diagnosis of oligohydramnios-related pulmonary hypoplasia (Potter syndrome): Value of portable voiding cystourethrography in newborns with respiratory distress. Radiology, 125:769, 1977.

Unilateral Renal Agenesis

Anders, J. M.: Congenital single kidney with report of a case. The practical significance of the condition with statistics. Am. J. Med. Sci., 139:313, 1910.

Anderson, E. E., and Harrison, J. H.: Surgical importance of the solitary kidney. N. Engl. J. Med., 273:683, 1965.

Ashley, D. J. B., and Mostofi, F. K.: Renal agenesis and dysgenesis. J. Urol., 83:211, 1960.

Barry, J. E., and Auldist, A. W.: The VATER Association. Am. J. Dis. Child., 128:769, 1974.

Beeby, D. I.: Seminal vesicle cysts associated with ipsilateral renal agenesis: Case report and review of literature. J. Urol., 112:120, 1974.

Biedel, C. W., Pagon, R. A., and Zapata, J. O.: Müllerian anomalies and renal agenesis: autosomal dominant urogenital adysplasia. J. Pediatr., 104:861, 1984.

Bryan, A. L., Nigro, J. A., and Counseller, V. S.: One hundred cases of congenital absence of the vagina. Surg. Gynecol. Obstet., 88:79, 1949.

Campbell, M. F.: Congenital absence of one kidney: Unilateral renal agenesis. Ann. Surg., 88:1039, 1928.

Charny, C. W., and Gillenwater, J. Y.: Congenital absence of the vas deferens. J. Urol., 93:399, 1965.

Collins, D. C.: Congenital unilateral renal agenesia. Ann. Surg., 95:715, 1932.

Cope, J. R., and Trickey, S. E.: Congenital absence of the kidney: problems in diagnosis and management. J. Urol., 127:10, 1982.

Currarino, G.: Single vaginal ectopic ureter and Gartner's duct cyst with ipsilateral renal hypoplasia and dysplasia (or agenesis). J. Urol., 128:988, 1982.

Curtis, J. A., Sadhu, V., and Steiner, R. M.: Malposition of the colon in right renal agenesis, ectopia and anterior nephrectomy. Am. J. Roentgenol., 129:845, 1977.

D'Alberton, A., Reschini, E., Ferrari, N., and Candiani, P.: Prevalence of urinary tract abnormalities in a large series of patients with uterovaginal atresia. J. Urol., 126:623, 1981.

Dees, J. E.: Prognosis of the solitary kidney. J. Urol., 83:550, 1960.

Donohue, R. E., and Fauver, H. E.: Unilateral absence of the vas deferens. JAMA, 261:1180, 1989.

Doroshow, L. W., and Abeshouse, B. S.: Congenital unilateral solitary kidney: Report of 37 cases and a review of the literature. Urol. Surv., 11:219, 1961.

Emanuel, B., Nachman, R., Aronson, N., and Weiss, H.: Congenital solitary kidney: A review of 74 cases. Am. J. Dis. Child., 127:17, 1974.

Fortune, C. H.: The pathological and clinical significance of congenital one-sided kidney defect with the presentation of three new cases of agenesis and one of aplasia. Ann. Intern. Med., 1:377, 1927.

Furtado, A. J. L.: The three cases of cystic seminal vesicle associated with unilateral renal agenesis. Br. J. Urol., 45:536, 1973.

Gilliland, B., and Dick, F.: Uterus didelphys associated with unilateral imperforate vagina. Obstet. Gynecol., 48:Suppl. 1, 5s, 1976.

Gutierrez, R.: Surgical aspects of renal agenesis: With special reference to hypoplastic kidney, renal aplasia and congenital absence of one kidney. Arch. Surg., 27:686, 1933.

Holt, S. A., and Peterson, N. E.: Ectopia of seminal vesicle: Associated with agenesis of ipsilateral kidney. Urology, 4:322, 1974.

Hynes, D. M., and Watkin, E. M.: Renal agenesis—roentgenologic problem. Am. J. Roentgenol., 110:772, 1970.

Jancu, J., Zuckerman, H., and Sudarsky, M.: Unilateral renal agenesis associated with multiple abnormalities. South. Med. J., 69:94, 1976.

Kenny, P. J., Robbins, G. L., Ellis, D. A., and Spert, B. A.: Adrenal glands in patients with congenital renal anomalies: Computed tomography appearance. Radiology, 155:181, 1985.

Kohn, G., and Borns, P. F.: The association of bilateral and unilateral renal aplasia in the same family. J. Pediatr., 83:95, 1973.

Kroovand, R. L.: Cystoscopy. In Kelalis, P. P., King, L. R., and Belman, A. B. (Eds.): Clinical Pediatric Urology. Philadelphia, W. B. Saunders Co., 1985.

Limkakeng, A. D., and Retik, A. B.: Unilateral renal agenesis with hypoplastic ureter: Observations on the contralateral urinary tract and report of four cases. J. Urol., 108:149, 1972.

Longo, V. J., and Thompson, G. J.: Congenital solitary kidney. J. Urol., 68:63, 1952.

Mace, J. W., Kaplan, J. M., Schanberger, J. E., and Gotlin, R. W.: Poland's syndrome: Report of seven cases and review of the literature. Clin. Pediatr., 11:98, 1972.

Magee, M. C., Lucey, D. T., and Fried, F. A.: A new embryologic classification for uro-gynecologic malformations: the syndromes of mesonephric duct induced mullerian deformities. J. Urol., 121:265, 1979.

Mascatello, V., and Lebowitz, R. L.: Malposition of the colon in left renal agenesis and ectopia. Radiology, 120:371, 1976.

McPherson, E., Carey, J., Kramer, A., Hall, J. G., Pauli, R. M., et al.: Dominantly inherited renal adysplasia. Am. J. Med. Genet., 26:863, 1987.

Nomura, S., and Osawa, G.: Focal glomerular sclerotic lesions in a patient with urinary oligomeganephronia and agenesis of the contralateral kidney: A case report. Clin. Nephrol., 33:7, 1990.

Ochsner, M. G., Brannan, W., and Goodier, E. H.: Absent vas deferens associated with renal agenesis. JAMA, 222:1055, 1972.

Phelan, J. T., Counseller, V. S., and Greene, L. F.: Deformities of the urinary tract with congenital absence of the vagina. Surg. Gynecol. Obstet., 97:1, 1953.

Radasch, H. E.: Congenital unilateral absence of the urogenital system and its relation to the development of the Wolffian and Muellerian ducts. Am. J. Med. Sci., 136:111, 1908.

Roodhooft, A. M., Birnholz, J. C., and Holmes, L. D.: Familial nature of congenital absence and severe dysgenesis of both kidneys. N. Engl. J. Med., 310:1341, 1984.

Rugui, C., Oldrizzi, L., Lupo, A., Valvo, E., et al.: Clinical features of patients with solitary kidneys. Nephron, 43:10, 1986.

Say, B., and Gerald, P. S.: A new polydactyly/imperforate-anus/vertebral anomalies syndrome? Lancet, 1:688, 1968.

Semmens, J. P.: Congenital anomalies of the female genital tract: functional classification based on review of 56 personal cases and 500 reported cases. Obstet. Gynecol., 19:328, 1962.

Shieh, C. P., Hung, C. S., Wei, C. F., and Lin, C. Y.: Cystic dilatations within the pelvis in patients with ipsilateral renal agenesis or dysplasia. J. Urol., 144:324, 1990.

Shumacker, H. B.: Congenital anomalies of the genitalia associated with unilateral renal agenesis. Arch. Surg., 37:586, 1938.

Smith, E. C., and Orkin, L. A.: A clinical and statistical study of 471 congenital anomalies of the kidney and ureter. J. Urol., 53:11, 1945.

Thompson, D. P., and Lynn, H. B.: Genital anomalies associated with solitary kidney. Mayo Clin. Proc., 41:538, 1966.

Uchida, S., Akiba, T., Sasaki, S., Imo, Y., et al.: Unilateral renal agenesis associated with various metabolic disorders in three siblings. Nephron, 54:86, 1990.

Vinstein, A. L., and Franken, E. A., Jr.: Unilateral hematocolpos associated with agenesis of the kidney. Radiology, 102:625, 1972.

Weiss, J. M., and Dykhuizen, R. F.: An anomalous vaginal insertion into the bladder: A case report. J. Urol., 98:60, 1967.

Whitaker, R. H., and Hunt, G. M.: Incidence and distribution of renal anomalies in patients with neural tube defects. Eur. Urol., 13:322, 1987.

Wiersma, A. F., Peterson, L. F., and Justema, E. J.: Uterine anomalies associated with unilateral renal agenesis. Obstet. Gynecol., 47:654, 1976.

Wilson, R. D., and Baird, P. A.: Renal agenesis in British Columbia. Am. J. Med. Genet., 21:153, 1985.

Woolf, R. B., and Allen, W. M.: Concomitant malformations: The frequent simultaneous occurrence of congenital malformations of the reproductive and urinary tracts. Obstet. Gynecol., 2:236, 1953.

Yoder, I. C., and Pfister, R. C.: Unilateral hematocolpos and ipsilateral renal agenesis: Report of two cases and review of the literature. Am. J. Roentgenol., 127:303, 1976.

Supernumerary Kidney

Campbell, M. F.: Anomalies of the kidney. In Campbell, M. F., and Harrison, J. H. (Eds.): Urology, Vol. 2, 3rd ed. Philadelphia, W. B. Saunders Co., 1970, p. 1422.

Carlson, H. E.: Supernumerary kidney: A summary of fifty-one reported cases. J. Urol., 64:221, 1950.

Exley, M., and Hotchkiss, W. S.: Supernumerary kidney with clear cell carcinoma. J. Urol., 51:569, 1944.

Geisinger, J. F.: Supernumerary kidney. J. Urol., 38:331, 1937.

Hoffman, R. L., and McMillan, T. E.: Discussion. Trans. South Central Sec., American Urology Assoc., 82, 1948.

Kaneoya, F., Botoh, B., and Yokokawa, M.: Unusual duplication of renal collecting system mimicking supernumerary kidney. Nippon Hinyokika Bakkai Zasshi, 80:270, 1989.

Kretschmer, H. L.: Supernumerary kidney. Report of a case with review of the literature. Surg. Gynecol. Obstet., 49:818, 1929.

McPherson, R. I.: Supernumerary kidney: Typical and atypical features. Can. Assoc. Radiol. J., 38:116, 1987.

N'Guessan, G., and Stephens, F. O.: Supernumerary kidney. J. Urol., 130:649, 1983.

Rubin, J. S.: Supernumerary kidney with aberrant ureter terminating externally. J. Urol., 61:405, 1948.

Sasidharan, K., Babu, A. S., Rao, M. M., and Bhat, H. S.: Free supernumerary kidney. Br. J. Urol., 48:388, 1976.

Shan, J. H.: Supernumerary kidney with vaginal ureteral orifice. J. Urol., 47:344, 1942.

Tada, Y., Kokado, Y., Hashinaka, Y., et al.: Free supernumerary kidney: a case report and review. J. Urol., 126:231, 1981.

Anomalies of Ascent

Simple Renal Ectopia

Abeshouse, B. S., and Bhisitkul, I.: Crossed renal ectopia with and without fusion. Urol. Int., 9:63, 1959.

Anderson, E. E., and Harrison, J. H.: Surgical importance of the solitary kidney. N. Engl. J. Med., 273:683, 1965.

Anderson, G. W., Rice, G. G., and Harris, B. A., Jr.: Pregnancy and labor complicated by pelvic ectopic kidney. J. Urol., 65:760, 1951.

Anderson, G. W., Rice, G. G., and Harris, B. A., Jr.: Pregnancy and labor complicated by pelvic ectopic kidney anomalies. A review of the literature. Obstet. Gynecol. Surv., 4:737, 1949.

Anson, B. J., and Riba, L. W.: The anatomical and surgical features of ectopic kidney. Surg. Gynecol. Obstet., 68:37, 1939.

Baggenstoss, A. H.: Congenital anomalies of the kidney. Med. Clin. North Am., 35:987, 1951.

Bell, E. T.: Renal Diseases. Philadelphia, Lea & Febiger, 1946.

Campbell, M. F.: Renal ectopy. J. Urol., 24:187, 1930.

D'Alberton, A., Reschini, E., Ferrari, N., and Candiani, P.: Prevalence of urinary tract abnormalities in a large series of patients with uterovaginal atresia. J. Urol., 126:623, 1981.

Delson, B.: Ectopic kidney in obstetrics and gynecology. N.Y. State J. Med., 75:2522, 1975.

Downs, R. A., Lane, J. W., and Burns, E.: Solitary pelvic kidney: Its clinical implications. Urology, 1:51, 1973.

Dretler, S. P., Olsson, C. A., and Pfister, R. C.: The anatomic, radiologic and clinical characteristics of the pelvic kidney, an analysis of 86 cases. J. Urol., 105:623, 1971.

Fowler, H. A.: Bilateral renal ectopia. A report of four additional cases. J. Urol., 45:795, 1941.

Hawes, C. J.: Congenital unilateral ectopic kidney: A report of two cases. J. Urol., 64:453, 1950.

Malek, R. S., Kelalis, P. P., and Burke, E. C.: Ectopic kidney in children and frequency of association of other malformations. Mayo Clin. Proc. 46:461, 1971.

McCrea, L. E.: Congenital solitary pelvic kidney. J. Urol., 48:58, 1942.

Stevens, A. R.: Pelvic single kidneys. J. Urol., 37:610, 1937.

Tabisky, J., and Bhisitkul, I.: Solitary crossed ectopic kidney with vaginal aplasia: A case report. J. Urol., 94:33, 1965.

Thompson, G. J., and Pace, J. M.: Ectopic kidney: A review of 97 cases. Surg.-Gynecol. Obstet., 64:935, 1937.

Ward, J. N., Nathanson, B., and Draper, J. W.: The pelvic kidney. J. Urol., 94:36, 1965.

Cephalad Ectopia

Pinckney, L. E., Moskowitz, P. S., Lebowitz, R. L., and Fritzsche, P.: Renal malposition associated with omphalocele. Radiology, 129:677, 1978.

Thoracic Kidney

Ang, A. H., and Chan, W. F.: Ectopic thoracic kidney. J. Urol., 108:211, 1972.

Barloon, J. W., and Goodwin, W. E.: Thoracic kidney: Case reports. J. Urol., 78:356, 1957.

Berlin, H. S., Stein, J., and Poppel, M. H.: Congenital superior ectopia of the kidney. Am. J. Roentgenol., 78:508, 1957.

Burke, E. C., Wenzl, J. E., and Utz, D. C.: The intrathoracic kidney. Report of a case. Am. J. Dis. Child., 113:487, 1967.

Campbell, M. F.: Renal ectopy. J. Urol., 24:187, 1930.

DeCastro, F. J., and Shumacher, H.: Asymptomatic thoracic kidney. Clin. Pediatr., 8:279, 1969.

DeNoronha, L. L., Costa, M. F. E., and Godinho, M. T. M.: Ectopic thoracic kidney. Am. Rev. Respir. Dis., 109:678, 1974.

Franciskovic, V., and Martincic, N.: Intrathoracic kidney. Br. J. Urol., 31:156, 1959.

Fusonie, D., and Molnar, W.: Anomalous pulmonary venous return, pulmonary sequestration, bronchial atresia, aplastic right upper lobe, pericardial defect and intrathoracic kidney. An unusual complex of congenital anomalies in one patient. Am. J. Roentgenol., 97:350, 1966.

Gray, S. W., and Skandalakis, J. E.: The diaphragm. In Embryology for Surgeons, pp. 359–366, Philadelphia, W. B. Saunders Co., 1972.

Hertz, M., and Shahin, N.: Ectopic thoracic kidney. Isr. J. Med. Sci., 5:98, 1969.

Hill, J. E., and Bunts, R. C.: Thoracic kidney: Case reports. J. Urol., 84:460, 1960.

Liddell, R. M., Rosenbaum, D. M., and Blumhagen, J. D.: Delayed radiologic appearance of bilateral thoracic ectopic kidneys. Am. J. Roentgenol., 152:120, 1989.

Lozano, R. H., and Rodriguez, C.: Intrathoracic ectopic kidney: Report of a case. J. Urol., 114:601, 1975.

Lundius, B.: Intrathoracic kidney. Am. J. Roentgenol., 125:678, 1975.

N'Guessan, G., and Stephens, F. D.: Congenital superior ectopic (thoracic) kidney. Urology, 24:219, 1984.

Paul, A. T. S., Uragoda, C. G., and Jayewardene, F. L. W.: Thoracic kidney with report of a case. Br. J. Surg., 47:395, 1960.

Robbins, J. J., and Lich, R., Jr.: Thoracic kidney. J. Urol., 72:133, 1954.

Shapira, E., Fishel, E., and Levin, S.: Intrathoracic kidney in a premature infant. Arch. Dis. Child., 40:86, 1965.

Spillane, R. J., and Prather, G. C.: Right diaphragmatic eventration with renal displacement. Case report. J. Urol., 68:804, 1952.

Williams, A. G., Christie, J. H., and Mettler, S. A.: Intrathoracic kidney on radionuclide renography. Clin. Nucl. Med., 8:408, 1983.

Anomalies of Form and Fusion

Crossed Renal Ectopia With and Without Fusion

Abeshouse, B. S.: Crossed ectopia with fusion: Review of literature and a report of four cases. Am. J. Surg., 73:658, 1947.

Abeshouse, B. S., and Bhisitkul, I.: Crossed renal ectopia with and without fusion. Urol. Int., 9:63, 1959.

Alexander, J. C., King, K. B., and Fromm, C. S.: Congenital solitary kidney with crossed ureter. J. Urol., 64:230, 1950.

Ashley, D. J. B., and Mostofi, F. K.: Renal agenesis and dysgenesis. J. Urol., 83:211, 1960.

Baggenstoss, A. H.: Congenital anomalies of the kidney. Med. Clin. North Am., 35:987, 1951.

Bauer, S. B.: Personal communication, 1977.

Bissada, N. K., Fried, F. A., and Redman, J. F.: Crossed-fused renal ectopia with a solitary ureter. J. Urol., 114:304, 1975.

Boatman, D. L., Culp, D. A., Jr., Culp, D. A., and Flocks, R. H.: Crossed renal ectopia. J. Urol., 108:30, 1972.

Caine, M.: Crossed renal ectopia without fusion. Br. J. Urol., 28:257, 1956.

Caldamone, A. A., and Rabinowitz, R.: Crossed fused renal ectopia, orthotopic multicystic dysplasia and vaginal agenesis. J. Urol., 126:105, 1981.

Campbell, M. F.: Renal ectopy. J. Urol., 24:187, 1930.

Cass, A. S., and Vitko, R. J.: Unusual variety of crossed renal ectopy with only one ureter. J. Urol., 107:1056, 1972.

Cook, W. A., and Stephens, F. D.: Fused kidneys: Morphologic study and theory of embryogenesis. In Bergsma, D., and Duckett, J. W. (Eds.): Urinary System Malformations in Children. New York, Allen R. Liss, Inc., 1977.

Currarino, G., and Weisbruch, G. J.: Transverse fusion of the renal pelves and single ureter. Urol. Radiol., 11:88, 1989.

Diaz, G.: Renal ectopy: Report of a case with crossed ectopy without fusion, with fixation of kidney in normal position by the extraperitoneal route. J. Int. Coll. Surg., 19:158, 1953.

Dretler, S. P., Olsson, C. A., and Pfister, R. C.: The anatomic, radiologic and clinical characteristics of the pelvic kidney: An analysis of eighty-six cases. J. Urol., 105:623, 1971.

Gerber, W. L., Culp, D. A., Brown, R. C., Chow, R. C., and Platz, C. E.: Renal mass in crossed-fused ectopia, J. Urol., 123:239, 1980.

Glenn, J. F.: Fused pelvic kidney. J. Urol., 80:7, 1958.

Greenberg, L. W., and Nelsen, C. E.: Crossed fused ectopia of the kidneys in twins. Am. J. Dis. Child., 122:175, 1971.

Hendren, W. H., Donahoe, P. K., and Pfister, R. C.: Crossed renal ectopia in children. Urology, 7:135, 1976.

Hertz, M., Rabenstein, Z. J., Shalrin, N., and Melzer, M.: Crossed renal ectopia: clinical and radiologic findings in 22 cases. Clin. Radiol., 28:339, 1977.

Hildreth, T. A., and Cass, A. S.: Cross renal ectopia with familial occurrence. Urology, 12:59, 1978.

Joly, J. S.: Fusion of the kidneys. Proc. R. Soc. Med., 33:697, 1940.

Kakei, H., Kondo, A., Ogisu, B. I., and Mitsuya, H.: Crossed ectopia of solitary kidney: A report of two cases and a review of the literature. Urol. Int., 31:40, 1976.

Kelalis, P. P., Malek, R. S., and Segura, J. W.: Observations on renal ectopia and fusion in children. J. Urol., 110:588, 1973.

Kretschmer, H. L.: Unilateral fused kidney. Surg. Gynecol. Obstet., 40:360, 1925.

Kron, S. D., and Meranze, D. R.: Completely fused pelvic kidney. J. Urol., 62:278, 1949.

Lee, H. P.: Crossed unfused renal ectopia with tumor. J. Urol., 61:333, 1949.

Looney, W. W., and Dodd, D. L.: An ectopic (pelvic) completely fused (cake) kidney associated with various anomalies of the abdominal viscera. Ann. Surg., 84:522, 1956.

Macksood, M. J., and James, R. E., Jr.: Giant hydronephrosis in ectopic kidney in a child. Urology, 22:532, 1983.

Magri, J.: Solitary crossed ectopic kidney. Br. J. Urol., 33:152, 1961.

Maizels, M., and Stephens, F. D.: Renal ectopia and congenital scoliosis. Invest. Urol., 17:209, 1979.

Malek, R. S., and Utz, D. C.: Crossed, fused, renal ectopia with an ectopic ureterocele, J. Urol., 104:665, 1970.

McDonald, J. H., and McClellan, D. S.: Crossed renal ectopia. Am. J. Surg., 93:995, 1957.

Miles, B. J., Moon, M. R., Bellville, W. D., and Keesling, V. J.: Solitary crossed renal ectopia. J. Urol., 133:1022, 1985.

Mininberg, D. T., Roze, S., Yoon, H. J., and Pearl, M.: Hypertension associated with crossed renal ectopia in an infant. Pediatrics, 48:454, 1971.

Nussbaum, A. R., Hartman, D. S., Whitley, N., McCauley, R. G., and Sanders, R. C.: Multicystic dysplasia and crossed renal ectopia. Am. J. Roentgenol., 149:407, 1987.

Pathak, I. C.: Crossed renal ectopia without fusion associated with giant hydronephrosis. J. Urol., 94:323, 1965.

Potter, E. L.: Pathology of the Fetus and the Newborn. Chicago, Year Book Medical Publishers, 1952.

Purpon, I.: Crossed renal ectopy with solitary kidney: A review of the literature. J. Urol., 90:13, 1963.

Rubinstein, Z. J., Hertz, M., Shahin, N., and Deutsch, V.: Crossed renal ectopia: Angiographic findings in six cases. Am. J. Roentgenol., 126:1035, 1976.

Shah, M. H.: Solitary crossed renal ectopia. Br. J. Urol., 47:512, 1975.

Srivastava, R. N., Singh, M., Ghai, O. P., and Sethi, U.: Complete renal fusion ("cake"/"lump" kidney). Br. J. Urol., 43:391, 1971.

Stubbs, A. J., and Resnick, M. I.: Struvite staghorn calculi in crossed renal ectopia. J. Urol., 118:369, 1977.

Tabrisky, J., and Bhisitkul, I.: Solitary crossed ectopic kidney with vaginal aplasia: A case report. J. Urol., 94:33, 1965.

Tanenbaum, B., Silverman, N., and Weinberg, S. R.: Solitary crossed renal ectopia. Arch. Surg., 101:616, 1970.

Thompson, G. J., and Allen, R. B.: Unilateral fused kidney. Surg. Clin. North Am., 14:729, 1934.

Wilmer, H. A.: Unilateral fused kidney: A report of five cases and a review of the literature. J. Urol., 40:551, 1938.

Winram, R. G., and Ward-McQuaid, J. N.: Crossed renal ectopia without fusion. Can. Med. Assoc. J., 81:481, 1959.

Yates-Bell, A. J., and Packham, D. A.: Giant hydronephrosis in a solitary crossed ectopic kidney. Br. J. Surg., 59:104, 1972.

Horseshoe Kidney

Advisory Committee to the Renal Transplant Registry: The twelfth report of Human Renal Transplant Registry. JAMA, 233:787, 1975.

Beck, W. C., and Hlivko, A. E.: Wilms' tumor in the isthmus of a horseshoe kidney. Arch. Surg., 81:803, 1960.

Bell, R.: Horseshoe kidney in pregnancy. J. Urol., 56:159, 1946.

Benjamin, J. A., and Schullian, D. M.: Observation on fused kidneys with horseshoe configuration: The contribution of Leonardo Botallo (1564). J. Hist. Med., 5:315, 1950.

Blackard, C. E., and Mellinger, G. T.: Cancer in a horseshoe kidney. Arch. Surg., 97:616, 1968.

Boatman, D. L., Cornell, S. H., and Kolln, C. P.: The arterial supply of horseshoe kidney. Am. J. Roentgenol., 113:447, 1971.

Boatman, D. L., Kolln, C. P., and Flocks, R. H.: Congenital anomalies associated with horseshoe kidney. J. Urol., 107:205, 1972.

Boyden, E. A.: Description of a horseshoe kidney associated with left inferior vena cava and disc-shaped suprarenal glands, together with a note on the occurrence of horseshoe kidneys in human embryos. Anat. Rec., 51:187, 1931.

Bridge, R. A. C.: Horseshoe kidneys in identical twins. Br. J. Urol., 32:32, 1960.

Buntley, D.: Malignancy associated with horseshoe kidney. Urology, 8:146, 1976.

Campbell, M. F.: Anomalies of the kidney. In Campbell, M. F., and Harrison, J. H. (Eds.): Urology, Philadelphia, W. B. Saunders Co., 1970, pp. 1447–1452.

Castor, J. E., and Green, N. A.: Complications of horseshoe kidney. Urology, 6:344, 1975.

Christoffersen, J., and Iversen, H. G.: Partial hydronephrosis in a patient with horseshoe kidney and bilateral duplication of the pelvis and ureter. Scand. J. Urol. Nephrol., 10:91, 1976.

Cook, W. A., and Stephens, F. D.: Fused kidneys: Morphologic study and theory of embryogenesis. In Bergsma, D., and Duckett, J. W. (Eds.): Urinary Systems Malformations in Children. New York, Allen R. Liss, Inc., 1977.

Correa, R. J., Jr., and Paton, R. R.: Polycystic horseshoe kidney. J. Urol., 116:802, 1976.

Dajani, A. M.: Horseshoe kidney: A review of twenty-nine cases. Br. J. Urol., 38:388, 1966.

Das, S., and Amar, A. D.: Ureteropelvic junction obstruction with associated renal anomalies. J. Urol., 131:872, 1984.

David, R. S.: Horseshoe kidney: A report of one family. Br. Med. J., 4:571, 1974.

Dees, J.: Clinical importance of congenital anomalies of upper urinary tract. J. Urol., 46:659, 1941.

Dische, M. R., and Johnston, R.: Teratoma in horseshoe kidneys. Urology, 13:435, 1979.

Eidelman, A., Yuval, E., Simon, D., and Sibi, Y.: Retrocaval ureter. Eur. Urol., 4:279, 1978.

Evans, W. P., and Resnick, M. I.: Horseshoe kidney and urolithiasis. J. Urol., 125:620, 1981.

Garg, R. K.: Personal communication, 1990.

Glenn, J. F.: Analysis of 51 patients with horseshoe kidney. N. Engl. J. Med., 261:684, 1959.

Grandone, C. H., Haller, J. O., Berdon, W. E., and Friedman, A. P.: Asymmetric horseshoe kidney in the infant: Value of renal nuclear scanning. Radiology, 154:366, 1985.

Gutierrez, R.: The Clinical Management of Horseshoe Kidney: A Study of Horseshoe Kidney Disease, Its Etiology, Pathology, Symptomatology, Diagnosis and Treatment. New York, Paul B. Hoeber, Inc., 1934.

Hefferman, J. C., Lightwood, R. G., and Snell, M. E.: Horseshoe kidney with retrocaval ureter: second reported case. J. Urol., 120:358, 1978.

Jarmin, W. D.: Surgery of the horseshoe kidney with a postaortic isthmus: Report of two cases of horseshoe kidney. J. Urol., 40:1, 1938.

Kolln, C. P., Boatman, D. L., Schmidt, J. D., and Flocks, R. H.: Horseshoe kidney: A review of 105 patients. J. Urol., 107:203, 1972.

Leiter, E.: Horseshoe kidney: Discordance in monozygotic twins. J. Urol., 108:683, 1972.

Lippe, B., Geffner, M. E., Dietrich, R. B., Boeschat, M. I., and Kangarloo, H.: Renal malformations in patients with Turner syndrome: Imaging in 141 patients. Pediatrics, 82:852, 1988.

Love, L., and Wasserman, D.: Massive unilateral nonfunctioning hydronephrosis in horseshoe kidney. Clin. Radiol., 26:409, 1975.

Meek, J. R., and Wadsworth, G. H.: A case of horseshoe kidney lying between the great vessels. J. Urol., 43:448, 1940.

Murphy, D. M., and Zincke, H.: Transitional cell carcinoma in the horseshoe kidney: report of 3 cases and review of the literature. Br. J. Urol., 54:484, 1982.

Nation, E. F.: Horseshoe kidney, a study of thirty-two autopsy and nine surgical cases. J. Urol., 53:762, 1945.

Novak, M. E., Baum, N. H., and Gonzales, E. T.: Horseshoe kidney with multicystic dysplasia associated ureterocele. Urology, 10:456, 1977.

Pitts, W. R., and Muecke, E. C.: Horseshoe kidneys: A 40 year experience. J. Urol., 113:743, 1975.

Roy, J. B., and Stevens, R. K.: Polycystic horseshoe kidney. Urology, 6:222, 1975.

Segura, J. W., Kelalis, P. P., and Burke, E. G.: Horseshoe kidney in children. J. Urol., 108:333, 1972.

Sharma, S. K., and Bapna, B. C.: Surgery of the horseshoe kidney—an experience of 24 patients. Aust. N. Zeal. J. Surg., 56:175, 1986.

Shoup, G. D., Pollack, H. M., and Dou, J. H.: Adenocarcinoma occurring in a horseshoe kidney. Arch. Surg., 84:413, 1962.

Silagy, J. M.: The horseshoe kidney and its disease. J. Mt. Sinai Hosp., 18:297, 1952.

Smith, D. W.: Recognizable patterns of human malformation; genetic embryologic and clinical aspects. Major Problems in Clinical Pediatrics. 7. Philadelphia, W. B. Saunders Co., 1970, p. 50.

Smith, E. C., and Orkin, L. A.: A clinical and statistical study of 471 congenital anomalies of the kidney and ureter. J. Urol., 53:11, 1945.

Voisin, M., Djernit, A., Morin, D., Grolleau, R., Dumas, R., and Jean, R.: Cardiopathies congenitales et malformations urinaires. Arch. Mal. Coeur, 81:703, 1988.

Walker, D.: Personal communication, 1977.

Whitaker, R. H., and Hunt, G. M.: Incidence and distribution of renal anomalies in patients with neural tube defects. Eur. Urol., 13:322, 1987.

Whitehouse, G. H.: Some urographic aspects of the horseshoe kidney anomaly—a review of 59 cases. Clin. Radiol., 26:107, 1975.

Zondek, L. H., and Zondek, T.: Horseshoe kidney in associated congenital malformations. Urol. Int., 18:347, 1964.

Anomalies of Rotation

Campbell, M. F.: Anomalies of the kidney. In Campbell, M. F. (Ed.): Urology, Vol. 2, 2nd ed. Philadelphia, W. B. Saunders Co., 1963, p. 1589.

Felix, W.: The development of the urogenital organs. In Keibel, F., and Mall, F. P. (Eds.): Manual of Human Embryology, Vol. 2. Philadelphia, J. B. Lippincott Co., 1912, p. 752.

Gray, S. W., and Skandalakis, J. E.: The kidney and ureter. In Embryology for Surgeons. Philadelphia, W. B. Saunders Co., 1972, p. 480.

Mackie, G. G., Awang, H., and Stephens, F. D.: The ureteric orifice: The embryologic key to radiologic status of duplex kidneys. J. Pediatr. Surg., 10:473, 1975.

Smith, E. C., and Orkin, L. A.: A clinical and statistical study of 471 congenital anomalies of the kidney and ureter. J. Urol., 53:11, 1945.

Weyrauch, H. M., Jr.: Anomalies of renal rotation. Surg. Gynecol. Obstet., 69:183, 1939.

Anomalies of the Renal Vasculature

Aberrant, Accessory, or Multiple Vessels

Anson, B. J., and Daseler, E. H.: Common variations in renal anatomy, affecting the blood supply, form and topography. Surg. Gynecol. Obstet., 112:439, 1961.

Anson, B. J., and Kurth, L. E.: Common variations in the renal blood supply. Surg. Gynecol. Obstet., 100:157, 1955.

Fraley, E. E.: Dismembered infundibulopyelostomy. Improved technique for correcting vascular obstruction of the superior infundibulum. J. Urol., 101:144, 1969.

Fraley, E. E.: Vascular obstruction of superior infundibulum causing nephralgia. A new syndrome. N. Engl. J. Med., 275:1403, 1966.

Geyer, J. R., and Poutasse, E. F.: Incidence of multiple renal arteries on aortography. JAMA, 182:118, 1962.

Graves, F. T.: The aberrant renal artery. J. Anat., 90:553, 1956.

Graves, F. T.: The anatomy of the intrarenal arteries and its application to segmental resection of the kidney. Br. J. Surg., 42:132, 1954.

Gray, S. W., and Skandalakis, J. E.: Anomalies of the kidney and ureter. In Embryology for Surgeons. Philadelphia, W. B. Saunders Co., 1972, p. 485.

Guggemos, E.: A rare case of an arterial connection between the left and right kidneys. Ann. Surg., 156:940, 1962.

Merklin, R. J., and Michele, N. A.: The variant renal and suprarenal blood supply with data on the inferior phrenic, ureteral and gonadal arteries. A statistical analysis based on 185 dissections and review of the literature. J. Int. Coll. Surg., 29:41, 1958.

Nathan, H.: Observation on aberrant renal arteries curving around and compressing the renal vein: Possible relationship to orthostatic proteinuria and to orthostatic hypertension. Circulation, 18:1131, 1958.

Pick, J. W., and Anson, B. J.: The renal vascular pedicle. J. Urol., 44:411, 1940.

White, R. R., and Wyatt, G. M.: Surgical importance of aberrant renal vessels in infants and children. Am. J. Surg., 58:48, 1942.

Renal Artery Aneurysms

Abeshouse, B. S.: Renal aneurysm: Report of two cases and review of the literature. Urol. Cutan. Rev., 55:451, 1951.

Cerny, J. C., Chang, C. Y., and Fry, W. J.: Renal artery aneurysms. Arch. Surg., 96:653, 1968.

Garritano, A. P.: Aneurysm of the renal artery. Am. J. Surg., 94:638, 1957.

Glass, P. M., and Uson, A. C.: Aneurysms of the renal artery: A study of 20 cases. J. Urol., 98:285, 1967.

Hageman, J. H., Smith, R. F., Szilagyi, D. E., and Elliot, J. P.: Aneurysms of the renal artery: problems of prognosis and surgical management. Surgery, 84:563, 1978.

Lorentz, W. B., Jr., Browning, M. C., D'Souza, V. J., Glass, T. A., and Formanek, A. G.: Intrarenal aneurysm of the renal artery in children. Am. J. Dis. Child., 138:751, 1984.

McKeil, C. F., Jr., Graf, E. C., and Callahan, D. H.: Renal artery aneurysms: A report of 16 cases. J. Urol., 96:593, 1966.

Poutasse, E. F.: Renal artery aneurysms. J. Urol., 113:443, 1975.

Poutasse, E. F.: Renal artery aneurysm: Report of 12 cases, two treated by excision of the renal aneurysm and repair of renal artery. J. Urol., 77:697, 1957.

Rhodes, J. F., and Johnson, G., Jr.: Renal artery aneurysm. J. Urol., 105:155, 1971.

Silvis, R. S., Hughes, W. F., and Holmes, F. H.: Aneurysm of the renal artery. Am. J. Surg., 91:339, 1956.

Stanley, J. C., Rhodes, E. L., Gewertz, G. L., Chang, C. Y., Walter, J. F., and Fry, W. J.: Renal artery aneurysms: significance of macroaneurysms exclusive of dissections and fibrodysplastic mural dilations. Arch. Surg., 110:1327, 1975.

Zinman, L., and Libertino, J. A.: Uncommon disorders of the renal circulation: renal artery aneurysm. In Breslin, D. J., Swinton, N. W., Libertino, J. A., and Zinman, L. (Eds.): Renovascular Hypertension. Baltimore, Williams & Wilkins, 1982, pp. 110–114.

Renal Arteriovenous Fistula

Bentson, J. R., and Crandall, P. H.: Use of the Fogarty catheter in arteriovenous malformations of the spinal cord. Radiology, 105:65, 1972.

Boijsen, E., and Kohler, R.: Renal arteriovenous fistulae. Acta Radiol., 57:433, 1962.

Bookstein, J. J., and Goldstein, H. M.: Successful management of post biopsy arteriovenous fistula with selective arterial embolization. Radiology, 109:535, 1973.

Cho, K. J., and Stanley, J. C.: Non-neoplastic congenital and acquired renal arteriovenous malformations and fistula. Radiology, 129:333, 1978.

Crummy, A. B., Jr., Atkinson, R. J., and Caruthers, S. B.: Congenital renal arteriovenous fistulas. J. Urol., 93:24, 1965.

DeSai, S. G., and DeSautels, R. E.: Congenital arteriovenous malformation of the kidney. J. Urol., 110:17, 1973.

Gunterberg, B.: Renal arteriovenous malformation. Acta Radiol., 7:425, 1968.

Maldonado, J. E., Sheps, S. G., Bernatz, P. E., DeWeerd, J. H., and Harrison, E. G., Jr.: Renal arteriovenous fistula. Am. J. Med., 37:499, 1964.

McAlhany, J. C., Jr., Black, H. C., Hanback, L. D., Jr., and Yarbrough, D. R., III: Renal arteriovenous fistula as a cause of hypertension. Am. J. Surg., 122:117, 1971.

Messing, E., Kessler, R., and Kavaney, P. B.: Renal arteriovenous fistula. Urology, 8:101, 1976.

Takaha, M., Matsumoto, A., Ochi, K., Takeuchi, M., Takemoto, M., and Sonoda, T.: Intrarenal arteriovenous malformation. J. Urol., 124:315, 1980.

Thomason, W. B., Gross, M., Radwin, H. M., Hulse, C. M., and Dobbs, R. M.: Intrarenal arteriovenous fistulas. J. Urol., 108:526, 1972.

Yazaki, T., Tomita, M., Akimoto, M., Konjiki, T., Kawai, H., and Kumazaki, T.: Congenital renal arteriovenous fistula: Case report, review of Japanese literature and description of nonradical treatment. J. Urol., 116:415, 1976.

Calyx and Infundibulum

Abeshouse, B. S.: Serous cysts of the kidney and their differentiation from other cystic diseases of the kidney. Urol. Cutan. Rev., 54:582, 1950.

Briner, V., and Thiel, G.: Hereditares Poland syndrom mit megacalicose der rechten niere. Schweitzerische Med. Wochenschr., 118:898, 1988.

Boyce, W. H., and Whitehurst, A. W.: Hypoplasia of the major renal conduits. J. Urol., 116:352, 1976.

Dacie, J. E.: The "central lucency" sign of low bar dysmorphism (pseudotumour of the kidney). Br. J. Radiol., 49:39, 1976.

Devine, C. J., Jr., Guzman, J. A., Devine, P. C., and Poutasse, E. F.: Calyceal diverticulum. J. Urol., 101:8, 1969.

Eisendrath, D. N.: Report of case of hydronephrosis in kidney with extrarenal calyces. J. Urol., 13:51, 1925.

Fraley, E. E.: Vascular obstruction of superior infundibulum causing nephralgia—new syndrome. N. Engl. J. Med., 275:1403, 1966.

Galian, P., Forest, M., and Aboulker, P.: La megacaliose. Nouv. Presse Med., 78:1663, 1970.

Gittes, R. F.: Congenital magacalices. Monogr. Urol., 5:(1):1, 1984.

Gittes, R. F., and Talner, L. B.: Congenital megacalyces vs. obstructive hydronephrosis. J. Urol., 108:833, 1972.

Harrison, R. B., Wood, J. L., and Gillenwater, J. Y.: A solitary calyx in a human kidney. Radiology, 121:310, 1976.

Johnston, J. H., and Sandomirsky, S. K.: Intrarenal vascular obstruction of the superior infundibulum in children. J. Pediatr. Surg., 7:318, 1972.

Kelalis, P. P., and Malek, R. S.: Infundibulopelvic stenosis. J. Urol., 125:568, 1981.

Kleeman, F. J.: Unilateral megacalicosis. J. Urol., 110:387, 1973.

Kozakewich, H. P. W., and Lebowitz, R. L.: Congenital megacalices. Pediatr. Radiol., 2:251, 1974.

Lister, J., and Singh, H.: Pelvicalyceal cysts in children. J. Pediatr. Surg., 8:901, 1973.

Malament, M., Schwartz, B., and Nagamatsu, G. R.: Extrarenal calyces: their relationship to renal disease. Am. J. Roentgenol., 86:823, 1961.

Mandell, G. A., Snyder, H. M., 3rd, Haymen, S., Keller, M., Kaplan, J. M., and Norman, M. E.: Association of congenital megacalycosis and ipsilateral segmental megaureter. Pediatr. Radiol., 17:28, 1987.

Mathieson, A. J. M.: Calyceal diverticulum: A case with a discussion and a review of the condition. Br. J. Urol., 25:147, 1953.

Middleton, A. W., Jr., and Pfister, R. C.: Stone-containing pyelocaliceal diverticulum: Embryogenic, anatomic, radiologic and clinical characteristics. J. Urol., 111:1, 1974.

Moore, T.: Hydrocalycosis. Br. J. Urol., 22:304, 1950.

Morimoto, S., Sangen, H., Takamatsu, M., et al.: Solitary calix in siblings. J. Urol., 122:690, 1979.

Neal, A., and Murphy, L.: Unipapillary kidney: an unusual developmental abnormality of the kidney. J. Coll. Radiol. Aust., 4:81, 1960.

Parker, J. A., Lebowitz, R., Mascatello, V., and Treves, S.: Magnification renal scintigraphy in differential diagnosis of septa of Bertin. Pediatr. Radiol., 4:157, 1976.

Patriquin, H., Lafortune, M., and Filiatrault, D.: Urinary milk of calcium in children and adults: Use of gravity-dependent sonography. Am. J. Roentgenol., 144:407, 1985.

Puigvert, A.: Megacaliosis: diagnostico diferencial con la hidrocaliectasia. Med. Clin., 41:294, 1963.

Puigvert, A.: Megacalicose—Diagnostic differentiel avec l'hydrocaliectasie. Helv. Chir. Acta, 31:414, 1964.

Rao, D. V. N., Sharma, S. K., Rao, N. S., and Bapna, B. C.: Extrarenal calyces with complications: A case report. Aust. N. Z. J. Surg., 42:178, 1972.

Sakatoku, J., and Kitayama, T.: Solitary unipapillary kidney: presentation of a case. Acta Urol. Jpn., 10:349, 1964.

Siegel, M. J., and McAlister, W. H.: Calyceal diverticula in children: unusual features and complications. Radiology, 131:79, 1979.

Timmons, J. W., Jr., Malek, R. S., Hattery, R. R., and DeWeerd, J.: Caliceal diverticulum. J. Urol., 114:6, 1975.

Toppercer, A.: Unipapillary human kidney associated with urinary and genital abnormalities. Urology, 16:194, 1980.

Uhlenhuth, E., Amin, M., Harty, J. I., and Howerton, L. W.: Infundibular dysgenesis: A spectrum of obstructive renal disease. Urology, 35:334, 1990.

Vela Navarrete, R., and Garcia Robledo, J.: Polycystic disease of the renal sinus: structural characteristics. J. Urol., 129:700, 1983.

Webb, J. A. W., Fry, I. K., and Charlton, C. A. C.: An anomalous calyx in the mid-kidney: An anatomical variant. Br. J. Radiol., 48:674, 1975.

Williams, D. I., and Mininberg, D. T.: Hydrocalycosis: Report of three cases in children. Br. J. Urol., 40:541, 1968.

Anomalies of the Ureteropelvic Junction

Allen, T. D.: Congenital ureteral stricture. J. Urol., 104:196, 1970.

Allen, T. D.: Congenital ureteral strictures. In Lutzeyer, W., and Melchior, H. (Eds.): Urodynamic. Upper and Lower Urinary Tract. Berlin, Springer-Verlag, 1973, pp. 137–147.

Amar, A. D.: Congenital hydronephrosis of lower segment in duplex kidney. Urology, 7:480, 1976.

Belis, J. A., Belis, T. E., Lai, J. C. W., Goodwin, C. A., and Gabrielle, O. F.: Radionuclide determination of individual kidney function in the treatment of chronic renal obstruction. J. Urol., 127:898, 1982.

Belman, A. B., Kropp, K. F., and Simon, N. M.: Renal pressor hypertension secondary to unilateral hydronephrosis. N. Engl. J. Med., 278:1133, 1968.

Bernstein, G. T., Mandell, J., Lebowitz, R. L., Bauer, S. B., Colodny, A. H., and Retik, A. B.: Ureteropelvic junction obstruction in the neonate. J. Urol., 140:1216, 1988.

Brown, T., Mandell, J., and Lebowitz, R. L.: Neonatal hydronephrosis in the era of ultrasonography. AJR, 148:959, 1987.

Cohen, B., Goldman, S. M., Kopilnick, M., Khurana, A. V., and Salik, J. O.: Ureteropelvic junction obstruction: its occurrence in 3 members of a single family. J. Urol., 120:361, 1978.

Colgan, J. R., III, Skaist, L., and Morrow, J. W.: Benign ureteral tumors in childhood: A case report and a plea for conservative management. J. Urol., 109:308, 1973.

Colodny, A. H., Retik, A. B., and Bauer, S. B.: Antenatal diagnosis of fetal urologic abnormalities by intrauterine ultrasonography; therapeutic implications. Presented at Annual Meeting of the American Urological Association, San Francisco, May 18, 1980.

Dejter, S. R., Jr., Eggli, D. F., and Gibbons, M. D.: Delayed management of neonatal hydronephrosis. J. Urol., 140:1305, 1988.

Dowling, K. J., Harmon, E. P., Ortenberg, J., Palanco, E., and Evans, B. B.: Ureteropelvic junction obstruction: The effect of pyeloplasty on renal function. J. Urol., 140:1227, 1988.

Ericsson, N. O., Rudhe, U., and Livaditis, A.: Hydronephrosis associated with aberrant renal vessels in infants and children. Surgery, 50:687, 1961.

Foote, J. W., Blennerhassett, J. B., Wiglesworth, F. W., and MacKinnon, K. J.: Observations on the ureteropelvic junction. J. Urol., 104:252, 1970.

Fourcroy, J. L., Blei, C. L., Glassman, L. M., and White, R.: Prenatal diagnosis by ultrasonography of genitourinary abnormalities. Urology, 22:223, 1983.

Grignon, A., Filiatrault, D., Homsy, Y., Robitaille, P., Fillion, R., Boutin, H., and Leblond, R.: Ureteropelvic junction stenosis: Antenatal ultrasonographic diagnosis, postnatal investigation and follow-up. Radiology, 160:649, 1986.

Grossman, I. C., Cromie, W. J., Wein, A. J., and Duckett, J. W.: Renal hypertension secondary to ureteropelvic junction obstruction. Urology, 17:69, 1981.

Gup, A.: Benign mesodermal polyp in childhood. J. Urol., 114:610, 1975.

Hanna, M. K., Jeffs, R. D., Sturgess, J. M., and Barkin, M.: Ureteral structure and ultrastructure. Part II. Congenital ureteropelvic junction obstruction and primary obstructive megaureter. J. Urol., 116:725, 1976.

Hutch, J. A., Hinman, F., Jr., and Miller, E. R.: Reflux as a cause of hydronephrosis and chronic pyelonephritis. J. Urol., 88:169, 1962.

Johnston, J. H.: The pathogenesis of hydronephrosis in children. Br. J. Urol., 41:724, 1969.

Johnston, J. H., Evans, J. P., Glassberg, K. I., and Shapiro, S. R.: Pelvic hydronephrosis in children: A review of 219 personal cases. J. Urol., 117:97, 1977.

Joseph, D. B., Bauer, S. B., Colodny, A. H., Mandell, J., Lebowitz, R. L., and Retik, A. B.: Lower pole ureteropelvic junction obstruction and incomplete duplication. J. Urol., 141:896, 1989.

Juskiewenski, S., Moscovici, J., Bouissou, F., Yayssi, P., and Guitard, J.: Le syndrome de la junction pyelo-ureterale chez l'enfant. A propos de 178 observations. J. d'Urologie, 89:173, 1983.

Kass, E. J., Majd, M., and Belman, A. B.: Comparison of the diuretic renogram and pressure profusion study in children. J. Urol., 134:92, 1985.

Kass, E. J., and Fink-Bennett, D.: Radioisotopic evaluation of the dilated urinary tract. Urol. Clin. North Am., 17:273, 1990.

Kelalis, P. P., Culp, O. S., Stickler, G. B., and Burke, E. C.: Ureteropelvic obstruction in children: Experiences with 109 cases. J. Urol., 106:418, 1971.

King, L. R., Coughlin, P. W. F., Bloch, E. C., Bowie, J. D., Ansong, K., and Hanna, M. K.: The case for immediate pyeloplasty in the neonate with ureteropelvic junction obstruction. J. Urol., 132:725, 1984.

Koff, S. A.: Ureteropelvic junction obstruction: role of newer diagnostic methods. J. Urol., 127:898, 1982.

Koff, S. A., Hayden, L. J., and Cirulli, C.: Pathophysiology of ureteropelvic junction obstruction: Experimental and clinical observations. J. Urol., 136:336, 1986.

Koff, S. A.: Pathophysiology of ureteropelvic junction obstructions. Urol. Clin. North Am., 17:263, 1990.

Krueger, R. P., Ash, J. M., Silver, M. M., Kass, E. J., et al.: Primary hydronephrosis: assessment of diuretic renography, pelvis perfusion pressure, operative findings and renal and ureteral histology. Urol. Clin. North Am., 7:231, 1980.

Lebowitz, R. L., and Blickman, J. G.: The coexistence of ureteropelvic junction obstruction and reflux. Am. J. Roentgenol., 140:231, 1983.

Lebowitz, R. I., and Griscom, N. T.: Neonatal hydronephrosis: 146 cases. Radiol. Clin. North Am., 15:49, 1977.

Leiter, E.: Persistent fetal ureter. J. Urol., 122:251, 1979.

Lowe, F. C., and Marshall, S. F.: Ureteropelvic junction obstruction in adults. Urology, 23:331, 1984.

Maizels, M., and Stephens, F. D.: Valves of the ureter as a cause of primary obstruction of the ureter: anatomic, embryologic and clinical aspects. J. Urol., 123:742, 1980.

Malek, R. S.: Intermittent hydronephrosis. The occult ureteropelvic junction obstruction. J. Urol., 130:863, 1983.

Mandell, J., Peters, C. A., and Retik, A. B.: Current concepts in the perinatal diagnosis and management of hydronephrosis. Urol. Clin. North Am., 17:247, 1990.

Manning, F. A.: Fetal surgery for obstructive uropathy: Rational considerations. Am. J. Kidney Dis., 10:259, 1987.

Mering, J. H., Steel, J. F., and Gittes, R. F.: Congenital ureteral valves. J. Urol., 107:737, 1972.

Munoz, A. I., Pascual y Baralt, J. F., and Melendez, M. T.: Arterial hypertension in infants with hydronephrosis. Am. J. Dis. Child., 131:38, 1977.

Murnaghan, G. F.: The dynamics of the renal pelvis and ureter with reference to congenital hydronephrosis. Br. J. Urol., 30:321, 1958.

Nesbit, R. M.: Diagnosis of intermittent hydronephrosis: Importance of pyelography during episodes of pain. J. Urol., 75:767, 1956.

Nixon, H. H.: Hydronephrosis in children: A clinical study of seventy-eight cases with special reference to the role of aberrant renal vessels and the results of conservative operations. Br. J. Surg., 40:601, 1953.

Notley, R. G.: Electron microscopy of the upper ureter and the pelviureteric junction. Br. J. Urol., 40:37, 1968.

O'Reilly, P. H., Lawson, R. S., Shields, R. A., and Testa, H. J.: Idiopathic hydronephrosis—the diuresis renogram: a new non-invasive method of assessing equivocal pelvioureteral junction obstruction. J. Urol., 121:153, 1979.

Osathanondh, V., and Potter, E. L.: Development of the kidney as shown by microdissection. Arch. Pathol., 76:271, 1963.

Ostling, K.: The genesis of hydronephrosis. Acta Chir. Scand., 86:Suppl. 72, 1942.

Parker, R. M., Rudd, T. G., Wonderly, R. K., and Ansell, J. S.: Ureteropelvic junction obstruction in infants and children: functional evaluation of the obstructed kidney preoperatively and post-operatively. J. Urol., 126:509, 1981.

Perlmutter, A. D., Kroovand, R. L., and Lai, Y. W.: Management of ureteropelvic obstruction in the first year of life. J. Urol., 123:535, 1980.

Ransley, P. G.: The continuing dilemma of the asymptomatic dilated urinary tract: The Great Ormond Street experience. Presented at the Annual Meeting of the Society for Pediatric Urology, New Orleans, May 12, 1990.

Robson, W. J., Rudy, S. M., and Johnston, J. H.: Pelviureteric obstruction in infancy. J. Pediatr. Surg., 11:57, 1976.

Roth, D. R., and Gonzales, E. J., Jr.: Management of ureteropelvic junction obstruction in infants. J. Urol., 129:108, 1983.

Ruano-Gil, D., Coca-Payeras, A., and Tejedo-Maten, A.: Obstruction and normal re-canalization of the ureter in the human embryo: its relation to congenital ureteric obstruction. Eur. Urol., 1:287, 1975.

Segura, J. W., Hattery, R. R., and Hartman, G. W.: Fluoroscopic evaluation of intermittent ureteropelvic junction obstruction after furosemide stimulation. J. Urol., 112:449, 1974.

Shopfner, C. E.: Ureteropelvic junction obstruction. Am. J. Roentgenol., 98:148, 1966.

Snyder, H. M., III, Lebowitz, R. L., Colodny, A. H., Bauer, S. B., and Retik, A. B.: Ureteropelvic junction obstruction in children. Urol. Clin. North Am., 7:273, 1980.

Squitieri, A. P., Ceccarelli, F. E., and Wurster, J. C.: Hypertension with elevated renal vein renins secondary to ureteropelvic junction obstruction. J. Urol., 111:284, 1974.

Stephens, F. D.: Ureterovascular hydronephrosis and the "aberrant" renal vessels. J. Urol., 128:984, 1982.

Thorup, J., Pederson, P. V., and Clausen, N.: Benign ureteral polyps as a cause of hydronephrosis in a child. J. Urol., 126:796, 1981.

Uehling, D. T., Gilbert, E., and Chesney, R.: Urologic implications of the VATER association. J. Urol., 129:352, 1983.

Ulmsten, U., and Diehl, J.: Investigation of ureteric function with simultaneous intraureteric pressure recordings and ureteropyelography. Radiology, 117:283, 1975.

Uson, A. C., Cox, L. A., and Lattimer, J. K.: Hydronephrosis in infants and children. I. Some clinical and pathological aspects. JAMA, 205:323, 1968.

Whitaker, R. H.: Methods of assessing obstruction in dilated ureters. Br. J. Urol., 45:15, 1973.

Whitaker, R. H.: Some observations and theories on the wide ureter and hydronephrosis. Br. J. Urol., 47:377, 1975.

Whitaker, R. H.: Reflux induced pelviureteric obstruction. Br. J. Urol., 48:555, 1976.

Williams, D. I., and Karlaftis, C. M.: Hydronephrosis due to pelviureteric obstruction in the newborn. Br. J. Urol., 38:138, 1966.

Williams, D. I., and Kenawi, M. M.: The prognosis of pelviureteric obstruction in childhood: A review of 190 cases. Eur. Urol., 2:57, 1976.

Williams, P. R., Fegetter, J., Miller, R. A., and Wickham, J. E. A.: The diagnosis and management of benign fibrous ureteric polyps. Br. J. Urol., 52:253, 1980.

Anomalies of the Ureter

General References

Arey, L. B.: Developmental Anatomy: A Textbook and Laboratory Manual of Embryology, 7th ed. Philadelphia, W. B. Saunders Co., 1974.

Campbell, M. F.: Anomalies of the ureter. In Campbell M. F., and Harrison, J. H. (Eds.): Urology, 3rd ed. Philadelphia, W. B. Saunders Co., 1970.

Ellerker, A. G.: The extravesical ectopic ureter. Br. J. Surg., 45:344, 1958.

Frazer, J. E.: The terminal part of the Wolffian duct. J. Anat., 69:455, 1935.

Glassberg, K. I., Braren, V., Duckett, J. W., Jacobs, E. C., King, L. R., Lebowitz, R. L., Perlmutter, A. D., and Stephens, F. D.: Suggested terminology for duplex systems, ectopic ureters and ureteroceles: Report of the Committee on Terminology, Nomenclature and Classification, Section on Urology, American Academy of Pediatrics. J. Urol., 132;1153, 1984.

Gray, S. W., and Skandalakis, J. E.: Embryology for Surgeons. The Embryological Basis for the Treatment of Congenital Defects. Philadelphia, W. B. Saunders Co., 1972.

Koyanagi, T., and Tsuji, I.: Experience of complete duplication of the collecting system. Int. Urol. Nephrol., 11:27, 1979.

Mackie, G. G., and Stephens, F. D.: Duplex kidneys: A correlation of renal dysplasia with position of the ureteral orifice. J. Urol., 114:274, 1975.

Mackie, G. G., Awang, H., and Stephens, F. D.: The ureteric orifice: The embryologic key to radiologic status of duplex kidneys. J. Pediatr. Surg., 10:473, 1975.

Meyer, R.: Normal and abnormal development of the ureter in the human embryo—a mechanistic consideration. Anat. Rec., 96:355, 1946.

Ruano-Gil, D., Coca-Payeras, A., and Tejedo-Mateu, A.: Obstruction and normal recanalization of the ureter in the human embryo. Its relation to congenital ureteric obstruction. Eur. Urol., 1:287, 1975.

Schwartz, R. D., Stephens, F. D., and Cussen, L. J.: The pathogenesis of renal dysplasia. II. The significance of lateral and medial ectopy of the ureteric orifice. Invest. Urol., 19:97, 1981.

Smith, E. C., and Orkin, L. A.: A clinical and statistical study of 471 congenital anomalies of the kidney and ureter. J. Urol., 53:11, 1945.

Stephens, F. D.: Congenital Malformations of the Rectum, Anus and Genito-urinary Tracts. London, E & S Livingstone Ltd., 1963.

Tanagho, E. A.: Embryologic basis for lower ureteral anomalies: A hypothesis. Urology, 7:451, 1976.

Wharton, L. R., Jr.: Double ureters and associated renal anomalies in early human embryos. Contrib. Embryol. Carnegie Inst. Wash., 33:103, 1949.

Anomalies of Number

Duplications of the Ureter

Ahmed, S., and Pope, R.: Uncrossed complete ureteral duplication with upper system reflux. J. Urol., 135:128–129, 1986.

Archangelskj, S.: Uerdoppelung der ureteren und ihre chirurgische bedeutung. Zentralorgan Fuer Die Gesamte Chirurgie Und Ihre Grenzgebeite., 37:137, 1927.

Atwell, J. D., Cook, P. L., Howell, C. J., et al.: Familial incidence of bifid and double ureters. Arch. Dis. Child., 49:390, 1974.

Barnes, D. G., and McGeorge, A. M.: The duplex ureter in Burnley, Pendle and Rossendale. Br. J. Urol., 64:345–346, 1989.

Beer, E., and Mencher, W. H.: Heminephrectomy in disease of the double kidney. Report of fourteen cases. Ann. Surg., 108:705, 1938.

Braasch, W. F.: The clinical diagnosis of congenital anomaly in the kidney and ureter. Ann. Surg., 56:756, 1912.

Christofferson, J., and Iversen, H. G.: Partial hydronephrosis in a patient with horseshoe kidney and bilateral duplication of the pelvis and ureter. Scand. J. Urol. Nephrol., 10:91, 1976.

Cohen, N., and Berant, M.: Duplications of the renal collecting system in the hereditary osteo-onychodysplasia syndrome. J. Pediatr., 89:261, 1976.

Colosimo, C.: Double and bifid ureters. Urologia, 5:239, 1938.

Cromie, W. J., Engelstein, M. S., and Duckett, J. W., Jr.: Nodular renal blastema, renal dysplasia and duplicated collecting systems. J. Urol., 123:100, 1980.

Dahl, D. S.: Bilateral complete renal duplication with total obstruction of both lower pole collecting systems. Urology, 6:727, 1975.

Hawthorne, A. B.: Embryologic and clinical aspect of double ureter. JAMA, 106:189, 1936.

Johnston, J. H.: Urinary tract duplication in childhood. Arch. Dis. Child., 36:180, 1961.

Kaplan, N., and Elkin, M.: Bifid renal pelves and ureters. Radiographic and cinefluorographic observations. Br. J. Urol., 40:235, 1968.

Kretschmer, H. L.: Hydronephrosis in infancy and childhood: Clinical data and a report of 101 cases. Surg. Gynecol. Obstet., 64:634, 1937.

Lenaghan, D.: Bifid ureters in children: An anatomical, physiological and clinical study. J. Urol., 87:808, 1962.

Meyer, R.: Normal and abnormal development of the ureter in the human embryo—a mechanistic consideration. Anat. Rec., 96:355, 1946.

Nation, E. F.: Duplication of the kidney and ureter: A statistical study of 230 new cases. J. Urol., 51:456, 1944.

Nordmark, B.: Double formations of the pelves of the kidneys and the ureters. Embryology, occurrence and clinical significance. Acta Radiol., 30:267, 1948.

O'Reilly, P. H., Shields, R. A., Testa, J., Lawson, R. S., and Edwards, E. C.: Ureteroureteric reflux. Pathological entity or physiological phenomenon? Br. J. Urol., 56:159–164, 1984.

Payne, R. A.: Clinical significance of reduplicated kidneys. Br. J. Urol., 31:141, 1959.

Pendergrass, T. W.: Congenital anomalies in children with Wilms' tumor: a new survey. Cancer, 37:403, 1976.

Phillips, D. I. W., Divall, J. M., Maskell, R. M., and Barker, J. P.: A geographical focus of duplex ureter. Br. J. Urol., 60:329–331, 1987.

Privett, J. T. J., Jeans, W. D., and Roylance, J.: The incidence and importance of renal duplication. Clin. Radiol., 27:521, 1976.

Stephens, F. D.: Anatomical vagaries of double ureters. Aust. N.Z. J. Surg., 28:27, 1958.

Timothy, R. P., Decter, A., and Perlmutter, A. D.: Ureteral duplication: Clinical findings and therapy in 46 children. J. Urol., 105:445, 1971.

Weigert, C.: Ueber einige Bildunsfehler der Ureteren. Virchows Arch. (Pathol. Anat.), 70:490, 1877.

Wharton, L. R., Jr.: Double ureters and associated renal anomalies in early human embryos. Contrib. Embryol. Carnegie Inst. Wash., 33:103, 1949.

Whitaker, J., and Danks, D. M.: A study of the inheritance of duplication of the kidney and ureters. J. Urol., 95:176, 1966.

Blind-Ending Duplication of the Ureter

Albers, D. D., Geyer, J. R., and Barnes, S. D.: Clinical significance of blind-ending branch of bifid ureter: Report of 3 additional cases. J. Urol., 105:634, 1971.

Albers, D. D., Geyer, J. R., and Barnes, S. D.: Blind-ending branch of bifid ureter: Report of 3 cases. J. Urol., 99:160, 1968.

Aragona, F., Passerini-Glazel, G., Zacchello, G., and Andreetta, B.: Familial occurrence of blind-ending bifid and duplicated ureters. Int. Urol. Nephrol. 19(2):137–139, 1987.

Barbalias, G. A., and DiGioacchino, R.: Rudimentary branched ureter. A report of four cases. Del. Med. J., 46:511, 1974.

Bergman, B., Hansson, G., and Nilson, A. E. V.: Duplication of the renal pelvis and blind-ending bifid ureter in twins. Urol. Int., 32:49, 1977.

Caller, C., Cendron, J., and Trotot, P.: Uretere double à branche borgne. J. Urol. Nephrol. (Paris), 85:473, 1979.

Campbell, M. F.: Diverticulum of the ureter. Am. J. Surg., 34:385, 1936.

Culp, O. S.: Ureteral diverticulum: Classification of the literature and report of an authentic case. J. Urol., 58:309, 1947.

de Filippi, G., dal Forno, S., and Bianchi, M.: Blind ureteric buds. Pediatr. Radiol., 5:160, 1977.

Dublin, A. B., Stadalnik, R. C., DeNardo, G. L., et al.: Scintigraphic imaging of a blind-ending ureteral duplication. J. Nucl. Med., 16:208, 1975.

Gray, S. W., and Skandalakis, J. E. (Eds.): Embryology for Surgeons. Philadelphia, W. B. Saunders Co., 1972.

Hanley, H. G.: Blind-ending duplication of the ureter. Br. J. Urol., 17:50, 1945.

Hansen, E. I., and Frost, B.: Multiple diverticula of the ureter. Scand. J. Urol. Nephrol., 12:93, 1978.

Harris, A.: Ureteral anomalies with special reference to partial duplication with one branch ending blindly. J. Urol., 38:442, 1937.

Holly, L. E., and Sumcad, B.: Diverticular ureteral changes: a report of four cases. AJR, 78:1053, 1957.

Jablonski, J. P., Voldman, C., and Bruéziere, J.: Duplication totale de la voie excrétrice dont un uretere est borgne. J. Urol. Nephrol. (Paris), 84:837, 1978.

Kontturi, M., and Kaski, P.: Blind-ending bifid ureter with ureteroureteral reflux. Scand. J. Urol. Nephrol., 6:91, 1972.

Kretschmer, H. L.: Duplication of the ureters at their distal ends, one pair ending blindly. So-called diverticula of the ureters. J. Urol., 30:61, 1933.

Lenaghan, D.: Bifid ureters in children: An anatomical and clinical study. J. Urol., 87:808, 1962.

Marshall, F. F., and McLoughlin, M. G.: Long blind-ending ureteral duplications. J. Urol., 120:626, 1978.

McGraw, A. B., and Culp, O. S.: Diverticulum of the ureter: Report of another authentic case. J. Urol., 67:262, 1952.

Miller, E. V., and Tremblay, R. E.: Symptomatic blindly ending bifid ureter. J. Urol., 92:109, 1964.

Norman, C. H., Jr., and Dubowy, J.: Multiple ureteral diverticula. J. Urol., 96:152, 1966.

Peterson, L. J., Grimes, J. H., Weinerth, J. L., et al.: Blind-ending branches of bifid ureters. Urology, 5:191, 1975.

Ponthieu, A., Anfossi, G., Guidicelli, C., and Boutboul, R.: Dedoublement segmentaire congenital de l'uretere lombaire. J. Urol. Nephrol. (Paris), 83:211, 1977.

Rank, W. B., Mellinger, G. T., and Spiro, E.: Ureteral diverticula: Etiologic considerations. J. Urol., 83:566, 1960.

Rao, K. G.: Blind-ending bifid ureter. Urology, 6:81, 1975.

Richardson, E. H.: Diverticulum of the ureter: A collective review with report of a unique example. J. Urol., 47:535, 1942.

Sarajlic, M., Durst-Zivkovic, B., Svoren, E., Vitkovic, M., Batinic, D., Bradic, I., et al.: Congenital ureteric diverticula in children and adults: classification, radiological and clinical features. Br. J. Radiol., 62(738):551–553, 1989.

Schultze, R.: Der blind endende Doppelureter. Z. Urol., 4:27, 1967.

Sharma, S. K., Malik, N., Kumar, S., and Bapna, B. C.: Bilateral incomplete ureteric duplication with a ureteric diverticulum. Aust. N.Z. J. Surg., 51:204, 1981.

Sharma, S. K., Subudhi, C. L., Kumar, S., Bapna, B. C., and Suri, S.: Ureteric diverticula: ureterodiverticular reflux and yo-yo effect. Br. J. Urol., 52:345, 1980.

Szokoly, V., Veradi, E., and Szporny, G.: Blind ending bifid and double ureters. Int. Urol. Nephrol., 6:174, 1974.

van Helsdingen, P. J. R. O.: A case of bifid ureter with blind-ending segment as the cause of chronic pain in the flank. Arch. Chir. Nederl., 27:277, 1975.

Youngen, R., and Persky, L.: Diverticulum of the renal pelvis. J. Urol., 94:40, 1965.

Inverted Y Ureteral Duplication

Beasley, S. W., and Kelly, J. H.: Inverted Y duplication of the ureter in association with ureterocele and bladder diverticulum. J. Urol., 136:899–900, 1986.

Bingham, J. G.: Duplicate segment within a single ureter. J. Urol., 135:1234, 1986.

Britt, D. B., Borden, T. A., and Woodhead, D. M.: Inverted Y ureteral duplication with a blind-ending branch. J. Urol., 108:387, 1972.

Ecke, M., and Klatte, D.: Inverted Y-ureteral duplication with a uterine ectopy as cause of ureteric enuresis. Urol. Int., 44:116–118, 1989.

Harrison, G. S. M., and Williams, R. E.: Inverted Y ureter in the male. Br. J. Urol., 58(5):564–565, 1986.

Hawthorne, A. B.: Embryologic and clinical aspect of double ureter. JAMA, 106:189, 1936.

Klauber, G. T., and Reid, E. C.: Inverted Y reduplication of the ureter. J. Urol., 107:362, 1972.

Mosli, H. A., Schillinger, J. F., and Futter, N.: Inverted Y duplication of the ureter. J. Urol., 135:126–127, 1986.

Suzuki, S., Tsujimura, S., and Sugiura, H.: Inverted Y ureteral duplication with a ureteral stone in atretic segment. J. Urol., 117:248, 1977.

Ureteral Triplication and Supernumerary Ureters

Arap, S., Lopes, R. N., Mitre, A. I., Menezes De Goes, G.: Triplicité urétérale complète associée à une urétérocèle ectopique. J. Urol. (Paris), 88:167, 1982.

Begg, R. C.: Sextuplicitas renum: A case of six functioning kidneys and ureters in an adult female. J. Urol., 70:686, 1953.

Blumberg, N.: Ureteral triplication. J. Pediatr. Surg., 11:579, 1976.

Delaere, K., and Debruyne, F.: Triplication and contralateral duplication of ureter. Urology, 19:302, 1982.

Fairchild, W. V., Solomon, H. D., Spence, C. R., and Gangai, M. P.: Case profile: unusual ureteral triplication. Urology, 14:95, 1979.

Finkel, L. I., Watts, F. B., Jr., and Corbett, D. P.: Ureteral triplication with a ureterocele. Pediatr. Radiol., 13:346–348, 1983.

Gill, R. D.: Triplication of the ureter and renal pelvis. J. Urol., 68:140, 1952.

Gilmore, O. J. A.: Unilateral triplication of the ureter. Br. J. Urol., 46:585, 1974.

Golomb, J., and Ehrlich, R. M.: Bilateral ureteral triplication with crossed ectopic fused kidneys associated with the vacteral syndrome. J. Urol., 141:1398–1399, 1989.

Juskiewenski, S., Soulie, M., Baunin, C., Moscovia, J., and Vaysse, P.: Ureteral triplication. Chir. Pediatr., 28:314–321, 1987.

MacKelvie, A. A.: Triplicate ureter: Case report. Br. J. Urol., 27:124, 1955.

Marc, J., Drouillard, J., Bruneton, J. N., and Tavernier, J.: La triplication urétérale. J. Radiol. Electrol. Med. Nucl., 58:427, 1977.

Parker, R. M., Pohl, D. R., and Robison, J. R.: Ureteral triplication with ectopia. J. Urol., 103:727, 1970.

Parvinen, T.: Complete ureteral triplication. J. Pediatr. Surg., 11:1039, 1976.

Patel, N. P., and Lavengood, R. W.: Triplicate duplicate ureters. Br. J. Urol., 54:436, 1982.

Patel, N. P., and Lavengood, R. W.: Triplicate ureter. Urology, 5:242, 1975.

Perkins, P. J., Kroovand, R. L., and Evans, A. T.: Triplication of ureter: A case report. Radiology, 108:533, 1973.

Pode, D., Shapiro, A., and Lebensart, P.: Unilateral triplication of the collecting system in a horseshoe kidney. J. Urol., 130:533–534, 1983.

Redman, J. F.: Triplicate ureter with contralateral ureteral duplication. J. Urol., 116:805, 1976.

Ringer, M. G., and MacFarlan, S. M.: Complete triplication of the ureter: A case report. J. Urol., 92:429, 1964.

Rodo Salas, R. J., Bishara, F., and Claret, I.: Triplication ureteral con reflujo y ureterocele. Arch. Esp. de Urol., 39(5):343–347, 1986.

Smith, I.: Triplicate ureter. Br. J. Surg., 34:182, 1946.

Soderdahl, D. W., Shiraki, I. W., and Schamber, D. T.: Bilateral ureteral quadruplication. J. Urol., 116:255, 1976.

Spangler, E. B.: Complete triplication of the ureter. Radiology, 80:795, 1963.

Wolpowitz, A., Evan, P., and Botha, P. A. G.: Triplication of ureter on one side and duplication on the other. Br. J. Urol., 47:622, 1975.

Anomalies of Structure

Atresia and Hypoplasia

Allen, T. D., and Husmann, D. A.: Ureteropelvic junction obstruction associated with ureteral hypoplasia. J. Urol., 142:353–355, 1989.

Campbell, M. F.: Anomalies of the ureter. In Campbell, M. F., and Harrison, J. H. (Eds.): Urology, 3rd ed., Philadelphia, W. B. Saunders Co., 1970, p. 1512.

Cussen, L. J.: The morphology of congenital dilatation of the ureter: Intrinsic ureteral lesions. Aust. N.Z. J. Surg., 41:185, 1971.

DeKlerk, D. P., Marshall, F. F., and Jeffs, R. D.: Multicystic dysplastic kidney. J. Urol., 118:306, 1977.

Dewolf, W. C., Fraley, E. E., and Markland, C.: Congenital hypoplasia of the proximal ureter. J. Urol., 113:236, 1975.

Gordon, M., and Reed, J. O.: Distal ureteral atresia. Am. J. Roentgenol., 88:579, 1962.

Griscom, N. T., Vawter, G. F., and Fellers, F. X.: Pelvoinfundibular atresia: The usual form of multicystic kidney: 44 unilateral and two bilateral cases. Semin. Roentgenol., 10:125, 1975.

Kornblum, K., and Ritter, J. A.: Retroperitoneal cyst with agenesia of the kidney. Radiology, 32:416, 1939.

Mackie, G. G.: Personal communication, 1977.

Slater, G. S.: Ureteral atresia producing giant hydroureter. J. Urol., 78:135, 1957.

Uson, A. C., Womack, C. E., and Berdon, W. E.: Giant ectopic ureter presenting as an abdominal mass in a newborn infant. J. Pediatr., 80:473, 1972.

Vinocur, L., Slovis, T. L., Perlmutter, A. D., Watts, F. B., Jr., Chang, C. H.: Follow-up studies of multicystic dysplastic kidneys. Radiology, 167:311–315, 1988.

Megaureters and Ureteral Stenosis and Stricture

Allen, T. D.: Discussion. In Bergsma, D., and Duckett, J. W., Jr. (Eds.): Urinary System Malformation in Children. Birth Defects: Original Article Series, Vol. 13, No. 5. New York, Alan R. Liss, 1977, p. 39.

Allen, T. D.: Congenital ureteral strictures. J. Urol., 104:196, 1970.

Bellman, A. B.: Megaureter—Classification, etiology, and management. Urol. Clin. North Am., 1:497, 1974.

Beseghi, U., Casolarie, E., Banchini, G., Ammenti, A., and Ghinelli, C.: Congenital stenosis of the mid ureter. Acta Biomed. Ateneo Parmense, 59(1–8):29–34, 1988.

Bischoff, P.: Observations on genesis of megaureter. Urol. Int., 11:257, 1961.

Blickman, J. G., and Lebowitz, R. L.: The coexistence of primary megaureter and reflux. AJR, 143:1053–1057, 1984.

Campbell, M.: Primary megalo-ureter. J. Urol., 68:584, 1952.

Caulk, J. R.: Megaloureter—The importance of the ureterovesical valve. J. Urol., 9:315, 1923.

Chwalle, R.: The process of formation of cystic dilations of the vesical end of the ureter and of diverticula at the ureteral ostium. Urol. Cutan. Rev., 31:499, 1927.

Creevy, C. D.: The atonic distal ureteral segment (ureteral achalasia). J. Urol., 97:457, 1970.

Cussen, L. J.: The morphology of congenital dilatation of the ureter: Intrinsic ureteral lesions. Aust. N.Z. J. Surg., 41:185, 1971.

Cussen, L. J.: The structure of the normal human ureter in infancy and childhood. J. Invest. Urol., 5:179, 1967a.

Cussen, L. J.: Dimensions of the normal ureter in infancy and childhood. J. Invest. Urol., 5:167, 1967b.

Gittes, R. F., and Talner, L. B.: Congenital megacalyces vs. obstructive hydronephrosis. J. Urol., 108:833, 1972.

Gregoir, W., and Debled, G.: L'etiologie du reflux congénital et du méga-uretère primaire. Urol. Int., 24:119, 1969.

Hanna, M. K., and Edwards, L.: Pressure perfusion studies of the abnormal uretero-vesical junction. Br. J. Urol., 44:331, 1972.

Hanna, M. K., and Wyatt, J. K.: Primary obstructive megaureter in adults. J. Urol., 113:328, 1975.

Hanna, M. K., Jeffs, R. D., Sturgess, J. M., et al.: Ureteral structure and ultrastructure. Part III. The congenitally dilated ureter (megaureter). J. Urol., 117:24, 1977.

Hanna, M. K., Jeffs, R. D., Sturgess, J. M., et al.: Ureteral structure and ultrastructure. Part 1. The normal human ureter. J. Urol., 116:718, 1976a.

Hanna, M. K., Jeffs, R. D., Sturgess, J. M., et al.: Ureteral structure and ultrastructure. Part II. Congenital ureteropelvic junction obstruction and primary obstructive megaureter. J. Urol., 116:725, 1976b.

Hertle, L., and Nawrath, H.: In vitro studies on human primary obstructed megaureters. J. Urol., 133:884–887, 1985.

Hofmann, J., Friedrich, U., Hofmann, B., and Gräbner, R.: Acetylcholinesterase activities in association with congenital malformation of the terminal ureter in infants and children. Z. Kinderchir, 41:32–34, 1986.

Huang, C. J.: Congenital giant megaureter. J. Pediatr. Surg., 22(3):235–239, 1987.

Hutch, J. A., and Tanagho, E. A.: Etiology of non-occlusive ureteral dilatation. J. Urol., 93:177, 1965.

Johnston, J. H.: Reconstructive surgery of mega-ureter in childhood. Br. J. Urol., 39:17, 1967.

Lewis, E. L., and Kimbrough, J. C.: Megalo-ureter. New concept in treatment. South. Med. J., 45:171, 1952.

MacKinnon, K. J., Foote, J. W., Wiglesworth, F. W., et al.: The pathology of the adynamic distal ureteral segment. J. Urol., 103:134, 1970.

Mandell, G. A., Snyder, H. M., III, Heyman, S., Keller, M., Kaplan, J. M., and Norman, M. E.: Association of congenital megacalycosis and ipsilateral segmental megaureter. Pediatr. Radiol., 17:28–33, 1986.

Mark, L. K., and Moel, M.: Primary megaloureter. Radiology, 93:345, 1969.

McGrath, M. A., Estroff, J., and Lebowitz, R. L.: The coexistence of obstruction at the ureteropelvic and ureterovesical junctions. AJR, 149:403–406, 1987.

McLaughlin, P., Pfister, R. C., III, Leadbetter, W. F., et al.: The pathophysiology of primary megaloureter. J. Urol., 109:805, 1973.

Murnaghan, G. F.: Experimental investigation of the dynamics of the normal and dilated ureter. Br. J. Urol., 29:403, 1957.

Notley, R. G.: The structural basis for normal and abnormal ureteric motility. The innervation and musculature of the human ureter. Ann. R. Coll. Surg. Engl., 49:250, 1971.

Notley, R. G.: Electron microscopy of the primary obstructive mega-ureter. Br. J. Urol., 44:229, 1972.

Nunn, I. N., and Stephens, F. D.: The triad syndrome: A composite anomaly of the abdominal wall, urinary system and testes. J. Urol., 86:782, 1961.

Palmer, J. M., and Tesluk, H.: Ureteral pathology in the prune belly syndrome. J. Urol., 111:701, 1974.

Pfister, R. C., McLaughlin, A. P., III, and Leadbetter, W. F.: Radiological evaluation of primary megaloureter. Radiology, 99:503, 1971.

Smith, D. E.: Report of Working Party to Establish an International Nomenclature for the Large Ureter. In Bergsma, D., and Duckett, J. W., Jr. (Eds.): Urinary System Malformations in Children. Birth Defects: Original Article Series, Vol. 13, No. 5. New York, Alan R. Liss, 1977, p. 3.

Stephens, F. D.: Idiopathic dilations of the urinary tract. J. Urol., 112:819, 1974.

Swenson, O., MacMahon, H. E., Jaques, W. E., et al.: A new concept of the etiology of megaloureters. N. Engl. J. Med., 246:41, 1952.

Tanagho, E. A., Smith, D. R., and Guthrie, T. H.: Pathophysiology of functional obstruction. J. Urol., 104:73, 1970.

Tatu, W., and Brennan, R. E.: Primary megaureter in a mother and daughter. Urol. Radiol., 3:185, 1981.

Tokunaka, S., and Koyanagi, T.: Morphologic study of primary nonreflux megaureters with particular emphasis on the role of ureteral sheath and ureteral dysplasia. J. Urol., 128:399, 1982.

Tokunaka, S., Gotoh, T., Koyanagi, T., and Miyabe, N.: Muscle dysplasia in megaureters. J. Urol., 131:383, 1984.

Tokunaka, S., Koyanagi, T., and Tsuji, I.: Two infantile cases of primary megaloureter with uncommon pathological findings: ultra-structural study and its clinical implication. J. Urol., 123:214, 1980.

Tokunaka, S., Koyanagi, T., Tsuji, I., and Yamada, T.: Histopathology of the nonrefluxing megaloureter: a clue to its pathogenesis. J. Urol., 127:238, 1982.

Von Niederhausern, W., and Tuchschmid, D.: A poorly known association: primary congenital megaureter and megacalyx kidney. Ann. D. Urol., 5:225, 1971.

Waltzer, W. C.: The association of congenital megaureter and ureteropelvic junction obstruction. Int. Urol. Nephrol. 15(3):237–244, 1983.

Whitaker, R. H.: Some observations and theories on the wide ureter and hydronephrosis. Br. J. Urol., 47:377, 1975.

Whitaker, R. H.: Methods of assessing obstruction in dilated ureters. Br. J. Urol., 45:15, 1973.

Whitaker, R. H., and Johnston, J. H.: A simple classification of wide ureters. Br. J. Urol., 47:781, 1975.

Williams, D. I.: The chronically dilated ureter. Ann. R. Coll. Surg. Engl., 14:107, 1954.

Williams, D. I., and Burkholder, G. V.: The prune belly syndrome. J. Urol., 98:244, 1967.

Williams, D. I., and Hulme-Moir, I.: Primary obstructive megaureter. Br. J. Urol., 42:140, 1970.

Ureteral Valves

Cussen, L. J.: Valves of the ureter. In Bergsma, D., and Duckett, J. W., Jr. (Eds.): Urinary System Malformations in Children. Birth Defects: Original Article Series. Vol. 13, No. 5. New York, Alan R. Liss, 1977, p. 19.

Cussen, L. J.: The morphology of congenital dilatation of the ureter: Intrinsic ureteral lesions. Aust. N.Z. J. Surg., 41:185, 1971.

Dajani, A. M., Dajani, Y. F., and Dahabrah, S.: Congenital ureteric valves—a cause of urinary obstruction. Br. J. Urol., 54:98, 1982.

Fitzer, P. M.: Congenital ureteral valve. Pediatr. Radiol., 8:54, 1979.

Foroughi, E., and Turner, J. A.: Congenital ureteral valve. J. Urol., 81:272, 1959.

Fried, A. M., Mulcahy, J. J., Bhathena, D. B., and Oliff, M.: Hydronephrosis with ureteral valve: diagnosis by ultrasonography and antegrade pyelography. J. Urol., 120:754, 1978.

Gosalbez, R., Garat, J. M., Piro, C., Martin, J. A., and Cortes, F.: Congenital ureteral valves in children. Urology, 21:237, 1983.

Kirks, D. R., Currarino, G., and Weinberg, A. G.: Transverse folds in the proximal ureter: a normal variant in infants. Am. J. Roentgenol., 130:463, 1978.

Maizels, M., and Stephens, F. D.: Valves of the ureter as a cause of primary obstruction of the ureter: anatomic, embryologic and clinical aspects. J. Urol., 123:742, 1980.

Noe, H. N., and Scaljon, W.: Case profile: ureteral valves. Urology, 14:411, 1979.

Passaro, E., Jr., and Smith, J. P.: Congenital ureteral valve in children: A case report. J. Urol., 84:290, 1960.

Reha, W. C., and Gibbons, D. M.: Neonatal ascites and ureteral valves. Urology, 33(6):468–471, 1989.

Reinberg, Y., Aliabadi, H., Johnson, P., and Gonzalez, R.: Congenital ureteral valves in children: Case report and review of the literature. J. Pediatr. Surg., 22(4):379–381, 1987.

Roberts, R. R.: Complete valve of the ureter: Congenital urethral valves. J. Urol., 76:62, 1956.

Simon, H. B., Culp, O. S., and Parkhill, E. M.: Congenital ureteral valves: Report of two cases. J. Urol., 74:336, 1955.

Tlili-Graiess, K., Allegue, M., Kraiem, C., Ben Romdhane, M. H., Bakir, D., et al.: Ureteral valves: report of a case diagnosed by antegrade pyelography. Pediatr. Radiol., 19:67–69, 1988.

Wall, B., and Wachter, H. E.: Congenital ureteral valve: Its role as a primary obstructive lesion: classification of the literature and report of an authentic case. J. Urol., 68:684, 1952.

Whiting, J. C., Stanisic, T. H., and Drach, G. W.: Congenital ureteral valves: report of 2 patients, including one with a solitary kidney and associated hypertension. J. Urol., 129:1222, 1983.

Williams, D. I.: Discussion. In Bergsma, D., and Duckett, J. W., Jr. (Eds.): Urinary System Malformations in Children. Birth Defects: Original Article Series. Vol. 13, No. 5. New York, Alan R. Liss, 1977, p. 39.

Spiral Twists and Folds of the Ureter

Campbell, M. F.: Anomalies of the ureter. In Campbell, M. F., and Harrison, J. H. (Eds.): Urology, 3rd ed. Philadelphia, W. B. Saunders Co., 1970.

Gross, R. E.: Uretero-Pelvic Obstruction. In The Surgery of Infancy and Childhood. Philadelphia, W. B. Saunders Co., 1953.

Östling, K.: The genesis of hydronephrosis. Acta Chir. Scand., 86:Suppl. 72, 1942.

Ureteral Diverticula

See *Anomalies of Number: Blind-Ending Duplication of the Ureter.*

Anomalies of Termination

Vesicoureteral Reflux

Ambrose, S. S., and Nicolson, W. P.: Ureteral reflux in duplicated ureters. J. Urol., 92:439, 1964.

Ambrose, S. S., and Nicolson, W. P., III: The causes of vesicoureteral reflux in children. J. Urol., 87:688, 1962.

Blickman, J. G., and Lebowitz, R. L.: The coexistence of primary megaureter and reflux. AJR, 143:1053–1057, 1984.

Privett, J. T. J., Jeans, W. D., and Roylance, J.: The incidence and importance of renal duplication. Clin. Radiol., 27:521, 1976.

Stephens, F. D., and Lenaghan, D.: The anatomical basis and dynamics of vesicoureteral reflux. J. Urol., 87:669, 1962.

Tanagho, E. A., Hutch, J. A., Meyers, F. H., et al.: Primary vesicoureteral reflux: Experimental studies of its etiology. J. Urol., 93:165, 1965.

Ectopic Ureter

Abeshouse, B. S.: Ureteral ectopia: Report of a rare case of ectopic ureter opening in the uterus and a review of the literature. Urol. Cutan. Rev., 47:447, 1943.

Alfert, H. J., and Gillenwater, J. Y.: Ectopic vas deferens communicating with lower ureter: Embryological considerations. J. Urol., 108:172, 1972.

Ayyat, F., Palmer, M. D., and Tingley, J. O.: Ectopic vas deferens communicating with lower ureter. Urology, 19:423, 1982.

Bard, R. H., and Welles, H.: Nonduplication of upper urinary tract associated with horseshoe kidney and bilateral ureteral ectopia. Urology, 5:784, 1975.

Borger, J. A., and Belman, A. B.: Uretero–vas deferens anastomosis associated with imperforate anus: An embryologically predictable occurrence. J. Pediatr. Surg., 10:255, 1975.

Brannan, W., and Henry, H. H., II: Ureteral ectopia: Report of 39 cases. J. Urol., 109:192, 1973.

Brown, D. M., Peterson, N. R., and Schultz, R. E.: Ureteral duplication with lower pole ectopia to the epididymis. J. Urol., 140:139–142, 1988.

Burford, C. E., Glenn, J. E., and Burford, E. H.: Ureteral ectopia: A review of the literature and 2 case reports. J. Urol., 62:211, 1949.

Cendron, J., and Bonhomme, C.: 31 cas d'uretere à abouchement ectopique sous-sphinctérien chez l'enfant du sexe féminin. J. Urol. Nephrol. (Paris), 74:1, 1968a.

Cendron, J., and Bonhomme, C.: Uretere à terminaison ectopique extra-vesicale chez des sujets de sexe masculin (à propos de 10 cas). J. Urol. Nephrol. (Paris), 74:31, 1968b.

Childlow, J. H., and Utz, D. C.: Ureteral ectopia in vestibule of vagina with urinary continence. South. Med. J., 63:423, 1970.

Cox, C. E., and Hutch, J. A.: Bilateral single ectopic ureter: A report of 2 cases and review of the literature. J. Urol., 95:493, 1966.

Cumes, D. M., Sanfelippo, C. J., and Stamey, T. A.: Single ectopic ureter masquerading as ureterocele in incontinent male. Urology, 17:60, 1981.

Currarino, G.: Single vaginal ectopic ureter and Gartner's duct cyst with ipsilateral renal hypoplasia and dysplasia (or agenesis). J. Urol., 128:988, 1982.

Das, S., and Amar, A. D.: Extravesical ureteral ectopia in male patients. J. Urol., 125:842, 1981.

Das, S., and Amar, A. D.: Ureteral ectopia into cystic seminal vesicle with ipsilateral renal dysgenesis and monorchia. J. Urol., 124:574, 1980.

Davis, D. M.: Urethral ectopic ureter in the female without incontinence. J. Urol., 23:463, 1930.

Deilmann, W., and Moormann, J. G.: Komplexe urogenital-missbildung im bereich der wolffschen gänge. Urologe A, 17:313, 1978.

DeWeerd, J. H., and Litin, R. B.: Ectopia of ureteral orifice (vestibular) without incontinence: Report of case. Proc. Staff Meet. Mayo Clin., 33:81, 1958.

Eisendrath, D. N.: Ectopic opening of the ureter. Urol. Cutan. Rev., 42:401, 1938.

Ellerker, A. G.: The extravesical ectopic ureter. Br. J. Surg., 45:344, 1958.

Feldman, S., and Ross, L.: Hydrocolpos with vaginal ureteral ectopia: a case report. J. Urol., 123:573, 1980.

Fuselier, H. A., and Peters, D. H.: Cyst of seminal vesicle with ipsilateral renal agenesis and ectopic ureter: Case report. J. Urol., 115:833, 1976.

Gibbons, M. D., and Duckett, J. W., Jr.: Single vaginal ectopic ureter: a case report. J. Urol., 120:493, 1978.

Gibbons, M. D., Cromie, W. J., and Duckett, J. W., Jr.: Ectopic vas deferens. J. Urol., 120:597, 1978.

Glenn, J. F.: Agenesis of the bladder. JAMA, 169:2016, 1959.

Gordon, H. L., and Kessler, R.: Ectopic ureter entering the seminal vesicle associated with renal dysplasia. J. Urol., 108:389, 1972.

Gotoh, T., Morita, H., Tokunaka, S., Koyanagi, T., and Tsuji, I.: Single ectopic ureter. J. Urol., 129:271, 1983.

Gravgaard, E., Garsdal, L., and Moller, S. H.: Double vas deferens and epididymis associated with ipsilateral renal agenesis simulating ectopic ureter opening into the seminal vesicle. Scand. J. Urol. Nephrol., 12:85, 1978.

Gray, S. W., and Skandalakis, J. E. (Eds.): Embryology for Surgeons. Philadelphia, W. B. Saunders Co., 1972.

Grossman, H., Winchester, P. H., and Muecke, E. C.: Solitary ectopic ureter. Radiology, 89:1069, 1967.

Honke, E. M.: Ectopic ureter. J. Urol., 55:460, 1946.

Johnston, J. H., and Davenport, T. J.: The single ectopic ureter. Br. J. Urol., 41:428, 1969.

Jona, J. Z., Glicklich, M., and Cohen, R. D.: Ectopic single ureter and severe renal dysplasia: an unusual presentation. J. Urol., 121:369, 1979.

Kesavan, P., Ramakrishnan, M. S., and Fowler, R.: Ectopia in unduplicated ureters in children. Br. J. Urol., 49:481, 1977.

Kittredge, R. D., and Levin, D. C.: Unusual aspect of renal angiography in ureteric duplication. Am. J. Roentgenol., 119:805, 1973.

Kjaeldgaard, A., and Fianau, S.: Classification and embryological aspects of ectopic ureters communicating with Gartner's cysts. Diagn. Gynecol. Obstet., 4:269, 1982.

Kjaeldgaard, A., Fianau, S., Thorgeirsson, T., and Ekman, P.: Single bifid ectopic left ureter presenting clinically as a vaginal cyst. Diagn. Gynecol. Obstet., 3:321, 1981.

Kondo, A., Sahashi, M., and Mitsuya, H.: A rare variant of ureteric ectopia: opening in vagina and vesico-uretero-vaginal communication. Br. J. Urol., 54:486, 1982.

Koyanagi, T., Hisajima, S., Sakashita, S., Goto, T., and Tsuji, I.: Ureteral ectopia in vestibule without urinary incontinence. Urology, 16:508, 1980.

Koyanagi, T., Takamatsu, T., Kaneta, T., Terashima, M., and Tsuji, I.: A spontaneous vesico-ectopic ureterovaginal fistula in a girl. J. Urol., 118:871, 1977.

Koyanagi, T., Tsuji, I., Orikasa, S., and Hirano, T.: Bilateral single ectopic ureter: report of a case. Int. Urol. Nephrol., 9:123, 1977.

Leef, G. S., and Leader, S. A.: Ectopic ureter opening into the rectum: A case report. J. Urol., 87:338, 1962.

Levisay, G. L., Holder, J., and Weigel, J. W.: Ureteral ectopia associated with seminal vesicle cyst and ipsilateral renal agenesis. Radiology, 114:575, 1975.

Lowsley, O. S., and Kerwin, T. J.: Clinical Urology, Vol. 1, 3rd ed. Baltimore, The Williams & Wilkins Co., 1956.

Lucius, G. F.: Klinik und Therapie der dystopen Hernleitermundungen in die Samenwege. Urologe, 2:360, 1963.

Malek, R. S., Kelalis, P. P., Stickler, G. B., et al.: Observations on ureteral ectopy in children. J. Urol., 107:308, 1972.

Mellin, H. E., Kjaer, T. B., and Madsen, P. O.: Crossed ectopia of seminal vesicles, renal aplasia and ectopic ureter. J. Urol., 115:765, 1976.

Mills, J. C.: Complete unilateral duplication of ureter with analysis of the literature. Urol. Cutan. Rev., 43:444, 1939.

Mogg, R. A.: The single ectopic ureter. Br. J. Urol., 46:3, 1974.

Moore, T.: Ectopic openings of the ureter. Br. J. Urol., 24:3, 1952.

Noseworthy, J., and Persky, L.: Spectrum of bilateral ureteral ectopia. Urology, 19:489, 1982.

Ogawa, A., Kakizawa, Y., and Akaza, H.: Ectopic ureter passing through the external urethral sphincter: Report of a case. J. Urol., 116:109, 1976.

Ostermayer, H., and Frei, A.: Nebenhoden und samenblase als mundungsort ektoper harnleiter. Urologe A, 20:389, 1981.

Prewitt, L. H., and Lebowitz, R. L.: The single ectopic ureter. Am. J. Roentgenol., 127:941, 1976.

Redman, J. F., and Sulieman, J. S.: Bilateral vasal-ureteral communications. J. Urol., 116:808, 1976.

Riba, L. W., Schmidlapp, C. J., and Bosworth, N. L.: Ectopic ureter draining into the seminal vesicle. J. Urol., 56:332, 1946.

Ritchey, M. L., Kramer, S. A., Benson, R. C., Jr., and Kelalis, P. P.: Bilateral single ureteral ectopia. Eur. Urol., 14:41–45, 1988.

Rognon, L., Brueziere, J., Soret, J. Y., et al.: Abouchement ectopique de l'ureter dans le tractus seminal: A propos de 10 cas. Chirurgie (Paris), 99:741, 1973.

Schnitzer, B.: Ectopic ureteral opening into seminal vesicle: A report of four cases. J. Urol., 93:576, 1965.

Schulman, C. C.: Fehlbildung des ureters und nierendysplasia—eine embryologische hypothese. Urologe A, 17:273, 1978.

Schulman, C. C.: The single ectopic ureter. Eur. Urol., 2:64, 1976.

Schulman, C. C.: Les implantations ectopiques de l'uretere. Acta Urol. Belg., 40:201, 1972.

Schwarz, R., and Stephens, F. D.: The persisting mesonephric duct: high junction of vas deferens and ureter. J. Urol., 120:597, 1978.

Scott, J. E. S.: The single ectopic ureter and the dysplastic kidney. Br. J. Urol., 53:300, 1981.

Seitzman, D. M., and Patton, J. F.: Ureteral ectopia: Combined ureteral and vas deferens anomaly. J. Urol., 84:604, 1960.

Sorenson, C. W., Jr., and Middleton, A. W., Jr.: The single ectopic ureter: 3 case reports. J. Urol., 129:132, 1983.

Uson, A. C., and Schulman, C. C.: Ectopic ureter emptying into the rectum: Report of a case. J. Urol., 108:156, 1972.

Uson, A. C., Womack, C. D., and Berdon, W. E.: Giant ectopic ureter presenting as an abdominal mass in a newborn infant. J. Pediatr., 80:473, 1972.

Vanhoutte, J. J.: Ureteral ectopia into a Wolffian duct remnant (Gartner's ducts or cysts) presenting as a urethral diverticulum in two girls. Am. J. Roentgenol., 110:540, 1970.

Varney, D. C., and Ford, M. D.: Ectopic ureteral remnant persisting as cystic diverticulum of the ejaculatory duct: Case report. J. Urol., 72:802, 1954.

Verbaeys, A., Oosterlinck, W., and Dhont, M.: Ureteric ectopia without incontinence in the female. Acta Urol. Belg., 48:366, 1980.

Weiss, J. P., Duckett, J. W., and Synder, H. M.: Single unilateral vaginal ectopic ureter: Is it really a rarity? J. Urol., 132:1177–1179, 1984.

Wesson, M. B.: Incontinence of vesical and renal origin (relaxed urethra and a vaginal ectopic ureter): A case report. J. Urol., 32:141, 1934.

Williams, D. I., and Lightwood, R. G.: Bilateral single ectopic ureters. J. Urol., 44:267, 1972.

Williams, D. I.: The ectopic ureter: Diagnosis problems. Br. J. Urol., 26:253, 1954.

Williams, D. I., and Royle, M.: Ectopic ureter in the male child. Br. J. Urol., 41:421, 1969.

Wilmarth, C. L.: Ectopic ureteral orifice within an urethral diverticulum: Report of a case. J. Urol., 59:47, 1948.

Ureterocele

Abrams, H. J., Sutton, A. P., and Buchbinder, M. I.: Ureteroceles in siblings. J. Urol., 124:135, 1980.

Ahmed, S.: Uncrossed complete ureteral duplication with caudal orthotopic orifice and ureterocele. J. Urol., 125:875, 1981.

Ambrose, S. S., and Nicolson, W. P.: Ureteral reflux in duplicated ureters. J. Urol., 92:439, 1964.

Androulakakis, P. A., Ossandon, F., and Ransley, P. G.: Intrinsic pathology of the lower moiety ureter in the duplex kidney with ectopic ureterocele. J. Urol., 125:873, 1981.

Arap, S., Arap-Neto, W., Chedid, E. A., Mitre, A. I., and de Góes, G. M.: Ureterocele of the lower pole ureter and an ectopic upper pole ureter in a duplex system. J. Urol., 129:1227, 1983.

Ayalon, A., Shapiro, A., Rubin, S. Z., and Schiller, M.: Ureterocele—a familial congenital anomaly. Urology, 13:551, 1979.

Babcock, J. R., Belman, A. B., Shkolnik, A., and Ignatoff, J.: Familial ureteral duplication and ureterocele. Urology, 9:345, 1977.

Bauer, S. B., and Retik, A. B.: The non-obstructive ectopic ureterocele. J. Urol., 119:804, 1978.

Bondonny, J. M., Diard, F., Bucco, P., Germaneu, J., and Cadier, L.: Les urétérocèles chez l'enfant: tentative de classification et de schéma thérapeutique à partir de l'etude de vingt-quatre dossiers. Ann. Pediatr. (Paris), 28:763, 1981.

Borden, T. A., and Martinez, A.: Vesicoureteral reflux associated with intact orthotopic ureterocele. Urology, 9:182, 1977.

Bruézière, J., Jablonski, J. P., and Frétin, J.: Les urétérocèles sur duplication pyélo-urétérale à développement intra-vesical chez l'enfant. J. Urol. Nephrol. (Paris), 85:704, 1979.

Campbell, M.: Ureterocele: A study of 94 instances in 80 infants and children. Surg. Gynecol. Obstet., 93:705, 1951.

Chwalle, R.: The process of formation of cystic dilatations of the vesical end of the ureter and of diverticula at the ureteral ostium. Urol. Cutan. Rev., 31:499, 1927.

Diard, F., Eklöf, O., Lebowitz, R., and Maurseth, K.: Urethral obstruction in boys caused by prolapse of simple ureterocele. Pediatr. Radiol., 11:139, 1981.

Eklöf, O., Löhr, G., Ringertz, H., and Thomasson, B.: Ectopic ureterocele in the male infant. Acta Radiol. [Diagn.] (Stockh), 19:145, 1978.

Eklöf, O., Parkkulainen, K., Thönell, S., and Wikstrom, S.: Ectopic ureterocele in the male. Ann. Radiol., 30(7):486–490, 1987.

Ericsson, N. O.: Ectopic ureterocele in infants and children. Acta Chir. Scand., Suppl. 197:8, 1954.

Farkas, A., Earon, J., and Firstater, M.: Crossed renal ectopia with crossed single ectopic ureterocele. J. Urol., 119:836, 1978.

Fenelon, M. J., and Alton, D. J.: Prolapsing ectopic ureteroceles in boys. Radiology, 140:373, 1981.

Fishman, M., and Borden, S.: Crossed fused renal ectopia with single crossed ectopic ureterocele. J. Urol., 127:117, 1982.

Friedland, G. W., and Cunningham, J.: The elusive ectopic ureteroceles. Am. J. Roentgenol., 116:792, 1972.

Gomez, F., and Stephens, F. D.: Cecoureterocele: Morphology and clinical correlations. J. Urol., 129:1017–1019, 1983.

Gross, R. E.: The Surgery of Infancy and Childhood. Its Principles and Techniques. Philadelphia, W. B. Saunders Co., 1953.

Gyllensten, L.: Contributions of the embryology of the human bladder. Part I. The development of the definitive relations between the openings of the Wolffian ducts and the ureters. Acta Anat., 7:305, 1949.

Johnson, D. K., and Perlmutter, A. D.: Single system ectopic ureteroceles with anomalies of the heart, testis and vas deferens. J. Urol., 123:81, 1980.

Kjellberg, S. R., Ericsson, N. O., and Rudhe, U.: The lower urinary tract in childhood; some correlated clinical and roentgenologic observations. Chicago, Year Book Publishers, Inc., 1957.

Klauber, G. I., and Crawford, D. B.: Prolapse of ectopic ureterocele and bladder trigone. Urology, 15:164, 1980.

Lachiewicz, A. M., Kogan, S. J., Levitt, S. B., and Weiner, R. L.: Concurrent agenesis of the corpus callosum and ureteroceles in siblings. Pediatrics, 75(5):904–907, 1985.

Leong, J., Mikhael, B., and Schillinger, J. F.: Refluxing ureteroceles. J. Urol., 124:136, 1980.

Lima, S. V. C., and Cavalcanti, A. C. C.: Case profile: ureterocele from lower pole. Urology, 17:286, 1981.

Malek, R. S., Kelalis, P. P., Burke, E. C., et al.: Simple and ectopic ureterocele in infancy and childhood. Surg. Gynecol. Obstet., 134:611, 1972.

Mandell, J., Colodny, A. H., Lebowitz, R., Bauer, S. B., and Retik, A. B.: Ureteroceles in infants and children. J. Urol., 123:921, 1980.

Orr, L. M., and Glanton, J. B.: Prolapsing ureterocele. J. Urol., 70:180, 1953.

Passerini-Glazel, G., Calabro, A., Aragona, F., Anvi, E. F., and Schulman, C. C.: Blind ureterocele. Eur. Urol., 12:331–333, 1986.

Perrin, E. V., Perksy, L., Tucker, A., et al.: Renal duplication and dysplasia. Urology, 4:660, 1974.

Prewitt, L. H., and Lebowitz, R. L.: The single ectopic ureter. Am. J. Roentgenol., 127:941, 1976.

Riba, L. W.: Ureterocele: with case reports of bilateral ureterocele in identical twins. Br. J. Urol., 8:119, 1936.

Sen, S., and Ahmed, S.: Single system ureteroceles in childhood. Aust. N.Z. Surg., 58:903–907, 1988.

Share, J. C., and Lebowitz, R. L.: Ectopic ureterocele without ureteral and calyceal dilatation: (Ureterocele disproportion): Findings on urography and sonography. AJR, 152:567–571, 1989.

Snyder, H. M., and Johnston, J. H.: Orthotopic ureteroceles in children. J. Urol., 119:543, 1978.

Stephens, F. D.: Etiology of ureteroceles and effects of ureteroceles on the urethra. Br. J. Urol., 40:483, 1968.

Stephens, F. D.: Congenital Malformations of the Rectum, Anus and Genito-urinary Tracts. London, E & S Livingstone Ltd., 1963.

Tanagho, E. A.: Embryologic basis for lower ureteral anomalies: A hypothesis. Urology, 7:451, 1976.

Tokunaka, S., Gotoh, T., Koyanagi, T., and Tsuji, I.: Morphological study of the ureterocele: a possible clue to its embryogenesis as evidenced by a locally arrested myogenesis. J. Urol., 126:726, 1981.

Uson, A. C., Lattimer, J. K., and Melicow, M. M.: Ureteroceles in infants and children: Report based on 44 cases. Pediatrics, 27:971, 1961.

Weiss, R. M., and Spackman, T. J.: Everting ectopic ureteroceles. J. Urol., 111:538, 1974.

Williams, D. I., and Royle, M.: Ectopic ureter in the male child. Br. Jr. Urol., 41:421, 1969.

Williams, D. I., and Woodard, J. R.: Problems in the management of ectopic ureteroceles. J. Urol., 92:635, 1964.

Williams, D. I., Fay, R., and Lillie, J. G.: The functional radiology of ectopic ureterocele. Br. J. Urol., 44:417, 1972.

Anomalies of Position

Preureteral Vena Cava

Bateson, E. M., and Atkinson, D.: Circumcaval ureter: A new classification. Clin. Radiol., 20.173, 1969.

Brooks, R. J.: Left retrocaval ureter associated with situs invertus. J. Urol., 88:484, 1962.

Cathro, A. J.: Section of the inferior vena cava for retrocaval ureter: A new method of treatment. J. Urol., 67:464, 1952.

Campbell, M. F.: Anomalies of the ureter. In Campbell, M. F., and Harrison, J. H. (Eds.): Urology, 3rd Ed. Philadelphia, W. B. Saunders Co., 1970, p. 1493.

Cendron, and Reis, C. F.: L'uretere retro-cave chez l'enfant. A propos de 4 cas. J. Urol. Nephrol., 78:375, 1972.

Clements, J. C., McLeod, D. G., Greene, W. R., and Stutzman, R. E.: A case report: duplicated vena cava with right retrocaval ureter and ureteral tumor. J. Urol., 119:284, 1978.

Crosse, J. E. W., Soderdahl, D. W., Teplick, S. K., et al.: Nonobstructive circumcaval (retrocaval) ureter. Radiology, 116:69, 1975.

Cukier, J., Aubert, J., and Dufour, B.: Uretere retrocave et rein en fer à cheval chez un garçon hypospade de 6 ans. J. Urol. Nephrol., 75:749, 1969.

Derrick, F. C., Jr., Price, R., Jr., and Lynch, K. M., Jr.: Retrocaval ureter. Report of a case and review of literature. J.S.C. Med. Assoc., 72:131, 1966.

Dreyfuss, W.: Anomaly simulating a retrocaval ureter. J. Urol., 82:630, 1959.

Duff, P. A.: Retrocaval ureter: Case report. J. Urol., 63:496, 1950.

Eidelman, A., Yuval, E., Simon, D., and Sibi, Y.: Retrocaval ureter: Eur. Urol., 4:279, 1978.

Gladstone, J.: Acardiac fetus (acephalus omphalositicus). J. Anat. Physiol., 40:71, 1905.

Goodwin, W. E., Burke, D. E., and Muller, W. H.: Retrocaval ureter. Surg. Gynecol. Obstet., 104:337, 1957.

Gray, S. W., and Skandalakis, J. E. (Eds.): Embryology for Surgeons. Philadelphia, W. B. Saunders Co., 1972.

Gruenwald, P., and Surks, S. N.: Pre-ureteric vena cava and its embryological explanation. J. Urol., 49:195, 1943.

Guarise, P., Cimaglia, M. L., Spata, F., Capellari, F., and Belloli, G.: Uretere retrotendineo. Una causa eccezionale di ostruzione del tratto urinario superiore. Ped. Med. Chir., 11:85–88, 1989.

Harrill, H. C.: Retrocaval ureter. Report of a case with operative correction of the defect. J. Urol., 44:450, 1940.

Hattori, N., Fujikawa, J., Kubo, K., Saga, T., Nagata, Y., et al.: CT diagnosis of periureteric venous ring. J. Comput. Assist. Tomogr., 10(6):1078–1079, 1986.

Heffernan, J. C., Lightwood, R. G., and Snell, M. E.: Horseshoe kidney with retrocaval ureter: second reported case. J. Urol., 120:358, 1978.

Hellsten, S., Grabe, M., and Nylander, G.: Retrocaval ureter. Acta Chir. Scand., 146:225, 1980.

Heslin, J. E., and Mamonas, C.: Retrocaval ureter: Report of four cases and review of literature. J. Urol., 65:212, 1951.

Hochstetter, F.: Entwicklungsgeschichte des Venen-systems der Amnioten. Morph. Jahrb., 20:543, 1893.

Hollinshead, W. H.: Anatomy for Surgeons, Vol. 2., New York, Hoeber Medical Division, Harper & Row, 1956.

Hradcova, L., and Kafka, V.: Retrocaval ureter in childhood. Urol. Int., 16:103, 1963.

Kellman, G. M., Alpern, M. B., Sandler, M. A., and Craig, B. M.: Computed tomography of vena caval anomalies with embryologic correlation. Radiographics, 8(3):533–556, 1988.

Kenawi, M. M., and Williams, D. I.: Circumcaval ureter: A report of four cases in children with a review of the literature and a new classification. Br. J. Urol., 48:183, 1976.

Kumeda, K., Takamatsu, M., Sone, M., Yasukawa, S., Doi, J., and Ohkawa, T.: Horseshoe kidney with retrocaval ureter: a case report. J. Urol., 128:361, 1982.

Lautin, E. M., Haramati, N., Frager, D., Friedman, A. C., Gold, K., et al.: CT diagnosis of circumcaval ureter. AJR, 150:591–594, 1988.

Lerman, I., Lerman, S., and Lerman, F.: Retrocaval ureter: Report of a case. J. Med. Soc. N.J., 53:74, 1956.

Lowsley, O. S.: Postcaval ureter, with description of a new operation for its correction. Surg. Gynecol. Obstet., 82:549, 1946.

Marcel, J. E.: Grosse hydronephrose par uretere retrocave. Arch. Franc. Pediat., 10:1, 1953.

Mayer, R. F., and Mathes, G. L.: Retrocaval ureter. South. Med. J., 51:945, 1958.

Mayo, J., Gray, R., St. Louis, E., Grosman, H., McLoughlin, M., et al.: Anomalies of the inferior vena cava. AJR, 140.339–345, 1983.

McClure, C. F. W., and Butler, E. G.: The development of the vena cava inferior in man. Am. J. Anat., 35:331, 1925.

Murphy, B. J., Casillas, J., and Becerra, J. L.: Retrocaval ureter: Computed tomography and ultrasound appearance. CT: J. Comput. Assist. Tomogr., 11:89–93, 1987.

Olson, R. O., and Austen, G., Jr.: Postcaval ureter. Report and discussion of a case with successful surgical repair. N. Engl. J. Med., 242:963, 1950.

Parks, R. E., and Chase, W. E.: Retrocaval ureter. Report of two cases diagnosed preoperatively in childhood. Am. J. Dis. Child., 82:442, 1951.

Peisojovich, M. R., and Lutz, S. J.: Retrocaval ureter: A case report and successful repair with a new surgical technique. Mich. Med., 68:1137, 1969.

Pick, J. W., and Anson, B. J.: Retrocaval ureter: Report of a case, with a discussion of its clinical significance. J. Urol., 43:672, 1940.

Psihramis, K. E.: Ureteral obstruction by a rare venous anomaly: A case report. J. Urol., 138:130–132, 1987.

Randall, A., and Campbell, E. W.: Anomalous relationship of the right ureter to the vena cava. J. Urol., 34:565, 1935.

Rowland, H. S., Jr., Bunts, R. C., and Iwano, J. H.: Operative correction of retrocaval ureter: A report of four cases and review of the literature. J. Urol., 83:820, 1960.

Salem, R. J., and Luck, R. J.: Midline ensheathed ureters. Br. J. Urol., 48:18, 1976.

Sasai, K., Sano, A., Imanaka, K., Nishizawa, S., Nagae, T., et al.: Right periureteric venous ring detected by computed tomography. J. Comput. Assist. Tomogr., 10(2):349–351, 1986.

Schaffer, R. M., Sunshine, A. G., Becker, J. A., Macchia, R. J., and Shih, Y. H.: Retrocaval ureter: sonographic appearance. J. Ultrasound Med., 4:199–201, 1985.

Taguchi, K., Shimada, K., Mori, Y., Ikoma, F.: A case of combined anomaly of horseshoe kidney, retrocaval ureter and pelviureteric stenosis. Hinyokika Kiyo, 32(5):745–750, 1986.

Voelkel, V. H. H.: Retrokavaler verlaut des rechten Ureters. Z. Urol., 56:49, 1963.

Preureteric Iliac Artery (Retroiliac Ureter)

Corbus, B. C., Estrem, R. D., and Hunt, W.: Retro-iliac ureter. J. Urol., 84:67, 1960.

Dees, J. E.: Anomalous relationship between ureter and external iliac artery. J. Urol., 44:207, 1940.

Gray, S. W., and Skandalakis, J. E. (Eds.): Embryology for Surgeons. Philadelphia, W. B. Saunders Co., 1972.

Hanna, M. K.: Bilateral retro-iliac artery ureters. Br. J. Urol., 44:339, 1972.

Iuchtman, M., Assa, J., Blatnoi, I., Ezagui, L., and Simon, J.: Urometrocolpos associated with retroiliac ureter. J. Urol., 124:283, 1980.

Jurascheck, F., Notter, A., Fernandez, R., Al Bati, R., and Schoenahl, C.: Anuria due to bilateral ureteral blockage by the iliac pedicles (retro-iliac ureters). Ann. Urol. (Paris), 19:355–357, 1985.

Nguyen, D. H., Koleilat, N., and Gonzalez, R.: Retroiliac ureter in a male newborn with multiple genitourinary anomalies: Case report and review of the literature. J. Urol., 141:1400–1403, 1989.

Radhrishnan, J., Vermillion, C. D., and Hendren, W. H.: Vasa deferentia inserting into retroiliac ureters. J. Urol., 124:746, 1980.

Seitzman, D. M., and Patton, J. F.: Ureteral ectopia: Combined ureteral and vas deferens anomaly. J. Urol., 84:604, 1960.

Taibah, K., Roney, P. D., McKay, D. E., and Wellington, J. L.: Retro-internal iliac artery ureter. Urology, 30(2):159–161, 1987.

Vascular Obstruction of the Distal Ureter

Campbell, M. F.: Anomalies of the ureter. *In* Campbell, M. F., and Harrison, J. H. (Eds.): Urology, 3rd ed., Philadelphia, W. B. Saunders Co., 1970.

Campbell, M. F.: Vascular obstruction of the ureter in children. J. Urol., 36:366, 1936.

Campbell, M. F.: Vascular obstruction of the ureter in juveniles. Am. J. Surg., 22:527, 1933.

Greene, L. F., Priestley, J. T., Simon, H. B., et al.: Obstruction of the lower third of the ureter by anomalous blood vessels. J. Urol., 71:544, 1954.

Hyams, J. A.: Aberrant blood vessels as factor in lower ureteral obstruction. Surg. Gynecol. Obstet., 48:474, 1929.

Scultety, S., and Varga, B.: Obstructions of the lower ureteral segment caused by vascular anomalies (author's transl.). Urologe (A), 14:144, 1975.

Young, J. D., Jr., and Kiser, W. S.: Obstruction of the lower ureter by aberrant blood vessels. J. Urol., 94:101, 1965.

Herniation of the Ureter

Beck, W. C., Baurys, W., Brochu, J., et al.: Herniation of the ureter into sciatic foramen ("curlicue ureter"). JAMA, 149:441, 1952.

Dourmashkin, R. L.: Herniation of the ureter. J. Urol., 38:455, 1937.

Jewett, H. J., and Harris, A. P.: Scrotal ureter: Report of a case. J. Urol., 69:184, 1953.

Lindblom, A.: Unusual ureteral obstruction by herniation of ureter into sciatic foramen; report of case. Acta Radiol., 28:225, 1947.

Oyen, R., Gielen, J., Baert, L., Van Poppel, H., and Baert, A. L.: CT demonstration of a ureterosciatic hernia. Urol. Radiol., 9:174–176, 1987.

Page, B. H.: Obstruction of ureter in internal hernia. Br. J. Urol., 27:254, 1955.

Powell, M. C., and Kapila, L.: Bilateral megaureters presenting as an inguinal hernia. J. Pediatr. Surg., 20:175–176, 1985.

Watson, L. F.: Hernia, 3rd ed. London, Henry Kimpton, 1948.

35
RENAL DYSPLASIA AND CYSTIC DISEASE OF THE KIDNEY

Kenneth I. Glassberg, M.D.

Renal dysgenesis is maldevelopment of the kidney that affects its size, shape, or structure. Dysgenesis is of three principal types: dysplastic, hypoplastic, and cystic. Imprecise language use has confused discussions of these disorders; to avoid perpetuating this confusion, I begin by outlining the terminology adopted in 1987 by the Section on Urology of the American Academy of Pediatrics, which provided precise definitions of dysgenesis, dysplasia, hypoplasia, hypodysplasia, aplasia, and agenesis (Table 35–1) that are in this chapter. Note particularly that whereas dysplasia is always accompanied by hypoplasia, the converse is not true; hypoplasia may occur in isolation. When both conditions are present, the term "hypodysplasia" is preferred (Schwarz et al., 1981a).

DYSPLASIA

A dysplastic kidney contains focal, diffuse, or segmentally arranged primitive structures, specifically primitive ducts, as a result of abnormal metanephric differentiation. "Dysplasia" is, therefore, a histologic diagnosis. The condition may affect all or only part of the kidney, and in a duplex system, one segment may be normal and the other dysplastic. The kidney may be of normal size or small and may be grossly normal or deformed. Cysts of various sizes may or may not be present. When they are present, the condition is called cystic dysplasia. When the entire kidney is dysplastic with a preponderance of cysts, that kidney is referred to as a "multicystic dysplastic kidney." This condition is discussed in a subsequent section of this chapter. Aplastic dysplasia is represented by a nubbin of nonfunctioning tissue, not necessarily of reniform shape, that meets the histologic criteria for dysplasia. In utero and postnatal follow-up by ultrasound has shown some

multicystic kidneys to shrink with time into such nubbins. Aplasia may thus represent the involuted stage of a multicystic kidney.

Dysplasia may be associated with an absent renal pelvis or ureter; atresia, stenosis, or tortuosity of the ureter; and a normal, atretic, or absent ureterovesical junction. The appearance of a grossly abnormal collecting system with or without ureteral anomalies on intravenous urography is sometimes described as "renal dysplasia," but such features may occur in the absence of dysplasia. Williams (1974) has suggested that the term "renal dysmorphism" rather than "renal dysplasia" be applied to abnormalities noted radiographically or grossly without histologic proof of primitive structures.

Etiology

The origin of renal dysplasia is unclear. Normal renal development is initiated by penetration of metanephric

Table 35–1. CLASSIFICATION OF HYPOPLASIA AND HYPODYSPLASIA

Hypoplasia
True ("oligonephronia")
  With normal ureteral orifice
  With abnormal ureteral orifice
Oligomeganephronia
Segmental (Ask-Upmark kidney)
Hypodysplasia
With normal ureteral orifice
  With obstruction
  Without obstruction
With abnormal ureteral orifice
  Lateral ectopia
  Medial or caudal ectopia with ureterocele
With urethral obstruction
Prune-belly syndrome

blastema by a ureteric bud at the proper time and place. According to the Mackie and Stephens (1975) "bud" theory, abnormal ureteric budding can lead not only to an ectopic orifice, but also to inappropriate penetration of the blastema, causing renal dysplasia. These investigators provided supportive evidence from studies of duplex systems, which showed a high correlation between the degree of lateral ectopia of the lower pole orifice and the extent of dysplasia of the lower pole segment.

Once renal function begins, obstruction can distort development secondary to the physical and chemical effects of poor drainage. It was long assumed that obstruction is a significant factor in dysplasia (Beck, 1971; Bernstein, 1971). Certainly, some evidence exists for the role of obstruction. For example, when both kidneys drain poorly, as in patients with posterior urethral valves, both kidneys may be dysplastic, whereas only the ipsilateral kidney is affected in cases of unilateral obstruction. Also in favor of a role for obstruction is the dysplasia observed in the upper pole of duplex systems when there is an associated obstructed ectopic ureter or ureterocele. The ipsilateral lower pole in such cases is not dysplastic, but the upper pole orifice is ectopic.

According to Mackie and Stephens (1975), an ectopic orifice is a sign of abnormal ureteric budding and metanephric development (i.e., dysplasia). However, some of these findings could also be explained as an embryologic abnormality that causes both obstruction and dysplasia. Moreover, one form of widespread dysplasia, namely, the type associated with multicystic disease, usually develops before urine formation. Potter suggested in 1972 that a teratogenic force acts at various sites to produce the combination of ureteral atresia and multicystic renal disease.

Growing awareness of the importance of the interactions between epithelial cells and mesenchyme in the control of normal development and growth has shed light on the origin of renal dysgenesis. In the chick embryo, simple ureteral ligation alone does not induce renal dysplasia (Berman and Maizel, 1982), whereas reduction of the condensed metanephrogenic mesenchyme is likely to lead to dysplasia (Maizel and Simpson, 1983). Moreover, ligation of the ureter seems to facilitate the dysplastic development of blastemas already deficient in mesenchyme (Maizel and Simpson, 1986). Spencer and Maizel (1987) found that inhibition of the glycosylation of extracellular matrix, which alters the interaction of epithelial and mesenchymal cells, can lead to dysplasia in the absence of obstruction.

The question of the etiology of dysplasia has assumed more than theoretical importance since the advent of fetal surgery. If obstruction is an epiphenomenon of dysplasia rather than its cause, then operations on a fetus to relieve obstruction are unlikely to be of value in preventing severe renal dysplasia or aplasia.

Histology

The histologic definition of renal dysplasia has evolved since the seminal work by Ericsson and Ivemark (1958a,

1958b), who sought to identify the structures that could arise only from embryonic maldevelopment, not from secondary events. They concluded that primitive ducts and cartilage were such unique features. Although the first part of their definition is still accepted, the second part is not. Ericsson and Ivemark (1958b), like some other investigators (Bernstein, 1971; Biglar and Killingsworth, 1949), considered all renal cartilage to be representative of aberrant development of the metanephric blastema and, thus, dysplastic. However, foci of hyaline cartilage have been found in normal kidneys (Potter, 1972) and in otherwise normal kidneys suffering from chronic inflammation (Taxy and Filmer, 1975). The present definition, therefore, does not specify nests of metaplastic cartilage as an absolute criterion for dysplasia.

Primitive ducts, which are lined by cuboidal or tall columnar epithelium (often ciliated) and surrounded by concentric rings of connective tissue containing collagen and a few smooth muscle cells but no elastin, are undeniable evidence of dysplasia (Fig. 35–1) (Bernstein, 1971; Ericsson and Ivemark, 1958b). The ducts are of various sizes and can be found in many sites, principally in the medulla and sometimes in the medullary rays. As a rule, the more severely deformed the kidney, the more extensive the primitive ducts (Ericsson, 1974), and in less severe cases, only the peripelvic area may be affected. These structures resemble the aberrant ductules of the fallopian tube and may be remnants of the mesonephric duct (E. endrath, 1935; Ericsson, 1954).

Several other histologic findings may (but need not) accompany the primitive ducts. Primitive ductules, which are smaller than the primitive ducts, are surrounded by connective tissue devoid of smooth muscle cells. Primitive tubules and glomeruli may be seen also; these resemble structures seen in human kidneys regenerating after neonatal renal necrosis (Bernstein and Meyer, 1961), in scars from renal biopsies (Bernstein, 1971), and in animal kidneys after trauma (Bernstein, 1966). Cysts and loose, disorganized mesenchyme and fibrous tissue are other possible features.

Familial Dysplasia

Although multicystic dysplasia is usually considered sporadic, a report by Squiers and associates (1987) suggests that some cases are part of a hereditary renal dysplasia syndrome, which is believed to be an autosomal dominant disease (Buchta et al., 1973). The renal abnormality in these patients might well be the result of a ureteric bud abnormality, but a primary defect of the metanephric blastema cannot be ruled out (Squiers et al., 1987).

HYPOPLASIA AND HYPODYSPLASIA

Hypoplasia and hypodysplasia have been subclassified as shown in Table 35–1. The subdivision according to the nature of the ureteral orifice acknowledges the bud theory, but it is not necessarily intended to be an endorsement of this theory. Hypodysplastic kidneys

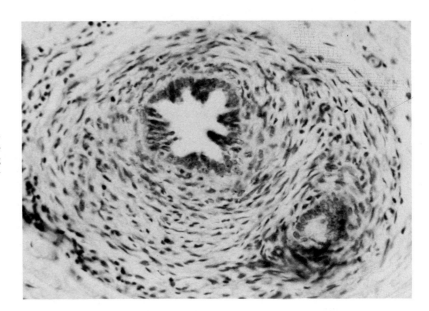

Figure 35–1. Primitive duct lined with columnar epithelial cells. Note concentric arrangement of spindle mesenchymal cells around the duct. Special staining is required to demonstrate smooth muscle cells. (Courtesy of C. K. Chen, M.D.)

most often occur in conjunction with ectopic ureteral orifices, with the extent of dysplasia correlating with the degree of ectopia (Schwarz et al., 1981a, 1981b, 1981c). However, hypodysplastic kidneys are seen in a few patients with normal ureteral orifices. In such cases, obstruction may or may not be present.

RENAL HYPOPLASIA

To avoid perpetuating the confusion that has attended the use of the term "hypoplasia," I restrict its use to describe those small kidneys that have less than the normal number of calyces and nephrons but that are not dysplasic or embryonic. The truly hypoplastic kidney may have a normal nephron density despite its small size.

Hypoplasia is not a specific condition; rather, it is a group of pathologic conditions with the same feature—an abnormally small kidney. It should be distinguished from renal aplasia, in which the kidney is rudimentary and the ureter atretic, and from renal agenesis, in which the kidney does not develop at all.

Hypoplasia may be bilateral or unilateral. In unilateral cases, the other kidney usually shows greater compensatory growth than is characteristic in patients with renal atrophy as a result of acquired disease. Hypoplasia can be associated with reflux, and the term "reflux nephropathy" is now applied to all types of abnormality associated with reflux. Segmental "hypoplasia" (Ask-Upmark kidney) probably is a type of reflux nephropathy.

Because of the similarity of the word "oligonephronia" (literally translated as a decreased number of nephrons) to "oligomeganephronia," which is a specific clinical entity (see following discussion), the former term should not be used.

True Hypoplasia

True hypoplasia is a congenital condition with no apparent familial tendency or gender predilection. The incidence is unknown, because many investigators fail to distinguish among the various causes of a small kidney. In a series of 2153 consecutive autopsies, Rubenstein and co-workers (1961) found a 2.5 per cent incidence of true hypoplasia.

Clinical Features

Clinical manifestations of true renal hypoplasia can be severe or absent. In patients with bilateral true hypoplasia or unilateral true hypoplasia with contralateral aplasia or agenesis, renal insufficiency, dehydration, or failure to thrive may be present. Often, these patients are premature infants who have developmental abnormalities of other organs, particularly the central nervous system. Respiratory problems are a common cause of death in these infants. At the other extreme, in patients with unilateral hypoplasia and contralateral hypertrophy, the diagnosis usually is made incidentally during an evaluation for some other urinary problem or for hypertension.

The urine is of low specific gravity when the condition is bilateral.

Histopathology

For the diagnosis of hypoplasia to be made, the renal parenchyma must be normal and without dysplasia, although Bernstein (1968) has described tubular degeneration, focal cortical scarring, and healed focal necrosis. The characteristic feature is the size of the kidney.

Evaluation

Ultrasound may be useful in demonstrating the presence and site of these kidneys, although it does not reveal the type of hypoplasia (Goldberg et al., 1975). Intravenous urography shows nonappearance or a small shadow; retrograde pyelography reveals a normal-caliber ureter and a reduced number of calyces. Reports by Porstman (1970) and Templeton and Thompson (1968) indicate the finding of a uniformly narrow renal artery on arteriography, in contrast to the tapered vessel seen in acquired atrophy, such as that secondary to pyelonephritis.

Differential diagnosis must take into account solid dysplasia (Potter's type IIB), segmental hypoplasia (Ask-Upmark kidney), oligomeganephronia, and acquired disease (chronic atrophic pyelonephritis, renal ischemia, and glomerulonephritis). Renal biopsy is the only way of proving the diagnosis.

Oligomeganephronia

The combination of a marked reduction in the number of nephrons and hypertrophy of each nephron was described independently by Habib and colleagues and Royer and colleagues in 1962. The latter group named the condition "oligomeganephronia." This condition, which is a specific histologic entity, has been reported in North America (Carter and Lirenman, 1970; Elfenbein et al., 1974; Morita et al., 1973; Scheinman and Abelson, 1970). It usually is bilateral, although a few instances of unilateral oligomeganephronia associated with contralateral renal agenesis have been reported (Lam et al., 1982).

Clinical Features

Oligomeganephronia is a congenital but nonfamilial disorder that affects boys more often than girls (3:1). It frequently is associated with low birthweight (<2500 g) and has been accompanied by ocular and auditory malformations, acral-renal syndrome with lobster-claw deformities of the hands and feet (Gruskin, 1977), and cyanotic congenital heart disease. However, other investigators note that the condition generally is not associated with other anomalies (Royer et al., 1962). In several cases, the mothers were older than 35 years at the time of the pregnancy (Royer et al., 1962). Whether "advanced" maternal age is still important today, 30 years later, is unknown.

The condition usually is discovered soon after the child's birth as a result of vomiting, dehydration, unexplained fever, intense thirst, and polyuria. The creatinine clearance is abnormal (10 to 50 ml/minute per 1.73^2), and the maximum specific gravity of the urine is 1.007 to 1.012. Moderate proteinuria may be present, but this is more likely to be a later finding.

Renal function remains below normal although stable for many years, but polydipsia and polyuria can worsen, and growth is severely retarded in many cases. As the patient enters his or her teens, the creatinine clearance begins to drop rapidly. Marked proteinuria (2 g/24 hours) is common, and the characteristic metabolic features of renal failure—disturbed acid-base balance and abnormal calcium and phosphorus metabolism—are seen. The blood pressure usually is normal. At this point, hemodialysis is required to maintain the patient's life.

Histopathology

The kidneys are smaller than normal (average weight at autopsy: 20 to 25 g) and are not always the same size.

Indeed, Griffel and associates (1972) described a unilateral case with contralateral renal agenesis, and Van Acker and colleagues (1971) reported a case with contralateral aplasia. The kidneys are pale and firm with a granular cortical surface and no clear distinction between the cortex and the medulla. The number of renal segments is reduced, generally five or six, although unirenicular and birenicular kidneys have been described (Bernstein, 1968). The renal artery is narrow.

The particular histologic features of a case depend on the duration of the disease. In patients 2 to 3 years of age, the characteristic findings are a reduced number of nephrons, enormously enlarged glomeruli (sevenfold to tenfold the normal volume), juxtaglomerular bodies, and proximal tubules elongated to four times their normal length (Fig. 35–2). In older children, interstitial fibrosis and atrophy become more prominent, and the glomeruli become increasingly hyalinized until they are destroyed. The end-stage kidney closely resembles that observed in glomerulonephritis except for persisting enlargement of the glomeruli. Dysplasia is not seen.

Evaluation

The kidneys may concentrate contrast medium adequately for an intravenous urogram, producing a picture of small kidneys, usually with normally formed calyces, although Morita and associates (1973) have described a case with dysmorphic calyces. The small kidneys also can be identified by sonography (Scheinman and Abelson, 1970).

Oligomeganephronia may resemble juvenile nephronophthisis–medullary cystic disease complex in its clinical features, but the latter condition generally appears later in life, and defects of tubular function precede glomerular insufficiency (Herdman et al., 1967). Moreover, juvenile nephronophthisis–medullary cystic disease is familial; other cases are found in the relatives of 50 to 80 per cent of affected persons (Habib, 1974).

Simple bilateral renal hypoplasia may be confused with oligomeganephronia (Carter and Lirenman, 1970). Segmental hypoplasia (Ask-Upmark kidney) is nearly always accompanied by severe hypertension, which is not seen in oligomeganephronia.

Treatment

High fluid intake and correction of salt loss and acidosis are the initial steps. Daily dietary protein should be limited to 1.5 g/kg during the stable phase (Royer et al., 1962). Frank renal failure is managed by dialysis and transplantation. The allograft may come from a living related donor, because the disease is not familial.

Ask-Upmark Kidney (Segmental "Hypoplasia")

In 1929, Ask-Upmark described distinctive small kidneys in eight patients, seven of whom had malignant hypertension. Six of these patients were adolescents.

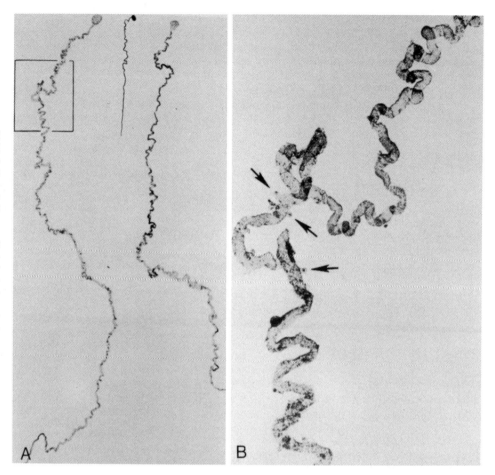

Figure 35–2. *A,* Mosaic photograph of two typical proximal tubules dissected from the kidney of a patient with oligomeganephronia. The silhouette in the top center is a diagrammatic representation to scale of an average proximal tubule from a kidney of an age-matched control.

B, Enlargement of the inset in *A,* showing the diverticula along the course of the nephron. (From Fetterman, G. H., and Habib, R.: Congenital bilateral oligonephronic renal hypoplasia with hypertrophy of nephrons (oligomeganephronic). Am. J. Clin. Pathol., 52:199–207, 1969. Reproduced with permission of the American Society of Clinical Pathologists.)

Etiology

Although the Ask-Upmark kidney was originally thought to be a developmental lesion because of the youth of the first patients, findings suggest otherwise. The presence of fibrotic glomeruli and chronic inflammatory cells, as described by Habib and associates (1965) and by Rauber and Langlet (1976), led both Johnston and Mix (1976) and Shindo and co-workers (1983) to suggest that the Ask-Upmark kidney is the result of reflux and ascending pyelonephritis. This hypothesis is supported by the data of Arant and co-workers (1979), who found that 16 of 17 affected patients had vesicoureteral reflux and that signs of reflux had been present in more than 50 per cent of the previously described cases in which appropriate studies had been done.

Chronic pyelonephritis secondary to reflux may be the cause even if no inflammatory cell infiltrates are found. For example, Heptinstall (1979) showed that such cells may disappear from the tissues with time. Hodson (1981) demonstrated in pigs that acute lesions of pyelonephritis may be followed by a histologic picture similar to that of Ask-Upmark kidney, in which glomeruli, collecting ducts, and inflammatory cells have disappeared. Hodson was able to produce histologically similar lesions with sterile high-pressure reflux. The presence of glomerular traces in periodic acid-Schiff (PAS)–stained sections of Ask-Upmark kidneys in areas grossly without glomeruli

is further evidence of an acquired rather than a developmental lesion.

Despite these data, the etiology of Ask-Upmark kidney is not yet clear. Some of these kidneys do contain dysplastic elements, indicating a developmental contribution (Bernstein, 1975).

Clinical Features

Most patients are 10 years or older at diagnosis, although the lesion has been reported in a premature infant (Valderrama and Berkman, 1979) and in a 13-month-old infant (Mozziconacci et al., 1968). Girls are twice as likely as boys to be affected (Arant et al., 1979; Royer et al., 1971).

Severe hypertension is a prominent symptom. Headache is common, either alone or together with hypertensive encephalopathy (Rosenfeld et al., 1973). Retinopathy is discovered in half the patients (Royer et al., 1971).

Proteinuria and some degree of renal insufficiency may be present if the disease is bilateral. Approximately half of the patients in the series described by Royer and associates (1971) had these signs at diagnosis.

Histopathology

The Ask-Upmark kidney is smaller than normal—12 to 35 g (Royer et al., 1971). Its distinctive feature is one or more deep grooves on the lateral convexity, underneath which the parenchyma consists of tubules resembling those in the thyroid gland. Usually, the hypoplastic segments are easily distinguished from adjacent areas. The medulla consists of a thin band, and remnants of the corticomedullary junction and arcuate arteries are seen. Arteriosclerosis is common, and juxtaglomerular hyperplasia may be seen (Arant et al., 1979; Bernstein, 1968; Kaufman and Fay, 1974; Meares and Gross, 1972).

Treatment

In unilateral disease, partial or total nephrectomy may control the hypertension (Meares and Gross, 1972; Royer et al., 1971). Failure of this measure suggests an unrecognized scar or generalized arteriosclerosis in the remaining kidney (Arant et al., 1979). Bilateral disease with renal insufficiency usually is managed medically, although dialysis and transplantation may be needed. Correction of reflux may prevent further renal damage but probably will have no effect on the hypertension.

RENAL HYPODYSPLASIA

Hypodysplasia may be associated with a normal or abnormal ureteral orifice, ureterocele, urethral obstruction, and prune-belly syndrome.

Hypodysplasia with Normal Ureteral Orifice

With Obstruction

Primary obstructive megaureter and ureteropelvic junction obstruction usually are associated with small but normal-appearing and normally situated ureteral orifices. Generally, this kidney has suffered diffuse damage because of hydronephrosis, although in a few cases, small areas or even the entire kidney is hypodysplastic or shows multicystic dysplasia (Fig. 35–3).

Without Obstruction

The "dwarf" kidney, although usually described as "hypoplastic," is, in fact, usually hypodysplastic. The calyces are normally cupped but generally fewer in number than would be expected from the size of the kidney. According to the bud theory, the dwarf kidney would be the result of deficient metanephric blastema rather than a budding abnormality (Stephens, 1983).

Hypodysplasia with Abnormal Ureteral Orifice

The small kidney associated with an abnormally positioned orifice usually is thin with ectatic calyces. The thin parenchyma is thought to reflect insufficient divisions of the ureteral bud, with a consequent reduction in the number of nephrons induced (Stephens, 1983).

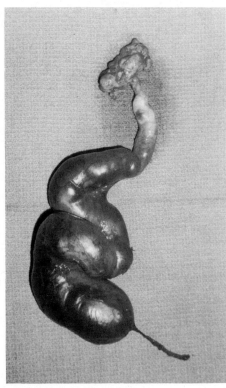

Figure 35–3. Small hypodysplastic kidney found in association with a severely obstructed primary megaureter. (From Glassberg, K. I., and Filmer, R. B.: Renal dysplasia, renal hypoplasia and cystic disease of the kidney. In Kelalis, P., King, L. R., and Belman, A. B. (Eds.): Clinical Pediatric Urology. Philadelphia, W. B. Saunders Co., 1985, pp. 922–971.)

The calyces generally are rounded, a picture characteristic of an earlier stage of development, before proliferating nephrons and papillary bulging indent the calyces to create the mature cup shape (Sommer and Stephens, 1981).

The radiographic appearance of rounded calyces should not be mistaken for the clubbing associated with reflux nephropathy, which is caused by parenchymal scars overlying the calyces rather than by the premature termination of calyceal development. On the basis of the view that abnormal budding leads to an ectopic ureteral orifice with thin renal parenchyma and ectatic calyces, Sommer and Stephens (1981) have designated the condition the "pan-bud anomaly." Their theory seems particularly applicable in duplex systems in which the thin renal segment with ectatic calyces is associated with a ureter draining ectopically into either a medial (often obstructed) or a lateral ureteric orifice.

Lateral Ectopia

Lateral ectopia generally is associated with reflux. If the pan-bud theory is correct, the rounded calyces found in the newborn infant with no history of infection would be the result of premature termination of calyceal development rather than of ballooning under the constant high-pressure assault by refluxing urine. Of course, infection leading to scarring and clubbing can confuse the picture, although pyelonephritic scars often create a characteristic indentation of the renal outline over the clubbed calyx (Hodson, 1981).

Medial or Caudal Ectopia and Ureteroceles

When the ureterovesical junction is displaced medially, the ureter and renal pelvis usually are dilated. The renal cortex may be thin, as in hydronephrosis, or severely dysplastic, perhaps with numerous small cysts (Fig. 35–4). When obstruction is complete, as in blind ureterocele, the upper pole segment may mimic the multicystic kidney histologically (Stephens, 1983).

Hypodysplasia with Urethral Obstruction

According to Osathanondh and Potter (1964), posterior urethral valves can be associated with two types of renal hypodysplasia. In the less severe form, there are small, generally subcapsular cysts and nearly normal renal function, a picture that could be caused by increased pressure secondary to urinary outflow obstruction. In the second form, the cysts are larger and more widely distributed, and numerous islands of cartilage are present. This form generally is associated with earlier onset and more severe obstruction and reflux (Fig. 35–5). Osathanondh and Potter (1964) believe that this highly abnormal condition has etiologic factors beyond urethral obstruction, and here again, abnormal budding appears to be involved.

In patients with posterior urethral valves, the position of the ureteral orifice correlates well with the extent of hypodysplasia, as shown by Henneberry and Stephens (1980) and by Schwarz and colleagues (1981b). When the orifice is normally positioned, the kidney is histolog-ically good but hydronephrotic, whereas a laterally placed orifice is associated with hypoplasia and an extremely lateral orifice with hypodysplasia. This correlation is present regardless of the presence or absence of reflux or the degree of urethral obstruction, suggesting that obstruction is not the only factor involved in creating the histologic picture. Further evidence for the role of factors beyond obstruction comes from cases of congenital ureteropelvic junction obstruction or primary obstructive megaureter, in which the ureteral orifices are almost always normally positioned, and the kidneys are rarely dysplastic.

Hypodysplasia Associated with Prune-Belly Syndrome

The features of the prune-belly syndrome (absent abdominal musculature; triad syndrome) include grossly deformed kidneys, which may have various degrees of dysplasia. The ureters are wide and tortuous, often with large and laterally placed orifices. Thus, the dysplasia in the kidneys of these patients is explainable by the abnormal budding theory of Mackie and Stephens (1975). Urethral obstruction or atresia may be present in the most severe cases, but patients usually have no lower urinary tract obstruction.

CYSTIC DISEASE

Classification

The kidney is one of the most common sites of cysts. Although the lesions themselves are histologically similar in the various cystic conditions—that is, microscopic or macroscopic sacs lined with epithelium—their num-

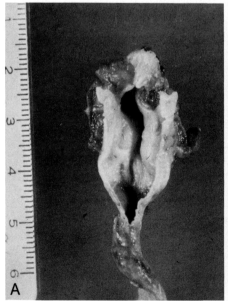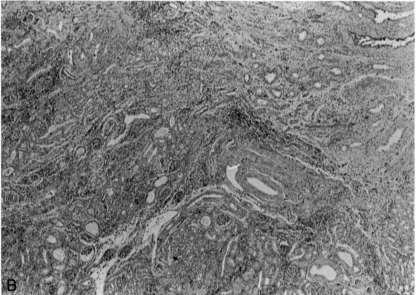

Figure 35–4. Upper pole of a duplex kidney associated with an ectopic ureterocele. *A,* Gross specimen had visible tiny cysts. *B,* On histology, primitive glomeruli are seen on left side and primitive ducts are seen in upper right corner ($\times$ 40).

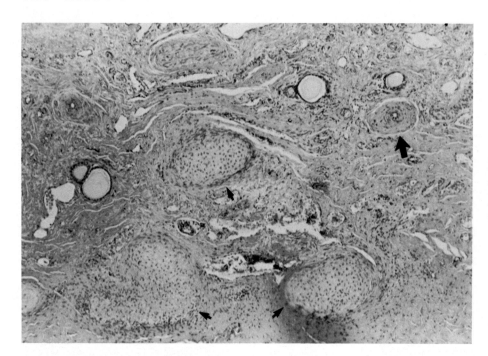

Figure 35–5. Histologic specimen of a nonfunctioning reflux kidney in a patient with posterior urethral valves. Note presence of nests of cartilage *(small arrows).* Primitive ducts are scattered throughout the specimen *(large arrow)* (× 100). The findings are compatible with dysplasia.

ber, location, and clinical features differ. For example, some renal cysts are ectatic collecting tubules continuous with the nephron, whereas others are saccular or fusiform structures resembling diverticula and located at various sites along the nephron. Cysts may or may not communicate with a glomerulus, collecting duct, or calyx. They may or may not be accompanied by dysplasia. Partly as a result of this diversity, several classifications have been proposed that are based on the clinical presentation, the supposed time of cyst appearance, the radiographic appearance, and the microscopic anatomy (Bernstein, 1973, 1976; Bernstein and Gardner, 1979a; Osthanondh and Potter, 1964; Spence and Singleton, 1972).

The best known classification may be that of Potter (1972), which is based on microdissection studies and considers principally the location of the cysts within the uriniferous tubule. Unfortunately, this system is difficult to apply clinically, and it groups together clearly dissimilar conditions, such as adult (autosomal dominant) polycystic disease and medullary sponge kidney.

In this chapter, the system used is based on the one proposed in 1987 by the Committee on Classification, Nomenclature and Terminology of the American Academy of Pediatrics (AAP) Section on Urology, in which the primary distinction is between genetic and nongenetic disease, and the various disorders are further classified according to their clinical, radiologic, and pathologic features (Table 35–2). A similar classification was offered by Stephens and Cussen (1983) and by Glassberg and Filmer (1985). Two discrete glomerulocystic entities have been added to the AAP classification; these are included in Table 35–2.

Etiology

Elucidation of the origin of renal cysts has been handicapped by the lack of suitable animal models.

Cysts can be induced in laboratory animals with various drugs and chemicals, such as lithium chloride, alloxan, lead acetate, and, especially, corticosteroids and diphenylamine (Filmer et al., 1973; Resnick et al., 1976). Diphenylamine also produces cysts in kidneys of the offspring when given to pregnant rats (Crocker et al., 1971). Hypokalemia secondary to long-acting corticosteroids also induces cysts in the absence of supplementary potassium (Filmer et al., 1973; Perey et al., 1967). Obstruction alone is not effective in inducing cysts (Carone et al., 1974; Filmer et al., 1973).

These results are compatible with a nephrotoxic theory of the origin of renal cysts with the proviso that the toxin may be a metabolite resulting from an inborn biochemical error as well as an external agent. Darmady and associates (1970) postulated that a toxic metabolite was the cause of adult polycystic kidney disease. Mongeau and Worthen (1967) suggested that the same was true of medullary cystic disease and juvenile nephro-

Table 35–2. CYSTIC DISEASES OF THE KIDNEY

Genetic
Autosomal recessive (infantile) polycystic kidneys
Autosomal dominant (adult) polycystic kidneys
Juvenile nephronophthisis–medullary cystic disease complex
  Juvenile nephronophthisis (autosomal recessive)
  Medullary cystic disease (autosomal dominant)
Congenital nephrosis (familial nephrotic syndrome) (autosomal recessive)
Familial hypoplastic glomerulocystic (cortical microcystic) disease (autosomal dominant)
Multiple malformation syndromes including renal cysts
Nongenetic
Multicystic kidney (multicystic dysplastic kidney)
Multilocular cystic kidney (multilocular cystic nephroma)
Simple cysts
Medullary sponge kidney (<5 per cent of cases inherited)
Sporadic glomerulocystic kidney disease
Acquired renal cystic disease
Calyceal diverticulum (pyelogenic cyst)

nophthisis. The occurrence and similar progression of the latter condition in monozygotic twins supports the view of a causative inborn error of metabolism. The attribution of some forms of cystic disease to infection is not at variance with this view, because organisms or their products could be nephrotoxic.

Carone and co-workers (1974) and Filmer and co-workers (1973) suggested that all cystic disease is the result of an imbalance between the intraluminal pressure and the resilience of the basement membrane. Again, this hypothesis is not at variance with the nephrotoxin theory of cyst origin. Basement membrane defects could result from genetically determined abnormal structural development or be acquired by either direct toxic action or a noxious influence on structures already inadequate.

Genetic Cystic Disease

Seven genetically determined forms of renal cystic disease are now recognized. Two types of polycystic kidney are known: autosomal recessive, often called "infantile," and autosomal dominant, often called "adult." Two types of medullary cystic disease complex are recognized: juvenile nephronophthisis, which is an autosomal recessive condition, and classic medullary cystic disease, which is autosomal dominant. Congenital nephrosis, the fifth type, is an autosomal recessive condition. Lastly, familial hypoplastic glomerulocystic disease, an autosomal dominant disorder, and cystic disease accompanying multiple malformation syndromes have also been identified. Polycystic kidneys do not demonstrate dysplasia and must not be confused with multicystic kidneys.

Autosomal Recessive ("Infantile") Polycystic Kidney Disease

In the past, the autosomal recessive type of cystic kidney disease often was referred to as the infantile form. This confusing and inaccurate age designation should be discarded.

Despite the attention it receives in the literature, this condition is rare. It was found in only 7 of nearly 109,000 pediatric admissions over a 13-year period in one series. Zerres and co-workers (1988) have estimated the frequency of autosomal recessive polycystic kidney disease at about 1 in 40,000 live births. The mode of inheritance is well established (Blyth and Ockenden, 1971; Lundin and Olow, 1961).

Autosomal recessive polycystic kidney disease (RPK) has a spectrum of severity, with the most severe forms appearing earliest in life. The cystic disease always becomes apparent during childhood (up to age 13; rarely, up to age 20) and is bilateral. Polycystic disease diagnosed in early childhood usually is of the recessive type (Cole et al., 1987).

According to Kissane and Smith (1975) and to Habib (1974), all cases of RPK involve the liver to some extent in the form of biliary ectasia or periportal fibrosis (Table 35–3).

CLINICAL FEATURES

Blyth and Ockenden (1971) subdivided RPK into four types, depending on the age at presentation and the severity of the renal abnormality (see Table 35–3). The earlier the age at which the patient is identified, the more severe the disease. These investigators thought that only one of the types—perinatal, neonatal, infantile, or juvenile—was present in a given family. However, numerous instances have subsequently been described that contradict the Blyth and Ockenden hypothesis.

The affected newborn usually has enormous kidney-shaped, nonbosselated flank masses that are hard and do not transilluminate. In some cases, the kidneys have been large enough to impede delivery. Oligohydramnios is common because of the lack of normal urine production by the fetus. The infant often displays Potter's facies and may have respiratory distress as a consequence of pulmonary hypoplasia. Oliguria is to be expected. Because of in utero "dialysis" by the placenta, the infant's serum creatinine and blood urea nitrogen (BUN) concentrations are normal at birth but soon begin to rise.

Table 35–3. BLYTH AND OCKENDEN CLASSIFICATION OF CHILDHOOD CYSTIC DISEASE

Feature	Perinatal	Neonatal	Infantile	Juvenile
Number of cases	9	6	5	5
Age at presentation	Birth	<1 mo	3–6 mo	6 wk (1) 1–5 y
Mode of presentation	Huge abdominal masses, normal liver	Large kidneys, hepatic enlargement	Large kidneys, hepatosplenomegaly	Variable renal enlargement, hepatomegaly
Typical course	Early death or rapid progression of uremia and death	Progressive renal failure	Chronic renal failure, systemic and portal hypertension	Portal hypertension, often necessitating portocaval shunt
Length of survival	All dead by 6 wk	Five dead by 8 mo	Two dead by 8 y, three alive at 18 mo, four alive at 10 y	One dead at 9 mo and another at 20 y, three alive after 12 y
Proportion of kidney affected*	>90%	60%	25%	<10%
Periportal fibrosis	Minimal	Mild	Moderate	Marked

*Dilated tubules; all patients had dilated and infolded bile ducts in the liver.
(Adapted from Blyth, H., and Ockenden, B. G.: Polycystic disease of kidneys and liver presenting in childhood. J. Med. Genet., 8:257, 1971.)

In infants in whom RPK is evident at birth, the usual clinical course is death within the first 2 months as a result of uremia or respiratory failure. However, if the infants survive their first 31 days, their chances of living at least a year are good if they receive proper supportive therapy. Cole and associates (1987) followed 17 such children for a mean of 6.1 years and found that eight were doing well with glomerular filtration rates of greater than 40 ml/minute per 1.73², although most were hypertensive. Moreover, three of the five who required hemodialysis had not done so until 7 years of age. In such survivors, the kidneys atrophy and shrink (Lieberman et al., 1971).

Children whose disease appears later in life develop renal failure and hypertension more slowly than those in whom RPK is manifest at birth. In general, their clinical problems are the consequence of liver disease rather than the renal condition, with hepatic fibrosis leading to portal hypertension, esophageal varices, and hepatosplenomegaly.

Some patients suffer from an intermediate type of disease, with both hepatic and renal failure appearing between the ages of 5 and 20 years (McGonigle et al., 1981). Neumann and associates (1988) described two sisters whose disease did not appear until their teens. The similarity of the clinical findings supports the view of Blyth and Ockenden that the type of disease tends to be similar within a family. The first case was identified as a result of abdominal pain when the girl was 14 years old. None of the cysts was larger than 3 to 4 cm. Blood pressure was 150/95, and all laboratory values were normal. When she was 18 years old, the serum creatinine level was 1.3 mg/dl, and at age 21 years, it was 1.6 mg/dl. Cystic kidneys were identified in the patient's 18-year-old sister as a result of family screening, and the serum creatinine level was 2.8 mg/dl. A liver biopsy revealed congenital hepatic fibrosis.

In contrast, Kaplan and co-workers (1988) described a family in which the index case was an infant who died at age 18 hours. Both RPK and congenital hepatic fibrosis were found in an asymptomatic 16-year-old sister. This girl and the two described by Neumann and associates (1988) may provide evidence for a fifth type of RPK in the Blyth and Ockenden system.

HISTOPATHOLOGY

The kidneys retain their fetal lobulation. Small sub-capsular cysts, representing generalized fusiform dilations of the collecting tubules, are grossly visible when the capsule is removed. In the sectioned kidney, the dilated tubules can be seen in a radial arrangement from the calyx outward to the capsule. The cortex is crowded with minute cysts. The renal pedicle is normal, as are the renal pelvis and ureter. In older children whose disease has been evident since birth, the cysts will be large and spherical, similar to those seen in the dominantly inherited disease (see following discussion). The nephron configuration is normal except for small dilatations, leading Potter (1972) to suggest that the abnormality appears late in gestation, with the dilatations of the collecting ducts and nephrons resulting from hyperplasia.

All children with RPK have lesions in the periportal areas of the liver (Habib, 1974; Kissane and Smith, 1975). Proliferation, dilatation, and branching of well-differentiated bile ducts and ductules accompany some degree of periportal fibrosis. Gross cysts are not found. Some have suggested that, just as all children with RPK have liver disease, all children with congenital hepatic fibrosis have RPK; however, it is not certain that this is the case. Darmis and associates (1970) found a 100 per cent incidence of RPK in children with congenital hepatic fibrosis; however, there are reports of children with hepatic but not renal disease. Kerr and colleagues (1962) found evidence of RPK in 60 per cent of children with congenital hepatic fibrosis using excretory urography. The kidneys were not studied histologically, however, so the true incidence of RPK in this series is unknown.

EVALUATION

The initial study should be sonography, which will show enormously enlarged kidneys bilaterally with uniformly increased medullary echogenicity (Sanders, 1979). It may be possible to identify small cysts. The kidneys will be more echogenic than the liver because of the return of sound waves from the enormous number of interfaces created by the tightly compacted and dilated ducts and tubules (Fig. 35–6). This noninvasive imaging study readily excludes severe bilateral hydronephrosis or multicystic kidney. Bilateral mesoblastic nephroma–Wilms' tumor will not appear as homogeneous masses, and the infant will have functioning kidneys. Bilateral renal vein thrombosis produces renal enlargement but hypoechogenic medullary areas. If the diagnosis remains in doubt, computed tomography (CT) is valuable, because it is more sensitive to inhomogeneity (and, thus, tumor) within abdominal masses. Macrocysts are rare in newborns but increase in frequency as the child gets older.

Intravenous urography with delayed films may show functioning kidneys with characteristic radial or medullary streaking (sunburst pattern) that is caused by dilated collecting tubules filled with contrast medium. This picture can persist for as long as 48 hours after the study (Fig. 35–7). The calyces, renal pelvis, and ureter generally are not visible. In a few cases, the kidneys will already be so dysfunctional that there will be no opacification, or only an increasingly dense nephrogram will appear.

Some investigators report cases of transient neonatal nephromegaly mimicking RPK. Avner and associates (1982) described a case in which an excretory urogram at age 2 days showed findings typical of RPK, whereas repeat studies at 6 weeks and 1 year showed normal renal architecture and size. They postulated that the radiographic findings were produced by transient intratubular obstruction. Berdon and co-workers (1969) presented a case of transient renal enlargement simulating RPK after an excretory urogram. Stapleton and colleagues (1981) described a similar case in which the sonographic findings were those expected in RPK. Therefore, one must remain aware of the possibility of transient nephromegaly, especially if a contrast study

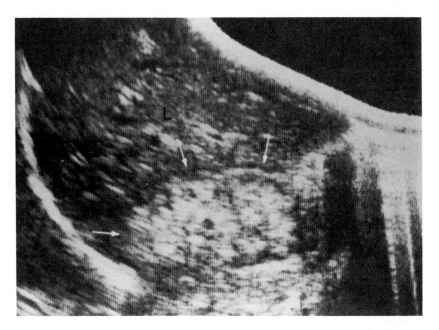

Figure 35–6. Sonogram of left kidney *(arrows)* in an infant with autosomal recessive polycystic kidney disease. Note homogeneously hyperechogenic kidneys, especially when seen in comparison with the less echogenic liver (L). Increased echogenicity is caused by the multiple interphases created by the dilated medullary ducts. (From Grossman, H., Rosenberg, E. R., Bowie, J. D., et al.: Sonographic diagnosis of renal cystic diseases. AJR, 140:81, 1983.)

has been performed, and not make a diagnosis of RPK prematurely. If necessary, a liver biopsy may be obtained.

A detailed family history covering at least three generations is needed when RPK is suspected. Once the diagnosis is confirmed, referral for genetic counseling is appropriate. Because this condition is transmitted in an autosomal recessive fashion, siblings of either sex have one chance in four of being affected.

Zerres and co-workers (1988) attempted prenatal diagnosis of RPK in 11 at-risk pregnancies and concluded that early identification was possible only in severe cases. In one instance, ultrasound scans at 18 and 22 weeks yielded normal findings, yet the child was born with enormous kidneys and soon died.

TREATMENT

No cure has been found for RPK. Respiratory care can ease or extend the child's life. Patients who survive may require treatment for hypertension, congestive heart failure, and renal and hepatic failure. Portal hypertension may be dealt with by end-to-side anastomosis of the left renal vein to the splenic vein. Esophageal varices may be managed at least temporarily by gastric section and reanastomosis. Transcatheter sclerotherapy has been employed in adults with chronically bleeding varices, but I am not aware of the use of this measure in children with RPK. Hemodialysis and renal transplantation must eventually be considered in many patients.

Autosomal Dominant ("Adult") Polycystic Kidney Disease

The autosomal dominant form of polycystic kidney disease (DPK) is an important cause of renal failure, accounting for approximately 9 to 10 per cent of the patients in Europe and the United States now receiving chronic hemodialysis (European Dialysis and Transplant Association, 1978; Grantham, 1979; Muther and Bennett, 1981). Approximately 600,000 Americans have DPK (Gabow et al., 1989). The gene has been localized to the short arm of chromosome 16 (Reeders et al., 1986a) and is not the one involved in RPK (Ramsey et al., 1988). The trait has 100 per cent penetrance, and because it is transmitted as an autosomal dominant trait, on average, 50 per cent of an affected individual's offspring will likewise be affected.

The traditional descriptor of "adult" polycystic disease is inaccurate. Although most cases are identified when the patients are between 30 and 50 years of age, the condition has been recognized in newborns. Presumably, the typical age at diagnosis will decline as more members of families at risk for the trait are screened by genetic testing and by ultrasound examination. All affected individuals will manifest the disease, although not necessarily symptomatically, if they live long enough, but renal failure is seldom seen before the age of 40.

A number of associated anomalies are common: cysts of the liver, pancreas, spleen, and lungs; aneurysms of the circle of Willis (berry aneurysms); colonic diverticula; and mitral valve prolapse.

ETIOLOGY

The genetically encoded defect responsible for DPK is the subject of several theories. One of these suggests that a defect in the basement membrane of the tubules accounts for cyst development. This theory is supported by the finding of abnormal basement membrane antigens (Carone et al., 1988).

A second theory, suggested by Grantham and co-workers (1987), holds that epithelial hyperplasia is an integral part of cyst formation. This theory is supported by the frequency of hyperplasia, polyps, and adenomas in DPK. Hyperplasia might cause tubular obstruction, resulting in weakening of the basement membrane and secondary proximal outpouching.

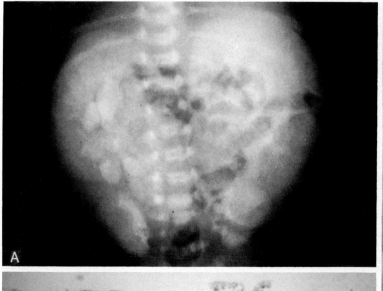

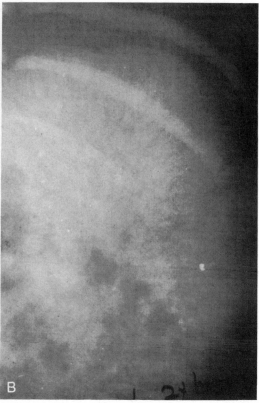

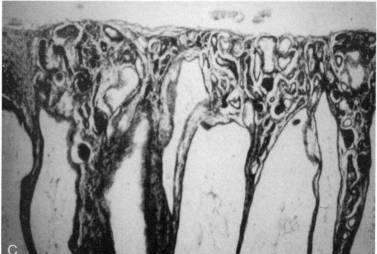

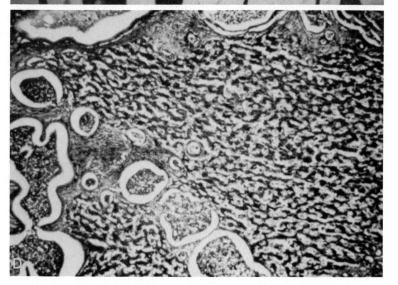

Figure 35–7. Newborn with abdominal mass and pulmonary hypoplasia.

A, On intravenous urography, 4 hours following injection of contrast medium, bilateral renomegaly is seen filling almost the entire abdomen with full and splayed out calyceal systems. Contrast medium can also be seen in right kidney as rays stretching from calyces to periphery of kidney.

B, Twenty-four hours later, contrast medium still is seen within the left kidney in radially oriented dilated ducts.

C, Renal histology also demonstrates dilated ducts radiating out to periphery of kidney.

D, On liver histology, ectatic biliary ducts are seen in left half of figure, and periportal fibrosis is seen at upper edge.

A third theory postulates a defect in one of the proteins of the supportive extracellular connective tissue matrix. Such an abnormality could account for both the basement membrane abnormalities (Gabow and Schrier, 1989) and the cysts found in other organs (Dalgaard and Norby, 1989). Support for this theory is provided by the association of DPK with mitral valve prolapse, colonic diverticula, and hepatic cysts (Gabow and Schrier, 1989), because similar constellations are seen in conditions known to involve defects of matrix proteins. Thus, diverticulosis, mitral valve prolapse, and berry aneurysms are common in patients with Ehlers-Danlos syndrome, and diverticulosis and mitral valve prolapse are seen in Marfan's syndrome.

CYTOGENETICS

Although the gene for DPK, sometimes referred to as PKD1, has not been isolated, it has been localized to chromosome 16 (Reeders et al., 1985; Ryynanen et al., 1987). Several nearby genes have been identified and shown to be linked in a similar fashion among members of an affected family but differ from one family to another. Therefore, one must find two individuals in the same family with the same linkages before one can say that an individual has the DPK gene.

The closer a genetic marker site is to a gene of interest, the more likely it is to be transmitted with that gene. If the flanking genes (i.e., those on either side of the DPK gene) can be identified, the accuracy of genetic diagnosis becomes even greater. In fact, closely linked sites have been uncovered on either side of the DPK gene, resulting in an accuracy of 99.004 per cent in identifying DPK in an asymptomatic family at risk (Mulley et al., 1990). Amniocentesis is now employed to make the diagnosis of DPK in utero (Reeders et al., 1986b), and in some of these cases, the families have elected abortion.

CLINICAL FEATURES

Neonates present mostly on the basis of renomegaly. When the disease is severe, stillbirth or significant respiratory distress can occur. For example, of the first 29 reported cases in newborns, seven were stillborn infants, four of whom died of dystocia (Begleiter et al., 1977; Bengtsson et al., 1975; Blyth and Ockenden, 1971; Euederink and Hogewind, 1978; Fellows et al., 1976; Fryns and van den Berghe, 1979; Kaplan et al., 1977; Kaye and Lewy, 1974; Loh et al., 1977; McClean et al., 1964; Mehrizi et al., 1964; Proesmans et al., 1982; Ritter and Siafarikas, 1976; Ross and Travers, 1975; Shokeir, 1978; Stickler and Kelalis, 1975; Stillaert et al., 1975; Wolf et al., 1978). Of the 20 patients who survived the neonatal period, 13 died within 9 months, eight of renal failure, usually in association with hypertension. Nevertheless, five of the seven patients who were alive at the time they were reported, at the ages of 3 months to 9 years, had good renal function.

In children who present after 1 year of age, the principal signs and symptoms are related to hypertension and enlarged and impaired kidneys (e.g., proteinuria,

hematuria). Now, with the families of DPK patients being screened by sonography, large numbers of asymptomatic children with renal cysts are being identified before full-blown disease develops.

Classically, DPK that manifests later in life takes two forms (Glassberg et al., 1981). In one form, patients present in the 4th decade of life with flank pain, hematuria, urinary tract infection, gastrointestinal symptoms, and renal colic (Table 35–4). The gastrointestinal problems are presumed to be caused by mechanical pressure exerted by the kidneys, and the renal colic is secondary to the passage of blood clots or stones. In the second type, the patient presents, usually in the 4th decade, with renal insufficiency and hypertension.

Various types of DPK may be found within a single family. As blood pressure screening has become more widespread, hypertension has become the principal form of presentation. For example, in a series from Heidelberg, Germany, 81 per cent of patients with DPK presented with hypertension (Zeier et al., 1988). In addition, among patients with a normal serum creatinine concentration, as many as 30 per cent were hypertensive. In this series, antihypertensive medication was instituted early, and as a result, fewer complications were seen, with only one cerebral hemorrhage occurring in 15 years.

As noted earlier, the polycystic condition in DPK is not confined to the kidneys. Hepatic cysts, usually identified incidentally by sonography, help in making the diagnosis of DPK. These cysts are more likely to be found in adults than in children. Such cysts were found by CT scanning in almost 60 per cent of one series of adults (mean age 49) (Thomsen and Thaysen, 1988). Hepatic cysts often grow, but they seldom produce any clinically important effects. New ones may appear as the patient grows older (Thomsen and Thaysen, 1988). In rare instances, enlargement of hepatic cysts leads to portal hypertension and bleeding esophageal varices (Campbell et al., 1958). When secondary portal hypertension appears, differentiating DPK from RPK can be difficult.

Approximately 10 to 40 per cent of patients have berry aneurysms, and approximately 9 per cent of these patients die because of subarachnoid hemorrhages (Grantham, 1979; Hartnett and Bennett, 1976; Ryu, 1990; Sedman and Gabow, 1984; Wakabayashi et al.,

Table 35–4. CLINICAL PRESENTATION OF AUTOSOMAL DOMINANT POLYCYSTIC KIDNEY DISEASE

	Frequency (%)	
Presenting Feature	Pittsburgh (Delaney et al., 1985)*	Heidelberg (Zeier et al., 1988)
Flank	30	13
Hypertension	21	81
Symptomatic urinary infection	19	23
Gross hematuria	19	23
Nephrolithiasis	34	15

*Delaney, V. B., Adler, S., Bruns, F. J., et al.: Autosomal dominant polycystic kidney disease: Presentation, complications and prognosis. Am. J. Kidney Dis., 5:104, 1985.

Adapted from Zeier, M., Gerberth, S., Ritz, E., et al.: Adult dominant polycystic kidney disease: Clinical problems. Nephron, 49:177, 1988. S. Karger AG, Basel.

1983). However, not all intracranial hemorrhages in patients with DPK are subarachnoid bleeding secondary to berry aneurysms; in some patients, hemorrhage follows the rupture of intracerebral arteries, the usual type of intracranial hemorrhage seen in patients with hypertension who do not have DPK. For example, in Ryu's series (1990), a cerebral artery rupture accounted for the hemorrhage in eight patients and a ruptured berry aneurysm in only three. In 10 of these 11 patients, hypertension was present, and fundoscopy suggested previous hypertension in the remaining one. Now, with earlier detection and treatment of the hypertension, one can expect fewer deaths from intracranial hemorrhage.

Intracerebral bleeding has been reported in at least one child with DPK. This child also had hypertrophic pyloric stenosis (Proesmans et al., 1982), a condition that has been reported in association with DPK in a set of identical twins and their father (Loh et al., 1977). Hypertrophic pyloric stenosis also has accompanied RPK (Gaisford and Bloor, 1968; Lieberman et al., 1971; McGonigle et al., 1981). Other abnormalities associated with DPK are mitral valve prolapse and colonic diverticulosis (Hossack et al., 1986; Kupin et al., 1987; Scheff et al., 1980). Patients who have diverticulosis are more likely to have hepatic cysts and symptomatic berry aneurysms (Kupin et al., 1987).

When DPK presents clinically, it usually is found with bilateral cysts. However, the disease can present asymmetrically, with cysts on only one side at first or with a unilateral renal mass (Fig. 35–8).

A variant form of DPK probably exists in which the renal cysts are primarily in Bowman's space. The cytogenetic study of Reeders and associates (1985) provided evidence that such a condition is a form of DPK. They found that a fetus with cystic disease predominantly of the glomeruli had the same genetic linkages on chromosome 16 as did its DPK-affected mother. Bernstein and Landing (1989) suggest that glomerulocystic kidneys in members of families with DPK are variants; the

glomerular cysts may be an early stage of DPK gene expression (Fig. 35–9). One caution: this condition should not be referred to as "glomerulocystic kidney disease" to avoid confusing it with sporadic glomerulocystic disease and other disorders associated with glomerular cysts, which are discussed later in this chapter.

HISTOPATHOLOGY

The renal cysts range from a few millimeters to a few centimeters in diameter and appear diffusely throughout the cortex and medulla with communications at various points along the nephron (Kissane, 1974). Frequently, the epithelial lining resembles the segment of the nephron from which the cyst is derived (Kaplan and Miller, unpublished data), and it often is active in secretion and reabsorption (Gardner, 1988).

Epithelial hyperplasia or even adenoma formation in the cyst wall is common, and the basement membrane of the wall is thickened. Arteriosclerosis is present in more than 70 per cent of patients with preterminal or terminal renal failure, and interstitial fibrosis, with or without infiltrates, is common (Zeier et al., 1988). This fibrosis may be secondary to infection or to an inflammatory reaction set off by spontaneously rupturing cysts.

Gregoire and co-workers (1987) found a 91 per cent incidence of hyperplastic polyps in kidneys removed from DPK patients either at autopsy or prior to transplantation. Some of the autopsies were performed on patients with normal renal function, yet polyps were still found. However, there was a greater predominance of polyps in patients with renal failure and in those on dialysis. Because hyperplastic epithelium is seen in both chronic renal failure and DPK, a uremic toxin not removed by dialysis might be involved.

Interestingly, the incidence of renal adenomas is just as high in DPK as in acquired renal cystic disease (ARCD), that is, approximately 1 in 4. The incidence of renal cell carcinoma probably is no higher in DPK

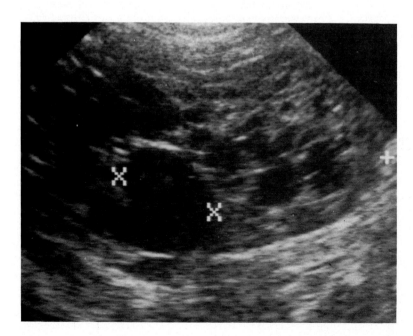

Figure 35–8. Asymmetric presentation of autosomal dominant polycystic kidney disease in a 9-year-old boy with hematuria. Sonogram demonstrates right kidney with multiple cysts. No cysts were identified in left kidney. Subsequently, the diagnosis was made in the patient's brother and mother. Cysts can be expected to develop in the right kidney with time.

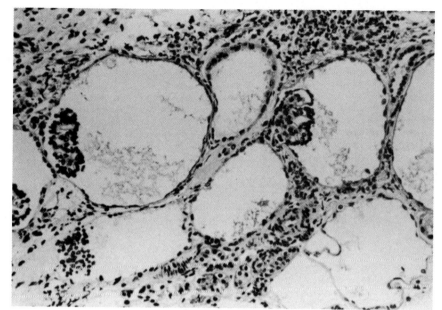

Figure 35–9. Glomerular cysts with a pattern compatible with that of autosomal dominant polycystic kidney disease in early childhood (× 190). (From Bernstein, J., and Gardner, K. D.: Cystic disease and dysplasia of the kidneys. *In* Murphy, W. M. (Ed.): Urological Pathology. Philadelphia, W. B. Saunders Co., 1989, pp. 483–524.)

than in the general population, whereas it is sevenfold the expected incidence in patients with ARCD (Gardner and Evan, 1984; Gregoire et al., 1987; Hughson et al., 1986). In the 87 kidneys examined by Gregoire and associates (1987), only one contained a renal cell carcinoma, whereas 19 demonstrated adenomas.

Three factors may have contributed to the impression of a higher incidence of renal cell carcinoma in DPK. First, the chance association of these two rather common lesions would be expected to be frequent. Second, some of the cases of simultaneous DPK and renal cell carcinoma probably, in fact, represented cancers in patients with von Hippel-Lindau disease or tuberous sclerosis. Third, the epithelial hyperplasia of DPK, which is a precancerous lesion in other conditions, might have been considered precancerous in DPK as well, although available data do not at present justify this view (Jacobs et al., 1979; Zeier et al., 1988).

Nevertheless, there is some evidence that DPK can be a precancerous lesion. In some patients with both DPK and renal cell carcinoma, the tumors were multiple or bilateral; and in ARCD, as well as in tuberous sclerosis and von Hippel-Lindau disease (two conditions known to be precancerous), renal cell carcinoma frequently is multiple, bilateral, or both (Gregoire et al., 1987; Ng and Suki, 1980; Torres et al., 1985).

Hepatic biopsy reveals cysts in approximately one third of patients.

EVALUATION

To make the diagnosis, it is important to have a history of the patient's family spanning at least three generations. Questions should be asked about renal disease, hypertension, and strokes. Cysts may be identifiable by sonography, but no readily available diagnostic test is specific for DPK.

When DPK is manifested in utero or in infancy, 50 per cent of affected kidneys are large with identifiable macrocysts (Pretorius et al., 1987). However, the kidneys may appear identical to those seen in RPK, having no apparent macrocysts and showing only enlargement and homogeneous hyperechoic features. In such situations, one must look for a parent with DPK to confirm the diagnosis.

On intravenous urography, the calyces may be stretched by cysts. However, the picture may simulate RPK, with medullary streaking of contrast medium. In adults, intravenous urography usually reveals bilateral renal enlargement, calyceal distortion, and a bubble or Swiss cheese appearance in the nephrogram phase. A CT scan may be helpful in some cases and often is superior to sonography in detecting cysts in organs other than the kidney (Fig. 35–10).

According to Gabow and associates (1989b), patients with DPK have a reduced maximum urine osmolality (680 ± 14 mOsm) after overnight water deprivation and administration of vasopressin. In cases where the diagnosis still is unclear, a liver biopsy may be warranted to rule out the specific portal lesion characteristic of RPK. A diagnosis of DPK may be confirmed by cytogenetic testing if an abnormality of chromosome 16 can be identified.

EXAMINATION OF FAMILY MEMBERS AND GENETIC COUNSELING

Because DPK is an autosomal dominant condition, 50 per cent of the children of affected adults will be affected. Therefore, when the disease is diagnosed, the patient's children should be examined by ultrasound. Before 1970, diagnosis of DPK before age 25 was rare. With ultrasound, the possibility of making the diagnosis in affected individuals before this age is at least 85 per cent (Table 35–5). When genetic studies are used, the diagnostic accuracy approaches 100 per cent.

Gabow and co-workers (1989a) identified DPK in 16 of 59 children under the age of 12, and the disease was

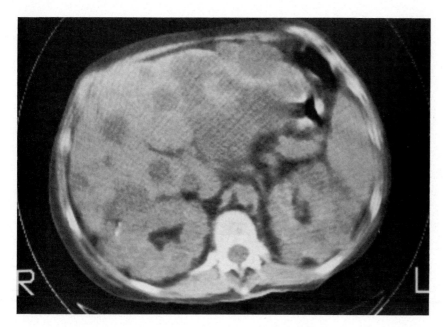

Figure 35–10. CT Scan of an adult male patient with autosomal dominant polycystic kidney disease. Bilateral renal cysts are seen in enlarged kidneys with calcification. Large asymptomatic cysts are seen throughout the liver as well.

suspected in another ten. Bear and colleagues (1984), who studied 61 children sonographically, found DPK in only 2 of 18 children younger than age 10 but in 14 of 43 children between 10 and 19 years of age. Similarly, Sahney and associates (1983) found only one of five children younger than age 15 but 16 of 19 aged 16 to 25 years to be affected. This last figure points out the fact that the 50 per cent incidence of affected offspring is an average, not a guarantee.

Bear and co-workers (1984) calculated that the chance that an asymptomatic relative between the ages of 10 and 19 years has DPK is 28 per cent if an ultrasound scan is negative and that, in a similar individual aged 20 to 29 years, the risk is 14 per cent. Other investigators have found rates of 32 to 50 per cent in siblings and children younger than age 20 (Sedman et al., 1987; Taitz et al., 1987; Walker et al., 1984).

At present, family members of an individual with DPK cannot obtain insurance before the age of 25 years because of the possibility of the disease (Dalgaard and Norby, 1989). Between the ages of 25 and 35, insurance is available but at higher rates, and after the age of 35, insurance can be obtained at normal rates if a sonogram has been negative. Now, with definitive cytogenetic

diagnosis available, it may be time for insurance companies to revise their criteria of insurability.

TREATMENT AND PROGNOSIS

More than 60 per cent of patients with DPK who do not yet have renal impairment have hypertension (Gabow et al., 1984), which can worsen renal function, cause cardiac disease, and predispose the patient to intracranial hemorrhage. The complications of DPK, thus, can be reduced significantly by controlling the blood pressure.

Upper tract urinary infections are common in patients with DPK, especially women. Schwab and co-workers (1987) divided these cases into parenchymal and cyst infections. In their series, 87 per cent of the cyst infections and 91 per cent of the parenchymal infections were in women. When a gram-negative enteric organism was the cause, 100 per cent of the infections were in women. Presumably, in women, the infection is an ascending one. Schwab and co-workers (1987) found that parenchymal infections responded better than cyst infections to treatment, even when the organism causing the cyst infection was proved to be sensitive to the antibiotic used. In their experience, the only dependable antibiotics were those that were lipid soluble, namely, trimethoprim-sulfa or chloramphenicol. Chloramphenicol produced better results.

The rate of renal deterioration seems to correlate with the rate of cyst growth, supposedly because the enlarging cysts cause pressure atrophy. However, histologic studies by Zeier and co-workers (1988) revealed no evidence of pressure atrophy, nor did these investigators find evidence of glomerular hyperperfusion, which had been theorized to damage the remaining glomeruli after some had been destroyed.

Because of the hypothesis that pressure atrophy was a cause of renal failure in patients with DPK, surgical unroofing of prominent cysts has been performed (Si-

Table 35–5. INCIDENCE OF RENAL CYSTS IN SIBLINGS AND OFFSPRING OF PATIENTS WITH DPK*

Reference	Age at Study (Years)	No. With Cysts/ No. Studied (%)
Bear et al.	< 10	2/18 (11)
Gabow et al.	< 12	26/59 (40)
Taitz et al.	< 14	10/22 (45)
Sahney et al.	< 15	1/5 (20)
Walker et al.	5–17	11/22 (50)
Bear et al.	10–19	14/43 (31)
Sedman et al.	< 19	49/154 (32)
Bear et al.	20–29	26/62 (42)
Sahney et al.	< 26	17/24 (70)

DPK, autosomal dominant polycystic kidney disease.

mon and Thompson, 1955). However, such surgery is not always effective, and some investigators point out that it removes functioning nephrons the patient can ill spare (Bricker and Patton, 1955; Milam et al., 1963).

When pain is significant, cyst decompression may be helpful. Bennett and co-workers (1987) suggest beginning with percutaneous aspiration, because it avoids the destruction of functioning tissue. However, they noted that the response to aspiration generally is less enduring than the response to surgery. Moreover, in their patients, no loss of renal function followed unroofing (in contrast to previous reports), and in five patients, the surgery also controlled hypertension. A similar observation was made by Yates-Bell in 1987. These reports make surgical unroofing more attractive. Ablation of the cysts with sclerosing agents probably is ill advised, because these lesions are more likely than are simple cysts to communicate with functioning nephrons or the pelvicalyceal system.

Symptomatic children generally are in the terminal stages of the disease, but their survival may be extended by supportive care for complications. As in affected adults, dialysis and transplantation may be appropriate. In the past, allografts from siblings were ruled out because of the frequency of DPK in such donors. However, now that siblings can be screened, this ban may no longer be appropriate.

Presymptomatic patients with DPK should be monitored with blood pressure measurements and tests of renal function. The advantages of such monitoring include the ability to prevent or control infection and hypertension, to identify potential kidney donors from among the family, to offer advice on marriage and childbearing, and to provide prenatal diagnosis. The question of abortion of an affected fetus is an issue that the parents and the physician must consider in view of the improved prognosis for such patients.

In earlier reports of DPK, the prognosis was quite poor, with the mean life expectancy ranging from 4 to 13 years after clinical presentation. Life expectancy was even shorter if the disease became apparent after the age of 50 years (Braasch and Schacht, 1933; Dalgaard, 1957; Rall and Odell, 1949). Death usually was attributable to uremia, heart failure, or cerebral hemorrhage (Dalgaard, 1957).

These data were based on the findings in symptomatic patients. From more recent data, Churchill and associates (1984) calculated that patients with sonographically identifiable DPK have a 2 per cent chance of developing end-stage renal failure by age 40, a 23 per cent chance by age 50, and a 48 per cent chance by age 73. Because of our greater ability to deal with problems such as urinary infection, calculi, hypertension, and renal failure, the outlook for the patient with DPK appears to be improving dramatically.

Juvenile Nephronophthisis–Medullary Cystic Disease Complex

Juvenile nephronophthisis was first described by Fanconi and colleagues in 1951. Medullary cystic disease was first reported by Smith and Graham in 1945. Although the two conditions are similar anatomically and clinically, they have a different mode of transmission and a different clinical onset.

Although either condition can occur sporadically, juvenile nephronophthisis usually is inherited as an autosomal recessive trait and becomes manifest between the ages of 6 and 20 years, whereas medullary cystic disease usually is inherited in autosomal dominant fashion and presents after the 3rd decade. The recessive transmission of juvenile nephronophthisis is supported by the frequency of consanguineous marriages among the parents of affected children (Bernstein and Gardner, 1979b; Cantani et al., 1986).

Although juvenile nephronophthisis is the more common condition and is responsible for approximately 10 to 20 per cent of the cases of renal failure in children (Cantani et al., 1986), this relatively high incidence does not appear to correlate with the low incidence (1 in 50,000 births) reported by Lirenman and associates (1974). A frequency of less than 1 in 100,000 has been reported for medullary cystic disease by Reeders (1990). Both conditions have been known by other names, such as uremic medullary cystic disease, salt-losing enteropathy, and uremic sponge kidney.

CLINICAL FEATURES

Juvenile nephronophthisis and medullary cystic disease both cause polydipsia and polyuria in more than 80 per cent of cases but not to the extent observed in patients with diabetes insipidus (Cantani et al., 1986; Gardner, 1984a). The polyuria is attributable to a severe renal tubular defect associated with an inability to conserve sodium. The polyuria is resistant to vasopressin, and a large dietary salt intake frequently is necessary. Proteinuria and hematuria usually are absent. In children, growth gradually slows, and malaise and pallor may appear in advanced disease. These latter findings are secondary to anemia, which may be attributable to a deficiency of erythropoietin production by the failing kidneys (Gruskin, 1977). Renal failure generally ensues 5 to 10 years after initial presentation (Cantani et al., 1986).

Juvenile nephronophthisis often is associated with disorders of the retina (particularly retinitis pigmentosa), skeletal abnormalities, hepatic fibrosis, and Bardet-Biedl syndrome—a combination of obesity, mental retardation, polydactyly, retinitis pigmentosa, and hypogenitalism. When renal and retinal disease coexist, the condition is referred to as renal-retinal syndrome (Gardner, 1984a). However, even within a family, not all those with renal disease have retinal disease. Alstrom's syndrome, a nephropathy accompanied by blindness, obesity, diabetes mellitus, and nerve deafness, may be a form of juvenile nephronophthisis (Bernstein, 1976).

Extrarenal abnormalities classically have been associated only with juvenile nephronophthisis. However, Green and co-workers (1990) described two sisters who presented with medullary cystic disease when they were in their mid-30s. Both had a history of congenital spastic quadriparesis.

HISTOPATHOLOGY

Early in the disease course, the kidneys may be of normal size (Cantani et al., 1986). In clinically manifest cases, the kidneys nearly always demonstrate interstitial nephritis, with round-cell infiltrates and tubular dilatation with atrophy. The corticomedullary junction is poorly defined. Atrophy begins in the cortex, but later, the entire organ becomes very small and has a granular surface.

Cysts are present in the kidneys of many patients, particularly those with medullary cystic disease (incidence: 85 per cent versus 40 per cent in patients with juvenile nephronophthisis) (Mongeau and Worthen, 1967). These cysts, which range in diameter from 1 mm to 1 cm, usually appear at the corticomedullary junction and, less often, in the medulla, generally within the distal convolutions and the collecting ducts (Fig. 35–11) (Cantani et al., 1986). Biopsies do not always reveal cysts, however, both because affected areas may be missed and because cysts tend to appear only with worsening disease (Cantani et al., 1986; Garel et al., 1984; Lirenman et al., 1974; Steele et al., 1980). Similar findings of tubulointerstitial nephritis with medullary cysts have been reported in Bardet-Biedl syndrome (or Laurence-Moon-Bardet-Biedl syndrome)—namely, obesity, mental retardation, hypogenitalism, polydactyly, and retinitis pigmentosa—as well as in Jeune's syndrome.

Some have suggested that the primary defect in juvenile nephronophthisis and medullary cystic disease is a defect of the tubular basement membrane (Cohen and Hoyer, 1986). These investigators described alternating areas of thickening and thinning of the basement membrane in the renal tubules in both of these conditions. They reported no abnormalities in the glomerular capillaries or Bowman's capsule and theorized that the interstitial damage was secondary to leakage of Tamm-Horsfall protein through the thin areas of the basement membrane. Kelly and Neilson (1990) were impressed by the number of inflammatory cells seen in the interstitium with medullary cystic disease. Particularly in the early stages, a heavy infiltrate of mononuclear cells is seen. The role of these cells is not clear. Do they represent a response to tubular leakage, antigen, or tissue damage, or do they play a primary role in the development of the cysts? Renal failure may be associated with a large mononuclear cell infiltrate and little evidence of cysts (Bernstein and Gardner, 1983; Neilson et al., 1985).

In some patients with juvenile nephronophthisis, especially those with hepatic disease, glomerular cysts have been detected. These lesions are rarely seen in other forms of nephronophthisis (Bernstein and Landing, 1989). Therefore, if glomerular cysts are discovered in a renal biopsy from a patient with juvenile nephronophthisis, hepatic biopsy is advisable. Hepatic biopsy is particularly important if renal transplantation is being considered, because hepatic fibrosis may lead to portal hypertension (Bernstein and Landing, 1989).

EVALUATION

In the early stages of the disease, intravenous urography may show a normal or slightly shrunken kidney (Chamberlin et al., 1977; Habib, 1974). Homogeneous streaking of the medulla may be found, presumably secondary to retention of contrast medium within dilated tubules, or ring-shaped densities at the bases of papillae, again perhaps representing contrast-filled tubules (Olsen et al., 1988). In the late stages of the disease, intravenous urography is of little value. Calcifications are not seen.

Sonography may show smaller than normal kidneys in juvenile nephronophthisis. Cysts may be imaged if they are large enough (Rosenfeld et al., 1977), but early in the disease, cysts are rarely visible. For example, Garel and associates (1984) demonstrated medullary cysts in 17 of 19 patients with end-stage disease but not in twins who had only mild uremia. The parenchyma may appear hyperechogenic secondary to tubulointerstitial fibrosis (Resnick and Hartman, 1990).

McGregor and Bailey (1989) described the CT appearance of juvenile nephronophthisis in a 19-year-old patient. In this case, cysts approximately 0.5 cm in diameter were apparent throughout the medulla, although no cysts were visible by sonography. These investigators recommended CT rather than sonography for investigating relatives of known cases. Even though the cysts may be prominent and help in diagnosis, renal failure probably results, not from the cysts, but from the tubulointerstitial changes.

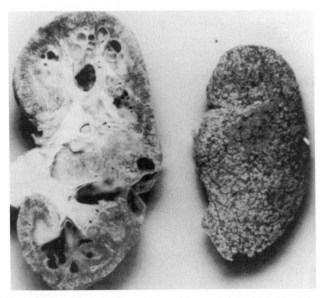

Figure 35–11. The gross appearance of the sectioned and subcapsular surface of a kidney from a patient with medullary cystic disease. Note that the cysts are concentrated at the corticomedullary junction, not at the papillae as in medullary sponge kidney. (From Kissane, J. M.: Pathology of Infancy and Childhood, Ed. 2. St. Louis, C. V. Mosby Co., 1975.)

TREATMENT

Sodium replacement is indicated early in the course of the disease. Later, dialysis and transplantation will need to be considered. Allografts apparently are not susceptible to the same process that destroyed the native kidney, because there is no evidence of serum antibodies to the basement membrane or other renal structural proteins (Cantani et al., 1986; Cohen and Hoyer, 1986).

Congenital Nephrosis (Microcystic Disease; Familial Nephrotic Syndrome)

Congenital nephrosis is predominantly of two types. The more common is referred to as the Finnish type (CNF) and has, as the name suggests, been reported principally in Finland, where the incidence is 1 in 8200 (Lanning et al., 1989; Norio, 1966). The other type, described by Habib and Bois in 1973, is referred to as diffuse mesangial sclerosis (DMS). The CNF type is recessive (Norio, 1966), whereas only 10 of the 30 reported cases of DMS were familial (Habib et al., 1989). Both conditions are associated with dilatation of the proximal convoluted tubules. The term "microcystic disease," is now rarely used.

CLINICAL FEATURES

CNF usually is discovered because of an enormously enlarged and edematous placenta, accounting for more than 25 per cent of the birthweight (Norio and Rapola, 1989). In DMS, the placenta usually is not enlarged.

In CNF, proteinuria is present in the first urinalysis. Edema usually develops within the first few days and always develops by the age of 3 months. Essentially, these infants starve because of their severe loss of protein in the urine; without treatment, they probably will die of sepsis before renal failure kills them. Without dialysis, half the patients die by the age of 6 months, and the rest die before their 4th birthday (Huttunen, 1976).

In DMS, the onset of symptoms is variable, with the diagnosis usually being made by 1 year of age. All children will have terminal renal failure by the age of 3 years.

Habib and colleagues (1985) have demonstrated that the nephropathy of Drash syndrome (nephrotic syndrome and Wilms' tumor with or without male pseudohermaphroditism) is, in fact, DMS. Of the 35 cases of DMS diagnosed by Habib and co-workers (1989), 13 were associated with Drash syndrome.

HISTOPATHOLOGY

CNF and DMS are both characterized by normalsized kidneys initially with pronounced proximal tubular dilatation. DMS is distinctive in that the glomeruli have an accumulation of PAS-positive and silver phosphate–staining mesangial fibrils. With advanced disease, the glomerular tufts sclerose and contract (Norio and Rapola, 1989; Habib et al., 1989). Diffuse hypertrophy of the podocytes is also found.

CNF is characterized by a proliferation of the glomerular mesangial cells. In both DMS and CNF, as in all types of nephrosis, there is fusion of the glomerular podocytes. Interstitial fibrosis is present in both conditions but is more pronounced in DMS (Norio and Rapola, 1989).

EVALUATION

The diagnosis of CNF can be made at about 6 weeks of gestation because of the greatly elevated levels of amniotic alpha-fetoprotein (AFP) secondary to fetal proteinuria. The use of AFP to diagnose DMS in utero has not been demonstrated.

In later stages of disease postnatally, ultrasonography has revealed enlarged kidneys with cortices that are more echogenic than the liver or spleen. The pyramids are small and hazy, and the corticomedullary junction is indistinct or absent. In one study, the kidneys continued to enlarge, and the corticomedullary junction became more effaced as the disease worsened (Lanning et al., 1989).

TREATMENT

After the kidneys have failed, transplantation is curative. Neither type of disease responds to steroids.

Familial Hypoplastic Glomerulocystic Kidney Disease (Cortical Microcystic Disease)

In 1982, Rizzoni and co-workers described two families in which a mother and two daughters were affected by what these investigators called "hypoplastic glomerulocystic disease." Melnick and associates (1984) described the same condition under the name "cortical microcystic disease," and Kaplan and colleagues (1989a) reported it in a mother and son. This condition is autosomal dominant.

The diagnosis of familial hypoplastic glomerulocystic disease requires four features. First, stable or progressive chronic renal failure must be present. Second, the kidneys must be small or of normal size with irregular calyceal outlines and abnormal papillae. Third, the condition must by present in two generations of a family. Lastly, histologic evidence of glomerular cysts must be found. These cysts are thin-walled and tend to be subcapsular. Tubular atrophy with some normal glomeruli and tubules in the deeper cortex is also observed. Marked prognathism has been present in some patients (Kaplan et al., 1989a; Rizzoni et al., 1982).

Multiple Malformation Syndromes Including Renal Cysts

Renal cysts are a feature of several syndromes characterized by multiple malformations (Table 35–6). Tuberous sclerosis and von Hippel-Lindau disease are autosomal dominant disorders and are the ones most likely to be encountered by urologists. Meckel's syndrome, Jeune's asphyxiating thoracic dystrophy, and Zellweger cerebrohepatorenal syndrome are some of the more common autosomal recessive syndromes. Many of these conditions involve glomerular cysts, and some have cystic dysplasia as a feature.

TUBEROUS SCLEROSIS

Bourneville described tuberous sclerosis in 1880. Since then, the disorder has been reported to be found in

Table 35–6. MULTIPLE MALFORMATION SYNDROMES
INCLUDING RENAL CYSTS

Mendelian (Single-Gene) Disorders
Autosomal dominant
   Tuberous sclerosis
   Von Hipple-Landau disease
Autosomal recessive
   Meckel's syndrome
   Jeune's asphyxiating thoracic dystrophy
   Zellweger cerebrohepatorenal syndrome
   Syndromes affecting the pancreas, liver, biliary system, and spleen*
   Syndromes affecting the brain*
   Syndromes affecting the cochlea*
   Syndromes affecting the skeletal system*
X-linked
   Orofaciodigital syndrome type I
Chromosomal Disorders
   Trisomy 13 (Patau's syndrome)
   Trisomy 18 (Edward's syndrome)
   Trisomy 21 (Down's syndrome)

*See text for list.

between 1 in 9000 and 1 in 170,000 infants (Kuntz, 1988). Although it is transmitted as an autosomal dominant trait in 15 to 25 per cent of cases, in the remainder, tuberous sclerosis is either sporadic or an example of the genetic condition with variable or incomplete penetrance.

Classically, tuberous sclerosis is described as part of a triad of epilepsy (80 per cent of cases), mental retardation (60 per cent of cases), and adenoma sebaceum (75 per cent of cases) (Lagos and Gomez, 1967; Pampigliana and Moynahan, 1976). The latter lesions are flesh-colored papules of angiofibroma, especially prevalent in the malar area. The hallmark lesion of the central nervous system is a superficial cortical hamartoma of the cerebrum, which sometimes looks like hardened gyri, lending the appearance of a tuber (root). Hamartomas often affect other organs as well, especially the kidneys and eyes. Periventricular subependymal nodules also occur frequently.

The kidneys of these patients may be free of lesions (approximately 50 per cent of cases) (Stillwell et al., 1987) or may display cysts, angiomyolipomas, or both (Fig. 35–12). It is not clear how common cysts are in these patients, because the cysts rarely exceed 3 cm in diameter, making them difficult to detect clinically. The cysts are of a unique histologic type, having a lining of hypertrophic, hyperplastic eosinophilic cells (Bernstein and Meyer, 1967; Stapleton et al., 1980). These cells have large, hyperchromatic nuclei, and mitoses are seen occasionally. The cells often aggregate into masses or tumorlets (Bernstein et al., 1986; Bernstein and Gardner, 1989). Later in the disease, the cyst walls may atrophy into a thickened, unidentifiable lining (Mitnick et al., 1983). In a few patients, predominantly glomerular cells have been seen (Bernstein and Gardner, 1989). The cystic disease can lead to renal failure with or without the presence of angiomyolipomas. The probable mechanism is compression of the parenchyma by the expanding cysts. Hypertension may also be present.

Angiomyolipomas occur in 40 to 80 per cent of patients (Chonko et al., 1974; Gomez, 1979). They are

rarely identified before the age of 6 years but are common after age 10 (Bernstein et al., 1986). By themselves, these lesions probably do not cause renal failure (Bernstein et al., 1986; Okada et al., 1982). Also, belying their aggressive histologic appearance, with pleomorphism and mitoses, no evidence of metastases has been presented.

Because more patients with tuberous sclerosis are surviving their central nervous system lesions now than in the past, the urologist is more likely to be called on for management of their renal problems (Stillwell et al., 1987). Cysts of the kidneys can be identified by sonography, the picture being very similar to that seen in DPK. Indeed, it may difficult to distinguish these two conditions. CT is helpful in demonstrating angiomyolipomas of the kidney or other organs, as well as in revealing cysts in other organs in patients with DPK. Scanning of the head may demonstrate the classic cranial calcifications associated with tubers or gliosis (Okada et al., 1982). Sometimes, both cysts and angiomyolipomas can be identified by sonography in tuberous sclerosis, the former lesions being sonolucent and the latter having a fluffy, white appearance.

The numerous reports of renal cell carcinoma in patients with tuberous sclerosis make it clear that this association is more than coincidental (Bernstein et al., 1986). These cancers appear in patients younger than would be expected (7 to 39 years) and may be single or multiple and unilateral or bilateral (Bernstein and Gardner, 1989). The karyotype of the cells near the tumor is similar to that of the tumor itself, and it is reasonable to suspect that the lining of the cysts evolves into the cancer (Ibrahim et al., 1989).

VON HIPPEL-LINDAU DISEASE

Von Hippel-Lindau disease is an autosomal dominant condition manifested by cerebellar hemangioblastomas; retinal angiomas; cysts of the pancreas, kidney, and epididymis; pheochromocytoma; and renal cell carcinomas. The penetrance probably is 100 per cent (Jennings and Gaines, 1988), and therefore, the condition can be expected to appear in 50 per cent of the offspring or siblings of affected persons.

Renal cysts are the most common malformation and are seen in 76 per cent of patients (Levine et al., 1982). Renal cell carcinoma occurs in 35 to 38 per cent of affected individuals (Fill et al., 1979; Levine et al., 1982). The renal cysts, as well as the tumors, usually are asymptomatic, although large tumors may cause pain or a mass. Hematuria may follow rupture of the tumor into the pelvicalyceal system.

Pheochromocytoma occurs in 10 to 17 per cent of individuals and appears to be confined to specific families (Horton et al., 1976; Levine et al., 1982). Patients may present with seizures or dizziness secondary to hemangioblastomas of the central nervous system. Cerebellar hemangioblastomas usually become symptomatic between 15 and 40 years of age (Jennings and Gaines, 1988). Some patients suffer blurred vision secondary to the retinal angiomas.

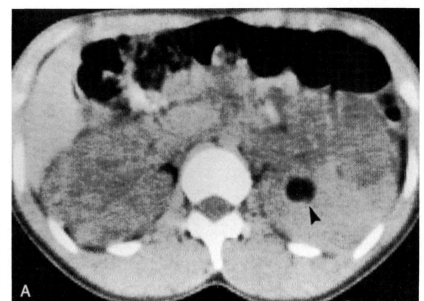

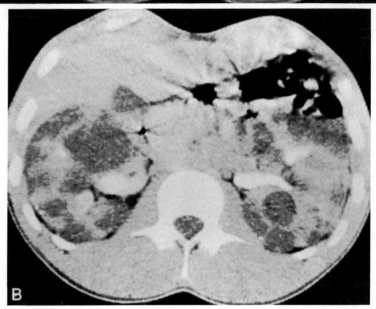

Figure 35–12. A 15-year-old girl with tuberous sclerosis and bilateral renal cystic disease has a history of seizures, cutaneous lesions, and moderate renal function impairment.

A, An unenhanced CT scan shows a 1.9-cm oval lesion *(arrowhead)* with a CT value of −110 HU, a value suggesting fat and compatible with diagnosis of a small angiomyolipoma.

B, Enhanced CT scan demonstrates fluid-filled renal cysts (4 to 6 HU). The CT findings are similar to those in autosomal dominant polycystic kidney disease, except for the finding of the small angiomyolipoma in *A,* which indicates the correct diagnosis. (From Mitnick, J. S., et al.: Cystic renal disease in tuberous sclerosis. Radiology, 147:85, 1983.)

When present, renal cysts and tumors often are multiple and bilateral. The cysts usually simulate simple benign cysts, with flattened epithelium that some investigators consider precancerous. Frank cancer usually appears between the ages of 20 and 50 years (Jennings and Gaines, 1988). Loughlin and Gittes (1986) found that the hyperplastic lining cells frequently resembled the clear-cell type of renal cell carcinoma, the most common type in these patients. Ibrahim and co-workers (1989) studied the cysts adjacent to carcinomas and found, much as in tuberous sclerosis, that the karyotype resembled that of the tumors. This similarity is evidence that the hyperplastic cells of the cyst lining are precursors of the carcinomas.

Solomon and Schwartz (1988) believe that a spectrum of pathology is found within the kidneys of patients with von Hippel-Lindau disease. At one extreme is a simple cyst with a single layer of bland epithelium. The next step is a typical proliferative cyst with layers of epithelial cells; in the ensuing step, there are complex neoplastic projections into the cyst lumen. If one agrees with the arbitrary distinction between adenoma and carcinoma on the basis of size, the next stage would be adenoma. Finally, there is the full-blown renal cell carcinoma. In some cases, one might stretch the spectrum two steps further: sclerosing renal cell carcinoma with residual foci of malignant epithelium, and completely hyalinized fibrotic nodules lacking epithelial foci. The latter condition may represent the endpoint of evolution of the renal cell carcinoma. All of these stages may be found within a single kidney (Solomon and Schwartz, 1988).

Sonography is useful in diagnosing the typical benign cystic features of von Hippel-Lindau disease: absence of internal echoes, well-defined margins, and acoustic enhancement. On CT, sharp, thin walls are seen around homogeneous contents without enhancement after contrast injection. Because multiple lesions (cysts, tumors, or both) are often present, CT frequently is more useful than sonography. CT often is useful in examining the adrenal glands for pheochromocytomas.

When lesions are small, it is impossible to distinguish tumors from cysts. In such cases, patients should have regular CT scans using narrow-screen collimation (Levine et al., 1982). With larger lesions, and whenever renal cell carcinoma is suspected, renal angiography with magnification or subtraction is advisable (Kadir et al., 1981; Loughlin and Gittes, 1986). This study will help reveal any additional tumors and will indicate the appropriateness of conservative surgery (Kadir et al., 1981; Loughlin and Gittes, 1986). Intra-arterial administration of epinephrine is sometimes helpful, because it causes vasoconstriction of the normal vessels but has no effect on tumor neovascularity.

Because of the high incidence of renal cell carcinoma in patients with von Hippel-Lindau disease, the urologist's primary role is careful surveillance so that small tumors can be identified and treated before they metastasize. Annual or perhaps biannual CT examinations are advised. Surgery should be as conservative as possible, with local resection or partial nephrectomy being preferable. Classically, the survival rate after nephrectomy has been only 50 per cent. However, in the closely monitored series of seven patients treated by Loughlin and Gittes (1986), six patients were followed for 4 months to 8 years, and only one death from metastatic disease was reported.

The genetic nature of this condition mandates examination of members of the patient's family. Ophthalmoscopic examination for retinal angiomas is useful, and an abdominal CT scan should be obtained between the ages of 18 and 20 years. If no disease is found, reevaluation is recommended at 4-year intervals (Levine et al., 1990). If cysts or small indeterminate lesions are identified, CT examination should be repeated every 2 years, perhaps with narrow-screen collimation (Levine et al., 1990). The goal is to identify any malignancies before they have metastasized.

MECKEL'S SYNDROME

Meckel's syndrome, an autosomal recessive condition, consists of microcephaly, polydactyly, posterior encephalocele, and cystic kidneys. The kidneys range from markedly enlarged to markedly hypoplastic with features suggesting dysplasia. Histologically, large cysts are observed, which appear to originate in the collecting ducts. The cysts have fibromuscular collars. A marked deficiency of glomeruli and poor corticomedullary development complete the picture. In severe cases, the kidney is nonfunctional.

JEUNE'S ASPHYXIATING THORACIC DYSTROPHY

Jeune's syndrome is an autosomal recessive disorder marked by generalized chondrodysplasia that predominantly affects the rib cage. Patients have short ribs and a small chest that restricts breathing, causing respiratory failure. Short limbs also are present. A wide spectrum of renal pathology is seen, including diffuse cystic dysplasia, cortical microcysts, and tubular interstitial disease with dilated medullary collecting ducts. The hepatic portal areas contain tortuous, interconnecting, and often dilated biliary ducts similar to those seen in RPK.

ZELLWEGER CEREBROHEPATORENAL SYNDROME

Zellweger syndrome, another autosomal recessive disorder, consists of hypotonia, a high forehead, and hepatosplenomegaly. Renal cysts are present in most patients and range from glomerular microcysts to 1-cm cortical cysts of glomerular or tubular origin (Smith et al., 1976). Smaller cysts are more prevalent, and cysts are seldom visible on intravenous urography. However, small (<5 mm) bilateral cortical cysts have been identified by sonography in two infants (Luisiri et al., 1988). Mild azotemia is present in some patients, but, as in trisomy 13 and 18, Zellweger syndrome may not have a definite feature of renal dysfunction.

OROFACIODIGITAL SYNDROME TYPE I

The type I form of orofaciodigital syndrome consists of hypertrophic lingular and buccal frenula; cleft lip, palate, and tongue; hypoplasia of the alinasal cartilage; bradydactyly; syndactyly; and alopecia. The syndrome is X-linked and dominant. In males, it is lethal, but affected girls may survive. Cystic kidneys were identified either late in the 1st decade or in the 2nd decade in six girls (Doege et al., 1964; Harrod et al., 1976; Mery et al., 1978; Stapleton et al., 1982). These cysts seem to develop as the patient grows, because in the patient described by Stapleton and associates (1982), no cysts were apparent by intravenous urography when the child was 1 year of age, whereas multiple cysts were identified by urography and sonography when the child presented 10 years later with hypertension and bilateral flank masses.

Because the cysts take some time to develop, it has been hypothesized that they represent the fortuitous appearance of DPK, a relatively common condition, rather than a true part of the orofaciodigital syndrome. Despite the similarities, however, Stapleton and colleagues (1982) thought that the pathologic features of the cyst and the differences in solute concentrations in the cyst fluid distinguished the lesions in orofaciodigital syndrome from those of DPK. These investigators found the osmolality and sodium concentration of the fluid aspirated from 20 cysts in one patient to be lower than those of the plasma, whereas in the kidneys of patients with DPK, two populations of cysts—with isotonic and hypotonic fluid—are found. Glomerular cysts are sometimes present, just as in DPK (Bernstein and Landing, 1989).

Once cysts become apparent, renal failure may develop.

SYNDROMES AFFECTING THE PANCREAS, LIVER, BILIARY SYSTEM, AND SPLEEN

The triad of hereditary bilateral renal cystic dysplasia, biliary dysgenesis with dilated intrahepatic ducts, and pancreatic dysplasia is known as renal-hepatic-pancreatic dysplasia or Ivemark syndrome (Bernstein et al., 1987; Ivemark et al., 1959). These three findings are associated with other conditions, such as the syndromes of Eljalde, Majewski, Saldino-Noonan, glutaric aciduria type II, and trisomy 9.

Bilateral cystic dysplasia and biliary dysgenesis without pancreatic abnormality can be associated with the syndromes of Zellweger, Robert, and Ellis–van Creveld (Bernstein, 1990). Bilateral cystic dysplasia without biliary or pancreatic dysplasia can be found in the Smith-Lemli-Opitz syndrome, which also includes mental retardation, growth retardation, microcephaly, micrognathia, and ambiguous genitalia. Franco and Aragona (1989) have hypothesized the existence of an autosomal recessive condition composed of polycystic renal disease or cystic dysplasia and hepatic and pancreatic fibrosis in association with situs inversus viscerum totalis and, frequently, splenic anomalies, such as small spleen or multiple spleens.

SYNDROMES AFFECTING THE BRAIN

Cystic dysplasia and other renal cystic abnormalities are part of several autosomal recessive disorders that involve the brain. One of these, Meckel's syndrome, has already been discussed. Others are the syndromes of Goldston (cerebral malformations, some of the Dandy-Walker type), Williams (supravalvular aortic stenosis, elfin facies, microcephaly, and mental retardation), Miranda, and Zellweger (already discussed) as well as lissencephaly (microcephaly, smoothness of the brain, internal hydrocephalus, minor facial abnormalities, and polydactyly).

SYNDROMES AFFECTING THE COCHLEA

Renal anomalies, including cystic dysplasia, are part of three syndromes associated with dysplasia of the cochlea (Mondini dysplasia): branchio-oto-renal (BOR) dysplasia, Klippel-Feil syndrome, and DiGeorge's syndrome. Animal studies have demonstrated immunologic similarities between the cochlea and the kidney, but it is not clear whether these data are applicable to human embryos (Arnold et al., 1976; Gimsing and Dyrmose, 1986; Quick et al., 1973). The BOR syndrome, which is transmitted in autosomal dominant fashion, usually is fairly benign, especially when it consists of preauricular pits, auricular deformities, or lateral cervical sinuses. Nevertheless, these signs should not be ignored, because some patients have severe hearing impairment or renal pathology (Gimsing and Dyrmose, 1986).

SYNDROMES AFFECTING THE SKELETON

Renal cysts are a feature of several other autosomal recessive multiple malformation syndromes, namely, chondrodysplasia punctata (rhizomelic type), short-rib polydactyly (Majewski and Saldino-Noonan types), and acrocephalopolydactylous dysplasia (Kissane, 1984). The nevoid basal-cell carcinoma syndrome, an autosomal dominant syndrome that includes cysts of the jaw, vertebral and rib abnormalities, and intracranial calcifications, has been reported to include renal cysts (Santis et al., 1983).

CHROMOSOMAL DISORDERS (TRISOMY 13, 18, AND 21)

Approximately one third of children with trisomy 13 have renal microcysts and segmental dysplasia. Other possible urinary abnormalities are duplication of the ureters, unilateral agenesis, and patent urachus (Potter, 1972). In trisomy 18, horseshoe kidney is a common anomaly. Usually, the cystic changes are microscopic and take the form of dysplastic, subcortical, and glomerular cysts without clinical sequelae.

Nongenetic Cystic Disease

Multicystic Kidney (Multicystic Dysplasia)

Historically, the terms "multicystic" and "polycystic" were used interchangeably in discussing the kidney. However, in 1955, Spence stressed that these terms designate completely different entities. He included them separately in his classification, and subsequent investigators have done likewise.

The multicystic kidney represents a severe form of dysplasia that is sometimes described as multicystic dysplasia. The kidney does not have a reniform configuration, and no calyceal drainage system is present. Typically, the kidney appears to be a "bunch of grapes," with little stroma between the cysts (Potter type IIA) (Fig. 35–13). Renal size is highly variable, from slightly less than normal to enormous, filling most of the abdomen. When the cysts are small, even microscopic, and stroma predominates, the condition is referred to as "solid cystic dysplasia" and is an example of Potter's type IIB cystic disease (Fig. 35–14).

ETIOLOGY

In the view of Felson and Cussen (1975), the multicystic kidney is an extreme form of hydronephrosis

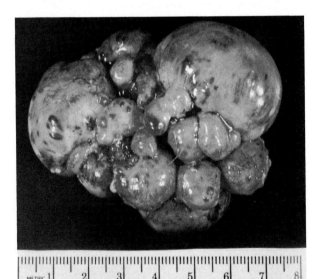

Figure 35–13. Multicystic dysplastic kidney having the typical appearance of a "bunch of grapes." The kidney was composed almost entirely of cysts and very little stroma.

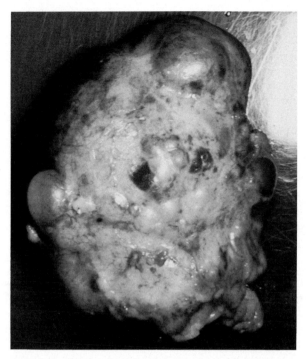

Figure 35–14. Nonfunctioning solid cystic dysplastic kidney, which differs from classic multicystic kidney by having smaller and fewer cysts and by being composed predominantly of stroma.

secondary to the atresia of the ureter or renal pelvis, which is a frequent concomitant. The fact that the left kidney is the one more often affected is supportive of this view, because this is the kidney more often associated with primary obstructive megaureter (Glassberg, 1977) and ureteropelvic junction obstruction (Johnston et al., 1977). In testing this hypothesis, several investigators have attempted to establish an animal model by ligation of the ureter at various points in gestation (Beck, 1971; Fetterman et al., 1974; Tanagho, 1972). This approach is not effective in mid or late gestation; early ligation of the fetal lamb ureter produces renal dysplasia, but not multicystic dysplasia (Beck, 1971). However, Berman and Maizel (1982) were unable to obtain similar results in the chick. Similarly, other investigators have been able to induce dysplasia, but no one as yet has been able to induce a multicystic dysplastic kidney.

Other theories have been offered by Hildebrandt (1894) and by Osathanondh and Potter (1964). Hildebrandt (1894) suggested that failure of the union between the ureteric bud and the metanephric blastema leads to cystic dilatation in the latter; this hypothesis, like the obstructive view, is supported by the high incidence of concomitant ureteral atresia. Osathanondh and Potter (1964) postulated that Potter type IIA kidneys, the type with large cysts, result from an ampullary abnormality in which the ampullae stop dividing early and, therefore, produce fewer generations of tubules. In this view, the last generation of tubules produced is cystic and does not induce metanephric differentiation, and the occasional normal or nearly normal nephron is

the result of a rare normal ampulla and collecting tubules.

CLINICAL FEATURES

Multicystic dysplasia is the most common type of renal cystic disease, and one of the most common causes of an abdominal mass, in infants (Griscom et al., 1975; Longino and Martin, 1958; Melicow and Uson, 1959). Widespread prenatal ultrasound evaluation has greatly increased the frequency with which the condition is identified. Although the pathogenetic process leading to a multicystic kidney probably is operative by the 8th week in utero, the mean age at the time of antenatal diagnosis is about 28 weeks, with a range of 21 to 35 weeks (Avni et al., 1987). The reason is not apparent. In less severely affected patients, the condition may be an incidental finding during evaluation of an adult for abdominal pain, hematuria, hypertension, or an unrelated condition. At any age, the condition is more likely to be found on the left (Fine and Burns, 1959; Friedman and Abeshouse, 1957; Griscom et al., 1975; Parkkulainen et al., 1959; Pathak and Williams, 1964) and is slightly more common in males.

In many cases, the contralateral upper tract also is abnormal. Common problems are ureteropelvic junction obstruction and obstructive megaureter (Greene et al., 1971; Pathak and Williams, 1964). For example, in a series of 13 patients with multicystic kidney, four had contralateral vesicoureteral reflux (Heikkinen et al., 1980). In another series, one third of the contralateral ureters had an irregular contour suggestive of fetal folds (Griscom et al., 1975; Johnston, 1969; Ostling, 1942). Although ureteral folds are a common transient finding in infants, the high incidence in the series of Griscom and associates (1975) suggests that folds are a factor in the contralateral multicystic disease.

Kleiner and co-workers (1986) found bilaterality of the multicystic pathology in 5 of 27 patients who were evaluated antenatally by ultrasound examination. In bilateral cases, the newborn has the classic abnormal facies and oligohydramnios of Potter's syndrome. This condition is incompatible with survival, although one infant survived for 69 days (Kishikawa et al., 1981). Another association is between multicystic kidney and contralateral renal agenesis, which is likewise incompatible with life.

Involution sometimes occurs in the multicystic kidney, either antenatally or postnatally (Avni et al., 1987; Hashimoto et al., 1986). This involution may be so severe that the affected kidney disappears from subsequent sonograms. In such cases, the kidney may be only a "nubbin," and the condition is referred to as "renal aplasia" or "aplastic dysplasia" (Bernstein and Gardner, 1989; Glassberg and Filmer, in press). Previously, aplastic kidneys, which often are associated with atretic ureters, were thought to be a separate entity. Now, with the experience of following multicystic kidneys sonographically, it is apparent that most aplastic kidneys represent involuted multicystic organs.

In a few cases, multicystic dysplasia has involved a

horseshoe kidney (Greene et al., 1971; Walker et al., 1978) or one pole of a duplex kidney.

HISTOPATHOLOGY

Multicystic kidneys with large cysts tend to be large with little stroma, whereas those with small cysts generally are smaller and more solid. The blood supply likewise is variable, ranging from a pedicle with small vessels to no pedicle at all (Parkkulainen et al., 1959). Usually, the ureter is partly or totally atretic, and the renal pelvis may be absent. Griscom and associates (1975) referred to the form without a renal pelvis as "pyeloinfundibular atresia" and reported finding no evidence of communication between the cysts. However, others have shown distribution of contrast medium among the cysts by means of connecting tubules (Saxton et al., 1981). Felson and Cussen (1975) referred to the variety with a renal pelvis as the "hydronephrotic type" and demonstrated connections between the cysts and the renal pelvis.

Microscopically, the cysts are lined by low cuboidal epithelium. They are separated by thin septa of fibrous tissue and primitive dysplastic elements, especially primitive ducts. Frequently, immature glomeruli are present, and on occasion, a few mature glomeruli are seen.

EVALUATION

Renal masses in infants most often represent either multicystic kidney disease or hydronephrosis, and it is important to distinguish the two, especially if the surgeon wishes to remove a nonfunctioning hydronephrotic kidney or repair a ureteropelvic junction obstruction while leaving a multicystic organ in situ. In newborns, ultrasonography generally is the first study. In a few cases, it will be difficult to distinguish multicystic kidney disease from severe hydronephrosis (Gates, 1980; Hadlock et al., 1981). In general, however, the multicystic kidney will have a haphazard distribution of cysts of various sizes without a larger central or medial cyst. In comparison, in cases of ureteropelvic junction obstruction, the cysts or calyces are organized around the periphery of the kidney, and connections usually can be demonstrated between the peripheral cysts and a central or medial cyst representing the renal pelvis (Fig. 35–15). When there is an identifiable renal sinus, the diagnosis is more likely to be hydronephrosis than multicystic kidney.

According to Stuck and associates (1982), who examined 15 patients, three ultrasound features are diagnostic of multicystic kidney: (1) visible interfaces between cysts, (2) nonmedial locations of larger cysts, and (3) absence of an identifiable renal sinus. However, absence of a renal sinus is an inconclusive finding, because even when a renal sinus is present, it can go unrecognized by the ultrasound examination. These investigators also noted absence of communication between the cysts in all but one of their patients and absence of identifiable parenchymal tissue in 11 cases.

A particular diagnostic problem arises in the unusual hydronephrotic form of multicystic kidney disease. Among 14 patients with multicystic kidneys, Felson and Cussen (1975) retrospectively identified four who, on intravenous urography, were found to have the calyceal crescents typical of severe hydronephrosis. This feature is thought to represent contrast medium in tubules compressed and displaced by dilated calyces (Dunbar and Nogrady, 1970). All four of these kidneys had small amounts of parenchyma and glomeruli, but no correlation could be made between the parenchymal tissue and the appearance of crescents. In all four kidneys, communications between the cysts were found, and communications with the renal pelvis were found in the three kidneys in which this structure was present.

In these difficult cases, radioisotope studies may be helpful. Hydronephrotic kidneys generally evidence some function on a dimercaptosuccinic acid (DMSA) scan, whereas renal concentration is seldom seen in multicystic kidneys. Angiography reveals an absent or small renal artery in the multicystic kidney, but this study is rarely indicated. Cystoscopy may reveal a hemitrigone and absent ureteral orifice on the affected side; however, more often, an orifice is present, but retrograde urography demonstrates ureteral atresia. Again, this study is seldom performed.

Percutaneous studies were performed by some investigators with the idea that the cysts do not communicate and, thus, injected contrast medium would remain localized in the injected cyst. This proved not to be true; in many of the reported cases and in one of ours, communication between cysts was apparent (Greene et al., 1971; Lang and Gershanik, 1978; Saxton et al., 1981; Summer et al., 1978).

In a few cases, diagnostic studies will not be performed until the patient is older. In these instances, the plain abdominal film often reveals renal calcifications. These deposits usually appear as annular or arcuate shadows (Felson and Cussen, 1975).

TREATMENT AND PROGNOSIS

It has often been stated that the multicystic kidney can be ignored unless its bulk is inconvenient (Griscom et al., 1975; Pathak and Williams, 1964) and that attention should be directed instead to identifying any abnormalities of the contralateral urinary tract. Certainly, the need in the past to explore some multicystic kidneys to rule out malignancy, such as cystic Wilms' tumor and congenital mesoblastic nephroma, has largely been erased by new diagnostic tools. Kidneys that do contain malignancies are likely to be explored because of the retention of some function as seen by excretory urography or nuclear medicine studies (Walker et al., 1984); therefore, routine exploration solely to rule out malignancy is inappropriate.

A nonfunctioning hydronephrotic kidney could be mistaken for a multicystic kidney, although complete nonfunction on a nuclear medicine study is unusual in kidneys affected by ureteropelvic junction obstruction. Even if the correct diagnosis is missed in such a case, however, it is unlikely to have significant consequences,

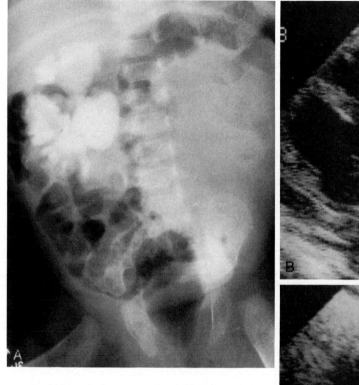

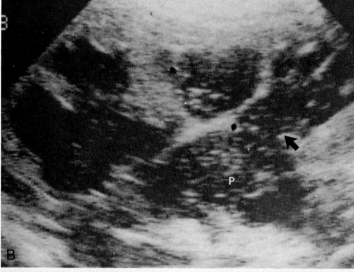

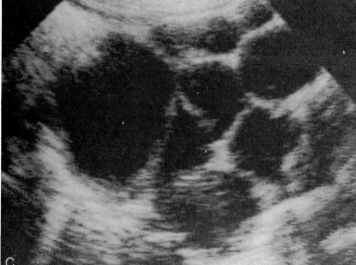

Figure 35–15. Female neonate with fetal alcohol syndrome.

A, Intravenous urogram reveals a right ureteropelvic junction obstruction and nonfunctioning left kidney.

B, Sonogram of right kidney demonstrates regular arrangement of peripheral calyces with infundibular connections *(arrow)* to a medial pelvis (P). Echogenic areas represent pelvicalyceal *Candida.*

C, In comparison, note the left contralateral multicystic kidney with large cysts arranged in a haphazard manner without any evidence of connections to or the presence of a large central or medial cyst. (Gross specimen appears in Figure 35–13.)

because a totally nonfunctioning hydronephrotic kidney is rarely salvageable and probably will cause no problems other than a predisposition to infection or hyperkalemia.

Of greater concern is the potential for malignant degeneration in a multicystic kidney. Seven patients have been described who developed cancers in previously unrecognized cystic dysplastic kidneys. Wilms' tumor was diagnosed in one patient at age 10 months (Raffensberger and Abouselman, 1968) and in another at age 4 years (Hartman et al., 1986). Renal cell carcinoma has been reported in four patients aged 15 to 68 years (Barrett and Wineland, 1980; Birken et al., 1985; Burgler and Hauri, 1983; Shirai et al., 1986), and another patient aged 68 years had an embryonal tumor (Gutter and Hermanek, 1957).

It is not clear, however, that all of these patients truly had multicystic kidneys. Although these tumors probably developed in the absence of normal renal tissue, the histologic pattern apparent in the various illustrations in some of these articles does not appear to represent the typical dysplasia seen in benign multicystic disease of

childhood. Also, the fact that these kidneys remained in situ suggests that none of the patients had a detectable mass early in life. Nevertheless, in a few reports, the ipsilateral ureter was either atretic or absent, suggesting that these were, indeed, examples of cystic dysplasia.

Did these patients have a more solid, less cystic form of renal dysplasia (Potter type IIB), or did a truly multicystic kidney involute? Is the Potter type IIA condition (classic multicystic kidney) less susceptible to malignant change? Defining the risk of malignancy in a multicystic kidney will require a prospective study, such as the one now in progress under the aegis of the AAP. Until such data are available, one must also consider whether a multicystic kidney that undergoes involution either prenatally or postnatally should be removed because of the possible risk of malignant degeneration. In the meantime, lifelong follow-up of multicystic kidneys left in situ will be essential.

Two reports in the literature might be interpreted as reinforcing the arguments in favor of prophylactic surgical removal. Dimmick and co-workers (1989) and Noe and co-workers (1989) described a total of 120 patients, of whom five had nephrogenic rests of nodular renal blastema. In addition, one of the patients in the series of Dimmick and co-workers (1989) had Wilms' tumorlets in the hilar region. Although these findings suggest a hazard in leaving a multicystic kidney in situ, one must realize that it is unusual for nodular renal blastema or even Wilms' tumorlets to develop into frank Wilms' tumor. For example, nodular renal blastema has been reported in approximately 0.25 to 0.5 per cent of normal kidneys (Beckwith, 1986; Bennington and Beckwith, 1975; Bove and McAdams, 1976), yet the incidence of Wilms' tumor in the general population is much lower. Thus, although nodular renal blastema and Wilms' tumorlets may be part of a nephroblastomatosis–Wilms' tumor spectrum, the majority of these lesions involute in time without ever becoming malignant.

Trying to predict what percentage of multicystic kidneys will develop Wilms' tumors, Noe and associates (1989) used Beckwith's estimated 1 per cent incidence of Wilms' tumor development in nodular renal blastema. They then calculated, using a 5 per cent incidence of nodular renal blastema in multicystic kidneys, that one would have to perform 2000 nephrectomies for multicystic kidney disease to prevent one Wilms' tumor. Accordingly, one must weigh the risk of surgery against that of Wilms' tumor. If one elects to monitor without surgery, the cost-benefit or even the effectiveness of long-term follow-up must be considered. Because nodular renal blastema occurs most often in the hilum (Dimmick et al., 1989), and because most kidneys that shrink lose only cyst fluid, leaving the dysplastic tissue, follow-up by sonography is unlikely to be helpful (Colodny, 1989).

In an effort to determine whether there is a relationship between multicystic dysplasia and neoplasia, Jung and co-workers (1990) performed flow cytometric analyses on specimens from 30 patients. No evidence of tetraploidy or aneuploidy, as would be expected in a preneoplastic condition, was found. This report is comforting to the surgeon who does not routinely remove multicystic kidneys. Still, one must be aware that some malignant cells retain a diploid karyotype.

Another management question in multicystic kidney is the frequency of hypertension. Gordon and associates (1988) have reviewed this topic in a thoughtful article. They noted that since 1966, only nine well-documented cases of hypertension in association with multicystic kidneys in situ have been published. In three of these cases, the hypertension resolved after nephrectomy (Burgler and Hauri, 1983; Chen et al., 1985; Javadpour et al., 1970). However, in a series of 20 patients older than 11 years who had multicystic disease, two had hypertension, and in neither of these patients was the blood pressure controlled by nephrectomy (Ambrose, 1976).

In summary, the available literature offers no proof that the incidence of either tumor or hypertension is higher in patients with retained multicystic kidneys than in normal persons. From Ambrose's experience, it appears that flank pain is the chief risk if such a kidney is left in situ. This pain can be relieved by nephrectomy. It is not clear whether these kidneys should be removed routinely.

Multilocular Cyst (Multilocular Cystic Nephroma)

A multilocular mass lesion in a child's kidney could be a benign multilocular cyst, a multilocular cyst with a partially differentiated nephroblastoma, a multilocular cyst with nodules of Wilms' tumor, or a cystic Wilms' tumor alone. These four lesions form a spectrum, with the multilocular cyst at one extreme and the cystic Wilms' tumor at the other (Beckwith, personal communication, 1986; Wood et al., 1982).

A multilocular cyst is not a renal segment affected by multicystic kidney disease, because these conditions differ clinically, histologically, and radiographically (Table 35–7). However, controversy continues concerning whether the multilocular cyst is a segmental form of renal dysplasia (Johnson et al., 1973; Osathanondh and Potter, 1964; Powell et al., 1951), a hamartomatous malformation (Arey, 1959), or a neoplastic disease (Boggs and Kimmelstiel, 1956; Christ, 1968; Fowler,

Table 35–7. COMPARISON OF MULTICYSTIC KIDNEY WITH MULTILOCULAR CYST

Feature	Multicystic Kidney	Multilocular Cyst
Age at presentation	Generally, in infancy	0–4 y (male)
		>4 (adult, female)
Mode of presentation	In utero sonography, abdominal or flank mass	Abdominal or flank mass, abdominal pain, hematuria
Other urologic anomalies	High incidence of contralateral abnormalities, especially UPJ obstruction; anomalies of lower urinary tract	Normal contralateral kidney
Intravenous urogram	Generally, nonappearance; little or no function on DMSA scan	Usually, distorted or displaced calyces
Ureter	Atretic or absent	Normal
Pathology		
Gross	Variable size and number of cysts, no recognizable normal renal tissue	Variable size; thick capsule, mass lesion usually polar; variable amount of normal parenchyma outside capsule
Microscopic	Dysplasia	Dysplastic tissue seen rarely in septa
Association with malignancy	Rare	Part of spectrum of neoplasia, little evidence of aggressiveness when malignant tissue present

Abbreviations: UPJ, ureteropelvic junction; DMSA, dimercaptosuccinic acid.

1971; Gallo and Penchansky, 1977). The confusion arises in part from the variability of the histologic picture; the appearance of the primitive stroma and the extent of stromal and epithelial atypia differ, not only from patient to patient, but within the same lesion. Beckwith and Kiviat (1981) reviewed these theories and proposed that there are three perspectives on the origin of these lesions. Two perspectives suggest that all the lesions are cystic neoplasms related to Wilms' tumor, or that they are either congenital or acquired non-neoplastic abnormalities of the parenchyma. The third perspective posits a heterogeneous spectrum of dysplastic, acquired, and neoplastic conditions.

Past use of many nonspecific terms, such as "lymphangioma," "partial" or "focal polycystic kidney," "multicystic kidney," and "cystic adenoma," makes it difficult to identify relevant published cases for review (Aterman et al., 1973). Edmunds used the term "cystic adenoma" in 1892 in what was probably the first published description of this lesion, and it has since become synonymous with "multicystic kidney." Terms frequently used today are "cystic nephroma" and "multilocular cystic nephroma," which I favor, because it encompasses the concepts of both multilocular cyst and neoplasm.

CLINICAL FEATURES

A gender difference has been observed in the usual age at presentation. The patient most likely is male if younger than 4 years but female if older than 4 years. For example, among the 58 patients described by Madewell and associates (1983), 75 per cent of the children younger than age 4 years at the time of diagnosis were male, and 89 per cent of those older than age 4 were female. In females, presentation is most common between 4 and 20 years and during the 40s and 50s (Madewell et al., 1983).

The signs and symptoms differ according to age at presentation. In children, an asymptomatic flank mass is the most common finding, whereas in adults, abdominal pain and hematuria are most likely. The bleeding is secondary to herniation of the renal mass through the transitional epithelium into the renal pelvis (Aterman et al., 1973; Madewell et al., 1983; Uson and Melicow, 1963). One patient had hypertension that resolved after nephrectomy.

Two cases of bilateral multilocular cysts of the kidney have been described (Chatten and Bishop, 1977; Geller et al., 1979), in one of which the lesion recurred after excision (Geller et al., 1979). Also, at least two instances are known in which multilocular cysts arose in kidneys known to have been normal previously (Chatten and Bishop, 1977; Uson and Melicow, 1963). Such cases support a neoplastic theory of the origin of this lesion.

HISTOPATHOLOGY

These lesions are bulky and are circumscribed by a thick capsule. Normal renal parenchyma adjacent to the lesion frequently is compressed by it. The lesion may extend beyond the renal capsule into the perinephric space or renal pelvis. The loculi, which range in diameter from a few millimeters to centimeters in diameter, do not intercommunicate. They contain clear straw-colored or yellow fluid and are lined by cuboidal or low columnar epithelial cells. In some cases, eosinophilic cuboidal cells project into the cyst lumen, creating a hobnail appearance (Madewell et al., 1983). The definition of multilocular cystic kidney given by Powell and co-workers (1951) and Boggs and Kimmelsteil (1956) requires a normal epithelial lining for the diagnosis. The septa do not contain nephrons or portions of nephrons (Boggs and Kimmelsteil, 1956; Powell et al., 1951), but spindle cells may be seen, along with collagen.

In 6 of the 58 patients in one series, one or more microscopic foci of Wilms' tumor were identified, with blastemal, epithelial, or mesenchymal elements, alone or in combination (Madewell et al., 1983). All of these patients were boys aged 3 to 15 months. Immature elements, such as embryonic mesenchyme and primitive tubules, may be seen. Such elements also may appear in multicystic kidney, but the two are different entities (see Table 35–7).

As noted earlier, some authorities consider multilocular cysts to be one end of a spectrum. When elements of immature blastema, stroma, or epithelial cells are found within the septa without evidence of nodules or a solid lesion, Joshi (1980) denotes the lesion a cystic, partially differentiated nephroblastoma (Fig. 35–16). When nodules of Wilms' tumor are present, Joshi (1980) designates the lesion a multilocular cyst with nodules of Wilms' tumor. The term "cystic Wilms' tumor" is reserved for the rare cases of tumor with cysts lined by epithelial cells. This entity should not be confused with Wilms' tumors having sonolucent or radiolucent cystlike spaces attributable to tumor necrosis.

Although there may be a continuum from multilocular cyst to cystic Wilms' tumor, and although all of these lesions may be derived from similar cells or tissues, no evidence suggests that one entity transforms into another. Interestingly, none of the genetically determined conditions associated with Wilms' tumor (e.g., hemihypertrophy, aniridia) has accompanied multilocular cysts (Banner et al., 1981).

EVALUATION

A number of tests may be useful including the following: intravenous urography, sonography, CT, cyst puncture with aspiration and double-contrast cystography, and arteriography. Ultrasound and CT can distinguish multicystic kidney and multilocular cyst, but neither study is sufficiently reliable to distinguish multilocular cyst, multilocular cyst with foci of Wilms' tumor or adenocarcinoma, mesoblastic nephroma, cystic Wilms' tumor, and clear cell sarcoma. Typically, the septa are highly echogenic with sonolucent loculi, although if there is debris in a loculus, it may appear more solid. On CT, the septa are less dense than normal parenchyma; when myxomatous material is present, the density is equal to that of solid structures (Wood et al., 1982). Calcification is rarely visible in such lesions in children (Madewell et al., 1983).

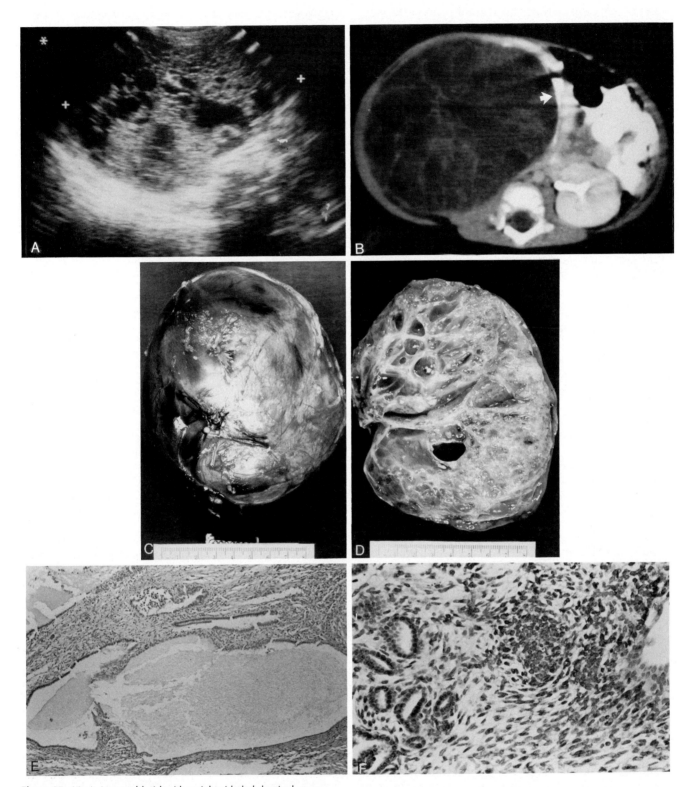

Figure 35–16. A 4-year-old girl with a right-sided abdominal mass.

A, Renal sonogram with multiple cysts throughout the left kidney.

B, On contrast-enhanced CT scan, a large, smoothly outlined left renal mass is seen with fine septae throughout the mass. Residual preserved parenchyma and pelvicalyceal system are compressed medially and pushed to the contralateral side (arrow).

C, Uncut gross specimen reveals a smooth-walled, encapsulated renal mass.

D, Cross section of mass reveals multiple noncommunicating loculations.

E, On histology, a hypocellular cystic area is seen with monotonous stroma (× 100).

F, Between loculi, nests of blastematous cells are visualized along with tubular elements (left), making the diagnosis of multilocular cyst with partially differentiated Wilms' tumor (× 200). (Courtesy of C. K. Chen, M.D.)

In the few cases in which angiography was performed, vascular, hypovascular, and hypervascular patterns have been seen (Davides, 1976; DeWall et al., 1986; Madewell et al., 1983). A tumor blush and neovascularity that sometimes was extensive have been apparent in some cases (Madewell et al., 1983).

Clear to yellow fluid is recovered by cyst puncture. Contrast will opacify only those loculi through which the needle has passed, because the loculi do not communicate (Madewell et al., 1983).

TREATMENT

Two questions must be answered in selecting the treatment for a multilocular cystic kidney: (1) Is the contralateral urinary tract normal? and (2) Is the abnormal kidney involved with Wilms' tumor? At least four of the cystic tumors in the National Wilms' Tumor Study (NWTS) metastasized (Beckwith and Palmer, 1978); thus, these lesions clearly have malignant potential, although they appear to be less aggressive than classic Wilms' tumor.

The treatment for a multilocular cyst is nephrectomy. If pathologic review shows cystic Wilms' tumor, further treatment should be given according to the NWTS recommendations for the appropriate stage of disease. However, if the focus of tumor does not exceed 2 cm, nephrectomy alone may be sufficient. If enucleation or partial nephrectomy is chosen, recurrence is possible. However, with more Wilms' tumors being treated by local excision, the case for enucleation or partial nephrectomy combined with close follow-up by sonography and CT is stronger, even if malignancy is found within the lesion. In comparison, if a clear cell sarcoma is found after enucleation, the remaining ipsilateral renal tissue should be removed because of the aggressiveness of this cancer. The recurrence of a multilocular cyst not containing malignancy probably reflects inadequate excision of the initial lesion.

Simple Cyst

The frequency of simple cysts increases with age. For example, Kissane and Smith (1975) found that more than half of adults older than age 50 had simple renal cysts at autopsy, and Laucks and McLachlan (1981), who used CT, demonstrated a 20 per cent incidence of cysts by the age of 40 years and approximately a 33 per cent incidence of cysts after age 60.

CLINICAL FEATURES

Simple cysts may present any time from soon after birth to old age. The mean age of presentation in children is approximately 4 years. Most reports show no gender predilection; however, in at least two studies, men were affected more frequently (Bearth and Steg, 1977; Tada et al., 1983). Cysts usually are solitary but can be multiple or bilateral.

In both children and adults, cysts rarely call attention to themselves. Instead, they are discovered incidentally on sonography, CT, or urography performed for a urinary tract or other pelvic or abdominal problem.

However, cysts can produce an abdominal mass or pain, hematuria secondary to rupture into the pyelocalyceal system, and hypertension secondary to segmental ischemia (Lüscher et al., 1986; Papanicolaou et al., 1986; Rockson et al., 1974). Cysts can cause calyceal or renal pelvic obstruction as well (Barloon and Vince, 1987; Evans and Coughlin, 1970; Hinman, 1978; Wahlqvist and Grumstedt, 1966).

Over an 18-year period, Papanicolaou and co-workers (1986) treated 25 patients who had suffered spontaneous or traumatic rupture of a known cyst, a large number of cases considering the rarity of cyst rupture. Most of these ruptures (21) were spontaneous; three followed blunt trauma, and one was iatrogenic. The cyst ruptured into a calyx in 12 patients. In one patient, the rupture was into the renal pelvis, through the parenchyma but not the capsule. In another, the cyst ruptured through the parenchyma and capsule. In five patients, the rupture was both calyceal and perinephric, and in the remaining four patients, the site of rupture could not be determined. In 21 patients, hematuria was present, and in 17 patients, flank pain was present. The diagnosis was made by high-dose drip infusion nephrotomography in 22 patients, by CT in two, and by retrograde pyelography in one. In 11 patients, the cyst communication closed spontaneously, and in eight, the cyst cavity was obliterated on follow-up studies. Two patients had persistent calyceal communication with 2 months or less of follow-up.

Cysts can rupture into the pelvicalyceal system, maintain a communication, and become a pseudocalyceal diverticulum. The reverse is also possible; closure of the communication of a diverticulum can create a simple cyst (Mosli et al., 1986; Papanicolaou et al., 1986). These two sequences of events can be distinguished only by histologic examination. Theoretically, diverticula should have linings of transitional epithelium, whereas simple cysts should be lined by a single layer of flattened or cuboidal epithelium.

Hypertension caused by cysts has been confirmed in several reports. For example, in two children with simple cysts and hypertension, the blood pressure normalized after surgical decompression of the cysts (Babka et al., 1974; Hoard and O'Brien, 1976). Also, Lüscher and co-workers (1986) identified 22 published cases of renal cysts and hypertension. Surgical removal or aspiration of the cyst was therapeutic in ten patients and yielded improvement in two others with a mean follow-up of 1 year. Ten of the 15 patients who were studied by renal vein renin assays had elevated activity, suggesting local tissue or arterial compression by the cyst. This hypothesis is easily believable if one realizes that a simple cyst can have a pressure as high as 57 cm H_2O and that the lesions in this series of cases generally were large, most exceeding 6 cm in diameter and containing several hundred milliliters of fluid (Amis et al., 1982; Lüscher et al., 1986).

HISTOPATHOLOGY

Simple cysts differ considerably in size, from less than 1 cm to greater than 10 cm. The majority are less than 2 cm in diameter, however (Tada et al., 1983). The wall is fibrous and of varying thickness and has no renal elements. The cyst lining is a single layer of flattened or cuboidal epithelium.

Because cysts are increasingly common with age, they have been considered an acquired lesion. Bearth and Steg (1977) found greater ectasia and cystic dilatation of the distal tubules and collecting ducts in patients over the age of 60 years and considered these changes to be precursors of macroscopic cysts.

EVALUATION

One can safely make the diagnosis of a classic benign simple cyst by sonography when the following criteria are met: (1) absence of internal echoes; (2) sharply defined, thin, distinct wall with a smooth and distinct margin; (3) good transmission of sound waves through the cyst with consequent acoustic enhancement behind the cyst; and (4) spherical or slightly ovoid shape (Goldman and Hartman, 1990). If all of these criteria are satisfied, the chances of malignancy being present are negligible (Fig. 35–17) (Lingard and Lawson, 1979; Livingston et al., 1981).

When some of these criteria are not met—for example, when there are septations, irregular margins, calcifications, or suspect areas—further evaluation by CT or perhaps needle aspiration or magnetic resonance imaging (MRI) is indicated (Bosniak, 1986). A cluster of cysts is another indication for further study, because they may be hiding a small carcinoma. CT is better than sonography in defining such a camouflaged lesion (Bosniak, 1986). Peripelvic cysts often require CT confirmation because they frequently are interspersed between structures of the collecting system and hilum, which can create artificial echoes (Bosniak, 1986).

The CT criteria for a simple cyst are similar to those of sonography: (1) sharp, thin, distinct, smooth walls and margins; (2) spherical or ovoid shape; and (3) homogeneous content. The density ranges from −10 to +20 Hounsfield units, similar to the density of water, and no enhancement should occur after the intravenous injection of contrast medium. Bosniak (1986) states that he has not seen a tumor with a density of less than 20 HU on a contrast-enhanced scan, but a truly benign cyst can have fluid with a density of greater than 20 HU. In these cases, intravenous contrast injection is particularly helpful.

Because cysts have no blood vessels and do not communicate directly with nephrons, they should not enhance; enhancement thus implies vascular tissue or contrast medium mixing with fluid. However, for several days after the injection of contrast medium, the fluid in a benign cyst may enhance (Hartman, 1990). Despite the diagnostic utility of contrast enhancement, the first scan should always be performed without enhancement, because contrast medium may obscure calcification, small amounts of fat, or recent hemorrhage (Bosniak, 1986). When the aforementioned criteria are respected, the accuracy of diagnosis of a simple cyst by CT approaches 100 per cent (Figs. 35–18, 35–19) (McClennan et al., 1979).

When sonographic or CT criteria are not met, such as when there is a thick wall, calcification, septation, nonhomogeneous or hyperdense fluid, or fluid with internal echoes, conditions other than simple cyst must be considered. Other possibilities are complicated cysts (i.e., those containing blood, pus, or calcification) and cystic neoplasms. One of the more common sources of confusion is the parenchymal beak classically seen on intravenous urography when the tissue partially engulfs the cyst margin. When seen in cross section on sonography or CT, this beak can create the appearance of a thick wall (Segal and Spitzer, 1979).

Cyst puncture and aspiration with or without contrast medium injection was popular in the 1960s and 1970s. Fluid from cystic renal cell carcinoma may be hemorrhagic or may contain elevated levels of protein, lactic dehydrogenase, or fat (Marotti et al., 1987). Today, with the improvements in sonography and CT, cyst puncture is less likely to be needed. The remaining

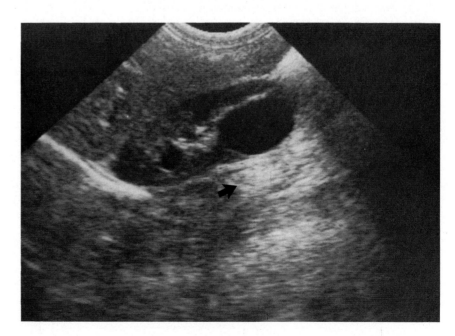

Figure 35–17. Two renal cysts in an 8-year-old boy. Note evidence of enhancement of sound wave transmission through the larger oval cyst by the hyperechogenicity (whiteness) of the image behind the cyst. Family history or even sonographic evaluation of family should be considered to rule out autosomal dominant polycystic kidney disease, especially when more than one cyst is present. In children, it is not unusual for autosomal dominant polycystic kidney disease to first present with one or two cysts.

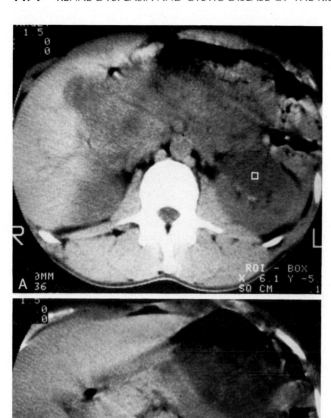

Figure 35–18. *A,* Hyperdense renal cysts on precontrast CT scan measuring +33 HU. *B,* Following contrast CT scan values were +30 HU. Absence of enhancement, spherical shape, and fine outline are findings compatible with the diagnosis of a simple cyst in spite of CT values greater than +20 HU.

indications are as follows: (1) suspected infection, in which case puncture may be therapeutic as well as diagnostic; (2) the presence of low-level echoes on sonography but a classic cyst on CT; and (3) a borderline lesion in a poor surgical candidate.

Bosniak (1986) believes that hyperdense cysts larger than 3 cm in diameter require further evaluation or close follow-up, because there are few data on the nature of hyperdense lesions of this size. In such cases, one might consider one of the following options, depending on the patient's age and general health: (1) cyst puncture with aspiration for cytologic study, (2) puncture and injection of contrast medium, or (3) follow-up by sonography or CT at progressively longer intervals.

When evaluating a possibly infected cyst, one must be aware that the wall may be thickened and sometimes calcified. Debris is often present (Hartman, 1990). Calcification may also be present in the absence of infection or malignancy; 1 to 3 per cent of renal cysts are calcified (Bree et al., 1984; Daniel et al., 1972). Such calcification is dystrophic and usually occurs secondary to hemorrhage, infection, or ischemia (Hartman, 1990). Also, 6

per cent of simple cysts can hemorrhage (Jackman and Stevens, 1974; Pollack et al., 1979). In 1971, 31 per cent of hemorrhagic cysts were reported to be malignant (Gross and Breach, 1971), but it was deemed necessary at that time to explore the majority of such cysts. Today, even if blood is present, the decision to operate usually can be made on the basis of sonographic or CT findings.

MRI offers little information beyond that available from sonography and CT, although it is more specific in identifying the nature of the cyst fluid. Marotti and co-workers (1987) found that if the fluid has low signal intensity (similar to that of urine) on T1-weighted images, the cyst is benign even if the wall is thick or septa are present. If this report is substantiated by additional studies, MRI may prove valuable in deciding which indeterminate cysts are benign and which should be considered for exploration. The T2-weighted images identify bloody fluid with an extremely bright image (Fig. 35–20).

Technical points need to be made about the evaluation of simple cysts by each of these imaging methods. First, when poor acoustic enhancement or low-level internal

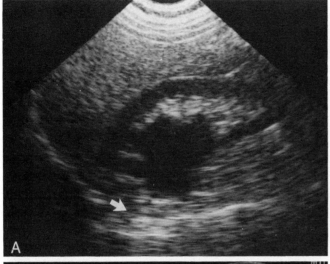

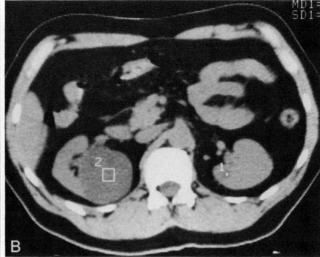

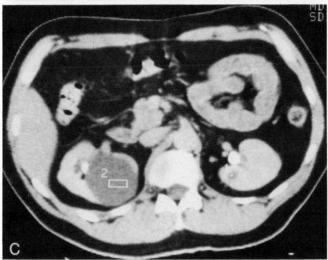

Figure 35–19. Fifty-six-year-old man with an indeterminate left renal cyst on renal sonography. *A,* Note the nonspherical, non–smoothly outlined sonolucent mass in left kidney. However, good sound wave transmission through the cysts (acoustic enhancement) is illustrated by the intensity (whiteness) of the sonogram image behind the cyst *(arrow). B,* On precontrast CT scan, a very small cyst (1) is seen in the left kidney. The right renal cyst (2) that was identified on sonography measures 17 HU. *C,* Following contrast, the CT values (2) were 16 HU, signifying no enhancement. CT values of between −10 and +20 HU are characteristic of cysts. No enhancement following contrast confirms the diagnosis of a simple renal cyst. The small cyst (1) is not large enough for determining accurate CT values. (Courtesy of G. Laungani, M.D.)

echoes are identified by real-time sonography, the findings may be an artifact of the method. Weinreb and co-workers (1986) suggest that, in these cases, a static ultrasound scan should be obtained to see if the findings are reproducible before performing CT. If no internal echoes are seen or if acoustic enhancement is clearly demonstrable, the contrary findings on the real-time scan can be considered artifactual, and CT can be avoided. Second, problems may occur in judging the density of cyst fluid by CT if the scanner is not regularly calibrated against gallbladder fluid or urine without contrast medium in the renal pelvis or bladder. These fluids should have densities near that of water (−10 to +20 HU). Third, with MRI, one must remember that ventilatory and bowel motions can degrade the signal intensity of cyst fluid, as well as lesion definition (Marotti et al., 1987).

To summarize, in most cases of simple cysts, the diagnosis is readily made. When the cyst is indeterminate, the most important diagnostic question is whether the cyst is a manifestation of malignancy. When the cysts are diffuse, multiple, or bilateral, one must consider the possibility of DPK. The sonographic and CT appearance of these two types of lesions can be identical.

Diagnosis then depends on identifying other family members with DPK or finding reduced renal function or other signs of DPK, such as hepatic cysts. One must keep in mind that, in its early stages, DPK is not always represented by multiple bilateral cysts; it may initially appear sonographically as a single renal cyst, multiple unilateral cysts, or cysts localized to one portion of the kidney.

TREATMENT AND PROGNOSIS

It is not clear what propensity simple cysts have to enlarge. Laucks and McLachlan (1981) found that cyst diameter increases with age. Contrary data were reported by Richter and associates (1983), who found an increase in cyst size in only 2 of 31 patients followed for as long as 10 years. Also, Dalton and co-workers (1986) followed 59 patients by sonography and found no significant changes in cyst size, although they did see an increase in the number of cysts in 20 per cent.

Before 1970, most cases of simple cysts in children were treated surgically. However, a number of large series published in the 1970s indicated that cysts could be managed much like those in adults, because they are

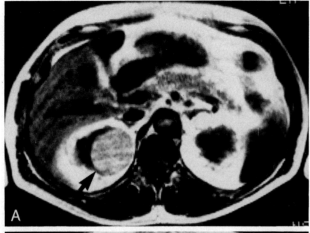

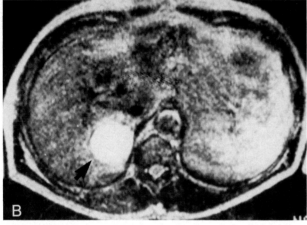

Figure 35–20. MRI scan of a hemorrhagic cyst. *A,* Blood is seen on T1 weighted images *(arrow). B,* Blood appears extremely white *(arrow)* on T2 weighted image because of the presence of methemoglobin.

the same type of lesion. Once malignancy has been ruled out, unroofing or removal of an asymptomatic cyst is not indicated (Bartholomew et al., 1980; Gordon et al., 1979; Ravden et al., 1980; Siegel and McAlister, 1980).

When a benign simple cyst causes pyelocalyceal obstruction or hypertension, one may choose to correct the problem either surgically, by unroofing the cyst, or percutaneously, by aspirating the fluid and perhaps injecting a sclerosing agent, particularly if fluid has reaccumulated after an earlier aspiration. Several sclerosing agents have been used, such as glucose, phenol, iophendylate (Pantopaque), and absolute ethanol, but none has been sufficiently impressive to become dominant (Holmberg and Hietala, 1989).

Holmberg and Hietala (1989) managed 156 patients who had simple cysts in one of three ways. In one group, no treatment was given; in 25 per cent of these patients, the cysts grew during a mean follow-up period of 3 years. In a second group, cyst aspiration was performed. In this group, the cysts disappeared in 10 per cent, and the mean size of the cysts in the remainder declined to 90 per cent of the original volume after 24 months. In the third group, cyst aspiration was followed by sclerotherapy with bismuth phosphate. In this group, the cysts disappeared in 44 per cent, and the mean size of the

cysts in the remainder was only 21 per cent of the original size after 3 to 4 years.

On the basis of this study and another study by Westberg and Zachrisson (1975), in which all bismuth-treated cysts shrank, it appears that, when treatment is needed for a simple cyst because of pain or compression effects, sclerosing the cyst lining with instilled bismuth phosphate is a method worthy of consideration. Newer approaches to recalcitrant cysts are percutaneous resection and intrarenal marsupialization (Hubner et al., 1990; Hulbert and Hunter, 1990; Meyer and Jonas, 1990).

Bosniak (1986) divides cysts and cystic lesions into four categories that have management implications. In this schema, type I cysts are single and benign and fulfill the sonographic or CT criteria for simple cysts.

Type II cysts are benign cystic lesions that are minimally complicated, such as by septations, small calcifications, infection, or high density, and will not require surgery. For example, when all the criteria for a simple cyst are fulfilled except that a fine line of calcium is seen in the wall, the lesion should be considered a benign cyst, and exploration is not required. Another example is the cyst with fine traversing strands, perhaps containing calcium. In this case, exploration is not required unless the septa are numerous, irregular, or thick.

Type III cysts are the more complicated lesions with radiologic features that also are seen in malignancy. One example is the lesion with more extensive calcification, especially if the wall is not pencil-point thin or is irregular. Other Type III cysts are those with septations, suggesting a multilocular cystic lesion and chronic infection with a thickened wall. These lesions are more problematic and require a surgical approach that is individualized. In some cases, one might consider violating Gerota's fascia to expose the kidney for examination of the lesion or partial nephrectomy.

Bosniak Type IV lesions are cystic malignant tumors and are dealt with as such, namely, by radical nephrectomy.

Medullary Sponge Kidney

The condition known as medullary sponge kidney was recognized by Beitzke in 1908, and its radiographic features were described by Lenarduzzi in 1939. The name of this disorder dates from a 1949 publication by Cacchi and Ricci.

The characteristic feature of medullary sponge kidney is dilatation of the collecting tubules with numerous associated cysts and clefts (Fig. 35–21). The condition resembles the medullary cystic disease–juvenile nephronophthisis complex only in that, in both, cysts are found in the medulla. Unlike medullary cystic disease, medullary sponge kidney does not appear to be an inherited condition and has occurred in more than one member of a family in less than 5 per cent of the published reports (Copping, 1967; Emmett and Witten, 1971; Kuiper, 1976a; Morris et al., 1965). Medullary sponge kidney has been associated with congenital hemihypertrophy (Alfonso and Oliviera, 1988; Sprayragen et al., 1973), Ehlers-Danlos syndrome (Levine and Mi-

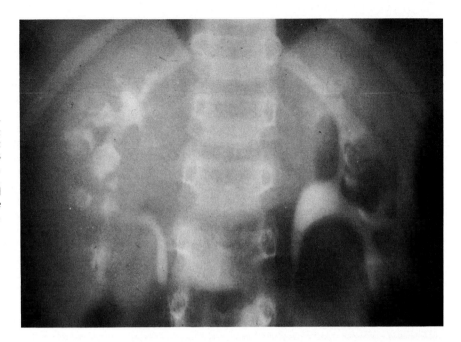

Figure 35–21. Intravenous urogram in a 9-year-old girl with hematuria. Characteristic puddling of contrast medium in the ectatic papillary collecting ducts makes the diagnosis of medullary sponge kidney. (From Glassberg, K. I., et al.: Congenital anomalies of kidney, ureter, and bladder. *In* Kendall, A. R., and Karafin, L. (Eds.): Harry S. Goldsmith's Practice of Surgery: Urology. New York, Harper & Row, 1981, pp. 1–82.)

chael, 1967; Morris et al., 1965), anodontia (Khoury et al., 1988), DPK (Abreo and Steele, 1982), and Caroli's disease (Mall et al., 1974).

A significant number of patients with medullary sponge kidney are asymptomatic, and their condition is never diagnosed. As a result, the true incidence of the condition is unknown. In patients undergoing intravenous urography for various indications, 1 in 200 is found to have medullary sponge kidney (Myall, 1970; Palubinskas, 1961). Bernstein and Gardner (1986), on the basis of a literature review, estimate the incidence in the general population to be between 1 in 5000 and 1 in 20,000.

CLINICAL FEATURES

Any clinical presentation usually is seen after age 20, although Hamberger and colleagues (1968) found, in more than 100 cases, that the first symptoms appear at ages ranging from 3 weeks to 71 years. The most common presentation is renal colic (50 to 60 per cent) followed by urinary tract infection (20 to 33 per cent) and gross hematuria (10 to 18 per cent) (Kuiper, 1976b). In many cases, the diagnosis is made when a patient is evaluated by intravenous urography for some unrelated problem, such as a renal mass, benign prostatic hyperplasia, or hypertension. Rarely is such hypertension attributable to the medullary sponge kidney unless there is pyelonephritis.

Another possible sign is the formation of urinary stones. Yendt (1990) found the incidence of medullary sponge kidney in patients who formed stones before age 20 to be twice as high as that in all other age groups combined. The incidence of medullary sponge kidney in stone-formers differs widely in the reported series, ranging from 2.6 per cent to 21 per cent. The incidence appears to be higher in female than in male stone-formers (Lavan et al., 1971; Palubinskas, 1961; Parks et al., 1982; Sage et al., 1982; Vagelli et al., 1988; Wiks-

trom et al., 1983; Yendt, 1990). Urinary tract infections likewise seem to be more common in female patients (Parks et al., 1982).

One third to one half of the patients with medullary sponge kidney have hypercalcemia (Ekstrom et al., 1959; Harrison and Rose, 1979; Parks et al., 1982; Yendt, 1990). The etiology does not appear to be the same in all cases. Maschio and co-workers (1982) found a renal calcium leak in eight patients and increased calcium absorption in two. Yendt (1990) found elevated parathyroid hormone levels in 2 of 11 patients with medullary sponge kidney.

In the absence of infections, the stones passed by patients with medullary sponge kidney are composed of calcium oxalate either alone or in combination with calcium phosphate.

HISTOPATHOLOGY

The principal finding is dilated intrapapillary collecting ducts and small medullary cysts, which range in diameter from 1 to 8 mm and give the cross-sectioned kidney the appearance of a sponge. The cysts are lined by collecting duct epithelium (Bernstein, 1990) and usually communicate with the collecting tubules. The cysts and the dilated collecting ducts may have concretions adherent to their walls. Ekstrom and co-workers (1959) found these concretions to be composed of pure apatite (calcium phosphate) in seven of ten patients and of apatite and calcium oxalate in the remaining three. The cysts contain a yellow-brown fluid and desquamated cells or calcified material.

DIAGNOSIS

In general, intravenous urography is more sensitive than CT in detecting mild cases of medullary sponge kidney. In 75 per cent of patients, the disease is bilateral (Kuiper, 1976); but, in some, only one pyramid may be affected. The urographic features of the disorder are as follows: (1) enlarged kidneys, sometimes with calcification, particularly in the papillae; (2) elongated papillary tubules or cavities that fill with contrast medium; and (3) papillary contrast blush and persistent medullary opacification (Gedroyc and Saxton, 1988). In some cases, the papillae resemble bunches of grapes or bouquets of flowers, whereas in others, discrete linear stripes appear that can be counted readily.

On occasion, the intravenous urogram of an older child or young adult with one of the milder forms of RPK mimics the appearance of medullary sponge kidney (Yendt, 1990). In these instances, one should evaluate the liver before making a diagnosis.

When nephrocalcinosis is found, one must rule out other hypercalciuric states, such as hyperparathyroidism, sarcoidosis, vitamin D intoxication, multiple myeloma, tuberculosis, and milk alkali syndrome. In these conditions, the calcium deposits are in collecting ducts of normal caliber, whereas in medullary sponge kidney, the calcifications occur in dilated ducts (Levine and Grantham, 1990).

Given that the cysts are small, sonography is not expected to be helpful. However, because children have less renal sinus fat and overlying muscle than adults, sonographic resolution is better, and hyperechoic papillae are seen on occasion (Patriquin and O'Regan, 1985). The hyperechogenicity is secondary to the multiple interfaces created by the dilated ducts and small cysts and to any intraductal calcification.

Gedroyc and Saxton (1988) described two groups of patients in whom additional renal anomalies were detected by ultrasound examination. One group had multiple cortical cysts; the other group had cavities deep in the medulla, which often communicated with the calyces.

Although, at present, urography generally is more sensitive in the detection of medullary sponge kidney than is CT, newer scanners can identify the tubular ectasia using bone-detail algorithms and window settings (Boag and Nolan, 1988). Thus, CT may be advantageous when bowel gas obscures the kidneys on urography or when renal function is poor.

TREATMENT AND PROGNOSIS

It is the complications of medullary sponge kidney that require management: calculus formation and infection. As noted earlier in this section, many of these patients have hypercalciuria. Thiazides are effective for lowering hypercalciuria and limiting stone formation. If thiazides cannot be used, inorganic phosphates may be appropriate. For those patients with renal lithiasis, thiazides should be administered even if hypercalciuria is not present (Yendt, 1990). Yendt (1990) reports that these drugs prevent calcium stones and arrest the growth of stones already present. If thiazides are ineffective or not tolerated, inorganic phosphates should be tried (Yendt, 1990). However, the latter should not be used in patients with urinary tract infections caused by urease-producing organisms because of the risk of struvite stones (Yendt, 1990).

Because infections are not unusual, especially if stones are present, cultures should be obtained frequently in patients with medullary sponge kidney, and long-term prophylaxis should be considered in some cases. Infections by coagulase-positive staphylococci are common in the setting of stones in these patients and should be treated even when the colony count in the cultures is less than 100,000/ml (Yendt, 1990).

Stones can now be removed by extracorporeal lithotripsy and percutaneous nephrolithotomy. Therefore, open surgery will rarely be necessary.

Kuiper (1976b) estimated that 10 per cent of symptomatic patients with medullary sponge kidney have a poor long-term prognosis because of nephrolithiasis, septicemia, and renal failure. However, this figure is probably lower now because of the more effective treatment available for hypercalciuria and renal lithiasis and because of the better antibiotics available and the selective use of prophylaxis.

Sporadic Glomerulocystic Kidney Disease

Glomerulocystic disease is a specific entity, but the term has often been applied as a catchall to include all conditions in which there are glomerular cysts. The term "glomerulocystic" means that cysts of the glomeruli or Bowman's space are present diffusely and bilaterally. However, cysts of the glomeruli are present in many forms of renal cystic disease, and they may or may not be the predominant pathology. Thus, the presence of glomerular cysts does not prove that the patient has glomerulocystic disease.

Table 35–8 shows the Bernstein and Landing classification of conditions with glomerular cysts as modified by Glassberg and Filmer (in press) to make it compatible with the AAP classification. The diagnosis of glomerulocystic disease should be made only when the disorder conforms to the 1941 definition of Roos and the 1976 definition of Taxy and Filmer. That is, glomerulocystic disease is a noninheritable condition producing bilaterally enlarged kidneys containing small cysts, predominantly of Bowman's space. Characteristically, no other family members are affected, and no associated anomalies are present, although in the case described by Taxy and Filmer (1976), subcapsular hepatic cysts were present.

Table 35–8. CONDITIONS ASSOCIATED WITH GLOMERULAR CYSTS

Sporadic glomerulocystic kidney disease
Familial hypoplastic glomerulocystic disease
Autosomal dominant polycystic disease
Juvenile nephronophthisis in association with hepatic fibrosis
Multiple malformation syndromes
    Zellweger syndrome
    Trisomy 13
    Meckel's syndrome
    Short-rib polydactyly (Majewski type)
    Tuberous sclerosis
    Orofaciodigital syndrome type I
    Brachymesomelia renal syndrome
    Renal-hepatic-pancreatic dysplasia

The patients evaluated by Bernstein and Landing (1989) after referral and those they found described in the literature differ in age of presentation, clinical course, and renal morphology. These investigators suggest that, in some of the published cases, features of other syndromes were overlooked or family members were inadequately screened for DPK. They have recommended the use of the term "sporadic glomerulocystic disease" to show that the condition is not genetic.

Acquired Renal Cystic Disease

In 1977, Dunhill and co-workers described acquired renal cystic disease (ARCD) in patients in renal failure. At first, ARCD was thought to be confined to patients receiving hemodialysis. However, it shortly became apparent that the disorder is almost as common in patients receiving peritoneal dialysis (Thompson et al., 1986) and that it may develop in patients with chronic renal failure who are being managed medically without any type of dialysis (Fisher and Horvath, 1972; Ishikawa et al., 1980; Kutcher et al., 1983; Miller et al., 1989). Thus, ARCD would appear to be a feature of end-stage kidneys rather than a response to dialysis. Ishikawa (1985) has suggested that the term "uremic acquired cystic disease" be applied to this entity (Fig. 35–22).

The incidence of ARCD differs among institutions, perhaps as a result of population differences or of the diagnostic criteria. For example, Feiner and co-workers (1981) require that at least 40 per cent of the kidney be affected by cysts, whereas Basile and co-workers (1988) require only 20 per cent involvement. Judging the extent of involvement is likewise subjective. Some reports include patients with only one cyst, whereas Thompson and co-workers (1986) grade ARCD according to the number of cysts involved, from grade 1 (less than 5 cysts bilaterally) to grade 4 (greater than 14 cysts bilaterally).

The importance of ARCD lies in two areas: (1) the symptoms it may produce (pain and hematuria), and (2) the high incidence of benign and malignant renal tumors accompanying the condition.

INCIDENCE

In 1984, Gardner identified 160 patients with ARCD among 430 patients receiving long-term hemodialysis, an incidence of 34 per cent (Gardner, 1984b). This incidence represents an overall figure, because the incidence of ARCD rises with time on dialysis and perhaps also with the duration of chronic renal failure and the age of the patient. For example, Ishikawa and co-workers (1980) found ARCD in 44 per cent of patients who had been receiving hemodialysis for less than 3 years but in 79 per cent of those who had been receiving hemodialysis for a longer time. In a later study, the same group found a higher incidence of ARCD with age, particularly in men (Ishikawa et al., 1985). We have identified ARCD in a 16-year-old boy. Miller and associates (1989) found ARCD in 58 per cent of autopsied dialysis patients, but, unlike other investigators, detected no correlation with the duration of dialysis.

The incidence of ARCD appears to be higher in patients with end-stage kidneys as a result of nephrosclerosis than in those in whom renal failure was the result of diabetes (Fallon and Williams, 1989; Miller et al., 1989). However, the lower incidence of ARCD in diabetic patients may well be a result of their shorter survival time on dialysis (Fallon and Williams, 1989).

Hughson and co-workers (1986) found a 2.9 to 1 male-to-female ratio for ARCD, which is striking when one considers that the number of male patients undergoing dialysis only slightly exceeds the number of female patients. Ishikawa and colleagues (1985) confirmed the higher incidence of ARCD in male patients. They suggested that a sex-related endogenous growth factor combined with a uremic metabolite was important.

The incidence of renal tumors warrants special consideration. Renal neoplasms, principally adenomas, oc-

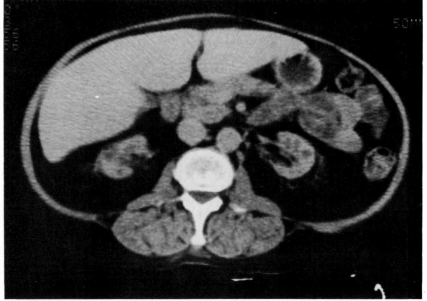

Figure 35–22. Small kidneys with multiple small cysts in a hemodialysis patient with acquired renal cystic disease.

cur in 10 per cent of patients receiving chronic hemodialysis, whereas the incidence in patients with ARCD is even higher, ranging from 20 per cent to 25 per cent (Gardner and Evan, 1984). The reported incidence of renal cell carcinoma in chronic dialysis patients ranges from 0.22 per cent to 1.5 per cent (Gardner and Evan, 1984; Gehrig et al., 1985; Ishikawa, 1988a, 1988b; MacDougall et al., 1987). In ARCD, the incidence of renal cell carcinoma is even more remarkably increased, ranging from 4 per cent to 5.8 per cent in some series (Basile et al., 1988; Gardner and Evans, 1984; Gehrig et al., 1985; Hughson et al., 1986; Ishikawa, 1985). Although the incidence of renal cell carcinoma is increased in chronic dialysis patients, particularly those with ARCD, compared with the general population, the extent of the increase has not been determined, because the incidence of renal cell carcinoma in age-matched individuals in the general population is not readily available.

Although most of these reports concern renal cell carcinoma found at autopsy or in kidneys removed for infection or hypertension, one should not minimize the risk of this cancer, because aggressive lesions do occur. Moreover, in patients with ARCD, renal cell carcinoma frequently occurs at an earlier age than in the general population, often in the 3rd or 4th decade. In these cases, the cysts are pronounced. When renal cell carcinoma appears after the age of 60 years, there usually are fewer cysts (Hughson et al., 1986).

Etiology

As noted earlier, the initial view that ARCD is a consequence of hemodialysis per se has been shown to be incorrect. However, if uremic toxins are the principal risk factor, why are there different incidences of ARCD at various institutions? It is possible that different durations of predialysis medical therapy or different dialysis regimens are important, but no data have been collected on this point.

A number of findings suggest a role for toxins. First, the cysts, adenomas, and carcinomas usually are multiple and bilateral, as are the carcinomas induced experimentally in rats by toxins. Second, there is a decline in the incidence of renal cell carcinoma and a regression of the cysts after successful transplantation (Ishikawa et al., 1983), suggesting that some cystogenic or carcinogenic toxin of uremia is being eliminated by the allograft. Third, if transplantation fails and dialysis is resumed, the cysts return.

Clinical Features

The most common presentation of ARCD is loin pain, hematuria, or both. Bleeding, whether into the kidney or into the retroperitoneum, may be secondary to renal cysts or to renal cell carcinoma. Feiner and co-workers (1981) suggested that cystic bleeding is secondary to rupture of unsupported sclerotic vessels in the wall. If the cyst communicates with the nephron, hematuria may result. In some patients, bleeding follows heparinization during dialysis. Also, in some cases, the serum hemoglobin concentration is elevated secondary to increased renal production of erythropoietin (Mickisch et al., 1984; Ratcliffe et al., 1983; Shalhoub et al., 1982).

Histopathology

The cysts develop predominantly in the cortex, although the medulla may be affected, and generally they are bilateral. They average 0.5 to 1.0 cm in diameter, but some have been reported to reach 5.0 cm (Miller et al., 1989). The cysts are filled with clear, straw-colored or hemorrhagic fluid and often contain calcium oxalate crystals (Miller et al., 1989). Some resemble simple retention cysts, with a flat epithelial lining.

The nuclei of the epithelial cells in these cases are round and regular, without prominent nucleoli (Hughson et al., 1980). However, some cysts (atypical or hyperplastic) are lined by epithelial cells with larger, irregular nuclei that contain prominent nucleoli and may show mitotic activity. This hyperplastic lining is thought by some workers to be a precursor of renal tumors. Moreover, some hyperplastic cysts have papillary projections, and to some observers, the distinction between cyst and neoplasm becomes blurred when papillary hyperplasia predominates.

Feiner and co-workers (1981) found that the cysts begin as dilatations or outpouchings of the nephrons. One theory suggests that calcium oxalate crystals precipitate along the nephron lining, disrupting it and causing outpouchings that dilate as they become obstructed by further crystallization (Hughson et al., 1986; Rushton et al., 1981). That oxalate crystals may be a factor in cyst formation is conceivable, because crystals have been implicated in the development of cysts in rats given ethylene glycol (Rushton et al., 1981).

The renal adenomas usually are multiple and often are bilateral. Miller and colleagues (1989) autopsied 155 cases with end-stage renal disease and found 25 to have small renal cortical nodules (adenomas). These nodules were multiple, and all were smaller than 2.5 cm in diameter. They usually arose from the walls of the atypical (hyperplastic) cysts.

The cells were either oriented into papillary projections or arranged as solid nodules with tubule formation. The cells were smaller than those found in renal cell carcinoma, with cytoplasm that was either granular and eosinophilic (oncocytes) or pale staining. The nuclei typically appeared small, rounded, and uniform with insignificant nucleoli. Anaplasia and mitosis were absent. In three of these cases, lesions of 3.0 to 3.5 cm were found, all of which were renal cell carcinoma. The cells in these lesions were usually of the clear cell type, with wrinkled nuclei and prominent nucleoli. They were arranged in solid or tubular patterns.

Differentiating these renal tumors into adenomas and carcinomas is arbitrary at times. In Bell's classic 1935 article, renal tumors larger than 3 cm in diameter were considered carcinomas, whereas the smaller ones were considered adenomas. However, even in Bell's work, tumors as small as 1 cm were associated with metastases in a few cases. Also, although the majority of renal cell carcinomas in patients with ARCD are larger than 2 to 3 cm, some have measured only 1.0 to 1.5 cm (Chung-Park et al., 1983; Feiner et al., 1981; Hughson et al., 1986). The smallest renal cell carcinoma associated with known metastases was 1.2 cm in diameter (Ishikawa, 1988a, 1988b). In sum, most renal nodules that are smaller than 1 cm in diameter are adenomas, and most that are more than 3 cm in diameter are carcinomas. Tumors between 1 and 3 cm in diameter must be considered a gray zone.

It is not clear whether renal adenomas undergo malignant transformation. The large incidence of renal adenomas in the general population and the even larger incidence in uremic patients, combined with the low incidence of renal cell carcinoma in both populations, suggest that the frequency of malignant transformation is low if, indeed, transformation occurs at all. However, because of the higher incidence of both renal cell carcinoma and adenomas in patients with ARCD, one cannot rule out malignant transformation.

Bretan and associates (1986) have postulated a continuum ranging from simple cysts to epithelial hyperplasia to carcinoma. In support of their hypothesis, they offered the finding of renal tumors in the hyperplastic epithelial lining of some cysts. However, no study we reviewed has demonstrated such a continuum. A curiosity is the morphologic similarity of the nuclei in the hyperplastic cells to those of renal cell carcinoma and the lack of similarity of the nuclei of the adenoma cells to those seen in either of the other lesions.

Hughson and co-workers (1986) believe that atypical hyperplastic epithelium occurs even without cyst formation and that it is these cells that are the precursors of both the atypical cysts and the adenomas. This theory accounts for the finding of end-stage kidneys with multiple adenomas without cysts. These investigators also believe that either hyperplastic cysts or adenomas can become renal cell carcinomas. Therefore, one must not ignore the native kidneys left in situ during a renal transplantation. Whereas the cysts as a precursor of renal cell carcinomas may disappear, the small adenomas probably persist, and these, too, may be premalignant lesions. Hyperplastic cyst epithelium has been considered a possible precursor of renal cell carcinoma in other cystic diseases, in particular, von Hippel-Lindau disease and tuberous sclerosis (Fayemi and Ali, 1980).

EVALUATION

In uremic patients with fever, one should consider the diagnosis of ARCD and the possibility of an infected cyst (Bonal et al., 1987). Sonography usually shows small, hyperechoic kidneys with cysts of various sizes. Cyst wall calcification may be visible but is more readily seen on CT. Infection should be suspected if sonographic examination shows internal echoes or a thickened wall. Cyst puncture can be used to confirm the diagnosis and to identify the infecting microorganism.

CT examination may identify cyst wall thickening in infected cases. If the patient is receiving dialysis, contrast medium can be given safely to see if it causes enhancement (Levine et al., 1984). In some cases, one will identify a metastatic retroperitoneal renal cell carcinoma but be unable to identify the primary lesion in the kidney.

In the differential diagnosis of ARCD, one must consider the etiology of the renal failure, in particular, the possibility of DPK. Usually, patients with ARCD have smaller kidneys and smaller cysts and are free of the extrarenal manifestations of DPK. In patients on hemodialysis, kidneys affected by ARCD usually are less than 300 g; DPK kidneys generally are greater than 800 g (Fig. 35–23) (Feiner et al., 1981).

The chief presentations of both cyst and tumor in patients on hemodialysis are abdominal or flank pain and gross hematuria. Gehrig and co-workers (1985) found 11 of 24 patients with ARCD and symptomatic bleeding to have renal tumors; 8 of these 11 proved to

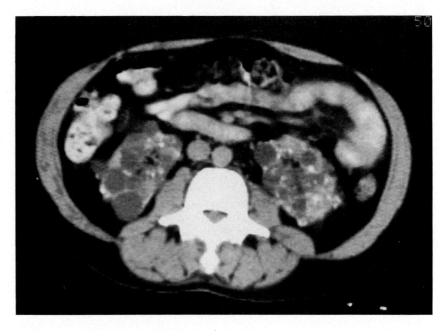

Figure 35–23. Bilateral multiple renal cysts and diffuse calcification in enlarged kidneys in a patient on chronic hemodialysis. The findings simulate those of autosomal dominant polycystic kidney disease. However, cystic disease was not the cause of the uremia and the diagnosis of acquired renal cystic disease was made. (Courtesy of D. Gordon, M.D.)

have renal cell carcinomas. The tumors themselves may be asymptomatic, revealing their presence only by metastases. The most common manifestation is loin pain, sometimes secondary to a retroperitoneal mass rather than to the primary tumor.

TREATMENT

If heparinization is associated with hematuria during hemodialysis, one may change to peritoneal dialysis. Other options are embolization and nephrectomy.

For an infected cyst, percutaneous drainage may be effective. When it is not, surgical drainage or nephrectomy should be considered.

Neumann and associates (1988) recommend that patients who have been receiving hemodialysis for longer than 3 years be screened by ultrasound and CT and then followed by ultrasonography every 6 months if the kidneys are without cysts and tumors or by both ultrasonography and CT on the same schedule if cysts or tumors smaller than 2 cm are identified.

A number of investigators have found that the cysts of ARCD regress after renal transplantation (Fig. 35–24) (Ishikawa et al., 1983; Kutcher et al., 1983; Thompson et al., 1986). In addition, Penn (1979) found renal cell carcinoma to be rare in patients who had received allografts; but at least three cases have been reported

(Arias et al., 1986; Faber and Kupin, 1987; Vaziri et al., 1984). The immunosuppression these patients receive by itself makes them vulnerable to carcinoma. Native kidneys account for 4.5 per cent of all malignancies in renal transplant recipients (Penn, 1979). The lower incidence of renal cell carcinoma in transplant recipients compared with those maintained on dialysis is further evidence of the importance of a toxic metabolite; one candidate is elevated levels of polyamines (Bagdade et al., 1979; Campbell et al., 1978; LaVoie et al., 1981).

Calyceal Diverticulum (Pyelogenic Cyst)

A calyceal diverticulum is a smoothly outlined intrarenal sac that communicates with the pelvicalyceal system by means of a narrow neck. Diverticula usually arise from the fornix of a calyx and most often affect upper pole calyces (Fig. 35–25). Some investigators reserve the term "calyceal diverticulum" for those lesions that communicate with a calyx or infundibulum and use "pyelogenic cyst" to designate lesions that communicate with the renal pelvis (Fig. 35–26). Other workers employ the term "pyelocal calyceal diverticulum" to encompass both entities (Fig. 35–27) (Friedland et al., 1990).

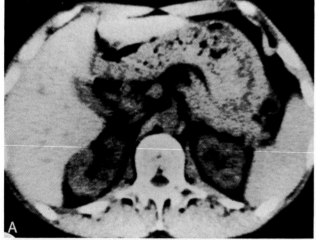
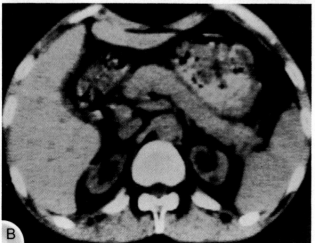

Figure 35–24. Effect of renal transplantation on acquired cystic kidney disease. *A,* CT scan obtained 1 month before renal transplantation in a patient who had been managed by dialysis for 7.5 years. Numerous bilateral renal cysts are present. *B,* Ten months after successful renal transplantation, almost all cysts, except one in the left kidney, have regressed. The kidney size has decreased considerably. (From Ishikawa, I., et al.: Regression of acquired cystic disease of the kidney after successful renal transplantation. Am. J. Nephrol., 3:310, 1983. S. Karger AG, Basel.)

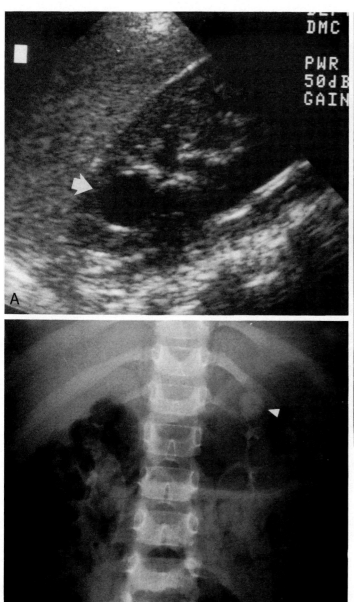

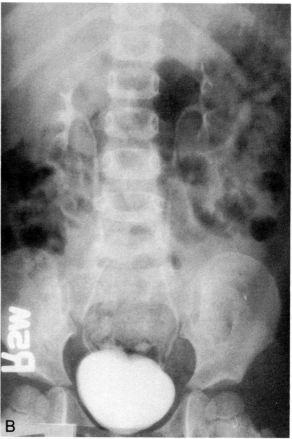

Figure 35–25. Calyceal diverticulum mimicking a simple cyst on sonography in a 5-year-old girl with recurrent urinary tract infections and no vesicoureteral reflux. *A*, Renal sonogram demonstrating a spherical mass in upper pole of left kidney *(arrow)* having the characteristics of a renal cyst. *B*, Early exposure on intravenous urogram reveals normal kidneys bilaterally. *C*, Exposure obtained 2 hours postinjection reveals contrast–filled upper pole calyceal diverticulum *(arrowhead)*.

Diverticula are lined by a smooth layer of transitional epithelium and covered by a thin patch of renal cortex. Most affected patients are adults. Timmons and colleagues (1975) found the incidence of calyceal diverticula on intravenous urograms in children to be 3.3 per 1000.

The etiology of these diverticula is unknown. Beneventi (1943) suggested that they are caused by achalasia of the calyceal neck, whereas Anderson (1963) thought that they arise from an inflammatory stricture of the infundibulum. Starer (1968) suggested that they are generated by anomalous vessels impinging on the infundibulum, and Amesur and Roy (1963) postulated rupture of a solitary cyst. However, solitary cysts are lined by a flat layer of epithelium, whereas diverticula have a transitional epithelial lining.

It is not clear how often a calyceal diverticulum becomes a simple cyst, although the possibility of such transformation has been suggested by Gordon and coworkers (1979). To date, only three confirmed cases of

the sealing of a diverticulum into a simple cyst have been published (Mosli et al., 1986; Nicholas, 1975). Because of the possibility of cyst formation, Mosli and associates (1986) recommended long-term ultrasound follow-up of patients with diverticula. However, such management would be costly and is unlikely to be tolerated by the patient.

Calyceal diverticula generally are asymptomatic and are discovered incidentally on an intravenous urogram. Any symptoms are often the result of a stone or infection.

Operation is seldom necessary. Either a partial nephrectomy or a wedge resection was often used in the past. Williams and associates (1969) described six cases treated by unroofing, ligation of the diverticular neck, and filling of the cavity with fat. Noe and Raghavaiah (1982) excised a diverticulum in toto through a nephrotomy incision.

In the past few years, some workers have described

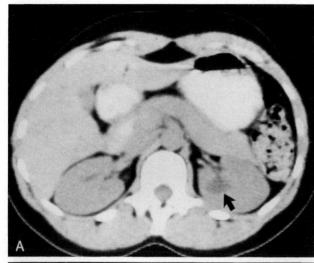

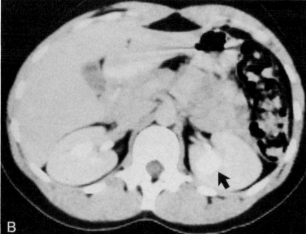

Figure 35–26. CT scans demonstrating pyelogenic cyst *(arrows)*. *A*, Precontrast scan. *B*, Postcontrast scan demonstrating communication to renal pelvis.

Figure 35–27. CT scan of the kidneys demonstrated a calyceal diverticulum *(arrow)* in the right kidney with contrast precipitating posteriorily because the patient is lying on his back. (Courtesy of D. Gordon, M.D.)

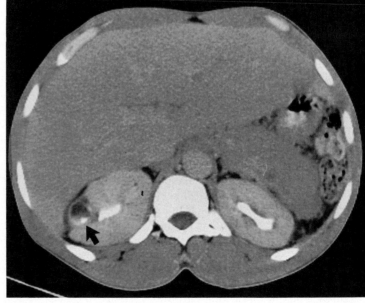

management of diverticula containing stones by a percutaneous procedure (Eshghi et al., 1987; Hulbert et al., 1986). The stone is removed with a nephroscope by way of a nephrostomy tract, and the infundibulum is incised with a cold knife or dilated. The lining of the diverticulum is fulgurated in some cases. Usually, the calyx is stented postoperatively. This essentially closed procedure probably is the best choice today in those few patients who require treatment.

Other Nongenetic Cysts

Intrarenal cysts may develop as a result of neoplastic disease, inflammation, or trauma.

PARAPELVIC AND RENAL SINUS CYSTS

Definitions

A number of terms have been used for cysts adjacent to the renal pelvis or within the hilum: "peripelvic cysts," "parapelvic cysts," "renal sinus cysts," "parapelvic lymphatic cysts," "hilus cysts," "cysts of the renal hilum," and "peripelvic lymphangiectasis." Some peripelvic cysts are, in fact, simple cysts that arise from the renal parenchyma but happen to abut the renal pelvis, with or without obstruction. Clearly, these are not cysts of the renal sinus. The terms "peripelvic" and "para-

pelvic" generally describe cysts around the renal pelvis or renal sinus. Those cysts derived from the renal sinus have no parenchymal etiology.

To avoid confusion, the terms "peripelvic" and "parapelvic" should be used only to describe location. I prefer to use these terms only as adjectives to describe simple parenchymal cysts adjacent to the renal pelvis or hilum, i.e., a peripelvic simple parenchymal cyst (Fig. 35–28). The term "renal sinus cyst" should be reserved for all other cysts in the hilum, i.e., those that are not derived from the renal parenchyma but rather from the other structures of the sinus, such as arteries, lymphatics, and fat.

Renal Sinus Cysts

The predominant type of renal sinus cyst appears to be one derived from the lymphatics. Most often, these cysts are multiple, and often, they are bilateral. The majority appear after the 5th decade, and they may be associated with inflammation, obstruction, or a calculus (Jordan, 1962; Kutcher et al., 1982).

One etiologic theory suggests that the lymphatic cyst is secondary to obstruction. Kutcher and associates (1982) note that lymphatic cysts or ectasia also can be found in other abdominal organs; these investigators refer to the condition in the renal sinus as peripelvic multicystic lymphangiectasia. In their patient, the cysts were lined by endothelial cells, and the fluid contained

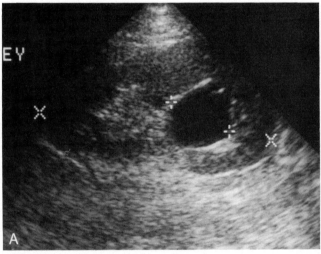
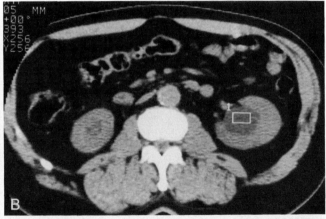
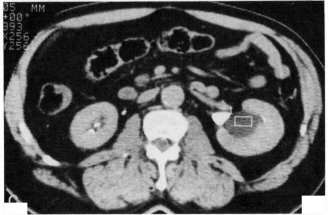

Figure 35–28. Simple cyst with peripelvic location. *A,* Renal sonogram reveals a centrally located left renal cyst. *B,* On precontrast CT scan, the cyst measures 3 HU. *C,* After contrast, the cyst calibrated to 2 HU. Note how the cyst is situated between a calyx and the renal pelvis. This is a simple parenchymal cyst in a peripelvic location and should not be confused with a renal sinus cyst.

lymphocytes. The intrarenal lymphatics also were dilated, with focal cyst formation. These cysts can cause obstruction or even extravasation of contrast medium during urography (Kutcher et al., 1982).

A condition previously described in the Spanish literature (Paramo, 1975; Paramo and Segura, 1972; Vela-Navarrete et al., 1974) but only recently described in the English literature has been called "polycystic disease of the renal sinus" (Vela-Navarrete and Robledo, 1983)—a problematic term because of the possible confusion with polycystic disease of the kidney. Vela-Navarrete and Robledo (1983) described 32 patients with this condition, some within multiple generations of a family (Vela-Navarrete personal communication, 1990). This entity sounds very much like the case reported by Kutcher and colleagues (1982) and is similar to others reported in association with renal calculi.

Vela-Navarrete and Robledo (1983) found nephrotomography and CT particularly useful in defining the lesions. Sonography was less helpful, perhaps because of limitations of the equipment then available. On nephrotomography, radiolucencies are identifiable in the renal sinus, along with stretching of the infundibula. Thus, the appearance is similar to that of renal sinus lipomatosis, leading Vela-Navarrete and Robledo (1983) to suggest that many cases of lipomatosis would be identified as polycystic disease of the renal sinus if CT were used (Fig. 35–29). On CT, the cysts can be seen

within the renal sinus as they displace the calyces peripherally (Fig. 35–30). The columns of Bertin may appear attenuated. In the Spanish series, 9 of the 32 patients had small renal calculi visible on plain film.

In five patients in the Spanish series, the lesions were explored. Multiple cysts were found, ranging in size from 2 to 4 cm in diameter and intertwined with stretched infundibula. The fluid was clear, with a plasma-like chemical composition. Histologically, the cyst walls were suggestive of a lymphatic vessel.

This entity has a benign natural history, except for the small calculi. These concretions may be secondary to stasis.

Serous cysts have also been reported in the renal sinus. Barrie (1953) suggested that these lesions are secondary to fatty tissue wasting in the renal sinus. Because the space left by the atrophied fat cannot collapse, it fills with transudate. However, no recent reports of serous cysts have been published, so I suspect that earlier cases were, in fact, lymphatic cysts.

Androulakakis and co-workers (1980) reported eight patients with parapelvic cysts, which they described as extraparenchymal. However, it is not clear how the cysts were identified as such. All lesions were said to be single cysts, but the description suggests that multiple cysts were present in some cases.

From a review of the literature, including CT findings in current cases, it appears that most multiple cystic

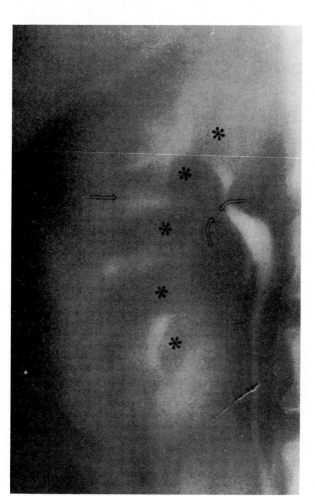

Figure 35–29. "Polycystic disease of the renal sinus" simulating renal pelvic lipomatosis. Nephrotomography demonstrating multiple renal lucencies in the renal sinus *(asterisks)* with medial displacement of the renal pelvis and elongation and stretching of infundibuli *(arrows)*. (From Vela-Navarrete, R., and Robledo, A. G.: Polycystic disease of the renal sinus: Structural characteristics. J. Urol., 129:700, 1983.)

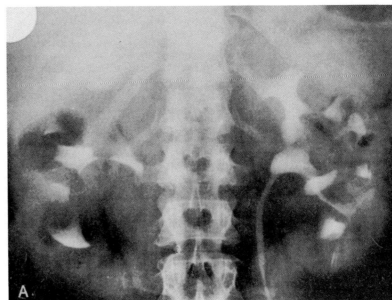

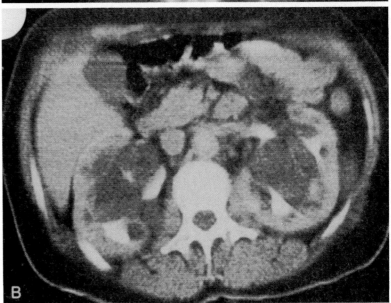

Figure 35–30. "Polycystic disease of the renal sinus," a form of renal sinus cysts. *A,* Intravenous urogram with enlargement of both kidneys, stretching of infundibuli, and trumpet-shaped calyces. *B,* CT scan in midportion of kidneys demonstrates multiple sinus cysts with peripheral displacement of renal pelvis and calyces. (From Vela-Navarrete, R., and Robledo, A. G.: Polycystic disease of the renal sinus: Structural characteristics. J. Urol., 129:700, 1983.)

structures in the area of the renal sinus will turn out to be lymphatic cysts, whereas most singular cysts will be found to be derived from the renal parenchyma. Continued study of cases by CT should clarify the nature of parapelvic and renal sinus cysts.

REFERENCES

Abreo, K., and Steele, H.: Simultaneous medullary sponge kidney and adult polycystic kidney. Arch. Intern. Med., 142:163, 1982.

Alfonso, D. N., and Oliviera, A. G.: Medullary sponge kidney and congenital hemihypertrophy. Br. J. Urol., 62:187, 1988.

Ambrose, S. S.: Unilateral multicystic renal disease in adults. Birth Defects, 13:349, 1976.

Amesur, N. R., and Roy, H. G.: Para-pelvic cyst of the kidney. Indian J. Surg., 25:45, 1963.

Amis, E. S., Jr., Cronan, J. J., Yoder, I. C., et al.: Renal cysts: Curios and caveats. Urol. Radiol., 4:199, 1982.

Anderson, J. C.: Hydronephrosis. Springfield, IL, Charles C. Thomas, 1963.

Androulakakis, P. A., Kirayiannis, B., and Deliveliotis, A.: The parapelvic renal cyst: A report of 8 cases with particular emphasis on diagnosis and management. Br. J. Urol., 52:342, 1980.

Arant, B. S., Sotelo-Auila, C., and Bernstein, J.: Segmental "hypoplasia" of the kidney (Ask-Upmark). J. Pediatr., 95:931, 1979.

Arey, J. B.: Cystic lesions of the kidney in infants and children. J. Pediatr., 54:429, 1959.

Arias, M., de Francisco, A. L. M., Ruiz, L., et al.: Acquired renal cystic disease and renal adenocarcinoma in a long term renal transplant patient. Int. J. Artif. Intern. Organs., 9:271, 1986.

Arnold, W., Weidaver, H., and Seelig, H. P.: Experimenteller Beweis einer gemeinsamen Antigenztat zwischen Innenohr und Niere. Arch Otorhinolaryngol., 212:99, 1976.

Ask-Upmark, E.: Über juvenile maligne Nephrosklerose und ihr Verhaltnis zu Störungen in der Nierenentwicklung. Acta Pathol. Microbiol. Scand., 6:383, 1929.

Aterman, K., Boustani, P., and Gillis, D. A.: Solitary multilocular cysts of the kidney. J. Pediatr. Surg., 8:505, 1973.

Avner, E. D., Ellis, D., Jaffe, R., et al.: Neonatal radiocontrast nephropathy simulating infantile polycystic kidney disease. J. Pediatr., 100:85, 1982.

Avni, E., Thova, Y., Lalmand, B., et al.: Multicystic dysplastic kidney: Natural history from in utero diagnosis and postnatal followup. J. Urol., 138:1420, 1987.

Babcock, D. S.: Medical diseases of the urinary tract and adrenal gland. *In* Haller, J. O., and Shkolnik, A. (Eds.): Ultrasound in Pediatrics. New York, Churchill Livingstone, 1981, p. 113.

Babka, J. C., Cohen, M. S., and Sode, J.: Solitary intrarenal cyst causing hypertension. N. Engl. J. Med., 291:343, 1974.

Bagdade, J. D., Subbaiah, P. V., Bartos, D., et al.: Polyamines: An unrecognized cardiovascular risk factor in chronic dialysis? Lancet, 1:412, 1979.

Banner, M. P., Pollack, H. M., Chatten, J., et al.: Multilocular renal cysts: Radiological-pathologic correlation. AJR, 136:239, 1981.

Barloon, J. T., and Vince, S. W.: Caliceal obstruction owing to a large parapelvic cyst: Excretory urography, ultrasound and computerized tomography findings. J. Urol., 137:270, 1987.

Barrett, D. M., and Wineland, R. E.: Renal cell carcinoma in multicystic dysplastic kidney. Urology, 15:152, 1980.

Barrie, J. H.: Paracalyceal cysts of the renal sinus. Am. J. Pathol., 29:985, 1953.

Bartholomew, T. H., Solvis, T. L., Kroovand, R. L., et al.: The sonographic evaluation and management of simple renal cysts in children. J. Urol., 123:732, 1980.

Basile, J. J., McCullough, D. L., Harrison, L. H., et al.: End stage renal disease associated with acquired cystic disease and neoplasia. J. Urol., 140:938, 1988.

Bear, J. C., McManamon, P., Morgan, J., et al.: Age at clinical onset and at ultrasonographic detection of adult polycystic disease. Am. J. Med. Genet., 18:45, 1984.

Bearth, K., and Steg, A.: On the pathogenesis of simple cysts in the adult: A microdissection study. Urol. Res., 5:103, 1977.

Beck, A. D.: The effect of intra-uterine urinary obstruction upon the development of the fetal kidney. J. Urol., 105:784, 1971.

Beckwith, J. B.: Wilms tumor and other renal tumors in childhood: An update. J. Urol., 136:320, 1986.

Beckwith, J. B., and Kiviat, N. B.: Multilocular renal cysts and cystic renal tumors [Editorial]. AJR, 136:435, 1981.

Beckwith, J. B., and Palmer, N. F.: Histopathology and prognosis of Wilms' tumor: Results from First National Wilms' Tumor Study. Cancer, 41:1937, 1978.

Begleiter, M. L., Smith, T. H., and Harris, D. J.: Ultrasound for genetic counselling in polycystic kidney disease. Lancet, 2:1073, 1977.

Beitzke, H.: Über Zysten in Nierenmark. Charite-Ann, 32:285, 1908.

Bell, E. T.: Cystic disease of the kidneys. Am. J. Pathol., 11:373, 1935.

Beneventi, F. A.: Hydrocalyx: Its relief by retrograde dilatation. Am. J. Surg., 61:244, 1943.

Bengtsson, U., Hedman, L., and Svalander, C.: Adult type of polycystic kidney disease in a newborn child. Acta Med. Scand., 197:447, 1975.

Bennett, W. M., Elzinga, L., Golper, T. A., et al.: Reduction of cyst volume for symptomatic management of autosomal dominant polycystic kidney disease. J. Urol., 137:620, 1987.

Bennington, J. L., and Beckwith, J. B.: Tumors of the kidney, renal pelvis and ureter. *In* Atlas of Tumor Pathology, Series 2, Fascicle 12. Washington, DC, Armed Forces Institute of Pathology, 1975, p. 33.

Berdon, W. E., Schwartz, R. H., Becker, J., et al.: Tamm-Horsfall proteinuria. Radiology, 92:714, 1969.

Berman, D. J., and Maizel, M.: Role of urinary obstruction in the genesis of renal dysplasia: A model in the chick embryo. J. Urol., 128:1091, 1982.

Bernstein, J.: Experimental study of renal parenchymal maldevelopment (renal dysplasia). Presented at the 3rd International Congress of Nephrology. Washington, DC, September, 1966.

Bernstein, J.: Developmental abnormalities of the renal parenchyma: Renal hypoplasia and dysplasia. Pathol. Annu., 3:213, 1968.

Bernstein, J.: The morphogenesis of renal parenchymal maldevelopment (renal dysplasia). Pediatr. Clin. North Am., 18:395, 1971.

Bernstein, J.: The classification of renal cysts. Nephron, 11:91, 1973.

Bernstein, J.: Developmental abnormalities of the renal parenchyma—renal hypoplasia and dysplasia. *In* Sommers, S. C. (Ed.): Kidney Pathology Decennial 1966–1975. New York, Appleton-Century-Crofts, 1975, pp. 11–17, 36–37.

Bernstein, J.: A classification of renal cysts. *In* Gardner, K. D., Jr. (Ed.): Cystic Disease of the Kidney. New York, John Wiley & Sons, 1976, p. 7.

Bernstein, J.: A classification of renal cysts. *In* Gardner, K. D., Jr.,

and Bernstein, J. (Eds.): The Cystic Kidney. The Netherlands, Kluwer Academic Publishers, 1990, p. 147.

Bernstein, J., Chandra, M., Creswell, J., et al.: Renal-hepatic-pancreatic dysplasia: A syndrome revisited. Am. J. Genet., 26:391, 1987.

Bernstein, J., and Gardner, K. D., Jr.: Cystic disease of the kidney and renal dysplasia. *In* Harrison, J. H., Gittes, R. F., Perlmutter, A. D., et al. (Eds.): Campbell's Urology, Ed. 4. Philadelphia, W. B. Saunders Co., 1979a, p. 1399.

Bernstein, J., and Gardner, K. D., Jr.: Familial juvenile nephronophthisis: Medullary cystic disease. *In* Edelman, C. M., Jr. (Ed.): Pediatric Kidney Disease. Boston, Little, Brown & Co., 1979b, p. 580.

Bernstein, J., and Gardner, K. D.: Hereditary tubulointerstitial nephropathies. *In* Cotran, R., Brenner, B., and Stein, J. (Eds.): Tubulointerstitial Nephropathies. New York, Churchill Livingston, 1983, pp. 335–357.

Bernstein, J., and Gardner, K. D., Jr.: Cystic disease of the kidney and renal dysplasia. *In* Walsh, P. C., Gittes, R. F., Perlmutter, A. D., et al. (Eds.): Campbell's Urology, Ed. 5. Philadelphia, W. B. Saunders Co., 1986, p. 1760.

Bernstein, J., and Gardner, K. D.: Cystic disease and dysplasia of the kidneys. *In* Murphy, W. M. (Ed.): Urological Pathology. Philadelphia, W. B. Saunders Co., 1989, p. 483.

Bernstein, J., and Landing, B. H.: Glomerulocystic kidney disease. Prog. Clin. Biol. Res., 305:27, 1989.

Bernstein, J., and Meyer, R.: Congenital abnormalities of the urinary system: II. Renal cortical and medullary necrosis. J. Pediatr., 59:657, 1961.

Bernstein, J., and Meyer, R.: Parenchymal maldevelopment of the kidney. *In* Kelley, V. C. (Ed.): Brennemann–Kelley, Practice of Pediatrics, Vol. 3. New York, Harper & Row, 1967, pp. 1–30.

Bernstein, J., Robbins, T. O., and Kissane, J. M.: The renal lesion of tuberous sclerosis. Semin. Diagn. Pathol., 3:97, 1986.

Biglar, J. A., and Killingsworth, W. P.: Cartilage in the kidney. Arch. Pathol., 47:487, 1949.

Birken, G., King, D., Vane, D., et al.: Renal cell carcinoma arising in a multicystic dysplastic kidney. J. Pediatr. Surg., 20:619, 1985.

Blyth, H., and Ockenden, B. G.: Polycystic disease of kidneys and liver presenting in childhood. J. Med. Genet., 8:257, 1971.

Boag, G. S., and Nolan, R.: CT visualization of medullary sponge kidney. Urol. Radiol., 9:220, 1988.

Boggs, L. K., and Kimmelstiel, P.: Benign multilocular cystic nephroma: Report of two cases of so-called multilocular cyst of the kidney. J. Urol., 76:530, 1956.

Bonal, J., Caralps, A., Lauzurica, R., et al.: Cyst infection in acquired renal cystic disease. Br. Med. J., 295:25, 1987.

Bosniak, M. A.: The current radiological approach to renal cysts. Radiology, 158:1, 1986.

Bourneville, D. M.: Sclérose tubereuse des circonvolutions cérébrales idote et épilepsie hémiplegique. Arch. Neurol. (Paris), 1:81, 1880.

Bove, K. E., and McAdams, A. J.: The nephroblastomatosis complex and its relationship to Wilms' tumor: A clinicopathologic treatise. Perspect. Pediatr. Pathol., 3:185, 1976.

Braasch, W. F., and Schacht, F. W.: Pathological and clinical data concerning polycystic kidney. Surg. Gynecol. Obstet., 57:467, 1933.

Bree, B. L., Raiss, G. J., and Schwab, R. E.: The sonographically ambiguous renal mass: Can surgery be avoided? Radiology, 153(Suppl.):212, 1984.

Bretan, P. N., Busch, M. P., Hricak, H., et al.: Chronic renal failure: A significant risk factor in the development of acquired renal cysts and renal cell carcinoma. Cancer, 57:1871, 1986.

Bricker, N. S., and Patton, J. F.: Cystic disease of the kidneys: A study of dynamics and chemical composition of cyst fluid. Am. J. Med., 18:207, 1955.

Bucciarelli, E., Sidoni, A., Alberti, P. F., et al.: Congenital nephrotic syndrome of the Finnish type. Nephron, 53:177, 1989.

Buchta, R. M., Viseskul, C., Gilbert, E. F., et al.: Familial bilateral renal agenesis and hereditary renal adysplasia. Z. Kinderheilkd., 115:111, 1973.

Burgler, W., and Hauri, D.: Vitale Komplikationen bei multizystischer Nierende Generation (multizystischer Dysplasie). Urol. Int., 38:251, 1983.

Cacchi, R., and Ricci, V.: Sur une rare maladie kystique multiple des pyramides rénales le "rein en éponge." J. Urol. Nephrol. (Paris), 55:497, 1949.

Campbell, G. S., Bick, H. D., and Paulsen, E. P.: Bleeding esophageal varices with polycystic liver: Report of three cases. N. Engl. J. Med., 259:904, 1958.

Campbell, R., Talwalker, Y. U., Bartos, D., et al.: Increased incidence of malignancy during chronic renal failure. Lancet, 1:883, 1978.

Cantani, A., Bamonte, G., Ceccoli, D., et al.: Familial nephronophthisis: A review and differential diagnosis. Clin. Pediatr., 25:90, 1986.

Carone, F. A., Maiko, H., and Kanwar, Y. S.: Basement membrane antigens in renal polycystic disease. Am. J. Pathol., 130:466, 1988.

Carone, F. A., Rowland, R. G., Perlman, S. G., et al.: The pathogenesis of drug-induced renal cystic disease. Kidney Int., 5:411, 1974.

Carter, J. E., and Lirenman, D. S.: Bilateral renal hypoplasia with oligomeganephronia: Oligomeganephronic renal hypoplasia. Am. J. Dis. Child., 120:537, 1970.

Chamberlin, B. C., Hagge, W. W., and Stickler, G. B.: Juvenile nephronophthisis and medullary cystic disease. Mayo Clin. Proc., 52:485, 1977.

Chatten, J., and Bishop, H. C.: Bilateral multilocular cysts of the kidney. J. Pediatr. Surg., 12:749, 1977.

Chen, Y. H., Stapleton, F. B., Roy, S., et al.: Neonatal hypertension from a unilateral multicystic dysplastic kidney. J. Urol., 133:664, 1985.

Cho, C., Friedland, G. W., and Swenson, R. S.: Acquired renal cystic disease and renal neoplasms in hemodialysis patients. Urol. Radiol., 6:153, 1984.

Chonko, A. M., Weiss, J. M., Stein, J. H., et al.: Renal involvement in tuberous sclerosis. Am. J. Med., 56:124, 1974.

Christ, M. L.: Polycystic nephroblastoma. J. Urol., 98:570, 1968.

Chung-Park, M., Ricanati, E., Lankerani, M., et al.: Acquired renal cysts and multiple renal cell and urothelial tumors. Am. J. Clin. Pathol., 141:238, 1983.

Churchill, D. N., Bear, J. C., Morgan, J., et al.: Prognosis of adult onset polycystic kidney disease re-evaluated. Kidney Int., 26:190, 1984.

Cohen, A. H., and Hoyer, J. R.: Nephronophthisis: A primary tubular basement membrane defect. Lab. Invest., 55:564, 1986.

Cole, B. R., Conley, S. B., and Stapleton, F. B.: Polycystic kidney disease in the first year of life. J. Pediatr., 111:693, 1987.

Colodny, A. H.: Comments in discussion. J. Urol., 142:489, 1989.

Copping, G. A.: Medullary sponge kidney: Its occurrence in a father and daughter. Can. Med. Assoc. J., 96:608, 1967.

Crocker, J. F., Brown, D. M., and Vernier, R. L.: Developmental defects of the kidney: A review of renal development and experimental studies of maldevelopment. Pediatr. Clin. North Am., 18:355, 1971.

Cussen, L. J.: Cystic kidneys in children with congenital urethral obstruction. J. Urol., 106:939, 1971.

Dalgaard, O. Z.: Bilateral polycystic disease of the kidneys: A followup of two hundred eighty-four patients and their families. Acta Med. Scand. [Suppl.], 38:1, 1957.

Dalgaard, O. Z., and Norby, S.: Autosomal dominant polycystic kidney disease in the 1980's. Clin. Genet., 36:320, 1989.

Dalton, D., Neiman, H., and Grayhack, J. J.: The natural history of simple renal cysts: A preliminary study. J. Urol., 135:905, 1986.

Daniel, W. W., Jr., Hartman, G. W., Witten, D. M., et al.: Calcified renal masses: A review of 10 years' experience at the Mayo Clinic. Radiology, 103:503, 1972.

Darmady, E. M., Offer, J., and Woodhouse, M. A.: Toxic metabolic defect in polycystic disease of kidney. Lancet, 1:547, 1970.

Darmis, F., Nahum, H., Mosse, A., et al.: Fibrose hépatique congénitale à progression clinique renal. Presse Med., 78:885, 1970.

Davides, K. C.: Multilocular kidney disease. J. Urol., 116:246, 1976.

Delaney, V. B., Adler, S., Bruns, F. J., et al.: Autosomal dominant polycystic kidney disease: Presentation, complications and progression. Am. J. Kidney Dis., 5:104, 1985.

Delano, B. G., Lazar, I. L., and Friedman, E. A.: Hypertension: Late consequences of kidney donation [Abstract]. Kidney Int., 23:168, 1983.

DeWall, J. G., Schroder, F. H., and Scholmeijer, R. J.: Diagnostic work up and treatment of multilocular cystic kidney: Difficulties in differential diagnosis. Urology, 28:73, 1986.

Dimmick, J., Johnson, H. W., Coleman, G. U., et al.: Wilms tumorlet, nodular renal blastema and multicystic renal dysplasia. J. Urol., 142:484, 1989.

Doege, T. C., Thuline, H. C., Priest, J. H., et al.: Studies of a family with the oral-facial-digital syndrome. N. Engl. J. Med., 271:1073, 1964.

Dunbar, J. S., and Nogrady, M. G.: The calyceal crescent: A roentgenographic sign of obstructive hydronephrosis. Am. J. Roentgenol., 110:520, 1970.

Dunhill, M. S., Milard, P. R., and Oliver, D. O.: Acquired cystic disease of the kidneys: A hazard of long-term intermittent maintenance hemodialysis. J. Clin. Pathol., 30:368, 1977.

Edmunds, W.: Cystic adenoma of kidney. Trans. Pathol. Soc. Lond., 43:89, 1892.

Eisendrath, D. N.: Clinical importance of congenital renal hypoplasia. J. Urol., 33:331, 1935.

Ekstrom, T., Engfeldt, B., Langergren, C., et al.: Medullary Sponge Kidney. Stockholm, Almquist and Wiksells, 1959.

Elfenbein, J. B., Baluarte, H. J., and Gruskin, A. B.: Renal hypoplasia with oligomeganephronia. Arch. Pathol., 97:143, 1974.

Emmett, J. L., and Witten, D. M.: Clinical Urography: An Atlas and Textbook of Roentgenologic Diagnosis, Ed. 3, Vol. 2. Philadelphia, W. B. Saunders Co., 1971, p. 1013.

Ericsson, N. O.: Ectopic ureterocele in infants and children: Clinical study. Acta Chir. Scand. [Suppl.], 97:1, 1954.

Ericsson, N. O.: Renal dysplasia. In Johnston, J. H., and Goodwin, W. E. (Eds.): Reviews in Paediatric Urology. Amsterdam, Excerpta Medica, 1974, p. 25.

Ericsson, N. O., and Ivemark, B. I.: Renal dysplasia and pyelonephritis in infants and children I. Arch. Pathol., 66:255, 1958a.

Ericsson, N. O., and Ivemark, B. I.: Renal dysplasia and pyelonephritis in infants and children: II. Primitive ductules and abnormal glomeruli. Arch. Pathol., 66:264, 1958b.

Eshghi, M., Tuong, W., Fernandez, R., et al.: Percutaneous (endo) infundibulotomy. J. Endourol., 1:107, 1987.

Euderink, F., and Hogewind, B. L.: Renal cysts in premature children: Occurrence in a family with polycystic kidney disease. Arch. Pathol. Lab. Med., 102:592, 1978.

European Dialysis and Transplant Association: Report. Proc. Eur. Dial. Transplant Assoc., 15:36, 1978.

Evans, A. T., and Coughlin, J. P.: Urinary obstruction due to renal cysts. J. Urol., 103:277, 1970.

Faber, M., and Kupin, W.: Renal cell carcinoma and acquired cystic disease after renal transplantation. Lancet, 1:1030, 1987.

Fallon, B., and Williams, R. D.: Renal cancer associated with acquired cystic disease of the kidney and chronic renal failure. Semin. Urol., 7:228, 1989.

Fanconi, G., Hanhart, E., Ailbertini, A., et al.: Die familiäre juvenile Nephronophthise (die idiopathische parenchymatose Schrumptniere). Helv. Paediatr. Acta, 6:1, 1951.

Fayemi, A. D., and Ali, M.: Acquired renal cysts and tumor superimposed on chronic primary diseases: An autopsy study of 24 patients. Pathol. Res. Pract., 68:73, 1980.

Feiner, H. D., Katz, L. A., and Gallo, G. R.: Acquired renal cystic disease of kidney in chronic hemodialysis patients. Urology, 17:260, 1981.

Fellows, R. A., Leonidas, J. C., and Beatty, E. C., Jr.: Radiologic features of "adult type" polycystic kidney disease in the neonate. Pediatr. Radiol., 4:87, 1976.

Felson, B., and Cussen, L. J.: The hydronephrotic type of congenital multicystic disease of the kidney. Semin. Roentgenol., 10:113, 1975.

Fetterman, G. H., Ravitch, M. M., and Sherman, F. E.: Cystic changes in fetal kidneys following ureteral ligation: Studies of microdissection. Kidney Int., 5:111, 1974.

Fill, W. L., Lamiel, J. M., and Polk, N. O.: The radiographic manifestations of von Hippel-Lindau disease. Radiology, 133:289, 1979.

Filmer, R. B., Carone, F. A., Rowland, R. G., et al.: Adrenal corticosteroid–induced renal cystic disease in the newborn hamster. Am. J. Pathol., 72:461, 1973.

Fine, M. G., and Burns, E.: Unilateral multicystic kidney: Report of six cases and discussion of the literature. J. Urol., 81:42, 1959.

Fisher, E. R., and Horvath, B.: Comparative ultrasound study of so-called renal adenoma and carcinoma. J. Urol., 108:382, 1972.

Fowler, M.: Differentiated nephroblastoma: Solid, cystic or mixed. J. Pathol., 105:215, 1971.

Franco, V., and Aragona, F.: Association of specific syndromes with renal cystic disease. Hum. Pathol., 20:496, 1989.

Friedland, G. W., deVries, P. A., Nino-Murcin, M., et al.: Congenital anomalies of the papillae, calyces, renal pelvis, ureter and ureteral orifice. *In* Pollack, H. M. (Ed.): Clinical Urography. Philadelphia, W. B. Saunders Co., 1990, p. 653.

Friedman, H., and Abeshouse, B. S.: Congenital unilateral multicystic kidney: A review of the literature and a report of three cases. Sinai Hosp. J. (Baltimore), 6:51, 1957.

Fryns, J. P., and van den Berghe, H.: "Adult" form of polycystic kidney disease in neonates. Clin. Genet., 15:205, 1979.

Gabow, P. A., Grantham, J. J., Bennett, W. N., et al.: Gene testing in autosomal dominant polycystic kidney disease: Results of National Kidney Foundation Workshop. Am. J. Kidney Dis., 13:85, 1989a.

Gabow, P. A., Ikle, W., and Holmes, J. H.: Polycystic kidney disease: Prospective analysis of non-azotemic patients and family members. Ann. Intern. Med., 101:238, 1984.

Gabow, P. A., Kaehny, W. D., Johnson, A. M., et al.: The clinical utility of renal concentrating capacity in polycystic kidney disease. Kidney Int., 35:675, 1989b.

Gabow, P. A., and Schrier, R. W.: Pathophysiology of adult polycystic kidney disease. Adv. Nephrol., 18:19, 1989.

Gaisford, W., and Bloor, K.: Congenital polycystic disease of kidney and liver: Portal hypertension, portacaval anastomosis. Proc. R. Soc. Med., 61:304, 1968.

Gallo, G. E., and Penchansky, L.: Cystic nephroma. Cancer, 39:1322, 1977.

Gardner, K. D., Jr.: Juvenile nephronophthisis and renal medullary cystic disease. *In* Gardner, K. D., Jr. (Ed.): Cystic Disease of the Kidney. New York, John Wiley & Sons, 1976, pp. 173–185.

Gardner, K. D., Jr.: Juvenile nephronophthisis—renal medullary cystic disease. Dialogues Pediatr. Urol., 7(5):3, 1984a.

Gardner, K. D., Jr.: Acquired renal cystic disease and renal adenocarcinoma in patients on long-term hemodialysis. N. Engl. J. Med., 310:390, 1984b.

Gardner, K. D., Jr.: Pathogenesis of human cystic renal disease. Annu. Rev. Med., 39:185, 1988.

Gardner, K. D., and Evan, A. P.: Cystic kidneys: An enigma evolves. Am. J. Kidney Dis., 3:403, 1984.

Garel, L. A., Habib, R., Pariente, D., et al.: Juvenile nephronophthisis: Sonographic appearance in children with severe uremia. Radiology, 151:93, 1984.

Gates, G. F.: Ultrasonography of the urinary tract in children. Urol. Clin. North Am., 7:215, 1980.

Gedroyc, W. M. W., and Saxton, H. M.: More medullary sponge variants. Clin. Radiol., 39:423, 1988.

Gehrig, J. J., Gottheiner, T. I., and Swenson, R. S.: Acquired cystic disease of the end-stage kidney. Am. J. Med., 79:609, 1985.

Geller, R. A., Pataki, K. I., and Finegold, R. A.: Bilateral multilocular renal cysts with recurrence. J. Urol., 121:808, 1979.

Gimsing, S., and Dyrmose, J.: Branchio-oto-renal dysplasia in three families. Ann. Otorhinolaryngol., 95:421, 1986.

Glassberg, K. I.: The dilated ureter: Classification and approach. Urology, 9:1, 1977.

Glassberg, K. I.: Cystic disease of the kidney. Probl. Urol., 2:157, 1988.

Glassberg, K. I., and Filmer, R. B.: Renal dysplasia, renal hypoplasia, and cystic disease of the kidney. *In* Kelalis, P. P., King, L. R., and Belman, A. B. (Eds.): Clinical Pediatric Urology. Philadelphia, W. B. Saunders Co., 1985, p. 922.

Glassberg, K. I., and Filmer, R. B.: Renal dysplasia, renal hypoplasia and cystic disease of the kidney. *In* Kelalis, P. P., King, L. R., Belman, A. B. (Eds.): Clinical Pediatric Urology, Ed. 3. Philadelphia, W. B. Saunders Co., 1991, In press.

Glassberg, K. I., Hackett, R. E., and Waterhouse, K.: Congenital anomalies of the kidney, ureter and bladder. *In* Kendall, A. R., and Karafin, L.: Harry S. Goldsmith's Practice of Surgery: Urology. Hagerstown, Harper & Row, 1981, p. 1.

Glassberg, K. I., Stephens, F. D., Lebowitz, R. L., et al.: Renal dysgenesis and cystic disease of the kidney: A report of the Committee on Terminology, Nomenclature and Classification, Section on Urology, American Academy of Pediatrics. J. Urol., 138:1085, 1987.

Goldberg, B. B., Kotler, M. M., Ziskin, M. C., et al.: Diagnostic Uses of Ultrasound. New York, Grune & Stratton, 1975.

Goldman, S. M., and Hartman, D. S.: The simple renal cysts. *In* Pollack, H. M. (Ed.): Clinical Urography. Philadelphia, W. B. Saunders Co., 1990, p. 1603.

Gomez, M. R.: Tuberous Sclerosis. New York, Raven Press, 1979.

Gordon, A. C., Thomas, D. F. M., Arthur, R. J., et al.: Multicystic dysplastic kidney: Is nephrectomy still appropriate? J. Urol., 140:1231, 1988.

Gordon, R. L., Pollack, H. M., Popky, G. L., et al.: Simple serous cysts of the kidney in children. Radiology, 131:357, 1979.

Grantham, J. J.: Polycystic renal disease. *In* Early, L. E., Gottschalk, C. W. (Eds.): Strauss and Welt's Disease of the Kidney, Ed. 3. Boston, Little, Brown & Co., 1979, p. 1123.

Grantham, J. J.: Polycystic kidney disease: A predominance of giant nephrons. Am. J. Physiol., 244:F3, 1983.

Grantham, J. J., Geiser, J. L., and Evan, A. P.: Cyst formation and growth in autosomal dominant polycystic kidney disease. Kidney Int., 31:1145, 1987.

Green, A., Kinirons, M., O'Meara, Y., et al.: Familial adult medullary cystic disease with spastic quadriparesis: A new disease association. Clin. Nephrol., 33:231, 1990.

Greene, L. F., Feinzaig, W., and Dahlin, D. C.: Multicystic dysplasia of the kidney: With special reference to the contralateral kidney. J. Urol., 105:482, 1971.

Gregoire, J. R., Torres, V. E., Hollen, K. E., et al.: Renal epithelial hyperplastic and neoplastic proliferation in autosomal dominant polycystic kidney disease. Am. J. Kidney Dis., 9:27, 1987.

Griffel, B., Pewzner, S., and Berandt, M.: Unilateral "oligomeganephronia" with agenesis of the contralateral kidney, studied by microdissection. Virchows Arch. [A], 357:179, 1972.

Griscom, N. T., Vawter, F. G., and Fellers, F. X.: Pelvoinfundibular atresia: The usual form of multicystic kidney; 44 unilateral and two bilateral cases. Semin. Roentgenol., 10:125, 1975.

Gross, M., and Breach, P. D.: The simultaneous occurrence of renal carcinoma and cyst: Problems in management. South. Med. J., 64:1059, 1971.

Gruskin, A. B.: Pediatric nephrology for the urologist. *In* Kendall, A. R., and Karafin, L. (Eds.): Harry S. Goldsmith's Practice of Surgery: Urology. Hagerstown, Harper & Row, 1977, p. 1.

Gutter, W., and Hermanek, P.: Maligner Tumor der Nierengegend unter dem Bilde der Knolleniere (nierenblastem Zysten). Urol. Int., 4:164, 1957.

Habib, R.: Renal dysplasia, hypoplasia and cysts. *In* Strauss, J. (Ed.): Pediatric Nephrology: Current Concepts in Diagnosis and Management. New York, Intercontinental Medical Book Corp., 1974, p. 209.

Habib, R., and Bois, E.: Heterogeneite des syndromes nephrotiques a debut precoce de nourisson (syndrome nephrotique "infantile"): Etude anatomoclinique et genetique de 37 observations. Helv. Paediatr. Acta 28:91, 1973.

Habib, R., Courtecuisse, V., Ehrensperger, J., et al.: Hypoplasie segmentaire du rein avec hypertension arterielle chez l'enfant. Ann. Pediatr. (Paris), 12:262, 1965.

Habib, R., Courtecuisse, V., Mathieu, H., et al.: Un type anatomo clinique particular, d'insuffisance renale chronique de l'enfant: l'Hypoplasie oligonephronique congenitale bilaterale. J. Urol. Nephrol. (Paris), 68:139, 1962.

Habib, R., Gubler, M., Niavdet, P., and Gagnadoux, M.: Congenital/infantile nephrotic syndrome with diffuse mesangial sclerosis: Relationships with Drash syndrome. *In* Bartsocas, C. S. (Ed.): Genetics of Kidney Disorders: Progress in Clinical and Biological Research, Vol. 305. New York, Alan R. Liss, 1989, p. 193.

Habib, R., Loirat, C., Gubler, M. D., et al.: The nephropathy associated with male pseudohermaphroditism and Wilson's tumor (Drash syndrome): A distinctive glanular lesion—report of 10 cases. Clin. Nephrol., 24:269, 1985.

Hadlock, F. P., Deter, R. L., Carpenter, P., et al.: Sonography of fetal urinary tract abnormalities. AJR, 137:261, 1981.

Hamberger, J., Richet, G., Crosnier, J., et al. (Eds.): Nephrology. Philadelphia, W. B. Saunders Co., 1968, p. 1087.

Harrison, A. R., and Rose, G. A.: Medullary sponge kidney. Urol. Res., 7:197, 1979.

Harrod, M. J. E., Stoker, J., Piede, L. F., et al.: Polycystic kidney disease in a patient with the oral-facial-digital syndrome–type I. Clin. Genet., 9:183, 1976.

Hartman, D. S.: Cysts and cystic neoplasms. Urol. Radiol., 12:7, 1990.

Hartman, G. E., Smolik, L. M., and Shochat, S. J.: The dilemma of the multicystic dysplastic kidney. Am. J. Dis. Child., 140:925, 1986.

Hartnett, M., and Bennett, W.: External manifestations of cystic renal disease. *In* Gardner, K. D., Jr. (Ed.): Cystic Disease of the Kidney. New York, John Wiley & Sons, 1976, pp. 201–219.

Hashimoto, B., Filly, R., and Cullen, P.: Multicystic dysplastic kidney in utero: Changing appearance on US. Radiology, 159:107, 1986.

Heikkinen, E. S., Herva, R., and Lanning, P.: Multicystic kidney: A clinical and histologic study of 13 patients. Ann. Chir. Gynaecol., 69:15, 1980.

Henneberry, M. O., and Stephens, F. D.: Renal hypoplasia and dysplasia in infants with posterior urethral valves. J. Urol., 123:912, 1980.

Heptinstall, R. H.: Discussion. *In* Hodson, J., and Kincaid-Smith, P. (Eds.): Reflux Nephropathy. New York, Masson, 1979, p. 253.

Herdman, R. C., Good, R. A., and Vernier, R. L.: Medullary cystic disease in two siblings. Am. J. Med., 43:335, 1967.

Hildebrandt, O.: Weiterer Beitrag zur patologischen Anatomie der Nierengeschwulste. Arch. Klin. Chir., 48:343, 1894.

Hinman, J. A. F.: Obstructive renal cysts. J. Urol., 119:681, 1978.

Hoard, T. D., and O'Brien, D. P., III: Simple renal cyst and high renin hypertension cured by cyst decompression. J. Urol., 115:326, 1976.

Hodson, C. R.: Reflux nephropathy: A personal historical review. AJR, 137:451, 1981.

Holmberg, G., and Hietala, S.: Treatment of simple renal cysts by percutaneous puncture and instillation of bismuth-phosphate. Scand. J. Urol. Nephrol., 23:207, 1989.

Horton, W. A., Wong, V., and Eldridge, R.: Von Hippel-Lindau disease: Clinical and pathological manifestations in nine families with 50 affected members. Arch. Intern. Med., 136:769, 1976.

Hossack, K. F., Leddy, C. L., Schrier, R. W., et al.: Incidence of cardiac abnormalities associated with autosomal dominant polycystic kidney disease (ADPKD) [Abstract]. Am. Soc. Nephrol., 19:46A, 1986.

Hubner, W., Pfaf, R., Porpaczy, P., et al.: Renal cysts: Percutaneous resection with standard urologic instruments. J. Endourol., 4:61, 1990.

Hughson, M. D., Buckwald, D., and Fox, M.: Renal neoplasia and acquired cystic kidney disease in patients receiving long term dialysis. Arch. Pathol. Lab. Med., 110:592, 1986.

Hughson, M. D., Henniger, G. R., and McManus, J. F.: Atypical cysts, acquired renal cystic disease, and renal cell tumors in end stage dialysis kidneys. Lab. Invest., 42:475, 1980.

Hulbert, J. C., and Hunter, D.: Percutaneous techniques for intrarenal marsupialization of difficult symptomatic renal cysts. Presented at the 85th Annual Meeting of the American Urological Association. New Orleans, May, 1990.

Hulbert, J. C., et al.: Percutaneous techniques for the management of caliceal diverticula containing calculi. J. Urol., 135:225, 1986.

Huttunen, J. R.: Congenital nephrotic syndrome of Finnish type: Study of 75 patients. Arch. Dis. Child., 51:344, 1976.

Ibrahim, R. E., Weinberg, D. S., and Weidner, N.: Atypical cysts and carcinomas of the kidneys in the phacomatoses: A quantitative DNA study using static and flow cytometry. Cancer, 63:148, 1989.

Ishikawa, I.: Uremic acquired cystic disease. Urology, 26:101, 1985.

Ishikawa, I.: Development of adenocarcinoma and acquired cystic disease of the kidney in hemodialysis patients. *In* Miller, R. W., et al. (Eds.): Unusual Occurrences as Clues to Cancer Etiology. Tokyo, Japan Scientific Society Press, 1988a, p. 77.

Ishikawa, I.: Adenocarcinoma of the kidney in chronic hemodialysis patients. Int. J. Artif. Organs, 11:61, 1988b.

Ishikawa, I., Onouchi, Z., Saito, Y., et al.: Sex differences in acquired cystic disease of the kidney on long term dialysis. Nephron, 39:336, 1985.

Ishikawa, I., Saito, Y., Onouchi, Z., et al.: Development of acquired cystic disease and adenocarcinoma of the kidney in glomerulonephrotic chronic hemodialysis patients. Clin. Nephrol., 14:1, 1980.

Ishikawa, I., Yuri, T., Kitada, H., et al.: Regression of acquired cystic disease of the kidney after successful renal transplantation. Am. J. Nephrol., 3:310, 1983.

Ivemark, B. I., Oldefelt, P., and Zetterstrom, B.: Familial dysplasia of kidneys, liver and pancreas: A probably genetically determined syndrome. Acta Paediatr., 48:1, 1959.

Jackman, R. J., and Stevens, J. M.: Benign hemorrhagic renal cyst: Nephrotomography, renal arteriography and cyst puncture. Radiology, 110:7, 1974.

Jacobs, C., Reach, I., and Degoulet, P.: Cancer in patients on hemodialysis. N. Engl. J. Med., 300:1279, 1979.

Javadpour, N., Chelouhy, E., Moncada, L., et al.: Hypertension in a child caused by a multicystic kidney. J. Urol., 104:918, 1970.

Jennings, C. M., and Gaines, P. A.: The abdominal manifestations of von Hippel-Lindau disease and a radiological screening protocol for an affected family. Clin. Radiol., 39:363, 1988.

Johnson, D. E., Ayala, A. G., Medellin, H., et al.: Multilocular renal cystic disease in children. J. Urol., 109:101, 1973.

Johnston, J. H.: The pathogenesis of hydronephrosis in children. Br. J. Urol., 41:724, 1969.

Johnston, J. H., Evans, J. P., Glassberg, K. I., et al.: Pelvic hydronephrosis in children: A review of 219 personal cases. J. Urol., 117:97, 1977.

Johnston, J. H., and Mix, L. W.: The Ask-Upmark kidney: A form of ascending pyelonephritis? Br. J. Urol., 48:393, 1976.

Jordan, W. P., Jr.: Peripelvic cysts of the kidney. J. Urol., 87:97, 1962.

Joshi, V. V.: Cystic partially differentiated nephroblastoma: An entity in the spectrum of infantile renal neoplasia. Perspect. Pediatr. Pathol., 5:217, 1980.

Jung, W. H., Peters, C. A., Mandell, J. A., et al.: Flow cytometric evaluation of multicystic dysplastic kidneys. J. Urol., 144:413, 1990.

Kadir, S., Kerr, W. S., and Athanasoulis, C. A.: The role of arteriography in the management of renal cell carcinoma associated with von Hippel-Lindau disease. J. Urol., 126:316, 1981.

Kangarloo, H., and Fine, R. N.: Ultrasonography of cystic renal dysplasia. Int. J. Pediatr. Nephrol., 4:205, 1973.

Kaplan, B. S., Gordon, I., Pincott, J., et al.: Familial hypoplastic glomerulocystic kidney disease: A definite entity with dominant inheritance. Am. J. Med. Genet., 34:569, 1989a.

Kaplan, B. S., Kaplan, P., de Chadarevian, J. P., et al.: Variable expression of autosomal recessive polycystic kidney disease and congenital hepatic fibrosis within a family. Am. J. Med. Genet., 29:639, 1988.

Kaplan, B. S., Kaplan, P., Rosenberg, H. K., et al.: Polycystic kidney disease in childhood. J. Pediatr., 115:867, 1989b.

Kaplan, B. S., Rabin, I., Nogrady, M. G., et al.: Autosomal dominant polycystic renal disease in children. J. Pediatr., 90:782, 1977.

Kaufman, J., and Fay, R.: Renal hypertension in childhood. *In* Johnston, J. H., and Goodwin, W. E. (Eds.): Reviews in Pediatric Urology. Amsterdam, Excerpta Medica, 1974, p. 201.

Kaye, C., and Lewy, P.: Congenital appearance of adult type (autosomal dominant) polycystic kidney disease. J. Pediatr., 85:807, 1974.

Kelly, C. J., and Neilson, E. G.: The interstitium of the cystic kidney. *In* Gardner, K. D., Jr., and Bernstein, J. (Eds.): The Cystic Kidney. The Netherlands, Kluwer Academic Publishers, 1990, pp. 43–53.

Kerr, D. N. S., Warrick, C. K., and Hart-Mercer, J.: A lesion resembling medullary sponge kidney in patients with congenital hepatic fibrosis. Clin. Radiol., 13:85, 1962.

Khoury, Z., Brezis, M., and Mogle, P.: Familial medullary sponge kidney in association with congenital absence of teeth (anodontia). Nephron, 48:231, 1988.

Kishikawa, T., Toda, T., Ito, H., et al.: Bilateral congenital multicystic dysplasia of the kidney. Jpn. J. Surg., 11:198, 1981.

Kissane, J. M.: Congenital malformations. *In* Heptinstall, R. H. (Ed.): Pathology of the Kidney, Ed. 2. Boston, Little, Brown & Co., 1974, p. 69.

Kissane, J. M.: Renal cysts associated with multiple malformation syndromes. Dialogues Pediatr. Urol., 7(May):7, 1984.

Kissane, J. M., and Smith, M. G.: Pathology of Infancy and Childhood, Ed. 2. St. Louis, C. V. Mosby, 1975, p. 587.

Kleiner, B., Filly, R., Mack, L., et al.: Multicystic dysplastic kidney: Observations of contralateral disease in the fetal population. Radiology, 161:27, 1986.

Kuiper, J. J.: Medullary sponge kidney. Perspect. Nephrol. Hypertens., 4:151, 1976a.

Kuiper, J. J.: Medullary sponge kidney. *In* Gardner, K. D. (Ed.): Cystic Diseases of the Kidney. New York, John Wiley & Sons, 1976b, p. 151.

Kuntz, M.: Population studies. *In* Gomez, M. R. (Ed.): Tuberous Sclerosis, Ed. 2. New York, Raven Press, 1988, p. 214.

Kupin, W., Norris, C., Levin, N. W., et al.: Incidence of diverticular disease in patients with polycystic kidney disease (PCKD). Presented at the 10th International Congress of Nephrology. London, July, 1987.

Kutcher, R., Amodio, J. R., and Rosenblatt, R.: Uremic renal cystic disease: Value of sonographic screening. Radiology, 147:833, 1983.

Kutcher, R., Manadevia, P., Nussbaum, M. K., et al.: Renal peripelvic multicystic lymphangiectasia. Urology, 30:177, 1982.

Lagos, J. C., and Gomez, M. R.: Tuberous sclerosis: Reappraisal of a clinical entity. Mayo Clin. Proc., 42:26, 1967.

Lam, M., Halverstadt, D., Altshuler, G., et al.: Congenital oligomeganephronia in a solitary kidney: Report of a case. Am. J. Kidney Dis., 1:300, 1982.

Lang, E. K., and Gershanik, J. B.: Multicystic dysplastic kidney: Diagnostic considerations and management. South. Med. J., 71:888, 1978.

Lanning, P., Uhari, M., Kouvalainan, K., et al.: Ultrasonic features of the congenital nephrotic syndrome of the Finnish type. Acta Paediatr. Scand., 78:717, 1989.

Laucks, S. P., Jr., and McLachlan, M. S. F.: Aging and simple renal cysts of the kidney. Br. J. Radiol., 54:12, 1981.

Lavan, J. N., Neale, F. C., and Posen, S.: Urinary calculi: Clinical, biochemical and radiological studies in 619 patients. Med. J. Aust., 2:1049, 1971.

LaVoie, E. J., Kolb, E., Rivenson, A., et al.: Carcinogenicity in Syrian golden hamsters of the N-nitrosamines formed during nitrosation of spermidine. Cancer Detect. Prev., 4:79, 1981.

Lenarduzzi, G.: Repert pielografico poco commune (dilatazione delle vie urinarie intrarenali). Radiol. Med., 26:346, 1939.

Levine, A. S., and Michael, A. F.: Ehlers-Danlos syndrome with renal tubular acidosis and medullary sponge kidney. J. Pediatr., 71:107, 1967.

Levine, E., Collins, D. L., Horton, W. A., et al.: CT screening of the abdomen in von Hippel-Lindau disease. AJR, 139:505, 1982.

Levine, E., and Grantham, J. J.: Radiology of cystic kidneys. *In* Gardner, K. D., Jr., and Bernstein, J. (Eds.): The Cystic Kidney. The Netherlands, Kluwer Academic Publishers, 1990, p. 171.

Levine, E., Grantham, J. J., Slusher, S. L., et al.: CT of acquired cystic disease and renal tumors in long-term dialysis patients. AJR, 142:125, 1984.

Levine, E., Hartmann, D. S., and Smirnidtopoulos, J. G.: Renal cystic disease associated with renal neoplasms. *In* Pollack, H. M. (Ed.): Clinical Urography. Philadelphia, W. B. Saunders Co., 1990, pp. 1126–1150.

Levine, E., Weigel, J. W., and Collins, D. L.: Diagnosis and management of asymptomatic renal cell carcinoma in von Hippel-Lindau syndrome. Urology, 21:146, 1983.

Lieberman, E., Salinas-Madrigal, L., Gwinn, J. L., et al.: Infantile polycystic disease of the kidneys and liver: Clinical, pathological and radiological correlations and comparison with congenital hepatic fibrosis. Medicine, 50:277, 1971.

Lingard, D. A., and Lawson, T. I.: Accuracy of ultrasound in predicting the nature of renal masses. J. Urol., 122:724, 1979.

Lirenman, D. S., Lowry, R. B., and Chase, W. H.: Familial juvenile nephronophthisis: Experience with eleven cases. Birth Defects, 10:32, 1974.

Livingston, W. D., Collins, T. L., and Novick, D. E.: Incidental renal masses. Urology, 17:257, 1981.

Loh, J. P., Haller, J. O., Kassner, E. G., et al.: Dominantly inherited polycystic kidneys in infants: Association with hypertrophic pyloric stenosis. Pediatr. Radiol., 6:27, 1977.

Longino, L. A., and Martin, L. W.: Abdominal masses in the newborn infant. Pediatrics, 21:596, 1958.

Loughlin, K. R., and Gittes, R. F.: Urological management of patients with von Hippel-Lindau disease. J. Urol., 136:789, 1986.

Luisiri, A., Sotelo-Avila, C., Silberstein, M. J., et al.: Sonography of Zellweger syndrome. J. Ultrasound Med., 7:169, 1988.

Lundin, P. M., and Olow, I.: Polycystic kidneys in newborns, infants and children: A clinical and pathological study. Acta Paediatr. Scand., 50:185, 1961.

Lüscher, T. F., Wanner, C., Siegenthaler, W., et al.: Simple renal cyst and hypertension: Cause or coincidence? Clin. Nephrol., 26:91, 1986.

MacDougall, M. L., Welling, L. W., and Wiegmann, T. B.: Renal adenocarcinoma and acquired cystic disease in chronic hemodialysis patients. Am. J. Kidney Dis., 9:166, 1987.

Mackie, G. G., and Stephens, F. D.: Duplex kidneys: A correlation of renal dysplasia with position of the ureteral orifice. J. Urol., 114:274, 1975.

Madewell, J. E., Goldman, S. M., and Davis, C. J., Jr.: Multilocular cystic nephroma: A radiographic pathologic correlation of 58 patients. Radiology, 146:309, 1983.

Mahony, B. S., Filly, R. A., Callen, P. W., et al.: Fetal renal dysplasia: Sonographic evaluation. Radiology, 152:143, 1984.

Maizel, M., and Simpson, S. B., Jr.: Primitive ducts in renal dysplasia induced by culturing ureteral buds denuded of condensed renal mesenchyme. Science, 209:509, 1983.

Maizel, M., and Simpson, S. B., Jr.: Ligating the embryonic ureter facilitates the induction of renal dysplasia. Dev. Biol., Part B:445, 1986.

Mall, J. C., Ghahremani, G. G., and Boyer, J. L.: Caroli's disease associated with congenital hepatic fibrosis and renal tubular ectasia. Gastroenterology, 66:1029, 1974.

Marotti, M., Hricak, H., Fritzche, P., et al.: Complex and simple cysts: Comparative evaluation with MR imaging. Radiology, 162:679, 1987.

Maschio, G., Tessitore, N., and D'Angelo, A.: Medullary sponge kidney and hyperparathyroidism: A puzzling association. Am. J. Nephrol., 2:77, 1982.

McClean, R. H., Goldstein, G., Conrad, F. U., et al.: Myocardial infarctions and endocardial fibro-elastosis in children with polycystic kidneys. Bull. Johns Hopkins Hosp., 115:92, 1964.

McClennan, B. L., Stanley, R. J., Melson, G. L., et al.: CT of the renal cyst: Is a cyst puncture necessary? AJR, 133:671, 1979.

McGonigle, R. J. S., Mowat, A. P., Benwick, M., et al.: Congenital hepatic fibrosis and polycystic kidney disease: Role of portacaval shunting and transplantation in three patients. Q. J. Med., 50:269, 1981.

McGregor, A. L., and Bailey, R.: Nephronophthisis-cystic medulla complex: Diagnosis by computerized tomography. Nephron, 53:70, 1989.

Meares, E. M., Jr., and Gross, D. M.: Hypertension owing to unilateral renal hypoplasia. J. Urol., 108:197, 1972.

Mehrizi, A., Rosenstein, B. J., Pusch, A., et al.: Myocardial and endocardial fibro-elastosis in children with polycystic kidneys. Bull. Johns Hopkins Hosp., 115:92, 1964.

Melicow, M. M., and Uson, A. C.: Palpable abdominal masses in infants and children: A report based on a review of 653 cases. J. Urol., 81:705, 1959.

Melnick, S. C., Brewer, D. B., and Oldham, J. S.: Cortical microcystic disease of the kidney with dominant inheritance: A previously undescribed syndrome. J. Clin. Pathol., 37:494, 1984.

Mery, J., Simon, P., Horuttle, T., et al.: À propos de deux observations de maladie polycystique rénale de l'adulte associée au syndrome oral-facial-digital. J. Urol. (Paris), 84:892, 1978.

Meyer, W. M., and Jonas, D.: Endoscopic percutaneous resection of renal cysts. Presented at the 8th World Congress on Endourology and ESWL. Washington, DC, August–September, 1990.

Mickisch, O., Bommer, J., Blackman, J., et al.: Multicystic transformation of kidneys in chronic renal failure. Nephron, 38:93, 1984.

Milam, J. H., Magee, J. H., and Bunts, R. C.: Evaluation of surgical decompression of polycystic kidneys by differential renal clearances. J. Urol., 90:144, 1963.

Miller, L. R., Soffer, O., Nasser, V. H., et al.: Acquired renal cystic disease in end stage renal disease: An autopsy study of 155 cases. Am. J. Nephrol., 9:322, 1989.

Mitnick, J. S., Bosniak, M. A., and Hilton, S.: Cystic renal disease in tuberous sclerosis. Radiology, 147:85, 1983.

Mongeau, J. G., and Worthen, H. G.: Nephronophthisis and medullary cystic disease. Am. J. Med., 43:345, 1967.

Morita, T., Wenzl, J., McCoy, J., et al.: Bilateral renal hypoplasia with oligomeganephronia: Quantitative and electron microscopic study. Am. J. Clin. Pathol., 59:104, 1973.

Morris, R. C., Yamauchi, H., Palubinskas, A. J., et al.: Medullary sponge kidney. Am. J. Med., 38:883, 1965.

Mosli, H., MacDonald, P., and Schillinger, J.: Caliceal diverticulum developing into simple renal cyst. J. Urol., 136:658, 1986.

Mozziconacci, P., Attal, C., Boisse, J., et al.: Hypoplasie segmentaire du rein avec hypertension artéielle. Ann. Pediatr., 15:337, 1968.

Mulley, J. C., Haan, A. H., Gedeon, A. K., and Sutherland, G. R.: Predictive diagnosis for polycystic kidney disease using DNA markers. Med. J. Aust. 152:287, 1990.

Muther, R. S., and Bennett, W. M.: Cyst fluid antibiotic concentration in polycystic kidney disease: Differences between proximal and distal cysts. Kidney Int., 20:519, 1981.

Myall, G. F.: The incidence of medullary sponge kidney. Clin. Radiol., 21:171, 1970.

Neilson, E. G., McCafferty, E., Mann, R., et al.: Murine interstitial nephritis III. J. Immunol., 134:2375, 1985.

Neumann, H. P. H., Zerres, K., Fischer, C. L., et al.: Late manifestations of autosomal-recessive polycystic kidney disease in two sisters. Am. J. Nephrol., 8:194, 1988.

Ng, R. C. K., and Suki, W. N.: Renal cell carcinoma occurring in a polycystic kidney of a transplant recipient. J. Urol., 124:710, 1980.

Nicholas, J. L.: An unusual complication of calyceal diverticulum. Br. J. Urol., 47:370, 1975.

Noe, H. N., Marshall, J. H., and Edwards, O. P.: Nodular renal blastema in the multicystic kidney. J. Urol., 127:486, 1989.

Noe, H. N., and Raghavaiah, N. V.: Excision of pyelocalyceal diverticulum under renal hypothermia. J. Urol., 127:294, 1982.

Norio, R.: Heredity in the congenital nephrotic syndrome: A genetic study of 57 Finnish families with a review of reported cases. Ann. Paediatr. (Finn.), 12(Suppl. 27):1, 1966.

Norio, R., and Rapola, J.: Congenital and infantile nephrotic syndromes. In Bartsocas, C. S. (Ed.): Genetics of Kidney Disorders: Progress in Clinical and Biological Research, Vol. 305. New York, Alan R. Liss, 1989, pp. 179–192.

Okada, R. D., Platt, M. A., and Fleischman, J.: Chronic renal failure in patients with tuberous sclerosis: Association with renal cysts. Nephron, 30:85, 1982.

Olsen, A., Hansen Hojhus, J., and Steffensen, G.: Renal medullary cystic disease. Acta Radiol., 29 (Fasc. 5):527, 1988.

Osathanondh, V., and Potter, E. L.: Pathogenesis of polycystic kidneys: Historical survey. Arch. Pathol., 77:459, 1964.

Ostling, K.: The genes of hydronephrosis. Acta Chir. Scand. [Suppl.], 72, 1942.

Palubinskas, A. J.: Medullary sponge kidney. Radiology, 76:911, 1961.

Pampigliana, G., and Moynahan, E. J.: The tuberous sclerosis syndrome: Clinical and EEG studies in 100 children. J. Neurol. Neurosurg. Psychiatry, 39:666, 1976.

Papanicolaou, N., Pfister, R. C., and Yoder, I. C.: Spontaneous and traumatic rupture of renal cysts: Diagnosis and outcome. Radiology, 160:99, 1986.

Paramo, P. G.: Patologia quística renal. Acta Assoc. Esp. Urol., 7:1, 1975.

Paramo, P. G., and Segura, A.: Hilioquisosis renal. Rev. Clin. Esp., 126:387, 1972.

Parkkulainen, K. V., Hjeldt, L., and Sirola, K.: Congenital multicystic dysplasia of kidney: Report of nineteen cases with discussion on the etiology, nomenclature and classification of cystic dysplasia of the kidney. Acta Chir. Scand. [Suppl.], 244:5, 1959.

Parks, J. H., Coe, F. L., and Strauss, A. L.: Calcium nephrolithiasis and medullary sponge kidney in women. N. Engl. J. Med., 306:1088, 1982.

Pathak, I. G., and Williams, D. I.: Multicystic and cystic dysplastic kidneys. Br. J. Urol., 36:318, 1964.

Patriquin, H. B., and O'Regan, S.: Medullary sponge kidney in childhood. AJR, 145:315, 1985.

Penn, I.: Tumor incidence in renal allograft recipients. Transplant Proc., 11:1047, 1979.

Perey, D. Y. E., Herdman, R. C., and Good, R. A.: Polycystic renal disease: A new experimental model. Science, 158:494, 1967.

Pollack, H. M., Banner, M. P., Arger, P. H., et al.: Comparison of computed tomography and ultrasound in the diagnosis of renal masses. In Rosenfeld, A. T. (Ed.): Genitourinary Ultrasonography. New York, Churchill Livingstone, 1979, p. 25.

Porstman, W.: Renal angiography in children. Prog. Pediatr. Radiol., 3:51, 1970.

Potter, E. L.: Normal and Abnormal Development of the Kidney. Chicago, Year Book Medical Publishers, 1972.

Powell, T., Schackman, R., and Johnson, H. D.: Multilocular cysts of the kidney. Br. J. Urol., 23:142, 1951.

Pretorius, D. H., Lee, M. E., Manco-Johnson, M. L., et al.: Diagnosis of autosomal dominant polycystic kidney disease in utero and in the young infant. J. Ultrasound Med., 6:249, 1987.

Proesmans, W., Van Damme, B., Basaer, P., et al.: Autosomal dominant polycystic kidney disease in the neonatal period: Association with a cerebral arteriovenous malformation. Pediatrics, 70:971, 1982.

Quick, C. A., Fish, A., and Brown, C.: The relationship between cochlea and kidney. Laryngoscope, 83:1469, 1973.

Raffensberger, J., and Abouselman, A.: Abdominal masses in children under one year of age. Surgery, 63:514, 1968.

Rall, J. E., and Odell, H. M.: Congenital polycystic disease of the kidney: Review of the literature and the data on 207 cases. Am. J. Med. Sci., 298, 394, 1949.

Ramsey, M., Reeders, S. T., Thomason, P. D., et al.: Mutations for the autosomal recessive and autosomal dominant forms of polycystic kidney disease are not allelic. Hum. Genet., 79:73, 1988.

Ratcliffe, P. J., Dunhill, M. S., and Oliver, D. O.: Clinical importance of acquired cystic disease of the kidneys in patients undergoing dialysis. Br. Med. J., 287:1855, 1983.

Rauber, G., and Langlet, M. L.: Hypoplasies segmentaires du rein: Distinction de deux formes histologiques. Nouv. Presse Med., 5:1759, 1976.

Ravden, M. I., Zuckerman, H. L., Kay, C. J., et al.: Evaluation of solitary simple renal cysts in children. J. Urol., 124:904, 1980.

Reeders, S. T.: The genetics of renal cystic disease. In Gardner, K. D., Jr., Bernstein, J. (Eds.): The Cystic Kidney. The Netherlands, Kluwer Academic Publishers, 1990, pp. 117–146.

Reeders, S. T., Breuning, M. H., Comey, G., et al.: Two genetic markers closely linked to adult polycystic kidney disease on chromosome 16. Br. Med. J., 292:851, 1986a.

Reeders, S. T., Bruening, M. H., Davies, K. E., et al.: A highly polymorphic DNA marker linked to adult polycystic kidney disease on chromosome 16. Nature, 317:542, 1985.

Reeders, S. T., Keeres, K., Gal, A., et al.: Prenatal diagnosis of autosomal dominant polycystic kidney disease with a DNA probe. Lancet, 2:6, 1986b.

Resnick, J. S., Brown, D. M., and Vernier, R. L., Jr.: Normal development and experimental models of cystic renal disease. In Gardner, K. D., Jr. (Ed.): Cystic Diseases of the Kidney. New York, John Wiley & Sons, 1976, p. 221.

Resnick, J. S., and Hartman, D. S.: Medullary cystic disease of the kidney. In Pollack, H. M. (Ed.): Clinical Urography. Philadelphia, W. B. Saunders Co., 1990, pp. 1178–1184.

Richter, S., Karbel, G., Bechar, L., et al.: Should a benign renal cyst be treated? Br. J. Urol., 55:457, 1983.

Ritter, R., and Siafarikas, K.: Hemihypertrophy in a boy with renal polycystic disease: Varied patterns of presentation of renal polycystic disease in his family. Pediatr. Radiol., 5:98, 1976.

Rizzoni, G., Loirat, C., Levy, M., et al.: Familial hypoplastic glomerulocystic kidneys: A new entity? Clin. Nephrol., 18:263, 1982.

Rockson, S. G., Stone, R. A., and Gunnels, J. C., Jr.: Solitary renal cyst with segmental ischemia and hypertension. J. Urol., 112:550, 1974.

Roos, A.: Polycystic kidney: Report of a case. Am. J. Dis. Child., 61:116, 1941.

Rosenfeld, A. T., Siegel, N. J., and Kappleman, M. B.: Grey scale ultrasonography in medullary cystic disease of the kidney and congenital hepatic fibrosis with tubular ectasia: New observations. AJR, 129:297, 1977.

Rosenfeld, J. B., Cohen, L., Garty, I., et al.: Unilateral renal hypoplasia with hypertension (Ask-Upmark kidney). Br. Med. J., 2:217, 1973.

Ross, D. G., and Travers, H.: Infantile presentation of adult-type polycystic kidney disease in a large kindred. J. Pediatr., 87:760, 1975.

Royer, P., Habib, R., Broyer, M., et al.: Segmental hypoplasia of the kidney in children. Adv. Nephrol., 1:145, 1971.

Royer, P., Habib, R., Mathieu, H., et al.: L'Hypoplasie renale bilaterale congenitale avec reduction du nombre et hypertrophie des nephrons chez l'enfant. Ann. Pediatr. (Paris), 38:133, 1962.

Rubenstein, M., Meyer, R., and Bernstein, J.: Congenital abnormalities of the urinary system: I. A postmortem survey of developmental anomalies and acquired congenital lesions in a children's hospital. J. Pediatr., 58:356, 1961.

Rushton, G. H., Spector, M., Rogers, A. L., et al.: Developmental aspects of calcium oxalate tubular deposits and calculi induced in rat kidneys. Invest. Urol., 19:52, 1981.

Ryynanen, M., Dolata, M. M., Lampainen, E., et al.: Localization of mutation producing autosomal dominant polycystic kidney disease without renal failure. J. Med. Genet., 24:462, 1987.

Ryu, S.: Intracranial hemorrhage in patients with polycystic kidney disease. Stroke, 21:291, 1990.

Sage, M. R., Lawson, A. D., Marshall, V. R., et al.: Medullary sponge kidney and urolithiasis. Clin. Radiol., 33:435, 1982.

Sahney, S., Sandler, M. A., Weiss, L., et al.: Adult polycystic disease: Presymptomatic diagnosis for genetic counseling. Clin. Nephrol., 20:89, 1983.

Sanders, R. C.: Renal cystic disease. In Resnick, M. I., and Sanders, R. C. (Eds.): Ultrasound in Urology. Baltimore, Williams & Wilkins, 1979, p. 97.

Santis, H. R., Nathanson, N. R., and Bauer, S. B.: Nevoid basal cell carcinoma syndrome associated with renal cysts and hypertension. Oral. Surg., 55:127, 1983.

Saxton, H. M., Golding, S. J., Chantler, C., et al.: Diagnostic puncture in renal cystic dysplasia (multicystic kidney): Evidence on the aetiology of the cysts. Br. J. Urol., 54:555, 1981.

Scheff, R. T., Zuckerman, G., Harter, H., et al.: Diverticular disease in patients with chronic renal failure due to polycystic kidney disease. Ann. Intern. Med., 92:202, 1980.

Scheinman, J. I., and Abelson, H. T.: Bilateral renal hypoplasia with oligonephronia. J. Pediatr., 76:369, 1970.

Schwab, S. J., Bander, S. J., and Klahr, S.: Renal infection in autosomal dominant polycystic kidney disease. Am. J. Med., 82:714, 1987.

Schwarz, R. D., Stephens, F. D., and Cussen, L. J.: The pathogenesis of renal hypodysplasia: I. Quantification of hypoplasia and dysplasia. Invest. Urol., 10:94, 1981a.

Schwarz, R. D., Stephens, F. D., and Cussen, L. J.: The pathogenesis of renal hypodysplasia: II. The significance of lateral and medial ectopy of the ureteric orifice. Invest. Urol., 19:97, 1981b.

Schwarz, R. D., Stephens, F. D., and Cussen, L. J.: The pathogenesis of renal hypodysplasia: III. Complete and incomplete urinary obstruction. Invest. Urol., 19:101, 1981c.

Sedman, A., Bell, P., Manco-Johnson, M., et al.: Autosomal dominant polycystic kidney disease in childhood: A longitudinal study. Kidney Int., 31:1000, 1987.

Sedman, A., and Gabow, P. A.: Autosomal dominant polycystic kidney disease. Dialogues Pediatr. Urol., 7:4, 1984.

Segal, A. J., and Spitzer, R. M.: Pseudo thick-walled renal cyst by CT. AJR, 132:827, 1979.

Shalhoub, R. J., Rajan, U., Kim, V. V., et al.: Erythrocytosis in patients on long-term hemodialysis. Ann. Intern. Med., 97:686, 1982.

Shindo, S., Bernstein, J., and Arant, B. S., Jr.: Evolution of renal segmental atrophy (Ask-Upmark kidney) in children with vesicoureteral reflux: Radiographic and morphologic studies. J. Pediatr., 102:847, 1983.

Shirai, M., Kitagawa, T., Nakata, H., et al.: Renal cell carcinoma originating from dysplastic kidney. Acta Pathol. Jpn., 36:1263, 1986.

Shokeir, M. H. K.: Expression of "adult" polycystic renal disease in the fetus and newborn. Clin. Genet., 14:61, 1978.

Siegel, M. J., and McAlister, W. H.: Simple renal cysts in children. J. Urol., 123:75, 1980.

Simon, H. B., and Thompson, G. J.: Congenital renal polycystic disease: A clinical and therapeutic study of three hundred sixty six cases. JAMA, 159:657, 1955.

Smith, C. H., and Graham, J. B.: Congenital medullary cysts of the kidneys with severe refractory anemia. Am. J. Dis. Child., 69:369, 1945.

Smith, D. W., Opitz, J. M., and Inhorn, S. L.: A syndrome of multiple developmental defects including polycystic kidneys and intrahepatic biliary dysgenesis in 2 siblings. J. Pediatr., 67:617, 1976.

Solomon, D., and Schwartz, A.: Renal pathology in von Hippel-Lindau disease. Hum. Pathol., 19:1072, 1988.

Sommer, J. T., and Stephens, F. D.: Morphogenesis of nephropathy with partial ureteral obstruction and vesicoureteral reflux. J. Urol., 125:67, 1981.

Spence, H. M.: Congenital unilateral multicystic kidney: An entity to be distinguished from polycystic kidney disease and other cystic disorders. J. Urol., 74:893, 1955.

Spence, H. M., and Singleton, R.: Cysts and cystic disorders of the kidney: Types, diagnosis, treatment. Urol. Surv., 22:131, 1972.

Spencer, J. R., and Maizel, M.: Inhibition of protein glycosylation causes renal dysplasia in the chick embryo. J. Urol., 138:94, 1987.

Sprayragen, S., Strasberg, Z., and Nadich, T. P.: Medullary sponge kidney and congenital hemihypertrophy. N.Y. State J. Med., 73:276, 1973.

Squiers, E. C., Morden, R. S., and Bernstein, J.: Renal multicystic dysplasia: An occasional manifestation of the hereditary renal adysplasia syndrome. Am. J. Med. Genet. [Suppl.], 3:279, 1987.

Stapleton, F. B., Bernstein, J., Koh, G., et al.: Cystic kidneys in a patient with oral-facial-digital syndrome, type I. Am. J. Kidney Dis., 1:288, 1982.

Stapleton, F. B., Hilton, S., Wilcox, J., et al.: Transient nephromegaly simulating infantile polycystic disease of the kidneys. Pediatrics, 67:554, 1981.

Stapleton, F. B., Johnson, D., Kaplan, G. W., et al.: The cystic renal lesion in tuberous sclerosis. J. Pediatr., 97:574, 1980.

Starer, F.: Partial hydronephrosis due to pressure from normal renal arteries. Br. Med. J., 1:98, 1968.

Steele, B. T., Lirenman, D. S., and Beattie, C. W.: Nephronophthisis. Am. J. Med., 68:531, 1980.

Stephens, F. D.: Congenital Malformations of the Urinary Tract. New York, Praeger Publishers, 1983.

Stephens, F. D., and Cussen, L. G.: Renal dysgenesis: A "urologic" classification. In Stephens, F. D. (Ed.): Congenital Malformations of the Urinary Tract. New York, Praeger Publishing, 1983, pp. 463–475.

Stickler, G. B., and Kelalis, P. P.: Polycystic kidney disease: A recognition of the "adult" form (autosomal dominant) in infancy. Mayo Clin. Proc., 50:547, 1975.

Stillaert, J., Baert, A., Van Damme, B., et al.: À propos du rein polykystique. In Kuss, R., and Legrain, M. (Eds.): Seminaries d'Uronephrologie in Pitiere-Salpetriere, 1975. Paris, Masson et Cie, 1975, p. 159.

Stillwell, T. J., Gomez, M. R., and Kelalis, P. P.: Renal lesions in tuberous sclerosis. J. Urol., 138:477, 1987.

Stuck, K. J., Koff, S. A., and Silver, T. M.: Ultrasonic features of multicystic dysplastic kidney: Expanded diagnostic criteria. Radiology, 143:217, 1982.

Summer, T., Friedland, G. W., Parker, B., et al.: Preoperative diagnosis of unilateral multicystic kidney with hydropelvis. Urology, 11:519, 1978.

Tada, S., Yamagishi, J., Kobayashi, H., et al.: The incidence of simple renal cyst by computed tomography. Clin. Radiol., 150:207, 1983.

Taitz, L. S., Brown, C. B., Blank, C. E., et al.: Screening for polycystic kidney disease: Importance of clinical presentation in the newborn. Arch. Dis. Child., 62:45, 1987.

Tanagho, E. A.: Surgically induced partial urinary obstruction in the fetal lamb: III. Ureteral obstruction. Invest. Urol., 10:35, 1972.

Taxy, J. B., and Filmer, R. B.: Metaplastic cartilage in nondysplastic kidneys. Arch. Pathol., 99:101, 1975.

Taxy, J. B., and Filmer, R. B.: Glomerulo-cystic kidney. Arch. Pathol. Lab. Med., 100:186, 1976.

Templeton, A. W., and Thompson, I. M.: Aortographic differentiation of congenital and acquired small kidneys. Arch. Surg., 97:114, 1968.

Thompson, B. J., Jenkins, D. A. S., Allan, P. L., et al.: Acquired cystic disease of the kidney: An indication for transplantation? Br. Med. J., 293:209, 1986.

Thomsen, H. S., and Thaysen, J. H.: Frequency of hepatic cysts in adult polycystic kidney disease. Acta Med. Scand., 224:381, 1988.

Timmons, J. W., Jr., Malek, R. S., Hattery, R. R., et al.: Calyceal diverticulum. J. Urol., 114:6, 1975.

Torres, V. E., Kolley, K. E., and Offord, P.: General features of autosomal dominant polycystic kidney disease: Epidemiology. In Grantham, J. J., and Gardner, K. D. (Eds.): Problems in Diagnosis and Management of Polycystic Kidney Disease. Proceedings of the 1st International Workshop on Polycystic Kidney Disease. Kansas City, PKD Foundation, 1985, p. 49.

Uson, A. C., and Melicow, M. M.: Multilocular cysts of the kidney with intrapelvic herniation of a "daughter" cyst: Report of 4 cases. J. Urol., 89:341, 1963.

Vagelli, G., Ferraris, V., Calbrese, G., et al.: Medullary sponge kidney and calcium nephrolithiasis [Abstract]. Urol. Res., 16:201, 1988.

Valderrama, E., and Berkman, J. I.: The Ask-Upmark kidney in a premature infant. Clin. Nephrol., 11:313, 1979.

Van Acker, K. J., Vincke, H., Quatacker, J., et al.: Congenital oligonephronic renal hypoplasia with hypertrophy of nephrons (oligonephronia). Arch. Dis. Child., 46:321, 1971.

Vaziri, N. D., Darwish, R., Martin, D. C., et al.: Acquired renal cystic disease in renal transplant patients. Nephron, 37:203, 1984.

Vela-Navarrete, R., Garcia de la Péna, E., Alverez Villalobos, C., et al.: Quistes nonefrogénicos del seno renal: Expreividad radiográphica y consideraciones diagnósticas. Rev. Clin. Esp., 132:29, 1974.

Vela-Navarrete, R., and Robledo, A. G.: Polycystic disease of the renal sinus: Structural characteristics. J. Urol., 129:700, 1983.

Wahlqvist, L., and Grumstedt, B.: Therapeutic effect of percutaneous puncture of simple renal cyst: Follow-up investigation of 50 patients. Acta Chir. Scand., 132:340, 1966.

Wakabayashi, T., Fujita, S., Onbora, Y., et al.: Polycystic kidney disease and intracranial aneurysms: Early angiographic diagnosis and early operation for the unruptured aneurysm. J. Neurosurg., 58:488, 1983.

Walker, F. C., Loney, L. C., Rout, E. R., et al.: Diagnostic evaluation of adult polycystic disease in childhood. AJR, 142:1273, 1984.

Walker, R. D., Fennell, R., Garin, E., et al.: Spectrum of multicystic renal dysplasia: Diagnosis and management. Urology, 11:433, 1978.

Weinreb, J. C., Arger, P. H., Coleman, B. G., et al.: Cystic renal mass evaluation: Real-time versus static imaging. J. Clin. Ultrasound, 14:29, 1986.

Westberg, G., and Zachrisson, L.: Proceedings of the Swedish Society of Medical Radiology, 4, 1975.

Wikstrom, B., Backman, U., and Danielson, B. G.: Ambulatory diagnostic evaluation of 38 recurrent renal stone formers: A proposal for clinical classification and investigation. Klin. Wochenschr., 61:85, 1983.

Williams, D. I.: Urology in Childhood. New York, Springer-Verlag, 1974, p. 79.

Williams, G., Blandy, J. P., and Tressider, G. C.: Communicating cysts and diverticula of the renal pelvis. Br. J. Urol., 41:163, 1969.

Wolf, B., Rosenfield, A. T., Taylor, K. J. W., et al.: Presymptomatic diagnosis of adult onset polycystic kidney disease by ultrasonography. Clin. Genet., 14:1, 1978.

Wood, B. P., Muurahainen, N., Anderson, V. M., et al.: Multicystic nephroblastoma: Ultrasound diagnosis (with a pathologic-anatomic commentary). Pediatr. Radiol., 12:43, 1982.

Yates-Bell, J. G.: Rovsing's operation for polycystic kidney. Lancet, 1:125, 1987.

Yendt, E. R.: Medullary sponge kidney. *In* Gardner, K. D., Jr., Bernstein, J. (Eds.): The Cystic Kidney. The Netherlands, Kluwer Academic Publishers, 1990, p. 379.

Zeier, M., Geberth, S., Ritz, E., et al.: Adult dominant polycystic kidney disease: Clinical problems. Nephron, 49:177, 1988.

Zerres, K., Hansmann, M., Mallman, R., et al.: Autosomal recessive polycystic kidney disease: Problems of prenatal diagnosis. Prenat. Diagn., 8:215, 1988.

36
EMBRYOLOGY OF THE GENITAL TRACT

Fredrick W. George, Ph.D.
Jean D. Wilson, M.D.

Sexual differentiation is a sequential process beginning with the establishment of chromosomal sex at fertilization, followed by the development of gonadal sex, and culminating with the appearance of anatomic characteristics, collectively termed the male and female sexual phenotypes (Fig. 36–1). Each step in this process is dependent on the preceding one, and under normal circumstances the chromosomal sex established at fertilization dictates gonadal development and, hence, the sexual phenotype of the embryo (George and Wilson, 1988; Jost, 1953). The process of gonadal differentiation does not begin immediately following fertilization, and the phenotypic development of the human male and female urogenital tract is identical prior to the 6th to 8th week of embryonic development. Only thereafter do anatomic and physiologic development diverge to result in the formation of the male and female anatomy. Although most aspects of this process are completed by the end of the first trimester, certain functional and structural parameters, including maturation of the genital tract and gonads, are not completed until postnatal life.

Probably no other aspect of embryonic development is understood as well as sexual differentiation. Normal sexual development, unlike most other embryonic processes, is not essential to the life of the individual. Consequently, a variety of naturally occurring disorders of sexual development are available for systematic study. These aberrations of sexual development occur at many levels and cause consequences that range from common defects, involving the terminal stages of male development (cryptorchidism and microphallus), to more fundamental abnormalities, involving hormone formation and action and resulting in various conditions of intersex.

In this chapter, attention is directed first to the normal sequence of events that results in development of the male and female phenotypes (Fig. 36–2) and then to the regulatory factors that control sexual differentiation. Complete sexual development involves the maturation of functional, as well as anatomic, processes. The former—which include the development of gender identity, the regulation of gonadotropin secretion by the hypothalamic-pituitary system, and certain aspects of behavior—are not considered here.

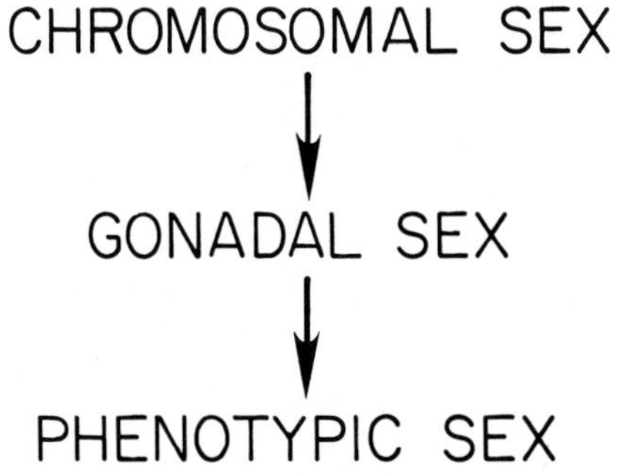

DEVELOPMENT OF CHROMOSOMAL SEX

Chromosomal sex is established at the moment of fertilization. If the fertilizing sperm contains an X chromosome, the zygote will be 46,XX—the genotype of the female. If the successful sperm carries a Y chromosome, the 46,XY karyotype that is characteristic of the male will result.

The Y chromosome is the third smallest human chromosome. Although it is thought to carry only a few functional genes (Goodfellow et al., 1985), the undisputed function of the mammalian Y chromosome is to serve as the repository for the genes that control testicular differentiation. For example, the presence of a

CHROMOSOMAL SEX

↓

GONADAL SEX

↓

PHENOTYPIC SEX

Figure 36–1. Successive events of sexual differentiation.

APPROXIMATE TIME AFTER FERTILIZATION		DEVELOPMENTAL PROCESS		
WEEKS	TRIMESTER	MALE	INDIFFERENT	FEMALE
3	First		• GERM CELLS BEGIN MIGRATION	
3.5–4.5			• WOLFFIAN DUCT APPEARS AS PRONEPHRIC DUCT	
5–6			• INDIFFERENT GONADS DEVELOP ON GENITAL RIDGES • MAMMARY LINES PRESENT	
6–7		• APPEARANCE OF TESTICULAR CORDS	• MULLERIAN DUCT DEVELOPMENT BEGINS	
7			• FORMATION OF UROGENITAL SINUS BEGINS	
7.5			• UROGENITAL TUBERCLE AND SWELLINGS COMPLETE • URETHRAL FOLD AND GROOVE COMPLETE	
9		• SERTOLI CELLS APPARENT • MULLERIAN DUCT REGRESSION BEGINS	• UROGENITAL SINUS, MULLERIAN AND WOLFFIAN DUCTS COMPLETE INDIFFERENT DEVELOPMENT	• FORMATION OF VAGINAL PLATE BEGINS • UTERINE DEVELOPMENT COMMENCES
9–10		• LEYDIG CELLS APPEAR IN TESTIS • ONSET OF TESTOSTERONE SYNTHESIS	• MULLERIAN DUCTS ATTACHED TO MULLERIAN TUBERCLE WITHOUT PENETRATING • WOLFFIAN DUCTS OPEN LATERALLY INTO UROGENITAL SINUS	
9–11		• LENGTHENING OF UROGENITAL DISTANCE • FUSION OF LABIO SCROTAL SWELLINGS • GROWTH OF WOLFFIAN DUCTS		
10		• FORMATION OF PROSTATE BEGINS		• CAUDAL FLEXION OF THE GENITAL TUBERCLE BEGINS
11		• MULLERIAN REGRESSION COMPLETE		• REGRESSION OF WOLFFIAN DUCT BEGINS • GERM CELLS ENTER MEIOSIS • CANALIZATION OF VAGINAL PLATE BEGINS
12–13	Second	• FORMATION OF SEMINAL VESICLES		
13–16		• FORMATION OF PROCESSUS VAGINALIS		
15		• PREPUCE FORMATION COMPLETE		• FOLLICLE FORMATION IN OVARY BEGINS
17		• TESTIS COMES TO REST AGAINST ANTERIOR ABDOMINAL WALL		• UTERINE DEVELOPMENT COMPLETE • VAGINAL DEVELOPMENT COMPLETE
28–37	Third	• TRUE TESTICULAR DESCENT BEGINS • GROWTH OF EXTERNAL GENITALIA		

Figure 36–2. Approximate sequence of events in sexual differentiation. (Data compiled from several sources, including Jirasek, J. E.: Development of the Genital System and Male Pseudohermaphroditism, Baltimore, Johns Hopkins Press, 1971; Koff, A. K.: Carnegie Contributions to Embryology, No. 140, 24:59–90, 1933; and Gillman, J.: Carnegie Contributions to Embryology, No. 210, 32:83–131, 1948.)

single Y chromosome in each cell ensures testicular differentiation and development of a predominantly male phenotype (Polani, 1981), even in situations in which multiple X chromosomes are present in each cell. The region of the Y chromosome thought to encode the human testis-determining factor (TDF) has been localized to the short arm of the Y chromosome between the centromere and the pseudoautosomal region (Page et al., 1987; Palmer et al., 1989). Extensive analysis of this region of the Y chromosome has identified a gene that is Y specific, conserved among a wide range of mammals, and encodes a testis-specific transcript (Gubbay et al., 1990; Sinclair et al., 1990). This transcript is homologous to two nuclear nonhistone proteins thought to play a role in chromosomal structure and gene activity. Conclusive proof that this gene regulates testis determination awaits further analysis. Even though the testis-determining region on the Y chromosome is ultimately responsible for male development, other genes essential for normal male development are also located on the X chromosome, and autosomal genes are also essential for the development of both the male and female phenotypes (Wilson and Goldstein, 1975). Consequently, the overall process of sexual differentiation is more correctly viewed as the result of interactions between genetic determinants on the X and Y chromosomes and autosomal genes rather than as the sole result of the sex chromosome composition.

DEVELOPMENT OF GONADAL SEX
Indifferent Development

The gonadal ridges (anlage) are formed during the 4th week of human development by proliferation of the coelomic epithelium and condensation of the underlying mesenchyme along the mesonephros. These primitive gonadal ridges are initially devoid of germ cells that, prior to the 2nd month of human gestation, are located in the endoderm of the yolk sac near the allantoic evagination (Peters, 1970; Witschi, 1948). During the 2nd month of gestation the germ cells leave the primitive gut and migrate by ameboid movement through the gut mesentery to the gonadal ridges (Fig. 36–3). Although it is not known what regulates this process, the fact that the germ cells migrate by pseudopodal movement to a specific location in the embryo suggests that the migration is directed by a chemotactic factor (McCarrey and Abbott, 1979). During migration the germ cells undergo many mitotic divisions, and their numbers are expanded several-fold by the time they come to rest in the gonadal ridges. Late in the 5th week of gestation, when germ cell migration is completed, the gonads of the male and female embryo are indistinguishable and are composed of three principal cell types: (1) germ cells, (2) supporting cells derived from the coelomic epithelium of the genital ridge that differentiate into either the Sertoli cells of the testis or the granulosa cells of the ovary, and (3) stromal (interstitial) cells derived from the mesenchyme of the gonadal ridge.

Differentiation

Phenotypic sexual differentiation is dependent on the differentiation of the fetal gonad and the subsequent onset of endocrine function of the fetal testis (Jost, 1953). The regulation of this important fundamental

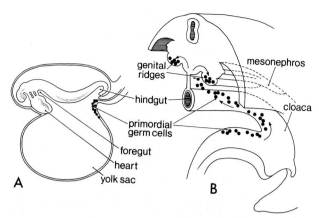

Figure 36–3. A, Schematic drawing showing the site of origin of the germ cells in the wall of the yolk sac in a 3-week-old embryo. B, Migratory path of the primordial germ cells along the wall of the yolk sac and dorsal mesentery and into the genital ridges. (From Langman, J.: Medical Embryology, 4th ed. Baltimore, Williams & Wilkins Co., 1981.)

process is not well understood. The first morphologic sign of sexual dimorphism in the gonads is the development of the primordial Sertoli cells and their aggregation into primitive spermatogenic cords in the fetal testis (Jost and Magre, 1984). In the human this process occurs around the 7th week of gestational development (Gillman, 1948). In contrast to early testicular development, ovarian epithelial components remain in irregular clusters around the primordial germ cells for many weeks. It is not until about the 4th month of gestation that the primitive granulosa cells organize around the dividing oocyte to form a single layer of follicular cells, thus establishing the primordial follicle (Gillman, 1948; Gondos et al., 1971). Gonadogenesis in other mammalian species is similar to that in humans in that the histologic differentiation of the fetal testis precedes that of the fetal ovary by days to weeks. In several species somatic cells of the gonadal ridge can organize into an ovary or a testis, irrespective of the presence or absence of germ cells (Handel and Eppig, 1979; Merchant, 1975; McCarrey and Abbott, 1978). Consequently, gonadal development and differentiation cannot be dependent solely on the presence or type of germ cell that migrates into the coelomic epithelium of the gonadal ridge.

Endocrine differentiation of the fetal ovary and testis is first detected soon after the histologic development of the spermatogenic tubules in the fetal testis at 7 weeks of gestation (Gillman, 1948). The formation of müllerian-inhibiting substance in the testis is associated with the appearance of the spermatogenic tubules (Josso, 1986). Thus, müllerian-inhibiting substance is the primordial hormone of the fetal testis. Consequently, regression of the müllerian ducts is the first event in male phenotypic development. Shortly thereafter, at approximately 8 to 9 weeks of gestation, Leydig's cells are recognized in the interstitium of the testis, and the testis begins to synthesize testosterone (Fig. 36–4) (Siiteri and Wilson, 1974). Although the histologic development of the ovary lags behind that of the testis, the onset of estrogen synthesis by the fetal ovary occurs at approximately the same time as the onset of testosterone

synthesis by the fetal testis (Fig. 36–4) (George and Wilson, 1978).

The endocrine differentiation of the fetal ovary and testis, studied in detail in the rabbit, appears to involve the differential expression of relatively few enzymes in the complex process of synthesizing testosterone and estradiol from cholesterol (George et al., 1979; Wilson et al., 1981). In the 18-day-old rabbit embryo, the activity of the rate-limiting enzyme for testosterone synthesis (3β-hydroxysteroid dehydrogenase-$\Delta^{4,5}$-isomerase) is greater in the testis than in the ovary, and the conversion of testosterone to estradiol (aromatase activity) is greater in the ovary than in the testis. All other enzyme activities in the steroidogenic pathway are initially equal in the ovary and testis (George et al., 1979). Thus, despite the overall complexity of the mechanisms of gonadal differentiation, variations in the activities of only a few enzymes have profound effects on the hormones formed and ultimately on sexual development.

Delineation of the factors that control the initiation of testosterone formation in the fetal testis is of paramount importance in understanding how genetic sex is translated into phenotypic sex. The enzymatic differentiation of the fetal rabbit gonad apparently does not require extragonadal hormones (George et al., 1978; George and Wilson, 1980), and the onset of testosterone secretion also appears to be independent of gonadotropin regulation, despite the fact that functional luteinizing

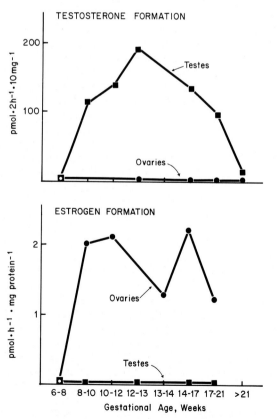

Figure 36–4. Endocrine differentiation of the human fetal ovary and testis. (From Siiteri, P. K., and Wilson, J. D.: J. Clin. Endocrinol. Metab., 38:113–125, 1974 and George, F. W., and Wilson, J. D.: J. Clin. Endocrinol. Metab., 47:550–555, 1978. © The Endocrine Society.)

hormone–human chorionic gonadotropin receptors are detectable in the fetal rabbit testis from the time of onset of testosterone synthesis (Catt et al., 1975; George et al., 1979).

The control of the onset of testosterone synthesis in the human embryo has not been studied in detail, and it is possible that gonadotropins from the placenta (chorionic gonadotropin) or fetal pituitary (luteinizing hormone) have important roles in initiating fetal testicular function in the human (Rabinovici and Jaffe, in press). Receptors for luteinizing hormone have been detected in the human fetal testis as early as the 12th week of gestation (Huhtaniemi et al., 1977; Molsberry et al., 1982), although the effect of the addition of human chorionic gonadotropin in vitro on testosterone synthesis by the fetal testis at this time is controversial (Abramovich et al., 1974; Huhtaniemi et al., 1977; Word et al., 1989). The suggestion that male pseudohermaphroditism can result from a defect in testicular gonadotropin receptors is in keeping with a role for gonadotropin regulation of testosterone synthesis at the time of male phenotypic development (Schwartz et al., 1981). However, until direct studies are done in the human fetal testis between 8 and 12 weeks of gestation, the question of whether gonadotropin plays a role in the initiation of testosterone synthesis in the human fetal testis remains open.

DEVELOPMENT OF PHENOTYPIC SEX

Indifferent Development

The internal accessory organs of both sexes, as well as the renal collecting ducts, are derived from cells of the mesonephric kidney (Fig. 36–5). The mesonephric kidney develops from intermediate mesoderm in the thoracolumbar region of the human embryo during the 4th week of gestation. Tubules form within the substance of the mesonephros and connect primitive capillary networks with a longitudinal mesonephric (wolffian) duct. Caudally, the wolffian duct empties into the primitive urogenital sinus. An outgrowth of the caudal wolf-

fian duct (ureteric bud) gives rise to the excretory ducts and collecting tubules of the permanent (metanephric) kidney. At approximately 6 weeks of development, the paramesonephric (müllerian) duct begins to develop in embryos of both sexes as an evagination in the coelomic epithelium just lateral to the mesonephric duct. This evagination develops into a tubular structure, the caudal end of which is intimately associated with the developing wolffian duct so that no basement membrane separates their epithelia (Fig. 36–6). Whether the müllerian duct "splits off" from the wolffian duct in its later caudal development to become an independent duct system that empties into the urogenital sinus or whether the wolffian duct simply acts as a guide for the subsequent evolution of the müllerian duct from the coelomic epithelium is uncertain. However, müllerian duct development cannot take place in the absence of the wolffian duct (Gruenwald, 1941). At the end of the indifferent phase of phenotypic sexual development (prior to 8 weeks), the dual duct system (wolffian and müllerian) constitutes the anlagen of the internal accessory organs of reproduction (Fig. 36–7).

The termination of the mesonephric ducts in the urogenital sinus divides the sinus into an upper and a lower portion. The upper portion, the vesicourethral canal, is involved in the development of the bladder neck. The lower portion contributes to the development of the prostate and external genitalia. Externally, the genital eminence is a rounded mass between the umbilical cord and the tail (Spaulding, 1921). This eminence is composed of a genital tubercle that is flanked by prominent genital swellings. The opening of the urogenital sinus between the genital swellings (urethral groove) is surrounded by genital folds (see Fig. 36–7). At 7 weeks of gestation the genital tubercle begins to elongate, and a shallow circular depression defines the glans of the tubercle. At this stage of development the external genitalia of male and female embryos are indistinguishable.

Male Development

The initial event in the virilization of the male urogenital tract is the onset of müllerian duct regression,

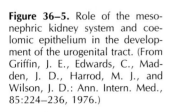

Figure 36–5. Role of the mesonephric kidney system and coelomic epithelium in the development of the urogenital tract. (From Griffin, J. E., Edwards, C., Madden, J. D., Harrod, M. J., and Wilson, J. D.: Ann. Intern. Med., 85:224–236, 1976.)

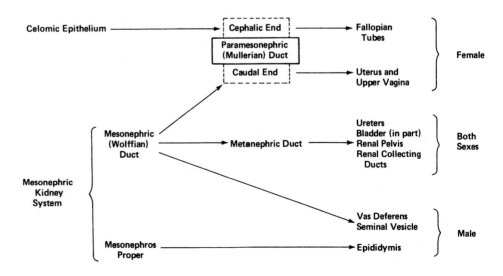

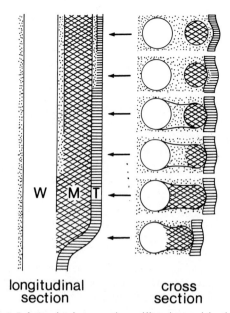

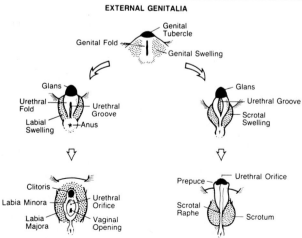

Figure 36–6. Relationship between the wolffian duct and the developing müllerian duct at about 8 weeks of development. The level of each cross-section is indicated by an arrow. M, müllerian duct; T, tubal ridge; W, wolffian duct. The mesenchyme is stippled. (From Gruenwald, P.: Anat. Rec., 81:1–19, 1941.)

which coincides with the development of the spermatogenic cords in the fetal testis between 7 and 8 weeks of gestation (see Fig. 36–2). As a consequence, the müllerian ducts of the male undergo almost complete regression, although a small cranial remnant persists as the nonfunctional appendix testis (Fig. 36–8A), and the extreme lower end can be recognized as the prostatic utricle (Glenister, 1962).

The transformation of the wolffian ducts into the male genital tract begins after müllerian duct regression has commenced. Although most of the mesonephric tubules regress, those adjacent to the testis (epigenital tubules) lose their primitive glomeruli and establish contact with the developing rete and spermatogenic tubules to form the efferent ducts of the testis (see Fig. 36–8A). The part of the wolffian duct that is cranial to the gonad becomes the vestigial appendix epididymis. The portion of the duct immediately distal to the efferent ducts becomes elongated and convoluted to form the epididymis (see Fig. 36–8A). The central portion of the duct develops thick muscular walls to become the vas deferens. At about the 13th week of gestation the seminal vesicles begin to develop as buds from the lower portions of the wolffian ducts (Watson, 1918). The terminal portions of the ducts between the developing seminal vesicles and the urethra become the ejaculatory ducts and the ampullae of the vas deferens. By the end of the 1st trimester of gestation, differentiation of the wolffian ducts of the male is largely complete.

The prostatic and membranous portions of the male urethra develop from the pelvic portion of the urogenital sinus. At about 10 weeks of gestation the endodermal lining of the urethra begins to bud into the surrounding mesenchyme (Bengmark, 1958; Kellokumpu-Lehtinen et al., 1980; Lowsley, 1912). These buds, which are the anlage of the prostatic epithelium, arise from all sides of the urethra but are most extensive in the area surrounding the entry of the wolffian ducts (ejaculatory ducts) into the male urethra (George and Peterson, 1988a). Although the initial differentiation of the prostate occurs early in embryogenesis, extensive growth and development of the gland continue into postnatal life.

Beginning in the 9th week of gestation and continuing through the 12th week, development of the external genitalia of the male and female diverges (see Fig. 36–7) (Spaulding, 1921). In the male, the genital swellings enlarge and migrate posteriorly to form the scrotum. Subsequently, the genital folds fuse over the urethral groove to form the penile urethra. The line of closure remains marked by the penile raphe. When the formation of the urethra is almost complete, the prepuce starts to develop, and by 15 weeks of gestation it completely covers the glans penis (Hunter, 1933). Incomplete fusion of the genital folds over the urethral groove results in various degrees of hypospadias.

The formation of the male genital tract is accomplished largely between 6 and 13 weeks of gestation. During the latter two thirds of gestation two additional

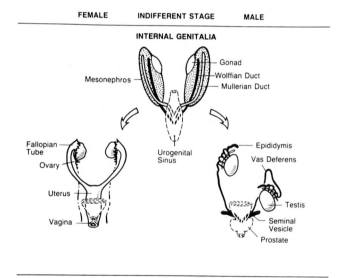

Figure 36–7. Differentiation of the internal and external genitalia of the human fetus.

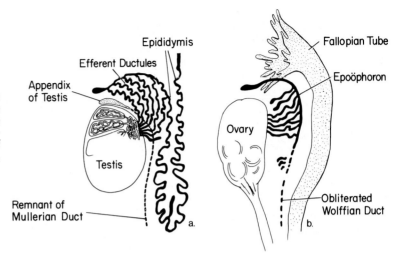

Figure 36–8. The diverse fates of the müllerian and wolffian ducts in the male (a) and female (b). The black areas denote wolffian duct-derived structures, and stippled areas denote müllerian duct derivatives. (From Arey, L. B.: Developmental Anatomy. A Textbook and Laboratory Manual of Embryology, 7th ed. Philadelphia, W. B. Saunders Co., 1974.)

anatomic processes are completed—descent of the testes and differential growth of the male external genitalia.

Testicular descent (Fig. 36–9) is a complex process (Backhouse, 1982). At about the 8th week of human gestation, the testis and the mesonephros are attached to the posterior abdominal wall by a broad peritoneal fold. Subsequently, as the mesonephros degenerates, the portion of this fold cranial to the testis also degenerates. The portion caudal to the testis, however, persists and becomes a narrow ligamentous attachment—the caudal genital ligament that is continuous in the inguinal region with the gubernaculum, a band of mesenchyme extending into the genital swellings (Fig. 36–9A). The gubernaculum anchors the fetal testis to the inguinal region and probably serves to prevent upward movement of the testis, as happens with the kidney, during the rapid elongation of the trunk. In the male embryo, the gubernacular mesenchyme expands. This expansion does not appear to be caused by an increase in cell number. The cells become more widely separated because of an increase in extracellular acid mucopolysaccharides (Backhouse, 1982).

During the 3rd month of gestation a herniation of the coelomic cavity (processus vaginalis) forms on each side of the midline, through the ventral abdominal wall along the course of the gubernaculum (Fig. 36–9B). Herniation probably results from the development of pressure within the abdominal cavity, which is intensified by rapid organ growth after closure of the umbilical cord. Intraabdominal pressure results in enlargement of the processus vaginalis around the gubernaculum and formation of an "inguinal canal."

The opening in the transversalis fascia produced by the processus vaginalis is termed the deep inguinal ring, and the opening in the external oblique aponeurosis is the superficial inguinal ring. In the human embryo, the testis does not move from the abdominal cavity through the inguinal canal and into the scrotum until after the 6th month of gestation. By this time, the gubernaculum has increased in thickness until the width of the inguinal canal approaches that of the testis (Fig. 36–9C). As the scrotum develops, the mesenchyme of the gubernaculum degenerates, and the testis slips through the inguinal canal assisted by abdominal pressure (Backhouse, 1982; Frey et al., 1983). The overall process is thought to be androgen-dependent (Elder et al., 1982; George, 1989; George and Peterson, 1988b; Rajfer and Walsh, 1977), although the precise role of androgen in the process is not well understood. After the testes are in the scrotum, continued development of the abdominal musculature causes closure of the deep and superficial inguinal rings and obliteration of the processus vaginalis.

When formation of the male urethra is largely complete at approximately 11 weeks of gestation, the size of the phallus in the male does not differ substantially from that of the female. However, during the last two trimesters the male external genitalia, prostate, and structures of the wolffian duct grow progressively so that at the time of birth the external genitalia of the male are larger than those of the female.

Female Development

The female reproductive tract is formed from the müllerian ducts. The wolffian ducts persist only in remnant form (epoöphoron) in the mesovarium. Remnants of the caudal wolffian duct are also occasionally found and are termed the Gartner ducts (see Fig. 36–8). The

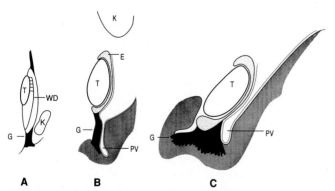

Figure 36–9. Testicular descent. A, Before transabdominal descent. B, Development of the processus vaginalis. C, Transinguinal descent. T, testis; WD, wolffian duct; K, kidney; E, epididymis; G, gubernaculum; and PV, processus vaginalis.

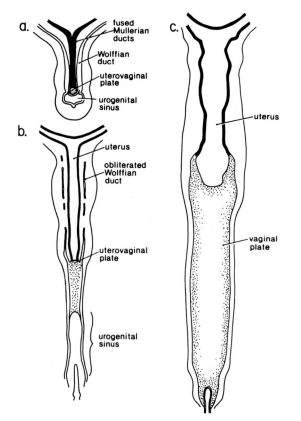

Figure 36–10. Development of the vagina. a, 7 to 8 weeks; b, 10 weeks; c, 20 weeks. (After Koff, A. K.: Carnegie Contributions to Embryology, No. 140, 24:59–90, 1933.)

cephalic ends of the müllerian ducts are the anlagen of the fallopian tubes, whereas the caudal portions fuse to form the uterus (Fig. 36–10). After fusion of the caudal portions of the ducts at 8 to 9 weeks of development, a septum divides the lumen of the uterus into two cavities. This septum subsequently disappears, and by 10 to 11 weeks of gestation, the uterus contains a single cavity lined by cuboidal epithelium. The junction of the body and cervix of the uterus can be recognized by 9 weeks of development, and the formation of the muscular walls of the uterus (myometrium) from the mesenchyme that surrounds the müllerian ducts is essentially completed at about 17 weeks of gestation.

Development of the vagina begins at approximately 9 weeks of gestation with the formation of a solid mass of cells (uterovaginal plate) between the caudal ends of the müllerian ducts and the dorsal wall of the urogenital sinus (see Fig. 36–10) (O'Rahilly, 1977). Although interaction between the müllerian and wolffian ducts and the urogenital sinus is thought to be essential for vaginal development (Acién et al., 1987; Bok and Drews, 1983; Bulmer, 1957; Gruenwald, 1941), the relative contributions of cells derived from these tissues to the development of the uterovaginal plate is not known. The cells of the uterovaginal plate subsequently proliferate, thus increasing the distance between the developing uterus and urogenital sinus (see Fig. 36–10). At 11 weeks of development a lumen begins to form in the caudal end of the vaginal plate; by 20 weeks of gestation canaliza-

tion of the vagina is complete (see Fig. 36–10) (Koff, 1933). The lumen of the vagina remains separated from the urogenital sinus by a thin membrane of mesodermal tissue (hymen).

The ovary also undergoes a partial transabdominal descent analogous to that of the testis. The caudal genital ligament forms the ligament of the ovary and the round ligament of the uterus. However, the gubernaculum and vaginal process remain poorly developed in female embryos, and transinguinal descent of the ovary does not occur. The permanent location of the ovary is just below the rim of the true pelvis.

After about 10 weeks of gestation the genital tubercle of the female bends caudally, the lateral portions of the genital swellings enlarge to form the labia majora, and the posterior portions of the genital swellings fuse to form the posterior fourchette. The urethral folds flanking the urogenital orifice do not fuse but persist as the labia minora (Fig. 36–7B). Thus, in contrast to the male in whom the phallic and perineal portions of the urogenital sinus are enclosed by fusion of the urethral folds and genital swellings, most of the urogenital sinus of the female remains exposed on the surface as a cleft into which the vagina and urethra open.

Breast Development

At 5 weeks of development, paired lines of epidermal thickening extend from the fore limb to the hind limb on the ventral surface of the embryo. Between 6 and 8 weeks of development these "mammary lines" disappear except for a single pair of buds that persist in the thoracic region. These rudimentary mammary buds undergo little development until the 5th month of gestation when secondary epithelial buds begin to appear and nipples develop. Proliferation of the ductules occurs throughout the remainder of gestation so that by the time of birth 15 to 25 separate glands are present, each of which is connected to the exterior through the nipple. Although in some species sexual dimorphism in breast development is apparent during embryogenesis, such dimorphism has never been documented in humans, and postnatal development of the breast in boys and girls is identical prior to the onset of puberty (Pfaltz, 1949).

ENDOCRINE CONTROL OF PHENOTYPIC DIFFERENTIATION

Jost (1953) established that differentiation of the sexual phenotype is ultimately dependent on the type of gonad that develops. The paradigm that chromosomal sex determines gonadal sex and that gonadal sex, in turn, determines phenotypic sex has now become the central dogma of sexual differentiation (see Fig. 36–1). This theory was based on the observation that removing the gonads from embryos of either sex prior to the onset of phenotypic differentiation resulted in the development of a female phenotype. As a consequence of this type of experiment as well as those involving transplantation of embryonic gonads or administration of hormones to embryos, Jost concluded that the male phenotype is induced by testicular secretions, whereas the female does not require hormones from the embryonic ovary. Furthermore, Jost recognized that two products of the fetal testis are essential to male development. The first, müllerian-inhibiting substance, causes regression of the müllerian ducts in the male. The second is an androgenic steroid that is responsible for virilization of the wolffian duct system and urogenital sinus and for formation of the male external genitalia.

Role of Testicular Hormones in Male Development

MÜLLERIAN DUCT REGRESSION. Regression of the müllerian ducts begins in male fetuses at 8 to 9 weeks of gestational age and is mediated by a large (>120 kD) dimeric glycoprotein that is synthesized and secreted by the Sertoli cells of the fetal testis (Blanchard and Josso, 1974; Hayashi et al., 1984; Josso, 1986). The protein has been purified (Picard and Josso, 1984), the complementary (c)DNA has been cloned (Cate et al., 1986; Picard et al., 1986), and the gene has been localized to the short arm of human chromosome 19 (Cohen-Haguenauer et al., 1987). Although the substance was formerly thought to act locally to suppress müllerian duct development (Vigier et al., 1981), the detection of müllerian-inhibiting substance in the serum of boys, but not girls, less than 10 years of age suggests that it may act as a hormone (Baker et al., 1990; Hudson et al., 1990; Josso et al., 1990).

The concept that müllerian duct regression is an active process in male development is supported by studies of males with persistence of müllerian ducts but no evidence of testosterone deficiency (Brook, 1981). The testes in this disorder are usually normal except for lesions associated with cryptorchidism, a common finding in those with persistence of the müllerian ducts. The persistent müllerian duct syndrome is an inherited disorder (Sloan and Walsh, 1976). Defects in both the testicular synthesis and peripheral action of the hormone have been proposed as etiologic factors to explain the persistence of müllerian derivatives in individual pa-

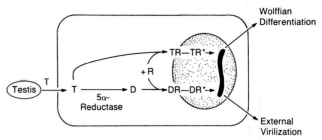

Figure 36–12. Androgen action. T, testosterone; D, dihydrotestosterone; R, androgen receptor.

tients, indicating that the disorder is genetically heterogeneous (Guerrier et al., 1989; Meyers-Wallen et al., 1989).

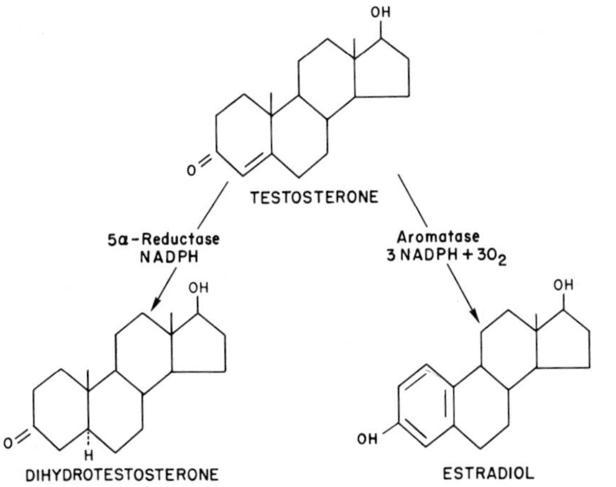

Although the precise mechanism of action of müllerian-inhibiting substance remains poorly understood, two main features of müllerian duct regression are dissolution of the basement membrane and condensation of mesenchymal cells around the müllerian duct (Dyche, 1979; Trelstad et al., 1982). A model, based largely on indirect evidence, proposes that müllerian-inhibiting substance acts by blocking phosphorylation of tyrosine residues on membrane proteins, possibly antagonizing the action of growth factors, such as epidermal growth factor (Cigarroa et al., 1989; Coughlin et al., 1987; Donahoe et al., 1987).

VIRILIZATION OF THE GENITAL TRACT. Virilization in the male fetus results from the action of androgen on specific target organs—the wolffian ducts, urogenital sinus, and external genitalia. Although testosterone is the principal androgen secreted by the fetal testis (George et al., 1987; Siiteri and Wilson, 1974) and adult testis (Hammond et al., 1977), testosterone is thought to have relatively few actions of its own but instead serves as a prohormone for two other potent hormones that are synthesized in target tissues (Fig. 36–11) (Wilson, 1975). Testosterone can undergo irreversible 5α-reduction to dihydrotestosterone, which mediates many of the differentiating, growth-promoting, and functional actions of the hormone. Alternatively, circulating androgens can be converted to estrogens in the peripheral tissues of both sexes. Estrogens in some instances act in concert with androgens to influence physiologic processes but may also exert independent effects on cellular function and on occasion exert effects that are in opposition to those of androgens. Thus, the physiologic consequences of circulating testosterone constitute the sum of the combined effects of testosterone itself and of its estrogenic and androgenic metabolites.

Role of the Androgen Receptor. The current formulation of how androgens act within target cells is depicted in Figure 36–12. Testosterone enters target cells passively by diffusion down an activity gradient. Inside the cell, testosterone binds directly to specific high affinity receptor proteins or undergoes 5α-reduction to dihydrotestosterone before binding to the androgen receptor. The hormone-receptor complex then undergoes a poorly understood "transformation" process in which it is believed to acquire the capacity to bind with high affinity

Figure 36–11. Role of testosterone as a circulating prohormone for the formation of other hormones.

TESTOSTERONE

5α-Reductase
NADPH

Aromatase
3 NADPH + 3O₂

DIHYDROTESTOSTERONE

ESTRADIOL

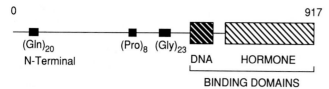

Figure 36–13. Schematic diagram of the androgen receptor.

to specific acceptor sites on the chromatin (Evans, 1988). As a consequence, an increase in transcription of specific messenger RNAs occurs, and ultimately new proteins are synthesized, giving rise to the phenotypic differentiation of the cell that we recognize as virilization.

The essential role of the androgen receptor in mediating the embryonic action of androgens was initially established as the result of studies of the testicular feminization (Tfm) mutation in the mouse. In this X-linked disorder, affected males have testes and normal testosterone production but are profoundly resistant to endogenous and exogenous androgens and develop as phenotypic females (Lyon and Hawkes, 1970). Dihydrotestosterone formation is normal, but the androgen receptor within the cell is not detectable (Bullock et al., 1971; Gehring et al., 1971; Goldstein and Wilson, 1972). Consequently, the hormone fails to interact with the chromosomes and elicit a hormone response. Total failure of androgen-mediated virilization of the wolffian duct, urogenital sinus, and external genitalia occurs. Müllerian duct derivatives (uterus and fallopian tubes) are not present in affected mice, indicating the müllerian-inhibiting function of the fetal testis is unimpaired. Abnormalities of the androgen receptor are also associated with resistance to androgens in humans (see Chapter 37).

The primary structure of the human androgen receptor was established from sequence data of DNA clones (Chang et al., 1988; Lubahn et al., 1988; Tilley et al., 1989; Trapman et al., 1988). The full length cDNA for the human androgen receptor predicts a protein of 917 amino acids and a molecular weight of 98,918. The androgen receptor shares structural similarities with other members of the steroid receptor family (Fig. 36–13). A centrally located DNA-binding domain is particularly well conserved (Carson-Jurica et al., 1990), and the hormone-binding domain is located on the carboxy-terminal end. The amino-terminal segment of the androgen receptor contains three separate homopolymeric segments of unknown function. This region of the molecule may be involved in the modulation of transcriptional activity (Evans, 1988).

Several disorders of the androgen receptor in humans have provided valuable insight into the mechanism of androgen action in embryonic virilization. These abnormalities range from a complete absence of receptor binding to more subtle structural defects in the receptor (Griffin and Wilson, 1989) (see Chapter 37) and cause a spectrum of phenotypic abnormalities ranging from women with the syndrome of complete testicular feminization (androgen insensitivity) to men with minor defects in virilization. In addition, abnormalities in androgen action have been identified in several patients despite the presence of apparently normal androgen binding (Griffin and Wilson, 1989). Not surprisingly, analysis of the various mutations of the androgen receptor at the molecular level has thus far indicated that many different defects in the androgen receptor exist. These mutations encompass deletion of the steroid-binding domain (Brown et al., 1988), deletion of a single nucleotide that results in a frame-shift (He et al., 1990), and point mutations that result in critical amino acid substitutions (Marcelli et al., 1990). Of these, the last is likely to be the most common cause of androgen resistance (Tilley et al., 1990).

Female embryos have the same androgen receptor system and the same ability to respond to androgens as do male embryos. As a consequence, female embryos virilize when exposed to androgens (Schultz and Wilson, 1974). The most common cause of female virilization in humans is congenital adrenal hyperplasia. Increased secretion of adrenal androgens virilize the external genitalia in affected females (New et al., 1989). Thus, differences in anatomic development between males and females are dependent on differences in the hormonal signals themselves and not on differences in the receptors for hormones.

Role of Dihydrotestosterone. In human development, the 5α-reductase enzyme that converts testosterone to dihydrotestosterone is present in anlagen of the external genitalia (genital tubercle and urogenital sinus and swellings) prior to the onset of phenotypic differentiation (Fig. 36–14) (Siiteri and Wilson, 1974). The wolffian duct, however, is incapable of converting testosterone to dihydrotestosterone until after male phenotypic differentiation is advanced and after the epididymis and seminal vesicle are formed. This difference between the human wolffian duct system, on the one hand, and the urogenital sinus and urogenital swellings and tubercle, on the other, is also true for other mammalian species. Thus, virilization of the external genitalia appears to be mediated by dihydrotestosterone, whereas testosterone itself appears to be responsible for virilization of the wolffian ducts. This view is substantiated by studies of humans with hereditary deficiency of the 5α-reductase enzyme in which the external genitalia fail to virilize because of the inability to form dihydrotestosterone in peripheral tissues. However, in affected individuals, the wolffian duct–derived structures—epididymis, vas deferens, and seminal vesicles—virilize normally (Walsh et al., 1974). Furthermore, the administration of specific 5α-reductase inhibitors to pregnant rats at the appropriate time during embryonic sexual differentiation causes undervirilized male offspring that are phenocopies of humans with 5α-reductase deficiency (George and Peterson, 1988a).

It is not clear why testosterone is responsible for one portion of virilization (wolffian duct differentiation) and dihydrotestosterone, for the remainder of the process. The fact that androgen-dependent tissues of wolffian duct origin fail to develop in animals and humans with single gene mutations that impair the androgen receptor is strong evidence that testosterone and dihydrotestosterone act via the same receptor. Because dihydrotestosterone binds with greater affinity to the androgen receptor than does testosterone (George and Noble,

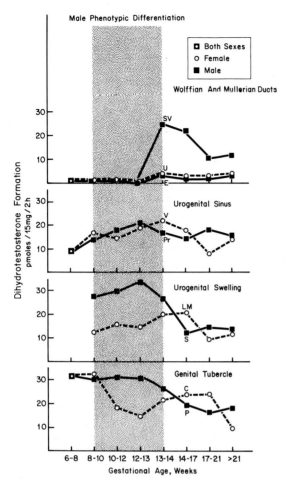

Figure 36–14. Dihydrotestosterone in urogenital tract tissues of the human fetus. SV, seminal vesicle; U, uterus; E, epididymis; V, vagina; Pr, prostate; LM, labia majora; S, scrotum; C, clitoris; P, penis. (From Siiteri, P. K., and Wilson, J. D.: J. Clin. Endocrinol. Metab., 38:113–125, 1974. © The Endocrine Society.)

Mesenchymal-Epithelial Interactions in Sexual Differentiation. Tissue recombination studies in mice indicate that the mesenchyme plays an important role in androgen-mediated differentiation of the urogenital tract (Cunha et al., 1983) and regression of the mammary bud (Kratochwil and Schwartz, 1976) in the male. For example, when tissue recombinants of embryonic urinary bladder epithelium and urogenital sinus mesenchyme are exposed to androgens, the epithelium develops prostatic buds. However, recombinants of epithelium from the urogenital sinus and mesenchyme from other embryonic sites are incapable of prostatic development under similar circumstances (Cunha et al., 1983). Furthermore, mesenchyme from the urogenital sinus of the androgen-insensitive Tfm mouse fails to mediate prostatic growth when recombined with normal urogenital sinus epithelium, whereas epithelium from the urogenital sinus of the Tfm mouse undergoes prostate formation in the presence of androgen when recombined with normal mesenchyme (Cunha and Lung, 1978; Lasnitzki and Mizuno, 1980). Similarly, androgen-mediated regression of the mammary bud in the male mouse requires an androgen-responsive mesenchyme. When normal, wild-type mouse mammary epithelium, containing a bud rudiment, is recombined with mammary mesenchyme from an androgen-resistant Tfm mouse, normal androgen-dependent regression of the bud does not occur, whereas mammary bud regression does occur in recombinants of wild-type mesenchyme and Tfm epithelium (Kratochwil and Schwartz, 1976).

These studies imply that the ability of a tissue to respond to androgenic stimulation resides in the mesenchyme of that tissue and emphasize the overall complexity of hormonal mediated events involved in morphogenesis and cellular differentiation of tissues. Understanding the nature of these mesenchymal-epithelial interactions is fundamental to understanding the hormonal control of sexual differentiation.

Role of Hormones in the Development of the Female Phenotype and the Breast

Embryogenesis takes place in a "sea" of steroid and nonsteroid hormones derived from the placenta, the maternal circulation, the fetal adrenal gland, the fetal testis, and possibly the fetal ovary. Because the embryo develops in the "female environment" of the mother, it has not been possible to devise a definitive experiment to determine whether any of these hormones is essential for female development. Even if not essential for the differentiation of the female urogenital tract, estrogens and progestogens are probably involved in the growth and maturation of the accessory reproductive organs of the female during the later phases of embryonic life.

Dimorphism in the development of the breast in human males and females has not been documented prior to puberty, and the transient milk secretion in the newborn male and female suggests no functional difference between the two sexes until later in life (Pfaltz, 1949). The endocrinologic control of female breast de-

1984; Wilbert et al., 1983) suggests that dihydrotestosterone formation may be an amplifying signal for androgen action in peripheral tissues. The wolffian ducts are in close proximity to the fetal testes, and the concentration of testosterone in the lumen of the wolffian ducts might be sufficiently high to overcome its low affinity for the androgen receptor, possibly mediating the virilization of the wolffian ducts. To substantiate this theory, it will be necessary to establish whether the concentration of testosterone in the wolffian ducts is substantially higher than in plasma and other androgen target tissues. A separate testosterone receptor may be transiently expressed in the embryonic wolffian duct.

In summary, three testicular hormones are thought to be involved in male phenotypic differentiation. The regression of the müllerian duct is mediated by müllerian-inhibiting substance, a hormone secreted by the Sertoli cells of the fetal testis. The other aspects of male phenotypic development of the embryo are accomplished by androgenic steroids. Testosterone, the androgen secreted by the fetal testis, causes virilization of the wolffian ducts prior to the development of their ability to form dihydrotestosterone. Dihydrotestosterone is responsible for virilization of the external genitalia and the male urethra.

velopment and milk formation in postembryonic life is complex. Estrogen plays a key role in the growth and maturation of the normal gland, and the administration of estrogen, or the alteration of the normal male ratio of androgen to estrogen, can result in profound breast development in the male at any phase in life. This supports the concept that embryonic development of the tissue in the male and female embryos is not fundamentally different (Wilson et al., 1980).

SUMMARY

Although genes located on the autosomes as well as on the sex chromosomes contribute to the establishment of genetic sex, determinants on the Y chromosomes in the male embryo are paramount in inducing differentiation of the indifferent gonadal primordia into testes. In the absence of the Y chromosome, the indifferent gonad develops into an ovary. The function of the embryonic gonads as endocrine organs determines the development of phenotypic sex. Specifically, the secretion by the fetal testis of two hormones—müllerian-inhibiting substance and testosterone—imposes male development on the indifferent fetus. Testosterone and its metabolite dihydrotestosterone act to virilize the male fetus via the same receptor machinery that mediates androgen action in the postnatal state. This receptor machinery is present in both male and female embryos. Consequently, normal phenotypic development is determined solely by the presence in males or absence in females of specific hormonal signals during a critical phase of embryonic development.

The characterization in humans and animals of several single gene defects that result in various forms of abnormal sexual development has aided in the elucidation of the genetic, molecular, and endocrine aspects of sexual differentiation. However, many of the most fundamental issues in sexual differentiation are still poorly understood. These include understanding the regulatory factors that control germ cell migration and gonadal differentiation and elucidation of the processes by which embryonic tissues acquire the ability to respond to a hormonal stimulus and, consequently, to undergo dimorphic anatomic and functional development.

Ultimately, these fundamental problems of embryology must be resolved before we can understand the overall program by which the myriad genetic and regulatory factors interact to cause differentiation of the sexual phenotypes.

REFERENCES

Abramovich, D. R., Baker, T. G., and Neal, P.: Effect of human chorionic gonadotropin on testosterone secretion by the human fetal testis in organ culture. J. Endocrinol., 60:179, 1974.

Acién, P., Arminana, E., and Garcia-Ontiveros, E.: Unilateral renal agenesis associated with ipsilateral blind vagina. Arch. Gynecol., 240:1, 1987.

Arey, L. B.: Developmental Anatomy: A Textbook and Laboratory Manual of Embryology, 7th ed. Philadelphia, W. B. Saunders Co., 1974.

Backhouse, K. M.: Embryology of testicular descent and maldescent. Urol. Clin. North Am., 9:315, 1982.

Baker, M. L., Metcalfe, S. A., and Hutson, J. M.: Serum levels of müllerian-inhibiting substance in boys from birth to 18 years, as determined by enzyme immunoassay. J. Clin. Endocrinol. Metab., 70:11, 1990.

Bengmark, S.: The Prostatic Urethra and Prostatic Glands. Lund, Sweden, Berlingska Boktryckeriet, 1958.

Blanchard, M. G., and Josso, N.: Source of the anti-müllerian hormone synthesized by the fetal testis: müllerian-inhibiting activity of the fetal bovine Sertoli cells in tissue culture. Pediatr. Res., 8(12):968, 1974.

Bok, G., and Drews, U.: The role of the wolffian ducts in the formation of the sinus vagina: an organ culture study. J. Embryol. Exp. Morphol., 73:275, 1983.

Brook, C. G. D.: Persistent müllerian duct syndrome. Pediatr. Adolesc. Endocrinol., 8:100, 1981.

Brown, T. R., Lubahn, D. B., Wilson, E. M., Joseph, D. R., French, F. W., and Migeon, C. J.: Deletion of the steroid-binding domain of the human androgen receptor gene in one family with complete androgen insensitivity syndrome: Evidence for further genetic heterogeneity in this syndrome. Proc. Natl. Acad. Sci. U S A, 85:8151, 1988.

Bullock, L. P., Bardin, C. W., and Ohno, S.: The androgen insensitive mouse: absence of intranuclear androgen retention in the kidney. Biochem. Biophys. Res. Commun., 44:1537, 1971.

Bulmer, D.: The development of the human vagina. J. Anat., 91:490, 1957.

Carson-Jurica, M. A., Schrader, W. T., and O'Malley, B. W.: Steroid receptor family: Structure and functions. Endocr. Rev., 11:201, 1990.

Cate, R. L., Mattaliano, R. J., Hession, C., Tizard, R., Farber, N. M., Cheung, A., Ninfa, E. G., Frey, A. Z., Gash, D. J., Chow, E. P., Fisher, R. A., Bertonis, J. M., Torres, G., Wallner, B. P., Ramachandran, K. L., Ragin, R. C., Manganaro, T. F., Maclaughlin, D. T., and Donahoe, P. K.: Isolation of the bovine and human genes for müllerian-inhibiting substance and expression of the human gene in animal cells. Cell, 45:685, 1986.

Catt, K. J., Dufau, M. L., Neaves, W. B., Walsh, P. C., and Wilson, J. D.: LH-hCG receptors and testosterone content during differentiation of the testis in the rabbit embryo. Endocrinology, 97:1157, 1975.

Chang, C., Kokontis, J., and Liao, S.: Structural analysis of complementary DNA and amino acid sequences of human and rat androgen receptors. Proc. Natl. Acad. Sci. U S A, 85:7211, 1988.

Ciagarroa, F. G., Coughlin, J. P., Donahoe, P. K., White, M. F., Uitvlugt, N., and MacLaughlin, D. T.: Recombinant human müllerian-inhibiting substance inhibits epidermal growth factor receptor tyrosine kinase. Growth Factors, 1:179, 1989.

Cohen-Haguenauer, O., Picard, J. Y., Mattéi, M.-G., Serero, S., Van Cong, N., de Tand, M.-F., Guerrier, D., Hors-Cayla, M.-C., Josso, N., and Frézal, J.: Mapping of the gene for anti-müllerian hormone to the short arm of human chromosome 19. Cytogenet. Cell Genet., 44:2, 1987.

Coughlin, J. P., Donahoe, P. K., Budzik, G. P., and MacLaughlin, D. T.: Müllerian-inhibiting substance blocks autophosphorylation of the EGF receptor by inhibiting tyrosine kinase. Mol. Cell. Endocrinol., 49:75, 1987.

Cunha, G. R., Chung, L. W. K., Shannon, J. M., Taguchi, O., and Fujii, H.: Hormone-induced morphogenesis and growth: role of mesenchymal-epithelial interactions. Recent Prog. Horm. Res., 39:559, 1983.

Cunha, G. R., and Lung, B.: The possible influence of temporal factors in androgenic responsiveness of urogenital tissue recombinants from wild-type and androgen-insensitive (Tfm) mice. J. Exp. Zool., 205:181, 1978.

Donahoe, P. K., Cate, R. L., MacLaughlin, D. T., Epstein, J., Fuller, A. F., Takahashi, M., Coughlin, J. P., Ninfa, E. G., and Taylor, L. A.: Müllerian-inhibiting substance: Gene structure and mechanism of action of a fetal regressor. Recent Prog. Horm. Res., 43:431, 1987.

Dyche, W. J.: A comparative study of the differentiation and involution of the müllerian duct and wolffian duct in the male and female mouse. J. Morphol., 162:175, 1979.

Elder, J. S., Isaacs, J. T., and Walsh, P. C.: Androgenic sensitivity of the gubernaculum testis: Evidence for hormonal/mechanical interactions in testicular descent. J. Urol., 127:170, 1982.

Evans, R. M.: The steroid and thyroid hormone receptor superfamily. Science, 240:889, 1988.

Frey, H. L., Peng, S., and Rajfer, J.: Synergy of abdominal pressure and androgens in testicular descent. Biol. Reprod., 29:1233, 1983.

Gehring, U., Tomkins, G. M., and Ohno, S.: Effect of the androgen-insensitivity mutation on a cytoplasmic receptor for dihydrotestosterone. Nature, 232:106, 1971.

George, F. W.: Developmental pattern of 5α-reductase activity in the rat gubernaculum. Endocrinology, 124:727, 1989.

George, F. W., Carr, B. R., Noble, J. F., and Wilson, J. D.: 5α-Reduced androgens in the human fetal testis. J. Clin. Endocrinol. Metab., 64:628, 1987.

George, F. W., Catt, K. J., Neaves, W. B., and Wilson, J. D.: Studies on the regulation of testosterone synthesis in the rabbit fetal testis. Endocrinology, 102:665, 1978.

George, F. W., and Noble, J. F.: Androgen receptors are similar in fetal and adult rabbits. Endocrinology, 115:1451, 1984.

George, F. W., and Peterson, K. G.: 5α-Dihydrotestosterone formation is necessary for embryogenesis of the rat prostate. Endocrinology, 122:1159, 1988a.

George, F. W., and Peterson, K. G.: Partial characterization of the androgen receptor of the newborn rat gubernaculum. Biol. Reprod., 39:536, 1988b.

George, F. W., Simpson, E. R., Milewich, L., and Wilson, J. D.: Studies on the regulation of steroid hormone biosynthesis in fetal rabbit gonads. Endocrinology, 105:1100, 1979.

George, F. W., and Wilson, J. D.: Conversion of androgen to estrogen by the human fetal ovary. J. Clin. Endocrinol. Metab., 47:550, 1978.

George, F. W., and Wilson, J. D.: Endocrine differentiation of the fetal rabbit ovary in culture. Nature, 283:861, 1980.

George, F. W., and Wilson, J. D.: Sex determination and differentiation. In Knobil, E., and Neill, J. (Eds.): The Physiology of Reproduction. New York, Raven Press, 1988, pp. 3–26.

Gillman, J.: The development of the gonads in man, with a consideration of the role of fetal endocrines and the histogenesis of ovarian tumors. Carnegie Contributions to Embryology, No. 210, 32:83, 1948.

Glenister, T. W.: The development of the utricle and of the so-called "middle" or "median" lobe of the human prostate. J. Anat., 96:443, 1962.

Goldstein, J. L., and Wilson, J. D.: Studies on the pathogenesis of the pseudohermaphroditism in the mouse with testicular feminization. J. Clin. Invest., 51:1647, 1972.

Gondos, B., Bhinaleus, P., and Habel, C. J.: Ultrastructural observations on germ cells in human fetal ovaries. Am. J. Obstet. Gynecol., 110:644, 1971.

Goodfellow, P. N., Ropers, H.-H., and Davis, K.: Report of the X and Y committee, human gene mapping 8. Cytogenet. Cell Genet., 40:296–352, 1985.

Griffin, J. E., Edwards, C., Madden, J. D., Harrod, M. J., and Wilson, J. D.: Congenital absence of the vagina. The Mayer-Rokitansky-Kuster-Hauser syndrome. Ann. Intern. Med., 85:224–236, 1976.

Griffin, J. E., and Wilson, J. D.: The androgen resistance syndromes: 5α-reductase deficiency, testicular feminization, and related disorders. In Scriver, C. R., Beaudet, A. L., Sly, W. S., and Valle, D. (Eds.): The Metabolic Basis of Inherited Disease, 6th ed. New York, McGraw-Hill, 1989, pp. 1919–1944.

Gruenwald, P.: The relation of the growing müllerian duct to the wolffian duct and its importance for the genesis of malformation. Anat. Rec., 81:1, 1941.

Gubbay, J., Collignon, J., Koopman, P., Capel, B., Economou, A., Münsterberg, A., Vivian, N., Goodfellow, P., and Levell-Badge, R.: A gene mapping to the sex-determining region of the mouse Y chromosome is a member of a novel family of embryonically expressed genes. Nature, 346:245–250, 1990.

Guerrier, D., Tran, D., Vanderwinden, J. M., Hideux, S., Outryve, L. V., Legeai, L., Bouchard, M., Vliet, G. V., de Laet, M. H., Picard, J. Y., Kahn, A., and Josso, N.: The persistent müllerian duct syndrome: A molecular approach. J. Clin. Endocrinol. Metab., 68:46, 1989.

Hammond, G. L., Ruokonen, A., Kontturi, M., Koskela, E., and Vihko, R.: The simultaneous radioimmunoassay of seven steroids in human spermatic and peripheral venous blood. J. Clin. Endocrinol. Metab., 45:16, 1977.

Handel, M. A., and Eppig, J. J.: Sertoli cell differentiation in the testes of mice genetically deficient in germ cells. Biol. Reprod., 20:1031, 1979.

Hayashi, M., Shima, H., Hayashi, K., Trelstad, R. L., and Donahoe, P. K.: Immunocytochemical localization of müllerian inhibiting substance in the rough endoplasmic reticulum and Golgi apparatus in Sertoli cells of the neonatal calf testis using a monoclonal antibody. J. Histochem. Cytochem., 32:649, 1984.

He, W. W., Young, C. Y.-F., and Tindall, D. J.: The molecular basis of the mouse testicular feminization (Tfm) mutation: A frame-shift mutation. Program and Abstracts, The Endocrine Society 72nd Annual Meeting, June 20–23, 1990, Atlanta, Abstract No. 862, 1990, p. 240.

Hudson, P. L., Dougas, I., Donahoe, P. K., Cate, R. L., Epstein, J., Pepinsky, R. B., and MacLaughlin, D. T.: An immunoassay to detect human müllerian inhibiting substance in males and females during normal development. J. Clin. Endocrinol. Metab., 70:16, 1990.

Huhtaniemi, I. T., Korenbrat, C. C., and Jaffe, R. R.: HCG binding and stimulation of testosterone biosynthesis in the human fetal testis. J. Clin. Endocrinol. Metab., 44(5):963, 1977.

Hunter, R. H.: Notes on the development of the prepuce. J. Anat., 70:68, 1933.

Jirasek, J. E.: Development of the Genital System and Male Pseudohermaphroditism. Baltimore, Johns Hopkins Press, 1971.

Josso, N.: Antimüllerian hormone: New perspectives for a sexist molecule. Endocr. Rev., 7:421, 1986.

Josso, N., Legeai, L., Forest, M. G., Chaussain, J.-L., and Brauner, R.: An enzyme-linked immunoassay for anti-müllerian hormone: A new tool for the evaluation of testicular function in infants and children. J. Clin. Endocrinol. Metab., 70:23, 1990.

Jost, A.: Problems of fetal endocrinology: The gonadal and hypophyseal hormones. Recent Prog. Horm. Res., 8:379, 1953.

Jost, A., and Magre, S.: Testicular developmental phases and dual hormonal control of organogenesis. In Serio, M., et al. (Eds.): Sexual Differentiation: Basic and Clinical Aspects. New York, Raven Press, 1984, pp. 1–15.

Kellokumpu-Lehtinen, P., Santti, R., and Pellíniemi, L. J.: Correlation of early cytodifferentiation of the human fetal prostate and Leydig cells. Anat. Rec., 196:253, 1980.

Koff, A. K.: Development of the vagina in the human fetus. Carnegie Contributions to Embryology, No. 140, 24:59, 1933.

Kratochwil, K., and Schwartz, P.: Tissue interaction in androgen response of embryonic mammary rudiment of the mouse: Identification of the target tissue for testosterone. Proc. Natl. Acad. Sci. U S A, 73:4041, 1976.

Langman, J.: Medical Embryology, 4th ed. Baltimore, Williams & Wilkins, 1981.

Lasnitzki, I., and Mizuno, T.: Prostate induction: Interaction of epithelium and mesenchyme from normal wild-type and androgen insensitive mice with testicular feminization. J. Endocrinol., 85:423, 1980.

Lowsley, O. S.: The development of the human prostate gland with reference to the development of other structures at the neck of the urinary bladder. Am. J. Anat., 13:299, 1912.

Lubahn, D. B., Joseph, D. R., Sullivan, P. M., Willard, H. F., French, F. S., and Wilson, E. M.: Cloning of human androgen receptor complementary DNA and localization to the X chromosome. Science, 240:327, 1988.

Lyon, M. F., and Hawkes, S. G.: X-linked gene for testicular feminization in the mouse. Nature, 227:1217, 1970.

Marcelli, M., Tilley, W. D., Wilson, C. M., Wilson, J. D., Griffin, J. E., and McPhaul, M. J.: A single nucleotide substitution introduces a premature termination codon into the androgen receptor gene of a patient with receptor-negative androgen resistance. J. Clin. Invest., 85:1522–1528, 1990.

McCarrey, J. R., and Abbott, U. K.: Chick gonad differentiation following excision of primordial germ cells. Dev. Biol., 66:256, 1978.

McCarrey, J. R., and Abbott, U. K.: Mechanisms of genetic sex determination, gonadal sex differentiation, and germ-cell development in animals. Adv. Genet., 20:217, 1979.

Merchant, H.: Rat gonadal and ovarian organogenesis with and without germ cells. An ultrastructural study. Dev. Biol., 44:1, 1975.

Meyers-Wallen, V. N., Donahoe, P. K., Ueno, S., Manganaro, T. F., and Patterson, D. F.: Müllerian-inhibiting substance is present in testes of dogs with persistent müllerian duct syndrome. Biol. Reprod., 41:881, 1989.

Molsberry, R. L., Carr, B. R., Mendelson, C. R., and Simpson, E. R.: Human chorionic gonadotropin binding to human fetal testes as a function of gestational age. J. Clin. Endocrinol. Metab., 55:791, 1982.

New, M. I., White, P. C., Pang, S., Dupont, B., and Speiser, P. W. The adrenal hyperplasias. In Scriver, C. W., Beaudet, A. L., Sly, W. S., and Valle, D. (Eds.): The Metabolic Basis of Inherited Disease, 6th ed. New York, McGraw-Hill, 1989, pp. 1881–1918.

O'Rahilly, R.: The development of the vagina in the human. In Blandau, R. J., and Bergsma, D. (Eds.): Morphogenesis and Malformation of the Genital System. Birth Defects Original Article Series. Vol. XIII, 1977, pp. 123–136.

Page, D. C., Mosher, R., Simpson, E. M., Fisher, E. M. C., Mardon, G., Pollack, J., McGillivray, B., de la Chapelle, A., and Brown, L. G.: The sex-determining region of the human Y chromosome encodes a finger protein. Cell, 51:1091, 1987.

Palmer, M. S., Sinclair, A. H., Berta, P., Ellis, N. A., Goodfellow, P. N., Abbas, N. E., and Fellous, M.: Genetic evidence that ZFY is not the testis-determining factor. Nature, 342:937, 1989.

Peters, H.: Migration of gonocytes into the mammalian gonad and their differentiation. Philos. Trans. R. Soc. Lond. (Biol.), 259:91, 1970.

Pfaltz, C. R.: Das embryonale and postnatale Verhalten den Männlichen Brustdruse beim Menschern. II. Das Mammanorgan in Kurder-, Junglings-Mannes-, und Greisenalten. Acta Anat., 8:293, 1949.

Picard, J. Y., Benarous, R., Guerrier, D., Josso, N., and Kahn, A.: Cloning and expression of cDNA for anti-müllerian hormone. Proc. Natl. Acad. Sci. U S A, 83:5464, 1986.

Picard, J. Y., and Josso, N.: Purification of testicular anti-müllerian hormone allowing direct visualization of the pure glycoprotein and determination of yield and purification factor. Mol. Cell. Endocrinol., 34:23, 1984.

Polani, P. E.: Abnormal sex development in man. I. Anomalies of sex determining mechanisms. In Austin, C. R., and Edwards, G. (Eds.): Mechanisms of Sex Differentiation in Animals and Man. London, Academic Press, 1981, pp. 465–547.

Rabinovici, J., and Jaffe, R. B.: Development and regulation of growth and differentiated function in humans and subhuman primate fetal gonads. Endocrinol. Rev., 11:532, 1990.

Rajfer, J., and Walsh, P. C.: Hormonal regulation of testicular descent: Experimental and clinical observations. J. Urol., 118:985, 1977.

Schultz, F. M., and Wilson, J. D.: Virilization of the wolffian duct in the rat fetus by various androgens. Endocrinology, 94:979, 1974.

Schwartz, M., Imperato-McGinley, J., Petersen, R. E., Cooper, G., Morris, P. L., MacGillivray, M., and Hensle, T.: Male pseudohermaphroditism secondary to an abnormality in Leydig cell differentiation. J. Clin. Endocrinol. Metab., 53:123, 1981.

Siiteri, P. K., and Wilson, J. D.: Testosterone formation and metabolism during male sexual differentiation in the human embryo. J. Clin. Endocrinol. Metab., 38:113, 1974.

Sinclair, A. H., Berta, P., Palmer, M. S., Hawkins, J. R., Griffiths, B. L., Smith, M. J., Foster, J. W., Frischauf, A.-M., Levell-Badge, R., and Goodfellow, P. N.: A gene from the human sex-determining region encodes a protein with homology to a conserved DNA-binding motif. Nature, 346:240–244, 1990.

Sloan, W. R., and Walsh, P. C.: Familial persistent müllerian duct syndrome. J. Urol., 115:459, 1976.

Spaulding, M. H.: The development of the external genitalia in the human embryo. Carnegie Contributions to Embryology, No. 61, 13:67, 1921.

Tilley, W. D., Marcelli, M., and McPhaul, M. J.: Recent studies of the androgen receptor: new insights into old questions. Mol. Cell. Endocrinol., 68:C7–C10, 1990.

Tilley, W. D., Marcelli, M., Wilson, J. D., and McPhaul, M. J.: Characterization and expression of a cDNA encoding the human androgen receptor. Proc. Natl. Acad. Sci. U S A, 86:327, 1989.

Trapman, J., Klaassen, P., Kniper, G. G. J. M., van der Korput, J. A. G. M., Faber, P. W., van Rooij, H. C. J., Geurts van Kessel, A., Voorhorst, M. M., Mulder, E., and Brinkmann, A. O.: Cloning, structure and expression of a cDNA encoding the human androgen receptor. Biochem. Biophys. Res. Comm., 153:241, 1988.

Trelstad, R. L., Hayashi, A., Hayashi, K., and Donahoe, P. K.: The epithelial-mesenchymal interface of the male rat müllerian duct: Loss of basement membrane integrity and ductal regression. Dev. Biol., 92:27, 1982.

Vigier, B., Picard, J. Y., Bezard, J., and Josso, N.: Anti-müllerian hormone: A local or long-distance morphogenetic factor? Hum. Genet., 58:85, 1981.

Walsh, P. C., Madden, J. D., Harrod, M. J., Goldstein, J. L., MacDonald, P. C., and Wilson, J. D.: Familial incomplete male pseudohermaphroditism, type 2: Decreased dihydrotestosterone formation is pseudovaginal perineoscrotal hypospadias. N. Engl. J. Med., 291:944, 1974.

Watson, E. M.: The development of the seminal vesicles in man. Am. J. Anat., 24:395, 1918.

Wilbert, D. M., Griffin, J. E., and Wilson, J. D.: Characterization of the cytosol androgen receptor of the human prostate. J. Clin. Endocrinol. Metab., 56:113, 1983.

Wilson, J. D.: Metabolism of testicular androgens. In Greep, R. O., and Astwood, E. G. (Eds.): Handbook of Physiology (Chapter 25, Section 7). Endocrinology, Vol. V. Male Reproductive System. Washington, D.C., American Physiological Society, 1975, pp. 491–508.

Wilson, J. D., Aiman, J., and MacDonald, P. C.: The pathogenesis of gynecomastia. Adv. Intern. Med., 25:1, 1980.

Wilson, J. D., and Goldstein, J. L.: Classification of hereditary disorders of sexual development. In Bergsma, D. (Ed.): Genetic Forms of Hypogonadism. Birth Defects Original Article Series, Vol. XI, 1975, pp. 1–16.

Wilson, J. D., Griffin, J. E., Leshin, M., and George, F. W.: Role of gonadal hormones in development of the sexual phenotypes. Hum. Genet., 58:78, 1981.

Witschi, E.: Migration of the germ cells of human embryos from the yolk sac to the primitive gonadal folds. Carnegie Contributions to Embryology, No. 209, 32:69, 1948.

Word, R. A., George, F. W., Wilson, J. D., and Carr, B. R.: Testosterone synthesis and adenylate cyclase activity in the early human fetal testis appear to be independent of human chorionic gonadotropin control. J. Clin. Endocrinol. Metab., 69:204, 1989.

37
DISORDERS OF SEXUAL DIFFERENTIATION

James E. Griffin, M.D.
Jean D. Wilson, M.D.

Normal sexual differentiation is a sequential and orderly process; chromosomal sex determines gonadal sex, and gonadal sex, in turn, determines phenotypic sex (see Chapter 36). Phenotypic sex encompasses the development of the male and female urogenital tracts and of the capacity to reproduce. Disturbances that impair any step in this process during embryonic life cause disorders of sexual differentiation.

Such disturbances can involve a variety of mechanisms: an environmental insult, as in the ingestion of a virilizing drug during pregnancy; nonfamilial aberrations of the sex chromosomes, as in 45,X gonadal dysgenesis; developmental birth defects of multifactorial origin, as in most cases of hypospadias; and hereditary disorders resulting from single-gene mutations, as in the syndromes of androgen resistance.

Pathophysiologically, abnormalities in sexual development can be categorized as resulting from derangements in any of the three principal processes involved in sexual differentiation, namely, disorders of chromosomal sex, disorders of gonadal sex, and disorders of phenotypic sex. This categorization is useful both conceptually and clinically, but two problems should be recognized. First, the manifestations of these disorders vary in severity from complete dissociation between genotype and phenotype, as in the testicular feminization syndrome, to inappropriate or impaired pubertal development to infertility in otherwise normal individuals (Table 37–1). This broad array of manifestations results from the fact that these disorders vary in the severity of their effects (e.g., the 47,XXY karyotype may predominantly impair fertility in men, whereas 46,XY/45,X mosaicism commonly results in sexual ambiguity). Second, because the process of sexual differentiation is sequential, specific manifestations of abnormal development such as hypospadias can result from the deviations that occur at any stage in the process.

Despite problems of variability and overlap, the correct diagnosis can usually be ascertained if all relevant clinical information is assembled, including analysis of the family history, delineation of the chromosomal complement, assessment of the endocrine status, and characterization of the anatomic features.

However, diagnosis can be difficult in the prepubertal and neonatal periods, when prediction of ultimate endocrine status may not be practical. Even in such instances, however, the combination of genetic, phenotypic, and chromosomal assessment usually restricts the diagnostic possibilities to a limited number of conditions so that appropriate gender assignment can be made and the phenotype can be suitably tailored.

DISORDERS OF CHROMOSOMAL SEX

Disorders of chromosomal sex occur when the number or structure of the X or Y chromosomes is abnormal (Table 37–2).

Klinefelter Syndrome

Klinefelter, Reifenstein, and Albright (1942) described a disorder in men characterized by small firm testes, varying degrees of impaired sexual maturation, azoospermia, gynecomastia, and elevated levels of urinary gonadotropins. The fundamental defect is the presence of an extra X chromosome in a male (Jacobs and Strong, 1959). The common karyotype is either a 47,XXY chromosomal pattern (the classic form) or 46,XY/47,XXY (the mosaic form). This disorder is the most common, major abnormality of sexual differentiation with an incidence of approximately 1 in 500 males.

CLINICAL FEATURES. Individuals with the Klinefelter syndrome usually come to medical attention after the time of expected puberty and often are diagnosed only incidentally. Prepubertally, patients have small testes with decreased numbers of spermatogonia,

Table 37–1. COMMON MANIFESTATIONS OF
ABNORMALITIES OF SEXUAL DIFFERENTIATION

Ambiguous Genitalia in the Newborn
True hermaphroditism
Mixed gonadal dysgenesis
The absent testes syndrome
Female pseudohermaphroditism
Male pseudohermaphroditism
Inappropriate Pubertal Development
Congenital adrenal hyperplasia due to 21- or 11- hydroxylase
deficiency
True hermaphroditism
Impaired Pubertal Development
Gonadal dysgenesis
Klinefelter syndrome
XX Male syndrome
Pure gonadal dysgenesis
Absent testes syndrome
Congenital adrenal hyperplasia due to 17-hydroxylase deficiency in
females
Male pseudohermaphroditism
Infertility
Klinefelter syndrome
XX Male syndrome
Infertile male with androgen resistance

but otherwise they appear normal. After puberty the disorder becomes manifest as infertility; gynecomastia; or, occasionally, underandrogenization (Fig. 37–1). The various clinical features are summarized in Table 37–3. Damage to the seminiferous tubules and azoospermia are consistent features of the 47,XXY variety. The small firm testes are characteristically less than 2 cm and always less than 3.5 cm in length (corresponding to 2 ml and 12 ml volume, respectively). Histologic findings in the testes include hyalinization of the tubules, absence of spermatogenesis, and increase in the Leydig cells.

The increased average body height in the disorder is the result of an increased lower body segment. Gynecomastia ordinarily develops during adolescence, is generally bilateral and painless, and may become disfiguring. Obesity and varicose veins occur in one third to one half of patients, and mild mental deficiency, social maladjustment, subtle abnormalities of thyroid function, diabetes mellitus, extragonadal germ cell tumors, and pulmonary disease may be more common than in the general population. The risk of breast cancer is 20 times that in normal men, although the incidence is only about one fifth that in women. Most patients have a male psychosexual orientation. They are capable of functioning sexually as normal men.

The variant with 46,XY/47,XXY mosaicism comprises about 10 per cent of the patients, as estimated by chromosomal karyotypes on peripheral blood leukocytes. The frequency of this variant may be underestimated, because chromosomal mosaicism may be demonstrable in only the testes, and the peripheral leukocyte karyotype may be normal. As summarized in Table 37–3, the mosaic form is usually not as severe as the 47,XXY, and the testes may be normal in size (Gordon et al., 1972). The endocrine abnormalities are also less severe, and gynecomastia and azoospermia are less common. Indeed, occasional patients with mosaicism may be fertile. In some, the diagnosis may not even be suspected because of the minor physical abnormalities.

Approximately 30 additional karyotypic varieties of the Klinefelter syndrome have been described, including those with uniform cell lines (such as XXYY, XXXY, and XXXXY) and a variety of mosaicisms of the X chromosome with or without associated structural abnormalities of the X chromosome. In general, the greater the degree of chromosomal abnormality and, in mosaic forms, the more cell lines that are abnormal, the more severe the manifestations.

PATHOPHYSIOLOGY. The classic form of the Klinefelter syndrome is caused by meiotic nondisjunction of the chromosomes during gametogenesis (Fig. 37–2). About 40 per cent of the responsible meiotic nondisjunctions occur during spermatogenesis, and 60 per cent occur during oogenesis. Advanced maternal age is a predisposing factor in the cases in which the defect occurs during oogenesis. In contrast, the mosaic form of the disorder is thought to result from chromosomal mitotic nondisjunction after fertilization of the zygote and can take place either in a 46,XY zygote (see Fig. 37–2) or in a 47,XXY zygote. The last defect or double nondisjunction (meiotic and mitotic) may be the usual cause of the mosaic form and may thus explain why the mosaic form is less common than the classic disorder.

Plasma levels of follicle-stimulating hormone (FSH) and luteinizing hormone (LH) are usually high; FSH shows the best discrimination, a consequence of the consistent damage to the seminiferous tubules (Leonard et al., 1979). The plasma testosterone level averages half that of normal, but the range of values overlaps the normal range. Mean plasma estradiol levels are elevated, the cause of which is not entirely clear. Early in the course of the disorder, the testes may secrete increased amounts of estradiol in response to the elevated plasma LH, but later in the course the testicular secretion of estradiol and testosterone declines. Elevated plasma estradiol levels in the older patient are probably due to the combined effects of a decreased rate of metabolic clearance and an increased rate of testosterone conversion to estradiol in extraglandular tissues (Wang et al., 1975). The net result, both early and late, is a variable degree of insufficient androgenization and enhanced feminization. Feminization, including the development of gynecomastia, is thought to depend on the ratio of circulating estrogen:androgen (relative or absolute), and it follows that individuals with the lower plasma testosterone and higher plasma estradiol levels are more likely to develop gynecomastia. After the age of expected puberty, the administration of luteinizing hormone-releasing hormone (LHRH) causes an exaggerated increase in plasma gonadotropin levels, and the normal feedback inhibition of testosterone on pituitary LH secretion is diminished. Older patients with untreated Klinefelter syndrome may have "reactive pituitary abnormalities" in the form of enlarged or abnormal sellae, presumably secondary to the persistent lack of gonadal feedback, and hypertrophy of gonadotropes in response to stimulation by LHRH (Samaan et al., 1979). It is not known whether actual adenomas can form.

MANAGEMENT. No therapy is available for reversing the infertility, and surgery is the only available means for effective treatment of the gynecomastia. Most pa-

Table 37–2. CLINICAL FEATURES OF THE DISORDERS OF CHROMOSOMAL SEX

Disorder	Common Chromosomal Complement	Gonadal Development	External Genitalia	Internal Genitalia	Breast Development	Comment
Klinefelter syndrome	47,XXY or 46,XY/47,XXY	Hyalinized testes	Normal male	Normal male	Gynecomastia	Most common disorder of sexual differentiation; tall stature.
XX Male	46,XX	Hyalinized testes	Normal male	Normal male	Gynecomastia	Shorter than normal men; increased incidence of hypospadias. Similar to Klinefelter syndrome. May be familial.
Gonadal dysgenesis (Turner syndrome)	45,X or 46,XX/45,X	Streak gonads	Immature female	Hypoplastic female	Immature Female	Short stature and multiple somatic abnormalities. May be 46,XX with structurally abnormal X chromosome.
Mixed gonadal dysgenesis	46,XY/45,X or 46,XY	Testis and streak gonad	Variable but almost always ambiguous; 60% reared as female	Uterus, vagina, and one fallopian tube	Usually male	Second most common cause of ambiguous genitalia in the newborn; tumors common.
True hermaphroditism	46,XX or 46,XY or mosaics	Testis and ovary or ovotestis	Variable but usually ambiguous; 75% reared as males	Usually a uterus and urogenital sinus; ducts correspond to gonad	Gynecomastia in 75%	May be familial.

From Petersdorf, R. G., Adams, R. D., Braunwald, E., et al.: Disorders of sexual differentiation. *In* Harrison's Principles of Internal Medicine, 10th ed. New York, McGraw-Hill Book Co., 1983, pp. 724–739.

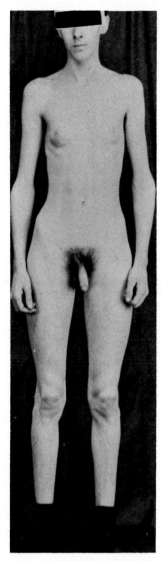

Figure 37–1. A patient with Klinefelter's syndrome. (Courtesy of Dr. Harry F. Klinefelter.)

tients benefit from supplemental androgen (Nielsen et al., 1988), but such treatment paradoxically may worsen the gynecomastia, presumably by providing increased androgen substrate for the extraglandular conversion to estrogens. Androgen should be administered in the form of injections of testosterone cypionate or testosterone enanthate (Snyder and Lawrence, 1980). Following the administration of testosterone, plasma LH levels return to normal, usually only after several months (Caminos-Torres et al., 1977).

XX Male Syndrome

The incidence of a 46,XX karyotype in phenotypic males is approximately one in 20,000 to 24,000 male births. More than 150 XX males have been reported. Affected individuals lack all female internal genitalia and have male psychosexual identification. The findings resemble those in the Klinefelter syndrome: the testes are small and firm (generally less than 2 cm); gyneco-

mastia is frequent; the penis is normal to small in size; azoospermia and hyalinization of the seminiferous tubules are usual. Mean plasma testosterone levels are low, plasma estradiol levels are elevated, and plasma gonadotropin levels are high (Perez-Palacios et al., 1981; Schweikert et al., 1982). Affected individuals differ from typical Klinefelter patients in that average height is less than in normal men, the incidence of mental deficiency is not increased, and hypospadias is more common (Roe and Alfi, 1977).

Four theories have been proposed to explain the pathogenesis of this disorder: (1) mosaicism in some cell lines for a Y-containing cell line or early loss of a Y chromosome; (2) single gene mutation on an autosome; (3) interchange of a portion of the Y chromosome with the X chromosome; and (4) deletion or inactivation of an X chromosomal gene or genes that normally have a negative regulatory effect on testis development (de-la-Chapelle, 1986). Mosaicism has not been documented, and no clear-cut evidence has been adduced for an autosomal gene mutation. The majority of XX males whose DNA is probed for Y-chromosome DNA fragments containing the testis-determining region contains Y-related DNA (Affara et al., 1986). The last candidate for the testis-determining gene, the SRY or sex-determining region Y, is present in all XX males tested (Sinclair et al., 1990). Thus, most of the individuals appear to have the Y-linked testis-determining factor, and in this group the etiology is presumably analogous to that in the *Sxr* mouse in which a critical fragment of the Y chromosome has been translocated to the X chromosome. The management of the disorder is similar to that of the Klinefelter syndrome.

Gonadal Dysgenesis (Turner Syndrome)

Gonadal dysgenesis is characterized by primary amenorrhea, sexual infantilism, short stature, multiple congenital anomalies, and bilateral streak gonads in phenotypic women with any of several defects of the X chromosome. This condition should be distinguished from three similar disorders: (1) mixed gonadal dysgen-

Table 37–3. CHARACTERISTICS OF PATIENTS WITH CLASSIC VERSUS MOSAIC KLINEFELTER SYNDROME*

	47,XXY (%)	46,XY/47,XXY (%)
Abnormal testicular histology	100	94†
Decreased length of testis	99	73†
Azoospermia	93	50†
Decreased testosterone	79	33
Decreased facial hair	77	64
Increased gonadotropins	75	33†
Decreased sexual function	68	56
Gynecomastia	55	33†
Decreased axillary hair	49	46
Decreased length of penis	41	21

*Table based on 519 XXY patients and 51 XY/XXY patients.
†Significantly different at P<.05 or better.
After Gordon, D. L., Krmpotic, E., Thomas, W., Gandy, H M., and Paulsen, C. A.: Pathologic testicular findings in Klinefelter's syndrome. Arch. Intern. Med., 130:726, 1972. Copyright 1972, American Medical Association.

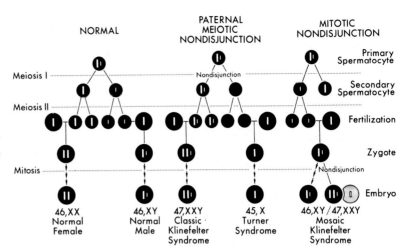

Figure 37–2. Schema for normal spermatogenesis and fertilization showing effects of meiotic and mitotic nondisjunction leading to the classic Klinefelter's syndrome, Turner's syndrome, and mosaic Klinefelter's syndrome. The schema would be similar if the abnormal events took place in oogenesis. (From Petersdorf. R. G., Adams, R. E., Braunwald, E., et al.: *In* Harrison's Principles of Internal Medicine. 10th ed. New York, McGraw-Hill Book Co., 1983, p. 727.)

esis, in which a unilateral testis and a contralateral streak gonad are present; (2) pure gonadal dysgenesis, in which bilateral streak gonads are associated with a normal 46,XX or 46,XY karyotype, normal stature, and primary amenorrhea; and (3) the Noonan syndrome, which is an autosomal dominant disorder characterized by the presence of webbed neck, short stature, congenital heart disease, cubitus valgus, and other congenital defects in both males and females with normal karyotypes and normal gonads. The eponym associated with gonadal dysgenesis stems from the description of seven patients with sexual infantilism, short stature, congenital webbed neck, and cubitus valgus (Turner, 1938). The term Turner's syndrome then came to be applied to such patients. Subsequently, a 45,X chromosomal complement was found to be present in typical patients (Ford et al., 1959). However, not all patients with bilateral streak gonads and an abnormality of the X chromosome have the characteristic somatic features or a 45,X chromosomal complement. Thus, gonadal dysgenesis is the preferred term whether or not the Turner features are present. This disorder is the most common cause of primary amenorrhea, accounting for as many as a third of all such patients (Ross et al., 1981).

CLINICAL FEATURES. The 45,X complement is the most common chromosomal abnormality in the disorder. It is found in 0.8 per cent of zygotes, but less than 3 per cent of 45,X embryos survive to term; therefore, the incidence of 45,X in newborns is about one in 2700 live females. However, this is an underestimate of the incidence because only about half of patients with gonadal dysgenesis have a 45,X chromosomal complement (see later discussion).

The diagnosis is made either at birth because of the associated anomalies or more commonly at puberty, when amenorrhea and failure of sexual development are noted in conjunction with the somatic anomalies (Fig. 37–3). The external genitalia are unambiguously female but immature, and no breast development occurs unless the patient is treated with exogenous estrogen. The internal urogenital tract consists of small but otherwise normal fallopian tubes and uterus and bilateral streak gonads located in the broad ligaments. Primordial germ cells are present transiently in the ovaries during embry-

ogenesis but disappear as the result of an accelerated rate of atresia (Singh and Carr, 1966). After the age of expected puberty, these streaks contain fibrous tissue that is indistinguishable from normal ovarian stroma and lack identifiable follicles and ova.

The associated somatic anomalies primarily affect tissues of mesodermal origin, that is, the skeleton and

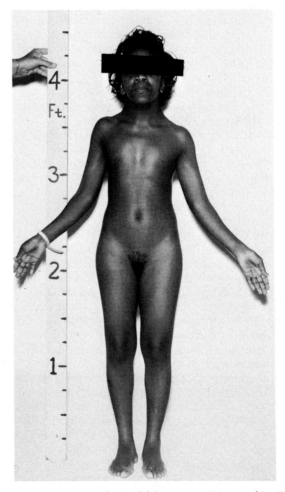

Figure 37–3. A patient with gonadal dysgenesis. (Courtesy of Dr. Peggy Whalley.)

connective tissue. Lymphedema of the hands and feet, webbing of the neck, low hair line, redundant skin folds on the back of the neck, shield-like chest with widely spaced nipples, and low birth weight are features that suggest the diagnosis in infancy. Characteristic facial features include micrognathia; epicanthal folds; prominent, low set or deformed ears; fish-like mouth, and ptosis. Short, fourth metacarpals are present in about 50 per cent, and 10 to 20 per cent have congenital cardiac abnormalities. Coarctation of the aorta (preductal or postductal) is the most common cardiac abnormality, especially in 45,X patients. Less common cardiac lesions include aortic valve disease, ventricular septal defect, atrial septal defect, dextrocardia, and hypoplastic left heart. Pulmonic stenosis (more typical of the Noonan syndrome) may occur in 45,X patients. Vascular malformations are infrequent but include intestinal telangiectasis, hemangiomas, and lymphangiectasis as potential causes of gastrointestinal bleeding. The average adult height rarely exceeds 150 cm. The short stature is primarily due to a decrease in the lower segment height. Associated conditions include renal malformations, pigmented nevi, hypoplastic nails, keloid formation tendency, perceptive hearing loss, unexplained hypertension, and certain autoimmune disorders.

The renal abnormalities are particularly common—about 60 per cent of patients have some renal structural abnormality compared with 10 per cent of normal individuals. Horseshoe kidneys, with or without duplication of the collecting ducts and malrotation of the kidney, are the most common abnormality. Ultrasonography may be useful as the initial screening technique to identify the presence of a renal abnormality (Lippe et al., 1988). The associated autoimmune disorders include primary hypothyroidism, inflammatory bowel disease, and diabetes mellitus. Frank hypothyroidism is seen in approximately 20 per cent of women with gonadal dysgenesis, but subtle evidence of thyroid dysfunction, including elevation of basal thyroid-stimulating hormone (TSH), enhanced response of TSH to thyrotropin-releasing hormone (TRH) stimulation, or the presence of antithyroid antibodies, is present in more than half of patients (Gruneiro de Papendieck et al., 1987). Both regional enteritis and ulcerative colitis appear to have an increased incidence in these patients as well. The association with diabetes mellitus is less clear.

PATHOPHYSIOLOGY. About half of patients have a 45,X karyotype. Approximately a fourth have mosaicism with no structural abnormality (46,XX/45,X), and the remainder have a structurally abnormal X chromosome with or without mosaicism (Simpson, 1979). On occasion, mosaicism may be limited to the streak gonad with a uniform 46,XX karyotype in peripheral blood and skin. The most frequent structural abnormality of the X chromosome is an isochromosome for the X long arm, or i(Xq), in which division of the centromere has occurred in the transverse rather than the longitudinal plane so that both arms of the chromosome are the same, with duplication of the long arm (Xq) and complete deletion of the short arm (Xp). This i(Xq) usually occurs in association with mosaicism for 45,X. Deletions of the X long arm [del (Xq)] or of the X short arm [del

(Xp)] are usually incomplete and less common. The 45,X variety may result from a chromosome loss during gametogenesis in either parent or from an error in mitosis during the early cleavage divisions of the fertilized zygote (see Fig. 37–2).

Short stature and other somatic features are due to loss of genetic material on the short arm of the X chromosome. Streak gonads result when genetic material is missing from either the long or short arm of the X chromosome. The region of the long arm of the X chromosome important for normal ovarian function has been localized to the Xq26-q27 region (Krauss et al., 1987). In individuals with mosaicism or with structural abnormalities of the X chromosome, the resulting phenotypes on average are intermediate in severity between those in the 45,X variety and the normal. In some patients with hypertrophy of the clitoris, an unidentified chromosomal fragment is present that is assumed to be an abnormal Y. Rarely, familial transmission of gonadal dysgenesis can be the result of a balanced X-autosome translocation (Leichtman et al., 1978).

Assessment of sex chromatin was previously used as a means of screening for abnormalities of the X chromosome. Sex chromatin in normal women (the Barr body) is the result of inactivation of one of two X chromosomes, and women with a 45,X chromosome composition, like normal men, are said to be chromatin-negative. However, only about half of the patients with gonadal dysgenesis (those with 45,X and those with the most extreme forms of mosaicism and structural abnormalities) are chromatin-negative, and karyotypic analysis is necessary both to establish the diagnosis and to identify the fraction of patients with Y-chromosome elements, who have as much as a 15 per cent chance of developing malignancy in the streak gonads.

Although sparse pubic and axillary hair develops at the time of expected puberty, the breasts usually remain infantile, and no menses occur. In contrast to individuals with the Klinefelter syndrome, who have no detectable endocrine abnormality prepubertally, patients with gonadal dysgenesis have elevations of plasma gonadotropin levels from the neonatal period to about 4 years of age (Conte et al., 1975). After this period, there is a decline to normal levels of plasma gonadotropins between 4 and 10 years of age, followed by a rise to high levels after 10 years of age. The degree of elevation of FSH is of greater magnitude than that of LH. This pattern of secretion is qualitatively similar to that of normal children, indicating that the program of gonadotropin secretion is inherent in the hypothalamic-pituitary axis and that only the amounts of gonadotropin secretion are modulated by gonadal function. As in the Klinefelter syndrome, mosaicism with a normal chromosomal complement lessens the severity of the gonadal abnormality. Thus, patients with gonadal dysgenesis who are past the age of expected puberty have a greater likelihood of menses and breast development if some cells have a normal 46,XX complement. Approximately 3 per cent of 45,X individuals and 12 per cent of patients with mosaicism have sufficient residual follicles to allow some menstruation. Moreover, although only 5 per cent of nonmosaic cases have spontaneous breast development, about a fifth of mosaic cases have some spontaneous feminization (Simpson, 1979).

Pregnancy occasionally occurs in the less severely affected individuals with spontaneous menses and secondary sex characteristics. About a dozen pregnancies in nonmosaic patients and more than 100 pregnancies in mosaic patients have been reported. A 50 per cent incidence of fetal miscarriage and a 33 per cent incidence of chromosomal abnormalities in newborn offspring are reported. The reproductive life of patients with gonadal dysgenesis who do menstruate is brief and is followed by early menopause.

MANAGEMENT. Recombinant human growth hormone (hGH) has been given alone and with the anabolic steroid oxandrolone during childhood in an effort to increase the final adult height of patients beyond the usual 142 to 144 cm. A 3-year, randomized controlled study in 70 patients has shown that hGH by itself causes a significant but modest increase in height and that the addition of oxandrolone results in a more marked acceleration of growth over a 3-year period (Rosenfeld et al., 1988). Although patients have not been studied to their final height as yet, more than half receiving combination therapy exceed the initially predicted height and are still growing. Whether such therapy will permit a significant number of patients to achieve a "normal" adult height of greater than 150 cm is unclear.

At the anticipated time of puberty, replacement therapy with estrogen should be instituted in those without spontaneous feminization. The aim of estrogen therapy is twofold—to induce maturation of the breasts, labia, vagina, uterus, and fallopian tubes and to minimize the development of osteoporosis. Linear growth and bone maturation rates are approximately doubled during the 1st year of treatment of girls of pubertal age with estrogen, but the eventual height of patients treated with estrogens only is low. Ultimate height is also not affected by the timing of the initiation of estrogen therapy (Martinez et al, 1987). Therapy should be initiated with low doses of conjugated estrogens: ethinyl estradiol or estradiol skin patches 25 days a month for the first 6 to 12 months with a subsequent increase in the dose to approximately 0.625 mg conjugated estrogen or its equivalent. It is customary to add medroxyprogesterone acetate during the last 10 of the 25 days to prevent the development of endometrial hyperplasia and possibly to decrease the long-term risk of endometrial cancer (Levine, 1978).

Gonadal tumors are rare in 45,X patients. However, gonadal malignancies do occur in patients with mosaicism involving the Y chromosome. Consequently, streak gonads should be removed in any patient with evidence of virilization or a Y-containing cell line.

Mixed Gonadal Dysgenesis

Mixed gonadal dysgenesis is a disorder in which phenotypic males or females have a testis on one side and a streak gonad on the other (Sohval, 1963). Most have 45,X/46,XY mosaicism, but the clinical entity is by no means confined to that chromosomal pattern. The true incidence is unknown, but in most hospitals it is the second most common cause of ambiguous genitalia reported in the neonate, after congenital adrenal hyperplasia.

CLINICAL FEATURES. About two thirds of patients are reared as females, and most phenotypic males are incompletely virilized at birth. The majority exhibit some degree of ambiguous genitalia, including phallic enlargement, urogenital sinus, and varying degrees of labioscrotal fusion (Fig. 37–4). In most, the testis is located intra-abdominally. Individuals with a testis in the inguinal or scrotal position are usually reared as males. A uterus, vagina, and at least one fallopian tube are almost invariably present in both phenotypic males and females (Fig. 37–5).

On histologic examination, the prepubertal testis appears relatively normal. The postpubertal testis contains abundant mature Leydig cells, but the seminiferous tubules contain Sertoli cells only and lack germinal elements. Frequently, the testis is undescended, and when descended it may appear in association with a hernia containing the uterus and fallopian tube. The streak gonad—a thin, pale, elongated structure located either in the broad ligament or along the pelvic wall—is composed of fibrous connective tissue that is often arranged in whorls so that it resembles ovarian stroma. At puberty, the testis secretes androgen, and both virilization and phallic enlargement occur. Feminization is rare. When it occurs, estrogen secretion from a gonadal tumor should be suspected.

Approximately a third of patients exhibit the somatic features of 45,X gonadal dysgenesis, namely, low posterior hairline, shield-like chest, multiple pigmented nevi, cubitus valgus, webbing of the neck, and short stature (height less than 150 cm).

Virtually all are chromatin-negative. About two thirds have the 45,X/46,XY karyotype. In the remainder, a 46,XY karyotype is present, and mosaicism might be

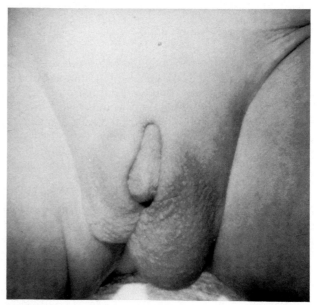

Figure 37–4. External genitalia of a patient with mixed gonadal dysgenesis.

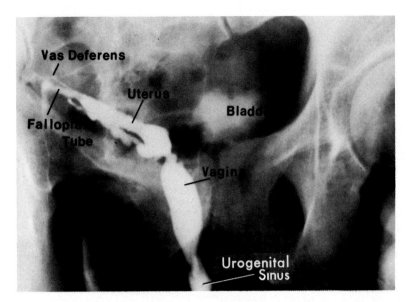

Figure 37–5. Retrograde genitogram, with a blunt-ended syringe placed in the urogenital sinus of a patient with mixed gonadal dysgenesis. The vagina, uterus, fallopian tube, and vas deferens are demonstrated.

present but undetected. The origin of 45,X/46,XY mosaicism is best explained by the loss of a Y chromosome during an early mitotic division of an XY zygote, similar to the postulated loss of the X chromosome in 46,XY/47,XXY mosaicism, as shown in Figure 37–2.

PATHOPHYSIOLOGY. It has been assumed that the 45,XY cell line stimulates testicular differentiation, whereas the 45,X leads to the development of the contralateral streak gonad, but actual comparisons between karyotype and phenotypic expression have failed to document such a relationship. Furthermore, no clear correlation has been found between the percentage of cells cultured from blood or skin containing 45,X or 46,XY and the degree of gonadal development or somatic anomalies.

Both masculinization and müllerian duct regression in utero are incomplete. Because Leydig cell function is normal at puberty, the inadequate virilization in utero may be the result of delay in the development of a testis that is ultimately capable of normal Leydig cell function. The capacity of the internal duct structures, the urogenital sinus, and the external genitalia to virilize completely in response to androgen is limited to a critical period between about 7 and 14 weeks of gestation. Consequently, a delayed but otherwise normal onset of endocrine function in the fetal testis would result in incomplete masculinization of the external genitalia and could explain the persistence of müllerian ducts. Alternatively, the fetal testis may simply be incapable of synthesizing normal amounts of müllerian-inhibiting substance and androgen.

MANAGEMENT. Several factors must be considered in the management of patients with mixed gonadal dysgenesis. For the older child or adult in whom gender assignment is not an issue, the principal consideration is the possibility of tumor development in the gonads. The overall incidence of gonadal tumors in patients with mixed gonadal dysgenesis is about 25 per cent. Seminomas occur more frequently than gonadoblastomas. The tumors may occur prior to puberty, develop most frequently in patients with a female phenotype who lack

the somatic features typical of 45,X gonadal dysgenesis, and are more common in intra-abdominal testes than in streak gonads. When the diagnosis of mixed gonadal dysgenesis is established in phenotypic females, early exploratory laparotomy and prophylactic gonadectomy should be undertaken for two reasons: (1) gonadal tumors may occur in childhood, and (2) testis secretes androgen at puberty and thus causes virilization. Such individuals like those with gonadal dysgenesis, are given estrogen beginning at the age of expected puberty to induce and maintain feminization.

When the diagnosis is established in phenotypic males during late childhood or adulthood, the management is more complicated. Phenotypic males with mixed gonadal dysgenesis are infertile (no germinal elements are present in the testes) and have a high risk of developing gonadal tumors. Which testes can be safely conserved? The following generalizations apply: (1) tumors develop in scrotal streak gonads but not in scrotal testes; (2) tumors that develop in intra-abdominal testes are always associated with ipsilateral müllerian duct structures; and (3) tumors in streak gonads are always associated with tumors in the contralateral abdominal testis. Based on these observations, it is recommended that (1) all streak gonads be removed; (2) scrotal testes be preserved; and (3) intra-abdominal testes be excised unless they can be relocated in the scrotum and unless no ipsilateral müllerian duct structures are present. Decisions as to reconstructive surgery of the phallus depend on the nature of the defect. Gender assignment is usually female in those who are identified because of ambiguous genitalia as newborns. Resection of the enlarged phallus and gonadectomy in such a patient can be accomplished in infancy, usually in one procedure.

True Hermaphroditism

True hermaphroditism is a condition in which both an ovary and a testis or a gonad with histologic features of both (ovotestis) is present. The incidence is unknown, but more than 400 cases have been reported (van Niekerk and Retief, 1981). To justify the diagnosis, there must be histologic documentation of both types of gonadal epithelium. The presence of ovarian stroma without oocytes is not sufficient. Three categories are recognized: (1) one fifth are bilateral (testicular and ovarian tissue, i.e., ovotestes, on each side); (2) two fifths are unilateral (an ovotestis on one side and an ovary or a testis on the other); and (3) two fifths are lateral (a testis on one side and an ovary on the other). The ovary occurs most commonly on the left side, whereas testicular tissue, occurring either as a testis or an ovotestis, is more frequent on the right side.

CLINICAL FEATURES. The external genitalia display all gradations of the male to female spectrum. Of patients, three fourths are sufficiently masculinized to be reared as males. However, less than one tenth have normal male external genitalia. Most have hypospadias, and more than half have incomplete labioscrotal fusion. Of phenotypic females, two thirds have an enlarged clitoris, and most have a urogenital sinus. Differentiation of the internal ducts usually corresponds to the adjacent gonad. Although an epididymis usually develops adjacent to a testis, a complete vas deferens is present in only a third of patients. Only one duct is usually present next to an ovotestis. On histologic examination, about two thirds of the ducts next to an ovotestis have the characteristics of a fallopian tube, and one third have the characteristics of a vas deferens. The more testicular tissue present in an ovotestis, the more likely that the adjacent duct will be a vas deferens (van Niekerk, 1981). A uterus is usually present, although it may be hypoplastic or unicornous. The last is characteristic of lateral true hermaphroditism with absence of the horn on the side of the testis. The ovary usually occupies the normal position, but the testis or ovotestis may be found at any level along the route of embryonic testicular descent and is frequently associated with an inguinal hernia. Testicular tissue is present in the scrotum or the labioscrotal fold in a third, in the inguinal canal in a third, and in the abdominal area in a third of patients.

At puberty, signs of variable feminization and virilization develop—three fourths of patients develop significant breast enlargement, and about half menstruate. In phenotypic men, menstruation usually presents as cyclic hematuria (Raspa et al., 1986). Ovulation occurs in approximately a fourth and is more common than spermatogenesis. In phenotypic men, ovulation may occur as testicular pain. Fertility has been reported in women following removal of an ovotestis. A man is reported who fathered two children. Congenital malformations of other systems are rare.

PATHOPHYSIOLOGY. About 70 per cent of patients have a 46,XX karyotype, 10 per cent have a 46,XY karyotype, and the remainder have chromosomal mosaicism. True hermaphroditism associated with chromosomal mosaicism falls into two categories. True hermaphroditism of 46,XX/46,XY is about as common as the 46,XY variety and is thought to arise most commonly from chimerism—the presence in a single individual of cells derived from two zygotes, as in the fertilization of both an ovum and its polar body. True hermaphroditism

has also been described in individuals with a 45,X/46,XY chromosome composition. However, neither ovulation nor spermatogenesis takes place, and it is likely that the disorder is a form of mixed gonadal dysgenesis, in which, as in other types of gonadal dysgenesis, atresia of ovarian follicles in the streak gonad is incomplete. True hermaphroditism has rarely been reported with other forms of mosaicism such as 46,XY/47,XXY, but these variants have not been characterized in detail.

The mechanism responsible for the gonadal asymmetry in true hermaphroditism is unknown. In general, the presence of a Y chromosome increases the likelihood of development of a true testis from about a fifth in the overall population of true hermaphroditism to three fifths. The most common gonadal pattern in 46,XX is an ovary on one side and an ovotestis on the other side. In those individuals who do not have a Y-containing line, it was assumed that testis development occurs as a result of the presence of genetic material derived from the Y chromosome. However, DNA hybridization studies using six Y-chromosome specific probes in ten 46,XX true hermaphrodites failed to detect any Y-related DNA (Ramsay et al., 1988). This finding suggests an etiologic difference between XX males and XX true hermaphrodites.

The rare instances of 46,XX true hermaphroditism associated with a positive family history seem to be most consistent with an autosomal recessive pattern of inheritance. A single family is reported with paternal transmission of an apparent autosomal gene leading to both XX males and XX true hermaphrodites in the offspring (Skordis et al., 1987). No studies of Y-chromosome related DNA were reported in this family.

Because corpora lutea are present in the ovaries of more than a fourth of patients, it can be deduced that a female neuroendocrine axis is present and functions normally. Feminization (gynecomastia and menstruation) is the result of the secretion of estradiol by the ovarian tissue that is present (Aiman et al., 1978). It is presumed that secretion of androgen predominates over secretion of estrogen in masculinized patients. The fact that some patients produce sperm is in keeping with this view.

MANAGEMENT. When the diagnosis is made in a newborn or young infant, gender assignment depends largely on the anatomic findings. In older children and adults, gonads and internal duct structures that are contradictory to the predominant phenotype and the gender of rearing should be removed. When necessary, the external genitalia should be modified appropriately. Although gonadal tumors are rare in true hermaphroditism, gonadoblastoma has been reported in an individual with an XY cell line. Consequently, the possibility of future tumor development in the gonad must be taken into consideration when the decision is made as to conservation of gonadal tissue.

DISORDERS OF GONADAL SEX

Disorders of gonadal sex result when chromosomal sex is normal but differentiation of the gonads is abnormal for any of several reasons. Thus, chromosomal sex does not correspond to gonadal and phenotypic sex.

Pure Gonadal Dysgenesis

The syndrome of "pure gonadel dysgenesis," as used here, is restricted to phenotypic females with gonads and genitalia identical to those with gonadal dysgenesis (bilateral streak gonads and, usually, sexual infantilism) but who have normal height, few if any somatic anomalies, and either a uniform 46,XX or 46,XY chromosomal complement. In one series, this disorder was about one third as common as gonadal dysgenesis (McDonough et al., 1977).

CLINICAL FEATURES. A clear-cut genetic basis exists for considering this syndrome to be a separate disorder from gonadal dysgenesis, but on clinical grounds it cannot be distinguished from those cases of gonadal dysgenesis associated with minimal somatic abnormalities. The height is normal or greater than normal, some individuals being more than 170 cm. Estrogen deficiency varies from profound, typical of classic 45,X gonadal dysgenesis, to that of some breast development and appearance of menses, which invariably terminate with an early menopause. As many as 40 per cent have some feminization (McDonough et al., 1977). Axillary and pubic hair are scanty, and internal genitalia consist solely of müllerian derivatives.

Tumors may develop in the streak gonads, particularly dysgerminoma or gonadoblastoma in the 46,XY disorder. Such tumors are frequently heralded by the appearance of virilizing signs or a pelvic mass.

PATHOPHYSIOLOGY. Although a variety of chromosomal mosaicisms have been described under this nosology, the designation of pure gonadal dysgenesis is here restricted to individuals with uniform 46,XX or 46,XY karyotypes. Those cases with mosaicism are actually variants of gonadal dysgenesis or mixed gonadal dysgenesis as already described. The rationale for this restricted definition is based on the fact that both the XX and XY varieties can result from separate types of single gene mutations. Several sibships have been reported in which more than one individual is affected with the 46,XX type of the disorder. Such patients are commonly the offspring of consanguineous matings, suggesting autosomal recessive inheritance. Furthermore, familial occurrence of the 46,XY variety has been described in which the mutation appears to be inherited either as an X-linked recessive mutation or as a male-limited autosomal recessive trait (Simpson et al., 1981). In both the 46,XX and the 46,XY forms the mutation prevents differentiation of the ovary and the testis, respectively, by an uncertain mechanism. Development of the female phenotype in the 46,XY disorder is the consequence of the failure of testicular development.

MANAGEMENT. Management of the estrogen deficiency is identical to that in gonadal dysgenesis. Appropriate estrogen replacement therapy is initiated at the time of expected puberty and is maintained in adult life. Because of the frequency of gonadal tumors in the 46,XY variety, exploratory surgery and removal of the streak gonads should be undertaken once the diagnosis is made (Olsen et al., 1988). The development of virilizing signs is indication for immediate surgery. The natural history of the gonadal tumors is uncertain, but the prognosis after surgical removal appears to be good.

Absent Testes Syndrome (Anorchia, Gonadal Agenesis, Testicular Regression, Agonadism)

A spectrum of phenotypes has been described in 46,XY males with absent or rudimentary testes and in whom unequivocal evidence exists that endocrine function of the testis (e.g., variable müllerian duct regression and variable testosterone synthesis) was present during embryonic life. This rare disorder can be distinguished from pure gonadal dysgenesis in which no evidence can be inferred for gonadal function during embryonic development. The disorder has been reported under a variety of eponyms and varies in its manifestations from complete failure of virilization to incomplete virilization of the external genitalia to otherwise normal males with bilateral anorchia (Bergada et al., 1962). An analogous disorder may occur in 46,XX phenotypic females in whom gonadal absence is associated with sexual infantilism and müllerian development (Medina et al., 1982).

CLINICAL FEATURES. The purest form of the syndrome is represented by 46,XY phenotypic females with absent testes, sexual infantilism, and concomitant absence of the müllerian duct derivatives and accessory organs of male reproduction. The syndrome in such individuals differs from the 46,XY form of pure gonadal dysgenesis in that no gonadal remnant can be identified—there are no streak gonads and no müllerian derivatives. In these women, testicular failure must have occurred during the interval between the onset of formation of müllerian-inhibiting substance and secretion of testosterone, that is, after development of the seminiferous tubules but before the onset of Leydig cell function. In others, the clinical features indicate that testicular failure occurred during later phases of gestation, and some of these cases constitute problems in gender assignment. In some, failure of müllerian regression occurs to a greater extent than failure of testosterone secretion, but none exhibit complete müllerian development. In individuals with more extensive virilization the external genitalia are phenotypically male, but rudimentary oviducts and vasa deferentia may coexist internally.

At the extreme is the syndrome of bilateral anorchia in phenotypic men with absence of müllerian structures and gonads but complete male development of the external genitalia and all of the wolffian system except the epididymis (Aynsley-Green et al., 1976). Microphallus in such patients implies that failure of androgen-mediated growth occurred during late embryogenesis after anatomic development of the male urethra was complete. Persistent gynecomastia may or may not occur after puberty.

PATHOPHYSIOLOGY. The pathogenesis of these disorders is not understood. The karyotype is 46,XY by definition. Whether the testicular regression is the result of mutant genes, teratogen, or trauma is unclear. Multiple instances of agonadism in the same family have been reported, and unilateral and bilateral agonadism can occur within the same family; consequently, it is necessary to obtain a careful family history. Five instances of discordance of anorchia in monozygotic twins have been reported, suggesting that nongenetic factors are also involved (Aynsley-Green et al., 1976; Glass, 1982).

The quantitative dynamics of gonadal steroid production have been studied in a few patients. In two phenotypic females who had primary amenorrhea, sexual infantilism, and no internal genital structures, androgen and estrogen kinetics were similar to those in gonadal dysgenesis. The daily production rates of estrogen were low, and no glandular secretion of testosterone could be documented, confirming the functional as well as the anatomic absence of the testes. In one phenotypic male with bilateral anorchia no glandular secretion of testosterone took place; total testosterone and estrogen production was accounted for by peripheral conversion from plasma androstenedione (Edman et al., 1977). However, some patients in whom no testes can be identified at laparotomy have blood testosterone values that are clearly above the range in castration, presumably derived from remnant testes (Kirschner et al., 1970). The pattern of gonadotropin secretion in children with congenital anorchism is similar to that in patients with gonadal dysgenesis (see previous mention) (Lustig et al., 1987).

MANAGEMENT. The management of the two extremes in this disorder is clear-cut. Sexually infantile, phenotypic females should be treated in the same manner as patients with gonadal dysgenesis; namely, they should be given adequate estrogen to ensure appropriate breast and female somatic development and any coexisting vaginal agenesis should be treated by either surgical or medical means. Likewise, phenotypic males with anorchia should be given adequate androgen replacement to allow normal male secondary sexual development. Patients with incomplete virilization or ambiguous development of the external genitalia require individual assessment as to whether surgery is appropriate for improving male or female phenotypes. In either case, appropriate hormonal therapy is mandatory at the time of expected puberty.

DISORDERS OF PHENOTYPIC SEX

Female Pseudohermaphroditism

In individuals with female pseudohermaphroditism, the ovaries and müllerian derivatives are normal, and abnormal sexual development is limited to the external genitalia. Since in the absence of testes the external genitalia feminize, masculinization of the female fetus implies the presence of androgen from either the maternal circulation or the fetal adrenal gland. The degree of masculinization is determined by two factors—the amount plus the potency of androgen and the stage of fetal development at the time of exposure. Late exposure to androgens (after the vagina has formed at about the 12th week) causes clitoral hypertrophy, whereas early exposure can cause hypospadias or rarely development of a true penile urethra. Even with severe masculinization of the external genitalia, the uterus and fallopian tubes remain normal, because the regression of their anlage, the müllerian ducts, requires the secretion of müllerian-inhibiting substance by the fetal testis. The two common causes of female pseudohermaphroditism are congenital adrenal hyperplasia and maternal virilizing syndromes.

Congenital Adrenal Hyperplasia

The pathways by which glucocorticoids are synthesized in the adrenal gland and androgens are formed in the testis and adrenal gland are summarized in Figure 37–6. A variety of syndromes result from hereditary defects in the enzymes of steroid hormone synthesis. Three processes are essential to the formation of glucocorticoids and androgens (20,22-desmolase, 3β-hydroxysteroid dehydrogenase, and 17α-hydroxylase). Deficiency of any of these enzymes results in deficiency of glucocorticoid and androgen syntheses and consequently results in both congenital adrenal hyperplasia due to enhanced adrenocorticotropic hormone (ACTH) levels and defective virilization of the male embryo (male pseudohermaphroditism).

Two reactions are involved exclusively in androgen formation (17,20-desmolase and 17β-hydroxysteroid dehydrogenase). A defect in either process results in pure male pseudohermaphroditism with normal glucocorticoid synthesis. Deficiency of either of the terminal reactions of glucocorticoid synthesis (21-hydroxylase and 11β-hydroxylase) results in defective formation of hydrocortisone. The compensatory increase in ACTH secretion causes enhanced formation of adrenal steroids proximal to the enzymatic defect and a secondary increase in androgen formation. As a consequence, the latter two disorders (21-hydroxylase and 11β-hydroxylase) result in adrenal hyperplasia and either virilization in the female embryo or precocious masculinization in the male. One disorder, 3β-hydroxysteroid dehydrogenase deficiency, can cause either male or female pseudohermaphroditism, but because the more common genital defect is incomplete virilization of the male, it is discussed under Male Pseudohermaphroditism.

CLINICAL FEATURES. The adrenal insufficiency in these disorders may produce equally severe and life-threatening problems in both sexes. The major features of the different forms of congenital adrenal hyperplasia are listed in Table 37–4. The management and diagnosis of the adrenal insufficiency in these disorders are reviewed elsewhere. The present discussion focuses on the sexual abnormalities. From the standpoint of abnormal sexual development it is helpful to consider separately those defects in steroidogenesis that cause female pseudohermaphroditism and those that cause male pseudohermaphroditism.

Congenital adrenal hyperplasia caused by *21-hydroxylase deficiency,* with an incidence of between one in

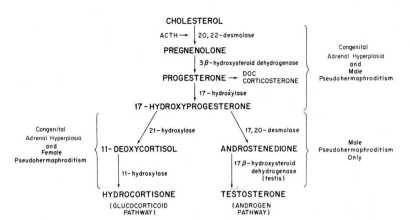

Figure 37–6. The relationship between the defects in steroid hormone biosynthesis and the development of male and female pseudohermaphroditism.

5000 and one in 15,000 in Europe and the United States, is the most common cause of ambiguous genitalia in the newborn. Virilization is usually apparent at birth in the female and within the first 2 to 3 years of life in the male. Approximately one fourth of the cases manifested in infancy are of the simple (virilizing) variety. More severe deficiency of the enzyme is associated with salt loss as well (see Table 37–4).

In the newborn female there is hypertrophy and ventral binding (chordee) of the clitoris, variable degrees of fusion of the labioscrotal folds, and virilization of the urethra (Fig. 37–7). The internal female structures and ovaries are unaltered. The wolffian ducts regress normally, probably because the onset of adrenal function occurs relatively late in embryogenesis. The labioscrotal folds are bulbous and rugated and resemble a scrotum. The external appearance of affected females is similar to that of boys with bilateral cryptorchidism and hypospadias. Rarely, the virilization is severe enough to cause development of a complete male penile urethra and prostate so that errors in sex assignment may occur at birth (see Fig. 37–7). Radiography following the injection of radiopaque dye into the external genital orifice is helpful in defining the internal structures and, in particular, in demonstrating the presence of vagina, uterus, and sometimes fallopian tubes. In a few cases,

virilization of the female is slight or absent at birth and becomes evident later in infancy, adolescence, or adulthood (i.e., so-called late onset or adult form of the disorder). The untreated female grows rapidly during the first year of life and has progressive virilization. At the time of expected puberty there is a failure of normal female sexual development and an absence of menstruation. In both sexes, rapid somatic maturation during childhood results in premature epiphyseal closure and short adult height.

Because male phenotypic differentiation is normal, the condition usually is not recognized in the newborn male in the absence of overt adrenal insufficiency. However, there is early growth and maturation of the external genitalia, and secondary sex characteristics, coarsening of the voice, frequent erections, and excessive muscular development may be noticeable in the first few years of life. Virilization in the male can follow either of two patterns. Excessive adrenal androgens can inhibit gonadotropin production so that the testes remain infantile in size despite the acceleration of masculinization. Such untreated adult men are capable of erection and ejaculation but have azoospermia. Alternatively, adrenal androgen secretion can activate a premature maturation of the hypothalamic-pituitary axis and initiate a true precocious puberty, including early

Table 37–4. FORMS OF CONGENITAL ADRENAL HYPERPLASIA

Deficiency	Cortisol	Aldosterone	Degree of Virilization of Females	Failure of Virilization of Males	Dominant Steroid Secreted	Comment
21-Hydroxylase, partial (simple virilizing or compensated)	Normal	↑	+ + + +	0	17-Hydroxyprogesterone	Most common type (~95% of total); from one third to two thirds salt losers
Severe (salt-losing)	↓	↓	+ + + +	0	17-Hydroxyprogesterone	
11β-Hydroxylase (hypertension)	↓	↓	+ + + +	0	11-Deoxycortisol and 11-deoxycycorticosterone	Hypertension
3β-Hydroxysteroid dehydrogenase	0	0	+	+ + + +	Δ⁵3β-OH compounds (dehydroepiandrosterone)	Probably second most common, usually salt loss
17α-Hydroxylase	↓	↓	0	+ + + +	Corticosterone and 11-deoxycorticosterone	No feminization of female, hypertension
20,22-Desmolase (lipoid adrenal hyperplasia)	0	0	0	+ + + +	Cholesterol (?)	Rare, usually salt loss

From Petersdorf, R. G., Adams, R. D., Braunwald, E., et al.: Disorders of sexual differentiation. *In* Harrison's Principles of Internal Medicine, 10th ed. New York, McGraw-Hill Book Co., 1983, pp. 724–739.

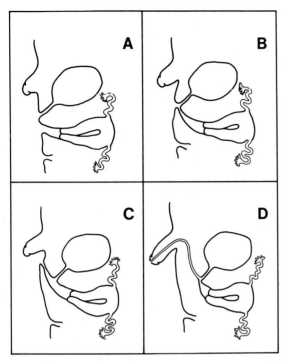

Figure 37–7. The spectrum of external virilization in congenital adrenal hyperplasia. *A,* Clitoromegaly. *B* and *C,* Progressive labioscrotal fusion. *D,* Complete virilization with penile urethra.

maturation of spermatogenesis. The untreated or undertreated male is also subject to the development of ACTH-dependent "tumors" of the testis composed of adrenal rest cells.

In 21-hydroxylase deficiency, which accounts for about 95 per cent of congenital adrenal hyperplasia, there is reduced activity of the 21-hydroxylase enzyme, which leads to decreased production of hydrocortisone and consequently to increased release of ACTH, enlargement of the adrenal glands, and partial or complete compensation of the defect in hydrocortisone formation. In patients with incomplete defects, cortisol secretion may be normal as the result of the adrenal enlargement. This form is termed "simple virilizing" or "compensated." In the remainder, the enzyme deficiency is more severe. The enlarged adrenal gland fails to produce adequate amounts of cortisol and aldosterone, leading to severe salt wastage with anorexia, vomiting, volume depletion, and collapse within the first few weeks of life, the so-called salt-losing form. In all untreated patients, the cortisol precursors prior to the 21-hydroxylase step are overproduced, leading to an increase in plasma progesterone and 17-hydroxyprogesterone. These steroids act at the receptor level as weak aldosterone antagonists and in the compensated form cause greater than normal aldosterone production to maintain normal sodium balance.

A rare form of congenital adrenal hyperplasia associated with female pseudohermaphroditism is *11β-hydroxylase deficiency* (see Fig. 37–6). In this disorder, a block in hydroxylation at the 11-carbon results in cortisol deficiency, increased ACTH secretion, and accumulation of 11-deoxycortisol and deoxycorticosterone (DOC). The latter is a potent mineralocorticoid that causes hypertension rather than salt loss. The clinical features that stem from glucocorticoid deficiency and androgen excess are similar to those in 21-hydroxylase deficiency.

PATHOPHYSIOLOGY. Both 21-hydroxylase and 11β-hydroxylase deficiencies are inherited as autosomal recessive disorders. The carrier frequency for 21-hydroxylase deficiency is about one in 50. At least three forms of 21-hydroxylase deficiency have been identified, all involving mutations of a gene on the sixth chromosome close to the HLA-B locus: simple virilizing disease associated with the HLA haplotype HLA-B5, the salt-wasting type associated with HLA-A3, Bw47, DR7, and Bw60, and nonclassic disease associated with HLA-B14, DR1. Patients with 21-hydroxylase deficiency and heterozygous carriers of the mutant genes within a given family can often be identified on the basis of the HLA haplotype. The 11β-hydroxylase gene is located on chromosome 8 and has no relation to the HLA system.

The gene that encodes 21-hydroxylase is adjacent to the C4B gene that encodes the fourth component of serum complement. This gene cluster is located between HLA-B and HLA-DR. About a third of the mutations responsible for 21-hydroxylase deficiencies studied to date result from major rearrangements and/or deletions of the gene, a third result from point mutations that impair enzyme function, and a third result from so-called gene conversions in which the normal gene is converted to a form similar to the pseudogene and thus is not transcribed. Considering the frequency of the disorder and its occurrence in patients with different ethnic backgrounds, elucidation of all the molecular defects that give rise to 21-hydroxylase deficiency is a major challenge.

Excretion of ketosteroids is elevated, as is the excretion of the major metabolites that accumulate proximal to the enzymatic blocks. In 21-hydroxylase deficiency, 17-hydroxyprogesterone accumulates in blood and is excreted predominantly as pregnanetriol. In 11-hydroxylase deficiency, 11-deoxycortisol accumulates in the blood and is excreted predominantly as tetrahydrocortexolone. Plasma ACTH levels are elevated in untreated patients with both disorders.

MANAGEMENT. Insofar as is possible, gender assignment in the newborn should correspond to the chromosomal and gonadal sex, and appropriate surgical correction of the external genitalia should be undertaken as early as is feasible. Adequate replacement therapy is of particular importance because appropriately treated men and women are capable of fertility. If the correct diagnosis is made late (after 2 years of age) gender assignment should be changed to correspond to chromosomal sex only after careful consideration of the psychosexual background.

Medical treatment with appropriate glucocorticoids prevents the consequences of hydrocortisone deficiency, arrests the rapid virilization, and prevents the premature somatic advancement and epiphyseal maturation. The suppression of the abnormal steroid secretion results in cure of the hypertension in patients with 11β-hydroxylase deficiency and allows normal onset of menses and development of female secondary sex characteristics in both disorders. In males, glucocorticoid therapy suppresses adrenal androgens and results in normal gonadotropin secretion, testicular development, and spermatogenesis. Measurements of plasma 17-hydroxy-progesterone, androstenedione, ACTH, and renin levels have all been used to assess the adequacy of replacement therapy. In severe forms of 21-hydroxylase deficiency associated with salt loss or elevated plasma renin activity, treatment with mineralocorticoids is also indicated. In such patients, the monitoring of plasma renin activity is of assistance in determining the adequacy of mineralocorticoid replacement.

Maternal Androgens and Progestogens

At present, nonadrenal causes of female pseudohermaphroditism are rare. In the past, the administration to pregnant women of progestational agents with androgenic side effects (e.g., ethisterone, medroxyprogesterone, and norethindrone) to prevent abortion resulted in masculinization of female fetuses. Such infants are usually virilized less severely than those with congenital adrenal hyperplasia. Female pseudohermaphroditism may also occur in babies of mothers with virilizing ovarian (e.g., arrhenoblastomas, luteomas of pregnancy) or adrenal tumors. Because of the exquisite sensitivity of embryos to the virilizing effects of androgens, the absence of virilization in the mother does not exclude a maternal source of androgen in female pseudohermaphroditism. Nevertheless, most infants born to mothers with virilizing tumors are not themselves virilized, probably because placental aromatization of androgens to estrogens protects the fetus from virilization. Female pseudohermaphroditism due to transfer of maternal androgens/progestogens is usually a self-limited disorder that does not progress after birth. No hormonal therapy is indicated, surgical correction of the external genitalia may or may not be required, and ovarian function at puberty is normal.

Congenital Absence of the Vagina (Müllerian Agenesis)

Congenital absence of the vagina in combination with some form of abnormal or absent uterus (the Mayer-Rokitansky-Küster-Hauser syndrome) is second only to gonadal dysgenesis as a cause of primary amenorrhea.

CLINICAL FEATURES. In most patients the disorder is ascertained after the time of expected puberty because of failure to menstruate and absence or hypoplasia of the vagina is found. Height and intelligence are normal. The breasts, axillary and pubic hair, and habitus are feminine in character. The uterus may vary from almost normal, lacking only a conduit to the introitus, to the more characteristic rudimentary bicornuate cords with or without a lumen (Fig. 37–8). In some patients, cyclic abdominal pain indicates that sufficient functional endometrium is present to result in retrograde menstruation or hematometra, or both.

Renal, skeletal, and other congenital anomalies are common (Griffin et al., 1976). About one third of patients have abnormal kidneys, most commonly agenesis or ectopy. Fused kidneys of the horseshoe type and solitary ectopic kidneys located in the pelvis also occur. Skeletal abnormalities are present in one tenth of patients. Two thirds of these abnormalities involve the spine. Limb and rib abnormalities account for most of the remainder. Specific bone abnormalities include wedge vertebrae, fusions, rudimentary or asymmetric vertebral bodies, and supernumerary vertebrae. The Klippel-Feil syndrome (congenital fusion of the cervical spine, short neck, low posterior hairline, and painless limitation of cervical movement) is a frequent association. In infants with the syndrome inguinal hernias may contain ovaries and müllerian remnants.

PATHOPHYSIOLOGY. The karyotype is 46,XX. Most cases are believed to be sporadic in nature, but several of familial occurrence have been described. The most extensive study of familial occurrence is the report by Shokeir (1978) of ten individuals with positive family histories. In eight of these ten families the pattern of inheritance was most consistent with a sex-limited autosomal dominant mutation. It is not known whether sporadic cases are representative of new mutations of the type responsible for the familial disorder or are multifactoral in etiology. In some familial cases variable expressivity of the defect occurs. Some affected family members have skeletal or renal abnormalities only, whereas others have müllerian derivative abnormalities, such as a double uterus (Griffin et al., 1976). Bilateral renal aplasia in stillborn infants is also commonly associated with absence of the uterus and vagina. Thus, the family histories should be probed for instances of isolated skeletal and renal abnormalities and for stillbirths that might result from the congenital absence of both kidneys.

Ovulatory peaks of plasma LH levels and biphasic temperature curves during the cycle suggest that ovarian function is normal. Successful pregnancies have been reported following corrective vaginal surgery in patients who have normal uteri.

MANAGEMENT. Vaginal agenesis can be treated by surgical or nonsurgical means. Surgical repair generally utilizes a split-thickness skin graft around a solid rubber mold for the creation of an artificial vagina. Medical treatment consists of the repeated application of pressure against the vaginal dimple with a simple dilator to cause development of adequate vaginal depth. In view of the overall complication rate of 5 to 10 per cent in surgical series, medical treatment should be attempted in most cases, and surgery should be reserved for patients in whom a well-formed uterus is present and the possibility of fertility exists. Continued coitus or instrumental dilation is probably essential for maintaining the neovagina formed by either the nonoperative method or the operative method.

Male Pseudohermaphroditism

Defective virilization of the male embryo (male pseudohermaphroditism) can result from defects in androgen synthesis, androgen action, and müllerian duct regression, and from other uncertain causes. Testosterone synthesis is normal in more than 80 per cent of patients

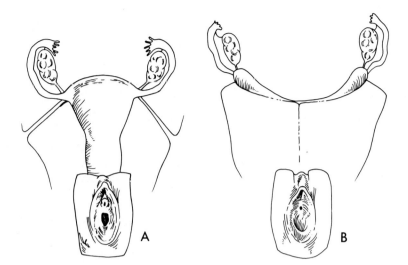

Figure 37–8. *A,* The normal female genital tract. *B,* The genital tract in congenital absence of the vagina. The blind-ending introitus, the replacement of the vagina and most of the uterus with fibrous tissue, and the bicornuate uterine remnants are characteristic findings.

with male pseudohermaphroditism (Campo et al., 1979, 1981; Savage et al., 1978).

Abnormalities in Androgen Synthesis

Five defects in testosterone synthesis (see Fig. 37–6) are known to cause incomplete virilization of the male embryo during embryogenesis (see Tables 37–4 and 37–5). Each of the disorders involves a critical enzymatic step in the conversion of cholesterol to testosterone. Three steps (20,22-desmolase, 3β-hydroxysteroid dehydrogenase, and 17α-hydroxylase) are common to the synthesis of other adrenal hormones as well. Consequently, their deficiency results in congenital adrenal hyperplasia (see Table 37–4) as well as male pseudohermaphroditism. The other two reactions (17,20-desmolase and 17β-hydroxysteroid dehydrogenase) are unique to the pathway of androgen synthesis, and their deficiency results in male pseudohermaphroditism only. Because 19-carbon androgens are obligatory precursors of estrogens, it likewise follows that in all but the terminal defect (17β-hydroxysteroid dehydrogenase deficiency) synthesis of estrogen is also low in affected individuals of both sexes.

CLINICAL FEATURES. In 46,XY individuals there is usually no trace of uterus or fallopian tubes, indicating that the müllerian-inhibiting function of the testis takes place normally during embryogenesis. However, the masculinization of the wolffian ducts, urogenital sinus, and urogenital tubercle and the degree of virilization at puberty vary from almost normal to absent. Therefore, the clinical findings range from phenotypic men who have mild hypospadias to phenotypic women who prior to puberty resemble patients with the complete testicular feminization syndrome. The extremes are presumed to be the consequence of the varying severity of the enzymatic defects in different patients and of the varying effects of the steroids that accumulate proximal to the metabolic blocks in each disorder. In patients with partial defects and normal plasma testosterone levels, the diagnosis can be made only by measuring the steroids that accumulate proximal to the metabolic block in question.

20,22-Desmolase deficiency (lipoid adrenal hyperplasia) is a form of congenital adrenal hyperplasia in which virtually no urinary steroids (either 17-ketosteroids or 17-hydroxycorticoids) can be detected and in which the enzyme deficiency occurs prior to the formation of pregnenolone. The abnormality is assumed to involve the 20,22-desmolase (side-chain cleavage) enzyme responsible for cleavage of cholesterol to form pregnenolone (P-450$_{SCC}$). However, no abnormalities of the gene for P-450$_{SCC}$ have been identified using the specific human DNA probe (Matteson et al., 1986). The syndrome is associated with salt wasting and profound adrenal insufficiency. Most affected individuals die during infancy, but one severely affected male was studied at 8 years of age (Kirkland et al., 1973). At autopsy the adrenal glands and the testes were enlarged and infiltrated with lipid. Another patient, diagnosed when a newborn, was reported to be successfully managed by replacement therapy to age 18 years (Haufa et al., 1985).

3β-Hydroxysteroid dehydrogenase deficiency is the second most common cause of congenital adrenal hyperplasia. In male infants it causes spectrum of defects from varying degrees of hypospadias to complete failure of masculinization associated with the presence of a vagina. Female infants may be modestly virilized at birth resulting from the weak androgenic potency of dehydroepiandrosterone, which is the major steroid secreted. In the mild form in women, the disorder may not be recognized until hirsutism develops at the expected time of puberty.

If the enzyme is absent in both the adrenal and the testis, no urinary steroids contain a Δ⁴-3-keto configuration. In patients in whom the defect is partial or affects only the testis, the urine may contain normal or even elevated levels of Δ⁴-3-keto steroids. Most patients have marked salt wasting and profound adrenal insufficiency. Long-term survival occurs only in states of partial deficiency. Reports have been made of several affected males who experienced otherwise normal male puberty except for pathologic gynecomastia (Parks et al., 1971). In these individuals the blood testosterone levels are in the low-normal range but accompanied by elevated Δ⁵-precursors (Rosenfield et al., 1974).

The enzyme in different tissues must be under complex genetic and regulatory control, because deficiency of the enzyme in the testis may be less severe than that in the adrenal gland and because enzyme activity in the liver may be normal in the presence of profound deficiency in the adrenal gland and the testis (Schneider et al., 1975).

Individuals with normal liver enzymes can be mistakenly identified as having 21-hydroxylase deficiency if an elevated ratio of Δ^5 to Δ^4 steroids is not documented (Cara et al., 1985). The 3β-hydroxysteroid dehydrogenase is not a P-450 cytochrome, and its gene has not been cloned.

17α-Hydroxylase deficiency characteristically results in hypogonadism, absence of secondary sex characteristics, hypokalemic alkalosis, hypertension, and virtually undetectable hydrocortisone secretion in phenotypic women (Biglieri et al., 1966). Secretion of both corticosterone and DOC by the adrenal gland is elevated, and urinary 17-ketosteroid levels are low. Aldosterone secretion is low, presumably as the result of high plasma DOC and depressed angiotensin levels, but it returns to normal after suppressive doses of hydrocortisone are administered. In 46,XX individuals, amenorrhea, lack of pubic hair, and hypertension are common, but since gonadal steroids are not required for female development during embryogenesis, the phenotype is that of a normal prepubertal woman. In 46,XY patients, however, the enzyme deficiency results in defective virilization that varies from complete male pseudohermaphroditism to ambiguous genitalia with perineoscrotal hypospadias (New, 1970). In males with presumed partial enzyme deficiency, severe gynecomastia may develop at puberty. Individuals with this disorder do not develop adrenal insufficiency, because the secretion of both corticosterone (a glucocorticoid and a mineralocorticoid) and DOC (a mineralocorticoid) is elevated. The hypertension and hypokalemia that are prominent features of the disorder even in the neonatal period remit after suppression of the DOC secretion by adequate glucocorticoid replacement.

A single P-450 cytochrome, P-450$_{C17}$, accomplishes both 17α-hydroxylation of progesterone and pregnenolone and cleavage of the side chain of C-21 steroids to form C-19 steroids (17,20-desmolase activity). It is not clear how a single P-450$_{C17}$ can possess both activities in vitro and yet cause the predominant formation of 19-carbon steroids in ovary and testis and 21-carbon steroids in the adrenal. Furthermore, some patients have clinical disorders characterized by deficiency of only 17,20-desmolase activity (see following discussion) and others by deficiency of both enzymatic activities. Studies using DNA probes have documented several distinct mutations in families with combined 17α-hydroxylase/ 17,20-desmolase deficiency including a premature stop codon and 4- and 7-base pair duplications in the gene (Yanase et al., 1990).

17,20-Desmolase deficiency has been described in 15 individuals from seven families. Affected males have a 46,XY chromosome pattern, a normal adrenocortical function, and a variable pattern of male pseudohermaphroditism (Zachmann et al., 1982). The defect leading to male pseudohermaphroditism involves a variable deficiency in the conversion of 17-hydroxyprogesterone to androstenedione. In the majority of patients genital ambiguity is observed at birth with some virilization at the time of expected puberty. However, two patients have had a female phenotype with no virilization at the time of expected puberty (Goebelsmann et al., 1976; Zachmann et al., 1982). The disorder has been recognized in one 46,XX woman with sexual infantilism (Larrea et al., 1983). DNA studies in families with the isolated deficiency of 17,20-desmolase activity have not been reported.

17β-Hydroxysteroid dehydrogenase deficiency involves the final step in androgen biosynthesis—reduction of the 17-keto group of androstenedione to form testosterone. This disorder is the most common enzymatic defect in testosterone synthesis causing male pseudohermaphroditism. Affected 46,XY males usually have a female phenotype with a blind-ending vagina and an absence of müllerian derivatives, but inguinal or abdominal testes and virilized wolffian duct structures are present. At the time of expected puberty, both virilization with phallic enlargement and development of facial and body hair and a variable degree of female breast development take place.

In one untreated individual in the United States and in a large Arab kindred, gender role reversal from female to male occurred at puberty (Imperato-McGinley et al., 1979; Rösler and Kohn, 1983). Androgen and estrogen dynamics have not been elucidated in detail, but the 17-keto reduction of estrone to estradiol by the gonads is also low. 17β-Hydroxysteroid dehydrogenase is normally present in many tissues in addition to the gonads, but only the gonadal enzyme appears to be defective in this disorder. Plasma testosterone concentration may be in the low-normal range, making it essential to document a significant elevation in plasma androstenedione concentration to make the diagnosis. Studies of the molecular defects causing the disorder have not been reported.

PATHOPHYSIOLOGY. The available data for the 17α-hydroxylase and 3β-hydroxysteroid dehydrogenase defects are compatible with autosomal recessive inheritance. The limited family data for 17,20-desmolase deficiency and 17β-hydroxysteroid dehydrogenase deficiency are compatible with either autosomal recessive or X-linked recessive mutations. Insufficient data are available for the 20,22-desmolase defect to warrant deduction as to the pattern of inheritance.

The pattern of steroid secretion and excretion depends on the site of the various metabolic blocks (see Fig. 37–6). In general, gonadotropin secretion is high. As a consequence, many individuals with incomplete defects are able to compensate so that the steady-state concentration of end products, such as testosterone, may be normal or almost normal.

Instances of male pseudohermaphroditism have been described in which testosterone formation is deficient for reasons other than a single enzyme defect in androgen synthesis. Included are disorders in which Leydig cell agenesis or unresponsiveness to gonadotropin (Berthezene et al., 1976) or the secretion of a biologically inactive LH molecule (Park et al., 1976) were thought to be the primary defects. In addition, as described, a spectrum of defects in testicular development have been characterized, including familial XY gonadal dysgenesis, sporadic dysgenetic testes, and absent testis syndrome in which deficient testosterone production is secondary to the impairment of gonadal development.

MANAGEMENT. Replacement therapy with glucocorticoids and, in some instances, mineralocorticoids is indicated in patients with those disorders that cause adrenal insufficiency. The decision as to the management of the genital abnormalities depends on the individual case. Fertility has not been reported, and its consideration does not enter into the decision of sex assignment. In genetic females there is no problem, except in diagnosis, in that affected individuals are raised appropriately as females, and suitable estrogen replacement is indicated at the time of expected puberty to promote development of normal female secondary sex characteristics.

The decision as to whether affected newborn males with ambiguous genitalia should be raised as males or females depends on the anatomic defect. In general, more severely affected individuals should be raised as females, and corrective surgery of the genitalia and removal of the testes should be undertaken as early as possible. In those raised as females, estrogen therapy is also indicated at the appropriate age to allow development of normal female secondary sex characteristics.

In individuals raised as males, corrective surgery is indicated for any coexisting hypospadias. Careful monitoring of values of plasma androgens and estrogens should be undertaken at the time of expected puberty to determine whether long-term supplemental testosterone therapy is appropriate.

Abnormalities in Androgen Action

Several disorders of male phenotypic development result from abnormalities of androgen action. The spectrum of phenotypes is described in Table 37–5. In these disorders, testosterone formation and müllerian regression are normal; however, male development is impaired to a variable degree as a result of resistance to androgen action in target cells (Griffin and Wilson, 1989).

5α-Reductase deficiency is a form of male pseudohermaphroditism that is inherited in an autosomal recessive fashion and is characterized by (1) a severe perineoscrotal hypospadias with a hooded prepuce, a ventral urethral groove, and opening of the urethra at the base of the phallus (Fig. 37–9A); (2) a blind vaginal pouch of variable size opening either into the urogenital sinus or more frequently onto the urethra immediately behind the urethral orifice; (3) a well-developed and histologically differentiated testes with normal epididymides, vasa deferentia, and seminal vesicles, and termination of the ejaculatory ducts into the blind-ending vagina (Fig. 37–9B); (4) a female habitus without female breast development but with normal axillary and pubic hair; (5) an absence of female internal genitalia; and (6) a normal male plasma testosterone level and masculini-

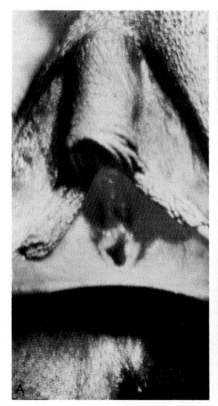
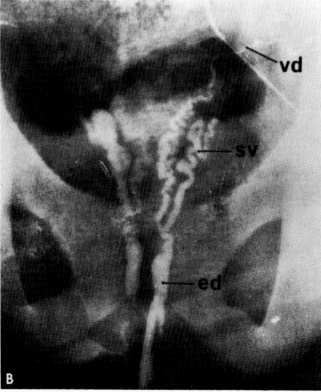

Figure 37–9. *A,* The external genitalia of a patient with 5α-reductase deficiency. *B,* Genitogram of the same patient (vd. vas deferens; sv, seminal vesicle: ed, ejaculatory duct). (From Walsh, P. C., Madden, J. D., Harrod, M. J., Goldstein, J. L., McDonald, P. C., and Wilson, J. D.: N. Engl. J. Med., 291:944, 1974.)

Table 37–5. ANATOMIC, GENETIC, AND ENDOCRINE PROFILE OF HEREDITARY MALE PSEUDOHERMAPHRODITISM

Disorder	Inheritance	Phenotype						Endocrine Profile Relative to Normal Male		
		Müllerian Ducts	Wolffian Ducts	Spermato-geneses	Urogenital Sinus	External Genitalia	Breast	Testosterone Production	Esterogen Production	LH
Defects in Testosterone Synthesis										
Five enzyme deficiencies	Autosomal or X-linked recessive	Absent	Variable development	Normal to decreased	Variable from male to female	Generally female	Usually male	Normal to decreased	Variable	High
Defects in Androgen Action										
5α-Reductase deficiency	Autosomal recessive	Absent	Male	Decreased	Female	Clitoromegaly	Male	Normal	Normal	Normal or increased
Receptor Disorders										
Complete testicular feminization	X-linked	Absent	Absent	Absent	Female	Female	Female	High	Hith	High
Incomplete testicular feminization	X-linked recessive	Absent	Male	Absent	Female	Clitoromegaly and posterior fusion	Female	High	High	High
Reifenstein syndrome	X-linked recessive	Absent	Variable development	Absent	Variable from male to female	Incomplete male development	Female	High	High	High
Infertile male syndrome	X-linked recessive	Absent	Male	Absent or decreased	Male	Male	Usually male	Normal or High	Normal or High	Normal or High
Undervirilized fertile male	X-linked recessive	Absent	Male	Variable	Male	Male	Female	Normal or High	Normal or High	Normal
Receptor-positive resistance	X-linked recessive	Absent	Variable	Absent or decreased	Variable	Female to male	Variable	Normal or High	Normal or High	Normal or High
Defects in Müllerian Regression										
Persistent müllerian duct syndrome	Autosomal or X-linked	Rudimentary uterus and fallopian tubes	Male	Normal	Male	Male	Male	Normal	Normal	Normal

Adapted from Petersdorf, R. G., Adams, R. D., Braunwald, E., et al.: Disorders of sexual differentiation. *In* Harrison's Principles of Internal Medicine. 10th ed. New York, McGraw-Hill Book Co., 1983, pp. 724–739 zation to a variable degree at the time of puberty (Imperato-McGinley et al., 1974; Walsh et al., 1974).

The fact that the defective virilization during embryogenesis is limited to the urogenital sinus and the anlage of the external genitalia provided insight into the nature of the fundamental abnormality. Testosterone, the androgen secreted by the fetal testis, is the intracellular mediator for differentiation of the wolffian duct into the epididymis, the vas deferens, and the seminal vesicle, whereas dihydrotestosterone is the functional intracellular hormone responsible for virilization of the urogenital sinus and the anlage of the external genitalia. Consequently, in a male embryo with normal testosterone synthesis and normal androgen receptors, a failure of dihydrotestosterone formation would be expected to result in the phenotype observed in this disorder, namely, normal male wolffian duct derivatives with defective masculinization of the structures originating from the urogenital sinus, genital tubercle, and genital swellings (Fig. 37–10). Because testosterone itself is the hormone that regulates LH secretion, plasma LH level is minimally if at all elevated. As a result, testosterone and estrogen production rates are those of normal men, and gynecomastia does not develop.

The fact that the 5α-reductase enzyme is deficient in this disorder was suspected on phenotypic and endocrine grounds and was established by direct enzymatic assay in biopsy tissues and in fibroblasts cultured from affected individuals (Walsh et al., 1974). Considerable genetic heterogeneity is noted. In most subjects, the 5α-reductase is either profoundly deficient or functionally absent; in others, the enzyme protein is synthesized at a normal rate but is structurally abnormal. It is not clear why virilization at puberty appears to be more normal than the virilization that takes place during sexual differentiation. The gene that encodes 5α-reductase has not been cloned.

Androgen receptor disorders may result in several distinct phenotypes (Fig. 37–11). Despite differences in clinical presentation and molecular pathology, these disorders are similar in regard to endocrinology, genetics, and basic pathophysiology. The major clinical features and issues of management of the disorders are considered first, followed by a discussion of the similar endocrinology and pathophysiology.

Complete testicular feminization is the most common form of male pseudohermaphroditism, estimates of frequency varying from one in 20,000 to one in 64,000 male births. It is the third most common cause of primary amenorrhea in phenotypic women after gonadal dysgenesis and congenital absence of the vagina. The clinical features are characteristic. A phenotypic female is usually seen by a clinician because of either inguinal hernia (prepubertal cases) or primary amenorrhea (postpubertal cases). The development of the breasts after puberty, the general habitus, and the distribution of body fat are female in character; therefore, many patients have a truly feminine appearance (Fig. 37–11A). Axillary and pubic hair is normal, and facial hair is absent. The external genitalia are unambiguously female (Fig. 37–12A). The clitoris is normal or small. The vagina is short and blind-ending and may be absent or rudimentary. All internal genitalia are absent except for the gonads, which have histologic features of undescended testes (normal or increased Leydig cells and seminiferous tubules without spermatogenesis).

The testes may be located in the abdomen, along the course of the inguinal canal, or in the labia majora. Occasionally, remnants of müllerian or wolffian duct origin can be identified in the paratesticular fascia or in fibrous bands extending from the testis. Patients tend to be rather tall. Bone age is normal, and intelligence is normal. The psychosexual development is unmistakably female in regard to behavior, outlook, and maternal instincts.

The major complication of undescended testes in this disorder, as in other forms of cryptorchidism, is the development of tumors. Because affected individuals undergo normal growth spurts at puberty and successful feminization at the time of expected puberty, and because testicular tumors rarely develop until after puberty in patients with intra-abdominal testes, it is usual to delay castration.

Surgical intervention is indicated in the prepubertal patient if the testes are present in the inguinal region or in the labia majora and result in discomfort or hernia formation. If prepubertal hernia repair is indicated, most physicians prefer to remove the testes at the same time to limit the number of operative procedures. When the testes are removed prepubertally, estrogen therapy is required at the appropriate age to ensure normal growth and breast development. When castration is performed postpubertally, menopausal symptoms and other evidence of estrogen withdrawal supervene and suitable estrogen replacement is indicated.

Figure 37–10. Deranged androgen physiology in 5α-reductase deficiency. T, testosterone; D, dihydrotestosterone; E, estradiol; LH, luteinizing hormone; R, androgen receptor.

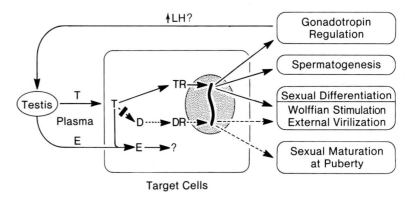

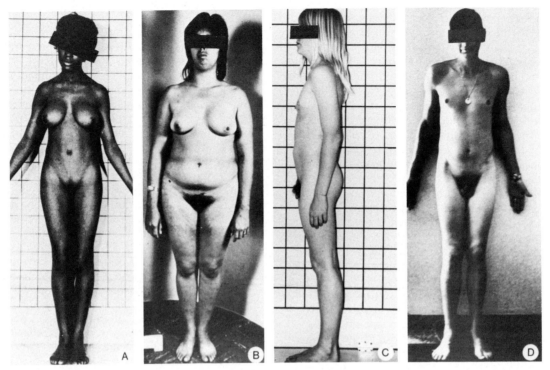

Figure 37–11. Patients with disorders of the androgen receptor. *A,* Complete testicular feminization. *B,* Incomplete testicular feminization. *C,* Reifenstein's syndrome. *D,* Infertile male syndrome. (*A* courtesy of Dr. Howard Jones, *C,* courtesy of Dr. Ronald Swerdloff, and *D* courtesy of Dr. James Aiman.)

Incomplete testicular feminization is about one tenth as frequent as the complete form. The disorders are similar except that in incomplete testicular feminization minor virilization of the external genitalia (partial fusion of the labioscrotal folds and some degree of clitoromegaly, Fig. 37–12*B*), normal pubic hair (Fig. 37–11*B*), and some virilization as well as feminization at the time of expected puberty occur. The vagina is short and blind-ending. In contrast to the complete form, the wolffian duct derivatives are often partially developed. The family history is usually uninformative. However, in several instances, multiple family members are affected in a pattern compatible with X-linkage.

The management of patients with the complete and the incomplete forms of testicular feminization differs. Because patients with the incomplete disorder experience virilization at the time of expected puberty, gonadectomy should be performed before that time with clitoromegaly or posterior labial fusion.

Reifenstein syndrome is the term applied to a variety of forms of incomplete male pseudohermaphroditism that were initially described by a number of other eponyms (Gilbert-Dreyfus syndrome, Lubs syndrome) (Wilson et al., 1974). Each of these phenotypes was originally assumed to be a distinct entity. Because several families have now been described in which affected members exhibit variable manifestations that span the phenotypes described using these terms, these syndromes probably constitute variable manifestations of a single mutation. The most common presentation is a child with perineoscrotal hypospadias (Fig. 37–12*C*) or a man with perineoscrotal hypospadias and gynecomastia (Figs. 37–11*C* and 37–12*D*). However, the spectrum of defective virilization in such families ranges from infertile men to men with gynecomastia and azoospermia to phenotypic women with pseudovaginas. Axillary and pubic hair are normal, but chest and facial hair are minimal. Cryptorchidism is common, the testes are usually small, and spermatogenesis is usually incomplete. Some individuals have defects in wolffian duct derivatives, such as absence or hypoplasia of the vas deferens.

Because psychologic development in most is unequivocally male, hypospadias and cryptorchidism should be corrected surgically. The only successful form of treatment of the gynecomastia is surgery.

The infertile male syndrome may be the most common disorder of the androgen receptor and, in contrast to the other disorders, is not actually a form of male pseudohermaphroditism (Aiman et al., 1979). Some are minimally affected individuals in families with Reifenstein syndrome. Azoospermia is the only manifestation of the receptor abnormality. More commonly, the individuals present with male infertility and have family histories that are negative. Evaluation of such men with normal external genitalia (Fig. 37–11*D*), apparently normal wolffian duct structures, and infertility due to azoospermia or severe oligospermia has shown that a disorder of the androgen receptor may be present in one fifth or more of those with idiopathic azoospermia (Aiman and Griffin, 1982). No treatment is available for the infertility in any of these disorders.

The least severely affected individual with an androgen receptor disorder is the *undervirilized fertile male* (Grino et al., 1988). Men in this family and similar families have gynecomastia, small phallus, and de-

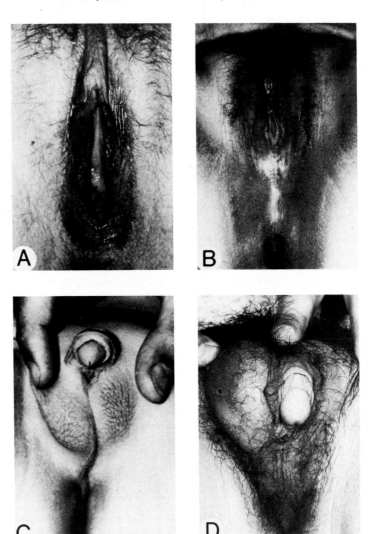

Figure 37–12. External genitalia of four patients with disorders of the androgen receptor. *A,* Complete testicular feminization. *B,* Incomplete testicular feminization. *C,* Reifenstein's syndrome in a prepubertal patient. *D,* Reifenstein's syndrome in a postpubertal patient.

creased beard and body hair but a normal sperm density and fertility in some affected individuals.

The endocrinology and pathophysiology of these five disorders of the androgen receptor are similar (Fig. 37–13). The karyotype is 46,XY, and the mutant gene is believed to be located on the X chromosome. The frequency of a positive family history varies from about two thirds of patients with testicular feminization and Reifenstein syndrome to only an occasional patient with infertile male syndrome. It is assumed the disorder in patients with a negative family history is the result of a new mutation.

Hormone dynamics have been best characterized in complete testicular feminization, but they are similar in all disorders of the androgen receptor. Plasma testosterone levels and rates of testosterone production by the testes are normal or higher than normal. The elevated rate of testosterone production is caused by the high mean plasma level of LH, which, in turn, is due to defective feedback regulation caused by resistance to

Figure 37–13. Deranged androgen physiology in receptor disorders. *T,* testosterone; *D,* dihydrotestosterone; *E,* estradiol; *LH,* luteinizing hormone; *R,* androgen receptor.

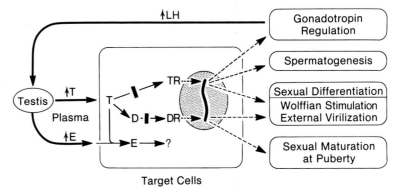

the action of androgen at the hypothalamic-pituitary level. Elevated LH concentration is probably also responsible for the increased estrogen production by the testes. In normal men, most estrogen is derived from peripheral formation from circulating androgens, but when plasma LH concentration is elevated, the testes secrete significant amounts of estrogen into the circulation. Thus, resistance to the feedback regulation of LH secretion by circulating androgen results in elevated plasma LH levels. This, in turn, results in the enhanced secretion of both testosterone and estradiol by the testes. Gonadotropin levels rise even higher and menopausal symptoms may develop when the testes are removed, indicating that gonadotropin secretion is under partial regulatory control. Presumably, in the steady state and in the absence of an androgen effect, estrogen alone regulates LH secretion, a control that is achieved at the expense of an elevated plasma estrogen concentration for a male.

Feminization in these disorders is the result of two interlocking phenomena. First, androgens and estrogens have antagonistic effects at the peripheral level, and normal virilization occurs in normal men when the ratio of androgen to estrogen is 100:1 or greater. In the absence of androgen action, the cellular effect of estrogen is unopposed. Second, the production of estradiol in these individuals is greater than that in the normal male, although it is less than that of the normal female (MacDonald et al., 1979). Different degrees of androgen resistance, coupled with variably enhanced estradiol production, results in different degrees of defective virilization and enhanced feminization in the four clinical syndromes. The defective virilization is most severe in complete testicular feminization, and the full feminizing effect of the increased estrogen is expressed. Estrogen production in the Reifenstein syndrome is increased to a similar or greater extent as that in testicular feminization, but a less severe androgen resistance results in a predominantly male phenotype with less pronounced feminization (Wilson et al., 1974). Only a few men with the infertile male syndrome have had evaluation of androgen-estrogen dynamics (Aiman et al., 1979). The hormonal changes seem to be similar to those in the other receptor disorders but less marked. Some men with this syndrome do not have elevation of plasma LH or plasma testosterone levels.

All of these syndromes are the result of an abnormality of the androgen receptor. Initially, fibroblasts cultured from the skin of some patients with complete testicular feminization were shown to have near absence of high-affinity dihydrotestosterone binding. Subsequently, other individuals with complete testicular feminization, as well as those with incomplete testicular feminization, Reifenstein syndrome, infertile male syndrome, and undervirilized fertile male, have been found to have either a decreased amount of an apparently normal receptor or a qualitatively abnormal androgen receptor. Absent or near-absent binding appears to be associated most commonly with complete testicular feminization. A qualitatively abnormal receptor has been detected in families with each of the five clinical phenotypes (Griffin and Wilson, 1989; Grino et al., 1988). Except for the lack of binding in complete testicular

feminization, no consistent correlation is noted between the receptor abnormality as demonstrated in cultured fibroblasts and the clinical severity of the androgen resistance in individual patients.

Receptor-positive resistance is a category of androgen resistance that does not appear to involve either the 5α-reductase or the androgen receptor. It was first identified in a family with the syndrome of testicular feminization (Amrhein et al., 1976). Subsequent patients, with a variety of phenotypes ranging from incomplete testicular feminization to findings similar to those in the Reifenstein syndrome, have been described. The hormonal profile is similar to that seen in the receptor disorders. The site of the molecular abnormality in these patients is unclear. It could be due to defects of the androgen receptor that are too subtle to be detected by the usual assay. If the defect is truly distal to the receptor, there could be failure of specific messenger RNA generation or an abnormality of RNA processing. Indeed, it is not established that a uniform defect is present, and the disorder may represent a heterogeneous group of molecular abnormalities. Studies designed to detect subtle qualitative abnormalities of the receptor are likely to decrease the number of patients in this category. At present they appear to amount to less than one fifth of patients with androgen resistance (Griffin and Wilson, 1989). Management of the patient depends on phenotype.

A number of families with disorders of the androgen receptor or apparent receptor-positive resistance have been studied using DNA probes. Most patients have had the phenotype of complete testicular feminization. A major deletion in the gene for the receptor has been found in one family. Most have had point mutations in the hormone-binding region or mutations leading to premature stop codons, partially truncating the hormone-binding region (Fig. 37–14). Two families with apparent receptor-positive resistance have had abnormalities in the DNA-binding region (McPhaul et al., 1991).

Persistent müllerian duct syndrome results in normal penile development and variable development of the vas deferens but, in addition, bilateral fallopian tubes, uterus, and upper vagina. These individuals commonly present with inguinal hernias that contain the uterus. Cryptorchidism is common. Most have uninformative family histories, but several pairs of siblings have been described in whom the condition must be inherited either as an autosomal recessive or an X-linked recessive mutation. Because the external genitalia are well developed and the patients masculinize normally at puberty, it is assumed that during the critical stage of embryonic sexual differentiation the fetal testes produced a normal amount of androgen. However, müllerian regression does not occur, possibly because of failure of the fetal testis to produce müllerian-inhibiting substance or possibly because of failure of the tissues to respond to this hormone (Guerrier et al., 1989).

The preservation of external male appearance and the maintenance of virilization are essential. A primary or staged orchiopexy should be performed. None of the reported patients has developed a malignancy in the uterus or vagina, and because the vas deferens is closely

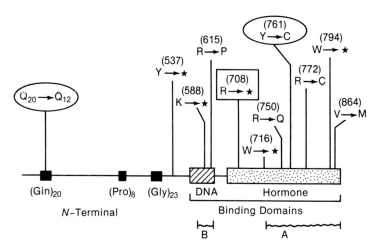

Figure 37–14. Schematic diagram of reported mutations in the androgen receptor. The horizontal line represents the 917 amino acid androgen receptor with the N-terminal region including homopolymeric repeats of glutamine (Gln), proline (Pro), and glycine (Gly)—the DNA and hormone-binding domains. The numbers in parentheses identify the amino acid positon. The letters before and after the arrows indicated the single-letter amino acid code. Asterisks donote stop codons. The regions indicated by A and B are the sites of deletions. The ovals identify two mutations in a single individual with a qualitatively abnormal receptor. The mutation enclosed in a box is a constitutively active artificial truncation mutation. (From McPhaul, M. J., Marcellis M., and Tilley, W. D.: FASEB J., 1991. In press.)

associated with the broad ligaments, the uterus and vagina should be left in place to avoid disruption of the vas deferens during removal and consequently to preserve possible fertility.

Microphallus

Microphallus is a congenital disorder in which the penis is small but otherwise anatomically normal and, specifically, in which the urethra is that of a normal male. By most criteria microphallus is defined as a penis that is below the 95 per cent confidence limits of penile size for age, as defined by Schonfeld and Beebe (1942). A nomogram that relates stretched penile length as a function of age for the Schonfeld data is useful in distinguishing true microphallus from normal (Fig. 37–15) (Lee et al., 1980). In the newborn, stretched penile length less than 1.9 cm is usually considered microphallus. A typical case of congenital microphallus is shown in Fig. 37–16. The condition is frequently associated with testicular maldescent.

Both the formation of the penile urethra and the phallic growth during embryogenesis are under the control of androgen. Formation of the male urethra is usually complete by the end of the 1st trimester of human embryogenesis, and differential growth of the male phallus takes place predominately during the 2nd and 3rd trimesters. Consequently, microphallus is generally considered the consequence of defective androgen secretion during the 2nd and 3rd trimesters. At the clinical level two broad categories of microphallus can be delineated.

One type is associated with other abnormalities involving either the hypothalamic-pituitary axis such as anencephaly, congenital absence of the pituitary, and the Prader-Willi syndrome, the testes themselves (Boyerson and Robinow syndromes), or the chromosomes. In these disorders, the diagnosis is a part of the overall clinical picture.

In the other type, microphallus appears to be an isolated finding, unassociated with other major abnormalities. The etiology may not be obvious in the prepubertal child. In some series hypogonadotropic hypogonadism is the most common cause of isolated

microphallus. The association of microphallus with disorders of the pituitary and of gonadotropin synthesis is in keeping with evidence suggesting that pituitary gonadotropins regulate testicular androgen production during the last 2 trimesters but not between weeks 8 and 12, when the male urethra is formed.

Primary hypogonadism is the second most common cause of isolated microphallus due to a variety of etiologies, most of which are poorly understood. Separation of the two causes of isolated microphallus is usually straightforward. Boys with hypogonadotropic hypogonadism have low plasma gonadotropin levels and respond normally to standard challenge with human chorionic gonadotropin (hCG) by increasing plasma testosterone levels, whereas boys with primary hypogonadism have elevated plasma gonadotropin levels, and do not respond normally to hCG. Furthermore, most patients with androgen resistance syndromes have more profound impairment of virilization, usually including hypospadias.

The initial management of microphallus is straightforward, namely, in patients younger than age 3 years, low-dosage, short-term systemic testosterone therapy (25 mg testosterone cypionate every 3 weeks for 3

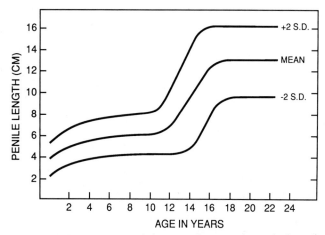

Figure 37–15. Nomogram of the normal range of stretched penile length in men as a function of age (S. D., standard deviation). (Redrawn from Lee, P. A., et al., Johns Hopkins Med. J. 146:156, 1980).

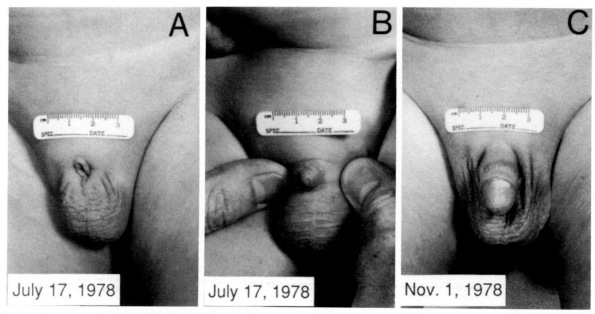

Figure 37–16. Effect on penile size of 25-mg testosterone cypionate intramuscularly every 3 weeks for 3 months in an infant with microphallus.

months) causes penile growth so that most eventually reach the normal range (see Fig. 37–16). On occasion, the regimen may be repeated a year later. Risk of acceleration of growth and bone age are minimal in this group. The long-term consequences of this therapy are not established. At puberty, boys with hypogonadotropic hypogonadism or primary hypogonadism must receive appropriate replacement therapy as indicated. Sometimes, late treatment of previously unrecognized hypogonadotropic hypogonadism with systemic testosterone esters can have profound effects on penile size (Fig. 37–17). The frequency with which early therapy combined with replacement therapy at the time of expected puberty will cause penile size to increase to within the adult normal range is not established. Inadequately treated adult patients remain below the 10th percentile in penile size, although vaginal penetration may be possible.

DIFFERENTIAL DIAGNOSIS AND EVALUATION OF SEXUAL AMBIGUITY

The evaluation of the newborn with ambiguous genitalia is one of the most complicated challenges of med-

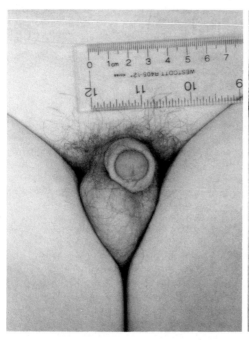

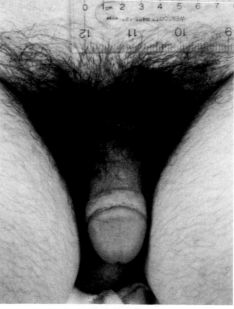

Figure 37–17. Effect on penile size of 200-mg testosterone cypionate intramuscularly every 2 weeks for 11 months in a previously untreated 22-year-old man with microphallus due to hypogonadotropic hypogonadism.

August 15, 1989   July 9, 1990

icine. Few decisions require a broader application of both theoretic and practical knowledge, and few decisions have greater social impact on the future of the patient. It is no exaggeration to say that the detection of sexual ambiguity in the newborn constitutes a true medical emergency. Untreated sexual ambiguity can lead to confusion about gender identity, role, or both, either because of uncorrected biologic abnormalities per se or because of uncertainty as to the correct sex assignment on the part of both the parents and the affected individual. Therefore, assignment of the sex of rearing should be made as early as possible, preferably in the newborn nursery, but not before all necessary diagnostic procedures have been performed.

In this section, the discussion centers on those disorders that most frequently occur with ambiguity of the external genitalia, thereby excluding disorders with clear-cut phenotypic sex, such as the Klinefelter syndrome, gonadal dysgenesis, testicular feminization, and so forth. This selection limits the differential diagnosis to the four most common causes of ambiguous genitalia: true hermaphroditism, mixed gonadal dysgenesis, female pseudohermaphroditism, and male pseudohermaphroditism.

While the infant with ambiguous genitalia is undergoing evaluation, the family should be informed that the development of the external genitalia is incomplete and that additional studies are necessary before the correct gender assignment can be made. The procedures employed for the investigation of patients with ambiguous genitalia include (1) a detailed history, including a pedigree analysis, with a physical examination; (2) an evaluation of the chromosomal sex, utilizing flourescent staining of the Y chromosome and karyotyping; (3) a biochemical evaluation of the urinary and plasma steroids before and after stimulation with hCG; (4) an evaluation of the urogenital sinus and internal duct structures utilizing endoscopy and radiography procedures; (5) an exploratory laparotomy and gonadal biopsy; and (6) when available, an assessment of androgen action utilizing cultured skin fibroblasts.

History and Physical Examination

Because many of these disorders are hereditary, the family history must be probed not only for identically affected individuals but also for variant forms of abnormal sexual development, unexplained death during infancy, infertility, amenorrhea, and hirsutism. If a similar disorder is present in a maternal aunt, uncle, or cousin, one of the disorders that is inherited as an X-linked recessive trait should be considered. For disorders inherited as autosomal recessive traits, the presence of parental consanguinity should be determined. In addition, the mother should be questioned about virilizing signs and about the ingestion of androgens, progestogens, or other drugs during pregnancy.

The most important finding on physical examination is the presence of a gonad in the labioscrotal fold or scrotum. Because ovaries rarely descend, the presence of a palpable gonad excludes the diagnosis of female pseudohermaphroditism. Other findings that are helpful on physical examination include (1) hyperpigmentation of the areola and labioscrotal folds, which is common in patients with congenital adrenal hyperplasia; (2) palpation of the uterus as a midline, thickened structure; (3) evidence of dehydration and failure to thrive; and (4) existence of other associated congenital anomalies. The size of the phallus and the location of the urethral meatus should be documented, and the contents of any hernias should be palpated carefully. Each infant with bilateral cryptorchidism or with unilateral cryptorchidism and hypospadias should be considered to have a disorder of sexual differentiation until proved otherwise.

Chromosomal Evaluation

A quick laboratory test in the differential diagnosis of intersexuality is the examination of buccal mucosal cells for the presence of chromatin clumps on the nuclear membrane—the Barr body. The Barr body, which represents the second X chromosome, is found in 20 per cent or more of the nuclei of normal females and in less than 2 per cent of the nuclei of normal males. Unfortunately, in practice, this assay has a high incidence both of false-positive and false-negative results and hence is of limited usefulness. Furthermore, in the female, counts may be lower during the first few days of life.

If buccal mucosal cells are stained with quinacrine or its mustard derivative and examined by fluorescence microscopy, the Y chromosome (the F body) can be identified because of its propensity to fluoresce. This phenomenon provides a more accurate, rapid means of obtaining insight into the chromosomal composition than other indirect means of estimating sex chromosomes. However, because the fluorescent portion of the Y chromosome is on the long arm of the chromosome and the male-determining factors are located on the short arm, the absence of a fluorescent Y must be interpreted with caution. Several reports have been made in which absence of the fluorescent portion has been associated with normal male sexual differentiation. DNA probes specific for different regions of the Y chromosome have also been utilized to characterize the DNA in individuals with structural abnormalities of the Y chromosome (Waibel et al., 1987).

The more direct and accurate means of determining the human chromosomal complement involves the culture of peripheral blood leukocytes in a medium that contains a mitogenic agent (phytohemagglutinin), which induces the lymphocytes to divide after a 3-day period of incubation at 37° C. A mitotic spindle poison such as colchicine that arrests mitosis at metaphase is added, and the cells are harvested and stained. The chromosomes of a number of cells in metaphase are assessed to establish the number and histologic characteristics. This technique is valuable in establishing the exact chromosomal complement, the presence of mosaicism, and the structural characteristics of the chromosomes. To determine mosaicism accurately, the study of multiple tissues may be necessary.

Biochemical Evaluation

Biochemical tests are most useful in identifying congenital adrenal hyperplasia and in determining whether the capacity to form testosterone is normal. In untreated patients with 21-hydroxylase deficiency, the common variety of congenital adrenal hyperplasia, morning plasma 17-hydroxyprogesterone levels are markedly elevated (usually >2000 ng/dl); the upper limit in control subjects of all ages is rarely >200 ng/dl (New et al., 1989). When plasma measurements are not available, the diagnosis of 21-hydroxylase deficiency can be established by measuring the urinary excretion of 17-ketosteroids and pregnanetriol. Caution must be exercised in interpreting values obtained from infants in the first 3 weeks of life. In normal infants, urinary 17-ketosteroid excretion may be as high as 2.5 mg per day in the first 3 weeks of life and thereafter fall to less than 0.5 mg per day. Pregnanetriol is a metabolic by-product of the hydrocortisone precursor 17-hydroxyprogesterone and is normally found in the urine in amounts less than 0.5 mg per day. Pregnanetriol excretion is increased in congenital virilizing adrenal hyperplasia, owing to the deficiency of 21-hydroxylase, and to a somewhat lesser extent in 11-hydroxylase deficiency.

In the rarer forms of defective steroid hormone biosynthesis, it may be necessary to document high levels of plasma pregnenolone and dehydroepiandrosterone (3β-hydroxysteroid dehydrogenase deficiency), profound deficiency of all C-21 and C-19 steroids (20,22-desmolase deficiency), high corticosterone and deoxycorticosterone levels (17-hydroxylase deficiency), or deficiency of C-19 steroids and elevation of C-21 precursor steroids (17,20-desmolase deficiency). Caution must be exercised in interpreting these measurements in the newborn as previously mentioned.

Although plasma testosterone level increases during the neonatal period in normal male infants, the diagnostic implication of plasma levels during this period has not been documented in pathologic states. Therefore, to evaluate the capacity for testosterone biosynthesis in infants with male pseudohermaphroditism, it is customary to measure plasma androgen values before and after the administration of hCG. Infants with possible androgen resistance can be distinguished from those with defective testosterone synthesis, caused either by single enzyme defects or by developmental defects in the testes by demonstrating that plasma testosterone level increases in the former group to greater than 2 ng per ml after treatment for 4 days with 2000 IU of hCG per day (Forest, 1979; Walsh et al., 1976). Plasma androstenedione levels should be measured simultaneously, because hCG causes a profound increase in individuals with 17β-hydroxysteroid dehydrogenase deficiency (Levine et al., 1980). Likewise, if the phenotype is suggestive of 5α-reductase deficiency, measurement of plasma dihydrotestosterone in the post-hCG plasma, and documentation that the ratio of plasma testosterone to plasma dihydrotestosterone is greater than 30, may establish the diagnosis of this condition (Peterson et al., 1977).

As is true for many other inborn errors of metabolism,

fibroblasts cultured from skin biopsy have been utilized to diagnose individuals affected with the syndromes of androgen resistance, and the measurement of steroid 5α-reductase activity or dihydrotestosterone binding in such fibroblasts may be useful in appropriate instances (Griffin and Wilson, 1989).

Endoscopy and Radiography

Radiographic and endoscopic procedures are of assistance in evaluating the status of the urogenital sinus, the internal duct structures, the adrenals, and the intra-abdominal gonads in patients with ambiguous genitalia. Genitography is accomplished with a blunt-ended syringe, positioned firmly at the opening of the urogenital sinus. While contrast medium is injected slowly, fluoroscopy is used to select spot films demonstrating the filling of the urogenital sinus and internal duct structures (Currarino, 1986) (Fig. 37–18). This method is superior to voiding cystourethrography. In addition, the location of the urogenital sinus, the size of the prostatic utricle, and the presence of a cervix can be confirmed on endoscopy.

At endoscopy the urogenital sinus or the prostatic utricle can be catheterized for retrograde contrast studies (Sloan and Walsh, 1976) (see Fig. 37–18). Although the lower vagina may be present in any of the common forms of intersexuality, the presence of a uterus and one fallopian tube excludes the diagnosis of male pseudohermaphroditism caused by a defect in androgen synthesis or androgen action.

When the urogenital sinus cannot be catheterized or when genitography is unsuccessful, pelvic ultrasonography is an ancillary means for documenting the presence and size of the uterus and fallopian tubes. Ultrasonography is also useful but not of diagnostic value in defining enlarged adrenal glands in some individuals with congenital adrenal hyperplasia (Bryan et al., 1988). Ultrasonography, computed tomography, and magnetic resonance imaging have been employed for the localization of nonpalpable testes, but failure to localize a testis with such techniques should not defer exploration when indicated (Kier et al., 1988).

At exploratory laparotomy, the status of the distal wolffian duct structures can be determined with anterograde vasography. The technique involves the exposure of the vas deferens and the insertion of a small blunt needle (20 to 25 gauge) through a transverse vasotomy. Following the injection of 1 ml of 50 per cent diatrizoate sodium, appropriate x-ray films are taken to document the character of the vas deferens, seminal vesicle, and ejaculatory duct (Walsh et al., 1974) (see Fig. 37–9B).

Exploratory Laparotomy and Gonadal Biopsy

In the newborn, exploratory laparotomy is occasionally undertaken for inspection and biopsy and occasional removal of gonadal tissue. Laparotomy is indicated only if gonadal biopsy will influence the sex of rearing. The

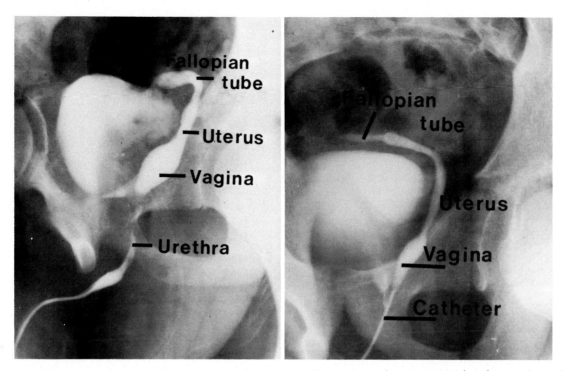

Figure 37–18. Radiograms performed after retrograde instillation of sodium diatrizoate into the prostatic utricles of two patients with familial persistent müllarian duct syndrome. (From Sloan, W. R., and Walsh, P. C.: J. Urol., 115:459, 1976. © 1976 Williams & Wilkins, Baltimore.)

major consideration in establishing the sex of rearing should be the achievement of functional genitalia. Fertility is of secondary importance. If the phallus is inadequate, there is no necessity for early exploration. Such children should be reared as females regardless of gonadal status. In the patient with both a vagina and a well-developed phallus, however, the findings on exploratory laparotomy and gonadal biopsy are occasionally of great importance in assigning the sex of rearing. In a 46,XX patient with a normal urinary steroid excretion, a negative family history, and no exposure to exogenous androgens, laparotomy is necessary to distinguish between female pseudohermaphroditism and true hermaphroditism. Similarly, in chromatin-negative patients with ambiguous genitalia (46,XY or mosaic), exploratory laparotomy is often necessary to distinguish among mixed gonadal dysgenesis, true hermaphroditism, and male pseudohermaphroditism.

Even when all available diagnostic criteria currently available are employed, including pedigree analysis, chromosomal studies, biochemical and molecular assessment, genitography, and exploratory laparotomy, it is not possible to establish the diagnosis in all instances of ambiguous genitalia. In such cases, the gender assignment and the decision regarding appropriate corrective surgery must be made empirically on the basis of the clinical findings and the psychosocial setting. However, it is imperative that a vigorous attempt be made to establish the exact cause in all cases of ambiguous genitalia, because the information may be invaluable in the genetic counseling of the families regarding the risks in subsequent children.

Working Scheme for the Evaluation of Ambiguous Genitalia

All the aforementioned procedures do not need to be utilized in the work-up of every patient. In practice, the design of the work-up is influenced by the physical examination (Fig. 37–19). The failure to find palpable gonads in a child with ambiguous genitalia suggests female pseudohermaphroditism, or, rarely, true hermaphroditism or male pseudohermaphroditism. The finding of two scrotal or inguinal gonads suggests that the infant is an incompletely virilized genetic male. A single palpable gonad suggests either mixed gonadal dysgenesis or rarely true hermaphroditism.

The second diagnostic procedure requires the establishment of chromosomal sex. If the infant is 46,XX without palpable gonads, it is necessary to determine whether congenital adrenal hyperplasia is present. It may be necessary to perform such tests prior to the availability of information about the karyotype if a suspicion exists as to the presence of a salt-losing form of congenital adrenal hyperplasia. Diagnosis of congenital adrenal hyperplasia in 46,XY males is reached by different means. Measurement of serum 17-hydroxyprogesterone level or urinary 17-ketosteroid excretion identifies 21-hydroxylase and 11β-hydroxylase deficiencies. Other hormonal assays are employed to identify the less common forms of the disorder. An infant with 46,XX female pseudohermaphroditism in the absence of congenital adrenal hyperplasia is rare and this is usually due to a maternal virilizing syndrome.

In the 46,XY infant with two palpable gonads, the

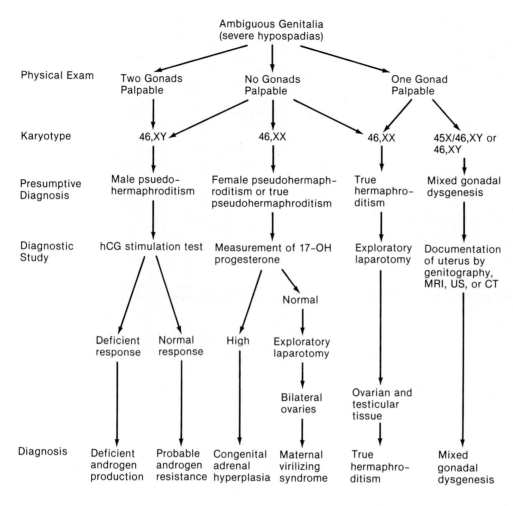

Figure 37–19. Diagnostic evaluation of the infant with ambiguous genitalia (17-OH progesterone, 17-hydroxyprogesterone; hCG, human chorionic gonadotropin; MRI, magnetic resonance imaging; US, ultrasound; CT, computer tomography).

differential diagnosis is between inadequate production of testosterone and resistance to the action of androgen. Normal response of plasma testosterone to hCG indicates that the diagnosis is androgen resistance or a temporary interference with androgen production during embryogenesis. Many individuals with profound androgen resistance virilize poorly at puberty and are candidates for female sex assignment. The diagnosis can sometimes be substantiated by measuring 5α-reductase and androgen receptor levels in fibroblasts cultured from genital skin. Defects in testosterone synthesis can be due either to hereditary defects in the enzymes required for testosterone biosynthesis or to a variety of developmental defects. In both types of deficient androgen production, virilization is usually satisfactory when androgen replacement is given at puberty.

A case of 46,XX karyotype and palpable gonads is fairly specific for true hermaphroditism; a 45,X/46,XY karyotype with one or no palpable gonads suggests mixed gonadal dysgenesis. Either combination provides an indication for genitography to define internal duct structures and eventually for gonadal biopsy to establish the definitive diagnosis.

Sex Assignment

Once the studies are complete, sex assignment should be made after careful consultation with the family. Some aspects of the problem are clear-cut. As mentioned previously, if the subject has an inadequate phallus, the individual should be reared as a female, regardless of the results of diagnostic tests. In the patient with an adequate phallus, however, as much information as possible should be obtained before a decision is made.

If a diagnosis of female pseudohermaphroditism is made, the patient should be reared as a female. The affected infant has ovaries, fallopian tubes, uterus, and upper vagina and is potentially fertile.

If a diagnosis of mixed gonadal dysgenesis is made, several factors favor rearing these patients as female. First, most of these patients are inadequately masculinized, and all have a uterus and vagina. Second, if they are reared as males, the testis in adulthood is infertile, and as many as a fourth with a testis may develop gonadal tumors. Third, approximately half the patients will be less than 150 cm in height.

In the true hermaphrodite with a vagina and a well-developed phallus, the sex of rearing should be based on the findings at exploratory laparotomy. If there is a normal testis that can be placed in the scrotum, the assignment should be male. If normal müllerian duct structures and a normal ovary are present on one side and either a testis or an ovotestis is present on the other side, the assignment should be female. These assignments provide the best prospects for future fertility, recognizing that the considerations of fertility are always of secondary importance. The primary decision should usually be based on the development of the external genitalia. The question of future fertility should never override this consideration.

In patients with male pseudohermaphroditism due to abnormalities of androgen synthesis or action, proper gender assignment is complicated because it may be impossible to predict what will occur at puberty. For example, will there be adequate growth of the phallus? Will the patient feminize? Will the patient be fertile? With further refinements in the understanding of male pseudohermaphroditism, it may someday be possible to predict these events accurately. At present, in the absence of a definitive diagnosis on genetic, endocrinologic, or biochemical grounds, the major criterion of sex assignment is the degree of masculinization of the external genitalia in utero. Presumably, if this was adequate, there will be sufficient masculinization at puberty, although in many instances the patient will not be fertile.

Gender assignment should be made as early as possible and only after involving the parents in the decision. When feasible, we prefer to complete diagnostic workups and perform plastic reconstructions before the infants are discharged from the newborn nursery. Orchidectomy during the neonatal period prevents the surge of androgen, in cases in which the decision is made to raise the child as a female. It is our assumption that the more normal the infant appears, the more favorably the parents usually react. Obviously, many therapeutic interventions make it necessary to plan lifetime medical follow-ups of patients, with institution of gonadal steroid treatment at the time of expected puberty. After a child has reached the period normally associated with well-differentiated psychosexual identity (1½ to 2 years), reassignment of gender is unwise and should be undertaken only after careful psychiatric, social, and endocrinologic evaluations.

REFERENCES

Klinefelter Syndrome

Caminos-Torres, R., Ma, L., and Snyder, P. J.: Testosterone-induced inhibition of the LH and FSH responses to gonadotropin-releasing hormone occurs slowly. J. Clin. Endocrinol. Metab., 44:1142, 1977.

Gordon, D. L., Krompotic, E., Thomas, W., Gandy, H. M., and Paulsen, C. A.: Pathologic testicular findings in Klinefelter's syndrome. 47,XXY vs. 46,XY/47,XXY. Arch. Intern. Med., 130:726, 1972.

Jacobs, P. A., Hassold, T. J., Whittington, E., Butler, G., Collyer, S., Keston, M., and Lee, M.: Klinefelter's syndrome: an analysis of the origin of the additional sex chromosome using molecular probes. Ann. Hum. Genet., 52:93, 1988.

Jacobs, P. A., and Strong, J. A.: A case of human intersexuality having a possible XXY sex-determining mechanism. Nature, 183:302, 1959.

Klinefelter, H. F., Jr., Reifenstein, E. C., Jr., and Albright, F.: Syndrome characterized by gynecomastia, aspermatogenesis without A-leydigism, and increased excretion of follicle-stimulating hormone. J. Clin. Endocrinol., 2:615, 1942.

Lee, M. W., and Stephens, R. L.: Klinefelter's syndrome and extragonadal germ cell tumors. Cancer, 60:1053, 1987.

Leonard, J. M., Paulsen, C. A., Ospina, L. F., and Burgess, E. C.: The classification of Klinefelter's syndrome. *In* Vallet, H. L., and Porter, I. H. (Eds.): Genetic Mechanisms of Sexual Development. New York, Academic Press, 1979, pp. 407–423.

Lubs, H. A., Jr.: Testicular size in Klinefelter's syndrome in men

over fifty. Report of a case with XXY/XY mosaicism. N. Engl. J. Med., 267:326, 1962.

Nielsen, J., Pelsen, B., and Sorensen, K.: Follow-up of 30 Klinefelter males treated with testosterone. Clin. Genet., 33:262, 1988.

Paulsen, C. A., Gordon, D. L., Carpenter, R. W., Gandy, H. M., and Drucker, W. D.: Klinefelter's syndrome and its variants: A hormonal and chromosomal study. Recent Progr. Horm. Res., 24:321, 1968.

Ratcliffe, S. G.: The sexual development of boys with the chromosome constitution 47,XXY (Klinefelter's syndrome). Clin. Endocrinol. Metab., 11:703, 1982.

Samaan, N. A., Stepanas, A. V., Danziger, J., and Trujillo, J.: Reactive pituitary abnormalities in patients with Klinefelter's and Turner's syndromes. Arch. Intern. Med., 139:198, 1979.

Snyder, P. R., and Lawrence, D. A.: Treatment of male hypogonadism with testosterone enanthate. J. Clin. Endocrinol. Metab., 51:1335, 1980.

Wang, C., Baker, H. W. G., Burger, H. G., De Kretser, D. M., and Hudson, B.: Hormonal studies in Klinefelter's syndrome. Clin. Endocrinol., 4:399, 1975.

XX Male Syndrome

Affara, N. A., Ferguson-Smith, M. A., Tolmie, J., Kwok, K., Mitchell, M., Jamieson, D., Cooke, A., and Florentin, L.: Variable transfer of Y specific sequence in XX males. Nucl. Acid Res., 14:5375, 1986.

de la Chapelle, A.: Nature and origin of males with XX sex chromosomes. Am. J. Hum. Genet., 24:71, 1972.

de la Chapelle, A.: Genetic and molecular studies on 46,XX and 45,X males. Cold Spring Harbor Symposia on Quantitative Biology, 51:249, 1986.

Perez-Palacios, G., Medina, M., Ullao-Aguirre, A., Chavez, B. A., Villareal, G., Dutrem, M. T., Cahill, L. T., and Wachtel, S.: Gonadotropin dynamics in XX males. J. Clin. Endocrinol. Metab., 53:254, 1981.

Roe, T. F., and Alfi, O. S.: Ambiguous genitalia in XX male children: Report of two infants. Pediatrics, 50:55, 1977.

Schweikert, H. U., Weissbach, L., Leyendecker, G., Schwinger, E., Wartenberg, H., and Kruck, F.: Clinical, endocrinological, and cytological characterization of two 46,XX males. J. Clin. Endocrinol. Metab., 54:745, 1982.

Sinclair, A. H., Berta, Ph., Palmer, M. S., Hawkins, J. R., Griffiths, B. L., Smith, M. J., Foster, J. W., Frischauf, A.-M., Lovell-Badge, R., and Goodfellow, P. N.: A gene from the human sex-determining region encodes a protein with homology to a conserved DNA-binding motif. Nature, 346:240, 1990.

Gonadal Dysgenesis (Turner Syndrome)

Brook, C. G. D., Murset, G., Zachmann, M., and Prader, A.: Growth in children with 45,XO Turner's syndrome. Arch. Dis. Child., 49:789, 1974.

Conte, F. A., Grumbach, M., and Kaplan, S. L.: A diphasic pattern of gonadotropin secretion in patients with the syndrome of gonadal dysgenesis. J. Clin. Endocrinol. Metab., 40:670, 1975.

Conte, F. A., Grumbach, M., Kaplan, S. L., and Reiter, E. O.: Correlation of luteinizing hormone-releasing factor-induced luteinizing hormone and follicle-stimulating hormone release from infancy to 19 years with the changing pattern of gonadotropin secretion in agonadal patients: Relation to the restraint of puberty. J. Clin. Endocrinol. Metab., 50:163, 1980.

Ford, C. E., Jones, K. W., Polani, P. E., De Almedia, J. C., and Briggs, J. H.: A sex-chromosome anomaly in a case of gonadal dysgenesis (Turner's syndrome). Lancet, 1:711, 1959.

Gruneiro de Papendieck, L., Iorcansky, S., Coco, R., Rivarola, M. A., and Bergada, C.: High incidence of thyroid disturbances in 49 children with Turner syndrome. J. Pediatr., 111:258, 1987.

Hall, J. G., Sybert, V. P., Williamson, R. A., Fisher, N. L., and Reed, S. D.: Turner's syndrome. West. J. Med., 137:32, 1982.

Krauss, C. M., Turksoy, R. N., Atkins, L., McLaughlin, C., Brown, L. G., and Page, D. C.: Familial premature ovarian failure due to an interstitial deletion of the long arm of the X chromosome. N. Engl. J. Med., 317:125, 1987.

Leichtman, D. A., Schmickel, R. D., Gelehrter, T. D., Judd, W. J.,

Woodbury, M. C., and Meilinger, K. L.: Familial Turner syndrome. Ann. Intern. Med., 89:473, 1978.

Levine, L. S.: Estrogen therapy in the young: Treatment of Turner's syndrome with estrogen. Pediatrics, 62:1178, 1978.

Lippe, B., Geffner, M. E., Dietrich, R. B., Boechat, M. I., and Kangarloo, H.: Renal malformations in patients with Turner syndrome: Imaging in 141 patients. Pediatrics, 82:852, 1988.

Martinez, A., Heinrich, J. J., Domene, H., Escobar, M. E., Jasper, H., Montuori, E., and Bergada, C.: Growth in Turner's syndrome: Long-term treatment with low dose ethinyl estradiol. J. Clin. Endocrinol. Metab., 65:253, 1987.

Rosenfeld, R. G., Hintz, R. L., Johanson, A. J., Sherman, B., Brasel, J. A., Burstein, S., Chernausek, S., Compton, P., Frane, J., Gotlin, R. W., Kuntze, J., Lippe, B. M., Mahoney, P. C., Moore, W. V., New, M. I., Saenger, P., and Syberg, V.: Three-year results of a randomized prospective trial of methionyl human growth hormone and oxandroline in Turner syndrome. J. Pediatr., 113:393, 1988.

Ross, G. T., Vande Wiele, R. L., and Frantz, A. G.: The ovaries and the breasts. Part I: The ovaries. In Williams, R. H. (Ed.): Textbook of Endocrinology. Philadelphia, W. B. Saunders Co., 1981, p. 355.

Samaan, N. A., Stepanas, A. V., Danziger, J., and Trujillo, J.: Reactive pituitary abnormalities in patients with Klinefelter's and Turner's syndromes. Arch. Intern. Med., 139:198, 1979.

Simpson, J. L.: Gonadal dysgenesis and sex chromosome abnormalities: Phenotypic-karyotypic correlations. In Vallet, H. L., and Porter, I. H. (Eds.): Genetic Mechanisms of Sexual Development. New York, Academic Press, 1979, p. 365.

Singh, R. P., and Carr, D. H.: The anatomy and histology of XO human embryos and fetuses. Anat. Rec., 155:369, 1966.

Turner, H. H.: A syndrome of infantilism, congenital webbed neck, and cubitus valgus. Endocrinology, 23:566, 1938.

Mixed Gonadal Dysgenesis

Davidoff, F., and Federman, D. D.: Mixed gonadal dysgenesis. Pediatrics, 52:727, 1973.

Donahoe, P. K., Crawford, J. D., and Hendren, W. H.: Mixed gonadal dysgenesis, pathogenesis and management. J. Pediatr. Surg., 14:287, 1979.

Kofman, S., Perez-Palacios, G., Medina, M., Escobar, N., Garcia, N., Ruz, L., Mutchinick, O., and Lisker, R.: Clinical and endocrine spectrum in patients with the 45,X/46,XY karyotype. Hum. Genet., 58:373, 1981.

Robboy, S. J., Miller, T., Donahoe, P. K., Jahre, C., Welch, W. R., Haseltine, F. P., Miller, W. A., Atkins, L., and Crawford, J. D.: Dysgenesis of testicular and streak gonads in the syndrome of mixed gonadal dysgenesis: Perspective derived from a clinicopathologic analysis of twenty-one cases. Hum. Pathol., 13:700, 1982.

Schellhas, H. F.: Malignant potential of the dysgenetic gonad. Part I. Obstet. Gynecol., 44:298, 1974a.

Schellhas, H. F.: Malignant potential of the dysgenetic gonad. Part II. Obstet. Gynecol., 44:455, 1974b.

Sohval, A. R.: "Mixed" gonadal dysgenesis: A variety of hermaphroditism. Am. J. Hum. Genet., 15:155, 1963.

Teter, J., and Boczkowski, K.: Occurrence of tumors in dysgenetic gonads. Cancer, 20:1301, 1967.

Zah, W., Kalderon, A. E., and Tucci, J. R.: Mixed gonadal dysgenesis. Acta Endocrinol., (Suppl.), 197:1, 1975.

True Hermaphroditism

Aiman, J., Hemsell, D. L., and MacDonald, P. C.: Production and origin of estrogen in two true hermaphrodites. Am. J. Obstet. Gynecol., 132:401, 1978.

Perez-Palacios, G., Carnevale, A., Escpbar, N., Villareal, G., Fernandez, E., and Medina, M.: Induction of ovulation in a true hermaphrodite with male phenotype. J. Clin. Endocrinol. Metab., 52:1257, 1981.

Ramsay, M., Bernstein, R., Zwane, E., Page, D. C., and Jenkins, T.: XX true hermaphroditism in Southern African blacks: An enigma of primary sexual differentiation. Am. J. Hum. Genet., 43:4, 1988.

Raspa, R. W., Subramaniam, A. P., and Romas, N. A.: True hermaphroditism presenting as intermittent hematuria and groin pain. Urology, 18:133, 1986.

Simpson, J. L.: True hermaphroditism: Etiology and phenotypic considerations. Birth Defects, 14(6C):9, 1978.

Skordis, N. A., Stetka, D. G., MacGillivray, M. H., and Greenfield, S. P.: Familial 46,XX males coexisting with familial 46,XX true hermaphrodites in same pedigree. J. Pediatr., 110:244, 1987.

van Niekerk, W. A.: True hermaphroditism. Pediatr. Adolesc. Endocrinol., 8:80, 1981.

van Niekerk, W. A., and Retief, A. E.: The gonads of human true hermaphrodites. Human. Genet., 58:117, 1981.

Pure Gonadal Dysgenesis

Aleem, F. A.: Familial 46,XX gonadal dysgenesis. Fertil. Steril., 35:317, 1981.

Carr, B. R., and Aiman, J.: Steroid production in a woman with gonadal dysgenesis, breast development, and clitoral hypertrophy. Obstet. Gynecol., 56:492, 1980.

German, J., Simpson, J. L., and Chaganti, R. S. K.: Genetically determined sex-reversal in 46,XY humans. Science, 202:53, 1978.

McDonough, P. C., Byrd, J. R., Tho, P. T., and Mahesh, V. B.: Phenotypic and cytogenetic findings in eighty-two patients with ovarian failure—changing trends. Fertil. Steril., 28:638, 1977.

Olsen, M. M., Caldamone, A. A., Jackson, C. L., and Zinn, A.: Gonadoblastoma in infancy: Indications for early gonadectomy in 46XY gonadal dysgenesis. J. Pediatr. Surg., 23:270, 1988.

Phansey, S. A., Satterfield, R., Jorgenson, R. J., Salinas, C. F., Yoder, F. E., Mathur, R. S., and Williamson, H. O.: XY gonadal dysgenesis in three siblings. Am. J. Obstet. Gynecol., 138:133, 1980.

Simpson, J. L., Blagowidow, N., and Martin, A. O.: XY gonadal dysgenesis: Genetic heterogeneity based upon clinical observations, H-Y antigen status and segragation analysis. Hum. Genet., 58:91, 1981.

Wilson, S. C., Oakey, R. E., and Scott, J. S.: In-vivo and in-vitro endocrine investigation of pure gonadal dysgenesis. Clin. Endocrinol., 29:485, 1988.

Absent Testes Syndrome

Aynsley-Green, A., Zachmann, M., Illig, R., Rampini, S., and Prader, A.: Congenital bilateral anorchia in childhood: A clinical, endocrine and therapeutic evaluation of twenty-one cases. Clin. Endocrinol., 5:381, 1976.

Bergada, C., Cleveland, W. E., Jones, H. W., Jr., and Wilkins, L.: Variants of embryonic testicular dysgenesis: Bilateral anorchia and the syndrome of rudimentary testes. Acta Endocrinol., 40:521, 1962.

Edman, C. D., Winters, A. J., Porter, J. C., Wilson, J., and MacDonald, P. C.: Embryonic testicular regression. A clinical spectrum of XY agonadal individuals. Obstet. Gynecol., 49:208, 1977.

Glass, A. R.: Identical twins discordant for the "rudimentary testes" syndrome. J. Urol., 127:140, 1982.

Hall, J. G., Morgan, A., and Blizzard, R. M.: Familial congenital anorchia. In Bergsma, D. (Ed.): Genetic Forms of Hypogonadism. Birth Defects: Original Article Series. Vol. XI, No. 4. Baltimore, Williams & Wilkins Co., 1975, pp. 115–119.

Kirschner, M. A., Jacobs, J. B., and Fraley, E. E.: Bilateral anorchia with persistent testosterone production. N. Engl. J. Med., 282:240, 1970.

Lustig, R. H., Conte, F. A., Kogan, B. A., and Grumbach, M. M.: Ontogeny of gonadotropin secretion in congenital anorchism: Sexual dimorphism versus syndrome of gonadal dysgenesis and diagnostic considerations. J. Urol., 138:587, 1987.

Medina, M., Kofman-Alfaro, S., and Perez-Palacios, G.: 46,XX gonadal absence: a variant of the XX pure gonadal dysgenesis? Acta Endocrinol., 99:585, 1982.

Congenital Adrenal Hyperplasia

Cunnah, D., Perry, L., Dacie, J. A., Grant, D. B., Lowe, D. G., Savage, M. O., and Besser, G. M.: Bilateral testicular tumours in congenital adrenal hyperplasia: A continuing diagnostic and therapeutic dilemma. Clin. Endocrinol., 30:141, 1989.

Dewailly, D., Vantyghem-Haudiquet, M.-C., Sainsard, C., Buvat, J., Cappoen, J. P., Ardaens, K., Racadot, A., Lefebvre, J., and

Fossati, P.: Clinical and biological phenotypes in late-onset 21-hyroxylase deficiency. J. Clin. Endocrinol. Metab., 63:418, 1986.

Glenthoj, A., Nielsen, M.D., and Starup, J.: Congenital adrenal hyperplasia due to 11B-hydroxylase deficiency: final diagnosis in adult age in three patients. Acta Endocrinol., 93:94, 1980.

Höller, W., Scholz, S., Knorr, D., Bidlingmaier, F., Keller, E., and Albert, E. D.: Genetic differences between the salt-wasting, simple virilizing, and nonclassical types of congenital adrenal hyperplasia. J. Clin. Endocrinol. Metab., 60:757, 1985.

Horrocks, P. M., and London, D. R.: Effects of long-term dexamethasone treatment in adult patients with congenital adrenal hyperplasia. Clin. Endocrinol., 27:635, 1987.

Kuttenn, F., Couillin, P., Girard, F., Billaud, L., Vincens, M., Coucekkine, C., Thalabard, J.-C., Maudelonde, T., Spritzer, P., Mowszowicz, I., Boue, A., and Mauvais-Jarvis, P.: Late-onset adrenal hyperplasia in hirsutism. N. Engl. J. Med., 313:224, 1985.

Lee, P. A., Rosenwaks, Z., Urban, M. D., Migeon, C. J., and Bias, W. D.: Attenuated forms of congenital adrenal hyperplasia due to 21-hydroxylase deficiency. J. Clin. Endocrinol. Metab., 55:866, 1982.

Levine, L. S., Dupont, B., Lorenzen, F., Pang, S., Pollack, M., Oberfield, S., Kohn, B., Lerner, A., Cacciarl, E., Mantero, F., Cassio, A., Scaroni, C., Chiumello, G., Rondanini, G. F., Garantini, L., Giovannelli, G., Virdis, R., Bartolotta, E., Migliori, C., Pintor, C., Tato, L., Barboni, F., and New, M. I.: Cryptic 21-hydroxylase deficiency in families of patients with classical congenital adrenal hyperplasia. J. Clin. Endocrinol. Metab., 51:1316, 1980.

Morel, Y., David, M., Forest, M. G., Betuel, H., Hauptman, G., Andre, J., Bertrand, J., and Miller, W. L.: Gene conversions and rearrangements cause discordance between inheritance of forms of 21-hydroxylase deficiency and HLA types. J. Clin. Endocrinol. Metab., 68:592, 1989.

Mulaikal, R. M., Migeon, C. J., and Rock, J. A.: Fertility rates in female patients with congenital adrenal hyperplasia due to 21-hydroxylase deficiency. N. Engl. J. Med., 316:178, 1987.

New, M. I., White, P. C., Pang, S., DuPont, B., and Speiser, P. W.: The adrenal hyperplasias. In Scriver, C. R., Beaudent, A. L., Sly, W. S., and Valle, D. (Eds.): The Metabolic Basis of Inherited Disease, 6th ed. New York, McGraw-Hill, 1989, p. 1881.

New, M. I., and Speiser, P. W.: Genetics of adrenal steroid 21-hydroxylase deficiency. Endocr. Rev., 7:331, 1986.

Newell, M. E., Lippe, B. M., and Ehrlich, R. M.: Testis tumors associated with congenital adrenal hyperplasia: A continuing diagnostic and therapeutic dilemma. J. Urol., 117:256, 1977.

Pang, S. Pollack, M. S., Marshall, R. N., and Immken, L.: Prenatal treatment of congenital adrenal hyperplasia due to 21-hydroxylase deficiency. N. Engl. J. Med., 322:111, 1990.

Rösler, A., Weshler, N., Leiberman, E., Hochberg, Z., Weidenfeld, J., Sack, J., and Chemke, J.: 11β-hydroxylase deficiency congenital adrenal hyperplasia: Update of prenatal diagnosis. J. Clin. Endocrinol. Metab., 66:830, 1988.

Speiser, P. W., New, M. I., and White, P. C.: Molecular genetic analysis of nonclassic steroid 21-hydroxylase deficiency associated with HLA-B14,DR1. N. Engl. J. Med., 319:19, 1988.

White, P. C., New, M. I., and DuPont, B.: Congenital adrenal hyperplasia. N. Engl. J. Med., 316:1519, 1987.

Nonadrenal Female Pseudohermaphroditism

Grumbach, M. M., and Conte, F. A.: Disorders of sexual differentiation. In Wilson, J. D., and Foster, D. W. (Eds.): Williams Textbook of Endocrinology, 7th ed. Philadelphia, W. B. Saunders Co., 1985, pp. 312–401.

Hensleigh, P. A., and Woodruff, J. D.: Differential maternal-fetal response to androgenizing luteoma or hyperreactio luteinalis. Obstet. Gynecol. Surv., 33:262, 1978.

Kirk, J. M., Perry, L. A., Shand, W. S., Kirby, R. S., Besser, G. M., and Savage, M. O.: Female pseudohermaphroditism due to a maternal adrenocortical tumor. J. Clin. Endocrinol. Metab., 70:1280, 1990.

Congenital Absence of the Vagina (Müllerian Agenesis)

Ataya, K. M., and Mroueh, A. M.: Urologic anomalies associated with an absent uterus. J. Urol., 127:1125, 1982.

Bryans, F. E.: Management of congenital absence of the vagina. Am. J. Obstet. Gynecol., 139:281, 1981.

Chryssikopoulos, A., and Grigoriou, O.: The etiology in 77 primary amenorrhea patients. Int. J. Fertil., 32:245, 1987.

Evans, T. N., Poland, M. L., and Boving, R. L.: Vaginal malformations. Am. J. Obstet. Gynecol., 141:910, 1981.

Fraser, I. S., Baird, D. T., Hobson, B. M., Michie, E. A., and Hunter, W.: Cyclical ovarian function in women with congenital absence of the uterus and vagina. J. Clin. Endocrinol. Metab., 36:634, 1973.

Griffin, J. E., Edwards, C., Madden. J. D., Harrod, M. J., and Wilson, J. D.: Congenital absence of the vagina. The Mayer-Rokitansky-Kuster-Hauser syndrome. Ann. Intern. Med., 85:224, 1976.

Jones, H. W., Jr., and Mermut, S.: Familial occurrence of congenital absence of the vagina. Am. J. Obstet. Gynecol., 114:1100, 1972

Rock, J. A., and Jones, Jr., H. W.: Construction of a neovagina for patients with a flat perineum. Obstet. Gynecol., 160:845, 1989.

Salvatore, C. A., and Lodovicci, O.: Vaginal agenesis: An analysis of ninety cases. Acta Obstet. Gynecol. Scand., 57:89, 1978.

Shokeir, M. H. K.: Aplasia of the müllerian system: Evidence for probable sex-limited autosomal dominant inheritance. In Summitt, R. L., and Bergsma, D. (Eds.): Sex Differentiation and Chromosomal Abnormalities. Birth Defects: Original Article Series, Vol. XIV, No. 6C. New York, Alan R. Liss, Inc., 1978, pp. 147–165.

Wright, J. E.: Failure of müllerian duct development. The Mayer-Rokitansky-Kuster-Hauser syndrome. Aust. Paediatr. J., 20:325, 1984.

Male Pseudohermaphroditism

Campo, S., Monteagudo, C., Nicolau, G., Pellizzari, E., Belgorosky, A., Stivel, M., and Rivarola, M.: Testicular function in prepubertal male pseudohermaphroditism. Clin. Endocrinol., 14:11, 1981.

Campo, S., Stivel, M., Nicolau, G., Monteagudo, C., and Rivarola, M.: Testicular function in postpubertal male pseudohermaphroditism. Clin. Endocrinol., 11:481, 1979.

Savage, M. O., Chaussain, J. L., Evain, D., Roger, M., Canlorbe, O., and Job, J. C.: Endocrine studies in male pseudohermaphroditism in childhood and adolescence. Clin. Endocrinol., 8:219, 1978.

Abnormalities in Androgen Synthesis

20,22-Desmolase

Camacho, A. M., Kowarski, A., Migeon, C. J., and Brough, A. J.: Congenital adrenal hyperplasia due to a deficiency of one of the enzymes involved in the biosynthesis of pregnenolone. J. Clin. Endocrinol., 28:153, 1968.

Haufa, B. P., Miller, W. L., Grumbach, M. M., Conte, F. A., and Kaplan, S. L.: Congenital adrenal hyperplasia due to deficient cholesterol side-chain cleavage activity (20,22 desmolase) in a patient treated for 18 years. Clin. Endocrinol. [Oxf.], 23:481, 1985.

Kirkland, R. T., Kirkland, J. L., Johnson, C. M., Horning, M. G., Librik, L., and Clayton, G. W.: Congenital lipoid adrenal hyperplasia in an eight-year-old phenotypic female. J. Clin. Endocrinol., 36:488, 1973.

Matteson, K. J., Chang, B.-C., Urdea, M. S., and Miller, W. L.: Study of cholesterol side chain cleavage (20,22-desmolase) deficiency causing congenital lipoid adrenal hyperplasia using bovine-sequence P450$_{scc}$ oligodeoxyribonucleotide probes. Endocrinology, 118:1296, 1986.

3β-Hydroxysteroid Dehydrogenase

Cara, J. F., Moshang, T., Bongiovanni, A. M., and Marx, B.: Elevated 17-hydroxyprogesterone and testosterone in a newborn with 3β-hydroxysteroid dehydrogenase deficiency. N. Engl. J. Med., 313:618, 1985.

Parks, G. A., Bermudez, J. A., Anast, C. S., Bongiovanni, A. M., and New, M. I.: Pubertal boy with the 3β-hydroxysteroid dehydrogenase defect. J. Clin. Endocrinol., 33:269, 1971.

Rosenfield, R. L., DeNiepomniszsze, A. B., Kenny, F. M., and Genel, M.: The response to human chorionic gonadotropin (hCG) administration in boys with and without Δ⁵-3β-hydroxysteroid dehydrogenase deficiency. J. Clin. Endocrinol. Metab., 39:370, 1974.

Schneider, G., Genel, M., Bongiovanni, A. M., Goldman. A. S., and Rosenfield, R. L.: Persistent testicular Δ⁵-isomerase-3β-hydroxysteroid dehydrogenase (Δ⁵-3β-HSA) deficiency in the Δ⁵-3β-HSD form of congenital adrenal hyperplasia. J. Clin. Invest., 55:681, 1975.

17α-Hydroxylase

Biglieri, E. G., Herron, M. A., and Brust, N.: 17-hydroxylation deficiency in man. J. Clin. Invest., 45:1946, 1966.

Griffing, G. T., Wilson, T. E., Holbrook, M. M., Dale, S. I., Jackson, T. K., Ullrich, I., and Melby, J. C.: Plasma and urinary 19-nor-deoxycortico-sterone in 17α-hydroxylase deficiency syndrome. J. Clin. Endocrinol. Metab., 59:1011, 1984.

New, M. I.: Male pseudohermaphroditism due to 17α-hydroxylase deficiency. J. Clin. Invest., 49:1930, 1970.

Winter, J. S. D., Couch, R. M., Muller J., Perry, Y. S., Ferreira, P., Baydala, L., and Shackleton, C. H. L.: Combined 17-hydroxylase and 17,20-desmolase deficiencies: evidence for synthesis of defective cytochrome P450$_{c17}$. J. Clin. Endocrinol. Metab., 68:309, 1989.

Yanase, T., Sanders, D., Shibata, A., Matsui, N., Simpson, E. R., and Waterman, M. R.: Combined 17α-hydroxylase/17,20-lyase deficiency due to a 7-base pair duplication in the N-terminal region of the cytochrome P450$_{17}$α(CYP17) gene. J. Clin. Endocrinol. Metab., 70:1325, 1990.

17,20-Desmolase

Forest, M. G., Lecornu, M., and DePeretti, E.: Familial male pseudohermaphroditism due to 17,20-desmolase deficiency. I. In vivo endocrine studies. J. Clin. Endocrinol. Metab., 50:826, 1980.

Goebelsmann, U., Zachmann, M., Davajan, V., Israel, R., Mestman, J. H., and Mishell, D. R.: Male pseudohermaphroditism consistent with 17,20-desmolase deficiency. Gynecol. Invest., 7:138, 1976.

Larrea, F., Lisker, R., Banuelos, R., Bermudez, J. A., Herrera, J., Rasilla, V. N., and Perez-Palacios, G.: Hypergonadotrophic hypogonadism in an XX female subject due to 17,20-steroid desmolase deficiency. Acta Endocrinol., 103:400, 1983.

Zachmann, M., Völlmin, J. A., Hamilton, W., and Prader, A.: Steroid 17, 20-desmolase deficiency: A new cause of male pseudohermaphroditism. Clin. Endocrinol., 1:369, 1972.

Zachmann, M., Werder, E. A., and Prader, A.: Two types of male pseudohermaphroditism due to 17,20-desmolase deficiency. J. Clin. Endocrinol. Metab., 55:487, 1982.

17β-Hydroxysteroid Dehydrogenase

Akesode, F. A., Meyer, W. J., III, and Migeon, C. J.: Male pseudohermaphroditism with gynecomastia due to testicular 17-ketosteroid reductase deficiency. Clin. Endocrinol., 7:443, 1977.

Givens, J. R., Wiser, W. L., Summitt, R. L., Kerber, I. J., Andersen, R. N., Pittaway, D. E., and Fish, S. A.: Familial male pseudohermaphroditism without gynecomastia due to deficient testicular 17-ketosteroid reductase activity. N. Engl. J. Med., 291:938, 1974.

Goebelsmann, U., Horton, R., Mestman, J. H., Arce, J. J., Nagata, Y., Nakamura, R. M., Thorneycroft, I. H., and Mishell, D. R., Jr.: Male pseudohermaphroditism due to testicular 17β-hydroxysteroids dehydrogenase deficiency. J. Clin. Endocrinol. Metab., 36:867, 1973.

Imperato-McGinley, J., Peterson, R. E., Stoller, R., and Goodwin, W. E.: Male pseudohermaphroditism secondary to 17β-hydroxysteroid dehydrogenase deficiency: Gender role change with puberty. J. Clin. Endocrinol. Metab., 49:391, 1979.

Rösler, A., and Kohn, G.: Male pseudohermaphroditism due to 17β-hydroxysteroid dehydrogenase deficiency: Studies on the natural history of the defect and effect of androgens on gender role. J. Steroid Biochem., 19:663, 1983.

Virdis, R., Saenger, P., Seniror, B., and New, M. I.: Endocrine studies in a pubertal male pseudohermaphrodite with 17-ketosteroid reductase deficiency. Acta Endocrinol., 87:212, 1978.

Leydig Cell Abnormalities

Berthezene, R., Forest, M. G., Grimaud, J. A., Claustrat, B., and Mornex, R.: Leydig-cell agenesis. A cause of male pseudohermaphroditism. N. Engl. J. Med., 295:969, 1976.

Lee, P. A., Rock, J. A., Brown, T. R., Fichman, K. M., Migeon, C. J., and Jones, H. W., Jr.: Leydig cell hypofunction resulting in male pseudohermaphroditism. Fertil. Steril., 37:675, 1982.

Park, I. J., Burnett, L. S., Jones, H. W., Jr., Migeon, C. J., and Blizzard, R. M.: A case of male pseudohermaphroditism associated with elevated LH, normal FSH and low testosterone possibly due to the secretion of an abnormal LH molecule. Acta Endocrinol., 83:173, 1976.

Perez-Palacios, G., Scaglia, H. E., Kofman-Alfaro, S., Saavedra, O. D., Ochoa, S., Larraza, O., and Perez, A. E.: Inherited male pseudohermaphroditism due to gonadotrophin unresponsiveness. Acta Endocrinol., 98:148, 1981.

Schwartz, M., Imperato-McGinley, J., Peterson, R. E., Cooper, G., Morris, P. L., MacGillivray, M., and Hensle, T.: Male pseudohermaphroditism secondary to an abnormality in Leydig cell differentiation. J. Clin. Endocrinol. Metab., 53:123, 1981.

Abnormalities in Androgen Action

5α-Reductase Deficiency

Griffin, J. E., and Wilson, J. D.: The androgen resistance syndromes: 5α-reductase deficiency, testicular feminization, and related syndromes. In Scriver, C. R., Beaudet, A. L., Sly, W. S., and Valle, D. (Eds.): The Metabolic Basis of Inherited Disease, 6th ed. New York, McGraw-Hill, 1989, pp. 1919–1944.

Imperato-McGinley, J., Gautier, T., Peterson, R. E., and Shackleton, C.: The prevalence of 5α-reductase deficiency in children with ambiguous genitalia in the Dominican Republic. J. Urol., 136:867, 1986.

Imperato-McGinley, J., Guerrero, L., Gautier, T., and Peterson, R. E.: Steroid 5α-reductase deficiency in man: An inherited form of male pseudohermaphroditism. Science, 186:1213, 1974.

Imperato-McGinley, J., Peterson, R. E., Gautier, T., Sturla, E.: Androgens and the evolution of male-gender identify among male pseudohermaphrodites with 5α-reductase deficiency. N. Engl. J. Med., 300:1233, 1979.

Peterson, R. E., Imperato-McGinley, J., Gautier, T., and Sturla, E.: Male pseudohermaphroditism due to steroid 5α-reductase deficiency. Am. J. Med., 62:170, 1977.

Price, P., Wass, J. A. H., Griffin, J. E., Leshin, M., Savage, M. O., Large, D. M., Bullock, D. E., Anderson, D. C., Wilson, J. D., and Besser, G. M.: High dose androgen therapy in male pseudohermaphroditism due to 5α-reductase deficiency and disorders of the androgen receptor. J. Clin. Invest., 74:1496, 1984.

Walsh, P. C., Madden, J. D., Harrod, M. J., Goldstein, J. L., MacDonald, P. C., and Wilson, J. D.: Familial incomplete male pseudohermaphroditism, type 2. Decreased dihydrotestosterone formation in pseudovaginal perineoscrotal hypospadias. N. Engl. J. Med., 291:944, 1974.

Receptor Disorders—Testicular Feminization, Reifenstein Syndrome, the Infertile Male Syndrome, and the Undervirilized Fertile Male

Aiman, J., and Griffin, J. E.: The frequency of androgen receptor deficiency in infertile men. J. Clin. Endocrinol. Metab., 54:725, 1982.

Aiman, J., Griffin, J. E., Gazak, J. M., Wilson, J. D., and MacDonald, P. C.: Androgen insensitivity as a cause of infertility in otherwise normal men. N. Engl. J. Med., 300:223, 1979.

Amrhein, J. A., Meyer, W. J., III, Jones, H. W., Jr., and Migeon, C. J.: Androgen insensitivity in man: Evidence for genetic heterogeneity. Proc. Natl. Acad. Sci. U S A, 73:891, 1976.

Bowen, P., Lee, C. S. N., Migeon, C. J., Kaplan, N. M., Whalley, P. J., McKusick, V. A., and Reinfenstein, E. C., Jr.: Hereditary male pseudohermaphroditism with hypogonadism, hypospadias, and gynecomastia (Reifenstein's syndrome). Ann. Intern. Med., 62:252, 1965.

Boyar, R. M., Moore, R. J., Rosner, W., Aiman, J., Chipman, J., Madden, J. D., Marks, J. F., and Griffin, J. E.: Studies of gonadotropin-gonadal dynamics in patients with androgen insensitivity. J. Clin. Endocrinol. Metab., 47:1116, 1978.

Griffin, J. E.: Testicular feminization associated with a thermolabile androgen receptor in cultured human fibroblasts. J. Clin. Invest., 64:1624, 1979.

Griffin, J. E., and Durrant, J. L.: Qualitative receptor defects in families with androgen resistance: Failure of stabilization of the fibroblast cytosol androgen receptor. J. Clin. Endocrinol. Metab., 55:465, 1982.

Griffin, J. E., and Wilson, J. D.: The androgen resistance syndromes: 5α-reductase deficiency, testicular feminization, and related syndromes. *In* Scriver, C. R., Beaudet, A. L., Sly, W. S., and Valle, D. (Eds.): The Metabolic Basis of Inherited Disease, 6th ed. New York, McGraw-Hill, 1989, pp. 1919–1944.

Grino, P. B., Griffin, J. E., Cushard, W. G., Jr., and Wilson, J. D.: A mutation of the androgen receptor associated with partial androgen resistance, familial gynecomastia, and fertility. J. Clin. Endocrinol. Metab., 66:754, 1988.

Hauser, G. A.: Testicular feminization. *In* Overzier, C. (Ed.): Intersexuality. London, Academic Press, 1963, pp. 255–276.

Imperato-McGinley, J., Peterson, R. E., Gautier, T., Cooper, G., Danner, R., Arthur, A., Morris, P. L., Sweeney, W. J., and Shackleton, C.: Hormonal evaluation of a large kindred with complete androgen insensitivity: Evidence for secondary 5α-reductase deficiency. J. Clin. Endocrinol. Metab., 54:931, 1982.

Keenan, B. S., Meyer, W. J., III, Hadjian, A. J., and Migeon, C. J.: Androgen receptor in human skin fibroblasts. Characterization of a specific 17β-hydroxy-5α-androstan-3-one-protein complex in cell sonicates and nuclei. Steroids, 25:535, 1975.

MacDonald, P. C., Madden, J. D., Brenner, P. F., Wilson, J. D., and Siiteri, P. K.: Origin of estrogen in normal men and in women with testicular feminization. J. Clin. Endocrinol. Metab., 49:905, 1979.

Madden, J. D., Walsh, P. C., MacDonald, P. C., and Wilson, J. D.: Clinical and endocrinologic characterization of a patient with the syndrome of incomplete testicular feminization. J. Clin. Endocrinol. Metab., 41:751, 1975.

McPhaul, M. J., Marcelli, M., and Tilley, W. D.: Androgen resistance caused by mutations in the androgen receptor gene. FASEB J., 1991, in press.

Reifenstein, E. C., Jr.: Hereditary familial hypogonadism. Clin. Res., 3:86, 1947.

Wilson, J. D., Harrod, M. J., Goldstein, J. L., Hemsell, D. L., and MacDonald, P. C.: Familial incomplete male pseudohermaphroditism, type I. Evidence for androgen resistance and variable clinical manifestations in a family with the Reifenstein syndrome. N. Engl. J. Med., 290:1097, 1974.

Persistent Müllerian Duct Syndrome

Brook, C. G. D., Wagner, H., Zachmann, M., Prader, A., Armendares, S., Frenk, P., Aleman, P., Najjar, S. S., Slim, M. S., Genton, N., and Bozic, C.: Familial occurrence of persistent müllerian structures in otherwise normal males. Br. Med. J., 1:771, 1973.

Guerrier, D., Tran, D., Vanderwinden, J. M., Hideux, S., Outryve, L. V., Legeai, L., Bouchard, M., Vliet, G. V., de Laet, M. H., Picard, J. Y., Kahn, A., and Josso, N.: The persistent müllerian duct syndrome: a molecular approach. J. Clin. Endocrinol. Metab., 68:46, 1989.

Sloan, W. R., and Walsh, P. C.: Familial persistent müllerian duct syndrome. J. Urol., 115:459, 1976.

Weiss, E. B., Kiefer, J. H., Rowlatt, U. T., and Rosenthal, I. M.: Persistent müllerian duct syndrome in male identical twins. Pediatrics, 61:797, 1978.

Microphallus

Burstein, S., Grumbach, M. M., and Kaplan, S. L.: Early determination of androgen-responsiveness is important in the management of microphallus. Lancet, 2:983, 1979.

Danish, R. K., Lee, P. A., Mazur, T., Amrhein, J. A., and Migeon, C. J.: Micropenis. II. Hypogonadotropic hypogonadism. Johns Hopkins Med. J., 146:177, 1980.

Guthrie, R. D., Smith, D. W., and Graham, C. B.: Testosterone treatment for micropenis during early childhood. J. Pediatr., 83:247, 1973.

Lee, P. A., Danish, R. K., Mazur, T., and Migeon, C. J.: Micropenis. III. Primary hypogonadism, partial androgen insensitivity syndrome, and idiopathic disorders. Johns Hopkins Med. J., 147:175, 1980.

Lee, P. A., Mazur, T., Danish, R., Amrhein, J., Blizzard, R. M., Money, J., and Migeon, C. J.: Micropenis. I. Criteria, etiologies, and classification. Johns Hopkins Med. J., 146:156, 1980.

Okuyama, A., Itatani, H., Aono, T., Matsumoto, K., Mizutani, S., and Sonoda, T.: Prognosis of sexual maturation in prepubertal boys with micropenis. Arch. Androl., 5:265, 1980.

Reilly, J. M., and Woodhouse, C. R. J.: Small penis and the male sexual role. J. Urol., 142:569, 1989.

Schonfeld, W. A., and Beebe, G. W.: Normal growth and variation in the male genitalia from birth to maturity. J. Urol., 48:759, 1942.

Vanelli, M., Bernasconi, S., Terzi, C., Bolondi, O., Boselli, E., Virdis, R., and Giovannelli, G.: Micropénis. Résultats du traitement par la testostérone. Arch. Fr. Pediatr., 41:473, 1984.

Walsh, P. C., Wilson, J. D., Allen, T. D., Madden, J. D., Porter, J. C., Neaves, W. B., Griffin, J. E., and Goodwin, W. E.: Clinical and endocrinological evaluation of patients with congenital microphallus. J. Urol., 120:90, 1978.

Chromosomal Evaluation

Simpson, J. L., Jirasek, J. E., Speroff, L., and Kase, N. G.: Disorders of Sexual Differentiation. New York, Academic Press, 1976, p. 466.

Surico, N., Messina, M., Ponzio, G., Libanori, E., Chiodo, F., Milani, P., and Folpini, E.: Limited diagnostic value of lymphocytic karyotype in primary amenorrhea with streak gonads. Eur. J. Obstet. Gynecol. Reprod. Biol., 26:145, 1987.

Waibel, F., Scherer, G., Fraccaro, M., Hustinx, T. W. J., Weissenbach, J., Wieland, J., Mayerová, A., Back, E., and Wolf, U.: Absence of Y-specific DNA sequences in human 46,XX true hermaphrodites and in 45,X mixed gonadal dysgenesis. Hum. Genet., 76:332, 1987.

Biochemical Evaluation

Forest, M. G.: Pattern of the response of testosterone and its precursors to human chorionic gonadotropin stimulation in relation to age in infants and children. J. Clin. Endocrinol. Metab., 49:132, 1979.

Griffin, J. E., and Wilson, J. D.: The androgen resistance syndromes: 5α-reductase deficiency, testicular feminization, and related syndromes. *In* Scriver, C. R., Beaudet, A. L., Sly, W. S., and Valle, D. (Eds.): The Metabolic Basis of Inherited Disease, 6th ed. New York, McGraw-Hill, 1989, p. 1919.

Levine, L. S., Lieber, E., Pang, S., and New, M. I.: Male pseudohermaphroditism due to 17-ketosteroid reductase deficiency diagnosed in the newborn period. Pediatr. Res., 14:480, 1980.

New, M. I., White, P. C., Pang, S., DuPont, B., and Speiser, P. W.: The adrenal hyperplasias. *In* Scriver, C. R., Beaudet, A. L., Sly, W. S., and Valle, D. (Eds.): The Metabolic Basis of Inherited Disease, 6th ed. New York, McGraw-Hill, 1989, p. 1881.

Peterson, R. E., Imperato-McGinley, J., Gautier, T., and Sturla, E.: Male pseudohermaphroditism due to steroid 5α-reductase deficiency. Am. J. Med., 62:170, 1977.

Walsh, P. C., Curry, N., Mills, R. C., and Siiteri, P. K.: Plasma androgen response to hCG stimulation in prepubertal boys with hypospadias and cryptorchidism. J. Clin. Endocrinol. Metab., 42:52, 1976.

Endoscopy and Radiography, Exploratory Laparoscopy

Bryan, P. J., Caldamone, A. A., Morrison, S. C., Yulish, B. S., and Owens, R.: Ultrasound findings in the adreno-genital syndrome (congenital adrenal hyperplasia). J. Ultrasound Med., 7:675, 1988.

Currarino, G.: Large prostatic utricles and related structures, urogenital sinus and other forms of urethrovaginal confluence. J. Urol., 136:1270, 1986.

Fritzsche, P. J., Hricak, H., Kogan, B. A., Winkler, M. L., and Tanagho, E. A.: Undescended testis: value of MR imaging. Radiology, 164:169, 1987.

Kier, R., McCarthy, S., Rosenfield, A. T., Rosenfield, N. S., Rapoport, S., and Weiss, R. M.: Nonpalpable testes in young boys: evaluation with MR imaging. Radiology, 169:429, 1988.

Sloan, W. R., and Walsh, P. C.: Familial persistent müllerian duct syndrome. J. Urol., 115:459, 1976.

Walsh, P. C., Madden, J. D., Harrod, M. J., Goldstein, J. L., MacDonald, P. C., and Wilson, J. D.: Familial incomplete male pseudohermaphroditism, type 2. Decreased dihydrotestosterone formation in pseudovaginal perineoscrotal hypospadias. N. Engl. J. Med., 291:944, 1974.

Weiss, R. M., Carter, A. R., and Rosenfield, A. T.: High resolution real-time ultrasonography in the localization of the undescended testis. J. Urol., 135:936, 1986.

Weiss, R. M., and Seashore, J. H.: Laparoscopy in the management of the nonpalpable testis. J. Urol., 138:382, 1987.

Wolverson, M. K., Jagannadharao, B., Sundaram, M., Riaz, M. A., Nalesnik, W. J., and Houttuin, E.: CT in localization of impalpable cryptorchid testes. AJR, 134:725, 1980.

Wright, J. E.: Impalpable testes: a review of 100 boys. J. Pediatr. Surg., 21:151, 1986.

Sex Assignment

Donahoe, P. K.: The diagnosis and treatment of infants with intersex abnormalities. Pediatr. Clin. North Am., 34:1333, 1987.

Lobe, T. E., Woodall, D. L., Richards, G. E., Cavallo, A., and Meyer, W. J.: The complications of surgery for intersex: changing patterns over two decades. J. Pediatr. Surg., 22:651, 1987.

Oesterling, J. E., Gearhart, J. P., and Jeffs, R. D.: A unified approach to early reconstructive surgery of the child with ambiguous genitalia. J. Urol., 138:1079, 1987.

Pagon, R. A.: Diagnostic approach to the newborn with ambiguous genitalia. Pediatr. Clin. North Am., 34:1019, 1987.

Sharp, R. J., Holder, T. M., Howard, C. P., and Grunt, J. A.: Neonatal genital reconstruction. J. Pediatr. Surg., 22:168, 1987.

38
CONGENITAL ANOMALIES OF THE TESTIS

Jacob Rajfer, M. D.

CRYPTORCHIDISM

Cryptorchidism means a hidden testis. This anomaly occurs when the testis fails to descend into its normal postnatal anatomic location, the scrotum. Because the testis develops originally in the abdominal region, its descent may be inhibited anywhere along its normal pathway. Alternatively, the testis may be diverted from this route into an ectopic location.

This apparently simple developmental anomaly represents one of the most common disorders of childhood. All races are affected, and there does not seem to be any geographic propensity. Although cryptorchidism may be associated with a number of chromosomal and hereditary disorders in which a specific defect can be identified, at the present time the majority of cases appear to be isolated, probably because relatively little is known about what actually causes the human testis to migrate from the abdomen into the scrotum. As technologic and scientific advances continue to be made in the fields of genetics, molecular biology, and reproductive endocrinology, the mechanisms involved in testicular migration will be ascertained. More clinical cases of cryptorchidism may therefore be identified as being the phenotypic expression of a more generalized systemic disorder.

WHY THE TESTIS DESCENDS

For the testis to produce viable and mature spermatozoa, in most mammalian species it must descend from the warmer intra-abdominal environment into the cooler scrotum (Cooper, 1929; Felizet and Branca, 1902; Moore and Quick, 1924; Pace and Cabot, 1936; Wangensteen, 1935). The slight temperature elevation of 1.5 to 2.0°C between these two locations is sufficient to inhibit spermatogenesis.

If the timing of testicular descent in various animal species is compared, interesting observations can be made regarding the thermoregulation of spermatogenesis. The primate is the only species in which the testis completely descends at or near the time of birth (Wislocki, 1933). In the monkey, the testes retract from the scrotum to the inguinal canal at about the 5th postnatal day only to return permanently to the scrotum between the 3rd and 5th years of life, which is the normal time of puberty in this species. In certain hibernating animals, the testes, which are intra-abdominal during the winter months, descend into the scrotum only during the breeding season (Bishop, 1945). In other animals, the testes remain intra-abdominal except during copulation, when they descend into the scrotum (Deming, 1936). In the whale, the testes are located intra-abdominally and are probably cooled by the animal's constant contact with cool water (Huberman and Israeloff, 1935). The testes of birds are located in the lumbar region and presumably are cooled by the air stream that constantly flows over them during flight. Therefore, cooling of the testes via migration into the scrotum appears to be a phylogenetic mechanism that man has retained in order to propagate the species.

EMBRYOLOGY OF TESTICULAR DESCENT

In order to comprehend how the testis migrates into the scrotum, a knowledge of the related embryology is essential (Arey, 1965; Hamilton et al., 1957). In the human, by the 6th week of gestation the primordial germ cells have migrated from the wall of the embryonic yolk sac along the dorsal mesentery of the hindgut to invade the genital ridges (Witschi, 1948). At this stage of development, the gubernaculum first appears as a ridge of mesenchymal tissue extending from the genital ridge through a gap in the anterior abdominal wall musculature to the genital swellings that are the site of the future scrotum (Backhouse, 1964). This gap in the anterior abdominal wall is the future inguinal canal.

1543

By 7 weeks of gestation, possibly under the influence of a protein that is most likely secreted by the XY primordial germ cells under the regulation of a gene located on the short arm of the Y chromosome (Page, et al., 1987), the indifferent gonad differentiates into the fetal testis. During the 8th week of gestation in the male embryo, the fetal testis begins to secrete two hormones, testosterone and müllerian-inhibiting factor (Jost, 1953 a and b). Testosterone, which is synthesized and secreted by the fetal Leydig cells (Payne and Jaffe, 1975; Siiteri and Wilson, 1974), is under the regulation of maternal human chorionic gonadotropin (hCG) at this stage of development (Clements et al., 1976) and induces the ipsilateral wolffian duct to form the epididymis and vas deferens.

Müllerian-inhibiting factor, which is secreted by the fetal Sertoli cells (Guerrier, et al., 1989; Josso, 1972, 1973), causes regression of the müllerian ducts, leaving only the appendix testis, a remnant of the müllerian ductal system. At this time, the processus vaginalis, an outpouching of peritoneum, may be seen ventral to the gubernaculum (Lemeh, 1960; Wyndham, 1943). The future muscle fibers of the cremaster may also appear at this time along the developing processus vaginalis. The processus vaginalis forms as a hernia in the weak triangle that consists of peritoneum backed only by the jelly of the gubernaculum (Gier and Marion, 1970). The margins of the triangle are formed dorsally by the internal iliac artery and vein and ventrolaterally by the most posterior bands of the transversus abdominis muscle.

Between the 8th and 16th weeks of gestation, the external genitalia develop (Jirasek et al., 1968). In the male embryo, testosterone, which is also secreted systemically by the fetal testis, is picked up by the tissues of the external genitalia and converted to dihydrotestosterone (DHT) by the 5-alpha reductase enzyme within the tissues of the external genitalia (Siiteri and Wilson, 1974). DHT is the active androgen that induces differentiation of the external genitalia in the male embryo (Siiteri and Wilson, 1974). After the development of the testis, ductal system, and external genitalia, the testis lies on top of the conically shaped gubernaculum, awaiting descent (Backhouse, 1981). The gubernaculum can be seen from the cauda epididymis distally through the inguinal canal toward the genital swellings. The growth of the gubernaculum is believed to be under the regulation of substances secreted by the fetal testis (Fentener Van Vlissingen et al., 1988). Under continued androgenic stimulation, the genital swellings are transformed into the scrotum. The testis has now assumed an intra-abdominal position right behind the internal inguinal ring. In reality, the testis is never more than 1.3 mm from the internal inguinal ring at any time during its development (Hutson, 1986; Wyndham, 1943).

The process of testicular descent remains relatively dormant between the 12th week and the 7th month of gestation. During this time, the processus vaginalis slowly extends into the scrotum (Wyndham, 1943). At about the 7th month of gestation, just prior to actual descent of the testis, rapid alterations occur simultaneously in the gubernaculum, processus vaginalis, and other surrounding structures. The size of the vas deferens and testicular vessels increases, the gubernaculum begins to swell, and the processus vaginalis now extends rapidly into the scrotum (Backhouse, 1964; Backhouse and Butler, 1960). A separation now occurs between the gubernaculum and the scrotal wall. As the scrotum and inguinal canal are stretched by the developing gubernaculum, the gonad, which sits on top of the gubernaculum, slips very rapidly into the scrotum (Backhouse, 1981; Schecter, 1963; Wyndham, 1943). During descent, the epididymis precedes the testis in its journey into the scrotum. After descent, the scrotal part of the processus vaginalis persists as the tunica vaginalis, and the upper part obliterates. The gubernaculum subsequently atrophies. If the processus vaginalis fails to obliterate, a hernia and/or hydrocele may form.

Incidence of Testis Descent

Cryptorchidism represents one of the most common disorders in man. The genitourinary system is well represented by the cryptorchid state in a multitude of congenital and hereditary abnormalities (Frey et al., 1981). In some premature babies, birth may occur prior to the onset of normal testicular descent during the last trimester of gestation. Scorer and Farrington (1971) found that of 1500 full-term (birth weight greater than 2500 g) infants examined at birth, 3.4 per cent had true undescended testes, whereas 30.3 per cent of 142 premature infants had undescended testes (Table 38–1). This differential in the incidence of testicular descent between full-term and premature infants has also been reported by other investigators (Buemann et al., 1961). Indeed, the smaller the birth weight of the infant, the greater the incidence of cryptorchidism. For example, 68.5 per cent of infants weighing less than 1800 g had undescended testes, whereas almost 100 per cent of infants weighing less than 900 g had bilateral cryptorchidism (Scorer, 1964). However, once these babies, particularly the premature ones, begin to gain weight and advance in age, the testes begin to descend.

By 1 year of age, the incidence of testicular descent is approximately 0.8 per cent, a marked decrease during this short time period (Scorer and Farrington, 1971; Villumsen and Zachau-Christiansen, 1966). Scorer and Farrington's data show that approximately 75 per cent of full-term cryptorchid testes and up to 95 per cent of premature cryptorchid testes will spontaneously descend by 1 year of age. Most of these testes that descend during the 1st year of life actually do so within the first

Table 38–1. INCIDENCE OF CRYPTORCHIDISM FROM BIRTH TO ADULTHOOD

Age	Incidence (%)
Preterm infant	30.3
Full-term infant	3.4
One year	0.8
Adulthood	0.8

Adapted from Scorer, G., and Farrington, G. H.: Congenital Deformities of the Testis and Epididymis. New York, Appleton-Century-Crofts, 1971.

Table 38–2. PLASMA TESTOSTERONE (ng%) IN HUMANS

	1–15 days	1–3 months	1 year	Prepuberty	Adulthood
Male	68 ± 60	208 ± 68	6.6 ± 4.6	6.6 ± 2.5	572 ± 135
Female	12 ± 6	9 ± 4	5.5 ± 2.8	6.6 ± 2.5	37 ± 10

Adapted from Forest, M. G., et al.: J Clin. Invest. 53:819, 1974.

3 months after birth. If descent had not occurred by this time, the testis descent was never complete. This testis remained relatively smaller than the contralaterally descended testis.

It is assumed, although not proved, that the reason the testis may descend within the first year is the elevated level of androgens in the plasma during the first 3 months of life (Table 38–2) (Forest et al., 1974; Scorer, 1964). The rise in the plasma testosterone level during the first 3 months in the male gradually falls to prepubertal levels (Forest et al., 1974; Winter et al., 1976). The Leydig cells, the source of the testosterone, become inactive and remain so until puberty. Despite the fact that the Leydig cells are inactive during the prepubertal years, they nevertheless retain the potential to respond to human chorionic gonadotropin (hCG) stimulation. This response to gonadotropin has been amply demonstrated in both prepubertal normal testes and prepubertal cryptorchid testes (Grant et al., 1976; Winter et al., 1972).

The cryptorchid state is most easily determined at birth, when the scrotum is relatively large, the minimal subcutaneous fat exists, and the cremasteric reflex is absent (Scorer and Farrington, 1971). However, the cremasteric reflex is most active between the 2nd and 7th years of age, and, as a result, a falsely high incidence of cryptorchidism may be obtained during childhood (McCutcheon, 1938; Ward and Hunter, 1960). In fact, in a number of studies, the incidence of cryptorchidism at or about the 5th year of age was estimated at about 10 per cent (Farrington, 1968). This high percentage was probably due to the inclusion of unrecognized cases of retractile testes. For example, if the incidence of cryptorchidism is the same at 1 year and at adulthood (0.8 per cent), this incidence cannot change at any time between these ages because human testes do not ascend permanently in the postnatal period. This ascent is what Farrington terms a retractile testis. Consequently, if there appears to be an increase in the incidence of cryptorchidism beyond 0.8 per cent at other ages, it must be due to testes that retract and then descend at a later date.

When Cour-Palais (1966) re-examined those cases of undescended testes of various age groups, the majority were indeed found to be retractile testes. In Cour-Palais's series, the true incidence of cryptorchidism was 0.76 per cent at age 5 years, 0.95 per cent at age 8 years, and 0.64 per cent at age 11 or thereafter.

In adults, Cour-Palais found the incidence of cryptorchidism to be in slightly less than 1 per cent of the male population. In addition to this careful study, other studies attest to the fact that the incidence of cryptorchidism at adulthood is less than 1 per cent. Baumrucker (1946) determined that the incidence of cryptorchidism in 10,000 consecutuve United States Army inductees

was 0.8 per cent. Others have noted similar incidences: 0.5 per cent in 10,000 Scottish recruits (Southam and Cooper, 1927), 0.7 per cent in male autopsies, and 0.55 per cent in almost 3 million United States Selective Service registrants between 1940 and 1944 (Campbell, 1959). The true incidence of cryptorchidism remains relatively constant from 1 year of age until adulthood, without any geographic distinction. The finding of Chilvers and co-workers (1984) that the incidence of cryptorchidism appears to be increasing could be due to the inclusion of retractile testes in their study population.

In surgical explorations for cryptorchidism, absence of one or both testes may be encountered in 3 to 5 per cent of cases (Goldberg et al., 1974). In 10 per cent of patients with cryptorchidism, the defect is bilateral; in 3 per cent, one or both testes are absent (Scorer and Farrington, 1971). A familial incidence is apparent in certain patients with cryptorchidism. Approximately 14 per cent of boys with undescended testes have family members with the same condition (Bishop, 1945; Brimblecomb, 1946; Wiles, 1934).

Mechanisms of Testicular Descent

Since Hunter's (1841) treatise, various mechanisms have been proposed to be responsible for the final placement of the testes into the scrotum (Table 38–3). Foremost are certain physical factors, which include (1) traction of the testis by the gubernaculum and/or cremaster muscle; (2) differential growth of the body wall in relation to a relatively immobile gubernaculum; (3) intra-abdominal pressure pushing the testis through an inguinal canal that is engorged by the swollen gubernaculum; and (4) development and maturation of the epididymis being responsible for testicular migration.

The traction theory adheres to the concept that the gubernaculum, or the cremaster muscle, or both, pulls the testis into the scrotum (Curling, 1840; Sonneland, 1925). Support for this concept comes from the observation that severance of the genitofemoral nerve, which innervates the gubernaculum, prevents testicular descent in rodents (Tayakkononta, 1963). However, severance of the gubernaculum in a variety of animal species did not prevent the testis from descending into the scrotum (Bergh et al., 1978; Wells, 1944). In addition, in the human fetus there is only a weak attachment between the gubernaculum and the scrotum and this is probably insufficient to support any traction on the testis (Bergh et al., 1978; Tayakkononta, 1963; Wyndham, 1943). Regarding the cremaster, it is well established that the sole function of this muscle is to retract the testis. Consequently, traction of the testis into the scrotum by the cremaster muscle is unlikely.

Table 38–3. MECHANISMS OF TESTIS DESCENT

Traction
Differential growth
Intra-abdominal pressure
Epididymal maturation
Hormonal

The differential growth theory adheres to the concept that as the body wall grows, the testis is kept in proximity to the internal inguinal ring. It is then pulled into the scrotum by the relatively immobile gubernaculum as a result of rapid growth of the body wall during the last trimester of pregnancy (Hunter, 1927; McMurrich, 1923). However, it has been demonstrated that the gubernaculum actually increases in size prior to descent and that it actually grows faster than the body as a whole (Hunter, 1927; Lemeh, 1960), thereby casting doubt on the validity of this theory.

The intra-abdominal pressure theory states that an increase in intra-abdominal pressure is the primary force that causes the testis to leave the abdomen and enter the inguinal ring (Bergin et al., 1970; Gier and Marion, 1970; Schechter, 1963). A number of investigators have provided theoretic and experimental evidence that appears to support the concept of intra-abdominal pressure as a promoter of testicular descent (Elder et al., 1982; Frey and Rajfer, 1984; Frey et al., 1983).

The epididymal theory of testicular descent (Hadziselomovic, 1981), which is based on the assumption that differentiation and maturation of the epididymis induce testicular descent, has been investigated in depth and may not be as important as initially thought (Frey and Rajfer, 1982).

Although it is difficult to refute unequivocally the aforementioned mechanical theories of testicular descent, and indeed all may play some role, it is generally accepted that endocrine factors somehow play the major role in promoting the descent of the testis into the scrotum. The endocrine regulation of testicular descent was initially inferred by Engle (1932), who induced premature testicular descent in the monkey with the use of gonadotropins. Thereafter, testosterone was found to be as efficacious as gonadotropins in inducing testicular descent in humans (Arnheim, 1938; Bigler et al., 1938; Goldman et al., 1926; Hamilton and Hubert, 1938; Hamilton, 1938; Thompson et al., 1937). Although it has been demonstrated that dihydrotestosterone, the 5-alpha reduced product of testosterone, appears to be the active androgen involved in testicular descent in at least two animal species (Rajfer and Walsh, 1977; Rajfer, 1982), inhibition of the 5-alpha reductase enzyme and the androgen receptor in rodents failed to retard descent (personal observation).

Endocrine Aspects of Cryptorchidism

If gonadotropins and androgens are necessary for testicular descent to occur, it follows that abnormalities in the hypothalamic-pituitary-testicular axis result in cryptorchidism. Indeed, in a variety of clinical syndromes characterized by defects in gonadotropin production, androgen synthesis, or androgen action, cryptorchidism may be observed (Fig. 38–1). In Kallmann's syndrome, in which there exists a deficiency in gonadotropin-releasing hormone (GnRH) secretion from the hypothalamus, cryptorchidism may be a presenting feature (Bardin et al., 1969; Santen and Paulsen, 1972). In anencephaly or developmental abnormalities of the pituitary gland, such as hypoplasia or aplasia, undescended testes are very common (Ch'in, 1938; Sadeghi-Nejad and Senior, 1974; Steiner and Boggs, 1965). In disorders of androgen synthesis or androgen action, cryptorchidism may also be a presenting feature (Grumbach and Van Wyk, 1974). In pseudovaginal perineoscrotal hypospadias, a condition in which there is an absence of the 5-alpha reductase enzyme that converts testosterone into dihydrotestosterone, cryptorchidism is frequent (Opitz et al., 1972; Walsh et al., 1974).

Although hormonal involvement in testicular descent appears clear-cut, there is nevertheless some discrepancy in the literature as to whether patients with cryptorchidism have discernible abnormalities in the hypothalamic-pituitary-testicular axes. Walsh and associates (1976) found no difference in plasma testosterone levels following hCG stimulation between children with cryptorchidism and normal children. In contrast, Cacciari and colleagues (1976) found a subnormal testosterone response to gonadotropin in children with cryptorchidism. When these workers used gonadotropin-releasing hormone (GnRH) to stimulate the hypothalamic-pituitary axis, they did not find any difference in pituitary leuteinizing hormone (LH) and follicle-stimulating hormone (FSH) secretion between the children with cryptorchidism and normal children. This finding was confirmed by Sizonenko and associates (1978), Van Vliet and associates (1980), and deMuinck Keizer-Schrama and associates (1986). However, the data of Hadziselimovic (1983) and Job and Gendrel (Gendrel et al., 1977, 1978, 1980a and b; Job et al., 1977) suggest that infants and children with cryptorchidism do indeed have abnormalities in the hypothalamic-pituitary-testicular axes, as evidenced by a decrease in the basal LH and testosterone levels and a blunted response of LH and testosterone to Gn-RH stimulation (Fig. 38–2). This deficiency in the secretion of LH and testosterone found in the infant with cryptorchidism persists through early puberty but disappears at midpuberty. No significant abnormality was seen in the FSH levels of these patients with cryptorchidism, although an occasional patient did demonstrate elevated basal FSH levels indicative of seminiferous tubular damage.

In spite of these data, the exact mechanism by which androgens act to promote testicular descent is still unknown. It is apparent, based on embryologic observations and some experimental data, that the gubernaculum is intimately involved with this important physiologic event. George and Peterson (1988) demonstrated some DHT binding within the gubernaculum of the postnatal rat, suggesting that the gubernaculum may be the androgen target tissue involved in testicular descent.

CLASSIFICATION OF UNDESCENDED TESTES

Based on its location, the cryptorchid testis can be classified as (1) abdominal-located, inside the internal inguinal ring; (2) canalicular-located, between the internal and external inguinal rings; (3) ectopic-located, away

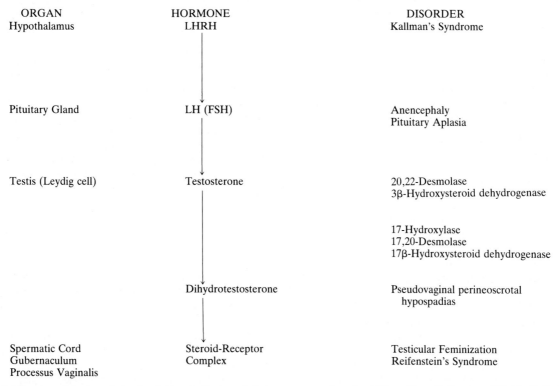

ORGAN	HORMONE	DISORDER
Hypothalamus	LHRH	Kallman's Syndrome
Pituitary Gland	LH (FSH)	Anencephaly Pituitary Aplasia
Testis (Leydig cell)	Testosterone	20,22-Desmolase 3β-Hydroxysteroid dehydrogenase 17-Hydroxylase 17,20-Desmolase 17β-Hydroxysteroid dehydrogenase
	Dihydrotestosterone	Pseudovaginal perineoscrotal hypospadias
Spermatic Cord Gubernaculum Processus Vaginalis	Steroid-Receptor Complex	Testicular Feminization Reifenstein's Syndrome

Figure 38–1. Disorders of the hypothalamic-pituitary-testicular axis in the presence of cryptorchidism. (From Rajfer, J. and Walsh, P. C.: Hormonal regulation of testicular descent: experimental and clinical observations. J. Urol., 118:985, 1977. © Williams & Wilkins.)

Figure 38–2. Age-dependent plasma testosterone and LH (mean ± SEM) values in newborn infants who presented at birth with undescended testes. One group (○) had spontaneous descent by 4 months, whereas the other group (●) had no testicular descent. (From Gendrel, D., et al.: J. Pediatr., 97:217, 1980.)

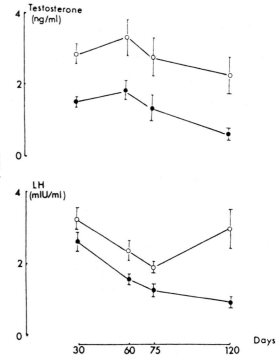

from the normal pathway of descent between the abdominal cavity and the bottom of the scrotum, and (4) retractile, the fully descended testis moves freely between the bottom of the scrotum and the groin, where it enters the superficial inguinal pouch (Browne, 1949). This pouch is actually a subcutaneous pocket lined by thin fibrous tissue situated in front of and lateral to the external inguinal ring.

The intra-abdominal testis, by definition, is impalpable. Very commonly, the testis is located just at the internal inguinal ring, and at the time of surgical exploration slight abdominal pressure usually causes the testis to pop into the inguinal canal. The canalicular testis is farther along the pathway of descent than the intra-abdominal testis. It may be located within the canal, or it may become emergent from within the canal to lie at the top of the scrotum. When it is located in the inguinal canal, the tension of the aponeurosis of the external oblique muscle may be too firm a barrier to allow the testis to become palpable (Scorer and Farrington, 1971).

On rare occasion, the testis may migrate from its normal pathway of movement between the abdominal cavity and the bottom of the scrotum and become located in an ectopic position. The five major sites of testicular ectopia are the perineum, the femoral canal, the superficial inguinal pouch, the suprapubic area, and the opposite scrotal compartment (Fig. 38–3). Testicular ectopia is believed to be directly related to the development of the gubernaculum. The gubernaculum is known to be divided into five branches, one each going to the aforementioned areas (Lockwood, 1888; Schechter, 1963). The scrotal area normally contains the bulk of the gubernaculum, and the testis normally follows this path during its descent. It has been suggested that when one of the other four branches contains the bulk of the gubernaculum, the testis is misdirected from its normal pathway of descent into the ectopic location. Experimental evidence to support this hypothesis comes from the data of Frey and Rajfer (1984). Clinically, the most common ectopic location is in the superficial inguinal pouch, which is a subcutaneous pocket lined by thin fibrous tissue situated in front of and lateral to the external ring (Browne, 1949). Transverse testicular ec-

topia is the rarest of all ectopic conditions but should be considered in any patient with an empty hemiscrotum and an additional mass in the contralateral hemiscrotum (Dajani, 1969; Davis, 1957; Muskerjee and Amesur, 1965).

The single most common factor that leads to an inaccurate diagnosis of an undescended testis is the presence of testicular retraction. Testicular retraction results from spontaneous or provoked activity of the cremaster muscle. It is most apparent in boys 5 to 6 years of age. In a survey of some 600 normal boys, Farrington (1968) found that in those under the age of 12 years, up to 20 per cent of the testes were in the superficial inguinal pouch at initial inspection. Between 6 months and 11 years of age, deliberate stimulation of the cremasteric reflex would result in withdrawal of up to 80 per cent of fully descended testes from their scrotal positions, leaving a seemingly empty hemiscrotum. Some 25% of these testes will retract fully into the superficial inguinal pouch, and the remainder will retract into the neck of the scrotum. From the 5th to 6th year of age until puberty, a gradual decline occurs in the number of testes that will fully retract out of the scrotum. At 11 years of age, with half of the boys who were showing evidence of the onset of puberty, only half of the testes retracted upon stimulation of the cremasteric reflex. At 13 years of age, the testis was usually found to be no longer retractile.

This retraction of the normal testis into the upper part of the scrotum or the superficial inguinal pouch during boyhood seems to be a protective reflex. Why this reflex appears to dissipate at the time of puberty is unknown. Therefore, it is of paramount importance to determine and record in an infant's chart whether the testes are palpable in the scrotum at birth or within the 1st year of life. In order to differentiate a retractile from a true cryptorchid testis, more than one visit to the physician may be necessary, and medical treatment with gonadotropins may be necessary (Rajfer et al., 1986b).

During the physical examination, manual traction is gently placed on the testis to try to bring it down to the bottom of the scrotum (Wylie, 1984). If it reaches the bottom of the scrotum, this is considered a retractile

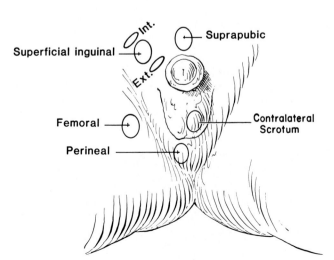

Superficial inguinal

Suprapubic

Int.

Ext.

Femoral

Contralateral Scrotum

Perineal

Figure 38–3. Schematic representation of sites of ectopic testes (int, internal inguinal ring; ext, external inguinal ring). (From Rajfer, J. Urol. Clin. North Am. 9:422, 1982.)

testis. If it does not, the patient returns on another visit for a second attempt at "milking the testis down." If it fails a second time, consideration is given to hormonal therapy.

If a testis is not palpable, it is intracanalicular, intra-abdominal, or absent (Scorer and Farrington 1971). The diagnosis of bilateral anorchia should always be considered in the presence of bilateral nonpalpable testes (Goldberg et al., 1974). Frequently, hCG stimulation tests are applied to distinguish bilateral anorchia from bilateral nondescent (Grant et al., 1976; Winter et al., 1972). A short course of hCG (2000 IU daily for 3 days) may be used to distinguish bilateral anorchia from bilateral cryptorchidism. In bilateral anorchia, basal gonadotropin levels may be extremely high and no response by testosterone to exogenous hCG takes place. If the basal gonadotropin levels are elevated in a boy less than 9 years of age, further work-up is not necessary to diagnose bilateral anorchia (Jarow et al., 1986).

The unilateral impalpable testis itself poses a unique diagnostic problem. Its presence must be verified and appropriate therapy taken either to make it palpable or to remove it. A variety of tests are employed in clinical practice to search for the impalpable testis. These include herniography, ultrasonography, computed tomography (CT) scanning, testicular arteriography and/or venography, and magnetic resonance imaging (MRI). Herniography is the oldest and least commonly practiced of these tests (White et al., 1970, 1973). It involves placement of contrast material intra-abdominally through a percutaneous catheter and radiologic demonstration of the presence of a hernia. Sometimes, it is possible to outline an undescended testis near the hernia sac, but, as can be expected, this procedure has an unacceptably high incidence of false-positive and false-negative results. For this reason, it is used rarely in routine clinical practice today.

Ultrasound scanning has been helpful in locating the testis only if it is located within the inguinal canal (Madrazo et al., 1979). If the testis is located underneath the aponeurosis of the external oblique muscle or is intra-abdominal, ultrasound is not very reliable.

CT scanning may be useful in bilateral impalpable testes to document their location (Fig. 38–4), but the test is expensive, emits radiation, and sometimes is difficult to perform in the young child (Lee et al., 1980; Pak et al., 1981; Rajfer et al., 1983; Wolverson et al., 1983).

MRI may be helpful in locating the impalpable testis (Fritzsche et al., 1987; Landa et al., 1987) but like CT scanning may be difficult in the young child. It is, however, the least invasive of all the current procedures (Fig. 38–5).

Angiography of the testicular vessels is technically difficult, and its complications (e.g., femoral thrombosis) may have disastrous consequences (Ben-Menachem et al., 1974; Vitale et al., 1974). Testicular venography has less morbidity than arteriography but is still an invasive procedure. Venography relies on the fact that when the pampiniform plexus of veins is present, the testis presumably is always present (Amin and Wheeler, 1976; Weiss et al., 1979). However, if the plexus is not visualized or if the testicular vein is blind-ending, one cannot unequivocally state that the testis is absent on that side (Weiss et al., 1979). For this reason, the test has its drawbacks.

Pediatric laparoscopy has evolved as an important tool in the search for the impalpable testis (Silber and Cohen, 1980). If the testicular vessels are seen ending blindly, it signifies that the testis is absent on that side and that no surgical exploration is necessary. If the vessels are seen entering the internal inguinal ring, an inguinal exploration is all that is required. When the testis is seen in the abdomen, a decision may be made to either perform an intra-abdominal exploration and attempt to place the testis in the scrotum (Naslund et al., 1989) or to clip the testicular vessels and perform an orchiopexy at a later date (Bloom et al., 1988; Ransley et al., 1984). Although laparoscopy requires an anesthetic, in most instances it can be combined with surgical exploration so that only one anesthetic is used for both localization and treatment (Naslund et al., 1989).

Histology

In 1929, Cooper published her classic paper on the histology of the cryptorchid testis. She noted that the longer a testis remained cryptorchid, the more likely it was to be histologically abnormal. The higher the testis resided away from the bottom of the scrotum, the more pronounced was the histologic abnormality. These histologic alterations in the cryptorchid testis appear by 1 1/2 years of age and include smaller seminiferous tu-

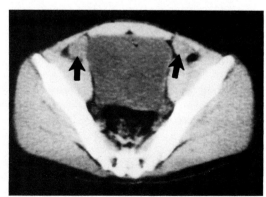

Figure 38–4. Computed tomographic scan of pelvis demonstrating bilateral undescended testes *(arrows)* at the internal inguinal rings (B, Bladder). (From Rajfer, J., et al.: The use of computerized tomography scanning to localize the impalpable testis. J. Urol., 129:978, 1983. © Williams & Wilkins.)

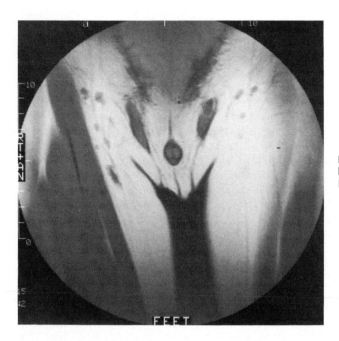

Figure 38–5. Magnetic resonance imaging scan of patient demonstrating bilateral cryptorchidism in the inguinal canals. (Courtesy of Dr. Jeffrey Phillips.)

bules, fewer spermatogonia, and more peritubular tissue. Since Cooper's work, a multitude of papers have appeared confirming these histologic alterations in the cryptorchid testis (Mack et al., 1961; Mengel et al., 1974; Scorer and Farrington, 1971; Sohval, 1954). Although the seminiferous tubules are definitely altered by the cryptorchid state, conflicting histologic evidence exists as to whether the Leydig cells are affected.

The electron microscope has been utilized to document certain ultrastructural changes in the seminiferous tubules as early as the 2nd year of life (Hadziselimovic, 1977; Hadziselimovic and Seguchi, 1973; Mengel et al., 1981; Zarzycki et al., 1977). These changes include (1) degeneration of the mitochondria, (2) loss of ribosomes in both the cytoplasm and the smooth endoplasmic reticulum, and (3) increase in the collagen fibers in the spermatogonia and Sertoli cells. Ultrastructural data are conflicting as to whether there are changes in the Leydig cells. It is still uncertain whether the known changes in the cryptorchid testis represent a primary defect or only an alteration secondary to the cryptorchid state. Support for the idea that the testis itself is defective lies in the observation that some of these histologic changes may also occur in the contralateral scrotal testis of the unilateral cryptorchid male (Mengel et al., 1974).

COMPLICATIONS

Neoplasia

A strong association exists between neoplasia and cryptorchidism. Approximately 10 per cent of testicular tumors arise from an undescended testis (Campbell, 1959; Gilbert, 1941; Gordon-Taylor and Wyndham, 1947). Statistically, the undescended testis is reported to be 35 to 48 times more likely to undergo malignant degeneration than the normal testis (Johnson et al., 1968; Jones and Scott, 1971; Martin and Menck, 1975).

The fact that neoplastic degeneration of an undescended testis is in itself a rare entity allows some surgeons to state that orchiectomy may not be the only choice of therapy in the postpubertal patient with cryptorchid testis (Welvaart and Tijssen, 1981).

Farrer and associates (1985) addressed this issue and, using updated statistical data, concluded that the true annual incidence of germ cell testis tumors in patients with cryptorchidism is one tumor per 2550. Employing the same statistical data, these investigators also concluded that after age 32, the patient with cryptorchidism is at greater risk of death from orchiectomy than testicular malignancy (Fig. 38–6). Therefore, we have modified our policy such that all impalpable testes are either removed or placed in a position to allow palpation. If a testis is undescended but palpable, we observe patients who are 32 years of age or older. For patients with palpable undescended testes less than 32 years of age, observation or orchiopexy is recommended depending on the patient's wishes.

With regard to location, an abdominal testis is four times more likely to undergo malignant degeneration than an inguinal testis (Campbell, 1959). Tumors in undescended testes occur mainly at the time of puberty or after, although some neoplasias have occurred in children and infants (Gordon-Taylor and Wyndham, 1947). For this reason, if surgical correction of the cryptorchid testis is to be performed, it should be carried out prepubertally.

In 1972, Skakkebaek reported the finding of carcinoma in situ in the testis of an infertile man with an undescended testis who developed a germ cell tumor 16 months later. Since 1972, the prevalence of carcinoma in situ has been determined to be 1.7 per cent in patients with cryptorchidism. All patients between 18 and 20 years of age with a history of cryptorchidism, treated or untreated, should be offered an open testis biopsy (Giwercman et al., 1987, 1989). If carcinoma in situ is not found on the biopsy, the risk of developing a future

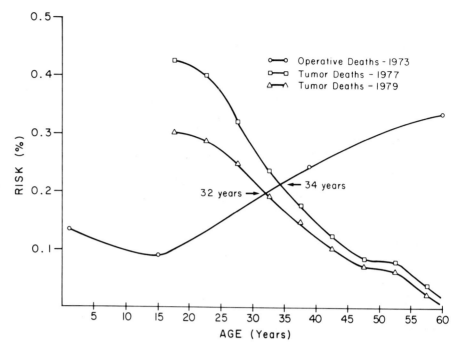

Figure 38–6. Lifetime risk of death from testis tumors for white male patients with cryptorchidism (1977 and 1979) compared with risk of death from surgery (age and American Society of Anesthesiology class-specific). (From Farrer, J. H., et al.: Management of the postpubertal cryptorchid testis: a statistical review. J. Urol., 134:1071, 1985. © Williams & Wilkins.)

testis cancer in that gonad is extremely low. If carcinoma in situ is discovered, the gonad is removed.

Because testicular tumors have occurred in patients who have undergone orchiopexy as early as 5 years of age (Altman and Malament, 1967), most workers currently recommend surgical correction between 1 and 1½ years of age, especially in light of the fact that ultrastructural changes begin to occur in the undescended testis at this early age (Mengel et al., 1974, 1981; Hadziselimovic, 1977). Whether this earlier surgical correction will deter the subsequent development of neoplasia in the undescended testis remains to be seen. Further support for the concept that there is an underlying pathologic process that affects both testes in the patient with unilateral cryptorchidism comes from the data of Johnson and associates (1986). They showed that one in five testicular tumors occurring in patients with cryptorchidism has developed in the contralateral, supposedly normal, scrotal testis.

In bilateral cryptorchidism, there is a 15 per cent chance of developing a tumor in the opposite testis if one of the testes becomes involved with a tumor (Gilbert and Hamilton, 1970). If both testes are intra-abdominal and one testis becomes malignant, there is a 30 per cent chance of the other testis becoming malignant. Seminoma followed by embryonal cell carcinoma are the two most frequent neoplasms encountered in cryptorchid testes (Batata et al., 1980; Gilbert and Hamilton, 1970; Martin, 1979). In patients with certain intersex disorders in which cryptorchidism is a presenting feature, gonadoblastoma is the most common tumor (Scully, 1970). Although gonadoblastomas themselves are nonmalignant tumors, they often coexist with germ cell tumors in the same gonad. Some evidence exists that gonadoblastomas develop because of a deletion of part of the long arm of the Y chromosome (Page, 1987).

TORSION

The increased susceptibility of the testis to undergo torsion is due to a developmental anatomic abnormality between the testis and its mesentery. If the testis is broader than its mesentery, it is more likely to twist on its stalk (Scorer and Farrington, 1971). Therefore, the incidence of torsion is greatest in the postpubertal period when the testis usually increases in size. Similarly, the undescended testis would be more susceptible to torsion by any mechanism causing an increase in testicular size, e.g., a tumor. In a review of the literature, Rigler (1972) found that 64 per cent of adults with torsion in an undescended testis had an associated germ cell tumor. The presentation of a patient with abdominal pain and an ipsilateral empty hemiscrotum should alert the physician to the possibility of torsion of a cryptorchid testis.

HERNIA

As stated in the previous section on embryology, the processus vaginalis is intimately associated with the structures involved in testicular descent. Following descent, which occurs at or about the 7th month of fetal life, the processus vaginalis, which connects the peritoneal cavity to the tunica vaginalis, closes between the 8th month of fetal life and the 1st month after birth. However, when the testis fails to descend, the processus vaginalis remains patent. This may permit some of the intra-abdominal contents to enter the tunica vaginalis through the processus vaginalis and appear clinically as a hernia or a hydrocele. Although the true incidence is unclear, hernia sacs may be found in greater than 90 per cent of patients with cryptorchidism (Scorer and Farrington, 1971).

INFERTILITY

Testicular maldescent retards the production of spermatozoa. Therefore, the fertility of patients with bilaterally retained testes is generally very poor (Albescu et al., 1971; Hansen, 1949; Mack, 1953; Scorer, 1967; Scott, 1962; Wolloch et al., 1980). The higher and longer the testis resides away from the bottom of the scrotum, the greater the likelihood of damage to the seminiferous tubules. The earlier the testis is brought down into the scrotum, the greater the potential for recovering spermatogenic activity. Consequently, it would seem prudent to perform orchiopexy at an age prior to degeneration of the seminiferous tubules (Ludwig and Potempa, 1975).

A defect may be present in the spermatogenic activity of the contralateral scrotal testis in the patient with unilateral cryptorchidism (Hecker and Heinz, 1967; Scorer, 1967; Woodhead et al., 1973). By comparing the sperm density of normal adults with that of adults who had undergone successful unilateral orchiopexy during childhood, Lipschultz and associates (1976) discovered that men with unilateral cryptorchidism had much lower than expected sperm counts. This observation further supports the hypothesis that there may be an inherent defect in both testes of the patient with unilateral cryptorchidism.

In addition to the defect in spermatogenesis, clinical and experimental evidence suggests that cryptorchidism may also affect the interstitial compartment of the testis. In cryptorchid animals, sex accessory tissue weight has been shown to be retarded, and the testicular enzymes necessary for testosterone synthesis may be inhibited (Clegg, 1960; Korenchevsy, 1931). It has also been demonstrated that the testosterone response of prepubertal children with cryptorchidism to exogenous hCG stimulation is retarded (Job et al., 1977; Gendrel et al., 1977, 1978, 1980a and b). Postpubertally, however, there appears to be no difference in the hCG response between children with cryptorchidism and normal children. If, indeed, cryptorchidism does have an adverse effect on testosterone synthesis, the defect is probably not clinically significant because most patients with bilateral cryptorchidism are normally androgenized both at birth and at adulthood.

ASSOCIATED ANOMALIES

Some question exists in the literature regarding the incidence of chromosomal abnormalities in patients with uncomplicated unilateral cryptorchidism (Dewald et al., 1977; Mininberg and Bragol, 1973). The genetic syndromes that are associated with the undescended testis are extremely rare and are associated with poor survival. Of these, the best known are Klinefelter's, Noonan's, and Prader-Willi's syndromes. Most patients with Klinefelter's syndrome are sterile, and the disease therefore cannot be passed to offspring. However, there is an occasional patient with a mosaic chromosomal constitution who may be potentially fertile. Noonan's syndrome, or male Turner's syndrome, is an endocrine disorder in which cryptorchidism is common (Redman, 1973). As in Klinefelter's syndrome, a patient with Noonan's syndrome may occasionally be fertile, but the disorder is usually not passed to offspring. Patients with Prader-Willi's syndrome, which is believed to be secondary to a hypothalamic defect, are usually obese, mentally retarded, hypotonic, and short in stature (Laurence, 1967). Treatment is currently directed at replacement of the deficient hypothalamic hormones.

Vasal and epididymal abnormalities have long been recognized as being associated with the undescended testis (Marshall, 1982). The epididymis may be extended in length, may undergo partial or total atresia, or may be totally disassociated from the testis (Scorer and Farrington, 1971). The same abnormalities may be seen with the vas deferens. Indeed, in the disorder cystic fibrosis, in which there is a very high incidence of congenital absence of the vas deferens, cryptorchidism is frequent (Holschaw et al., 1971; Landing et al., 1969; Shwachman et al., 1977; Toussig et al., 1972).

Epididymal defects have also been described in the male offspring of women exposed to diethylstilbestrol during pregnancy (Cosgrove et al., 1977; Bibbo et al., 1975; McLachlan et al., 1975). The most common abnormalities in these patients are cryptorchidism and cystic dilatations of the epididymis. Although this finding may suggest that some cases of cryptorchidism may be due to elevated in utero levels of estrogen, which may act either via the hypothalmic-pituitary-testicular axis or via a direct effect on the tissues themselves, all fetuses are normally bathed in estrogen during the entire gestational period.

TREATMENT

The reasons for correcting the undescended testis are as follows: (1) a defect that is obvious and visible to both parents and patient is permanently corrected; (2) certain psychopathologic tendencies that surface initially around the 5th year of age, when the child enters school, may be prevented or alleviated (Cytryn et al., 1967); (3) the undescended testis has an increased susceptibility to malignant degeneration, and, consequently, it seems wise to place the testis in a site where it can be palpated easily; and (4) fertility is improved.

Because the prognosis for fertility in patients with bilateral cryptorchidism is extremely poor, every conceivable effort should be made to salvage at least one, or preferably both, of the testes and place them into the scrotum. The placement of the testis should be accomplished as early as 12 to 18 months of age. In the unilateral cryptorchid male, a determined effort should be made to deliver the retained testis into the scrotum, in light of reports that suggest that fertility may be impaired. It is our policy at the present time to salvage all testes, if at all possible, and position them at a site where they are readily palpable. Otherwise, an orchiectomy is performed. Orchiectomy is also reserved for the older postpubertal male patient (Farrer et al., 1985), if the patient so desires, and for the patient with certain intersex disorders in which the testis is dysgenetic and prone to malignant degeneration (Scully, 1970).

Two avenues of therapy are available for placing the cryptorchid testis into the scrotum: hormonal and surgical. The optimal time for attempting to place the retained testis into the scrotum is debatable. It appears, from the data concerning the changes in the seminiferous tubules by the 2nd year of age and from the observation that a testis not descended by 1 year of age will probably remain undescended, that treatment probably should be rendered as early as possible, preferably during or prior to the 2nd year of age.

Hormonal Therapy

Hormonal therapy is the only medical therapy available for the undescended testis. At present, there are two types of hormonal therapy: hCG and Gn-RH (luteinizing hormone-releasing factor, or LH-RH). The hormone hCG is given under the premise that stimulation of the Leydig cells will result in an increase in plasma testosterone, which will promote testicular descent. Gn-RH is used under the premise that children with cryptorchidism have an abnormality in the secretion of Gn-RH (LH-RH) from the hypothalamus, as evidenced by a decrease in basal LH levels. Replacement therapy with exogenous Gn-RH should reverse this defect or deficiency.

A number of studies have been done in which hCG has been given parenterally to induce testicular descent in children with cryptorchidism, and the success rate has varied between 14 per cent and 50 per cent (Bigler et al., 1938; Ehrlich et al., 1969; Job et al., 1982). The hormone hCG has been given in a total dose varying from 3000 IU to more than 40,000 IU. The frequency of injection has ranged from daily to weekly, and the duration of treatment has ranged from a few days to several months.

Job and associates (1982) have demonstrated that in order to obtain a maximal stimulation of the Leydig cells from hCG, a total dose of at least 10,000 IU is needed; however, above 15,000 IU of hCG, side effects may occur. Under 15,000 IU of hCG, testicular histology does not change and bone age is not affected. Rarely, there is a transient increase in the size of the penis, which regresses following cessation of therapy.

The less than ideal results with exogenous hCG and the fact that it has to be given parenterally along with the data of Job and colleages (1977) that gonadotropin levels are deficient in infants with cryptorchidism led European investigators to initiate studies using exogenous Gn-RH as a form of therapy. The dosage of native Gn-RH that has been used and is found to be effective in stimulating LH is 1.2 mg per day as a pernasal spray for 4 weeks (Rajfer et al., 1986a). The efficacy of this form of hormonal therapy in cryptorchidism has been reported to be successful in up to 70 per cent of patients treated (Bartsch and Frick, 1974; Hadziselimovic, 1982; Happ et al., 1975, 1978a; Illig et al., 1977, 1980; Job et al., 1974; Pirazzoli et al., 1978; Spona et al., 1979; Zabransky, 1981). However, in other clinics (deMuinck

Keizer-Schrama et al., 1986; Rajfer et al., 1986b), the success rate in inducing descent with Gn-RH is, at best, 6 to 18 per cent.

This low success rate with Gn-RH is not due to defective LH and testosterone secretion by the hypothalamus and testis, respectively (Rajfer, et al., 1986b). Synthetic, long-lasting analogues of Gn-RH, which may have a paradoxical effect on serum LH concentration, have also been used, but results are reported to be less effective than those of native Gn-RH (Frick et al., 1980; Happ et al., 1978b). No side effects, such as precocious growth, have been reported with native Gn-RH, although the relapse rate after 6 months of therapy approximates 10 per cent. In addition, there does not appear to be a difference in the success rate between unilateral and bilateral cryptorchidism. Some evidence suggests that hCG injections subsequent to Gn-RH therapy may have an additional effect in promoting descent in the testes (Hadziselimovic, 1982), but this use has never been accepted as standard. Indeed, the serum testosterone levels during therapy for cryptorchidism are much higher with hCG than those with Gn-RH (Fig. 38–7).

One explanation for the markedly different success rates with Gn-RH among various investigators may be due to the fact that retractile testes were not carefully excluded. Of the 56 patients who were referred to us for treatment of undescended testis with either hCG or Gn-RH, 13 (23 per cent) were found to have retractile testes rather than true cryptorchid testes (Rajfer et al., 1986b). Because these boys were examined and referred to us by competent urologists and pediatricians, the proportion of boys (23 per cent) with retractile testes may in actuality have been much lower when compared with earlier study populations, which used primary physician referrals as a source of patients. We believe that this may explain the high success rate of Gn-RH therapy in earlier studies compared with later data from our group and others.

The term retractile testes refers to those testes that migrate freely between the bottom and upper parts of the scrotum and/or superficial inguinal pouch. They are most common between 5 and 7 years of age (Farrington, 1968). In 1949, Browne observed that for every five patients referred to him for surgery, four actually had retractile testes and were misdiagnosed by the referring physician. Puri and Nixon (1977) later demonstrated that children with retractile testes do not require any interventional therapy such as surgery because at adulthood these testes are of normal volume and fertility. Wylie (1984) recommended that if a testis can be milked down on physical examination into the bottom of the scrotum, it was a retractile testis and did not require therapy. However, when the testis could be milked down only to the upper scrotum, this testis at adulthood had a smaller volume that a normal descended testis and should therefore be treated as a true undescended testis.

It has been proposed that a significant number of patients with retractile testes are still misdiagnosed as having true undescended testes and are being treated surgically. As an example, Chilvers and colleagues (1984) reported that between 1962 and 1981 the diagnosis of cryptorchidism and the rate of orchiopexy

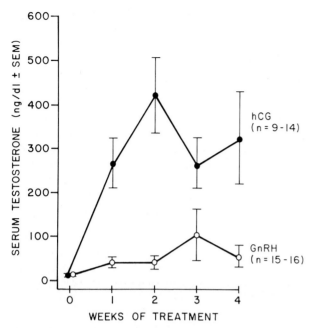

Figure 38–7. Mean serum testosterone levels among boys with cryptorchidism treated with weekly parenteral human chorionic gonadotropin or daily intranasal gonadotropin-releasing hormone. (From Rajfer, J., et al.: N. Engl. J. Med., 314:466–470, 1986.)

increased tenfold, during a time when the incidence of cryptorchidism in the general population remained stable at 0.8 per cent of all boys. Cooper and Little (1985) reported that in Nottingham, England, where the population and incidence of cryptorchidism have remained stable for decades, approximately five times the expected amount of orchiopexies per year are performed. Approximately 14,070 orchiopexies were actually performed annually instead of the expected 3150. These data would tend to suggest that the inclusion of retractile testes into population groups of true cryptorchid testes is very common among both primary physicians and specialists.

Therefore, if a simple diagnostic test could be made available to these primary physicians and specialists to allow the accurate distinction of retractile from true undescended testes, a huge number of children may be spared the trauma, morbidity, and expense of orchiopexy. Some data in the literature suggest that retractile testes treated with hCG almost always descend (Cooper and Little, 1985; Deming, 1936; Rajfer et al., 1986b). Intranasal Gn-RH has never been used to help in this differentiation of retractile from true undescended testes. As a result, it has been proposed that hCG should be given to all children with palpable but undescended testes to help differentiate retractile (those that descend) from true undescended testes (those that do not descend). However, hCG requires a series of injections and this itself is traumatic to both parent and child. If intranasal Gn-RH were found to be as effective as hCG in promoting descent of retractile testis, this would provide a simple and nontraumatic avenue of differentiating a retractile from a true cryptorchid testis. In turn, such a result would encourage its utilization by all primary physicians, urologists, and surgeons as the preliminary step in the diagnosis and work-up of a patient with a testis outside the scrotum (Hazebroek et al., 1987). Until this occurs, we recommend hCG to help in this differentiation (Rajfer et al., 1986b).

INGUINAL HERNIA IN INFANCY AND CHILDHOOD

In clinical practice, the majority of infantile inguinal hernias appear in the 1st year, the diagnosis being made most commonly in the 1st month after birth. New cases are less frequent in older children.

The overall incidence in the pediatric population has been variously reported as being from 1.0 to 4.4 per cent. In immature infants, those weighing less than 2000 g at birth, the incidence rises to over 13 per cent. The condition affects boys nine times more frequently than girls.

BILATERAL INGUINAL HERNIAS

Controversy has arisen with regard to the desirability of routine bilateral exploration in cases of apparent unilateral inguinal hernia. For instance, Gunnlaugsson and colleagues (1967) reported that 60 per cent of such patients were found, on surgical exploration, to also have a clinically undiagnosed hernial sac on the contralateral side.

While accepting that these and other workers have shown it to be likely that a patent sac is present on the opposite side in early childhood, it seems pertinent to inquire whether this is of practical significance, as long as the sac does not accept abdominal viscera. A follow-up study performed by Hamrick and Williams (1962) on 229 patients showed that only 15 patients (6.55 per cent) developed a clinical hernia on the contralateral unexplored side. The majority of these appeared in children operated on when under the age of 6 years. Of these patients, only one child in ten developed a second hernia. Hence, it may reasonably be argued that routine operation on the second side of a younger child may be unnecessary in up to 90 per cent of cases. When additional consideration is given to the close association of the spermatic vessels and vas deferens to the patent processus vaginalis, routine exploration cannot be done without risk to the testicular apparatus. Indeed, there is an incidence of testicular atrophy of approximately 0.5 per cent following infantile hernia repair. Occasionally, a vas deferens is seen by the pathologist in the resected hernia sac. We recommend that no attempt be made in this case to reconstruct or reconnect the vas, but the patient's family should be made aware of the situation should a problem with infertility arise later during adulthood.

Diagnosis

The majority of patients with infantile inguinal hernias present to the physician within the first 3 months of life. The parent describes the sudden appearance of a bulge in the child's groin, often after a period of crying, coughing, or straining at stool. The swelling is generally absent in the morning, becoming more noticeable later in the day.

The diagnosis is sometimes simple to make—a fullness is visible in one groin as compared with the other, and a cough or cry makes the swelling briefly more obvious. Gentle pressure on the abdomen may provoke the child to grunt and cause the swelling to reappear. Palpation reveals an indistinct swelling in the area, accompanied by an impulse on coughing or crying. On occasion, there is no immediately visible abnormality, yet the child's parents are convinced that they have seen a swelling, that the child was distressed at the time, but that the swelling has since disappeared. Careful synchronous palpation, in which both spermatic cords are rolled gently over the pubic tubercles, may reveal that the cord on the suspected side is more bulky and more tangible than the more delicate structure on the other side. The presence of a patent processus does seem to impart a palpable thickness and substance to the spermatic cord. Such a finding gives reliable confirmation to the parent's account. To complete the examination, it is important to inspect the scrotum, ensuring that both testes are fully descended, because up to 6 per cent of congenital inguinal hernias are associated with incomplete descent.

INGUINAL HERNIA IN GIRLS

Some 1.6 per cent of girls with inguinal hernias prove to have a 46,XY genotype with intra-abdominal testes but with female external genitalia and female endocrine function (i.e., the testicular feminization syndrome). Karyotypes should routinely be performed on all female infants presenting with inguinal hernias, particularly if these are bilateral. The importance lies in the realization that the hernial sac may contain not an ovary (as is commonly the case with girls with inguinal hernias) but a testis. If a testis is found, there is some support based on endocrinology that it should not be excised during childhood. When a decision is made, a simple herniotomy should be performed with excision of the processus vaginalis but placement of the testis to the abdomen.

After the patient has passed puberty and growth and feminization are complete, the testis should be excised, as it is liable to malignant change like any other undescended testis.

Support for leaving the testis in situ until puberty has passed lies in the endocrine alterations that ensue during puberty (Griffin and Wilson, 1980). As gonadotropins are secreted at puberty, the testes begin to secrete testosterone and some estrogen. Because the androgen receptor is absent or defective in these patients, the serum testosterone cannot inhibit gonadotropin secretion from the pituitary gland thereby allowing the serum LH level to remain remarkably elevated, along with the serum testosterone level. The high circulating testosterone is converted to 17β-estradiol by the aromatase enzyme found in the peripheral fatty tissues. The high serum 17β-estradiol level coupled with a totally ineffective serum testosterone level provides for the feminization that these individuals undergo at puberty. In adult life, these patients become normal women in build. Anatomically normal female external genitalia develop, although the vagina tends to be hypoplastic. They have normal breast development and female social behavior. Because the uterus and ovaries are absent, there is a consequent primary amenorrhea, which may be the presenting feature that brings some of these patients to clinical recognition at the time of puberty.

INFANT HYDROCELE

A hydrocele is a collection of fluid between the parietal and visceral layers of the tunica vaginalis. Hydroceles usually occur during infancy or at adulthood. During infancy, it is believed that a patent processus vaginalis contributes to the collection of peritoneal fluid in the tunica vaginalis (Fig. 38–8). In adulthood, some theoretic evidence exists that an imbalance in the secretory and absorptive capacities of the parietal and visceral layers of the tunica vaginalis is responsible for the collection of fluid within the tunic (Ozdilek, 1957; Rinker and Allen, 1951).

Clinical Presentation

A hydrocele is very common after birth, occurring in about 6 per cent of full-term boys (Scorer and Farrington, 1977). It occurs as a transilluminating, painless, oval, scrotal swelling that may extend along the spermatic cord. Because a hydrocele at birth is almost universally secondary to a patent processus vaginalis, therapy should be delayed until after the processus closes, which may occur spontaneously within the 1st year of life. The patent processus vaginalis also explains why the size of the infant hydrocele may vary in size daily. Although this would suggest that the hydrocele fluid can be manually reduced back into the peritoneal cavity, this is usually not the case. The presence of mesenteric adenitis may also accentuate the size of a hydrocele.

Occasionally, an inguinal hernia or a torsion (if a

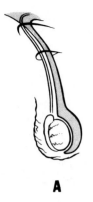
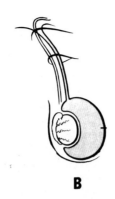
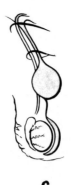

A   **B**   **C**

Figure 38–8. Causes of infant hydrocele. *A*, Completely open processus vaginalis, which may also allow herniation of bowel contents. *B*, Incomplete closure of the processus vaginalis, which allows peritoneal fluid, but not bowel contents, to enter. *C*, Hydrocele of spermatic cord as a result of complete closure of lower end of processus vaginalis.

testis cannot be palpated) may be suspected in a patient with a hydrocele. A history of no previous scrotal pain or swelling and an adequate physical examination will usually rule out torsion or an inguinal hernia.

Therapy involves observation during the 1st year of life, but thereafter surgical intervention is necessary. In the pediatric age group, surgery involves ligation of the patent processus vaginalis (McKay et al., 1958). Sclerosing agents are not to be used in children because the patent processus vaginalis will allow the agent to pass freely into the peritoneal cavity and produce chemical peritonitis. Aspiration of the hydrocele fluid from the tunic is usually an unsuccessful procedure, because the fluid recollects, owing to the patency between the peritoneum and the tunic. Occasionally, aspiration is necessary in order to carefully palpate the testis. However, a risk exists of introducing infection and possible peritonitis when aspiration is performed.

TESTICULAR TORSION

Torsion or twisting of the testis is considered a surgical emergency because the gonad may be lost. When torsion occurs, obstruction to the venous blood supply, with secondary edema and hemorrhage and subsequent arterial obstruction, results. This ultimately leads to necrosis of the entire gonad. Although testicular torsion is possible at any age, it is most common during adolescence (between the ages of 12 and 18 years), after which the incidence slowly decreases (Scorer and Farrington, 1971). The incidence is estimated to be approximately one in 4000 male patients less than 25 years of age (Barada et al., 1989). A few cases also appear during the neonatal period (Scorer and Farrington, 1971).

Although a variety of predisposing factors have been mentioned as etiology for testicular torsion, Scorer and Farrington believe that torsion occurs because of a narrow mesenteric attachment from the cord onto the testis and epididymis (Fig. 38–9). This narrow mesenteric attachment allows the testis to fall forward. Within the vaginal cavity, the testis is free to rotate like a clapper in a bell. When the mesenteric attachment to the testis and epididymis is broad, the testis does not fall forward but attains a more upright position, thereby making it less likely to rotate on its axis. This characteristic explains why the pubertal testis has more of a propensity for undergoing torsion than its prepubertal

counterpart, for at puberty the testis increases in volume approximately fivefold to sixfold (Marshall and Tanner, 1980). This ability also explains why the onset of torsion in an undescended testis may signal the development of a tumor, because this will also increase the size of the testis in relation to its mesentery (Rigler, 1972). This anatomic abnormality is usually bilateral. For this reason, when torsion of the testis is confirmed at operation, the contralateral testis should also be fixed to the scrotum.

Differential Diagnosis

The classic presentation of testicular torsion is pain and swelling on the affected side. In order to make the diagnosis, one must first be aware of the disorder. In the infant, symptoms may be absent such that the patient may present only with irritability, restlessness, and lack of appetite (Scorer and Farrington, 1971). Usually, the body temperature is normal and the urinalysis is clear.

The most common misdiagnosis of testicular torsion is acute epididymitis. Acute epididymitis may appear with similar symptoms except that the patient may have an elevated temperature or a urethral discharge. The urinalysis demonstrates pyuria or bacteriuria. Strangulated hernia, hematocele, hydrocele, testicular tumor, and idiopathic scrotal edema are to be considered in the differential diagnosis. Usually, the history and physical examination will help in arriving at the correct diagnosis.

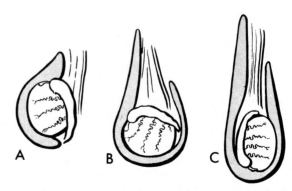

A   **B**   **C**

Figure 38–9. Attachment of testicular mesentery to testis. *A*, The normal peritoneal disposition around the testis. *B*, A capacious tunica vaginalis surrounding the cord; the testis lies horizontally. *C*, The inverted testis, which most easily twists because of its narrow attachment.

However, in those instances when the diagnosis is in doubt, a Doppler study (Levy, 1975; Thompson et al., 1975) or a nuclear perfusion study (Holder et al., 1977; Datta and Mishkin, 1975) may be helpful (Fig. 38–10).

Neonatal Testicular Torsion

In the newborn period, the testis has just descended into the scrotum and the gubernaculum has still not become completely attached to the scrotal wall (Backhouse, 1982). Therefore, the testis and gubernaculum are free to rotate within the neonatal scrotum. In this age group, the entire testis, epididymis, and tunica vaginalis may twist together in a vertical axis on the spermatic cord above. This condition is known as extravaginal torsion of the testis. The more common form of testicular torsion that occurs after puberty is classified as intravaginal torsion. Clinically, the neonate presents with a firm, hard, and large scrotal mass that does not transilluminate. Usually, the mass is not tender and the child does not appear to be disturbed by it. Occasionally, the child may appear restless and may be reluctant to take feedings. Although early exploration has been the rule in this situation, most testes are gangrenous at the time of exploration. Logic would dictate that unless a pyogenic infection is present, surgical exploration need not be undertaken in the newborn with testicular torsion because the testis is already necrotic and there is no basis for contralateral orchiopexy at this time. However, experimental evidence suggests that immunologic damage to the contralateral testis may occur if a necrotic testis that has undergone torsion is left in situ (Krarup, 1978). Reports have been made of delayed torsion of the contralateral testis in patients who had a neonatal testicular torsion. As a result of this observation, contralateral orchiopexy is recommended in these patients.

Pubertal Testicular Torsion

It is a wise axiom that an acutely painful swollen testis in an adolescent is due to torsion until proved otherwise at surgery. In this form of torsion, the testis twists intravaginally, because the gubernaculum is fixed to the scrotal wall. The testis is therefore free to rotate because of its short peritoneal attachment (see Fig. 38–9). The onset of pain is sudden. Scrotal edema occurs very soon thereafter. Scrotal exploration should be performed if the diagnosis is considered at all. Contralateral orchiopexy with at least two distinct sutures is done simultaneously, because of the propensity for the disorder to occur with at least two distinct sutures bilaterally (Burton, 1972; Chapman and Walton, 1972; Macnicol, 1974). If a torsion is reduced manually, surgical fixation should be performed because recurrent torsion and testicular loss may occur even before the patient leaves the hospital (Korbel, 1974; Sparks, 1972). It is recommended that nonabsorbable suture coupled with a three-point fixation can be used for the orchiopexy (Barada et al., 1989).

TORSION OF TESTICULAR APPENDAGES

The most common testicular appendage susceptible to torsion is the appendix testis, which is a remnant of the müllerian duct. The clinical picture is not different from that in a patient with true testicular torsion. Usually, the patients are adolescents, and they present with the sudden onset of testicular pain. If scrotal swelling has not developed, it may allow one to palpate the twisted appendage as a 3- to 5-mm tender mass near the upper pole of the testis; a characteristic blue dot sign may be seen on the skin of the scrotum (Dresner,

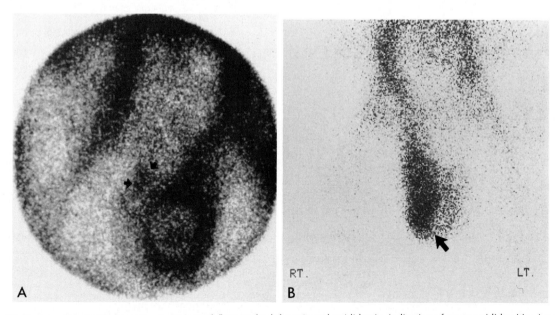

Figure 38–10. Radionuclide testicular scan. *A,* Increased flow to the left testis and epididymis, indicative of acute epididymitis. Arrows point to normal right testis next to large left testis. *B,* Absence of testicular flow is characteristic of a right testicular torsion. Left testis *(arrow)* is normally perfused.

1973). Once edema occurs, palpation of the appendage becomes impossible. Occasionally, a local anesthetic may be administered to the cord near the external inguinal ring to allow a more definitive examination. If any doubt exists as to the reason for testicular pain and swelling, scrotal exploration is recommended.

Prognosis

The prognosis for torsion is good if the patient is operated on within 4 to 6 hours and contralateral orchiopexy is performed (Krarup, 1978). In the operating room, an injection of fluorescein may be given and the testis may be observed under Wood's lamp (ultraviolet) if testicular viability is in doubt. If the fluorescein perfuses the testis, testicular viability is almost certain and the testis is left in situ. If a necrotic testicular mass is found, the testis should be removed. A testicular prosthesis may be inserted at the same time or at a later date.

Some data suggest that if testicular torsion occurs and the testis is left in situ, an abnormal sperm count at adulthood is more common than if the affected testis has been excised (Bartsch et al., 1980; Krarup, 1978). It is believed that when the testis undergoes torsion, certain proteins may be liberated within the systemic circulation, with the development of antitesticular antibodies that theoretically may damage the normal contralateral testis. This autoimmune theory of torsion is at present hypothetic, and further investigation must be conducted to verify this assumption. However, it has been shown that the testicular dysfunction may antedate the onset of torsion and that the histologic alterations may be due to an inherent abnormality of these testes (Hadzieselimovic et al., 1986).

REFERENCES

Cryptorchidism

Albescu, J. Z., Bergada, C., and Cullen, M.: Male fertility in patients treated for cryptorchidism before puberty. Fertil. Steril., 22:829, 1971.

Altman, B. L., and Malament, M.: Carcinoma of the testis following orchiopexy. J. Urol., 97:498, 1967.

Amin, M., and Wheeler, C. S.: Selective testicular venography in abdominal cryptorchidism. J. Urol., 115:760, 1976.

Arey, L. B.: The genital system. In Arey, L. B. (Ed.): Developmental Anatomy, 7th ed. Philadelphia, W. B. Saunders Co., 1965, pp. 315–341.

Arnheim, R. E.: The treatment of undescended testes with gonadotropic hormones. J. Mt. Sinai Hosp., 4:1036, 1938.

Backhouse, K. M.: The gubernaculum testis in hunteri: testicular descent and maldescent. Ann. R. Coll. Surg. (Engl.), 35:15, 1964.

Backhouse, K. M.: Embryology of the normal and cryptorchid testis. In Fonkalsrud, E. W., and Mengel, W. (Eds.): The Undescended Testis. Chicago, Year Book Medical Publishers, 1981, p. 5.

Backhouse, K. M., and Butler H.: The gubernaculum testis of the pig (Sus scropha). J. Anat., 94:107, 1960.

Bardin, C. W., Ross, G. T., Rifkind, A. B., and Cargille, C.: Studies of the pituitary-leydig. Cell axis in young men with hypogonadotropic hypogonadism and hyposmia: comparison with normal men, prepubertal boys and hypopituitary patients. J. Clin. Invest., 48:2046–2056, 1969.

Bartsch, G., and Frick, J.: Therapeutic effects of luteinizing hormone-releasing hormone (LH-RH) in cryptorchidism. Andrologia, 6:197, 1974.

Batata, M. A., Whitmore, W. F., Jr., Chu, F. C. H., Hilaris, B., Loh, J., Grabstald, H., and Golbey, R.: Cryptochidism and testicular cancer. J. Urol., 124:382, 1980.

Baumrucker, G. O.: Incidence of testicular pathology. Bull. U. S. Army Medical Dept., 5:312, 1946.

Ben-Menachem, Y., deBarardinis, M. D. C., and Salinas, R.: Localization of intra-abdominal testes by selective testicular arteriography: a case report. J. Urol., 112:493, 1974.

Bergh, A., Helander, H. F., and Wahlquist, L.: Studies on factors governing testicular descent in the rate—particularly the role of the gubernaculum testis. Int. J. Androl., 1:342, 1978.

Bergin, W. C., Gier, H. T., Marion, G. B., and Coffman, J. R.: A developmental concept of equine cryptorchidism. Biol. Reprod., 3:82, 1970.

Bibbo, M., Al-Nageeb, M., Baccarini, L., Gill, W., Newton, M., Sleeper, K. M., Sonek, M., and Wied, G.: Follow-up study of male and female offspring of DES-treated mothers. A preliminary report. J. Reprod. Med., 15:129, 1975.

Bidlingmaier, F., Dörr, H. G., Eisenmenger, W., Kuhnie, U., and Knorr, D.: Testosterone and androstenedione concentrations in human testis and epididymis during the first two years of life. J. Clin. Endocrinol. Metab., 57:311, 1983.

Bigler, J. A., Hardy, L. M., and Scott, H. V.: Cryptorchidism treated with gonadotropic principle. Am. J. Dis. Child., 55–273, 1938.

Bishop, P. M. F.: Studies in clinical endocrinology vs. the management of the undescended testicle. Guys Hospital Rep., 94:12, 1945.

Bloom, D. A., Ayers, J. W. T., and McGuire, E. J.: The role of laparoscopy in management of nonpalpable testes. J. d'Urol., 94:465, 1988.

Brimblecomb, S. L.: Bilateral cryptorchidism in three brothers. Br. Med. J., 1:526, 1946.

Browne, D.: Treatment of undescended testicle. Proc. R. Soc. Med., 42–643, 1949.

Buemann, B., Henriksen, H., and Villumsen, A. L.: Incidence of undescended testis in the newborn. Acta Chir. Scand. (Suppl.), 238–289, 1961.

Cacciari, E., Cicognani, A., Pirazzoli, P., Zappulla, F., Tassoni, P., Bernardi, F., and Salardi, S.: Hypophysogonadal function in the cryptorchid child: differences between unilateral and bilateral cryptorchids. Acta Endocrinol., 83–182, 1976.

Campbell, H. E.: The incidence of malignant growth of the undescended testicle: a reply and re-evaluation. J. Urol., 81–563, 1959.

Chilvers, C., Pike, M. C., Forman, D., Fogelman, K., and Wadsworth, M. E. J.: Apparent doubling of frequency of undescended testis in England and Wales in 1962–1981. Lancet, 2:330, 1984.

Ch'in, K. Y.: The endocrine glands of anecephalic foetuses. Chin. Med. J., 2:63, 1938.

Clegg, E. J.: Some effects of artificial cryptochidism on the accessory reproductive organs of the rat. J. Endocrinol., 10:210, 1960.

Clements, K. A., Reyes, F. I., Winter, J. S. D., and Faiman, C.: Studies on human sexual development. III. Fetal pituitary and amniotic fluid concentration of LH, CG and FSH. J. Clin. Endocrinol. Metab., 42:9, 1976.

Cooper, B. J., and Little, T. M.: Orchiopexy theory and practice. Brt. Med. J., 291:706–707, 1985.

Cooper, E. R.: The histology of the retained testis in the human subject at different ages and its comparison with the testis. J. Anat., 64:5, 1929.

Cosgrove, M. D., Benton, B., and Henderson, B. W.: Male genitourinary abnormalities and maternal diethylstilbestrol. J. Urol., 117:220, 1977.

Cour-Palais, I. J.: Spontaneous descent of the testicle. Lancet, 1:1403, 1966.

Curling, J. B.: Observations on the structure of the gubernaculum and on the descent of the testis in the foetus. Lancet, 2:70, 1840.

Cytryn, L., Cytryn, E., and Reger, R. E.: Physchological implications of cryptorchidism. J. Am. Acad. Child Psychiatr., 6:131, 1967.

Dajani, A. M.: Transverse ectopia of the testis. Br. J. Urol., 41:80, 1969.

Davis, J. E.: Transverse aberrant testicular maldescent. U. S. Armed Forces Med. J., 8:1046, 1957.

Deming, C. L.: The gonadotropic factor as an aid to surgery in the treatment of the undescended testicle. J. Urol., 36:274, 1936.

deMuinck Keizer-Schrama, S. M. P. F., Hazebroek, F. W. J., Matroos, A. W., Drop, S. L. S., Molenaar, J. C., and Visser, H. K. A.: Double-blind, placebo-controlled study of luteinizing hormone-releasing hormone nasal spray in treatment of undescended testes. Lancet, 1:876, 1986.

Dewald, G. W., Kelalis, P. P., and Gordon, H.: Chromosomal studies in cryptorchidism. J. Urol., 117:110, 1977.

Ehrlich, R. M., Dougherty, L. M., Tomashefsky, P., and Lattimer, J. K.: Effect of gonadotropin cryptorchidism. J. Urol., 102:793, 1969.

Elder, J. S., Isaacs, J. T., and Walsh, P. C.: Androgenic sensitivity of the gubernaculum testis: evidence for hormonal/mechanical interactions in testicular descent. J. Urol., 127:170, 1982.

Engle, E. T.: Experimentally induced descent of the testis in the *Macaca* monkey by hormones from the anterior pituitary and pregnancy urine. Endocrinology, 16:513, 1932.

Farrer, J. H., Walker, A. H., and Rajfer, J.: Management of the postpubertal cryptorchid testis: a statistical review. J. Urol., 134:1071, 1985.

Farrington, G. H.: The position and retractability of the normal testis in childhood, with reference to the diagnosis and treatment of cryptorchidism. J. Pediatr. Surg., 3:53, 1968.

Felizet, G., and Branca, A.: Sur le testicule en ectopie. J. L'Anat., 38:329, 1902.

Fentener Van Vlissengen, J. M., Van Zoelen, E. J. J., Ursem, P. J. F., and Wensing, C. J. G.: In vitro model of the first phase of testicular descent: identification of a low molecular weight factor from fetal testis involved in proliferation of gubernaculum testis cells and distinct from specified polypeptide growth factors and fetal gonadal hormones. Endocrinology, 123:2868, 1988.

Firor, H. V.: Two-stage orchiopexy. Arch. Surg., 102:598, 1971.

Forest, M. G., Sizonenko, P. C., Cathard, A. M., and Bertrand, J.: Hypophysogonadal function in humans during the first year of life. J. Clin. Invest., 53:819, 1974.

Frey, H. L., Blumberg, B., and Rajfer, J.: Genetics for the urologist. *In* Goldsmith, H. S. (Ed.): Practice of Surgery, Vol. 1. New York, Harper & Row, 1981, p. 1.

Frey, H. L., and Rajfer, J.: Epididymis does not play an important role in the process of testicular descent. Surg. Forum, 23:617, 1982.

Frey, H. L., and Rajfer, J.: The role of the gubernaculum and intra-abdominal pressure in the process of testicular descent. J. Urol., 131:574, 1984.

Frey, H. L., Peng, S., and Rajfer, J.: Synergy of androgens and abdominal pressure in testicular descent. Biol. Reprod., 29:1233, 1983.

Frick, J., Danner, C., Kunit, G., Glavan, G., and Bernroider, G.: The effect of chronic administration of a synthetic LH-RH analogue intranasally in cryptorchid boys. Int. J. Androl., 3:469, 1980.

Fritzsche, P. J., Hricak, H., Kogan, B. A., Winkler, M. L., and Tanagho, E. A.: Undescended testis value of MR imaging. Radiology, 164:169, 1987.

Gendrel, D., Chaussain, J. L., Roger, M., and Job, J. C.: Simultaneous postnasal rise of plasma LH and testosterone in male infants. J. Pediatr., 97:600, 1980a.

Gendrel, D., Job, J. C., and Roger, M.: Reduced postnatal rise of testosterone in plasma of cryptorchid children. Acta Endocrinol., 89:372, 1978.

Gendrel, D., Roger, M., Chaussain, J. L., Canlorbe, P., and Job, J. C.: Correlation of pituitary and testicular responses to stimulation tests in cryptorchid children. Acta Endocrinol., 86:641, 1977.

Gendrel, D., Roger, M., and Job, J. C.: Plasma gonadotropin and testosterone values in infants with cryptorchidism. J. Pediatr., 97:217, 1980b.

George, F. W., and Peterson, K. G.: Partial characterization of the androgen receptor of the newborn rat gubernaculum. Biol. Reprod., 39:536, 1988.

Gier, H. T., and Marion, G. B.: Development of the mammalian testis. *In* Johnson, A. D., and Gomes, W. R. (Eds.): The Testis. New York, Academic Press, 1970, pp. 1–45.

Gilbert, J. B.: Studies in malignant testis tumors. V. Tumors developing after orchiopexy. J. Urol., 46:740, 1941.

Gilbert, J. B., and Hamilton, J. B.: Incidence and nature of tumors in ectopic testes. Surg. Gynecol. Obstet., 71:731, 1970.

Giwercman, A., Bruun, E., Frimodt-Moller, C., and Skakkebaek, N.: Prevalence of carcinoma in situ and other histopathological abnormalities in testes of men with a history of cryptorchidism. J. Urol., 1989.

Giwercman, A., Grinsted, J., Hansen, B., Jensen, O., and Skakkebaek, N.: Testicular cancer risk in boys with maldescended testis: a cohort study. J. Urol., 138:1214, 1987.

Goldberg, L. M., Skaist, L. B., and Morrow, J. W.: Congenital absence of testis: anorchia and monorchism. J. Urol., 111:840, 1974.

Goldman, A., Stein, L., and Lapin, J.: The treatment of undescended testes by the anterior pituitary–like principle. N. Y. State J. Med., 36:15, 1926.

Gordon-Taylor, G., and Wyndham, N. R.: On malignant tumors of the testis. Br. J. Surg., 35:6, 1947.

Grant, D. B., Laurence, B. M., Atherden, S. M., and Ryness, J.: hCG stimulation test in children with abnormal sexual development. Arch. Dis. Child., 51:596, 1976.

Grumbach, M. M., and Van Wyk, J. J.: Disorders of sex differentiation. *In* Williams, R. H. (Ed.): Textbook of Endocrinology, 4th ed. Philadelphia, W. B. Saunders Co., 1974, p. 481.

Guerrier, D. T., et al.: The persistent müllerian duct syndrome: a molecular approach. J. Clin. Endocrinol. Metab., 68:46, 1989.

Hadziselimovic, F.: Cryptorchidism: ultrastructure of cryptorchid testes development. Adv. Anat. Embryol. Cell Biol., 53:3, 1977.

Hadziselimovic, F.: Pathogenesis of cryptorchidism. Clin. Androl., 7:147, 1981.

Hadziselimovic, F.: Treatment of cryptorchidism with GnRH. Urol. Clin. North Am., 9:413, 1982.

Hadziselimovic, F.: Cryptorchidism. Management and Implications. Heidelberg, Springer-Verlag, 1983.

Hadziselimovic, F., and Seguchi, H.: Electron microscope investigations in cryptorchidism (elektronen mikroskopische untersuchungen beim kryptorchismus). Z. Kinderchir., 12:376, 1973.

Hadziselimovic, F., Snyder, H., Duckett, J., and Howards, S.: Testicular histology in children with unilateral testicular torsion. J. Urol., 136:208, 1986.

Hamilton, J. B.: The effect of male hormone upon the descent of the testes. Anat. Rec., 70:533, 1938.

Hamilton, J. B., and Hubert, G.: Effect of synthetic male hormone substance on descent of testicles in human cryptorchidism. Proc. Soc. Exp. Biol. Med., 39:4, 1938.

Hamilton, W. J., Boyd, J. D., and Mossman, J. D.: Human Embryology. Cambridge, England, W. Heffer and Sons, 1957, pp. 255–256.

Hansen, T. S.: Fertility in operatively treated and untreated cryptorchidism. Proc. R. Soc. Med., 42:645, 1949.

Happ, J., Kollmann, F., Krawehl, C., Neubauer, M., and Beyer, J.: Intranasal GnRH therapy of maldescended testes. Horm. Metab. Res., 7:440, 1975.

Happ, J., Kollmann, F., Krawehl, C., Neubauer, M., Krause, U., Demisch, K., Sandow, J., Von Rechenberg, W., and Beyer, J.: Treatment of cryptorchidism with perinasal gonadotropin-releasing hormone therapy. Fertil. Steril., 29:546, 1978a.

Happ, J., Weber, T., Callnesee, W., Ermert, J. A., Esckol, A., and Beyer, J.: Treatment of cryptorchidism with a potent analog of gonadotropin-releasing hormone. Fertil. Steril., 29:552, 1978b.

Hazebroek, F. W. J., deMuinck Keizer-Schrama, S. M. P. F., van Maarschalkerweerd, M., Visseer, H. K. A., and Molenaar, J. C.: Why luteinizing hormone-releasing-hormone nasal spray will not replace orchiopexy in the treatment of boys with undescended testes. J. Pediatr. Surg., 22:1177–1182, 1987.

Hecker, W. C., and Heinz, H. A.: Cryptorchidism and fertility. J. Pediatr. Surg., 2:513, 1967.

Holschaw, D. S., Perlmutter, A. D., Joclin, H., and Shwachman, H.: Genital abnormalities in male patients with cystic fibrosis. J. Urol., 106:568, 1971.

Huberman, J., and Israeloff, H.: The application of recent theories in the treatment of undescended testes. J. Pediatr., 7:759, 1935.

Hunt, J. B., Witherington, R., and Smith, A. D.: The midline approach to orchiopexy. Am. Surg., 47:184, 1981.

Hunter, J. A.: A description of the situation of the testis in fetus with its descent into the scrotum. *In* Observations on Certain Parts of the Animal Oeconomy. New Orleans, John J. Haswell and Co., 1841, pp. 42–50.

Hunter, P. A.: The etiology of congenital inguinal hernia and abnormally placed testes. Br. J. Surg., 14:125, 1927.

Hutson, J. M.: Testicular feminization: a model for testicular descent in mice and men. J. Pediatr. Surg., 21:195, 1986.

Illig, R., Bucher, H., and Prader, A.: Success, relapse and failure after intranasal LH-RH treatment of cryptorchidism in 55 prepuberal boys. Eur. J. Pediatr., 133:147, 1980.

Illig, R., Kollman, F., Borkenstein, M., Kuber, W., Exner, G. U., Kellerer, K., Lunglmayr, L., and Prader, A.: Treatment of cryptorchidism by intranasal synthetic luteinizing-hormone releasing hormone. Lancet, 2:518, 1977.

Imperato-McGinley, J., Binienda, Z., Gendey, J., and Vaughn, Jr., E. D.: Nipple differentiation in fetal male rats treated with an inhibitor of the enzyme 5-reductase: definition of a selective role for dihydrotestosterone. Endocrinology, 118:132, 1986.

Jarow, J. P., Berkovitz, G. D., Migeon, C. J., Gearhart, J. P., and Walsh, P. C.: Elevation of serum gonadotropins establishes the diagnosis of anorchism in prepubertal boys with belated cryptorchidism. J. Urol., 136:277, 1986.

Jirasek, J. E., Raboch, J., and Uher, J.: The relationship between the development of the gonads and external genitals in human fetuses. Am. J. Obstet. Gynecol., 101:803, 1968.

Job, J. C., Canlorbe, P., Garagorri, J. M., and Toublanc, J. E.: Hormonal therapy of cryptorchidism with human chorionic gonadotropin (hCG). Urol. Clin. North Am., 9:405, 1982.

Job, J. C., Garnier, P. E., Chaussain, J. L., Toublanc, J. E., and Canlorbe, P.: Effect of synthetic luteinizing hormone-releasing hormone on the release of gonadotropins in hypophyseal disorders of children and adolescents. IV. Undescended testes. J. Pediatr., 84:371, 1974.

Job, J. C., Gendrel, D., Safar, A., Roger, M., and Chaussain, J. L.: Pituitary LH and FSH and testosterone secretion in infants with undescended testes. Acta Endocrinol., 85:644, 1977.

Johnson, D. E., Woodhead, D. M., Pohl, D. R., and Robinson, J. R.: Cryptorchidism and testicular tumorigenesis. Surgery, 63:919, 1968.

Jones, H. W., and Scott, W. W.: Cryptorchidism. *In* Jones, H. W., and Scott, W. W. (Eds.): Hermaphroditism, Genital Anomalies and Related Endocrine Disorders, 2nd ed. Baltimore, Williams & Wilkins, 1971, p. 363.

Josso, N.: Evolution of the müllerian-inhibiting activity of the human testis. Biol. Neonate, 20:368, 1972.

Josso, N.: In vitro synthesis of müllerian-inhibiting hormone by seminiferous tubules isolated from the calf fetal testis. Endocrinology, 93:829, 1973.

Jost, A.: A new look at the mechanisms controlling sex differentiation in mammals. Johns Hopkins Med. J., 130:8, 1953a.

Jost, A.: Problems of fetal endocrinology: the gonadal and hypophyseal hormones. Rec. Prog. Horm. Res., 8:379, 1953b.

Kaplan, L. M., Koyle, M. A., Kaplan, G. W., Farrer, J. H., and Rajfer, J.: Association between abdominal wall defects and cryptorchidism. J. Urol., 136:645, 1986.

Korenchevsy, V.: The influence of cryptorchidism and of castration on body-weight, fat deposition, the sexual and endocrine organs of male rats. J. Pathol. Bacteriol., 33:607, 1931.

Landa, H. M., Gylys-Morin, V., Mattrey, R. F., Krous, H. F., Kaplan, G. W., and Packer, M. G.: Magnetic resonance imaging of the cryptorchid testis. Eur. J. Pediatr., 146 [Suppl 2]:S16, 1987.

Landing, B. H., Wells, T. R., and Wong, C. I.: Abnormality of the epididymis and vas deferens in cystic fibrosis. Arch. Pathol., 88:569, 1969.

Laurence, B. M.: Hypotonia, mental retardation, obesity, cryptorchidism associated with dwarfism and diabetes in children. Arch. Dis. Child., 42:126, 1967.

Lee, J. K., McClennan, B. L., Stanley, R. J., and Sagel, S. S.: Utility of computed tomography in the localization of the undescended testis. Radiology, 135:121, 1980.

Lemeh, C. N.: A study of the development and structural relationships of the testis and gubernaculum. Surg. Gynecol. Obstet., 110:164, 1960.

Levitt, S. B., Kogan, S. J., Engel, R. M., Weiss, R. M., Martin, D. C., and Ehrlich, R. M.: The impalpable testis: a rational approach to management. J. Urol., 120:515, 1978.

Lipschultz, L. I., Caminos-Torres, R., Greenspan, C. S., and Snyder, P. J.: Testicular function after orchiopexy for unilaterally undescended testis. N. Engl. J. Med., 195:15, 1976.

Lockwood, C. G.: Development and transition of the testis, normal and abnormal. J. Anat. Physiol., 22:505, 1888.

Ludwig, G., and Potempa, J.: Der optimale Zeipunkt der Bahandlung des Kryptorchismus. Dtsch. Med. Wochenschr., 100:680, 1975.

Mack, W. S. L.: Discussion on male fertility. Proc. R. Soc. Med., 46:840, 1953.

Mack, W. S., Scott, L. S., Ferguson-Smith, M. A., and Lennox, B.: Ectopic testis and true undescended testis: a histological comparison. J. Pathol. Bacteriol., 82:439, 1961.

Madrazo, B. L., Klugo, R. C., Parks, J. A., and DiLoreto, R.: Ultrasonographic demonstration of undescended testes. Radiology, 123:181, 1979.

Marshall, F. F.: Anomalies associated with cryptorchidism. Urol. Clin. North Am., 9:339, 1982.

Martin, D. C.: Germinal cell tumors of the testis after orchiopexy. J. Urol., 121:422, 1979.

Martin, D. C., and Menck, H. R.: The undescended testis: Management after puberty. J. Urol., 114:77, 1975.

McCutcheon, A. B.: Further observations on delayed testis. Med. J. Aust., 1:654, 1938.

McLachlan, J. A., Newbold, R. R., and Bullock, B.: Reproductive tract lesions in male mice exposed prenatally to diethylstilbestrol. Science, 90:991, 1975.

McMurrich, J. P.: The Development of the Human Body. A Manual of Human Embryology, 7th ed. Philadelphia, P. Blakiston's Son and Co., 1923, pp. 374–376.

Mengel, W., Heinz, H. A., Sippe, W. G., and Hecker, W. C. H.: Studies on cryptorchidism: A comparison of histological findings in the germinal epithelium before and after the second year of life. J. Pediatr. Surg., 9:445, 1974.

Mengel, W., Wronecki, K., and Zimmerman, F. A.: Comparison of the morphology of normal cryptorchid testes. *In* Fonkaslrud, E. W., and Mengal, W. (Eds.): The Undescended Testis. Chicago, Year Book Medical Publishers, 1981, p. 72.

Mininberg, D. T., and Bragol, N.: Chromosomal abnormalities in undescended testis. Urology, 1:98, 1973.

Moore, C. R., and Quick, W. J.: The scrotum as a temperature regulator for the testes. Am. J. Physiol., 68:70, 1924.

Mukerjee, S., and Amesur, N. R.: Transverse testicular ectopia with unilateral blood supply. Ind. J. Surg., 27:547, 1965.

Naslund, M. J., Gearhart, J. P., and Jeffs, R. D.: Laparoscopy: its selected use in patients with unilateral nonpalpable testis after human chorionic gonadotropin stimulation. J. Urol., 142:108, 1989.

Optitz, J. M., Simpson, J. L., Sarto, G. E., Summitt, R. L. New, M., and German, J.: Pseudovaginal perineoscrotal hypospadias. Clin. Genet., 3:1026, 1972.

Pace, J. M., and Cabot, M.: A histological study in 24 cases of retained testes in the adult. Surg. Gynecol. Obstet., 63:16, 1936.

Page, D. C.: Hypothesis: a Y-chromosomal gene causes gonadoblastoma in dysgenetic gonads. Development 101[Suppl]:157, 1987.

Page, D. C., Mosher, R., Simpson, E. M., Fisher, E. M. C., Mardon, G., Pollack, J., McGillivray, B., de la Chapelle A. and Brown, L. G.: The sex determining region of the human Y chromosome encodes a finger protein. Cell 51:1091–1104, 1987.

Pak, K., Sakaguchi, N., Takeuchi, H., and Tomoyoshi, T.: Computed tomography of carcinoma of the intra-abdominal testis: a case report. J. Urol., 125:253, 1981.

Payne, A. H., and Jaffe, R. B.: Androgen formation from pregnenolone sulfate by fetal neonatal adult human testes. J. Clin. Endocrinol. Metab., 40:102, 1975.

Pirazzoli, P., Zappulla, F., Bernardi, F., Villa, M. P., Aleksandrowitz, D., Scandola, A., Stancari, P., Cicognani, A., and Cacciari, E.: Luteinizing hormone-releasing hormone nasal sprays as therapy for undescended testicle. Arch. Dis. Child., 53:235, 1978.

Puri, P., and Nixon, M. H.: Bilateral retractile testes—subsequent effects on fertility. J. Pediatr. Surg., 12:563–1566, 1977.

Rajfer, J.: An endocrinological study of testicular descent in the rabbit. J. Surg. Res., 33:158, 1982.

Rajfer, J., Handelsman, D. J., Swerdloff, R. S., Hurwitz, R., Kaplan, H., Vandergast, T., and Ehrlich, R. M.: Hormonal therapy of cryptorchidism. N. Engl. J. Med., 312:466, 1986b.

Rajfer, J., Handelsman, D. J., Swerdloff, R. S., et al.: Luteinizing hormone follicle-stimulating hormone responses to intranasal gonadotropin-releasing hormone. Fert. Steril., 45:794–99, 1986a.

Rajfer, J., Tauber, A., Zinner, N., Naftulin, E., and Worthen, N.: The use of computerized tomography scanning to localize the impalpable testis. J. Urol., 129:978, 1983.

Rajfer, J., and Walsh, P. C.: Hormonal regulation of testicular descent: experimental and clinical observations. J. Urol., 118:985, 1977.

Ransley, P. G., Vordermark, J. S., Caldamone, A. A., and Bellinger, M. F.: Preliminary ligation of the gonadal vessels prior to orchiopexy for the intra-abdominal testicle: a staged Fowler-Stephens procedure. World J. Urol., 2:266, 1984.

Redman, J.: Noonan's syndrome and cryptorchidism. J. Urol., 109:909, 1973.

Rigler, H. C.: Torsion of intra-abdominal testes. Surg. Clin. North Am., 52:371, 1972.

Sadeghi-Nejad, A., and Senior, B.: A familial syndrome of isolated aplasia of the anterior pituitary. J. Pediatr., 84:79, 1974.

Santen, R. J., and Paulsen, C. A.: Hypogonadotropic eunochoidism. Gonadal responsiveness to exogenous gonadotropins. J. Clin. Endocrinol. Metab., 36:47, 1972.

Schechter, J.: An investigation of the anatomical mechanisms of testicular descent. (Thesis for Master of Arts degree.) Baltimore, Johns Hopkins University, 1963.

Scorer, C. G.: The descent of the testis. Arch. Dis. Child., 39:605, 1964. Scorer, C. G.: Early operation for the undescended testis. Br. J. Surg., 54:694, 1967.

Scorer, G., and Farrington, G. H.: Congenital Deformities of the Testis and Epididymis. New York, Appleton-Century-Crofts, 1971.

Scott, L. S.: Unilateral cryptorchidism; subsequent effects on fertility. J. Reprod. Fertil., 2:54, 1961.

Scott, L. S.: Fertility in cryptorchidism. Proc. R. Soc. Med., 55:1047, 1962.

Scully, R. E.: Gonadoblastoma. A review of 74 cases. Cancer, 25:1340, 1970.

Shwachman, H., Kowlski, M., and Khaw, K.: Cystic fibrosis: a new outlook. Medicine, 56:129, 1977.

Siiteri, P. K., and Wilson, J. D.: Testosterone formation and metabolism during male sexual differentiation in the human embryo. J. Clin. Endocrinol. Metab., 38:113, 1974.

Silber, S. J., and Cohen, R.: Laparoscopy for cryptorchidism, J. Urol., 124:928, 1980.

Sizonenko, P. C., Schindler, R. A., Roland, W., Paunier, L., and Cuendet, A.: FSH III: evidence for a possible prepubertal regulation of its secretion by the seminiferous tubules in cryptorchid boys. J. Clin. Endocrinol. Metab., 46:301, 1978.

Skakkebaek, N. E.: Possible carcinoma in situ of the testis. Lancet, 1:516, 1972.

Sohval, A. R.: Histopathology of cryptorchidism. Am. J. Med., 16:346, 1954.

Sonneland, C. G.: Undescended testicle. Surg. Gynecol. Obstet., 40:535, 1925.

Southam, A. H., and Cooper, E. R. A.: Hunterian lecture on the pathology and treatment of the retained testis in childhood. Lancet, 1:805, 1927.

Spona, J., Gleispach, H., Happ, J., et al.: Changes of serum testosterone and of LH-RH test after treatment of cryptorchidism by intranasal LH-RH. Endocrinol. Exp., 13:204, 1979.

Steiner, M. D., and Boggs, J. D.: Absence of the pituitary gland, hypothyroidism, hypoadrenalism and hypogonadism in a 17-year-old dwarf. J. Clin. Endocrinol. Metab., 25:1591, 1965.

Tayakkononta, K.: The gubernaculum testis and its nerve supply. Aust. N. Z. J. Surg., 33:61, 1963.

Toussig, L. M., Lobeck, L. C., DiSant'Aznese, P. A., Ackerman, D. R., and Kattwinkel, J.: Fertility in males with cystic fibrosis. N. Engl. J. Med., 287:586, 1972.

Van Vliet, G., Caufriez, A., Robyn, C., and Wolter, R.: Plasma gonadotropin values in prepubertal cryptorchid boys: similar increase of FSH in unilateral and bilateral cases. J. Pediatr., 97:253, 1980.

Villumsen, A. L., and Zachau-Christiansen, B.: Spontaneous alterations in position of the testis. Arch. Dis. Child., 41:198, 1966.

Vitale, P. J., Khademi, M., and Seebode, J. H.: Selective gonadal angiography for testicular localization in patients with cryptorchidism. Surg. Forum, 25:538, 1974.

Walsh, P. C., Curry, N., Mills, R. C., and Siiteri, P. K.: Plasma androgen response to hCG stimulation in prepubertal boys with hypospadias and cryptorchidism. J. Clin. Endocrinol. Metab., 42:52, 1976.

Walsh, P. C., Madden, J. D., Harrod, M. J., Goldstein, J. L., MacDonald, P. C., and Wilson, J. D.: Familial incomplete male pseudohermaphroditism, type 2. Decreased dihydrotestosterone formation in pseudovaginal perineoscrotal hypospadias. N. Engl. J. Med., 291:944, 1974.

Wangensteen, O. H.: The undescended testis. Ann. Surg., 102:875, 1935.

Ward, B., and Hunter, W. M.: The absent testicle, a report on a survey carried out among schoolboys in Nottingham. Br. Med. J., 1:2220, 1960.

Weiss, R. M., Glickman, M. G., and Lytton, B.: Clinical implications of gonadal venography in the management of the non-palpable undescended testis. J. Urol., 121:745, 1979.

Wells, L. J.: Descent of the testis. Anatomical and hormonal considerations. Surgery, 14:436, 1943.

Wells, L. J.: Descensus testiculorum: descent after severance of the gubernaculum. Anat. Rec., 88:465, 1944.

Welvaart, K., and Tijssen, J. P. G.: Management of the undescended testis in relation to the development of cancer. J. Surg. Oncol., 17:218, 1981.

White, J. J., Haller, Jr., J. A., and Dorst, J. P.: Congenital inguinal hernia and inguinal herniography. Surg. Clin. North Am., 50:823, 1970.

White, J. J., Shaker, I. J., and Oh, K. S.: Herniography: a diagnostic refinement in the management of cryptor'chidism. Ann. Surg., 39:624, 1973.

Wiles, P.: Family tree showing hereditary undescended right testis and associated deformities. Proc. R. Soc. Med., 28:157, 1934.

Winter, J. S. D., Hughes, I. A., Reyes, F. I., and Faiman, C.: Pituitary-gonadal relations in infancy: 2. Patterns of serum gonadal steroidal concentrations in man from birth to two years of age. J. Clin. Endocrinol. Metab., 42:679, 1976.

Winter, J. S. D., Teraska, S., and Faiman, C.: The hormonal response to hCG stimulation in male children and adolescents. J. Clin. Endocrinol. Metab., 34:348, 1972.

Wislocki, G. B.: Observation on the descent of the testes in the macaque and in the chimpanzee. Anat. Rec., 57:133, 1933.

Witschi, E.: Migration of the germ cells of human embryos from the yolk sac to the primitive gonadal folds. Contrib. Embryol. Carnegie Inst., 32:67, 1948.

Wollach, Y., Shaher, E., Schachter, A., and Dintsman, M.: Fertility and sexual development after bilateral orchiopexy for cryptorchidism. Isr. J. Med. Sci., 16:707, 1980.

Wolverson, M. K., Jagannadharao, B., Sundaram, M., Riaz, M. A., Nalesnik, W. J., and Houttiun, E.: CT localization of impalpable cryptorchid testes. Am. J. Roentgenol., 134:725, 1980.

Woodhead, D. M., Pohl, D. R., and Johnson, D. E.: Fertility of patients with solitary testes. J. Urol., 100:66, 1973.

Wylie, G. C.: The retractile testis. Med. J. Aust., 140:403–405, 1984.

Wyndham, N. R.: A morphological study of testicular descent. J. Anat., 77:179, 1943.

Zabransky, S.: LH-RH-Nasal spray (Kryptocur), ein neur Aspekt in der hormonellen Behandlung des Hodenhoch-Standes. Klin. Paediatr., 193:382, 1981.

Zarzycki, J., Szroeder, J., and Michaelowski, W. L.: Ultrastructure of seminiferous tubule cells and interstitial cells in cryptorchid human testicles. Acta Med. Pol., 18:38, 1977.

Inguinal Hernia in Infancy and Childhood

Griffin, J. E., and Wilson, J. D.: The syndromes of androgen resistance. N. Engl. J. Med., 302:198, 1980.

Gunnlaugsson, G. H., Dawson, B., and Lynn, H. B.: Treatment of inguinal hernia in infants and children: Experience with contralateral exploration. Mayo Clin. Proc., 42:129, 1967.

Hamrick, L. C., and Williams, J. O.: Is contralateral exploration indicated in children with unilateral inguinal herniae? Am. J. Surg., 104:52, 1962.

Infant Hydrocele

McKay, D. G., Fowler, R., and Barnett, J. S.: The pathogenesis and treatment of primary hydroceles in infancy and childhood. Aust. N. Z. Surg., 28:2, 1958.

Ozdilek, S.: The pathogenesis of idiopathic hydrocele and a simple operative technique. J. Urol., 77:282, 1957.

Rinker, J. R., and Allen, L.: Lymphatic defect in hydrocele. Am. Surg., 17:681, 1951.

Scorer, G. C., and Farrington, G. H.: Congenital anomalies of the testis. In Harrison, J. H., Gittes, R., Perlmutter, A., Stamey, T. A., and Walsh, P. C. (Eds.): Campbell's Urology, vol. 2. Philadelphia, W. B. Saunders Co., 1977, p. 1564.

Testicular Torsion

Backhouse, K. M.: Embryology of testicular descent and maldescent. Urol. Clin. North Am., 9:315, 1982.

Barada, J. H., Weingarten, J. L., and Cromie, W. J.: Testicular salvage and age-related delay in the presentation of testicular torsion. J. Urol., 142:746, 1989.

Bartsch, G., Frank, S., Marberger, H., and Mikuz, G.: Testicular torsion: late results with special regard to fertility and endocrine function. J. Urol., 124:375, 1980.

Burton, J. A.: Atrophy following testicular torsion. Br. J. Surg., 59:422, 1972.

Chapman, R. H., and Walton, A. J.: Torsion of the testis and its appendages. Br. Med. J., 1:164, 1972.

Datta, N. S., and Mishkin, F.: Radionuclide imaging and intrascrotal lesions. JAMA, 231:1060, 1975.

Dresner, M.: Torsed appendage: blue dot sign. Urology, 1:63, 1973.

Holder, L. E., Martine, J. R., Holmes, E. R., and Wagner, H. N.: Testicular radionuclide angiography and static imaging: Anatomy, scinitigraphic interpretation, and clinical indications. Radiology, 125:739, 1977.

Korbel, E. I.: Torsion of the testis. J. Urol., 111:521, 1974.

Krarup, T.: The testes after torsion. Br. J. Urol., 50:43, 1978.

Levy, B. J.: The diagnosis of torsion of the testicle using the Doppler ultrasonic stethoscope. J. Urol., 113:63, 1975.

Macnicol, M. F.: Torsion of the testis in childhood. Br. J. Surg., 61:905, 1974.

Marshall, J. C., and Tanner, J. M.: Variations in pattern of pubertal changes in boys. Arch. Dis. Child., 45:13, 1980.

Rigler, H. C.: Torsion of intra-abdominal testes. Surg. Clin. North Am., 52:371, 1972.

Scorer, C. G., and Farrington, G. H.: Congenital Deformities of the Testis and Epididymis. London, Butterworth and Co., 1971.

Sparks, J. P.: Torsion of the testis in adolescents and young adults. Clin. Pediatr., 11:484, 1972.

Thompson, I. M., Latourette, H., Chadwick, S., Ross, G., and Lichti, E.: Diagnosis of testicular torsion using Doppler ultrasonic flowmeter. Urology, 6:706, 1975.

39

PRENATAL AND POSTNATAL DIAGNOSIS AND MANAGEMENT OF CONGENITAL ABNORMALITIES

James Mandell, M.D.
Craig A. Peters, M.D.
Alan B. Retik, M.D.

DETECTION OF CONGENITAL UROPATHIES

The indications for evaluation of possible congenital urologic abnormalities in utero remain at this time purely speculative. Maternal fetal sonography is performed in certain areas as a routine examination during pregnancy, or in some countries, it is incorporated into the standard health care practice system as a mandatory procedure. In this and many other countries, however, the clinical application of maternal/fetal ultrasound as part of routine gestational care is dependent on such divergent factors as the type of the available third-party payment plan, the presence of in-office or nearby center-based ultrasound technology, and the availability of health care providers familiar with the usage of this technology. Given this lack of consensus for routine screening, the question arises as to whether specific indications exist for genitourinary evaluation in utero.

Divergence from the expected fundal height for age is one indication for further evaluation. A reduction in the normal amount of amniotic fluid may be due to renal agenesis, dysgenesis, or severe obstructive uropathy. The finding of a persistent breech presentation may also be associated with oligohydramnios and warrants further examination (Neal and Andrassy, 1984). Conversely, the presence of an increased amount of amniotic fluid (polyhydramnios) has also been reported to be associated with unilateral hydronephrosis and is re-flected as an elevated height of the fundus compared with height of the fundus for known gestational age (Broecker et al., 1988; Ray et al., 1982; Seeds and Bowes, 1986). In rare instances, maternal renal failure may occur in this setting (Seeds et al., 1984; Skovbo and Smith-Jensen, 1981). Maternal serum alpha-fetoprotein (AFP) has become a common screening test during pregnancy. Abnormally elevated AFP levels in mid-trimester are most commonly associated with neural tube defects, fetal death, or multiple fetuses. Elevated levels of AFP have also been reported with genitourinary anomalies (Gardner et al., 1981; Koontz et al., 1983).

A history of urinary developmental abnormalities in a sibling or other family member represents another indication for maternal fetal ultrasonography. The degree of risk involved is fairly small; however, we have seen patients for whom a history of fetuses with bladder outlet obstruction has been associated with a similar anatomic defect in subsequent pregnancies. However, the most common source of referral in diagnosing genitourinary defects is the routine gestational examination. In a large series of patients, the majority of patients were seen in a referral center following an abnormality detected on a screening evaluation in the primary obstetric office (Mandell et al., 1991a).

To appreciate the potential of ultrasound examination, one needs to understand the principles of ultrasound technology. The ultrasound transducer generates a series of high-pressure zones emanating concentrically from the source. Sound passes through the soft tissues, and at interfaces of dissimilar tissues a portion of the sound beam is reflected as an echo. Those echoes that come from a surface perpendicular to the axis of the sound beam are reflected back at the transducer. Given the physical properties of the speed of the sound wave and the time generation, a composite image of the soft tissue anatomy is constructed (Seeds and Bowes, 1986).

The echo contrast between inhomogeneous tissues, such as solid and fluid surfaces, provides most of the visibility for diagnosing congenital malformations. An ideal context for this would be the dilated fluid-filled collecting system of the fetal genitourinary tract as seen by the ultrasound observer. The presence or absence of amniotic fluid surrounding the fetus is also an ideal contrast for this technology.

The fetal genitourinary system can be observed at several different stages of development with reasonable clarity. The fetal kidney itself is reliably detected after about 15 weeks of gestation (Lawson et al., 1981). The images are not very clear, however, until about 20 weeks, at which time the internal renal architecture appears distinct. This change is presumably due to the deposition of fat in the perirenal space (Bowie et al., 1983). Renal growth can be measured from that time on, and standards have been published for normal values according to gestational age (Jeanty et al., 1982).

In general, normal renal architecture is very comparable to that of the newborn, with the presence of sonolucent pyramids and a relatively distinct cortico-medullary junction. The calyces and collecting system are rarely seen in detail in the absence of minimal degrees of fullness. It is not unusual, however, to see what has previously been termed mild or transitory hydronephrosis in the late first and early second trimester (Mandell et al., 1991a). The fetal bladder may also be detected about the same time as the kidney and can be seen to empty and fill over time. If, over time, the bladder is not seen, an abnormality must be suspected (Hobbins et al., 1984). Bladder volume rarely exceeds 4 to 5 ml, and the typical fetus appears to void on an hourly cycle (Wladimiroff and Campbell, 1974).

After 16 weeks, amniotic fluid volume reflects mainly contributions from fetal urine. Therefore, evaluation of amniotic fluid is part of the routine evaluation of the genitourinary system. The relationship between amniotic fluid and fetal mass does change during gestation with a relative decrease in this ratio after 23 weeks (Quennan et al., 1972). Polyhydramnios has been defined as an amniotic fluid volume greater than 2000 ml, although the definition obviously depends on the observer's qualitative measurement. Oligohydramnios, when severe, usually reflects the absence of any single area of fluid measuring 2 cm in greatest dimension on ultrasound (Manning et al., 1981).

Prenatal ultrasound is extremely operator dependent and, despite the improved technical aspects of this modality, the reliability of examinations may differ considerably among the operators involved. The level of sophistication in technology at referring centers makes it mandatory that any fetus with a previously suspected urinary tract abnormality undergo a further examination at what is termed a "level two" center. We have found that, although a majority of cases referred for a more thorough evaluation will have some abnormality, the specific anatomy and degree of involvement vary greatly; both overestimation and underestimation of the importance of abnormalities have occurred. In general, prenatal ultrasound is an extremely sensitive tool for determining the presence of an abnormality, but deciding on the overall implications of these findings requires a great deal of experience.

Other diagnostic modalities available for the overall evaluation of the fetus are chorionic villous sampling and percutaneous umbilical blood sampling (PUBS). These procedures have become relatively standard aspects of prenatal diagnosis and management. Chorionic villous sampling has the advantage of allowing detection of chromosomal abnormalities at 8 to 10 weeks of gestation, permitting early diagnosis of genetic diseases. PUBS has become a safe and standard method for fetal diagnosis and allows assessment as early as 14 to 16 weeks of gestation. In addition, PUBS allows direct access to the bloodstream of the fetus, thereby providing a mode of therapy. New, experimental techniques are continuing to evolve, which will allow the assessment and care of the fetus to be expanded. These techniques include direct in utero tissue biopsy, amnioinfusion, and in utero cardiac catheterization and valvuloplasty.

DIAGNOSTIC CATEGORIES

The spectrum of structural genitourinary defects detected in utero represents a large portion of those congenital anomalies that may or may not be detectable on neonatal examination. Because of the large number of upper urinary tract anomalies that are not detectable on routine neonatal examination, the importance of the prenatal findings has become increasingly apparent.

In a large series of patients with genitourinary defects detected in utero, the majority (87 per cent) had hydronephrosis (Table 39–1). The remainder of the anomalies included multicystic dysplastic kidney, autosomal reces-

Table 39–1. PRENATAL DIAGNOSIS OF HYDRONEPHROSIS

	Number	%
Hydronephrosis	154	87
Bilateral hydronephrosis	73	41
Unilateral hydronephrosis	61	34
Bladder outlet obstruction with oligohydramnios	9	5
Duplex/hydronephrosis	9	5
Prune-belly syndrome	2	1
Multicystic dysplastic kidney	10	6
Autosomal recessive polycystic kidney disease	5	3
Potter's syndrome	4	2
Renal agenesis	2	1
Hypodysplasia	1	1
Echogenic kidney	1	1
Total number of patients	177	

Adapted from Mandell, J., Blyth, B., Peters, C. A., Retik, A. B., Estroff, J. A., and Benacerraf, B. R.: The natural history of structural genitourinary defects detected in utero. Radiology, 178:194, 1991.

sive polycystic kidney disease, renal agenesis, and hypodysplasia (Mandell et al., 1991a). Other abnormalities that have been described include bladder exstrophy, adrenal hyperplasia, imperforate anus, cloacal abnormalities, neuroblastoma, mesoblastic nephroma, and genital abnormalities. These abnormalities will be discussed in further detail.

With hydronephrosis, the simple finding of dilatation of the urinary collecting system does not, in itself, imply obstructive uropathy or a significant functional abnormality. When characterizing hydronephrosis detected in the prenatal period, one must assess several important findings. A description of the degree of dilatation either by subjective severity (mild, moderate, or severe) or by accurate measurements of anteroposterior diameter of the pelvis is critical. This parameter must be correlated with the age of gestation at diagnosis, because it has been shown to vary during gestation.

Studies evaluating the threshold of fetal hydronephrosis associated with significant postnatal problems have been reported (Arger et al., 1985; Grignon et al., 1986; Gruenwald et al., 1984; Kleiner et al., 1987). In most cases, postnatal renal abnormalities of significance are observed in those fetuses with renal pelvic diameters greater than 10 mm. However, earlier in pregnancy, pelvic diameters as low as 5 to 8 mm may imply functional significance postnatally (Mandell et al., 1991a).

One must also determine whether the hydronephrosis is unilateral or bilateral, and if it is bilateral, whether it is symmetric. The absence or presence of ureteral dilatation must be noted. The size of the fetal bladder, its emptying, and the presence or absence of posterior urethral dilatation should also be noted. Special attention should be given to the presence or absence of any type of cystic changes or hyperechogenicity in the renal parenchyma. Determination of the presence and absence as well as relative volume of amniotic fluid should be noted, not only in general, but specifically in relation to the presence of hydronephrosis. This observation also applies to the presence or absence of other anatomic abnormalities, the overall growth and development of the fetus, and its gender (Table 39–2).

Table 39–2. EVALUATION OF PRENATAL HYDRONEPHROSIS

Renal parenchyma: thickness, echogenicity, cystic changes
Degree of upper urinary tract dilatation
Unilateral or bilateral
Ureteral dilatation
Variation in degree of hydronephrosis during or between
    examinations
Bladder: size, thickness, emptying
Posterior urethral dilatation
Amniotic fluid volume
Extrarenal fluid collections
Other anatomic abnormalities
Gender
Overall growth and development

Adapted from Mandell, J., Peters, C. A., and Retik, A. B.: Current concepts in the perinatal diagnosis and management of hydronephrosis. Urol. Clin. North Am. 17(2):249, 1990.

The most common finding of hydronephrosis on fetal ultrasound examination is dilatation of the pelvis of the kidney. This finding is often seen on both sides with some degree of asymmetry. As was mentioned, the degree of fetal renal pelvic diameter varies throughout gestation, and the diagnosis of hydronephrosis in these situations is often arbitrary. Therefore, if one discusses "significant" hydronephrosis, the most common cause is ureteropelvic junction obstruction (Fig. 39–1), and it is represented by those fetuses at greater than 20 weeks of gestation with renal pelvic diameters of more than 8 mm. The presence of caliectasis, however, increases the importance of the finding of hydronephrosis and should be considered significant even with smaller degrees of pelvic diameter.

In the classic findings of ureteropelvic junction obstruction, the renal parenchyma appears normal in texture but may be thinned. One can see, however, varying degrees of cystic dysplasia in the most severe cases. The ureters should not be seen during the ultrasound examination, and the bladder should fill and empty with regularity. On repeated fetal examinations, the degree of dilatation most often remains fairly constant; however, at times, there is significant worsening of the findings. In cases involving pelvic dilatation of less than 8 to 10 mm after 20 weeks of gestation, the minimal pelviectasis often regresses (Hoddick et al., 1985; Mandell et al., 1991a).

The presence of ureteral dilatation in association with pelvic dilatation is the next most frequent abnormality seen with hydronephrosis. This dilatation is most often unilateral and also presents with a range of severity. A dilated ureter is more difficult to see ultrasonographically, but it may be visible just at the ureterovesical or ureteropelvic junction. In the presence of a normal bladder, this finding most often represents either mild-to-moderate reflux or ureterovesical junction obstruction. The distinction between these conditions is difficult. In the presence of a dilated bladder, however, the differential diagnosis includes either massive reflux with a so-called megacystis-megaureter syndrome or bladder outlet obstruction secondary to posterior urethral valves. In our experience, in the presence of a very dilated, apparently thin-walled bladder, significant hydroureteronephrosis, normal renal parenchymal architecture, and normal amounts of amniotic fluid, the most likely diagnosis is massive reflux (Fig. 39–2).

The diagnosis of posterior urethral valves can be made with relative assurance with findings of early onset bilateral hydroureteronephrosis; a thick-walled, slightly dilated bladder; incomplete bladder emptying; the suggestion of a dilated posterior urethra; and a male sex identification (Fig. 39–3). Oftentimes, if this condition presents early in gestation, significant hyperechogenicity or cystic changes will be present in the renal parenchyma. In addition, varying degrees of oligohydramnios may be present depending on the severity of the obstructed lesions. The outcome of such lesions is fairly dismal, and in a review of prenatally diagnosed cases, only two out of nine fetuses with these findings were ultimately viable (Mandell et al., 1991a). This outcome is similar to those previously reported (Nakayma et al.,

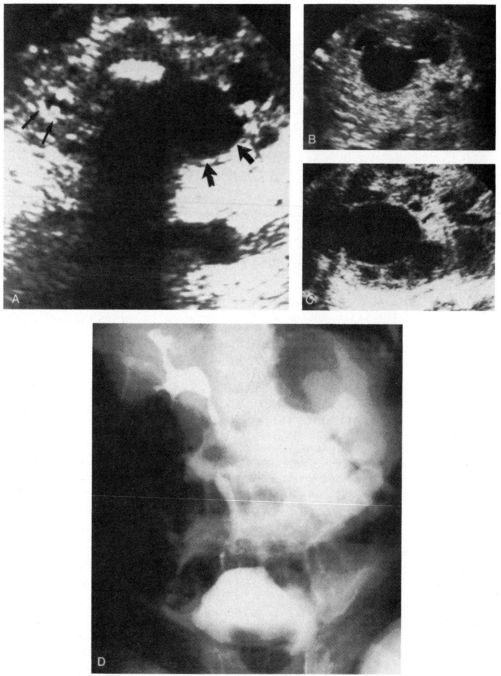

Figure 39–1. Prenatal diagnosis of ureteropelvic junction obstruction. *A,* Ultrasound scan at 29 weeks of gestation, axial view, shows left hydronephrosis and a large dilated pelvis due to ureteropelvic junction obstruction *(large arrows).* Right kidney is normal *(small arrows).* Vertebral body in midline casts an echo shadow. *B,* Left kidney at 31 weeks of gestation; ureteropelvic junction obstruction with dilated pelvis and calyces. *C,* Three weeks later, increased pelvic and calyceal dilatation. Renal cortex has not been significantly atrophied. *D,* Intravenous urogram, 5 weeks after birth, showing mild right dilatation and significant obstruction at the left ureteropelvic junction. The pelvic and calyceal dilatation is comparable to that seen on the prenatal ultrasound *(C).* (From Mandell, J., Peters, C. A., and Retik, A. B.: Current concepts in the perinatal diagnosis and management of hydronephrosis. Urol. Clin. North Am., 17(2):250, 1990.)

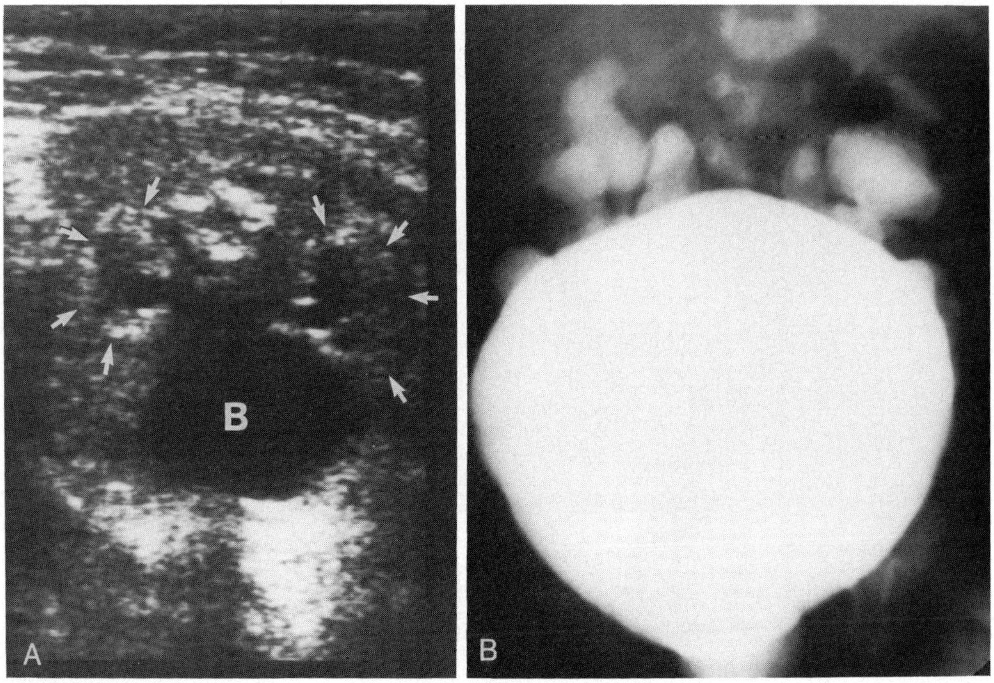

Figure 39–2. Prenatal diagnosis of massive reflux with megacystis-megaureter syndrome. *A,* Ultrasound scan at 34 weeks of gestation, axial view, showing large, thin-walled bladder (B) and bilateral hydroureteronephrosis *(arrows around kidneys). B,* Voiding cystourethrogram at 1 day of age shows large-capacity, smooth-walled bladder and reflux into dilated, tortuous collecting systems.

1986) and will be discussed later in relation to its significance for therapy.

Duplication anomalies of the upper tract should be suspected in the presence of hydroureteronephrosis and either an asymmetrically nondilated portion of the kidney or ureterocele (Fig. 39–4). In most cases, however, the ultrasound findings are nonspecific, and the diagnosis of duplication anomalies is determined postnatally after the prenatal finding of hydronephrosis (Winters and Lebowitz, 1990).

Prune-belly syndrome which presents with renal and collecting system abnormalities, undescended testicles, and deficient abdominal wall musculature, is most often

seen in utero as bilateral hydroureteronephrosis and a large bladder. In the absence of urethral atresia or obstruction, amniotic fluid is normal. One of the difficulties with prune-belly syndrome is that it can mimic posterior urethral valves, and in previous reports, fetuses with prune-belly syndrome have had prenatal intervention (Golbus et al., 1982; Manning et al., 1986). The majority of patients with prune-belly syndrome do not have bladder outlet obstruction; therefore, this constitutes a diagnostic dilemma. Clues to the presence of prune-belly syndrome include significant ureteral dilatation out of proportion to the renal pelvic dilatation, and, in one instance, the diagnosis has been made

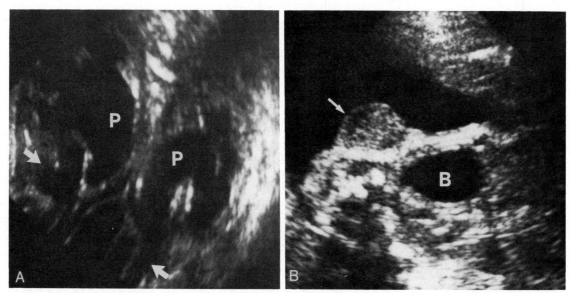

Figure 39–3. Prenatal diagnosis of posterior urethral valves. *A,* Ultrasound examination at 37 weeks of gestation showing marked bilateral hydroureteronephrosis (P, renal pelvis) with tortuous ureters *(arrows). B,* View of fetal pelvis with distended, thick-walled bladder (B) and testes in scrotum *(arrow).* Note ample amniotic fluid.

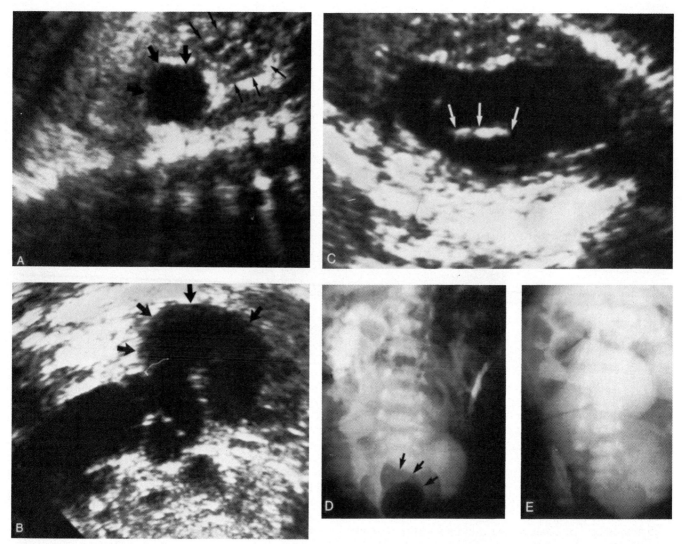

Figure 39–4. Prenatal diagnosis of duplex system with ureterocele. *A,* Ultrasound examination at 36 weeks of gestation demonstrating a dilated upper pole segment of the left kidney *(large arrows).* The normal lower pole is indicated by the smaller arrows. *B,* Earlier ultrasound at 29 weeks of gestation showing the dilated and tortuous ureter draining the hydronephrotic left upper pole, which ends in a ureterocele. *C,* Prenatal ultrasound examination of the bladder showing the ureterocele within the bladder *(arrows). D,* Postnatal intravenous urogram at age 1 week with early films showing right hydronephrosis due to obstruction by the contralateral ureterocele, and a nonobstructed but laterally displaced left lower pole. *E,* Delayed films demonstrating the massively dilated upper pole segment from the left with contrast medium entering due to reflux. (From Mandell, J., Peters, C. A., and Retik, A. B.: Current concepts in the perinatal diagnosis and management of hydronephrosis. Urol. Clin. North Am., 17(2):252–253, 1990.)

prenatally by detection of a megalourethra (Fig. 39–5) (Benacerraf et al., 1989).

Hydronephrosis is known to be part of many different anomaly complexes. The presence of significant pyelectasis should alert the examiner to specifically screen for chromosomal anomalies (Benacerraf et al., 1990).

Renal cystic dysplasias are readily seen by ultrasound examination of the fetus. A multicystic dysplastic kidney is characterized by multiple cysts of various sizes and shapes with no evidence of communication with a collecting system (Fig. 39–6). The spectrum of multicystic dysplasia, however, runs from the most overt cases to the smaller hypodysplastic kidneys, which are more difficult to distinguish.

In three of our patients, the previous presence of ureteropelvic junction obstruction and the occurrence of a perinephric urinoma led to the ultimate finding of a nonfunctioning, small, dysplastic kidney postnatally (Fig. 39–7) (Benacerraf et al., 1991). We have also seen severely dysplastic kidneys associated with ureteropelvic junction obstruction. Autosomal recessive polycystic disease has been noted prenatally as large, echogenic kidneys often associated with oligohydramnios. We and others (Mahoney et al., 1984) have noted that the prenatal course of this disease ranges from some fetuses with severe involvement during the first trimester to others in whom normal-sized, questionably hyperechogenic kidneys were seen initially, which then progressed during the second trimester to enlarge and become obviously very bright on ultrasound with the delayed onset of oligohydramnios (Fig. 39–8). This situation has occurred even when a previous history of autosomal recessive polycystic kidney disease prompted us to carefully look for early changes.

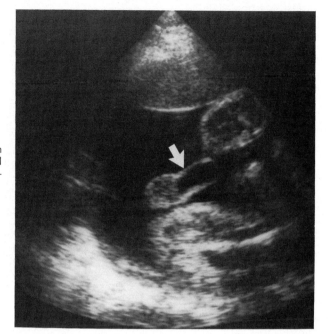

Figure 39–5. Prenatal diagnosis of megalourethra. Ultrasound examination at 33 weeks of gestation showing fluid-filled penile urethra *(arrow)*, normal scrotum, and normal amniotic fluid. The patient had some features of prune-belly syndrome.

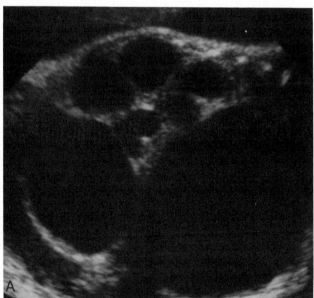

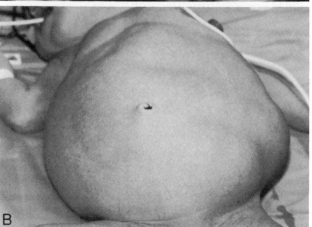

Figure 39–6. Prenatal diagnosis of multicystic dysplastic kidney. *A,* Ultrasound examination at 38 weeks of gestation showing huge multcystic kidney filling entire cross section of the fetal abdominal cavity. *B,* Picture of neonate with grossly distended abdomen and renal mass visible through the anterior abdominal wall. Infant had moderate respiratory distress from compression of the diaphragm.

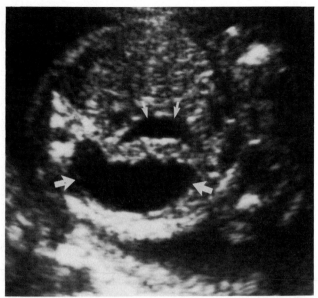

Figure 39–7. Prenatal diagnosis of perinephric urinoma. Ultrasound examination at 30 weeks of gestation with mildly hydronephrotic renal pelvis *(small arrows)* and large perinephric urinoma *(large arrows)*. The kidney did not function postnatally.

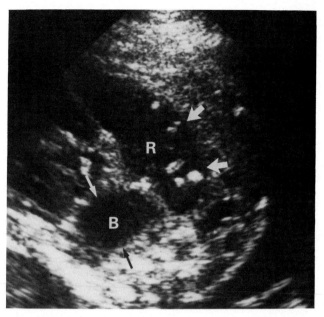

Figure 39–9. Prenatal diagnosis of imperforate anus with rectourinary fistula. Ultrasound examination at 36 weeks of gestation showing dilated rectum (R) *(large arrows)* with intraluminal calcifications posterior to full bladder (B) *(small arrows)*. (From Mandell, J., Lillehei, C. W., Greene, M., and Benacerraf, B.: Prenatal diagnosis of imperforate anus with rectourinary fistula: Dilated fetal colon with enterolithiasis. J. Pediatr. Surg. In press.)

Anomalies in the exstrophy/cloaca/imperforate anus complex have been diagnosed prenatally. Intraluminal intestinal calcifications seen in utero should immediately suggest the presence of an anorectal malformation (Fig. 39–9) (Harris et al., 1987; Mandell et al., 1991b; Shalev et al., 1983).

Genital anomalies have also been diagnosed prenatally, usually in the last trimester of gestation. Cases of prenatal sonographic findings of hydroceles (Thomas et al., 1985), chordee (Benacerraf et al., 1991), and

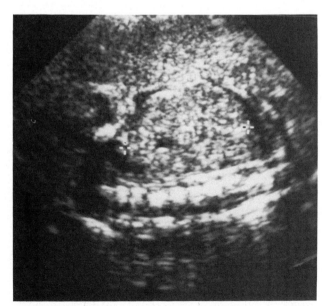

Figure 39–8. Prenatal diagnosis of autosomal recessive polycystic kidney disease. Ultrasound examination at 25 weeks of gestation showing enlarged (37.6 mm), echogenic kidney. Normal kidney length is 30 to 32 mm. Amniotic fluid was diminished.

ambiguous genitalia (Cooper et al., 1985) have been reported.

Another condition that warrants mention is congenital adrenal hyperplasia, which is an important issue in the management of those fetuses who have the potential for inheriting the masculinizing, salt-losing types of endocrinopathy. Diagnosis of this disorder is not readily made with ultrasound, but it has been diagnosed by HLA typing, allowing fetal endocrine manipulation or therapeutic termination as potential options (Pang et al., 1990).

Neuroblastoma has been diagnosed prenatally (Guilian et al., 1986; Janetschek et al., 1984). A variant of neuroblastoma termed cystic neuroblastoma has also been noted prenatally with postnatal confirmation (Peters et al., 1989a). Other tumors that have been noted prenatally include teratoma (Teal et al., 1988) and mesoblastic nephroma (Guilian, 1984).

NATURAL HISTORY

Although there is a great deal of information yet to be gained about the natural history of genitourinary defects diagnosed in utero, much has been learned in recent years. Based on routine ultrasound screening programs, the overall incidence of genitourinary defects appears to be between 0.2 and 0.9 per cent (Helin and Persson, 1981; Scott and Renwick, 1987). In general, genitourinary anomalies represent about 50 per cent of all sonographically detectable lesions. Hydronephrosis accounts for about two thirds of the genitourinary lesions seen. As previously discussed, the significance of these findings has been somewhat difficult to determine retrospectively. In cases of hydronephrosis, pelvicalyceal dilatation at specific gestational ages seems to be the single most reliable factor in predicting ultimate outcome.

Not only are more infants being diagnosed with genitourinary defects because of ultrasound screening, but the overall incidence of various abnormalities seen postnatally has changed. In one review, ureteropelvic junction obstruction was the most common entity; however, distal ureteral obstruction and vesicoureteral reflux replaced posterior urethral valves and ureteral ectopia as the next leading causes of hydronephrosis detected in the perinatal period (Brown et al., 1987).

The rate of occurrence of these lesions is related in great part to the accuracy of in utero diagnosis. Several studies have reviewed this topic and the relationship between pre- and postnatal diagnosis (Avni et al., 1985; Blane et al., 1983; Bruno et al., 1985; Sholder et al., 1988). The error rate expressed as false-positive diagnoses has ranged between 9 and 22 per cent (Reznik et al., 1988; Scott and Renwick, 1987). This overestimation may be due, in part, to the lack of criteria for the diagnosis of hydronephrosis. Other reasons include transient vesicoureteral reflux or prolapsing ureterocele in the female. The degree of dilatation does not appear to be related to maternal-fetal hydration (Allen et al., 1987; Hoddick et al., 1985).

The postnatal outcome for identified fetal genitourinary anomalies is difficult to assess. In several surveys, survival rates and postnatal treatment frequency are variable. One explanation for this variability is that perinatal mortality rates vary from center to center, depending on the population mix and the level of medical sophistication. In one series with a 72 per cent perinatal mortality, urethral atresia and renal dysplasia were present in a majority of the fetuses examined (Reuss et al., 1988). Another series identified 69 infants, 29 of whom died in the perinatal period. Of those that survived, half had bilateral obstruction with a postnatal surgical rate of 90 per cent (Reznik et al., 1988). In another series of 162 prenatally identified cases, 32 deaths occurred, and a surgical procedure was performed in 75 per cent of the remaining patients (Scott and Renwick, 1987). Other reports have shown much lower mortality and surgical rates (Arnold and Rickwood, 1990; Sanders and Graham, 1982; Thon et al., 1987). The pre- and postnatal bias of the physicians and centers involved plays an important role in the variation seen in these figures.

The outcome of these lesions is, of course, related to the occurrence of nonrenal congenital anomalies. This association is much higher in those infants who ultimately die in the perinatal period. One report shows 52 per cent with nonrenal anomalies who died versus 17 per cent without other abnormalities present (Reuss et al., 1988). The strongest negative indicators of overall prognosis include early onset of severe renal parenchymal changes, oligohydramnios, severe nonrenal congenital anomalies, and bladder outlet obstruction. The majority of cases of hydronephrosis, even with bilateral involvement, fall within a moderate degree of obstruc-tion and are not associated with these severe parameters. The overall prognosis for patients with other types of bilateral renal disease, whether it be hypoplasia, dysplasia, or cystic disease, is similarly linked to the presence of oligohydramnios.

PRENATAL INTERVENTION

The natural consequence of the evolution in prenatal diagnosis in terms of sophistication and usage has led to the issue of intervention before birth to reverse potentially life-threatening processes. One must be aware that the concept of prenatal intervention itself is not new. Both medical and surgical therapies have been used with varying degrees of success in the treatment of the fetus. Examples of medical treatment, which necessarily involve exposing the mother to the risks of therapy, include exogenous thyroid hormone supplementation for hypothyroidism (Redding et al., 1972), corticosteroid supplementation for affected females with congenital adrenal hyperplasia to diminish in utero virilization (Pang et al., 1990), and corticosteroid administration to improve fetal lung maturity (Depp et al., 1980).

The concept of an interventional approach requiring actual physical transgression of the mother and the fetus is also not new. In 1963, Liley reported the first intra-uterine fetal transfusion for severe erythroblastosis. The technical aspects of this approach involved the use of fluoroscopy with about a 50 per cent accuracy of delivery. Since that time, with further modifications of technique, including ultrasound guidance and direct fetal umbilical vessel cannulation, the accuracy of this therapy has improved dramatically with reduction of risk to the mother and fetus (Seeds and Bowes, 1986). Open hysterotomy was also advocated for exchange transfusion in the 1960s (Ascensio et al., 1966; Freda and Adamsons, 1964), but, over time, the percutaneous approach has proven more beneficial in terms of both risk and benefit.

Some types of direct intervention have already fallen into disfavor, and others are in their infancy. Fetal ventricular shunting for hydrocephalus (Glick et al., 1984b) has had no proven benefit over time with multiple applications. The application of open intrauterine surgery for congenital diaphragmatic hernia has emerged into both the scientific and the lay press (Harrison et al., 1990). It is unclear whether this procedure will prove to be of benefit in the long run, despite the quite remarkable technical aspects of this approach.

The interest in intervention for congenital hydrone-phrosis began in the early 1980s. The San Francisco Fetal Treatment Program reported the percutaneous placement of a vesicoamniotic shunt in one of twins at 32 weeks of gestation (Golbus et al., 1982). This fetus was later delivered and found to have prune-belly syndrome. The report stated that the child did well with subsequent postnatal therapy. Additionally, the same group reported on the use of open hysterotomy for fetal urinary diversion in a 20-week-old fetus with obstructive uropathy. The pregnancy was able to be continued to 35 weeks; however, the infant had pulmonary hypoplasia and did not survive (Harrison et al., 1981). As a result of the recognized feasibility of this approach, a large number of interventions were carried out in the next several years. Vesicoamniotic shunting was performed for apparent bladder outlet obstruction with and without oligohydramnios. Many cases of intervention involved unilateral obstructive disease (Kirkinen et al., 1982; Newnham et al., 1987; Vintzileos et al., 1983).

The interventions performed for unilateral obstructive disease, in retrospect, had no justification except for those rare cases of maternal impairment. The approach to suspected bladder outlet obstruction also varied in terms of usage criteria and applicability. An international fetal registry was established in 1982 and, in 1986, published its first survey of contributing specialists involved in intervention for genitourinary disorders (Manning et al., 1986). These data have been analyzed and reviewed by many groups.

In the initial publication, the perinatal mortality rate was 52 per cent. The overall incidence of complications was 43 per cent. Ninety-two per cent of the patients required between two and seven separate attempts at catheter placement. The difficulty of evaluating the efficacy of this series was enhanced by the fact that there was no overall protocol or specifications for the diagnosis, time of gestation, or the procedure itself; 14 of 20 contributing institutions reported only one case. More importantly, 45 per cent of the reported cases had hydronephrosis of unknown origin.

The number of interventions reported has dropped dramatically. The review by Manning (1990) reveals that 87 cases have been registered as of June, 1987. In comparison, the initial series of 73 cases was collected between 1982 and 1985 (Manning et al., 1986). An issue that remains to be determined is the postnatal follow-up, which often is ambiguous and incomplete. Another continuing problem is that the diagnosis of prune-belly syndrome is frequently used in association with bladder outlet obstruction when, in most cases, obstruction in prune-belly syndrome is not present postnatally (Greskovich and Nyberg, 1988). Review of this and other series (Harrison et al., 1987) has produced skepticism about the overall results (Colodny, 1987; Elder et al., 1987; Sholder et al., 1988).

Technical innovations are still being made in this field. Improvements in the techniques and types of catheters used for vesicoamniotic shunting have allowed longer term diversion with less repeated procedures (Rodeck, personal communication). Open fetal vesicostomy has also been shown to be technically feasible with maintenance of the pregnancy (Crombleholme et al., 1990). In this instance, as in others, however, the reported details of the pre- and postnatal diagnosis as well as long-term outcome leave one uncertain of the overall results.

The risks of intervention involve the mother and the fetus. Reported complications include chorioamnionitis, premature delivery (Elder et al., 1987), and fetal bowel herniation (Robichaux et al., 1991). The additional risk factors associated with open hysterotomy remain of concern.

One of the major issues relates to the ability to prognosticate which fetuses might benefit from intervention. The role of prognostic indicators is also in the stage of evolution. Some reports have indicated that fetal urinary electrolytes correlate well with ultimate outcome (Crombleholme et al., 1990; Glick et al., 1985; Grannum et al., 1989). Others, however, have found fetal urinary electrolytes to be of much less help in prognostication (Reuss et al., 1987; Wilkins et al., 1987).

Other indications for potential fetal renal function include sonographic findings related to the degree of echogenicity of the renal parenchyma. This feature provides some estimation of the potential for renal development after relief of obstruction (Mahoney et al., 1984). This finding, however, is not always present and, in our experience, does not uniformly predict irreversible fetal renal damage.

Other ultrasonographic findings include bladder refilling and emptying as a corollary to overall urine flow rate. This finding, of course, does not reflect the quality of glomerular or tubular function. The presence of oligohydramnios is the end stage of bladder outlet obstruction and implies a fairly far advanced degree of renal shutdown. The issue in these cases then relates to whether, after relief of the obstruction, amniotic fluid will return to allow lung development, and more critically, whether the degree of renal impairment is irreversible. Further investigations into renal tubular enzymes and metabolites as well as other potential molecular markers may prove to be beneficial.

What then are the potential indications for prenatal intervention? The options for intervention include elective abortion before fetal viability. Certainly, the availability of this modality rests ultimately on its legality; however, as long as this option remains accessible, it must be presented as an alternate strategy. Other categories of intervention include simple aspiration of dilated urinary structures in late gestation to relieve dystocia (Colodny, 1987). Rarely, alleviation of the maternal effects of fetal renal obstruction has been documented, and intervention has proved efficacious (Broecker et al., 1988; Seeds et al., 1984).

The most common situation in which one might entertain the concept of intervention involves the male fetus with bilateral hydroureteronephrosis, enlarged bladder, and some degree of oligohydramnios on ultrasound examination. The difficult issues of assessment of potential fetal renal function must be addressed in the best way possible. Currently, this assessment would include aspiration of the bladder and/or kidneys to determine fetal electrolytes and osmolality. Chromosomal analysis of the fetus as well as overall ultrasound examination for other somatic congenital anomalies must be thorough. If, based on these findings, it is decided that the fetus is without other lethal anomalies and is at risk for progressive renal and pulmonary damage from the presumed obstructive uropathy, then detailed discussion with the parents should be undertaken. This discussion should include the potential risks and benefits of the maternal-fetal interventional procedure, the personal experience of the physicians involved, and the experimental nature of the undertaking.

If the gestational age is such that the fetus could be potentially viable if delivered, then early delivery is an option. Whether or not steroid supplementation should be given rests on the evaluation of the lecithin/sphingomyelin ratio (Krieglsteiner et al., 1986). If the gestational stage is before this period of viability, then either percutaneous or open shunting should be entertained.

One must realize that renal reversibility is present for only a short window. We have found that, in those infants with early onset of high-grade obstructive uropathy, oligohydramnios may ensue any time after 16 weeks. Despite initially favorable urine electrolytes, within several weeks, these indices have been seen to dramatically change to suggest a poorer prognosis for the patient.

ETHICAL CONSIDERATIONS

Because of the availability of fetal diagnosis and therapy, a previously uncharted area of medical/legal issues has been raised. The issues of what is best for the mother and the fetus have been raised by many groups, and this has been helpful in evaluating what is available and what is justifiable. Inherent to this discussion is the status of the rights of the fetus as a person. Virtually none of the cases in our experience has involved an adversarial relationship between the mother and the fetus. This is not, however, the case with other situations (Fletcher, 1985).

The controversy over the moral and legal implications of abortion continues to evolve. Judicial and legislative impact on this decision will certainly occur in the next several years. Other legal issues include the obligatory informed consent of the mother in terms of risks to her as well as to the fetus. In a situation in which the emotional outlook is extremely heightened, one must bring to the discussion additional people who are knowledgeable but not directly involved with the therapy. This would imply a multidisciplinary committee involved in both the clinical and the scientific issues.

An issue that is often last to be raised is that of incomplete therapy. Clinical and research studies have been reasonably convincing that reversal of the oligohydramnios can prevent or minimize the associated pulmonary hypoplasia. Whether the renal function parameters are changed remains to be elucidated. Certainly, there are patients in whom, after in utero drainage, postnatal lung function is reasonable but renal function cannot sustain life. The proper informed consent regarding this possibility is important.

POSTNATAL MANAGEMENT

Many of the issues of prenatal diagnosis are related to the fact that the parents and the physicians involved need to be informed of the congenital anomalies so that postnatal evaluation and treatment can commence. We believe that one of the most important issues is the early use of low-dose prophylactic antibiotics in those with significant hydronephrosis. Because one cannot determine whether definite obstruction exists and further-

more, whether vesicoureteral reflux is present, the prevention of infection is extremely important. We do not recommend that ultrasound examination be performed immediately unless bladder outlet obstruction is suspected. Neonatal oliguria may mask a moderately obstructive lesion (Laing et al., 1984).

In the presence of marked bilateral hydronephrosis and a thick-walled bladder on prenatal ultrasound examination, postnatal evaluation, especially in the male infant, is performed within the first 24 hours. This evaluation consists primarily of ultrasound examination and voiding cystourethrogram. If posterior urethral valves are confirmed, then catheter placement and early surgical therapy are performed expeditiously.

In the usual case of prenatally diagnosed hydronephrosis, ultrasound examination is performed after the first few days of life. The postnatal ultrasound examination often is crucial in determining whether further studies should be done. The issue of whether voiding cystourethrography should be done on every patient with mild degrees of fullness of the collecting system remains unanswered. Our policy is that if the pre- and postnatal ultrasound findings show only mild degrees of renal pelvic fullness without ureteric dilatation, voiding cystourethrograms are not routinely performed. Others, however, might disagree with this.

The issue of how long one needs to follow children with mild hydronephrosis that is clearly not obstructive on initial evaluation remains a fascinating problem. We have previously thought that if the postnatal ultrasound showed mild renal pelvic fullness at birth and on subsequent follow-up at 1 to 2 years, the risk of subsequent deterioration was negligible. However, we have seen two children with prenatally diagnosed hydronephrosis and mild renal pelvic fullness on postnatal scans who developed high-grade obstruction at 4 and 6 years of age (Fig. 39–10). We now recommend follow-up of these children through puberty.

With more severe degrees of hydronephrosis, a voiding cystourethrogram and upper urinary tract imaging study are performed at 4 to 6 weeks. The latter routinely includes intravenous urography and/or diuretic renal scan at our institution. The decision as to what constitutes "significant" obstruction and what is the optimal management of these children remains controversial. The controversy arises because there is no "gold standard" in the diagnosis of obstruction. The majority of centers use a combination of ultrasound and renal scan findings on which to base their conclusion.

There are many ways to perform, interpret, and define information gained from the renal scan. The specific radionuclide, the dose and timing of the diuretic, and the data collection software vary from one institution to another. Utilization of individual kidney function (Ransley et al., 1987), washout curves (Thrall et al., 1981), and renal transit time (Whitfield et al., 1978) have all been championed as the best method for determining management decisions. Pressure perfusion studies (Whitaker, 1979) are also used in this determination, although they are usually reserved for indeterminate situations in most institutions.

The management is no more clearly defined or agreed

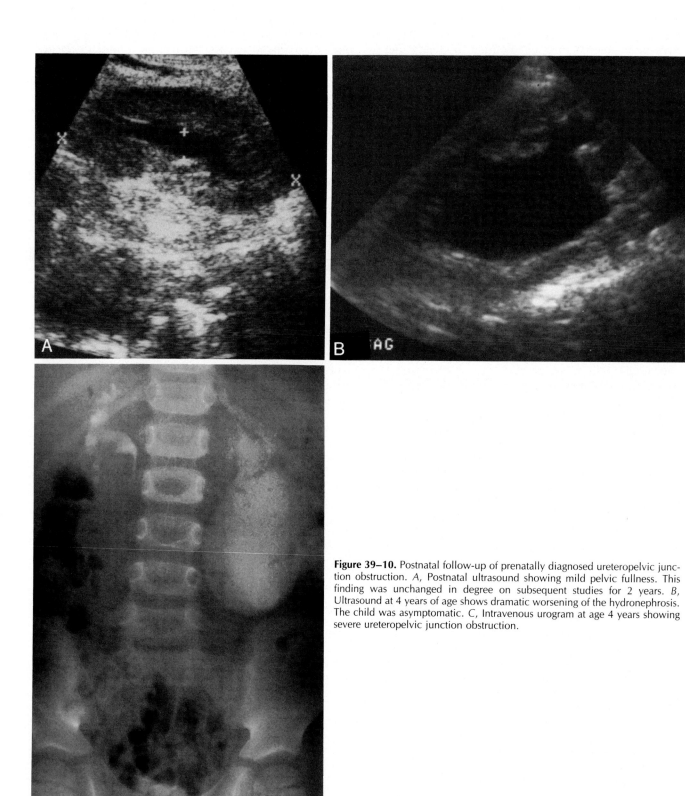

Figure 39–10. Postnatal follow-up of prenatally diagnosed ureteropelvic junction obstruction. *A,* Postnatal ultrasound showing mild pelvic fullness. This finding was unchanged in degree on subsequent studies for 2 years. *B,* Ultrasound at 4 years of age shows dramatic worsening of the hydronephrosis. The child was asymptomatic. *C,* Intravenous urogram at age 4 years showing severe ureteropelvic junction obstruction.

upon. Early neonatal correction of obstruction can be performed successfully and safely (Bernstein et al., 1988; Peters et al., 1989b). The question as to whether this results in the best outcome is unanswered. Ransley has advocated waiting until a marked decrease in differential function is seen before operating (Ransley et al., 1987). Experimental and clinical data suggest that early relief of obstruction, before diminution in function, is beneficial (Chevalier and El Dahrs, 1988).

What has become clear in postnatal follow-up of prenatally diagnosed hydronephrosis is that the natural history of primary obstructive megaureter may be different than that of ureteropelvic junction obstruction. Whereas the excellent results from surgical repair of ureteropelvic junction obstruction (Fig. 39–11) may warrant early operation, primary megaureter will sometimes improve spontaneously (Fig. 39–12) (Keating et al., 1989). It is difficult, however, to predict the ultimate outcome of these infants, and management remains controversial (Keating and Retik, 1990). Many of these infants who maintain good renal function may be followed with renal scans and ultrasound examinations in the first years of life.

The care of infants with urologic abnormalities, including multicystic dysplastic kidney, obstructive uropathy, hydronephrosis, cystic renal diseases, and other abnormalities, has been dramatically changed by the evolution of prenatal diagnosis. The number of patients presenting with urosepsis has diminished markedly. No longer do we see the ravages of postnatal infection in the presence of congenital anomalies in the same volume that was previously seen. This improvement has allowed the managed care of congenital uropathies in a way that will ultimately improve the quality of life and health in these children.

RESEARCH PERSPECTIVES

The emergence of the clinical aspects of prenatal diagnosis and management has led to the further development of research efforts to answer various questions raised in this area. Enormous opportunity exists for multiple levels of investigation that can address clinical concerns while integrating many new and exciting developments in the areas of cell biology and molecular biology. This is an opportune time for such investigation because the tools of molecular biology are becoming

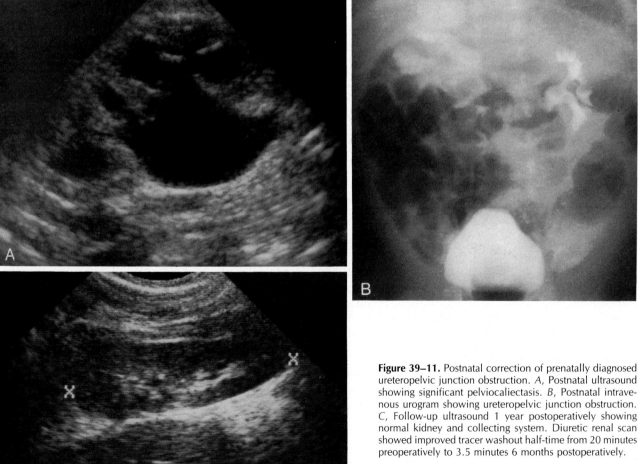

Figure 39–11. Postnatal correction of prenatally diagnosed ureteropelvic junction obstruction. *A,* Postnatal ultrasound showing significant pelviocaliectasis. *B,* Postnatal intravenous urogram showing ureteropelvic junction obstruction. *C,* Follow-up ultrasound 1 year postoperatively showing normal kidney and collecting system. Diuretic renal scan showed improved tracer washout half-time from 20 minutes preoperatively to 3.5 minutes 6 months postoperatively.

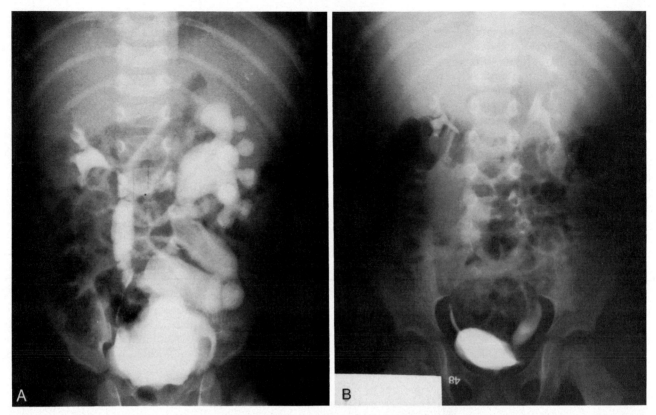

Figure 39–12. Postnatal follow-up of prenatally diagnosed megaureter. *A,* Initial postnatal intravenous urogram showing left hydroureteronephrosis and a tortuous ureter. Renal scan showed no diminution in function. *B,* Follow-up intravenous urogram 20 months later, with no surgery, showing normal upper collecting system with mild distal ureteral dilation.

widely accessible and the knowledge base associated with them is similarly expanding. Although research in the various aspects of this field is truly in its infancy, it is useful to review the major topics being considered. In the following section, we discuss the current status of this research, review some of the controversies, and present the horizons in this area.

Renal Development

Much of the previous research in this area has involved clinically related questions regarding renal development as linked to obstruction. The more basic question of what the underlying mechanisms of renal development are needs renewed analysis because it relates to many of the clinical renal malformations that are seen. In addition, the effects of obstructive lesions that are imposed on developing kidneys are certainly influenced by the state of development.

Understanding the principles underlying renal development involves basic embryology, for which several exciting areas of investigation are evolving. The mechanisms of inductive agents are being investigated, including retinoic acids (Smith et al., 1989; Thaller and Eichele, 1987) and growth factors (Liu and Nicoll, 1988; Rappolee et al., 1988; Paik et al., 1989) and their regulation (Roberts et al., 1990).

Within the kidney, the mechanisms of ureteral bud induction of the metanephric blastema have been inten-

sively studied, and many pieces of the puzzle have been placed; yet much remains to be clarified (Ekblom et al., 1990; Grobstein, 1953; Risau and Ekblom, 1986; Saxén, 1987). One of the critical aspects of this process is the phenomenon of mesenchymal to epithelial transformation that occurs in the developing nephron (Aufderheide et al., 1987; Hay, 1989a). This process may be amenable to examination in a tissue cell line that permits detailed manipulation and examination of the regulation of this transformation (Freeman et al., 1990).

The role of the extracellular matrix in regulating the differentiation of the embryonic and fetal kidney continues to be explored (Ekblom et al., 1982; Hay, 1989b; Holthöfer et al., 1984; Spencer and Maizels, 1987). On the horizon, one can envision identification of the signaling mechanisms that interact in a regulatory system to control cell growth and differentiation and the means by which various signals are transduced to the intrinsic regulatory mechanisms of specific cells. Although this may seem to be drifting somewhat away from the topic of a dysplastic kidney, an understanding of the detailed mechanisms of renal development is essential to eventually understand the maldevelopment seen clinically.

Inheritable Renal Abnormalities

Development may also be examined within the paradigm of a specific disease model, one of the more extensively investigated being autosomal recessive polycystic kidney disease. This disorder involves both developmental and genetic issues. An additional impetus for urologists to become specifically interested in autosomal recessive polycystic kidney disease relates to evaluating the potentially affected fetus of a family with a history of this lethal condition. As noted previously, several incidents of late identification of this disease have occurred, heightening the need for a specific prenatal marker.

Autosomal recessive polycystic kidney disease is being explored in a mouse model system *(cpk)* (Fry et al., 1985; Preminger et al., 1982), originated at the Jackson Laboratories. This model is an autosomal recessive condition in a C57/Bl6 mouse, which has been identified and described for 10 years now. It has permitted detailed investigation of the pathogenesis of the renal cysts in tissue culture by Avner and co-workers (1987, 1988), whose work suggests that cystogenesis may be related to a sodium-potassium ion pump in the tubular cells (Holthöfer et al., 1990). Others have described basement membrane changes (Ebihara et al., 1988), disordered regulation of epidermal growth factor gene expression (Gattone et al., 1990; Horikoshi et al., 1991), and induction of the c-*myc* proto-oncogene in the polycystic mice (Cowley et al., 1987).

A more direct approach is being taken by Davisson and associates (1991), who have localized the gene to mouse chromosome 12 and are attempting to specifically map the gene both in the mouse and in humans. Following mapping, cloning of the gene may permit identification of a gene product, which could lead to a specific marker. Genetic information such as this may facilitate characterization of mechanisms of the disease.

Obstruction

The kidney has been the primary focus of attention in genitourinary maldevelopment, particularly the area of congenital obstructions of the kidney. The pathophysiology of congenital obstructive uropathy, in its broadest context, remains unknown. This issue touches on a wide spectrum of pediatric urologic disease, including ureteropelvic junction obstruction, obstructive megaureter, and posterior urethral valves.

At one end of the spectrum, it is important to understand whether dysplasia is a product of the obstruction or a primary condition (Maizels and Simpson, 1983; Schwarz et al., 1981). In less severe cases, it is important to identify reliable clinical markers of congenital obstructive uropathy that can predict salvageable renal function (Huland et al., 1988; Kühl and Seyberth, 1990; Lenz et al., 1985; Steinhardt et al., 1990b). At the mildest end of the spectrum, one needs to know whether any therapeutic intervention is necessary at all. Clinical benefits will be yielded by this information regarding the proper evaluation of obstructive uropathies in the pre- and postnatal period, as well as decisions regarding intervention.

Postnatal Models of Obstruction

For the postnatal period, several models have been described looking at obstructive uropathy produced in the neonatal period in small animals (Chevalier and Kaiser, 1984; Chevalier et al., 1987a; Josephson et al., 1980). In general, these studies have involved creation of an obstructive lesion with later assessment of structure as well as function of the kidney. Partial obstructions have been induced in a number of ways, including burying of the ureter within the psoas muscle (Josephson et al., 1980). This technique produces an obstructive lesion that changes with growth of the animal. It does have the drawback of being unpredictable.

Long-term functional evaluations have been conducted with these models of partial obstruction. Several of these evaluations have demonstrated stable hydronephrosis and apparently stable renal function. These models have usually assessed only glomerular filtration rate, and few have specifically addressed tubular function. Concentrating defects, acid excretion, and sodium handling may be significantly impaired in congenital obstruction, even in the absence of diminished glomerular filtration rate. Josephson and associates (1990) have identified age-related differences in sensitivity to postnatal obstruction, reflected in the degree of sodium retention and hypertension.

An increased sensitivity of the neonate to effects of obstruction has been identified in the work of Chevalier and colleagues using models of partial ureteral obstruction in the guinea pig. The modifying influences of the renal vascular autoregulatory system, renal sympathetic nerves, and renal counterbalance have been shown to play a role in the global response to obstruction (Chevalier et al., 1988; Chevalier and Jones, 1986; Chevalier and Kaiser, 1984; Chevalier and Peach, 1985; Chevalier et al., 1987b; Purkerson and Klahr, 1989). As in the adult, decreases in renal blood flow, mediated by means of the renin-angiotensin system, have been associated with the pathophysiology of obstructive uropathy in the neonate. The issue of whether such alterations are responsible for the changes associated with obstructive uropathy or are secondary phenomena remains unsettled.

Attention has also been focused on the immunologic response of the obstructed kidney. Inflammatory infiltrates have been identified in postnatal models of obstruction. Several mechanisms of damage have been investigated, including the role of endotoxins, bradykinin, prostaglandin E_2 and thromboxane A_2 (Kühl and Seyberth, 1990), as well as macrophages, eosinophils, and leukocytes (Harris et al., 1989; Schreiner et al., 1988). Manipulation of the interactions of these elements has provided some tentative models for the mechanisms of damage. These models suggest some overlap with renal vascular autoregulatory mechanisms, indicating that the actual mechanisms will be complex.

Although renal obstruction has been investigated extensively in the postnatal animal, it is becoming evident that these conclusions may not be universally applicable to the prenatally obstructed kidney. It remains unanswered whether the outcomes seen in these experimental preparations are influenced by the fact that the obstruction is imposed upon an entirely normal neonatal kidney. This situation is not analogous to the actual clinical condition seen with a prenatally identified obstruction that is being evaluated in the postnatal period. For this reason, prenatal models have been investigated, and it seems reasonable that these models may be more valid overall in the consideration of congenital obstructive uropathy.

Prenatal Models of Obstruction

Prenatal congenital obstructive uropathy is not the same as postnatal obstruction. This premise is supported by the fact that the prenatal kidney is undergoing rapid growth and development with formation of new structures as well as significant structural and functional maturation of previously formed elements. The fetal kidney is in an environment where the placenta performs virtually all of the dialysis of the fetal circulation. The principal activity of the fetal kidney is growth and development rather than function. Although the fetal kidney is certainly an excretory organ, this role is relatively minor and largely limited to excretion of excess water (Lumbers, 1983; Smith and Robillard, 1989).

Renal blood flow in the fetal kidney is approximately 7 per cent of cardiac output at 10 weeks of gestation and 3 per cent at 20 weeks, in contrast to 20 to 30 per cent of cardiac output in the postnatal period (Rudolph and Heyman, 1970). The entire environment of the fetal kidney is distinct from that of the postnatal kidney. Oxygen tension is markedly reduced and the hormonal environment is different in terms of both levels of various hormones effecting renal circulation and the renal sensitivity to their effects. This feature has been documented with regard to the renin-angiotensin system as well as aldosterone (Smith and Robillard, 1989). Atrial natriuretic peptide has also been studied, and levels are distinctly higher in the fetus than in the postnatal animal; the sensitivity to its natriuretic effects is less (Robillard et al., 1988).

Although creating an in utero obstruction would more closely mimic the clinical condition, inherent difficulties exist in developing models of prenatal obstructive uropathy besides the technical ones of operating on a pregnant animal (Adzick and Harrison, 1986). The obstructions produced are usually acute, which may have a different effect on a developing kidney than one of gradual onset. Systemic effects of fetal manipulation occur, and these must be rigorously controlled. Despite these difficulties, determination of relevant postnatal outcomes can only be effectively carried out with reproducible prenatal models.

Prenatal models have been described in a number of situations, ranging from the chick embryo to large animals, such as sheep. Early obstructions have been induced in the chick embryo at the metanephric stage, which allow investigation of the production of renal dysplastic lesions (Berman and Maizels, 1982; Maizels and Simpson, 1983). These models have the advantage of permitting manipulation very early in renal development. It is extremely difficult, however, to create a precise lesion that is completely reproducible. The avian

kidney is distinct from that of the mammal, which may have significance in the interpretation of this data.

Congenital obstruction of the fetal rabbit kidney may be produced as early as 23 days out of 32 days in gestation (McVary and Maizels, 1989; Thomasson et al., 1970). The rabbit continues glomerulogenesis until age 2 weeks postnatally, which has made it attractive for consideration of the effects of obstruction on nephronogenesis. It must be borne in mind that the postnatal kidney, even though it is undergoing nephronogenesis, is distinct from the prenatal kidney; this may markedly influence its response to obstruction and decompression. The small size of the rabbit limits the range of experimental manipulations possible.

A novel approach to studying congenital obstruction has been exploited in the opossum, a marsupial (Steinhardt et al., 1988, 1990b). The opossum pups are "born" into the marsupium of the mother at a developmental stage approximately equivalent to 8 weeks of gestation in the human. At this point, metanephric development is just beginning. Obstructions induced several days later are comparable to those at the 12th to 14th week in the human, and these have been achieved. This system has the advantage of not requiring surgical violation of the uterus, which may precipitate preterm labor.

The fetal sheep has been used for many years to investigate the fetal kidney (Alexander et al., 1958; Beck, 1971; Tanagho, 1972). This animal offers the advantage of having a long gestation similar to that of the human, as well as being manipulable for experimental preparations without excessive fetal loss. Multiple procedures may be performed on a given fetal sheep to explore the dynamics of renal response to obstruction (Figs. 39–13 and 39–14) (Glick et al., 1984a; Peters et al., 1990c).

At the foundation of the conclusions of the many investigations into congenital obstruction of the kidneys is the fact that fetal manipulation in an experimental system is indeed feasible, practical, and reproducible in a number of animal systems, which may be applied to specific questions regarding congenital uropathies. The response of the fetal kidney to obstruction can be completely distinct from that in the postnatal animal. Postnatally induced renal obstruction has never been reported to produce changes consistent with renal dysplasia or to produce the growth effects seen with prenatally obstructed kidney. The response of the fetal kidney to obstruction is determined to various degrees by (1) the time of onset of obstruction during gestation, (2) the duration of the obstruction, and (3) the severity of the obstruction. The status of the contralateral kidney has also been shown to have a significant role in the response of the affected kidney to obstruction (Beck, 1971).

Renal Function and Congenital Obstruction

Several studies have demonstrated that in utero functional differences produced by prenatal obstruction are much less distinct than those seen postnatally (Adzick

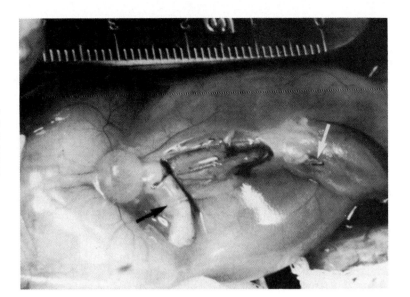

Figure 39–13. Operative photograph of experimental creation of bladder outlet obstruction in a fetal lamb at 60 days of gestation (term = 140 days). The penile urethra has been mobilized and clipped. The urachus, between the paired umbilical arteries, has been clipped. The animal is approximately 12 cm in length. (From Peters, C. A., and Mandell, J.: Experimental congenital obstructive uropathy. Urol. Clin. North Am., 17(2):442, 1990.)

et al., 1985; Bellinger et al., 1986; Ward et al., 1990). This finding is a logical reflection of the fact that the fetal kidney is not primarily involved in function; consequently, even significant damage may only be seen as small increments of change in function.

Postnatal renal functional assessment following prenatal obstruction has been carried out in a number of models (Glick et al., 1983, 1984a; Hawtrey et al., 1985). The nature of the defects observed reflects those seen clinically in the postnatal period in the child with obstructive uropathy, including reduced glomerular filtration, impaired acid excretion, and reduced sodium and water reabsorption (Hutcheon et al., 1976; Mayor et al., 1975; McCrory et al., 1971).

No studies have followed these functional parameters beyond either the late prenatal or very early postnatal period. It is, therefore, difficult to assess the applicability of the currently available prenatal models to the clinical spectrum of disease.

Renal Blood Flow and Congenital Obstruction

Postnatal renal blood flow in congenital obstruction has not been evaluated extensively. In a model of spontaneous congenital obstruction in the rat, renal blood flow has been demonstrated to be an important factor in the renal response to obstruction (Boineau et al., 1987; Friedman et al., 1979). In prenatally induced partial ureteral obstruction, reductions in blood flow were demonstrated, but the variability in the degree of obstruction precluded identification of specific relationships (Hawtrey et al., 1985). This finding is consistent with the observations from postnatal models, but it still remains unclear whether these changes are a secondary phenomenon or are directly related to the causes of the functional impairments. Investigation of a variety of vasoactive compounds has also demonstrated changes in response to obstruction, which may be either causa-

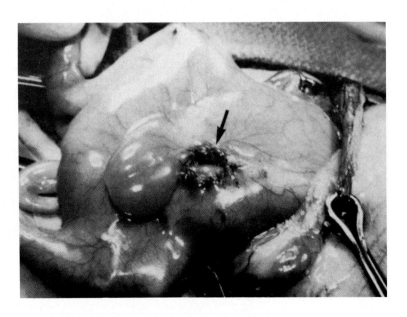

Figure 39–14. In utero urinary decompression of an experimentally obstructed fetal lamb at 95 days of gestation (term = 140 days). Obstruction was created 5 weeks before. On ultrasound, this animal had a dilated bladder, hydronephrosis, and oligohydramnios. Decompression is accomplished using a cutaneous vesicostomy as shown. (From Peters, C. A., and Mandell, J.: Experimental congenital obstructive uropathy. Urol. Clin. North Am., 17(2):443, 1990.)

tive or reactive (Chevalier and Jones, 1986; Chevalier and Peach, 1985; Kühl and Seyberth, 1990). These issues will be important facets of the pathophysiology of congenital obstruction.

The effect of congenital obstruction on renal blood flow in utero has not been examined. This problem is further complicated by the relatively low rate of normal renal blood flow in utero, reminding the investigator that the dynamics and regulatory mechanisms of renal blood flow in utero, and therefore in prenatal obstruction, may be significantly different than those occurring postnatally.

Renal Growth and Development and Congenital Obstruction

Renal structural abnormalities have been produced with prenatal obstruction. Impaired nephrogenesis has been reported in the fetal rabbit (McVary and Maizels, 1989). This effect was apparently reversed with early postnatal decompression, before nephronogenesis is complete in the rabbit. Assessments of glomerular number must be interpreted in light of the methodology of counting (Cruz-Orive, 1980; Elias and Hyde, 1980), and these conclusions need confirmation. The issue of the potential for reversal of changes produced by in utero obstruction is important and requires careful continued investigation.

Kidney obstruction in the opossum has produced histologic dysplasia. It remains entirely unknown, however, whether the marsupial kidney, although mammalian, behaves in a similar fashion to a kidney that remains on placental dialysis. It is unclear how the marsupial pup handles fluids and solutes from the maternal milk. This approach, however, has many attractions and hopefully will be developed further.

Dysplastic changes have been reported by several investigators in sheep with early gestational obstructions (Figs. 39–15 and 39–16) (Beck, 1971; Glick et al., 1983; Gonzalez et al., 1990; Peters et al., 1990c; Pringle and Bonsib, 1988). This dysplasia is characterized by primitive ductal epithelium, peritubular mesenchymal collars, cystic changes, and disorganized architecture. In the avian kidney, similar results were only achieved with

obstruction in combination with mesenchymal stripping. Definitive production of heterotopic tissue has not been documented.

Controversy remains concerning whether the dysplasia seen in human situations is always a primary or inductive dysplastic change or whether some may be due to the obstructive lesion (Bernstein, 1968). As with much of biology, it is probable that many instances are a combination of these two factors. The fact that a histopathologic condition virtually indistinguishable from classic renal dysplasia can be produced by experimental prenatal obstruction strongly suggests that this may occur in nature. Because functional assessments in utero may be less distinct in terms of outcome differences, effects on growth or differentiation may yield more reproducible indicators of the effects of obstruction (Peters et al., 1991a).

The occurrence of in utero compensatory renal hypertrophy has been documented with prenatal nephrectomy (Moore et al., 1979) and in the setting of unilateral prenatal obstructive uropathy (see Fig. 39–15) (Steinhardt et al., 1990b; Peters et al., 1990c). It remains unknown what the specific mechanisms of in utero compensatory hypertrophy are and whether they are the same as those that occur postnatally (Fine, 1986; Malt, 1983; Nomura et al., 1985; Sawczuk et al., 1989; Wesson, 1989).

These observations are important to indicate that the responses of the fetal kidney to obstruction include alterations in the patterns and pathways of growth and differentiation. Whereas investigation of developmental parameters may provide critical markers of the progression of congenital uropathy, functional changes and ultimate outcome must be related to these developmental markers. This relationship would allow us to relate human clinical cases seen in the early neonatal period to experimental preparations and their developmental "signposts" of the progression of congenital uropathy. The functional consequences of the experimental preparations could then be related to their human counterparts.

At the present time, the significant issues that remain to be settled in our attempt to understand congenital obstructive uropathy include identification of the actual

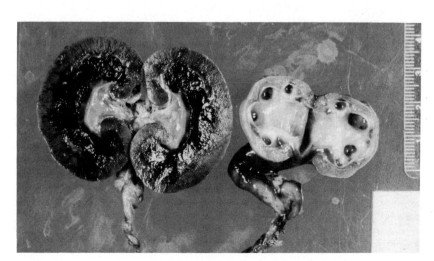

Figure 39–15. Photograph of the kidneys from a fetal lamb at term following in utero unilateral complete ureteral ligation at 60 days of gestation (term = 140 days). The obstructed kidney *(right)* is smaller than its mate: 5 g versus 16 g. The contralateral kidney is larger than normal (normal term kidney weight, 10.5 g). The obstructed kidney shows marked cortical and medullary thinning and has a coarse, fibrous texture. The pelvis is dilated. The contralateral mate has a normal gross appearance.

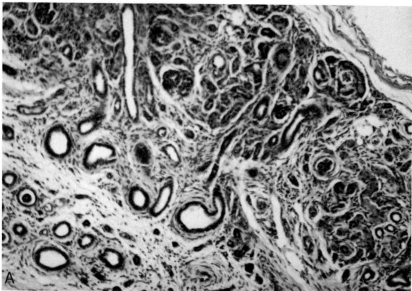

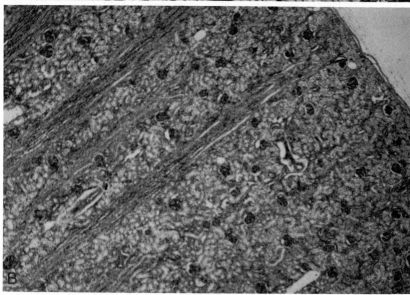

Figure 39–16. Photomicrographs of sheep kidneys at term (× 250, hematoxylin and eosin). *A*, Section of the unilaterally obstructed kidney shown in Figure 39–15. Complete obstruction at 60 days of gestation produced marked structural changes and evidence of dysplasia. Tubules have cuboidal to columnar epithelium and are surrounded by mesenchymal collars. Glomerulogenesis was impaired, and abnormal glomeruli are evident. The relative amount of interstitial tissue compared with the tubular and glomerular elements was increased above that in the normal kidney. *B*, Normal-term sheep kidney showing the corticomedullary rays and glomeruli in the outer cortex.

mediators of the obstructive effect or injury. Hydrostatic pressure is involved, but the precise mechanism of renal effect remains unknown. Renal blood flow is a likely candidate for involvement in the kidney's response to prenatal obstruction, as well as inflammatory and immunologic responses. The initiating factors of these responses remain to be identified. As the mediators of obstructive uropathy become known, it will be important to relate them to functional parameters and to develop specific markers of the natural history of congenital obstructive uropathies.

The long-term aim of such investigation is the integration of an understanding of congenital obstructive uropathy with an understanding of the mechanisms of renal growth and development. A more precise understanding of the underlying mechanisms will permit better correlation of the in utero effects with postnatal functional parameters. With an improved ability to follow and measure the effects of prenatal obstruction, both in experimental and subsequently in human situations, the

possible means with which to prevent or reduce the damage should be suggested. The long-range goal is to improve the ability to determine the need for, and best method of, intervention that may permit a more rational and less empiric approach to this common condition.

Bladder Responses to Congenital Obstruction

The effect of congenital bladder outlet obstruction may be seen perinatally in terms of the renal and pulmonary injury. However, this effect may continue long after correction of the obstruction in the form of bladder dysfunction. A variety of patterns of bladder dysfunction are seen in the postobstructive bladder (Peters et al., 1990a), yet it is unclear what differentiates these patterns in terms of etiology. The ability to predict the specific pattern of dysfunction that a given patient

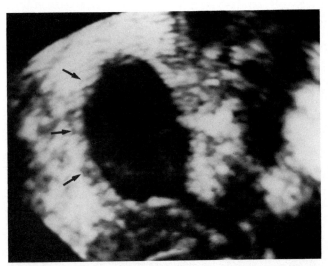

Figure 39–17. In utero ultrasound of obstructed fetal lamb bladder at 95 days of gestation. Obstruction had been produced at 60 days of gestation (term = 140 days). Bladder wall is thicker than normal for age (arrows). Oligohydramnios was present.

is at risk for would be clinically valuable, but this is not yet possible.

Whereas the significant long-term consequences of prenatal bladder obstruction have been recognized for almost a decade, the investigation into the nature of congenital bladder obstruction is barely beginning (Workman and Kogan, 1990). Most of the models are in postnatal animals and, despite a variety of experimental approaches, no consistent picture has yet appeared to help explain the clinical patterns seen in

children with bladder obstruction (Elbadawi et al., 1989; Kato et al., 1988; Speakman et al., 1987).

Several new models of prenatally induced obstructions are being developed (Figs. 39–17 and 39–18) (Vasavada et al., 1990). Partial bladder outlet obstructions are more common clinically but are difficult to predictably induce. In a model of complete early gestation bladder outlet obstruction, a marked increase in the mass of bladder smooth muscle is seen, approximately five and a half times normal. Morphometric data suggest this is mostly muscle cell hypertrophy, but it is possible that some degree of hyperplasia is present (Dator et al., 1991).

Connective tissue elements are increased to a lesser degree than the smooth muscle mass. Patterns of collagen subtypes within the bladder have been shown to be altered in human cases of prenatal obstruction (Kim et al., 1991a, 1991b). This finding is consistent with the fact that the fetal bladder is actively involved in growth and development during the period of obstruction.

Using indicators of muscle differentiation as well as neuromuscular integration, some have suggested that the dynamics of the fetal bladder influence its development (Peters et al., 1990b, 1991b). The ratios of myosin heavy chain isoforms, which have been well described to progress in a predictable fashion during development (Boone et al., 1989; McConnell et al., 1988), and which may have physiologic consequences (McConnell et al., 1990), are affected by in utero obstruction in which a prematurely accelerated pattern is seen. These ratios are also affected by in utero defunctionalization, as are the levels of muscarinic cholinergic receptor, when normalized to smooth muscle mass. No significant change

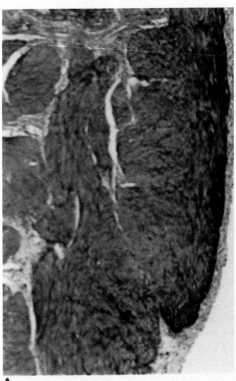

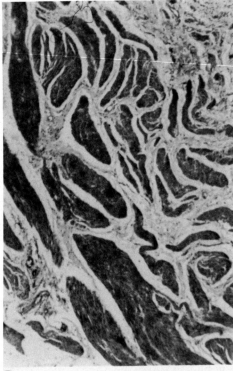

Figure 39–18. Photomicrographs of lamb bladders at term (× 140, Giemsa trichrome staining). A, Obstructed bladder (obstruction at 60 days of gestation, no decompression). The relative increase in the amount of smooth muscle to connective tissue is evident. The individual smooth muscle bundles are larger. The total volume of smooth muscle increased about five times, whereas that of the connective tissue increased two times. Total bladder weight increased four times over normal. B, Normal bladder with darker staining bundles of smooth muscle interspersed by connective tissue.

A

B

in receptor density was seen with obstruction, however, despite a marked increase in the amount of smooth muscle mass.

Further investigation of the pharmacologic sensitivities of prenatal bladder as well as the smooth muscle physiologic effects of partial bladder outlet obstruction in the fetal bladder is ongoing (Kogan and Iwamato, 1989). Another important area of investigation has been in studying the normal development of the urinary smooth muscle. Its physiologic behavior as well as its biochemical relationships to various effects change during development. This research may help shed light on certain patterns of neonatal urinary tract abnormalities as well as different patterns of response to obstruction (Zedric et al., 1990). It is hoped that reproducible models of prenatal obstruction of the bladder will be readily applicable to the assessment of obstructed human bladders with the well-known attendant functional abnormalities.

Pulmonary Effects of Congenital Obstructive Uropathy

The relationship of congenital uropathies to maldevelopment of the lungs has been recognized for nearly 40 years and remains an important example of the unique relationships of organ systems in utero. This relationship has taken on further clinical significance with the increasing frequency of detection of severe obstructive uropathies associated with risk for pulmonary hypoplasia on maternal/fetal ultrasound examination, as well as the ability to perform fetal surgical interventions (Crombleholme et al., 1990; Manning, 1987). Because the prognosis of a fetus with apparent bladder outlet obstruction with oligohydramnios is extremely poor, largely due to pulmonary complications (Nakayama et al., 1986), it is important to be able to determine the status and potential salvageability of lung function.

No diagnostic measures are available to specifically predict the degree of pulmonary compromise, largely because of the lack of understanding of the pulmonary lesion and the mechanisms of injury in the setting of obstructive uropathy with oligohydramnios. The differences in the pulmonary effects of oligohydramnios due to varying degrees of obstructive uropathy between early and late gestation remain to be determined, making accurate clinical prognosis even more difficult. It has, therefore, become important to develop an understanding of the disease mechanisms as well as the potentials for intervening and altering the course of the disease. Study of this unique system may provide a means for developing a basic understanding of the relationship between the kidney and lung by revealing the complex relationships of regulatory mechanisms that occur in the developing fetus.

The relationship of the kidney and amniotic fluid in pulmonary development has been investigated in several model systems. In the rabbit, oligohydramnios has been produced by bladder outlet obstruction as well as by amniotic shunting (Nakayama et al., 1983). In both

situations, in the last one third of gestation, lung size is decreased. The specific structural differences in these lungs have not been carefully studied.

In the guinea pig, a number of investigations have been carried out with regard to lung fluid, including drainage and ligation of the trachea (Moessinger et al., 1986). It is evident that lung growth and development are modulated by lung fluid dynamics. Increased lung growth can be produced by retention of the lung fluid (Adzick et al., 1984; Alcorn et al., 1977; Scurry et al., 1989), providing support to the concept of a simple mechanical factor relating the kidneys and lungs through the amniotic fluid. It has been suggested that the drainage of lung fluid is more rapid in the setting of oligohydramnios, when amniotic pressure is less than when amniotic fluid (from urine) is present (Nicolini et al., 1989). Some support for this concept has been reported in experimental preparations looking at rates of lung fluid production and drainage depending on volume and pressure status of the amniotic fluid (Dickson and Harding, 1989).

It remains to be explained why a significant impairment of lung growth in humans can be induced by kidney damage that occurs in the first trimester before the absence of urine would produce oligohydramnios (Seeds, 1980). In cases of renal agenesis or bilateral dysplasia, airway branching is diminished. Embryologically, branching is known to occur only up to 14 weeks of gestation, a time when the kidneys have not yet begun to contribute significantly to the amniotic fluid volume (Hislop et al., 1979). This finding raises the strong possibility of a very specific kidney factor being necessary for normal lung airway branching (Clemmons, 1977). The balance between the roles of the kidney and the amniotic fluid in later gestation remains to be clarified. These observations are interesting in light of anecdotal cases of monoamniotic twins in which one twin is anephric yet has normal pulmonary function, presumably due to some contribution by its twin with normal kidneys.

The most detailed experimental models used to investigate the clinically relevant relationship of the kidney and lung have been in the fetal sheep. A model to recreate the lesion of pulmonary hypoplasia was produced by Harrison's group in San Francisco with creation of a bladder outlet obstruction in the fetal sheep during the last one third of gestation (Harrison et al., 1982, 1983). In those sheep, pulmonary function was compromised and lung sizes were found to be smaller than normal. In utero decompression of these obstructed and oligohydramnic fetuses later in gestation produced an improvement in initial postnatal pulmonary function as well as larger lungs. Detailed analysis of pulmonary function was not performed nor were pulmonary morphometric analyses performed.

Earlier preparations of bladder outlet obstruction, in the fetal sheep before five-tenths of gestation, also produced a significant pulmonary lesion with pulmonary volumes being approximately one half of normal (Docimo et al., 1989, 1991). Morphometric analysis in these sheep demonstrated not only the diminished size but also an immature structural pattern in the lungs, com-

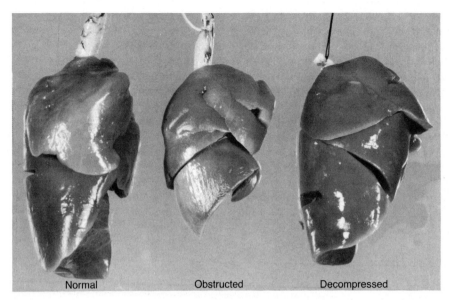

Figure 39–19. Gross photograph of lungs from term lambs (140 days) inflated to 25 cm H₂O pressure. Normal lung on left. Middle lung is from animal with bladder outlet obstruction created at 60 days of gestation and left in place until term. Lung was smaller than normal and histologic structure was age-inappropriate, being comparable to that of a 120-day fetus. Right lung is from animal with identical bladder obstruction created at 60 days of gestation but decompressed in utero at 95 days. At the time of decompression, the animal had a dilated bladder, hydronephrosis, and oligohydramnios. Lung volume was increased compared with that of the animal with obstruction left in place until term, and histology was age-appropriate. (From Peters, C. A., Docimo, S. G., Luetic, T., Reid, L. M., Retik, A. B., and Mandell, J.: Effect of in utero vesicostomy on pulmonary hypoplasia in the fetal lamb with bladder outlet obstruction and oligohydramnios: A morphometric analysis. J. Urol., 1991. In press.)

parable to those at approximately 120 days out of 140 days in gestation. In utero decompression of this early gestation model demonstrated the potential for preventing the severe hypoplastic condition, but reversal of size differences was only partial in most animals (Fig. 39–19). Structural maturity appeared to be complete in all animals where some degree of return of amniotic fluid volume was noted.

In several preparations, when the kidneys were irreversibly damaged by the initial bladder outlet obstruc-

tion, severe pulmonary hypoplasia was seen, despite urinary decompression (Peters et al., 1991c). Evaluation of the contributions of the kidney and amniotic fluid to lung growth and structural maturity seemed to support the concept of an early role of the kidney for basic growth and a later role of amniotic fluid for structural maturity, as in normal alveolarization (Peters et al., 1991d).

Experimental models have thus demonstrated that bladder outlet obstruction producing oligohydramnios

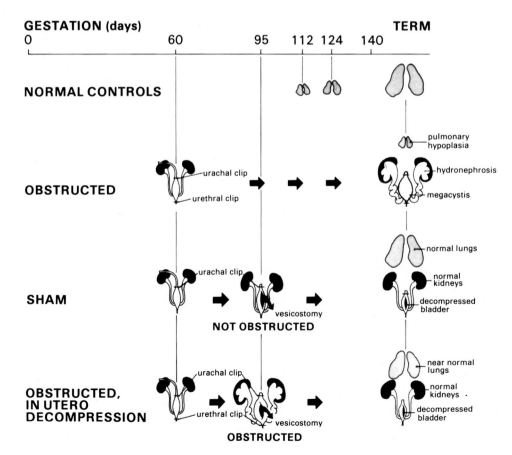

Figure 39–20. Diagram showing experimental scheme of study of the pulmonary effects of in utero bladder outlet obstruction and decompression. The first step included morphometric assessment of the alveolar stage of lung development (112 to 140 days of gestation). Bladder outlet obstruction at 60 days of gestation produced small lungs at term that were histologically immature. In utero sham vesicostomy at 95 days of gestation did not affect lung volume or histology. In utero urinary decompression of experimentally obstructed animals produced lungs of near normal size and normal maturity. This study has demonstrated that in utero decompression of bladder outlet obstruction can prevent the expected pulmonary hypoplasia from obstruction with oligohydramnios.

can cause a pulmonary hypoplastic lesion consistent with that seen in humans. This finding may also be observed with bilateral nephrectomy in utero prior to eight-tenths of gestation (Peters, unpublished data). The degree of pulmonary hypoplasia is clearly dependent on gestational age. With in utero decompression of obstructive lesions, partial prevention of pulmonary hypoplasia is achieved (Fig. 39–20). This partial prevention has also been accomplished in rabbits with amnio infusion, although structural analyses are not available. It has also been shown that prevention of lung fluid loss by tracheal ligation accompanying oligohydramnios can not only prevent growth impairment but can actually produce larger than normal lungs (Alcorn et al., 1977; Peters, unpublished data). Maturity appears satisfactory from histologic analysis, yet the actual biochemical maturity as reflected by surfactant levels has not been demonstrated.

At the present time, the primary questions relate to the identity of the mediators of this unique relationship. Lung fluid appears important, and the role of the kidney may be earlier in gestation, during the major growth period for the lung, possibly as a source of a significant growth substrate or metabolite (Wigglesworth et al., 1981). As with the studies of the kidney, it is clear that reproducible markers of normal and abnormal lung growth and maturation need to be identified and characterized. These markers may enhance our ability to assess experimental models investigating the nature and reversal of the lung lesions and improve our ability to prognosticate in the clinical setting.

REFERENCES

Adzick, N. S., and Harrison, M. R.: Surgical techniques in the fetal rabbit. *In* Nathanielsz, P. W. (Ed.): Animal Models in Fetal Medicine, Vol. 4. Ithaca, NY, Perinatology Press, 1986, p. 67.

Adzick, N. S., Harrison, M. R., Flake, A. W., and Laberge, J. M.: Development of a fetal renal function test using endogenous creatinine clearance. J. Pediatr. Surg., 20:602, 1985.

Adzick, N. S., Harrison, M. R., Glick, P. L., Villa, R. L., and Finkbeiner, W.: Experimental pulmonary hypoplasia and oligohydramnios: Relative contributions of lung fluid and fetal breathing movements. J. Pediatr. Surg., 19:658, 1984.

Alcorn, D., Adamson, T. M., Lambert, T. F., Maloney, J. E., Ritchie, B. C., and Robinson, P. M.: Morphological effects of chronic tracheal ligation and drainage in the fetal lamb lung. J. Anat., 123:649, 1977.

Alexander, D. P., Nixon, D. A., Widdas, W. F., and Wohlzogen, F. X.: Renal function in the sheep foetus. J. Physiol., 140:14, 1958.

Allen, K. S., Arger, P. H., Mennuti, M., et al.: Effects of maternal hydration on fetal renal pyelectasis. Radiology, 163:807, 1987.

Arger, P. H., Coleman, B. G., Mintz, M. C., et al.: Routine fetal genitourinary tract screening. Radiology, 156:485, 1985.

Arnold, A. J., and Rickwood, A. M. K.: Natural history of pelviureteric obstruction detected by prenatal sonography. Br. J. Urol., 65:91, 1990.

Ascensio, S. H., Figueroa-Longo, J. G., and Pelegrina, I. A.: Intrauterine exchange transfusion. Am. J. Obstet. Gynecol., 95:1129, 1966.

Aufderheide, E., Chiquet-Ehrismann, R., and Ekblom, P.: Epithelial-mesenchymal interactions in the developing kidney lead to expression of tenascin in the mesenchyme. J. Cell Biol., 105:599, 1987.

Avner, E. D., Studnicki, F. E., Young, M. C., Sweeney, W. E., Jr., Piesco, N. P., Ellis, D., and Fetterman, G. H.: Congenital murine polycystic kidney disease: I. The ontogeny of tubular cyst formation. Pediatr. Nephrol., 1:587, 1987.

Avner, E. D., Sweeney, W. E., Jr., Young, M. C., and Ellis, D.: Congenital murine polycystic kidney disease: II. Pathogenesis of tubular cyst formation. Pediatr. Nephrol., 2:210, 1988.

Avni, E. F., Rodesch, F., and Schulman, C. C.: Fetal uropathies: Diagnostic pitfalls and management. J. Urol., 134:921, 1985.

Beck, A. D.: The effect of intra-uterine urinary obstruction upon the development of the fetal kidney. J. Urol., 105:784–789, 1971.

Bellinger, M. F., Ward, R. M., Boal, D. K., Zaino, R. J., Sipio, J. C., and Wood, M. A.: Renal function in the fetal lamb: A chronic model to study the physiologic effects of ureteral ligation and deligation. J. Urol., 136:225–228, 1986.

Benacerraf, B. R., Mandell, J., Estroff, J. A., et al.: Fetal pyelectasis: A possible association with Down syndrome. Obstet. Gynecol., 76:58, 1990.

Benacerraf, B. R., Peters, C. A., and Mandell, J.: The prenatal evolution of renal cystic dysplasia in the setting of obstructive hydronephrosis and urinoma formation followed sonographically. J. Clin. Ultrasound, 1991. In press.

Benacerraf, B. R., Saltzman, D. H., and Mandell, J.: Sonographic diagnosis of abnormal fetal genitalia. J. Ultrasound Med., 8:613, 1989.

Berman, D. J., and Maizels, M.: The role of urinary obstruction in the genesis of renal dysplasia: A model in the chick embryo. J. Urol., 128:1091, 1982.

Bernstein, G. T., Mandell, J., Lebowitz, R. L., et al.: Ureteropelvic junction obstruction in the neonate. J. Urol., 140:1216, 1988.

Bernstein, J.: Developmental abnormalities of the renal parenchyma: Renal hypoplasia and dysplasia. Pathol. Annu., 3:213, 1968.

Blane, C. E., Koff, S. A., Bowerman, R. A., et al.: Nonobstructive fetal hydronephrosis: Sonographic recognition and therapeutic implications. Radiology, 147:95, 1983.

Boineau, F. G., Vari, R. C., and Lewy, J. E.: Reversible vasoconstriction in rats with congenital unilateral hydronephrosis. Pediatr. Nephrol., 1:498, 1987.

Boone, T. B., Ewalt, D. H., and McConnell, J. D.: Effects of sympathetic denervation and thyroid hormone on myosin heavy chain isoforms in the neonatal rabbit bladder [Abstract 620]. J. Urol., 141:324A, 1989.

Bowie, J. D., Rosenberg, E. R., Andreotti, R. F., et al.: The changing appearance of fetal kidneys during pregnancy. J. Ultrasound Med., 2:505, 1983.

Broecker, B. H., Redwine, F. O., and Petres, R. E.: Reversal of acute polyhydramnios after fetal decompression. Urology, 31:60, 1988.

Brown, T., Mandell, J., and Lebowitz, R. L.: Neonatal hydronephrosis in the era of sonography. AJR, 148:959, 1987.

Bruno, A. N., Lavin, J. P., and Nasrallah, P. F.: Ultrasound experience with prenatal genitourinary abnormalities. Urology, 26:196, 1985.

Cendron, M., Horton, C. E., Karim, O. M., Mostwin, J. L., Jeffs, R. D., and Gearhart, J. P.: A fetal lamb model of partial urethral obstruction: Effects on the developing bladder. Presented at the European Society of Pediatric Urology, April, 1991.

Chevalier, R. L., and El Dahrs, S.: The case for early relief of obstruction in young infants. *In* King, L. R. (Ed.): Urologic Surgery in Neonates and Young Infants. Philadelphia, W. B. Saunders Co., 1988, p. 95.

Chevalier, R. L., Gomez, R. A., and Jones, C. E.: Release of neonatal unilateral chronic partial ureteral obstruction reciprocally alters angiotensin-mediated vascular tone of both kidneys. Pediatr. Res., 21:473A, 1987a.

Chevalier, R. L., Gomez, R. A., and Jones, C. E.: Developmental determinants of recovery after relief of partial ureteral obstruction. Kidney Int., 33:775, 1988.

Chevalier, R. L., and Jones, C. E.: Contribution of endogenous vasoactive compounds to renal vascular resistance in neonatal chronic partial ureteral obstruction. J. Urol., 136:532, 1986.

Chevalier, R. L., and Kaiser, D. L.: Chronic partial ureteral obstruction in the neonatal guinea pig: I. Influence of uninephrectomy on growth and hemodynamics. Pediatr. Res., 18:1266, 1984.

Chevalier, R. L., and Peach, M. J.: Hemodynamic effects of enalapril on neonatal chronic partial ureteral obstruction. Kidney Int., 28:891, 1985.

Chevalier, R. L., Sturgill, B. C., Jones, C. E., and Kaiser, D. L.:

Morphologic correlates of renal growth arrest in neonatal partial ureteral obstruction. Pediatr. Res., 21:338, 1987b.

Claesson, G., Josephson, S., and Robertson, B.: Experimental partial ureteric obstruction in newborn rats: IV. Do the morphological effects progress continuously? J. Urol., 130:1217, 1983.

Claesson, G., Josephson, S., and Robertson, B.: Experimental partial ureteric obstruction in newborn rats: VII. Are the long-term effects on renal morphology avoided by release of the obstruction? J. Urol., 136:1330, 1986.

Claesson, G., Josephson, S., and Robertson, B.: Renal recovery after release of experimental neonatal ureteric obstruction. Urol. Int., 42:353, 1987.

Claesson, G., Svensson, L., Robertson, B., Josephson, S., and Cederlund, T.: Experimental obstructive hydronephrosis in newborn rats: XI. A one-year follow-up study of renal function and morphology. J. Urol., 142:1602, 1989.

Clemmons, J. J. W.: Embryonic renal injury: A possible factor in fetal malnutrition [Abstract]. Pediatr. Res., 11:404, 1977.

Colodny, A. H.: Antenatal diagnosis and management of urinary abnormalities. Pediatr. Clin. North Am., 34:1365, 1987.

Cooper, C., Mahoney, B. S., Bowie, J. D., et al.: Prenatal ultrasound diagnosis of ambiguous genitalia. J. Ultrasound Med., 4:443, 1985.

Cowley, B. D., Jr., Smardo, F. L., Jr., Grantham, J. J., and Calvet, J. P.: Elevated c-myc protooncogene expression in autosomal recessive polycystic kidney disease. Proc. Natl. Acad. Sci. USA, 84:8394, 1987.

Crombleholme, T. M., Harrison, M. R., Golbus, M. S., Longaker, M. T., Langer, J. C., Callen, P. W., Anderson, R. L., Goldstein, R. B., and Filly, R. A.: Fetal intervention in obstructive uropathy: Prognostic indicators and efficacy of intervention. Am. J. Obstet. Gynecol., 162:1239, 1990.

Cruz-Orive, L. M.: On the estimation of particle number. J. Microsc., 120:1, 1980.

Dator, D. P., Peters, C. A., Retik, A. B., and Mandell, J.: The effect of congenital bladder obstruction on bladder smooth muscle nuclear number and size. J. Urol., 145:218A, 1991.

Davisson, M. T., Guay-Woodford, L. M., Harris, H. W., and D'Eustachio, P.: The mouse polycystic kidney disease mutation (cpk), is located on proximal chromosome 12. Genomics, 9:778, 1991.

Depp, R., Boehm, J. J., Nosek, J. A., et al.: Antenatal corticosteroids to prevent neonatal respiratory distress syndrome: Risk vs benefit considerations. Am. J. Obstet. Gynecol., 137:338, 1980.

Dickson, K. A., and Harding, R.: Decline in lung liquid volume and secretion rate during oligohydramnios in fetal sheep. J. Appl. Physiol., 67:2401, 1989.

Docimo, S. G., Crone, R. K., Davies, P., Reid, L., Retik, A. B., and Mandell, J.: Pulmonary development in the fetal lamb: Morphometric study of the alveolar phase. Anat. Rec., 229:495, 1991.

Docimo, S. G., Luetic, T., Crone, R. K., Davies, P., Reid, L. M., Retik, A. B., and Mandell, J.: Pulmonary development in the fetal lamb with severe bladder outlet obstruction and oligohydramnios: A morphometric study. J. Urol., 142 (Part 2):657, 1989.

Ebihara, I., Killen, P. D., Laurie, G. W., Huang, T., Yamada, Y., Martin, G. R., and Brown, K. S.: Altered mRNA expression of basement membrane components in a murine model of polycystic kidney disease. Lab. Invest., 58:262, 1988.

Ekblom, M., Klein, G., Mugrauer, G., Fecker, L., Deutzmann, R., Timpl, R., and Ekblom, P.: Transient and locally restricted expression of laminin A chain mRNA by developing epithelial cells during kidney organogenesis. Cell, 60:337, 1990.

Ekblom, P., Saxén, L., and Timpl, R.: The extracellular matrix and kidney differentiation. Prog. Clin. Biol. Res., 91:429, 1982.

Elbadawi, A., Meyer, S., Malkowicz, S. B., Wein, A. J., Levin, R. M., and Atta, M. A.: Effects of short-term partial bladder outlet obstruction on the rabbit detrusor: An ultrastructural study. Neurourol. Urodyn., 8:89, 1989.

El Dahr, S. S., Gomez, R. A., Gray, M. S., Peach, M. J., Carey, R. M., and Chevalier, R. L.: In situ localization of renin and its mRNA in neonatal ureteral obstruction. Am. J. Physiol., 258:F854, 1990.

Elder, J. S., Duckett, J. W., and Synder, H. M.: Intervention for fetal obstructive uropathy: Has it been effective? Lancet, 2:1007, 1987.

Elias, H., and Hyde, D. M.: An elementary introduction to stereology (quantitative microscopy). Am. J. Anat., 83:412, 1980.

Fine, L.: The biology of renal hypertrophy. Kidney Int., 29:619, 1986.

Fletcher, J. C.: Ethical considerations in and beyond experimental fetal surgery. Semin. Perinatol., 9:130, 1985.

Freda, V. J., and Adamsons, K.: Exchange transfusion in utero: Report of a case. Am. J. Obstet. Gynecol., 89:817, 1964.

Freeman, M. R., Song, Y., Carson, D., Guthroe, P. D., and Chung, L. W. K.: Alterations in gene expression and biochemical properties following spontaneous transformation of a prostatic fibroblast cell line [Abstract 149]. J. Urol., 143:226A, 1990.

Friedman, J., Hoyer, J. R., McCormick, B., and Lewy, J. E.: Congenital unilateral hydronephrosis in the rat. Kidney Int., 15:567, 1979.

Fry, J. L., Jr., Koch, W. E., Jennette, J. C., McFarland, E., Fried, F. A., and Mandell, J.: A genetically determined murine model of infantile polycystic kidney disease. J. Urol., 134:828, 1985.

Gardner, S., Burton, B. K., and Johnson, A. M.: Maternal serum alpha-fetoprotein screening: A report of the Forsyth County project. Am. J. Obstet. Gynecol., 140:250, 1981.

Gattone, V. H., II, Andrews, G. K., Fu-Wen, N., Chadwick, L. J., Klein, R. M., and Calvet, J. P.: Defective epidermal growth factor gene expression in mice with polycystic kidney disease. Dev. Biol., 138:225, 1990.

Glick, P. L., Harrison, M. R., Adzick, N. S., Noall, R. A., and Villa, R. L.: Correction of congenital hydronephrosis in utero: IV. In utero decompression prevents renal dysplasia. J. Pediatr. Surg., 19:649, 1984a.

Glick, P. L., Harrison, M. R., Golbus, M. S., et al.: Management of the fetus with congenital hydronephrosis: II. Prognostic criteria and selection for treatment. J. Pediatr. Surg., 20:376, 1985.

Glick, P. L., Harrison, M. R., and Nakayama, D. K.: Management of ventriculomegaly in the fetus. J. Pediatr., 105:97, 1984b.

Glick, P. L., Harrison, M. R., Noall, R. A., and Villa, R. L.: Correction of congenital hydronephrosis in utero: III. Early midtrimester ureteral obstruction produces renal dysplasia. J. Pediatr. Surg., 18:681, 1983.

Golbus, M. S., Harrison, M. R., Filly, R. A., et al.: In utero treatment of urinary tract obstruction. Am. J. Obstet. Gynecol., 142:383, 1982.

Gonzalez, R., Reinberg, Y., Burke, B., Wells, T., and Vernier, R. L.: Early bladder outlet obstruction in fetal lambs induces renal dysplasia and the prune-belly syndrome. J. Pediatr. Surg., 25:342, 1990.

Grannum, P. A., Ghidini, A., Scioscia, A., et al.: Assessment of fetal renal reserve in low level obstructive uropathy. Lancet, 1:281, 1989.

Greskovich, F. J., III, and Nyberg, L. M., Jr.: Prune belly syndrome: Review of its etiology, defects, treatment and prognosis. J. Urol., 140:707, 1988.

Grignon, A., Filion, R., Filatrault, et al.: Urinary tract dilatation in utero: Classification and clinical applications. Radiology, 160:645, 1986.

Grobstein, C.: Inductive epithelio-mesenchymal interaction in cultured organ rudiments of the mouse. Science, 118:52, 1953.

Gruenwald, S. M., Crocker, E. F., Walker, A. G., et al.: Antenatal diagnosis of urinary tract abnormalities: Correlation of ultrasound appearance with postnatal diagnosis. Am. J. Obstet. Gynecol., 148:278, 1984.

Guilian, B. B.: Prenatal ultrasonic diagnosis of fetal renal tumors. Radiology, 152:69, 1984.

Guilian, B. B., Chang, C. C. N., and Yoss, B. S.: Prenatal ultrasonographic diagnosis of fetal adrenal neuroblastoma. J. Clin. Ultrasound, 14:225, 1986.

Harris, K. P., Schreiner, G. F., and Klahr, S.: Effect of leukocyte depletion on the function of the postobstructed kidney in the rat. Kidney Int., 36:210, 1989.

Harris, R. D., Nyberg, D. A., Mack, L. A., et al.: Anorectal atresia: Prenatal sonographic diagnosis. AJR, 149:395, 1987.

Harrison, M. R., Filly, R. A., Parer, J. T., et al.: Management of the fetus with a urinary tract malformation. JAMA, 246:435, 1981.

Harrison, M. R., Golbus, M. S., Filly, R. A., et al.: Fetal hydronephrosis: Selection of surgical repair. J. Pediatr. Surg., 22:556, 1987.

Harrison, M. R., Langer, J. C., Adzick, N. S., et al.: Correction of congenital diaphragmatic hernia in utero: V. Initial clinical experience. J. Pediatr. Surg., 25:47, 1990.

Harrison, M. R., Nakayama, D. K., Noall, R. A., and deLorimer, A. A.: Correction of congenital hydronephrosis in utero: II. Decompression reverses the effects of obstruction on the fetal lung and urinary tract. J. Pediatr. Surg., 17:965, 1982.

Harrison, M. R., Ross, N., Noall, R. A., and deLorimer, A. A.: Correction of congenital hydronephrosis in utero: I. The model: Fetal urethral obstruction produces hydronephrosis and pulmonary hypoplasia in fetal lambs. J. Pediatr. Surg., 18:247, 1983.

Hawtrey, C. E., VanVoohis, B., and Robillard, J. E.: Experimental congenital unilateral hydronephrosis in fetal lambs, an anatomic and physiologic assessment [Abstract 66]. J. Urol., 133 (Part 2):130A, 1985.

Hay, E. D.: Theory for epithelial-mesenchymal transformation based on the "fixed cortex" cell motility model. Cell Motil. Cytoskeleton, 14:455, 1989a.

Hay, E. D.: Extracellular matrix, cell skeletons, and embryonic development. Am. J. Med. Genet., 34:14, 1989b.

Helin, I., and Persson, P.: Prenatal diagnosis of urinary tract abnormalities by ultrasound. Pediatrics, 78:879, 1981.

Heyman, S., and Duckett, J. W.: The "extraction factor": An estimate of single kidney function in children during routine radionuclide renography with Tc-99m DTPA. J. Urol., 140:780, 1988.

Hislop, A., Hey, E., and Reid, L. M.: The lungs in congenital bilateral renal agenesis and dysplasia. Arch. Dis. Child., 54:32, 1979.

Hobbins, J. C., Romero, R., Grannum, P., et al.: Antenatal diagnosis of renal anomalies with ultrasound: I. Obstructive uropathy. Am. J. Obstet. Gynecol., 148:868, 1984.

Hoddick, W. K., Filly, R. A., Mahoney, B. S., et al.: Minimal fetal renal pyelectasis. J. Ultrasound Med., 4:85, 1985.

Holthöfer, H., Kumpulainen, T., and Rapola, J.: Polycystic disease of the kidney: Evaluation and classification based on nephron segment and cell-type specific markers. Lab. Invest., 62:363, 1990.

Holthöfer, H., Miettinen, A., Lehto, V.-P., Lehtonen, E., and Virtanen, I.: Expression of vimentin and cytokeratin types of intermediate filament proteins in developing and adult human kidneys. Lab. Invest., 50:552–559, 1984.

Horikoshi, S., Kubota, S., Martin, G. R., Yamada, Y., and Klotman, P. E.: Epidermal growth factor (EGF) expression in the congenital polycystic mouse kidney. Kidney Int., 39:57, 1991.

Huland, H., Gonnermann, D., Werner, B., and Possin, U.: A new test to predict reversibility of hydronephrotic atrophy after stable partial unilateral ureteral obstruction. J. Urol., 140:1591, 1988.

Hutcheon, R. A., Kaplan, B. S., and Drummond, K. N.: Distal renal tubular acidosis in children with chronic hydronephrosis. J. Pediatr., 89:372, 1976.

Janetschek, G., Weitzel, D., and Stern, W.: Prenatal diagnosis of neuroblastoma by sonography. Urology, 24:397, 1984.

Jeanty, P., Dramaix-Wilmet, M., Elkhazen, N., Hubinont, C., and van Regemorter, N.: Measurement of the fetal kidney growth on ultrasound. Radiology, 144:159, 1982.

Josephson, S.: Experimental obstructive hydronephrosis in newborn rats: III. Long-term effects on renal function. J. Urol., 129:396, 1983.

Josephson, S.: Experimental obstructive hydronephrosis in newborn rats: V. Long-term effects on renal tissue solute content. J. Urol., 133:1099, 1985a.

Josephson, S., Aperia, A., Lännergren, K., and Eklöf, A.-C.: Partial unilateral ureteral obstruction in weanling rats: Hypertension and sodium retention [Abstract 43]. In Programs and Abstracts of the American Academy of Pediatrics Meeting, 1990.

Josephson, S., Ericson, A. C., and Sjoquist, M.: Experimental obstructive hydronephrosis in newborn rats: VI. Long-term effects on glomerular filtration and distribution. J. Urol., 134:391, 1985b.

Josephson, S., Robertson, B., Claesson, G., and Wikstad, I.: Experimental obstruction in hydronephrosis in newborn rats: I. Surgical technique and long-term morphologic effects. Invest. Urol., 17:478, 1980.

Josephson, S., Wolgast, M., and Ojteg, G.: Experimental obstructive hydronephrosis in newborn rats: II. Long-term effects on renal blood flow distribution. Scand. J. Urol. Nephrol., 16:179, 1982.

Kato, K., Wein, A. J., Kitada, S., Haugaard, N., and Levin, R. M.: The functional effect of mild outlet obstruction on the rabbit urinary bladder. J. Urol., 140:880, 1988.

Keating, M. A., Escala, J., Snyder, H. M., et al.: Changing concepts in management of primary obstructive megaureter. J. Urol., 142:636, 1989.

Keating, M. A., and Retik, A. B.: Management of the dilated obstructed ureter. Urol. Clin. North Am., 17:291, 1990.

Kekomaki, M., Wehle, M., and Walker, R. D.: The growing rabbit with a solitary, partially obstructed kidney: Analysis of an experimental model with reference to the renal concentrating ability. J. Urol., 133:870, 1985.

Kim, K. M., Kogan, B. A., and Massas, C. A.: Collagen and elastin in normal fetal bladder. J. Urol., 146:524, 1991a.

Kim, K. M., Kogan, B. A., and Massas, C. A.: Collagen and elastin in the obstructed fetal bladder. J. Urol., 146:528, 1991b.

Kirkinen, P., Jouppila, P., Tuononen, S., et al.: Repeat transabdominal renocentesis in a case of fetal hydronephrotic kidney. Am. J. Obstet. Gynecol., 142:1049, 1982.

Kleiner, B., Callen, P. W., and Filly, R. A.: Sonographic analysis of the fetus with ureteropelvic junction obstruction. AJR, 148:359, 1987.

Kogan, B. A., and Iwamato, H. S.: Lower urinary tract function in the sheep fetus: Studies of autonomic control and pharmacologic responses of the fetal bladder. J. Urol., 141:1019, 1989.

Koontz, W. L., Seeds, J. W., Adams, N. J., Johnson, A. M., and Cefalo, R. C.: Elevated maternal serum alpha-fetoprotein, second trimester oligohydramnios and pregnancy outcome. Obstet. Gynecol., 62:301, 1983.

Krieglsteiner, H. P., Lohninger, A., Riedl, R., Kolak, H., and Kaiser, E.: The assessment of foetal lung maturity by chemical analysis of amniotic fluid. J. Clin. Chem. Clin. Biochem., 24:705, 1986.

Kühl, G. P., and Seyberth, H. W.: Increased biosynthesis of PGE$_2$ and TxB$_2$ in human congenital obstructive uropathy. Pediatr. Res., 27:130, 1990.

Laing, F. C., Burke, V. D., Wing, V. W., Jeffrey, R. B., Jr., and Hashimoto, B.: Postpartum evaluation of fetal hydronephrosis: Optimal timing for follow-up sonography. Radiology, 152:423, 1984.

Lawson, T. L., Foley, W. D., Berland, L. I., and Clark, K. E.: Ultrasonic evaluation of fetal kidneys: Analysis of normal size and frequency of visualization as related to stage of pregnancy. Radiology, 138:153, 1981.

Leahy, A. L., Ryan, P. C., McEntee, G. M., Nelson, A. C., and Fitzpatrick, J. M.: Renal injury and recovery in partial ureteric obstruction. J. Urol., 142:199, 1989.

Lenz, S., Lund-Hansen, T., Bang, J., and Christensen, E.: A possible prenatal evaluation of renal function by amino acid analysis on fetal urine. Prenat. Diagn., 5:259, 1985.

Liley, A. W.: Intrauterine transfusion of foetus in haemolytic disease. Br. Med. J., 2:1107, 1963.

Liu, M., and Nicoll, C. S.: Evidence for a role of basic fibroblast growth factor in rat embryonic growth and differentiation. Endocrinology, 123:2027, 1988.

Lumbers, E. R.: A brief review of fetal renal function. J. Dev. Physiol., 6:1, 1983.

Mahoney, B. S., Filly, R. A., Callen, P. W., et al.: Fetal renal dysplasia: Sonographic evaluation. Radiology, 152:143, 1984.

Maizels, M., and Simpson, S. B.: Primitive ducts of renal dysplasia induced by culturing of ureteral buds denuded of condensed renal mesenchyme. Science, 219:509, 1983.

Malt, R. A.: Humoral factors in regulation of compensatory renal hypertrophy. Kidney Int., 23:611, 1983.

Mandell, J., Blyth, B., Peters, C. A., Retik, A. B., Estroff, J. A., and Benacerraf, B. R.: The natural history of structural genitourinary defects detected in utero. Radiology, 178:193, 1991a.

Mandell, J., Lillehei, C. W., Greene, M., et al.: Prenatal diagnosis of imperforate anus with rectourinary fistula: Dilated fetal colon with enterolithiasis. J. Pediatr. Surg., 1991b. In press.

Manning, F. A.: Fetal surgery for obstructive uropathy: Rational considerations. Am. J. Kidney Dis., 10:259, 1987.

Manning, F. A.: The fetus with obstructive uropathy: The fetal surgery registry. In Harrison, M. R., Golbus, M. S., and Filly, R. A. (Eds.): The Unborn Patient. Philadelphia, W. B. Saunders Co., 1990, p. 394.

Manning, F. A., Harrison, M. R., and Rodeck, C.: Catheter shunts for fetal hydronephrosis and hydrocephalus. N. Engl. J. Med., 315:336, 1986.

Manning, F. A., Hill, L. M., and Platt, L. D.: Qualitative amniotic fluid volume determination by ultrasound: Antepartum detection of intrauterine growth retardation. Am. J. Obstet. Gynecol., 139:254, 1981.

Mayor, G., Genton, N., Torrado, A., et al.: Renal function in obstructive nephropathy: Long-term effect of reconstructive surgery. Pediatrics, 56:740, 1975.

McConnell, J. D., Lin, V. K., and Cher, M. L.: Myosin heavy chain expression in bladder obstruction [Abstract 78]. In Programs and Abstracts of Neurourology and Urodynamics, the 20th Meeting of the International Continence Society, 1990.

McConnell, J. D., Robertson, J. B., Abernathy, B. B., and Limmer, R. L.: Myosin heavy chain heterogeneity in the developing rabbit bladder [Abstract 383]. J. Urol., 139:258A, 1988.

McCrory, W. W., Shibuya, M., Leumann, E., et al.: Studies of renal function in children with chronic hydronephrosis. Pediatr. Clin. North Am., 18:445, 1971.

McVary, K., and Maizels, M.: Urinary obstruction reduces glomerulogenesis in the developing kidney: A model in the rabbit. J. Urol., 142 (Part 2):646, 1989.

Moessinger, A. C., Collins, M. H., Blanc, W. A., Rey, H. R., and James, L. S.: Oligohydramnios-induced lung hypoplasia: The influence of timing and duration in gestation. Pediatr. Res., 20:951, 1986.

Moore, E. S., deLeon, L. B., Weiss, L. S., MacMann, B. J., and Ocampo, M.: Compensatory renal hypertrophy in fetal lambs. Pediatr. Res., 13:1125, 1979.

Nakayama, D. K., Glick, P. L., Harrison, M. R., Villa, R. L., and Noall, R. A.: Experimental pulmonary hypoplasia due to oligohydramnios and its reversal by relieving thoracic compression. J. Pediatr. Surg., 18:347, 1983.

Nakayama, D. K., Harrison, M. R., and deLorimer, A. A.: Prognosis of posterior urethral valve syndrome presenting at birth. J. Pediatr. Surg., 21:43, 1986.

Neal, R., and Andrassy, R.: Fetal surgery in utero. Tex. Med., 80:40, 1984.

Newnham, J. P., Thomson, M. R., Murphy, A., et al.: Successful placement of a pyeloamniotic shunt catheter for ureteropelvic junctional obstruction in utero. Med. J. Aust., 146:587, 1987.

Nicolini, U., Fisk, N. M., Rodeck, C. H., Talbert, D. G., and Wigglesworth, J. S.: Low amniotic pressure in oligohydramnios—is this the cause of pulmonary hypoplasia? Am. J. Obstet. Gynecol., 161:1098, 1989.

Nomura, K., Mizuhira, V., Shiihashi, M., et al.: Renotropic stimulation of DNA synthesis of proximal tubules and endothelial cells in the outer medulla. Nephron, 39:255, 1985.

Paik, S., Rosen, N., Jung, W., You, J. M., Lippman, M. E., Perdue, J. F., and Yee, D.: Expression of insulin-like growth factor-II mRNA in fetal kidney and Wilms' tumor: An in situ hybridization study. Lab. Invest., 61:522, 1989.

Pang, S., Pollack, M. S., Marshall, R. N., et al.: Prenatal treatment of congenital adrenal hyperplasia due to 21-hydroxylase deficiency. N. Engl. J. Med., 322:111, 1990.

Peters, C. A., Atala, A., Freeman, M. R., Retik, A. B., and Mandell, J.: Molecular indicators of abnormal renal differentiation in an animal model of congenital obstruction of the kidney. J. Urol., 145:244A, 1991a.

Peters, C. A., Bolkier, M., Bauer, S. B., Hendren, W. H., Colodny, A. H., Mandell, J., and Retik, A. B.: The urodynamic consequences of posterior urethral valves. J. Urol., 144:122, 1990a.

Peters, C. A., Lepor, H., Shapiro, E., Retik, A. B., and Mandell, J.: Changes in muscarinic cholinergic receptor densities in obstructed and decompressed fetal sheep bladders. J. Urol., 145:309A, 1991b.

Peters, C. A., Luetic, T., Docimo, S. G., Reid, L. M., Retik, A. B., and Mandell, J.: Effect of in utero vesicostomy on pulmonary hypoplasia in the fetal lamb with bladder outlet obstruction and oligohydramnios: A morphometric analysis. J. Urol., 1991c. In press.

Peters, C. A., Luetic, T., Hendren, W. H., et al.: Congenital cystic neuroblastoma presenting as an intrauterine sonolucent suprarenal mass. J. Urol., 141:248A, 1989a.

Peters, C. A., Mandell, J., Lebowitz, R. L., et al.: Congenital obstructed megaureters in early infancy: Diagnosis and treatment. J. Urol., 142:641, 1989b.

Peters, C. A., McConnell, J. D., Vasavada, S. P., Carr, M. C., Retik, A. B., and Mandell, J.: Changes in myosin heavy chain (MHC) composition in the prenatally obstructed sheep bladder [Abstract 8]. In Programs and Abstracts of the 59th Annual Meeting of the American Academy of Pediatrics, 1990b.

Peters, C. A., Reid, L. M., Docimo, S. G., Luetic, T., Carr, M. C., Retik, A. B., and Mandell, J.: The role of the kidney in lung growth and maturation in the setting of obstructive uropathy and oligohydramnios. J. Urol., 146:597, 1991d.

Peters, C. A., Whitcomb, W., Kozakewich, H., Carr, M. C., Retik, A. B., and Mandell, J.: The fetal kidney: Morphologic responses to obstruction and decompression. J. Urol., 143:253A, 1990c.

Preminger, G. M., Koch, W. E., Fried, F. A., McFarland, E., Murphy, E. D., and Mandell, J.: Murine congenital polycystic kidney disease: A model for studying development of cystic disease. J. Urol., 127:556, 1982.

Pringle, K. C., and Bonsib, S. M.: Development of fetal lamb lung and kidney in obstructive uropathy: A preliminary report. Fetal Ther., 3:118, 1988.

Purkerson, M. L., and Klahr, S.: Prior inhibition of vasoconstrictors normalizes GFR in postobstructed kidneys. Kidney Int., 35:1305, 1989.

Quennan, J. T., Thompson, W., Whitfield, C. R., et al.: Amniotic fluid volumes in normal pregnancies. Am. J. Obstet. Gynecol., 114:34, 1972.

Ransley, P. G., Duffy, P. G., Manzoni, G. A., et al.: The postnatal management of hydronephrosis diagnosed by antenatal ultrasound. Proceedings of the American Academy of Pediatrics, 1987, p. 28.

Rappolee, D. A., Brenner, C. A., Schultz, R., Mark, D., and Werb, Z.: Developmental expression of PDGF, TGF-alpha, and TGF-beta genes in preimplantation mouse embryos. Science, 241:1823, 1988.

Ray, D., Berger, N., and Ensor, R.: Hydramnios in association with unilateral fetal hydronephrosis. J. Clin. Ultrasound, 10:82, 1982.

Redding, R. A., Douglas, W. H. J., and Stern, M.: Thyroid hormone influence upon lung surfactant metabolism. Science, 175:994, 1972.

Reuss, A., Wladimiroff, J. W., Pijpers, L., et al.: Fetal urinary electrolytes in bladder outlet obstruction. Fetal Ther., 2:148, 1987.

Reuss, A., Wladimiroff, J. W., Scholtmeyer, R. J., Stewart, P. A., Sauer, P. J. J., and Niermeijer, M. F.: Prenatal evaluation and outcomes of fetal obstructive uropathies. Prenat. Diagn., 8:93, 1988.

Reznik, V. M., Kaplan, G. W., Murphy, J. L., et al.: Follow-up of infants with bilateral renal disease detected in utero. Am. J. Dis. Child., 142:453, 1988.

Risau, W., and Ekblom, P.: Growth factors and the embryonic kidney. Prog. Clin. Biol. Res., 226:147, 1986.

Roberts, A. B., Flanders, K. C., Heine, U. I., Jakowlew, S., Kondaiah, P., Kim, S.-J., and Sporn, M. B.: Transforming growth factor-β: Multifunctional regulator of differentiation and development. Philos. Trans. R. Soc. Lond. [Biol], 327:145, 1990.

Robichaux, A. G., III, Mandell, J., Green, M., et al.: Fetal abdominal wall defect: A new complication of vesico-amniotic shunting. Fetal Diagn. Ther., 1991. In press.

Robillard, J. E., Nakamura, K. T., Varille, V. A., Andresen, A. A., Matherne, G. P., VanOrden, D. E.: Ontogeny of the renal response to natriuretic peptide in sheep. Am. J. Physiol., 254:F634, 1988.

Rudolph, A. M., and Heyman, M. A.: Circulatory changes during growth in the fetal lamb. Circ. Res., 26:289, 1970.

Sanders, R., and Graham, D.: Twelve cases of hydronephrosis in utero diagnosed by ultrasonography. J. Ultrasound Med., 1:341, 1982.

Sawczuk, I. S., Hoke, G., Olsson, C. A., Connor, J., and Buttyan, R.: Gene expression in response to acute unilateral ureteral obstruction. Kidney Int., 35:1315, 1989.

Saxén, L.: Organogenesis of the Kidney. Cambridge, Cambridge University Press, 1987.

Schreiner, G. F., Harris, K. P. J., Purkerson, M. L., and Klahr, S.: Immunological aspects of acute ureteral obstruction: Immune cell infiltrates in the kidney. Kidney Int., 34:487, 1988.

Schwarz, R. D., Stephens, F. D., and Cussen, L. J.: The pathogenesis of renal dysplasia: I. Quantification of hypoplasia and dysplasia. Invest. Urol., 19:94, 1981.

Scott, J. E. S., and Renwick, M.: Antenatal diagnosis of congenital abnormalities in the urinary tract. Br. J. Urol., 62:295, 1987.

Scurry, J. P., Adamson, T. M., and Cussen, L. J.: Fetal lung growth in laryngeal atresia and tracheal agenesis. Aust. Paediatr. J., 25:47, 1989.

Seeds, A. E.: Current concepts of amniotic fluid dynamics. Am. J. Obstet. Gynecol., 138:575, 1980.

Seeds, J. W., and Bowes, W. A.: Ultrasound guided fetal intravascular transfusion in severe rhesus immunization. Am. J. Obstet. Gynecol., 154:1105, 1986.

Seeds, J. W., Cefalo, R. C., Herbert, W. N., and Bowes, W. A., Jr.: Hydramnios and maternal renal failure: Relief with fetal surgery. Obstet. Gynecol., 64:26S, 1984.

Shalev, E., Weiner, E., and Zuckerman, H.: Prenatal ultrasound diagnosis of intestinal calcifications with imperforate anus. Acta Obstet. Gynecol., 65:95, 1983.

Sholder, A. J., Maizels, M., Depp, R., et al.: Caution in antenatal intervention. J. Urol., 139:1026, 1988.

Skovbo, P., and Smith-Jensen, S.: Ultrasonic scanning and fetography at polyhydramnios. Acta Obstet. Gynecol. Scand., 60:51, 1981.

Smith, F. G., and Robillard, J. E.: Pathophysiology of fetal renal disease. Semin Perinatol., 13:305, 1989.

Smith, S. M., Pang, K., Sundin, O., Wedden, S. E., Thaller, C., and Eichele, G.: Molecular approaches to vertebrate limb morphogenesis. Development, 107(Suppl.):121, 1989.

Speakman, M. J., Brading, A. F., Gilpin, C. J., Dixon, J. S., Gilpin, S. A., and Gosling, J. A.: Bladder outflow obstruction: A cause for denervation supersensitivity. J. Urol., 138:1461, 1987.

Spencer, J. R., and Maizels, M.: Inhibition of protein glycosylation causes renal dysplasia in chick embryo. J. Urol., 138(Part 2):984, 1987.

Steinhardt, G., Salinas-Madrigal, L., Farber, R., Lynch, R., and Vogler, G.: Experimental urinary obstruction in the pouch young of *Didelphis virginiana*. J. Urol., 143:237A, 1990a.

Steinhardt, G. F., Salinas-Madrigal, L., Farber, R., Lynch, R., and Vogler, G.: Experimental ureteral obstruction in the fetal opossum: I. Renal functional assessment. J. Urol., 144(Part 2):564, 1990b.

Steinhardt, G. F., Vogler, G., Salinas-Madrigal, L., and LaRegina, M.: Induced renal dysplasia in the young pouch opossum. J. Pediatr. Surg., 23:1127, 1988.

Tanagho, E. A.: Surgically induced partial urinary obstruction in the fetal lamb: III. Ureteral obstruction. Invest. Urol., 10:35, 1972.

Teal, L. N., Angtuaco, T. L., Jimenex, J. F., et al.: Fetal teratoma: Antenatal diagnosis and clinical management. J. Clin. Ultrasound, 16:329, 1988.

Thaller, C., and Eichele, G.: Identification and spatial distribution of retinoids in the developing chick limb bud. Nature, 327:625, 1987.

Thomas, D. F. M., Irving, H. C., and Arthur, R. J.: Prenatal diagnosis: How useful is it? Br. J. Urol., 57:784, 1985.

Thomasson, B. H., Esterly, J. R., and Ravitch, M. M.: Morphologic changes in the fetal rabbit kidney after intrauterine ureteral ligation. Invest. Urol., 8:261, 1970.

Thon, W., Schlickenrieder, J. H. M., Thon, A., et al.: Management and early reconstruction of the urinary tract abnormalities detected in utero. Br. J. Urol., 59:214, 1987.

Thrall, J. H., Koff, S. A., and Keyes, J. W., Jr.: Diuretic radionuclide renography and scintigraphy in the differential diagnosis of hydroureteronephrosis. Semin. Nucl. Med., 11:89, 1981.

Vasavada, S. P., Peters, C. A., Carr, M. C., Retik, A. B., and Mandell, J.: The effects of infravesical obstruction on the bladder of the fetal lamb [Abstract 717]. J. Urol., 143:368A, 1990.

Vintzileos, A. M., Nochimson, D. J., and Walzak, M. P.: Unilateral fetal hydronephrosis: Successful in utero surgical management. Am. J. Obstet. Gynecol., 145:885, 1983.

Ward, R. M., Starr, N. T., Snow, B. W., Bellinger, M. F., Pysher, T. J., and Zaino, R. J.: Serial renal function in an ovine model of unilateral fetal urinary tract obstruction. J. Urol., 142(Part 2):652, 1990.

Wesson, L. G.: Compensatory growth and other growth responses of the kidney. Nephron, 51:149, 1989.

Whitaker, R. H.: The Whitaker test. Urol. Clin. North Am., 6:529, 1979.

Whitfield, H. N., Britton, K. E., Hendry, W. F., et al.: The distinction between obstructive uropathy and nephropathy by radioisotope transit times. J. Urol., 50:433, 1978.

Wigglesworth, J. S., Desai, R., and Guerrini, P.: Fetal lung hypoplasia: Biochemical and structural variations and their possible significance. Arch. Dis. Child., 56:606, 1981.

Wilkins, I. A., Chitkara, V., Lynch, L., et al.: The nonpredictive value of fetal urinary electrolytes: Preliminary report of outcomes and correlations with pathologic diagnosis. Am. J. Obstet. Gynecol., 157:694, 1987.

Winters, W. D., and Lebowitz, R. L.: Importance of prenatal detection of hydronephrosis of the upper pole. AJR, 155:125, 1990.

Wladimiroff, J. W., and Campbell, S.: Fetal urine production rates in normal and complicated pregnancy. Lancet, 1:151, 1974.

Workman, S. J., and Kogan, B. A.: Fetal bladder histology in posterior urethral valves and the prune belly syndrome. J. Urol., 144:337, 1990.

Zedric, S. A., Duckett, J. W., Snyder, H. M., III, Wein, A. J., and Levin, R. M.: Ontogeny of bladder compliance. Neurourol. Urodynamics, 9:595, 1990.

40

NEONATAL AND PERINATAL EMERGENCIES

John R. Woodard, M.D.
Rafael Gosalbez, M.D.

Neonate is the term generally applied to the newborn infant during his or her 1st and most critical month of life (Behrman, 1973). Whereas approximately two thirds of all infant deaths occur during the 1st year of life, most are during the neonatal period, with the 1st day of life being the most hazardous. Between 10 and 15 per cent of all neonatal deaths are attributable to gross congenital malformations (Schaffer and Avery, 1977). In a series of 543 autopsies performed on neonates and stillborn infants, 264 different urologic abnormalities were discovered in 91 infants or fetuses. That is, 17 per cent had one or more urologic abnormalities (Woodard, 1986).

We have witnessed increasingly specialized expertise in the management of urologic problems in the perinatal period. The urgency of diagnosis and treatment of infants with congenital abnormalities depends on the risks associated with that abnormality. A disorder that produces the most marked abnormality of form may not be as urgent a problem as one that produces a major abnormality of function (Keay and Morgan, 1974). Because the least easily recognizable urologic abnormality may be the one that requires the most urgent attention, an awareness of the possibilities is important.

A neonatal urologic emergency is any genitourinary condition during the 1st month of life that jeopardizes the gonads, the kidneys, or the life of the infant if there is a delay in either diagnosis or treatment. Therefore, it is crucial that urologists involved in the care of newly born infants be alert to the perinatal clues of underlying genitourinary abnormalities or diseases in the neonate and be acutely aware of those conditions requiring immediate attention. Because the pathophysiology and management of many of these conditions are dealt with extensively elsewhere in this text, this chapter will emphasize early detection and initial management.

CLUES TO THE PRESENCE OF UROLOGIC DISORDERS

Pregnancy

A family history or past history in the mother of *fetal wastage* should alert one to an increased likelihood of malformation, as should a family history of *chromosomal abnormalities*, such as translocation. Although severe obstructive uropathy, prune-belly syndrome, or renal agenesis might be signaled by the presence of *oligohydramnios*, neonatal ovarian cysts are said to be more common in pregnancies characterized by *polyhydramnios*. A pregnancy complicated by *bleeding*, especially in the first trimester, is more likely to produce a baby with congenital malformation.

Illnesses in the mother during pregnancy, particularly rubella and diabetes, are known to be associated with abnormalities in the baby; as are certain *drugs* administered during the period of gestation. Intrauterine growth retardation should further alert one to the possibility of an abnormality. As the *age of the prospective mother* passes 35 years, perinatal mortality more than doubles (Behrman, 1973; Keay and Morgan, 1974; Schaffer and Avery, 1977; Vulliamy, 1972).

The advent of diagnostic real-time ultrasonography and its widespread obstetric use in prenatal management has totally revolutionized the detection of urologic disease, particularly obstructive uropathy, in the fetus. Although technologic improvements are still occurring, the important role of diagnostic ultrasonography—prenatal and postnatal—in pediatric urology is now obvious. The impact of fetal ultrasonography is mind boggling. The idea of 4 or 5 months' prior warning of a neonatal patient, its sex, and its diagnosis, would have been virtually unthinkable even a few years ago.

Our concept of congenital obstructive urologic disease and its pathogenesis must now be altered to accommodate this elongated natural history. Because the patient is now presented to the urologist on the 1st day of life (or before) with a diagnosis (Fig. 40–1) rather than a symptom, the management of congenital obstructive uropathy requires the surgeon to be proficient in the care of neonates. These developments are tremendously exciting and theoretically offer the potential for improved therapeutic results. Thus far, however, attempts to alter the course of events in favor of improved renal function or improved infant survival by prenatal intervention in certain selected cases have been disappointing.

Strong evidence relates the occurrence of renal dysplasia to the presence of ureteral obstruction in fetal life. Yet, to prevent either renal dysplasia or pulmonary hypoplasia by an intrauterine drainage procedure, the obstruction would have to be detected earlier than is usually possible. Because morphogenesis and differentiation of the fetal kidney are achieved by 20 weeks in utero, intervention to decompress an obstructed kidney must be accomplished in the 1st trimester to preserve renal function (Abni et al., 1985; Bellinger et al., 1983; Kleiner et al., 1987).

The relationship between oligohydramnios and pulmonary hypoplasia is also well documented. Although renal factors, such as proline production, may play a role in fetal pulmonary development, the pulmonary hypoplasia associated with obstruction of the urinary tract appears to be due to oligohydramnios per se, which results in a lack of intraluminal stenting fluid for the developing fetal lung (Docimo et al., 1989; Reid, 1977). Fetal urine is the main source of amniotic fluid, especially in the third trimester. A severely obstructed urinary system may result in a marked decrease in the volume of amniotic fluid that is readily detected by ultrasound (Colodny, 1987).

Improvements in ultrasound technology have in-creased our ability to detect even subtle abnormalities. The fetal urinary tract may be evaluated not only for obstruction but also for renal dysplasia and other abnormalities, such as bladder exstrophy. Sites of obstruction and, at times, the exact cause of obstruction may be deduced (Cohen and Haller, 1987). Fetal urinary tract dilatation has been diagnosed in utero as early as 14 weeks of gestation. Although this case may be exceptional, the fetal urinary tract can often be delineated as early as 15 weeks of gestational age, and the kidney is routinely imaged between 17 and 22 weeks (Cohen and Haller, 1987).

An ultrasound examination at some stage during pregnancy is now common practice. Indeed, interval ultrasound examinations during pregnancy are a standard part of prenatal care in some countries (Hellstrom et al., 1984). A structural fetal abnormality is detected in 1 per cent of pregnancies, and 20 per cent of these are genitourinary in origin (Cohen and Haller, 1987; Colodny, 1987; Seeds et al., 1986). Most of these abnormalities are discovered in infants of women not known to be at increased risk to produce a child with such a malformation.

Labor and Delivery

If the mother is given *magnesium sulfate* for toxemia during labor, the neonate may have neuromuscular blockade with generalized hypotonia and bladder distension (Cockburn and Drillien, 1974). Asphyxia from a *traumatic delivery* can result not only in renal cortical or tubular necrosis but also in inappropriate antidiuretic hormone (ADH) secretion, leading to generalized edema. Congenital malformations are almost twice as likely to occur in babies born by *breech delivery* (Schaffer and Avery, 1977).

Approximately 0.9 per cent of all babies are born with a *single umbilical artery*, and controversy exists

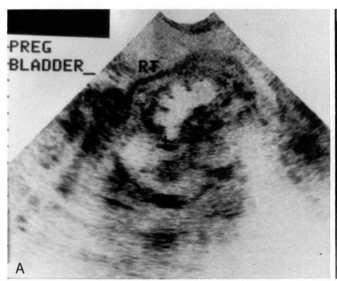 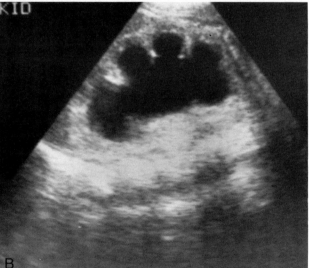

Figure 40–1. *A*, Fetal/maternal ultrasound at 28 to 30 weeks of gestation showing hydronephrotic right kidney. *B*, One day after birth, neonatal ultrasound confirming right hydronephrosis in otherwise healthy infant.

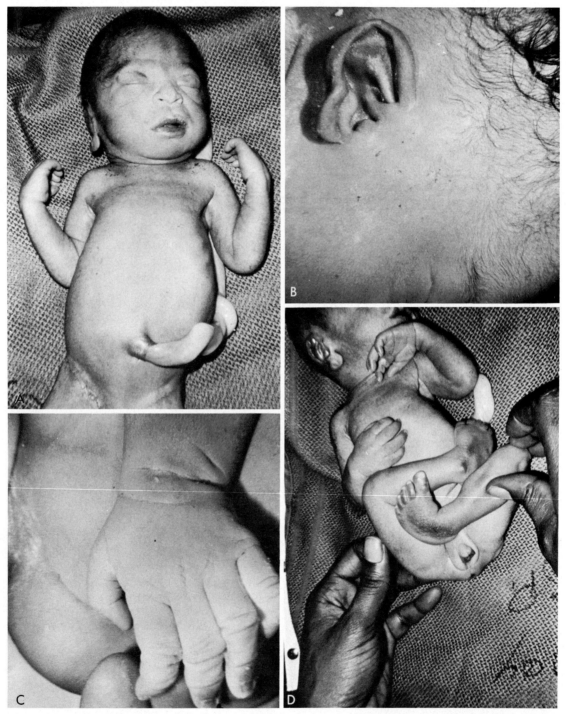

Figure 40–2. This newborn with bilateral multicystic kidneys was born of a pregnancy characterized by oligohydramnios, and he died from pulmonary hypoplasia. He illustrates the features of Potter's syndrome: *(A)* flattened face, "beaked" nose, apparent hypertelorism, skin fold below the eye, and micrognathia; *(B)* low-set, abnormally shaped ears with large lobes; *(C)* abnormally large hands with flabby digits; and *(D)* bowed legs with clubbed feet.

regarding its urologic significance. The mortality rate in infants born with single umbilical arteries is almost four times that of newborns in general, and of those who die, approximately 28 per cent have genitourinary malformations. However, in babies not having single umbilical arteries but born with malformations, the instance of genitourinary abnormalities almost equals 28 per cent as well. From the information currently available, it appears that surviving infants with a history of a single umbilical artery are suspect for having a urologic malformation, which should be investigated (Altshuler et al., 1975; Bryan and Kohler, 1975; Feingold et al., 1964; Froehlich and Fugikura, 1973; Gellis, 1975; Lemtis and Klemme, 1971).

External Features of the Neonate

Despite the foregoing discussion, many clues to the existence of urologic abnormalities are still derived from actual examination of the newborn baby. *Potter's facies*, characterized by large, low-set flabby ears and widely spaced eyes, is now well known as a sign of renal agenesis (Fig. 40–2) (Potter, 1946). These facies might also occur in some infants with prune-belly syndrome or bilateral multicystic kidneys (Williams, 1974).

Abnormalities of the external ear may signal the presence of a uropathy. Many syndromes in which urologic defects are a major feature are also characterized by *widely spaced nipples*. *Deficiency of the abdominal musculature* is a reliable indication of prune-belly uropathy (Fig. 40–3) and cryptorchidism. *Renal enlargements* are usually detectable during the initial examination of the newborn, and *abnormalities of the genitalia and anus* should also be obvious. Subtle clues, such as a *sacral dermal sinus*, may indicate either a spinal abnormality or a teratoma. Although this list could be expanded, Smith (1976) states that, if as many as three minor abnormalities are found, a 90 per cent likelihood of a major abnormality exists.

FETAL INTERVENTION

With the ability to detect obstructive uropathy in the fetus and the availability of interventional radiologic techniques to establish *in utero* drainage of the obstructed urinary tract, an opportunity is afforded that might both decompress the urinary tract and replenish amniotic fluid. The theoretic basis for in utero decompression of bilateral fetal hydronephrosis by means of a shunting catheter between the urinary tract and the amniotic space is obvious. Decompression should ameliorate potentially fatal pulmonary hypoplasia caused by oligohydramnios and, if it is accomplished early enough in renal development, prevent dysmorphogenesis of the kidney and preserve renal function.

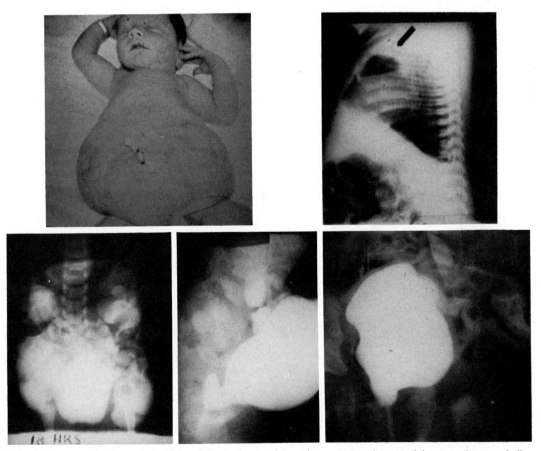

Figure 40–3. Infant with congenital hypoplasia of the abdominal musculature demonstrating the typical features of "prune-belly uropathy" and pneumomediastinum.

Table 40–1. ALGORITHM FOR RADIOGRAPHIC EVALUATION OF PRENATALLY DIAGNOSED HYDRONEPHROSIS

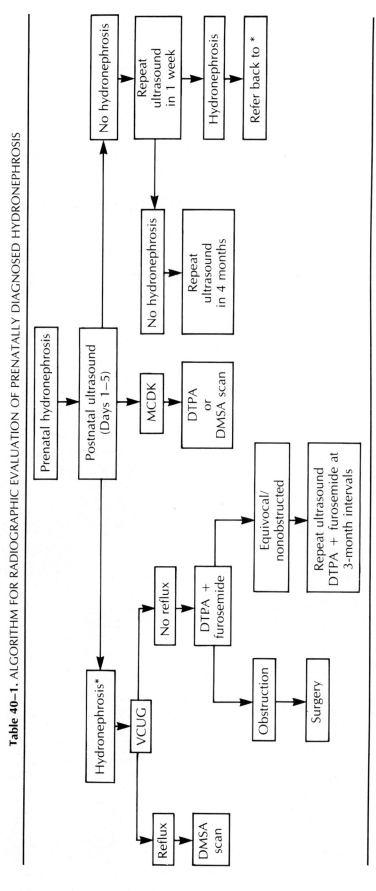

Abbreviations: DMSA, dimercaptosuccinic acid; DTPA, diethylenetriamine penta-acetic acid; MCDK, multicystic dysplastic kidney; VCUG, voiding cystourethrogram.

Despite early enthusiasm for fetal intervention engendered by these theoretic benefits, the efficacy of in utero decompression is yet to be established (Woodard, 1990). Furthermore, severely affected fetuses with associated oligohydramnios diagnosed prior to 24 weeks of gestation generally have not survived even when technically successful decompression was accomplished. In fact, in utero decompression at 20 or 21 weeks has failed to prevent either renal dysplasia or pulmonary hypoplasia. Lastly, and most importantly, one cannot operate upon the fetus without transgressing the mother (Colodny, 1987; Crombleholme et al., 1988; Dowling et al., 1988).

Because the risks of such intervention include injury to any of the fetal organs, life-threatening sepsis of either fetus or mother, premature labor, chorioamnionitis, urinary ascites, intestinal perforation, and possibility of an incorrect diagnosis, it is now generally agreed that *in utero* therapy for urinary tract decompression should be limited to an extremely small number of highly selected cases and performed in a few medical centers as clinical investigation (Crombleholme et al., 1988; Elder et al., 1987).

An understanding of the embryology of renal dysplasia and hydronephrosis as well as the development of pulmonary hypoplasia is basic to the management of the fetus with hydronephrosis. Fetal intervention rarely seems effective because early obstructive uropathy results in renal dysplasia that is irreversible. Thus, the fetus with urethral valves and associated oligohydramnios identified at 18 to 20 weeks of gestation has little or no expectation of recoverable renal function even if pulmonary development could be satisfactory.

Pulmonary hypoplasia is responsible for the high neonatal death rate resulting from oligohydramnios. The most important prognostic feature in the fetus with bilateral hydronephrosis and distended bladder is the volume of amniotic fluid. A normal volume indicates a level of renal function sufficient to allow normal pulmonary development. Such a fetus should be monitored every few weeks to ascertain that the volume of amniotic fluid remains normal. Early delivery is reserved for those rare cases in which diminishing amniotic fluid might conceivably have an adverse effect on later stages of pulmonary development (Elder and Duckett, 1988; Flake et al., 1986). Early delivery should not be performed in the fetus with unilateral hydronephrosis. Plans should simply be made to evaluate the fetus following term delivery (Table 40–1). In addition, decompression of the fetal urinary tract should not be performed for unilateral hydronephrosis unless the renal dilatation is massive enough to cause dystocia.

In most cases, intervention has been used for presumed posterior urethral valves characterized by bilateral hydronephrosis and distended bladder. The procedure involves ultrasound-guided percutaneous placement of a one-way catheter shunt between the fetal bladder and the amniotic sac. The International Fetal Surgery Registry reported 73 cases in which this type of vesicoamniotic shunt was placed. Survival was 40 per cent, both in those with oligohydramnios and in those with normal amniotic fluid. In 28 patients with bilateral hydronephrosis and oligohydramnios, who underwent a

Table 40–2. FINAL DIAGNOSIS IN 203 CASES OF FETAL HYDRONEPHROSIS

Neonatal Diagnosis	Number of Cases	%
Normal	41	20
Ureteropelvic obstruction	53	26
Ureterovesical obstruction	22	11
Multicystic kidney	29	14
Posterior urethral valves	13	6
Prune-belly syndrome	9	4
Ectopic ureteroceles	8	4
Vesicoureteral reflux	9	4
Other	19	9
Total	203	98

Adapted from Woodard, J. R.: Postgrad. Med. J., 66 (Suppl. 1):37, 1990.

corrective procedure, intervention failed to improve renal function; however, in one or two patients, it may have allowed more normal pulmonary development to occur (Manning et al., 1986).

Another problem concerning the feasibility of fetal intervention is lack of accuracy in urologic diagnosis. Although accuracy increases as the pregnancy progresses toward term, some reports indicate a rate of diagnostic error as high as 30 to 40 per cent (Colodny, 1987; Thon et al., 1987). Table 40–2 shows the nature of the lesion in 203 cases of fetal hydronephrosis compiled from several reports in the literature (Woodard, 1990).

The most common obstructive lesion was ureteropelvic junction obstruction; however, 20 per cent of those thought to have hydronephrosis were found "normal" at birth. In some instances, this finding may be transient fetal hydronephrosis. However, some newly born infants who have a history of fetal hydronephrosis will have normal findings on ultrasound at birth only to turn up several months later with hydronephrosis again. This phenomenon can be explained by the relative oliguria in the neonate period (Baker et al., 1985). Accordingly, re-examination is recommended for all infants with a history of fetal hydronephrosis not confirmed on neonatal ultrasonography or renal scan (see Table 40–1).

When a genitourinary anomaly is discovered prenatally, it is essential that the obstetrician, pediatrician, and pediatric urologist work together to maximize the chances for a successful outcome. Knowing that a fetus has a potential abnormality produces extreme anxiety in the prospective parents, and a team approach is helpful in providing not only optimal medical care but also emotional support.

SIGNS AND SYMPTOMS OF GENITOURINARY EMERGENCIES IN NEONATES

Abdominal Mass

An abdominal mass is the most common sign or symptom leading to urologic surgery in the neonate and requires immediate evaluation (Woodard and Parrott,

Table 40–3. FREQUENCY OF CAUSES OF NEONATAL ABDOMINAL MASSES IN 115 PATIENTS

Site and Cause	No. of Patients
Kidney	
Hydronephrosis	33
Multicystic kidney	35
Polycystic kidney	2
Renal vein thrombosis	3
Solid tumors	2
Retroperitoneum	
Neuroblastoma	7
Teratoma	2
Hemangioma	1
Bladder	
Urethral valves	1
Female genital tract	
Hydrometrocolpos	7
Ovarian cyst	5
Gastrointestinal tract	
Duplications	5
Giant cystic mecomium peritonitis	2
Mesenteric cyst	1
Volvulus if ileum	1
Teratoma of stomach	1
Leiomyoma of colon	1
Hepatic or biliary tract	
Hemangioma of liver	2
Solitary cyst of liver	1
Hepatoma	1
Distended gallbladder	1
Choledochal cyst	1

Data from Longino, L. A., and Martin, L. W.: Pediatrics, 21:596, 1958; Raffensperger, J., and Abousleiman, A.: Surgery, 63:514,1968; and Wedge, J. J., et al.: J. Urol., 106:770, 1971.

1976). Approximately one half of neonatal abdominal masses arise in the kidney, and one should not assume that a mass presenting anteriorly cannot arise from the retroperitoneal area. Table 40–3, a composite inventory derived from three published series reporting on abdominal masses, shows the relative frequency of various entities that are likely to present in the neonate as an abdominal mass (Longino and Martin, 1958; Raffensperger and Abousleiman, 1968; Wedge et al., 1971).

Disorders of the kidney accounted for more than 50 per cent of these abdominal masses, with hydronephrosis and multicystic kidney being approximately equal in frequency. Later data derived from fetal ultrasonography show the incidence of ureteropelvic junction obstruction to be significantly greater than the incidence of multicystic kidney (Brown et al., 1987). Of all masses recorded, 83 per cent originated in the kidney, retroperitoneal area, or female genital tract. Only 17 per cent were related to the liver or the gastrointestinal tract. Consequently, diagnostic evaluations should seldom begin with barium studies of the gastrointestinal tract (Longino and Martin, 1958; Raffensperger and Abousleiman, 1968; Wedge et al., 1971).

The most important aspect of managing the neonate with an abdominal mass is accurate diagnosis, and Table 40–3 lists most of the diagnostic possibilities. The evaluation of such a mass should proceed in a logical and

systematic fashion, beginning with careful abdominal palpation, which will usually provide important information. The size, contour, location, and mobility of the mass help to determine its site of origin. For example, a mass in the epigastrium that moves with respiration is likely to be hepatic, omental, or gastric in origin. When masses are bilateral, they are more often of renal origin, with hydronephrosis and polycystic kidneys (Fig. 40–4) being the more likely lesions. A smooth midline abdominal mass could represent a distended bladder; but in the female patient, it might be of uterine or ovarian origin (Figs. 40–5 and 40–6).

Following abdominal palpation, the simplest and often useful diagnostic tool prior to the ultrasound era was transillumination. This examination is still useful and should be carried out in a completely darkened room with a powerful light source, such as a fiberoptic system. It is most useful in white infants and helps to distinguish the solid from the cystic or fluid-filled lesion.

In the past, radiographic examination was considered the most definitive diagnostic modality. Plain films of the abdomen would usually confirm the presence of a mass and help localize it by showing displacement of the abdominal viscera with shifting of the intestinal gas pattern. Films were made in the anteroposterior and lateral projections with penetration sufficient to allow the detection of subtle calcifications that might occur in patients with meconium peritonitis, neuroblastoma, or teratoma.

The initial plain radiograph was often followed by excretory urography with infants tolerating up to 4 ml/kg contrast material, which usually produced satisfactory visualization of the urinary tract. The immature neonatal nephron, however, excreted slowly and concentrated poorly. A high dose of contrast material and delayed filming (Fig. 40–7) was required for maximum information, and the quality of excretory urography was usually better by the 3rd week of life (Martin et al., 1975). If opacification was inadequate on excretory urography, radionuclide renal scan would often yield complementary information, but it was generally agreed that the intravenous pyelogram was the single most important diagnostic tool in the evaluation of neonatal abdominal masses.

The introduction of real-time ultrasound has revolutionized the diagnostic approach to neonatal abdominal masses. Abdominal ultrasonography has become the most widely used and most important diagnostic study. With modern equipment, ultrasonography provides highly accurate and reproducible images. The machines

Table 40–4. SONOGRAPHIC CRITERIA FOR THE DIAGNOSIS OF MULTICYSTIC DYSPLASTIC KIDNEY

Presence of interfaces between cysts
Nonmedial location of largest cyst
Absence of identifiable renal sinus
Multiple noncommunicating cysts
Absence of parenchymal rim

Adapted from Peters, C. A., and Mandell, J.: The multicystic dysplastic kidney. AUA update series, VIII (70):50, 1989.

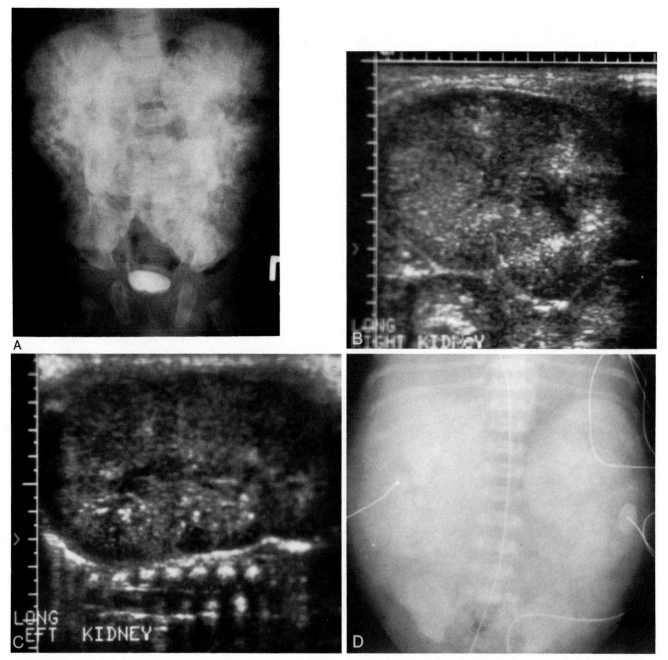

Figure 40–4. *A,* Excretory urogram (4 hours after contrast injection) in a neonate having bilateral abdominal masses. The film illustrates the "sunburst" appearance typical of infantile polycystic kidney disease. *B, C,* A more recent case investigated initially on day of birth with renal ultrasound showing right and left kidney markedly enlarged with heterogeneous echogenicity typical of infantile polycystic kidneys. *D,* Plain film of the abdomen on 1st day of life in same infant showing magnitude of renal enlargement.

are portable and are usually available in neonatal intensive care units and newborn nursery areas, avoiding the necessity of transporting sick neonates to the radiology department for examination. In most instances, an experienced ultrasonographer can determine whether the abdominal mass is cystic or solid and describe its exact location in relation to surrounding structures.

In addition, ultrasonography may distinguish between the two most common fluid-filled renal masses—hydronephrosis and multicystic dysplastic kidney (Sanders and Hartman, 1984). The sonographic criteria for diagnosis

of multicystic kidney have been described and are included in Table 40–4 (Peters and Mandell, 1989). When the differential diagnosis between multicystic dysplastic kidney and hydronephrosis remains in doubt, however, a radionuclide renal scan will often help to resolve the dilemma. The absence of tracer uptake with dimercaptosuccinic acid (DMSA) or early diethylenetriamine penta-acetic acid (DTPA) images supports the diagnosis of multicystic kidney (Sty et al., 1980). Once the diagnosis of upper tract distention is confirmed by ultrasound, evaluation is completed with a voiding cystoure-

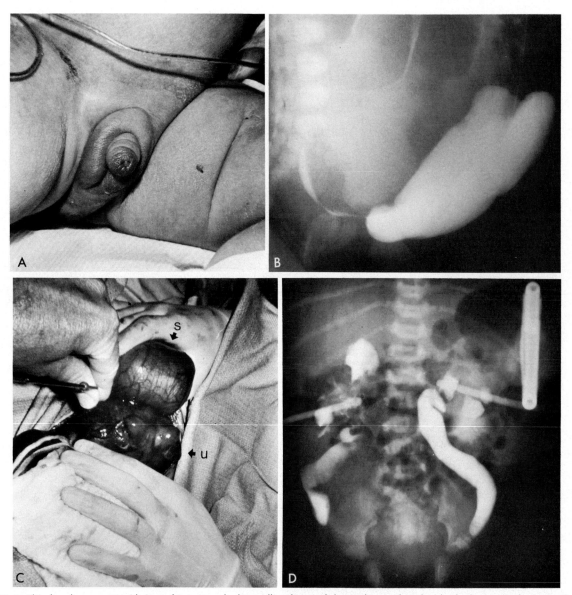

Figure 40–5. This female neonate with imperforate anus had a midline lower abdominal mass found to be hydrometrocolpos. *A,* The external genitalia appear ambiguous. *B,* The mass displaces the ureter posterolaterally and the bladder anteriorly. *C,* At operation, the distended uterus (u) is seen adjacent to the sigmoid (s). *D,* Postoperative antegrade pyelograms show lower ureteral obstruction persisting despite catheter drainage of the uterus. The baby died of sepsis.

throgram to rule out vesicoureteral reflux or bladder outlet obstruction. Table 40–5 is a listing of the most common cystic and solid abdominal masses.

Table 40–5. POSSIBLE ETIOLOGIES OF ABDOMINAL MASSES IN NEONATES BASED ON ULTRASOUND CHARACTERISTICS

Cystic	Solid
Hydronephrosis	Renal vein thrombosis
Multicystic dysplastic kidney	Neuroblastoma
Adrenal hemorrhage	Teratoma
Hydrometrocolpos	Congenital mesoblastic nephroma
Ovarian cyst	Wilms' tumor
Mesenteric, choledocal, or pancreatic cysts	Liver hemangioma
	Infantile polycystic kidneys

The evaluation of solid or mixed density abdominal masses may require further biochemical and radiologic tests. Studies should include serum levels of alpha-fetoprotein and human chorionic gonadotropin, and urinary determinations of vanillylmandelic acid and homovanillic acid (Hartman and Shochat, 1989). Additional radiographic examinations, such as radionuclide scans, excretory urography, computed tomographic (CT) scans, magnetic resonance imaging (MRI), arteriography, and venography, may occasionally be necessary to determine the exact nature of a particular abdominal mass, although the availability of ultrasonography has markedly reduced the need for these additional studies. Lastly, barium studies are indicated for the evaluation of bowel obstruction or intestinal duplications. A careful physical examination followed by appropriate diagnostic imaging should allow a correct diagnosis of a neonatal abdominal

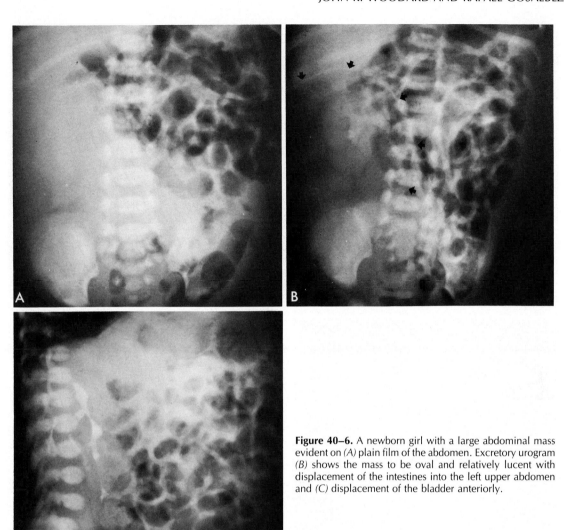

Figure 40–6. A newborn girl with a large abdominal mass evident on (A) plain film of the abdomen. Excretory urogram (B) shows the mass to be oval and relatively lucent with displacement of the intestines into the left upper abdomen and (C) displacement of the bladder anteriorly.

mass in most instances, so that a surgical procedure for diagnosis is seldom necessary.

Hematuria

An axiom of urologic practice is that either microscopic or gross hematuria must be fully evaluated in all patients. This axiom also applies to the neonate, for whom the need for evaluation may be more urgent. Possible renal and nonrenal causes of neonatal hematuria are listed in Table 40–6. Gross hematuria in the newborn is rare as evidenced by only 35 neonatal admissions to the Children's Memorial Hospital in Chicago for that reason between 1950 and 1967 (Emanuel and Aronson, 1974). Table 40–7 lists the narrow spectrum of causes of gross hematuria found in those 35

neonates. In the 11 undiagnosed cases, the possibilities included neonatal glomerular nephritis, hemorrhagic disease of the newborn, traumatic delivery, in utero vascular coagulation, and renal necrosis.

Table 40–6. CAUSES OF NEONATAL HEMATURIA

Renal	Nonrenal
Renal vein thrombosis	Adrenal hemorrhage
Obstructive uropathy	Endocarditis
Polycystic kidney disease	Air embolus
Renal artery thrombosis	Hemorrhagic disease of the
Nephrolithiasis	newborn
Medullary sponge kidney	Drugs
Wilms' tumor	
Glomerulonephritis	
Renal cortical necrosis	

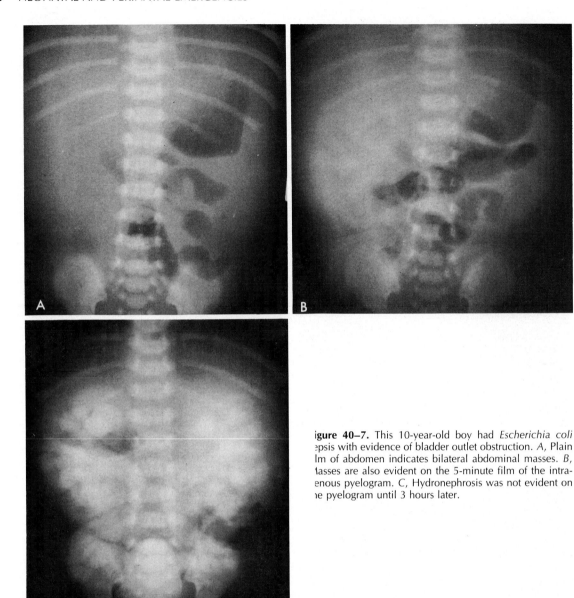

Figure 40–7. This 10-year-old boy had *Escherichia coli* sepsis with evidence of bladder outlet obstruction. *A,* Plain film of abdomen indicates bilateral abdominal masses. *B,* Masses are also evident on the 5-minute film of the intravenous pyelogram. *C,* Hydronephrosis was not evident on the pyelogram until 3 hours later.

In our experience, the neonate is vulnerable to three lethal conditions in which hematuria is likely to be a prominent sign or symptom (Table 40–8). These conditions require immediate recognition and prompt and appropriate therapy if survival is to be expected. The management of these three entities is discussed later in this chapter. Not discussed here are a variety of birth traumas, such as rupture of a distended bladder or hydronephrotic kidney during a difficult or traumatic delivery. In these circumstances, hemoperitoneum may be more prominent than hematuria (Cywes, 1967; Ravitch and Schell, 1961).

The increased use of umbilical artery catheters for monitoring purposes in neonatal units increased the incidence of renal artery thrombosis, the first sign of which might be hematuria (Bloch, 1988; Burdick et al., 1982; Caeton and Goetzman, 1985; O'Neill et al., 1981). Certain drugs, including indomethacin (Corazza et al., 1984), quinone, and 8-quinolinol (Bajoghli, 1982), have also been implicated in the etiology of neonatal hematuria. In addition, the use of furosemide (Lasix) may induce renal calculus formation in premature infants, resulting in gross hematuria (Gilsanz et al., 1985; Hufnagle et al., 1982).

Table 40–7. FINDINGS IN 35 NEONATES HOSPITALIZED FOR HEMATURIA

Cause	No. of Patients
Renal vein thrombosis	7
Obstructive uropathy	7
Polycystic kidney disease	6
Sponge kidney	3
Wilms' tumor	1
Undiagnosed	11

Adapted from Emanuel, B., and Aronson, N.: Neonatal Hematuria. Am J. Dis. Child., 128:204, 1974. Copyright 1974, American Medical Association.

Table 40–8. EMERGENCY CONDITIONS PRESENTING IN THE NEONATE AS HEMATURIA

Renal artery thrombosis
Renal vein thrombosis
Renal cortical necrosis

Hypertension

Arterial hypertension is a rare condition in the neonate, which requires prompt diagnosis and immediate treatment. The risk for developing potentially devastating complications, such as congestive heart failure and cerebrovascular accidents, is high at this age. The blood pressure at birth is normally low with a mean systolic pressure of 76± 10 mm Hg (Swiet et al., 1980). The blood pressure in the legs should be within 20 mm Hg of the pressure in the arms as measured by flush or Doppler techniques (Lees, 1973).

Hypertension may be congenital or acquired. Table 40–9 is a listing of renal and nonrenal causes of neonatal hypertension (Guignard et al., 1989). The most common cause of hypertension in the neonate is coarctation of the aorta; nephrogenic causes are second in frequency (Lees, 1973). Coarctation of the aorta proximal to the ductus arteriosus will result in hypertension, whereas coarctation distal to the ductus will likely produce congestive heart failure. Among the nephrogenic causes of hypertension, perhaps the most urgent is renal artery thrombosis, which has been observed more frequently since the introduction of umbilical artery catheterization for neonatal monitoring (Krueger et al., 1985; Neal et al., 1972; O'Neill et al., 1981; Plummer et al., 1976). Renal artery thrombosis may produce severe hypertension, rapidly leading to congestive heart failure (Woodard et al., 1967). The position of the tip of the umbilical artery catheter above L1, prolonged catheterization, injection of highly osmotic or irritating solutions, and infection are known risk factors of renal artery thrombosis due to umbilical artery catheters (Guignard, 1989).

Although adrenal hypertension in the neonate is rare, adrenal hemorrhage associated with hypertension secondary to renal artery compression has been reported (Bensman et al., 1982). Hypertension has also been associated with cases of the adrenogenital syndrome, in which a deficiency of 11-hydroxylase causes an accumulation of deoxycorticosterone, a potent mineralocorticoid, as well as of 11-deoxycortisol. The 17-α-hydroxylase defect also results in hypertension. However, hypertension in these forms of adrenogenital syndrome is inconsistent, and it is not certain whether this actually occurs during the neonatal period (Avery, 1975; Eberlein and Bongiovanni, 1956). Other rare causes of hypertension in the neonate include pheochromocytoma, Cushing's disease, primary hyperaldosteronism, and neuroblastoma.

The morbidity and mortality of uncontrolled hypertension in the neonate are considerable (Adelman, 1987; Levin et al., 1978; Rosendahl et al., 1980). Immediate medical treatment with antihypertensive drugs and prompt surgical treatment, when indicated, is essential to ensure a favorable outcome (Burdick et al., 1982; Guignard et al., 1989; Woodard et al., 1967). In a significant number of patients, the medication may be discontinued in the ensuing months following successful treatment (Adelman, 1987).

Abnormal Micturition

Oliguria, anuria, or a poor urinary stream in the neonate may be an indication of a urologic emergency. As seen in Table 40–10, most infants will void within the first 12 hours of life, and more than 90 per cent will void by 24 hours (Clark, 1977; Sherry and Kramer, 1955). Failure of micturition to occur during the first 24 hours of life should arouse concern, and the problem should be evaluated.

Urinary output in the term infant is approximately 1 to 2 ml/kg/hour. In the preterm infant, urinary output is signficantly higher, approximately 4 ml/kg/hour. With an abnormally low urine output, volume depletion should be considered as well as acute renal failure or severe structural renal abnormality. Lower urinary tract obstruction, such as posterior urethral valves, should also be considered in the presence of delayed micturition or a weak urinary stream, especially with a palpable lower abdominal mass. In our experience, a weak urinary stream was the presenting sign in 15 per cent of neonates requiring major urologic surgery (Woodard and Parrott, 1976).

One must also remember that a neuropathic bladder may be distended in the neonatal period and that a

Table 40–9. POSSIBLE ETIOLOGIES OF NEONATAL ARTERIAL HYPERTENSION

Renal	Nonrenal
Renal artery stenosis–hypoplasia	Coarctation of the aorta
Renal artery–aortic thrombosis	Bronchopulmonary dysplasia
Reflux and obstructive nephropathy	Hyperthyroidism
Polycystic kidney disease	Central nervous system disorders
Acute oliguric renal failure	Prematurity
Neuroblastoma	Adrenal hyperplasia
	Drug induced (heroin- and methadone-addicted mothers)

Adapted from Guignard, J. P., et al.: Biol. Neonate, 55:77, 1989. S. Karger AG, Basel.

Table 40–10. TIME TO FIRST MICTURITION IN 500 NEONATES

	Cumulative Percentage (%)		
Hours	*Term (n = 395)*	*Preterm (n = 80)*	*Postterm (n = 25)*
0–8	51.1	83.7	38
9–16	91.1	98.7	84
17–24	100.0	100.0	100

Adapted from Clark, D. A.: Pediatrics, 60:457, 1977.

palpable bladder may be the initial sign of the subtle neurologic deficit.

The infant with anuria and Potter's facies is likely to have renal agenesis. Oliguria and hematuria may signal a vascular catastrophy, such as renal vein thrombosis, renal artery thrombosis, or renal cortical necrosis. However, less ominous causes may be responsible for delayed voiding and bladder distention, such as drugs administered to the mother during delivery that cross the placental barrier and affect bladder function in the neonate. For instance, magnesium sulphate or ritodrine may result in transient bladder atony of the neonate requiring catheterization (Gross et al., 1985).

Scrotal Mass

Any firm enlargement of the testis in the neonate must be considered a possible torsion of the spermatic cord until proven otherwise. Unlike torsion of the cord in older children, which occurs intravaginally in a "bell clapper" situation, prenatal and neonatal torsion almost always occurs extravaginally, occasionally even intra-abdominally (Campbell and Schneider, 1976; Hcyden-rych, 1974; Watson, 1974).

In addition to torsion of the spermatic cord, the differential diagnosis of a testicular or scrotal mass in the older child includes epididymitis, incarcerated inguinal hernia, torsion of the appendix testis or epididymis, orchitis, and testicular tumor. These various conditions may also occur in the neonate, although they are considerbly less common at this age (Gierup et al., 1975; Qvist, 1955). However, hemorrhage into the testicle resulting from birth trauma might be found in the neonate.

Testicular tumors also occur in the neonate. In fact, approximately one fourth of all pediatric testicular teratomas are detected at or shortly after birth (Giebink and Ruymann, 1974). Other testicular tumors, such as yolk sac tumors and gonadal stromal tumors, have been described in the neonate (Kaplan, 1984; Lawrence et al., 1985; Uehling et al., 1987). No useful tumor markers for gonadal stromal tumors or teratomas have been found. The alpha-fetoprotein is often elevated in yolk sac tumors; but this marker may be misleading, because the level may also be elevated in the normal neonate (Kaplan et al., 1986).

Incarcerated inguinal hernia in the neonate is associated with a high incidence of testicular ischemia secondary to cord compression, and urgent surgical correction is indicated in this situation (Sloman and Mylius, 1963).

Ambiguous Genitalia

The embryology, pathophysiology, and management of abnormalities of the genitalia are dealt with in other sections of this text. However, infants born with ambiguous genitalia constitute at least a "social emergency" and require urgent evaluation.

The most common cause of sexual ambiguity is congenital adrenal hyperplasia. The typical patient is a genetic female subjected to excessive androgen exposure prior to the 12th week of gestation, resulting in a variable degree of masculinization of the external genitalia. If unrecognized, the salt-losing form of this disorder carries a high mortality rate. Therefore, such infants should first be evaluated for congenital adrenal hyperplasia and monitored with appropriate blood and urine studies. Second, the actual sex of the infant and the plan of management must be determined as soon as reasonably possible to minimize the trauma to the parents and the problems of dealing with relatives and with the community.

A diagnosis should not be forthcoming and corrective surgery should not be performed until the evaluation is completed. Such an evaluation might include serum electrolyte determinations, blood and urine steroid studies, x-ray examination of the urogential sinus (Fig. 40–8), possibly cystoscopy and vaginoscopy, x-ray studies to determine bone age, buccal mucosal smear for Barr and Y body studies, and karyotype. In the occasional case, diagnostic laparotomy with gonadal biopsies may be indicated. Data obtained from any or all of these studies plus evaluation of the potential of the external organs allow for a diagnosis and a proposed therapeutic plan.

Gender assignment follows diagnosis. Individuals considered at birth to have severe hypospadias should be more thoroughly evaluated to avoid erroneous assignment and to delay complications (Aarskog, 1971).

Ascites

Ascites is the abnormal accumulation of fluid within the peritoneal cavity. An infant with ascites has a bulging abdomen in which fluctuation, fluid wave, and shifting dullness can be elicited on physical examination. Radiographic examination demonstrates gas-filled loops of small bowel floating in a densely opaque background (Fig. 40–9), and abdominal ultrasound examination demonstrates free fluid in the abdominal cavity. This disorder is relatively rare in neonates, in whom the various forms include chylous ascites, ascites caused by syphilis, hepatobiliary obstruction with bile ascites, ascites caused by meconium peritonitis, and urinary ascites. Ascites might also occur with the nephrotic syndrome, for which the fluid is a transudate having a protein content usually less than 500 mg/dl (Spitzer et al., 1973). In approximately 15 per cent of the cases of neonatal ascites, the etiology remains unknown (Griscom et al., 1977).

Urine is the fluid most commonly found in neonatal ascites (Moncada et al., 1973), and obstructive uropathy is the usual underlying cause (Garrett and Franken, 1969; Krane and Retik, 1974; Mann et al., 1974; Parker, 1974; Reha and Gibbons, 1989; Scott, 1976; Wasnick, 1987; Williams and Eckstein, 1965). Although, in the past, this was considered a lethal condition with a mortality rate approximating 45 per cent, reports indicate that early aggressive treatment and improved neo-

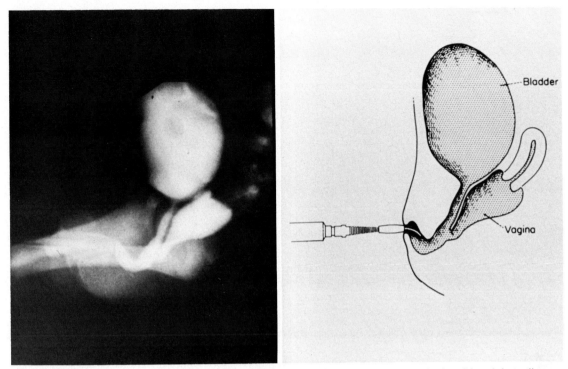

Figure 40–8. This artist's drawing and corresponding radiograph of a female neonate with congenital adrenal hyperplasia illustrate the simple radiographic technique for examining infants with urogenital sinus and cloacal anomalies.

natal care have decreased the mortality figures to 0 to 12 per cent (Greenfield et al., 1982; Tank et al., 1980).

Urinary ascites occurs seven times more often in male patients with the common primary obstructive lesion being posterior urethral valves. The second most common cause of urinary ascites is hydronephrosis due to congenital ureteropelvic junction obstruction. In lesser numbers, ascites has been reported to occur as a result of urethral stricture, urethral atresia, other bladder outlet obstruction, ectopic ureterocele, neurogenic bladder, hydrocolpos, sacrococcygeal teratoma, bladder perforation secondary to traumatic delivery, and urachal lacerations secondary to umbilical artery catheterization (Mata et al., 1987; Reha and Gibbons, 1989; Tank et al., 1980; Trulock et al., 1985; Wasnick, 1987).

The urine may enter the peritoneal cavity by several mechanisms. Although the site of extravasation is often undetected, urine may accumulate in the retroperitoneum from a leak in a ruptured calyceal fornix. From the retroperitoneum, it may enter the peritoneum either by direct rupture or by transudation. In other cases, urine enters the peritoneum from the bladder, renal pelvis, or urachus by direct rupture. The true incidence of urinary ascites in association with posterior urethral valves has been difficult to determine. Garrett and Franken (1969) reported ascites in one third of their valve cases, whereas Williams and Eckstein (1965) found only one example among 104 patients.

Some cases of ascites are now detected by prenatal ultrasound examination. In others, ascites is detected by physical examination or by radiographic studies that have distinguished the ascites from intestinal obstruction. A paracentesis will yield a urine-colored fluid that may have an elevated creatinine and urea content. However, because absorption of urine from the peritoneal cavity is rapid, equilibration of creatinine and urea contents of the peritoneal fluid and plasma occurs promptly. This mechanism may raise the blood urea and creatinine to levels disproportionate to the actual level of renal function. A high ratio of urea to creatinine in the ascitic fluid (30:1) has been described as a clue that ascites is urinary (Sullivan, 1972); however, lower ratios usually occur because of the rapid equilibration factor.

Because of its morbidity and potentially high mortality, urinary ascites must be detected promptly, evaluated quickly, and treated expeditiously. An immediate abdominal ultrasound examination should not only confirm the presence of ascites but also serve as a highly useful initial examination of the urinary tract, because obstructive uropathy is to be anticipated. A voiding cystourethrogram should also be done.

With this initial evaluation, treatment begins immediately with correction of fluid and electrolyte imbalance, keeping the patient under close observation for respiratory distress. Paracentesis may be necessary to combat respiratory embarrassment, which is common in severe neonatal ascites. Antibiotics are usually given. Prompt and appropriate urinary drainage is then indicated.

In the past, prompt upper urinary tract diversion or drainage was instrumental in improving the previously poor record of survival. It has been suggested that the surgical approach be the simplest one, appropriate to the problem, and that lower urinary tract drainage by means of bladder catheter may be satisfactory in some instances. Whatever the type of urinary drainage, it

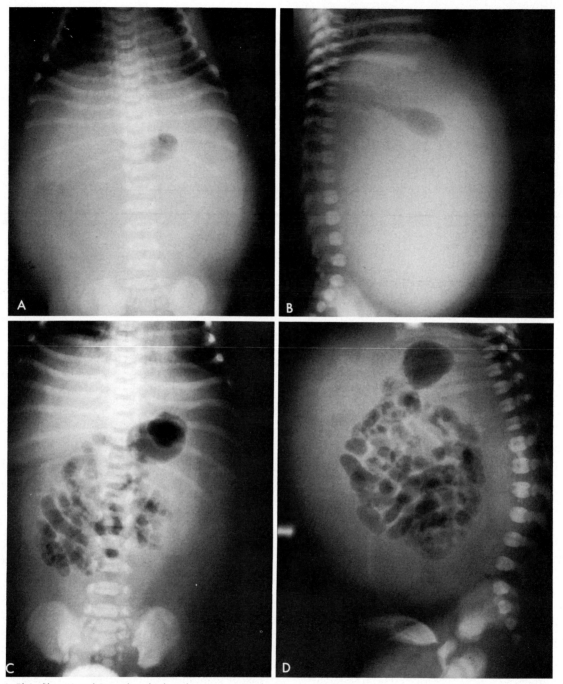

Figure 40–9. Plain films *(A and B)* made at birth and intravenous pyelograms *(C and D)* made several hours after birth in a female infant born with severe ascites. These films show the typical appearance of ascites with intestines "floating" toward the center of the abdomen. This child did not have an obstructive uropathy, and ascites subsided.

must be effective in decompressing the upper urinary tracts satisfactorily. If urinary leakage persists with reaccumulation of ascites, more proximal urinary diversion, such as placement of a nephrostomy tube, must be considered.

Early institution of proximal urinary drainage has significantly improved the outlook for these patients (Tank et al., 1980). This is particularly true in those cases resulting from ureteropelvic junction obstruction, for which percutaneous nephrostomy may be both diagnostic and therapeutic with subsequent antegrade pyelogram demonstrating the site of obstruction and extravasation (Wasnick, 1987). Bladder perforations and urachal lacerations require primary repair and urinary diversion by way of suprapubic cystostomy or vesicostomy.

After suitable correction of fluid and electrolyte problems and satisfactory drainage of the urinary tract, the infant is allowed to recover and stabilize before definitive treatment of the primary obstructive disorder is begun. Surprising, and paradoxic as it may seem, the development of urinary ascites may actually improve the long-term prognosis in many of these patients by decompressing the upper urinary tract in utero and by preserving the integrity of the upper urinary tracts.

Other Signs and Symptoms of Genitourinary Emergencies

Infants born with *cloacal exstrophy*, the most extreme variation in the exstrophy-epispadias complex, present an early problem in management. They are apt to have multiple system involvement in addition to a markedly shortened intestinal tract, resulting in poor potential for survival. Many will have an omphalocele requiring immediate attention. Some will have myelodysplasia. These infants are likely to have anomalous upper urinary tracts as well. In addition, practically all of these patients should be assigned as female at the outset (Diamond and Jeffs, 1985; Hurwitz et al., 1987; Marshall and Muecke, 1962; Mitchell et al., 1990; Tank and Lindenauer, 1970).

Infants born with *classic exstrophy* of the bladder, however, are usually not acutely ill and present no immediate problem. Associated anomalies of the upper urinary tract and other organ systems are infrequent. Most of these infants are amenable to primary functional closure of the bladder, and it is desirable that this procedure be performed within the first 24 to 48 hours of life, during which time the bony pelvis can be brought together anteriorly without osteotomy. Therefore, these babies require immediate urologic consultation. One should cover the exstrophied bladder with plastic wrap (Saran) to protect it from the abrasive and damaging effects of porous material, such as gauze (Jeffs et al., 1982).

Congenital absence of the abdominal musculature is readily apparent in the newborn. It signals the typical prune-belly uropathy (see Fig. 40–3). Such infants require immediate evaluation and close monitoring. Although some will have pulmonary hypoplasia or extreme degrees of renal dysplasia that make survival impossible, others will have no problems whatsoever.

Between these two extremes are the majority, who may have some pulmonary difficulties resulting from either pneumomediastinum or pneumothorax and severe urinary stasis making them vulnerable to bacteriuria with the possibility of increasing azotemia. These infants will require antibiotic prophylaxis and close monitoring of pulmonary function, renal function, and urine bacteriology. Instrumentation of the urinary tract should be avoided insofar as possible until a management plan is formulated. The role of early drainage and reconstructive procedures in these patients has been controversial and is discussed in Chapter 48 (Williams and Parker, 1974; Woodard, 1978; Woodard and Zucker, 1990).

It is common knowledge that a male infant with *imperforate anus* is likely to have a fistula connecting the distal gastrointestinal tract with the prostatic urethra or bladder and that an affected female infant is likely to have a rectovaginal fistula. It is also true that infants with imperforate anus are likely to have other major internal genitourinary abnormalities (Belman and King, 1972; Parrott, 1977; Parrott and Woodard, 1979; Puckner et al., 1975). At our institution, among 40 neonates evaluated because of imperforate anus, 21 urogenital abnormalities were found exclusive of rectourinary fistulae. These abnormalities included 10 instances of vesicoureteral reflux and/or hydronephrosis, and three fused or ectopic kidneys (Parrott and Woodard, 1979). Other studies indicate that between 25 and 50 per cent of all infants with imperforate anus will have associated urogenital abnormalities other than fistulae. Renal agenesis is frequently reported. All patients with imperforate anus should have voiding cystourethrograms and upper urinary tract imaging studies as part of their initial evaluations.

Persistent cloaca warrants special consideration because of the extent and severity of both the primary and the associated abnormalities. The "cloacogram," in addition to endoscopic examination, is helpful in delineating the abnormal anatomy. A much higher incidence of genital and urinary abnormalities is reported in patients with persistent cloaca than in those with other forms of imperforate anus (Parrott and Woodard, 1979). Such infants are prone to have hydrometrocolpos (Cheney et al., 1974; Raffensperger and Ramenofsky, 1973). Various degrees of vaginal and uterine duplication are also common.

SPECIFIC DISORDERS REQUIRING PROMPT UROLOGIC MANAGEMENT

Hydronephrosis

The evaluation and management of hydronephrosis are dealt with extensively elsewhere in this text. It is, nonetheless, the most common cause of a neonatal abdominal mass and one of the most common abnormalities in the neonate requiring surgical correction, and thus, it is discussed at some length in this section.

In the past, neonatal hydronephrosis usually presented as a palpable abdominal mass, for which the differential diagnosis has already been discussed. Currently, most neonates with hydronephrosis have had abnormal findings on fetal ultrasound study (see Fig. 40–1A), so the anomaly is expected to be present whether or not an abdominal mass is easily palpable. The most common site of obstruction is the ureteropelvic junction, being slightly more common in male infants and occurring bilaterally in 6 to 20 per cent of the cases (Brown et al., 1987; Elder and Duckett, 1988; Kleiner et al., 1987).

Once hydronephrosis has been confirmed by means of postnatal ultrasonography (see Fig. 40–1B), the presence of obstruction must be documented. Its site and severity requires delineation so that the proper type and

timing of treatment may be determined. Table 40–1 is a guideline for evaluating neonates with suspected hydronephrosis.

Although ultrasound and radionuclude studies are clearly the most important, excretory urography and retrograde pyelograms are still necessary in selected cases. Once the evaluation is complete, treatment should be directed toward preservation of renal substance. Pyeloplasty and other reconstructive procedures in the newborn can be very successful, and a kidney should be preserved even in the presence of a thin rim of recognizable renal parenchyma (Fig. 40–10).

In any neonate with a solitary kidney, bilateral ureteropelvic junction obstruction, or an obstructed kidney contributing less than 40 per cent of overall function by

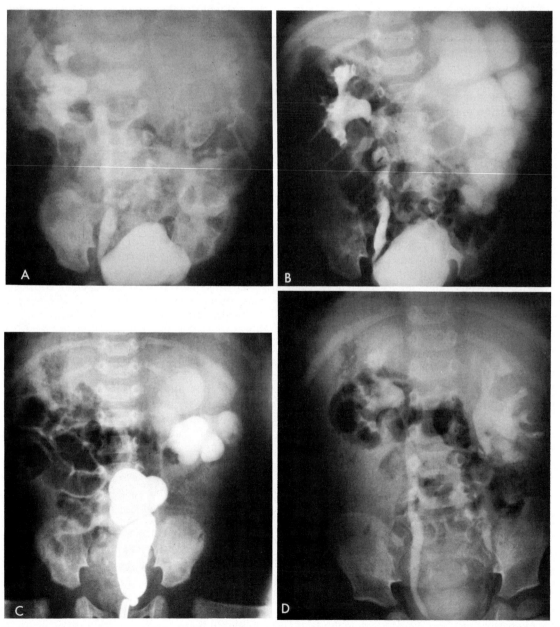

Figure 40–10. These excretory urograms at (A) 1 minute and (B) 2 hours in an infant with a left flank mass show massive left hydronephrosis with extremely thin renal parenchyma. Retrograde pyelogram (C) localizes the obstruction at the ureterovesical junction. An intravenous pyelogram (D) 2 years after tailoring and reimplanting the left ureter demonstrates the remarkable recovery potential of the neonatal obstructed kidney.

DTPA scan, early pyeloplasty is indicated. However, controversy exists over the management of neonates with otherwise asymptomatic unilateral ureteropelvic junction obstruction. Some prefer early surgical repair of the demonstrably obstructed ureteropelvic junction regardless of the degree of function of the involved kidney. Others defer surgical repair until such time as loss of renal function in the involved kidney can be demonstrated.

When indicated, however, pyeloplasty in the young infant can be done with minimal morbidity and excellent results (King et al., 1984; Wolpert et al., 1989). When hydronephrosis is not severe and the degree of obstruction appears equivocal, delaying surgical intervention to allow interval re-evaluation and better documentation of the degree of obstruction is the proper approach. Such a delay also allows for stronger maternal/infant bonding and perhaps improved anesthetic risks.

Ureterovesical junction obstruction is the second most common cause of prenatally diagnosed hydronephrosis (Brown et al., 1987). Formerly, primary obstruction at the ureterovesical junction was less likely to be recognized during infancy; but, with the advent of prenatal ultrasonography, the diagnosis is now usually made at birth. The postnatal evaluation of these patients follows the same protocol outlined earlier. However, obstruction at this site may be more difficult to quantitate than obstruction at the ureteropelvic junction.

The difficulty of assessing obstruction at the ureterovesical junction is partly due to increased compliance of the neonatal ureter, which complicates the interpretation of the diuretic renogram. Because, in the past, many of these patients did not become symptomatic until they were much older, and some improved spontaneously, some uncertainty exists concerning the natural history of congenital megaureter. At the present time, the surgeon is obligated to identify and select those patients having obstruction sufficient to require early corrective surgery and to carefully follow the other patients long enough to determine if the obstruction is significant or if the process is improving with time.

Serial radionuclide scans and ultrasound studies are necessary in many of these patients. Prophylactic antibiotics, at least initially, may also be appropriate in those patients selected for surveillance. Tailored ureteral reimplantation, either by surgical tapering or by folding technique, has proven highly successful in those patients demonstrating severe or progressive findings (Parrott et al., 1990). Treatment of this condition poses a dilemma; one report suggested that 77 per cent of patients with primary megaureters be followed conservatively, whereas another report indicated that 87 per cent of such patients were candidates for surgical repair (Keating et al., 1989; Peters, 1989).

Ectopic ureterocele is probably the third most common cause of neonatal obstructive hydronephrosis (Brown et al., 1987). Because it is a lesion that presented primarily because of urinary infection in the past, incidental discovery by fetal ultrasound may actually lead to earlier treatment with significantly improved results.

The standard surgical treatment for ectopic ureterocele consists of upper pole partial nephrectomy with or without excision of the ureterocele itself. Perhaps the incidental discovery of ectopic ureteroceles on fetal ultrasonography will lead to an increased salvageability of the upper pole segment. This, in fact, appears to be the case. Upper pole salvage has increased from 6 to 31 per cent in some series (Woodard, 1990). Some have suggested that initial treatment of the incidentally discovered ectopic ureterocele should be cystoscopic incision to relieve the obstruction prior to the initial infection. This procedure has produced gratifying results in early reports (Monfort et al., 1985).

Posterior urethral valves are the most common lower urinary tract obstruction in male infants and the third or fourth most common cause of fetal hydronephrosis (Brown et al., 1987). The neonatal ultrasound study usually demonstrates a thickened bladder wall and dilated ureters. Reflux may or may not be present, and the diagnosis is made by demonstrating the characteristic dilation of the prostatic urethra.

This disorder occurs in a spectrum and may produce a severe degree of obstruction with markedly damaged renal function. The mortality has been quite high in the past, and the outlook in severe cases must still be considered guarded. Because the high mortality in the past was at least partly attributable to urinary infection and electrolyte imbalance (Williams and Eckstein, 1965), incidental detection of posterior urethral valves in the fetus may afford an opportunity to treat this problem before the occurrence of either of these complications.

When the diagnosis is made, a small urethral catheter is placed in the bladder, prophylactic antibiotics are instituted, and careful attention is given to fluid and electrolyte management. The initial treatment of the infant with posterior urethral valves in many cases is simple endoscopic ablation of the valves, whereas other cases require a urinary diversion procedure, such as vesicostomy or ureterostomy. This disorder is discussed in detail elsewhere in this text.

Prenatal ultrasound imaging allows for the identification of some fetuses with *vesicoureteral reflux* (Scott, 1987; Seeds et al., 1986). This early identification offers a new opportunity to investigate the natural history of reflux and the pathogenesis of renal scarring. Patients discovered to have vesicoureteral reflux require the initiation of prophylactic antibiotic treatment. The definitive treatment of the reflux itself is discussed extensively in Chapter 44.

It has been shown that even severe degrees of hydronephrosis and hydroureter in the neonate can result from *sepsis* and that complete reversal may occur with proper antibiotic treatment (Alton, 1977; Lebowitz and Griscom, 1977; Uson et al., 1968). This possibility must be borne in mind when evaluating an infant with hydronephrosis and urinary sepsis (Pais and Retik, 1975).

Multicystic Kidney

Multicystic dysplastic kidney (MCDK) represents an extreme form of dysplasia associated with atresia of the ureter, which is classified as Potter type II (Potter,

1972). On histologic examination, renal dysplasia is apparent with reduction in the number of nephrons and no normal renal parenchyma. In most instances, MCDK is a unilateral phenomenon, although bilateral cases have been reported in association with Potter's facies (Williams, 1974). The cysts are variable in number, heterogeneous in size, and loosely bound together.

MCDK is the second most frequent cause of neonatal abdominal mass. Although it typically presented as an abdominal mass in the past, reports indicate that the majority of cases of MCDK are now being diagnosed in utero by prenatal ultrasonography (Arger et al., 1985; Avni et al., 1987; Hadlock et al., 1981). This change has produced a large number of patients with asymptomatic MCDK in whom the indications for surgical excision remain unclear. Although most patients were previously operated on and the MCDK removed, many reports now advocate conservative management with long-term surveillance (Avni et al., 1987; Belman, 1987; Gordon et al., 1988).

The natural history of MCDK has not yet been determined, but some have undergone spontaneous involution (Avni et al., 1987; Pedicelli et al., 1986). The possible complications of MCDK include pain, infection, hypertension, and neoplasia (Ambrose et al., 1982; Barrett and Wineland, 1980; Birken et al., 1985; Gordon et al., 1988; Hartman et al., 1986; Susskind and King, 1987). In addition, Snyder and co-workers (1986) noted neuroblastoma elements in several dysplastic segments of MCDK specimens. These reports emphasize the need for close follow-up surveillance of nonoperated patients and for inclusion of these patients in a national MCDK registry (Wacksman, 1987).

Although in most neonates with MCDK, the condition has been detected prenatally, a palpable abdominal mass is usually present, which is typically nontender, mobile, and irregular in shape. In addition to the previously discussed sonographic criteria for the diagnosis of MCDK, renal scan (DTPA or DMSA) (Fig. 40–11) will show no evidence of functioning renal tissue on the affected side (Sty et al., 1980). There appears to be a significant likelihood of an associated urologic anomaly, with a reported incidence of up to 33 per cent, including contralateral renal agenesis, horseshoe kidney, contralateral ureteropelvic junction obstruction, obstructed megaureter, and vesicoureteral reflux.

Treatment alternatives include surgical excision or surveillance. Clearly, surgical exploration is indicated when the diagnosis is less than certain or when the MCDK constitutes a large abdominal mass that might produce secondary respiratory or gastrointestinal complaints. Surgery has also been advocated when follow-up surveillance is deemed to be unreliable or when the parents are unwilling to make that commitment. If surgical removal is to be done on an elective basis, it should probably be done when anesthetic risk is minimal, such as after age 2 months.

Renal Vein Thrombosis

Although uncommon, renal vein thrombosis (RVT) is the cause of approximately 20 per cent of the cases of gross hematuria occurring in the 1st month of life and is a prominent cause of renal enlargement (Emanuel and Aronson, 1974; Longino and Martin, 1958; Parrott and Woodard, 1976; Raffensperger and Abousleiman, 1968; Wedge et al., 1971). It implies a serious prognosis,

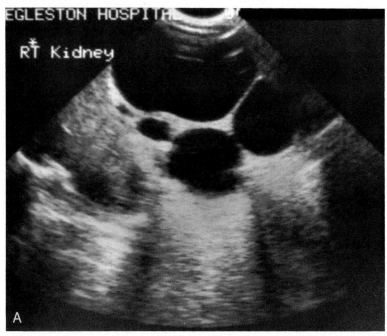

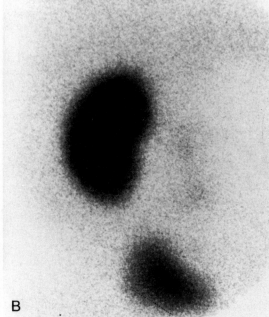

Figure 40–11. *A,* Ultrasound image of right kidney in 4-day-old female infant with a history of abnormal right kidney on fetal ultrasound study during third trimester. She had an easily palpable mass in the right flank. *B,* Dimercaptosuccinic acid renal scan in same infant 4 days later showing a normal-appearing left kidney with no evidence of isotope uptake on right side.

especially when bilateral. In the pediatric age group, approximately 65 per cent of cases of RVT occur in the neonatal period with the majority presenting during the first 2 weeks of life (Lloyd, 1986). RVT has also been diagnosed in utero (Evans et al., 1981; Tank et al., 1974).

The arterial pressure in the neonate is uniformly low and is reflected in a low venous pressure. The nature of renal circulation, with a double capillary network, results in further slowing of the bloodstream in the renal vein. This sluggish renal perfusion in the normally polycythemic neonate, especially if combined with trauma, dehydration, infection, vascular endothelial damage, or dehydrating effects of a diabetic mother, creates an ideal situation for RVT to occur (Belman et al., 1970; McFarland, 1965; Verhagen et al., 1965).

RVT has also been reported in otherwise healthy neonates (Fielding et al., 1986). Up to 20 per cent of cases are said to be bilateral, in which the thrombosis may be bilateral and caval in origin or in which the thrombosis may be caval in origin, with involvement of both renal veins, or bilateral, with simultaneous renal vein thrombosis in the absence of caval involvement. It is generally believed, however, that a unilateral renal vein thrombosis does not propagate to become bilateral renal vein thrombosis (Belman et al., 1970; Thompson et al., 1974).

Primary RVT occurs suddenly in a previous healthy neonate, whereas secondary RVT results from a known cause, such as diarrhea with dehydration. Secondary RVT carries a poorer prognosis for the patient (McFarland, 1965). The site of origin of the thrombotic process is variable. However, in unilateral RVT, the thrombus usually originates peripherally in the small intrarenal branches of the renal vein.

The clinical features of RVT are listed in Table 40–11. Although the typical clinical picture is that of a firm, enlarging kidney accompanied by hematuria and proteinuria in a sick infant, the constitutional disturbance may be very mild. Gross hematuria is a consistent finding and is due to hemorrhagic infarction. Anemia, secondary to hemolysis, hematuria, or the trapping of erythrocytes in the thrombotic process, may occur, and blood transfusion is occasionally necessary.

Thrombocytopenia secondary to trapping of platelets within the thrombotic process is also a remarkably consistent finding. However, it has generally not resulted in bleeding problems from other sites or during operation. Thrombocytopenia is such a consistent feature of this disorder that, when it is absent, one suspects the RVT to have occurred sometime earlier and to be in the resolving stage. The renal enlargement is readily apparent, smooth, and firm. Initially, the mass enlarges, but it can be felt to diminish as the process resolves.

Although proteinuria occurs in neonatal RVT, it is not as prominent a feature as it is in the adult type of thrombosis, in which it may be massive. Shock or a sepsis-like clinical picture is variable and may be in part due to the predisposing factors as well as to the infarction itself. Such a septic picture can be confusing until the renal mass is detected. Azotemia is usually present, even in unilateral thrombosis (Belman et al., 1970; McFarland, 1965). Lower extremity edema may be present with inferior vena cava thrombosis, and pulmonary embolus is a potential complication (Duncan et al., 1977).

Abdominal ultrasonography is very helpful in establishing the diagnosis of RVT in the neonate (Metreweli and Pearson, 1984). A renal vein thrombus can usually be demonstrated along with enlargement of the ipsilateral kidney. In addition, this study allows evaluation of the inferior vena cava. Nonfunction of the involved kidney, either on intravenous pyelogram or on DTPA renal scan, helps confirm the diagnosis. Although a CT scan may be helpful in determining the extent of the thrombus when the vena cava is involved, it is usually unnecessary. The role of MRI in this setting is also yet to be determined. Cavography/venography may occasionally be necessary, particularly in evaluating the bilateral cases.

The treatment of RVT should begin with hydration and correction of the electrolyte imbalance. Antibiotics are also recommended. Beyond that, treatment is still slightly controversial. Heparin has been recommended because of its activity against thrombin formation and platelet aggregation and its success in treating disseminated intravascular clotting.

When heparin is used, the dose schedule usually starts with 100 U/kg every 4 hours, with the aim of keeping the clotting time to 1 to 2 times normal. Treatment with heparin should last for 1 to 2 weeks (Belman et al., 1970; Seeler et al., 1970). Selective intravenous thrombolytic therapy with low-dose streptokinase (50 U/kg/hour) has been used in infants and children with success and with acceptable morbidity (LeBlanc et al., 1986; Pritchard et al., 1985). Potential complications associated with systemic use of streptokinase include major hemorrhage (Bell and Meek, 1979) and severe allergic reactions (Dotter et al., 1974). These complications are uncommon, however, with selective low-dose therapy. Although fibrolytic therapy for RVT in the neonate is still evolving, reports in the literature indicate that it may be a viable alternative, which deserves continued investigation. Early nephrectomy in the treatment of unilateral RVT is rarely necessary and should be done only for difficult-to-control hemorrhage or infection.

Bilateral RVT, a more serious problem, requires more aggressive management (Fig. 40–12). Renal failure, pulmonary embolus, and death are possible complications (Duncan et al., 1977). The initial management might be the same as in the unilateral case. When the primary process is caval thrombosis, surgical thrombectomy is an option. At operation, both kidneys should be pre-

Table 40–11. CLINICAL FEATURES OF RENAL VEIN THROMBOSIS

Renal enlargement
Hematuria
Thrombocytopenia
Anemia
Azotemia
Nonfunction on intravenous pyelogram
Proteinuria
"Shock-sepsis"

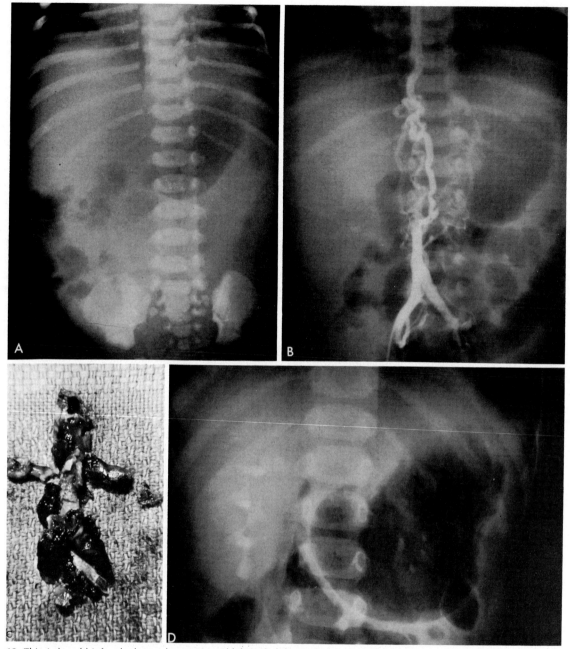

Figure 40–12. This 1-day-old infant had gross hematuria and bilateral abdominal masses. *A,* The excretory urogram failed to show any excretion at 4 hours. *B,* An inferior venacavogram demonstrated caval obstruction at the level of the renal veins with collateral venous return by way of the azygous system. *C,* At operation, the thrombus was extracted from the cava and both renal veins, with subsequent renal vein "back bleeding." Three years later, the child was normotensive with normal blood urea nitrogen and creatinine values. *D,* An intravenous pyelogram shows bilateral renal function but a small left kidney.

served, whether or not good back bleeding is achieved after extraction of the thrombi. Vigorous postoperative care, which may include peritoneal dialysis, is required. Aggressive supportive therapy, including peritoneal dialysis, plus fibrinolytic therapy to restore rapid renal vein patency has resulted in an excellent survival rate among this high-risk group of patients (Bromberg and Firlit, 1990; Pritchard et al., 1985).

Following RVT, the involved kidney may recover completely or may show evidence of damage. The result may be nonfunction with complete fibrosis, partial fibrosis with diminished function, renal hypertension, ne-

phrotic syndrome, or chronic renal infection. Chronic renal tubular dysfunction may also result (Stark and Geiger, 1973). If sufficiently severe, these late complications may necessitate delayed nephrectomy.

Adrenal Hemorrhage

Small hemorrhages into the adrenal glands of neonates are surprisingly frequent; they are found in 1 to 2 per cent of cases undergoing autopsy examination (Black and Williams, 1973; DeSa and Nicholls, 1972). Massive adrenal hemorrhage (Fig. 40–13), however, is an entirely different entity. It is an uncommon occurrence that, as reported in the older literature, carried a high mortality. For instance, before 1965, only three cases were reported in which the diagnosis was made prior to death (Sober and Hirsch, 1965). Until 1970, only 13 cases had been accurately diagnosed and successfully treated during the neonatal period (Eklof et al., 1975). Improved neonatal care and wide use of diagnostic ultrasonography seem to have led to the more frequent discovery of less serious adrenal hemorrhages during the 1st week of life. Although uniform diagnostic and therapeutic guidelines are still evolving, it appears that most of these cases can be managed conservatively.

It has been speculated that a sudden increase in pressure in the inferior vena cava is readily transmitted to the right adrenal gland by way of a short adrenal vein, whereas it is blunted by the longer renal vein on the left side, thus placing the right adrenal gland at higher risk of hemorrhage. Approximately 10 per cent of cases are bilateral (Hartman and Shochat, 1989).

The traumatic events of childbirth, prolonged labor, difficult or traumatic delivery, and possible resuscitative efforts appear to be leading etiologic factors with large birthweight, perinatal anoxia, bradycardia, sepsis, and hypoprothrombinemia possibly being additional contributing factors (Emery and Zachary, 1952). These events tend to produce prolonged abdominal compression, which renders the neonate susceptible to massive adrenal hemorrhage, especially when coupled with or in combination with hypoprothrombinemia, increased vascular fragility, and disseminated thromboembolic lesions with possible thrombocytopenia.

The clinical features of massive adrenal hemorrhage include the presence of a mass in one or both flanks; signs of blood loss, such as anemia, paleness, shock, or lethargy; jaundice; and urinary infections or sepsis. Azotemia may be present. Whereas gross hematuria usually occurs with RVT, microscopic hematuria is likely in adrenal hemorrhage. Ultrasound is presently the most valuable radiologic tool for confirming the diagnosis.

The sonographic appearance of adrenal hemorrhage

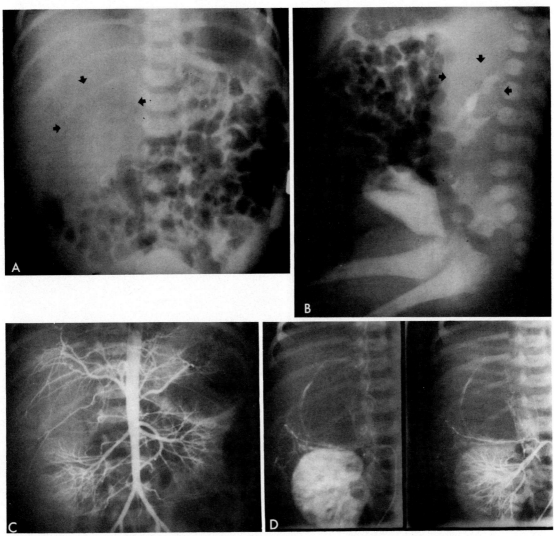

Figure 40–13. *A* and *B,* Excretory urograms in an infant with massive adrenal hemorrhage, showing a mass above the right kidney. Aortogram *(C)* and selective renal arteriograms *(D)* confirm that the mass is of adrenal origin with an avascular center. *Note:* Studies such as these are seldom necessary since the advent of high-resolution real time ultrasonography as shown in Figure 40–14.

(Fig. 40–14) is variable (Eklof et al., 1986). Although, initially, the mass tends to be highly echogenic and irregular, complex and cystic masses are also commonly identified (Cohen et al., 1986). Serial ultrasound examinations will show a progressive diminution in size and a cystic appearance of the mass because of liquefaction and reabsorption of the hematoma (Eklof et al., 1986). Calcifications will also be identified and have been reported as early as 7 days after the hemorrhage (Smith and Middleton, 1979).

The ultrasonographer should make a special effort to image the ipsilateral kidney. Enlargement of the ipsilateral kidney and the presence of microscopic or gross hematuria may indicate concomitant RVT. This finding has been reported by several investigators and demands further work-up with a functional renal study (Bowen and Smazal, 1981; Eklof et al., 1986; Khuri et al., 1980; Lebowitz and Belman, 1983). On plain x-ray film, pe-

ripheral shell-like calcifications of the mass are typical of adrenal hemorrhage, whereas stippled calcifications and widening of the paravertebral soft tissues are suggestive of neuroblastoma (Galatius-Jensen and Damgaard-Pedersen, 1981). Excretory urography is not often indicated in the evaluation of adrenal hemorrhage, and CT scan and angiography are also seldom required.

The differential diagnosis should include neuroblastoma, adrenal cyst, renal tumor, and ureteral duplication anomalies. Special consideration must be given to neuroblastoma, because it accounts for 50 per cent of all neonatal malignancies; approximately 65 per cent of these arise in the adrenal gland/retroperitoneum (Hartman and Shochat, 1989). Concomitant adrenal hemorrhage and neuroblastoma have also been reported (Eklof et al., 1986). Sonographic appearance of neuroblastoma may actually be indistinguishable from that of adrenal hemorrhage, and serial ultrasound examinations

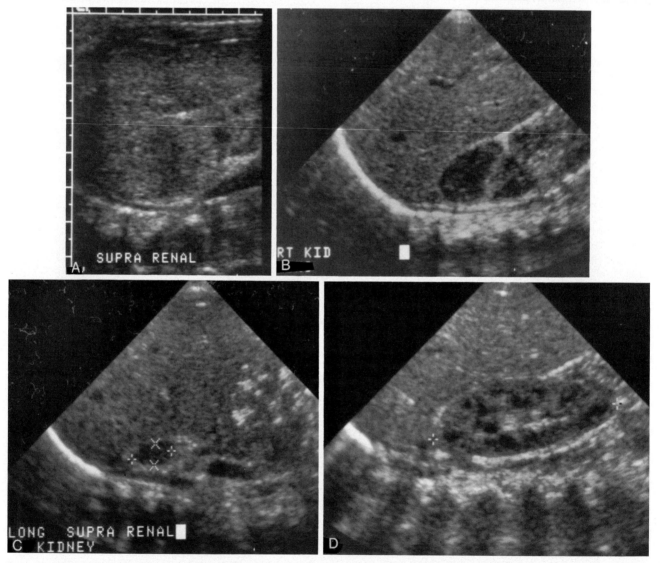

Figure 40–14. *A,* Large adrenal hemorrhage in a 6-day-old female infant presenting with right flank mass. Note the echodense homogeneous mass lesion extending from the upper pole of the right kidney. *B,* A repeat ultrasound in the same patient 11 days later showing marked decrease in size of mass lesion with decreasing echogenicity, indicating liquefaction. *C,* Sonogram in same patient at 6 weeks of age showing still further resolution of the adrenal hemorrhage. *D,* One year later, an ultrasound study of the right kidney shows complete disappearance of the adrenal hemorrhage.

demonstrating decreasing size of the mass with changing echogenic pattern are the cornerstone of the differential diagnosis. In addition, determinations of serum catecholamine levels, and urinary vanillylmandelic and homovanillic acid levels are mandatory. Elevation of these markers has been reported in up to 94 per cent of neuroblastomas (Eklof et al., 1986).

Conservative treatment of adrenal hemorrhage is warranted in most cases. The process is usually self-limiting and will resolve spontaneously. Careful surveillance with serial ultrasounds (see Fig. 40–14), hematocrits, and bilirubin determinations along with supportive measures, including adequate hydration, blood replacement when indicated, antibiotic treatment, and steroid replacement in selected cases will prove sufficient. Surgical intervention may be necessary when the diagnosis is in doubt or when complications such as uncontrollable hemorrhage or abscess formation occur (Atkinson et al., 1985; Black and Williams, 1973; Glenn, 1962; Gross et al., 1967).

Renal Tumors

The most common renal tumor in childhood is nephroblastoma (Wilms' tumor). Although Wilms' tumors have been reported to occur in the fetus and neonate (Hartenstein, 1949), it is now apparent that most solid tumors in the neonate are not true Wilms' tumors. Rather, they have different morphologic and clinical characteristics (Richmond and Dougall, 1970; Waisman and Cooper, 1970; Wigger, 1969). It is important that these predominantly mesenchymal tumors be recognized as an entity separate from Wilms' tumor to avoid the hazards of overtreatment. The benign nature of this tumor is now widely known and although occasionally referred to as fetal hamartoma, it is best known as mesoblastic nephroma.

The presentation is usually that of an incidentally discovered palpable mass with pyelographic features of a renal mass lesion and ultrasound characteristics of a solid renal tumor (Fig. 40–15). Typically, the cut surface of the tumor has a whorled pattern with interlacing bundles of mature fibrocytes seen microscopically. A very cellular spindle cell growth is seen. Although it may recur locally with tumor spill at operation, distant metastases are exceptional (Steinfeld et al., 1984). Patients are generally cured by surgical removal of the tumor (metastases are not reported). Further treatment with irradiation or chemotherapy is contraindicated, because the few reported fatalities have resulted from the treatment rather than the disease (Richmond and Dougall, 1970; Waisman and Cooper, 1970; Wigger, 1969).

Renal Cortical Necrosis

Symmetric renal cortical necrosis may occur early in the neonatal period as the result of hypoxia, dehydra-

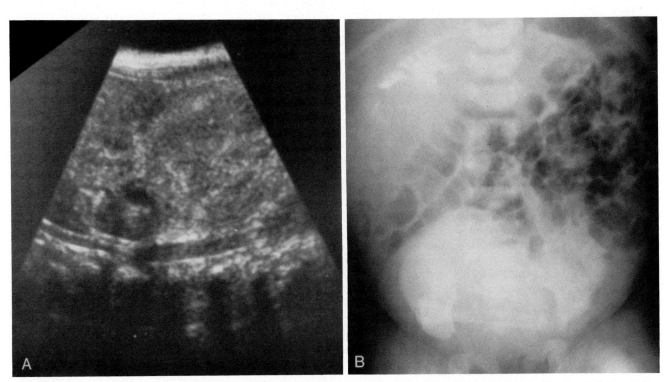

Figure 40–15. *A,* Sonogram in 1-day-old female infant presenting with large, right-sided abdominal mass. Sonogram shows normal upper pole to the right kidney below, which is a large, relatively homogeneous, echogenic oval mass filling the right flank. *B,* An intravenous pyelogram performed the next day shows a normal left kidney, largely obscured by intestinal gas. On the right side, there is upward displacement and some dilatation of the upper pole calyces with a large lower pole renal mass lesion. The following day she was operated on and her kidney was removed, revealing a mesoblastic nephroma.

tion, sepsis, or blood loss; it may also be caused by birth trauma or intrauterine distress of sufficient severity and duration to lead to renal ischemia (Reisman and Pathole, 1966). The clinical features include pallor, flaccidity, and cyanosis. In the acute stage, the kidneys are enlarged; thrombocytopenia, anemia, azotemia, and hematuria may be present. Accordingly, renal cortical necrosis may be easily confused with bilateral RVT. Although renal biopsy may be necessary to confirm the diagnosis of renal cortical necrosis, inferior vena cavography is useful in distinguishing it from bilateral RVT. Ultrasonography may also be helpful.

Renal cortical nephrosis is generally fatal. The treatment is supportive and includes management of renal failure (Bernstein and Mayer, 1961; Reisman and Pathole, 1966).

Renal Artery Thrombosis

Until the 1970s, renal artery thrombosis was regarded as a rare disorder in neonates, and most reported cases were based on autopsy studies (Waisman and Cooper, 1970). Thrombosis of the ductus arteriosus with subsequent embolism to the renal artery was considered the most likely etiology in the majority of cases.

Currently, the widespread use of umbilical artery catheterization in newborn management has resulted in an increased number of renal artery and aortic thromboses reported as a complication of this invasive procedure (Burdick et al., 1982; Caeton and Goetzman, 1985; Flanigan et al., 1982; O'Neill et al., 1981; Plummer et al., 1976; Pritchard et al., 1985). The incidence of renal artery thrombosis following umbilical artery catheterization increases when the tip of the catheter is located above L1. Other risk factors include traumatic arterial catheterization, injection of hyperosmotic and irritating solutions, low perfusion status, sepsis, infection, and prolonged maintenance of the arterial catheter (Guignard et al., 1989).

The clinical features (Table 40–12) of this disorder include hematuria, proteinuria, azotemia, lower extremity ischemia (when associated with aortic thrombosis), and severe hypertension often leading to congestive heart failure (Woodard et al., 1967). In a report of ten young infants with hypertension, five had renal artery thrombosis and two others had thrombosis of the abdominal aorta. Eight of these ten infants had histories of umbilical artery catheterization (Plummer et al., 1975). Traditionally, the diagnosis has been established by arteriography and radionuclide studies, although

Table 40–12. CLINICAL FEATURES OF RENAL ARTERY THROMBOSIS

Hematuria
Proteinuria
Azotemia
Hypertension
Congestive heart failure
Nonfunction on intravenous pyelogram or
   diethylenetriamine penta-acetic acid scan

high-resolution ultrasonography has become an equally effective and noninvasive method of establishing the diagnosis. Color Doppler ultrasonography should be particularly helpful.

The treatment of renal artery thrombosis varies depending on the clinical setting. Aggressive medical management with diuretics, antihypertensives, and peritoneal dialysis when indicated has proved effective in some cases (Malin et al., 1985). Surgical treatment may be appropriate in some cases. Revascularization by placement of an aortorenal graft (Burdick et al., 1982) and thrombectomy in case of aortic occlusion (Flanigan et al., 1982; Krueger et al., 1985) has been reported with good results. Nephrectomy, which seemed to produce the most survivors in the past (Fig. 40–16), is indicated when hypertension is refractory to intensive medical treatment.

Selective intra-arterial thrombolytic therapy with streptokinase and urokinase is becoming a viable treatment alternative in infants with major vessel thrombosis. Successful treatment with acceptable morbidity has been reported by several workers (Bromberg and Firlit, 1990; LeBlanc et al., 1986; Pritchard et al., 1985). Concern remains, however, regarding the use of thrombolytic agents when hypertension has not been adequately controlled.

Hydrometrocolpos

Although rare, hydrometrocolpos is an important abdominal mass occurring in the neonate. It is produced by fluid distention of the vagina and uterus. Circumstances necessary for its development are vaginal obstruction and excessive secretion of cervical glands in response to circulating maternal estrogen. It is less common than hematocolpos that occurs at menarche. Although imperforate hymen can produce the vaginal obstruction, vaginal atresia is more common and has been shown to be inherited as a simple autosomal recessive disorder (McKusick et al., 1964).

Hydrometrocolpos produces a mass that is large, firm, and midline in position and that arises from the pelvis (see Fig. 40–5). On rectal examination or on plain lateral radiograph of the abdomen, it is easily seen to be anterior to the rectum and posterior to the bladder. An abdominal ultrasound study should localize the lesion and demonstrate fluid-debris levels within the mass (Russ et al., 1986). Because hydrometrocolpos commonly produces ureteral obstruction with hydronephrosis, an excretory urogram has been considered an essential part of the evaluation in the past. This information can now be obtained with ultrasonography. Intestinal or vascular obstruction might also result from the mass.

When hydrometrocolpos is secondary to imperforate hymen, the diagnosis is made from external examination. However, in the more frequently encountered vaginal atresia, a vaginal examination might be confusing. As is so often true in clinical practice, an accurate diagnosis depends on an awareness of the condition by the examiner. In one series of 49 cases, only one half

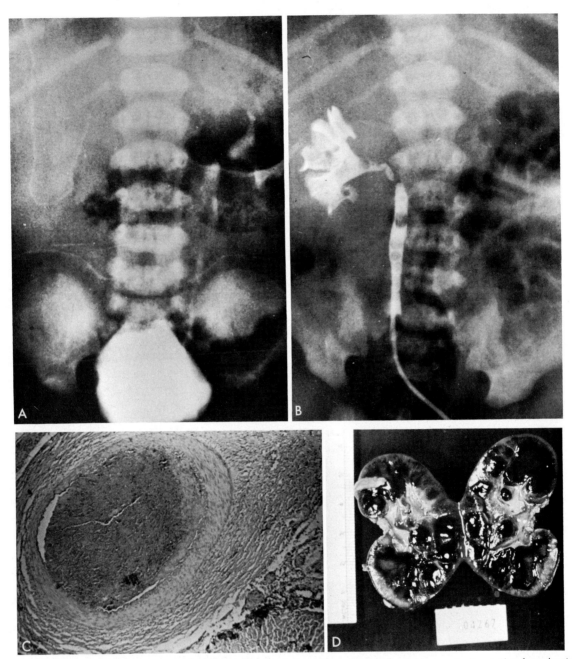

Figure 40–16. *A,* Excretory pyelogram in a 1-week-old boy with hematuria and hypertension showing no contrast excretion from the right kidney. *B,* On retrograde study, the kidney is not obstructed. *C,* Operation revealed an organizing thrombus completely occluding the main renal artery, and there was diffuse hemorrhagic medullary necrosis of the kidney. *D,* The infant was cured by nephrectomy. (From Woodard, J. R., Patterson, J. H., and Brinsfield, D.: Am. J. Dis. Child., 114:191, 1967. Copyright 1967, American Medical Association.)

were diagnosed correctly, one third were operated upon with an inadequate diagnosis, and one half of those were subjected to hysterectomy (Cook and Marshall, 1964).

The knowledge that hydrometrocolpos is likely to occur in female infants with imperforate anus or cloacal anomalies is essential, because rectal palpation is not possible in these instances, and the external genitalia may actually have an ambiguous appearance (see Fig. 40–5A) (Parrott and Woodard, 1976).

The treatment of hydrometrocolpos should be aggressive (Ramenofsky and Raffensperger, 1971). Whereas

imperforate hymen can usually be managed by simple incision, the more common vaginal atresia requires a major surgical correction. The distended uterus is opened through a lower abdominal incision. Incision of the obstructing vaginal septum by a combined vaginal and abdominal approach with indwelling catheter drainage of the uterus has been used in the past, but this form of treatment has been followed by an excessive number of deaths from sepsis and is considered inadequate (Ramenofsky and Raffensperger, 1971). Accordingly, the vaginal pull-through operation (Fig. 40–17) as described by Snyder (1966) is recommended. This pro-

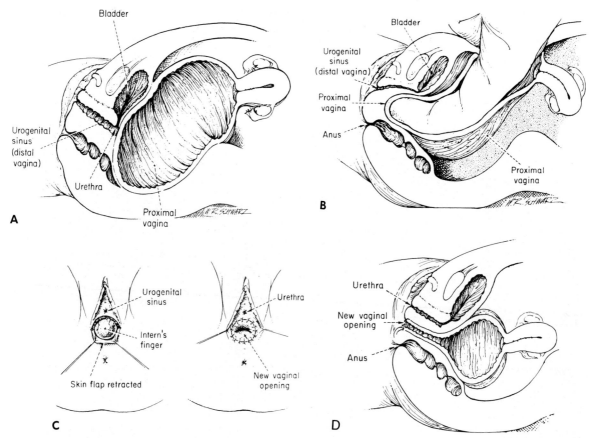

Figure 40–17. Artist's drawings showing (A) the basic anatomy of hydrometrocolpos and (B, C, D) the pull-through operation. The abdomen is opened through a transverse incision. The anterior vaginal wall is opened, and its contents are evacuated and cultured. With a finger in the vagina (B), an incision is made behind the urogenital sinus in the perineum, raising an inverted U flap of skin (C). The incision is deepened to meet the posterior wall of the vagina, which is being pushed down by the finger. When the back wall of the vagina is completely mobilized through the perineum, it is opened and sutured to the perineal skin behind the urogenital sinus (C and D). (From Ramenofsky, M. I., and Raffensperger, J. G.: J. Pediatr. Surg., 6:381, 1971.)

cedure adequately separates the genital and urinary tract.

In general, the obstructive uropathy can be expected to resolve following satisfactory drainage of the uterus. Occasionally, however, surgical intervention for upper tract drainage will be necessary, either for persistent urinary obstruction or for the occurrence of urinary sepsis.

Torsion of the Spermatic Cord

Torsion of the spermatic cord resulting in testicular infarction can occur at any age and constitutes one of the true urologic emergencies. Animal studies indicate that complete occlusion of the spermatic circulation results in some damage to the spermatogenic cells after 2 hours, severe damage after 4 hours, and complete loss after 6 hours (Smith, 1955). The Leydig cells are severely damaged after 8 hours and are completely lost after 10 hours. Immediate surgical intervention is, therefore, necessary if one is to salvage a functional testis.

As already stated, neonatal torsion is typically of the extravaginal type (Frederick et al., 1967). Extravaginal torsion may occur both in utero and in the neonatal period, but the former seems to be more frequent with the problem simply becoming apparent at birth (Das and Singer, 1990). Accordingly, the testis may be non-salvageable at the time of initial neonatal examination.

The tunica vaginalis has loose attachments to the scrotum at birth (Campbell and Schneider, 1976), and this condition may persist for the first several weeks of life. During this period of time, a spermatic cord may twist proximal to the reflection of the tunica vaginalis. Neonatal torsion does not appear to be related to prematurity, low birthweight, or traumatic delivery (Kaplan and Silber, 1988). Although uncommon, extravaginal testicular torsion may occur bilaterally; both synchronous and asynchronous torsion have been described. Asynchronous torsion is much less common, however (Atallah et al., 1975; Frederick et al., 1967; Gertsmann and Marble, 1980; Kay et al., 1980; La-Quaglia, 1987; Weingarten et al., 1990).

The physical findings are rather typical with induration and enlargement of the scrotal contents. Anatomic detail may be obscured, and the testicular mass may be several times the normal size with hard consistency and some overlying ecchymosis. These findings, although suggestive of birth trauma, may reflect failure of the infarction and extravasation to be contained within the tunic. The right and left testes are affected with equal frequency, and a number of bilateral cases have been reported (Auldist and Ferguson, 1975; Papadatos and Monsouris, 1967). The differential diagnosis of extravaginal torsion of the spermatic cord should include hydrocele, hematocele, incarcerated inguinal hernia, thrombosis of the spermatic cord, and neoplasia.

The treatment, if testicular salvage is to be hoped for, is immediate surgical intervention, barring some contraindication to operation. Manipulative reduction has no place in the management of this condition. The testicular salvage rate in neonatal torsion is very low, perhaps as low as 5 to 10 per cent (Kaplan and Silber, 1988). This finding is, in large part, due to the high incidence of in utero torsion and has led some investigators to question the need for surgical exploration at all. If we are to increase the salvage rate, however, early intervention is mandatory.

Some controversial aspects of the management of neonatal torsion include whether the exploration should be by means of the inguinal or scrotal approach and whether the contralateral testis should be subjected to fixation orchiopexy (Das and Singer, 1990; Kaplan and Silber, 1988). If the infant is otherwise healthy and no contraindication to general anesthesia exists, operation should be undertaken to attempt salvage of the testis. If significant question exists regarding the diagnosis, the inguinal approach should be used. Otherwise, scrotal exploration is feasible.

If a nonviable testis is found, it is removed. With any evidence of viability, the testis can be fixed to the scrotal wall and left in place. Extravaginal torsion does not have the strong predisposition to a similar occurrence on the contralateral side that is known to exist in intravaginal torsion. However, many surgeons elect to perform fixation orchiopexy on the contralateral side, largely because it represents a solitary testis, which might be amenable to subsequent torsion.

REFERENCES

Aarskog, D.: Intersex conditions masquerading as simple hypospadias. Birth Defects, 7:122, 1971.

Abni, E. F., Rodesch, F., and Shulman, C. C.: Fetal uropathies: Diagnostic pitfalls and management. J. Urol., 134:921, 1985.

Adelman, R. D.: Long-term follow-up of neonatal reno-vascular hypertension. Pediatr. Nephrol., 1:35, 1987.

Alton, D. J.: Pelviuretic obstruction in childhood. Radiol. Clin. North Am., 15:61, 1977.

Altshuler, G., Tsang, R. C., and Ermocilla, R.: Single umbilical artery. Am. J. Dis. Child., 129:697, 1975.

Ambrose, S. S., Gould, R. A., Trulock, T. S., and Parrott, T. S.: Unilateral multicystic renal disease in adults. J. Urol., 128:366, 1982.

Arger, P. H., Coleman, B. G., Mintz, M. C., Snyder, H. P., Canardese, T., Arenson, R. L., Gabbe, S. G., and Arvino, L.: Routine fetal genitourinary tract screening. Radiology, 156:485, 1985.

Atallah, M. W., Ippolito, J. J., and Rubin, B. W.: Intrauterine bilateral torsion of the spermatic cord. J. Urol., 116:128, 1975.

Atkinson, G. O., Jr., Kodroff, M. D., Gay, B. B., Jr., and Ricketts, R. R.: Adrenal abscess in the neonate. Radiology, 155:101, 1985.

Auldist, A. W., and Ferguson, R. F.: Torsion of the testicle in the newborn. Aust. N. Z. J. Surg., 45:14, 1975.

Avery, G. B.: Endocrine disorders. In Moshang, T., Bongiovanni, A. M. (Eds.): Neonatology. Philadelphia, J. B. Lippincott Co., 1975, pp. 945–971.

Avni, E. F., Thoua, Y., Lalmand, B., Dedier, F., Droulle, P., and Schulman, C. C.: Multicystic dysplastic kidney: Natural history from in utero diagnosis and post natal follow-up. J. Urol., 138:1420, 1987.

Bajoghli, M.: Gross hematuria of newborns and infants induced by quinone and 8-quinolinol (mexaform) [Letter]. Eur. J. Pediatr. (European), 138:359, 1982.

Baker, M. E., Rosenberg, E. R., Bowie, J. D., and Gall, S.: Transient in utero hydronephrosis. J. Ultrasound Med., 4:51, 1985.

Barrett, D. M., and Wineland, R. E.: Renal cell carcinoma in multicystic dysplastic kidney. Urology, 15:152, 1980.

Behrman, R. E.: The higher risk infant. In Behrman, R. E. (Ed.): Neonatology. St. Louis, C. V. Mosby Co., 1973, pp. 1–49.

Bell, W. R., and Meek, A. G.: Guidelines for the use of thrombolytic agents. N. Engl. J. Med., 301:1266, 1979.

Bellinger, M. F., Cromstock, C. H., and Grosso, D.: Fetal posterior urethral valves and renal dysplasia at 15 weeks gestational age. J. Urol., 129:1238, 1983.

Belman, A. B.: Nonoperative management in management of multicystic dysplastic kidney. Dialogues Pediatr. Urol., 10:6, 1987.

Belman, A. B., and King, L. R.: Urinary tract abnormalities associated with imperforate anus. J. Urol., 108:823, 1972.

Belman, A. B., Susmano, D. F., Burden, J. J., and Kaplan, G.: Nonoperative treatment of unilateral renal vein thrombosis in the newborn. J.A.M.A., 211:1165, 1970.

Bensman, A., Nevenschwander, S., Lavollay, B., and Gruner, M.: Hypertension arterialle et compression du pedicule vasculaire renal par un hematome de la surrenal chez un nouveau-ne. Ann. Pediatr., 29:670, 1982.

Bernstein, J., and Meyer, R.: Congenital anomalies of the urinary system. II. Renal cortical and medullary necrosis. J. Pediatr., 59:687, 1961.

Birken, G., Vane, D., King, D., et al.: Adenocarcinoma arising in a multicystic dysplastic kidney. Pediatr. Surg., 20:619, 1985.

Black, J., and Williams, D. I.: Natural history of adrenal hemorrhage in the newborn. Arch. Dis. Child., 48:183, 1973.

Bloch, E. C.: Anesthetic consideration in the neonate. In King, L. R. (Ed.): Urologic Surgery in Neonates and Young Infants. Philadelphia, W. B. Saunders Co., 1988, p. 119.

Bowen, A. D., and Smazal, S. F.: Ultrasound of coexisting right renal vein thrombosis and adrenal hemorrhage in a newborn. J. Clin. Ultrasound, 9:511, 1981.

Bromberg, W. D., and Firlit, C. R.: Fibrinolytic therapy for renal vein thrombosis in the child. J. Urol., 143:86, 1990.

Brown, T., Mandell, J., and Lebowitz, R. L.: Neonatal hydronephrosis in the era of sonography. Am. J. Radiol., 148:959, 1987.

Bryan, E. M., and Kohler, H. G.: The missing umbilical artery: II. Pediatric follow-up. Arch. Dis. Child., 50:714, 1975.

Burdick, J. F., Helikson, M. A., Judak, M. L., et al: Revascularization for bilateral renal artery occlusion after umbilical artery catheterization. Surgery, 91:650, 1982.

Caeton, A. J., and Goetzman, B. W.: Risky business: Umbilical artery catheterization. Am. J. Dis. Child., 139:120, 1985.

Campbell, J. R., and Schneider, C. P.: Intrauterine torsion of an intraabdominal testis. Pediatrics, 57:262, 1976.

Campbell, M. F., and Matthews, W. F.: Renal thrombosis in infancy. J. Pediatr., 20:604, 1942.

Cheney, G. K., Fisher, J. H., O'Hare, K. H., Retik, A. B., and Darling, D. B.: Anomaly of the persistent cloaca in female infants. Am. J. Roentgenol., 120:413, 1974.

Clark, D. A.: Times of first void and first stool in 500 newborns. Pediatrics, 60:457, 1977.

Cockburn, F., and Drillien, C. M.: Pharmacology. In Cockburn, F., and Drillien, C. M. (Eds.): Neonatal Medicine. Oxford, Blackwell Scientific Publishers, 1974, pp. 752–787.

Cohen, E. K., Daneman, A., Stringer, D. A., Soto, G., and Thorner, P.: Focal adrenal hemorrhage: A new ultrasound appearance. Radiology, 161:631, 1986.

Cohen, H. H., and Haller, D. O.: Diagnostic sonography of the fetal genitourinary tract. Urol. Radiol., 9:88, 1987.

Colodny, A. H.: Antenatal diagnosis and management of urinary abnormalities. Pediatr. Clin. North Am., 34:1365, 1987.

Cook, G. T., and Marshall, V. F.: Hydrocolpos causing urinary obstruction. J. Urol., 92:127, 1964.

Corazza, M. S., Davis, R. F., Merritt, T. A., et al.: Prolonged bleeding time in preterm infants receiving indomethacin for patent ductus arteriosus. J. Pediatr., 105:292, 1984.

Crombleholme, T. M., Harrison, M. R., Langer, J. C., et al.: Early experience with early fetal surgery for congenital hydronephrosis. J. Pediatr. Surg., 23:1114, 1988.

Cywes, S.: Haemoperitoneum in the newborn. S. Afr. Med. J., 41:1063, 1967.

Das, S., and Singer, A.: Controversies of perinatal torsion of the spermatic cord: A review, survey and recommendations. J. Urol., 143:231, 1990.

DeSa, D. J., and Nicholls, S.: Haemorrhagic necrosis of the adrenal gland in perinatal infants. A clinical-pathological study. J. Pathol., 106:133, 1972.

Diamond, D. A., and Jeffs, R. D.: Cloacal exstrophy: A 22-year experience. J. Urol., 133:779, 1985.

Docimo, S. G., Luetic, T., Crone, R. K., et al.: Pulmonary development in the fetal lamb with severe bladder outlet obstruction and oligohydramnios: A morphometric study. J. Urol., 142:657, 1989.

Dotter, C. T., Rasch, J., and Seaman, A. J.: Selective clot lysis with low dose streptokinase. Radiology, 111:31, 1974.

Dowling, K. J., Harmon, E. P., Ortenberg, J., Polanco, E., and Evans, B. B.: Ureteropelvic junction obstruction: The effect of pyeloplasty on renal function. J. Urol., 140:1227, 1988.

Duncan, R. E., Evans, A. T., and Martin, L. W.: Natural history and treatment of renal vein thrombosis in children. J. Pediatr. Surg., 12(5):639, 1977.

Eberlein, W. R., and Bongiovanni, A. M.: Plasma and urinary corticosteroids in hypertensive forms of congenital adrenal hyperplasia. J. Biol. Chem., 223:85, 1956.

Eklof, O., Grotte, G., Garulf, H., Lohr, G., and Ringerts, H.: Perinatal hemorrhagic necrosis of the adrenal gland. Pediatr. Radiol., 4:31, 1975.

Eklof, O., Mortensson, W., and Sandstedt, B.: Suprarenal hematoma versus neuroblastoma complicated by hemorrhage—a diagnostic dilemma in the newborn. Alta Radiol. Diagnosis, 27:3, 1986.

Elder, J. S., and Duckett, J. W.: Management of the fetus and neonate with hydronephrosis detected by prenatal ultrasonography. Pediatr. Ann., 17:19, 1988.

Elder, J. S., Duckett, J. W., and Snyder, H. M.: Intervention for fetal obstructive uropathy: Has it been effective? Lancet II:1007, 1987.

Emanuel, B., and Aronson, N.: Neonatal hematuria. Am. J. Dis. Child., 128:204, 1974.

Emery, J. L., and Zachary, R. B.: Hematoma of adrenal gland in newborn. Br. Med. J., 2:857, 1952.

Evans, D. J., Silverman, M., and Bowley, N. B.: Congenital hypertension due to unilateral renal vein thrombosis. Arch. Dis. Child., 56:306, 1981.

Fielding, G. A., Masel, J., and Leditschke, J. F.: Spontaneous neonatal renal vein thrombosis. Aust. N. Z. J. Surg., 56:485, 1986.

Feingold, M., Fine, R. M., and Ingall, D.: Intravenous pyelography in infants with single umbilical artery. N. Engl. J. Med., 270:1178, 1964.

Flake, A. W., Harrison, M. R., Sauer, N., Adzick, N. S., and d'Lorimier, A. A.: Ureteropelvic junction obstruction in the fetus. J. Pediatr. Surg., 21:1058, 1986.

Flanigan, D. P., Stolar, C. J. H., Pringle, K. C., et al.: Aortic thrombosis after umbilical artery catheterization. Arch. Surg., 117:371, 1982.

Frederick, P. L., Dusha, N., and Eralkis, A. J.: Simultaneous bilateral torsion of the testes in a newborn infant. Arch. Surg., 94:299, 1967.

Froehlich, L. A., and Fugikura, T.: Follow-up of infants with single umbilical artery. Pediatrics, 52:6, 1973.

Galatius-Jensen, F., and Damgaard-Pedersen, K.: Malignant versus benign paravertebral widening in children. Pediatr. Radiol., 11:193, 1981.

Garrett, R. A., and Franken, E. A., Jr.: Neonatal ascites: Perirenal extravasation and bladder outlet obstruction. J. Urol., 102:627, 1969.

Gellis, S. S.: Editorial comment. In Gellis, S. S. (Ed.): Yearbook of Pediatrics. Chicago, Year Book Medical Publishers, Inc., 1975, p. 42.

Gertsmann, D. R., and Marble, R. D.: Bilaterally enlarged testicles in a newborn: An atypical presentation of intrauterine spermatic cord torsion. Am. J. Dis. Child., 134:992, 1980.

Giebink, G. S., and Ruymann, F. B.: Testicular tumors in childhood. Am. J. Dis. Child., 127:433, 1974.

Gierup, J., Hedenberg, C., and Osterman, A.: Acute nonspecific epididymitis in boys. Scand. J. Urol. Nephrol., 9:5, 1975.

Gilsanz, N., Fernal, W., Reid, B. S., et al.: Nephrolithiasis in premature infants. Radiology, 154:107, 1985.

Glenn, J. F.: Neonatal adrenal hemorrhage. J. Urol., 87:639, 1962.

Gordon, A. C., Thomas, D. F. M., Arthur, R. J., and Irving, H. C.: Multicystic dysplastic kidney: Is nephrectomy still appropriate? J. Urol., 140(Part 2):1231, 1988.

Greenfield, S. P., Hensle, T. W., Berdon, W. E., et al.: Urinary extravasation in the newborn male with posterior urethral valves. J. Pediatr. Surg., 17:751, 1982.

Griscom, N. T., Colodny, A. H., Rosenberg, H. K., Fliegael, C. P., and Hardy, B. E.: Diagnostic aspects of neonatal ascites: Report of 27 cases. Am. J. Roentgenol., 128:961, 1977.

Gross, M., Kittmeier, P. K., and Waterhouse, J.: Diagnosis and treatment of neonatal hemorrhage. J. Pediatr. Surg., 2:308, 1967.

Gross, T. L., Kuhnert, B. R., Kuhnert, P. M., et al.: Maternal and fetal plasma concentrations of ritodrine. Obstet. Gynecol., 65:793, 1985.

Guignard, J. P., Gouyon, J. B., and Adelman, R. D.: Arterial hypertension in the newborn infant. Biol. Neonate, 55:77, 1989.

Hadlock, F. P., Deter, R. L., Carpenter, R., Gonzales, E. T., and Park, S. K.: Sonography of fetal urinary tract anomalies. Am. J. Roentgenol., 137:261, 1981.

Hartenstein, H.: Wilms' tumor in a newborn infant. J. Pediatr., 35:381, 1949.

Hartman, G. E., and Shochat, S. S.: Abdominal mass lesions in the newborn: Diagnosis and treatment. Clin. Perinatol., 16(1):123, 1989.

Hartman, G. E., Smolik, L. M., and Shochat, S. S.: The dilemma of the multicystic dysplastic kidney. Am. J. Dis. Child., 140:925, 1986.

Hellstrom, W. J. G., Kogan, B. A., Jeffrey, R. B., and McAninch, J. W.: The natural history of prenatal hydronephrosis with normal amounts of amniotic fluid. J. Urol., 132:947, 1984.

Heydenrych, J. J.: Haemoperitoneum and associated torsion of the testicle in the newborn. S. Afr. Med. J., 48:2221, 1974.

Hufnagle, K. G., Khan, S. N., Penn, D., et al.: Renal calcifications: A complication of long-term furosemide therapy in preterm infants. Pediatrics, 70:360, 1982.

Hurwitz, R. S., Mansoni, G. A. M., Ransley, P. G., and Stephens, F. D.: Cloacal exstrophy: A report of 34 cases. J. Urol., 138:1060, 1987.

Jeffs, R. D., Guice, S. L., and Oesch, I.: The factors in successful exstrophy closure. J. Urol., 127:974, 1982.

Kaplan, G. W.: Prepubertal testicular tumors. World J. Urol., 2:283, 1984.

Kaplan, G. W., Cromie, W. J., Kelalis, P. P., et al.: Gonadal stromal tumors: A report of the prepubertal testicular tumor registry. J. Urol., 136:300, 1986.

Kaplan, G. W., and Silber, I.: Neonatal torsion—to pex or not? In King, L. R. (Ed.): Urologic Surgery in Neonates and Young Infants. Philadelphia, W. B. Saunders Co., 1988, p. 386.

Kay, R., Strong, D. W., and Tank, E. S.: Bilateral spermatic cord torsion in the neonate. J. Urol., 123:293, 1980.

Keating, M. A., Escala, J., Snyder, H. M., Heyman, S., and Duckett, J. W.: Changing concepts in the management of primary obstructive megaureter. J. Urol., Part 2, 142:636, 1989.

Keay, A. J., and Morgan, D. M.: Congenital anomalies. In Keay, A. J., and Morgan, D. M. (Eds.): Craig's Care of the Newly Born Infant. Edinburgh, Churchill Livingstone, 1974, pp. 191–262.

Khuri, F. J., Alton, D. J., Hardy, B. E., Cook, G. T., and Churchill, B. M.: Adrenal hemorrhage in neonates: Report of 5 cases and review of the literature. J. Urol., 124:684, 1980.

King, L. R., Coughlin, P. W. F., Bloch, E. C., Ansong, K., and Hannah, M. K.: The case for immediate pyeloplasty and the neonate with ureteropelvic junction obstruction. J. Urol., 132:725, 1984.

Kleiner, B., Callen, P. W., and Filly, R. A.: Sonographic analysis of the fetus with ureteropelvic junction obstruction. J. Am. Radiol., 148:359, 1987.

Krane, R. J., and Retik, A. B.: Neonatal perirenal urinary extravasation. J. Urol., 111:96, 1974.

Krueger, T. C., Neblett, W. W., III, O'Neill, J. A., et al.: Management of aortic thrombosis secondary to umbilical artery catheters in neonates. J. Pediatr. Surg., 20:328, 1985.

LaQuaglia, M. P., Bauer, S. B., Eraklis, A., Feins, N., and Mandell, S.: Bilateral neonatal torsion. J. Urol., 138:1051, 1987.

Lawrence, W. D., Young, R. H., and Scully, R. E.: Juvenile granulosa cell tumor of the infantile testis: A report of 14 cases. Am. J. Surg. Pathol., 9:87, 1985.

LeBlanc, J. G., Wilham, J. A. G., Chan, K. W., Patterson, M. W., Tipple, M., and Sandor, G. G.: Treatment of grafts and major vessel thrombosis with low dose streptokinase in children. Ann. Thorac. Surg., 41:630, 1986.

Lebowitz, J. M., and Belman, A. B.: Simultaneous idiopathic adrenal hemorrhage and renal vein thrombosis in the newborn. J. Urol., 129:574, 1983.

Lebowitz, R. L., and Griscom, N. T.: Neonatal hydronephrosis: 146 Cases. Radiol. Clin. North Am., 15:49, 1977.

Lees, M. H.: Disease of the cardiovascular system. In Behrman, R. E. (Ed.): Neonatology. St. Louis, C. V. Mosby Co., 1973, pp. 241–344.

Lemtis, H. G., and Klemme, G.: Is there any correlation between aplasia of one umbilical artery and other congenital malformations? In Proceedings of the Second European Congress of Perinatal Medicine. Basel, S. Karger, 1971, pp. 308–309.

Levin, D. L., Hyman, A. I., Heymann, M. A., et al.: Fetal hypertension and the development of increased pulmonary vascular smooth muscle: A possible mechanism for persistent pulmonary hypertension in the newborn infant. J. Pediatr., 92:265, 1978.

Lloyd, D. A.: Renal vein thrombosis. In Welch, K. J., Randolph, J. G., Ravitch, M. M., et al. (Eds.): Pediatric Surgery, Vol. 2, Ed. 4. Chicago, Year Book Medical Publishers, 1986, p. 1146.

Longino, L. A., and Martin, L. W.: Torsion of the spermatic cord in the newborn infant. N. Engl. J. Med., 253:695, 1955.

Longino, L. A., and Martin, L. W.: Abdominal masses in the newborn infant. Pediatrics, 21:596, 1958.

Malin, S. W., Baumgart, S., Rosenberg, H. K., et al.: Nonsurgical management of obstructive aortic thrombosis complicated by renovascular hypertension in the neonate. J. Pediatr., 106:630, 1985.

Mann, C. M., Leape, L. L., and Holden, T. M.: Neonatal urinary ascites: A report of two cases of unusual etiology and a review of the literature. J. Urol., 111:124, 1974.

Manning, F. A., Harrison, M. R., Rodeck, C., et al.: Catheter shunts for fetal hydronephrosis: Report of the International Fetal Surgery Registry. N. Engl. J. Med., 315:336, 1986.

Marshall, V. F., and Muecke, E. C.: Variations in exstrophy of the bladder. J. Urol., 88:766, 1962.

Martin, D. J., Gilday, D. L., and Reilly, B. J.: Evaluation of the urinary tract in the neonatal period. Radiol. Clin. North Am., 13:359, 1975.

Mata, J. A., Livne, R. M., and Gibbons, D. M.: Urinary ascites: A complication of umbilical artery catheterization. Urology, 30:375, 1987.

McFarland, J. B.: Renal venous thrombosis in children. Q. J. Med., 34:269, 1965.

McKusick, V. A., Bauer, R. L., Koop, C. E., and Scott, R. B.: Hydrometrocolpos as a simply inherited malformation. J.A.M.A., 189:813, 1964.

Metreweli, C., and Pearson, R.: Echographic diagnosis of neonatal renal vein thrombosis. Pediatr. Radiol., 14:105, 1984.

Mitchell, M. E., Bito, C. G., and Rink, R. C.: Cloacal exstrophy reconstruction for urinary continence. J. Urol., 144:554, 1990.

Moncada, R., Cooper, R. A., Reynes, C. J., and Greene, R.: Neonatal urine ascites associated with urinary outlets obstruction: Another survivor. Br. J. Radiol., 46:1005, 1973.

Monfort, G., Morisson-Lacombe, G., and Coquet, M.: Endoscopic treatment of ureteroceles revisited. J. Urol., 133:1031, 1985.

Neal, W. A., Reynolds, J. W., Jarvis, C. W., et al.: Umbilical artery catheterization: Demonstration of arterial thrombosis by aortography. Pediatrics, 50:6, 1972.

O'Neill, J. A., Jr., Neblet, W. W., III, and Born, M. L.: Management of major thromboembolic complications of umbilical artery catheters. J. Pediatr. Surg., 16:972, 1981.

Pais, V. M., and Retik, A. B.: Reversible hydronephrosis in the neonate with urinary sepsis. N. Engl. J. Med., 192:465, 1975.

Papadatos, C., and Monsouris, C.: Bilateral testicular torsion in the newborn. J. Pediatr., 71:249, 1967.

Parker, R. M.: Neonatal urinary ascites. Urology, 3:589, 1974.

Parrott, T. S.: Urologic implications of imperforate anus. Urology, 10:407, 1977.

Parrott, T. S., and Woodard, J. R.: Urologic surgery in the neonate. J. Urol., 116:506, 1976.

Parrott, T. S., and Woodard, J. R.: Importance of cystourethrography in neonates with imperforate anus. Urology, 13:607, 1979.

Parrott, T. S., Woodard, J. R., and Wolpert, J. J.: Ureteral tailoring: A comparison of wedge resection with infolding. J. Urol., 144:328, 1990.

Pedicelli, G., Jequier, S., Bowen, A., and Boisvert, J.: Multicystic dysplastic kidney: Spontaneous regression demonstrated with ultrasound. Radiology, 160:23, 1986.

Peters, C. A., and Mandell, J.: The multicystic dysplastic kidney. AUA Update Series, VIII(70):50, 1989.

Peters, C. A., Mandell, J., Lebowitz, R. L., Colodny, A. H., Bauer, S. B., Hendren, H. W., and Retik, A. B.: Congenital obstructed megaureters in early infancy: Diagnosis and treatment. J. Urol., Part 2, 142:641, 1988.

Plummer, L. B., Kaplan, G. W., and Mendoza, S. A.: Hypertension in infants—a complication of umbilical artery catheterization. J. Pediatr., 89:802, 1976.

Plummer, L. B., Mendoza, S. A., and Kaplan, J. W.: Hypertension in infancy: The case for aggressive management. J. Urol., 113:555, 1975.

Potter, E. L.: Bilateral renal agenesis. J. Pediatr., 29:68, 1946.

Potter, E. L.: Normal and Abnormal Developments of the Kidney. Chicago, Year Book Medical Publishers, 1972, pp. 1–305.

Pritchard, S. L., Culham, J. A. G., and Rogers, P. C. J.: Low dose fibrinolytic therapy in infants. J. Pediatr., 106:594, 1985.

Puckner, P. J., Santulli, T. B., and Lattimer, J. K.: Urological problems associated with imperforate anus. Urology, 6:205, 1975.

Qvist, O.: Swelling of the scrotum in infants and children and nonspecific epididymitis. Acta Chir. Scand., 110:418, 1955.

Raffensperger, J., and Abousleiman, A.: Abdominal masses in children under one year of age. Surgery, 63:514, 1968.

Raffensperger, J. G., and Ramenofsky, M. L.: The management of a cloaca. J. Pediatr. Surg., 8:647, 1973.

Ramenofsky, M. L., and Raffensperger, J. G.: An abdomino-perineal vaginal pull-through for definitive treatment of hydrometrocolpos. J. Pediatr. Surg., 6:381, 1971.

Ravitch, L., and Schell, N. B.: Rupture of the kidney and the newborn infant. N.Y. State Med., 61:2823, 1961.

Reha, W. C., and Gibbons, M. D.: Neonatal ascites and ureteral valves. Urology, 33:468, 1989.

Reid, L.: The lung: Its growth and remodeling in health and disease. Am. J. Roentgenol., 129:777, 1977.

Reisman, L. E., and Pathole, A.: Bilateral renal cortical necrosis in the newborn. Am. J. Dis. Child., 111:541, 1966.

Richmond, H., and Dougall, A. J.: Neonatal renal tumors. J. Pediatr. Surg., 5:413, 1970.

Rosendahl, W., Ranke, M., and Mentzel, H.: Sodium loss as leading symptom of renovascular hypertension in the newborn. Klin. Wochenschr., 58:953, 1980.

Russ, P. D., Zavitz, W. R., Pretorium, D. H., Manco-Johnson, M. L., Rumack, C. M., Pfister, R. R., and Greenholz, S. K.: Hydrometrocolpos, uterus didelphys, and septate vagina: An antenatal sonographic diagnosis. J. Ultrasound Med., 5:211, 1986.

Sanders, R. C., and Hartman, D. S.: The sonographic distinction between neonatal multicystic kidney and hydronephrosis. Radiology, 151:621, 1984.

Schaffer, A. J., and Avery, M. E.: Introduction. In Schaffer, A. J., and Avery, M. E. (Eds.): Diseases of the Newborn. Philadelphia, W. B. Saunders Co., 1977, pp. 1–13.

Scott, J. E. S.: Fetal ureteric reflux. Br. J. Urol., 59:291, 1987.

Scott, T. W.: Urinary ascites secondary to posterior urethral valves. J. Urol., 116:87, 1976.

Seeds, J. W., Mittlestaedt, C. A., and Mandell, J.: Pre and post natal ultrasonographic diagnosis of congenital obstructive uropathies. Urol. Clin. North Am., 13:131, 1986.

Seeler, R. A., Kapadia, P., and Moncada, R.: Non-surgical management of thrombosis of bilateral renal veins and inferior vena cava in a newborn infant. Clin. Pediatr., 9:543, 1970.

Sherry, S. N., and Kramer, I.: The time of passage of first stool and first urine by the newborn infant. J. Pediatr., 46:158, 1955.

Sloman, J. G., and Mylius, R. E.: Testicular infarction in infancy: Its association with irreducible inguinal hernia. In Stephens, F. D. (Ed.): Congenital Malformations of the Rectum, Anus, and Genitourinary Tract. Edinburgh, E & S Livingstone, 1963, p. 321.

Smith, D. W.: Introduction. *In* Smith, D. W. (Ed.): Recognizable Patterns of Human Malformation. Philadelphia, W. B. Saunders Co., 1976, pp. 1–5.

Smith, G. I.: Cellular changes from graded testicular ischemia. J. Urol., 73:355, 1955.

Smith, J. A., Jr., and Middleton, R. G.: Neonatal adrenal hemorrhage. J. Urol., 122:674, 1979.

Snyder, H. M., Duckett, J. W., and Elder, J. S.: Nodular renal blastema in a multicystic dysplastic kidney. Soc. Pediatr. Urol. Newsletter, April, 1986.

Snyder, W. H., Jr.: Some unusual forms of imperforate anus in female infants. Am. J. Surg., 111:319, 1966.

Sober, I., and Hirsch, M.: Unilateral massive adrenal hemorrhage in the newborn infant. J. Urol., 93:430, 1965.

Spitzer, A., Bernstein, J., and Edelman, C. M., Jr.: Diseases of the kidney and urinary tract. *In* Behrman, R. E. (Ed.): Neonatology. St. Louis, C. V. Mosby Co., 1973, pp. 485–513.

Stark, H., and Geiger, R.: Renal tubular dysfunction following vascular accidents to the kidney in the newborn period. J. Pediatr., 83:933, 1973.

Steinfeld, A. D., Crowley, C. A., O'Shea, P. A., and Tefft, M.: Recurrent and metastatic mesoblastic nephroma in infancy. J. Clin. Oncol., 2:956, 1984.

Sty, J. R., Babbitt, D. P., and Oechler, H. W.: Evaluating the multicystic kidney. Clin. Nucl. Med., 5:457, 1980.

Sullivan, M. J., Lackner, L. H., and Banowsky, L. H. W.: Intraperitoneal extravasation of urine, BUN/serum creatinine disproportion. J.A.M.A., 221:491, 1972.

Susskind, M. R., and King, L. R.: Hypertension and the multicystic kidney. Presented at the 82nd Annual Meeting of the American Urologic Association. Anaheim, CA, May 17, 1987.

Swiet, M. de, Fayers, P., and Shinebourne, C. A.: Systolic blood pressure in a population of infants in the first year of life: The Brompton Study. Pediatrics, 65:1028, 1980.

Tank, E. S., Bessette, P. L., and Heidelberger, K. P.: The definition and diagnosis of antenatal renal vein thrombosis. J. Urol., 111:242, 1974.

Tank, E. S., Carey, T. C., and Seifert, A. L.: Management of neonatal urinary ascites. Urology, 16:270, 1980.

Tank, E. S., and Lindenauer, S. M.: Principles of management of exstrophy of the cloaca. Am. J. Surg., 119:95, 1970.

Thompson, I. M., Schneider, R., and Lababidi, Z.: Thrombectomy for renal vein thrombosis. J. Urol., 113:396, 1974.

Thon, W., Schlickenrieder, J. H. M., Thon, A., and Altwien, J. E.: Management and early reconstruction of urinary tract abnormalities detected in utero. Br. J. Urol., 59:214, 1987.

Trulock, T. S., Finnerty, D. P., and Woodard, J. R.: Neonatal bladder rupture: Case report and review of the literature. J. Urol., 133:271, 1985.

Uehling, D. T., Smith, J. E., Logan, R., and Hafez, G. R.: Newborn granulosa cell tumor of the testis. J. Urol., 138:385, 1987.

Uson, A. C., Cox, L. A., and Lattimer, J. K.: Hydronephrosis in infants and children. J.A.M.A., 205:323, 1968.

Verhagen, A. D., Hamilton, J. P., and Genel, M.: Renal vein thrombosis in infants. Arch. Dis. Child., 49:214, 1965.

Vulliamy, D. G.: Congenital anomalies and deformities with some genetic disorders. *In* Vulliamy, D. G. (Ed.): The Newborn Child. Baltimore, Williams & Wilkins, 1972, pp. 142–180.

Wacksman, J.: Multicystic kidney registry in management of multicystic dysplastic kidney. Dialog. Pediatr. Urol., 10:4, 1987.

Waisman, J., and Cooper, P. H.: Renal neoplasms of the newborn. J. Pediatr. Surg., 5:407, 1970.

Wasnick, R. J.: Neonatal urinary ascites secondary to ureteropelvic junction obstruction. Urology, 30:470, 1987.

Watson, R. A.: Torsion of the spermatic cord in the neonate. Urology, 5:439, 1974.

Wedge, J. J., Grosfeld, J. L., and Smith, J. P.: Abdominal masses in the newborn: 63 Cases. J. Urol., 106:770, 1971.

Weingarten, J. L., Garofalo, F. A., and Cromie, W. J.: Bilateral synchronous neonatal torsion of spermatic cord. Urology, 35:135, 1990.

Wigger, H. J.: Fetal hamartoma of the kidney. Am. J. Clin. Pathol., 51:323, 1969.

Williams, D. I.: Renal anomalies. *In* Williams, D. I. (Ed.): Urology in Childhood. New York, Springer-Verlag, 1974, pp. 70–80.

Williams, D. I., and Eckstein, H. R.: Obstructive valves in the posterior urethra. J. Urol., 92:236, 1965.

Williams, D. I., and Parker, R. M.: The role of surgery in the prune belly syndrome. *In* Johnston, H., and Goodwin, W. E. (Eds.): Reviews in Pediatric Urology, Amsterdam, Excerpta Medica, 1974, pp. 315–331.

Wolpert, J. J., Woodard, J. R., and Parrott, T. S.: Pyeloplasty in the young infant. J. Urol., 142:573, 1989.

Woodard, J. R.: The prune belly syndrome. Urol. Clin. North Am., 5:75, 1978.

Woodard, J. R.: Neonatal and perinatal emergencies. *In* Walsh, P., Gittes, B., Perlmutter, A., and Stamey, T. (Eds.): Campbell's Urology. Philadelphia, W. B. Saunders Co., 1986, pp. 2217–2243.

Woodard, J. R.: The impact of fetal diagnosis on the management of obstructive uropathy. Postgrad. Med. J., 66 (Suppl. 1):37, 1990.

Woodard, J. R., and Parrott, T. S.: Urologic surgery in the neonate. J. Urol., 116:506, 1976.

Woodard, J. R., Patterson, J. H., and Brinsfield, D.: Renal artery thrombosis in newborn infants. Am. J. Dis. Child., 114:191, 1967.

Woodard, J. R., and Zucker, I.: Current management of the dilated urinary tract in prune belly syndrome. Urol. Clin. North Am., 17:407, 1990.

41
ENURESIS

Stephen A. Koff, M.D.

Enuresis (from the Greek *enourein*, to void urine) has been defined as an involuntary discharge of urine. The term is often used alone, imprecisely, to describe wetting that occurs only at night during sleep. It is more accurate, however, to refer to nighttime wetting as nocturnal enuresis and to distinguish it from daytime wetting, which is called diurnal enuresis. Because incontinence is normal in young children, the age at which enuresis becomes inappropriate depends on the statistics of developing urinary control, the pattern of wetting, and the sex of the child. Approximately 15 per cent of normal children still wet at night at age 5 years. Nocturnal enuresis occurring after the age of 5 or by the time the child enters grade school is generally considered a cause for concern. With a spontaneous resolution rate of about 15 per cent per year, 99 per cent of children are dry by the age of 15 years (Forsythe and Redmond, 1974). In contrast, diurnal enuresis that persists much after toilet training may be a problem. A larger proportion of girls than boys are dry both day and night by the age of 2 years, and nocturnal enuresis is 50 per cent more common in boys than in girls.

More than 80 per cent of enuretics wet only at night. The remainder have variable and varying patterns of nocturnal and diurnal incontinence. Most nocturnal enuretics have never been dry and are termed primary enuretics. However, the development of urinary control is not always final, and approximately 25 per cent of children who attain initial nighttime dryness by age 12 will relapse and wet for a period averaging 2.5 years. These children are termed secondary enuretics, and in many, emotional stress that occurred during a vulnerable period in their development may be recognized. Children who develop initial daytime dryness by age 12 are less prone to relapse, but at least 10 per cent will redevelop daytime wetting for periods averaging 1.2 years (Oppel et al., 1968).

THE DEVELOPMENTAL BIOLOGY OF URINARY CONTROL

In the infant, micturition occurs spontaneously as a spinal cord reflex. When increasing amounts of urine distend the bladder and sufficiently stimulate the afferent limb of the reflex arc, the detrusor contracts. Even at this young age, the periurethral striated muscles that compose the voluntary (external) urinary sphincter are fully integrated into the voiding reflex so that as the bladder fills, the urinary sphincter constricts progressively to prevent incontinence. During micturition, the striated muscle sphincter relaxes reflexly to allow low-pressure bladder emptying.

The young infant sleeps nearly 60 per cent of the day, and approximately 40 per cent of voidings occur during sleep. In the first year of life, the number of voidings per day remains fairly constant at about 20. Thereafter, during the first 3 years of life, the frequency of urinations per day decreases to about 11, while the mean voided volume increases nearly fourfold (Goellner et al., 1981). This progressive reduction in bladder responsiveness has been presumed to be due to the unconscious inhibition of the micturition reflex (Yeates, 1973). It appears that these changes in voided volume and frequency of voidings may instead reflect changes in the volume of fluid intake and alterations in the size of the infant's bladder. Daily urine volume correlates closely with oral intake and, when expressed as a percentage of intake, does not change appreciably during the first 3 years of life. Similarly, when mean voided volumes are expressed per unit of body weight, voiding size changes little with age. However, the volume of urine produced per unit of body weight per day decreases and bladder capacity increases during this period (Goellner et al., 1981; Koff, 1983). It thus appears that the reduction in voiding frequency observed during the first 3 years of life is due primarily to a growth-related increase in bladder capacity that is proportionately greater than is the increase in urine volume produced.

As a child matures, the success of toilet training and the development of an adult type of urinary control depend on the outcome of at least three separate events in the development of bladder form and bladder-sphincter function (Nash, 1949). First, the capacity of the bladder must increase to permit it to function as an adequate reservoir. The capacity of the newborn's bladder is approximately 1 to 2 ounces. Each year until nearly age 12, the bladder enlarges by about 1 ounce per year. As a consequence, bladder capacity in childhood can be accurately estimated and expressed by the formula: bladder capacity (in ounces) equals age (in years) plus 2 (Koff, 1983). Second, voluntary control over the periurethral striated muscle sphincter must occur to permit the decisive initiation and termination of micturition. As with other acquired striated muscle skills, sphincter control fits into an orderly scheme of developmental landmarks and usually is complete by the age of 3 years. Third, direct volitional control over the spinal micturition reflex must develop in order for the child to initiate or inhibit detrusor contraction voluntarily. This last phase in the development of urinary control is the most complex, but once accomplished, the ability to void or inhibit voiding voluntarily at any degree of bladder filling sets the child apart from all other mammals (except the canine). Although voluntary control over the bladder smooth muscle is somewhat perplexing from a physiologic standpoint, its occurrence has been well documented (Lapides et al., 1957; Muellner, 1960).

Eventually, by the age of 4 years, most children will have developed an adult pattern of urinary control and will be continent day and night. This adult pattern is characterized by the absence of spontaneous uncontrolled infant-type or so-called uninhibited bladder contractions. Urodynamic studies have confirmed that even at bladder capacity, when the desire to void is strongest, the detrusor will not contract unless voluntarily initiated (Diokno et al., 1974). During bladder filling, the striated muscles of the urinary sphincter will be reflexly activated, and their constriction will become maximal at bladder capacity. This is a guarding reflex that prevents urinary incontinence. However, when detrusor contraction is voluntarily initiated, simultaneous reflex relaxation of the striated muscle sphincter will afford low-pressure bladder emptying.

The ultimate maturation of bladder control depends on more than reservoir size and spinal cord reflex modulation. It also requires a decrease in the nocturnal urine volume excreted by the kidneys as a result of acquiring a circadian rhythm in the secretion of pituitary hormones, which generally occurs by about age 3 or 4 years (George et al., 1975; Mandell et al., 1966; Winter et al., 1976). Current studies by Norgaard and co-workers (1989b) demonstrate that enuretic patients have stable levels of antidiuretic hormone (ADH) throughout the day and night, whereas normal controls display an increase in ADH secretion during the night. This low nighttime ADH level in enuretics leads to low urine osmolality and results in high urinary output, which over the course of the night can exceed daytime bladder capacity by several hundred per cent. This high nocturnal urinary output does not itself cause enuresis and, as a result, antidiuretic treatment with 1-deamino-(8-D-arginine)-vasopressin (DDAVP) is only moderately effective in curing or improving enuresis. It does suggest, however, that delayed maturation of all components that ultimately affect bladder control is extremely important in the genesis of nighttime wetting.

The development of urinary control thus fits into an orderly scheme of overall bowel and bladder control that follows a typical sequence of development: (1) control of bowel function at night; (2) control of bowel function by day; (3) control of bladder function by day; and (4) finally, after a lag of several months or more, control of bladder function by night. However, this sequence of achieving urinary control is malleable and can be overridden by external forces. Consequently, there is a marked individual variability in the age of achieving nighttime urinary control (Stein and Susser, 1967).

ETIOLOGY

As a group, nocturnal enuretic children are basically similar, biologically and psychologically, to normal children; however, they do not awaken when the bladder is full. The explanation for this phenomenon is not yet apparent.

A variety of theories have been proposed to explain enuresis. These include developmental delay, sleep abnormalities, genetic factors, stress and psychologic factors as well as organic urinary tract disease. Because enuresis is, in fact, a symptom rather than a true disease state, it is likely that no single hypothesis will explain all cases and that, in each individual instance, multiple factors may be operative. However, the vast majority of nocturnal enuretics do not suffer from obvious or treatable psychiatric disease, neurologic abnormalities, or urologic disturbances. As a result, causal analysis is often frustratingly difficult and unrewarding.

Urodynamic Factors

The single most important static urodynamic observation in children with enuresis is a reduced bladder capacity compared with normals (Esperanca and Gerrard, 1969a; Hallman, 1950; Muellner, 1960; Starfield, 1967; Wu et al., 1988). The magnitude of this reduction is often in excess of 50 per cent of bladder capacity. Measurements of bladder capacity in enuretics under anesthesia indicate that total bladder capacity is not actually reduced and that the disturbance causing a reduction in capacity is functional rather than anatomic (Troup and Hodgson, 1971). This finding is supported by the results of intravenous anticholinergic therapy for enuresis, which effects an increase in functional bladder capacity of 25 to 600 per cent (Johnstone, 1972).

In addition to small functional bladder capacity, a number of enuretics have diurnal symptoms of frequency, urgency, and incontinence. These diurnal symptoms suggest and, in fact, are predictive of the presence of uninhibited bladder contractions (Wu et al., 1988); this may represent involuntary and insuppressible detrusor activity, which may occur in children who have failed to gain complete voluntary control over the micturition reflex (Koff et al., 1979; Lapides and Diokno, 1970). Although they represent the normal mechanism for infant micturition, the precise cause for persistence of these contractions after toilet training is unknown. They are believed to represent either a delay in central nervous system maturation or a developmental regression (Nash, 1949).

In childhood enuresis, uninhibited contractions have been documented in more than 50 per cent of unselected patients (Booth et al., 1983; Linderholm, 1966; McGuire and Savastanes, 1984; Pompeius, 1971; Wu et al., 1988). Current studies suggest, however, that this incidence may be underestimated because, when cystometry is performed in only the supine position, it may fail to identify correctly up to two thirds of children with uninhibited contractions. When provocative tests aimed at eliciting uninhibited contractions are performed, such as sitting or standing cystometry or micturition stop testing, a much higher incidence (78 to 84 per cent) of uninhibited bladder activity is discovered (Giles et al., 1978; Mahony et al., 1981). These findings suggest that uninhibited bladder contractions may be much more common in enuresis than is generally appreciated. However, reliance on symptoms to predict which child will have this problem may be misleading because nearly a third of children with uninhibited contractions have no incontinence at all; conversely, 20 per cent of children with daytime symptoms will have normal cystometric studies (Koff and Murtagh, 1983).

Urodynamic studies performed during sleep or under anesthesia using artificial bladder filling confirm the presence of bladder hyperactivity in a number of enuretics. Whereas deep anesthesia will depress bladder contractility, bladder contractions can be recorded in more than 90 per cent of susceptible children under light anesthesia although the threshold volume at which the contraction occurs may be different from when awake (Grossman et al., 1977). Sleep cystometrograms recorded from enuretics show spontaneous bladder contractions that are more frequent and of greater amplitude than those of controls. Intravesical pressure during contractions may reach 50 cm H_2O or higher. These contractions may occur spontaneously or be secondary either to internal stimuli associated with autonomic changes and alterations in the electroencephalogram (EEG) or to external stimuli, such as loud noise.

Gastaut and Broughton characterized a typical enuretic wetting episode as a series of high-pressure bladder contractions culminating in micturition. Enuretics who happen not to wet during sleep studies will still display the same bladder hyperactivity, but pressures will be lower and frequency of contractions less than those preceding an enuretic event. In contrast, normal, nonenuretic individuals will display few, if any, low-pressure bladder contractions during sleep cystometrography (Gastaut and Broughton, 1965; Broughton, 1968).

More currently, Norgaard and co-workers (1989a) found that enuretic wetting episodes were nearly identical to voluntary daytime voiding with a single bladder contraction leading to enuresis. Although unstable contractions were observed in half of the cystometric studies, these contractions did not necessarily lead to incontinence; about 45 per cent of the time, the children awakened to void. The differences between wetting and voluntary voiding were slight; the bladder was usually full when it contracted, the detrusor contraction time was longer, and bladder pressure was higher with sleep wetting. Interestingly, pelvic floor muscle activity signaled arousal and led to voluntary voiding, whereas a silent pelvic floor was associated with sleep wetting (Norgaard et al., 1989a; Norgaard et al., 1989b).

In summary, these findings suggest that bladder contractions that produce nocturnal enuresis are potentially inhibitable even during sleep, and that the ability to suppress bladder hyperactivity while awake and asleep is essential for the successful development of day and nighttime urinary control. Although uninhibited contractions appear to be much more common and more intimately associated with the pathophysiology of nocturnal enuresis than has been generally appreciated, there does not appear to be a direct causal relationship between uninhibited bladder contractions and nighttime wetting for most enuretics. Cure of enuresis, therefore, does not necessarily depend on elimination of uninhibited contractions but simply on converting them to awake voiding. Thus, it is not surprising that anticholinergic therapy aimed at eliminating uninhibited contractions is quite ineffective for nocturnal enuresis (Lovering et al., 1988).

Developmental Delay

In a sense, nocturnal and diurnal enuresis represent an arrest in development because both occur normally in young children. Consequently, the hypothesis that enuresis represents a developmental delay or maturational lag in central nervous system development is both attractive and well supported by a number of diverse clinical observations.

The aforementioned urodynamic abnormalities of functional bladder capacity and bladder hyperactivity, which occur so commonly in enuresis, tend to improve with time and to resolve spontaneously. Children displaying these abnormalities do not manifest obvious neuropathy, and neurologic disease is rarely identified. It is most likely that these phenomena are merely an expression of neurophysiologic immaturity and reflect a delay in development.

A developmental cause for enuresis is also supported by the observation that a number of nonorganic disturbances, such as social factors and stress, can modify the attainment of urinary control and influence the timing and duration of enuresis. Bedwetting is more common in lower socioeconomic groups and occurs twice as often among unskilled workers as compared with professionals (Essen and Peckham, 1976).

In families undergoing stress, the likelihood of enuresis occurring is increased threefold (Miller et al., 1960). MacKeith (1968) has pointed out that the second to the fourth year is a particularly sensitive period in the development of nocturnal bladder control and is a time when a high proportion of the population develops enuresis. Consequently, children with a significant anxiety-producing episode in this period have a much increased chance for developing enuresis. Young and Morgan (1973) have suggested further that the difference between primary and secondary enuresis is simply related to the timing of stressful events, with primary enuresis resulting from stress during the sensitive period and secondary enuresis being due to stresses occurring after the sensitive developmental period. Although these stressful episodes are typically transient, they may prevent the child from developing nocturnal urinary control at the appropriate point in time and allow the child to pass into a later developmental stage where spontaneous control is less likely to occur.

The negative effect of stress on maturation of urinary control is further evidenced by the increased prevalence of enuresis in children from deprived environments, from broken homes, and with a background of temporary institutional habitation. In considering the effect of stress on urinary control, one must recognize that another potential form of stress facing the young child is insuppressible uninhibited bladder activity, which renders the child incontinent during this critical developmental period of toilet training. The occurrence of daytime incontinence at this time may be sufficiently disturbing to further delay the acquisition of nocturnal urinary control.

Critics of developmental delay argue that this hypothesis is not anatomically correct or physiologically valid and point out that the occurrence of a single dry day and night in an enuretic child is proof that the neurologic pathways are intact and operative (Apley and MacKeith, 1968; MacKeith, 1972). They suggest, instead, that both primary and secondary enuresis are entirely stress-related phenomena, recognizing that in secondary enuresis these stressful events are usually much more obvious. However, to counter these views, it is apparent that despite the fact that neuroanatomic pathways are intact, their successful integration and the acquisition of behavioral skills necessary for nighttime urinary control may be adversely affected by developmental immaturity. This is reflected in the tendency for encopresis to occur more commonly (10 to 25 per cent) in enuretics and supports the generally apparent clinical observation that children who are retarded in one aspect of sphincter control tend to be retarded in another. In addition, a significantly higher proportion of bedwetting is observed in children who are also delayed in walking and in talking, and a significant number of children with primary enuresis display retardation in skeletal maturation (bone age), which may reflect delayed maturation of regulatory central nervous system functions (Mimouni et al., 1985).

These findings all suggest that achieving dryness is a sequential part of the child's general development and that when the overall rate of maturation is delayed, the delay appears in most of the individual aspects of development (Stein and Susser, 1967).

Sleep Factors

Objective evaluation of the relationship between sleep and enuresis required the development of sleep laboratories capable of monitoring all night the physiologic variables during sleep. Such studies demonstrated that sleep is not simply the progressive and passive slowing of body and brain processes. Normal sleep begins with so-called nonrapid eye movement (NREM) sleep, which is divisible into four progressively deep sleep stages

(Stages 1–4), each characterized by specific EEG changes. In addition, a particularly light stage of sleep is recognized and characterized by bursts of conjugate rapid eye movements (REM). REM sleep is associated with increased autonomic activity, generalized muscle atonia, and dreaming. Normal sleep structure is composed of cycles of NREM sleep, REM sleep, and occasional awakenings. In older children and adults, these cycles last about 1 to 1.5 hours, and the percentage of time spent in REM sleep increases as the cycles progress (Rechtschaffen and Kales, 1968).

Historically, enuresis has been considered a disorder of sleep and more precisely a consequence of deep sleep, recognizing that some enuretics appear to be deep sleepers (Anders and Weinstein, 1972; Broughton, 1968; Kales and Kales, 1974; Lowy, 1970). Early sleep studies supported this view by demonstrating that enuresis occurred during deep sleep and that adult enuretics were often very deep sleepers who required amphetamines to lighten their sleep (Strom-Olsen, 1950). However, the observation that enuretics are often deep sleepers may be biased and partially invalidated by the fact that parents do not regularly attempt to arouse their nonenuretic children from sleep (Boyd, 1960; Graham, 1973; Hallgren, 1957; McKendry et al., 1968). When children are aroused from deep stage 4 sleep, they may be hard to awaken and appear confused and disoriented. It has been suggested that the degree of "sleep drunkenness" may be more deeply observed in enuretics, and this finding might account in part for the perception that enuretics sleep more soundly than do normals (Lowy, 1970).

Although depth of sleep may be a factor for some enuretic children, currently accumulated evidence has suggested that previously hypothesized relationships between enuresis and sleep may be erroneous. Controlled sleep research studies indicate that children with enuresis sleep no more soundly than do normals and that a proportion of enuretics actually wet during very light sleep or while awake (Ritvo et al., 1969). Findings such as these encouraged the notion that enuresis was a disorder of arousal, implying that enuresis might correlate better with a transition from one level of sleep to another than with an inability to awaken from deep sleep (Broughton, 1968).

Two large sleep studies have demonstrated that neither of these hypotheses—deep sleep or arousal—is an accurate description of enuretic sleep structure. Enuretics were observed to sleep no more deeply than age-matched controls, and enuretic events were associated neither with deep sleep nor with a transition between sleep stages or arousal signs. Instead, enuretic episodes were noted throughout the night on a random basis and occurred in each stage of sleep in proportion to the actual amount of time spent in that stage (Inouie et al., 1987; Kales et al., 1977; Mikkelson et al., 1980; Norgaard et al., 1989a).

These findings indicate that enuretic sleep patterns are not appreciably different from the sleep patterns of normal children, and that most enuretics do not wet as a consequence of sleeping too deeply.

Genetic Factors

It is an old but valid observation that enuresis tends to run in families. In multiple series, over a third of fathers and a fifth of mothers of enuretics have an enuretic history themselves (Frary, 1935; Hallgren, 1957). Bakwin (1971, 1973) showed further that, when both parents had enuresis, 77 per cent of children were enuretic, whereas when one parent was enuretic, 44 per cent of children developed wetting. These figures contrast with a 15 per cent incidence of enuresis in children from nonenuretic parents. Studies in twins indicate as well that, when one twin has enuresis, the other is predisposed to develop wetting (Bakwin, 1971).

Organic Urinary Tract Disease

Children with enuresis, particularly girls, are predisposed to develop urinary tract infections (Dodge et al., 1970). However, many of these children will have diurnal symptoms due to uninhibited bladder contractions. The mechanism for their infection is voluntary constriction of the urinary sphincter muscles in an attempt to maintain continence during the uninhibited bladder contraction. This produces obstruction with high intravesical pressures of a degree comparable to an anatomic urinary tract obstruction. Not all children will have both day and night wetting, but characteristically their symptoms will persist after the infection is eradicated and they will continue to display a small functional bladder capacity. In contrast to girls, boys with enuresis seem less prone to develop urinary tract infections even if they have associated uninhibited bladder activity (Koff et al., 1979; Koff and Murtagh, 1983; Lapides and Diokno, 1970).

Excluding uninhibited bladder activity, most children with nocturnal enuresis do not have an organic urinary tract cause for their wetting; the incidence of organic disease is less than 10 per cent and probably closer to 1 per cent (Forsythe and Redmond, 1974; Hallgren, 1957; McKendry and Stewart, 1974). However, prior to a decade ago, diseases that nowadays would be classified as normal variants or minor abnormalities were regularly invoked as common causes for enuresis, and many children underwent some type of surgical procedure (Arnold and Ginsberg, 1973; Fisher and Forsythe, 1954; Mahony, 1971). It is now generally appreciated that these minor disorders, such as meatal stenosis, do not cause enuresis, and in only a small percentage of children will relief of symptoms follow an operation, such as meatotomy (Kunin et al., 1970). In contrast to pure nocturnal enuresis, Cutler and colleagues (1978) found an increased incidence of organic abnormalities in children with diurnal symptoms, although not all series have substantiated this finding (Redman and Seibert, 1979).

Psychologic Factors

The occurrence of emotional disturbances in enuretic children is probably slightly higher than in the general population, but most enuretics do not suffer from sig-

nificant psychologic disease (Fergusson et al., 1986; Werry, 1967). From a psychodynamic viewpoint, if enuresis were the somatic expression of an emotional disorder, its elimination might prove undesirable and result either in a worsening of the psychopathologic disturbance or in the development of substitute symptoms (Young and Morgan, 1973). Such a hypothesis is insupportable by clinical observation and most therapists find precisely the opposite, that childhood adjustment tends to improve rather than worsen after successful treatment of enuresis (Baker, 1969). Bindelglas and Dee (1978) reported the fate of enuretics who had been successfully treated with imipramine 10 years earlier. They convincingly put to rest the notion that enuresis was a symptom of severe psychopathologic disturbance by demonstrating that treatment of enuresis did not produce psychologic decomposition, inhibition of learning, or, in fact, any negative effect on adolescent health, growth, or development. In most instances, enuresis should be considered a disturbance unrelated to psychopathologic abnormality, and its symptomatic treatment is therefore perfectly justifiable.

In some instances, enuresis and a psychopathologic disorder may coexist, although disturbed children are not particularly prone to enuresis. Occasionally, emotional disturbance may actually be due to or exacerbated by enuresis because wetting places an additional burden on the child suffering from multiple difficulties (Young and Morgan, 1973).

Miscellaneous Factors

Although there is no objective evidence relating allergy to enuresis for most patients, in a small number of selected individuals, such an association may exist. Zaleski and associates (1972) have shown that food allergy may cause bladder hyperactivity and a reduced functional bladder capacity. Both of these were observed to improve convincingly after elimination of the offending dietary allergen. However, no differences were observed in the level of immunoglobulins often associated with allergenic phenomena (IgE) in enuretics as compared with controls (Kaplan, 1973).

Enuretics have a higher incidence of EEG abnormalities compared with normal children (Campbell and Young, 1966; Fermaglich, 1969; Kajtor et al., 1967). This finding has been alternately interpreted as demonstrating mild degrees of cerebral dysfunction in these children or, more probable, as providing evidence for delayed functional maturation of the central nervous system because many of these described abnormalities were nonspecific and minor.

Sudden onset enuresis and urinary frequency in little girls may be due to *Enterobius vermicularis* (pinworm) infestation without perineal itching. Diagnosis is made by recovery of characteristic eggs in feces, from perianal skin, or from under fingernails. Immediate and dramatic relief of symptoms will follow appropriate antihelminthic therapy (Sachdev and Howards, 1975).

EVALUATION

The enuretic child and family seek medical attention to find cause or cure. Unfortunately, it is often difficult to pinpoint the etiologic factor and to eliminate the symptoms. Out of frustration, the physician may be tempted to perform overly invasive diagnostic testing or to attach pathologic significance to minor anatomic variations and treat them aggressively. Such an approach is unwarranted for childhood enuresis and is unjustifiable.

Most children with enuresis do not have an organic lesion and those who do are readily detected by routine evaluation. A careful history, physical examination, and urinalysis with culture are needed for all children with bedwetting and are all that is needed for the child with purely nocturnal enuresis. Routine radiographic studies, such as intravenous pyelography or voiding cystourethrography, are not indicated for enuretics who have a normal physical examination, a negative urine, and no obvious neuropathy. This is a view supported by the American Academy of Pediatrics (1980). Likewise, endoscopic evaluation is unwarranted, and urologists must resist the compulsion to inspect and manipulate the lower urinary tracts of children with enuresis simply because they are referred for evaluation. In the vast majority of enuretics, the diagnostic yield from cystourethroscopy is nil, as is the prospect for influencing symptoms by altering urethral caliber or by fulgurating prominent urethral folds.

The nature and extent of the history, physical examination, and urinary examination are important because they will permit wetting pattern recognition, which allows segregation of patients into useful diagnostic and therapeutic categories. Specific features in the voiding history should include the age and success of toilet training, the pattern of urinary incontinence (such as day, night, urgency), maneuvers that are used to stay dry (such as squatting), and the results of prior therapeutic trials. It is often helpful to interview the patient and family privately to assess their perceptions of the problem, to measure the child's maturity and motivation for cure, and to establish rapport. In addition to routine physical examination, neurologic examination is required. Careful palpation and inspection of the lumbosacral spine may reveal hairy patches, lipomata, tracts, or bony irregularities, which suggest occult spinal dysraphism. After a check for rectal sphincter tone and perineal sensation, assessment of the sensory, motor, and reflex functions of the lower extremities is needed to exclude neuropathy. Examination for abnormalities of gait and bony alterations in the lower extremities, such as deformed feet, may reveal evidence of occult neurologic disease. In addition, a complete urinalysis requires a check for proteinuria and for fixed low specific gravity in addition to microscopic examination and urine culture.

The aforementioned evaluation will separate children with only nocturnal enuresis and no infection, who require no additional diagnostic studies, from those with urinary infection or overt neuropathy, who require full urologic investigation. It will also identify those children without infection who either have both daytime and nighttime incontinence or display a variety of dysfunctional voiding symptoms, which may suggest more complicated micturitional disturbances. The majority of these children ultimately prove not to have an underlying anatomic urinary tract abnormality but instead display urodynamic disturbances, such as uninhibited bladder activity. In this group of patients, urinary tract anatomy should be screened and this can be accomplished noninvasively and satisfactorily with an ultrasound examination of the kidneys, ureters, and bladder before and after voiding. This study will effectively exclude even mild degrees of hydroureteronephrosis and will assess the completeness of bladder emptying. Any positive findings can be pursued with conventional urologic studies. When ultrasonography is normal, consideration should be given to an empirical therapeutic trial of pharmacologic agents, such as anticholinergic drugs, aimed at the suspected urodynamic disturbance. This approach is generally satisfactory provided that the patient continues to be followed closely. If symptoms of wetting persist, complete urodynamic studies are indicated to exclude neuropathy and to identify treatable voiding disturbances.

TREATMENT

A variety of different programs have been used in the treatment of enuresis. They range from home remedies and nonspecific measures, such as decreasing fluids and awakening the child during the night, to sophisticated medical regimens. Because almost all children will eventually outgrow enuresis on their own, it has been genuinely difficult to objectively evaluate even seemingly well controlled treatment programs in order to determine which are effective. This difficulty is compounded by the fact that the yearly spontaneous remission rate is approximately 15 per cent and that the placebo improvement effect may be as high as 68 per cent (Forsythe and Redmond, 1974; Mishra et al., 1980). Despite this analytic handicap, reproducibly proven and effective therapy does exist for enuresis and has evolved along two main lines: pharmacologic therapy and modification of behavior.

Before initiating therapy, the physician must realize, once the parents are reassured that organic causes are excluded, that not all families will desire medical treatment or will accept any risks, inconveniences, or responsibility; some may lack the motivation and intelligence needed to execute and sustain a behavior-oriented therapy. Surprisingly, although most parents generally believe that children should be dry at a much younger age than do physicians, only 63 per cent of parents believe that medical therapy is appropriate treatment for enuresis, as opposed to 87 per cent of physicians. Likewise, the vast majority of parents (93 per cent) do not consider drugs a good form of treatment for bedwetting (Haque et al., 1981). It is necessary in developing a treatment plan for the physician to recognize that wide differences exist between parental and physician attitudes and perceptions toward enuresis. For most nocturnal enuretics, therapy should be discouraged before the age of 5 or 6 years. However, for children with significant day and night symptoms, pharmacotherapy may be required at an even younger age (see following discussion).

Pharmacotherapy

Autonomic Agents

Effective pharmacologic therapy exists for enuresis but not in the form of sedatives, stimulants, or sympathomimetic agents (Blackwell and Currah, 1973). Overall, anticholinergic drug therapy has been disappointing. Its effectiveness has been in the range of 5 to 40 per cent, and in some series, therapy was unappreciably different from placebo (Harrison and Albino, 1970; Kunin et al., 1970; Leys, 1956; Lovering et al., 1988; Rapoport et al., 1980). Although anticholinergic drugs have been shown to increase the functional capacity of the bladder in enuretic children, clinical improvement does not follow in about one half of cases (Johnstone, 1972). However, because these agents are very useful in eliminating uninhibited contractions, they may be effective for subgroups of enuretics with this urodynamic disturbance. Indeed, Kass and co-workers (1979) found anticholinergic therapy to be very effective (87.5 per cent) in treating enuretic patients with symptoms of bladder hyperactivity, such as urgency, frequency, and day and night incontinence, and highly effective (90.6 per cent) in those with proven uninhibited bladder contractions. The success rate was much less (50 per cent) in patients with pure nocturnal enuresis and was only 11 per cent in those with normal cystometrograms. It is apparent that by tailoring pharmacotherapy to clinical symptoms or urodynamic findings that indicate urodynamic disturbances, the results of anticholinergic therapy for enuresis can be improved.

Agents Affecting Urinary Output

Reduction of urine output at night is theoretically attractive for treating bedwetting. However, simply limiting fluids or using diuretics during the daytime to produce relative dehydration at night has not been particularly effective (Scott and Morrison, 1980). In contrast, manipulation of antidiuretic hormone levels (ADH, vasopressin) offers a prospect for treatment. Measurements of urinary and serum vasopressin demonstrate an absence or reversal of the normal circadian rhythm in enuretics who have lower than normal excretion levels of vasopressin during the night (Norgaard et al., 1989b; Puri, 1980).

Until recently, however, any preparation containing natural vasopressin was not useful for enuresis control because the drug effect was too short or was associated with unpleasant smooth muscle side effects. With the development of desmopressin (DDAVP), an analog of vasopressin, wide potential application for treating enuresis became available. This drug can be given intranasally, has no pressor or smooth muscle activity in the effective dose range, and has an effect lasting 7 to 10 hours. It can also be given in an oral form with an equal effect (Fjellestad-Paulsen et al., 1987).

In double-blind studies, DDAVP has been shown to be more effective than placebo in treating enuresis. Its mechanism of action is believed to be due to its antidiuretic effect, which has been reported to achieve a 30 to 60 per cent reduction in wet nights and up to a 50 per cent cure rate. After treatment, most children resume wetting, unfortunately. The usual clinical dose ranges between 20 and 40 μg and responses are dose dependent. A large multicenter U.S. clinical trial showed a 24 per cent reduction in wet nights at 20 μg and a 40 per cent reduction at 40 μg compared with a 14 per cent placebo effect (Klauber, 1989). Better results have occurred in older children with no appreciable side effects or alterations in serum electrolytes or osmolality being observed. The drug may be safely used for longer periods, but it is relatively expensive and, upon discontinuation, less than one third of cured patients stay dry (Aladjem et al., 1982; Birkasova et al., 1978; Dimson, 1977; Harris, 1989; Miller et al., 1989; Pedersen et al., 1985; Rew and Rundle, 1989; Tuvemo, 1978).

Imipramine

Imipramine, typical of a class of tricyclic antidepressants, is probably the most effective and most widely studied of all antienuretic agents. Since its effect on enuresis was first observed in 1960 (MacLean), it has proved to be significantly effective in large numbers of well-controlled clinical studies. Overall, enuresis can be cured in more than 50 per cent of children and will be improved in another 15 to 20 per cent. However, discontinuation of medication will cause up to 60 per cent of patients to relapse (Blackwell and Currah, 1973; Esperanca and Gerrard, 1969b; Hagglund and Parkkulainen, 1965; Harrison and Albino, 1970; Kardash et al., 1968; Kunin et al., 1970; Liederman et al., 1969; Martin, 1971; Miller et al., 1968; Milner and Hills, 1968; Poussaint et al., 1966; Shaffer et al., 1968). Although imipramine (Tofranil) is the most widely used agent, other drugs in this class, such as nortriptyline (Aventyl), amitriptyline (Elavil), and desipramine (Pertofrane), have similar effects.

Imipramine possesses several pharmacologic actions on the central and peripheral nervous system that could be responsible for its effect in enuresis, although its precise mechanism of action remains unknown. Its peripheral effects include (1) weak anticholinergic activity that is $\frac{1}{157}$ as active as atropine on bladder smooth muscle (Sigg, 1959) but that is ineffective in abolishing uninhibited detrusor contractions (Diokno et al., 1972); (2) direct in vitro antispasmodic activity on bladder smooth muscle that is inapparent at clinically effective antienuretic doses (Labay and Boyarsky, 1973; Stephenson, 1979); and (3) a complex effect on sympathetic input to the bladder, which prevents norepinephrine action on alpha receptors and enhances its effect on beta receptors by inhibiting norepinephrine reuptake (Labay and Boyarsky, 1973; Stephenson, 1979). Combined, these peripheral actions of imipramine produce significant increase in bladder capacity. It has been observed that successful clinical improvement in enuresis correlates with an average 34 per cent increase in bladder functional capacity (Hagglund, 1965), whereas those children who have no change in bladder capacity are generally not cured (Esperanca and Gerrard, 1969b).

Imipramine effects on the central nervous system include its antidepressant activity and its action on sleep. It is unlikely that antienuretic effect is related to antidepressant activity because the time course of action in enuresis is immediate, whereas the effect on depression requires higher dosage and is often delayed for a period of time (Rapoport et al., 1980). Imipramine significantly alters sleep patterns by decreasing the time spent in REM sleep and increasing the time spent in light NREM sleep. This REM sleep suppression occurs primarily during the first two thirds of the night, and as a result, there are less enuretic events in this period of sleep and more during the last third. In sleep studies, imipramine can be shown to reduce the total number of wetting episodes, but it does not appreciably alter the time at which wetting occurs. Incontinence seems to occur in each sleep stage roughly in proportion to the time spent in that stage (Kales et al., 1977; Rapoport et al., 1980; Ritvo et al., 1969). Compared with placebo, no more frequent night wakenings occur during imipramine therapy and the occurrence of wakenings does not correlate with clinical response. This indicates that imipramine does not work by converting enuresis to nocturia and further supports the observation that its effect on sleep stage is independent of its effect on enuresis (Kales et al., 1977; Rapoport et al., 1980).

In some studies, the clinical response to imipramine has been shown to correlate with plasma levels; this has provided a better understanding of drug action and a more rational approach to therapy (DeGatta et al., 1984; Jorgensen et al., 1980; Rapoport et al., 1980).

Imipramine is generally prescribed as a single dose of 25 mg for children between 5 and 8 years of age and 50 mg for older children. On a weight basis, the usual recommended dosage is 0.9 to 1.5 mg/kg/day (Maxwell and Seldrup, 1971). Unfortunately, this dosage results in an optimal therapeutic plasma concentration in only 30 per cent of patients (Jorgensen et al., 1980). This finding may explain the variability in clinical effect noted in early reports. An increase of three to five fold in dose would be required to achieve a therapeutic level in all patients, but this cannot be justified because nearly toxic levels would result for a significant number of patients (Stephenson, 1979). However, even high plasma levels will not ensure a response in all instances because true nonresponders can be identified as well as patients who have developed a tolerance to the antienuretic effect of the drug. Likewise, clinical response does not always correlate directly with serum concentration of imipramine, and some patients have been observed to respond when their serum concentration was markedly below optimal levels. As a result, routine measurement of the concentration of imipramine or its metabolites does not appear to be clinically useful for response monitoring (DeVane et al., 1984).

Imipramine is generally given once per day and usually shortly before bedtime. The exact time of administration does not appear critical, although some children who wet very early at night may benefit from late afternoon administration (Alderton, 1970). A 2-week trial is generally adequate to assess drug responsiveness. Thereafter, adjustments in the dosage and time can be made if necessary. It is not entirely clear how long a satisfactorily responding child should be kept on drug therapy. Because the long-term effects of tricyclic therapy in children are unknown, continued medication is difficult to justify except in instances where the child is extremely distressed or when all other therapies have been exhausted and are unsuccessful. When the decision is made to stop medication, it may be advisable to wean the drug rather than to discontinue therapy abruptly because some studies have shown a reduced tendency for a relapse using this withdrawal technique (Martin, 1971).

Imipramine drug therapy has two potentially hazardous consequences. The first is a manifestation of drug toxicity. Side effects, although infrequent, include personality changes, adverse effects on sleep and appetite, gastrointestinal symptoms, and nervousness (Kardash et al., 1968; Shaffer et al., 1968). Because of the low ratio between beneficial effect and toxic effect, toxic overdose is a potential hazard. At greatest risk are the younger siblings of enuretics who unwarily ingest the medication in large amounts. Poisoning is characterized by severe myocardial depression and electrocardiographic changes that are not observed at therapeutic levels (Fouron and Chicoine, 1971; Koehl and Wenzel, 1971; Martin, 1973; Rohner and Sanford, 1975). Should a toxic reaction occur, careful attention must be given to specific therapeutic protocols aimed at drug effect reversal (Green and Cromie, 1981).

The second effect of imipramine that is potentially problematic is its ability to improve wetting symptoms not only in cases of enuresis but also when the incontinence is due to an organic abnormality, such as neuropathy (Cole and Fried, 1972; Epstein and DeQuevedo, 1964). As a result, the use of imipramine as a therapeutic test to distinguish organic from nonorganic incontinence is not advisable.

Behavior Modification

Modification of behavior to control enuresis has met with varying success. Although generalized supportive measures designed to improve self-confidence and provide encouragement are unpredictably effective, certain specific approaches, when determinedly applied to a motivated child, produce the most effective rate of sustained cure and should be considered a first-line approach to the management of enuresis.

Techniques that have been used include bladder training, responsibility reinforcement, and classical conditioning therapy. Often, a successful treatment program for enuresis combines aspects of each specific technique that may be used in conjunction with pharmacotherapy.

Bladder Training

Bladder training, or so-called retention control training, (Kimmel and Kimmel, 1970) was developed as specific therapy for the reduced functional bladder capacity that characterizes most enuretics. Because an increase in the functional capacity of the bladder correlates positively with reduced bedwetting, the rationale for this treatment is well founded and the initial results were promising.

The goal of therapy is to increase progressively the time interval between voidings so that the bladder capacity is effectively enlarged. Positive reinforcement is provided as the child goes for longer intervals and demonstrates larger recorded urine volumes. With retention control therapy, mean bladder capacity can be increased sizably in enuretic subjects compared with controls (approximately 35 per cent). However, as a cure for enuresis, this method has not met clinical expectations because the frequency of bedwetting does not appear to decrease significantly in many children so treated. Although enlargement in bladder capacity generally accompanies cure of enuresis, treatments aimed only at bladder capacity, such as retention control therapy and anticholinergic therapy, are not effective for most nocturnal wetters (Doleys, 1977; Harris and Purohit, 1977). However, when retention control is combined with conditioning therapy using the urinary alarm (see following discussion), results can be highly successful both in the initial arrest of wetting (92 per cent) and in ultimate cure (Geffken et al., 1986).

Responsibility Reinforcement

Behavior modification techniques are successful in treating enuresis, but they require a motivated child, conscientious parents, and rapport between the physician and family. The components of a successful responsibility reinforcement program include motivation, reward, response shaping, and reinforcement. The program aims to motivate the child to assume both the responsibility for wetting and the credit for dryness. The child keeps a progress record or "gold star" chart, and by trying to determine what factors are responsible for wetting, attempts to reduce enuresis and to keep totally dry. Progressively longer dry intervals and dry nights are rewarded by stars or an equivalent. The consequence of these stepwise rewards for changes in behavior results in a generalized molding of responses and progressive attainment of continence.

The results of a responsibility reinforcement program may be difficult to evaluate on a controlled basis because better results are observed when the child takes an active role in therapy compared with a passive role. For selected children, improvement may be more rapid and the relapse rate lower than with other types of programs (Marshall et al., 1973).

Conditioning Therapy

At least four randomized controlled trials have shown that conditioning is the most effective means of eliminating bed wetting (DeLeon et al., 1966; McKendry et al., 1975; Moffatt et al., 1987; Werry and Cohrsen, 1965). Conditioning using the urinary alarm has evolved from the bell and pad popularized by Mowrer and

Mowrer in 1938. It originally consisted of a battery-operated detector upon which the child sleeps. The detector is activated by urine and the child is awakened by a bell, turns off the alarm, then gets up and completes voiding in the toilet. The success of the urinary alarm method has been explained by classical conditioning theory. If the alarm that awakens the child and initiates inhibition of micturition is repeatedly followed by the onset of normal voiding, then ultimately those factors causing the reflex micturition at night, such as bladder distention, would produce the same inhibition response as the alarm and awaken the child before enuresis occurs (Doleys, 1977). Although not all investigators agree with the precise mechanism of effect (Lovibond, 1963), conditioning therapy using an alarm appears to be the most statistically effective available therapy for enuresis.

In its modern form—a small transistorized battery-powered device attached either to the collar or wrist and connected by a fine wire to underclothes—the urinary alarm is well accepted, safe, and relatively inexpensive.

The single most important cause for failure of the alarm has been lack of parental understanding and cooperation. This can be prevented by proper instruction and supervision. However, before embarking on this program, parents and child must be motivated and well selected and must recognize that the period of therapy is long, often lasting approximately 4 months. In addition, there must be no delay between the alarm sounding and the child getting up to void. As a result, parents may have to awaken their child at variable times throughout the night; this no doubt leads to the high dropout rate observed with conditioning therapy. Once enuresis has been converted to nocturia or cured completely, relapse can be prevented in many instances by using overlearning techniques (Young and Morgan, 1972). These involve forcing fluids prior to bedtime to promote bladder overdistention in order to provide a stronger conditioning stimulus. The likelihood for relapse can also be reduced by having the alarm sound intermittently on some nights but not others.

In controlled studies, the urinary alarm is superior to drug therapy, imipramine and DDAVP, with a cure rate of 60 to 100 per cent. Compared to DDAVP, the alarm cure rate was 86 per cent versus 70 per cent for DDAVP; however, after therapy, the relapse rate with DDAVP was ten times greater (Wagner et al., 1982; Wille, 1986). Although as many as 25 per cent of patients may relapse with the alarm, in many instances, this is preventable and retreatment will effect a cure in a significant proportion (Doleys, 1977; Forsythe and Redmond, 1970; Young and Morgan, 1973). Conditioning therapy is effective under a variety of circumstances; age and intelligence are not factors in achieving dryness, nor is the amount of incontinence.

Conditioning therapy using the urinary alarm may be combined with pharmacotherapy or behavioral modification to create an individually tailored approach to treatment. With this approach, the prospect for enhanced results both in decreasing wet nights and in totally eliminating bedwetting is excellent (Geffken et al., 1986; Sukhai et al., 1989).

Miscellaneous Therapy

In addition to the aforementioned programs, numerous other treatments have been used for enuresis. Hypnotherapy and psychotherapy are highly effective for selected patients who have a stressful emotional cause for their wetting or in whom enuresis accompanies psychologic disturbance. However, for most enuretics who have no significant psychopathologic disorder, these approaches would be inappropriate and inefficient (Fraser, 1972).

Certain children will show a marked improvement following recognition and elimination of dietary ingredients that enhance enuresis. The approach to diagnosis is similar to that used to identify food allergens, which involves serial elimination of foods such as chocolate, dairy products, and red-dye–containing substances (Esperanca and Gerrard, 1969b). Of course, foods and drinks that contain caffeine may enhance enuresis by producing a diuresis that overwhelms the small functional capacity bladder and should be omitted.

ADULT ENURESIS

Enuresis occurring in adults is seen in two contexts: persistent primary enuresis, which occurs in more than 1 per cent of the population (Levine, 1943; Miller et al., 1973); and adult onset enuresis. Unlike the situation in children, a high proportion (greater than 70 per cent) of adults with persistent primary enuresis will display overt urodynamic abnormalities, generally in the form of uninhibited bladder activity (Torrens and Collins, 1975; Whiteside and Arnold, 1975). These abnormalities are not due to a neuropathic process, and once identified, may persist for many years as fixed urodynamic disturbances. Although symptoms from uninhibited bladder dysfunction usually depend on the frequency of detrusor contraction and on the opposing forcefulness of sphincteric constriction, the presence of diurnal symptoms and urge incontinence are often useful predictors of which patient has uninhibited bladder activity and may be a guide to empiric pharmacologic therapy (Hindmarsh and Byrne, 1980).

In the absence of overt neuropathy, urinary infection, or obstructive symptoms, the incidence of organic disease does not appear to be appreciably greater for adults with persistent nocturnal enuresis than for children (Torrens and Collins, 1975). Even though the presence of diurnal symptoms may increase the likelihood of urodynamic disturbance in these patients, it is not clear that such symptoms increase the possibility of organic disease. Consequently, it is a matter of clinical judgment in each individual case to determine the need for and the extent of investigation in excess of the evaluation required for childhood enuresis. Once a dignosis of primary enuresis has been established, treatment may follow the general guidelines described for children. It is noteworthy, however, that caffeine withdrawal significantly reduces bedwetting in adult enuretics, suggesting that caffeine intake should first be reduced before other forms of treatment are initiated (Edelstein et al., 1984; Karacan et al., 1976).

Acquired or adult onset enuresis is not generally a solitary symptom but occurs more commonly in association with generalized bladder hyperactivity and with other disturbances of micturition and continence. Even in the absence of urinary infection, patients usually require a thorough anatomic evaluation as well as a careful neurologic and urodynamic study, recognizing that occult neurologic dysfunction and anatomic disease can masquerade as a disturbance of genitourinary tract function and present as adult onset enuresis.

SUMMARY

The physician evaluating and treating enuresis must keep in perspective its medical significance and recognize that, for the vast majority of patients, the condition is medically benign and subject to a high spontaneous cure rate. Because an organic cause for enuresis is rare, and such patients can usually be readily diagnosed by a systematic history, physical examination, and urinalysis, the evaluation of most enuretics can be accomplished in the office at the first visit. The so-called urologic workup consisting of an intravenous pyelogram, voiding cystogram, and cystoscopy has no place in the routine evaluation of childhood enuretics. Such studies should be considered only after less invasive tests, such as ultrasonography, incriminate structural disease.

For certain enuretics, no therapy is necessary because none will be successful; all involved must wait frustratingly until spontaneous cure occurs. Assessment of the motivation of the family and particularly the child is important in determining whether therapy more than reassurance alone is actually being sought and in deciding which treatment is likely to succeed.

Conditioning therapy using the urinary alarm is the most statistically effective treatment available, but it is not suitable for all patients. It can only be effective if it is properly supervised and continued sufficiently long in highly receptive and motivated individuals. Considering the potential and unknown risks of long-term pharmacotherapy, drugs such as imipramine probably should be reserved for failures of other therapy or when short-term dry periods are essential. A trial of DDAVP may be considered appropriate therapy for older individuals, especially mature teenagers who are eager to achieve rapid results, with the recognition that the medication is not inexpensive and that discontinuation is regularly associated with relapse.

REFERENCES

Aladjem, M., Wohl, R., Boichis, H., et al.: Desmopressin in nocturnal enuresis. Arch. Dis. Child., 57:137, 1982.
Alderton, H. R.: Imipramine in childhood enuresis: Further studies on the relationship of time of administration to effect. Can. Med. Assoc. J., 102:1179, 1970.
American Academy of Pediatrics, Committee on Radiology: Excretory urography for evaluation of enuresis. Pediatrics, 65:644, 1980.
Anders, T. F., and Weinstein, P.: Sleep and its disorders in infants: A review. Pediatrics, 50:312, 1972.

Apley, J., and MacKeith, R.: The Child and His Symptoms, ed. 2. Philadelphia, F. A. Davis Co., 1968.

Arnold, S. J., and Ginsberg, A.: Enuresis, incidence and pertinence of genitourinary disease in healthy enuretic children. Urology, 2:437, 1973.

Baker, B. L.: Symptom treatment and symptom substitution in enuresis. J. Abnorm. Psychol., 74:42, 1969.

Bakwin, H.: Enuresis in twins. Am. J. Dis. Child., 121:222, 1971.

Bakwin, H.: The genetics of enuresis. In Kolvin, I., MacKeith, R. C., and Meadow, S. R. (Eds.): Bladder Control and Enuresis. London, W. Heinemann Medical Books Ltd., 1973, pp. 73–77.

Bindelglas, P. M., and Dee, G.: Enuresis treatment with imipramine hydrochloride: A 10-year follow-up study. Am. J. Psychiatry, 135:12, 1978.

Birkasova, M., Birkas, O., Flynn, M. J., et al.: Desmopressin in the management of nocturnal enuresis in children: A double blind study. Pediatrics, 62:970, 1978.

Blackwell, B., and Currah, J.: The psychopharmacology of nocturnal enuresis. In Kolvin, I., MacKeith, R. C., and Meadow, S. R. (Eds.): Bladder Control and Enuresis. London, W. Heinemann Medical Books Ltd., 1973, pp. 231–257.

Booth, C. M., and Gosling, J. A.: Histologic and urodynamic study of the bladder in enuretic children. Br. J. Urol., 55:367–370, 1983.

Boyd, M. M.: The depth of sleep in enuretic school children and nonenuretic controls. J. Psychosom. Res., 4:274, 1960.

Broughton, R. J.: Sleep disorders: Disorders of arousal? Science, 159:1070, 1968.

Campbell, E. W., Jr., and Young, J. D., Jr.: Enuresis and its relationship to electroencephalographic disturbances. J. Urol., 96:947, 1966.

Cole, A. T., and Fried, F. A.: Favorable experiences with imipramine in the treatment of neurogenic bladder. J. Urol., 107:44, 1972.

Cutler, C., Middleton, A. W., and Nixon, G. W.: Radiographic findings in children surveyed for enuresis. Urology, 11:480, 1978.

DeGatta, M. F., Garcia, M. J., and Acosta, A.: Monitoring of serum levels of imipramine and desipramine and individualization of dose in enuretic children. J. Ther. Drug Monit., 6:438–443, 1984.

DeLeon, G., and Mandell, A. J.: A comparison of conditioning and psychotherapy and the treatment of functional enuresis. J. Clin. Psychol., 22:326–330, 1966.

DeVane, C. L., Walker, R. D., Sawyer, W. P., and Wilson, J. A.: Concentrations of imipramine and its metabolites during enuresis therapy. Pediatr. Pharmacol., 4:245–251, 1984.

Dimson, S. B.: Desmopressin as treatment for enuresis. Lancet, 1:1260, 1977.

Diokno, A. C., Hyndman, C. W., Hardy, D. A., and Lapides, J.: Comparison of action of imipramine (Tofranil) and propantheline (Probanthine) on detrusor contractions. J. Urol., 107:42, 1972.

Diokno, A. C., Koff, S. A., and Bender, L.: Periurethral striated muscle activity in neurogenic bladder dysfunction. J. Urol., 112:743, 1974.

Dodge, W. F., West, E. F., Bridgforth, E. B., and Travis, L. B.: Nocturnal enuresis in 6 to 10 year-old children: Correlation with bacteriuria, proteinuria and dysuria. Am. J. Dis. Child., 120:32, 1970.

Doleys, D. M.: Behavioral treatments for nocturnal enuresis in children: A review of the recent literature. Psychol. Bull. 1:30, 1977.

Edelstein, B. A., Keaton-Brasted, C., and Burd, M. M.: Effects of caffeine withdrawal on nocturnal enuresis, insomnia, and behavioral restraints. J. Consult. Clin. Psychol., 52:857–862, 1984.

Epstein, S. J., and DeQuevedo, A.: The control of enuresis with imipramine in the presence of organic bladder disease. Am. J. Psychiatry, 120:908, 1964.

Esperanca, M., and Gerrard, J. W.: Nocturnal enuresis: Studies in bladder function in normal children and enuretics. Can. Med. Assoc. J., 101:324, 1969a.

Esperanca, M., and Gerrard, J. W.: Nocturnal enuresis. Comparison of the effect of imipramine and dietary restriction on bladder capacity. Can. Med. Assoc. J., 101:721, 1969b.

Essen, J., and Peckham, C.: Nocturnal enuresis in childhood. Dev. Med. Child Neurol., 18:577, 1976.

Fergusson, D. M., Horwood, L. J., and Shannon, F. T.: Factors related to the age of attainment of nocturnal bladder control: An eight-year longitudinal study. Pediatrics, 78(5):884–890, 1986.

Fermaglich, J. L.: Electroencephalographic study of enuretics. Am. J. Dis. Child., 118:473, 1969.

Fisher, O. D., and Forsythe, W. I.: Micturating cystourethrography in the investigation of enuresis. Arch. Dis. Child., 29:460, 1954.

Fjellestad-Paulsen, A., Wille, S., and Harris, A. S.: Comparison of intranasal and oral desmopressin for nocturnal enuresis. Arch. Dis. Child. 62:674–677, 1987.

Forsythe, W. I., and Redmond, A.: Enuresis and the electric alarm: Study of 200 cases. Br. Med. J., 1:211, 1970.

Forsythe, W. I., and Redmond, A.: Enuresis and spontaneous cure rate: Study of 1129 enuretics. Arch. Dis. Child., 49:259, 1974.

Fouron, J., and Chicoine, R.: ECG changes in fatal imipramine (Tofranil) intoxication. Pediatrics, 48:777, 1971.

Frary, L. G.: Enuresis: A genetic study. Am. J. Dis. Child., 49:553, 1935.

Fraser, M. S.: Nocturnal enuresis. Practitioner, 208:203, 1972.

Gastaut, H., and Broughton, R.: A clinical and polygraphic study of episodic phenomena during sleep. In Wortis, J. (Ed.): Recent Advances in Biological Psychiatry. New York, Plenum Press, 1965, pp. 197–221.

Geffken, G., Johnson, S. B., and Walker, D.: Behavioral interventions for childhood nocturnal enuresis: The differential effect of bladder capacity on treatment, progress and outcome. Health Psychol., 5(3):261–272, 1986.

George, C. P. L., Messeril, F. H., Gennest, J., et al.: Diurnal variation of plasma vasopressin in man. J. Endocrinol. Metab., 41:332, 1975.

Giles, G. R., Light, K., and Van Blerk, P. J. P.: Cystometrogram studies in enuretic children. S. Afr. J. Surg., 16:33, 1978.

Goellner, M. H., Ziegler, E. E., and Fomon, S. J.: Urination during the first three years of life. Nephron, 28:174, 1981.

Graham, P.: Depth of sleep and enuresis: A critical review. In Kolvin, I., MacKeith, R. C., and Meadow, S. R. (Eds.): Bladder Control and Enuresis. London, W. Heinemann Medical Books Ltd., 1973, pp. 78–83.

Greaves, M. W.: Hazards of enuresis alarms. Arch. Dis. Child., 44:285, 1969.

Green, A. S., and Cromie, W. J.: Treatment of imipramine overdose in children. Urology, 18:314, 1981.

Grossman, H. B., Koff, S. A., and Diokno, A. C.: Cystometry in children. J. Urol., 117:646, 1977.

Hagglund, T. B.: Enuretic children treated with fluid restriction or forced drinking: A clinical and cystometric study. Ann. Paediatr. Fenn., 11:84, 1965.

Hagglund, T. B., and Parkkulainen, K. V.: Enuretic children treated with imipramine (Tofranil). Ann. Paediatr. Fenn., 11:53, 1965.

Hallgren, B.: Enuresis: A clinical and genetic study. Acta Psychiatr. Neurol. Scand. [Suppl.], 114:1, 1957.

Hallman, N.: On the ability of enuretic children to hold urine. Acta Paediatr., 39:87, 1950.

Haque, M., Ellerstein, N. S., Gundy, J. H., et al.: Parental perceptions in enuresis, a collaborative study. Am. J. Dis. Child., 135:809, 1981.

Harris, A. S.: Clinical experience with desmopressin: Efficacy and safety in central diabetes insipidus and other conditions. J. Pediatr., 114:711–718, 1989.

Harris, L. S., and Purohit, A. P.: Bladder training and enuresis: A controlled trial. Behav. Res. Ther., 15:485, 1977.

Harrison, J. S., and Albino, V. J.: An investigation into the effects of imipramine hydrochloride on the incidence of enuresis in institutionalized children. S. Afr. Med. J., 44:253, 1970.

Hindmarsh, J. R., and Byrne, P. O.: Adult enuresis—a symptomatic and urodynamic assessment. Br. J. Urol., 52:88, 1980.

Inoue, M., Shimojima, H., Shiba, H., et al.: Rhythmic slow wave observed on nocturnal sleep encephalogram in children with idiopathic nocturnal enuresis. J. Sleep, 10(6):570–579, 1987.

Johnstone, J. M. S.: Cystometry and evaluation of anticholinergic drugs in enuretic children. J. Pediatr. Surg., 7:18, 1972.

Jorgensen, O. S., Lober, M., Christiansen, J., et al.: Plasma concentration and clinical effect in imipramine treatment of childhood enuresis. Clin. Pharmacokinet., 5:386, 1980.

Kajtor, F., Ovary, I., and Zsadanyi, O.: Nocturnal enuresis: Electroencephalographic and cystometric examinations. Acta Med. Acad. Sci. Hung., 23:153, 1967.

Kales, A., and Kales, J. D.: Sleep disorders: Recent findings in the diagnosis and treatment of disturbed sleep. N. Engl. J. Med., 290:487, 1974.

Kales, A., Kales, J. D., Jacobson, A., Humphrey, F. J., and Soldatos,

C. R.: Effect of imipramine on enuretic frequency and sleep stages. Pediatrics, 60:431, 1977.

Kaplan, G.: Serum IgE and allergy in enuresis. Presented at Section on Urology, American Academy of Pediatrics, Oct. 22, 1973.

Karacan, I., Thornby, J. I., Anch, A. M., et al.: Dose-related sleep disturbances induced by coffee and caffeine. Clin. Pharmacol. Ther., 20:682–689, 1976.

Kardash, S., Hillman, E. S., and Werry, J.: Efficacy of imipramine in childhood enuresis: A double blind control study with placebo. Can. Med. Assoc. J., 99:263, 1968.

Kass, E. J., Diokno, A. C., and Montealegre, A.: Enuresis: Principles of management and result of treatment. J. Urol., 121:794, 1979.

Kimmel, H. D., and Kimmel, E. C.: An instrumental conditioning method for the treatment of enuresis. J. Behav. Ther. Exp. Psychiatry, 1:121, 1970.

Klauber, G. T.: Clinical efficacy and safety of desmopressin in the treatment of nocturnal enuresis. J. Pediatr., 114:719–722, 1989.

Koehl, G. W., and Wenzel, J. E.: Severe postural hypotension due to imipramine therapy. Pediatrics, 47:71, 1971.

Koff, S. A.: Estimating bladder capacity in children. Urology, 21:248, 1983.

Koff, S. A., Lapides, J., and Piazza, D. H.: The uninhibited bladder in children: A cause for urinary tract infection, obstruction and reflux. In Hodson, J., and Kincaid-Smith, P. (Eds.): Reflux Nephropathy. New York, Masson Publishing, 1979, pp. 161–170.

Koff, S. A., and Murtagh, D. S.: The uninhibited bladder in children: Effect of treatment on recurrence of urinary infection and on vesicoureteral reflux resolution. J. Urol., 130:1138, 1983.

Kunin, S. A., Limbert, D. J., Platzker, A. C. G., and McGinley, J.: The efficacy of imipramine in the management of enuresis. J. Urol., 104:612, 1970.

Labay, P., and Boyarsky, S.: The action of imipramine on the bladder musculature. J. Urol., 109:385, 1973.

Lapides, J., and Diokno, A. C.: Persistence of the infant bladder as a cause of urinary infection in girls. J. Urol., 103:243, 1970.

Lapides, J., Sweet, R. B., and Lewis, L. W.: Role of striated muscle in urination. J. Urol., 77:247, 1957.

Levine, A.: Enuresis in the Navy. Am. J. Psychiatry, 100:320, 1943.

Leys, D.: Value of propantheline bromide in treatment of enuresis. Br. Med. J., 1:549, 1956.

Liederman, P. C., Wasserman, D. H., and Liederman, V. R.: Desipramine in the treatment of enuresis. J. Urol., 101:314, 1969.

Linderholm, B. E.: The cystometric findings in enuresis. J. Urol., 96:718, 1966.

Lovering, J. S., Tallett, S. E., and McKendry, J. B. J.: Oxybutynin efficacy and the treatment of primary enuresis. Pediatrics, 82:104–106, 1988.

Lovibond, S. H.: The mechanism of conditioning treatment of enuresis. Behav. Res. Ther., 1:17, 1963.

Lowy, F. H.: Recent sleep and dream research: Clinical implications. Can. Med. Assoc. J., 102:1069, 1970.

MacKeith, R. C.: A frequent factor in the origins of primary nocturnal enuresis: Anxiety in the third year of life. Dev. Med. Child Neurol., 10:465, 1968.

MacKeith, R. C.: Is maturation delay a frequent factor in the origins of primary nocturnal enuresis? Dev. Med. Child Neurol., 14:217, 1972.

MacLean, R. E. G.: Imipramine hydrochloride (Tofranil) and enuresis. Am. J. Psychiatry, 117:551, 1960.

Mahony, D. T.: Studies of enuresis: I. Incidence of obstructive lesions and pathophysiology of enuresis. J. Urol., 106:951, 1971.

Mahony, D. T., Laferte, R. O., and Blais, D. J.: Studies on enuresis: IX. Evidence of a mild form of compensated detrusor hyperreflexia in enuretic children. J. Urol., 126:520, 1981.

Mandell, A. J., Chaffey, B., Brill, P., Mandell, M. P., et al.: Dreaming sleep in man: Changes in urine volume and osmolality. Science, 151:1558–1560, 1966.

Marshall, S., Marshall, H. H., and Lyon, R. P.: Enuresis: An analysis of various therapeutic approaches. Pediatrics, 52:813, 1973.

Martin, G. I.: Imipramine pamoate in the treatment of childhood enuresis: A double-blind study. Am. J. Dis. Child., 122:42, 1971.

Martin, G. I.: ECG monitoring of enuretic children given imipramine. JAMA, 244:902, 1973.

Maxwell, C., and Seldrup, J.: Imipramine in the treatment of childhood enuresis. Practitioner, 207:809, 1971.

McGuire, E. J., and Savastanes, J. A.: Urodynamic studies in enuresis and the non-neurogenic bladder. J. Urol., 132:229–302, 1984.

McKendry, J. B. J., and Stewart, D. A.: Enuresis. Pediatr. Clin. North Am., 21:1019, 1974.

McKendry, J. B. J., Stewart, D. A., Kahnna, F., and Netley, C.: Primary enuresis: Relative success of three methods of treatment. Can. Med. Assoc. J., 113:953–955, 1975.

McKendry, J. B. J., Williams, H. A. L., and Broughton, C.: Enuresis—a study of untreated patients. Appl. Ther., 10:815, 1968.

Mikkelsen, E. J., Rapoport, J. L., Nee, L., et al.: Childhood enuresis: I. Sleep patterns and psychopathology. Arch. Gen. Psychiatry, 37:1139, 1980.

Miller, F. J. W., Court, S. D. M., Walton, N. G., and Knox, E. G.: Growing-up in Newcastle upon Tyne. London, Oxford University Press, 1960.

Miller, F. J. W., Knox, E. G., and Brandon, S.: Children who wet the bed. In Kolvin, I., MacKeith, R. C., and Meadow, S. R. (Eds.): Bladder Control and Enuresis. London, W. Heinemann Medical Books Ltd., 1973, pp. 47–52.

Miller, K., Goldberg, S., and Atkin, B.: Nocturnal enuresis: Experience with long-term use of intranasally administered desmopressin. J. Pediatr., 114:723–726, 1989.

Miller, P. R., Champelli, J. W., and Dinello, F. A.: Imipramine in the treatment of enuretic school children. Am. J. Dis. Child., 115:17, 1968.

Milner, G., and Hills, N. F.: A double-blind assessment of antidepressants in the treatment of 212 enuretic patients. Med. J. Aust., 1:943, 1968.

Mimouni, M., Schuper, A., Mimouni, F., et al.: Retarded skeletal maturation in children with primary enuresis. J. Pediatr., 144:234–235, 1985.

Mishra, P. C., Agarwal, V. K., and Rahman, H.: Therapeutic trial of amytriptiline in the treatment of nocturnal enuresis—a controlled study. Indian Pediatr., 17:279, 1980.

Moffatt, M. E. K., Kato, C., and Pless, I. B.: Improvements in self-concept after treatment of nocturnal enuresis: Randomized controlled trial. J. Pediatr., 110:647–652, 1987.

Mowrer, O. H., and Mowrer, W. M.: Enuresis—a method for its study and treatment. Am. J. Orthopsychiatry, 8:436, 1938.

Muellner, S. R.: Development of urinary control in children. JAMA, 172:1256, 1960.

Nash, D. F. E.: The development of micturition control with special reference to enuresis. Ann. R. Coll. Surg. Engl., 5:318, 1949.

Neal, B. W., and Coote, M. A.: Hazards of enuresis alarms. Arch. Dis. Child., 44:651, 1969.

Norgaard, J. P., Hansen, J. H., and Willdschiotz, G.: Cystometries in children with nocturnal enuresis. J. Urol., 141:1156, 1989a.

Norgaard, J. P., Pederson, E. B., and Djurhuus, J. C.: Diurnal antidiuretic hormone levels in enuretics. J. Urol., 134:1029, 1985.

Norgaard, J. P., Rittig, S., and Djurhuus, J. C.: Nocturnal enuresis: An approach to treatment based on pathogenesis. J. Pediatr., 114:705–710, 1989b.

Oppel, W. C., Harper, P. A., and Rider, R. V.: The age of attaining bladder control. Pediatrics, 42:614, 1968.

Pedersen, P. S., Hejl, M., and Kjoller, S. S.: Desamino-D-arginine vasopressin in childhood nocturnal enuresis. J. Urol., 133:65–66, 1985.

Pompeius, R.: Cystometry in pediatric enuresis. Scand. J. Urol., 5:222, 1971.

Poussaint, A. F., Ditman, K. S., and Greenfield, R.: Amitriptyline in childhood enuresis. Clin. Pharmacol. Ther., 7:21, 1966.

Puri, V. N.: Urinary levels of antidiuretic hormone in nocturnal enuresis. Indian Pediatr., 17:675, 1980.

Rapoport, J. L., Mikkelsen, E. J., Zavodil, A., et al.: Childhood enuresis. II. Arch. Gen. Psychiatry, 37:1146, 1980.

Rechtschaffen, A., and Kales, A. (Eds.): A Manual of Standardized Terminology, Techniques and Scoring System for Sleep Stages of Human Subjects. Los Angeles, Brain Information Service/Brain Research Institute, UCLA, 1968, pp. 1–12.

Redman, J. F., and Seibert, J. J.: The uroradiographic evaluation of the enuretic child. J. Urol., 122:799, 1979.

Rew, D. A., and Rundle, J. S. H.: Assessment of the safety of regular DDAVP therapy in primary nocturnal enuresis. Br. J. Urol., 63:352–353, 1989.

Ritvo, E. R., Ornitz, E. M., Gottlieb, F., Poussaint, A. F., Maron, B. J., Ditman, K. S., and Blinn, K. A.: Arousal and non-arousal enuretic events. Am. J. Psychiatry, 126:115, 1969.

Rohner, T. J., and Sanford, E. J.: Imipramine toxicity. J. Urol., 114:402, 1975.

Sachdev, Y. V., and Howards, S. S.: *Enterobius vermicularis* infestation and secondary enuresis. J. Urol., 113:143, 1975.

Scott, R., and Morrison, L. H.: Diuretic treatment of enuresis: Preliminary communication. J. R. Coll. Surg. Edinb., 25:470, 1980.

Shaffer, D., Costello, A. J., and Hill, I. D.: Control of enuresis with imipramine. Arch. Dis. Child., 43:665, 1968.

Sigg, E. B.: Pharmacological studies with Tofranil. Can. Psychiatr. Assoc. J., 4:75, 1959.

Starfield, B.: Functional bladder capacity in enuretic and non-enuretic children. J. Pediatr., 5:777, 1967.

Stein, Z. M., and Susser, M. W.: Social factors in the development of sphincter control. Dev. Med. Child Neurol., 9:692, 1967.

Stephenson, J. D.: Physiological and pharmacological basis for the chemotherapy of imipramine. Psychol. Med., 9:249, 1979.

Strom-Olsen, R.: Enuresis in adults and abnormality of sleep. Lancet, 2:133, 1950.

Sukhai, R. N., Mol, J., and Harris, A. S.: Combined therapy of enuresis alarm and desmopressin in the treatment of nocturnal enuresis. Eur. J. Pediatr., 148:465–467, 1989.

Torrens, M. J., and Collins, C. D.: The urodynamic assessment of adult enuresis. Br. J. Urol., 47:433, 1975.

Troup, C. W., and Hodgson, N. B.: Nocturnal functional bladder capacity in enuretic children. J. Urol., 129:132, 1971.

Tuvemo, T.: DDAVP in childhood nocturnal enuresis. Acta Pediatr. Scand., 67:753, 1978.

Wagner, W., Johnsson, S. S., Walker, D., et al.: A controlled comparison of two treatments for nocturnal enuresis. J. Pediatr., 101:302–307, 1982.

Werry, J. S.: Enuresis—a psychosomatic entity? Can. Med. Assoc. J., 97:319, 1967.

Werry, J. S., and Cohrsen, J.: Enuresis: An etiologic and therapeutic study. J. Pediatr., 67:423–431, 1965.

Whiteside, C. G., and Arnold, E. P.: Persistent primary enuresis: A urodynamic assessment. Br. Med. J., 1:364, 1975.

Wille, S.: Comparison of desmopressin and enuresis alarm for nocturnal enuresis. Arch. Dis. Child., 61:30–33, 1986.

Winter, J. S. D., Hughes, I. E., Rayes, F. I., and Famin, C.: Pituitary-gonadal relations in infancy: Serum gonadal steroid concentrations in man from birth to two years of age. J. Endocrinol. Metab., 42:679–686, 1976.

Wu, H. H. H., Chen, M.-T., Lee, Y.-H.: Urodynamics studies and primary nocturnal enuresis. Chin. Med. J. [Taipei], 41:227–232, 1988.

Yeates, W. K.: Bladder function in normal micturition. *In* Kolvin, I., MacKeith, R. C., and Meadow, S. R. (Eds.): Bladder Control and Enuresis. London, W. Heinemann Medical Books Ltd., 1973, pp. 28–36.

Young, G. C., and Morgan, R. T. T.: Overlearning in the conditioning treatment of enuresis. Behav. Res. Ther., 10:147–151, 1972.

Young, G. C., and Morgan, R. T. T.: Conditioning technics and enuresis. Med. J. Aust., 2:329, 1973.

Zaleski, A., Shokeir, M. K., and Gerrard, J. W.: Enuresis: Familial incidence and relationship to allergic disorders. Can. Med. Assoc. J., 106:30, 1972.

42
NEUROGENIC VESICAL DYSFUNCTION IN CHILDREN

Stuart B. Bauer, M.D.

At least 25 per cent of the clinical problems in pediatric urology are the result of neurologic lesions that affect lower urinary tract function. In the past, urinary diversion was the mainstay of treatment for these children with either intractable incontinence or abnormal upper urinary tracts (Smith, 1972). The advent of clean intermittent catheterization (CIC) in the early 1970s by Dr. Jack Lapides (Lapides et al., 1972) and the refinements in the techniques of urodynamic studies in children (Blaivas, 1979; Blaivas et al., 1977; Gierup and Ericsson, 1970) dramatically changed the way this pediatric population had been traditionally managed. Along with this change came a greater understanding of the pathophysiology of the many diseases that affect children primarily.

With the increased reliability of data collection, the applicability of urodynamic testing has expanded to the point where most pediatric urologic centers now believe that functional assessment of the lower urinary tract is an essential element in the evaluation process and is as important as x-ray visualization in characterizing and managing these abnormal conditions (McGuire et al., 1981). Because urodynamic testing is such an integral part of any discussion on the subject, this chapter will first define the testing process as it applies to children, describe its pitfalls and advantages, and then elaborate on the various neurourologic abnormalities that are prevalent in children.

URODYNAMIC EVALUATION

Before a urodynamic study is performed, it is important that the child and the family have full knowledge of the procedure. An explanation of the test and a questionnaire are sent to each family before the appointment. A booklet is provided so that parents know what to expect and can explain the test to their child. If old enough, the child can read about it. Attempts are made to minimize the anxiety level in those children who are

old enough to understand what will happen. The questionnaire elicits information about the child's birth and development, his or her current bladder and bowel habits, and any other information that might be pertinent to know at the time of the procedure.

Sometimes, in very anxious children over 1 year of age, meperidine, 1 mg/kg body weight, is administered intramuscularly to reduce the discomfort and anxiety level; this dose does not alter the child's cooperativeness or responsiveness (Ericsson et al., 1971). If at all feasible, however, no medication is given. The child is conscientiously attended to, in order to minimize his or her fears. If possible, the child is instructed to come to the urodynamic suite with a full bladder to obtain an initial, representative uroflowmetry. In addition, it enables the nurse to record a reliable residual urine volume when catheterizing the child after voiding. The flowmeter is located in a private bathroom, which contains a one-way mirror so that voiding can be viewed unobtrusively. This arrangement allows the investigator to see if Credé or a Valsalva maneuver is employed by the individual to help empty the bladder.

Next, the nurse reviews the test and shows the child all the equipment in an attempt to make him or her as comfortable as possible. The child is catheterized with either a 7 or an 11 French triple-lumen urodynamic catheter (Bard Urologic, Murray Hill, NJ) after a small amount of liquid xylocaine is injected into the urethra and held in place for a moment or two. Then the residual urine is carefully measured. Sometimes, it is necessary to aspirate the catheter to get an accurate volume of residual urine, especially if the bladder is hypotonic (particularly if the child is taking anticholinergic medication) or if it has been previously augmented and secretes mucus, for it may not drain completely following insertion.

A small balloon catheter is passed into the rectum at this time to measure intra-abdominal pressure during the cystometrogram to identify artifacts of motion and to monitor increases in abdominal pressure during the filling and emptying phases of the study (Bates et al., 1970; Bauer, 1979). Uninhibited contractions can be clearly differentiated by this maneuver.

Before filling the bladder, a urethral pressure profile is sometimes obtained by infusing saline through the side-hole channel at a rate of 2 ml/minute as the catheter is withdrawn at a rate of 2 mm/sec (Yalla et al., 1980). Some urodynamicists advocate using a balloon or micro-tipped transducer catheter to measure urethral resistance instead of a saline infusion (Tanagho, 1979). When the maximum resistance is known, the catheter is positioned so that the urethral pressure port is located at that or any other point of interest. This area can then be monitored throughout the urodynamic study.

Urethral pressure profilometry (UPP) measures the passive resistance of a particular point within the urethra to stretch (Gleason et al., 1974). Many factors contribute to this resistance, including the elastic properties of the tissues surrounding the lumen and the tension generated by the smooth and skeletal muscles of the urethra, which are constantly changing during the micturition cycle (Fig. 42–1) (Abrams, 1979; Evans et al., 1979). Thus, the static urethral pressure profile is a measure of the resistance under a specific set of circumstances (Yalla et al., 1979). It is difficult to extrapolate data from when the bladder is empty and apply it to a time when the bladder is full, when it responds to increases in abdominal pressure, or when bladder emptying takes place (Fig. 42–2). Failure to recognize this will lead to false assumptions and improper treatment.

External urethral sphincter electromyography (EMG) is recorded using a 24-gauge concentric needle electrode (Blaivas et al., 1977a; Diokno et al., 1974) inserted perineally in males or paraurethrally in females, and advanced into the skeletal muscle component of the sphincter until individual motor unit action potentials are seen or heard on a standard EMG recorder. Alternatively, perineal (Maizels and Firlit, 1979) or abdominal patch electrodes (Koff and Kass, 1982), or anal plugs (Bradley et al., 1974) have been used to record the bioelectric activity in the sphincter muscle. Disagreements exist concerning the accuracy of these surface electrode measurements versus those of needle electrodes, particularly during voiding. The intactness of sacral cord function is easily measured with needle electrodes by (1) looking at the characteristic wave form of individual motor unit action potentials when the patient is relaxed and the bladder empty, (2) performing and recording responses to bulbocavernosus and anal stimulation, and Credé and Valsalva maneuvers, (3) asking the patient to voluntarily contract and relax the external sphincter, and (4) seeing the reaction of the sphincter to filling and emptying of the bladder (Fig. 42–3) (Blaivas, 1979b; Blaivas et al., 1977a).

The rate of bladder filling is usually set by determining the child's predicted capacity—average capacity (ml) = [age (years) + 2] × 30 (Koff, 1983)—and dividing by 10. It has been shown that more rapid filling rates may yield falsely low levels of detrusor compliance and minimize uninhibited contractions (Joseph and Duggan, 1991; Turner-Warwick, 1975). In an attempt to avoid this, the bladder is filled slowly with saline solution

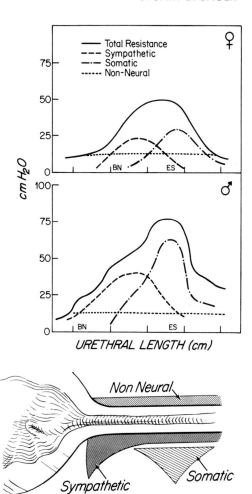

Figure 42–1. Components of urethral wall tension according to their geographic distribution and effect along the urethra in males and females (BN, bladder neck; ES, external sphincter.) (From Bauer, S. B.: Urodynamic evaluation and neuromuscular dysfunction. *In* Kelalis, P. P., King, L. R., and Belman, A. B. (Eds.): Clinical Pediatric Urology, Ed. 2, Vol I. Philadelphia, W. B. Saunders Co., 1985, pp. 283–310.)

warmed to 37°C. When it is important to determine very mild degrees of hypertonicity, even slower rates of filling are employed. During filling, it is helpful to try to divert the child's attention by asking unrelated questions, reading him or her a story, or showing a videotape cartoon. If the examiner wishes to elicit uninhibited contractions, the child is asked to cough; alternatively, a cold solution may be instilled at a rapid rate.

The study is not considered complete unless the child urinates and the voiding pressures are measured. The small size of the urodynamic catheter does not seem to adversely affect the micturition pressures, even in very young children. The normal voiding pressure in boys varies between 55 and 80 cm H_2O, and between 30 and 65 cm H_2O in girls (Blaivas, 1979a; Blaivas et al., 1977b; Gierup et al., 1969). Sometimes, it is difficult to get the child to void; patience and a great deal of time are needed to accomplish this. Placing a bedpan under the buttocks, if the child is supine, or dripping tepid water on the genital area will often stimulate the child sufficiently to begin urinating. Having the child listen to the audio channel of the EMG amplifier machine while he

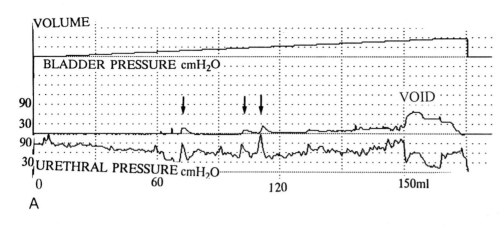

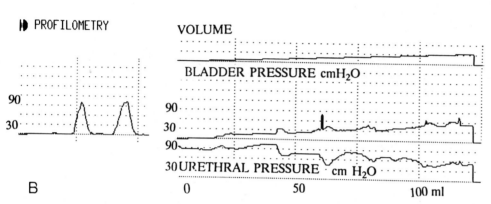

Figure 42–2. *A,* Urodynamic study in an 8-year-old boy with enuresis with the urethral pressure profilometry (UPP) port of the multichannel urodynamic catheter positioned in the mid-urethra. Note that urethral resistance is adequate at the start of filling, but it decreases just before and then increases with each uninhibited contraction *(arrows).* At capacity, the resistance is very high, but then it equals bladder pressure during voiding. *B,* A 7-year-old girl with myelomeningocele has a very good level of resistance when a urethral pressure profile is performed initially. During bladder filling, with the catheter positioned in the mid-urethra, urethral resistance drops from 90 to 58 cm H_2O at capacity.

tightens and relaxes the sphincter provides a means of biofeedback training to encourage him to void. Once the child has voided, analyzing the pressure curve to see if it is sustained until voiding is complete, determining if abdominal pressure has been used to facilitate the emptying process, listening to the change in EMG activity of the sphincter, noting the flow rate characteristics and voided volume, and observing for after-contractions are all important factors to consider.

Oftentimes, it is appropriate to see the effects of drug administration, so studies are repeated under similar circumstances several weeks to months later. This is especially true when one is trying to medically treat detrusor hypertonicity. To determine its maximum ef-

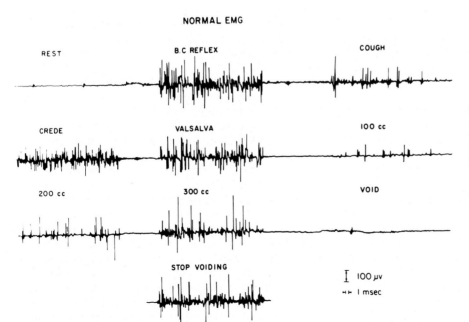

Figure 42–3. Normal reaction of the external urethral sphincter on electromyogram (EMG) to all the sacral reflexes and to bladder filling and emptying. (From Bauer, S. B.: Urodynamic evaluation and neuromuscular dysfunction. *In* Kelalis, P. P., King, L. R., and Belman, A. B. (Eds.): Clinical Pediatric Urology, Ed. 2, Vol I. Philadelphia, W. B. Saunders Co., 1985, pp. 283–310.)

Table 42–1. DRUG THERAPY IN NEUROPATHIC BLADDER DYSFUNCTION

Type	Dosage	
	Minimum	*Maximum*
Cholinergic		
Bethanechol (Urecholine)	0.7 mg/kg tid	0.8 mg/kg qid
Anticholinergic		
Propantheline (Pro-Banthine)	0.5 mg/kg bid	0.5 mg/kg qid
Oxybutynin (Ditropan)	0.2 mg/kg bid	0.2 mg/kg qid
Glycopyrrolate (Robinul)	0.01 mg/kg bid	0.03 mg/kg tid
Hyoscyamine (Levsin)	0.03 mg/kg bid	0.1 mg/kg qid
Sympathomimetic		
Phenylpropanolamine (alpha)	2.5 mg/kg bid	2.5 mg/kg tid
Ephedrine (alpha)	0.5 mg/kg bid	1.0 mg/kg tid
Pseudoephedrine (alpha)	0.4 mg/kg bid	0.9 mg/kg tid
Sympatholytic		
Prazosin (alpha) (Minipress)	0.05 mg/kg bid	0.1 mg/kg tid
Phenoxybenzamine (alpha)	0.3 mg/kg bid	0.5 mg/kg tid
Propanolol (beta)	0.25 mg/kg bid	0.5 mg/kg bid
Smooth muscle relaxant		
Flavoxate (Urispas)	3.0 mg/kg bid	3.0 mg/kg tid
Dicyclomine (Bentyl)	0.1 mg/kg tid	0.3 mg/kg tid
Other		
Imipramine (Tofranil)	0.7 mg/kg bid	1.2 mg/kg tid

Table 42–2. FAMILIAL RISK OF MYELODYSPLASIA IN THE UNITED STATES PER 1000 LIVE BIRTHS

Relationship	Incidence
General population	0.7–1.0
Mother with one affected child	20–50
Mother with two affected children	100
Patient with myelodysplasia	40
Mother older than 35 years	30
Sister of mother with affected child	10
Sister of father with affected child	3
Nephew who is affected	2

fect, the usual dose of most drugs is taken 2 to 3 hours before the test is performed a second time. The most commonly used drugs that affect lower urinary tract function are listed in Table 42–1 along with their appropriate dose ranges.

NEUROSPINAL DYSRAPHISMS

Myelodysplasia

The most common etiology of neurogenic bladder dysfunction in children is secondary to abnormal spinal column development. Formation of the spinal cord and vertebrae begin about the 18th day of gestation. The canal closes in a caudal direction from the cephalad end and is complete by 35 days. The exact mechanism causing the dysraphism is unknown at present, but numerous factors have been implicated. The incidence has been reported to be 1 per 1000 births in the United States (Stein et al., 1982), but there has been a definite decrease in this occurrence in the last 10 years (Laurence, 1989). If spina bifida is already present in one member of a family, there is a 2 to 5 per cent chance of a second sibling being born with the same condition (Scarff and Fronczak, 1981). The incidence doubles when more than one family member has a neurospinal dysraphism (Table 42–2).

Pathogenesis

Myelodysplasia is an all-inclusive term used to describe the various abnormal conditions of the vertebral column that affect spinal cord function. More specific labels regarding each abnormality include the following. A *meningocele* occurs when just the meninges extend beyond the confines of the vertebral canal without any

neural elements contained inside of it. A *myelomeningocele* implies that neural tissue, either nerve roots and/or portions of the spinal cord, have evaginated with the meningocele (Fig. 42–4). A *lipomyelomeningocele* denotes that fatty tissue has developed with the cord structures and both are protruding into the sac.

Myelomeningocele accounts for more than 90 per cent of all the open spinal dysraphic states (Stark, 1977). Most spinal defects occur at the level of the lumbar vertebrae, with the sacral, thoracic, and cervical areas affected in decreasing order of frequency (Table 42–3) (Bauer et al., 1977). An overwhelming number of meningoceles are directed posteriorly; but, on rare occasions, the meningocele may protrude anteriorly, particularly in the sacral area. Usually, the meningocele is made up of a flimsy covering of transparent tissue, but it may be open and leaking cerebrospinal fluid. It is for

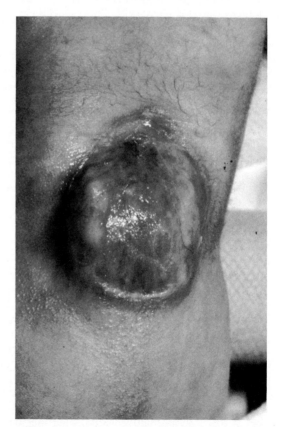

Figure 42–4. Typical appearance of a newborn with an open myelomeningocele.

Table 42–3. SPINAL LEVEL OF MYELOMENINGOCELE

Location	Incidence (%)
Cervical–High thoracic	2
Low thoracic	5
Lumbar	26
Lumbosacral	47
Sacral	20

this reason that urgent repair is necessary, with sterile precautions being followed in the interval between birth and closure. In 85 per cent of affected children there is an associated Arnold-Chiari malformation, in which the cerebellar tonsils have herniated down through the foramen magnum, obstructing the fourth ventricle and preventing the cerebrospinal fluid from entering the subarachnoid space surrounding the brain and the spinal cord.

The neurologic lesion that this condition produces can be quite variable. It depends on what neural elements, if any, have everted with the meningocele sac. The bony vertebral level often gives little or no clue as to the exact neurologic level or lesion that is produced. The height of the bony level and the highest extent of the neurologic lesion may vary from one to three vertebrae in one direction or another (Bauer et al., 1977). Differences in function may be found from one side of the body to the other at the same neurologic level, and from one neurologic level to the next, due to asymmetry of affected neural elements. In addition, 20 per cent of affected children have a vertebral bony or intraspinal abnormality occurring more cephalad from the vertebral defect and meningocele, which can affect function in those additional portions of the cord as well.

Children with thoracic and upper lumbar meningoceles often have complete reconstitution of their spine in the sacral area, and these individuals will frequently have intact sacral reflex arc function involving the sacral spinal roots. In fact, it is more likely for children with upper thoracic or cervical lesions to have just a meningocele and no myelocele. Lastly, the differential growth rates between the vertebral bodies and the elongating spinal cord add a factor of dynamicism in the developing fetus, which further complicates the picture. Superimposed on all this is the Arnold-Chiari malformation; this deformity may have profound effects on the brain stem and pontine center, which are involved in control over lower urinary tract function.

Thus, the neurologic lesion that this condition produces influences lower urinary tract function in a variety of ways and its effects cannot be predicted just by looking at the spinal abnormality or the neurologic function of the lower extremities. Even careful assessment of the sacral area may not provide sufficient information to make a concrete inference. As a result, urodynamic evaluation in the neonatal period is now recommended at most pediatric centers in the United States, because it not only provides a clear picture of the function of the sacral spinal cord and lower urinary tract, but it also has predictive value regarding babies at risk for future urinary tract deterioration and pro-

gressive neurologic change (Bauer et al., 1984; McGuire et al., 1981; Sidi et al., 1986; VanGool et al., 1982).

Newborn Assessment

Ideally, it would be best to perform urodynamic testing immediately after the baby is born, but the risk of spinal infection and the exigency for closure have not made this a viable option. One study, however, was able to accomplish this and has shown that less than 5 per cent of children experience a change in their neurologic status as a result of the spinal canal closure (Kroovand et al., 1990). Therefore, renal ultrasonography and a measure of residual urine are performed as early as possible after birth, either before or immediately after the spinal defect is closed, with urodynamic studies being delayed until it is safe to transport the child to the urodynamic suite and place him on his back or side for the test.

If the infant cannot empty his bladder following a spontaneous void or with a Credé maneuver, then intermittent catheterization is begun, even before urodynamic studies are conducted. If use of the Credé maneuver is effective in emptying the bladder, it is performed instead of CIC on a regular basis. The normal bladder capacity in the newborn period is between 10 and 15 ml; thus, an acceptable residue of urine is less than 5 ml. Other tests that should be performed in the neonatal period include a urine analysis and culture, and serum creatinine levels.

Once the spinal closure has healed sufficiently, an excretory urogram, or renal ultrasonogram and renal scan are performed to reassess upper urinary tract architecture and function. Following this, a voiding cystourethrogram and urodynamic study are conducted. These studies fulfill several objectives. They provide baseline information about the radiologic appearance of the upper and lower urinary tract, as well as the condition of the sacral spinal cord and the central nervous system; the studies can then be compared with later assessments, so that early signs of deteriorating urinary tract drainage and function or of progressive neurologic denervation can be detected. They help to identify babies at risk for urinary tract deterioration as a result of detrusor hypertonicity or outflow obstruction from detrusor sphincter dyssynergy, which then allows prophylactic measures to be initiated before the changes actually take place. Lastly, these studies help the physician to counsel parents with regard to their child's future bladder and sexual function (Bauer, 1984b; Bauer et al., 1984; McGuire et al., 1981; Sidi et al., 1986).

Findings

Ten to 15 per cent of newborns have an abnormal radiologic appearance to their urinary tract when first evaluated (Bauer, 1985). Three per cent have hydroureteronephrosis secondary to spinal shock, probably caused by the closure procedure (Chiaramonte et al., 1986), whereas 10 per cent have abnormalities that developed in utero as a result of abnormal lower urinary tract function in the form of outlet obstruction.

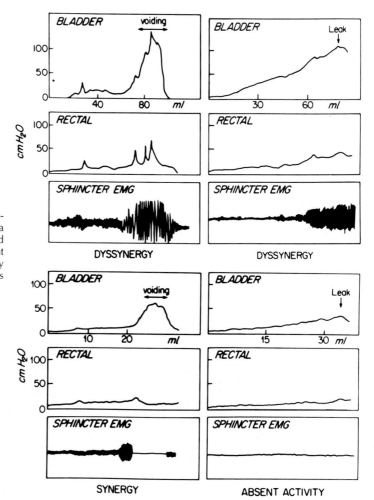

Figure 42–5. Various patterns of urodynamic findings on electromyogram (EMG) in newborns with myelodysplasia. Note that a hypertonic detrusor with a nonrelaxing sphincter is also labeled dyssynergy. (From Bauer, S. B.: Early evaluation and management of children with spina bifida. *In* King, L. R. (Ed.): Urologic Surgery in Neonates and Young Infants. Philadelphia, W. B. Saunders Co., 1988, pp. 252–264.)

Urodynamic studies in the newborn period have shown that 57 per cent of infants have bladder contractions. This finding is especially true in children with upper lumbar or thoracic lesions who have sparing of the sacral spinal cord, 83 per cent of whom have detrusor contractions (Keating et al., 1987). Forty-three per cent have an areflexic bladder; compliance during bladder filling is either good (25 per cent) or poor (18 per cent) in this subgroup (Bauer et al., 1984). EMG assessment of the external urethral sphincter demonstrates an intact sacral reflex arc with no evidence of lower motor neuron denervation in 47 per cent of newborns, whereas partial denervation is seen in 24 per cent and complete loss of sacral cord function is noted in 29 per cent (Spindel et al., 1987).

Combining bladder contractility and external sphincter activity results in three categories of lower urinary tract dynamics: synergic; dyssynergic, with and without detrusor hypertonicity; and complete denervation (Fig. 42–5) (Bauer et al., 1984; Sidi et al., 1986). Dyssynergy occurs when the external sphincter fails to decrease or actually increases its activity during a detrusor contraction or a sustained increase in intravesical pressure, as the bladder is filled to capacity (Blaivas et al., 1986). Frequently, a poorly compliant bladder with high intravesical pressure is seen in conjunction with a dyssynergic sphincter resulting in a bladder that empties only

at high intravesical pressures (Sidi et al., 1986; VanGool et al., 1982). Synergy is characterized by complete silencing of the sphincter during a detrusor contraction or when capacity is reached at the end of filling. Voiding pressures are usually within a normal range. Complete denervation is noted when no bioelectric potentials are detectable in the region of the external sphincter at any time during the micturition cycle or in response to a Credé maneuver or sacral stimulation.

Categorizing lower urinary tract function in this way has been extremely useful because it has revealed which children are at risk for urinary tract changes, which should be treated prophylactically, which need close surveillance, and which can be followed at greater intervals. Of newborns with dyssynergy, 71% had, on initial assessment or on subsequent studies, urinary tract deterioration within the first 3 years of life; whereas only 17 per cent of synergic children and 23 per cent of completely denervated individuals developed similar changes (Fig. 42–6). The infants in the synergic group who deteriorated did so only after they converted to a dyssynergic pattern of sphincter function. Among the infants with complete denervation, the ones who deteriorated were those who had elevated levels of urethral resistance, presumably due to fibrosis of the skeletal muscle component of the external sphincter. Thus, it appears that outlet obstruction is a major contributor to

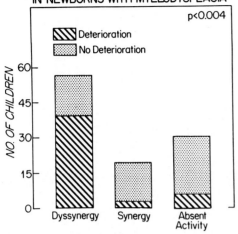

URINARY TRACT CHANGES IN RELATION TO
EXTERNAL URETHRAL SPHINCTER FUNCTION
IN NEWBORNS WITH MYELODYSPLASIA

Figure 42–6. Urinary tract deterioration is related to outflow obstruction and is most often associated with dyssynergy. Children with synergy converted to dyssynergy and patients with complete denervation developed fibrosis with a fixed high outlet resistance in the external sphincter, before any changes occurred in the urinary tract. (From Bauer, S. B.: Early evaluation and management of children with spina bifida. *In* King, L. R. (Ed.): Urologic Surgery in Neonates and Young Infants. Philadelphia, W. B. Saunders Co., 1988, pp. 252–264.)

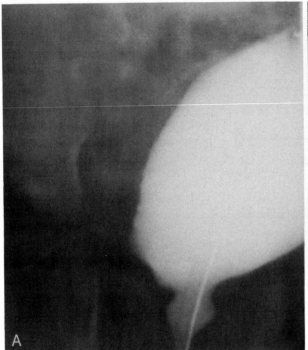

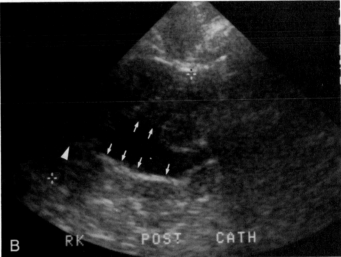

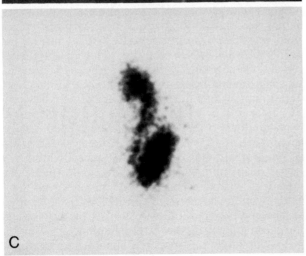

Figure 42–7. *A,* A voiding cystourethrogram in a newborn girl with dyssynergy and elevated voiding pressures demonstrates no reflux and a smooth-walled bladder. Her initial renal echogram was normal. She was started on clean intermittent catheterization and oxybutynin chloride (Ditropan) but did not respond. Within 1 year, she developed right hydronephrosis *(B) (white arrows)* and severe reflux on a radionuclide cystogram *(C).*

the development of urinary tract deterioration in these children (Fig. 42–7).

Bladder tonicity plays an important but somewhat less critical role in this regard (McGuire et al., 1981), although detrusor compliance seems to be worse in children with high levels of outlet resistance (Ghoniem et al., 1989). Bloom and co-workers (1990) noted an improvement in compliance when outlet resistance was lowered following gentle urethral dilation in these children; however, the reasons for this finding are unclear, and the long-term effect of this maneuver remains uncertain.

Recommendations

Because expectant treatment has revealed that infants with outlet obstruction in the form of detrusor sphincter dyssynergy are at considerable risk for urinary tract deterioration, the idea of prophylactically treating the children has emerged as an important alternative. When CIC is begun in the newborn period, it becomes easy for parents to master, even in uncircumcised boys, and for children to accept as they grow older (Joseph et al., 1989). Complications of meatitis, epididymitis, or urethral injury are rarely encountered, whereas urinary infection occurs in less than 30 per cent (Kasabian et al., 1990).

CIC alone or in combination with anticholinergic agents, when detrusor filling pressures are greater than 40 cm H_2O and voiding pressures reach levels higher than 80 to 100 cm H_2O has resulted in only an 8 to 10 per cent incidence of urinary tract deterioration (Geraniotis et al., 1988; Kasabian et al., 1990). This figure represents a significant drop in the occurrence of detrimental changes when compared with the group of children followed expectantly (Bauer et al., 1984; McGuire et al., 1981; Sidi et al., 1986).

Oxybutynin hydrochloride is administered in a dose of 1.0 mg per year of age, every 12 hours, to help lower detrusor filling pressure. In neonates or children less than 1 year of age, the dose is lowered to below 1.0 mg in relation to the child's age at the time and increased proportionately as he or she approaches 1 year. Side effects have not manifested themselves when oxybutynin has been administered according to this schedule (Joseph et al., 1989; Kasabian et al., 1990). When a hyperreflexic or hypertonic bladder fails to respond to these measures, a cutaneous vesicostomy may need to be performed (Fig. 42–8) (Duckett, 1974; Mandell et al., 1981).

Neurologic Findings and Recommendations

Although it has been suspected for a long time, it has not been well documented until recently, that the neurourologic lesion in myelodysplasia is a dynamic disease process with changes taking place throughout childhood (Epstein, 1982; Reigel, 1983; Venes and Stevens, 1983), especially in early infancy (Spindel et al., 1987), and then at puberty (Begger et al., 1986), when the linear growth rate accelerates again. When a change is noted

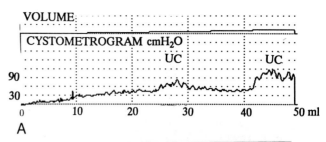

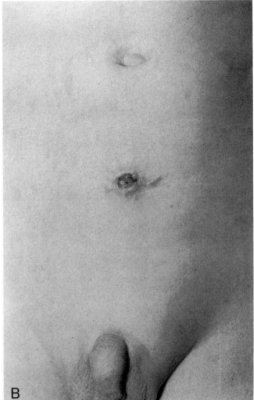

Figure 42–8. *A,* A 6-month-old boy with a myelomeningocele and detrusor sphincter dyssynergy fails to lower bladder filling and detrusor contractile pressures on oxybutynin. *B,* Because the lower ureters showed increasing dilation on ultrasonography and this poor response to medication in lowering intravesical pressure, a vesicostomy was performed. (UC, uninhibited contraction.)

on neurologic, orthopedic, or urodynamic assessment, radiologic investigation of the central nervous system often reveals (1) tethering of the spinal cord (Fig. 42–9), (2) a syrinx or hydromyelia of the cord, (3) increased intracranial pressure due to a shunt malfunction, or (4) partial herniation of the brain stem and cerebellum. Children with completely intact or only partially denervated sacral cord function are particularly vulnerable to progressive changes. Today, magnetic resonance imaging (MRI) is the test of choice because it reveals beautiful anatomic details of the spinal column and central nervous system. However, it is not a functional study, and when used alone, it cannot provide exact information with regard to a changing neurologic lesion.

Sequential urodynamic testing on a yearly basis, beginning in the newborn period and continuing until 5 years of age, provides the means for carefully following these children to detect signs of change, thus offering

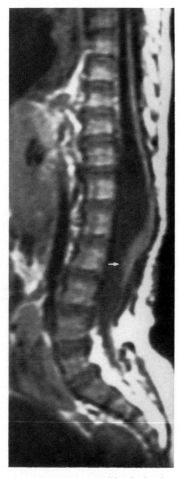

Figure 42–9. An MRI scan in a 9-year-old girl who developed a tethered cord after myelomeningocele repair reveals the conus opposite the L3–4 vertebrae *(arrow)*.

the hope that early detection and neurosurgical intervention may help arrest or even reverse a pathologic process that is progressive. Changes occurred in a group of newborns followed in this manner that involved both the sacral reflex arc as well as the pontine-sacral reflex

Table 42–4. SURVEILLANCE IN INFANTS WITH MYELODYSPLASIA*

Sphincter Activity	Recommended Tests	Frequency
Intact–synergic	Postvoid residual volume	q 4 mo
	IVP or renal echo	q 12 mo
	UDS	q 12 mo
Intact–dyssynergic†	IVP or renal echo	q 12 mo
	UDS	q 12 mo
	VCUG or RNC‡	q 12 mo
Partial denervation	Postvoid residual volume	q 4 mo
	IVP or renal echo	q 12 mo
	UDS§	q 12 mo
	VCUG or RNC‡	q 12 mo
Complete denervation	Postvoid residual volume	q 6 mo
	Renal echo	q 12 mo

*Until age 5.
†Patients on intermittent catheterization and anticholinergic agents.
‡If detrusor hypertonicity or reflux is already present.
§Depending on degree of denervation.
Abbreviations: IVP, intravenous pyelogram; echo, sonogram; UDS, urodynamic study; VCUG, voiding cystourethrogram; RNC, radionuclide cystogram.

interaction (Fig. 42–10) (Spindel et al., 1987). Most children who change tend to do so in the first 3 years of life (Fig. 42–11). Of 15 children who exhibited a worsening in their neurologic picture, seven underwent a second neurosurgical procedure. Most had a beneficial effect from the surgery with four of these seven showing improvement in urethral sphincter function (Spindel et al., 1987).

As a result of these developments, all babies with myelodysplasia should be followed according the guidelines set forth in Table 42–4. It is not enough to look at just the radiologic appearance of the urinary tract; critical scrutiny of the functional status of the lower urinary tract is important as well. In addition to the reasons cited above, it may be necessary to repeat a urodynamic study when the upper urinary tract dilates secondary to impaired drainage from a hypertonic detrusor.

Management of Reflux

Vesicoureteral reflux occurs in 3 to 5 per cent of newborns with myelodysplasia, usually in association with detrusor hypertonicity and/or dyssynergia. It is rare to find reflux in any neonate without dyssynergy or poor compliance (Bauer, 1984b; Geraniotis et al., 1988). If left untreated, the incidence of reflux in these infants at risk increases with time until 30 to 40 per cent are afflicted by 5 years of age (Bauer, 1984a).

In children with reflux, grades 1 to 3 (international classification), who void spontaneously or who have complete lesions with little or no outlet resistance and empty their bladders completely, management consists of antibiotic prophylaxis to prevent recurrent infection. When these children have high-grade reflux, grade 4 or 5, intermittent cahterterization is begun to insure complete emptying. Children who cannot empty their bladder spontaneously, regardless of the grade of reflux, are catheterized intermittently to efficiently empty their bladder. Children with detrusor hypertonicity with or without hydroureteronephrosis, are also started on oxybutynin to lower intravesical pressure and to insure adequate upper urinary tract decompression. When reflux has been managed in this manner, there has been a dramatic response with reflux resolving in 30 to 55 per cent of individuals (Bauer, 1984a; Joseph et al., 1989; Kass et al., 1981). Bacteriuria can be seen in as many as 56 per cent of children on intermittent catheterization; generally, it is not harmful, except in the presence of high-grade reflux, because symptomatic urinary infection and renal scarring rarely occurs with the lesser grades of reflux (Kass et al., 1981).

Credé voiding is to be avoided in children with reflux, especially those with a reactive external sphincter. Under these conditions, the Credé maneuver results in a reflex response in the external sphincter, which increases urethral resistance and raises the pressure needed to expel urine from the bladder (Fig. 42–12) (Barbalias et al., 1983). This maneuver aggravates the degree of reflux and accentuates the water hammer effect of regurgitation on the kidneys. Vesicostomy drainage (Duckett, 1974; Mandell et al., 1981) is reserved for those infants

PONTINE-SACRAL REFLEX ARC CHANGES

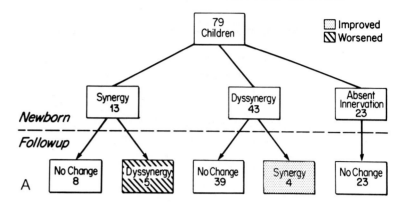

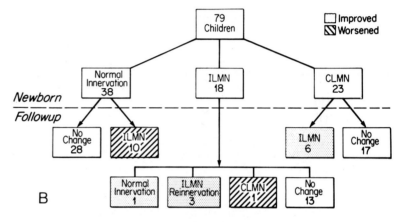

Figure 42–10. The changes in innervation of the pontine-sacral *(A)* and purely sacral *(B)* reflex arc pathways that occurred in a group of children with myelodysplasia followed with sequential urodynamic studies between the newborn period and a subsequent time. (ILMN, incomplete lower motor neuron lesion; CLMN, complete lower motor neuron lesion.) (From Bauer, S. B.: Early evaluation and management of children with spina bifida. *In* King, L. R. (Ed.): Urologic Surgery in Neonates and Young Infants. Philadelphia, W. B. Saunders Co., 1988, pp. 252–264.)

(1) who have such severe reflux that intermittent catheterization and anticholinergic medication fail to improve upper urinary tract drainage, or (2) whose parents cannot adapt to the catheterization program.

The indications for antireflux surgery today are not very different from those for children with normal bladder function and include the following: (1) recurrent symptomatic urinary tract infection while on adequate antibiotic therapy and appropriate catheterization techniques, (2) persistent hydroureteronephrosis despite effective emptying of the bladder and lowering of intravesical pressure, (3) severe reflux with an anatomic abnormality at the ureterovesical junction, and (4) reflux persisting into puberty. In addition, children with any grade of reflux who are being considered for implantation of an artificial urinary sphincter or any other pro-

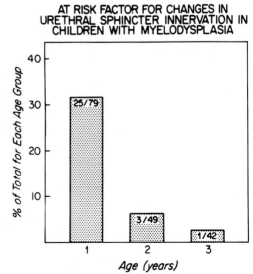

Figure 42–11. The propensity for a change in urethral sphincter innervation is greatest in the 1st year of life. (From Bauer, S. B.: Early evaluation and management of children with spina bifida. *In* King, L. R. (Ed.): Urologic Surgery in Neonates and Young Infants. Philadelphia, W. B. Saunders Co., 1988, pp. 252–264.)

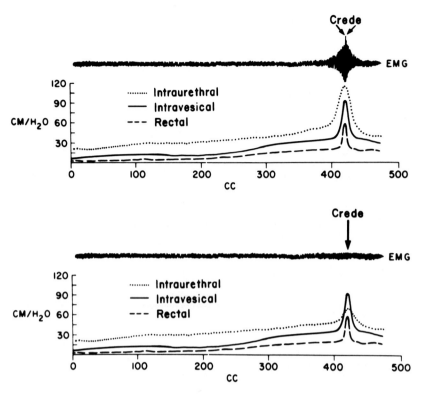

Figure 42–12. When the external sphincter is reactive, a Credé maneuver produces a reflex increase in electromyographic (EMG) activity of the sphincter and a concomitant rise in urethral resistance resulting in high "voiding" pressure. A child whose sphincter is denervated and nonreactive will not have a corresponding rise in EMG activity, urethral resistance, or voiding pressure. A Credé maneuver here will not be detrimental. (From Bauer, S. B.: Early evaluation and management of children with spina bifida. *In* King, L. R. (Ed.): Urologic Surgery in Neonates and Young Infants. Philadelphia, W. B. Saunders Co., 1988, pp. 252–264.)

cedure designed to increased bladder outlet resistance should have the reflux corrected at the time or before the anti-incontinence surgery.

Jeffs and associates (1976) noted that antireflux surgery can be very effective in children with neurogenic bladder dysfunction as long as it is combined with measures to insure complete bladder emptying. Before this observation was made, the results of ureteral reimplantation were so dismal that most physicians treating these children advocated urinary diversion as a means of managing their reflux (Cass, 1976; Smith, 1972). Since the advent of intermittent catheterization, success rates for antireflux surgery have approached 95 per cent (Bauer et al., 1982; Kaplan and Firlit, 1983; Kass et al., 1981; Woodard et al., 1981).

Continence

Urinary continence is becoming an increasingly important issue to deal with at an early age as parents try to mainstream their handicapped children. Initial attempts at achieving continence include CIC and drug therapy designed to maintain low intravesical pressure and a reasonable level of urethral resistance (Figs. 42–13 and 42–14). Although this approach can be conducted on a trial and error basis, it is more efficient to have exact treatment protocols based on specific urodynamic findings. As a result, urodynamic testing is performed if initial attempts with CIC and oxybutynin fail to achieve continence. Without urodynamic studies it is hard to know whether (1) a single drug is effective, (2) it should be increased, or (3) a second drug should be added or exchanged to the regimen.

At this point, if detrusor hypertonicity or uninhibited contractions have not been effectively dealt with (see

Table 42–1) another anticholinergic agent may be combined with or given instead of the oxybutynin. Glycopyrrolate is the most potent oral anticholinergic drug available today, but it may have the typical belladonna-like side effects common to all these drugs. Hyoscyamine, although less effective, seems to produce fewer side effects.

If urodynamic testing reveals that urethral resistance is inadequate to maintain continence because there is either a failure of the sphincter to react to increases in abdominal pressure or a drop in resistance with bladder filling (see Fig. 42–2*B*), then alpha-sympathomimetic agents are added to the regimen (see Table 42–1); phenylpropanolamine is the most effective drug in this regard.

Surgery becomes a viable option when this program fails to achieve continence. In general, this alternative is not undertaken until the child is about 5 years of age and ready to start school. Persistent hypertonicity and/or hyperreflexia may be treated with either enterocystoplasty (Mitchell and Piser, 1987; Sidi et al., 1987) or autoaugmentation (Cartwright and Snow, 1989a, 1989b). First, sigmoid; then, cecum; and lastly, small intestine has been used to enlarge the bladder. Although the ileocecal segment is a favored source for bladder replacement in adults, it is avoided here because removing it might aggravate the bowel dysfunction that is so often a factor in these children already. Detubularization of the bowel is needed to minimize intrinsic contractions of the segment from causing intractable incontinence once it has been added to the bladder (Goldwasser et al., 1987; Hinman, 1988). Recently, gastrocystoplasty has been advocated when considering a bowel augment because it has fewer intrinsic contractions, provides an acid milieu, and is free of mucus secretions, which help reduce the incidence of urinary tract infection (Adams et al., 1988).

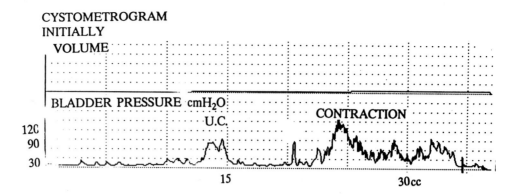

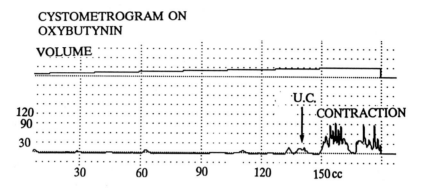

Figure 42–13. Oxybutynin is a potent anticholinergic agent, which dramatically delays detrusor contractions and lowers contraction pressure as demonstrated on these two graphs. (U.C., uninhibited contraction.)

If bladder neck or urethral resistance is insufficient to allow for an adequate storage capability, several operations are available to improve this continence mechanism. Bladder neck reconstruction can be undertaken in a variety of ways, including the Young-Dees (Dees, 1949; Young, 1919) and Leadbetter (Leadbetter, 1964) procedures, and the operation described by Kropp (Kropp and Angwafo, 1986). Fascial sling operations to suspend the bladder neck and buttress it up against the undersurface of the pubis have been advocated with enthusiasm by several individuals (McGuire et al., 1986; Peters et al., 1989; Raz et al., 1988). Each of these operations necessitate the use of CIC to empty the bladder postoperatively. The artificial sphincter (Barrett and Furlow, 1982; Light et al., 1983) also increases bladder outlet resistance, but its mechanism of action allows for emptying at low urethral pressures. Any person who could empty his bladder before the device was implanted should be able to do so afterwards without the need for CIC. Long-term results with the sphincter are lacking (Bosco et al., 1991); as a result, many people do not find this option a viable alternative for children.

Diversion and Undiversion

Urinary diversion, once considered a panacea for children with myelodysplasia, has turned out to be a Pandora's box of new clinical problems (Schwarz and Jeffs, 1975; Shapiro et al., 1975). Pyelonephritis and renal scarring, calculi, ureterointestinal obstruction, strictures of the conduit, and stomal stenosis are problems often encountered in children who are followed on a long-term basis. Although antirefluxing colon conduits seem to have fewer complications, they are still not ideal. In the last 10 years, very successful attempts have been made to undivert the urinary tract in those children who probably would not be diverted today (Hendren, 1973, 1976). Few, if any, are undergoing urinary diversion now; if they are, it is in the form of a continent stoma.

Several operations have been devised, but the ones that have achieved the most publicity are the Kock pouch in adults (Kock, 1971; Skinner et al., 1987) and the Indiana reservoir in children (Rowland et al., 1987). Mitrofanoff (1980) created a continence mechanism by tunneling one end of the vermiform appendix into the bladder just as one would reimplant the ureter to

Figure 42–14. Alpha-sympathomimetic agents potentially have their greatest effect in the bladder neck region, where the highest concentration of alpha receptor sites exists. They can raise outlet resistance and improve continence in many individuals. (BN, bladder neck; ES, external sphincter.)

prevent reflux, with the other end being brought to the skin as a catheterizable stoma. This principle has been extended to the ureter, which is transected at approximately the pelvic brim. Following this, a proximal transureteroureterostomy is performed, while the cut end of the distal segment is brought to the skin as a stoma (Duckett and Snyder, 1986); again, the continence mechanism is provided for, by the intramural tunnel of the ureter.

Other narrow structures, such as a fallopian tube, a rolled strip of stomach, or a tapered ileal segment, have been implanted either into the native bladder or along the tinea of a detubularized portion of sigmoid or cecum acting as a urinary reservoir (Bihrle et al., 1991; Riedmiller et al., 1990; Woodhouse et al., 1989). The success rate for achieving continence has been excellent due primarily to the flap valve effect of the intramural tunnel (Hinman, 1990) and to active peristalsis of the conduit itself (Tutrone et al., 1991).

Sexuality

Sexuality in this population is becoming an increasingly important issue to deal with as more and more individuals are reaching adulthood and wanting to either marry or have meaningful long-term relationships with the opposite sex (Cromer et al., 1990). Investigators are looking into the concerns, fears, and desires of emerging teenagers and the ability of males to procreate and females to bear children. Few studies are available, however, that critically look at sexual function in these patients.

In one study, researchers interviewed a group of teenagers and reported that at least 28 per cent of them had one or more sexual encounters, whereas almost all had a desire to marry and ultimately bear children (Cromer et al., 1990). Another study revealed that 70 per cent of myelodysplastic women were able to get pregnant and have an uneventful pregnancy and delivery, although urinary incontinence in the latter stages of gestation and cesarean section were common in many (Cass et al., 1986). In the same study, 17 per cent of males claimed they were able to father children. It is more likely for males to have problems with erectile and ejaculatory function because of the frequent neurologic involvement of the sacral spinal cord; reproductive function in the female, which is under hormonal control, is not affected.

As important as knowing what the precise sexual function is in an individual, sexuality or the ability to interact with the opposite sex in a meaningful and lasting way is just as important. Until recently, however, this subject was not addressed. Sexual identity, education, and social mores are issues that have been taken out of the realm of secrecy and are now openly discussed and taught to handicapped people. Boys reach puberty at an age similar to that for normal males, whereas breast development and menarche tend to start as much as 2 years earlier than usual in myelodysplastic females. The etiology of this early hormonal surge is uncertain, but it may be related to pituitary function changes in girls secondary to their hydrocephalus (Hayden, 1985).

Bowel Function

No unanimity exists regarding the ideal bowel management program for myelodysplastic children. The external anal sphincter is innervated by the same or similar nerves that modulate the external urethral sphincter, whereas the internal anal sphincter is influenced by more proximal nerves from the sympathetic nervous system. As a result, the internal anal muscle reflexively relaxes in response to anal distention. Consequently, bowel incontinence is frequently unpredictable; it is often related to the consistency of fecal material and how rapidly the anal area refills after it is evacuated.

A majority of pediatricians believe that a regular and efficient bowel emptying regimen is mandatory. Most programs begin at about 1 year of age, but the best method of attaining these objectives is still controversial. Usually, the children are placed on diets that try to create formed but not severely constipated stool. Roughage in the form of fruits and bran and stool softeners (in older children) are given to achieve this goal. Suppositories to help evacuate the rectum are used on a regular basis to help train the lower bowel to fill and empty. Some physicians believe that enemas may be more effective in evacuating a greater portion of the lower bowel, but one problem with administering them is the difficulty in retaining the fluid when the anal sphincter muscle is lax.

Biofeedback training programs to strengthen the external anal sphincter are no more effective than a good bowel management program in attaining fecal continence (Loening-Baucke et al., 1988). When a carefully constructed bowel regimen is adhered to, most children with myelomeningocele can achieve some degree of fecal continence (Myers, 1984), but the uncertainty of accidents always makes this a tenuous situation. Often, the urinary incontinence is effectively managed with CIC, drugs, and/or surgery; but episodes of bowel incontinence remain a problem, particularly in socially minded adolescents (Hayden, 1985).

Lipomeningocele and Other Spinal Dysraphisms

Diagnosis

Certain congenital defects affect the formation of the spinal column but do not result in an open vertebral canal (Table 42–5) (James and Lassman, 1972). These lesions may be very subtle with no obvious outward signs; but, in more than 90 per cent of these children, a

Table 42–5. TYPES OF OCCULT SPINAL DYSRAPHISMS

Lipomeningocele
Intradural lipoma
Diastematomyelia
Tight filum terminale
Dermoid cyst/sinus
Aberrant nerve roots
Anterior sacral meningocele
Cauda equina tumor

cutaneous abnormality overlying the lower spine is found (Anderson, 1975). This abnormality may vary from a small dimple or skin tag to a tuft of hair, a dermal vascular malformation, or a very noticeable subcutaneous lipoma (Fig. 42–15). In addition, one may note, on careful inspection of the legs, a high arched foot or feet, alterations in the configuration of the toes with hammer or claw digits, a discrepancy in muscle size and strength between the legs with weakness at the ankle, and/or a gait abnormality—especially in older

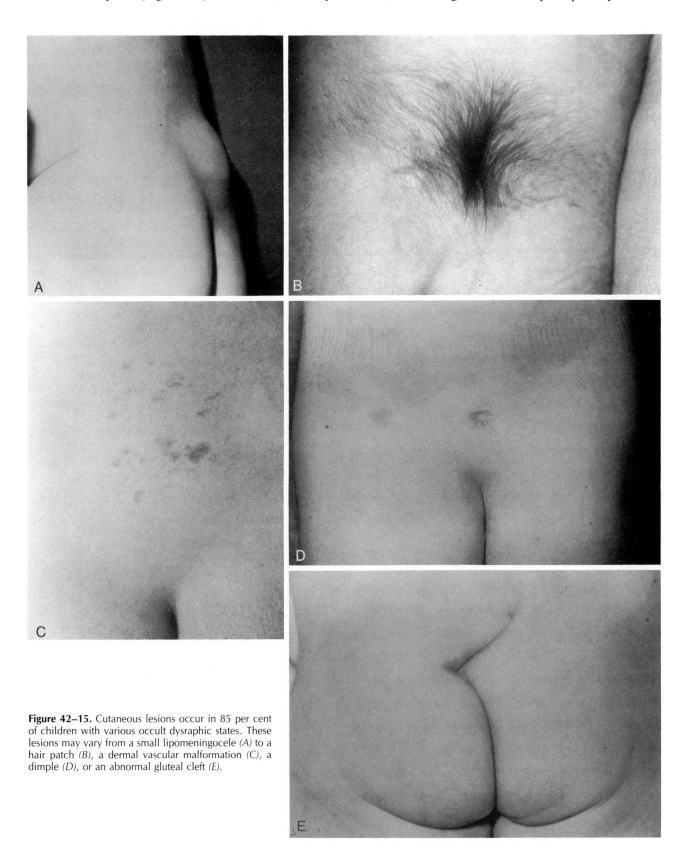

Figure 42–15. Cutaneous lesions occur in 85 per cent of children with various occult dysraphic states. These lesions may vary from a small lipomeningocele (A) to a hair patch (B), a dermal vascular malformation (C), a dimple (D), or an abnormal gluteal cleft (E).

children—due to shortness of one leg (Dubrowitz et al., 1965; Weissert et al., 1989).

Absent perineal sensation and back pain are not uncommon symptoms in older children or young adults (Linder et al., 1982; Weissert et al., 1989; Yip et al., 1985). Lower urinary tract function is abnormal in 40 per cent of affected individuals (Mandell et al., 1980). The child may experience difficulty with training, urinary incontinence after an initial period of dryness following toilet training (especially during the pubertal growth spurt), recurrent urinary infection, and fecal soiling.

Findings

When these children are evaluated in the newborn or early infancy period, the majority have a perfectly normal neurologic examination. Urodynamic testing, however, will reveal abnormal lower urinary tract function in about one third of the babies under the age of 1½ years (Fig. 42–16) (Keating et al., 1988). In fact, these studies may provide the only evidence for a neurologic injury involving the lower spinal cord (Foster et al., 1990; Keating et al., 1988). When present, the most likely abnormality is an upper motor neuron lesion characterized by detrusor hyperreflexia and/or hyperactive sacral reflexes, with mild forms of detrusor sphincter dyssynergy being rarely noted. Lower motor neuron signs with denervation potentials in the sphincter or detrusor areflexia occur in only 10 per cent of young children.

In contrast, practically all individuals over 3 years of age who have not been operated on or who have been belatedly diagnosed as having an occult dysraphism will have an upper motor neuron lesion or a lower motor neuron lesion on urodynamic testing (92 per cent) (Fig. 42–16), or neurologic signs of lower extremity dysfunction (Keating et al., 1988; Kondo et al., 1986; Yip et al., 1985). There does not seem to be a preponderance for one type of lesion over the other (upper versus lower motor neuron); either one occurs with equal frequency, and often the child manifests signs of both (Hellstrom et al., 1986; Kondo et al., 1986).

Pathogenesis

The reason for this difference in neurologic findings may be related to (1) compression on the cauda equina or sacral nerve roots by an expanding lipoma or lipomeningocele (Yamada et al., 1983), or (2) tension on the cord from tethering secondary to differential growth rates between the bony and neural elements (Dubrowitz et al., 1965). Under normal circumstances, the conus medullaris ends just below the L2 vertebra at birth and should recede upward to T12 by adulthood (Barson, 1970). When the cord does not "rise" secondary to one of these lesions, ischemic injury may ensue (Yamada et al., 1981).

Correction of the lesion in infancy has resulted in not only stabilization but also improvement in the neurologic picture in some instances (Fig. 42–17). Sixty per cent of the babies with abnormal urodynamic findings preoperatively revert to normal postoperatively, with improvement noted in 30 per cent; whereas 10 per cent worsen with time. In the older child, there is a less dramatic change following surgery, with only 27 per cent becoming normal, 27 per cent improving, 27 per cent stabilizing, and 19 per cent worsening with time (Fig. 42–17) (Keating et al., 1988). Older individuals with hyperreflexia tend to improve, whereas those with areflexic bladders do not (Flanigan et al., 1989; Hellstrom et al., 1986; Kondo et al., 1986). Lastly, less than 5 per cent of the children operated on in early childhood develop secondary tethering when followed for several years, suggesting that early surgery has both a beneficial and sustaining effect with these conditions.

As a result of these findings, it is apparent that urodynamic testing may be the only way to document that an occult spinal dysraphism is actually affecting lower spinal cord function (Keating et al., 1988; Khoury et al., 1990). Some investigators have shown that posterior tibial somatosensory evoked potentials are even a more sensitive indicator of tethering and should be an integral part of the urodynamic evaluation (Roy et al., 1986). The implication of this lies in the fact that early detection and intervention has both a reversibility to the lesion, which is lost in the older child (Kaplan et al., 1988; Tami et al., 1987; Yamada et al., 1983), and a degree of protection from subsequent tethering, which seems to be a frequent occurrence when the lesion is not dealt with expeditiously in infancy (Seeds and Jones, 1986).

Recommendations

Consequently, in addition to MRI (Tracey and Hanigan, 1990) urodynamic testing should be conducted in everyone who has a questionable skin or bony abnormality of the lower spine (Campobasso et al., 1988; Hall et al., 1988; Packer et al., 1986). If the child is less than 4 to 6 months of age, ultrasound may be useful to image the spinal canal before the vertebral bones have had a chance to ossify (Fig. 42–18) (Raghavendra et al., 1983; Scheible et al., 1983).

In the past, these conditions were usually treated by removing only the superficial skin lesions without delving further into the spinal canal to remove or repair the entire abnormality. Today, most neurosurgeons advocate laminectomy and removal of the intraspinal process as completely as possible without injuring the nerve

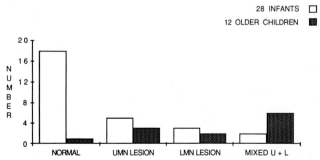

Figure 42–16. Most newborns with a covered spinal dysraphism have normal lower urinary tract function, whereas older children tend to have both upper (UMN) and lower motor neuron (LMN) lesions.

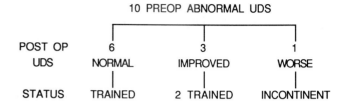

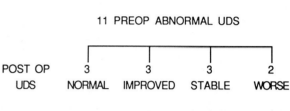

Figure 42–17. The potential for recoverable function is greatest in infants (6 of 10, 60 per cent) and less so in older children (3 of 11, 27 per cent). The risk of damage to neural tissue at the time of exploration to those with normal function is small (2 of 19, 11 per cent). (UDS, urodynamic study.)

roots or cord to release the tether and to prevent further injury with subsequent growth (Foster et al., 1990; Kaplan et al., 1988; Kondo et al., 1986; Linder et al., 1982).

Sacral Agenesis

Sacral agenesis has been defined as absence of part or all of two or more lower vertebral bodies. The etiology of this condition is still uncertain, but teratogenic factors may play a role because insulin-dependent mothers have a 1 per cent chance of giving birth to a child with this disorder. Conversely, 16 per cent of children with sacral agenesis have an affected mother (Guzman et al., 1983; Passarge and Lenz, 1966). Oftentimes, the mothers may only have gestational, insulin-dependent diabetes. The disease was reproduced in chicks when their embryos were exposed to insulin (Landauer, 1945; White and Klauber, 1976). Maternal

Figure 42–18. *A,* During the first few months of life, ultrasound can clearly demonstrate intravertebral anatomy because the posterior arches have not completely ossified. Note that the spinal cord along with its central canal is displaced anteriorly *(white arrows)* beginning at L-3 because of an intradural lipoma. *B,* The MRI is juxtaposed to confirm the ultrasound findings. The longitudinal white intraspinal mass is the lipoma; the longitudinal gray mass is the spinal cord.

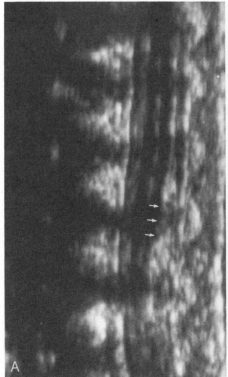

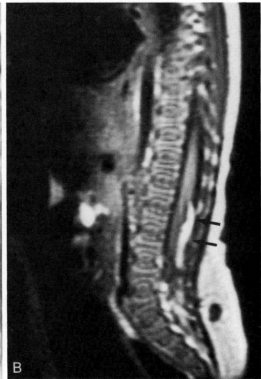

insulin-antibody complexes have been noted to cross the placenta, and their concentration in the fetal circulation is directly correlated with macrosomia (Menon et al., 1990). It is possible that a similar cause-and-effect phenomenon is occurring in sacral agenesis.

Diagnosis

The diagnosis is often delayed until failed attempts at training bring the child to the attention of a physician. Sensation, including sensation in the perianal dermatomes, is usually intact, and lower extremity function is normal (Jakobson et al., 1985; Koff and DeRidder, 1977). Because these children have normal sensation and little or no orthopedic deformity involving the lower extremities (although high-arched feet and claw or hammer toes may be present), the underlying lesion is often overlooked. In fact, 20 per cent of children escape detection until age 3 or 4 (Guzman et al., 1983), when parents begin to question their inability to toilet-train their child.

The only clue, besides a high index of suspicion, is flattened buttocks and a low, short gluteal cleft (Fig. 42–19) (Bauer, 1990). Palpation of the coccyx will detect the absent vertebrae (White and Klauber, 1977). The diagnosis is most easily confirmed with a lateral film of the lower spine, because this area is often obscured by the overlying gas pattern on an anteroposterior (AP) projection (Fig. 42–20) (Guzman et al., 1983; White and Klauber, 1976). MRI has been used to visualize the spinal cord in these cases, and a sharp cutoff of the conus opposite T-12 vertebra seems to be a consistent finding (Fig. 42–21).

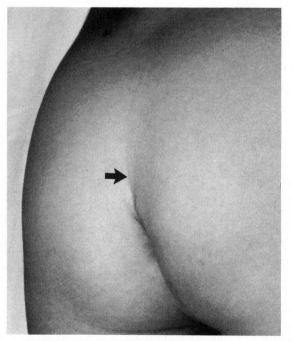

Figure 42–19. Characteristically, the gluteal crease is short and seen only inferiorly *(below arrow)* because of the flattened buttocks in sacral agenesis.

Findings

When urodynamic studies are undertaken, almost an equal number of individuals will manifest an upper or a lower motor neuron lesion (35 per cent versus 40 per cent, respectively), whereas 25 per cent have no signs of denervation at all (Guzman et al., 1983). The upper motor neuron lesion is characterized by detrusor hyperreflexia, exaggerated sacral reflexes, absence of voluntary control over sphincter function, detrusor-sphincter dyssynergy, and no EMG evidence of denervation potentials in the sphincter (Guzman et al., 1983; Koff and DeRidder, 1977; White and Klauber, 1976). A lower motor neuron lesion is noted when detrusor areflexia and partial or complete denervation of the external urethral sphincter with diminished or absent sacral reflexes are seen. The number of affected vertebrae does not seem to correlate with the type of motor neuron lesion present (Fig. 42–22). The injury appears to be stable without signs of progressive denervation.

Recommendations

Management depends on the specific type of neurourologic dysfunction observed on urodynamic testing. Anticholinergic agents should be given to those children with upper motor neuron findings of uninhibited contractions, whereas intermittent catheterization and alpha-sympathomimetic medication may need to be initiated in individuals with lower motor neuron deficits who cannot empty their bladder or stay dry between catheterizations. The bowels manifest a similar picture of dysfunction and need as much characterization and treatment as the lower urinary tract. It is important to identify these individuals as early as possible so that they can be rendered continent and out of diapers at an appropriate age, thus avoiding the social stigmata of fecal and urinary incontinence.

Associated Conditions

Imperforate Anus

Imperforate anus is a condition that can occur alone or as part of a constellation of anomalies that has been called the VATER or VACTERL syndrome (Barry and Auldist, 1974). This mnemonic stands for all the organs that can possibly be affected: V = vertebral, A = anal, C = cardiac, TE = tracheoesophageal fistula, R = renal, and L = limb). Urinary incontinence is not common unless the spinal cord is involved or the pelvic floor muscles and/or nerves are injured during the imperforate anus repair. A plain film of the abdomen and an ultrasound of the spine and kidneys are obtained in the neonatal period in all children, regardless of the level of rectal atresia, once the child has either stabilized or had a colostomy performed (Karrer et al., 1988; Tunnell et al., 1987).

Vertebral bony anomalies often signify an underlying spinal cord abnormality. Because the vertebral segments

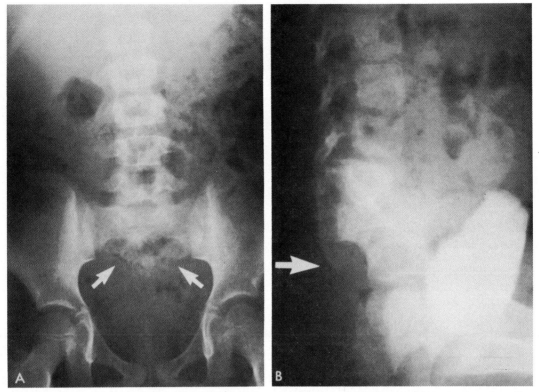

Figure 42–20. The diagnosis of partial or complete sacral agenesis is easily confirmed on an anteroposterior *(A)* or lateral *(B)* film of the spine (if bowel gas obscures the sacral area). (From Bauer, S. B.: Urodynamic evaluation and neuromuscular dysfunction. *In* Kelalis, P. P., King, L. R., and Belman, A. B. (Eds.): Clinical Pediatric Urology, Ed. 2, Vol. I. Philadelphia, W. B. Saunders Co., 1985, pp. 283–310.)

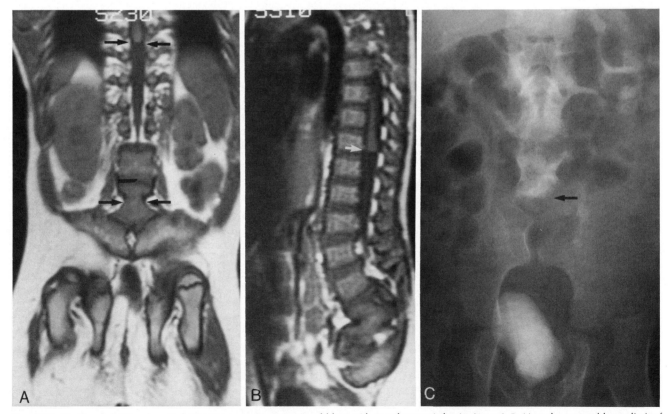

Figure 42–21. Coronal *(A)* and sagittal *(B)* MR images in a 10-year-old boy with sacral agenesis beginning at L-5. Note the squared lower limit of the cord adjacent to T-11 *(upper arrows in* A and *white arrow in* B) and the two sacroiliac joints *(lower arrows in* A), which are in the midline because of absence of the sacrum. *C*, An anteroposterior radiograph from an excretory urogram shows no vertebral bodies below L-4 *(arrow).*

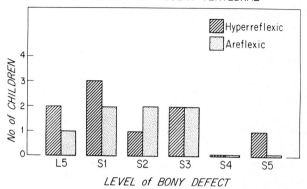

COMPARISON OF TYPE OF BLADDER FUNCTION TO HEIGHT OF ABSENT VERTEBRAE

Figure 42–22. Bladder contractility is unrelated to the number of absent vertebrae. (From Bauer, S. B.: Urodynamic evaluation and neuromuscular dysfunction. *In* Kelalis, P. P., King, L. R., and Belman, A. B. (Eds.): Clinical Pediatric Urology, Ed. 2, Vol. I. Philadelphia, W. B. Saunders Co., 1985, pp. 283–310.)

have not fully calcified at this time, ultrasound can readily image the spinal cord. Any hint of an abnormality on these studies or the presence of a lower midline skin lesion overlying the spine warrants an MRI to delineate any pathologic intraspinal process (Fig. 42–23) (Barnes et al., 1986). If the radiologic images demonstrate an abnormality, urodynamic studies are conducted in the first few months of life. Urodynamic studies are also indicated before repair in the child with a high imperforate anus who has undergone an initial colostomy. These studies serve two functions: (1) they provide a reason to explore and treat any intraspinal abnormality in order to improve the child's chances at becoming continent of both feces and urine, and (2) they provide a baseline for comparison, especially if incontinence should become a problem in the future, particularly in those children needing extensive repair of their imperforate anus.

EMG studies of the perianal musculature at this time help to define the exact location of the future anus. Before the Pena operation (which uses a posterior midline approach) was developed to correct the high imperforate anus, rectal incontinence was thought to be due to an injury involving the pelvic nerves that innervate the levator ani muscles (Parrott and Woodard, 1979; Pena, 1986; Williams and Grant, 1969). Because the dissection is confined to the midline area, this procedure has reduced the chance of traumatizing the nerve fibers that course laterally and around the bony pelvis from the spine to the sphincter muscles. Urodynamic and perianal EMG studies are repeated after the imperforate anus repair if fecal or urinary continence has not been achieved by a reasonable age or if incontinence develops secondarily.

Thirty to 45 per cent of these children have a spinal abnormality even though they may not have any other associated anomalies (Carson et al., 1984; Uehling et al., 1983). This abnormality may range from tethering of the spinal cord secondary to an intraspinal dysraphism, which produces an upper motor neuron type of dysfunction involving the bladder and external urethral sphincter (see Fig. 42–23), to an atrophic abnormality of the conus medullaris, which leads to a partial or complete lower motor neuron lesion involving the lower urinary tract (Greenfield and Fera, 1990). In these circumstances, urinary and fecal incontinence might be the child's only complaints. Lower extremity function may be totally normal, so an examination of just the legs can be misleading (Carson et al., 1984).

CENTRAL NERVOUS SYSTEM INSULTS

Cerebral Palsy

Etiology

Cerebral palsy is a nonprogressive injury to the brain in the perinatal period that produces a neuromuscular disability or a specific symptom complex of cerebral dysfunction. Its incidence is approximately 1.5 per 1000 births but may be increasing because many smaller and younger premature infants are surviving in intensive care units. It is usually due to a perinatal infection or a period of anoxia or hypoxia that affects the central nervous system (Naeye et al., 1989; Nelson and Ellenberg, 1986). It most commonly appears in babies who were premature, but it may be seen following seizures, infections, or intracranial hemorrhage in the neonatal period.

Diagnosis

Affected children have delayed gross motor development, abnormal fine motor performance, altered muscle tone, abnormal stress gait, and exaggerated deep tendon reflexes. These findings can vary substantially from being very obvious to being exquisitely subtle with no discernible lesion present unless a careful neurologic examination is performed. Among the more overtly affected individuals, spastic diplegia is the most common of the five types of dysfunction that characterize this disease, accounting for nearly two thirds of the cases.

Findings

Most children with cerebral palsy develop total urinary control. Incontinence is a feature in some, but the exact incidence has never been truly determined (Decter et al., 1987; McNeal et al., 1983). The presence of incontinence is not related to the extent of the physical impairment, although the physical handicap may prevent the individual from getting to the bathroom before he or she has an episode of wetting. A number of children have such a severe degree of mental retardation that they are not trainable, but the majority have sufficient intelligence to learn basic societal protocol with patient and persistent handling. Oftentimes, continence is achieved at a later-than-expected age. Therefore, urodynamic evaluation is reserved for children who appear trainable and do not seem to be hampered too much by their physical impairment, but who have not achieved continence by late childhood or early puberty.

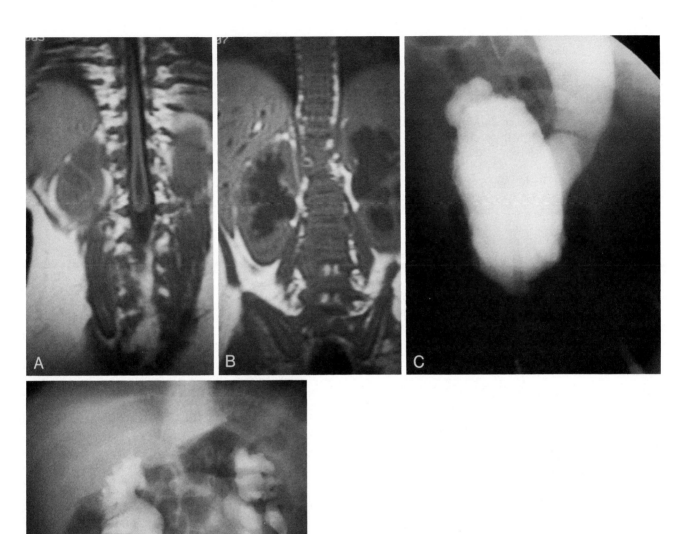

Figure 42–23. *A* and *B*, A 1-year-old girl with an imperforate anus and bony vertebral abnormalities has a tethered cord and bilateral hydronephrosis on MRI. *C*, Voiding cystourethrogram reveals significant trabeculation and reflux on the left. *D*, Excretory urogram demonstrates bilateral hydronephrosis secondary to the reflux on the left and a ureterovesical junction obstruction on the right. Subsequent urodynamic study manifested detrusor hypertonicity and dyssynergy.

Table 42–6. LOWER URINARY TRACT FUNCTION IN CEREBRAL PALSY

	Number	%
Upper motor neuron lesion	49	86
Mixed upper + lower motor neuron lesion	5	9.5
Incomplete lower motor neuron lesion	1	1.5
No urodynamic lesion	2	3

Adapted from Decter, R. M., et al.: J. Urol., 138:1110, 1987.

Table 42–7. URODYNAMIC FINDINGS IN CEREBRAL PALSY*

Upper Motor Neuron	
Uninhibited contractions	35
Detrusor sphincter dyssynergy	7
Hyperactive sacral reflexes	6
No voluntary control	3
Small-capacity bladder	2
Hypertonia	2
Lower Motor Neuron	
Excessive polyphasia	5
↑ Amplitude + ↑ duration potentials	4

*Some had more than one finding.
Adapted from Decter, R. M., et al.: J. Urol., 138:1110, 1987.

In a review of this subject, urodynamic studies were performed in 57 children with cerebral palsy (Table 42–6) (Decter et al., 1987). Forty-nine (86 per cent) had the expected picture of a partial upper motor neuron type of dysfunction with exaggerated sacral reflexes, detrusor hyperreflexia, and/or detrusor-sphincter dyssynergia (Fig. 42–24), even though they manifested voluntary control over voiding. Six of the 57 (11 per cent), however, had evidence of both upper and lower motor neuron denervation with detrusor areflexia or abnormal motor unit potentials on sphincter EMG assessment (Table 42–7). Most of the children who exhibited these latter findings were discovered to have had an episode of cyanosis in the perinatal period when their records were analyzed on a retrospective basis (Table 42–8). Thus, a lower motor neuron lesion may be seen in addition to the expected upper motor neuron dysfunction.

Recommendations

Treatment usually centers around abolishing the uninhibited contractions with anticholinergic medication, but residual urine volumes must be monitored closely

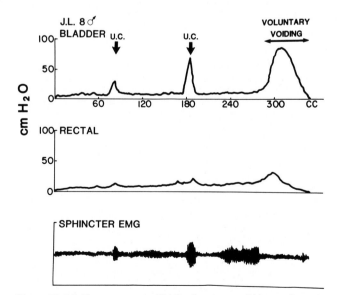

Figure 42–24. Electromyogram (EMG) of an 8-year-old boy with spastic diplegia shows a typical partial upper motor neuron type bladder with uninhibited contractions (U.C.) associated with increased sphincter activity but normal voiding dynamics at capacity. Wetting is due to these contractions when they are unaccompanied by the heightened sphincter activity.

to insure complete evacuation with each void. Intermittent catheterization may be required for those who cannot empty their bladder.

Traumatic Injuries to the Spine

Despite the exposure and potential for a traumatic spinal cord injury, this condition is rarely encountered in children. When an injury does occur, it is most likely to happen as a result of a motor vehicle accident, a gunshot wound, or a diving incident (Cass et al., 1984). It has also occurred iatrogenically following surgery to correct scoliosis, kyphosis, or other intraspinal processes as well as congenital aortic anomalies or patent ductus arteriosus (Cass et al., 1984). Newborns are particularly prone to hyperextension injuries during high forceps delivery (Adams et al., 1988; Lanska et al., 1990).

The lower urinary tract dysfunction that ensues is not likely to be an isolated event; rather, it is usually associated with loss of sensation and paralysis of the lower limbs. Radiologic investigation of the spine may not reveal any bony abnormality even though momentary subluxation of osseus structures due to elasticity of vertebral ligaments can result in a neurologic injury (Pollack et al., 1988). Myelography and computed tomography (CT) will show swelling of the cord below the level of the lesion (Adams et al., 1988; Lanska et al., 1990). Many times, what appears as a permanent lesion initially, turns out to be a transient phenomenon instead. Although sensation and motor function in the lower

Table 42–8. PERINATAL RISK FACTORS IN CEREBRAL PALSY

Factor	UMN	LMN
Prematurity	10	1
Respiratory distress/arrest/apnea	9	2
Neonatal seizures	5	
Infection	5	
Traumatic birth	5	
Congenital hydrocephalus	3	
Placenta previa/abruption	2	2
Hypoglycemia ± seizures	2	
Intracranial hemorrhage	2	
Cyanosis at birth	1	3
No specific factor noted	15	

UMN, upper motor neuron lesion; LMN, lower motor neuron lesion.
Adapted from Decter, R. M., et al.: J. Urol., 138:1110, 1987.

extremities may be restored relatively soon, the dysfunction involving the bladder and rectum may persist for a considerable period of time.

If urinary retention occurs immediately following the injury, an indwelling Foley catheter is passed into the bladder and left in place for as short a time as possible, until intermittent catheterization can be started safely on a regular basis (Barkin et al., 1983; Guttmann and Frankel, 1966). When the child starts voiding again, the timing of catheterization can be such that it is used as a means of measuring the residual urine volume after a spontaneous void. Residual urine volumes of 25 ml or less are considered safe enough to allow for reducing the frequency and even stopping the catheterization program (Barkin et al., 1983). After 2 to 3 weeks, however, if there is no improvement in lower urinary tract function, urodynamic studies are conducted to determine if this condition is the result of spinal shock or actual nerve root or spinal cord injury. Detrusor areflexia is not uncommon under these circumstances (Iwatsubo et al., 1985). In comparison, EMG recording of the sphincter often reveals normal motor units without fibrillation potentials but absent sacral reflexes and a nonrelaxing sphincter with bladder filling, a sign that transient spinal shock has occurred (Iwatsubo et al., 1985). The outcome from this event is guarded but good, because most cases resolve completely as edema of the cord in response to the injury subsides, leaving no permanent damage (Fanciullacci et al., 1988; Iwatsubo et al., 1985).

Most permanent traumatic injuries involving the spinal cord produce an upper motor neuron type lesion with detrusor hyperreflexia and detrusor-sphincter dyssynergia. The potential danger from this outflow obstruction is obvious (Donnelly et al., 1972). Substantial residual urine volumes, high-pressure reflux, and urinary tract infections and their sequelae are the leading causes of long-term morbidity and mortality in spinal cord–injured patients. Urodynamic studies will identify those patients at risk (Barkin et al., 1983). Early identification and proper management may prevent the signs and effects of outlet obstruction before they become apparent on x-ray examination of the urinary tract (Ogawa et al., 1988; Pearman, 1976).

FUNCTIONAL VOIDING DISORDERS

Enuresis is defined as inappropriate voiding at an age when urinary control is expected. It is difficult, however, to say when urinary control should occur. Studies of large groups of children have provided some guidelines for expectations, but there are no absolute milestones for the individual child (Bellman, 1966; Fergusson et al., 1986). Girls tend to become trained before boys, and daytime continence is achieved before nighttime control. Although the possibility exists, it is rare to achieve control before 1½ years of age (Yeats, 1973). From that time onward, urinary control is gained by approximately 20 per cent of children for each year of life up to 4½ years, with a smaller percentage of the population attaining complete continence every year

after that. By age 10, about 5 per cent of children still have urinary incontinence; this diminishes, however, to 2 per cent after puberty (MacKeith et al., 1973).

The evaluation of the incontinent child begins with a comprehensive history, including details of the mother's pregnancy and delivery, family history of enuresis, developmental milestones, school performance, fine and gross motor coordination, previous continence, social setting and sibling interaction, parental expectations, and characterization of the wetting episodes. If there is a suspicion of an ectopic ureter in a girl (someone who voids normally but is constantly damp both day and night), then an excretory urogram (preferably) or a renal ultrasound is performed. Boys who have a question of outflow obstruction (urgency or urge incontinence and enuresis beyond age 5) are subjected to a voiding cystogram.

The indications for performing urodynamic studies are as follows: any suspicion of a neurologic condition, diurnal incontinence with no associated pathology, nocturnal enuresis in a pubertal child who is resistant to conventional therapy, fecal and urinary incontinence at any age, persistent voiding difficulties long after an infection has been treated, recurrent urinary tract infection despite continuous antibiotics, and bladder trabeculation or "sphincter spasm" on voiding cystography (Fig. 42–25).

When urodynamic studies are performed on a group of children who have these findings without an obvious neurologic or systemic disorder, a spectrum of voiding pattern abnormalities emerge (Table 42–9) (Bauer et al., 1980). Classification of these disorders helps one to understand and treat each condition specifically. The

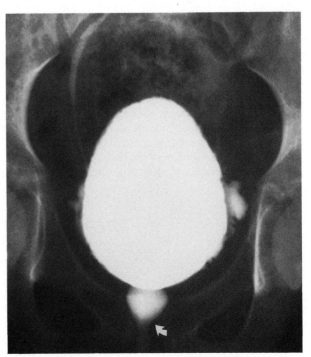

Figure 42–25. A 10-year-old girl with recurrent urinary tract infection has spasm of the sphincter during voiding with "narrowing" in the distal urethra on voiding cystourethrogram *(arrow)*.

Table 42–9. PATTERNS OF VOIDING DYSFUNCTION IN NEUROLOGICALLY NORMAL CHILDREN

Small-capacity bladder
Detrusor hyperreflexia
Infrequent voider—lazy bladder syndrome
Psychologic non-neuropathic bladder (Hinman syndrome)

following discussion will elaborate these different entities.

Small-Capacity Hypertonic Bladder

Children with recurrent urinary tract infection without an anatomic abnormality may have symptoms of voiding dysfunction, including frequency, urgency, urge incontinence, staccato voiding, nocturia and/or enuresis, and dysuria, long after the infection has cleared. Sometimes, persistence of these symptoms with their associated abnormal voiding dynamics can lead to repeated infections (Hansson et al., 1990).

An inflammatory reaction in the bladder wall may produce an irritability that affects the sensory threshold and increases the need to void sooner than anticipated. If the detrusor muscle is affected as well, the increased irritability may lead to instability of the muscle and eventually to poor compliance (Mayo and Burns, 1990). When the child attempts to hold back urination because it is either painful or inappropriate to void, he or she may actually tighten, or only partially or intermittently relax the external sphincter muscle during voiding, producing a form of outflow obstruction and disrupting the laminar flow pattern that normally exists (Figs. 42–26 and 42–27) (Hansson et al., 1990; Tanagho et al., 1971; VanGool and Tanagho, 1977).

The stop-and-start voiding leads to recurrent infection because bacteria can be carried back up into the bladder from the meatus as a result of the "milk back" phenomenon occurring within the urethra when urination is interrupted in this manner (Webster et al., 1984). Theoretically, if unrecognized or left untreated in young girls, this condition may become the forerunner of interstitial cystitis seen in many adult females and may even be the precursor of prostatitis in males.

Radiologic investigation often reveals a normal upper urinary tract, but the bladder may be small and have

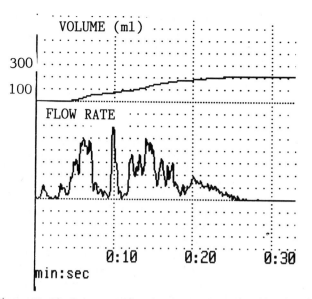

Figure 42–26. Staccato voiding is seen in an 8-year-old girl with recurrent infection.

varying degrees of trabeculation on routine excretory urography or a thickened wall on ultrasonography (Bauer et al., 1980; Lebowitz and Mandell, 1987). During the voiding phase of the cystourethrogram, the posterior urethra may show signs of intermittent dilation at its upper end with a uniform narrowing occurring toward the external sphincter region. In girls, this "spinning top" deformity has raised the question of an obstructed meatus (see Fig. 42–25) (Tanagho et al., 1971; VanGool and Tanagho, 1977); in boys, it has often been mistaken for posterior urethral valves. This appearance is due to failure of complete relaxation of the external sphincter and persistence of a relative obstruction at the distal end of the posterior urethra in an attempt by the child to suppress voiding (Saxton et al., 1988).

Urodynamic studies demonstrate a bladder of small capacity (when adjusted for age) and elevated detrusor pressure during filling (Fig. 42–28) (Bauer et al., 1980; VanGool and Tanagho, 1977). At capacity, the child has an uncontrolled urge to void and, sometimes, cannot suppress urination despite contraction of the external sphincter. The bladder contraction is usually sustained with pressures reaching higher than normal values. Emp-

INTERMITTENCY

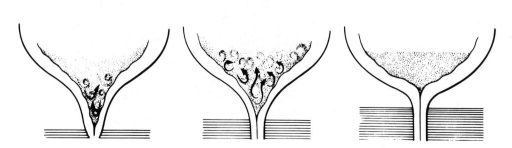

Figure 42–27. Nonlaminar flow secondary to periodic tightening and relaxation of the external sphincter leads to eddy currents and the "milk back" phenomenon, which can carry bacteria colonized at the urethral meatus up into the bladder and cause infection of the residual urine.

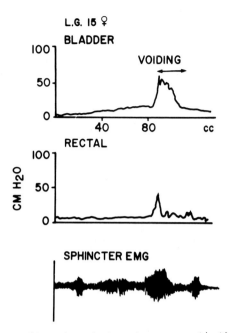

Figure 42–28. This urodynamic picture in a teenage girl with recurrent infections reveals a small-capacity hypertonic bladder and a hyperactive sphincter, which relaxes only partially during voiding.

tying may not always be complete despite these high pressures. The baseline sphincter EMG activity is normal at rest, but complex repetitive discharges (pseudomyotonia) (Dyro et al., 1983) or periodic relaxation of the muscle during filling may occur, contributing to the sense of urgency or actual incontinent episodes. During voiding, the sphincter may relax intermittently or even completely at first, but then contract in response to discomfort, preventing complete emptying (Fig. 42–28) (Hansson et al., 1990; Rudy and Woodside, 1991).

Treatment is based on trying to eliminate the recurrent infections, to minimize any possible environmental influences that predispose the individual to infection, and to improve both the child's voiding pattern and bathroom habits. Girls should learn to take showers instead of baths, or at least bathe alone without other siblings, wipe from front to back, try to completely relax when they void so that a steady stream is produced, and take the time to completely empty the bladder each time they urinate (Hansson et al., 1990). In addition to antibiotics, antispasmodic agents (flavoxate, hyoscyamine, dicyclomine) are administered. On rare occasions when cystoscopy is performed, an intense inflammatory reaction, which contributes to the symptomatology, may be noted in the trigone region. If present, fulguration of this area will prove beneficial in some children (personal observation).

Detrusor Hyperreflexia

Children with long-standing symptoms of daytime frequency, urgency, or sudden incontinence and squatting, in addition to nocturia and/or enuresis, may have detrusor hyperreflexia. Vincent's curtsy, a characteristic

posturing by these children in an attempt to prevent voiding, is a commonly described behavior pattern (Kondo et al., 1983; Vincent, 1966). Oftentimes, the child's parents or siblings relate a history of delayed control over micturition. These affected family members may be compensating for their abnormality currently by having continued daytime frequency or nocturia.

The child's physical examination may be normal, but hyperactive deep tendon reflexes in the lower or upper extremities, ankle clonus, posturing with a stress gait, or difficulty with tandem walking and mirror movements (similar motion in the contralateral hand when the individual is asked to rapidly pronate and supinate one hand) may be evident. Left-handedness, -footedness, or -eyedness in a family in which all other members are right-handed may signify crossed dominance from a previously unrecognized perinatal insult. Carefully questioning the parents about perinatal events may uncover such an insult, which has affected the central nervous system and caused these findings.

X-ray evaluation usually reveals no abnormality other than a mildly trabeculated or thick-walled bladder. Urodynamic studies demonstrate uninhibited contractions of the bladder during filling, which the child may or may not sense or abolish by increasing the activity of the external urethral sphincter (Fig. 42–29) (Bauer et al., 1980; Rudy and Woodside, 1991). During filling, capacity may be reached sooner than expected, at which time a normal detrusor contraction occurs with a sustained relaxation of the sphincter, resulting in complete emptying. Some children will not be able to suppress this contraction even though the bladder has not been filled to capacity. Sometimes, uninhibited contractions may only be elicited following a cough or strain, or when the child assumes a change in posture (Kondo et al., 1983). The uninhibited contractions are thought to be responsible for the symptoms (McGuire and Savastano, 1984).

These findings may be the result of a cerebral insult, however mild, in the neonatal period; but, more commonly, they are linked to delayed maturation of the reticulospinal pathways and the inhibitory centers in the mid-brain and cerebral cortex. Thus, total control over vesicourethral function may be lacking (MacKeith et al., 1973; Mueller, 1960; Yeats, 1973). Several investigators have found a similar urodynamic picture in a significant number of adults with nocturnal enuresis and/or daytime symptoms (Torrens and Collins, 1975). Parents who exhibit the same behavior pattern as their children may have a genetically determined delayed rate of central nervous system maturation.

On occasion, children with profound constipation develop uninhibited contractions of the bladder and urinary incontinence secondary to them (O'Regan et al., 1985). The etiology of this condition is unclear, but treatment of the bowel distention has resulted in a dramatic improvement in the bladder dysfunction (O'Regan et al., 1986).

Sometimes, repeated urinary infection may produce an identical urodynamic picture. Detrusor hyperreflexia occurs as a result of the inflammatory response in the bladder wall that irritates the receptors located in the submucosa and/or detrusor muscle layers (Koff and

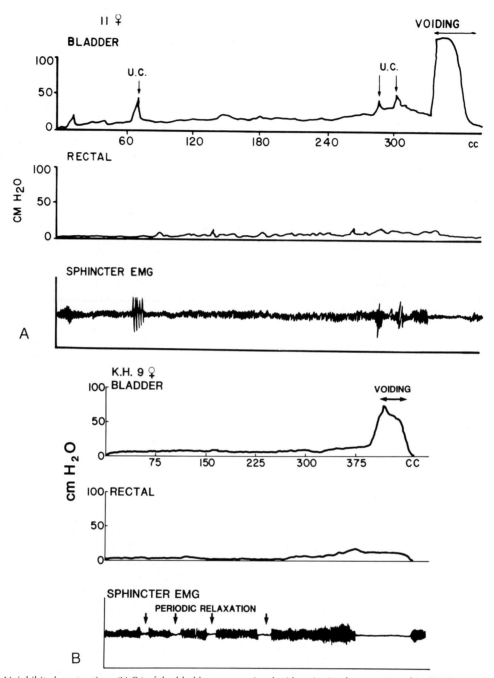

Figure 42–29. *A,* Uninhibited contractions (U.C.) of the bladder are associated with a rise in electromyographic (EMG) activity. During voluntary voiding, a coordinated vesicourethral unit exists. (From Bauer, S. B.: Urodynamic evaluation and neuromuscular dysfunction. *In* Kelalis, P. P., King, L. R., and Belman, A. B. (Eds.): Clinical Pediatric Urology, Ed. 2, Vol I. Philadelphia, W. B. Saunders Co., 1985, pp. 283–310.) *B,* Some children only manifest periodic relaxation of the sphincter without a rise in detrusor pressure as an early phase of a hyperreflexic bladder, producing urgency and incontinence.

Murtagh, 1983). Therefore, all children with these findings should be screened for infection. It has been postulated that a hyperactive detrusor may lead to inappropriate voiding. When the child realizes what is happening, he or she tightens the sphincter to reverse this process, which shuts the distal urethra first and the bladder neck second, causing the column of urine to be "milked back" into the bladder (Webster et al., 1984). This has the effect of carrying bacteria from the meatal opening up into the bladder, setting up the potential for

infection in the residual volume of urine, especially if the child does not immediately make an attempt to empty the bladder (Koff and Murtagh, 1983).

Anticholinergic medication (oxybutynin, propantheline, glycopyrrolate, and imipramine) alone or in combination has been used successfully to manage this condition (Kondo et al., 1983). If infection is present, it should be treated simultanously (Bauer et al., 1980; Buttarazzi, 1977; Firlit et al., 1978; Kass et al., 1979; Mayo and Burns, 1990).

The Infrequent Voider—Lazy Bladder Syndrome

Most children urinate four to five times per day and defecate daily or at least every other day. Some children, primarily girls, may void only twice a day, once in the morning (either at home or after they are in school), and again at night (DeLuca et al., 1962). It is not unusual to find children who do not void at all while in school. These children had normal voiding patterns as infants, but after toilet training, they learned to withhold micturition for extended periods of time. Their parents may have instilled in them, however unintentionally, the idea that it is bad to wet or soil themselves. As a result, a few develop a fear of strange bathrooms or mimic their mother's pattern of infrequent urination and defecation (Bauer et al., 1980). Others have experienced an aversive event or had an infection associated with dysuria around the time of training, which lead to the infrequent pattern of micturition. Some children are excessively neat or have a fetish for cleanliness which causes them to avoid bathrooms. Often they only void enough to relieve the pressure to urinate and do not empty their bladder completely.

The infrequent voiding and incomplete emptying produce an ever-increasing bladder capacity and a dimished stimulus to urinate (Webster et al., 1984). The chronically distended bladder is prone to urinary infection and overflow or stress incontinence. Sometimes, these signs are the first manifestations of the abnormal voiding pattern. When the child is carefully questioned, the aberrant micturition is easily detected. More often, the problem is diagnosed following a voiding cystourethrogram when a larger-than-normal capacity (for age) is noted and the residual urine volume on initial catheterization is measured, with the child being questioned afterwards about his or her voiding habits (Fig. 42–30) (Webster et al., 1984). In addition, the cystogram usually reveals a smooth-walled bladder without reflux.

Urodynamic studies demonstrate a very large capacity, highly compliant bladder with normal, unsustained, or absent detrusor contractions (Fig. 42–31A) (Bauer et al., 1980). Straining to void is a common form of emptying. Sphincter EMG reveals normal motor unit potentials at rest and normal responses to various sacral reflexes, bladder filling, and attempts at emptying. The urinary flow rate may be intermittent with sudden peaks coinciding with straining, or it may be normal but short-lived secondary to an unsustained detrusor contraction (Webster et al., 1984). Unless strongly encouraged, the child will not completely empty his or her bladder during voiding (Fig. 42–31B) (Bauer et al., 1980). This picture is consistent with myogenic failure from chronic distention (Koefoot et al., 1981).

Changing the child's voiding habits is the first approach to therapy. Keeping to a rigid schedule of toileting and encouraging the child to empty each time he or she voids is mandatory (Masek, 1985). Behavioral therapy techniques to get the child to comply are helpful. Occasionally, bethanechol chloride is administered to increase the sensitivity to regular voiding. Rarely, intermittent catheterization may be necessary to allow the detrusor muscle to regain its contractility and ability to empty. Antibiotics are needed when urinary tract infection is present; they are continued until the voiding pattern improves.

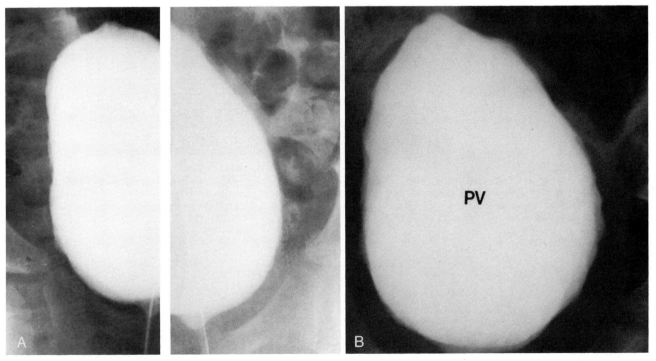

Figure 42–30. *A,* A large-capacity bladder with no reflux is noted in a 10-year-old girl with an infrequent voiding pattern. *B,* The postvoid (PV) residual volume is quite large.

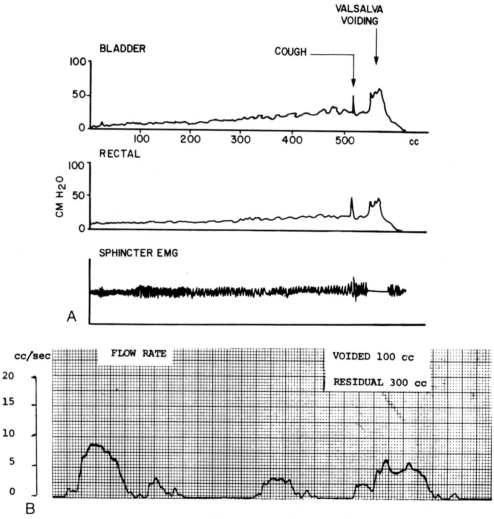

Figure 42–31. *A,* Urodynamic evaluation reveals a very large capacity bladder with no voiding contraction. The child empties by straining after relaxing the sphincter. *B,* The flow rate is characteristic of this effort to empty and leads to a considerable volume of residual urine. (From Bauer, S. B.: Urodynamic evaluation and neuromuscular dysfunction. *In* Kelalis, P. P., King, L. R., and Belman, A. B. (Eds.): Clinical Pediatric Urology, Ed. 2, Vol I. Philadelphia, W. B. Saunders Co., 1985, pp. 283–310.)

Psychologic Non-Neuropathic Bladder (Hinman Syndrome)

Some children have an apparent "syndrome" of voiding dysfunction that mimics neuropathic bladder disease, but which may be a learned disorder. At first, it was believed to be an isolated neurologic lesion (Johnston and Farkas, 1975; Mix, 1977; Williams et al., 1975), but now it is thought to be an acquired abnormality (Allen, 1977; Allen and Bright, 1978; Bauer et al., 1980; Hinman, 1974). It is produced by an active contraction of the sphincter during voiding, which creates a degree of outflow obstruction. Some investigators think this may be the result of persistence of the transitional phase of gaining control, whereby the child learns to prevent voiding by voluntarily contracting the external sphincter (Allen, 1977; Rudy and Woodside, 1991). Others think this pattern results from the child's normal response to uninhibited contractions (McGuire and Savastano, 1984). This behavior becomes habitual because the child has difficulty distinguishing between involuntary and voluntary voiding; as a consequence, the inappropriate sphincter activity occurs all the time (Bauer et al., 1980).

These children have urgency, urge and/or stress incontinence, infrequent voluntary voiding, intermittent urination associated with straining, recurrent urinary tract infection, and irregular bowel movements with fecal soiling in-between times (Bauer et al., 1980). What is most striking is the similarity in the pattern of family dynamics, which is disclosed upon carefully observing and carefully questioning of the family (Table 42–10) (Allen and Bright, 1978). The parents, especially the father, tend to be domineering, exacting, unyielding, and intolerant of weakness or failure. Delayed training or continued wetting is viewed as such a characteristic. Divorce and alcoholism are common threads that only exacerbate the situation.

Wetting is perceived as immature, defiant, and purposeful behavior, which the parents believe must be counteracted with stern reprimands. The children are often punished, both mentally and physically, for their ineptness. Confusion, depression, and withdrawal for fear of wetting with its added punitive response become the child's prevalent attitude, because he or she does not know how to nor can he or she prevent this provocative behavior. The child tries to further withhold urination and defecation by keeping the sphincter muscle tight, aggravating the situation. Thus, wetting becomes more commonplace and abdominal pain from chronic constipation is not unusual.

Table 42–10. FEATURES OF PSYCHOLOGIC NON-NEUROPATHIC BLADDER

Daytime and nighttime wetting
Encopresis, constipation, fecal impaction
Recurrent urinary tract infection
Parental characteristics
Domineering, exacting
Divorce
Alcoholism
Punishments (mental and physical) inflicted for wetting

Radiologic evaluation reveals profound changes within the urinary tract. Hydroureteronephrosis with or without pyelonephritic scarring from recurrent infection occurs in two thirds of the children (Fig. 42–32*A*) (Bauer et al., 1980). Fifty per cent have severe vesicoureteral reflux. Nearly every child has a grossly trabeculated, large-capacity bladder with a considerable postvoid residual urine volume (Fig. 42–32*B, C*). Voiding films show either persistent or intermittent narrowing in the region of the external sphincter in almost half the children (Fig. 42–32*B, C*). Finally, the scout film from the excretory urogram displays considerable fecal material in the colon consistent with chronic constipation.

Urodynamic studies demonstrate a large-capacity bladder with poor compliance, uninhibited contractions, and either high-pressure or ineffective detrusor contractions during voiding (Fig. 42–33*A*) (Bauer et al., 1980; Kass et al., 1979). Sometimes, Valsalva voiding is needed to empty the bladder. The urinary flow rate is often intermittent as a result of the failure of the external sphincter to relax (Fig. 42–33*B*). The bethanechol supersensitivity test may be positive; in the past, it was this response which lead to the belief that these children had neuropathic bladder dysfunction (Williams et al., 1975).

EMG recordings, however, reveal normal external urethral sphincter innervation and exclude the possibility of a sacral spinal cord lesion. The sphincter fails to completely relax and may actually tighten episodically once voiding commences (Rudy and Woodside, 1991); this finding along with the uninhibited contractions suggest an upper motor neuron lesion, but usually no other signs are present to confirm this urodynamic hypothesis. Spinal canal imaging with magnetic resonance has failed to reveal any intraspinal process as a cause for the voiding dysfunction in these children (Fig. 42–32*D*) (Hinman, 1986).

The dyssynergy created by the incoordination between the bladder and sphincter muscles leads to high voiding pressures initially and, later, to ineffective detrusor contractions (Rudy and Woodside, 1991). Depending on which point of the spectrum one is at, a low or intermittent flow rate and either a significant or a minimal postvoid residual urine volume are noted.

Before this "syndrome" was recognized and the pathophysiology elucidated, many children underwent multiple operations to improve bladder emptying and correct vesicoureteral reflux. Failure of these procedures to succeed led to urinary diversion in a number of instances. Some of these individuals were eventually able to be undiverted at an older age after they outgrew the conditions that caused their dysfunction in the first place.

Today, an entirely different approach is taken. Treatment is focused on improving the child's ability to empty the bladder and bowel and alleviating the psychosocial pressures that contribute to the aggravation of the voiding dysfunction (Table 42–11) (Hinman, 1986; Masek, 1985). A frequent emptying schedule accompanied by biofeedback techniques to relax the sphincter during voiding, anticholinergic drugs to abolish uninhibited contractions, and improved bowel emptying regimens

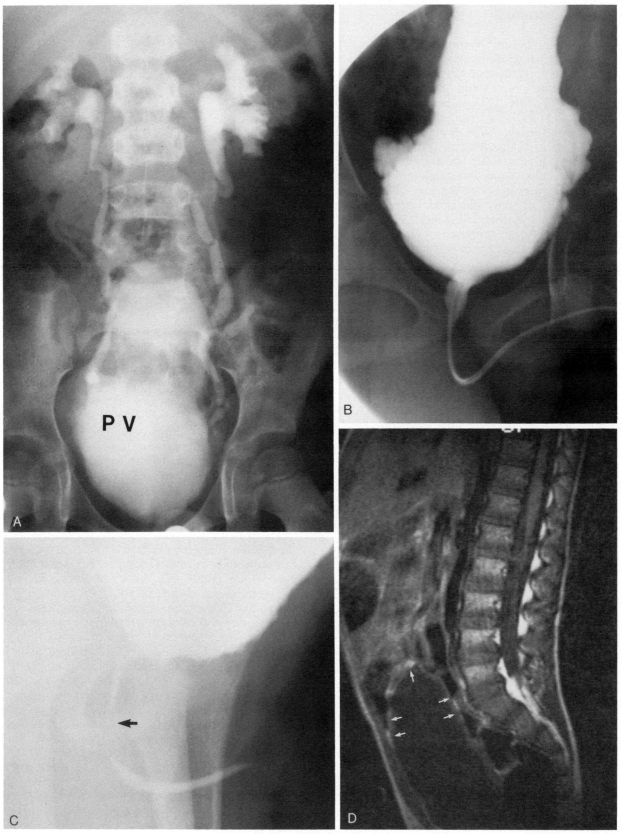

Figure 42–32. *A,* An excretory urogram in a 7-year-old boy with day and nighttime wetting and fecal soiling demonstrates bilateral hydronephrosis and a large bladder with incomplete emptying. *B* and *C,* Voiding cystogram reveals no reflux, but severe trabeculation and a weak, narrow urine stream. *D,* An MRI scan of the spine is normal, but note the large bladder *(arrows).* (PV, postvoid.)

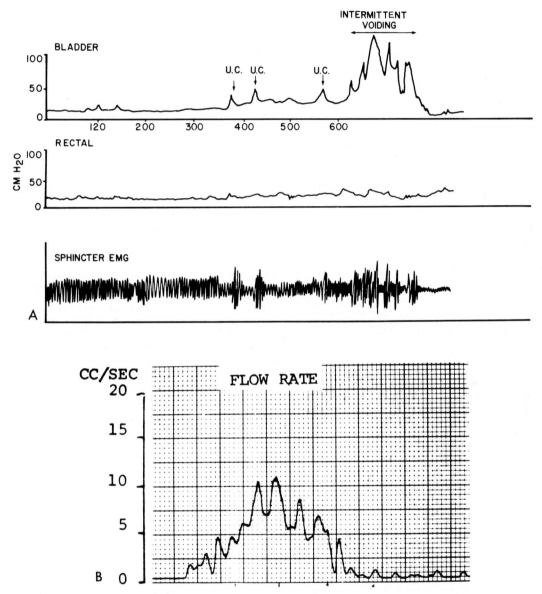

Figure 42–33. *A*, The urodynamic picture reveals both uninhibited contractions (U.C.) and high voiding pressures with a nonrelaxing sphincter. *B*, The urinary flow rate reflects the voiding pattern seen on urodynamic evaluation. (From Bauer, S. B.: Urodynamic evaluation and neuromuscular dysfunction. *In* Kelalis, P. P., King, L. R., and Belman, A. B. (Eds.): Clinical Pediatric Urology, Ed. 2, Vol I. Philadelphia, W. B. Saunders Co., 1985, pp. 283–310.)

Table 42–11. TREATMENT OF PSYCHOLOGIC NON-
NEUROPATHIC BLADDER

Psychotherapy
Behavioral modification
Biofeedback
Drugs
    Oxybutynin
    Flavoxate
    Bethanechol
    Diazepam
Antibiotics
Intermittent catheterization
Bowel re-regulation program
    Stool softeners
    Bulking agents
    Laxatives, enemas

are instituted (Bauer et al., 1980). Bethanechol chloride and prazosin (an alpha blocking agent) may be added if the detrusor exhibits poor contractility. Despite these measures, intermittent catheterization may be needed in children who fail to respond and in those individuals who require immediate decompression of the upper urinary tract (Snyder et al., 1982). In some cases, the outflow obstruction may have produced severe renal damage and even chronic kidney failure, which must be managed accordingly.

Psychotherapy is an integral part of the rehabilitative process to re-educate both the child and the parents in appropriate voiding habits. Punishments are stopped, and a reward system is initiated to improve the child's self-image and confidence (Masek, 1985).

REFERENCES

Blaivas, J. G.: A critical appraisal of specific diagnostic techniques. *In* Krane, R. J., and Siroky, M. B. (Eds.): Clinical Neurourology. Boston, Little, Brown & Co., 1979, pp. 69–110.

Blaivas, J. G., Labib, K. B., Bauer, S. B., and Retik, A. B.: Changing concepts in the urodynamic evaluation of children. J. Urol., 117:777, 1977.

Gierup, J., and Ericsson, N. O.: Micturition studies in infants and children: Intravesical pressure, urinary flow and urethral resistance in boys with intravesical obstruction. Scand. J. Urol. Nephrol., 4:217, 1970.

Lapides, J., Diokno, A. C., Silber, S. J., and Lowe, B. S.: Clean intermittent self-catheterization in the treatment of urinary tract disease. J. Urol., 107:458, 1972.

McGuire, E. J., Woodside, J. R., Borden, T. A., and Weiss, R. M.: The prognostic value of urodynamic testing in myelodysplastic patients. J. Urol., 126:205, 1981.

Smith, E. D.: Urinary prognosis in spina bifida. J. Urol., 108:115, 1972.

Urodynamic Evaluation

Abrams, P. H.: Perfusion urethral profilometry. Urol. Clin. North Am., 6:103, 1979.

Bates, C. P., Whiteside, C. G., and Turner-Warwick, R. T.: Synchronous cine/pressure/flow/cystourethrography with special reference to stress and urge incontinence. Br. J. Urol., 42:714, 1970.

Bauer, S. B.: Pediatric neurourology. *In* Krane, R. J., and Siroky, M. B. (Eds.): Clinical Neurourology. Boston, Little, Brown & Co., 1979, pp. 275–294.

Blaivas, J. G.: A critical appraisal of specific diagnostic techniques. *In* Krane, R. J., and Siroky, M. B. (Eds.): Clinical Neurourology. Boston, Little, Brown & Co., 1979a, pp. 69–110.

Blaivas, J. G.: EMG: Other uses. *In* Barrett, D. M., and Wein, A. J. (Eds.): Controversies in Neuro-urology. New York, Churchill Livingstone, 1979b, pp. 103–116.

Blaivas, J. G., Labib, K. B., Bauer, S. B., and Retik, A. B.: A new approach to electromyography of the external urethral sphincter. J. Urol., 117:773, 1977a.

Blaivas, J. G., Labib, K. B., Bauer, S. B., and Retik, A. B.: Changing concepts in the urodynamic evaluation of children. J. Urol., 117:777, 1977b.

Bradley, W. E., Timm, G. W., and Scott, F. B.: Sphincter electromyography. Urol. Clin. North Am., 1:69, 1974.

Diokno, A. C., Koff, S. A., and Bender, L. F.: Periurethral striated muscle activity in neurogenic bladder dysfunction. J. Urol., 112:743, 1974.

Ericsson, N. O., Hellstrom, B., Negardth, A., and Rudhe, U.: Micturition urethrocystography in children with myelomeningocele. Acta Radiol. Diagn., 11:321, 1971.

Evans, A. T., Felker, J. R., Shank, R. A., and Sugarman, S. R.: Pitfalls of urodynamics. J. Urol., 122:220, 1979.

Gierup, J., Ericsson, N. O., and Okmain, L.: Micturition studies in infants and children. Scand. J. Urol. Nephrol., 3:1, 1969.

Gleason, D. M., Reilly, R. J., Bottacini, M. R., and Pierce, M. J.: The urethral continence zone and its relation to stress incontinence. J. Urol., 112:81, 1974.

Joseph, D. B., and Duggan, M. L.: The effects of fast and slow saline infusion on hypertonicity and peak/leak pressure during cystometrogram evaluation of infants and children with myelodysplasia. J. Urol., 1991. In press.

Koff, S. A., and Kass, E. J.: Abdominal wall electromyography: A noninvasive technique to improve pediatric urodynamic accuracy. J. Urol., 127:736, 1982.

Koff, S. A.: Estimating bladder capacity in children. Urology, 21:248, 1983.

Maizels, M., and Firlit, C. F.: Pediatric urodynamics: Clinical comparison of surface vs. needle pelvic floor/external sphincter electromyography. J. Urol., 122:518, 1979.

Tanagho, E. A.: Membrane and microtransducer catheters: Their effectiveness for profilometry of the lower urinary tract. Urol. Clin. North Am., 6:110, 1979.

Turner-Warwick, R. T.: Some clinical aspects of detrusor dysfunction. J. Urol., 113:539, 1975.

Yalla, S. V., Rossier, A. B., and Fam, B.: Vesico-urethral pressure recordings in the assessment of neurogenic bladder functions in spinal cord injury patients. Urol. Int., 32:161, 1979.

Yalla, S. V., Sharma, G. V. R. K., and Barsamian, E. M.: Micturitional static urethral pressure profile method of recording urethral pressure profiles during voiding and implications. J. Urol., 124:649, 1980.

Neurospinal Dysraphisms

Myelodysplasia

Adams, M. C., Mitchell, M. E., and Rink, R. C.: Gastrocystoplasty: An alternative solution to the problem of urological reconstruction in the severely compromised patient. J. Urol., 140:1152, 1988.

Barbalias, G. A., Klauber, G. T., and Blaivas, J. G.: Critical evaluation of the Credé maneuver: A urodynamic study of 207 patients. J. Urol., 130:720, 1983.

Barrett, D. M., and Furlow, W. L.: The management of severe urinary incontinence in patients with myelodysplasia by implantation of the AS791/792 urinary sphincter device. J. Urol., 128:44, 1982.

Bauer, S. B.: Vesico-ureteral reflux in children with neurogenic bladder dysfunction. *In* Johnston, J. H. (Ed.): International Perspectives in Urology, Vol. 10. Baltimore, Williams & Wilkins, 1984a, pp. 159–177.

Bauer, S. B.: Myelodysplasia: Newborn evaluation and management. *In* McLaurin, R. L. (Ed.): Spina Bifida: A Multidisciplinary Approach. New York, Praeger, 1984b, pp. 262–267.

Bauer, S. B.: The management of spina bifida from birth onwards. *In* Whitaker, R. H., and Woodard, J. R. (Eds.): Paediatric Urology. London, Butterworth & Co., 1985, pp. 87–112.

Bauer, S. B.: Early evaluation and management of children with spina bifida. *In* King, L. R. (Ed.): Urologic Surgery in Neonates and Young Infants. Philadelphia, W. B. Saunders Co., 1988, pp. 252–264.

Bauer, S. B.: Bladder neck reconstruction. *In* Glenn, J. F., Graham, S. D. (Eds.): Urologic Surgery. Philadelphia, J. B. Lippincott Co., 1990, pp. 509–522.

Bauer, S. B.: Evaluation and management of the newborn with myelomeningocele. *In* Gonzales, E. T., Roth, D. R. (Eds.): Common Problems in Urology. Chicago, Mosby Year Book Inc., 1991. In press.

Bauer, S. B., Colodny, A. H., and Retik, A. B.: The management of vesico-ureteral reflux in children with myelodysplasia. J. Urol., 128:102, 1982.

Bauer, S. B., Hallet, M., Khoshbin, S., Lebowitz, R. L., Colodny, A. H., and Retik, A. B.: The predictive value of urodynamic evaluation in the newborn with myelodysplasia. JAMA, 152:650, 1984.

Bauer, S. B., Labib, K. B., Dieppa, R. A., et al.: Urodynamic evaluation in a boy with myelodysplasia and incontinence. Urology, 10:354, 1977.

Bauer, S. B., Reda, E. F., Colodny, A. H., and Retik, A. B.: Detrusor instability: A delayed complication in association with the artificial sphincter. J. Urol., 135:1212, 1986.

Begger, J. H., Meihuizen de Regt, M. J., Hogen Esch, I., et al.: Progressive neurologic deficit in children with spina bifida aperta. Z. Kinderchir., 41(Suppl. 1):13, 1986.

Bihrle, R., Klee, L. W., Adams, M. C., Steidle, S. P., and Foster, R. S.: The transverse colon-gastric tube urinary reservoir. Transverse Colon-Gastric Tube Composite Reservoir. Urology, 37:36–40, 1991.

Blaivas, J. G., Sinka, H. P., Zayed, A. H., et al.: Detrusor-sphincter dyssynergia: A detailed electromyographic study. J. Urol., 125:545, 1986.

Bloom, D. A., Knechtel, J. M., and McGuire, E. J.: Urethral dilation improves bladder compliance in children with myelomeningocele and high leak point pressures. J. Urol., 144:430, 1990.

Bosco, P. J., Bauer, S. B., Colodny, A. H., Mandell, J., and Retik, A. B.: The long-term follow-up of artificial urinary sphincters in children. Long-Term Results of Artificial Urinary Sphincters in Children. J. Urol., 146:396–399, 1991.

Cartwright, P. C., and Snow, B. W.: Bladder autoaugmentation: Early clinical experience. J. Urol., 142:505, 1989a.

Cartwright, P. C., and Snow, B. W.: Bladder autoaugmentation: Partial detrusor excision to augment bladder without use of bowel. J. Urol., 142:1050, 1989b.

Cass, A. S.: Urinary tract complications of myelomeningocele patients. J. Urol., 115:102, 1976.

Cass, A. S., Bloom, B. A., and Luxenberg, M.: Sexual function in adults with myelomeningocele. J. Urol., 136:425, 1986.

Chiaramonte, R. M., Horowitz, E. M., Kaplan, G. A., et al.: Implications of hydronephrosis in newborns with myelodysplasia. J. Urol., 136:427, 1986.

Cromer, B. A., Enrile. B., McCoy, K., Gerhardstein, M. J., Fitzpatrick, M., and Judis, J.: Knowledge, attitudes and behavior related to sexuality in adolescents with chronic disability. Dev. Med. Child Neurol., 32:602, 1990.

Dees, J. E.: Congenital epispadias with incontinence. J. Urol., 62:513, 1949.

Duckett, J. W.: Cutaneous vesicostomy in childhood. Urol. Clin. North Am., 1:485, 1974.

Duckett, J. W., and Snyder, H. M., III: Continent urinary diversion: Variations of the Mitrofanoff principle. J. Urol., 136:58, 1986.

Epstein, F.: Meningocele: Pitfalls in early and late management. Clin. Neurosurg., 30:366, 1982.

Geraniotis, E., Koff, S. A., and Enrile, B.: Prophylactic use of clean intermittent catheterization in treatment of infants and young children with myelomeningocele and neurogenic bladder dysfunction. J. Urol., 139:85, 1988.

Ghoniem, G. M., Bloom, D. A., McGuire, E. J., and Stewart, K. L.: Bladder compliance in meningocele children. J. Urol., 141:1404, 1989.

Goldwasser, B., Barrett, D. M., Webster, G. D., and Kramer, S. A.: Cystometric properties of ileum and right colon after bladder augmentation, substitution and replacement. J. Urol., 138:1007, 1987.

Hayden, P.: Adolescents with meningomyelocele. Pediatr. Rev., 6:245, 1985.

Hendren, W. H.: Reconstruction of the previously diverted urinary tracts in children. J. Pediatr. Surg., 8:135, 1973.

Hendren, W. H.: Urinary diversion and undiversion in children. Surg. Clin. North Am., 56:425, 1976.

Hinman, F., Jr.: Selection of intestinal segments for bladder substitution: Physical and physiological characteristics. J. Urol., 139:519, 1988.

Hinman, F., Jr.: Functional classification of conduits for continent diversion. J. Urol., 144:27, 1990.

Jeffs, R. D., Jones, P., and Schillinger, J. F.: Surgical correction of vesico-ureteral reflux in children with neurogenic bladder. J. Urol., 115:449, 1976.

Joseph, D. B., Bauer, S. B., Colodny, A. H., Mandell, J., and Retik, A. B.: Clean intermittent catheterization in infants with neurogenic bladder. Pediatrics, 84:78, 1989.

Kaplan, W. E., and Firlit, C. F.: Management of reflux in myelodysplasic children. J. Urol., 129:1195, 1983.

Kasabian, N. G., Bauer, S. B., Dyro, F. M., Colodny, A. H., Mandell, J., and Retik, A. B.: The value of prophylactic therapy in neonates and infants with myelodysplasia at risk for urinary tract deterioration [Abstract 11]. Presented at the Annual Meeting of the Urology Section of the American Academy of Pediatrics. Boston, October 6, 1990.

Kass, E. J., Koff, S. A., and Lapides, J.: Fate of vesico-ureteral reflux in children with neuropathic bladders managed by intermittent catheterization. J. Urol., 125:63, 1981.

Keating, M. A., Bauer, S. B., Krarup, C., et al.: Sacral sparing in children with myelodysplasia. Presented at the Annual Meeting of the American Urological Association. Anaheim, May 18, 1987.

Khoury, A. E., Hendrick, E. B., McLorie, G. A., Kulkarni, A., and Churchill, B. M.: Occult spinal dysraphism: Clinical and urodynamic outcome after division of the filum terminale. J. Urol., 144:426, 1990.

Kock, N. G.: Ileostomy without external appliances: A survey of 25 patients provided with intra-abdominal intestinal reservoir. Ann. Surg., 173:545, 1971.

Kroovand, R. L., Bell, W., Hart, L. J., and Benfeld, K. Y.: The effect of back closure on detrusor function in neonates with myelodysplasia. J. Urol., 144:423, 1990.

Kropp, K. A., and Angwafo, F. F.: Urethral lengthening and reimplantation for neurogenic incontinence in children. J. Urol., 135:533, 1986.

Laurence, K. M.: A declining incidence of neural tube defects in U. K. Z. Kinderchir., 44(Suppl. 1):51, 1989.

Leadbetter, G. W., Jr.: Surgical correction for total urinary incontinence. J. Urol., 91:261, 1964.

Light, J. K., Hawila, M., and Scott, F. B.: Treatment of urinary incontinence in children: The artificial sphincter vs. other methods. J. Urol., 130:518, 1983.

Light, J. K., and Scott, F. B.: Use of the artificial urinary sphincter in spinal cord injury patients. J. Urol., 130:1127, 1983.

Loening-Baucke, V., Desch, L., and Wolraich, M.: Biofeedback training for patients with myelomeningocele and fecal incontinence. Dev. Med. Child Neurol., 30:781, 1988.

Mandell, J., Bauer, S. B., Colodny, A. H., and Retik, A. B.: Cutaneous vesicostomy in infancy. J. Urol., 126:92, 1981.

McGuire, E. J., Wang, C. C., Usitalo, H., and Savastano, J.: Modified pubovaginal sling in girls with myelodysplasia. J. Urol., 135:94, 1986.

McGuire, E. J., Woodside, J. R., Borden, T. A., and Weiss, R. M.: The prognostic value of urodynamic testing in myelodysplastic patients. J. Urol., 126:205, 1981.

McLorie, G. A., Perez-Morero, R., Csima, A. L., and Churchill, B. M.: Determinants of hydronephrosis and renal injury in patients with myelomeningocele. J. Urol., 140:1289, 1986.

Mitchell, M. E., and Piser, J. A.: Intestinocystoplasty and total bladder replacement in children and young adults: Follow-up of 129 cases. J. Urol., 138:1140, 1987.

Mitrofanoff, P.: Cystometrie continente trans-appendiculaire dans le traitement de vessies neurologiques. Chir. Pediatr., 21:297, 1980.

Myers, G. J.: Myelomeningocele: The medical aspect. Pediatr. Clin. North Am., 31:165, 1984.

Peters, C. A., Bauer, S. B., Colodny, A. H., Mandell, J., and Retik, A. B.: The use of rectus fascia to manage urinary incontinence. J. Urol., 142:516, 1989.

Raz, S., Ehrlich, R. M., Ziedman, E. J., Alarcon, A., and McLaughlin, S.: Surgical treatment of the incontinent female patient with myelomeningocele. J. Urol., 139:524, 1988.

Reigel, D. H.: Tethered spinal cord. Concepts Pediatr. Neurosurg., 4:142, 1983.

Riedmiller, H., Burger, R., Muller, S., Thuroff, J., and Hoffenfellner, R.: Continent appendix stoma: A modification of the Mainz Pouch technique. J. Urol., 143:1115, 1990.

Rinck, C., Berg, J., and Hafeman, C.: The adolescent with myelomeningocele: A review of parent experiences and expectations. Adolescence, 24:699, 1989.

Roth, D. R., Vyas, P. R., Kroovand, R. L., and Perlmutter, A. D.: Urinary tract deterioration associated with the artificial urinary sphincter. J. Urol., 135:528, 1986.

Rowland, R. G., Mitchell, M. E., Birhle, R., Kahnoski, R. J., and Piser, J. E.: Indiana continent urinary reservoir. J. Urol., 137:1136, 1987.

Scarff, T. B., and Fronczak, S.: Myelomeningocele: A review and update. Rehabil. Lit., 42:143, 1981.

Schwarz, G. R., and Jeffs, R. D.: Ileal conduit urinary diversion in children: Computer analysis of follow-up from 2 to 16 years. J. Urol., 114:285, 1975.

Shapiro, S. R., Lebowitz, R. L., and Colodny, A. H.: Fate of 90 children with ileal conduit urinary diversion a decade later: Analysis of complications, pyeloplasty, renal function and bacteriology. J. Urol., 114:289, 1975.

Sidi, A. A., Aliabadi, H., and Gonzalcz, R.: Encrocystoplasty in the management and reconstruction of the pediatric neurogenic bladder. J. Pediatr. Surg., 22:153, 1987.

Sidi, A. A., Dykstra, D. D., and Gonzalez, R.: The value of urodynamic testing in the management of neonates with myelodysplasia: A prospective study. J. Urol., 135:90, 1986.

Skinner, D. G., Lieskovsky, G., Boyd, S. D.: Construction of a continent ileal reservoir (Kock pouch) as an alternative to cutaneous urinary diversion: An update after 250 cases. J. Urol., 137:1140, 1987.

Smith, E. D.: Urinary prognosis in spina bifida. J. Urol., 108:115, 1972.

Spindel, M. R., Bauer, S. B., Dyro, F. M., Krarup, C., Khoshbin, S., Winston, K. R., Lebowitz, R. L., Colodny, A. H., and Retik, A. B.: The changing neuro-urologic lesion in myelodysplasia. JAMA, 258:1630, 1987.

Stark, G. D.: Spina bifida: Problems and management. Oxford, Blackwell Scientific Publications, 1977.

Stein, S. C., Feldman, J. G., Freidlander, M., et al.: Is myelomeningocele a disappearing disease? Pediatrics, 69:511, 1982.

Steinhardt, G. F., Goodgold, H. M., and Samuels, L. D.: The effect of intravesical pressure on glomerular filtration rates in patients with myelmeningocele. J. Urol., 140:1293, 1986.

Torrens, M., and Abrams, P.: Cystometry. Urol. Clin. North Am., 6:79, 1979.

Tutrone, R. F., Bauer, S. B., Peters, C. A., Mandell, J., Colodny, A. H., and Retik, A. B.: Physiologic basis for continence in the Mitrofanoff principle. Presented at the Annual Meeting of the American Urological Association. Toronto, June 3, 1991.

VanGool, J. D., Kuijten, R. H., Donckerwolcke, R. A., and Kramer, P. P.: Detrusor-sphincter dyssynergia in children with myelomeningocele: A prospective study. Z. Kinderchir., 37:148, 1982.

Venes, J. L., and Stevens, S. A.: Surgical pathology in tethered cord secondary to meningomyelocele repair. Concepts Pediatr. Neurosurg., 4:165, 1983.

Woodard, J. R., Anderson, A. M., and Parrott, T. S.: Ureteral reimplantation in myelodysplastic children. J. Urol., 126:387, 1981.

Woodhouse, C. R. J., Malone, P. R., Cumming, J., Reilly, T. M.: The Mitrofanoff principle for continent urinary diversion. Br. J. Urol., 63:53, 1989.

Woodside, J. R., and McGuire, E. J.: Techniques for detection of detrusor hypertonia in the presence of urethral sphincter incompetence. J. Urol., 127:740, 1982.

Young, H. H.: An operation for the cure of incontinence of urine. Surg. Gynecol. Obstet., 28:84, 1919.

Lipomeningocele and Other Spinal Dysraphisms

Anderson, F. M.: Occult spinal dysraphism: A series of 73 cases. Pediatrics, 55:826, 1975.

Barson, A. J.: The vertebral level of termination of the spinal cord during normal and abnormal development. J. Anat., 106:489, 1970.

Campobasso, P., Galiani, E., Verzerio, A., Spata, F., Cimaglia, M.

L., and Belloli, G.: A rare cause of occult neuropathic bladder in children: The tethered cord syndrome. Pediatr. Med. Chir., 10:641, 1988.

Dubrowitz, V., Lorber, J., and Zachary, R. B.: Lipoma of the cauda equina. Arch. Dis. Child., 40:207, 1965.

Flanigan, R. F., Russell, D. P., and Walsh, J. W.: Urologic aspects of tethered cord. Urology, 33:80, 1989.

Foster, L. S., Kogan, B. A., Cogan, P. H., and Edwards, M. S. B.: Bladder function in patients with lipomyelomeningocele. J. Urol., 143:984, 1990.

Hall, W. A., Albright, A. L., and Brunberg, J. A.: Diagnosis of tethered cord by magnetic resonance imaging. Surg. Neurol., 30(Suppl. 1):60, 1988.

Hellstrom, W. J., Edwards, M. S., and Kogan, B. A.: Urologic aspects of the tethered cord syndrome. J. Urol., 135:317, 1986.

James, C. M., and Lassman, L. P.: Spinal dysraphism: Spina bifida occulta. New York, Appleton-Century-Krofts, 1972.

Kaplan, W. E., McLone, D. G., and Richards, I.: The urologic manifestations of the tethered spinal cord. J. Urol., 140:1285, 1988.

Keating, M. A., Rink, R. C., Bauer, S. B., Krarup, C., Dyro, F. M., Winston, K. R., Shillito, J., Fischer, E. G., Retik, A. B.: Neuro-urologic implications of changing approach in management of occult spinal lesions. J. Urol., 140:1299, 1988.

Khoury, A. E., Hendrick, E. B., McLorie, G. A., Kulkarni, A., Churchill, B. M.: Occult spinal dysraphism: Clinical and urodynamic outcome after diversion of the filum terminale. J. Urol., 144:426, 1990.

Kondo, A., Kato, K., Kanai, S., and Sakakibara, T.: Bladder dysfunction secondary to tethered cord syndrome in adults: Is it curable? J. Urol., 135:313, 1986.

Linder, M., Rosenstein, J., and Sklar, F. H.: Functional improvement after spinal surgery for the dysraphic malformations. Neurosurgery, 11:622, 1982.

Mandell, J., Bauer, S. B., Hallett, M., Khoshbin, S., Dyro, F. M., Colodny, A. H., and Retik, A. B.: Occult spinal dysraphism: A rare but detectable cause of voiding dysfunction. Urol. Clin. North Am., 7:349, 1980.

Packer, R. J., Zimmerman, R. A., Sutton, L. N., Bilaniuk, L. T., Bruce, D. A., and Schut, L.: Magnetic resonance imaging of spinal cord diseases of childhood. Pediatrics, 78:251, 1986.

Raghavendra, B. N., Epstein, F. J., Pinto, R. S., Subramanyam, B. R., Greenberg, J., and Mitnick, J. S.: The tethered spinal cord: Diagnosis by high-resolution real-time ultrasound. Radiology, 149:123, 1983.

Roy, M. W., Gilmore, R., and Walsh, J. W.: Evaluation of children and young adults with tethered spinal cord syndrome: Utility of spinal and scalp recorded somatosensory evoked potentials. Surg. Neurol., 26:241, 1986.

Scheible, W., James, H. E., Leopold, G. R., and Hilton, S. W.: Occult spinal dysraphism in infants: Screening with high-resolution real-time ultrasound. Radiology, 146:743, 1983.

Seeds, J. W., and Jones, F. D.: Lipomyelomeningocele: Prenatal diagnosis and management. Obstet. Gynecol., 67(Suppl.):34, 1986.

Tami, S., Yamada, S., and Knighton, R. S.: Extensibility of the lumbar and sacral cord: Pathophysiology of the tethered cord in cats. J. Neurosurg., 66:116, 1987.

Tracey, P. T., and Hanigan, W. C.: Spinal dysraphism: Use of magnetic resonance imaging in evaluation. Clin. Pediatr., 29:228, 1990.

Weissert, M., Gysler, R., Sorensen, N.: The clinical problem of the tethered cord syndrome: A report of 3 personal cases. Z. Kinderchir., 44:275, 1989.

Yamada, S., Knierim, D., Yonekura, M., Schultz, R., and Meada, G.: Tethered cord syndrome. J. Am. Paraplegia Soc., 6(Suppl. 3):58, 1983.

Yamada, S., Zincke, D. E., and Sanders, D.: Pathophysiology of "tethered cord syndrome." J. Neurosurg., 54:494, 1981.

Yip, C. M., Leach, G. E., Rosenfeld, D. S., Zimmern, P., and Raz, S.: Delayed diagnosis of voiding dysfunction: Occult spinal dysraphism. J. Urol., 124:694, 1985.

Sacral Agenesis

Bauer, S. B.: Urodynamics in children. *In* Ashcraft, K. W. (Ed.): Pediatric Urology. Orlando, Grune & Stratton, Inc., 1990, pp. 49–76.

Guzman, L., Bauer, S. B., Hallett, M., et al.: The evaluation and management of children with sacral agenesis. Urology, 23:506, 1983.

Jakobson, H., Holm-Bentzen, M., and Hald, T.: Neurogenic bladder dysfunction in sacral agenesis and dysgenesis. Neurourol. Urodynam., 4:99, 1985.

Koff, S. A., and DeRidder, P. A.: Patterns of neurogenic bladder dysfunction in sacral agenesis. J. Urol., 118:87, 1977.

Landauer, W.: Rumplessness of chicken embryos produced by the injection of insulin and other chemicals. J. Exp. Zool., 98:65, 1945.

Menon, R. K., Cohen, R. M., Sperling, M. A., Cutfield, W. S., Mimoui, F., and Khoury, J. C.: Transplacental passage of insulin in pregnant women with insulin-dependent diabetes mellitus. N. Engl. J. Med., 323:309, 1990.

Passarge, E., and Lenz, K.: Syndrome of caudal regression in infants of diabetic mothers: Observations of further cases. Pediatrics, 37:672, 1966.

White, R. I., and Klauber, G. T.: Sacral agenesis: Analysis of twenty-two cases. Urology, 8:521, 1976.

Imperforate Anus

Barnes, P. D., Lester, P. D., Yamanashi, W. S., and Prince, J. R.: MRI in infants and children with spinal dysraphism. Am. J. Radiol., 147:339, 1986.

Barry, J. E., and Auldist, A. W.: The Vater syndrome. Am. J. Dis. Child., 128:769, 1974.

Carson, J. A., Barnes, P. D., Tunell, W. P., Smith, E. I., and Jolley, S. G.: Imperforate anus: The neurologic implication of sacral abnormalities. J. Pediatr. Surg., 19:838, 1984.

Greenfield, S. P., and Fera, M.: Urodynamic evaluation of the imperforate anus patient: A prospective study. Presented at the Annual Meeting of the American Academy of Pediatrics. Boston, October 6, 1990.

Karrer, F. M., Flannery, A. M., Nelson, M. D., Jr., McLone, D. G., and Raffensperger, J. G.: Anal rectal malformations: Evaluation of associated spinal dysraphic syndromes. J. Pediatr. Surg., 23:45, 1988.

Parrott, T., and Woodard, J.: Importance of cystourethrography in neonates with imperforate anus. Urology, 13:607, 1979.

Peña, A.: Posterior saggital approach for the correction of anal rectal malformations. Adv. Surg., 19:69, 1986.

Tunnell, W. P., Austin, J. C., Barnes, T. P., and Reynolds, A.: Neuroradiologic evaluation of sacral abnormalities in imperforate anus complex. J. Pediatr. Surg., 22:58, 1987.

Uehling, D. T., Gilbert, E., and Chesney, R.: Urologic implications of the VATER syndrome. J. Urol., 129:352, 1983.

Williams, D. I., and Grant, J.: Urologic complications of imperforate anus. Br. J. Urol., 41:660, 1969.

Central Nervous System Insults

Cerebral Palsy

Decter, R. M., Bauer, S. B., Khoshbin, S., Dyro, F. M., Krarup, C., Colodny, A. H., and Retik, A. B.: Urodynamic assessment of children with cerebral palsy. J. Urol., 138:1110, 1987.

McNeal, D. M., Hawtrey, C. E., Wolraich, M. L., and Mapel, J. R.: Symptomatic neurogenic bladder in a cerebral-palsied population. Dev. Med. Child Neurol., 25:612, 1983.

Naeye, R. L., Peters, E. C., Bartholomew, M., and Landis, R.: Origins of cerebral palsy. Am. J. Dis. Child., 143:1154, 1989.

Nelson, K. B., and Ellenberg, J. H.: Antecedents of cerebral palsy. N. Engl. J. Med., 315:81, 1986.

Traumatic Injuries to the Spine

Adams, C., Babyn, P. S., and Logan, W. J.: Spinal cord birth injury: Value of computed tomographic myelography. Pediatr. Neurol., 4:109, 1988.

Barkin, M., Dolfin, D., Herschorn, S., Bharatwal, N., and Comisarow, R.: The urologic care of the spinal cord injury patient. J. Urol., 129:335, 1983.

Cass, A. S., Luxenberg, M., Johnson, C. F., and Gleich, P.: Management of the neurogenic bladder in 413 children. J. Urol., 132:521, 1984.

Donnelly, J., Hackler, R. H., and Bunts, R. C.: Present urologic status of the World War II paraplegic: 25-year follow-up comparison

with status of the 20-year Korean War paraplegic and 5-year Vietnam paraplegic. J. Urol., 108:558, 1972.

Fanciullacci, F., Zanollo, A., Sandri, S., and Catanzaro, F.: The neuropathic bladder in children with spinal cord injury. Paraplegia, 26:83, 1988.

Guttmann, L., and Frankel, H.: The value of intermittent catheterization in the early management of traumatic paraplegia and tetraplegia. Paraplegia, 4:63, 1966.

Iwatsubo, E., Iwakawa, A., Koga, H., Imamura, A., Yamashita, H., and Komine, S.: Functional recovery of the bladder in patients with spinal cord injury—prognosticating programs of an aseptic intermittent catheterization. Acta Urol. Japonica, 31:775, 1985.

Lanska, M. J., Roessmann, U., and Wiznitzer, M.: Magnetic resonance imaging in cervical cord birth injury. Pediatrics, 85:760, 1990.

Ogawa, T., Yoshida, T., and Fujinaga, T.: Bladder deformity in traumatic spinal cord injury patients. Acta Urol. Japonica, 34:1173, 1988.

Pearman, J. W.: Urologic follow-up of 99 spinal cord injury patients initially managed by intermittent catheterization. Br. J. Urol., 48:297, 1976.

Pollack, I. F., Pang, D., and Sclabassi, R.: Recurrent spinal cord injury without radiographic abnormalities in children. J. Neurosurg., 69:177, 1988.

Functional Voiding Disorders

Bauer, S. B., Retik, A. B., Colodny, A. H., Hallett, M., Khoshbin, S., and Dyro, F. M.: The unstable bladder of childhood. Urol. Clin. North Am., 7:321, 1980.

Bellman, N.: Encopresis. Acta Paediatr. Scand., 70(Suppl. 1):1, 1966.

Fergusson, D. M., Hons, B. A., Horwood, L. J., and Shannon, F. T.: Factors related to the age of attainment of nocturnal bladder control: An eight year longitudinal study. Pediatrics, 78:884, 1986.

MacKeith, R. L., Meadow, S. R., and Turner, R. K.: How children become dry. In Kolvin, I., MacKeith, R. L., Meadow, S. R. (Eds.): Bladder Control and Enuresis. Philadelphia, J. B. Lippincott Co., 1973, pp. 3–15.

Yeats, W. K.: Bladder function in normal micturition. In Kolvin, I., MacKeith, R. C., Meadow, S. R. (Eds.): Bladder Control and Enuresis. Philadelphia, J. B. Lippincott Co., 1973, pp. 28–41.

Small-Capacity Hypertonic Bladder

Bauer, S. B., Retik, A. B., Colodny, A. H., Hallett, M., Khoshbin, S., and Dyro, F. M.: The unstable bladder of childhood. Urol. Clin. North Am., 7:321, 1980.

Dyro, F. M., Bauer, S. B., Hallett, M., and Khoshbin, S.: Complex repetitive discharges in the external urethral sphincter in a pediatric population. Neurourol. Urodynam., 2:39, 1983.

Hansson, S., Hjalmas, K., Jodal, U., and Sixt, R.: Lower urinary tract dysfunction in girls with untreated asymptomatic or covert bacteriuria. J. Urol., 143:333, 1990.

Lebowitz, R. L., and Mandell, J.: Urinary tract infection in children: Putting radiology in its place. Radiology, 165:1, 1987.

Mayo, M. E., and Burns, M. W.: Urodynamic studies in children who wet. Br. J. Urol., 65:641, 1990.

Rudy, D. C., and Woodside, J. R.: Non-neurogenic neurogenic bladder: The relationship between intravesical pressure and the external sphincter EMG. Neurourol. Urodynam., 10:169–176, 1991.

Saxton, H. M., Borzyskowski, M., Mundy, A. R., and Vivian, G. C.: Spinning top deformity: Not a normal variant. Radiology, 168:147, 1988.

Tanagho, E. A., Miller, E. A., and Lyon, R. P.: Spastic striated external sphincter and urinary tract infection in girls. Br. J. Urol., 43:69, 1971.

VanGool, J. D., and Tanagho, E. A.: External sphincter activity and recurrent urinary tract infection in girls. Urology, 10:348, 1977.

Webster, G. D., Koefoot, R. B., and Sihelnik, S.: Urodynamic abnormalities in neurologically normal children with micturition dysfunction. J. Urol., 132:74, 1984.

Hyperreflexic Bladder

Bauer, S. B., Retik, A. B., Colodny, A. H., Hallett, M., Khoshbin, S., and Dyro, F. M.: The unstable bladder of childhood. Urol. Clin. North Am., 7:321, 1980.

Buttarazzi, P. J.: Oxybutinin chloride (Ditropan) in enuresis. J. Urol., 118:46, 1977.

Firlit, C. F., Smey, P., and King, L. R.: Micturition: Urodynamic flow studies in children. J. Urol., 119:250, 1978.

Kass, E. J., Diokno, A. C., and Montealegre, A.: Enuresis: Principles of management and results of treatment. J. Urol., 121:794, 1979.

Koff, S. A., and Murtagh, D. S.: The uninhibited bladder in children: Effect of treatment on recurrence of urinary infection and vesico-ureteral reflux. J. Urol., 130:1158, 1983.

Kondo, A., Kobayashi, M., Otani, T., Takita, T., and Mitsuya, H.: Children with unstable bladder: Clinical and urodynamic observation. J. Urol., 129:88, 1983.

MacKeith, R. L., Meadow, S. R., and Turner, R. K.: How children become dry. *In* Kolvin, I., MacKeith, R. L., Meadow, S. R. (Eds.): Bladder Control and Enuresis. Philadelphia, J. B. Lippincott Co., 1973, pp. 3–15.

Mayo, M. E., and Burns, M. W.: Urodynamic studies in children who wet. Br. J. Urol., 65:641, 1990.

McGuire, E. J., and Savastano, J. A.: Urodynamic studies in enuresis and non-neurogenic bladder. J. Urol., 132:299, 1984.

Mueller, S. R.: Development of urinary control in children. JAMA, 172:1256, 1960.

O'Regan, S., Yazbeck, S., Hamburger, B., and Schick, E.: Constipation: A commonly unrecognized cause of enuresis. Am. J. Dis. Child., 140:260, 1986.

O'Regan, S., Yazbeck, S., and Schick, E.: Constipation, unstable bladder, urinary tract infection syndrome. Clin. Nephrol., 5:154, 1985.

Rudy, D. C., and Woodside, J. R.: Non-neurogenic neurogenic bladder: The relationship between intravesical pressure and the external sphincter EMG. Neurourol. Urodynam., 10:169–176, 1991.

Torrens, M. J., and Collins, C. D.: The urodynamic assessment of adult enuresis. Br. J. Urol., 47:433, 1975.

Vincent, S. A.: Postural control of urinary incontinence: The curtsy sign. Lancet, 2:631, 1966.

Webster, G. D., Koefoot, R. B., and Sihelnik, S.: Urodynamic abnormalities in neurologically normal children with micturition dysfunction. J. Urol., 132:74, 1984.

Yeats, W. K.: Bladder function in normal micturition. *In* Kolvin, I., MacKeith, R. C., and Meadow, S. R. (Eds.): Bladder Control and Enuresis. Philadelphia, J. B. Lippincott Co., 1973, pp. 28–41.

The Infrequent Voider—Lazy Bladder Syndrome

Bauer, S. B., Retik, A. B., Colodny, A. H., Hallett, M., Khoshbin, S., and Dyro, F. M.: The unstable bladder of childhood. Urol. Clin. North Am., 7:321, 1980.

DeLuca, F. G., Swenson, O., Fisher, J. H., and Loutfi, A. H.: The dysfunctional "lazy" bladder syndrome in children. Arch. Dis. Child., 37:117, 1962.

Koefoot, R. B., Webster, G. D., Anderson, E. E., and Glenn, J. F.: The primary megacystis syndrome. J. Urol., 125:232, 1981.

Masek, B. J.: Behavioral management of voiding dysfunction in neurologically normal children. Dialog. Pediatr. Urol., 8:7, 1985.

Webster, G. D., Koefoot, R. B., and Sihelnik, S.: Urodynamic abnormalities in neurologically normal children with micturition dysfunction. J. Urol., 132:74, 1984.

Psychologic Non-Neuropathic Bladder (Hinman Syndrome)

Allen, T. D.: The non-neurogenic bladder. J. Urol., 117:232, 1977.

Allen, T. D., and Bright, T. C.: Urodynamic patterns in children with dysfunctional voiding problems. J. Urol., 119:247, 1978.

Bauer, S. B., Retik, A. B., Colodny, A. H., Hallett, M., Khoshbin, S., and Dyro, F. M.: The unstable bladder of childhood. Urol. Clin. North Am., 7:321, 1980.

Hinman, F.: Urinary tract damage in children who wet. Pediatrics, 54:142, 1974.

Hinman, F.: Non-neurogenic bladder (the Hinman Syndrome) fifteen years later. J. Urol., 136:769, 1986.

Johnston, J. H., and Farkas, A.: Congenital neuropathic bladder: Practicalities and possibilities of conservational management. Urology, 5:719, 1975.

Kass, E. J., Diokno, A. C., and Montealegre, A.: Enuresis: Principles of management and results of treatment. J. Urol., 121:794, 1979.

Masek, B. J.: Behavioral management of voiding dysfunction in neurologically normal children. Dialog. Pediatr. Urol., 8:7, 1985.

McGuire, E. J., and Savastano, J. A.: Urodynamic studies in enuresis and non-neurogenic bladder. J. Urol., 132:299, 1984.

Mix, L. W.: Occult neuropathic bladder. Urology, 10:1, 1977.

Rudy, D. C., and Woodside, J. R.: Non-neurogenic neurogenic bladder: Its relationship between intravesical pressure and the external sphincter EMG. Neurol. Urodynam., 10:169–176, 1991.

Snyder, H. McC., Caldamone, A. A., Wein, A. J., and Duckett, J. W., Jr.: The Hinman syndrome—alternatives for treatment. Presented at the Annual Meeting of the American Urological Association. Kansas City, May 16, 1982.

Williams, D. I., Hirst, G., and Doyle, D.: The occult neuropathic bladder. J. Pediatr. Surg., 9:35, 1975.

43
URINARY TRACT INFECTIONS IN INFANTS AND CHILDREN

Linda M. Dairiki Shortliffe, M.D.

CHILDHOOD URINARY TRACT INFECTIONS

Urinary tract infections are not uncommon in children or adults, yet their evaluation and management may differ widely depending on age, because urinary infections in children seem to be more likely to damage the kidney than those in adults (Hodson, 1965). In children, the goal of managing urinary tract infections is prevention of renal damage. To achieve this, the mechanisms by which bacteria gain access to and damage the kidney and the identification of children who may be at risk for renal damage need to be understood. During the last decade, research has started to clarify these areas. The importance of identifying short- and long-term complications of renal infection, such as hypertension, recurrent infections, and progressive renal dysfunction, has, furthermore, been recognized. This chapter focuses on host and bacterial factors responsible for causing bacteriuria and initial and progressive renal damage in children and the means needed to prevent this damage.

Diagnosis

In infants younger than 1 year, urinary tract infections may be difficult to diagnose. The symptoms may be generalized: elevated temperature, irritability, poor feeding, vomiting and diarrhea, and ill appearance (Ginsburg and McCracken, 1982) (Table 43–1). Older children, also, may show few signs referable to the urinary tract when they have urinary infections. Other symptoms, such as intermittent voiding dysfunction, dysuria, suprapubic pain, or incontinence, may be vague. For this reason, one needs to be suspicious of a urinary infection in any ill child without localizing signs or a child with symptoms only vaguely referable to the urinary tract. A urinary specimen should be obtained.

Urinalysis and Urinary Culture

The diagnosis of urinary infection is usually made from urinalysis and culture findings. These specimens may be difficult to obtain in young children. In a child, urinary specimens may be obtained by attachment of a plastic bag to the perineum— a "bagged specimen," midstream void, catheterization, or suprapubic aspiration of the bladder. Even after extensive cleaning of the skin, a plastic bag specimen usually reflects the perineal and rectal flora and is useful only if a few or no organisms grow. Although a midstream-voided specimen in a circumcised boy, older girl, or older, uncircumcised boy who can retract his foreskin may reliably reflect bacteriuria, such specimens obtained in young girls and young uncircumcised boys usually reflect periurethral and preputial organisms. A catheterized specimen is reliable if the first portion of urine, which may contain urethral organisms, is discarded, and the specimen is taken from later flow through the catheter; however, this technique has the disadvantages of being traumatic and potentially introducing urethral organisms into a sterile bladder.

The most reliable specimen is obtained by suprapubic

Table 43–1. SYMPTOMS OF URINARY TRACT INFECTION IN 100 INFANTS WITH ACUTE URINARY TRACT INFECTIONS

Symptom	Percentage (%)
Fever	67
≥38° C	100
≥39° C	57
Irritable	55
Poor feeding	38
Vomiting	36
Diarrhea	31
Abdominal distention	8
Jaundice	7

Adapted from Ginsburg, C. M., and McCracken, G. H., Jr.: Urinary tract infections in young infants. Pediatrics, 69(4):409–412, 1982. Reproduced by permission of Pediatrics.

bladder aspiration. This technique can be performed in a child with a full bladder by introducing a 21- or 22-gauge needle 1 to 2 cm above the pubic symphysis until urine is obtained by aspiration into a sterile syringe. Because the urine does not cross the urethra, urethral or periurethral organisms are absent. Organisms present in a suprapubic aspirate are pathognomonic of bacteriuria. The main drawback of suprapubic aspiration is that the needle may be frightening to older children or their parents.

Detection of Bacteria

The exact number of organisms that causes a "significant" urinary infection is unknown. Although greater than or equal to 100,000 colony-forming units/ml of voided urine has been used to define a clinically significant urinary infection (Kass and Finland, 1956), other studies have shown that fewer organisms may cause a significant infection (Bollgren et al., 1984; Stamm et al., 1982). A lower number of organisms may be due to urinary dilution of bacteria by increased hydration and frequent voiding, preventing bacterial multiplication within the bladder.

Because organisms from urinary cultures may take 24 to 48 hours to grow, and urinalyses may be misleading, more rapid tests to detect the presence of bacteria have been examined. These tests vary in reliability depending on the number and types of bacteria present. When a urinary culture showing greater than or equal to 100,000 bacteria/ml is used to define an infection, other more rapid but less specific tests, such as urinary nitrite, have been utilized to diagnose infection (Hallender et al., 1986; Powell et al., 1987). Employing this definition of infection, one study demonstrated (Hallender et al., 1986) that, 93 per cent of the time, bacteria were seen in a spun high-power microscopic field; 92 per cent of the time, the nitrite test findings were positive [this correlation was lower in other studies (Powell et al., 1987)]; and 87 per cent of the time, leukocytes were seen in spun high-power microscopic fields. When the bacterial count is lower than 100,000 organisms/ml, these tests are even less reliable for detecting bacteriuria.

Classification of Urinary Infections

Many systems of classifying urinary tract infections, such as complicated versus uncomplicated, upper tract versus lower tract, and persistent infections versus reinfections, have been described. For practical purposes, urinary infections may be categorized based on the source of infection (Stamey, 1975): (1) first infections, (2) unresolved bacteriuria during therapy, (3) bacterial persistence at an anatomic site, and (4) reinfections. In children, all first urinary tract infections are "complicated" because children require radiologic evaluation to look for anatomic anomalies.

A urinary infection may remain unresolved because of inadequate therapy, bacterial resistance to the therapeutic agent selected, inadequate urinary concentration of the drug due to poor renal concentration or gastrointestinal malabsorption, or a multiple organism infection. Unresolved infections can usually be treated successfully with appropriate antimicrobial agents after proper culture and antimicrobial sensitivity studies have been done. Because radiologic studies are obtained early in the evaluation of children with infections, sources of bacterial persistence, such as poor functioning duplicated renal segments, infection stones, papillary necrosis, urethral diverticula, and areas of obstruction, are detected and may be surgically corrected (Table 43–2). The majority of infections are, however, reinfections with the same or a different organism.

Incidence of Bacteriuria

Childhood urinary tract infections are more common in girls than in boys at all ages except the first few months of life (Asscher, 1975; Winberg et al., 1974). Although the reasons are not entirely known, the prepuce may be involved. In a study screening infants for urinary tract infections during the first year of life, 2.7 per cent of boys and 0.7 per cent of girls were found to have bacteriuria (Wettergren et al., 1980). The incidence of infections was highest during the first few months and afterwards decreased to less than 1 per cent in boys (ranging between 0.03 and 1.2 per cent during the school years) while rising to 1 to 3 per cent during these years in girls (Asscher, 1975; Bailey, 1979a; Savage, 1975).

Bacterial Factors

Most organisms that infect the urinary tract are gram-negative Enterobacteriaceae; of these, *Escherichia coli* are the most common (Bergström, 1972; Kunin et al., 1964; Winberg et al., 1974). During the past 20 years, various bacterial traits that may cause virulence for the urinary tract have been explored. Particular bacterial cell wall O-antigens, identified by serotyping (e.g., 01, 02, 04, 06, 07, and 075), have been associated with urinary tract infections in children (Kunin et al., 1964; Winberg et al., 1974).

The contribution of bacterial fimbriae to urinary tract virulence has been clarified during the past decade. Several investigators demonstrated that bacterial adherence and agglutination are mediated by bacterial fimbriae or pili and that these fimbriae can be classified by their characteristic agglutination of red blood cells. This

Table 43–2. SURGICALLY CORRECTABLE CAUSES OF BACTERIAL PERSISTENCE IN CHILDREN

Infection stones
Infected nonfunctioning or poorly functioning kidneys or renal segments
Infected ureteral stumps following nephrectomy
Vesicointestinal or urethrorectal fistula
Vesicovaginal fistula
Infected necrotic papillae in papillary necrosis
Unilateral medullary sponge kidney
Infected urachal cyst
Infected urethral diverticulum or periurethral gland

hemagglutination can be blocked by different sugars (Duguid et al., 1978; Svanborg Edén and Hanson, 1978). Källenius and associates (1981) recognized that the *E. coli* commonly causing pyelonephritis in children also seemed to cause mannose-resistant hemagglutination (MRHA) of human red blood cells. This work led to the finding that the terminal glycolipid of the P blood group antigen on the human red blood cell is a receptor for binding the P-fimbriae on *E. coli* that commonly cause pyelonephritis.

In 1981, Väisänen and associates and Källenius and co-workers (1981) reported that the two best markers for virulence in pyelonephritogenic *E. coli* were MRHA characteristics and P blood group–specific adhesins (P-fimbriae or P-pili). Of 32 strains isolated from childhood pyelonephritic episodes, 91 per cent (29/32) had MRHA and 81 per cent had P-fimbriae (Väisänen et al., 1981). Källenius and associates (1981) then examined *E. coli* that had caused urinary tract infections in 97 different children and *E. coli* that were isolated from the feces of 82 healthy controls. They found P-fimbriae on 94 per cent (33/35) of *E. coli* causing acute pyelonephritis; 19 per cent (5/26), causing acute cystitis; 14 per cent (5/36), causing asymptomatic bacteriuria; and 7 per cent (6/82), from the feces of healthy children.

The characteristic of increased adherence is also associated with the acute ureteral dilation noted to accompany some episodes of acute pyelonephritis in children without obstruction or reflux (Måarild et al., 1989). Although less well characterized, hydrophobic properties of *E. coli* and Aerobactin production (associated with an iron-binding capability of the bacteria) may also relate to urinary tract virulence (Jacobson et al., 1988; Jacobson et al., 1989).

Host Factors

Host factors causing susceptibility to urinary tract infections have also been examined (Table 43–3). From epidemiologic data, it is known that, during the first few weeks of life, all babies have an increased incidence of urinary tract infections. During this time, the periurethral area of healthy girls and boys is massively colonized with aerobic bacteria, especially *E. coli*, enterococci, and staphylococci (Bollgren and Winberg, 1976a). This colonization decreases during the first year and is unusual in children who do not get recurrent infections after age 5. After this period, only those women and children who suffer repeated urinary tract infections routinely remain more colonized by periurethral gram-negative bacteria than those who do not get infections (Bollgren

Table 43–3. HOST FACTORS AFFECTING BACTERIURIA

Age
Immune status
Availability of receptors (blood group antigens)
Vesicoureteral reflux
Genitourinary anomalies
Sex
Fecal colonization

and Winberg, 1976a; Bollgren and Winberg, 1976b; Stamey and Sexton, 1975). Increased periurethral colonization has, therefore, been associated with increased risk of infection.

The factors causing increased colonization were unclear until bacterial adherence was recognized to be related to colonization. When bacterial P-fimbriae were identified as a virulence factor, it was realized that glycolipids characterizing the P blood group system are found on host uroepithelial cells and may serve as bacterial receptors. Because hosts with many of these receptors (i.e., P blood group phenotype) might have special susceptibility for infection, children with recurrent infections were examined for the P blood group phenotype (Lomberg et al., 1983). Whereas the P_1 blood group phenotype was found in 97 per cent (35/36) of girls with recurrent pyelonephritis with minimal (grade 1) or no reflux, it was found in only 75 per cent (63/84) of controls without infections. Of girls with pyelonephritis and reflux (grades 2 to 5), 84 per cent (27/32) had the P_1 blood group phenotype; this is not significantly different from the incidence in individuals without infection. The investigators found, moreover, that bacteria binding to glycolipid receptors (bacteria with P-fimbriae) were more likely to be found in girls with the P_1 blood group who were without reflux than those with the P_1 blood group who had reflux, further suggesting that host vesicoureteral reflux contributes more to getting bacteria into the kidney than virulence related to fimbriae; whereas, in children with minimal or no reflux, P-fimbriae and blood group antigens may be the major contributing factors.

Other blood group antigens on the urothelial surface (ABO, Lewis, and secretor phenotypes) also appear to influence susceptibility to urinary tract infections. Women with Le(a−b−) and Le(a+b−) blood phenotypes have a three times greater risk of recurrent urinary infections than women with Le(a−b+) phenotype, and epithelial cells from nonsecretors have more bacterial receptors than cells from secretors (Sheinfeld et al., 1989).

In a group of 72 children with various anatomic abnormalities (ureteropelvic junction obstruction, vesicoureteral reflux, ureteroceles, and primary obstructive megaureters), immunohistochemical analysis to characterize H, A, B, Le^a, and Le^b antigens was performed (Sheinfeld et al., 1990). These data suggest that children with anatomic abnormalities and presumed nonsecretor phenotype (minimal or undetectable ABO and Le^b immunoreactivity) are more likely to have a history of urinary infections (16/17, 94.1 per cent) than secretors (16/30, 53.3 per cent), whose tissue had intense ABO and Le^b staining. In children without a history of urinary infections, 23 of 24 (95.8 per cent) were secretors and had intense ABO and/or Le^b immunoreactivity. In summary, nonsecretor status may allow structures that serve as bacterial receptors to be more available for binding and result in greater susceptibility to urinary infections.

Age also seems to affect the incidence of bacteriuria. The incidence of bacteriuria for both boys and girls younger than the age of 1 is higher than at other times during childhood. The causes for this age-dependent relationship are unknown, but the immune status may contribute. Serum levels of IgG are lowest between ages 1 and 3 months (Robbins, 1972) when periurethral colonization is high in normal children. Secretory IgA, moreover, is an important human immunoglobulin at the secretory and mucosal surface and may be transferred to the newborn in colostrum if the child is breast fed. Serum IgA is found in diminished concentrations for the first several months and is either absent or almost absent at the secretory surfaces of the nasopharynx, gut, and urothelium during this time (Fliedner et al., 1986; Svanborg Edén et al., 1985; Yoder and Polin, 1986). Furthermore, even when IgA levels in the urine of infants and children with acute pyelonephritis are comparatively elevated, these levels are far below those found in adults.

The IgA from the urine of infants, moreover, occurs in the monomeric rather than the secretory form normally found in adults, thus suggesting that urinary IgA in infants results from systemic immunoglobulin that reaches the urine because of tubular damage during infection rather than by secretion (Svanborg Edén et al., 1985). Children with recurrent urinary tract infections are also reported to have lower urinary concentrations of secretory IgA than children without infections (Fliedner et al., 1986).

Lower Versus Upper Tract Infections

Efforts to differentiate cystitis and pyelonephritis by either clinical symptoms or simple noninvasive tests have been unsuccessful. Clinical symptoms alone are not reliable markers of upper versus lower tract infections. In 1984, Busch and Huland localized urinary tract infections to upper or lower tract infections using the Fairley technique and found that clinical symptoms were poor predictors of whether a urinary tract infection was confined to the bladder or involved the kidney. When patients (the majority of whom were children) had a urinary tract infection characterized by flank pain and fever, it was found that only 46.6 per cent (34/73) of infection localized to the upper tracts with the remainder localized to the bladder. In comparison, when the patient had bladder symptoms and/or enuresis, 15.1 per cent (27/179) still had supravesical localization of bacteria; moreover, 17.5 per cent (83/473) of episodes of asymptomatic bacteriuria also localized to the upper tracts. This poor correlation between severity of symptoms and site of bacteriuria implies that diagnosis based on clinical symptoms alone is inadequate.

Invasive tests may determine when bacteria involve either the lower or upper urinary tract. The standard means of differentiating between the two is the technique described by Stamey and associates (Stamey, 1980; Stamey and Pfau, 1963), which obtains upper tract urinary specimens by bilateral ureteral catheterization. Through this technique, the source of bacteria can be determined to be renal pelvis or bladder; however, this does not necessarily imply that an upper tract localization of bacteria is always associated with renal inflammation and acute pyelonephritis. When risk factors have been sought to identify children likely to have treatable

urologic problems, only fever (>38°C rectal or >37°C oral) in 10 of 24 children (41.7 per cent) could be correlated (Johnson et al., 1985). Other single tests diagnosing renal infection through radionuclide scans, radiographic studies, erythrocyte sedimentation rates, C-reactive protein, urinary concentrating ability, urinary tubular enzymes, antibody-coated bacteria, and urinary antibodies, have also not proven to be totally reliable in differentiating upper and lower tract infection.

In spite of the inadequacies of diagnosing pyelonephritis on the basis of clinical symptoms and signs alone, this is probably the most common means of diagnosis for management. When bacteria enter the upper urinary collecting system and cause inflammation of the renal pelvis and kidney, this is defined as pyelonephritis. In the child, the diagnosis is usually made clinically, but as discussed previously, the clinical symptoms may not necessarily reflect upper tract bacteria. Most of the time, however, fever and abdominal or flank pain accompanied by dysuria, frequency, and urgency are employed to characterize clinical acute pyelonephritis. The urinary sediment usually shows increased white and sometimes red blood cells, white blood cell casts, rods, or chains of cocci. The urine culture grows bacteria.

The term chronic pyelonephritis has been used to refer to a variety of renal findings, including focal coarse renal scarring, reflux nephropathy, chronic atrophic pyelonephritis, and interstitial nephritis. Most often, it is diagnosed radiographically in a scarred, shrunken kidney with pathologic, histologic evidence of chronic inflammation. No signs of active bacterial infection may be evident.

Primary Vesicoureteral Reflux

Vesicoureteral reflux allows bladder urine to pass retrograde into the ureter and renal pelvis and calyces and does not occur in most healthy children. This reflux probably occurs because of a more lateral position of the vesicoureteral orifice (Stephens, 1977) and may be affected by immature bladder dynamics (Koff et al., 1979). Reflux may be graded by severity and has been separated into five categories according to the International Reflux Study, from minimal ureteral reflux alone (grade 1) to gross pyelocalyceal reflux with major distortion and dilation of the collecting system, and loss of the papillary impression (grade 5) (Fig. 43–1). When bacteriuria occurs, reflux allows bladder bacteria rapid ureteral and renal access.

In the asymptomatic pediatric population, the incidence of primary congenital vesicoureteral reflux is 0.4 to 1.8 per cent (Bailey, 1979b); the incidence correlates inversely with age—that is, the younger the child, the higher the incidence of reflux. When Kollerman and Ludwig (1984) examined the incidence of reflux in 102 children without urinary infections, they found that greater than 60 per cent of children younger than 6 months experienced reflux, whereas almost none older than 5 years did. This study has been criticized because cystograms were performed with high-pressure injection, and this is the only study to show such high rates

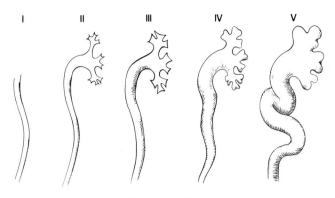

I   II   III   IV   V

GRADES OF REFLUX

Figure 43–1. International Reflux Study Classification of grades of vesicoureteral reflux. Grade I, into the ureter only; Grade II, into the ureter, renal pelvis, and calices; Grade III, mild or moderate dilation of the ureter and renal pelvis with no or minimal forniceal blunting; Grade IV, moderate dilation and tortuosity of ureter and pelvis with blunting of the fornices but maintenance of the papillary impressions; Grade V, gross dilation and tortuosity of the ureter and pelvis with absence of the papillary impressions. (From Report of the International Reflux Study Committee: Medical versus surgical treatment of primary vesicoureteral reflux: a prospective international reflux study in children. J. Urol. 125:277–283, 1981.)

of reflux in normal children. However, this study is still important because it demonstrates the correlation with age and the tendency for the ureterovesical junction to decompensate under high pressures, permitting reflux.

Roberts (1978) has shown similarly that primary vesicoureteral reflux in young primates tends to resolve spontaneously with time even if there are intervening urinary tract infections. Similarly, in children, the vesicoureteral reflux may disappear spontaneously with time depending on its extent and severity (Edwards et al., 1977; Lenaghan and Cussen, 1968; Lenaghan et al., 1976; Roberts, 1978). Whether this disappearance is related to an anatomic change with bladder maturation or is related to bladder dynamics alone is unclear.

Although the finding of vesicoureteral reflux in normal asymptomatic children is rare, it is commonly found in children who have had a urinary tract infection. Epidemiologic surveys have shown that 21 to 57 per cent of children who have had bacteriuria are subsequently found to have vesicoureteral reflux (Abbott, 1972; Asscher et al., 1973; Kunin et al., 1964; Newcastle Asymptomatic Bacteriuria Research Group, 1975). This reflux may also resolve spontaneously (Bellinger and Duckett, 1984; Skoog et al., 1987). One study found that when urinary infections are prevented, 87 per cent of grade 1, 63 per cent of grade 2, 53 per cent of grade 3, and 33 per cent of grade 4 vesicoureteral reflux resolved spontaneously over about 3 years (Bellinger and Duckett, 1984). Others have estimated that the rate of spontaneous resolution in patients who experience resolution of reflux is about 30 to 35 per cent each year (Skoog et al., 1987) (Fig. 43–2). The finding of bacteriuria in a child, therefore, serves as a marker for a possible genitourinary anatomic abnormality requiring treatment as well as further radiologic evaluation.

When symptomatic and asymptomatic siblings of children with vesicoureteral reflux have been screened for reflux, 8 to 45 per cent have been identified to have

reflux, 8 to 45 per cent have been identified to have reflux (Van den Abbeele et al., 1987). Although these data show that reflux has a familial association, the genetics are unknown. This high familial incidence found in some of these studies has led some investigators to recommend screening even asymptomatic siblings of children with reflux who are younger than 10 years with a nuclear voiding cystourethrogram (Lebowitz, 1986; Van den Abbeele et al., 1987).

Uninhibited Bladder and Vesicoureteral Reflux

Although abnormal bladder dynamics have been cited as a source of acquired vesicoureteral reflux for some time (Hutch, 1952), the concept that bladder dynamics in the neurologically "normal" child may be involved in persistent reflux and urinary tract infections has only been documented more currently (Homsy et al., 1985; Koff et al., 1979; Koff and Murtagh, 1983; Koff and Murtagh, 1984).

In 1979, Koff and associates hypothesized that increased intravesical pressure resulting from voluntary urethral sphincteric contraction during involuntary uninhibited bladder contraction may contribute to the initiation or persistence of vesicoureteral reflux in children. In 1983, Koff and Murtagh identified 62 neurologically normal children with vesicoureteral reflux (mainly grades 2 to 4) and treated 26 patients (43 refluxing ureters) with uninhibited bladder contractions and voluntary sphincteric contractions with anticholinergic agents; no medications were given to eight patients (12 refluxing ureters) with uninhibited bladder contractions

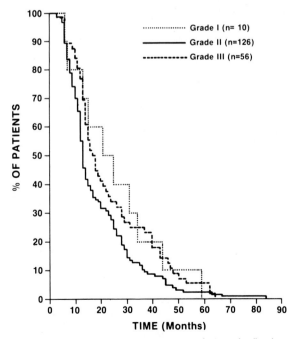

Figure 43–2. Time course to spontaneous resolution of reflux by grade of reflux (n, number of patients). The majority of those who experienced resolution of reflux had a resolution rate of 30 to 35 per cent per year of observation. (From Skoog, S. J., Belman, A. B., and Majd, M.: A nonsurgical approach to the management of primary vesicoureteral reflux. J. Urol., 138:941–946, 1987.)

and 28 patients (47 refluxing ureters) with normal uro-dynamic studies.

After an average of 3.9 years of follow-up, these investigators found that reflux resolved in 44 per cent of ureters treated with anticholinergics regardless of reflux severity. Reflux resolved in 33 per cent of refluxing ureters associated with uninhibited contractions without anticholinergic medication, whereas only 17 per cent of those ureters in bladders with normal urodynamics untreated by anticholinergics ceased refluxing. The increased reflux resolution of ureters treated with anticholinergic agents over that of ureters in urodynamically normal bladders is statistically significant.

In addition, fewer children treated with prophylactic antimicrobial agents and anticholinergics had a breakthrough infection than those treated with prophylactic agents alone. Because uninhibited bladder contractions have been found in many young children with recurrent urinary tract infections, and these contractions may be responsible for perpetuating vesicoureteral reflux, bladder dynamics may be an important consideration in the treatment of children with vesicoureteral reflux.

COMPLICATIONS OF URINARY TRACT INFECTIONS

Reflux Nephropathy

Most focal renal scarring in children is related to a combination of vesicoureteral reflux and bacteriuria. This kind of scarring, to differentiate it from renal scarring caused by other injuries, has been termed *reflux nephropathy* and occurs in varying degrees of severity (Fig. 43–3). In general, the greater the degree of reflux, the higher the incidence of renal scarring and associated impaired renal growth (Filly et al., 1974; Smellie et al., 1981). Without infections, no association between the severity of vesicoureteral reflux and impaired renal growth has been demonstrated in an otherwise normal urinary tract (Smellie et al., 1981).

The coarse renal scarring associated with reflux nephropathy may be detected radiologically by calyceal deformity and renal parenchymal thinning over localized or multiple calyces. The small, shrunken, irregular kidney represents the end stage of severe vesicoureteral reflux and infections.

The radiologic appearance of these small kidneys may, however, be confused with congenitally small, dysplastic, poorly functioning or nonfunctioning kidneys. This distinction—one that is difficult and sometimes impossible to make radiologically—is important because dysplastic kidneys are histologically abnormal congenitally and are not the result of urinary infections after birth even though they may be associated with such infections. Although these gross renal changes may be detected radiologically, lesser lesions that may be related to infectious insult, such as cortical pitting and mild global renal shrinkage, will not be detected by radiologic tests, and yet may affect renal function. Evidence suggests that even acute pyelonephritis is associated with tubular defects, such as reduced urinary concentrating ability, and these functional renal defects are more severe when associated with renal parenchymal damage and reflux (Walker, 1990).

Approximately 17 per cent of children who are bacteriuric on screening urine cultures have renal scarring (Asscher et al., 1973; Newcastle Asymptomatic Bacteriuria Research Group, 1975; Savage, 1975). Children with asymptomatic urinary tract infections, thus, are as likely to experience damage to their kidneys as are children with symptomatic infections. Winberg and colleagues (1974) have documented, moreover, that renal scarring will increase with subsequent symptomatic urinary infections. They found that, after the symptoms of a first urinary tract infection, 4.5 per cent of children have radiologic renal scars, and after the second symptomatic infection, 17 per cent have scars.

If children with renal scarring are then evaluated for radiologic evidence of vesicoureteral reflux, 60 per cent still have it (Asscher et al., 1973; Newcastle Asymptomatic Bacteriuria Research Group, 1975; Savage, 1975). The majority of renal scars are found on the first radiologic evaluation of children with urinary tract infections; it is hypothesized that these scars result from early urinary infections in the neonate or child younger than 4 or 5 years when the kidney seems to be more susceptible to scarring. The worse the grade of reflux, the greater the risk of scarring. Investigation has shown renal scarring in 5 to 20 per cent of kidneys with grade 1 vesicoureteral reflux and scarring in 50 per cent or

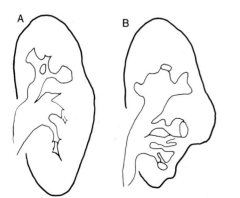
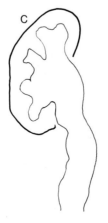
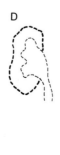

Figure 43–3. Grades of renal parenchymal scarring (*a*, loss of a papillary impression and thinning of the parenchyma over the papilla; *b*, multiple lower pole scars plus medial compensatory hypertrophy; *c*, generalized calicectasis and generalized parenchymal thinning; *d*, a small atrophic kidney with little parenchyma). (From Smellie, J. D., Edwards, N., Hunter, I. C. S., Normand, C. S., and Prescod, N.: Vesicoureteric reflux and renal scarring. Kidney Int. 8(Suppl):S65, 1975.)

more of kidneys with grade 5 reflux (Govan et al., 1975; Ozen and Whitaker, 1987; Skoog et al., 1987).

Although old renal scars may progress, new scarring occurs less frequently after a child is more than 10 years old. The kidneys in children younger than 5 years seem to be particularly vulnerable to scarring from infection; current studies suggest that this vulnerability persists until a child is 10 years old. In girls younger than 10 years with vesicoureteral reflux and recurrent urinary tract infections, 43 per cent (17/40) of kidneys had renal scars progress (developed clubbing or scarring in an area that was previously normal or developed a focal parenchymal decrease of at least 3 mm between examinations), and two of 16 normal kidneys developed new scarring (Filly et al., 1974). Some of the scars took up to 2 years from the episode of pyelonephritis to evolve maximally.

When children in a large English collaborative study were sought specifically for the development of a new renal scar or a scar in a previously normal area, 87 kidneys (in 74 children) were found; 34 (46 per cent) of which developed the scar when the child was between 5 and 10 years old (Smellie et al., 1985). Almost all the episodes of new scars were associated with symptomatic infections or persistent bacteriuria, and 72 of the 87 kidneys refluxed. Most of the children were not taking prophylactic antimicrobial agents. In adults who have normal genitourinary tracts, however, focal renal cortical scarring from infection is rarely seen, but papillary and calyceal distortion or generalized renal shrinkage may occur rarely after acute nonobstructive pyelonephritis (Davidson and Talner, 1978).

The reason why children's kidneys scar and adult's kidneys rarely scar is not entirely known. Whether or not a renal scar will occur when infection and vesicoureteral reflux are present appears to be affected by at least four factors: the intrarenal reflux, the pressure or "water-hammer" effect of reflux, the host immune response to infection and reflux, and the individual's age. In 1974, Rolleston and associates found that areas of renal scarring were associated with foci of intrarenal reflux (pyelotubular backflow) observed on voiding cystourethrography in children who had vesicoureteral reflux and were younger than age 4.

Further investigation revealed that the calyces allowing reflux contained papillae fused with adjacent papillae that caused the papillary ducts to open at right angles rather than at the oblique angles more resistant to reflux (Ransley and Risdon, 1974) (Fig. 43–4). Supporting the

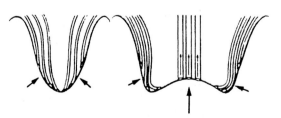

Figure 43–4. Papillary anatomy (a, a schematic drawing of a simple convex papilla that does not normally allow intrarenal reflux; b, a concave papilla that allows intrarenal reflux). (From Ransley, P. G.: Intrarenal reflux: anatomical, dynamic, and radiological studies. Part 1. Urol. Res. 5:61, 1977.)

importance of this finding, these compound papillae were found most commonly at the renal poles, the areas in which renal scarring is most commonly observed clinically. In pigs with vesicoureteral reflux and even intrarenal reflux, however, renal scarring did not develop unless both vesicoureteral reflux and bacteriuria were present (Ransley and Risdon, 1978). Renal scarring with reflux alone without bacteriuria could be created only if the urethra was partially obstructed, resulting in abnormally high voiding pressures (Hodson et al., 1975; Ransley et al., 1984). Experimentally, therefore, the water-hammer effect of vesicoureteral and intrarenal reflux caused renal scarring only if reflux occurred with abnormally high bladder and renal pressures.

Once bacterial access to the kidney from the bladder has been attained, the bacterial infection stimulates both humoral and cellular immune responses. With infection, the kidney is infiltrated by inflammatory cells. In rat models of pyelonephritis, maximal renal suppuration and exudation occurs 3 to 5 days after the infection starts, and collagen infiltration and scarring occurs afterward (Glauser et al., 1978; Miller and Phillips, 1981; Miller et al., 1979; Roberts et al., 1981; Shimamura, 1981; Slotki and Asscher, 1982). If antimicrobial treatment is started within the first few days of infection, the acute suppurative response to the bacteria is prevented and renal scarring can be lessened or prevented (Glauser et al., 1978; Miller and Phillips, 1981; Shimamura, 1981; Slotki and Asscher, 1982).

Other studies suggest that the bactericidal activity of the neutrophils with the release of enzymes, superoxide, and oxygen radicals causes the renal tubular damage observed in pyelonephritis. Inhibition of superoxide production may decrease renal inflammation and tubular damage (Roberts et al., 1982).

Clinical studies show that the young child is at greatest risk of renal scarring from bacterial pyelonephritis. Several factors contribute to this risk. First, the neonatal kidney may respond to urinary back pressure, the water-hammer effect, in different ways and at different thresholds than the adult kidney. Autopsy studies on neonates less than 1 month old reveal that intrarenal reflux into compound calyces may be created at low pressures of 2 mm Hg, whereas the same reflux in a child 1 year old occurs at 20 mm Hg. Furthermore, autopsy studies of cadavers under 12 years of age demonstrate that intrarenal reflux occurs in all calyces, even simple ones, at 50 mm Hg (Funston and Cremin, 1978). This finding suggests that physiologically normal urinary intrapelvic pressures in normal, living adults or older children may be abnormally high in normal, living neonates.

In addition, very young children have incompletely developed immune and neurologic systems. A depressed or incompletely mature immune system may allow bacteria rapid colonization of the bladder and kidney because of decreased local and systemic defenses. It may also kill or eliminate bacteria less efficiently once bacteriuria occurs. Moreover, neurologic immaturity of the bladder may allow frequent uninhibited bladder contractions to transmit their pressures to the upper tracts in even the apparently normal child (Koff and Murtagh, 1984). Bacteriuria combined with reflux in such a child may result in greater susceptibility to renal damage. Furthermore, neonatal symptoms of urinary infection and pyelonephritis are often vague and nonspecific, resulting in delayed or inadequate treatment and a kidney that may respond to bacterial invasion with an inflammatory response characterized by later scarring and loss of renal parenchyma (Winberg et al., 1974). For these reasons, the theory that most renal scarring develops after a single bad infection in the neonate or young child, and, therefore, is present when the genitourinary tract is first evaluated is popular.

The incidence of hypertension in childhood depends on age and sex and has been cited as between 1 and 11 per cent with a renal etiology being most common (Dillon, 1979). Children with reflux nephropathy, in particular, have at least a 10 to 20 per cent risk of future hypertension (Holland et al., 1975; Jacobson et al., 1989; Smellie and Normand, 1979; Wallace et al., 1978) with risks of later progressive deterioration in renal function and other complications of hypertension. Wallace and associates (1978) found that 12.8 per cent of 141 patients with urinary infections and surgically corrected vesicoureteral reflux developed hypertension during the next 10 years. Of those who had renal scarring, 17 per cent became hypertensive; none were hypertensive when they underwent operation. In another series, Smellie and Normand (1979) followed 83 children with reflux nephropathy. Eleven were hypertensive initially, six with malignant hypertension, and another 14 became hypertensive over the next 4 to 20 years. Therefore, 30 per cent were or became hypertensive from reflux nephropathy. Similarly, in Sweden, Jacobson and associates (1989) found that seven of 30 children (23 per cent) with nonobstructive focal renal scarring developed hypertension after 27 years; 10 per cent had developed end-stage renal disease. Of the children followed by Smellie and Normand (1979), 11 had hypertension initially, whereas none of the children in Wallace's group (1978) or Jacobson's group (1989) did, probably indicating that the group of Smellie and Normand had more severe renal damage initially. In all series, however, hypertension occurred whether renal scarring was segmental, focal, unilateral, or bilateral, and was, therefore, independent of the degree of scarring.

The etiology of this hypertension is poorly understood. Some investigators suggest that the renin-angiotensin system is involved. In 1978, the plasma renin activity was measured in children with reflux nephropathy that had been corrected surgically 1 to 10 years before (Savage et al., 1978). In all 15 children who were hypertensive when studied, plasma renin activities were above the normal mean; nine of these children had levels above normal for their age. Of 100 children who were normotensive after surgery, eight had plasma renin levels that were elevated above the normal range for their age. When 85 of these 100 children were traced 5 years later, four had developed serious hypertension and four others had borderline hypertension (Savage et al., 1987). A single elevated plasma renin activity in 1978 did not, however, predict hypertension 5 years later. By 1987, 19 per cent (16/85) of the children had elevated plasma renin activity. In this study, moreover, the normal tendency for the plasma renin activity to decrease with age was not seen and instead the opposite was observed. Plasma renin activity increased with age, and the standard deviation also increased. No direct correlation among blood pressure, degree of scarring, plasma renin activity, or creatinine levels could be made, however.

The value of selective renal vein renin measurements in the management of children with hypertension from reflux nephropathy is controversial (Bailey et al., 1984; Bailey et al., 1978; Dillon et al., 1984; Holland et al., 1975; Stecker et al., 1977) even though segmental renal vein renins have been useful in some for localizing sources of renin production (Dillon et al., 1984). Further indirect evidence of the role of renin in reflux nephropathy has been the successful treatment of hypertension with agents specifically aimed at blocking the renin-angiotensin system. In those children who have been examined with renal arteriography, normal main renal arteries are found to proceed into scarred kidneys with vascular changes limited to small interlobular arterial branches (Holland et al., 1975; Stecker et al., 1977).

Progressive Deterioration of Renal Function in Reflux Nephropathy

Children with reflux nephropathy may develop delayed hypertension and progressive renal dysfunction without apparent further urinary infections. For more than a decade, glomerular lesions and progressive proteinuria have been observed in patients who have reflux nephropathy (Kincaid-Smith, 1975; Torres et al., 1980). Significant proteinuria (> 1 g/24 hours) has been a routine finding in the patient with vesicoureteral reflux and progressive deterioration in renal function (Torres et al., 1980). Certain investigators, moreover, have found glomerular sclerosis in the nonscarred, radiologically normal kidney in cases of unilateral reflux nephropathy (Bailey et al., 1984; Kincaid-Smith, 1975; Kincaid-Smith, 1984). Two theories, one involving progressive renal damage from hyperfiltration of remaining nephrons and the other involving progressive immunologic damage to the kidney, have been postulated to cause this condition.

Micropuncture studies of rat renal tubules allow measurement of single nephron glomerular filtration rates. These investigations show that removal of a kidney or loss of a majority of functioning nephrons results in hyperfiltration in the remaining nephrons and increased glomerular plasma flow. From rat studies in which one kidney and two thirds of the other kidney are removed (a five-sixths nephrectomy model), increases in glomerular plasma flow, mean net glomerular transcapillary hydraulic pressure, and single nephron glomerular filtration rates are measured in the remnant nephrons. Later, as an apparent consequence, these rats develop focal segmental glomerulosclerosis (Hostetter et al., 1981; Hostetter et al., 1982). The glomerulosclerosis is thought to result from vascular injury caused by renal hyperfiltration. Rats maintained on a low-protein diet failed to show the pressure of pathologic changes, and, indeed, rats maintained on a high-protein diet had greater degrees of glomerular sclerosis and more rapid renal death than those on normal diets (Brenner et al., 1982). This sequence of progression has not been proven to occur in reflux nephropathy even though it has been hypothesized.

Another explanation for the progressive renal dysfunction involves a chronic inflammatory response that develops as an autoimmune phenomenon. Tamm-Horsfall protein is produced in the renal tubular cells of the loop of Henle and distal convoluted tubules and is secreted into the urine. Whether it has any specific physiologic role is unknown, but it does appear to affect bacterial adherence to the mucosa and may serve some protective role (Duncan, 1988). Although Tamm-Horsfall protein normally is found only in the urine and on the luminal side of the tubules, both clinically and experimentally, the protein has been detected in interstitial deposits in kidneys that have been subject to infection or reflux and has been associated with mononuclear cell infiltrates and renal scarring (Andriole, 1985).

In addition, even though antibodies (autoantibodies) to Tamm-Horsfall protein are widespread, the immunologic response to Tamm-Horsfall protein after a urinary tract infection may be disturbed in children with reflux nephropathy (Fasth et al., 1980). This protein may account for findings of renal dysfunction or scarring associated with urinary vesicoureteral reflux without known infections, and the autoimmune response related to it may also provide a reason why chronic or progressive renal damage occurs long after cessation of reflux or active infections (Andriole, 1985).

Children at Risk of Renal Damage from Urinary Tract Infections

Although any child who suffers an untreated urinary infection caused by a virulent bacteria may risk renal damage, some children are more prone to infection and subsequent renal damage than others. For this reason, specific host characteristics that may relate to situations of increased risk of renal damage are discussed.

Vesicoureteral Reflux

As discussed, vesicoureteral reflux is present in the majority of children who have renal scarring and urinary tract infections. The reflux appears to be a major mechanism allowing bacterial access to the kidney.

Elevated Bladder Pressure

A neurogenic bladder with chronically or intermittently elevated bladder pressures may cause secondary vesicoureteral reflux because of decompensation of the ureterovesical junction due to the elevated pressure (Hutch, 1952). If this reflux does not occur, the elevated bladder pressures associated with a neurogenic bladder may also cause effective ureterovesical obstruction. This obstruction enhances the risk of renal damage associated with urinary tract infections. As discussed previously in this chapter, intermittent elevations in bladder pressure

associated with physiologic bladder dynamics in the immature bladder may exacerbate vesicoureteral reflux and the risks associated with it.

Peripubertal Girls with Persistent Vesicoureteral Reflux

The question of whether girls approaching puberty who have persistent vesicoureteral reflux risk greater renal damage is problematic. If primary vesicoureteral reflux persists as a girl approaches puberty, it becomes statistically less likely to resolve spontaneously each year. For this reason, some have recommended that girls approaching puberty undergo surgical correction of reflux to avoid the risks of pyelonephritis during future pregnancies. Whether these girls are actually at increased risk of morbidity and should undergo routine correction of reflux is unclear.

Although the prevalence of bacteriuria in pregnant women is the same as that in nonpregnant women (Shortliffe and Stamey, 1986), the likelihood that the bacteriuria may progress to pyelonephritis is greater. Of pregnant women who test as bacteriuric on a screening urinary culture, 13.5 to 65 per cent will develop pyelonephritis during pregnancy if left untreated (Sweet, 1977), whereas an uncomplicated cystitis in a nonpregnant woman rarely progresses to pyelonephritis.

The reason for this increased risk of pyelonephritis may be related to the hydronephrosis of pregnancy, which occurs from hormonal and mechanical changes. Elevated progesterone levels produce smooth muscle atony of the collecting system and bladder, and the enlarging uterus probably causes some mechanical obstruction of the ureters. Although there is little data about vesicoureteral reflux during pregnancy, there are none to suggest that pregnancy causes vesicoureteral reflux.

In one series in which 321 women had a single-film voiding cystourethrogram during the 3rd trimester of pregnancy or immediately post partum, only nine (2.8 per cent) had vesicoureteral reflux (Heidrick et al., 1967). Although 6.2 per cent (20/321) of these women had asymptomatic bacteriuria, only one of these 20 had vesicoureteral reflux. Therefore, few of the pregnant women with bacteriuria who risked pyelonephritis had reflux. Of the nine women who were detected to have reflux, in comparison, three had had a documented episode of pyelonephritis during a pregnancy.

In another series, 21 of 100 pregnant women (27 refluxing renal units in 21 patients) with asymptomatic bacteriuria were found to have vesicoureteral reflux post partum, mostly low grade (67 per cent into the ureter only), and 17 per cent of these women also had renal scarring (Williams et al., 1968).

Although some clinicians have inferred that this scarring was related to the bacteriuria during pregnancy, this percentage is similar to that found when children with asymptomatic bacteriuria are examined for scars radiologically (Asscher et al., 1973; Newcastle Asymptomatic Bacteriuria Research Group, 1975; Savage, 1975). Because these women were not evaluated radiologically before their pregnancy, it is unknown when they developed the scars, and it is most likely that the scars were present since childhood. These data suggest that postpubertal females who have vesicoureteral reflux and predisposition for frequent urinary tract infections will continue to have this predisposition for infections into adulthood and pregnancy.

Although ureteral reimplantation to prevent vesicoureteral reflux may decrease the likelihood of ascending pyelonephritis in normal circumstances, the physiologic changes during pregnancy may allow pyelonephritis to develop even if vesicoureteral reflux has been corrected. Whether the postsurgical nonrefluxing ureteral orifice is less likely to allow pyelonephritis during pregnancy than the normal nonrefluxing ureteral orifice seems unlikely. Therefore, not only the persistent reflux but also the predisposition for bacteriuria needs to be assessed when surgical correction of reflux is considered. Moreover, if vesicoureteral reflux is surgically corrected, these girls still should not be assured that pyelonephritis during pregnancy is impossible, because the majority of pyelonephritis cases during pregnancy are associated with nonrefluxing kidneys. In these patients, urine should still be screened for bacteriuria during pregnancy.

Before a woman with known reflux nephropathy and possible renal insufficiency is counseled about pregnancy, renal function should be evaluated carefully. Although data on the outcome of pregnancies with varying degrees of renal insufficiency is limited, a normal pregnancy is rare if the preconception serum creatinine level exceeds 3 mg/dl (about 30 ml/minute clearance) (Davison and Lindheimer, 1978). Other data documenting the pregnancy complications of prematurity, hypertension, and worsening renal insufficiency have caused some to recommend that conception is ill-advised in women with less than 50 per cent of normal renal function (serum creatinine level > 1.7 mg/dl or < 50 ml/minute clearance) (Bear, 1976).

Boys with Increased Preputial Bacterial Colonization

The reasons for and against circumcision have made routine neonatal circumcision a controversial issue. During the 1970s, however, the association of the foreskin and neonatal urinary tract infections has heightened this controversy (Hallett et al., 1976). This association has resulted in numerous editorials and recommendations by the American Academy of Pediatrics (Cunningham, 1986; King, 1982; Lohr, 1989; Poland, 1990; Roberts, 1986; Schoen, 1990; Schoen et al., 1989; Winberg et al., 1989).

Bollgren and Winberg (1976a) documented in a group of mainly uncircumcised boys that preputial aerobic bacterial colonization is highest during the first months after birth, decreases after 6 months, and is uncommon after age 5 years. Subsequently, Wiswell and associates (1988) have compared the periurethral bacterial flora (using intraurethral and glanular cultures) during the first year of life in circumcised and uncircumcised boys and found that periurethral uropathogenic organisms were cultured more frequently from the periurethral area in uncircumcised than circumcised boys during the

first 6 months of life. They and others have concluded that the foreskin is responsible for this finding (Glennon et al., 1988; Hallett et al., 1976; Wiswell et al., 1988).

Although the reasons for this neonatal bacterial colonization of the foreskin may be related to a number of factors, including early immune status, unusual nosocomial colonization, breast-feeding (Winberg et al., 1989), and other characteristics mediating bacterial adherence (Fussell et al., 1988), higher colonization does appear to be associated with a higher number of neonatal urinary tract infections. Obviously, not all infants who are colonized become infected, but the majority of urinary infections in boys appear to occur in those younger than 3 months, and the frequency appears to be increased in uncircumcised versus circumcised boys.

In a series of retrospective reviews of 55 worldwide United States Army Hospitals, Wiswell and Roscelli (1986) examined the incidence of urinary tract infections in male infants hospitalized for urinary infection diagnosed by catheterization or suprapubic aspirate during 1974 to 1983. They found that the incidence of infections in circumcised male infants was 0.11 per cent (193/175, 317); in uncircumcised male infants, 1.12 per cent (468/41, 799); and in female infants, 0.57 per cent (1164/205, 212). The majority of infections were during the first 3 months of life. When the incidence of infections during the first and the final years of the study were compared, the total number of urinary tract infections increased as the circumcision rate decreased (Wiswell et al., 1987; Wiswell and Roscelli, 1986). Although there may be difficulties with these data related to retrospective analysis and selection bias from studying boys hospitalized for urinary tract infections, periurethral colonization has been associated with increased risk of urinary tract infection in girls and women as well.

Because long-term data are missing from these studies, the importance of detecting urinary tract infections as harbingers of urinary tract abnormalities in these boys is unknown. From epidemiologic studies by Winberg and associates (1974) of symptomatic infections in largely uncircumcised boys, approximately 10 per cent (18/174) had radiologic evidence of obstruction (vesicoureteral reflux not included) and 30 per cent had vesicoureteral reflux. In another study examining urinary infections in male infants, 95 per cent of whom were uncircumcised, 75 per cent of infections occurred during the first 3 months of life; only 11 per cent of infections occurred between 3 and 8 months, and 7 per cent of those infected had genitourinary abnormalities (Ginsburg and McCracken, 1982).

The natural history of an infection in an uncircumcised boy can be determined from the study by Winberg and co-workers (1974) in which the majority of boys were uncircumcised. They found that boys who had a urinary tract infection during the first year of life had an 18 per cent recurrence rate, but recurrences later than 1 year were rare. If a boy had a urinary tract infection when he was older than 1 year (when the incidence is lower), the recurrence rate was 32 per cent. This finding suggests that boys who have urinary infections after the neonatal period may be more likely to have a biologic predisposition for these infections.

From these data, it appears that the association between the foreskin, bacterial colonization, and urinary tract infections is strongest during the first few months of life. These boys may still have a 7 to 40 per cent incidence of genitourinary abnormalities on radiologic evaluation. If the urinary tract is normal, recurrent infection, especially after a year, is unusual.

Acute Hemorrhagic Cystitis

Acute hemorrhagic cystitis accompanied by frequency, urgency, and dysuria in children has been associated with urinary tract infections caused by adenovirus 11 (Manolo et al., 1971; Mufson et al., 1973; Numazaki et al., 1973; Numazaki et al., 1968) and, occasionally by *E. coli* (Loghman-Adham et al., 1988–1989). In a series of 69 infants and children with acute hemorrhagic cystitis, adenovirus 11 was recovered from the urine in ten (14.5 per cent); adenovirus 21, in two (2.9 per cent); and *E. coli*, in 12 (17.4 per cent). However, the remainder (more than 60 per cent) had no infectious agents isolated from the urine (Mufson et al., 1973). Because viral cultures are rarely done, children with symptoms of acute hemorrhagic cystitis most commonly have no growth on routine urinary culture. Although no antimicrobial treatment is indicated with viral cystitis, radiologic evaluation should still be performed to eliminate other causes for hematuria.

MANAGEMENT OF URINARY TRACT INFECTIONS

Rapid recognition of a urinary tract infection and rapid, appropriate antimicrobial treatment are key factors in preventing renal damage. As discussed, most clinical and experimental data show that early antimicrobial treatment appears to be the most effective means of preventing renal scarring and subsequent complications. Treatment varies depending on the age of the child and the severity of the illness. The neonate or infant who has a urinary infection; the child who has an elevated temperature, flank or abdominal pain, and is unable to take fluids; the immunocompromised child; or the child who has a highly resistant organism should be treated with parenteral broad-spectrum antimicrobial agents (e.g., aminoglycoside and ampicillin) until bacterial sensitivities are obtained to allow treatment with an agent with a narrower antimicrobial spectrum. Parenteral treatment should be continued for 7 to 10 days in the neonate or immunocompromised child. Parenteral treatment in the older child should continue until he or she is afebrile and well for 48 hours. Then the child may be given an oral agent so that a total of 10 to 14 days of treatment has been received. In a child 1 year or older who does not appear systemically ill and has clinical cystitis, many oral broad-spectrum antimicrobial agents that are well tolerated will probably cure the infection in a course of 3 to 5 days (Lohr et al., 1981). After this initial treatment, the child should be given a daily prophylactic antimicrobial agent (e.g., low-dose trimethoprim-sulfamethoxazole, nitrofurantoin, and

cephalexin), and the full radiologic evaluation may be performed when convenient within the next few days to weeks. A renal and bladder ultrasound should be performed more immediately, if the child is seriously ill; has newly diagnosed azotemia; has a poor response to appropriate antimicrobials after 3 to 4 days; has an unusual organism (tuberculosis or urea-splitting bacteria, such as *Proteus*); has congenital urinary tract abnormalities that may cause potential obstruction, such as a ureterocele, ureteropelvic junction obstruction, megaureters, and nonfunctioning or poorly functioning renal units; or has diabetes, papillary necrosis, or neuropathic bladder.

Radiologic Evaluation and Follow-Up

A radiologic evaluation of the urinary tract should be performed on a child with well-documented bacteriuria. Although there is some controversy whether studies need to be performed after the first or recurrent episode, if reflux occurs in 21 to 57 per cent of bacteriuric children (Abbott, 1972; Asscher et al., 1973; Kunin et al., 1964; Newcastle Asymptomatic Bacteriuria Research Group, 1975), early detection of vesicoureteral reflux merits radiologic evaluation after the first infection in young children. Bacteriuria in a child, therefore, serves as a marker for a possible genitourinary anatomic abnormality, most commonly vesicoureteral reflux.

Although some have advocated the need for immediate radiologic evaluation to try to determine if a urinary tract infection is an upper or lower tract infection, the findings of enlarged kidneys, focal enlargement from edema, and ureteral widening may be subtle (Conway, 1988; Hellström et al., 1987; Johansson et al., 1988; Silver et al., 1976). Therefore, radiologic evaluation is not generally performed to determine if the kidney is involved in infection. Radiologic evaluation is performed, however, to disclose structural abnormalities that may affect management and treatment.

The timing and mode of the radiologic evaluation of the child with a urinary tract infection is controversial. Most of the time, renal ultrasonography may be performed as soon as convenient after the diagnosis of urinary tract infection. The voiding cystourethrogram (VCUG) may be performed as soon as the urine is sterile. Studies have shown that reflux is not caused by urinary infection and even if it were associated with inflammation, this would be important information for management (Lebowitz, 1986). The voiding cystourethrogram will show urethral and bladder abnormalities and vesicourethral reflux, but the detection of vesicoureteral reflux may be dependent on the technical performance of the VCUG (Fairley and Roysmith, 1977; Lebowitz, 1986; Macpherson and Gordon, 1986). Whether these studies are performed during treatment, immediately following treatment, or a few weeks afterwards may not be important, as long as the child responds rapidly to antimicrobial treatment, has normal renal function, and is maintained on prophylactic antimicrobial treatment, with the urine sterile in the interval between the herald infection and the radiologic evaluation.

When the VCUG is performed as the initial radiologic study, future radiologic studies may be planned (Hellström et al., 1989). If the VCUG shows no apparent abnormalities or low-grade vesicoureteral reflux, an ultrasound examination of the kidney and bladder will usually demonstrate other structural abnormalities or anomalies of the urinary collecting system, such as dysplasia or obstruction, if they exist. In comparison, if the VCUG shows a possible ureterocele, reflux, or other abnormalities, an intravenous urogram (IVU) may be more likely than ultrasound to show more detailed abnormalities of the collecting systems, such as duplication, renal scarring, or other collecting system abnormalities. In general, renal and bladder ultrasound will detect those who may need urgent urologic surgery (Alon et al., 1989; Alon et al., 1986; Honkinen et al., 1986; Lindsell and Moncrieff, 1986; Macpherson and Gordon, 1986).

Ultrasound examination may also be more useful than IVU in the neonate in whom contrast material may not yet concentrate and in whom preparation and prevention of movement may be difficult or impossible. Renal and bladder ultrasound in the pediatric population is, however, often dependent on the skill and experience of the radiologist with children.

When vesicoureteral reflux has been detected on VCUG and surveillance on prophylactic antimicrobial agents is planned, an IVU with select tomograms or ^{99m}Tc–dimercaptosuccinic acid (^{99m}Tc-DMSA) scan may document renal scarring that may not be apparent on ultrasound (Conway, 1988; Gordon, 1986; Lindsell and Moncrieff, 1986). Baseline renal studies may need to be performed several months after an acute urinary infection because renal studies performed at the time of or within the first several months after acute pyelonephritis may show generalized or focal renal enlargement from inflammation and may not show scars that develop after this acute inflammation (Conway, 1988; Filly et al., 1974; Gordon, 1986; Johansson et al., 1988). An acute study may cause overestimation of renal size or lack of appreciation of renal scarring that may be misinterpreted when later studies performed for comparison show a smaller or scarred kidney.

After initial radiologic studies have been used to diagnose reflux, a nuclear voiding cystourethrogram (nuclear VCUG) may be used to assess the presence of reflux and ultrasound may be used to re-evaluate renal morphology and annual growth (Troell et al., 1984). Although the nuclear VCUG may not allow definition of reflux grade, it is more sensitive for the detection of reflux than fluoroscopic examination (Kogan et al., 1986; Macpherson and Gordon, 1986). If, for example, vesicoureteral reflux is still suspected in a patient after a VCUG showing no reflux, a nuclear VCUG may reveal reflux (Kogan et al., 1986; Macpherson and Gordon, 1986).

These examinations will allow adequate surveillance and minimize future radiation to the kidneys and gonads (Gustafson and Mortensson, 1980; Macpherson and Gordon, 1986). Although nuclear VCUG and ultrasound may be performed annually in young children, re-examinations may be delayed for longer intervals if no clinical infections have occurred and the child is older than 8 years. In the older child, scarring from pyelonephritis becomes unlikely (Smellie et al., 1985; Winter et al., 1983), and frequent radiologic surveillance and antimicrobial prophylaxis may be unnecessary. In children in whom severe renal scarring has occurred and the glomerular filtration rate may need to be estimated, the ^{99m}Tc-DTPA renogram gives an accurate estimate of glomerular filtration rate, even in young children (Gates, 1982; Rehling et al., 1989; Shore et al., 1984).

Obstruction and other anatomic abnormalities demonstrated by radiography may require other evaluation specific to their diagnosis before definitive management is decided. Each patient needs to be evaluated and treated individually.

Management of Vesicoureteral Reflux and Bacteriuria

The long-term management of vesicoureteral reflux should be designed to prevent bladder and subsequent renal bacteriuria. Upper tract bacteriuria can usually be prevented either by daily antimicrobial treatment to maintain a sterile urine until the child is no longer at great risk of scarring (i.e., reflux ceases, predilection for infection stops, risk of severe scarring decreases—the child is older than 8 to 10 years) or by surgical treatment of the vesicoureteral reflux. Because it has been shown that vesicoureteral reflux may resolve spontaneously about 80 per cent of the time, depending on its extent and degree, in many situations with low or moderate reflux, antimicrobial prophlaxis and surveillance are worthwhile. If antimicrobial treatment is selected, the urinary tract should be re-evaluated for reflux and new scarring annually, and the urine should be cultured at intervals to ensure that it remains sterile. Re-examinations may be delayed for longer intervals if no clinical infections have occurred and the child is older.

In children with persistent and/or severe vesicoureteral reflux, consideration of bladder function and dynamics may be worthwhile. Some children with recurrent infections and persistent reflux may also have frequent involuntary uninhibited bladder contractions manifest by long-term nocturnal enuresis, urgency, urgency incontinence, squatting, and leg-crossing, and even resulting in a thickened bladder. As discussed previously in this chapter, bladder activity may be a factor in causing or perpetuating vesicoureteral reflux, and this factor may need further evaluation before operative correction or further long-term surveillance is considered.

Prophylactic Antimicrobial Agents

Although a number of agents may be used for treatment of a urinary infection, fewer agents have been used for low-dose prophylaxis. The ideal prophylactic agent should have low serum levels and high urinary levels, have minimal effect on the normal fecal flora, be well tolerated, and be low in cost. The potency of these antimicrobial agents is based on the general susceptibility of most fecal Enterobacteriaceae to these agents at urinary levels. Because the urinary drug levels are much higher than serum, gut, or tissue levels, antimicrobial resistance patterns in the gut should not develop. One problem associated with starting antimicrobial prophylaxis after several days of full-dose parenteral or oral drug treatment of a urinary tract infection is that by the time a prophylatic agent is started, the fecal flora may already have developed resistance to it. This accounts for early breakthrough infection on prophylactic antimicrobial agents and the reason why the treating antimicrobial agent should not necessarily be the prophylactic agent.

NITROFURANTOIN. Nitrofurantoin is an effective urinary prophylactic agent because its serum levels are low, urinary levels are high, and it produces minimal effect on the fecal flora (Winberg et al., 1973). Its effectiveness is based on maintaining a sterile urine by excretion of antimicrobial once a day, and it has been found to be effective in girls at doses of 1.2 to 2.4 mg/kg each evening (Lohr et al., 1977). When renal function is reduced to less than half that of normal, the efficacy of nitrofurantoin may be reduced.

The majority of nitrofurantoin drug reactions occur in adults; it has caused acute allergic pneumonitis, neuropathy, and liver damage (Holmberg et al., 1980). Long-term treatment has been associated with rare cases of pulmonary fibrosis. It should not be used in children with glucose-6-phosphate dehydrogenase deficiencies because it is an oxidizing agent and can cause hemolysis. About 10 per cent of blacks in the United States, Sardinians, non-Ashkenazi Jews, Greeks, Eti-Turks, and Thais may have a glucose-6-phosphate dehydrogenase deficiency and in these people, regeneration of glutathione, which is partially responsible for maintaining red blood cell integrity, is impaired by the enzyme deficiency. When nitrofurantoin is given, it oxidizes the hemoglobin to methemoglobin, which is degraded (Thompson, 1969).

CEPHALEXIN. Cephalexin has been studied in adults as a prophylactic agent. Although resistance to fecal Enterobacteriaceae has developed in many patients taking full-dose cephalexin (500 mg four times a day), patients taking low doses (one-quarter to one-eighth the adult daily dose, 250 to 125 mg/day) do not appear to daily develop resistance. Cephalexin at one quarter of the routine treatment dose per weight given once a day may then be a useful prophylactic agent.

TRIMETHOPRIM-SULFAMETHOXAZOLE. Trimethoprim-sulfamethoxazole has been a successful combination drug in the treatment of urinary tract infections and is useful for prophylaxis at a dose of approximately 2 mg/kg of trimethoprim once a day (Grüneberg et al., 1976; Stamey et al., 1977). The trimethoprim has the unusual characteristic that it diffuses into the vaginal fluid and, therefore, decreases vaginal bacterial colonization (Stamey and Condy, 1975). Because trimethoprim-sulfamethoxazole contains a sulfonamide, it probably should not be given for the first few months of life; sulfonamides may compete for bilirubin binding sites on albumin and cause neonatal hyperbilirubinemia and kernicterus.

TRIMETHOPRIM. Although most of the studies have been done in women, trimethoprim (approximately 2 mg/kg once nightly) has been found to be as effective as trimethoprim-sulfamethoxazole and nitrofurantoin in preventing recurrent urinary infections (Stamm et al., 1980).

NALIDIXIC ACID. Nalidixic acid had been administered to treat children before the advent of more powerful quinolones; however, testing of the quinolones (norfloxacin, cinoxacin) has shown that these drugs may be contraindicated in prepubertal children because they have caused cartilage erosion in weight-bearing joints and arthropathy in immature animals.

Surgical Treatment of Vesicoureteral Reflux

Although the majority of low- to moderate-grade vesicoureteral reflux cases may resolve spontaneously, operative correction by reimplantation or some other antireflux procedure, such as periureteral polytetrafluoroethylene or collagen injection, may be indicated under individual circumstances (Table 43–4). These procedures may be indicated with severe grades of reflux (g 4 and 5) that are less likely to resolve spontaneously, when multiple documented reinfections have occurred while the patient has been maintained on an appropriate antimicrobial agent, when long-term antimicrobial prophylaxis is impossible or ineffective for medical or social reasons, when reflux has failed to improve or resolve after multiple years of appropriate surveillance and the patient continues to be prone to reinfections, when open bladder surgery to correct other urinary anomalies is required, and when new or significant new progressive renal scarring, usually associated with an infection, is observed. Because renal scarring from an episode of pyelonephritis may take up to 2 years to evolve maximally, it is important that a renal scar resulting from acute pyelonephritis and apparent for the first time a few months after the episode is not interpreted as new scarring.

Treatment of Recurrent Urinary Infections Without Reflux

If the radiologic evaluation following the first urinary tract infection shows no urinary tract structural abnor-

Table 43–4. POSSIBLE INDICATIONS FOR ANTIREFLUX PROCEDURES

Severe grade of reflux (grade 4 or 5)
Multiple breakthrough infections while on appropriate antimicrobial prophylaxis
Long-term antimicrobial prophylaxis is impossible for social or medical reasons
Reflux fails to improve or resolve after multiple years of appropriate surveillance
Open bladder surgery to correct other anomalies is required
New or significant progression of renal scarring is observed

mality, no routine tests can predict which patients will continue to have a biologic predisposition for recurrent urinary tract infections. If the child, however, has recurrent infections, urinary prophylactic antimicrobial treatment over a limited period may be worthwhile because the child has then proved to have a biologic susceptibility for infections. When women highly susceptible to urinary infections were studied, it was found that one who had two or more infections without 6 months elapsing between any two of them has a 66 per cent chance of having another infection during the next 6-month period (Kraft and Stamey, 1977). Although children who take prophylactic antimicrobial agents for extended periods may experience a decrease in infections during the time of prophylaxis, the rate of infection returns to the pretreatment rate after prophylaxis is stopped. Even long interruptions in the pattern of recurrence, therefore, do not appear to alter a patient's basic susceptibility to infections.

Treatment of Asymptomatic Bacteriuria

The treatment of asymptomatic bacteriuria is problematic. Not only is the definition of asymptomatic bacteriuria difficult because symptoms may vary with time, but the natural history is not completely known. The incidence of recurrent bacteriuria after treatment of asymptomatic bacteriuria, is, however, greater than 50 per cent (Hansson et al., 1989c; Shortliffe, 1986). *E. coli* causing asymptomatic bacteriuria may belong to specific strains of *E. coli*, some of which are self-agglutinating, are less likely to have P-pili, and are less pathogenic. Although symptomatic or asymptomatic urinary infections in children have usually been treated, especially with vesicoureteral reflux, some evidence exists that nontreatment of asymptomatic bacteriuria in the child older than 3 years who has recurrent infections may result in decreased risk of *symptomatic* attacks of acute pyelonephritis (Hansson et al., 1989c). These studies suggest that urinary tract colonization with a strain of *E. coli* causing asymptomatic bacteriuria may prevent later symptomatic occurrences of pyelonephritis, and treatment, in fact, may predispose the patient to a later acute symptomatic pyelonephritis (Hansson et al., 1989a; Hansson et al., 1989b). Although these conclusions need to be confirmed, they suggest that under certain circumstances, consideration should be given to not treating asymptomatic bacteriuria.

Renal Function and Estimation of Glomerular Filtration Rate

Plasma creatinine levels cannot give the same estimation of renal function in a child that they can in an adult because the plasma creatinine level changes with age and size (Donckerwolcke et al., 1970; Schwartz et al., 1976b). In comparison, glomerular filtration rate, when corrected for body surface area, does not change appreciably after age 2 years (Counahan et al., 1976). For this reason, several estimates of glomerular filtration rate from plasma creatinine level and body height have been developed for use in following serial renal function in children and calculating drug doses of nephrotoxic agents (Counahan et al., 1976; Morris et al., 1982; Schwartz et al., 1976a). The following formula provides an estimate of glomerular filtration rate in children: glomerular filtration rate (in ml/minute/1.73 m^2) = 0.55 × body length (in cm)/plasma creatinine (in mg/dl) (Schwartz et al., 1976a). This formula has compared favorably with inulin and creatinine clearances performed simultaneously. Normal values for plasma creatinine and urea for children of various ages are presented in Tables 43–5 and 43–6.

Treatment Considerations for Children with Bacteriuria and Renal Scarring

After a child with bacteriuria and renal scarring has been identified, management consists of preventing further renal damage. This is usually achieved by preventing further bacteriuria and subsequent pyelonephritis by either antimicrobial prophylaxis or ureteral reimplantation. After the vesicoureteral reflux resolves, whether surgically or spontaneously, the urologist needs to make the patient and his or her parents aware that bacteriuria may still occur in the future.

When a renal scar has been identified, the child and parents need to be educated about future possibilities of hypertension, proteinuria, and progressive nephropathy. In moderate to severe reflux nephropathy with renal insufficiency, early nephrologic consultation for evaluation and surveillance for hypertension, proteinuria, acid-base balance, and dietary counseling about protein restriction may improve or stabilize renal function and improve body growth.

Table 43–5. DISTRIBUTION OF PLASMA CREATININE CONCENTRATIONS FOR BOYS AND GIRLS BY AGE

Age (years)	Females			Males			P
	n	x̄	s	n	x̄	s	
1	8	0.35	0.05	9	0.41	0.10	<.2
2	13	0.45	0.07	18	0.43	0.12	<.7
3	24	0.42	0.08	30	0.46	0.11	<.1
4	28	0.47	0.12	49	0.45	0.11	<.5
5	44	0.46	0.11	50	0.50	0.11	<.1
6	44	0.48	0.11	62	0.52	0.12	<.1
7	50	0.53	0.12	59	0.54	0.14	<.9
8	61	0.53	0.11	60	0.57	0.16	<.1
9	61	0.55	0.11	52	0.59	0.16	<.1
10	46	0.55	0.13	58	0.61	0.22	<.1
11	57	0.60	0.13	56	0.62	0.14	<.5
12	54	0.59	0.13	67	0.65	0.16	<.1
13	41	0.62	0.14	53	0.68	0.21	<.2
14	30	0.65	0.13	44	0.72	0.24	<.2
15	22	0.67	0.22	40	0.76	0.22	<.2
16	16	0.65	0.15	24	0.74	0.23	<.2
17	12	0.70	0.20	22	0.80	0.18	<.2
18–20	15	0.72	0.19	19	0.91	0.17	<.005

n, sample number; x̄, mean plasma creatinine concentration (mg/dl); s, standard deviation; P, significance of difference between male and female means.
From Schwartz, G. J., Haycock, M. B., and Spitzer, A: Plasma creatinine and urea concentration in children: Normal values for age and sex. J. Pediatr., 88:828–830, 1976.

Table 43–6. DISTRIBUTION OF PLASMA UREA CONCENTRATIONS FOR BOYS AND GIRLS BY AGE

Age (years)	Females			Males			P
	n	$\bar{x}$	s	n	$\bar{x}$	s	
1	8	4.91	1.23	9	4.82	1.71	<.9
2	13	6.23	2.47	18	4.93	2.12	<.2
3	24	5.08	1.29	30	5.07	1.58	<.9
4	28	4.57	2.02	49	4.78	1.40	<.6
5	44	4.68	1.36	50	5.52	1.74	<.02
6	44	4.81	1.63	62	5.23	1.56	<.2
7	50	4.67	1.39	59	5.44	1.74	<.02
8	61	5.02	1.61	60	4.84	1.69	<.6
9	61	5.16	1.85	52	5.60	2.68	<.4
10	46	4.67	1.82	58	5.55	3.00	<.1
11	57	4.51	1.62	56	5.04	1.73	<.1
12	54	4.23	1.18	67	5.18	1.46	<.001
13	41	4.82	1.71	53	5.24	1.65	<.3
14	30	5.38	2.18	44	5.11	1.90	<.7
15	22	4.87	2.11	40	5.35	1.62	<.4
16	16	4.77	1.59	24	5.18	1.48	<.5
17	12	4.56	1.64	12	5.67	1.59	<.1
18–20	15	5.41	1.46	19	5.48	1.26	<.9

n, sample number; $\bar{x}$, mean plasma urea concentration (mM/l); s, standard deviation; P, significance of difference between male and female means.

From Schwartz, G. J., Haycock, M. B., and Spitzer, A.: Plasma creatinine and urea concentration in children: Normal values for age and sex. J. Pediatr., 88:828–830, 1976.

In addition, the young female patient with reflux nephropathy and renal insufficiency may desire pregnancy counseling. Although familial screening for vesicoureteral reflux may not be routine at all medical institutions, families in which a member has vesicoureteral reflux or reflux nephropathy must be made aware of the familial occurrence of vesicoureteral reflux and the need for early diagnosis, treatment, and evaluation of urinary tract infections.

REFERENCES

Abbott, G. D.: Neonatal bacteriuria: A prospective study in 1460 infants. Br. Med. J. 1:267, 1972.

Alon, U., Berant, M., and Pery, M.: Intravenous pyelography in children with urinary tract infection and vesicoureteral reflux. Pediatrics, 83(3):332–336, 1989.

Alon, U., Pery, M., Davidai, G., and Berant, M.: Ultrasonography in the radiologic evaluation of children with urinary tract infection. Pediatrics, 78(1):58–64, 1986.

Andriole, V. T.: The role of Tamm-Horsfall protein in the pathogenesis of reflux nephropathy and chronic pyelonephritis. Yale J. Biol. Med., 58:91–100, 1985.

Asscher, A. W.: Urinary tract infection: The value of early diagnosis. Kidney Int., 7:63–67, 1975.

Asscher, A. W., McLachlan, M. S. F., Verrier-Jones, R., Meller, S., Sussman, M., and Harrison, S.: Screening for asymptomatic urinary-tract infection in schoolgirls. Lancet, 2:1, 1973.

Bailey, R. R.: An overview of reflux nephropathy. In Hodson, J. J., and Kincaid-Smith, P. (Eds.): Reflux Nephropathy. New York, Masson Publishing U.S.A., Inc., 1979a, pp. 3–13.

Bailey, R. R.: Vesicoureteric reflux in healthy infants and children. In Hodson, J., and Kincaid-Smith, P. (Eds.): Reflux Nephropathy. New York, Masson Publ., 1979b, pp. 59.

Bailey, R. R., Lynn, K. L., and McRae, C. U.: Unilateral reflux nephropathy and hypertension. In Hodson, C. J., Heptinstall, R. H., and Winberg, J. (Eds.): Reflux Nephropathy Update: 1983. New York, S. Karger, 1984, pp. 116–125.

Bailey, R. R., McRae, C. U., Maling, T. M. J., Tisch, G., and Little,

P. J.: Renal vein renin concentration in the hypertension of unilateral reflux nephropathy. J. Urol., 120:21–23, 1978.

Bailey, R. R., Swainson, C. P., Lynn, K. L., and Burry, A. F.: Glomerular lesions in the "normal" kidney in patients with unilateral reflux nephropathy. Contrib. Nephrol., 39:126–131, 1984.

Bear, R. A.: Pregnancy in patients with renal disease: A study of 44 cases. Obstet. Gynecol., 48:13–18, 1976.

Bellinger, M. F., and Duckett, J. W.: Vesicoureteral reflux: A comparison of non-surgical and surgical management. Contrib. Nephrol., 39:81–93, 1984.

Bergström, T.: Sex differences in childhood urinary tract infection. Arch. Dis. Child., 47:227–232, 1972.

Bollgren, I., Engström, C. F., Hammarlind, M., Källenius, G., Ringertz, H., and Svenson, S. B.: Low urinary counts of P-fimbriated Escherichia coli in presumed acute pyelonephritis. Arch. Dis. Child., 59:102–106, 1984.

Bollgren, I., and Winberg, J.: The periurethral aerobic bacterial flora in healthy boys and girls. Acta Paediatr. Scand., 65:74–80, 1976a.

Bollgren, I., and Winberg, J.: The periurethral aerobic flora in girls highly susceptible to urinary infections. Acta Paediatr. Scand., 65:81–87, 1976b.

Brenner, B. M., Meyer, T. W., and Hostetter, T. H.: Dietary protein intake and the progressive nature of kidney disease. N. Engl. J. Med., 307:652–659, 1982.

Busch, R., and Huland, H.: Correlation of symptoms and results of direct bacterial localization in patients with urinary tract infections. J. Urol., 132:282–285, 1984.

Conway, J. J.: The role of scintigraphy in urinary tract infection. Sem. Nucl. Med., XVIII(4):308–319, 1988.

Counahan, R., Chantler, C., Ghazali, S., Kirkwood, B., Rose, F., and Barratt, T. M.: Estimation of glomerular filtration rate from plasma creatinine concentration in children. Arch. Dis. Child., 51:875–878, 1976.

Cunningham, N.: Circumcision and urinary tract infections. Pediatrics, 77:267–269, 1986.

Davidson, A. J., and Talner, L. B.: Late sequelae of adult-onset acute bacterial nephritis. Radiology, 127:367–371, 1978.

Davison, J. M., and Lindheimer, M. D.: Renal disease in pregnant women. Clin. Obstet. Gynecol., 21:411, 1978.

Dillon, M. J., Gordon, I., and Shah, V.: Tc(99m)-DMSA scanning and segmental renal vein renin estimations in children with renal scarring. In Hodson, C. J., Heptinstall, R. H., and Winberg, J. (Eds.): Reflux Nephropathy Update: 1983. New York, S. Karger, 1984, pp. 28–35.

Dillon, M. J.: Recent advances in evaluation and management of childhood hypertension. Eur. J. Pediatr., 132:133–139, 1979.

Donckerwolcke, R. A., Sander, P. C., van Stekelenburg, G. J., Stoop, J. W., and Tiddens, H. A. W. M.: Serum creatinine values in healthy children. Acta Paediatr. Scand., 59:399–402, 1970.

Duguid, J. P., Clegg, S., and Wilson, M. I.: The fimbrial and nonfimbrial hemagglutinins of Escherichia coli. J. Med. Microbiol., 12:213, 1978.

Duncan, J. L.: Differential effect of Tamm-Horsfall protein on adherence of Escherichia coli to transitional epithelial cells. J. Infect. Dis., 158(6):1379–1382, 1988.

Edwards, D., Norman, I. C. S., Prescod, N., and Smellie, J. M.: Disappearance of vesicoureteric reflux during long-term prophylaxis of urinary tract infection in children. Br. Med. J., 2:285–288, 1977.

Fairley, K. F., and Roysmith, J.: The forgotten factor in the evaluation of vesicoureteric reflux. Med. J. Aust., 2(11):10–12, 1977.

Fasth, A., Bjure, J., Hellström, M., Jacobsson, B., and Jodal, U.: Autoantibodies to Tamm-Horsfall glycoprotein in children with renal damage associated with urinary tract infections. Acta Paediatr. Scand., 69:709–715, 1980.

Filly, R., Friedland, G. W., Govan, D. E., and Fair, W. R.: Development and progression of clubbing and scarring in children with recurrent urinary tract infections. Pediatr. Radiol., 113:145–153, 1974.

Fliedner, M., Mehls, O., Rauterberg, E.-W., and Ritz, E.: Urinary sIgA in children with urinary tract infection. J. Pediatr., 109:416–421, 1986.

Funston, M. R., and Cremin, B. J.: Intrarenal reflux—papillary morphology and pressure relationships in children's necropsy kidneys. Br. J. Urol., 51:665–670, 1978.

Fussell, E. N., Kaack, M. B., Cherry, R., and Roberts, J. A.: Adherence of bacteria to human foreskins. J. Urol., 140:997–1001, 1988.

Gates, G. F.: Glomerular filtration rate: Estimation from fractional renal accumulation of 99m Tc-DTPA (stannous). AJR, 138:565–570, 1982.

Ginsburg, C. M., and McCracken, G. H., Jr.: Urinary tract infections in young infants. Pediatrics, 69(4):409–412, 1982.

Glauser, M. P., Lyons, J. M., and Braude, A. I.: Prevention of chronic experimental pyelonephritis by suppression of acute suppuration. J. Clin. Invest., 61:403, 1978.

Glennon, J., Ryan, P. J., Keane, C. T., and Rees, J. P. R.: Circumcision and periurethral carriage of *Proteus mirabilis* in boys. Arch. Dis. Child., 63:556–557, 1988.

Gordon, I.: Use of Tc-99m DMSA and Tc-99m DTPA in reflux. Semin. Urol., IV(2):99–108, 1986.

Govan, D. E., Fair, W. R., Friedland, G. W., and Filly, R. A.: Management of children with urinary tract infections: The Stanford experience. Urology, VI(3):273–286, 1975.

Grüneberg, R. N., Smellie, J. M., Leaky, A., et al.: Long-term low-dose cotrimoxazole in prophylaxis of childhood urinary tract infection: Bacteriological aspects. Br. Med. J., 2(2):206, 1976.

Gustafsson, M., and Mortensson, W.: Radiation doses to children at urologic radiography. Acta Radiol. (Diagn.) (Stockh.), 22:337–348, 1981.

Hallander, H. O., Kallner, A., Lundin, A., and Österberg, E.: Evaluation of rapid methods for the detection of bacteriuria (screening) in primary health care. Acta Pathol. Microbiol. Immunol. Scand., 94:39–49, 1986.

Hallett, R. J., Pead, L., and Maskell, R.: Urinary infection in boys: A three-year prospective study. Lancet, 2:1107–1110, 1976.

Hansson, S., Caugant, D., Jodal, U., and Svanborg-Edén, C.: Untreated asymptomatic bacteriuria in girls: I. Stability of urinary isolates. Br. Med. J., 298:853–855, 1989a.

Hansson, S., Jodal, U., Lincoln, K., and Svanborg-Edén, C.: Untreated asymptomatic bacteriuria in girls: II. Effect of phenoxymethylpenicillin and erythromycin given for intercurrent infections. Br. Med. J., 298:856–859, 1989b.

Hansson, S., Jodal, U., Norén, L., and Bjure, J.: Untreated bacteriuria in asymptomatic girls with renal scarring. Pediatrics, 84(6):964–968, 1989c.

Heidrick, W. P., Mattingly, R. F., and Amberg, J. R.: Vesicoureteral reflux in pregnancy. Obstet. Gynecol., 29:571–578, 1967.

Hellström, M., Jacobsson, B., Mårild, S., and Jodal, U.: Voiding cystourethrography as a predictor of reflux nephropathy in children with urinary-tract infection. AJR, 152:801–804, 1989.

Hellström, M., Jodal, U., Mårild, S., and Wettergren, B.: Ureteral dilatation in children with febrile urinary tract infection or bacteriuria. AJR, 148:483–486, 1987.

Hodson, C. J.: Natural history of chronic pyelonephritic scarring. Br. Med. J., 2:191–194, 1965.

Hodson, J., Maling, T. M. J., McManamon, P. J., and Lewis, M. G.: Reflux nephropathy. Kidney Int., 8(Suppl.):50–58, 1975.

Holland, N. H., Kotchen, T., and Bhathena, D.: Hypertension in children with chronic pyelonephritis. Kidney Int. [Suppl.], Sept.:243–251, 1975.

Holmberg, L., Boman, G., Bottiger, L. E., Eriksson, B., Spross, R., and Wessling, A.: Adverse reactions to nitrofurantoin: Analysis of 921 reports. Am. J. Med., 69(5):733–738, 1980.

Homsy, Y. L., Nsouli, I., Hamburger, B., Laberge, I., and Schick, E.: Effects of oxybutynin on vesicoureteral reflux in children. J. Urol., 134:1168–1171, 1985.

Honkinen, O., Ruuskanen, O., Rikalainen, H., Mäkinen, E., and Välimäki, I.: Ultrasonography as a screening procedure in children with urinary tract infection. Pediatr. Infect. Dis., 5(6):633–635, 1986.

Hostetter, T. H., Olson, J. L., Rennke, H. G., Venkatachalam, M. A., and Brenner, B. M.: Hyperfiltration in remnant nephrons: A potentially adverse response to renal ablation. Am. J. Physiol., 10:F85–93, 1981.

Hostetter, T. H., Rennke, H. G., and Brenner, B. M.: Compensatory renal hemodynamic injury: A final common pathway of residual nephron destruction. Am. J. Kidney Dis., 5:310–314, 1982.

Hutch, J. A.: Vesico-ureteral reflux in the paraplegic: Cause and correction. J. Urol., 68(2):457–467, 1952.

Jacobson, S. H., Eklöf, O., Eriksson, C. G., Lins, L.-E., Tidgren, B., and Winberg, J.: Development of hypertension and uraemia after pyelonephritis in childhood: 27-year follow-up. Br. Med. J., 299:703–706, 1989.

Jacobson, S. H., Hammarlind, M., Lidefeldt, K. J., Österberg, E., Tullus, K., and Brauner, A.: Incidence of Aerobactin-positive *Escherichia coli* strains in patients with symptomatic urinary tract infection. Eur. J. Clin. Microbiol. Infect. Dis., 7(5):630–634, 1988.

Jacobson, S. H., Tullus, K., and Brauner, A.: Hydrophobic properties of *Escherichia coli* causing acute pyelonephritis. J. Infect., 19:17–23, 1989.

Johansson, B., Troell, S., and Berg, U.: Renal parenchymal volume during and after acute pyelonephritis measured by ultrasonography. Arch. Dis. Child., 63:1309–1314, 1988.

Johnson, C. E., Shurin, P. A., Marchant, C. D., Strieter, C. M., Murdell-Panek, D., Debaz, B. P., Shah, Z. R., Scillian, J. J., and Hall, P. W.: Identification of children requiring radiologic evaluation for urinary infection. Pediatr. Infect. Dis., 4(6):656–663, 1985.

Källenius, G., Möllby, R., Svenson, S. B., Helin, I., Hultberg, H., Cedergren, B., and Winberg, J.: Occurrence of P-fimbriated *Escherichia coli* in urinary tract infections. Lancet, 2:1369–1372, 1981.

Kass, E. H., and Finland, M.: Asymptomatic infections of the urinary tract. Trans. Assoc. Am. Physicians, 69:56–64, 1956.

Kincaid-Smith, P.: Glomerular lesions in atrophic pyelonephritis and reflux nephropathy. Kidney Int., 8:S81–83, 1975.

Kincaid-Smith, P. S.: Diffuse parenchymal lesions in reflux nephropathy and the possibility of making a renal biopsy diagnosis in reflux nephropathy. *In* Hodson, C. J., Heptinstall, R. H., and Winberg, J. (Eds.): Reflux Nephropathy Update: 1983. New York, S. Karger, 1984, pp. 111–115.

King, L. R.: Neonatal circumcision in the United States in 1982. J. Urol., 128:1135–1136, 1982.

Koff, S. A., Lapides, J., and Piazza, D. H.: Association of urinary tract infection and reflux with uninhibited bladder contractions and voluntary sphincteric obstruction. J. Urol., 122:373–376, 1979.

Koff, S. A., and Murtagh, D. S.: The uninhibited bladder in children: Effect of treatment on recurrence of urinary infection and on vesicoureteral reflux resolution. J. Urol., 130:1138–1141, 1983.

Koff, S. A., and Murtagh, D. S.: The uninhibited bladder in children: Effect of treatment on vesicoureteral reflux resolution. *In* Hodson, C. J., Heptinstall, R. H., and Winberg, J. (Eds.): Reflux Nephropathy Update: 1983. New York, S. Karger, 1984, pp. 211–220.

Kogan, S. J., Sigler, L., Levitt, S. B., Reda, E. R., Weiss, R., and Greifer, I.: Elusive vesicoureteral reflux in children with normal contrast cystograms. J. Urol., 136:325–328, 1986.

Kollerman, M. W., and Ludwig, H.: The current status of vesicoureteral reflux: A review. Monogr. Urol., 5:155–173, 1984.

Kraft, J. K., and Stamey, T. A.: The natural history of symptomatic recurrent bacteriuria in women. Medicine, 56:55, 1977.

Kunin, C. M., Deutscher, R., and Paquin, A.: Urinary tract infection in school children: An epidemiologic, clinical and laboratory study. Medicine, 43:91–130, 1964.

Lebowitz, R.: The detection of vesicoureteral reflux in the child. Invest. Radiol., 21(7):519–531, 1986.

Lenaghan, D., and Cussen, L. J.: Vesicoureteral reflux in pups. Invest. Urol., 5:449–461, 1968.

Lenaghan, D., Whitaker, J. G., Jensen, F., and Stephens, F. D.: The natural history of reflux and long-term effects of reflux on the kidney. J. Urol., 115:728–730, 1976.

Lindsell, D., and Moncrieff, M.: Comparison of ultrasound examination and intravenous urography after a urinary tract infection. Arch. Dis. Child., 61:81–82, 1986.

Loghman-Adham, M., Tejero, H. T., and London, R.: Acute hemorrhagic cystitis due to *Escherichia coli*. Child Nephrol. Urol., 9:29–32, 1988–1989.

Lohr, J. A.: The foreskin and urinary tract infections. J. Pediatr., 114(3):502–504, 1989.

Lohr, J. A., Hayden, G. F., Kesler, R. W., Gleason, C. H., Wood, J. B., Ford, R. F., Perrillo, V. A., Benjamin, J. T., and Dickens, M. D.: Three-day therapy of lower urinary tract infections with nitrofurantoin macrocrystals: A randomized clinical trial. Pediatrics, 99(6):980–983, 1981.

Lohr, J. A., Nunley, D. H., Howards, S. S., and Ford, R. F.: Prevention of recurrent urinary tract infections in girls. Pediatrics, 59(4):562–565, 1977.

Lomberg, H., Hanson, L. Å., Jacobsson, B., Jodal, U., Leffler, H., and Svanborg Edén, C.: Correlation of P blood group, vesicoureteral reflux, and bacterial attachment in patients with recurrent pyelonephritis. N. Engl. J. Med., 308:1189–1192, 1983.

Macpherson, R. I., and Gordon, L.: Vesicoureteric reflux: Radiologic aspects. Semin. Urol., IV(2):89–98, 1986.

Manolo, D., Mufson, M. A., Zollar, L. M., and Mankad, V. N.: Adenovirus infection in acute hemorrhagic cystitis: A study of 25 children. Am. J. Dis. Child., 121(4):281–285, 1971.

Mårild, S., Hellström, M., Jacobsson, B., Jodal, U., and Svanborg Edén, C.: Influence of bacterial adhesion on ureteral width in children with acute pyelonephritis. J. Pediatr., 115(2):265–268, 1989.

Miller, T., and Phillips, S.: Pyelonephritis: The relationship between infection, renal scarring, and antimicrobial therapy. Kidney Int., 19:654–662, 1981.

Miller, T. E., Stewart, E., and North, J. D. K.: Immunobacteriological aspects of pyelonephritis. Contrib. Nephrol., 16:11–15, 1979.

Morris, M. C., Allanby, C. W., Toseland, P., Haycock, G. B., and Chantler, C.: Evaluation of a height/plasma creatinine formula in the measurement of glomerular filtration rate. Arch. Dis. Child., 57:611–615, 1982.

Mufson, M. A., Belshe, R. B., Horrigan, T. J., and Zollar, L. M.: Cause of acute hemorrhagic cystitis in children. Am. J. Dis. Child., 26:605–608, 1973.

Newcastle Asymptomatic Bacteriuria Research Group: Asymptomatic bacteriuria in schoolchildren in Newcastle upon Tyne. Arch. Dis. Child., 50:90, 1975.

Numazaki, Y., Kumasaka, T., Yano, N., Yamanaka, M., Miyazawa, T., Takai, S., and Ishida, N.: Further study on acute hemorrhagic cystitis due to adenovirus type 11. N. Engl. J. Med., 289:344–347, 1973.

Numazaki, Y., Shigeta, S., Kumasaka, T., Miyazawa, T., Yamanaka, M., Yano, N., Takai, S., and Ishida, N.: Acute hemorrhagic cystitis in children: Isolation of adenovirus type 11. N. Engl. J. Med., 278(13):700–704, 1968.

Ozen, H. A., and Whitaker, R. H.: Does the severity of presentation in children with vesicoureteric reflux relate to the severity of the disease or the need for operation? Br. J. Urol., 60:110–112, 1987.

Poland, R. L.: The question of routine neonatal circumcision. N. Engl. J. Med., 322(18):1312–1315, 1990.

Powell, H. R., McCredie, D. A., and Ritchie, M. A.: Urinary nitrite in symptomatic and asymptomatic urinary infection. Arch. Dis. Child., 62:138–140, 1987.

Ransley, P. G.: Intrarenal reflux: Anatomical, dynamic, and radiologic studies–part 1. Urol. Res., 5:61, 1977.

Ransley, P. G., and Risdon, R. A.: Renal papillae and intrarenal reflux in the pig. Lancet, ii:1114, 1974.

Ransley, P. G., and Risdon, R. A.: Reflux and renal scarring. Br. J. Radiol., 51(Suppl.):1–35, 1978.

Ransley, P. G., Risdon, R. A., and Godley, M. L.: High pressure sterile vesicoureteral reflux and renal scarring: An experimental study in the pig and minipig. In Hodson, C. J., Heptinstall, R. H., and Winberg, J. (Eds.): Reflux Nephropathy Update: 1983. New York, S. Karger, 1984, pp. 320–343.

Rehling, M., Jensen, J. J., Scherling, B., Egeblad, M., Lønborg-Jensen, H., Kanstrup, I. K., and Dige-Petersen, H.: Evaluation of renal function and morphology in children by ^{99m}Tc-DTPA gamma camera renography. Acta Paediatr. Scand., 78:601–607, 1989.

Report of the International Reflux Study Committee: Medical versus surgical treatment of primary vesicoureteral reflux: A prospective international reflux study in children. J. Urol., 125:277–283, 1981.

Robbins, J. B.: Immunologic mechanisms, Chap. 10. In Barnett, H. L. (Ed.): Pediatrics. New York, Appleton-Century-Crofts, 1972.

Roberts, J. A.: Studies of vesicoureteral reflux: A review of work in a primate model. South Med. J., 71:28–30, 1978.

Roberts, J. A.: Does circumcision prevent urinary tract infection. J. Urol., 135:991–992, 1986.

Roberts, J. A., Domingue, G. J., Martin, L. N., et al.: Immunology of pyelonephritis in the primate model: Live versus heat-killed bacteria. Kidney Int., 19:297, 1981.

Roberts, J. A., Roth, J. K., and Domingue, G. J.: Immunology of pyelonephritis in the primate model: V. Effect of superoxide dismutase. J. Urol., 128:1394, 1982.

Rolleston, G. L., Maling, T. M. J., and Hodson, C. J.: Intrarenal reflux and the scarred kidney. Arch. Dis. Child., 49:531–539, 1974.

Savage, D. C. L.: Natural history of covert bacteriuria in schoolgirls. Kidney Int., 8:S90–S95, 1975.

Savage, J. M., Dillon, M. J., Shah, V., Barratt, T. M., and Williams, D. I.: Renin and blood pressure in children with renal scarring and vesicoureteric reflux. Lancet, 2:441–444, 1978.

Savage, J. M., Koh, C. T., Barratt, T. M., and Dillon, M. J.: Five-year prospective study of plasma renin activity and blood pressure in patients with longstanding reflux nephropathy. Arch. Dis. Child., 62:678–682, 1987.

Schoen, E. J.: The status of circumcision of newborns. N. Engl. J. Med., 322(18):1308–1312, 1990.

Schoen, E. J., Anderson, G., Bohon, C., Hinman, F., Poland, R. L., and Wakeman, E. M.: Report of the Task Force on Circumcision. Pediatrics, 84(4):388–391, 1989.

Schwartz, G. J., Haycock, M. B., Edelmann, C. M., and Spitzer, A.: A simple estimate of glomerular filtration rate in children derived from body length and plasma creatinine. Pediatrics, 58(2):259–263, 1976a.

Schwartz, G. J., Haycock, M. B., and Spitzer, A.: Plasma creatinine and urea concentration in children: Normal values for age and sex. J. Pediatr., 88:828–830, 1976b.

Sheinfeld, J., Cordon-Cardo, C., Fair, W. R., Wartinger, D. D., and Rabinowitz, R.: Association of type 1 blood group antigens with urinary tract infections in children with genitourinary structural abnormalities. J. Urol., 144(2, part 2):469–473, 1990.

Sheinfeld, J., Schaeffer, A. J., Cordon-Cardo, C., Rogatko, A., and Fair, W. R.: Association of the Lewis blood-group phenotype with recurrent urinary tract infections in women. N. Engl. J. Med., 320(12):773–777, 1989.

Shimamura, T.: Mechanisms of renal tissue destruction in an experimental acute pyelonephritis. Exp. Mol. Pathol., 34:34, 1981.

Shore, R. M., Koff, S. A., Mentser, M., Hayes, J. R., Smith, S. P., Smith, J. P., and Chesney, R. W.: Glomerular filtration rate in children: Determination from the Tc-99m-DTPA renogram. Radiology, 151:627–633, 1984.

Shortliffe, L. M. D.: Asymptomatic bacteriuria: Should it be treated? Urology, XXVII(2):19–25, 1986.

Shortliffe, L. M. D., and Stamey, T. A.: Urinary infections in adult women. In Walsh, P. C., Gittes, R. F., Perlmutter, A. D., and Stamey, T. A. (Eds.): Campbell's Urology. Philadelphia, W. B. Saunders, 1986, pp. 797–830.

Silver, T. M., Kass, E. J., Thornbury, J. R., Konnak, J. W., and Wolfman, M. G.: The radiological spectrum of acute pyelonephritis in adults and adolescents. Radiology, 118:65–71, 1976.

Skoog, S. J., Belman, A. B., and Majd, M.: A nonsurgical approach to the management of primary vesicoureteral reflux. J. Urol., 138:941–946, 1987.

Slotki, I. N., and Asscher, A. W.: Prevention of scarring in experimental pyelonephritis in the rat by early antibiotic therapy. Nephron, 30:262, 1982.

Smellie, J., Edwards, D., Hunter, N., Normand, I. C. S., and Prescod, N.: Vesicoureteric reflux and renal scarring. Kidney Int., 8(Suppl.):S65, 1975.

Smellie, J. M., Edwards, D., Normand, I. C. S., and Prescod, N.: Effect of vesicoureteric reflux on renal growth in children with urinary tract infection. Arch. Dis. Child., 56:593–600, 1981.

Smellie, J. M., and Normand, I. C. S.: Reflux nephropathy in childhood. In Hodson, J., and Kincaid-Smith, P. (Eds.): Reflux Nephropathy. New York, Masson Publishing U.S.A., Inc., 1979, pp. 14–20.

Smellie, J. M., Ransley, P. G., Norman, I. C. S., Prescod, N., and Edwards, D.: Development of new renal scars: A collaborative study. Br. Med. J., 290:1957–1960, 1985.

Stamey, T. A.: Editorial: A clinical classification of urinary tract infections based upon origin. South. Med. J., 68:934, 1975.

Stamey, T. A.: Pathogenesis and Treatment of Urinary Tract Infections. Baltimore, Williams & Wilkins, 1980.

Stamey, T. A., and Condy, M.: The diffusion and concentration of trimethoprim in human vaginal fluid. J. Infect. Dis., 131:261, 1975.

Stamey, T. A., Condy, M., and Mihara, G.: Prophylactic efficacy of nitrofurantoin macrocrystals and trimethoprim-sulfamethoxazole in urinary infections. N. Engl. J. Med., 296:780, 1977.

Stamey, T. A., and Pfau, A.: Some functional, pathological bacteriologic, and chemotherapeutic characteristics of unilateral pyelonephritis in man: II. Bacteriologic and chemotherapeutic characteristics. Invest. Urol., 1:162, 1963.

Stamey, T. A., and Sexton, C. C.: The role of vaginal colonization with Enterobacteriaceae in recurrent urinary infections. J. Urol., 113:214, 1975.

Stamm, W. E., Counts, G. W., Running, K. R., Fihn, S., Turck, M., and Holmes, K. K.: Diagnosis of coliform infection in acutely dysuric women. N. Engl. J. Med., 307:463–468, 1982.

Stamm, W. E., Counts, G. W., Wagner, K. F., Martin, D., Gregory, D., McKevitt, M., Turck, M., and Holmes, K. K.: Antimicrobial prophylaxis of recurrent urinary tract infections. Ann. Intern. Med., 92:770–775, 1980.

Stecker, J. F., Read, B. P., and Poutasse, E. F.: Pediatric hypertension as a delayed sequela of reflux-induced chronic pyelonephritis. J. Urol., 118:644–646, 1977.

Stephens, F. D.: Correlation of ureteral orifice position with renal morphology. Trans. Am. Assoc. G. U. Surg., 68:53–55, 1977.

Svanborg Edén, C., and Hanson, L. A.: *Escherichia coli* pili as possible mediators of attachment to human urinary tract epithelial cells. Infect. Immun., 21:229, 1978.

Svanborg Edén, C., Kulhavy, R., Mårild, S., Prince, S. J., and Mestecky, J.: Urinary immunoglobulins in healthy individuals and children with acute pyelonephritis. Scand. J. Immunol., 21:305–313, 1985.

Sweet, R. L.: Bacteriuria and pyelonephritis during pregnancy. Semin. Perinatol., 1:25–40, 1977.

Thompson, R. B.: A Short Textbook of Haematology. Philadelphia, J. B. Lippincott Co., 1969.

Torres, V. E., Velosa, J. A., Holley, K. E., Kelalis, P. P., Stickler, G. B., and Kurtz, S. B.: The progression of vesicoureteral reflux nephropathy. Ann. Intern. Med., 92:776–784, 1980.

Troell, S., Berg, U., Johansson, B., and Wikstad, I.: Ultrasonographic renal parenchymal volume related to kidney function and renal parenchymal area in children with recurrent urinary tract infections and asymptomatic bacteriuria. Acta Radiol. [Diagn.] (Stockh), 25(5):411–416, 1984.

Väisänen, V., Elo, J., Tallgren, L. G., Siitonen, A., Mäkelä, P. H., Svanborg-Edén, C., Källenius, G., Svenson, S. B., Hultberg, H., and Korhonen, T.: Mannose-resistant haemagglutination and P antigen recognition are characteristic of *Escherichia coli* causing primary pyelonephritis. Lancet, 2:1366–1369, 1981.

Van den Abbeele, A. D., Treves, S. T., Lebowitz, R. L., Bauer, S., Davis, R. T., Retik, A., and Colodny, A.: Vesicoureteral reflux in asymptomatic siblings of patients with known reflux: Radionuclide cystography. Pediatrics, 79(1):147–153, 1987.

Walker, R. D.: Renal functional changes associated with vesicoureteral reflux. Urol. Clin. North Am., 17(2):307–316, 1990.

Wallace, D. M. A., Rothwell, D. L., and Williams, D. I.: The long-term follow-up of surgically treated vesicoureteric reflux. Br. J. Urol., 50:479–484, 1978.

Wettergren, B., Fasth, A., Jacobsson, B., Jodal, U., and Lincoln, K.: UTI during the first year of life in a Göteborg area 1977–79. Pediatr. Res., 14:981, 1980.

Williams, G. L., Davies, D. K. L., Evans, K. T., and Williams, J. E.: Vesicoureteric reflux in patients with bacteriuria in pregnancy. Lancet, 2:1202–1205, 1968.

Winberg, J., Anderson, H. J., Bergström, T., Jacobsson, B., Larson, H., and Lincoln, K.: Epidemiology of symptomatic urinary tract infection in childhood. Acta Paediatr. Scand., S252:1–20, 1974.

Winberg, J., Bergström, T., Lidin-Janson, G., and Lincoln, K.: Treatment trials in urinary tract infection (UTI) with special reference to the effect of antimicrobials on the fecal and periurethral flora. Clin. Nephrol., 1:142, 1973.

Winberg, J., Bollgren, I., Gothefors, L., Herthelius, M., and Tullus, K.: The prepuce: A mistake of nature? Lancet, 1:598–599, 1989.

Winter, A. L., Hardy, B. E., Alton, D. J., Arbus, G. S., and Churchill, B. M.: Acquired renal scars in children. J. Urol., 129:1190–1194, 1983.

Wiswell, T. E., Enzenauer, R. W., Holton, M. E., Cornish, J. D., and Hankins, C. T.: Declining frequency of circumcision: Implications for changes in the absolute incidence and male to female sex ratio of urinary tract infections in early infancy. Pediatrics, 79(3):338–342, 1987.

Wiswell, T. E., Miller, G. M., Gelston, H. M., Jones, S. K., and Clemmings, A. F.: Effect of circumcision status on periurethral bacterial flora during the first year of life. J. Pediatr., 113(3):442–446, 1988.

Wiswell, T. E., and Roscelli, J. D.: Corroborative evidence for the decreased incidence of urinary tract infections in circumcised male infants. Pediatrics, 78(1):96–99, 1986.

Yoder, M. C., and Polin, R. A.: Immunotherapy of neonatal septicemia. Pediatr. Clin. North Am., 33:481–501, 1986.

XI
PEDIATRIC UROLOGIC SURGERY

44
VESICOURETERAL REFLUX, MEGAURETER, AND URETERAL REIMPLANTATION

Lowell R. King, M.D.

VESICOURETERAL REFLUX

The recognition of vesicoureteral reflux as an abnormal phenomenon in humans, often associated with urinary infection and signalling both developmental and acquired renal abnormalities, has led to the study of the embryology, anatomy, and physiology of the ureterovesical junction. From a gradual understanding of the causes, consequences, and natural history of vesicoureteral reflux, generally accepted principles of patient management have evolved. The gap has narrowed between the proponents of surgical and "conservative" (i.e., nonoperative) management of patients with reflux. Specific indications for antireflux surgery have been defined, and surgical techniques have been improved to the point at which operative correction, when necessary, is relatively safe and reliable. Progressive renal damage occurs in only about 2 per cent of patients with uncomplicated reflux, whether they are treated by early surgery or by antibacterials and surveillance until the reflux stops with growth.

Historical Perspective

Semblinow observed reflux of urine stained with methylene blue from the bladder into the ureters of both dogs and rabbits in 1883. Pozzi reported the first case of vesicoureteral reflux in humans in 1893. He noted the appearance of urine from the distal end of a ureter divided during a transabdominal gynecologic procedure. In experiments with human cadavers, Young was unable to make urine flow backward from the bladder into the ureter, irrespective of the pressure used in filling. In 1929, Gruber noted that the structure of the trigone and ureterovesical junction varied in different animal species and that the incidence of vesicoureteral reflux varied directly with the length of the intravesical ureter and

the muscular development of the trigone. Kretschmer (1916) and Bumpus (1924) presented early observations on the clinical use of cystography and the occurrence of vesicoureteral reflux.

Partly because reflux is normal in many mammals, its presence in humans was not always considered to be abnormal until Hutch (1958) convincingly demonstrated that acquired periureteral diverticula commonly resulted in reflux, which led to renal damage from hydronephrosis or supraimposed infection. The cystogram came into general use as a clinical tool through the 1950's and with it the recognition that reflux was not uncommon and had several specific causes.

Anatomy and Function of the Ureter

The ureter is a muscular conduit that contracts in response to the stretch reflex to transport a bolus of urine to the bladder. Distally, it passes through a hiatus in the posterolateral aspect of the bladder wall. The spiral muscle fibers of the ureter, which transmit peristaltic waves, terminate at this point, and only longitudinal muscle fibers continue in the intravesical ureter, covered by bladder mucosa and buttressed by the underlying detrusor muscle. As the intravesical ureter passes from the hiatus to its orifice, these longitudinal fibers decussate, passing medially to form Mercier's bar and inferiorly to form Bell's muscle, the borders of the superficial trigone. Thus, the musculature of the ureter and the trigone is in continuity because the ureteral muscular coat passes through the hiatus and fans out on the floor of the bladder to form the superficial trigone (Figs. 44–1 and 44–2).

The adventitia of the juxtavesical ureter is composed of a superficial and a deep periureteral sheath, the former derived from the bladder and the latter derived

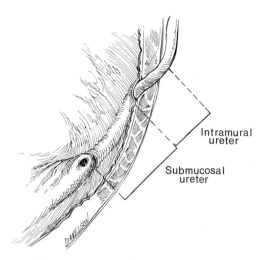

Figure 44–1. Normal ureterovesical junction.

from the ureter. A plane of cleavage occupied by loose connective tissue, the space of Waldeyer, separates the superficial from the deep periureteral sheath (Fig. 44–3).

When a bolus of urine passes down the ureter, several factors operate to facilitate its passage through the intravesical segment into the bladder. The longitudinal muscle of the intravesical ureter contracts as the bolus appears at the hiatus. This shifts the orifice cranially and laterally toward the hiatus, shortening and widening the intravesical ureter and reducing resistance to the passage of the bolus into the lumen of the bladder.

After the bolus has passed, the intrinsic ureteral musculature relaxes, permitting the intravesical ureter to resume its resting configuration beneath the bladder mucosa. The intravesical ureter is a delicate structure. The normally low pressure in the resting bladder (8 to

15 mm Hg) is sufficient to passively compress the roof of the intravesical ureter against the underlying detrusor to prevent reflux. Peristaltic pressure in the extravesical ureter, between 20 and 35 mm Hg, is sufficient to propel a bolus of ureteral urine rapidly and forcefully into the bladder in an abrupt spurt. Thus, the normal compliance and elasticity of the intravesical ureter are crucial, and inflammation of the overlying bladder mucosa may alter the function of the ureterovesical junction significantly.

Critical to the normal absence of reflux in humans are the length of the intravesical ureter relative to its diameter and the intrinsic longitudinal muscular coat of the submucosal ureter that inserts onto the superficial trigone (Fig. 44–4) (Paquin, 1959). These factors are reflected in the appearance of the ureteral orifice, described by Lyon and co-workers (1969) as normally resembling a cone, but sometimes resembling a stadium, horseshoe, or golf hole with increasing tendency toward laterality and reflux (Fig. 44–5).

Ambrose and Nicolson (1962), Stephens and Lenaghan (1962), and others also noted that as the orifice becomes more abnormal in appearance, it usually occupies a more lateral position (ureteral ectopia lateralis), and more of the intravesical ureter is missing. As a result, the more lateral the orifice, the more likely it is that reflux will occur. Such reflux is congenital and often familial and has been termed primary reflux (Garret et al., 1963).

Reflux is a radiographic sign (typically detected by instilling radiographic contrast material into the bladder), which can be caused by one of several different mechanisms (Table 44–1). For example, the lack of an adequate detrusor buttress under the intravesical ureter may result in reflux. If the ureterovesical junction is of marginal competence intrinsically, infection may reduce the compliance of the roof of the intravesical ureter and permit reflux to occur. Although such reflux is often

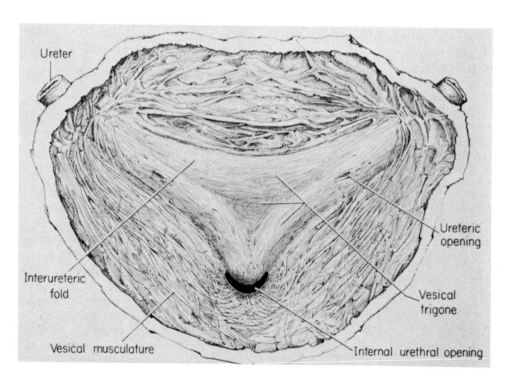

Figure 44–2. Interior of posterior-inferior portion of bladder: vesical trigone and ureteric and urethral apertures. (From Woodburne, R. T.: J. Urol., 92:431, 1964.)

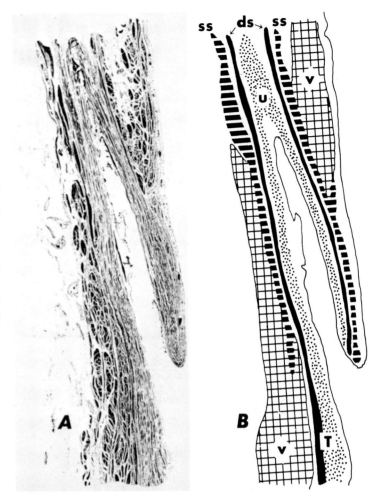

Figure 44–3. Ureterovesical junction in longitudinal section. *A,* Photomicrograph. *B,* Diagrammatic representation. Ureteral muscularis *(u)* is surrounded by superficial *(ss)* and deep *(ds)* periureteral sheaths, which extend in the roof of the submucosal segment and continue beyond the orifice into trigonal muscle *(T).* Relationship of superficial sheath to vesical muscularis *(v)* is clearly seen. Transverse fascicles in superior lip of ureteral orifice belong to superficial and deep sheaths. No true space can be seen separating ureter from bladder. Plane between the two sheaths is occupied by loose connective tissue. Modified trichrome stain, reduced from × 9 (muscle, black; connective tissue, gray). Diagram was drawn by tracing muscular elements of 12 serial sections, including section shown in photomicrograph. (From Elhadaiwi, A.: J. Urol., 107:224, 1972.)

transient or inconsistent, it must be understood and recognized as such so that it can be categorized in each patient. This occurrence will have major therapeutic implications, particularly in deciding whether operative correction is likely to be needed.

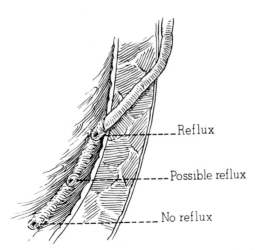

Figure 44–4. Refluxing ureterovesical junction. Same anatomic features as nonrefluxing orifice, except for inadequate length of intravesical submucosal ureter, are shown. Some orifices reflux intermittently with borderline submucosal tunnels. (From Glenn, J. (Ed.): Urologic Surgery, 2nd ed. New York, Harper & Row, 1975.)

Incidence and Epidemiology of Reflux

The incidence of reflux in individuals without urologic symptoms is quite low, varying from 0 to 2 per cent in reported series, including those with premature infants and adults of both sexes (Estes and Brooks, 1970; Gibson, 1949; Leadbetter et al., 1960; Lich et al., 1964; McGovern et al., 1960; Peters et al., 1967; Ransley, 1978). Such studies suggest that the incidence of reflux in healthy children is less than 1 per cent.

When urinary infection is the reason for investigation, reflux has been discovered in 20 to 50 per cent of children (Shopfner, 1970; Smellie and Normand, 1966; Walker et al., 1977). In children with urinary tract infection the prevalence of reflux seems directly proportional to age (Baker et al., 1966; Smellie, 1975b). Infants in particular seem prone to develop reflux in association with infection. With growth, the submucosal ureter elongates and the ratio between the length and diameter of the submucosal tunnel increases (King, 1976; Lenaghan et al., 1976; Stephens, 1976), making noncompliance of the valve mechanism less likely as a cause of reflux.

A high prevalence of reflux in siblings of children with known reflux is noted. Dwoskin (1976) found reflux in approximately 30 per cent of siblings. In a review by Jenkins and Noe (1982), 104 siblings of 78 patients with

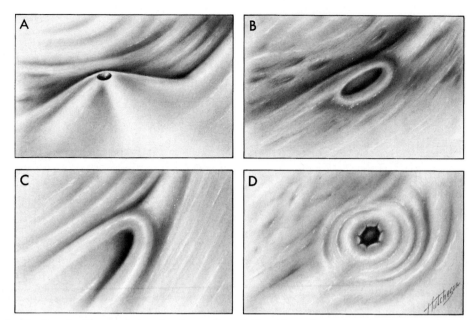

Figure 44–5. Lyon classification of orifice morphology in primary reflux. *A,* Normal or volcano-shaped orifice at cystoscopy by the right-angle lens system. *B,* Stadium orifice. Usually slightly more lateral than the normal orifice and sometimes associated with reflux. The intravesical ureter, however, is usually well developed, and reflux associated with such orifices will usually stop with growth. *C,* Horeshoe orifice. Part or most of the intravesical ureter is represented by the longitudinal muscle in the ridges above and below the orifice. The proximal submucosal ureter may be well fused but is usually short, and reflux will often persist, at least for several years. *D,* A golf-hole orifice is most lateral in position and lacks any vestige of an intravesical ureter. Associated reflux is quite persistent and usually continues after full growth is achieved. (From Kelalis, P. P., and King L. R. (Eds.): Clinical Pediatric Urology. Philadelphia, W. B. Saunders Co., 1976.)

reflux were screened by cystogram without anesthesia. Of these, 24 (33 per cent) were found to have reflux. Of this group, 73 per cent had no history of infection or any abnormal voiding symptoms.

Noe updated this experience in 1986. Reflux was found in over 30 per cent of siblings. Of these, two thirds have no history of urinary tract infections (UTI) or urinary symptoms. Interestingly, when the index patient exhibits dysfunctional voiding—incontinence due to bladder hyperactivity or sphincter dyssynergia—the incidence of reflux in siblings drops to 20 per cent

compared with 38 per cent in siblings of those without symptoms of bladder dysfunction (Noe, 1988). Reflux was more likely to occur in the siblings of patients with urographic evidence of renal damage, irrespective of the sex of the patient. Prevalence of both reflux and renal scarring is therefore estimated to be at least ten times greater in siblings of school-aged children with known reflux than in an unselected age-matched population (Lancet editorial, 1978).

Because the high incidence of reflux in the siblings of patients with reflux is now well established, some type of sibling screening is recommended (Van den Abbeele, et al., 1987). A cystogram will detect all grades of reflux. Those with grades 2 and 3 reflux may then be maintained on antibacterial prophylaxis until the reflux stops. Children with more severe reflux can be more fully evaluated. Alternately, sonography may be utilized to screen the siblings. The presence of hydroureteronephrosis suggests high-grade reflux, which should be confirmed with a cystogram. Similarly, ureterectasis after voiding suggests reflux. If ultrasound is used to screen, reflux of grades 1 to 3 and possibly some higher grades will be missed. A conventional cystogram should then be performed if even a single infection occurs.

A review of 88 families at Christchurch Hospital revealed increased frequency of the genes HLA A9 and B12 in patients with end-stage renal disease due to renal scarring associated with reflux (Bailey and Wallace, 1978). In addition, Torres et al. (1980a), have found HLA B8 and BW15 more frequently in such patients. These genes may become "markers" for reflux. However, the pattern of genetic transmission remains undetermined. Most investigators favor a polygenic or mul-

Table 44–1. CAUSES OF REFLUX

Primary Cause	Mechanisms Resulting in Reflux
Short or absent intravesical ureter (primary reflux, ureteral ectopia lateralis, gaping or golf-hole orifice)	End on opening between ureter and bladder
Absence of adequate detrusor buttress	Congenital paraureteral bladder diverticulum
	Acquired paraureteral diverticulum (urethral obstruction)
	Weak and thin detrusor, as in flaccid neurogenic bladder or closed exstrophy
Cystitis-inflammation of the intravesical ureter	Alone, this probably rarely results in reflux, but it operates with any of the factors listed above when the ureterovesical junction is of marginal competence
Ectopic ureter High intravesical pressure Iatrogenic reflux	Mechanisms described in text

tifactorial mode of inheritance (King, 1976; Lancet editorial, 1982). However, an autosomal dominant or a sex-linked mode of inheritance is suggested in some families (Lewy and Belman, 1975). Also of interest from a genetic standpoint is the observation that reflux is perhaps only one tenth as common in black American girls with infection compared with white American girls (Askari and Belman, 1981).

Reflux can be intermittent, unilateral, or bilateral. Failure to demonstrate reflux during a single cystogram does not preclude its presence. Conversely, the observation of minor degrees of transient reflux on a single examination is of limited significance.

Diagnosis of Reflux

Reflux can be detected at the time of cystoscopy by filling the bladder with a solution containing methylene blue or indigo carmine and then noting the color of the efflux from each ureteral orifice after the bladder is emptied and refilled with clear sterile water (Amar, 1966). Sonography can be employed to detect severe reflux, as the ureter will appear more dilated during and immediately after voiding.

Reflux may be suspected from the appearance of the kidneys and ureters on intravenous urography. In particular, a dilated lower ureter, a ureter visible for its entire length, ureteral or pelvic striations from redundant mucosa, vascular markings on the ureter, hydronephrosis, calyceal distortion, and renal scarring may be clues to the presence of vesicoureteral reflux or its existence in the past. With the aid of fluoroscopy during voiding after intravenous pyelography, it is often possible to detect vesicoureteral reflux with a high degree of certainty. However, retrograde cystography remains the most sensitive and accurate study to detect or exclude reflux.

Cystography

Cystography is performed prior to intravenous pyelography in order to avoid confusion about the source of contrast material in the upper tracts. Cystography involves the insertion of a catheter into the bladder after a preliminary radiograph of the abdomen has been obtained; the bladder is filled with a radiopaque solution from a drip chamber approximately 60 to 80 cm above the pubic symphysis. Radiographs are taken with the patient in the supine position and the right and left lateral oblique projections. Additional films are exposed during and after voiding. Fluoroscopy and cineradiographic equipment facilitate the voiding portion of the study and maximize the amount of information obtainable. In particular, observation of the presence of posterior urethral valves and dynamic changes in the configuration of ureteroceles, bladder diverticula, and ureteral duplications during voiding are critical to proper patient management when these related anomalies are present.

Variations in the technique of cystography are numerous. Delayed films are useful when reflux is intermittent or when the patient is unable to void during the examination. Expression cystography using anesthesia may demonstrate reflux in patients who do not demonstrate reflux while awake (Woodard and Filardi, 1976) and vice versa (Timmons et al., 1977; Vlahakis et al., 1971).

Timmons found that in 23 of 67 refluxing ureters, reflux was detected only with the patient awake. In five instances, however, reflux was detected only with the patient anesthetized. Depending upon the filling pressure and volume, reflux using anesthesia may not be representative of the usual behavior of the ureterovesical junction being studied. Various anesthetic agents may influence bladder tone and capacity (Doyle and Briscoe, 1976). Nevertheless, this technique can be of assistance with the uncooperative patient.

A distinction is often made between reflux seen during the filling phase and that seen only during voiding. The implication is that reflux seen only during voiding is occurring at higher intravesical pressures and is therefore less likely to be associated with a relatively severe degree of derangement of the ureterovesical junction than is reflux seen in the filling phase. Because the child is in very abnormal surroundings during cystography, however, this is not necessarily the case. The patient is likely to contract the bladder to resist filling, and usually he or she then can develop a high intravesical pressure—higher than that at which voiding normally occurs if no urethral obstruction is present.

Conway and Kruglik (1976), using isotope techniques for cystography in which the entire urinary tract is visualized throughout the examination, found that reflux occurring only during the filling phase is three times as common as reflux occurring only during the voiding phase. Thus, in many children the intravesical pressure is higher during the filling phase than during the voiding phase. Unless the intravesical pressure is monitored during the cystogram, cystoscopic evaluation of the refluxing ureterovesical junction (to determine orifice position and morphology and to permit estimation of the length of the intravesical ureter) is a more accurate means to gauge the prognosis for spontaneous cessation of reflux.

Timing of the cystogram in relationship to the presence of infection must be taken into consideration, because inflammation of the intravesical ureter or the overlying mucosa may reduce the compliance of the roof of the ureter and result in transient reflux at normal voiding pressures. Some evidence exists that intravesical pressure is sometimes elevated during acute infections (Van Gool and Tanagho, 1977). Therefore, an infection-free interval of 2 to 4 weeks is often recommended before the cystogram is performed.

When the severity of the infection is worrisome, or when the patient may not be followed after discharge, earlier cystography is not harmful. Transient reflux is usually not severe in degree and does not suggest the need for surgical correction. Additionally, once reflux is detected antibacterial therapy is continued, reducing the risk of re-infection after the therapy is discontinued. Mild reflux resulting from cystitis usually resolves quickly after the infection is eliminated. Reflux of higher grades will require further evaluation.

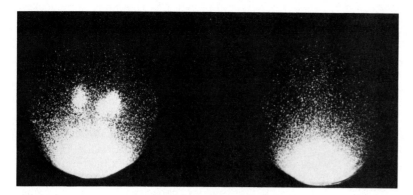

Figure 44–6. Preoperative and postoperative nuclear cystograms. Bilateral reflux, evident on the initial study *(left)* is absent 6 months following surgery.

Radionuclide Scanning

Radionuclide cystography in the detection of vesicoureteral reflux is an attractive alternative to conventional cystography (Conway et al., 1972, 1975; Conway and Kruglik, 1976; Winter, 1959). Approximately 1 μC of ^{99m}Tc-pertechnetate is instilled into the bladder through a catheter, and the bladder is filled slowly with normal saline. The urinary tract is continuously monitored on a persistence scope attachment to the scintillation camera. Images are recorded on Polaroid film at intervals. The special advantage of this technique is that it allows continuous monitoring of the patient with minimal radiation exposure. The limitation of radionuclide cystography is that the resolution of the image does not approach that of roentgenography. Abnormalities of the urethra and bladder, or reflux into the distal ureter only, may not be appreciated.

Nuclear cystography is especially useful in following patients with known reflux and in verifying that reflux is indeed absent after antireflux surgery (Fig. 44–6). In following patients with reflux, radioactive emissions are counted continuously over various areas of the abdomen, allowing ready calculation of the bladder volume at which reflux begins or ceases, the volume of the reflux, the rate of upper tract drainage (renogram), and the residual urine after voiding. A real benefit occurs in recording these parameters, because the bladder volume at which reflux begins is significant in predicting when reflux will cease (Fig. 44–7).

Classification and Grading of Reflux

Classification of the degree of reflux is as important clinically as determination of its presence. Reflux as demonstrated by cystography can be readily graded on a scale of increasing severity of 1 to 4 (Dwoskin and Perlmutter, 1973). Grade 1 represents lower ureteral filling only; grade 2A represents ureteral and pelvicalyceal filling without dilatation; grade 2B represents pelvicalyceal filling with mild calyceal blunting; grade 3 represents ureteral and pelvicalyceal filling, calyceal clubbing, and minor to moderate pelvic dilatation without extreme ureteral tortuosity; and grade 4 represents massive ureteral dilatation and tortuosity. In general, the lower the grade of reflux, the greater the chance of spontaneous cessation (Fig. 44–8).

Several other grading systems have been proposed based on the severity of reflux judged from the cystogram (Heikel and Parkkulainen, 1966; Rolleston et al., 1975). Some have emphasized ureteral caliber as well as the degree of pelvicalyceal dilatation (Bridge and Roe, 1969; Howerton and Lich, 1963; Edelbrook and Mickelson, 1970), whereas other investigators have graded reflux according to bladder pressure (i.e., filling vs.

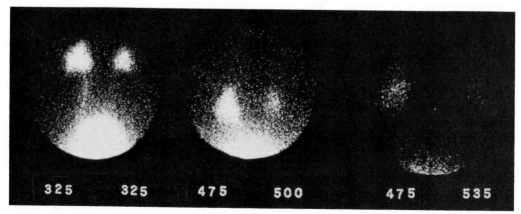

Figure 44–7. Nuclear cystograms are usually employed to follow children with known reflux. In this sequence, bilateral reflux was noted when the bladder had been filled to 325 ml. One year later, reflux did not begin on the right until 475 ml had been instilled. Mild reflux was noted on the left with 500 ml in the bladder. The next year, reflux was minimal. Increasing bladder volume before reflux occurs indicates growth of the intravesical ureter, as does a reduced volume of refluxed urine.

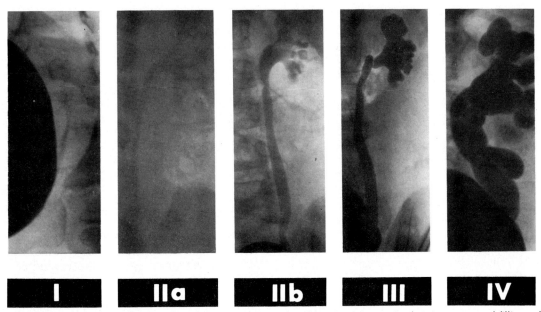

Figure 44–8. Classification of reflux according to the volume of urine seen to reflux on cystogram. Grade I: Lower ureteral filling only. Grade IIa: Ureteral and pelviocalyceal filling, without dilatation. Grade IIb: Ureteral and pelviocalyceal filling with mild calyceal blunting but without clubbing and without dilatation of the pelvis or tortuosity of the ureter. Grade III: Ureteral and pelviocalyceal filling, calyceal clubbing, and minor-to-moderate pelvic dilatation without tortuosity of the ureter. Grade IV: Massive ureteral dilatation and tortuosity. (From Dwoskin, J. Y., and Perlmutter, A. D.: J. Urol., 109:888, 1973.)

voiding) (Lattimer et al., 1963; Melick et al., 1962; Smellie et al., 1968).

An international grading system has come into general use and provides a common standard for the assessment of the severity of reflux, thereby allowing for more objective comparison of therapeutic modalities. This international grading system is based primarily on the appearance of the calyx on the cystogram (Fig. 44–9). Although the degree of dilatation of the ureter usually parallels the degree of dilatation of the pyelocalyceal system, this is not always the case. In the awake child, the intravesical pressure may be considerably higher than the normal voiding pressure during the cystogram. Reflux may therefore at times be overgraded in systems of this type.

The overall prognostic factors of importance in grading reflux are (1) the degree of hydronephrosis seen on the cystogram; (2) the degree of laterality of the orifice within the bladder; (3) the morphology of the orifice in the Lyon classification (1969); (4) the estimated length and width of the intravesical ureter; (5) the age of the patient, reflecting potential for growth of the intravesical ureter; and (6) the presence or absence of other factors that may cause or contribute to reflux, such as bladder outlet obstruction or neurogenic bladder (see Table 44–1).

Any of these factors may be used as guides in deciding whether reflux is likely to persist after full growth has been achieved. Any one factor may at times be misleading, so it is safest to assess several factors in deciding whether a trial of nonoperative therapy is warranted. The exception is mild reflux in an infant or a younger child, in whom cystoscopic evaluation is now usually deemed unnecessary.

Steele and colleagues (1989) followed 13 neonates in whom hydronephrosis during fetal development was found after birth to be due to severe reflux. One baby with bilateral grade 4 reflux developed a breakthrough infection and underwent ureteral reimplantations at 1 year of age. Of these patients, 12 did not have surgery. In nine, the reflux stopped completely before 2 years of age. Reflux resolved in four of seven with grade 5 reflux, and in four of five with grade 4 reflux. A similar experience was reported by Bloom and Bennett (1986).

These observations emphasize how quickly reflux may subside with growth of the intravesical ureter, particularly in infants.

The cystogram, particularly a single cystogram, may fail to detect primary reflux. The degree of ureterectasis, which influences grading, is subject to variation because of the bladder pressure at the time of each film and therefore may be quite inconsistent. The degree of orifice laterality is a fairly dependable concept but is difficult to judge at cystoscopy because of the absence of local landmarks. It may be determined in conjunction with an estimation of the length and diameter of the intravesical ureter. These, however, are also subjective measurements, made by inserting a ureteral catheter

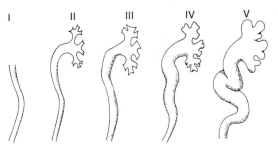

Figure 44–9. International classification of reflux.

into the orifice and estimating the length of intravesical ureter elevated by the catheter until it passes through the hiatus (Fig. 44–10). Because a 4:1 or 5:1 ratio of length to width in the intravesical ureter is necessary to prevent reflux (Paquin, 1959), diameter must be estimated also.

The morphology of the refluxing orifice is simpler to determine, although the appearance of the orifice may change with the degree of bladder filling. Many horseshoe and stadium orifices do not reflux. Age is important in the equation because the more growth potential remains (the younger the child), the more likely it is that defects in the ureterovesical junction will eventually correct themselves. Although small paraureteral diverticula may vanish with time, larger diverticula and ureters entering such diverticula will require surgical correction. Although an obstruction, such as a urethral valve, may be relieved, resulting in cessation of reflux, recurrent cystitis may dictate early antireflux surgery in a not always successful attempt (Govan et al., 1975) to protect the kidneys from pyelonephritic scarring and atropy.

In general, the classification of reflux and the decision to recommend or withhold ureteral reimplantation depend on an assessment of all the foregoing factors. The presence of pyelonephritic scarring, as distinct from a thin renal parenchyma, is considered by some as an indication for early surgery. This guideline is not recommended. If renal scarring is already present, the increased risk of late hypertension is established. Such kidneys may be hydronephrotic and reflux tends to be high grade. Both are relative indications for antireflux surgery. However, reflux is probably as likely to stop with growth in the presence of such scars as in instances in which the kidneys are normal (King, 1983).

Residual urine predisposes the patient to UTI. Urine that refluxes during voiding soon returns to the bladder and makes continuous antibacterial therapy necessary, if recurrent infection are to be prevented.

Relative indications for early surgery are grade 4 or grade 5 reflux (international classification) in an older child; lateral, golf-hole, or horseshoe orifice with a short (2 to 5 mm) or absent intravesical ureter or refusal to take long-term antibacterial prophylaxis. Recurrences of infection or progressive renal scarring mandate antireflux surgery.

Factors suggesting that reflux will cease with growth and will not impede renal development or function include grade 3 reflux or less; orifice in the "B" or "C" position with a stadium or horseshoe configuration; intravesical ureter more than 5 mm in length; relatively young child; and freedom from obstruction or infection. The need for a safe chemotherapeutic agent to keep the urine clear is not viewed as a contraindication to nonoperative management, but those children with a tendency toward asymptomatic reinfection must be followed very carefully. Home urine cultures, such as those done with Uricult tubes, are a great help in this regard.

Primary Reflux

If the normal position of the ureteral orifice on the corner of the trigone is designated as the "A" position, orifices that are progressively more lateral than normal can be designated as "B," "C," and "D," in order of increasing laterality (Lyon et al., 1969; Mackie and Stephens, 1975). The "D" position represents an orifice that opens on the edge of (D_1) or into (D_2) a diverticulum. In general, the more lateral the orifice, the more gaping and abnormal its appearance cystoscopically; the shorter its effective submucosal course, the more prone it is to reflux (Fig. 44–11).

Such lateral ectopia has been explained in two ways:

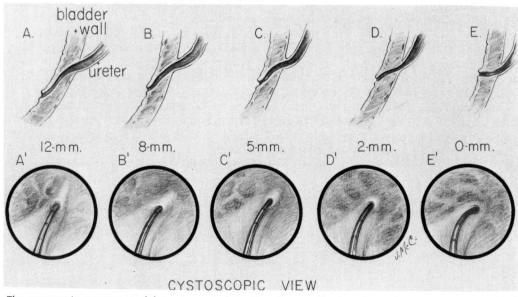

Figure 44–10. The cystoscopic appearance of the ureterovesical junction. A ureteral catheter is used to estimate the length of the submucosal tunnel. The ureter is drawn as normal in diameter to emphasize the appearance of the flap elevated by the catheter. (From Kelalis, P. P., and King, L. R. (Eds.): Clinical Pediatric Urology. Philadelphia, W. B. Saunders Co., 1976.)

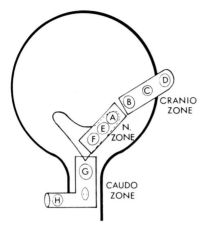

Figure 44–11. Diagram of bladder and urethra showing three zones of ureteral orifices. A, E, and F, Normal zone. B, C, and D, Lateral in cranio zone (D in diverticulum). G and H, Caudo zone with G in urethra and H in sex ducts. (From Mackie, G. G., and Stephens, F. D.: J. Urol., 114:274, 1975.)

first, as a result of intrinsic weakness in the muscular attachment of the terminal ureter to the trigone (Tanagho, 1976), and second, as a consequence of an abnormality in the location of the ureteral bud on the wolffian duct (Ambrose and Nicolson, 1964; Stephens, 1976). The first explanation is a functional one based on physiologic observations and animal experimentation. The second is a pathoembryologic explanation based on the correlation of clinical and post-mortem observations with the embryology of the ureter.

Both provide a framework for viewing the phenomenon of reflux as a manifestation of a primary abnormality of the ureterovesical junction caused by a deficiency in the longitudinal muscle of the submucosal ureter. Because the incidence of reflux decreases with age, it is apparent that certain defects that allow reflux to occur in childhood may correct themselves with growth and development. This concept of primary reflux and the knowledge that it may subside spontaneously form the foundation for the nonoperative management of vesicoureteral reflux.

Further considerations in formulating a program of patient care include whether or not reflux itself poses a threat to renal function, either directly or indirectly. The potential coexistence of reflux with urinary tract infection, lower urinary obstruction or dysfunction, and renal hypoplasia or dysplasia contributes to the complexity of this problem. Each aspect must be reviewed before a rational plan of treatment can be outlined.

Embryology and Association Between Primary Reflux and Abnormal Renal Morphology and Function

The embryology of the urinary tract is described in Chapter 32. Stephens in 1976, particularly, and again in 1980 described how an abnormal ureteral bud site may result in reflux or obstruction and abnormal development or dysgenesis of the kidney or renal segment subtended by the displaced ureteral bud. The association of segmental renal hypoplasia and dysplasia in kidneys with total duplication of the ureters that arise from cranially or caudally ectopic ureteral buds supports the view that the position at which the ureteral bud contacts the metanephric blastema determines the quality of the kidney that results (Fig. 44–12).

Sommer and Stephens (1981) examined the role of the position of the orifice associated with dysplasia and renal scarring in children with reflux compared with those with partial ureteral obstruction but no reflux. The groups had comparable degrees of calycectasis. Histologic examination of the kidneys of those with partial obstruction revealed obstructive atrophy but not dysplasia. Only refluxing renal units with abnormal orifice sites contained dysplastic elements. The investigators believe that these findings support the concept of renal parenchymal maldevelopment occurring pari passu with reflux, and they concluded that the renal changes seen in patients with reflux are developmental or secondary to superimposed infection but not to hydrodynamic effects of the reflux.

In this sense, therefore, primary reflux results from

Figure 44–12. Relationship of orifice zones in bladder and urethra and points of origin from wolffian duct is shown, as well as relationship of bud positions on wolffian duct and nephrogenic blastema. (From Mackie, G. G., and Stephens, F. D.: J. Urol., 114:274, 1975.)

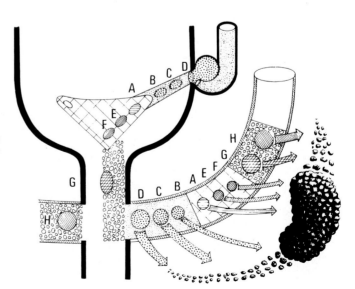

the site of the ureteral bud, determined in the 4th week of gestation. Further, the reflux itself probably has little or no effect on the kidney, as faulty induction of the metanephros is ordained when the displaced ureteral bud fails to contact the renal blastema near enough to the normal junction site to permit formation of a normal kidney.

These embryologic studies explain the association between reflux and renal anomalies that result in poor renal function at birth or progressive renal deterioration in later life in the absence of any history of urinary infection or obstruction as an obvious cause. Such faulty kidneys may be adequate to support life in childhood and even to sustain nearly normal growth and development for a time, but they remain abnormal and may be unable to grow to meet the load imposed by an ever-increasing body mass. Renal failure is not uncommon in these patients at puberty or when nearly full growth has been achieved. Anemia, hypertension, lethargy, or growth arrest results in the discovery of the problem, and the reflux may then be detected for the first time.

Other factors may operate to produce acquired vesicoureteral reflux or to increase voiding pressure, which markedly worsens the degree of existing reflux. Sphincter dyssynergia and forceful inappropriate involuntary voiding contractions are two commonly acquired conditions that may have this effect.

Hyperactive Bladder and Detrusor-Sphincter Dyssynergia

Hinman and Baumann described reflux voiding dysfunction and renal damage in boys without anatomic obstruction or abnormal bladder innervation in 1973. Allen expanded upon these observations in 1977, naming the syndrome the "non-neurogenic neurogenic bladder."

This condition clearly seems to be acquired and has not been recognized in neurologically intact infants or very young children. It may result from early and forceful efforts at toilet training or from dysurea accompanying urinary infection. Such a syndrome is also often recognized in children in very dysfunctional family situations. Most commonly, such children present with inappropriate wetting during the day, but some present with only a history of urinary infections. Upon investigation, they are often found to have vesicoureteral reflux, frequently associated with otherwise unexplained bladder trabeculation with or without bladder decompensation and residual urine. The diagnosis is partly one of exclusion of infravesical obstruction and is confirmed by the persistent presence of spontaneous bladder contractions on cystometric studies, failure of one or both sphincters to open during voiding, or both. Sphincter dyssynergia especially is associated with high intravesical pressures, at least during voiding, and if reflux is present, these pressures may be transmitted to the upper tract, causing increased dilatation. If reflux is initially absent, the resultant detrusor hypertrophy and elevated intravesical pressures may result in periureteral diverticula breaking down the normal antireflux mechanism and

resulting in reflux, which becomes progressively worse if the condition persists.

Bladder hyperreflexia, instability, and noncompliance are other causes of relatively elevated intravesical pressures. The pressure may rise quite rapidly as the resting bladder begins to fill (Glassberg, 1982; Koff and Murtagh, 1983). If reflux is present, these pressures are transmitted to the kidney, increasing the degree of hydronephrosis.

In 1983, King reported on several patients in whom sphincter dyssynergia superimposed upon mild reflux resulted in renal damage when breakthrough UTI occurred. Bladder dysfunction was noted to prejudice the result of anti-reflux surgery, as reported by Allen (1977, 1978).

Koff and Murtagh (1983) followed 32 neurologically intact children with reflux and uninhibited bladder contractions and dyssynergia for 2 to 6 years. These investigators compared them to age-matched controls with reflux and normal bladder function. All but eight with uninhibited contractions were treated with anticholinergics, and all were maintained on antibacterial prophylaxis. Reflux resolved in 44 per cent of those with treated uninhibited bladder contractions but in only 17 per cent of controls, over this time span. Grades 4 and 5 reflux resolved only in those with uninhibited contractions. Further, anti-reflux surgery, performed for breakthrough infections, was required in only 33 per cent of those with impairment of bladder function versus 57 per cent of the control group.

Homsy and associates (1985) randomly selected 40 children with persistent reflux for full urodynamic assessment, and all had some degree of hyperreflexia with or without vesicoperineal dyssynergia. Of these children, 37 could be treated with oxybutynin for 3 to 18 months and were followed for at least 30 months. Reflux disappeared in 51 per cent of ureters and improved to grade 1 in 11.3 per cent. In 27 children with obvious incontinence initially, reflux resolved in 68.4 per cent and became grade 1 in 10.2 per cent. In seven of the children in whom reflux disappeared, incontinence recurred after medication was stopped. Mild reflux recurred as well. These findings particularly underscore the role of bladder hyperactivity in at least some patients with reflux.

Griffiths and Scholtmeijer (1987) found two contrasting patient populations with reflux in a review of 458 children who were evaluated urodynamically. One type exhibited bladder instability with strong spontaneous contractions and usually unilateral reflux. It was as if the unilateral reflux served as a "blow-off valve," perhaps lowering intravesical pressure and preventing contralateral reflux as seen in many children with urethral valves. Reflux nephropathy was measured in this group. The other patient population tended to have stable bladders with poor continuity and hyperactive sphincters. Reflux was usually bilateral, and reflux nephropathy or hydronephrosis was common.

Seruca (1989) evaluated 53 neurologically intact children with reflux urodynamically. All patients had elevated bladder pressures during filling or voiding, and many exhibited abnormal perineal muscle activity (vesicoperineal incoordination). They were treated with baclofen, flavoxate, dicyclomine, and diazepam according to the urodynamic abnormalty, as well as with antibacterial prophylaxis. Of these children, 39 had frequency, urgency, hesitancy, or discomfort on voiding, and ten were too young to permit evaluation of symptoms. Children were followed for 2 to 5 years. Reflux stopped in 91.8 per cent of refluxing ureters and decreased in the remainder. Repeated urodynamic studies at the end of treatment documented normal bladder function in 46 of the children. This group did much better than a previous cohort, in whom reflux stopped in only 53.7 per cent, while they were followed with antibacterial therapy only.

These observations suggest that bladder hyperreflexia with or without sphincter dyssynergia is common in the younger child after toilet training has apparently been achieved. Elevated intravesical pressure worsens the degree of reflux and may even produce reflux when the intravesical ureter is only marginally competent. Such children clearly benefit from appropriate pharmacotherapy. Clinically, the presence of incontinence, without infection, or unexplained bladder trabeculation, should lead the urologist to suspect bladder dysfunction in any case. Urodynamic evaluation may be difficult in the younger child, but trials of anticholinergic or alpha-adrenergic agents may result in symptomatic improvement as well as in the cessation of reflux.

The increased rate of surgical complications—recurrent reflux and obstruction—when refluxing ureters are reimplanted into the overt neurogenic or non-neurogenic neurogenic bladder is an additional incentive to pursue appropriate medical therapy to normalize bladder function. If significant reflux persists, antireflux surgery can then be accomplished without the greater risk of an unfavorable result.

Urinary Tract Infection

Urinary tract infection is the problem most closely associated with vesicoureteral reflux. Reflux is more commonly diagnosed in boys during infancy and in girls during early childhood, peaking at 3 to 7 years of age. Reflux, usually mild in degree, has been noted to occur clinically in association with acute urinary tract infection and to disappear when the urine becomes sterile. Thus, inflammation of the ureterovesical junction can contribute to the occurrence of reflux.

Conversely, severe reflux predisposes the patient to urinary infection, because it provides a reservoir of residual urine. Thus, although infection causes the transient occurrence of reflux when the ureterovesical junction is marginally competent, it does not play a crucial role in reflux in the majority of cases, especially in those with more severe degrees of reflux and with hydronephrosis as seen on the intravenous urogram. It is not uncommon to find the marginal ureterovesical junction refluxing during episodes of acute cystitis. This is not an important cause of reflux, because the kidneys are normal as seen on intravenous pyelograms; ureterectasis is slight; and reflux abates soon after infection is eliminated.

The incidence of recurrent urinary tract infection in children without reflux or in children in whom reflux has been surgically corrected does not differ greatly from that in children with reflux. However, the incidence of clinical pyelonephritis is greatly reduced by the correction of rcflux in children prone to recurrent infection. The danger posed by vesicoureteral reflux is its potential to convert lower urinary tract infection into pyelonephritis with consequent renal damage (Fair and Govan, 1976; Govan et al., 1975).

Infection, superimposed on vesicoureteral reflux, may arrest the normal development of the kidney. Sequential measurements of renal length alone may be employed to assess renal growth, but the length of normal kidneys has been shown to be affected by numerous factors (Hernandez et al., 1979). Hypertrophy of the intervening normal renal parenchyma and the predominantly polar distribution of renal scars make interpretation of renal size using length alone inaccurate and somewhat unreliable. Most studies of renal growth in kidneys with reflux suffer from this deficient methodology (Redman et al., 1974).

Claësson et al. (1980, 1981) critically addressed the question of how to best measure renal parenchymal volume. They devised a nomogram to compare observed and expected renal mass derived from several measurements taken from the urogram. Further work by the same group has produced a technique of computerized planimetry to measure total renal parenchymal area in units of square centimeters. Such measurements provide considerable anatomic detail, as areas of compensatory hypertrophy are indexed and sequential measurements can be accurately compared.

Renal scans can also be utilized to estimate the function of the individual kidney. The function can be calculated from the uptake of Hippuran I131, measuring effective renal plasma flow, or ^{99m}Tc DTPA (technetium-99m-diethylenetriaminepentacetic acid), estimating glomerular filtration rate. 2,3 Dimercaptosuccinic acid (DMSA) provides good anatomic detail when compared with the aforementioned compounds and can reveal small areas of diminished renal function that are not detectable on conventional urography. In addition, DMSA uptake can be utilized to calculate unilateral renal function. At present, however, no ideal technique for the measurement of renal mass is available.

On the one hand, given the shortcomings of bipolar renal length measurements, Lyon (1973) and Redman and co-workers (1974) observed a subnormal rate of renal growth in the presence of reflux without documented urine infection. Kelalis (1971), on the other hand, reported resumption of growth in kidneys with reflux after infection alone had been eliminated.

Longitudinal measurements of bipolar renal length were used by Smellie and associates (1981) to monitor the effects of reflux on the kidney in a series of 76 children with persistent reflux of varying grades. Renal growth was impaired (bipolar length less than half the increment expected for the child's linear growth) in only five of 93 kidneys drained by undilated ureters. Of the 18 kidneys drained by a dilated ureter, six had growth impairment; however, five were already scarred at the time of clinical presentation. The sixth developed new renal scarring. All patients had episodes of documented infection. The overall relationship among the grade of reflux, the presence of infection, and the rate of renal growth can be summarized as follows: If no infection or obstruction is present, normal renal growth can be expected. Renal growth is retarded in about half the refluxing cases with chronic or recurrent episodes of infection. The more severe the reflux, the greater the likelihood of renal growth impairment.

The effect of antireflux surgery on renal growth has been examined by several investigators. McRae and colleagues (1974) reported accelerated growth after successful surgery. Babcock and co-workers (1976), considering the effects of unilateral reflux, observed neither a radiographic improvement nor a change in the ratio of size in the refluxing kidney compared with the normal contralateral kidney after elimination of reflux. In comparison, Willscher and associates (1976a) demonstrated normal rates of growth in nonscarred kidneys with severe reflux. However, these kidneys showed accelerated growth after surgical elimination of the reflux. Where renal scarring was present, this accelerated pattern of growth following surgery was seen only in patients with bilateral scarring. Murnaghan (1980) observed significant focal nodular parenchymal hypertrophy in two postpubertal patients following successful

antireflux surgery. In addition, somatic growth of prepubertal children with reflux has been observed to accelerate after successful surgical correction (Merrell and Mowad, 1979). However, physical growth alone, particularly during puberty, may account for the increased renal growth rate that has been observed (Claësson et al., 1981).

In 1960, Hodson and Edwards studied the association between reflux and renal scarring. Such renal damage takes three forms on urography: (1) characteristic focal pyelonephritic scarring, in which the contracted parenchyma is seen as a dimple on the outer perimeter of the renal shadow, the clubbed calyx being directly beneath; (2) generalized calyceal dilatation and parenchymal atrophy (Fig. 44–13); and (3) failure of renal growth with the kidney smaller than expected, often associated with either focal scarring or generalized atrophy. *Reflux nephropathy* has been suggested as a preferable term for the scarred kidney associated with reflux. Hypertension, proteinuria, reduced renal function, or any combination of these may also be present.

Radiographic evidence of scarring is almost always accompanied by reflux. In some instances, the scars may be evidence of reflux that has subsequently stopped because of growth of the intravesical ureter. Conversely, between 30 and 60 per cent of children with reflux are found to have renal scarring. The higher figure is derived

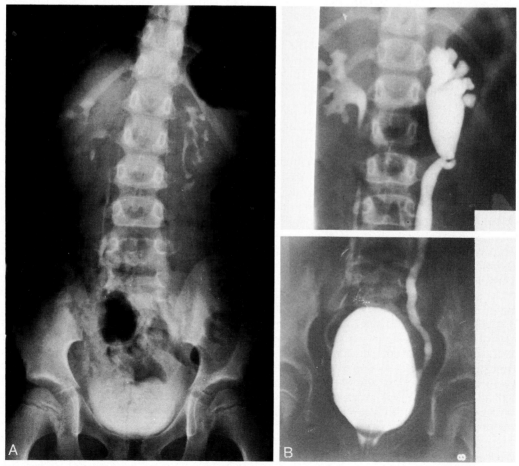

Figure 44–13. *A,* Small atrophic-appearing kidney with clubbed calyces on intravenous pyelography. This appearance is almost invariably associated with reflux and a history of superimposed infection. *B,* The reflux is demonstrated on cystogram.

from data originating in surgical clinics (Williams and Eckstein, 1965), the lower from medical surveys (Smellie and Normand, 1979). Sterile reflux alone may be sufficient to cause renal scarring (Rolleston et al., 1975). Nevertheless, the appearance of fresh scars or the extension of established scars in the absence of obstruction, neuropathic bladder, or sphincter dyssynergia has been documented only in children with urinary infection. Smellie (1975b) reported no new scars in 150 normal or scarred kidneys in children with uncomplicated primary reflux in whom low-dose chemoprophylaxis was successful in maintaining sterile urine. In an additional group of 121 normal or scarred kidneys with reflux, only two developed a new scar when the children were maintained on continuous low-dose therapy for a 7- to 15-year follow-up period (Edwards et al., 1977). Both cases were associated with breakthrough infections. Both had a moderate-to-severe degree of reflux.

Lenaghan and co-workers (1976) used intermittent short courses of antibacterial drugs for the treatment of recurrent infection in 102 children with reflux. In 76 kidneys that were initially normal, scarring developed in 16 (21 per cent). Of 44 kidneys with established scars, 29 worsened (66 per cent). Filly and colleagues (1974) observed two new scars in 16 initially normal kidneys with reflux while the children were on "intermittent" therapy. However, scars also developed in two of 15 (13 per cent) initially normal kidneys in which reflux was not demonstrated. Cystoscopic examination of these latter cases demonstrated poorly muscularized ureteral orifices, suggesting that reflux may have been present at some time in the past. Some 15 of 24 (62 per cent) initially scarred kidneys showed progression of scarring. Intermittent antibacterial therapy does not protect against renal scarring; thus, the need for safe, low-dose, continuous antibacterial therapy seems clear in the follow-up of children with known reflux.

A history of bacteriuria can often be elicited in children with reflux and scarring. The higher the grade of reflux, the more likely is the occurrence of new or progressive scarring associated with recurrent urinary infection (Rolleston et al., 1970). The radiographic appearance of renal scarring develops over a period of at least 8 months (Hodson et al., 1975). It is sometimes difficult to determine whether earlier scars actually worsen or simply become more obvious as the surrounding healthy renal parenchyma hypertrophies.

If renal scars occur in conjunction with reflux, they are usually present at the time of the initial intravenous pyelogram. Some investigators believe that scars rarely occur in kidneys after infancy and that, when present, they seldom progress even when reflux and infection coexist (Ransley and Risdon, 1981). Older children who have sphincter dyssynergia, bladder instability, or noncompliant bladders are at risk for renal scarring when reflux is also present, however (Koff et al., 1979b). If reflux is present together with unrecognized obstruction, progressive renal damage is the rule.

Experimental Studies

Reflux is always present in the rat and is normal in many other rodents. Reflux is also often observed in rabbits and dogs (Winter, 1959). When absent, it can be induced by incising the trigone (Tanagho et al., 1965); by crushing a part of the bladder and introducing bacteria causing chronic cystitis (Schoenberg et al., 1964); or by interfering with the innervation of the trigone as is sometimes seen clinically following lumbar sympathectomy (Tanagho, 1976). Resection of the roof of the submucosal tunnel will also consistently result in reflux. The adage that "reflux, if present, may be demonstrated only intermittently" is probably even more true in animals than in humans (Winter, 1959). Jeffs and Allen (1962) as well as Kaveggia and associates (1966) induced acute pyelonephritis by the introduction of bacteria through a nephrostomy tube. They were able to produce reflux without direct manipulation of the normal ureteral vesical junction in puppies and dogs. Contralateral reflux often occurred as well. These investigations suggest that reflux can be caused by pyelonephritis and bacteria in the absence of disease of the bladder or urethra. Boyarsky's demonstration of the toxic effect of bacteria on the ureter, with consequent interference with normal peristalsis, may explain this effect, because normal peristalsis is known to be one of the defense mechanisms that protects against reflux in the human (Boyarsky and Labay, 1972). Grana and co-workers (1965) found *Escherichia coli* exotoxins particularly effective in ablating peristalsis.

Experimental work in the pathogenesis of renal scarring has centered on the concept of intrarenal reflux (IRR). This is defined as reflux of urine into the collecting tubules and parenchyma. IRR provides a readily apparent mechanism whereby urinary microorganisms can gain access to the renal parenchyma and produce renal scarring. Roberts and colleagues (1982) produced IRR in primates with a bacterial inoculum in order to define the precise mechanism of tubular damage secondary to bacterial infection. Phagocytosis of bacteria by invading neutrophils produces superoxide, an enzyme toxic to renal tubular cells. Administration of superoxide dismutase, an antagonist of superoxide, seemed successful in preventing renal tubular cell damage histologically but did not interfere with phagocytosis. Thus, the work of these investigators suggests that the inflammatory response itself, while eliminating invading bacteria by neutrophil phagocytosis, also produces the irreversible damage in the renal tissue.

Besides inflammation of the parenchyma due to bacterial infection, other mechanisms have been proposed to explain the pathogenesis of scar formation. Cotran and colleagues (1981) have investigated the role of Tamm-Horsfall protein (THP). This mucoprotein is produced in high concentration by the tubular epithelial cells in the loop of Henle and distal nephron. THP is a primary constituent of renal tubular casts. Immunofluorescent techniques have demonstrated extratubular THP in the interstitium of kidneys with intrarenal reflux. Extratubular THP, therefore, may serve as a marker of urinary extravasation.

Experimental studies by Ransley and Risdon (1978) and Tamminen and Kaprio (1977) indicate that the areas of renal parenchyma susceptible to intrarenal reflux and subsequent scarring are drained by flat, concave, or compound papillae, which occur predominantly in the

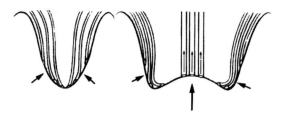

Figure 44–14. Papillary factors in intrarenal reflux. *A,* Convex papilla (nonrefluxing papilla)—crescentic or slit-like openings of collecting ducts opening obliquely onto the papilla. *B,* Concave or flat papilla (refluxing papilla)—collecting ducts opening at right angles onto flat papilla. (From Ransley, P. G., and Risdon, R. A.: Br. J. Radiol. [Suppl.], 14:1, 1978.)

polar regions of the human kidney (Fig. 44–14). Among experimental animals, only pigs possess renal papillary morphology similar to that of humans. Thus, this animal has been used to study the mechanism of intrarenal reflux and renal scarring. Studies suggest that in the presence of infected urine, intrarenal reflux results in the development of scarring in less than 4 weeks. However, antimicrobial treatment, introduced after 1 week of urine infection in models that are prone to such scar formation, significantly reduces the extent of the scarring (Ransley and Risdon, 1981).

Hodson and co-workers (1975), also working with the pig model, demonstrated that focal scarring can be produced by sterile reflux but only in the presence of a sustained increase in intravesical pressure produced by incorporating ureteral obstruction into the refluxing model. Ransley and Risdon (1981), using three strains of pigs and sophisticated urodynamic monitoring, found that parenchymal scarring occurred only with sufficient bladder outlet obstruction, produced by a partially occluding urethral ring, which resulted in bladder decompensation. They concluded that during the relatively brief interval of high intravesical pressure without bladder decompensation, no lesions were produced. Once bladder decompensation supervened, scarring was induced. Thus, if these results can be extrapolated to humans, it seems unlikely that sterile reflux results in renal damage in the absence of significant obstruction. This conclusion correlates with almost all clinical observations.

Clinical Correlation

In the clinical context, intrarenal reflux has been defined radiographically as the appearance of contrast material in the renal parenchyma during the voiding cystourethrogram. However, visualization of intrarenal reflux may be difficult when the upper tracts are dilated and filled with nonopacified urine that dilutes the contrast material. Radiographic detection of intrarenal reflux almost certainly underestimates its true prevalence. Such reflux has been observed in 5 to 15 per cent of neonates and infants with reflux (Rolleston et al., 1974; Rose et al., 1975). Rolleston and associates (1975) reviewed the cystograms of several hundred children with reflux. Intrarenal reflux was detected only in chil-

dren under the age of 5 years and only in conjunction with moderate or severe degrees of reflux. A significant correlation was found between the presence of intrarenal reflux and the subsequent development of renal scarring in the affected area.

The more frequent detection of intrarenal reflux in neonates and infants with vesicoureteral reflux can be explained by the relatively large size of the collecting ducts, which allows better visualization of contrast material in the renal parenchyma. In older children in whom scarring has already occurred, parenchymal fibrosis may prevent intrarenal reflux into the affected segments. Studies of papillary morphology in human kidneys indicate that at least two thirds possess papillae of the type that may permit intrarenal reflux. Controversy exists concerning the clinical significance of intrarenal reflux in predicting the production of renal scars, however, as some infants who exhibit such reflux never develop scars.

The "big bang" theory of Ransley and Risdon (1978) attempts to reconcile the clinical, radiologic, and pathologic features of intrarenal reflux–related renal scarring in the majority of infants and children in whom the scars are already present on the initial urogram. These investigators suggest that the initial infection in the child with reflux and nonconical papillae results in pyelonephritic scarring of one or both poles. Because all susceptible segments of the kidney are generally affected simultaneously, sequential scar formation with subsequent infections is unusual. However, on occasion, marginally refluxing papillae may be transformed into the refluxing variety, accounting for new scarring with new infections as opposed to progressive contraction of the renal parenchyma following the initial insult.

Despite the very impressive evidence that the combination of moderate-to-severe vesicoureteral reflux, intrarenal reflux, and bacteriuria may result in pyelonephritic scarring, at least 30 to 40 per cent of patients investigated for renal insufficiency and found to have the radiographic features of reflux nephropathy have no history of a urinary infection. Family surveys of index patients with reflux regularly report other individuals with advanced reflux nephropathy who have no history of urinary tract symptomatology or infection. In addition, reflux nephropathy is often detected during the course of diagnostic evaluation for hypertension or proteinuria in the older child or young adult. Several mechanisms exist by which reflux nephropathy and end-stage renal disease associated with reflux may be produced, and it seems likely that each predominates in some patients.

From a clinical point of view, four possible explanations are made for renal failure in these patients without history of infection to account for severe reflux nephropathy: (1) asymptomatic infections in conjunction with reflux resulted in renal damage; (2) sterile reflux persisting over many years damaged the kidneys permanently; (3) renal damage occurred when an episode of sphincter dyssynergia or bladder hyperreflexia resulted in elevated voiding pressures, worsening reflux, and initiating or compounding of parenchymal damage; and (4) renal dysgenesis was present at birth, resulting in a relatively fixed renal mass, with renal failure occurring only when the kidneys were overwhelmed by ever-increasing body mass.

The embryologic studies cited earlier indicate that the last explanation is often the correct one. Children or adults may harbor urinary infections that cause so few symptoms that they are not perceived as infections. Most patients with such infections, however, will admit to some symptoms when closely questioned (unexplained fevers, urgency, enuresis, episodic incontinence, and the like), and the majority of such patients have no renal impairment. Similarly, functional urodynamic abnormalities that can result in elevated voiding pressure are not silent but are manifested by diurnal enuresis and poor urinary control. Usually, at least a few random urine specimens have been examined in childhood. If these were normal, it is difficult to imagine that intercurrent infections could often produce profound kidney damage without symptoms. Indirect evidence for this statement is derived from monitoring children with known reflux. Renal arrest, failure of the kidney to develop as expected (let alone atrophy), or onset of renal scarring is unknown in prospective studies in children, unless infection has recurred or obstruction was overlooked at the time of the initial evaluation.

Alternatively, even though primary reflux has been reported as an incidental finding in septuagenarians with normal for age renal function, the lifelong effect of reflux on renal function in the human is unknown and probably cannot be studied except in retrospect. It seems possible that when the ureter is of normal or nearly normal caliber, retrograde peristalsis damps the bladder pressure at which reflux occurs. When ureterectasis prevents coaptation of the ureter, renal dilatation and damage may occur very gradually, over a period of years.

Because the follow-up of patients with reflux is costly and time-consuming over a very long time, persistent reflux in the adult should usually be treated by anti-reflux surgery once the diagnosis has been established (Hawtrey et al., 1983).

The embryologic study of primary reflux implies that the common clinical association of abnormal renal structure and function with abnormal ureteral orifice position may represent faulty development of the derivatives of the nephrotome rather than progressive pathologic change secondary to hydrostatic effects or intervening infection.

Associated Anomalies

Neuropathic Bladder

An increased incidence of reflux occurs in individuals of any age with congenital or acquired neuropathic bladder. Although evidence exists in animals that interference with either the sympathetic or the parasympathetic innervation of the trigone and distal ureter can predispose an individual to reflux, clinically a combination of factors usually seems to be operative. In the presence of elevated intravesical pressure, trabeculation and paraureteral diverticulum formation associated with

functional bladder outlet obstruction can render the ureterovesical junction incompetent. The incomplete bladder emptying commonly associated with neuropathic bladder predisposes the patient to chronic urinary tract infection and the development of bladder calculi. These conditions promote edema and inflammation of the ureterovesical junction and may also alter its function, thus permitting reflux. In myelodysplasia there is also an increased incidence of concomitant urinary tract malformations, including the primary abnormalities of the ureterovesical junction associated with reflux (Hutch, 1962).

Bauer and associates (1984) have shown that babies with neurogenic bladder are at very high risk for reflux if sphincter dyssynergia is present on screening urodynamic studies.

Ureteropelvic Junction Obstruction Associated with Reflux

King reported nine children with reflux in whom an ipsilateral obstruction was also present at the ureteropelvic junction (UPJ). Lebowitz and Blickman (1983) point out that since both UPJ obstruction and reflux are relatively frequent, it is not surprising that these entities coexist. It is also possible that severe reflux occasionally causes disproportionate hypertrophy of the smooth muscle cells at the UPJ and secondary obstructions by this mechanism. Blickman observed such obstruction in 21 children over a 10-year period during which time about 2800 children were found to have reflux and 200 to have UPJ obstruction alone. About 10 per cent of children with UPJ obstructions, therefore, will be found to have reflux.

Significant UPJ obstruction in association with mild reflux can mimic severe reflux when viewed on the cystogram, but the operation needed is obviously not ureteral reimplantation but pyeloplasty. Conversely, when UPJ obstruction coexists with significant reflux, both operations may be necessary and can be done together. In this situation, I prefer to do the pyeloplasty first, leaving a catheter in the bladder for a few days postoperatively. If surgical correction of the reflux is deemed necessary, the reimplantation can be done safely during the same anesthetic procedure, by an intravesical ureteral advancement technique when the pyeloplasty proceeds well.

Cystography with appropriate films of postvoid drainage and an excretory urography or a renal scan with a catheter draining the bladder to prevent reflux are both necessary to quantitate the severity of each problem.

Associated Anomalies of the Ureterovesical Junction

Ureteral Duplication

An increased incidence of vesicoureteral reflux occurs in patients with complete duplication of the ureters. Following the Weigert-Meyer rule, in 97 per cent of cases the ureter draining the upper pole of the kidney opens into the vesicourethral canal, medial and caudal to the ureter draining the lower pole. Although reflux may affect either ureter, it is much more common in the ureter draining the lower pole because of the more lateral orifice of that ureter and its tendency to have only a short or absent submucosal tunnel. When the upper pole ureter demonstrates reflux despite its usually longer submucosal course, the defect often proves to be one of deficient muscularization of the submucosal ureter, or the orifices may be juxtaposed, both lacking sufficient intravesical ureteral length.

Although the presence of duplication does not preclude the spontaneous cessation of reflux, the orifice draining the middle and lower pole calyces is apt to be lateral and to have a golf-hole appearance; early surgical correction is often elected (King, 1976).

The study of total duplication of the ureters has illuminated the role of the ureteral bud in the differentiation of the kidney to a considerable degree.

Bladder Diverticulum

The other trigonal abnormality that is at times associated with reflux is vesical diverticulum. A diverticulum can be congenital or acquired and can occur anywhere in the bladder. An acquired diverticulum represents herniation of mucosa through an area of relatively deficient muscularization in the bladder wall in the presence of elevated intravesical pressure and bladder outlet obstruction. A congenital diverticulum, which is observed more commonly in children, is a similar herniation caused by incomplete muscularization in the presence of normal intravesical pressure, in an otherwise normal urinary tract. An acquired diverticulum is associated with gross trabeculation of the bladder and is secondary to anatomic or functional obstruction of the vesicourethral outlet, e.g., urethral valve, sphincter dyssynergia, neurogenic bladder, and similar entities.

The ureteral hiatus represents a potential weak spot in the posterolateral wall of the bladder and is analogous in this respect to the inguinal canal. This hiatus is the most common site of congenital and acquired diverticula. A diverticulum at or near the hiatus predisposes the patient to reflux, if it is large enough to impinge upon muscular support of the intravesical ureter. Spontaneous cessation of reflux in the presence of such a diverticulum is unusual. Early surgical correction of both lesions is generally indicated. However, small diverticula and associated reflux have been noted to disappear with growth during childhood (Colodny, 1983; King, 1976). Occasionally, a diverticulum may interfere with drainage of the ureter in addition to or instead of predisposing the individual to reflux. Surgical repair is indicated in such instances, unless renal function is so poor in the affected unit that nephroureterectomy, as well as diverticulectomy, becomes the treatment of choice.

Reflux and Renal Function

When reflux is relatively severe in degree and marked ureterectasis is present, the voiding pressure is transmitted more or less directly to the renal pelvis (Ong et al., 1974). It has been suggested that such intermittent elevation of the intrapelvic pressure during voiding acts as a water hammer and in certain instances produces progressive renal damage. Support for the supposition that sterile reflux interferes with intrarenal circulation is derived from animal models in which glomerular and tubular function decreased following the creation of surgical reflux (Helin, 1975).

Although this mechanism may play a role in renal atrophy secondary to bladder outlet obstruction when the intravesical pressures generated during voiding are much higher than normal, any water hammer effect has not been observed to cause progressive parenchymal thinning in patients with unobstructed and uninfected bladders who are followed prospectively. Perhaps the pressures generated during voiding by the normal unobstructed bladder are simply not high enough or sustained enough to cause a measurable increase in calyceal dilatation. The retrograde peristaltic wave in the relatively undilated ureter will probably damp such pressure somewhat. An alternative explanation for the calycectasis seen with severe but uncomplicated reflux is that the faulty ureteral bud was able to induce only a thin kidney that is deficient in renal pyramid development and is unable to concentrate the urine to a normal degree (see previous discussion).

Uehling (1971) and Walker (1990) have made use of the diminished concentrating ability seen in children with reflux and hydronephrosis by following such children with overnight concentration tests to assess the severity of the reflux. When medical surveillance is elected as the primary form of treatment in the expectation that reflux may stop with growth, concentrating ability improves as the severity of the reflux diminishes. Failure of the concentrating ability to improve is seen in patients with fixed calycectasis and those with reflux that does not decrease with age. If sequential concentration tests for a period of 2 or 3 years demonstrate no improvement, cystoscopic reevaluation is indicated, as the refluxing orifice may not have improved with growth as initially anticipated. Clinically, correction of reflux may result in improved concentrating ability (Uehling and Wear, 1976) and renal growth (Willscher et al., 1976a), but calycectasis is often fixed in patients in whom surgical correction is necessary (Babcock et al., 1976). Some permanent diminution in overall concentrating ability is the rule.

Management

In practice, children who demonstrate vesicoureteral reflux require classification of the type and degree of reflux, as outlined previously, as well as measurement of renal size and cortical thickness and study of the calyceal architecture. These abnormalties may indicate primary renal malformation or acquired renal damage. Ureteral duplication, bladder diverticula, and other abnormalities of the genitourinary tract and the skeletal, nervous, and gastrointestinal systems are noted. Urinalysis and urine culture and sensitivity tests should be performed. Urinary infection should be treated with specific antibiotic therapy. The medical history should be obtained, with particular attention paid to bladder and bowel habits and to family history.

When reflux is marked in degree, cystoscopy may be done to evaluate the vesicourethral outlet, the appearance of the interior of the bladder, and the architecture and location of the ureteral orifices. The length of the submucosal course of the ureter when the bladder is full is the single most useful guideline in estimating the probability that reflux will subside spontaneously (Fig. 44–15). It normally measures approximately 5 mm at birth, 10 mm by age 10 years, and 13 mm in adulthood (Hutch, 1962). Many studies have shown that in at least 50 to 60 per cent of cases, primary reflux will cease spontaneously, particularly if the submucosal tunnel is more than 5 mm at the time of diagnosis. If the submucosal tunnel is between 2 and 5 mm, the probability that reflux will stop is about 33 per cent. If no submucosal tunnel is present, the chances that reflux will subside spontaneously, particularly if the child is older than 2 years of age, is less than 10 per cent (see Fig. 44–9). Conversely, the younger child at diagnosis, the more likely it is that the intravesical ureter will elongate enough to prevent reflux before full growth is achieved.

Prompt eradication and prevention of urinary tract infection are necessary if a trial of nonoperative management is elected. This entails regular examination and culture of the urine at intervals of 8 weeks to exclude asymptomatic reinfection. Home culture kits are useful. The urine should also be tested whenever the child becomes ill.

Recurrence of urinary tract infection, despite appropriate, specific chemotherapy and long-term prophylactic chemotherapy, is unequivocally the major indication for surgical correction of reflux in the child in whom a trial of nonoperative management was elected.

If the child remains healthy, intravenous pyelograms should be obtained at intervals of 1 to 3 years. The development of renal scarring during the period of surveillance is likewise generally an indication for surgery. Cystograms should be obtained at yearly intervals to follow the degree of reflux. The radionuclide cystogram is advantageous in this situation for the reasons outlined earlier. Poor parental cooperation in administering prescribed medication and in keeping follow-up appointments may become a factor in electing early surgical intervention.

It had been suggested that spontaneous resolution of reflux is most likely to occur within the first months or years following diagnosis, but it now seems that the rate at which reflux disappears remains relatively constant throughout childhood, being approximately 20 per cent in each 2-year period (Normand and Smellie, 1979). Reflux was as likely to disappear in children who had recurrent infections as in those without further infections. Puberty is not associated with an increased rate of spontaneous cessation (Edwards et al., 1977).

Even reflux associated with paraureteral diverticula has been observed to undergo spontaneous cessation. Colodny (1983) reported eight children, all with grade 3 or 4 (international classification) reflux and periureteral diverticula up to 2 cm in diameter, who each experienced cessation of reflux without surgery. In seven of the eight instances the diverticula also disappeared, as judged by follow-up cystogram. However, when the ureter actually enters the diverticulum, associated reflux cannot be expected to resolve spontaneously.

Persistence of reflux into the teenage years is a relative indication for corrective surgery, because reflux cannot be expected to stop after growth is completed. Surgery will allow the patient to avoid an indefinite period of surveillance as an adult.

Anti-reflux surgery in patients with advanced reflux nephropathy remains controversial. Torres and col-

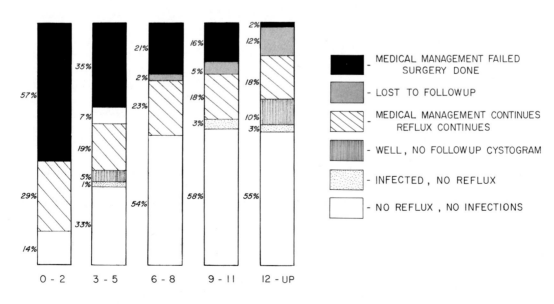

LENGTH OF INTRAMURAL URETER IN MILLIMETERS

Figure 44–15. This graft depicts the relationship between the estimated length of the intravesical ureter at the time of diagnosis and the outcome of a trial of nonoperative management in 247 refluxing units in which the tunnel length was estimated in patients followed 4 to 10 years. A nearly linear relationship exists between original tunnel length and eventual cessation of reflux, indicating the importance of this parameter. (From Kelalis, P. P., and King, L. R. (Eds.): Clinical Pediatric Urology. Philadelphia, W. B. Saunders Co., 1976.)

leagues (1980b) reported continuing renal deterioration in 11 patients with bilateral reflux and renal scars. Mean creatinine values were greater than 2.75 mg/dl prior to surgery. Progression of renal failure occurred despite successful surgical correction of the reflux. In children with severe bilateral reflux, Burger and Smith (1971) have suggested that proteinuria and a creatinine clearance of less than 25 ml/m^2 portend progressive renal insufficiency, regardless of therapy.

Salvatierra and Tanagho (1977) recommend anti-reflux surgery even in children and adolescents with advanced renal insufficiency. Although protection of the already compromised renal parenchyma from the risk of offending infection is of obvious benefit, surgical reimplantation has implications in the future management of end-stage renal disease. In particular, bilateral nephroureterectomy is performed for severe reflux with ureteral dilatation in preparation for a renal transplant, because of the risk of recurrent pyelonephritis in patients receiving immunosuppressive therapy after the transplantation. Although no firm evidence exists that reimplantation will delay progression of end-stage renal failure, the success rate of anti-reflux surgery is high. A succesful procedure may obviate the need for pretransplant bilateral nephroureterectomy, making management during periods of dialysis less complex in terms of fluid balance and anemia (Malek et al., 1983b).

Continued surveillance is necessary after reflux stops spontaneously or after successful anti-reflux surgery, because urinary infections may occur and require recognition and treatment. Late obstruction of the ureterovesical junction is seen in 0.25 to 0.5 per cent of patients after successful anti-reflux surgery (Weiss and Lytton, 1974). Pyelography or sonography should be repeated every 2 to 3 years, even in asymptomatic postoperative patients, until the child is fully grown.

Hypertension

Hypertension is a well-known, long-term complication encountered in children and adults with reflux and renal scarring. A review of 100 children with severe hypertension (diastolic blood pressure greater than 100 mm Hg) revealed 14 with reflux nephropathy, all presenting between the ages of 6 and 15 years (Gill et al., 1976). Pyelonephritic scarring was second in frequency only to chronic glomerulonephritis as the etiology of the high blood pressure. Holland (1979) has reviewed 177 cases of hypertension with scarred atrophic kidneys under various diagnostic terms in 16 series. She suggests that all these terms, in fact, refer to the same pathologic entity, namely, reflux nephropathy.

Smellie's long-term study of a large population of children with reflux showed progression of renal damage in the patients who developed hypertension (Smellie and Normand, 1979). The prevalence of high blood pressure in patients with such scarring is unknown, but hypertension was a significant feature of those developing end-stage renal failure. In Smellie's series, hypertension was detected in 20 per cent of the children with established scars. Of the 17 hypertensive children six

had severe hypertension and eight had some degree of renal insufficiency. However, at least half had normal or near-normal renal function, indicating that the appearance of hypertension is not necessarily related to the development of renal failure but probably associated with vascular lesions within the kidney (Kincaid-Smith, 1975). In favor of such a mechanism is the finding of a high plasma renin activity in two girls with hypertension and reflux nephropathy in whom serum creatinine levels were 0.6 and 1.2 mg/dl, respectively (Siegler, 1976).

Savage and associates (1978) studied 100 normotensive children with reflux nephropathy and found eight with increased plasma renin levels. After 5 years of follow-up, two of the eight children had developed high blood pressure (Dillon, 1982). An additional 51 patients with hypertension at the same medical center were found on examination to have coarse renal scarring. Almost all those studied had evidence of reflux; 36 had elevated plasma renin activity. Smellie (1975b) has suggested that hypertension associated with reflux and renal scarring is age-related, with increasing risk above age 15 years. Thus, the long-term outcome of patients with renal scarring needs to be accurately defined. Wallace and colleagues (1978) reported hypertension in 18.5 per cent of children with bilateral renal scars and in 11.3 per cent with unilateral renal scars more than 10 years following surgery for reflux. Stecker and co-workers (1977) reported hypertension in three of 70 children 1 to 19 years after ureteral reimplantation and state that elimination of reflux did not protect against the development of hypertension. No improvement in hypertension occurred in two patients following successful correction of reflux.

In addition to pharmacologic antihypertensive therapy, unilateral nephrectomy has been advocated for relief of hypertension associated with reflux when the affected kidney has very poor function. Dillon (1982) performed 46 renal vein renin studies in 44 hypertensive patients with renal scarring. Ten patients with unilateral scars, in nine of whom the renal vein renin ratio was greater than 1.5, underwent nephrectomy. Of these, eight were cured, and two were improved. Six patients with asymmetric bilateral involvement, with renal vein renin ratios greater than 1.5, also underwent surgery. Five had unilateral nephrectomy, and one had unilateral nephrectomy with contralateral partial nephrectomy. Three were cured, and three were improved. Of special interest is the observation that approximately half these 44 patients required segmental renal vein renin determinations in order to define the source of their hypertension. Bailey (1979a) described two patients who had unilateral renal scarring and hypertension with renal vein renin ratios of greater than 1.5, yet with low peripheral renin levels. This report confirms the importance of segmental renal vein renin sampling.

Wallace and associates (1978) found that more than 10 per cent of children with renal scarring become hypertensive within 10 years. All such patients should have blood pressure determinations yearly. The incidence of hypertension is very likely to increase with age. If not detected, hypertension can evolve into a malignant phase and cause further deterioration of kidney function. The complications of hypertension are completely prevented with early detection and treatment.

Reflux and Pregnancy

Surgical correction of reflux is generally recommended when the reflux persists beyond puberty. An additional rationale is the protection of the sexually active and potentially pregnant woman from pyelonephritic episodes, thereby reducing the risk of maternal renal damage, premature delivery, and increased fetal or perinatal loss. Hutch (1958) demonstrated reflux during pregnancy in five of 12 women whose gestation was complicated by pyelonephritis. He also reported a disproportionately high incidence of pyelonephritis during pregnancy among 23 women known to have recurrent bacteriuria and chronic pyelonephritis with reflux.

Heidrick and co-workers (1967) performed 200 cystograms in the last trimester of pregnancy in an unselected population. Seven studies revealed reflux (3.5 per cent). An additional 121 women underwent cystography within 30 hours of delivery; two of these also experienced reflux. Three of these nine women with reflux developed pyelonephritis earlier in their pregnancy compared with only 4.8 per cent in those without reflux. Thus, it appears that reflux is a significant risk factor predisposing a patient to pyelonephritis during pregnancy.

Williams and associates (1968) evaluated 100 women with asymptomatic coliform bacteriuria during pregnancy. All were treated with a standard course of antibiotic therapy. They were studied radiographically 4 to 6 months post partum. Cystography demonstrated reflux in 21. Bacteriuria was again found at the time of the study in 13 of these women (62 per cent) compared with only 16 per cent of women without reflux. Ten of the 21 patients with reflux (48 per cent) had renal scarring compared with only 9 per cent without reflux. Two thirds of those with reflux required two or more courses of antibiotics to clear the infection compared with less than a fourth of those without reflux. These data suggest that in pregnant women bacteriuria with reflux is more difficult to eradicate than bacteriuria without reflux. Moreover, persistent bacteriuria during pregnancy while receiving antibacterial therapy appears to identify a population of women with a high incidence of reflux nephropathy.

Other workers have noted that bacteriuria with reflux in pregnancy tends to persist post partum. Pyelonephritis, which is observed in only 1 to 3 per cent of all pregnancies, occurs in about 30 per cent of pregnant women with otherwise asymptomatic bacteriuria (Whalley and Cunningham, 1977). Although a strong suspicion exists that reflux during pregnancy predisposes the patient to bacteriuria, lack of a longitudinal study in a population of pregnant women with known reflux does not allow a definite conclusion. Because one cannot predict which women will develop bacteriuria during pregnancy, surgical correction of reflux is still recommended when it persists beyond puberty.

Austenfeld and Snow (1988) followed 67 women who had undergone anti-reflux surgery more than 15 years earlier. Of these, 30 patients had a total of 64 pregnancies. Some 57 per cent of these women had at least one UTI during gestation and 5 (17 per cent) had clinical pyelonephritis. There were eight spontaneous abortions and one severe ureteral obstruction requiring proximal renal drainage until delivery. Clearly there seems to be an increased risk of urine infection and fetal loss in women who had anti-reflux surgery as children. Those with renal scarring seem most susceptible to these occurrences.

Clinical Trials of Medical Versus Surgical Treatment

Only a randomized prospective clinical trial can determine whether spontaneous cessation of reflux, when it occurs, is preferable to surgery, and which course of therapy has the best potential in terms of renal growth. Moreover, the issue of sterile reflux in conjunction with ureterectasis and its possible eventual deleterious effect on the kidney can be resolved only by such a study. In the only prospective randomized trial yet published, Scott and Stansfeld (1968) compared the results of early surgical correction of reflux with prophylactic antibiotic therapy and observed that the renal growth in children in whom the reflux was surgically cured exceeded that observed in children in whom the reflux was still present. The population sampled was small, however, and the follow-up period was short.

In 1980, an international prospective randomized clinical trial was instituted among a group of major teaching hospitals in the United States and Europe. Because children with moderate-to-severe reflux experience the most difficult problems to manage, particularly regarding the choice of therapy, this was the group that was selected for study. All patients less than 9 years of age with primary grade 4 (international classification) reflux are accepted into the trial as well as patients with grade 3 reflux persisting beyond infancy (the latter in the European branch only). The aim of the study is to compare the effects of successful anti-reflux surgery performed at the time of diagnosis with effective, continuous, low-dose antibiotic prophylaxis. This therapeutic trial is designed to test whether sterile high-grade reflux is harmful in and of itself and whether a difference exists between early successful surgery and effective medical management in preventing the possible deleterious effects of reflux on renal growth, creatinine clearance, development of new renal scars, or progression of established scars. In addition, this study will establish the true incidence of recurrent urine infections and hypertension in surgically and medically treated patients.

This prospective approach employs random allocation. Precise criteria are used to select patients, and the standardization of diagnostic, therapeutic, and follow-up procedures should permit an accurate comparison of the two therapeutic modalities. Preliminary results may be available shortly, but as yet they only indicate that those in the medication group have a higher risk of infection.

Summary

Vesicoureteral reflux is most often a manifestation of a congenital abnormality of the ureterovesical junction. Depending on the degree of derangement, primary reflux may subside spontaneously during childhood or may persist after full growth has been achieved. However, the presence of reflux places the kidney at risk to deleterious effects from urinary tract infections. Therefore, diligent surveillance for and prevention of urinary tract infection are mandatory in children with reflux. Judicious operative intervention is required to correct vesicoureteral reflux in those patients with severe derangement of the ureterovesical junction or intractable recurrent urinary tract infection. The surgical techniques employed are described later in this chapter.

MEGAURETER

Much of the debate surrounding the diagnosis and treatment of "megaureter" stems from confusion in nomenclature, the term meaning a single specific disease to some and carrying a more general connotation to others. Caulk (1923) first used the term to denote the condition of a 32-year-old woman with distal ureterectasis without pyelectasis or calycectasis. The word itself is simply a combination of *mega,* meaning "big," and ureter. Thus, it may be argued that the term can be applied to any dilated ureter.

Cussen (1967) has established normal measurements of ureteral diameter in infants and children from 30 weeks of gestation to 12 years of age. Any ureter outside these norms, e.g., 7 mm at age 12 years, is abnormal and could be considered a megaureter. However, in the clinical setting, megaureter usually denotes more than minimal ureterectasis. The term has been expanded to include dilated ureters with or without pyelocalycectasis, which may or may not be associated with demonstrable obstruction. Debate centers on precise differentiation of the obstructed from the nonobstructed megaureter. The practical reason for differentiating these causes is that obstructed ureters require surgical correction, whereas dilated ureters without reflux or obstruction can generally be successfully managed with a modicum of surveillance only or, at most, antibacterial prophylaxis. In addition, nonobstructed but dilated ureters do not often improve after successful reimplantation but seem prone to surgical complications, which may result in increased hydronephrosis. The furosemide (Lasix)–assisted intravenous pyelogram and renogram and the Whitaker test help in differentiating the obstructed from the nonobstructed state and have advanced the understanding of the causes of ureterectasis.

The purposes of this discussion are to define megaureter in a reasonable way and to establish guidelines for differential diagnosis that are of practical use to clinicians. Emphasis is placed on the classification of megaureter so that the various causes will quickly come to mind when one is managing such a case. The various anatomic causes of obstructed meagureter are described, but once the diagnosis is made, techniques of successful surgical correction become much more important than considerations of etiology, which may remain unclear in individual cases.

All dilated ureters have characteristics in common, especially lack of effective peristalsis caused by inability of the walls of the dilated ureter to coapt. However, lack of peristalsis does not itself result in renal damage or in failure of the kidney to grow. Therefore, to stop the evaluation at the diagnosis of "big ureter" or to advise ureteral tailoring and reimplantation is to do the patient a disservice. Furthermore, the congenital nonobstructed megaureter is often associated with megacalycosis, which is calyceal dilatation without obstruction. Thus, the presence of ureteral dilatation and calycectasis is not in itself absolutely indicative of ureterovesical junction (UVJ) obstruction. Both may be the residual of obstruction during fetal development, which resolved spontaneously. It is safest to initially consider megaureter a radiographic finding and to proceed systematically to exclude reflux or UVJ obstruction as causes.

Classification of Megaureter

All modern attempts to classify megaureter have been in response to the practical need to differentiate the obstructed from the unobstructed variety. Whitaker (1973) and others have pointed out that relatively severe reflux may result in the appearance of megaureter on intravenous pyelography. Further classifications have attempted to start with ureterectasis, with or without calycectasis, and to include all possible causes. The international classification of Smith and co-workers (1977) is the most comprehensive (Table 44–2). In this scheme, megaureter may be due to obstruction or reflux, or it may be idiopathic—that is, developmental—and not associated with either reflux or obstruction. Each of these major categories may then be subdivided into a primary and secondary group. Thus, the cause of primary obstructive megaureter is obstruction at or just above the ureterovesical junction. In secondary obstructive megaureter, the ureterectasis is due to intravesical obstruction from valves, prolapsing ureterocele, and the like.

Primary refluxing megaureter is due to a short or absent intravesical ureter, congenital paraureteral diverticulum, or other derangement of the ureterovesical

Table 44–2. INTERNATIONAL CLASSIFICATION OF MEGAURETER

	Primary	Secondary
Obstructed	Intrinsic ureteral obstruction	To urethral obstruction or extrinsic lesions
Reflux	Reflux is only abnormality	Associated with bladder outlet obstruction or neurogenic bladder
Nonrefluxing, nonobstructed	Idiopathic ureteral dilation	To polyuria (diabetes inspidus) or infection (?)

junction. In secondary refluxing megaureter, reflux is present together with another anomaly, such as neuropathic bladder or infravesical obstruction.

In primary nonobstructive, nonrefluxing megaureter there is no juxtavesical obstruction, reflux, bladder anomaly, or outlet obstruction. The ureterectasis is isolated or associated with calycectasis, but upper tract drainage is good by all functional parameters. In children, such systems tend to improve in radiographic appearance with growth, although some ureterectasis usually persists. In secondary nonrefluxing, nonobstructive megaureter the dilatation of the upper tract is due to urinary infection, diabetes insipidus, or other rare causes of very high rates of urine formation.

This classification is exhaustive. The main advantage is that all patients with ureterectasis can be classified within the system. Glassberg (1977) and others have found its use cumbersome, however, when dealing with what most consider typical megaureter. They argue that in general use the term "megaureter" is not applied to hydroureter caused by overt neuropathic bladder or typical bladder outlet obstruction with bladder trabeculation and residual urine. Megaureter is usually reserved for more mystifying conditions in which the bladder and bladder outlet are normal but the ureter is dilated to some extent (Figs. 44–16 and 44–17).

Dilated ureters of the prune-belly syndrome are given a category of their own. However, it must be recognized that in this syndrome the ureterectasis commonly associated may be due to reflux or ureterovesical junction obstruction or may be of the nonobstructive variety and can be categorized according to these characteristics. Glassberg and associates (1982) have also addressed the cause of residual ureterectasis commonly seen after successful resection of urethral valves.

My practical classification of megaureter is given in Table 44–3. I tend to agree that the international classification is more complex than necessary and that megaureter means ureteral dilatation in the absence of another overt disease to most urologists. The prune-belly and iatrogenic megaureters can be categorized,

Table 44–3. SIMPLIFIED CLASSIFICATION OF PRIMARY MEGAURETER

1. Nonobstructing, nonrefluxing megaureter—without obstruction or reflux
2. Obstructive megaureter—due to ureterovesical obstruction
3. Refluxing megaureter
4. Megaureter due to ureterovesical obstruction masked by reflux

This simplified system is useful when there is not intravesical obstruction, reflux, or overt abnormality of the urinary tract except for hydroureteronephrosis. Megaureter can then be due to UVJ obstruction or reflux. Category 4 is included to remind the clinician that these lesions can coexist.

Ureterectasis not associated with obstruction or reflux is also a variety of primary megaureter (category 1).

after evaluation, into one of the four groups, as appropriate diagnostic studies need to be done in nearly every case to rule out obstruction.

The "reflux with UVJ obstruction" category was added to call attention to the fact that reflux and obstruction can coexist in a small proportion of patients. In these instances, the reflux is often the most obvious finding, and concomitant obstruction may not be considered unless the possibility of dual lesions is kept in mind. If a delayed film is obtained after the cystogram, poor drainage of one or both upper tracts may suggest associated UVJ obstruction (Fig. 44–18). This can be confirmed or excluded by further evaluation. In a series of over 400 refluxing renal units, Weiss and Lytton (1974) found concomitant UVJ obstruction in nine. Lebowitz and Blickman (1983) also reported nine cases. This can be an important observation, because proven obstruction generally requires early surgical correction, whereas reflux is often treated by surveillance, at least for a time.

The clinician should employ the system of megaureter classification that seems most useful. Ureterectasis does not always mean obstruction, even when calycectasis is also present. Primary megaureter is an inherently compound term and usually includes both primary obstructed megaureter and primary nonobstructive megaureter.

APERISTALTIC DISTAL URETERAL SEGMENT (PRIMARY MEGAURETER)

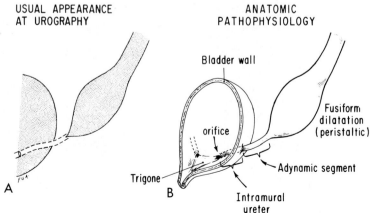

USUAL APPEARANCE AT UROGRAPHY

ANATOMIC PATHOPHYSIOLOGY

Figure 44–16. Artist's conception of megaureter. Ureteral dilatation begins above the ureterovesical junction, usually a few millimeters or more above the bladder. (Courtesy of Dr. A. P. McLaughlin, III.)

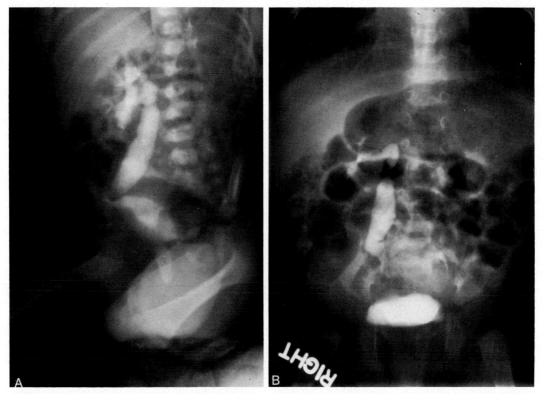

Figure 44–17. Megaureter with calycectasis was diagnosed on fetal ultrasound. *A,* At 1 week of age, an intravenous pyelography revealed ureteral dilatation but less calycectasis than was suggested by the degree of ureterectasis. There was no reflux. A renogram showed an obstructive curve with prompt drainage after furosemide administration. *B,* The calycectasis has resolved 3 months later.

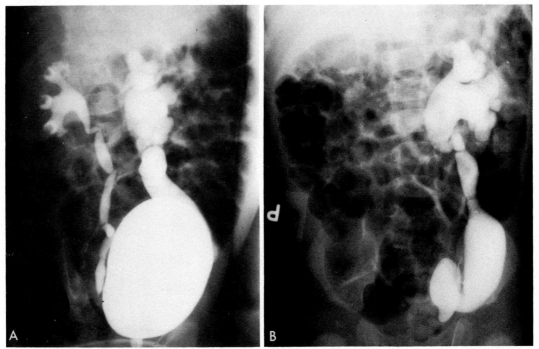

Figure 44–18. *A,* Child with bilateral reflux, dilated collecting system with significant calycectatic changes. *B,* Six-hour drainage film. Note right side completely empty and sharp cutoff on left at ureterovesical junction. This left side combines the worst features of two problems—reflux and obstruction.

Etiology

Nonobstructive, Nonrefluxing Megaureter

The cause of isolated nonobstructed megaureter is not clear, but it may be the result of UVJ obstruction that resolved during development. There is usually no stenosis of the juxtavesicular ureter, but the ureter is usually dilated beginning at a point just above the bladder. The dilatation may involve the entire ureter or may be segmental. The lowermost ureter is often the widest and is bulbous in appearance, with a sharp cutoff and little tortuosity. Rarely, only the midportion of the ureter may be dilated. This configuration is sometimes reminiscent of the dilated ureters often seen in boys with the prune-belly syndrome; therefore, a primary abnormality of the ureteral musculature has been a suspected cause.

Refluxing Megaureter

This term implies that the appearance of megaureter on intravenous pyelography, minimally some ureterectasis, is due to reflux. The presence of reflux is usually noted on cystogram. Any of the various causes of reflux maybe responsible. The reflux can be managed according to the etiology, that is, by surveillance or by early operative correction. The choice of therapy in such instances is discussed earlier in this chapter.

Obstructed Megaureter

The juxtavesical ureter may be normal in caliber and yet be the site of functional obstruction, causing proximal ureterectasis. In such instances, the undilated segment does not conduct the peristaltic wave, usually owing to a deficiency in the muscle fibers that are oriented in spiral fashion. Occasionally, circular muscle bundles are hypertrophied and appear to cause obstruction. The presence of a narrowed juxtavesicular ureteral segment is the most important cause of primary obstructive megaureter, however. The narrow segment measures from 0.5 to 4 cm in length.

Gregoir and Debled (1969) described four histologic types, the majority (60 per cent) exhibiting increased collagenous tissue in the terminal 3 to 4 cm of the ureter. A band of circumferential tissue devoid of muscle in the most distal portion of the narrowed segment is another cause (MacKinnon, 1977). At times a band of thickened muscle is arranged in a nearly circular pattern and seems to be the site of obstruction. It is postulated that such obstruction is initially caused by focal congenital absence of the spiral musculature of the lowermost ureter and that consequent local secondary muscular hypertrophy compounds the problem.

McLaughlin and colleagues (1973) reviewed the histopathology of 32 typical primary megaureters (obstructed and nonobstructed). Four anatomic varieties could be distinguished. The most common type (69 per cent) was characterized by pronounced muscular hypoplasia and atrophy of the muscle fibers, which were separated by sheets of fibrotic tissue (Fig. 44–19). These workers concluded that obstruction had two causes: (1) absence of muscle fibers, which prevents transmission of peristalsis, and (2) fibrotic rigidity of the ureteral wall, which prevents expansion and free passive urine egress.

Tanagho (1973) presented an explanation of these changes, based on embryologic studies in the fetal lamb. He noted that the distal ureter is the last portion to develop its muscular coat and that early muscular differentiation is primarily of the muscle with circular orientation. This observation suggests that arrest late in development results in absence of the longitudinally oriented musculature that conducts the peristaltic wave, and that this, in turn, results in obstruction by the circular muscle fibers, which then often undergo hypertrophy.

When conveying a bolus of urine, each muscular component of a ureteral segment or spindle contracts to force the fluid into the adjacent spindle (Murnaghan, 1957). Obstruction at the terminal ureter causes partial retrograde emptying. Ureteral dilatation is potentially dependent on the rate of urine flow, in that all ureters become dilated if their volume capacity is exceeded (Hutch and Tanagho, 1965). The retrograde flow of urine from the most distal ureter combined with newly excreted urine produces an excessive load, resulting in dilatation of the normal ureter proximal to the stenotic segment. Vesicoureteral reflux, in quantity, evokes a similar response. Ureterectasis occurs when refluxed bladder urine exceeds the ureter's normal carrying capacity.

Several electron microscopic studies of the lower ureter in nonrefluxing megaureter confirm the variable nature of the lesion (Hanna and Jeffs, 1975; Pagano and Passerini, 1977; Tokunaka et al., 1982). Moreover, pathologic studies of the narrow ureteral segment have not yet been correlated in adequate numbers of patients with the findings on diuretic renogram or Whitaker test to define which lesions are truly obstructive.

Ureterectasis without obstruction must occur by a different mechanism, or obstruction might be present during early development, which results in residual ureterectasis even though the obstruction itself somehow resolves. At the time of his original description, Caulk (1923) equated megaureter and Hirschsprung's disease, a concept supported by Swenson and Fisher (1955) and Grana and Swenson (1965). Absence of ureteral parasympathetic ganglia, as in Hirschsprung's disease, has not been noted in children with ureterectasis, however (Gregoir and Debled, 1969; Leibowitz and Bodian, 1963; Notley, 1972).

Radiographic Appearance

In obstructive megaureter the narrow, most distal segment is so close to the bladder wall that this segment is usually obscured by the overlying contrast-filled bladder. It was visualized on the initial intravenous pyelogram in only three of 38 megaureters reviewed by Pfister and Hendren (1978). The chances of visualizing the

Hypoplasia

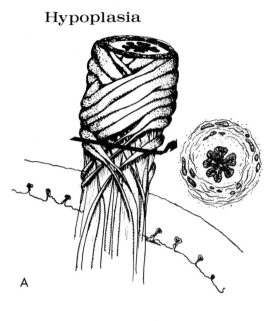

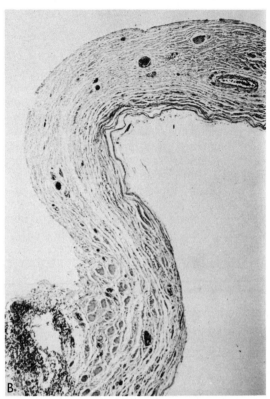

Figure 44–19. *A,* Hypoplasia and atrophy of ureteral muscle as seen in 22 patients in McLaughlin's series. *B,* Photomicrograph from section of ureter. (From McLaughlin, A. P., III, Pfister, R. C., Leadbetter, W. F., et al.: J. Urol., 109:805, 1973. © 1973, Williams & Wilkins, Baltimore.)

obstructing segment are improved by obtaining oblique views or postvoiding films (Fig. 44–20). Distal ureteral dilatation may be so severe that the bulbous lower ureter prolapses below the proximal portion of the narrowed segment so that the distal dilated portion and the narrow

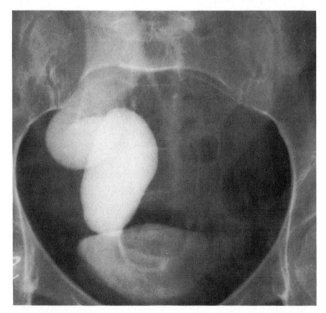

Figure 44–20. A retrograde ureterogram demonstrates that the obstruction of the ureter in primary obstructed megaureter is extravesical. The ureterovesical junction is normal. When the intravesical ureter is short, reflux will also be present.

lowermost ureter appear side by side. This observation has given birth to the term "ureteral valve," which is quite descriptive but sometimes misleading. First, the term "ureteral valve" is too easily confused with "urethral valve" phonetically. More important, the septum or valve between the dilated portion of the ureter and the narrow part is seldom, if ever, the primary cause of the obstruction, which seems clearly due in these instances to intrinsic stenosis of the most distal segment. The valve-like flap may compound the obstruction but rarely, if ever, occurs without a very narrow, more distal juxtavesical segment, which is the hallmark of obstructed megaureter.

Regardless of the severity of upper ureteral dilatation, active movement of the ureteral wall is seen on cineradiographic studies in almost all cases. Effective peristalsis is absent when the walls of the ureter cannot coapt, and, like ureteral peristalsis generally, this movement is reduced by bacterial exotoxins during some infections. Usually, the ureteral movements convey the contrast medium to the narrowed segment, where most of the bolus simply floods back up the ureter. If the upper ureter is of normal or near-normal caliber, this "refluxed" urine will initiate a wave of retrograde peristalsis. It seems likely that such peristalsis damps the pressure and prevents dilatation of the pelvis. When only the lower ureter is dilated, the pelvis is usually normal in size. When the entire ureter is dilated, some pelvic dilatation is often present also.

McGarth and co-workers (1987) reported 14 children in whom obstructive megaureter was associated with ipsilateral UPJ obstruction. The preoperative diagnosis of both conditions may be difficult. When UPJ obstruction is present, the ipsilateral ureter is seldom seen on intravenous urography. The diagnosis is not made until a retrograde ureterogram is performed when the child is under anesthesia for a pyeloplasty or when the ureter is seen to be dilated at the time of the pyeloplasty. A preoperative renal scan is more helpful in this regard, as the obstructed ureter usually fills and is visualized as the obstructed pelvis drains.

Van Niederhaursen and Tuchschmid (1971) found nonobstructed megaureter frequently in patients with megacalycosis. They pointed out that neither the ureteral dilatation nor the calycectasis was associated with obstruction. Vargas and Lebowitz (1986) reported six children with this combination, now thought probably to be caused by obstruction during fetal life that resolved spontaneously. I have managed three patients who have been followed more than 15 years without progression of calycectasis. The megaureter has become less pronounced with growth, as is the rule when the dilatation is not associated with obstruction.

Mode of Presentation

Most patients now present because hydronephrosis was noted on fetal sonography. An older child with megaureter with or without calycectasis presents with urinary infection, which may be cystitis and unrelated to the upper tract anomaly; with hematuria, or with otherwise unexplained abdominal pain. It is not unusual for the dilated ureter to be noted at the time of appendectomy or other abdominal surgery. Uremia, anemia, renal rickets, failure to thrive, or other signs of renal failure are, fortunately, rare presenting complaints. Megaureter is bilateral in about 25 per cent of patients. Children presenting prior to 1 year of age are more apt to have bilateral megaureter than are older patients (Williams and Hulme-Moir, 1970). The incidence in males is 1.5 to 4.8 times greater than in females. The left ureter is involved 1.6 to 4.5 times more often than the right. The incidence of contralateral renal agenesis is about 9 per cent (see Table 44–3). The condition is not known to be hereditary, but families with more than one member with megaureter have been described.

Methods for the Differential Diagnosis of Obstructive Versus Nonobstructive Megaureter

Because reflux of moderate or severe degree is usually diagnosed without difficulty on cystogram, this discussion centers on differentiating obstructed from nonobstructed megaureters. Many tests are clinically useful in this regard, and these are summarized later. The child with megaureter usually presents with antenatal or postnatal hydronephrosis, urinary tract infection, hematuria, or a flank mass. Ureterectasis without reflux or infravesical obstruction is observed on cystogram. Renal scans

usually provide better visualization than excretory urography in the neonate. These scans are used to try to differentiate nonobstructive dilatation from obstruction. Williams and Holme-Moir (1970) noted that when only the distal ureter is dilated, all patients remain stable or improved. The patients that require further evaluation are those with dilatation of the entire ureter and calycectasis.

Furosemide Renogram

The next evaluation is commonly a renogram using furosemide (Lasix) to stimulate washout of the dilated collecting system if the renogram curve appears obstructive. This test is in wide use, but normal parameters that rule out obstruction have not yet been clearly established. The reason for difficulty in interpretation is that if the hydronephrosis is very severe, even a relatively well-functioning kidney may not be able to perform diuresis fast enough to clearly demonstrate good drainage after the administration of furosemide. A poorly functioning kidney may not be able to excrete enough urine under any conditions to clear the radioactivity at a "normal" rate.

Differences in the degree of hydroureteronephrosis mean that varying degrees of diuresis will dilute the radioactive isotope already excreted by varying amounts; therefore, a spectrum of unobstructed drainage patterns is to be expected. Therefore, the furosemide renogram allows various interpretations, e.g., severely and unequivocally obstructed, unobstructed, and a group in which the diagnosis is not certain. This last group needs further definition. However, some guidelines for the test can be summarized.

The child should have no prior dehydration or enemas. Technetium-labeled DPTA is utilized to estimate renal blood flow. Hippuran I 131 is given, and images of the kidney and ureter are made at 2, 5, 10, 15, 20, 25, and 30 minutes. The counting crystals should be centered over the area where the isotope is pooled, and a catheter should be indwelling to keep the bladder empty. The Hippuran I 131 renogram is a sensitive test; the initial renogram curve will usually look obstructed in most cases of collecting system dilatation of any etiology. If a catheter is not in place, the child is asked to void, or is catheterized, to determine the effect of bladder emptying on the curve. If the curve continues to appear obstructed, a standard dose, 1 mg of furosemide per kg of body weight is administered. If the amount of radioactivity is reduced by half in less than 10 minutes, the study findings are normal and UVJ obstruction is not present. When the half-time clearance is 10 to 20 minutes, the study is equivocal and further tests are needed. A half-time clearance of radioactivity requiring longer than 20 minutes is indicative of obstruction unless renal function is very poor or hydronephrosis is extreme, as described earlier.

Some potential pitfalls associated with the furosemide renogram can be avoided by careful attention to test conditions. Accidental dehydration may minimize the diuresis effect. The technician may accidentally alter the "Y" axis of the renogram curve. The furosemide dose must be standardized and weight-related, as the diuretic effect increases with larger doses. Hippuran, not DTPA, must be used to gauge the furosemide response. Furosemide affects tubular function; hippuran is secreted by the tubules, and hippuran is cleared faster than DPTA. Furosemide administration less than 30 minutes after DTPA administration may result in the collecting system being washed out by "hot," i.e., radioactive, urine, which would produce a false-positive test result. The child's position during the test should be standardized, as this may affect drainage of the dilated collecting system. If only the ureter is dilated, the counting crystal should be placed over the area of ureterectasis, not over the kidney.

In spite of these qualifications, the furosemide renogram is a useful test. In fact, Kass and associates (1982) compared it with the more invasive Whitaker test and found the results to be as accurate. Patients with hydroureter without obstruction are spared more invasive investigations. Also, even though some furosemide renograms are equivocal in some patients with megaureters, such tests are quite reproducible in the same patients when performed in exactly the same manner. Therefore, if the results fall into the equivocal range, a follow-up study done several months after the first may demonstrate improved drainage and thereby exclude obstruction.

Other Studies

In children who continue to appear to have possible ureteral obstruction, an equivocal or obstructed furosemide renogram is often an indication for further diagnostic studies. These include (1) cystoscopy with ureteral catheterization, to see if a "hydronephrotic drip" is present, and (2) measurement of the renal pelvic pressure at which fluid flows into the bladder across the site of possible obstruction (Whitaker test) (Fig. 44–21). It is difficult to make a firm rule as to which of these examinations should be performed first. Many children with megaureters have had previous cystoscopic examinations to rule out urethral obstructions; therefore, a Whitaker test often seems the more pertinent. If cystoscopy has not been done, one may choose to do that first. The anterior urethra is calibrated with bougies and is inspected for an anterior or a posterior valve. More than mild bladder trabeculation suggests outflow obstruction. Because the voiding cystogram was normal in these children, the urethra will usually be normal. Outlet obstruction, however, may be caused by sphincter dyssynergia, and the hydroureter may be the result of the neurogenic/non-neurogenic bladder syndrome. Urodynamics are then indicated.

Attention is next turned to the ureteral orifices. Are they normal, or do their size and position suggest reflux, which is occasionally not detected on cystogram? Is there a small ureterocele? If the orifice is normal, the next step is to pass a 4 or 5 F. ureteral catheter, the caliber depending on the size of the child. At least a 4 F. is preferred, so that a hydronephrotic drip can be detected. Occasionally, the ureteral catheter will not pass. This may be due to technical factors, e.g., a difficult angle, or to ureteral meatal stenosis, which is an uncommon cause of ureterectasis but usually susceptible to dilatation or to transurethral or percutaneous meatotomy. Usually, in primary obstructive megaureter the point of obstruction is above the ureteral hiatus, about 5 to 15 mm from the bladder. The ureteral

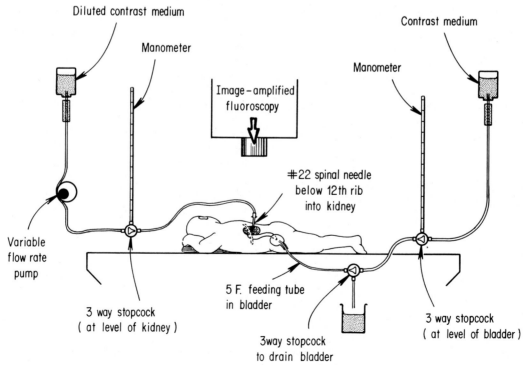

Figure 44–21. Schematic diagram of antegrade pyelography with pressure-perfusion study (Whitaker test).

catheter may stop at that point but will usually pass. If a large volume of urine then comes out of the ureteral catheter in a steady drip (hydronephrotic drip), obstruction is deemed likely.

Contrast material is introduced, and drainage films are made. The normal rate of drainage from a dilated collecting system in a dehydrated child has not been quantitated, but persistence of contrast material in the ureter for 6 hours is usually indicative of obstruction. Conversely, complete drainage within an hour or two is usually most compatible with the diagnosis of nonobstructed, nonrefluxing megaureter. If obstruction is absent, the total volume of the continuous hydronephrotic drip is also apt to be less than one would expect from the size of the dilated collecting system on intravenous pyelography. These cystoscopic tests to differentiate obstructed from nonobstructed megaureter are all subjective, and yet the results seem fairly accurate. It is difficult to conceive that a dilated ureter that produces 20 ml immediately after catheterization and retains contrast material for several hours after filling is not an obstructed ureter.

Whitaker Test

The other method permitting more complete evaluation of the dilated ureter is measurement of the renal pelvic pressure at which a high volume of fluid, 10 ml per minute, passes the site of possible obstruction. This is a well thought out physiologic test that has the great advantage of being quantitative. A number, the maximum renal pressure during sustained flow minus the bladder pressure, is produced. The drawbacks are that the test is relatively invasive and usually requires a general anesthetic in children. Similar to the furosemide renogram, it is at times difficult to interpret with certainty. Nonetheless, it can differentiate hydroureteronephrosis due to obstructive causes from the nonobstructive causes of ureterectasis or calycectasis.

The test requires a nephrostomy or pyelostomy or, most commonly, insertion of long percutaneous needles under fluoroscopic control. Needles of 20 or 22 gauge are usually employed, although some prefer a larger bore. The needle resistance is subtracted from the renal pressure. A urethral catheter is inserted. A pump capable of delivering a constant flow perfuses the renal pelvis at a standard rate, 10 ml per minute. Manometers or strain gauges are attached to the perfusion catheter and bladder outflow tubing. Perfusion is maintained until the collecting system is filled and the renal pressure reaches a plateau or is obviously increasing and is far above the physiologic range, indicating obstruction. Maximum renal relative pressures (renal pelvis pressure minus needle resistance minus bladder pressure) below 15 cm of H_2O are considered to indicate an absence of obstruction. Conversely, higher pressures are regarded as indicative of obstruction, although some cases of marginal elevation may remain equivocal, as discussed later.

In typical UPJ obstructions, the relative renal pressure may be very elevated during the test; however, most UPJ obstructions are readily diagnosed by the typical appearance of the dilated pelvis and calyces on intravenous pyelogram or ultrasound. Megacalycosis, defined as underdevelopment of the renal pyramids in the absence of obstruction, may occur with ipsilateral nonobstructed megaureter (Talner and Gittes, 1974; Von Niederhausern and Tuchschmid, 1971; Whitaker and Flower, 1981), as noted earlier. In this situation, further evaluation is generally needed, as it is when pyelocalycectasis is combined with typical megaureter. A Whitaker test is usually diagnostic in this situation and yields relative renal pressures in the normal (usually low normal) or the unequivocally obstructed range. Patients with obstruction are operated upon, while those without obstruction are followed with an occasional intravenous pyelogram or diuretic renogram to make absolutely certain that the upper tracts do not deteriorate.

Witherow and Whitaker (1981) reported on 21 patients, all but four of whom were children, evaluated by the Whitaker test in 1973. Patients were divided into four groups. Nine of 11 with elevated pressures who underwent corrective surgery exhibited improved pyelograms or clearances, or both, more than 5 years later. In five children with elevated relative renal pressure, no operation was performed. Four of these patients were boys with valves, in whom the hydroureteronephrosis persisted after valve resection and in whom reimplantation was deferred. In two, the bladder pressures indicated a noncompliant bladder. This elevated pressure was reflected in the kidney, although the relative renal perfusion pressure (renal pressure minus bladder pressure) was not elevated. Renal function deteriorated with time in both patients. One of the patients with valves was studied soon after valve resection. The relative renal pressures were elevated. This boy improved. It is surmised that the ureters were obstructed by the hypertrophied detrusor and that as the hypertrophy subsided, the obstruction was relieved.

In seven patients, the pressure-flow study was normal and no operation was performed. After 5 to 9 years, all upper tracts were stable in appearance and function. In four patients, a low relative pressure was found, but operation was performed on clinical grounds.

The Whitaker test was introduced in 1973, but its accuracy was uncertain; therefore, these four patients were treated surgically. Two had bilateral and two had unilateral megaureters. A good surgical result was obtained in each instance. However, after 5 to 8 years, the pyelographic appearance of the kidneys had not changed, except that the tailored lowermost ureter looked less dilated, and renal function was stable. One must conclude that these were patients with nonobstructed megaureters and that ureteral tailoring and reimplantation could not improve them even though an optimal surgical result was achieved.

The false-positive test finding in the boy with valves, alluded to earlier, is illustrative of problems in interpretation, which are not uncommon. Two groups of children seem particularly prone to misleading or uninterpretable test results. Some are boys with residual hydroureteronephrosis after relief of bladder outlet obstruction, and others are children of either sex with persistent or worsened ureterectasis after ureteral reimplantation.

The vagaries of the Whitaker test in boys with residual hydronephrosis after valve resection are so great that Glassberg and associates (1982) use the test results to define four different types of megaureters observed in such patients. They consider relative renal pressures between 15 and 20 cm of H_2O to be inherently equivocal; three of 14 renal units studied fell into this marginal category. Only four of the kidneys had low pressures with the bladder both full and empty and were clearly unobstructed. No evaluated patients had unequivocally high relative renal pressures, but in seven of 14 renal units the test was difficult to interpret. The reason was that renal pressures were normal with the bladder empty but rose quickly into the pathologic range when the bladder began to fill. Thus, strictly speaking, the Whitaker test is normal if done as originally described, with a catheter draining the bladder. However, since some boys with noncompliant bladders after valve ablations develop progressive renal damage, it seems that this observation is important. Also, it seems futile to reimplant such ureters into the bladder with the expectation that drainage will be improved or that the bladder will then somehow function more normally. Glassberg and colleagues (1982) advise following such patients for at least 6 months. If the upper tracts do not improve and renal pressures remain elevated when the bladder fills, these investigators, and Mitchell (1981), advocate augmentation ileocecocystoplasty to reduce the bladder pressure. Only a small proportion of boys with residual hydronephrosis and no reflux after valve resection need further intervention, and loss of bladder compliance, rather than ureteral obstruction, is the major indication for such surgery.

Other common problems with interpretation of the Whitaker test are seen in children who have persistent or worsening hydronephrosis after ureteral reimplantation in whom renal perfusion pressures are normal. The ureter may be "hooked" as it passes into the vesical hiatus, often around the obliterated umbilical artery, or by the peritoneum. In this situation, the ureter may drain well with the bladder empty. However, as the bladder fills, the entrapped extravesical ureter is immobilized. As the intravesical ureter is shifted laterally, the ureter is angulated at the ureterovesical junction, producing obstruction (Mayo and Ansell, 1980). Such children may also exhibit noncompliant bladders, with renal pressure rising sharply as the bladder begins to fill. Most of these children have normal relative renal pressures with the bladder empty, and most do well over the long term. The bladder seems usually to recover with time, and the child does well, although interval vesicostomy or intermittent catheterization may be required if ureterectasis increases.

Occasionally, specific children will have a completely normal test result with a compliant bladder and a low relative renal pressure. In spite of this, hydronephrosis may occasionally increase dramatically, even over only a few months. The reason for this appears to be that, as scar matures, the once unobstructed ureter becomes obstructed, usually at the new hiatus as it passes through the detrusor. This is not a common sequence of events, but it occurs often enough to warn that the Whitaker test must be interpreted with caution in postoperative patients. A negative test finding does not necessarily mean that obstruction will not occur in the future.

Woodburg and co-workers (1989) have modified the Whitaker test, using renal pelvic perfusion at a constant low physiologic pressure (7 to 12 cm H_2O) in dogs and pigs). These investigators reason that constant pressure perfusion is independent of the effects of upper tract compliance and that such pressure normally results in flows of 1 to 5 ml per minute. When employing constant pressure perfusions in systems with partial ureteral obstructions, flow rates are diminished or nil. Obstruction was defined in the same systems by constant flow, but sometimes the renal pelvic pressure was in the 15 to 20 cm H_2O range, which is often deemed equivocal.

Even with all these provisos, renal pressure-flow measurements have become the most accurate test to differentiate obstructed from nonobstructed megaureter. The test is most accurate in patients who have not been operated upon and who have compliant bladders. It may be performed intraoperatively to document obstruction, although at that point it is too late if obstruction is not found. The dilated ureters in the prune-belly syndrome may be obstructed or nonobstructed, just as in other types of megaureter, and can be accurately categorized employing the Whitaker test.

The only potential problem caused by nonobstructed megaureter is due to stasis caused by the inability of the walls of the ureter to coapt. This loss of effective peristalsis clearly seems not to prevent renal growth, either in children or in animal models, but such ureterectasis occasionally seems to be the reason for susceptibility to urine infection.

Management of Primary Obstructed Megaureter

History of Surgical Treatment

Caulk treated his initial patient with transurethral endoscopic meatotomy in 1923. The patient did well clinically, but, of course, it is not certain whether the surgeon was dealing with an obstructed or a nonobstructed megaureter. Lewis and Kimbrough (1952) performed ureteral meatotomy after ureteral dilations and nephroureterolysis failed to result in improvement, but reflux resulted. In 1954, in view of the poor surgical results up to that time, Nesbit and Withycombe concluded that megaureter should not be treated surgically. In retrospect, it seems that ureteral meatotomy was doomed to fail, since the obstruction, when present, is extravesical. In fact, the intravesical ureter is seldom involved, although an occasional child will have severe stenosis at the ureteral meatus without a ureterocele.

The use of a tapered, isolated portion of small bowel to replace the ureter in patients with extreme hydronephrosis was reported by Swenson and colleagues (1956). No attempt was made to form an anti-reflux anastomosis with the bladder. Also in 1956, Lewis and Cletsoway reported using a ureteral nipple similar to that fashioned in a Paquin ureteral reimplantation for reflux. The ureter was not tapered, but the lower extremely dilated portion was excised. Good surgical results were achieved, and reflux was not demonstrable postoperatively in any of 12 ureters so treated.

Goodwin and associates (1957) also replaced the dilated ureter with isolated ileal segments. Partial extravesical intussusception of the upper ileum into the lower for a distance of 1 to 2 inches was the anti-reflux mechanism employed. Good long-term results have been achieved. Politano (1972) also successfully utilized small bowel to replace megaureters. He incorporated a long everted nipple of the distalmost ileal segment through the bladder anastomosis as the antireflux mechanism. All investigators have emphasized the need to remove a disc of bladder equal in size to the lumen of the bowel to prevent obstruction when an ileal segment is employed to replace the ureter. The orientation of the bowel loop must always be isoperistaltic. Hirschhorn (1964) and Politano (1972) sought to restore ureteral peristalsis in the patient with megaureter by wrapping the dilated ureter with an isolated segment of small bowel from which the mucosa had been removed. The bowel segment must always run the full length of the ureter, preferably from the renal hilum to the bladder, as ureteral dilatation may increase postoperatively above the wrapped segment.

Creevy (1967) was the first to report extensive ureteral tailoring combined with a Politano type of anti-reflux reimplantation. He clearly defined the radiographic characteristics of the different types of megaureter and believed that ureteral reimplantation was generally indicated when calycectasis was present. Thus, some of his patients probably had nonobstructed megaureters with megacalycosis. Bischoff (1957) advocated tapering of only the lowermost ureter in most instances in order to achieve an anti-reflux reimplantation.

Current Therapy

Peters and co-workers (1989) reported on 42 infants with primary obstructive megaureters operated upon before 8 months of age. The mean age at the time of surgery was 1.8 months in those detected prenatally and 3.8 months in those detected postnatally. Function in the obstructed kidney improved in all patients. Eight had postoperative reflux that subsided with time in three, continues to be followed in two, and required repeated reimplantation in three. Five patients had mild postoperative obstructions that were managed without surgery, whereas two underwent reoperations. These investigators concluded that correction of the obstruction in early infancy improved drainage and prevented renal damage from infection. With proper attention to detail, excellent results may be achieved.

Keating and associates (1989) followed 44 hydronephrotic renal units in neonates who were diagnosed as having primary obstructed megaureters on the basis of renal scans alone soon after birth. None had deterioration of renal function over time. In 15 of 16 with moderately to severely dilated systems, the degree of hydronephrosis improved, sometimes dramatically.

Twelve of 21 primary obstructed ureters discovered in older infants were also followed. At the time of the report, only two of these required surgical corrections. These workers concluded that primary obstructed megaureters diagnosed at birth because of antenatal hydronephrosis may be distinct entities, which carry little risk of subsequent deterioration in renal function.

This experience also underscores how difficult it is to make the diagnosis of obstruction on objective grounds. Some experimental ureteral narrowings are known to be nonobstructive at low rates or volumes of urine production but to compromise flow at high rates or volumes. This observation is the basis for the Whitaker test and the "diuretic-enhanced" renogram. It seems best to employ these tools aggressively to diagnose obstruction. Surgical correction of obstructive megaureter is usually successful, and infection superimposed on obstruction rapidly results in renal damage.

The majority of patients who present with primary megaureter, particularly older children or adults, prove clearly to have the nonobstructed variety and do not require surgical intervention. The ureter generally becomes less dilated as the child grows.

Surgery should be reserved for patients with progressive ureterectasis or extreme generalized hydroureteronephrosis, with parenchymal loss, and for those with lesser degrees of dilatation in whom diagnostic tests indicate obstruction.

Another indication for surgery in a child with megaureter is recurrent or persistent infection that can be localized to the hydronephrotic system by culturing samples taken from the upper tracts. The urine can be obtained by ureteral catheterization or percutaneous aspiration. This group may include some with nonobstructed megaureter but severe stasis. As noted earlier, nonobstructed upper tracts seldom improve after surgery in function or appearance, but the infection may be eliminated. It is in this group with persistent infection that the strongest case can be made for tailoring the dilated ureter above the bladder, wrapping the ureter with denuded bowel, or replacing the ureter with a bowel segment to restore peristalsis.

Summary

The diagnosis of primary megaureter is fulfilled under the following conditions:

1. The bladder and bladder outlet appear normal.
2. Ureterectasis begins above a narrow, usually short, distal ureteral segment, which may be difficult to visualize on the intravenous pyelogram. The ureter is dilated for a varying length above but is usually not as tortuous as one would expect, given the degree of ureterectasis. Calycectasis may or may not be present.
3. Vesicoureteral reflux is absent, except in refluxing megaureter.
4. The ureteral orifice has a normal appearance endoscopically.

Such ureters must then be further studied to differentiate obstructed from nonobstructed megaureter. If intrinsic obstruction is present, a ureteral catheter may not pass through the narrow juxtavesicular ureter. When it does pass, a large volume of urine comes out steadily in a hydronephrotic drip. Contrast material instilled for retrograde pyelography will remain in an obstructed system for several hours. The renogram curve on hydrated renal scan has an obstructed pattern that does not normalize with the administration of a diuretic. Renal pressures are elevated when the pelvis or upper ureter is perfused with fluid at 10 ml per minute (Whitaker test).

In primary nonobstructive megaureter, a ureteral catheter will pass without difficulty unless technical problems are present. Although some urine may come out in a steady drip, the volume is less than would be expected considering the volume of the system. Similarly, contrast material instilled through the catheter tends to drain more quickly, although this is still a function of the volume of the hydroureteronephrosis or ureterectasis. The diuretic renogram findings may be equivocal, but the Whitaker test results will show low relative renal pressures. When marked calycectasis is present with nonobstructed megaureter, this is usually due to megacalycosis. A clue may be that the renal pelvis is usually not as dilated as one would expect with apparent calycectasis of severe degree.

Although the diagnosis of no obstruction can be established with relative certainty, a child with nonobstructive megaureter should be followed to be certain that the upper tracts are stable or improve as expected with growth.

The treatment of refluxing megaureter, or the appearance of a typical megaureter on intravenous pyelogram that turns out to be due to reflux, depends on the etiology of the reflux and the chance that the reflux may subside spontaneously. Reflux can occur in conjunction with obstructive megaureter—they are different lesions—and this possibility should be considered when the reflux is severe in grade and the ureter drains poorly.

Megaureter of iatrogenic cause, following prior ureteral reimplantation, or ureterectasis seen in boys with prune-belly syndrome can be evaluated and categorized according to whether or not ureteral obstruction is present.

Secondary obstructive megaureter is initially treated by correcting the primary problem. When bladder outlet obstruction is the cause, the hydroureter usually improves as detrusor hypertrophy regresses. When ureterectasis persists in such circumstances, re-evaluation will permit differentiation of the megaureters into the obstructed or nonobstructed category or detection of a noncompliant bladder. Hydrated, diuretic augmented renograms and Whitaker test findings may indicate obstruction until the detrusor hypertrophy has had time— 6 months to a year—to subside. However, the results of ureteral reimplantation are usually better when the detrusor is normal. Partly for this reason, such ureterectasis should be given a chance to improve after the outlet obstruction is relieved. Reimplantation into a noncompliant bladder should be avoided and alternatives, such as bladder augmentation or ileocecal cystoplasty considered, as discussed in the section on urethral valves.

Neuropathic bladder is another common cause of secondary megaureter. Reflux and obstruction may be combined. When urine is retained in the bladder, the keystone of therapy has become intermittent catheterization on a regular timed basis, although ureteral reimplantation or bladder augmentation may be needed.

Other causes of acquired obstructed megaureter include calculus, granulomatous disease, and a rare ureteral valve or midureteral stricture.

URETERAL REIMPLANTATION

Ureteroneocystostomy

In 1900, Bovee reviewed ureteral surgery and credited Tauffer with performing the first ureteroneocystostomy in 1877. Eighty cases had been reported, most of which were performed after accidental division of the ureter at the time of laparotomy or during surgery for ureteral fistulas following difficult labor or forceps delivery. Bovee mentions several operations for "abnormal congenital ureteral openings" but none for vesicoureteral reflux. Concerning the technique of ureteroneocystectomy, he commented that a transabdominal extraperitoneal approach was appropriate and noted that "an effort has been made to imitate the normal oblique bladder implantation of the ureter to prevent reflux." Ancillary techniques to correct the difficult clinical situation of inadequate ureteral length that were mentioned in this early article include the psoas hitch, transureteroureterostomy, and inferior nephropexy!

In 1934, Vermooten and Neuswanger described a "submucous" technique of ureteral reimplantation in dogs that lessened the incidence of vesicoureteral reflux postoperatively compared with direct ureterovesical anastomosis. In 1943, Stevens and Marshall reported ten patients in whom a similar technique had been employed. Dodson (1946) reviewed the techniques of ureteroneocystostomy and mentioned the "advantage of mobilizing or straightening the ureter to lengthen it and lessen the distance that it must traverse to reach the bladder," when the ureter was dilated and tortuous.

Pioneering studies of patients with spinal cord injury after World War II demonstrated that reflux was the most common cause of hydronephrosis and led to progressive renal deterioration in the presence of urinary tract infection. Talbot and Bunts (1949) suggested that ureteral reimplantation to correct vesicoureteral reflux would be beneficial in such cases. In 1952, Hutch reported success in eight of 11 ureteral reimplantations for vesicoureteral reflux in nine paraplegic patients. Hutch employed a combined extravesical and intravesical approach to the distal ureter. Hutch also reported satisfactory results in 11 of 13 ureteral reimplantations in seven children, four of whom had myelodysplasia.

In 1958, Politano and Leadbetter described their technique of intravesical mobilization of the terminal ureter with subsequent reimplantation through a new vesical hiatus and submucosal tunnel. They reported the elimination of reflux in 14 patients requiring a total of 21 ureteral reimplantations. One case of postoperative ureteral obstruction required reoperation. The four patients reported in detail in this series were children who did not have overt neuropathic bladders (Fig. 44–22).

Paquin (1959) summarized the fundamental requirements of a satisfactory anti-reflux operation. These include a tension-free anastomosis between the ureter and bladder, a submucosal tunnel that is five times as long as the diameter of the ureter, and firm support for the intravesical ureter from the underlying bladder muscle. The ureter should be straightened when necessary to secure proper drainage, but care should be taken to preserve its blood supply. The terminal 3 to 4 cm of ureter should be tapered if its diameter is greater than 8 to 10 mm in order to restore the proper ratio of length to width in the intramural ureter.

Paquin also reported a technique of ureteroneocystostomy that included both extravesical and intravesical dissection to create the new vesical hiatus and submucosal tunnel as well as formation of an everted nipple at the ureterovesical anastomosis. This technique has also remained in general use, except that formation of the intravesical nipple is now generally omitted.

Lich and co-workers (1961) described an extravesical approach to create a submucosal tunnel for the ureter and a new hiatus in the muscular wall of the bladder. This technique does not disturb the continuity of the ureterovesical mucosa, nor does it alter the position of the ureteral orifice (Fig. 44–23). It is employed primarily in situations involving little ureterectasis, as the amount of lengthening of the intravesical ureter that can be obtained without angulation is limited.

Williams (1961), Hutch (1963), and Glenn and Anderson (1967) all described intravesical ureteral advance-

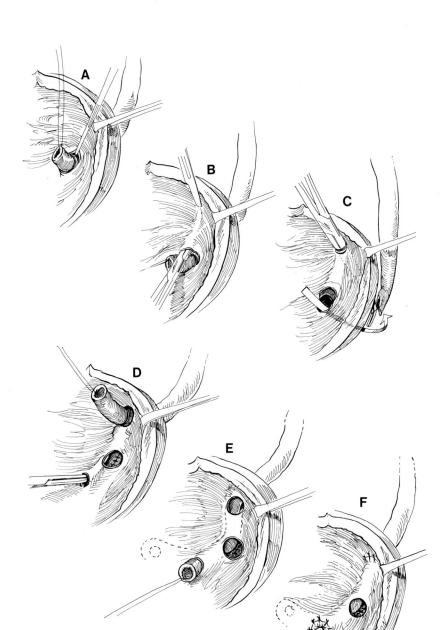

Figure 44–22. Politano-Leadbetter technique of ureteroneocystostomy.

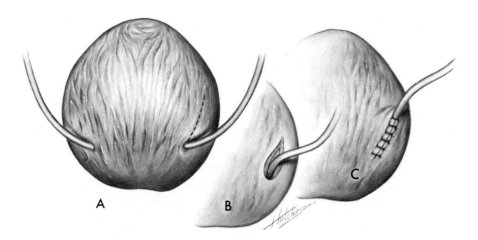

Figure 44–23. Lich's technique of vesicoureteroplasty. (From Kelalis, P. P., and King, L. R. (Eds.): Clinical Pediatric Urology, Philadelphia, W. B. Saunders Co., 1976.)

ment procedures. Each requires mobilization of the ureter from its attachments as it traverses the muscular wall of the bladder, with advancement of its orifice to a new location on the floor of the bladder in order to secure a longer intravesical segment. These procedures are also originally limited to patients in whom the ureter is of relatively normal caliber and in whom there is sufficient room for advancement of the ureter on the floor of the bladder (Fig. 44–24).

Stephens (1977) and Glenn and Anderson (1967) later refined the intravesical advancement technique. After mobilization of the ureter within the deep periureteral

sheath, the bladder wall at the superior margin of the vesical hiatus is incised for a distance of 2 to 3 cm. The hiatus is closed inferiorly in order to buttress the intravesical ureter, displace the hiatus superiorly, and gain more length for the submucosal tunnel. The orifice is then advanced to a new location on the floor of the bladder. Utilizing the exposure obtained by initially enlarging the hiatus, a dilated, tortuous ureter can be satisfactorily shortened and tapered from within the bladder prior to reimplantation. This technique is also applicable to the reimplantation of double ureters.

Cohen (1975) modified the advancement technique

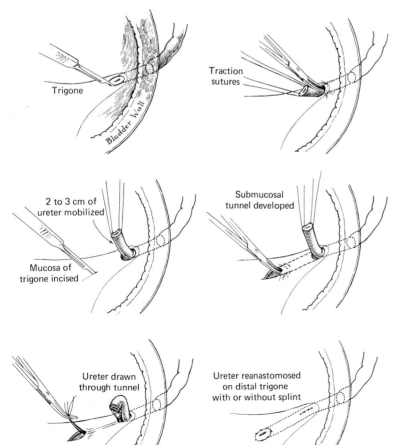

Figure 44–24. Glenn-Anderson distal tunnel ureteral reimplantation. Mobilization of distal tunnel and development of submucosal tunnel distally across trigone obviates some of the potential difficulties of ureteral advancement procedures. (From Glenn, J. F. (Ed.): Urologic Surgery, 2nd ed. New York, Harper & Row, 1975.)

and obtained additional length for creation of an adequate submucosal tunnel by leading the reimplanted ureter across the midline (Fig. 44–25). The Cohen operation has become very popular because of its versatility. It must be employed when the trigone is tubularized to form a sphincter in incontinence operations, and the results achieved after conventional anti-reflux surgery have been very good. Perhaps because the original urinary hiatus is usually maintained, there is a very low incidence of obstruction following reimplantation with this technique. One often cited drawback to the Cohen procedure is that the reimplanted orifices tend to face laterally, as each ureter commonly crosses the midline. Subsequent instrumentation through a cystoscope may be difficult. However, it is possible to fill the bladder and puncture the anterior wall percutaneously with a Cystocath sheath under direct cystoscopic visualization. The sheath of the Cystocath is placed opposite the lateral facing reimplanted orifice, and a ureteral catheter is then passed percutaneously (Lamesch, 1981). This method of retrograde catheterization following a Cohen reimplant seems very safe. Catheter drainage after bladder puncture is generally unnecessary, as the puncture wound in the bladder usually seals almost immediately. An additional advantage is that adult-sized instruments that will not pass through pediatric cystoscopes can be introduced in this way. For instance, a stone basket can often be inserted into such a ureter by percutaneous puncture, whereas the instrument will not pass through a cystoscope that can be employed in boys. Transurethral scissors are also occasionally helpful to incise an ischemic stricture of the distalmost ureter following reimplantation.

When ureteral reimplantation is performed on a young infant, primarily for obstructive megaureter, the need to leave a postoperative cystostomy in the bladder

Figure 44–25. Cross trigone reimplantation technique. (From Hendren, W. H.: *In* Smith, R. B., and Skinner, D. G. (Eds.): Complications of Urologic Surgery: Prevention and Management. Philadelphia, W. B. Saunders Co., 1976.)

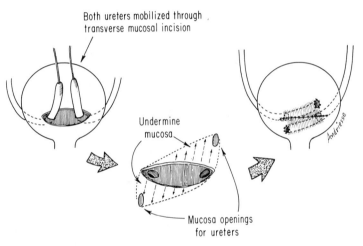

CROSS TRIGONE REIMPLANT

Both ureters mobilized through transverse mucosal incision

Undermine mucosa

Mucosa openings for ureters

CROSS TRIGONE REIMPLANT
in small bladder and / or trigone

ONE OF TWO URETERS

2–3 cm tunnel

SOLITARY URETER

Closure original hiatus

BOTH URETERS

2 separate tunnels

Each ureter in original hiatus

may result in intractable bladder spasms. Infants seem resistant to anticholinergics, and it is difficult to control postoperative pain and spasms. Belladonna and opium suppositories, given every 4 to 6 hours, are recommended as prophylaxes. They will not, however, generally control bladder spasms once begun.

Another approach, which began in infants only, but which now is used almost routinely, is to leave a stent in the reimplanted ureter or ureters. This stent is sutured to the bladder with 5–0 catgut. The bladder is closed in three layers, with a reliable watertight closure as is employed after renal transplantation. Drains are left alongside the bladder as the wound is closed. No catheter is left in the bladder.

This technique obviates the risk of severe postoperative bladder spasms. Additionally, even if all ureters are stented, the children void some urine, and thus dysuria is alleviated before they leave the hospital. A sonogram is performed before discharge to be sure there is no perivesical urinoma, although this has not been a problem. The stent-and-drain technique (no catheter) definitely prevents postoperative bladder spasms.

Surgical Correction of Megaureter

The standard surgical therapy for primary obstructive megaureter derives from the work of Politano and Leadbetter (1958), Paquin (1959), Creevy (1967), and Hendren (1968). Creevy (1967) and Bischoff (1972) advocated tapering only that portion of the wide ureter that would become the new intravesical ureter after reimplantation but would permit a reliable type of antireflux anastomosis. Hendren (1968) showed that, with care, more of the lower ureter could be narrowed without devascularizing the most distal portion. The key to success is atraumatic manipulation of the ureter and preservation of the blood vessels that enter the wall of the dilated ureter on its medial aspect (Fig. 44–26). If dilatation of the upper ureter persists or infection ensues, the upper ureter is occasionally narrowed in a similar fashion 6 to 8 weeks later.

The simpler, limited approach has proved to be adequate in most children with obstructed megaureters. If obstruction is relieved and reflux prevented, the dilated ureter above the bladder will narrow and straighten as the child grows. Tailoring long ureteral segments, with an increased risk of distal ureteral ischemia and stenosis even when care is taken to preserve the blood supply, is unnecessary. In practice, we find that modeling or tailoring the lowermost 5 cm of ureter, which is to be retained and to serve mainly as the new intravesical ureter after reimplantation, is adequate. This tapered segment, about 12 Fr. in diameter, is reimplanted into the bladder medial to and above the original hiatus so that a 4-cm intravesical course can be achieved, with care taken so that the medial blood supply of the justavesical ureter is not disrupted (Hendren, 1969).

Alternatively, a cross-trigone method of implantation can be employed. This also permits a relatively long intravesical course. Hensley and co-workers (1982), Ahmed (1980), and Cohen (1975) believe that intraves-

ical tailoring and preservation of the original hiatus reduces the risk of distal ureteral ischemia or obstruction due to angulation outside the bladder.

An alternative to tailoring of the lower ureter to achieve an adequate length-to-width ratio to prevent reflux has been described by Kalicinski and associates (1977) and evaluated by Starr (1979), Politano (1981), and Ehrlich (1982) (Figs. 44–27 and 44–28). In their view, the risks of devascularization of the distalmost remaining ureter following straightening and tapering of the dilated ureter are best avoided by leaving intact the full circumference of the distal dilated ureter.

Bakker and colleagues (1987, 1988) studied ureteral tapering, with excision of the lateral aspect of the dilated ureter and ureteral modeling (folding), using the Kalicinski technique. These investigators found both procedures successful in preventing reflux without producing obstruction. Microangiograms, however, showed consistently better preservation of the blood supply in the tapered, folded ureters. The slight risk of a fistula from the proximal portion of a tapered ureter to the bladder, which would result in reflux, is also avoided.

Technique of Ureteral Modeling

The ureter, in its collapsed state, should not be more than about 2 cm in diameter. If it is wider, tapering will be required, as such ureters are too bulky when folded to achieve an adequate tunnel length to reliably prevent reflux. An 8 Fr. stent is passed into the ureter. The ureteral lumen is then segregated with a longitudinal running mattress suture of 3–0 chromic, placed to divide the ureter into two longitudinal openings of more or less equal calibre. If the ureter is less than 14 mm collapsed, the lumen containing the stent is then larger. Care is taken not to narrow the lumen containing the stent to less than a uniform 8 to 10 mm diameter. One portion of the dilated ureter is then rolled over the lumen and the stent. Interrupted adventitial sutures hold the rolled segment in place. The result of such "modeling" results in less ureteral bulk than might be expected, and an antireflux anastomosis through a long submucosal tunnel is readily accomplished. The new orifice is anchored to the detrusor and overlying mucosa with interrupted sutures, as in the more standard techniques. We have not seen obstruction or persistence of reflux in approximately 30 patients in whom this procedure was employed, and Ehrlich (1982) reports over 100 consecutive successes.

Surgical Alternatives

Very good results (99 per cent success) have been obtained with Lich's operation (Gregoir, 1964; Marberger et al., 1978; McDuffie et al., 1977), but it is difficult to quantitate the degree to which the extravesical ureter is compressed, and perhaps compromised, by closing the bladder muscle behind the ureter. Also, this operation is not applicable when the ureter is dilated to more

Text continued on page 1729

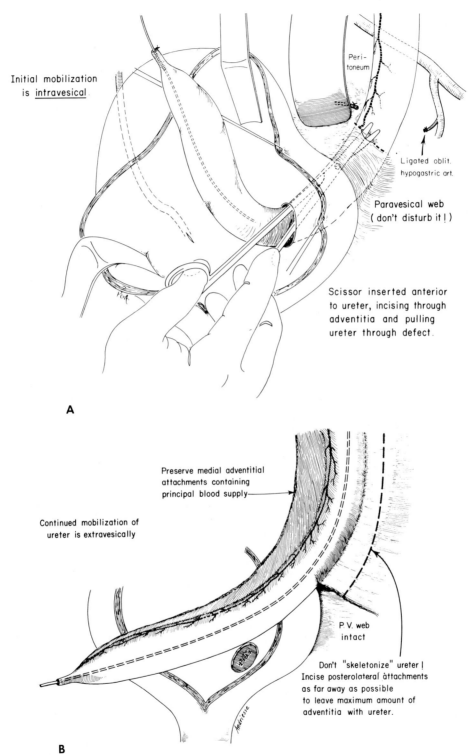

Initial mobilization
is <u>intravesical</u>.

Peri-
toneum

Ligated oblit.
hypogastric art.

Paravesical web
(don't disturb it !)

Scissor inserted anterior
to ureter, incising through
adventitia and pulling
ureter through defect.

A

Preserve medial adventitial
attachments containing
principal blood supply

Continued mobilization of
ureter is extravesically

P. V. web
intact

Don't "skeletonize" ureter !
Incise posterolateral attachments
as far away as possible
to leave maximum amount of
adventitia with ureter.

B

Figure 44–26. Hendren's technique of reimplantation of the megaureter. *A,* Initial mobilization of the ureter from inside the bladder. *B,* Continued extravesical mobilization of bladder after dividing obliterated hypogastric ligament. (From Hendren, W. H.: *In* Smith, R. B., and Skinner, D. G. (Eds.): Complications of Urologic Surgery: Prevention and Management. Philadelphia, W. B. Saunders Co., 1976.)

Illustration continued on following page

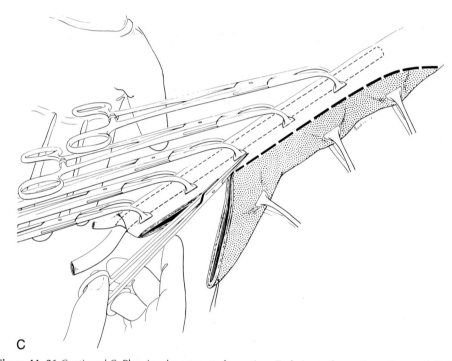

C

Figure 44–26 *Continued* C, Planning the amount of resection. Technique of resection using special clamps.

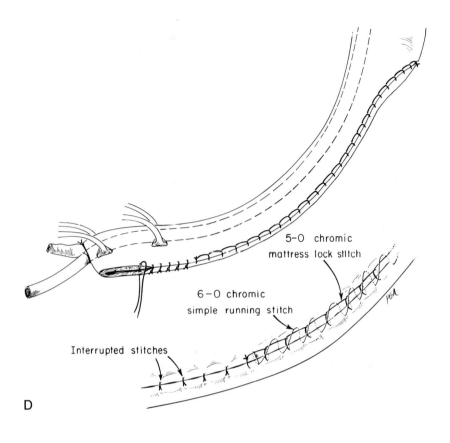

5-0 chromic
mattress lock stitch

6-0 chromic
simple running stitch

Interrupted stitches

D

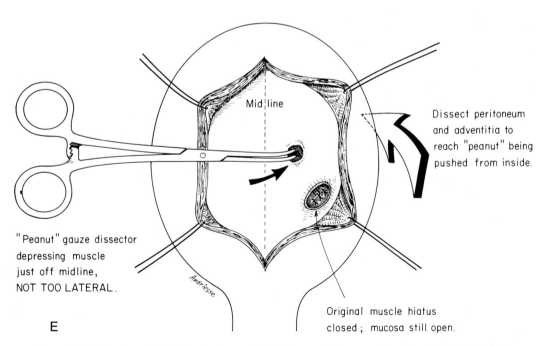

Mid line

Dissect peritoneum
and adventitia to
reach "peanut" being
pushed from inside.

"Peanut" gauze dissector
depressing muscle
just off midline,
NOT TOO LATERAL.

Original muscle hiatus
closed; mucosa still open.

E

Figure 44–26 *Continued D,* Details of closure. *E,* Selecting new hiatus, craniad and medial to original one.

Illustration continued on following page

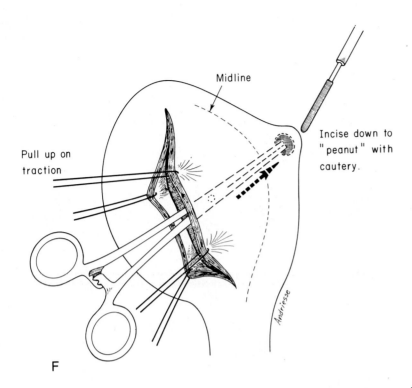

Midline

Pull up on traction

Incise down to "peanut" with cautery.

F

Figure 44–26 *Continued F,* Opening hiatus after carefully selecting suitable point. *G,* Incising mucosa to construct-tunnel.

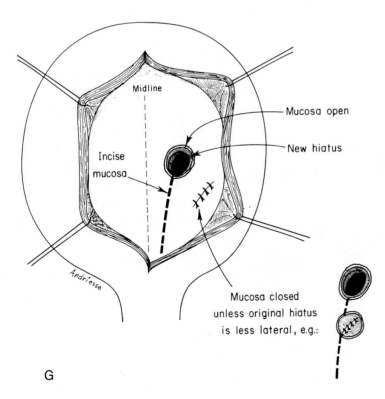

Midline

Mucosa open

New hiatus

Incise mucosa

Mucosa closed unless original hiatus is less lateral, e.g.:

G

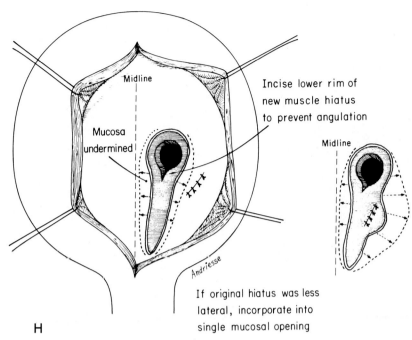

Incise lower rim of
new muscle hiatus
to prevent angulation

Midline

Mucosa
undermined

If original hiatus was less
lateral, incorporate into
single mucosal opening

H

Figure 44–26 *Continued H,* Elevating mucosal flaps.
I, Resecting excess length.
Illustration continued on following page

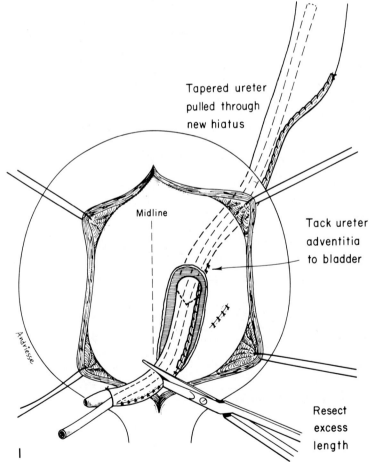

Tapered ureter
pulled through
new hiatus

Tack ureter
adventitia
to bladder

Midline

Resect
excess
length

I

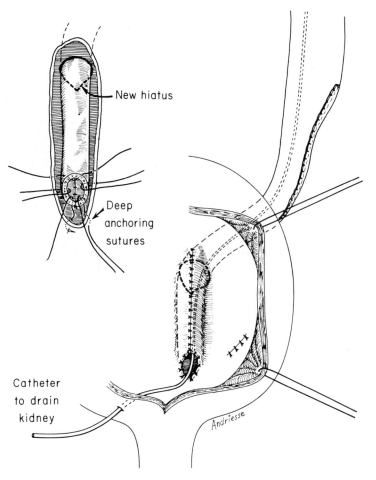

New hiatus

Deep anchoring sutures

Catheter to drain kidney

Andriesse

J

Figure 44–26 *Continued J,* Completing repair. Ureteral suture line lies posteriorly.

Figure 44–27. Kalicinski's method of "modeling" the lower portion of a dilated ureter as modified by Ehrlich. The caliber of the ureter is reduced to facilitate antireflux ureteral reimplantation. The lower 5 cm of ureter is divided longitudinally by a running absorbable suture. Interrupted sutures are used distally so that excessive length can be resected if necessary. The ureter is then folded with interrupted sutures, preserving both lumens. Folding only the portion that becomes the new intravesical ureter makes subsequent ischemic stenosis unlikely.

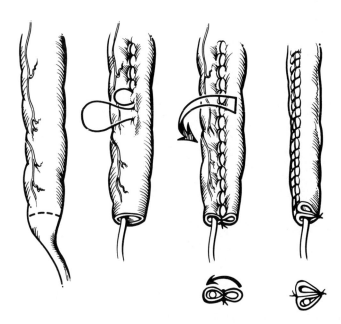

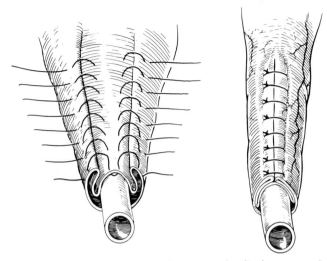

Figure 44–28. The Starr method of narrowing the distalmost ureter is performed by placing interrupted sutures to plicate the ureter. Considerable reduction in bulk can be achieved. This method is favored when the dilated ureter is thin walled.

than one or two times its normal diameter. Perhaps for these reasons the procedure is not in very general use.

The procedures in common use today are those of Politano and Leadbetter (1958) and Cohen (1975), and the advancement operations, particularly as modified by Glenn and Anderson (1967) and modified by Stephens (1977), to recess the hiatus and permit a greater increase in the length of the intravesical ureter. The Politano-Leadbetter procedure can be made more versatile by incorporating an extravesical approach to mobilize the distal ureter and to free the posterolateral wall of the bladder in order to create the new vesical hiatus under direct vision. This manuever reduces the risk of kinking the lower ureter, facilitates the tapering or modeling what will become the new intravesical ureter when needed, and obviates any risk of perforating the peritoneum or adjacent viscera, because these structures are all then visualized directly (Fig. 44–29).

A ureteral stent is employed postoperatively if tapering of the reimplanted ureter is required. A feeding tube or soft Silastic tubing (No. 5 or 8 Fr) is ideal for this purpose. It can be readily brought through the bladder through a stab wound and connected to dependent drainage. If extensive modeling or tapering has been performed, the stent is left in place for 7 to 10 days, or until urine begins to drain into the bladder around the stents as edema subsides. Use of a stent, at least on one side, during the first 24 to 72 hours after bilateral reimplantation without tapering is also often beneficial to avoid any risk of oliguria during the period of maximal postoperative edema. The bladder is usually drained by a suprapubic catheter in males and a urethral catheter in females for 4 to 6 days after simple reimplantations, or until all stents are removed after more complicated procedures.

Technique of Ureteral Implantation without a Catheter

We employ stents and a drain in infants and in most older girls undergoing ureteral implantations. Infants are very intolerant to catheters, which induce painful spontaneous bladder contractions. Anticholinergics are not very successful in preventing or ablating such spasms. Stents are placed in the ureter after reimplantation and are sutured to the adjacent bladder with 5–0 chromic catgut. The stents exit through the anterior bladder wall and a stab wound in the abdomen. The bladder is closed in a watertight fashion in three layers, as after a renal transplant. Drains are left down to the ureteral hiatus.

Voiding is often painful at first, but infrequent until most of the urine begins to drain around the stent or until the stent is removed about 3 days postoperatively. Twelve babies did well and did not develop urinomas or any complications requiring prolonged hospitalization.

We now utilize this technique routinely in females of all ages. We continue to use suprapubic Malecot catheters in most boys, unless the bladders can be completely re-epithelialized, because the relatively small catheters that can be inserted transurethrally are often not very helpful when clots must be evacuated. A suprapubic rather than a urethral catheter almost obviates the risk of postoperative epididymitis in males.

Uncomplicated implantations may not require such a prolonged period of bladder drainage. Gonzales and associates (1978) have often been able to discharge patients 2 to 4 days after such surgery. Often, however, there is considerable persistence of dysuria when the catheter is removed so soon. Early discharge is most often feasible when the Lich type of reimplantation has been performed, in which the bladder was unopened.

Reoperations

Patients who have had previous anti-reflux surgery should undergo a combined intravesical-extravesical approach if they require reoperation. It is often convenient to utilize a low midline incision and open the peritoneum and identify the dilated ureters at the pelvic brim. The lower ureters are mobilized toward the bladder, and extreme care is taken to preserve the adventitial blood supply and the entire length of ureter that is not involved in stricture or ischemic stenosis. The umbilical arteries are divided if this has not already been done, so that they will not angulate the ureter after reimplantation. If ureteral length is adequate for an anti-reflux reimplantation without tension, this is carried out using the open Politano-Leadbetter, Cohen, or Paquin technique. The portion of the ureter that will become intravesical is tapered or folded, if necessary, to achieve a 4:1 or 5:1 ratio of length to width. The suture line in the ureter after tapering is oriented against the detrusor and away from the bladder lumen to minimize the risk of a fistula between the ureter above the new orifice and the bladder

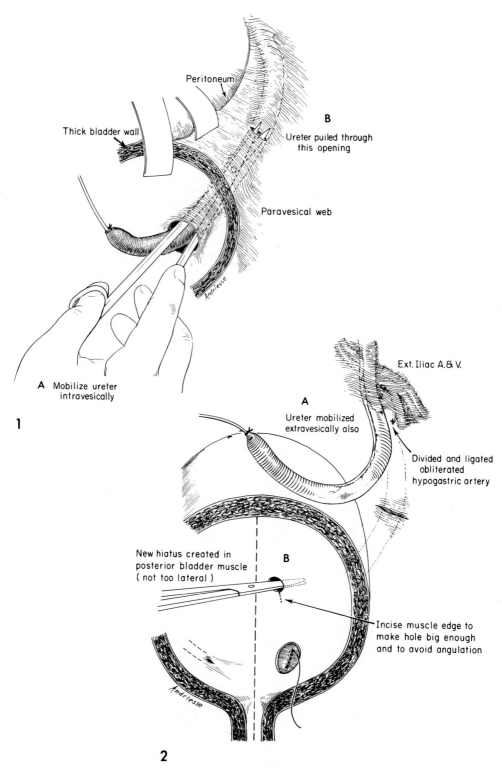

Figure 44–29. Combined intravesical-extravesical reimplantation technique. (From Hendren, W. H.: *In* Smith, R. B., and Skinner, D. G.: Complications of Urologic Surgery: Prevention and Management. Philadelphia, W. B. Saunders Co., 1976.)

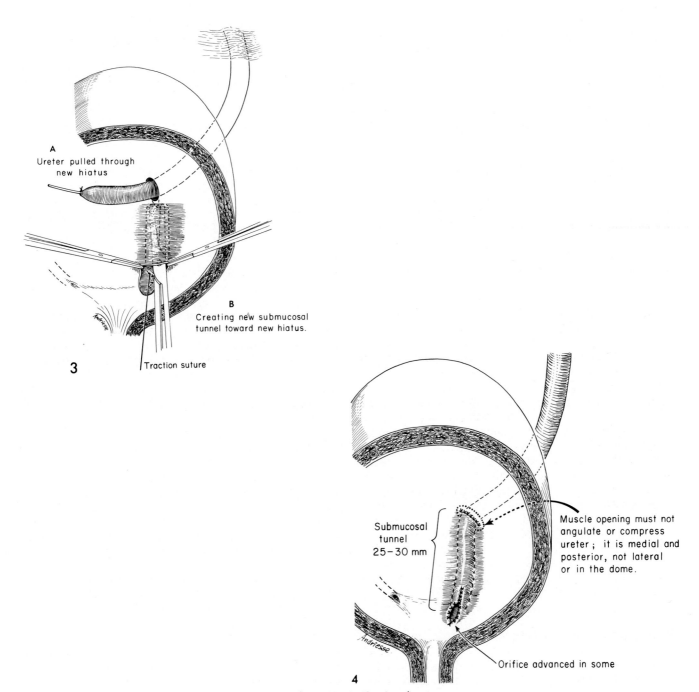

A
Ureter pulled through
new hiatus

B
Creating new submucosal
tunnel toward new hiatus.

Traction suture

3

Submucosal
tunnel
25–30 mm

Muscle opening must not
angulate or compress
ureter; it is medial and
posterior, not lateral
or in the dome.

Orifice advanced in some

4

Figure 44–29. (Continued)

lumen. The ureter is anchored in place with three or four absorbable sutures, generally 4–0 chromic catgut, between the muscle of the trigone and all layers of the ureter on either side of the posterior ureteral suture line that results from tapering. If available, bladder mucosa is drawn over the reimplanted ureter, but if mucosa is friable and has been torn, the intravesical surface of the ureter will quickly epithelialize.

If the ureter will not reach the trigone without tension, several alternatives may be satisfactory. The bladder may be mobilized and drawn over to the ureter by sewing the superolateral aspect of the bladder to the psoas muscle with heavy absorbable sutures, a psoas hitch.

If the contralateral ureter is functioning normally and is neither obstructed nor refluxing, transureteroureterostomy is an attractive alternative, provided that the discrepancy in the diameter of the ureters is not too great. A ureter 1 cm in diameter, or a little more in its collapsed state, may be anastomosed to a ureter of little more than normal caliber with great reliability. If the recipient ureter is more than twice the normal caliber, anastomosis of a transposed ureter of any size can be accomplished without difficulty. Transureteroureterostomy should not be performed when retroperitoneal inflammation is present. The technique of transureteroureterostomy is described elsewhere in this text.

The Boari bladder flap is often an alternative to transureteroureterostomy when a psoas hitch alone will not make up the needed deficiency in ureteral length. This procedure is described elsewhere in this text. The anterior bladder flap is rotated upward toward the mobilized ureter, where a submucosal tunnel is developed in the flap. The ureter is reimplanted as in the Politano-Leadbetter procedure. The flap is closed in two layers; it encloses the submucosal tunnel and, in effect, provides an extension of the bladder into which a shortened ureter can be implanted without tension in the bladder by an anti-reflux technique.

When the ureter is extremely dilated, straightening and resection of excessive tortuous redundant ureteral length improve drainage and lessen residual urine in the upper tracts. Tapering or folding of the remaining distal portion of the ureter that becomes the new intravesical segment is necessary to secure an adequate submucosal tunnel to prevent reflux.

Reflux and ureteral obstruction can coexist in megaureter, but antireflux ureteral reimplantation is designed to correct both conditions.

Reimplantation in Ureteral Duplication

When the ureters are completely duplicated, reflux into only the lower pole segment is the most common associated anomaly that may require surgical correction. Because double ureters are usually joined by a common sheath just before they reach the bladder, it is not difficult to mobilize and reimplant the ureters as one, in a common tunnel. The drawback to this approach is that if the upper pole ureter does not reflux it is often very small, and it may subtend only a few calyces. Thus,

it is probably slightly more likely to become obstructed than a ureter of normal caliber after reimplantation.

An alternative that I often prefer is to identify both ureters extravesically. The refluxing ureter is mobilized distally to the common sheath. The refluxing ureter only is transected, ligating the distal stump. The transected ureter is passed medially below the upper pole ureter and implanted into the bladder above the trigone using the transverse Cohen technique.

Ipsilateral ureteroureterostomy is another alternative (Bockrath et al., 1983). The refluxing ureter is transected obliquely 2 to 3 cm above the bladder and anastomosed to the lateral aspect of the upper pole ureter. A stent is employed postoperatively. This alternative method should not be used when the upper pole ureter is very delicate.

Results

Satisfactory results are obtainable in more than 95 per cent of operations overall for primary vesicoureteral reflux and in over 98 per cent of patients without severe hydronephrosis or infection. The most frequent complication of ureteroneocystostomy is persistence of reflux in the reimplanted ureter. Failure to correct reflux is more common in those who have had previous ureterovesical surgery and in those with dilated ureters or scarred and noncompliant bladders. The most frequent reason for continued reflux is failure to create an adequate length of submucosal tunnel. The minimal acceptable ratio of tunnel length to ureteral diameter is about 4:1. However, a ratio of 5:1 is ideal. Another common reason for persistent reflux, especially after surgery for obstructive megaureter, is that the wall of the ureter is too thick to be collapsed by urine at normal intravesical pressure. Such ureters need to be reimplanted with long submucosal courses.

The failure to taper a very dilated ureter adequately is another cause of persistent reflux. An adequate flap-valve mechanism is not obtained.

Reflux is also much more prone to recur when the patient has a noncompliant bladder or an untreated sphincter dyssynergia. The good results reported after reimplantation into a neuropathic bladder suggest that prompt reinstitution of anticholinergics and intermittent catheterization after surgery minimizes the risk of failure.

The other frequent complication is obstruction of the ureter. This may be extrinsic or intrinsic. The former is due to angulation of the ureter proximal to its entry into the bladder or failure to create a large enough hiatus in the bladder wall, so that the ureter is compressed as it enters the bladder. Stenosis of the reimplanted ureter implies ischemia caused by vascular compromise or tension on the anastomosis.

Drainage by ureteral catheter for a few days is advised, if a catheter can be passed. If not, and when hydronephrosis persists, a percutaneous nephrostomy is inserted. The nephrostomy is maintained until free drainage of fluid can be demonstrated into the bladder at normal pressures, i.e., Paquin's buret test. If after 2 or 3 months the obstruction has not resolved, cystoscopy is performed. Ureteral meatotomy alone will suffice to correct meatal stenosis at times, but, more often, resection of the narrowed terminal ureter and another reimplantation are required after more adequate mobilization of the ureter.

Sonography performed during the first few weeks after ureteroneocystostomy may demonstrate a mild-to-moderate increase in hydronephrosis, which generally improves over time as postoperative edema resolves and healing progresses. In postoperative films, one expects to see no more evidence of hydroureteronephrosis than was noted on the preoperative cystogram. This degree of dilatation is probably physiologic and represents "ureteral memory," in that the once dilated ureter will often look dilated on intravenous urogram with a high fluid load (Lebowitz, 1983). However, delayed visualization, particularly if accompanied by febrile urinary tract infection, is an indication for nephrostomy drainage in order to prevent irreversible kidney damage.

If the postoperative patient is doing well, sonography may be deferred until 1 to 2 months after surgery. A nuclear cystogram is performed 3 to 6 months postoperatively. If a cystogram is performed in the immediate postoperative period, reflux is often present owing to edema and inflammation secondary to surgery and incomplete healing. At 3 months, reflux is usually absent, but its occurrence at this time does not mean that it will persist. In 30 per cent of patients with postoperative reflux, such reflux is not present on a second cystogram made 6 to 9 months after surgery. If reflux persists this long, reoperation is generally necessary because healing is complete and the scar at the site of reimplantation precludes improvement with further growth.

If the initial intravenous pyelogram or ultrasound is satisfactory and the upper tracts are normal or improved, imaging is repeated every 2 to 3 years until full growth is achieved, to monitor kidney growth and because of the slight risk of late ureteral obstruction due to scar maturation or changing anatomic relationships. Once reflux is demonstrated to be absent on an adequate cystogram, cystography is not repeated unless the child suffers recurrent infections or unless hydronephrosis is detected.

Ideally, urinary tract infection should be eradicated prior to anti-reflux surgery, and prophylactic chemotherapy should be administered during the immediate postoperative period while catheter drainage is employed. The urine is recultured after all catheters and drains are removed, and specific antibacterial therapy is started if infection is present. If the urine is sterile, prophylactic chemotherapy such as nitrofurantoin, sulfa, or nalidixic acid is continued during the first 6 to 8 weeks after hospitalization.

The development of reflux in the contralateral ureter after unilateral ureteroneocystostomy has been noted to occur in as many as 15 to 20 per cent of patients (Warren et al., 1972), especially in children with neuropathic bladders (Johnston et al., 1976). If the ureteral orifice is normally developed and has an adequate submucosal tunnel, this reflux subsides spontaneously with the resolution of postoperative edema. However, if this ureterovesical junction possessed only borderline compe-

tency initially, reflux may not subside and a second operative procedure is occasionally necessary. For this reason, if a nonrefluxing orifice appears gaping and has a short or absent submucosal tunnel, "prophylactic" reimplantation is at times indicated when the contralateral ureter is reimplanted, even though bilateral reflux was not demonstrated on the preoperative cystogram.

ENDOSCOPIC CORRECTION OF REFLUX

O'Donnell and Puri described the use of Teflon paste (polytef) injected endoscopically to correct vesicoureteral reflux in 1988. Polytef is the generic name for pyrolyzed Teflon particles suspended in an equal volume of glycerin, which has long been employed in otolaryngology for injection into a paralyzed vocal cord (Arnold, 1962). Its use in treating incontinent patients was described in the early 1970s by Politano and by Berg. For incontinence, 14 to 20 ml is commonly injected around the bladder neck and urethra to provide needed resistance. Politano has reported this indication for polytef in over 600 patients and has noted no significant complications.

In 1983, Mittleman and Marraccini reported the autopsy findings in a 76-year-old man who had committed suicide. He had become incontinent after a radical prostatectomy 4 years earlier but had undergone periurethral polytef injections twice, with good restoration of continence. He was apparently in good physical health at the time of suicide. At autopsy, there were small granulomas in the lungs, often a single Teflon granule encased in a giant cell. This case report triggered a debate as to whether polytef injections are safe over the long term in humans, especially in children. Malizia found that Teflon granules result in a granulomatous reaction after periurethral injection and migrate to at least the regional lymph nodes.

Subsequently, many studies have confirmed the propensity of Teflon particles to migrate to distant parts of the body. Claesh and associates (1989) reported a 22-year-old female who developed fever and right upper lobe lung inflammation after the third periurethral Teflon injection. Bronchoscopy revealed numerous sites of inflammation. Biopsy specimens showed mainly intravascular particles of Teflon. These investigators warned against the use of polytef in children.

Politano, however, argues that polytef is safe. He has not found changes in blood chemistry, liver function, chest radiographs, or urine content during the follow-up of patients who had periurethral injections. Because injections of less than 1 ml of paste under the ureteral orifice are adequate to correct reflux, versus an average of perhaps 15 ml to treat incontinence, many believe that intravesical Teflon in small amounts is safe.

Approval of polytef for the treatment of reflux in the United States appears unlikely at this writing; therefore, its use is limited. Several investigators have sought alternative substances. Collagan of bovine origin, autologous cartilage, and ground-up Ivalon foam have been investigated, but these materials are reabsorbed in large measure over time. An acceptable biologically inert alternative has not yet been found.

Results of Teflon Injection

O'Donnell and Puri reported their experience in treating 91 ureters in 61 patients in 1988: 76 renal units had no reflux after a single injection, eight were corrected after a second injection, one after a third injection, and one after a fourth. Six ureters showed reduction in the grade of reflux, and two were unchanged.

The experience of these workers has markedly increased subsequently. They do not advocate treating grade 1 or grade 2 reflux but do so when such reflux is occurring in a child with contralateral reflux of a more severe degree. In order to address the criticism that the endoscopic treatment worked best in those with mild reflux, and presumably more normal intravesical ureters, they have reported patients with grades 4 and 5 reflux separately. In 42 ureters, reflux stopped after a single injection in 28 and after a second in six. Reflux disappeared after three injections in three ureters and after a fourth injection in one ureter. Reflux was downgraded in two patients after a second injection and did not change in two. Six to 30 months later, reflux was absent in 84 per cent but had recurred in 16 per cent. Three patients exhibited emergent contralateral reflux.

Some have argued that the need for multiple anesthetics and the relative uncertainty of the results outweigh the advantages of endoscopic treatment. Brown (1989), for instance, was able to correct reflux in all but one of 76 ureters by open surgery but was successful in only 70 per cent of 40 comparable ureters employing endoscopic treatment. Children receiving polytef paste, on average, need significantly more anesthetics and cystograms. In his view, the cumulative morbidity and stress equals that of an open operation. Kaplan and co-workers (1987) and Schulman and co-workers (1987) reported initial success rates over 80 per cent in stopping reflux but with some subsequent recurrence.

Kaplan and associates (1987) and Quinn and associates (1988) point out the advantages of polytef in children with heavily trabeculated and noncompliant neurogenic bladders in whom less than optimal results can be expected from conventional reimplantation. In my view, Teflon paste is the best treatment when reflux persists after surgery and when the submucosal tunnel is very long. In this situation, the cause of the reflux is a thick-walled ureter, which is not collapsed by urine stored at normal intravesical pressure. Making the submucosal course of such ureters even longer may still be ineffective, but polytef injected under the orifice is usually effective.

Technique of Polytef Injection

Polytef is very viscous. A special injection system or Teflon "gun" is required to prevent movement of the needle tip during injection. O'Donnell and Puri (1988) employ a needle, manufactured by Storz, with a 21-gauge tip bonded to a 5-Fr. flexible shaft. The needle is inserted endoscopically through the bladder mucosa at 6 o'clock, just below the refluxing orifice, for a distance of about 5 mm. Wolff manufactures a cystoscope with an offset lens through which a rigid needle can be inserted. Injection converts the orifice to an inverted crescent. A sphere of polytef is placed below the intravesical ureter. Because 50 per cent of the volume of the polytef is glycerin, which will be reabsorbed, enough paste is injected to nearly cause the edges of the orifice to coapt. Less than 1 ml of polytef is required. A cystogram is performed with the patient still under anesthesia. The filled bladder is forcibly compressed. If reflux persists, additional paste is injected, usually just medial to the site of the first injection.

Absorption of the glycerin takes several weeks. A definitive cystogram is obtained 1 month later, before the child stops antibacterial therapy. If reflux has recurred, the treatment can be repeated.

Obstruction from Teflon injection has been reported once; therefore, the risk is slight. However, a postoperative sonogram that images the kidney and detects hydronephrosis is recommended.

Summary

Surgical correction of reflux has become quite reliable. Techniques of ureteral tailoring or modeling can be incorporated into each of the commonly used methods of ureteral reimplantation to enable a 5:1 ratio of length to width in the intravesical ureter to be achieved. The transverse Cohen method of implantation is quite versatile and has become the most commonly selected operation.

The risk of new scars and renal damage in children with known reflux treated by antibacterial prophylaxis is 1.2 to 2.8 per cent. These problems occur because of relatively asymptomatic reinfections, which are not treated in a timely fashion. The success rate of antireflux surgery—when implanting the ureter into a normal bladder—is now 98 per cent or 99 per cent in many series. Therefore, it is often reasonable to present both alternatives to parents. Some will elect early surgery in order to avoid long-term medication. There is a minimal risk with this approach. Particularly in infants, severe reflux may stop or improve significantly very quickly. The clearest indication for ureteral implantation is the infection that occurs when a child is already on antibacterial prophylaxis, particularly when the child does not become obviously symptomatic.

REFERENCES

Vesicoureteral Reflux

Allen, T. D., and Bright, T. C., III: Urodynamic patterns in children with dysfunctional voiding problems. J. Urol., 142:448–494, 1978.

Allen, T. D.: The non-neurogenic neurogenic bladder. J. Urol., 117:232, 1977.

Allen, T. D.: Vesicoureteral reflux as a manifestation of dysfunctional voiding. In Hodson, C. J., and Kincaid-Smith, P. (Eds.): Reflux Nephropathy. New York, Masson Publishing USA, 1979, pp. 171–180.

Al-Magousy, A., Hanafy, M. H., Saad, S. M., El-Rifaie, M., and Al-Ghorab, J. M.: Early Arabian medicine. Urology, 8:63, 1976.

Amar, A. D.: Calicotubular backflow with vesicoureteral reflux. JAMA, 213:293, 1970.

Amar, A. D.: Cystoscopic demonstration of vesicoureteral reflux: Evaluation in 250 patients. J. Urol., 95:776, 1966.

Ambrose, S. S.: Reflux pyelonephritis in adults secondary to congenital lesions of the ureteral orifice. J. Urol., 102:302, 1969.

Ambrose, S. S., and Nicolson, W. P.: The causes of vesicoureteral reflux in children. J. Urol., 87:688, 1962a.

Ambrose, S. S., and Nicolson, W. P.: Vesicoureteral reflux secondary to anomalies of the ureterovesical junction: Management and results. J. Urol., 87:695, 1962b.

Ambrose, S. S., and Nicolson, W. P.: Ureteral reflux in duplicated ureters. J. Urol., 92:439, 1964.

Ambrose, S. S., Parrott, T. S., Woodard, J. R., and Campbell, W. G., Jr.: Observations on the small kidney associated with vesicoureteral reflux. J. Urol., 123:349, 1980.

Aperia, A., Broberger, O., Ericsson, N. O., and Wikstad, I.: Effect of vesicoureteral reflux on renal function in children with recurrent urinary infection. Kidney Int., 9:418, 1976.

Apperson, J. W., Atkins, II., and Fleming, R.: The value of the isotope cystogram in determining pressure and volume at which ureteral reflux occurs. J. Urol., 89:405, 1963.

Arant, B. S., Jr., Sotelo-Avila, C., and Bernstein, J.: Segmental "hypoplasia" of the kidney (Ask-Upmark). J. Pediatr., 95:931, 1979.

Ashcraft, K. W. (Ed.): Vesicoureteral Reflux in Pediatric Urology. Philadelphia, J. B. Lippincott Co., 1990, pp. 165–166.

Askari, A., and Belman, A. B.: Vesicoureteral reflux in black girls. J. Pediatr. Nephrol. Urol., 1:11, 1981.

Ask-Upmark, E.: Uber juvenile maligne nephrosklerose und ihr verhöltnis zu störungen in der nierenen twicklung. Acta Pathol. Microbiol. Scand., 7:383, 1929.

Atwell, J. D., Cook, P. L., Strong, L., and Hyde, I.: The interrelationship between vesicoureteral reflux, trigonal abnormalities and a bifid collection system: A family study. Br. J. Urol., 49:97, 1977.

Auer, J., and Seager, L. D.: Experimental local bladder edema causing urine reflux into ureter and kidney. J. Exp. Med., 66:741, 1937.

Austenfeld, M. S., and Snow, B. W.: Complications of pregnancy in women after reimplantation for vesicoureteral reflux. J. Urol., 140:1103–1106, 1988.

Babcock, J. R., Keats, G. K., and King, L. R.: Renal changes after uncomplicated antireflux operation. J. Urol., 115:720, 1976.

Bailey, M., and Wallace, M.: HLA-BIZ as a genetic marker for vesicoureteral reflux? (Letter). Br. Med. J., 1:48, 1978.

Bailey, R. R.: Reflux nephropathy and hypertension. In Hodson, C. J., and Kincaid-Smith, P. (Eds.): Reflux Nephropathy. New York, Masson Publishing USA, 1979a, pp. 263–267.

Bailey, R. R.: Sterile reflux: Is it harmless? In Hodson, C. J., and Kincaid-Smith, P. (Eds.): Reflux Nephropathy. New York, Masson Publishing USA, 1979b, pp. 334–339.

Baker, R., and Barbaris, H. T.: Comparative results of urological evaluation of children with initial and recurrent urinary tract infection. J. Urol., 116:503, 1976.

Baker, R., Masted, W., Maylath, J., and Shuman, I.: Relation of age, sex, and infection to reflux: Data indicating high spontaneous cure rate in pediatric patients. J. Urol., 95:26, 1966.

Barrett, D. M., Malek, R. S., and Kelalis, P. P.: Problems and solutions in surgical treatment of 100 consecutive ureteral duplications in children. J. Urol., 114:126, 1975.

Bauer, S. B., Hallett, M., Khoshoin, S., et al.: Predictive valve of urodynamic evaluation in newborns with myelodysplasia. JAMA, 232:650, 1984.

Bell, C.: Account of the muscles of the ureters and their effects in irritable states of the bladder. Trans. Med. Chir. (Lond.), 3:171, 1812.

Berger, R. E., Ansell, J. S., Shurtleff, D. B., and Hickman, R. O.: Vesicoureteral reflux in children with uremia. JAMA, 246:56, 1981.

Birmingham Reflux Study Group: Prospective trial of operative vs. non-operative treatment of severe vesicoureteral reflux—two years observation in 96 children. Br. Med. J., 187:171, 1983.

Blank, E.: Caliectasis and renal scars in children. J. Urol., 110:255, 1973.

Blaufox, M. D., Gruskin, A., Sandler, P., Goldman, H., Ogwo, J. E., and Edelmann, C. M., Jr.: Radionuclide scintigraphy for detection of vesicoureteral reflux in children. J. Pediatr., 79:239, 1971.

Boyarsky, S., and Labay, P.: Ureteral dynamics. Baltimore, The Williams & Wilkins Co., 1972, p. 354.

Blickman, J. G., and Leboqitz, R. L.: The coexistence of primary megaureter and reflux. Am. J. Roentgen., 143:1053, 1984.

Bloom, D. A., and Bennett, C. J.: Nonoperative management of vesicoureteral reflux. Semin. Urol., 4:74–79, 1986.

Bredin, H. C., Winchester, P., McGovern, J. H., and Degan, M.: Family study of vesicoureteral reflux. J. Urol., 113:623, 1975.

Bridge, R. A. C., and Roe, C. W.: The grading of vesicoureteral reflux: A guide to therapy. J. Urol., 101:831, 1969.

Brenner, B. M.: Nephron adaptation to renal injury or ablation. Am. J. Physiol., 249:F324, 1985.

Brenner, B. M., Meyer, T. W., and Hostetler, T. H.: Dietary protein intake and the progressive nature of kidney disease. N. Engl. J. Med., 307:52–59, 1982.

Bumpus, H. C.: Urinary reflux. J. Urol., 12:341, 1924.

Bunge, R. G.: Delayed cystograms in children. J. Urol., 70:729, 1953.

Bunts, R. C.: Vesicoureteral reflux in paraplegic patients. J. Urol., 79:747, 1958.

Burger, R. H.: A theory on the nature of the transmission of congenital vesicoureteral reflux. J. Urol., 108:249, 1972.

Burger, R. H., and Smith, C.: Hereditary and familial vesicoureteral reflux. J. Urol., 106:845, 1971.

Claësson, I., Jacobsson, B., Jodal, U., and Winberg, J.: Compensatory kidney growth in children with UTI and unilateral renal scarring: an epidemiologic study. Kidney Int., 20:759, 1981.

Claësson, I., Jacobsson, B., Olsson, T., and Ringertz, H.: Assessment of renal parenchymal thickness in normal children. Acta Radiol. Diagn., 97:291, 1980.

Colodny, A. H., and Lebowitz, R. L.: The importance of voiding during a cystourethrogram. J. Urol., 111:838, 1974a.

Colodny, A. H., et al.: Disappearance of Periureteral Diverticula and Reflux. Presented at Section on Urology, American Academy of Pediatrics. San Francisco, October 1983.

Conway, J. J., and Kruglik, G. D.: Effectiveness of direct and indirect radionucleotide cystography in detecting vesicoureteral reflux. J. Nucl. Med., 17:81, 1976.

Conway, J. J., Belman, A. B., and King, L. R.: Direct and indirect cystography. Semin. Nucl. Med., 4:197, 1974.

Conway, J. J., Belman, A. B., King, L. R., and Filmer, R. B.: Direct and indirect radionucleotide cystography. J. Urol., 113:689, 1975.

Conway, J. J., King, L. R., Belman, A. B., and Thorson, T.: Detection of vesicoureteral reflux with radionucleotide cystography. Am. J. Roentgenol. Radium Ther. Nucl. Med., 115:720, 1972.

Corriere, J. N., Lipshutz, L. I., Judson, F. N., and Murphy, J. J.: Autoradiographic localization of refluxed live and dead E. coli and sulfur colloid particles in the rat kidney. Invest. Urol., 6:364, 1969.

Corriere, J. N., Sanders, T. P., Kuhl, D. E., Schoenberg, H. W., and Murphy, J. J.: Urinary particle dynamics and vesicoureteral reflux in the human. J. Urol., 103:599, 1970.

Cotran, R. S., and Pennington, J. E.: Urinary tract infection, pyelonephritis, and nephropathy. In Brenner, B. M., and Rector, F. C., Jr. (Eds.): The Kidney. Vol. II. 2nd ed. Philadelphia, W. B. Saunders Co., 1981, pp. 1571–1632.

Cunningham, F. G., Morris, G. B., and Mickal, A.: Acute pyelonephritis of pregnancy: a clinical review. Obstet. Gynecol. 42:112, 1973.

Damanski, M.: Vesicoureteric reflux in paraplegia. Br. J. Surg., 52:168, 1965.

Decter, R. M., Roth, D. R., and Gonzales, E. T., Jr.: Vesicoureteral reflux in boys. J. Urol., 140:1089–1091, 1988.

Deture, F. A., and Walker, R. D.: Measurement of the distance from the ureteral orifice to the bladder neck: Additional objective data in the cystoscopy of patients with reflux. J. Urol., 112:326, 1974.

De Vargas, A., Evans, K., Ransley, P., et al.: A family study of vesicoureteric reflux. J. Med. Genet., 15:85, 1978.

Dillon, M. J.: Personal communication, 1982.

Doyle, P. T., and Briscoe, C. E.: The effects of drugs and anesthetic agents on the urinary bladder and sphincters. Br. J. Urol., 48:329, 1976.

Duckett, J. W., and Bellinger, M. F.: A plea for standardized grading of vesicoureteral reflux. Eur. Urol., 8:74, 1982.

Dwoskin, J. Y.: Sibling uropathology. J. Urol., 115:726, 1976.

Dwoskin, J. Y., and Perlmutter, A. D.: Vesicoureteral reflux in children: A computerized review. J. Urol., 109:888, 1973.

Edelbrook, H. H., and Mickelson, J. C.: Selection of children for vesicoureteroplasty. J. Urol., 104:342, 1970.

Edwards, D., Nomand, I. C. S., Prescod, N., et al.: Disappearance of reflux during long-term prophylaxis of urinary tract infection in children. Br. Med. J., 2:285, 1977.

Ehrlich, R.: Success of the transvesical advancement technique for VUR. J. Urol., 128:554, 1982a.

Ekman, H., Jacobsson, B., Kock, N. G., et al.: High diuresis: a factor in preventing vesicoureteral reflux. J. Urol., 95:511, 1966.

Elbadawi, A.: Anatomy and function of the ureteral sheath. J. Urol., 107:224, 1972.

Ellis, G. V.: An account of the arrangement of the muscular substance in the urinary and certain of the generative organs. Trans. Med. Chir. (Lond.), 39:327, 1856.

Estes, R. C., and Brooks, R. T.: Vesicoureteral reflux in adults. J. Urol., 103:603, 1970.

Fair, W. R., and Govan, D. E.: Influence of vesicoureteral reflux on the response to treatment of urinary tract infections in female children. Br. J. Urol., 48:111, 1976.

Filly, R. F., Friedland, G. W., Govan, F., et al.: Development and progression of clubbing and scarring in children with recurrent urinary tract infection. Radiology, 113:145, 1974.

Friedland, G. W.: The voiding cystourethrogram: an unreliable examination. In Hodson, C. J., and Kincaid-Smith, P. (Eds.): Reflux Nephropathy. New York, Masson Publishing USA, 1979, pp. 93–99.

Fryjordet, A.: Sympathectomy and ureteral reflux. Scand. J. Urol. Nephrol., 2:196, 1968.

Galen: Cited in Polk, H. C., Jr.: Notes on Galenic urology. Urol. Surv., 15:2, 1965.

Garrett, R. A., Rhamy, R. K., and Newman, D.: Management of nonobstructive vesicoureteral reflux. J. Urol., 90:167, 1963.

Gibson, H. M.: Ureteral reflux in the normal child. J. Urol., 62:40, 1949.

Gilbert, B. R., and Vaughan, D.: A urologist's view of renal pathophysiology. II. AUA Update Series, 7:202, 1988.

Gill, D. G., Mendes da Costa, B., Cameron, J. S., Joseph, M. C., Ogg, C. S., and Chantler, C.: Analysis of 100 children with severe and persistent hypertension. Arch. Dis. Child., 51:951, 1976.

Govan, D. E., and Palmer, J. M.: Urinary tract infection in children: the influence of successful antireflux operations in morbidity from infection. Pediatrics, 44:677, 1969.

Govan, D. E., Fair, W. R., Friedland, G. W., and Filly, R. H.: Management of children with urinary tract infections. Urology, 6:273, 1975.

Grana, L., Kidd, J., and Idriss, F.: Effect of chronic urinary tract infection on ureteral peristalsis. J. Urol., 94:652, 1965.

Graves, R. C., and Davidoff, L. M.: Studies on the bladder and ureters with especial reference to regurgitation of the vesical contents. J. Urol., 14:1, 1925.

Griffiths, D. J., and Scholtmeijer, R. J.: Vesicoureteral reflux and lower urinary tract dysfunction: Evidence for two different reflux/dysfunction complexes. J. Urol., 137:240–244, 1987.

Gruber, G. M.: A comparative study of the intravesical ureter in man and in experimental animals. J. Urol., 21:567, 1929.

Harrison, R.: On the possibility and utility of washing out the pelvis of the kidney and the ureters through the bladder. Lancet, 1:463, 1888.

Hawtrey, C. E., Culp, D. A., Loening, S., et al.: Ureterovesical reflux in an adolescent and adult population. J. Urol., 130:1067, 1983.

Hay, A. M., Norman, W. J., Rice, M. L., and Steventon, R. D.: A comparison between diuresis renography and the Whitaker text in 64 kidneys. Br. J. Urol., 56:561, 1984.

Heidrick, W. P., Mattingly, R. F., and Amberg, J. R.: Vesicoureteral reflux in pregnancy. Obstet. Gynecol., 29:571, 1967.

Heikel, P. E., and Parkkulainen, K. V.: Vesico-ureteric reflux in children: A classification and results of conservative treatment. Ann. Radiol., 9:37, 1966.

Helin, I.: Clinical and experimental studies on vesicoureteral reflux. Scand. J. Urol. Nephrol. (Suppl.) 28:1, 1975.

Hernandez, R. J., Poznanski, A. K., Kuhns, L. R., et al.: Factors affecting measurement of renal length. Radiology, 130:653, 1979.

Hicks, C. C., Woodard, J. R., Walton, K. W., et al.: Hypertension

as complication of vesicoureteral reflux in children. Urology, 7:587, 1976.

Hinman, F., Jr., and Baumann, F. W.: Vesical and ureteral damage from voiding dysfunction in boys without neurogenic or obstructive disease. J. Urol., 109:727, 1973.

Hinman, F., Jr.: Non-neurogenic neurogenic bladder (the Hinman syndrome)—15 years later. J. Urol., 136:769, 1986.

Hinman, F., and Baumann, F. W.: Vesical and ureteral damage from voiding dysfunction in boys without neurologic or obstructive disease. J. Urol., 109:727, 1973.

Hinman, F., and Hutch, J. A.: Atrophic pyelonephritis from ureteral reflux without obstructive signs (reflux pyelonephritis). J. Urol., 87:230, 1962.

Hodson, C. J.: The radiological contribution toward the diagnosis of chronic pyelonephritis. Radiology, 88:857, 1967.

Hodson, C. J., and Edwards, D.: Chronic pyelonephritis and vesicoureteric reflux. Clin. Radiol., 11:219, 1960.

Hodson, C. J., Maling, T. M. J., McManaman, P. H., et al.: Pathogenesis of reflux nephropathy. Br. J. Radiol. (Suppl.), 13:1, 1975.

Holland, N.: Reflux nephropathy and hypertension. In Hodson, C. J., and Kincaid-Smith, P. (Eds.): Reflux Nephropathy. New York, Masson Publishing USA, 1979, pp. 257–262.

Homsy, Y. L., Nsouli, I., Hamburger, B., Laberge, I., and Schick, E.: Effects of oxybutynin on vesicoureteral reflux in children. J. Urol., 134:1168, 1985.

Howerton, L. W., and Lich, R., Jr.: The cause and correction of ureteral reflux. J. Urol., 89:762, 1963.

Huland, H., and Busch, R.: Chronic pyelonephritis as a cause of end stage renal disease. J. Urol., 127:642, 1982.

Huland, H., and Busch, R.: Pyelonephritic scarring in 213 patients with upper and lower tract infections: Long-term followup. J. Urol., 132:936, 1984.

Hutch, J. A.: The Ureterovesical Junction. Berkeley, University of California Press, 1958.

Hutch, J. A.: Theory of maturation of the intravesical ureter. J. Urol., 86:534, 1961.

Hutch, J. A.: The role of the ureterovesical junction in the natural history of pyelonephritis. J. Urol., 88:354, 1962.

Hutch, J. A.: Ureteric advancement operation: anatomy, technique and early results. J. Urol., 89:180, 1963.

Hutch, J. A., and Tanagho, E. A.: Etiology of nonocclusive ureteral dilatation. J. Urol., 93:177, 1965.

Iannaccone, G., and Panzironi, P. E.: Ureteral reflux in normal infants. Acta Radiol., 44:451, 1955.

Ireland, G. W., and Cass, A. S.: The clinical measurement of the intravesical pressure during voiding. Invest. Urol., 2:303, 1965.

Jeffs, R. D., and Allen, M. S.: The relationship between ureterovesical reflux and infection. J. Urol., 88:691, 1962.

Jenkins, G. R., and Noe, H. N.: Familial vesicoureteral reflux: A prospective study. J. Urol., 128:774, 1982.

Johnston, J. H.: Vesical diverticula without urinary obstruction in childhood. J. Urol., 84:535, 1960.

Johnston, J. H.: Vesicoureteral reflux: its anatomical mechanism, causation, effects and treatment in the child. Ann. R. Coll. Surg. Engl., 30:324, 1962.

Johnston, J. H.: Vesicoureteral reflux with urethral valves. Br. J. Urol., 51:100, 1979.

Johnston, J. H., and Mix, L. W.: The Ask-Upmark kidney: a form of ascending pyelonephritis? Br. J. Urol., 48:393, 1976.

Jones, B. W., and Headstream, J. W.: Vesicoureteral reflux in children. J. Urol., 80:114, 1958.

Jones, K. V., Asscher, W., Jones, R. V., et al.: Renal functional changes in school girls with correct asymptomatic bactiurea. Cont. Nephrol., 39:152, 1984.

Kaplan, W. E., Nasrallah, P., and King, L. R.: Reflux in complete duplication in children. J. Urol., 120:220, 1978.

Kass, E. J., Koff, S. A., and Diokno, A. C.: Fate of vesicoureteral reflux in children with neuropathic bladders managed by intermittent catheterization. J. Urol., 125:63, 1981.

Kaveggia, L., King, L. R., Grana, L., and Idriss, F. S.: Pyelonephritis: A cause of vesicoureteral reflux? J. Urol., 95:158, 1966.

Kelalis, P. P.: Subject review: Proper perspective on vesicoureteric reflux. Mayo Clin. Proc., 46:807, 1971.

Kincaid-Smith, P.: Glomerular and vascular lesions in chronic atrophic pyelonephritis and reflux nephropathy. Adv. Nephrol., 5:3, 1975.

King, L. R., and Idriss, F. S.: The effect of vesicoureteral reflux on renal function in dogs. Invest. Urol., 4:419, 1967.

King, L. R.: Apparent ureteropelvic junction obstruction caused by vesicoureteral reflux. Illinois Med. J., 133:711–715, 1968.

King, L. R.: Vesicoureteral reflux: History, etiology and conservative management. *In* Kelalis, P. P., and King, L. R. (Eds.): Clinical Pediatric Urology. Vol. 1. Philadelphia, W. B. Saunders Co., 1976, pp. 342–365.

King, L. R.: Sphincter dyssynergia in children with reflux. J. Urol., 129:217–218, 1983.

King, L. R., Kazmi, S. O., and Belman, A. B.: Natural history of vesicoureteral reflux. Urol. Clin. North Am., 1:441, 1974.

King, L. R., Mellens, H. A., and White, H.: Measurement of the intravesical pressure during voiding. Invest. Urol., 2:303, 1965.

King, L. R., and Sellards, H. G.: The effects of vesicoureteral reflux on renal growth and development in puppies. Invest. Urol., 9:95, 1971.

King, L. R., Surian, M. A., Wendel, R. M., and Burden, J. J.: Vesicoureteral reflux: The importance of etiology in management. Trans. Am. Assoc. Genitourin. Surg., 59:110, 1967.

Koff, S. A., and Murtagh, D. S.: The uninhibited bladder in children: Effect of treatment on recurrence of urinary infection and on vesicoureteral reflux resolution. J. Urol., 120:1138, 1983.

Koff, S. A., Lapides, J., and Piazza, D. H.: Association of urinary tract infection and reflux with uninhibited bladder contractions and voluntary sphincter obstruction. J. Urol., 122:373, 1979a.

Koff, S. A., Lapides, J., and Piazza, D. H.: The uninhibited bladder in children: A cause for urinary obstruction, infection and reflux. *In* Reflux Nephropathy. Hodson, J., and Kincaid-Smith, P. (Eds.): New York, Masson Publishing, 1979, Section 5, Chapter 17.

Kogan, S. J., and Freed, S. W.: Postoperative course of vesicoureteral reflux associated with benign obstructive prostatic disease. J. Urol., 112:322, 1974.

Kogan, S. J., Sigler, L., Levitt, S. B., Reda, E. F., Weiss, R., and Griefer, I.: Elusive vesicoureteral reflux in children with normal contrast cystograms. J. Urol., 136:325–328, 1986.

Kretschmer, H. L.: Cystography, its value and limitations in surgery of the bladder. Surg. Gynecol. Obstet., 23:709, 1916.

Kunin, C. M., Deutscher, R., and Paquin, A.: Urinary tract infection in school children. Medicine, 43:91, 1964.

Lancet editorial. Screening for reflux. 2:23, 1978.

Lancet editorial, 2:44, 1982.

Langworthy, O. R., and Kolb, L. C.: Histological changes in the vesical muscle following injury of the peripheral innervation. Anat. Rec., 71:249, 1938.

Lattimer, J. K., Apperson, J. W., Gleason, D. M., Baker, D., and Fleming, S. S.: The pressure at which reflux occurs: An important indicator of prognosis and treatment. J. Urol., 89:395, 1963.

Laverson, P. L., Hankins, G. D. V., and Quirk, J. G.: Ureteral obstruction during pregnancy. J. Urol., 131:327, 1984.

Leadbetter, G. W., Danbury, J. H., and Dreyfuss, J. R.: Absence of vesicoureteral reflux in normal adult males. J. Urol., 84:69, 1960.

Lebowitz, R. L., and Blickman, J. G.: The coexistence of ureteropelvic junction obstruction and reflux. Am. J. Roentgenol., 140:231–238, 1983.

Lenaghan, D., Whitaker, J. G., Jensen, F., and Stephens, F. D.: The natural history of reflux and long-term effects of reflux on the kidney. J. Urol., 115:738, 1976.

Lewy, P. R., and Belman, A. B.: Familial occurrence of non-obstructive, non-infectious vesicoureteral reflux with renal scarring. J. Pediatr., 86:851, 1975.

Lich, R., Howerton, L. W., Goode, L. S., and Davis, L. A.: The uretero-vesical junction of the newborn. J. Urol., 92:436, 1964.

Lines, D.: 15th century ureteric reflux. Lancet, 2:1473, 1982.

Lupton, E. W., Richards, D., Testa, H. J., Gilpin, S. A., Gosling, J. A., and Barnard, R. S.: A comparison of diuresis renography, the Whitaker test, and renal pelvis morphology in idiopathic hydronephrosis. Brit. J. Urol., 57:119, 1985.

Lyon, R. P.: Renal arrest. J. Urol., 109:707, 1973.

Lyon, R. P., Halverstadt, D., Tank, E. S., et al.: Vesicoureteral reflux. *In* Dialogues in Pediatric Urology. Vol. I. New York, Wm. J. Miller Assoc., 1977, pp. 1–8.

Lyon, R. P., Marshall, S., and Tanagho, E. A.: The ureteric orifice: Its configuration and competency. J. Urol., 102:504, 1969.

Mackie, C. G., and Stephens, F. S.: Duplex kidneys: a correlation of renal dysplasia with position of the ureteral orifice. J. Urol., 114:274, 1975.

Malek, R. S., Svensson, J., and Torres, V. E.: Vesicoureteral reflux in the adult. I. Factors in pathogenesis. J. Urol., 130:37, 1983a.

Malek, R. S., Svensson, J., Neves, R. J., and Torres, V. E.: Vesicoureteral reflux in the adult. III. Surgical correction: Risks and benefits. J. Urol., 130:882, 1983b.

Marshall, F. C.: Excretory urographic changes in children which suggest occurrence of reflux. J. Urol., 87:681, 1962.

Mattingly, R. F., and Borkowf, H. I.: Clinical implications of ureteral reflux in pregnancy. Clin. Obstet. Gynecol., 21:863, 1978.

Mazze, R. I., Schwartz, F. S., Slocum, H. C., and Barry, K. G.: Renal function during anesthesia and surgery. Anesthesiology, 24:279, 1963.

McGovern, J. H., Marshall, V. F., and Paquin, A. J.: Vesicoureteral regurgitation in children. J. Urol., 83:122, 1960.

McRae, C. U., Shannon, F. T., and Utley, W. L. F.: Effect on renal growth of reimplantation of refluxing ureters. Lancet, 1:1310, 1974.

Mebust, W. K., and Foret, J. D.: Vesicoureteral reflux in identical twins. J. Urol., 108:635, 1972.

Melick, W. F., Brodeur, A. E., and Karellos, D. N.: A suggested classification of ureteral reflux and suggested treatment based on cineradiographic findings and simultaneous pressure recordings by means of the strain gauge. J. Urol., 83:35, 1962.

Mendoza, J. M., and Roberts, J. A.: Effects of sterile high pressure vesicoureteral reflux on the monkey. J. Urol., 130:602, 1983.

Merrell, R. W., and Mowad, J. J.: Increased physical growth after successful antireflux operation. J. Urol., 122:523, 1979.

Middleton, G. W., Howards, S. S., and Gillenwater, J. Y.: Sex-linked familial reflux. J. Urol., 114:36, 1975.

Murnaghan, G. F.: Urologists' correspondence club letter. March 1980.

Noe, H. N.: Screening for familial reflux: An update. Semin. Urol., 4:86–87, 1986.

Noe, H. N.: The relationship of sibling reflux to index patient dysfunctional voiding. J. Urol., 140:119–120, 1988.

Normand, C., and Smellie, J.: Vesicoureteral reflux: The case for conservative management. *In* Hodson, C. J., and Kincaid-Smith, P. (Eds.): Reflux Nephropathy. New York, Masson Publishing USA, 1979, pp. 281–286.

Ong, T. H., Ferguson, R. S., and Stephens, F. D.: The pattern of intrapelvic pressure during vesicoureteral reflux in the dog with normal caliber ureter. Invest. Urol., 11:347, 1974.

Paquin, A. J.: Ureterovesical anastomosis: The description and evaluation of a technique. J. Urol., 82:573, 1959.

Paulsen, E. U., Frokjaer, J., Taegehoj-Jensen, F., Jorgensen, T. M., and Djurhaus, J. C.: Diuresis renography and simultaneous renal pelvic pressure in hydronephrosis. J. Urol., 138:272, 1987.

Peters, P. C., Johnson, D. E., and Jackson, J. H.: The incidence of vesicoureteral reflux in the premature child. J. Urol., 97:259, 1967.

Pinter, A. B., Jaszai, V., and Dober, I.: Medical treatment of vesicoureteral reflux detected in infancy. J. Urol., 140:121–124, 1988.

Politano, V. A.: Ureterovesical junction. J. Urol., 107:239, 1972.

Pollet, J. E., Sharp, P. F., Smith, R. W., Davidson, A. I., and Miller, S. S.: Intravenous radionuclide cystography for the detection of vesicorenal reflux. J. Urol., 125:75, 1981.

Poznanski, E., and Poznanski, A. K.: Psychogenic influences on voiding: observations from voiding cystourethrography. Psychosomatics, 10:339, 1969.

Pozzi, S.: Ureteroverletzung bei laparatomie. Zbl. Gynack., 17:97, 1893.

Prather, G. C.: Vesicoureteral reflux, report of a case cured by operation. J. Urol., 52:437, 1944.

Quinby, W. C.: Observations on the physiology and pathology of the ureter. J. Urol., 7:259, 1922.

Ransley, P. G.: Vesicoureteral reflux: Continuing surgical dilemma. Urology, 3:246, 1978.

Ransley, P. G., and Risdon, R. A.: Renal papillae and intra-renal reflux in the pig. Lancet, 2:1114, 1974.

Ransley, P. G., and Risdon, R. A.: Reflux and renal scarring. Br. J. Radiol. (Suppl.), 14:1, 1978.

Ransley, P. G., and Risdon, R. A.: Reflux nephropathy: Effects of antimicrobial therapy on the evolution of the early pyelonephritic scar. Kidney Int., 20:733, 1981.

Redman, J. F., Scriber, L. J., and Bissad, N. K.: Apparent failure of renal growth secondary to vesicoureteral reflux. Urology, 3:704, 1974.

Report of the International Reflux Study Committee: Medical versus surgical treatment of primary vesicoureteral reflux. Pediatrics, 67(3):392, 1981.

Roberts, J. A., Roth, J. K., Jr., Domingue, G., Lewis, R. W., Kaack, B., and Baskin, G.: Immunology of pyelonephritis in the primate model. V. Effect of superoxide dismutase. J. Urol., 128:1394, 1982.

Rolleston, G. L., Maling, T. M. J., and Hodson, C. J.: Intrarenal reflux and the scarred kidney. Arch. Dis. Child., 49:531, 1974.

Rolleston, G. L., Shannon, F. J., and Utley, W. L. F.: Relationship of infantile vesicoureteral reflux to renal damage. Br. Med. J., 1:460, 1970.

Rolleston, G. L., Shannon, F. T., and Utley, W. L. F.: Follow up of vesicoureteric reflux in the newborn. Kidney Int., 8:59, 1975.

Rose, J. S., Glassberg, K. I., and Waterhouse, K.: Intrarenal reflux and its relationship to renal scarring. J. Urol., 113:400, 1975.

Ryan, P. C., and Fitzpatrick, J. M.: Partial ureteric obstruction: A new variable canine experimental model. J. Urol., 137:1034, 1987.

Salvatierra, O., and Tanagho, E. A.: Reflux as a cause of end stage kidney disease: Report of 32 cases. J. Urol., 117:441, 1977.

Sampson, J. A.: Ascending renal infection, with special reference to the reflux of urine from the bladder into the ureters as an etiological factor in its causation and maintenance. Bull. Johns Hopkins Hosp., 14:334, 1903.

Satani, Y.: Histologic study of the ureter. J. Urol., 3:247, 1919.

Savage, D. C. L., Wilson, M. I., Ross, E. M., et al.: Asymptomatic bacteriuria in girl entrants to Dundee Primary School. Br. Med. J., 3:75, 1969.

Savage, J. M., Shah, V., Dillon, M. J., et al.: Renin and blood pressure in children with renal scarring and vesicoureteric reflux. Lancet, 2:441, 1978.

Schmidt, J. D., Hawtry, C. E., and Flocks, R. H.: Vesicoureteral reflux: an inherited lesion. JAMA, 220:821, 1972.

Schoenberg, H. W., Beisswanger, P., Howard, W. J., et al.: Effect of lower urinary tract infection upon ureteral function. J. Urol., 92:107, 1964.

Schulman, C. C., Duarte-Escalante, O., and Boyarsky, S.: The ureterovesical innervation. Br. J. Urol., 44:698, 1972.

Scott, J. E. S.: The management of ureteric reflux in children. Br. J. Urol., 49:109, 1977.

Scott, J. E. S., and Stansfeld, J. M.: Ureteric reflux and kidney scarring in children. Arch. Dis. Child., 43:468, 1968.

Semblinow, V. I.: Zur Pathologie der duech Bacterien bewinkten ambsteifenden Nephritis. 1883 Dissertation. Cited by Alksne, J.: Folia Urol., 1:338, 1907.

Shopfner, C. E.: Vesicoureteral reflux. Radiology, 95:637, 1970.

Seruca, H.: Vesicoureteral reflux and voiding dysfunction: A prospective study. J. Urol., 142:494–498, 1989.

Shimada, K., Matsui, T., Ogino, T., Arima, M., Mori, Y., and Ikoma, F.: Growth and progression of reflux nephropathy in children with vesicoureteral reflux. J. Urol., 140:1097–1100, 1988.

Siegler, R. L.: Renin dependent hypertension in children with reflux nephropathy. Urology, 7:474, 1976.

Smellie, J. M.: The disappearance of reflux in children with urinary tract infection during prophylactic chemotherapy. In Proceedings of the 4th International Congress on Nephrology (Stockholm). Vol. 3. Basel, S. Karger, 1969, p. 357.

Smellie, J. M., and Normand, C.: Reflux nephropathy in childhood. In Hodson, C. J., and Kincaid-Smith, P. (Eds.): Reflux Nephropathy. New York, Masson Publishing, 1979, pp. 14–20.

Smellie, J. M., and Normand, I. C. S.: Experience of follow-up of children with urinary tract infection. In O'Grady, F., and Brumditte, W. (Eds.): Urinary Tract Infection. London, Oxford University Press, 1968, p. 123.

Smellie, J. M., and Normand, I. C. S.: Bacteriuria, reflux and renal scarring. Arch. Dis. Child., 50:581, 1975.

Smellie, J. M., and Normand, I. C. S.: The clinical features and significance of urinary infection in childhood. Proc. R. Soc. Lond., 59:415, 1966.

Smellie, J. M., Edwards, D., Hunter, N., et al.: Vesicoureteric reflux and renal scarring. Kidney Int., 8:565, 1975a.

Smellie, J., Edwards, D., Hunter, N., Normand, I. C. S., and Prescod, N.: Vesicoureteric reflux and renal scarring. Kidney Int. (Suppl.), 8:65, 1975b.

Smellie, J. M., Edwards, D., Normand, I. C. S., and Prescod, N.: Effect of VUR on renal growth in children with UTI. Arch. Dis. Child., 56:593, 1981.

Smith, A. M.: Comparison of standard and cinecystography for detecting vesicoureteral reflux. J. Urol., 96:49, 1966.

Sommer, J. T., and Douglas, F. D.: Morphogenesis of nephropathy with partial ureteral obstruction and vesicoureteral reflux. J. Urol., 125:67, 1981.

Sommer, J. T., and Stephens, F. D.: Morphogenesis of nephropathy with partial ureteral obstruction and vesicoureteral reflux. J. Urol., 125:67, 1981.

Stamey, T. A.: The question of residual urine. In Stamey, T. A. (Ed.): Urinary Infections. Baltimore, The Williams & Wilkins Co., 1972, pp. 230–231.

Stecker, J. F., Jr., Read, B. P., and Poutasse, E. F.: Pediatric hypertension as a delayed sequela of reflux induced pyelonephritis. J. Urol., 118:644, 1977.

Steele, B. T., Robitaille, P., DeMaria, J., and Grignon, A.: Followup evaluation of prenatally recognized vesicoureteric reflux. J. Pediatr. 115:95–96, 1989.

Stephens, F. D.: Correlation of ureteric orifice position with renal morphology. Trans. Am. Assoc. Genitourin. Surg., 1976, p. 53.

Stephens, F. D.: Ureteric configurations and cystoscopy schema. Soc. Pediatr. Urol. Newsletter, Jan. 23, 1980, p. 2.

Stephens, F. S., and Lenaghan, D.: Anatomical basis and dynamics of vesicoureteral reflux. J. Urol., 87:669, 1962.

Stewart, C. M.: Delayed cystograms. J. Urol., 70:588, 1953.

Stickler, G. B., Kelalis, P. P., Burke, E. C., et al.: Primary interstitial nephritis with reflux—A cause of hypertension. Am. J. Dis. Child., 122:144, 1971.

Talbot, H. S., and Bunts, R. C.: Late renal changes in paraplegia: Hydronephrosis due to vesicoureteral reflux. J. Urol., 61:870, 1949.

Tamminen, T. E., and Kaprio, E. A.: The relation of the shape of renal papillae and of collecting duct openings to intrarenal reflux. Br. J. Urol., 49:345, 1977.

Tanagho, E. A.: Embryologic basis for lower ureteral anomalies: A hypothesis. Urology, 7:451, 1976.

Tanagho, E. A., and Hutch, J. A.: Primary reflux. J. Urol., 93:158, 1965.

Tanagho, E. A., and Puch, R. C. B.: The anatomy and function of the ureterovesical junction. Br. J. Urol., 35:151, 1963.

Tanagho, E. A., Hutch, J. A., Meyers, F. H., et al.: Primary vesicoureteral reflux: Experimental studies of its etiology. J. Urol., 93:165, 1965.

Timmons, J. W., Watts, F. B., and Perlmutter, A. D.: A comparison of awake and anesthesia cystography. Birth Defects: Original Articles Series (New York), 13:364, 1977.

Tokunaka, S., Koyanagi, T., Matsuno, T., Gotoh, T., and Tsuji, I.: Paraureteral diverticula: Clinical experience with 17 cases with associated renal dysmorphism. J. Urol., 124:791, 1980.

Torbey, K., and Leadbetter, W. F.: Innervation of the bladder and lower ureter: Studies on pelvic nerve section and stimulation in the dog. J. Urol., 90:395, 1963.

Torres, V. E., Moore, S. B., Kurtz, S. B., Offord, K. P., and Kelalis, P. P.: In search of a marker for genetic susceptibility to reflux nephropathy. Clin. Nephrol., 14:217, 1980a.

Torres, V. E., Velosa, J. A., Holley, K. E., Kelalis, P. P., Stickler, G. B., and Kurtz, S. B.: The progression of vesicoureteral nephropathy. Ann. Intern. Med., 92:776, 1980b.

Tremewan, R. N., Bailey, R. R., Little, T. M. J., Peters, T. M., and Tait, J. J.: Diagnosis of gross vesico-ureteric reflux using ultrasonography. Br. J. Urol., 48:431, 1976.

Uehling, D. T.: Effect of vesicoureteral reflux on concentrating ability. J. Urol., 106:947, 1971.

Uehling, D. T., and Wear, J. B., Jr.: Concentrating ability after antireflux operation. J. Urol., 116:83, 1976.

Van den Abbeele, A., Treves, S. T., Lebowitz, R. L., Bauer, S., Davis, R. T., Retik, A., and Colodny, A.: Vesicoureteral reflux in asymptomatic siblings of patients with known reflux: Radionuclide cystography. Pediatrics, 79:147, 1987.

Van Gool, J. D.: Bladder infection and pressure. In Hodson, C. J., and Kincaid-Smith, P. (Eds.): Reflux Nephropathy. New York, Masson Publishing USA, 1979, pp. 181–189.

Van Gool, J., and Tanagho, E. A.: External sphincter activity and recurrent urinary tract infections in girls. Urology, 10:348, 1977.

Vargas, B., and Lebowitz, R. L.: The coexistence of congenital megacalyces and primary megaureter. Am. J. Radiol., 147:313–316, 1986.

Vermillion, C. D., and Heale, W. F.: Position and configuration of the ureteral orifice and its relationship to renal scarring in adults. J. Urol., 109:579, 1973.

Vermooten, V., and Neuswanger, C. H.: Effects on the upper urinary tract in dogs of an incompetent ureterovesical valve. J. Urol., 32:330, 1934.

Vlahakis, E., Hartman, G. W., and Kelalis, D. D.: Comparison of voiding cystourethrography and expression cystourethrography. J. Urol., 106:414, 1971.

Walker, D., Richard, G., and Dobson, D.: Maximum urine concentration: early means of identifying patients with reflux who may require surgery. Urology, 1:343, 1973.

Walker, D., Richard, G., and Fennell, V. I. M.: Renal growth and scarring in kidneys with reflux and concentrating defect. J. Urol., 129:748, 1983.

Walker, R. D.: Renal functional changes associated with vesicourethral reflux. Urol. Clin. North Am., 17:307–317, 1990.

Walker, R. D., Duckett, J., Bartone, F., et al.: Screening school children for urologic disease. Pediatrics, 60:239, 1977.

Wallace, D. M. A., Rothwell, D. L., and Williams, D. I.: The long-term followup of surgically treated vesicoureteral reflux. Br. J. Urol., 50:479, 1978.

Warren, M. M., Kelalis, P. P., and Stickler, G. B.: Unilateral ureteroneocystostomy: The fate of the contralateral ureter. J. Urol., 107:466, 1972.

Warshaw, B. L., Edelbrock, H. H., Ettenger, R. B., et al.: Renal transplantation in children with obstructive uropathy. J. Urol., 123:737, 1980.

Wein, H. A., and Schoenberg, H. W.: A review of 402 girls with recurrent urinary tract infections. J. Urol., 107:329, 1972.

Weiss, R. M., and Lytton, B.: Vesicoureteral reflux and distal ureteral obstruction. J. Urol., 111:245, 1974.

Weiss, R. M., Schiff, M., Jr., and Lytton, B.: Late obstruction after ureteroneocystostomy. J. Urol., 106:144, 1971.

Wesson, M. B.: Anatomical, embryological and physiological studies of the trigone and neck of the bladder. J. Urol., 4:297, 1920.

Whalley, P. J., and Cunningham, F. G.: Short-term vs. continuous antibiotic therapy for asymptomatic bacteriuria in pregnancy. Obstet. Gynecol., 49:292, 1977.

Williams, D. I.: The ureter, the urologist and the pediatrician. Proc. R. Soc. Lond., 63:595, 1970.

Williams, D. I., and Eckstein, H. B.: Surgical treatment of reflux in children. Br. J. Urol., 37:12, 1965.

Williams, G. L., Davies, D. K. L., Evans, K. T., and Williams, J. E.: Vesicoureteral reflux in patients with bacteriuria in pregnancy. Lancet, 2:1202, 1968.

Willscher, M. K., Bauer, S. B., Zammuto, P. J., and Retik, A. B.: Renal growth and urinary infection following antireflux surgery in infants and children. J. Urol., 115:722, 1976a.

Willscher, M. K., Bauer, S. B., Zammuto, P. J., et al.: Infection of the urinary tract after antireflux surgery. J. Pediatr., 89:743, 1976b.

Winter, C. C.: A new test for vesicoureteral reflux: An external technique using radioisotopes. J. Urol., 81:105, 1959.

Woodard, J. R., and Filardi, G.: The demonstration of vesicoureteral reflux under anesthesia. J. Urol., 116:501, 1976.

Woodburg, P. W., Mitchell, M. E., Scheidler, D. M., Adams, M. C., Rink, R. C., and McNulty, A.: Constant pressure perfusion: A method to determine obstruction in the upper urinary tract. J. Urol., 142:632–635, 1989.

Woodburne, R. T.: Anatomy of the ureterovesical junction. J. Urol., 92:431, 1964.

Young, H. H.: Johns Hopkins Hosp. Bull., 9:100, 1898.

Young, H. H., and Wesson, M. B.: The anatomy and surgery of the trigone. Arch. Surg., 3:1, 1921.

Zinner, N. R., Foster, E. A., Spaulding, B. H., and Paquin, A. J.: Experimental vesicoureteral reflux: Comparison of three cystographic techniques. J. Urol., 90:405, 1963.

Megaureter

Albertson, K. W., and Talner, L. B.: Valves of the ureter. Radiology, 103:91, 1972.

Allen, T. D.: Congenital ureteral strictures. J. Urol., 104:196, 1970.

Bakker, H. H. R.: The primary obstructive megaureter in children. A clinical and experimental study, 1987. Thesis, University of Amsterdam, the Netherlands.

Bakker, H. H. R., Scholtmeijer, R. J., and Klopper, P. J.: Compar-
ison of two different tapering techniques in megaureter. J. Urol., 140:1237–1239, 1988.

Belman, A. B.: Megaureter classification, etiology, and management. Urol. Clin. North Am., 1:497, 1974.

Bischoff, P. F.: Megaureter. Br. J. Urol., 29:46, 1957.

Boxer, R. J., Fritsche, P., Skinner, D. F., et al.: Replacement of the ureter by small intestine: clinical application and results of the ileal ureter in 89 patients. J. Urol., 121:728, 1979.

Caine, M., and Hermann, G.: The return of peristalsis in the anastomosed ureter: A cine-radiographic study. Br. J. Urol., 42:164, 1970.

Caulk, J. R.: Megaloureter: the importance of the ureterovesical valve. J. Urol., 9:315, 1923.

Considine, J.: Retrocaval ureter: A review of the literature with a report on two new cases followed for fifteen years and two years, respectively. Br. J. Urol., 38:412, 1966.

Creevy, C. D.: The atonic distal ureteral segment (ureteral achalasia). J. Urol., 97:457, 1967.

Cussen, L. J.: Dimensions of normal ureter in infancy and childhood. Invest. Urol., 5:164, 1967.

Cussen, L. J.: The morphology of congenital dilatation of the ureter: intrinsic ureteral lesions. Aust. N. Z. J. Surg., 41:185, 1971.

Deter, R. L., Hadlock, F. P., Gonzales, E. T., and Wait, R. B.: Prenatal detection of primary megaureter using dynamic image ultrasonography. Obstet. Gynecol., 56:759, 1980.

Ehrlich, R. M.: The ureteral folding technique for megaureter surgery. J. Urol., 134:668, 1985.

Fitzer, P. M.: Congenital ureteral valve. Pediatr. Radiol., 8:54, 1979.

Flatmark, A. L., Maurseth, K., and Knutrud, O.: Lower ureteric obstruction in children. Br. J. Urol., 42:431, 1970.

Garrett, W. J., Kossoff, G., and Osborn, R. A.: The diagnosis of fetal hydronephrosis, megaureter and urethral obstruction by ultrasonic echography. Br. J. Obstet. Gynaecol., 82:115, 1975.

Glassberg, K. I.: Dilated ureter: Classification and approach. Urology, 9:1, 1977.

Glassberg, K. I., Schneider, M., Haller, D. O., et al.: Observations on persistently dilated ureter after posterior urethral valve ablation. Urology, 20:20, 1982.

Goodwin, W. E., Burke, D. E., and Muller, W. H.: Retrocaval ureter. Surg. Gynecol. Obstet., 104:337, 1957.

Gosling, J. A., and Dixon, J. S.: Functional obstruction of the ureter and renal pelvis. A histological and electron microscopic study. Br. J. Urol., 50:145, 1978.

Grana, L., and Swenson, O.: A new surgical procedure for the treatment of aperistaltic megaloureter. Am. J. Surg., 109:532, 1965.

Gregoir, W., and Debled, G.: L'etiologie du reflux congenital et du mega-uretere primaire. Urol. Int., 24:119, 1969.

Hanani, Y., Goldwasser, B., Jonas, P., et al.: Management of unilateral reflux by ipsilateral ureteroneocystostomy—Is it sufficient? J. Urol., 129:1022–1023, 1983.

Hanna, M. K.: Early surgical correction of massive refluxing megaureter in babies by total ureteral reconstruction and reimplantation. Urology, 18:562, 1981.

Hanna, M. K., and Jeffs, R. D.: Primary obstructive megaureter in children. Urology, 6:419, 1975.

Heal, M. R.: Primary obstructive megaureter in adults. Br. J. Urol., 45:490, 1973.

Hensley, T. W., Berdon, W. E., Baker, D. H., and Goldstein, H. R.: The ureteral "J" sign: radiographic demonstration of iatrogenic distal ureteral obstruction after ureteral reimplantation. J. Urol., 127:766, 1982.

Hirschhorn, R. C.: The ileal sleeve. II. Surgical technique in clinical application. J. Urol., 92:120, 1964.

Hodgson, N. B., and Thompson, L. W.: Technique of reductive ureteroplasty in the management of megaureter. J. Urol., 113:118, 1975.

Hurst, A. F., and Gaymer-Jones, J.: A case of megaloureter due to achalasia of the ureterovesical sphincter. Br. J. Urol., 3:43, 1931.

Hutch, J. A.: Nonobstructive dilatation of the upper urinary tract. J. Urol., 71:412, 1954.

Hutch, J. A., and Tanagho, E. A.: Etiology of nonocclusive ureteral dilatation. J. Urol., 93:177, 1965.

Jeffs, R. D., Jonas, P., and Schillinger, J. F.: Surgical correction of vesicoureteral reflux in children with neurogenic bladders. J. Urol., 115:449, 1976.

Johnston, J. H.: Reconstructive surgery of mega-ureter in childhood. Br. J. Urol., 39:17, 1967.

Johnston, J. H.: Hydro-ureter and mega-ureter. *In* Williams, D. I. (Ed.): Pediatric Urology. London, Butterworth and Co., 1968, pp. 160–174.

Johnston, J. H., and Farkas, A.: The congenital refluxing megaureter: Experiences with surgical reconstruction. Br. J. Urol., 47:153, 1975.

Kass, E. J., Massond, M., and Belman, A. B.: Comparison of the diuretic renogram and the pressure perfusion study in children. J. Urol., 134:92–96, 1985.

Keating, M. A., Escala, J., Snyder, H. McC., III, Heyman, S., and Duckett, J. W.: Changing concepts in the management of primary obstructive megaureter. J. Urol., 142:636–640, 1989.

Keating, M. A., and Retik, A. B.: Management of the dilated obstructed ureter. Urol. Clin. North Am., 17:291–306, 1990.

King, L. R.: Megaloureter: definition, diagnosis and management (Editorial). J. Urol., 123:222, 1980.

Koff, S. A., Thrall, J. H., and Keyes, J. W., Jr.: Assessment of hydroureteronephrosis in children using diuretic radionuclide urography. J. Urol., 123:531, 1980.

Leibowitz, S., and Bodian, M.: A study of the vesical ganglia in children and the relationship to the megaureter megacystis syndrome and Hirschsprung's disease. J. Clin. Pathol., 16:342, 1963.

Lewis, E. L., and Cletsoway, R. W.: Megaloureter. J. Urol., 75:643, 1956.

Lewis, E. L., and Kimbrough, J. C.: Megaloureter: New concept in treatment. South. Med. J., 45:171, 1952.

Lockhart, J. L., Singer, A. M., and Glenn, J. F.: Congenital megaureter. J. Urol., 122:310, 1979.

MacKinnon, K. J.: Primary megaureter. Birth Defects, 13:15, 1977.

Mayo, M. E., and Ansell, J. S.: The effect of bladder function on the dynamics of the ureterovesical junction. J. Urol., 123:229, 1980.

McGrath, M. A., Estroff, J., and Lebowitz, R. L.: The coexistence of obstruction at the ureteropelvic and ureterovesical junctions. Am. J. Radiol., 149:403–406, 1987.

McLaughlin, A. P., Pfister, R. C., Leadbetter, W. F., et al.: The pathophysiology of primary megaloureter. J. Urol., 109:805, 1973.

Mitchell, M. E.: The rate of bladder augmentation in undiversion. J. Pediatr. Surg., 16:790, 1981.

Mesrobian, H. G. J., Kramer, S. A., and Kelalis, P. P.: Reoperative ureteroneocystomy: Review of 69 patients. J. Urol., 133:388–390, 1985.

Mollard, P., and Paillot, J. M.: Primary megaureter (pathogenesis and treatment of 104 patients—131 ureters). Prog. Pediatr. Surg., 5:113, 1973.

Murnaghan, G. F.: Experimental investigation of the dynamics of the normal and dilated ureter. Br. J. Urol., 29:403, 1957.

Nesbit, R. M., and Withycombe, J. F.: The problem of primary megaloureter. J. Urol., 72:162, 1954.

Notley, R. G.: Electron microscopy of the primary obstructive megaureter. Br. J. Urol., 44:229, 1972.

Ohl, D. A., Konnak, J. W., Campbell, D. A., Dafoe, D. C., Merion, R. M., and Turcotte, J. G.: Extravesical ureteroneocystostomy in renal transplantation. J. Urol., 139:499–502, 1988.

Pagano, P., and Passerini, G.: Primary obstructed megaureter. Br. J. Urol., 49:469, 1977.

Passaro, E., and Smith, J. P.: Congenital ureteral valve in children: a case report. J. Urol., 84:290, 1960.

Peters, C. A., Mandell, J., Lebowitz, R. L., Colodny, A. H., Bauer, S. B., Hendren, W. H., and Retik, A. B.: Congenital obstructed megaureters in early infancy: Diagnosis and treatment. J. Urol., 142:641–645, 1989.

Pfister, R. C., and Hendren, W. H.: Primary megaureter in children with adults. Clinical and pathophysiologic features of 150 ureters. Urology, 12:160, 1978.

Pitts, W. R., and Muecke, E. C.: Congenital megaloureter: A review of 80 patients. J. Urol., 111:468, 1974.

Politano, V. A.: Ureterovesical junction. J. Urol., 107:239, 1972.

Rabinowitz, R., Barkin, M., Schillinger, J. F., Jeffs, R. D., and Cook, G. T.: Salvaging the iatrogenic megaureter. J. Urol., 121:330, 1979.

Retik, A. B., McEvoy, J. P., and Bauer, S. B.: Megaureters in children. Urology, 11:281, 1978.

Skinner, D. G., and Goodwin, W. E.: Indications for the use of intestinal segments in management of nephrocalcinosis. Trans. Am. Assoc. Genitourin. Surg., 66:158, 1974.

Smith, E. D., et al.: Report of Working Party to Establish an International Nomenclature for the Large Ureter. *In* Bergsma, D., and Duckett, J. W. (Eds.): Birth Defects. Original Articles Series. Vol. 13, No. 5, 1977, pp. 3–8.

So, E. P., Brock, W. A., and Kaplan, G. W.: Ureteral reimplantation without catheters. J. Urol., 125:551, 1981.

Starr, A.: Ureteral plication: A new concept in ureteral tailoring for megaureter. Invest. Urol., 17:153, 1979.

Swenson, O., and Fisher, J. H.: The relation of megacolon and megaloureter. N. Engl. J. Med., 253:1147, 1955.

Swenson, O., Fisher, J. H., and Cendron, J.: Megaloureter: Investigation as to the cause and report on the results of newer forms of treatment. Surgery, 40:223, 1956.

Talner, L. B., and Gittes, R. F.: Megacalyces: Further observation and differentiation from obstructive renal disease. Am. J. Roentgenol., 121:473, 1974.

Tanagho, E. A.: Ureteral tailoring. J. Urol., 106:194, 1971.

Tanagho, E. A.: Intrauterine fetal ureteral obstruction. J. Urol., 109:196, 1973.

Tatu, W., and Brennan, R. E.: Primary megaureter in a mother and daughter. Urol. Radiol., 3:185, 1981.

Tokunaka, S., and Koyanagi, T.: Morphologic study of primary nonreflux megaureters with particular emphasis on the role of ureteral sheath and ureteral dysplasia. J. Urol., 128:399, 1982.

Tokunaka, S., Koyanagi, T., Tsuji, I., and Yamade, T.: Histopathology of the nonrefluxing megaloureter: A clue to its pathogenesis. J. Urol., 17:238, 1982.

Tscholl, R., Tettamatti, F., and Singg, E.: Ileal substitutes of ureter with reflux-plasty by terminal intussusception of bowel. Urology, 9:385, 1977.

Turner, R. D., and Goodwin, W. E.: Experiments with intussuscepted ileal valve in ureteral substitution. J. Urol., 81:526, 1959.

Tveter, K. J., and Goodwin, W. E.: The use of ileum as substitute for the ureter. *In* Resnick, M. I. (Ed.): Current Trends in Urology. Vol. 2. Baltimore, Williams & Wilkins Co., 1982, pp. 1–51.

Uson, A. C., Braham, S. B., Abrams, C. A., et al.: Retrocaval ureter in a child with Turner's syndrome. Am. J. Dis. Child., 119:267, 1970.

Vargas, B., and Lebowitz, R. L.: The coexistence of congenital megacalyces and primary megaureter. Am. J. Roentgenol., 147:313–316, 1986.

Von Niederhausern, W., and Tuchschmid, D.: Une association mal connue: le mega-uretere congenital primaire et le rein a megacalices. Ann. Urol., 5:225, 1971.

Weiss, R. M., and Lytton, B.: Vesicoureteral reflux and distal ureteral obstruction. J. Urol., 111:245, 1974.

Weiss, R. M., Schiff, M., Jr., and Lytton, B.: Late obstruction after ureteroneocystostomy. J. Urol., 106:144, 1971.

Whitaker, R. H.: Methods of assessing obstruction in dilated ureter. Br. J. Urol., 45:15, 1973.

Whitaker, R. H., and Flower, C. D.: Megacalices—how broad a spectrum? Br. J. Urol., 53:1, 1981.

Williams, D. I., and Hulme-Moir, I.: Primary obstructive megaureter. Br. J. Urol., 42:140, 1970.

Witherow, R. O., and Whitaker, R. H.: The predictive accuracy of antigrade pressure flow studies in equivocal upper tract obstruction. Br. J. Urol., 53:496, 1981.

Woodard, J. R., Anderson, A. M., and Parrott, T. S.: Ureteral reimplantation in myelodysplastic children. J. Urol., 126:387, 1981.

Woodbury, P. W., Mitchell, M. E., Scheidler, J. M., Adams, M. C., Rink, R. C., and McNulty, A.: Constant pressure perfusion: A method to determine obstruction in the upper tract. J. Urol., 142:632–635, 1989.

Ureteral Reimplantation

Ahmed, S., and Boucaut, H. A.: Vesicoureteral reflux in complete ureteral duplication: Surgical options. J. Urol., 140:1092–1094, 1988.

Ahmed, S.: Transverse advancement ureteral reimplantation: pull-through alternative in megaureter. J. Urol., 123:218, 1980.

Ahmed, S., and Tan, H.: Complications of transverse advancement ureteral reimplantation: Diverticulum formation. J. Urol., 127:970, 1982.

Arap, S., Abrao, E. G., and Menezes de Goes, G.: Treatment and prevention of complications after extravesical antireflux technique. Eur. Urol., 7:263, 1981.

Bellinger, M. F.: The management of vesicoureteric reflux. Urol. Clin. North Am., 12:23, 1985.

Bischoff, P. F.: Problems in treatment of vesicoureteral reflux. J. Urol., 107:133, 1972.

Bishop, M. C., Askew, A. R., and Smith, J. C.: Reimplantation of the wide ureter. Br. J. Urol., 50:383, 1978.

Bjordal, R. I., Stake, G., and Knutrud, O.: Surgical treatment of megaureter in the first few months of life. Ann. Chir. Gynaecol. Fenn., 69:10, 1980.

Bockrath, J. M., Maizels, M., and Firlit, C. F.: The use of lower ipsilateral ureteroureterostomy to treat vesicoureteral reflux or obstruction in children with duplex ureters. J. Urol., 129:543, 1983.

Bovee, J. W.: A critical survey of ureteral implantation. Ann. Surg., 31:165, 1900.

Burkowski, A.: Operative treatment of megaureter in adults. Int. Urol. Nephrol., 9:105, 1977.

Caine, M., and Hermann, G.: The return of peristalsis in the anastomosed ureter: a cine-radiographic study. Br. J. Urol., 42:164, 1970.

Carlson, H. E.: The intrapsoas transplant of megalo-ureter. J. Urol., 72:172, 1954.

Clark, P., and Hosmame, R. U.: Reimplantation of the ureter. Br. J. Urol., 48:31, 1976.

Cohen, S. J.: Ureterozystoneostome: Eine neue antirefluxtechnik. Aktuel. Urol., 6:1, 1975.

Creevy, C. D.: The atomic distal ureteral segment (ureteral achalasia). J. Urol., 97:457, 1967.

Dodson, A. I.: Some improvements in the technique of ureterocystostomy. J. Urol., 55:225, 1946.

Ehrlich, R. M.: Ureteral folding technique for megaureter surgery. Soc. Pediatr. Urol. Newsletter, May 5, 1982, pp. 56–57.

Filly, R. A., Friedland, G. W., Fair, W. R., and Govan, D. E.: Late ureteric obstruction following ureteral reimplantation for reflux. Urology, 4:540, 1974.

Garrett, R. A., and Schlueter, D. P.: Complication of antireflux operations: Causes and management. J. Urol., 109:1002, 1973.

Gearhart, J. P., and Woolfenden, K. A.: The vesicopsoas hitch as an adjunct to megaureter repair in childhood. J. Urol., 127:505, 1982.

Gibbons, M. D., and Gonzales, E. T., Jr.: Complications of antireflux surgery. Urol. Clin. North Am., 10:489, 1983.

Glenn, J. F., and Anderson, E. E.: Distal tunnel ureteral reimplantation. J. Urol., 97:623, 1967.

Gonzales, E. T., Caffarena, E., and Carlton, C. E.: The advantages of short-term vesical drainage after antireflux operation. J. Urol., 119:817, 1978.

Gregoir, W.: Le traitement chirurgical du reflux vesicoureteral congenital. Acta Chir. Belg., 63:431, 1964.

Gregoir, W., and Schulman, C. C.: Die extravesikale antireflux plastik. Urologie, A16:124, 1977.

Gregoir, W., and Van Regemorter, G.: Le reflux vésicourétéral congénital. Urol. Int., 18:122, 1964.

Hampel, N., Richter-Levin, D., and Gersh, I.: Extravesical repair of primary vesicoureteral reflux in children. J. Urol., 117:335, 1977.

Hanna, M. K.: New surgical method for one stage total remodeling of massively dilated and tortuous ureter: tapering in situ technique. Urology, 14:453, 1979.

Hendren, W. H.: Ureteral reimplantation in children. J. Pediatr. Surg., 3:649, 1968.

Hendren, W. H.: Operative repair of megaureter in children. J. Urol., 101:491, 1969.

Hendren, W. H.: Complications of megaureter repair in children. J. Urol., 113:238, 1975.

Hendren, W. H.: Tapered bowel segment for ureteral replacement. Urol. Clin. North Am., 5:697, 1978.

Hensley, T. W., Berdon, W. E., Baker, D. H., and Goldstein, H. R.: The ureteral "J" sign: radiographic demonstration of iatrogenic distal ureteral obstruction after ureteral reimplantation. J. Urol., 127:766, 1982.

Hutch, J. A.: Vesicoureteral reflux in the paraplegic: Cause and correction. J. Urol., 68:457, 1952.

Hutch, J. A., Smith, D. R., and Osborne, R.: Review of a series of ureterovesicoplasties. J. Urol., 100:285, 1968.

Jeffs, R. D., Jonas, P., and Schillinger, J. F.: Surgical correction of vesicoureteral reflux in children with neurogenic bladder. J. Urol., 115:449, 1976.

Johnston, J. H., and Heal, M. R.: Reflux in complete duplicated ureters in children: Management and technique. J. Urol., 105:881, 1971.

Johnston, J. H., Shapiro, S. R., and Thomas, G. G.: Antireflux surgery in the congenital neuropathic bladder. Br. J. Urol., 48:639, 1976.

Kalicinski, Z. H., Kansy, J., Kotarbinska, B., and Juszt, W.: Surgery of megaureters—modification of Hendren's operation. J. Pediatr. Surg., 12:183, 1977.

Kelalis, P. P., and Kramer, S. A.: Complications of megaureter surgery. Urol. Clin. North Am., 10:417, 1983.

Lamesch, A. J.: Retrograde catheterization of the ureter after antirefluxplasty by the Cohen technique of transverse advancement. J. Urol., 125:73, 1981.

Lebowitz, R. L.: Section on Urology. American Academy of Pediatrics Annual Meeting. San Francisco, October 1983.

Lich, R., Howerton, L. W., and Davis, L. A.: Recurrent urosepsis in children. J. Urol., 86:554, 1961.

Marberger, M., Altwein, J. E., Straub, E., Wulff, H. D., and Hohenfellner, R.: The Lich-Gregoir antireflux plasty: experiences with 371 children. J. Urol., 120:216, 1978.

Mayo, M. E., and Ansell, J. S.: The effect of bladder function on the dynamics of the ureterovesical junction. J. Urol., 123:229, 1980.

McDuffie, R. W., Litin, R. B., and Blundon, K. E.: Ureteral reimplantation: Lich method. Urology, 10:19, 1977.

Nanninga, J., King, L. R., Downing, J., et al.: Factors affecting the outcome of 100 ureteral reimplantations done for vesicoureteral reflux. J. Urol., 72:162, 1954.

Paquin, A. J.: Ureterovesical anastomosis: The description and evaluation of a technique. J. Urol., 82:573, 1959.

Paquin, A. J.: Surgery of the ureterovesical junction. In Glenn, J. F., and Boyce, W. H. (Eds.): Urologic Surgery. New York, Harper & Row, 1969, pp. 191–252.

Politano, V.: Poster session, American Urological Association. Boston, 1981.

Politano, V. A., and Leadbetter, W. F.: An operative technique for the correction of vesicoureteral reflux. J. Urol., 79:932, 1958.

So, E. P., Brock, W. A., and Kaplan, G. W.: Ureteral reimplantation without catheters. J. Urol., 125:551, 1981.

Starr, A.: Ureteral plication: A new concept in ureteral tailoring for megaureter. Invest. Urol., 17:153, 1979.

Stephens, F. D.: A new technique of ureteral reimplantation based on anatomical principles. Presented at the meeting of the Society for Pediatric Urology, 1977.

Stevens, A. R., and Marshall, V. F.: Reimplantation of the ureter into the bladder. Surg. Gynecol. Obstet., 77:585, 1943.

Talbot, H. S., and Bunts, R. C.: Late renal changes in paraplegia: Hydronephrosis due to vesicoureteral reflux. J. Urol., 61:810, 1949.

Tocci, P. E., Politano, V. A., Lynne, C. M., and Carrion, H. M.: Unusual complications of transvesical ureteral reimplantation. J. Urol., 115:1731, 1976.

Udall, D. A., Hodges, C. V., Pearse, H. M., et al.: Transureterostomy: Experience in pediatric patient. Urology, 2:401, 1973.

Vermooten, V., and Neuswanger, O. H.: Effects on the upper urinary tract in dogs of an incompetent ureterovesical valve. J. Urol., 32:330, 1934.

Warren, M. M., Kelalis, P. P., and Stickler, G. B.: Unilateral ureteroneocystostomy: The fate of the contralateral ureter. J. Urol., 107:466, 1972.

Weiss, R. M., Schiff, M., and Lytton, B.: Late obstruction after ureteroneocystostomy. J. Urol., 106:144, 1971.

Whitaker, R. H.: Diagnosis of obstruction in dilated ureters. Ann. R. Coll. Surg., 53:153, 1973.

Williams, D. I., and Eckstein, H. B.: Surgical treatment of reflux in children. Br. J. Urol., 37:13, 1965.

Woodard, J. R., and Keats, G.: Ureteral reimplantation: Paquin's procedure after 12 years. J. Urol., 109:819, 1973.

Endoscopic Correction of Reflux

Arnold, G. E.: Further experiences with intrachordal Teflon injection. Laryngoscope, 74:802, 1964.

Berg, S.: Polytef augmentation urethroplasty. Correction of surgically incurable incontinence by injection technique. Arch. Surg., 107:379, 1973.

Brown, S.: Open vs. endoscopic surgery in the treatment of vesicoureteral reflux. J. Urol., 142:499–500, 1989.

Claesh, J., Stroobants, D., VanMeerbeek, J., Verbeken, E., Knockaert, D., and Baert, L.: Pulmonary migration following periurethral polytetrafluoroethylene injection for urinary incontinence. J. Urol., 142:821–822, 1989.

Kaplan, W. E., Dalton, D. P., and Firlit, C. F.: The endoscopic correction of reflux by polytetrafluoroethylene injection. J. Urol., 138:953–955, 1987.

Malizia, A. A., Jr., Reiman, H. M., Myers, R. P., Sonde, J. R., Borham, S. S., Benson, R. C., Jr., Devanjee, M. K., and Utz, W. J.: Migration and granulomatous reaction after periuretheral injection of Polytef (Teflon). JAMA, 251:3277, 1984.

Malizia, A. A., Rushton, H. G., Woodard, J. R., Newton, N. E., Reiman, H. M., and Lopez, O. F.: Migration and granulomatous reaction after intravesical/subureteric injection of Polytef. J. Urol., Part 2, 137:122A, Abstract 74, 1987.

Merguerian, P. A., McLorie, G. A., Khoury, A., and Churchill, B. M.: Submucosal injection of polyvinyl alcohol foam (Ivalon) and autologous cartilage in rabbit bladder. J. Urol., 144:531–533, 1990.

Mittleman, R. E., and Marraconi, J. V.: Pulmonary Teflon granulo-mas following periurethral injection for urinary incontinence. Arch Pathol. Labs. Med, 107:611, 1983.

O'Donnell, B., and Puri, P.: Technical refinements in endoscopic correction of vesicoureteral reflux. J. Urol., 140:1101–1102, 1988.

Politano, V. A., Small, M. P., Harper, J. M., and Lynne, C. M.: Periurethral Teflon injection for urinary incontinence. J. Urol., 111:180, 1974.

Puri, P., and O'Donnell, B.: Endoscopic correction of grades IV and V primary vesicoureteric reflux: 6- to 30-month follow-up in 42 ureters. J. Pediatr. Surg., 22:1087, 1987.

Quinn, F. M., Diamond, T., and Boston, V. E.: Endoscopic management of vesicoureteral reflux in children with neuropathic bladder secondary to myelomeningocele. Zectschrift fur Kinderchirurgie 43, Suppl. 2, pp. 43–45, 1988.

Schulman, C. C., Simon, J., Pamart, D., and Avni, E. E.: Endoscopic treatment of vesicoureteral reflux in children. J. Urol., 138:950–952, 1987.

45
ECTOPIC URETER AND URETEROCELE

Alan B. Retik, M.D.
Craig A. Peters, M.D.

ECTOPIC URETER

A ureter that opens anywhere except on the trigone of the bladder is considered to be ectopic. In girls, the usual sites for an ectopic orifice are the bladder neck, proximal or distal urethra, and vestibule. Because the ectopic ureteral orifice, during embryonic growth, is occasionally incorporated into the structures derived from the müllerian ducts, the ureter may empty into the vagina, uterus, or cervix. Therefore, in the female, an ectopic ureteral orifice may be either within or outside the urinary sphincter, making ectopic ureters one of the more important causes of urinary incontinence in girls (Fig. 45–1). Infection may also be the presenting sign of an ectopic ureter in girls, whereas it is almost always so in boys. In the male, ectopic ureters usually drain into the prostatic urethra, prostatic utricle, seminal vesicle, vas deferens, or ejaculatory duct. Openings into the rectum occur rarely in both sexes. In the male, the ureter, even if ectopic, will be proximal to the verumontanum and will not cause urinary incontinence.

Embryology

Embryologically, an ectopic ureteral orifice results when a ureteral bud or, more often, a second or an accessory ureteral bud arises from the mesonephric (wolffian) duct more craniad than is usual and is not incorporated into the trigone but is only "carried" to a point more inferior and caudad, often within the urethra, through the common excretory duct. In general, abnormally located ectopic ureteral orifices within the bladder produce no symptoms. Ectopic ureters opening into the bladder neck and urethra are the most common causes of the clinical problems due to ureteral ectopia. Should the ureter arise from the mesonephric duct at a still higher level, it will completely fail to become incorporated into the lower urinary tract and will remain confluent with the mesonephric duct in the male (seminal vesicle or vas deferens) or with its vestiges in the female (Gartner's duct, upper vagina, cervix, uterus, fallopian tubes) (Tanagho, 1976); this type of ureter will invariably cause symptoms.

The incidence of ectopic ureters has been reported to be higher in females than in males by at least 4 to 1 (Mandell et al., 1981). This difference is less pronounced with nonduplicated ureteral ectopia. Because ureteral ectopia usually produces incontinence in females, its discovery at an earlier age is far more likely.

Ectopic Ureter in Girls

Ectopic ureteral orifices in girls are most often associated with renal duplication and may be an important cause of urinary incontinence. In the Japanese literature, however, ureteral ectopia is more frequently associated with single systems (see below) (Gotoh et al., 1983).

Clinical Manifestations

Continuous incontinence in a girl with an otherwise normal voiding pattern after toilet training is the classic sign of an ectopic ureteral orifice. Such incontinence will occur if the ectopic orifice is located in the distal urethra, vagina, or vestibule. If the urine drains only when the child assumes the erect position, incontinence may be diurnal when the renal unit drained by the ectopic ureter is dysplastic and poorly functioning. On occasion, incontinence becomes apparent at a later age and may be confused with stress incontinence, incontinence associated with neurogenic bladder dysfunction, or psychogenic incontinence. A persistent vaginal discharge from an ectopic orifice located in the vagina is another clinical sign. Most ectopic ureters are associated

Female

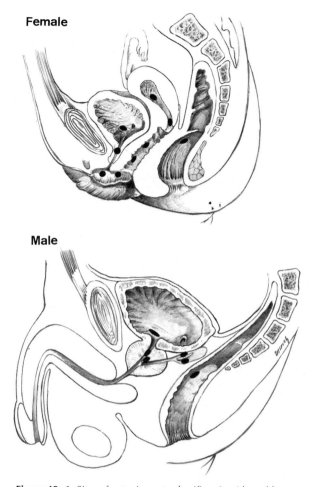

Male

Figure 45–1. Sites of ectopic ureteral orifices in girls and boys.

In most instances, the diagnosis of an ectopic ureter is confirmed by excretory urography. The usual radiographic feature is a nonvisualizing or poorly visualizing upper pole of a duplex system that may be massively hydronephrotic. The upper pole displaces the lower pole downward and outward—the so-called drooping flower appearance (Fig. 45–3). The calyces of the lower pelvis are fewer in number than in the normal kidney, the axis of the lowest to uppermost calyx is deviated away from the midline, and the uppermost calyx is usually farther from the upper limit of the renal border than is the lowest calyx from the corresponding lower limit. In addition, this pelvis and the upper portion of its ureter may be farther from the spine than on the contralateral side, and the lower pole ureter may also be scalloped and tortuous secondary to a markedly dilated upper pole ureter wrapped around it. When an ectopic ureter drains a nonvisualizing, diminutive, dysplastic renal unit, the typical radiologic features as mentioned may not be demonstrated. Particular attention should be paid to the contralateral kidney on excretory urography to avoid missing bilateral ureteral ectopia (Fig. 45–4). This is reported to occur in 5 to 15 per cent of cases (Malek et al., 1972b; Mandell et al., 1981) but was noted in 25 per cent of cases in one series (Campbell, 1951).

The functional status of the upper pole renal segment of duplex systems may be evident on excretory urography, but more precise assessment may become important if upper pole salvage is considered. Isotopic renal scanning using ^{99m}technetium–dimercaptosuccinic acid (^{99m}Tc-DMSA) has proved to be the most adequate, although differentiating between the function of the upper and lower poles may be difficult.

with acute or recurrent urinary tract infection. A patient may also present with failure to thrive and chronic infection. Ectopic ureters draining into the proximal urethra often reflux, and urge incontinence is common. On occasion, an ectopic ureter may be severely obstructed, causing massive hydronephrosis and hydroureter, and it may occur as an abdominal mass (Uson et al., 1972) or be detected on prenatal ultrasonographic evaluation.

Diagnosis

Prenatal ultrasonographic diagnosis of ectopic ureters has become common. The condition is identifiable by virtue of the hydronephrosis produced by obstruction. If this is isolated to the upper pole of a duplex system and the bladder is normal, the diagnosis is straightforward. In other situations, prenatal findings will serve to initiate a postnatal evaluation, which will specifically identify the condition.

In a girl, the diagnosis of an ectopic ureter can sometimes be made by history and physical examination. Direct visualization of the vulva may reveal continuous urinary dribbling or wetness. Often, a punctum or orifice is apparent in the urethrovaginal septum (Fig. 45–2). In the absence of neurogenic vesical dysfunction or a urethral sphincter defect, an ectopic ureter is likely.

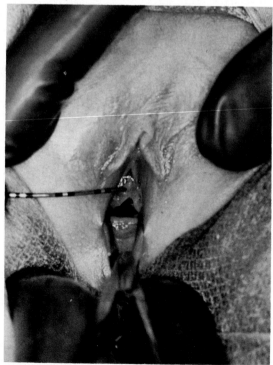

Figure 45–2. Photograph at the time of cystoscopy of an ectopic ureteral orifice in the urethrovaginal septum. A ureteral catheter is in the orifice.

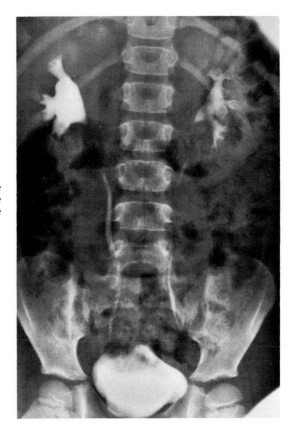

Figure 45–3. Excretory urogram in a 5-year-old girl with urinary incontinence shows a nonvisualizing upper pole on the right side displacing the lower pole downward and outward. Also note the right renal pelvis and upper ureter to be farther from the spine than on the left.

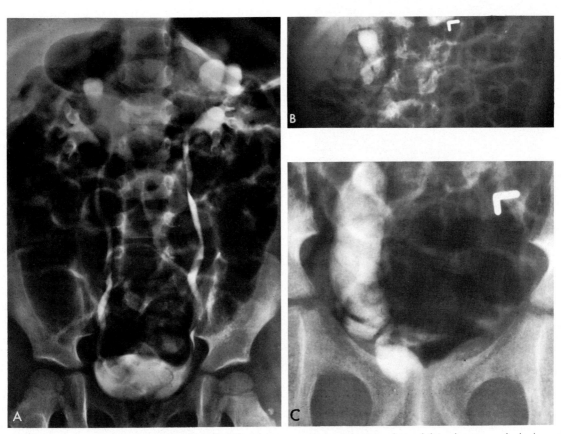

Figure 45–4. A, Excretory urogram in a 3-year-old girl with two severe urinary infections shows bilateral upper pole hydronephrosis and hydroureter. B and C, Voiding cystourethrography demonstrates reflux to the ectopic right upper pole ureter.

The ultrasonographic findings of an ectopic ureter include the dilated pelvis and collecting system of the upper pole or, occasionally, the entire renal unit and a dilated ureter behind an otherwise normal bladder. Occasionally, the renal parenchyma is difficult to locate owing to dysplasia or atrophy. The dilated ureter is clearly extravesical with a thick septum of bladder muscle between the ureteral lumen and bladder lumen. This finding is in contrast to a ureterocele where the septum is thin and delicate and the ureteral lumen is partially intravesical (Fig. 45–5). The renal parenchyma associated with the ectopic ureter is often thinner than that of the normally draining lower pole (Nussbaum et al., 1986).

Voiding cystourethrography will demonstrate reflux into the lower pole ureter frequently, in at least half of the cases (Fig. 45–6). More importantly, reflux may be demonstrated into the ectopic ureter at different phases of voiding, providing evidence of the location of the orifice (Fig. 45–7). If reflux into the ectopic ureter is seen before voiding, the orifice is proximal to the bladder neck; reflux only with voiding suggests an orifice in the urethra. The last finding may be evident only with several cycles of voiding monitored fluouroscopically (Wyly and Lebowitz, 1984). Sphincteric orifices may not reflux at all. A large ectopic ureter may press against the bladder and create an indentation appearing much like a ureterocele and termed a "pseudoureterocele" (Diard et al., 1987).

In unusual cases, in which an ectopic ureter is strongly suspected because of incontinence, yet no definite evidence of the upper pole renal segment is found (Simms and Higgins, 1975), computed tomography has demonstrated the small poorly functioning upper pole segment (Fig. 45–8).

Ectopic ureteral orifices may be identified at the time of cystourethroscopy and vaginoscopy. Careful inspection of the vestibule, urethra, and vagina will sometimes reveal the ectopic orifice. We have not found the intravenous injection of indigo carmine to be particularly helpful because of the very poor function of the segment drained by the ectopic ureter. Two oral doses of phenazopyridine (Pyridium) given the night before and morning of cystoscopy have been suggested to improve visualization of the ectopic ureter (Weiss et al., 1984). Filling the bladder with a dye solution, such as methylene blue or indigo carmine, is sometimes helpful in detecting the elusive ectopic orifice. If a clear fluid continues to drain into the vulva, one can be certain that an ectopic orifice is present.

Sometimes, the diagnosis must be made by exclusion, i.e., the vestibule is damp, no orifice is found, the excretory urogram shows subtle changes suggesting a tiny dysplastic upper segment of a duplex system, and the patient is cured by an upper pole nephrectomy! With current imaging techniques and an appropriate index of suspicion, the diagnosis is usually made before surgery.

Treatment

The usual treatment for an ectopic ureter associated with a poorly visualizing or nonvisualizing upper pole of a renal duplication is upper pole nephrectomy and ureterectomy through a standard flank incision. The entire kidney is mobilized, and both ureters are identified (Fig. 45–9). Usually, two or three small arteries with corresponding veins supply the upper pole; these are divided. Although the renal capsule is often markedly adherent to the scarred upper pole parenchyma, it is usually possible to strip the capsule well back onto the normal lower pole parenchyma. The ectopic ureter is then isolated and divided at the lower pole of the kidney, passed behind the vessels, and used to lift the upper pole away from the lower pole. The inferior aspect of the upper pole pelvis also provides the plane of access between the two renal segments, and this may be developed bluntly.

In most instances, it is helpful to place an atraumatic vascular clamp on the main renal artery prior to incising the renal parenchyma. Before the renal circulation is occluded, mannitol is injected intravenously (25 per cent solution; dose, 0.5 ml/kg) and a brisk diuresis should

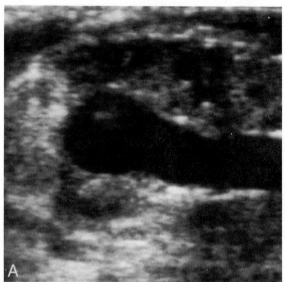
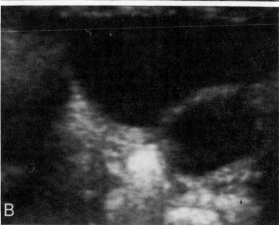

Figure 45–5. Ultrasound appearance of an ectopic ureter. *A,* Upper pole hydronephrosis with substantial renal parenchyma. *B,* Bladder view demonstrating the dilated distal ureter with a thick echodense bladder wall between the bladder and ureteral lumena. (Compare with Figure 45–22.)

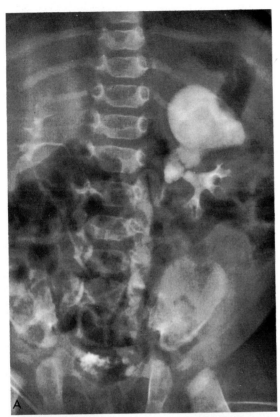

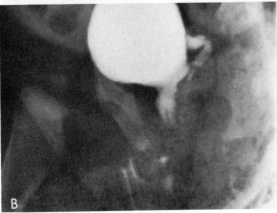

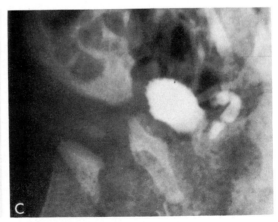

Figure 45–6. *A,* Excretory urogram in a 4-month-old girl with a urinary tract infection reveals a left renal duplication with hydronephrosis and hydroureter of the upper pole system. *B* and *C,* Voiding cystourethrogram demonstrates reflux to the ectopic ureter, whose orifice was located in the proximal urethra.

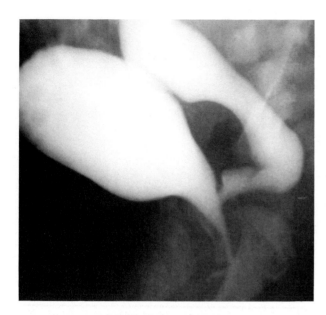

Figure 45–7. Cyclic voiding cystourethrogram in a 1-month-old boy, with prenatal detection of upper pole hydronephrosis, demonstrating reflux into a ureter ectopic to the prostatic urethra. Several cycles of voiding and filling were performed to identify the reflux.

Figure 45–8. *A,* Excretory urogram in 10-year-old girl with constant wetting. No definite evidence for an upper pole segment is present. *B,* Left renal ultrasound in the same patient, also without a clear indication of the presence of an upper pole segment. *C,* Contrast-enhanced computed tomography image in this girl specifically demonstrating the small upper pole segment (*arrow*) associated with the ectopic ureter. Upper pole nephrectomy cured wetting.

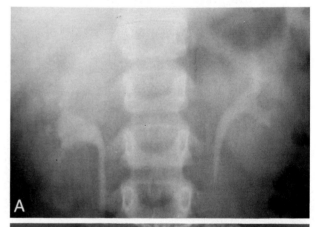
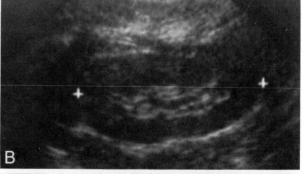
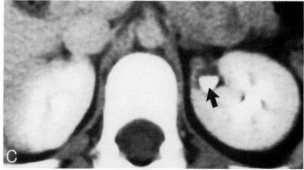

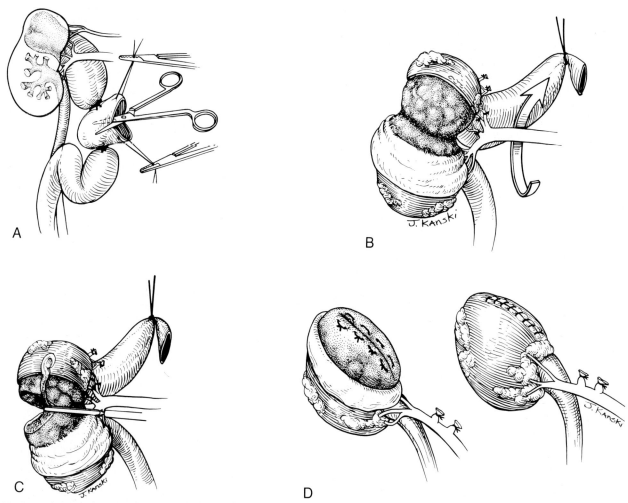

Figure 45–9. Technique of upper pole nephrectomy. *A,* The upper pole ureter is usually very dilated and tortuous and can be identified readily at the lower pole of the kidney. It is separated carefully from the lower pole ureter, divided, and used to improve access to the upper pole moiety.

B, The upper pole ureter is passed beneath the hilar renal vessels and retracted upward. Small feeding vessels to the upper pole are individually ligated and divided. Any larger vessels that may be supplying the upper pole may be temporarily clamped to determine the extent of their distribution. The capsule of the upper pole is bluntly stripped away, exposing the often coarse and cystic parenchyma of the upper pole. This can usually be distinguished from the smooth texture of the normal lower pole. Often, an indented demarcation is seen between the two poles.

C, With traction being applied to the lower pole ureter, the upper pole is excised using electrocautery. Vascular control is achieved by temporary clamping of the lower pole vessels. This may also be performed by gentle finger compression of the lower pole. Individual vessels are identified and ligated during this part of the procedure.

D, The parenchyma of the lower pole is approximated at the site of removal of the upper pole using broad mattress sutures. The redundant capsule is then brought over the site of repair and sewn together with a running suture.

ensue. With any manipulation of the renal vessels, particularly in small babies, one should have agents to reverse vasospasm readily available. These include lidocaine 0.25 per cent (2.5 mg/ml, maximum dose 7 mg/kg—use half of this dose) and papaverine (15 mg) on a small cotton pledget (Gearhart and Jeffs, 1985). Usually, a rather clear-cut demarcation occurs between the dysplastic, hydronephrotic upper pole and the lower pole. Electrocautery is very useful to incise the thin rim of parenchyma connecting the upper pole to the lower after the pelvis has been dissected free. After the upper pole is removed, the parenchyma is reapproximated with mattress sutures of 3-0 chromic catgut. The capsule is then closed over the repair with a running suture. Occasionally, when a large hydronephrotic upper pole has been removed and the lower pole is excessively mobile, nephropexy is performed to provide improved renal fixation. The remaining upper pole ureter is dissected carefully away from the lower pole ureter and excised at a level below the iliac vessels. It is important in this dissection not to injure the blood supply of the lower pole ureter, taking care to sweep all periureteral adventitia toward the remaining ureter, which should not be dissected from its bed. The cut edges of the distal ureteral stump are cauterized and left open, and the flank is drained.

Complete distal ureterectomy is not usually necessary unless reflux into the ectopic ureter is present. Rarely will the retained segment cause symptoms and require subsequent surgical excision (Belman, Filmer, and King, 1974; Mandell et al., 1981). If the ectopic ureter refluxes, its distal portion should be excised through a separate suprapubic or groin incision. A Robinson catheter inserted into the distal ureteral stump at the time of partial nephrectomy makes the ectopic ureter more readily identifiable through the small second incision. It is usually very difficult to separate the distal 2.5 cm of the upper pole ureter from the lower pole ureter. The ectopic ureter can be completely excised up to this point, and its outer wall is then incised or excised only down to the level of the bladder, where a transfixing suture will obliterate its lumen (Fig. 45–10). Care should be taken not to ligate the lumen of the lower pole ureter. Refluxing ureters ectopic to the urethra may be very difficult to remove entirely, and a small residual stump may need to be left in place.

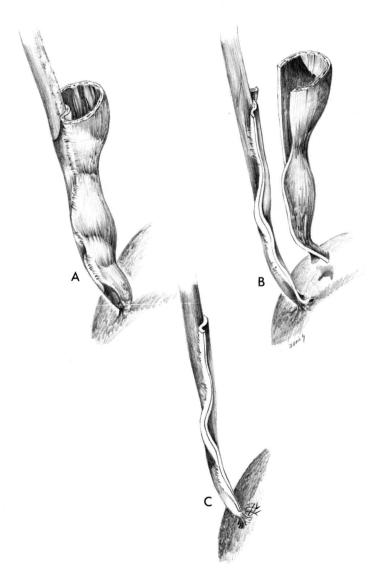

Figure 45–10. Surgical management of the refluxing ureteral stump. *A,* It is difficult to completely separate the distal 2 to 3 cm of the upper pole ureter from the lower pole ureter. The ectopic ureter is excised to this point. *B,* The outer wall of the ectopic ureter is excised to the bladder level. *C,* A transfixing suture obliterates its lumen, with care being taken not to injure the orthotopic ureter.

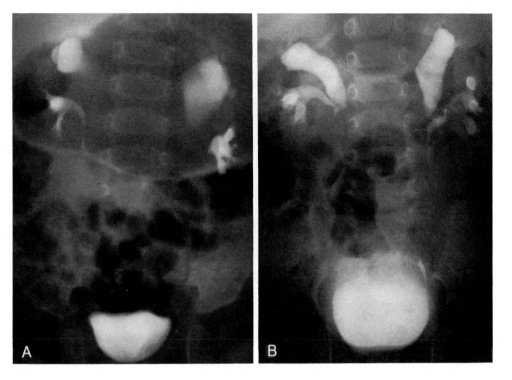

Figure 45–11. *A,* Excretory urogram in a 6-month-old girl with a urinary infection showing bilateral duplicated systems with bilateral upper pole function with obstruction. She underwent bilateral proximal ureteroureterostomies. *B,* Postoperative excretory urogram showing prompt function and drainage in both upper and lower systems bilaterally.

In a minority of cases, when the upper pole is not markedly hydronephrotic and has not suffered significant parenchymal loss, the upper pole ureter can be anastomosed to the lower pole pelvis or to the proximal lower pole ureter when it is of adequate caliber (Fig. 45–11) (Heloury et al., 1988). The distal upper pole ureter is then removed as previously described. Smith and associates (1989) reported a series using this procedure to salvage the upper pole in 15 of 35 children.

Common sheath ureteral reimplantation may be performed in instances when reflux to the lower pole ureter is significant, and when the ectopic ureter is not severely dilated and drains a renal unit worth saving. The ectopic ureter may be readily identified, deep and slightly lateral, during the dissection of the orthotopic lower pole ureter. Ureteral tailoring or tapering may be required to ensure adequate reimplantation. Even with one dilated ureter, results of this method have been good (Weinstein et al., 1988). The functional contribution of the upper pole renal segment may be difficult to determine precisely but is most effectively demonstrated by ^{99m}Tc-DMSA.

A high incidence of postoperative reflux has been cited in common sheath ureteral reimplantation, particularly when one ureter is dilated (Huisman et al., 1987). Distal ureteroureterostomy has been advocated as an alternative. A second alternative, reported in the unusual situation without lower pole reflux, is to reimplant only the ectopic ureter (Marshall, 1986).

Ectopic Ureter in Boys

Ectopic ureter is not as common in boys and is more often associated with a single renal unit than with renal duplication. Because ectopic ureters in boys always drain proximal to the external urinary sphincter, dribbling incontinence is not a presenting feature unless there is an associated sphincter abnormality. In general, the more distant the ectopic orifice is located from the trigone, the more likely the involved kidney is to be dysplastic. The majority of single ectopic ureters in the male open into the prostatic urethra or into the genital tract. The presenting symptoms are those of urinary infection when the orifice drains into the prostatic urethra and those of epididymo-orchitis when drainage involves the genital tract (Hernanz-Schulman et al., 1989; Rajfer et al., 1978; Squadrito et al., 1987; Zaontz and Kass, 1987). The ureter may enter the seminal vesicle or ejaculatory duct, but in some instances the ureter and vas deferens join to share a common terminal duct, as in the embryo. Reflux of urine into the ureter, seminal vesicles, or vas deferens is common during voiding cystourethrography (Fig. 45–12). Excretory urography often reveals a nonvisualizing kidney on the affected side. At cystoscopy, the ectopic orifice is usually just distal to the bladder neck or adjacent to the verumontanum.

Because the kidney is generally dysplastic, treatment of an ectopic ureter associated with a single renal system usually consists of nephrectomy, and, if reflux is present, total ureterectomy. When the ureter enters the genital tract, even if reflux is not present, total ureterectomy, excision of the common duct, and ligation of the vas are necessary to prevent subsequent epididymitis and pyoureter. Surgical access to the ectopic ureter as it enters the genital tract may be facilitated by a transtrigonal approach. Treatment of the ectopic ureter associated with renal duplication is the same as that described previously in the female.

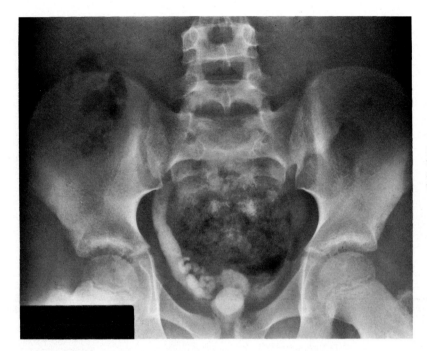

Figure 45–12. Postvoiding film following cystoure-thrography demonstrates reflux of urine into the ureter and seminal vesicle in a 5-year-old boy with a urinary tract infection.

Single System Ectopic Ureter

The single system ectopic ureter is more common in males than in females, as discussed in the previous section. The Japanese literature, however, reports that 70 per cent of ectopic ureters are associated with single systems, completely reversed from the 70 to 80 per cent association with duplex systems in the European and American literature (Gotoh et al., 1983). In girls, too, it is very likely to be associated with a dysplastic, poorly visualizing, or nonvisualizing kidney on excretory urography (Fig. 45–13). Occasionally, an ectopic ureter is associated with an ectopic kidney that may be fused with the contralateral organ. Uncommonly, a single ectopic ureter in the female opens in or just distal to the bladder neck and drains a relatively normal ureter and kidney (this appears to be contrary to the Mackie-Stephens theory of greater ectopia being associated with greater degrees of dysplasia)(Mackie and Stephens, 1975). Reflux in this type of situation is common (Fig. 45–14).

A subset of single system ectopic ureters connecting to Gartner's duct cysts has been presented in the Japanese literature. These are contrasted to ectopic ureters connecting to the vagina or to dilated Gartner's ducts. Connection with a Gartner's duct cyst was associated with a high frequency of uterine abnormalities, a renal agenesis, and a greater degree of renal dysplasia as judged by the Mackie-Stephens hypodysplasia score, when the kidney was present. It is suggested that these represent wolffian duct defects or fusion anomalies of the müllerian duct (Gotoh and Koyanagi, 1987).

The diagnosis of a single ectopic ureter in the female may be difficult, especially if the orifice drains outside the sphincter mechanism and the associated kidney is nonvisualizing by excretory urography. Diagnostic ultra-sound or computed tomography may sometimes be helpful in locating the kidney. Some reports have noted an apparent increase in the frequency of diagnosis of single system vaginal ectopic ureters (Weiss et al., 1984), possibly due to improved imaging techniques. Rarely, exploratory laparotomy is indicated when the diagnosis cannot be made by conventional methods.

Treatment depends on the function of the kidney. In most instances, treatment consists of nephrectomy or nephroureterectomy. When the ectopic ureter opens just distal to the bladder neck, is refluxing, and is associated with a relatively normal kidney, antireflux surgery is indicated. The proximity of the ureteral orifice to the bladder neck adds to the difficulty of ureteral mobilization, and combined intra- and extra-vesical dissection may be necessary.

Bilateral Single System Ectopic Ureters

Bilateral single system ectopic ureters are fortunately rare, as they present a complex therapeutic problem. In this condition, the ureters usually drain into the prostatic urethra in the male and into the distal urethra in the female. Embryologically, the portion of the urogenital sinus between the orifices of the wolffian duct and the ureter develops into the bladder neck musculature. This development does not occur if both ureters remain in the position of the wolffian duct orifice. Because there is no formation of the trigone and base plate, a very wide, poorly defined, incompetent vesical neck results. In rare instances, bilateral single ectopic ureters are associated with agenesis of the bladder and urethra. This condition is usually but not always incompatible with life (Glenn, 1959).

Commonly, the involved kidneys are dysplastic or

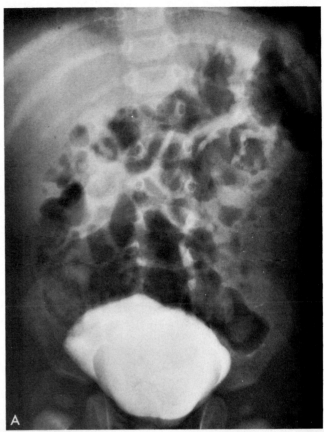

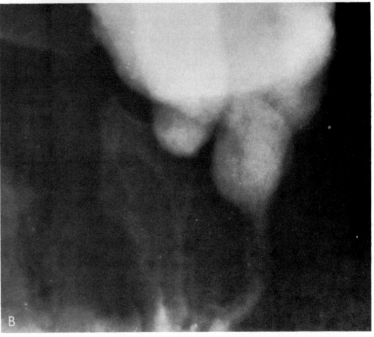

Figure 45–13. *A,* Excretory urogram in a 3-year-old girl reveals a poorly visualizing right kidney. *B,* Voiding cystourethrography demonstrates severe reflux into an ectopic ureter whose orifice was in the proximal urethra.

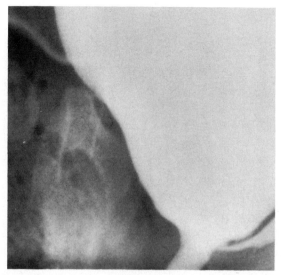

Figure 45–14. Voiding cystogram in a 2-year-old girl shows a refluxing ectopic ureter associated with a single system. The intravenous pyelogram was normal.

display varying degrees of hydronephrosis (Fig. 45–15). The ureters are usually dilated, and reflux is usually present. The bladder neck is incompetent and the bladder has a small capacity; therefore, the child dribbles continuously. In the male, incontinence is not as severe, and bladder capacity may be better because the external sphincter provides a variable degree of control.

At cystoscopy, the ureteral orifices can be identified in the male, usually just distal to the bladder neck. The lax bladder neck and small bladder are clearly evident. In the female, it can be difficult to find both ureteral orifices, which are usually located in the distal urethra but occasionally enter the genital tract.

The abnormality is akin to epispadias, with the basic defect being a short urethra and incompetent bladder neck. However, unlike epispadias, there is a high incidence of renal and ureteral abnormalities with this condition as well as the small bladder capacity.

Treatment usually consists of ureteral reimplantation and reconstruction of the bladder neck for continence by one of the tubularization procedures, e.g., the Young-Dees procedure. It is often helpful to employ vesicourethral suspension at the same time. Increased exposure using symphyseal splitting has been helpful during these reconstructions. The success rate is higher in boys than in girls. Bladder capacity in the child who gains satisfactory control will often increase. An enterocystoplasty to increase bladder capacity may be necessary in selected cases.

Ectopic Ureter with Renal Triplication

This is one of the rarest of all anomalies. The incidence is higher in females. In two patients seen by one of us (A.R.), both young adult females, one had mild incontinence and the other, a persistent vaginal discharge. The ureteral configuration has been described by Prantl and Tewes (1988), compiled from previous

studies. Complete triplication was noted in one fourth of patients, confluence of the two lower ureters in one fourth, and confluence of all three ureters in one third. An inverted Y was seen in 3 per cent, involving the lower two ureters.

Similar to other forms of ureteral ectopy, treatment depends on the functional status of the kidneys and the specifics of each case (Golomb and Ehrlich, 1989; Perkins et al., 1973; Smith, 1946; Spangler, 1963).

URETEROCELES

Ureterocele is a cystic dilatation of the terminal ureter within the bladder, urethra, or both. Strictly interpreted, the term "simple" or "orthotopic" ureterocele means that the ureterocele is located on the trigone at the usual location of the ureteral orifice. In the "ectopic" type, the ureterocele is located distal to the trigone and may project well into the urethra. The ectopic orifice is located at the bladder neck or in the urethra. In common usage, however, "ectopic ureterocele" often means any ureterocele associated with a duplex system, even if not strictly ectopic. Simple ureteroceles, often also called "adult-type," usually suggest those associated with a single system. In the pediatric population, ureteroceles associated with duplex systems are the most common and usually the most problematic, whether they are indeed ectopic or not.

Simple or Orthotopic Ureterocele

Simple or orthotopic ureteroceles are more commonly detected in adults. They usually occur as a normally placed ureter on the trigone, associated either with a single collecting system or, very rarely, with an upper pole ureter of a complete duplication. The etiology of simple ureteroceles is debatable and may be similar to that of ectopic ureteroceles discussed subsequently. Although most simple ureteroceles have obstructing pinpoint orifices, nonobstructed ureteroceles do exist. The degree of obstruction is probably not significant in most adult cases.

The ureterocele may vary in size from a tiny cystic dilatation of the submucosal ureter to that of a large balloon that fills the bladder. Histologically, the wall of the ureterocele contains varying degrees of attenuated smooth muscle bundles and fibrous tissue. The ureterocele is covered by vesical mucosa and lined with ureteral mucosa.

Most children with simple ureteroceles present with symptoms of urinary tract infections. Prenatal ultrasonography has detected these asymptomatic cases. Stasis and infection predispose the patient to stone formation in the ureterocele and upper urinary tract. Rarely, large simple ureteroceles prolapse through the bladder neck, causing urinary obstruction.

Excretory urography often demonstrates the characteristic "cobra-head" (or "spring-onion") deformity—an area of increased density similar to the head of a cobra with a halo or less dense shadow around it. Larger

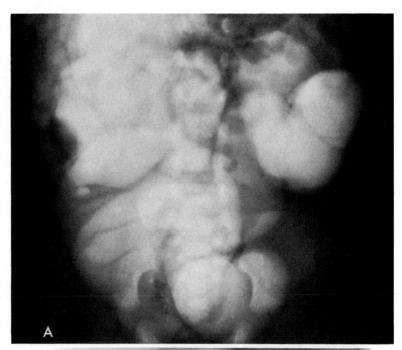

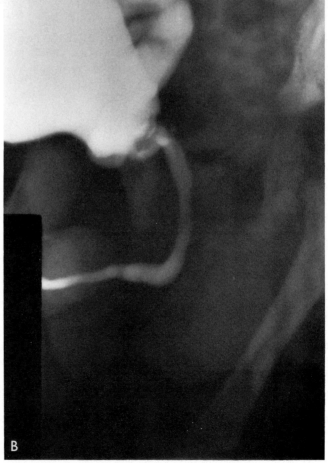

Figure 45–15. *A,* Excretory urogram in a 6-day-old boy shows very severe bilateral hydronephrosis and hydroureter. *B,* A voiding cystourethrogram demonstrates refluxing ectopic ureters draining into the prostatic urethra.

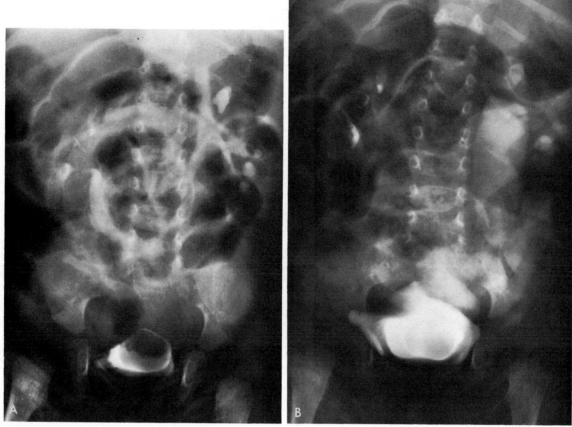

Figure 45–16. *A,* This 15-minute excretory urogram film reveals a filling defect in the bladder, which was a simple ureterocele. *B,* Severe left hydronephrosis and hydroureter are seen on a delayed film.

ureteroceles often fail to fill early with contrast material, resulting in a sizable filling defect in the bladder (Fig. 45–16). These findings are associated with varying degrees of hydronephrosis and hydroureter. The upper urinary tract changes associated with a simple ureterocele are usually not as severe as those associated with an ectopic ureterocele. Vesicoureteral reflux is rarely seen with a simple ureterocele. At cystoscopy, the ureterocele usually will expand rhythmically with each peristaltic wave of urine that fills it and then shrink as a thin jet of urine drains, usually continuously, through the small orifice.

Transurethral *resection* of simple ureteroceles, previously recommended as a method of decompression, invariably results in vesicoureteral reflux and the risk of upper urinary tract infection. Transurethral *incision* of small simple ureteroceles, making a tiny transverse slit with a Bugbee electrode, often is therapeutic and leaves the intravesical hood of the ureter intact. Reflux is not the usual result, and if it occurs a secondary elective ureteral reimplantation can be done when required (Rich et al., 1990). However, in most instances, primary excision of the ureterocele with reimplantation of the involved ureter is the surgical procedure of choice. If the lower ureter is extremely dilated, it may have to be tapered as well. In rare instances, when kidney damage is very severe, nephroureterectomy is indicated.

In the uncommon situation of a simple ureterocele associated with a duplication, treatment depends on the obstructive effects of the ureterocele and whether or not reflux to the lower pole is present. At times, the ureterocele is associated with minimal dilatation of the upper pole ureter, and surgery may not be indicated (Fig. 45–17). The choices of management are essentially those of a duplex "ectopic" ureterocele (discussed subsequently). Surgery for obstruction or reflux in this case is similar to that for a single ureter, i.e., excision of the ureterocele and distal portions of both ureters, with common sheath reimplantation of both ureters by advancement (Politano and Leadbetter, 1958), or cross-trigonal technique (Cohen, 1975).

Ectopic Ureterocele

Ectopic ureterocele is one of the more serious anomalies of the urinary tract in infancy and childhood. It is one of the most common causes of lower urinary tract obstruction in girls. Ectopic ureterocele is far more common in girls than in boys (at least 2:1). The reasons for this finding are unknown. Approximately 10 per cent of ectopic ureteroceles are bilateral. An increased incidence of duplication is noted on the contralateral side (Caldamone et al., 1984; Mandell et al., 1980). Rarely, ectopic ureteroceles occur without duplication, usually in males (Johnson and Perlmutter, 1980).

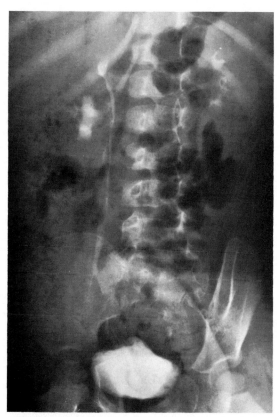

Figure 45–17. Excretory urogram in a 4-year-old girl with two urinary tract infections characterized by irritative symptoms shows the cobrahead deformity of a right ureterocele. Note the lack of dilatation of the upper pole ureter.

Classification

One classification popularized of late is that of Stephens (1958a, 1964, 1971, 1983), largely an anatomic and descriptive one (Figs. 45–18 through 45–20).

A stenotic ectopic ureterocele, which occurs in about 40 per cent of cases, is characterized by a small orifice located at the tip of the cystic dilatation of the ureter or on the superior or inferior surface of the ureterocele (Fig. 45–18).

A sphincteric ectopic ureterocele, found in about 40 per cent of cases terminates within the internal sphincter. The orifice may be normal or large and may open either in the posterior urethra in the male or distal to the external sphincter in the female (Fig. 45–19).

With the sphincterostenotic ectopic ureterocele, found in about 5 per cent of cases, the stenotic ureteral orifice is located in the floor of the urethra or beyond.

In the cecoureterocele (rare, <5 per cent), the lumen extends distal to the orifice as a long tongue or "cecum" beneath the urethral submucosa; the orifice communicates with the lumen of the bladder and is large and incompetent (Fig. 45–20).

Other types of ureteroceles that have been described are the blind ectopic ureterocele (rare, <5 per cent), with atrophy of the portion of ureter extending distal to the ureterocele and no orifice, and the nonobstructed ectopic ureterocele (rare, <5 per cent) with terminal expansion of the ureter, which has a large orifice in the bladder.

Embryology

A number of theories have evolved to explain the formation of an ectopic ureterocele. In Chwalle's theory (1927), a membrane covering the ureteral orifice persists for a prolonged period of time, leading to the formation of a ureterocele. Ericsson (1954) proposed that there was a failure of reabsorption of a membrane between the wolffian duct and the vesicourethral canal, with the subsequent formation of a caudal opening in this membrane. The ectopic ureteral orifice is buried beneath this membrane. The most popular theory, which can account for all of the various types of ureteroceles including the unobstructed ones, is that of a primary embryologic maldevelopment put forth by Stephens (1971). It is theorized that a ureterocele forms when an ectopic ureter is affected by the stimulus to expansion that transforms the bladder into a globular shape, creating an expanded, thin-walled distal ureter. If the ureteral orifice is not affected by virtue of its position, it may remain small and stenotic. Obstruction may be a contributory factor to the formation of the ureterocele, particularly in maintaining distention, but is not thought to be a primary cause. A cecoureterocele is suggested as being the result of the position of the dilated terminal ureter co-migrating distally with the müllerian duct. The ultimate configuration of the ureterocele is seen as the product of the timing of abnormal ureteral budding; the effect of aberrant local stimuli on structural development of the distal ureter; and, to a minor degree, the consequence of obstruction. Tanagho (1976) has suggested a higher block with defective canalization. A localized embryonic arrest has also been hypothesized as the cause of ureteroceles (Tokunaka et al., 1981).

As in simple ureteroceles, the cystic submucosal dilatation is lined by ureteral mucosa. Similarly, the wall of the ureterocele has varying degrees of attenuated smooth muscle bundles arranged longitudinally, circularly, or their combination.

Clinical Manifestations

The patient often presents during the first few months of life with symptoms of urinary infection or failure to thrive. As previously mentioned in girls, ureteroceles may prolapse intermittently through the urethra (Fig. 45–21). Urinary retention is uncommon but occurs when an ectopic ureterocele prolapses through the bladder neck. Some degree of urinary incontinence may occur in a girl with a large intraurethral ectopic ureterocele that has rendered the external urinary sphincter lax and inefficient.

Prenatal ultrasonographic detection of ectopic ureteroceles has permitted early antibiotic prophylaxis and prevention of the usual infection and its risks of renal damage. Formal evaluation of the pathologic anatomy is conducted at an early age, usually 2 to 6 weeks, with the safety of antibiotic coverage.

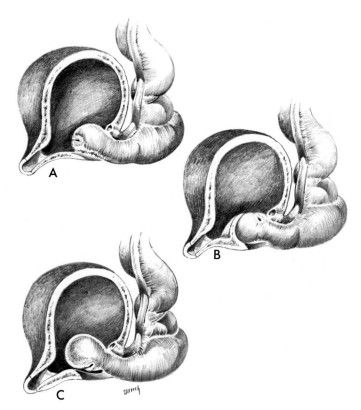

Figure 45–18. *A* to *C,* Stenotic ectopic ureteroceles—orifice may be located at the tip or at the superior or inferior surface of the ureterocele.

Figure 45–19. *A* and *B,* Sphincteric ectopic ureteroceles. *C,* Sphincterostenotic ectopic ureterocele.

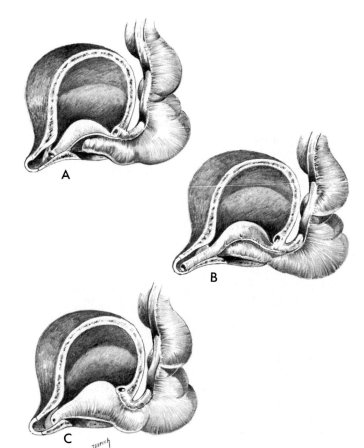

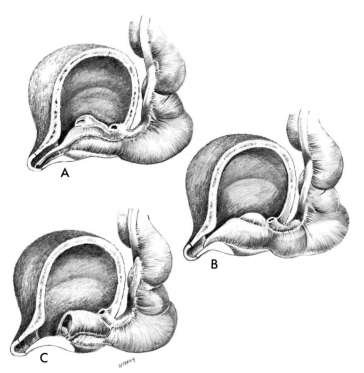

Figure 45–20. *A,* Cecoureterocele—lumen extends distal to the orifice as a long tongue beneath the urethral submucosa. The orifice communicates with the lumen of the bladder and is large and incompetent. *B,* Blind ectopic ureterocele—atrophy of the ureter distal to the ureterocele, which ends blindly. *C,* Nonobstructed ectopic ureterocele—terminal expansion of the ureter, which has a large orifice in the bladder.

Diagnosis

The renal unit associated with an ectopic ureterocele is commonly dysplastic and has little or no function. The radiologic findings are related to the effect of the ureterocele on the ipsilateral and contralateral ureters and renal units. Large ectopic ureteroceles may obstruct the ipsilateral lower pole ureter and, on occasion, are large and tense enough to obstruct the contralateral side as well. More often, the ureterocele distorts the ipsilat-

eral lower pole ureteral orifice, effectively shortening the submucosal course of this ureter and producing vesicoureteral reflux.

Ultrasonographic evaluation is often the first study obtained in the patient with prenatally detected hydronephrosis (with or without the suspicion of a ureterocele) and with infection. The degree of hydronephrosis in the involved kidney is usually distinct between the upper and lower pole, in addition to thinning of the upper pole parenchyma. It is unusual, but not unheard

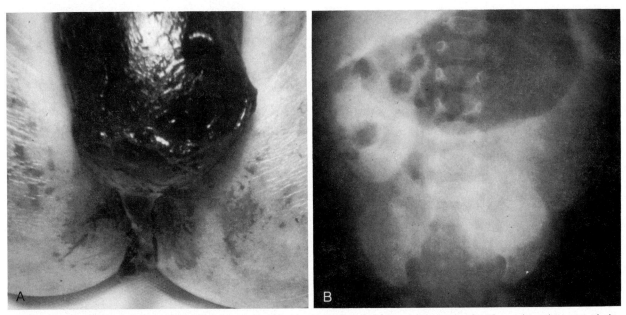

Figure 45–21. *A,* Appearance of the perineum of a 5-month-old girl with prolapse of an ectopic ureterocele. The prolapsed tissue is dusky and congested. *B,* Excretory urogram at presentation of the same patient showing delayed visualization and hydroureteronephrosis of the contralateral kidney due to obstruction by the prolapsed ureterocele, and nonvisualization of the ipsilateral kidney.

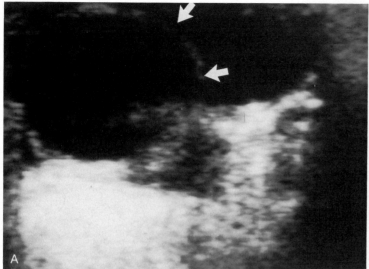

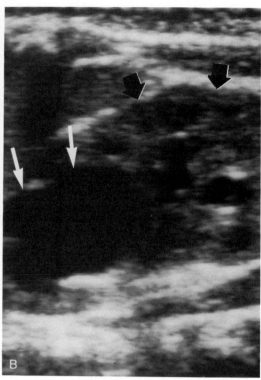

Figure 45–22. Ultrasound images in a 3-month-old girl with urinary infection and a large ectopic ureterocele. *A,* Bladder image demonstrating the large, thin-walled ureterocele (*arrows*), with a mostly intravesical location. *B,* Kidney image showing the dilated left upper pole (*white arrows*) above the normal parenchyma of the lower pole (*dark arrows*).

of, to be unable to detect the presence of a duplicated system with discrepant degrees of hydronephrosis. Examination of the course of the ureter is essential and often reveals the dilated upper pole ureter, particularly as it enters the posterior bladder wall. The typical sonographic appearance of a ureterocele within the bladder may be present (Fig. 45–22) but depends on the degree of bladder filling and the pressure within the ureterocele itself. If the bladder is overdistended, the ureterocele may collapse and only a dilated ureter may be seen entering the bladder. In the setting of a clear duplication at the level of the kidney, an ectopic ureter rather than an actual ureterocele would be suggested. If the duplication were not recognized, a primary mega-ureter would be suggested. If the bladder is not full, the dilated ureterocele may fill the entire bladder, giving the impression of a partially full bladder without a ureterocele. It is clear that a high index of suspicion and an experienced examiner are essential to permit an accurate diagnosis (Nussbaum et al., 1986).

The findings on excretory urography are similar to those described for ectopic ureter but, with ureterocele, the upper pole is generally more dilated. Most upper poles are nonvisualizing or show severe hydronephrosis. On occasion, no evidence of an upper pole system will be seen, suggesting the existence of "ureterocele dispro-portion" with a small dysplastic upper pole (see following discussion). Characteristically, a nonopaque filling defect of varying size in the bladder is usually situated off center and always appears on the bladder outline rather than as a complete circle within the bladder shadow as in a simple ureterocele (Fig. 45–23). The filling defect may extend behind or into the prostatic urethra in the male or the entire urethra in the female, thus causing obstruction. Trigonal cysts, which are mentioned in the earlier literature, probably represent sub-

trigonal extensions of these ureteroceles. The typical filling defect in the bladder associated with an ectopic ureterocele is usually diagnostic. In unusual circum-stances, it can be confused with similar defects caused

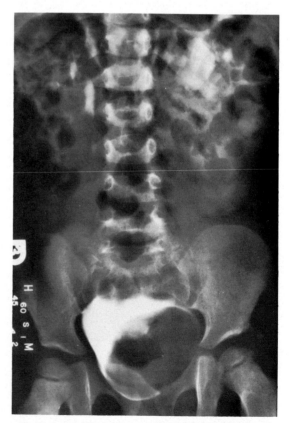

Figure 45–23. Large filling defect in the bladder of an ectopic uretero-cele associated with the upper pole of a left renal duplication. A voiding cystogram demonstrated severe reflux to the lower pole.

by rhabdomyosarcoma of the bladder or prostate, or very severe cystitis cystica.

In addition to outlining the ectopic ureterocele (Fig. 45–24), voiding cystourethrography with diluted contrast medium is important for demonstrating the tension in, and compressibility of, the ureterocele, the presence of reflux, and the degree of detrusor backing of the ureterocele. The information thus gained has important therapeutic implications.

Reflux into the ureterocele is rare but may occur, especially in the cecoureterocele. Reflux into the ipsilateral lower pole ureter, in comparison, occurs in almost 50 per cent of these patients. Ectopic ureteroceles may change size during voiding, and this, to a large extent, depends on their compressibility. Tense ureteroceles will remain the same size during micturition, and the filling defect on the voiding cystogram will not change. However, when the ectopic ureteral orifice is wide and the ureteral contents are at low pressure, the ureterocele is compressed during voiding and its contents either pass into the urethra or empty back into the ureter. In addition, reflux to the lower pole ureter is much more common with a compressible ureterocele than with a tense one. Cystography also demonstrates

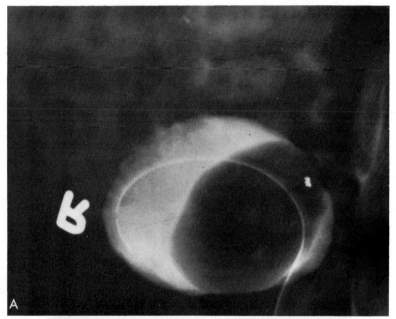

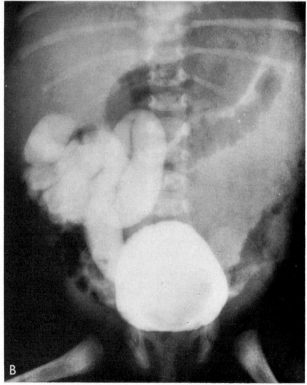

Figure 45–24. A, Cystogram outlines a *left* ectopic ureterocele. B, Postvoiding film shows reflux to the *right* lower pole. This girl had *bilateral* ectopic ureteroceles, the right being a small subtrigonal one, which was not demonstrated on the cystogram.

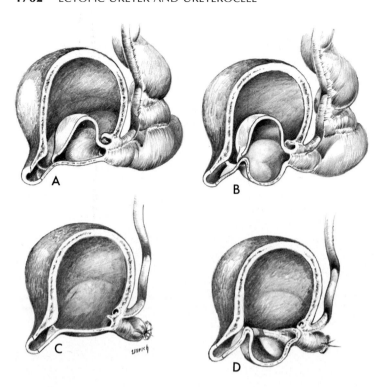

Figure 45–25. *A* and *B*, Ectopic ureterocele with poor backing is displaced outward during voiding. *C* and *D*, If the ureterocele is only uncapped, a wide-mouthed diverticulum results, whose distal lip at the bladder neck may be obstructive.

whether the detrusor backing is poor or even absent (Fig. 45–25). In the last situation, filling of the bladder everts the ureterocele, simulating the appearance of a bladder diverticulum. Koyanagi (1980) reported that eight of 24 extravesical ureteroceles everted on voiding studies.

A ureterocele may be ruptured either spontaneously or following instrumentation. Radiologically, an irregular cavity lying outside the bladder outline with an edge forming a filling defect within the bladder shadow is characteristically demonstrated. Here, reflux into the ectopic ureter as well as into the ipsilateral lower pole ureter usually occurs.

Cystourethroscopy can confirm the radiologic findings. It is often very difficult to find the ectopic ureteral orifice, and it may not be clinically important to find it preoperatively by endoscopy. Large ureteroceles will often make visualization difficult and confusing. If the bladder is overfilled at endoscopy, the ureterocele may be effaced and missed; if it everts, the endoscopist may erroneously diagnose a wide-mouthed diverticulum. It is extremely important to ascertain whether a small ureterocele is present on the contralateral side as well. When the typical radiologic features of a renal duplication are not apparent, it is sometimes helpful to inject the ureterocele with contrast medium through a fine-gauge endoscopic needle to delineate the characteristics of the upper pole kidney and ureter (Fig. 45–26). Assessing the configuration of this renal segment is often important in choosing therapy (see following discussion).

Treatment

Ureteroceles have a broad spectrum of presentation, anatomy, and pathophysiology; thus, each child must be treated individually. No single method of surgical repair will suffice for all. The goals of therapy should be clearly defined and factored into the clinical decisions. The primary concern is the preservation of renal parenchyma, including the lower pole of the affected

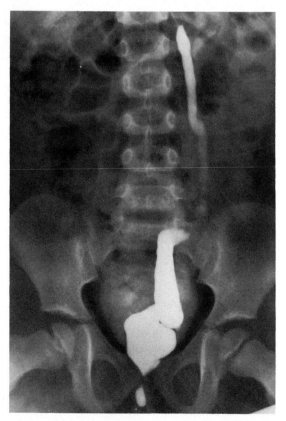

Figure 45–26. Endoscopic injection of a ureterocele outlines the upper pole and the distal extent of the ureterocele.

kidney. This preservation may be achieved by correcting obstruction and preventing reflux with its risks of renal parenchymal damage from infection. It is at times necessary to balance one against the other in that relieving the obstruction of a ureterocele may induce reflux in the lower pole moiety; yet, at other times, the same action may cause existing lower pole reflux to resolve. Minimizing surgical morbidity is a goal that must also be included in this consideration. Several means of achieving these goals of therapy are available.

Transurethral incision of an ectopic ureterocele may lead to reflux into the upper pole collecting system and require additional procedures. It is, however, a minor procedure and, on occasion, initial transurethral incision of the ureterocele may be indicated as a temporizing measure in the extremely ill infant with sepsis. Several nonvisualizing kidneys, after decompression, have been observed to function and have thus been salvaged. Transurethral incision may also permit assessment of the effect of ureterocele decompression on lower pole reflux or obstruction in cases in which a combined upper and lower procedure is being contemplated. This practice may avoid the need for a combined procedure and, on occasion, may even obviate the need for any further procedures (Fig. 45–27). Of 40 patients who underwent transurethral incision as reported by Tank (1986), 20 demonstrated functional improvement and only two patients needed surgery later. The risk involved in transurethral incisions of ureteroceles is the conversion of a nonrefluxing to a refluxing renal unit, which may necessitate surgery at the bladder as well as at the kidney level in some cases.

The treatment of choice, therefore, in the majority of children who have ectopic ureteroceles associated with nonvisualizing or poorly functioning upper renal segments should be upper pole nephrectomy with partial ureterectomy alone (Mandell et al., 1980). In most cases, this is the only procedure necessary to decompress the ureterocele, to provide adequate drainage of the ipsilateral as well as the contralateral collecting systems, and to control infection. The ureterocele is decompressed from above with a fine feeding tube at the time of upper pole nephrectomy and partial ureterectomy (as described in the previous section on ectopic ureter, Figures 45–9 and 45–10). The distal stump is left open at the time of surgery to avoid pyoureter. During the next several months, the ureterocele will diminish in size as seen on follow-up ultrasonography or excretory urography, often to the extent that no evidence of the ureterocele remains (Fig. 45–28). Failure of the ureterocele to collapse may be the result of inadequate decompression. In such a case, transurethral aspiration to decompress the ureterocele may be successful.

Lower pole reflux will develop, where it had previously not been detected, in a certain number of cases. Caldamone and co-workers (1984) report a high incidence of persisting new onset reflux following upper pole heminephrectomy compared with that reported by Mandell and co-workers (1980). This variance may be the result of differences in selection of the patient to undergo the limited procedure.

Total excision of the ureter to the level of the bladder wall has been advocated by Kroovand and Perlmutter (1979) to prevent pyoureter or alternating diverticulum and possible surgical complications from an intravesical procedure in small children with large distorting ureteroceles. However, it is our experience that surgery for the retained ureteral stump and ureterocele per se is most often not necessary (Mandell et al., 1980).

Milder degrees of reflux into the ipsilateral and even contralateral ureters usually subside after the ureterocele has been decompressed from above. More severe reflux into the lower pole collecting system, in association with a nonfunctioning upper pole moiety, warrants consideration for repair at the kidney and bladder levels. These severe degrees of reflux are less likely to disappear, especially if the muscular backing of the ureterocele is deficient. In this instance, excision of the ureterocele and ipsilateral lower pole reimplantation, with or without tapering, may be necessary in addition to upper pole nephrectomy. The cross-trigonal technique may be used in this situation to reimplant the ureter away from the area of detrusor repair. Our preference, however, is the Politano-Leadbetter ureteral reimplantation with ureteral advancement. This entire dissection can often be tedious and time-consuming. The trigonal musculature is reapproximated to reconstitute a strong bladder wall before the reimplantation is completed.

In the unusual cases in which massive reflux into the lower pole is associated with a large, everting ureterocele and a nonfunctioning upper pole, consideration should be given to a single-stage total repair. This would involve upper pole nephrectomy, ureterectomy, and ureterocele resection with ureteral reimplantion. Usually performed using two incisions, this strategy provides for definitive correction of the defect. Although this method is technically more demanding, results have been satisfactory (Hendren and Mitchell, 1979; Scherz et al., 1989). In one series, total correction was performed on 28 patients; four (14 per cent) required a second procedure—in all cases, for reflux. Scherz and co-workers recommend ureterocele marsupialization rather than excision and trigonal reconstruction. Although their results are good, it is unclear how many of their cases included everting or prolapsing ureteroceles with deficient muscular backing.

Gotoh and colleagues (1988) have reported on using the presence or absence of radiographic eversion of the ureterocele, the separation between the upper and lower orifices, and the upper pole function to determine the means of correction. In cases with eversion and separation of the orifices, upper pole function was always absent. When the orifices were adjacent, function was absent in one third of cases. Upper pole nephrectomy was performed with an extravesical resection of the ureterocele and repair of the bladder wall, without lower pole reimplantation.

Determining the most appropriate means of treatment, however, remains difficult (Decter et al., 1989). It has not been possible to definitively predict which ureterocele system will be completely treated with just an upper pole nephrectomy. In some instances, reflux develops following upper pole nephrectomy, often necessitating a subsequent bladder repair. Although it is

Text continued on page 1768

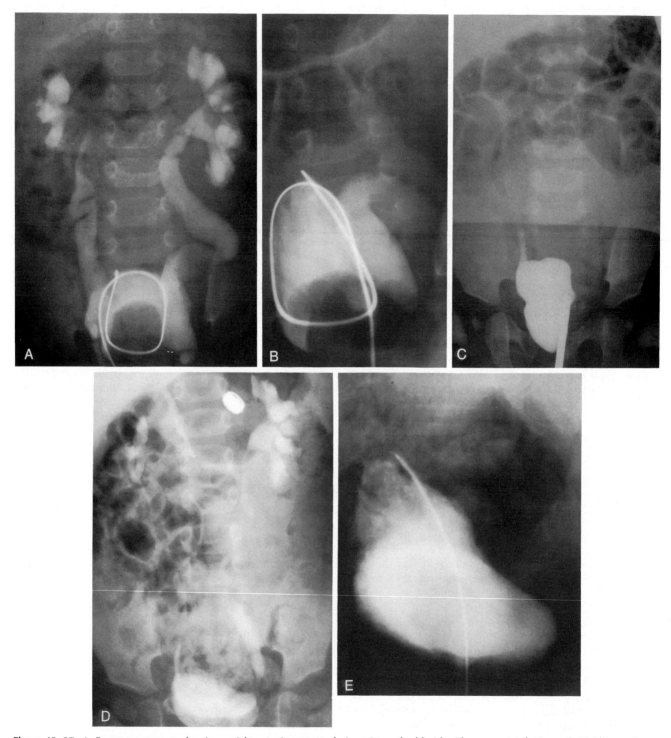

Figure 45–27. *A,* Excretory urogram showing a *right* ectopic ureterocele in a 6-month-old girl with recurrent infections. *B,* Voiding cystogram demonstrates *left* grade 5 reflux. *C,* Transurethral endoscopic injection of the ureterocele demonstrates connection to a small atretic ureter and a small dysplastic renal segment. Transurethral incision of the ureterocele was performed. *D,* Postoperative excretory urogram demonstrating improvement of obstruction of the right lower pole and the left kidney. *E,* Resolution of the left-sided reflux was demonstrated on a postoperative voiding cystogram.

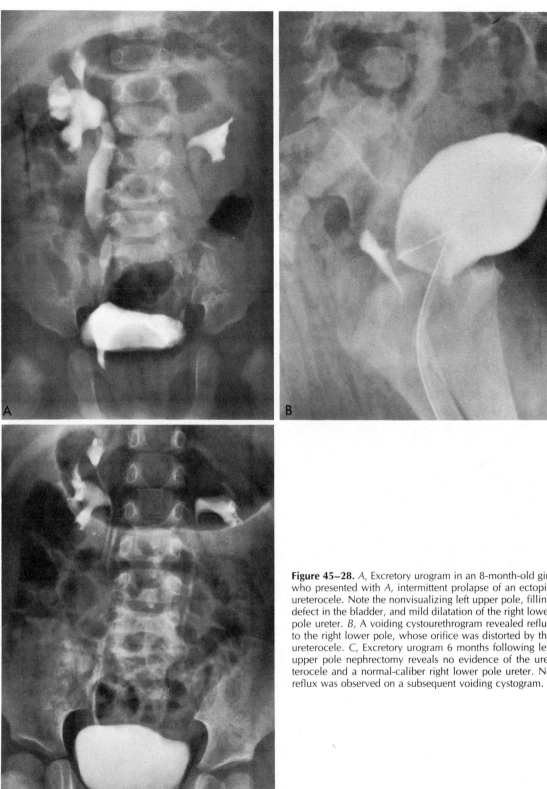

Figure 45–28. *A,* Excretory urogram in an 8-month-old girl who presented with *A,* intermittent prolapse of an ectopic ureterocele. Note the nonvisualizing left upper pole, filling defect in the bladder, and mild dilatation of the right lower pole ureter. *B,* A voiding cystourethrogram revealed reflux to the right lower pole, whose orifice was distorted by the ureterocele. *C,* Excretory urogram 6 months following left upper pole nephrectomy reveals no evidence of the ureterocele and a normal-caliber right lower pole ureter. No reflux was observed on a subsequent voiding cystogram.

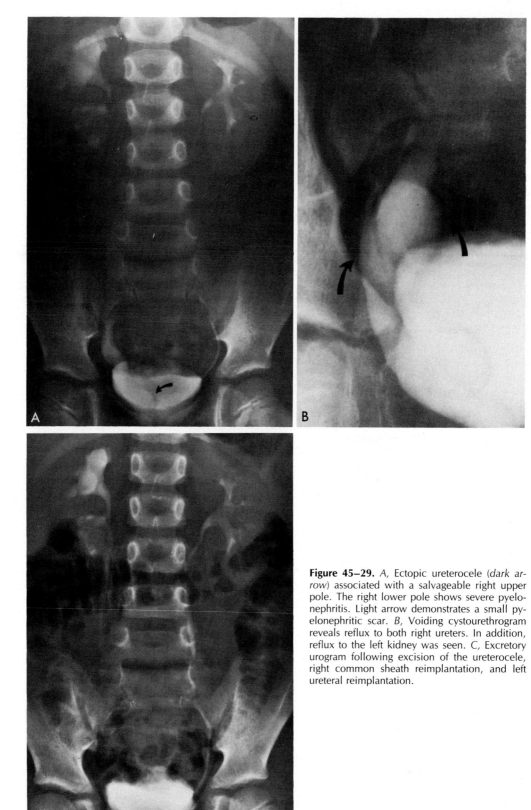

Figure 45–29. *A,* Ectopic ureterocele (*dark arrow*) associated with a salvageable right upper pole. The right lower pole shows severe pyelonephritis. Light arrow demonstrates a small pyelonephritic scar. *B,* Voiding cystourethrogram reveals reflux to both right ureters. In addition, reflux to the left kidney was seen. *C,* Excretory urogram following excision of the ureterocele, right common sheath reimplantation, and left ureteral reimplantation.

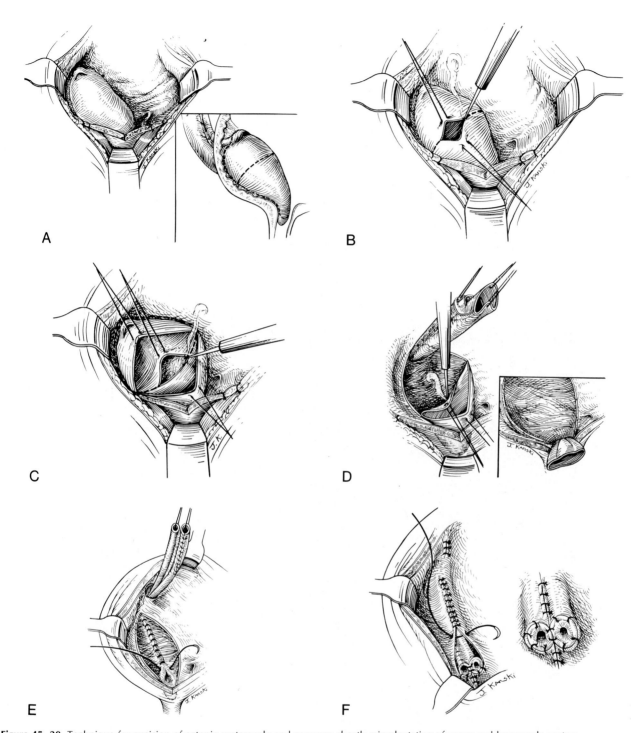

Figure 45–30. Technique for excision of ectopic ureterocele and common sheath reimplantation of upper and lower pole ureters.

A, Appearance of right-sided ureterocele with open bladder, viewed from below. Note proximity of the contralateral ureteral orifice. *Inset,* Cutaway side view demonstrating the close association of the two polar ureters with a common vascular supply. The dotted line indicates the planned initial incision of the ureterocele.

B, After stay sutures are placed, the ureterocele is incised with electrocautery in a transverse direction, exposing the inner cavity of the ureterocele.

C, The posterior mucosal wall of the ureterocele is incised transversely, revealing the often thinned posterior muscular wall of the bladder. This incision will then be continued around the bladder mucosal edge of the ureterocele, including the orifice of the lower pole ureter. Stay sutures are important to provide adequate exposure.

D, The upper and lower pole ureters have been mobilized and are retracted into the bladder. The distal aspect of the ureterocele is being mobilized in a similar fashion. The bladder mucosal surface will also be incised around the edge of the ureterocele to permit complete removal of the ureterocele. *Inset,* The fully mobilized distal ureterocele is retracted caudally revealing its narrowing attachment at the bladder neck.

E, The dilated upper pole ureter associated with the ureterocele has been tapered and remains in continuity with the lower pole ureter. Both have been brought into the bladder through a newly formed muscular hiatus to provide adequate tunnel length for the ureteral reimplantation. The thinned-out posterior bladder wall has been repaired with multiple interrupted sutures to provide adequate muscular backing for the ureters. The bladder mucosa surrounding the ureterocele defect has been mobilized to permit covering of the ureters.

F, Left, The ureters have been reimplanted into the new ureteral tunnel, sutured distally after spatulation, and are being covered with bladder mucosa. The lower pole orifice is medial. *Right,* Final appearance of the ureteral orifices following completion of the reimplantation.

not possible to unequivocally predict the response of a given system to upper pole nephrectomy, careful diagnostic evaluation can provide important information regarding the pathologic anatomy of the ureterocele. A large defect in the bladder wall is unlikely to permit the normal antireflux function of the ureter and is expected to demonstrate persistent reflux after ureterocele decompression. Of course, a planned two-stage procedure is completely reasonable, and in some patients may be the most appropriate therapy.

In a few children with massive lower pole ureteral reflux and nonvisualization of both upper and lower renal segments, excision of the ureterocele and complete nephroureterectomy are indicated.

When the upper renal segment demonstrates reasonable function on the basis of an excretory urogram or radionuclide renal scan (^{99m}Tc-DMSA), consideration should be given to preserving this portion of the kidney. If the upper pole ureter is not greatly dilated, excision of the ureterocele and common sheath reimplantation should be considered, especially if significant lower pole reflux is present (Figs. 45–29 and 45–30). In the absence of severe lower pole reflux and in the presence of a marked discrepancy between the size of the duplicate ureters, the procedure of choice is either ureteroureterostomy or pyeloureterostomy with partial ureterectomy.

In some instances, an ectopic ureterocele drains a tiny, almost atretic ureter attached to a small dysplastic renal segment (Fig. 45–31)—so-called ureterocele disproportion (Bauer and Retik, 1978; Share and Lebowitz, 1989). Ipsilateral lower pole reflux frequently accompanies these findings. In this situation, too, excision of

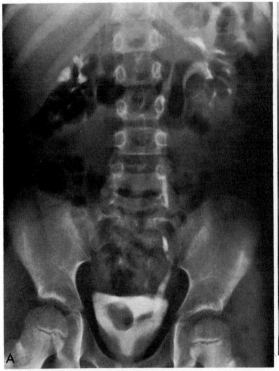

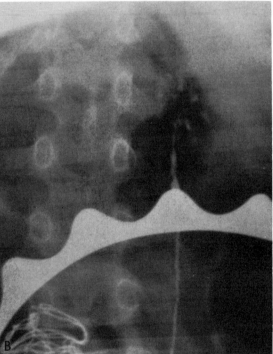

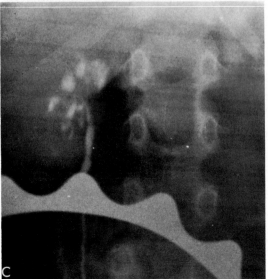

Figure 45–31. *A,* Excretory urogram in a 5-year-old girl shows bilateral ureteroceles. *B* and *C,* Bilateral ureterograms at the time of surgery demonstrate small upper pole dysplastic kidneys.

the ureterocele combined with common sheath reimplantation of both ureters has been employed. In our experience, subsequent upper pole nephrectomy because of infection or hypertension has not been necessary, although the renal unit left behind is dysplastic and presumably nonfunctioning. The issue of the safety of leaving the dysplastic tissue remains unsettled. Nodular renal blastema, a possibly premalignant pathologic state, has been identified in some cases of renal duplication with dysplasia (Cromie et al., 1980; Crower et al., 1986; Gaddy et al., 1985). We have not considered this to be a contraindication to leaving the upper pole, because this approach avoids additional surgery at the kidney level and takes care of the more important problem—i.e., ipsilateral lower pole reflux—with minimal risk to the patient. Transurethral incision to decompress the ureterocele may also be successful in these cases, provided that the ureterocele is not extremely large or without muscular backing.

REFERENCES

Aas, T. N.: Ureterocele: A clinical study of 68 cases in 52 adults. Br. J. Urol., 32:133, 1960.

Abeshouse, B. S.: Ureteral ectopia: Report of a rare case of ectopic ureter opening in the uterus and review of the literature. Urol. Cutan. Rev., 47:447, 1943.

Ahmed, S.: Ureteral duplication with ectopic ureterocele: Report of a case presenting with peritonitis. J. Urol., 106:287, 1971.

Alfert, H. J., and Gillenwater, J. Y.: Ectopic vas deferens communicating with lower ureter: Embryological considerations. J. Urol., 108:172, 1972.

Amar, A. D.: Ureteropyelostomy for relief of single ureteral obstruction in cases of ureteral duplication. Arch. Surg., 101:379, 1970.

Amar, A. D.: Lateral ureteral displacement: Sign of non-visualized duplication. J. Urol., 105:638, 1971a.

Amar, A. D.: Simple ureterocele at the distal end of a blind-ending ureter. J. Urol., 106:423, 1971b.

Amar, A. D.: The management of urinary calculus disease in patients with duplicated ureters. Br. J. Urol., 44:541, 1972.

Anhalt, M. A., and Guthrie, T. H.: Management of ectopic ureterocele. J. Urol., 107:856, 1972.

Arey, L. B.: Developmental Anatomy: A Textbook and Laboratory Manual of Embryology, 7th ed. Philadelphia, W. B. Saunders Co., 1974.

Asaad, E. I., Badawi, Z. H., and Gaballah, M. F.: Nature and fate of the ureteric membrane closing the primitive ureterovesical opening. Acta Anat., 92:524, 1975.

Barrett, D. M., Malek, R. S., and Kelalis, P. P.: Problems and solutions in surgical treatment of 100 consecutive ureteral duplications in children. J. Urol., 114:126, 1975.

Bauchard, J.: Un cas de trifidité urétérale bilaterale avec volumineuse hydronephrose. J. Urol. Nephrol. (Paris), 65:476, 1978.

Bauer, S. B., and Retik, A. B.: The non-obstructive ureterocele. J. Urol., 119:804–807, 1978.

Beck, A. D.: The effect of intrauterine urinary obstruction upon the development of the fetal kidney. J. Urol., 105:784, 1971.

Belman, A. B., Filmer, R. B., and King, L. R.: Surgical management of duplication of the collecting system. J. Urol., 112:316–321, 1974.

Bengmark, S., Nilsson, S., and Romanus, R.: Ectopic ureter draining into a seminal megavesicle causing defecation troubles: Report of a case and review of the literature. Acta Chir. Scand., 123:471, 1962.

Berdon, W. E., Levitt, S. B., Baker, D. H., Becker, J. A., and Uson, A. C.: Ectopic ureterocele. Radiol. Clin. North Am., 6:205, 1968.

Boatwright, D. C.: Ureterocele: Surgical treatment. J. Urol., 106:48, 1971.

Boijsen, E.: Angiographic studies of the anatomy of single and multiple renal arteries. Acta Radiol. (Suppl.), 183:1, 1959.

Brannan, W., and Hector, H. H.: Ureteral ectopia: Report of 39 cases. J. Urol., 109:192, 1973.

Brown, T., Mandell, J., and Lebowitz, R. L.: Neonatal hydronephrosis in the era of sonography. AJR, 148:959–963, 1987.

Burford, C. E., Glen, J. E., and Burford, E. H.: Ureteral ectopia: Review of literature and two case reports. J. Urol., 62:211, 1949.

Caldamone, A. A., Snyder, H. McC., III, and Duckett, J. W.: Ureteroceles in children: Follow-up of management with upper tract approach. J. Urol., 131:1130–1132, 1984.

Campbell, M.: Ectopic ureteral orifice. Surg. Gynecol. Obstet., 64:22–29, 1937.

Campbell, M.: Ureterocele. J. Urol., 45:598–611, 1941.

Campbell, M.: Ureterocele: A study of 94 instances in 80 infants and children. Surg. Gynecol. Obstet., 93:705, 1951.

Cendron, J., and Bonhomme, C.: 31 cas d'urètre à abouchement ectopique sous-sphinctérien chez l'enfant du sexe feminin. J. Urol. Nephrol. (Paris), 74:1, 1968a.

Cendron, J., and Bonhomme, C.: Uretère à terminaison ectopique extravésicale chez des sujets de sexe masculin (à propos de 10 cas). J. Urol. Nephrol. (Paris), 74:1, 1968b.

Chidlow, J. H., and Uts, D. C.: Ureteral ectopia in vestibule of vagina with urinary continence. South. Med. J., 63:423, 1970.

Chwalle, R.: The process of formation of cystic dilatations of the vesicle end of the ureter and of diverticula at the ureteral ostium. Urol. Cutan. Rev., 31:499, 1927.

Cibert, J., Cibert, J., Gilloz, A., et al.: Triplicite ureterale. J. Urol. Nephrol. (Paris), 71:429, 1965.

Clark, C. W., and Leadbetter, G.: General treatment, mistreatment and complications of ureterocele. J. Urol., 106:518, 1971.

Cohen, S. J.: Ureterozystoneostomie. Eine neue antirefluxtechnik. Aktuel Urol., 6:1, 1975.

Constantian, H. M.: Ureteral ectopia, hydrocolpos, and uterus didelphys. JAMA, 197:54, 1966.

Cromie, W. J., Engelstein, M. S., and Duckett, J. W., Jr.: Nodular renal blastema, renal dysplasia and duplicated collecting systems. J. Urol., 123:100–102, 1980.

Crower, R., Dimmick, J., Johnson, H., and Nigro, M.: Congenital obstructive uropathy and nodular renal blastema. J. Urol., 136:305–307, 1986.

Culp, O. S.: Heminephro-ureterectomy: Comparison of one-stage and two-stage operations. J. Urol., 83:369, 1960.

Cussen, L. J.: The structure of the human ureter in infancy and childhood. Invest. Urol., 5:179, 1967.

Decter, R. M., Roth, D. R., and Gonzales, E. T.: Individualized treatment of ureteroceles. J. Urol., 142 (part 2):535–537, 1989.

DeWeerd, J. H., and Feeney, D. P.: Bilateral ureteral ectopia with urinary incontinence in a mother and daughter. J. Urol., 98:335, 1967.

DeWeerd, J. H., and Litin, R. B.: Ectopia of ureteral orifice (vestibular) without incontinence: Report of a case. Proc. Staff Meet. Mayo Clin., 33:81, 1958.

Diament, M. J., and Stanley, P.: Two unusual duplication anomalies of the urinary tract: Use of percutaneous urography. Urol. Radiol., 9:185–187, 1987.

Diard, F., Chateil, J. F., Bondonny, J. M., Nicolau, A., and DeLambilly, C.: "Pseudo-ureterocele": Buckling of an ectopic megaureter imprinting the urinary bladder. J. Radiol., 68:177–184, 1987.

Diaz-Ball, F. L., Finak, A., Moore, C. A., et al.: Pyeloureterostomy and ureteroureterostomy: Alternative procedures to partial nephrectomy for duplication of the ureter with only one pathological segment. J. Urol., 102:621, 1969.

Dorst, J. P., Cussen, G. H., and Silverman, F. N.: Ureteroceles in children, with emphasis on the frequency of ectopic ureteroceles. Radiology, 74:88–89, 1960.

Eklof, O., and Makinen, E.: Ectopic ureterocele: A radiological appraisal of 66 consecutive cases. Pediatr. Radiol., 2:111–120, 1974.

Eklof, O., Parkkulainen, K., Thonell, S., and Wilkstrom, S.: Ectopic ureterocele in the male. Ann. Radiol., 30:486–490, 1987.

Emery, J. G., and Gill, G.: A classification and quantitative histological study of abnormal ureters in children. Br. J. Urol., 46:69, 1974.

Ericsson, N. O.: Ectopic ureterocele in infants and children: A clinical study. Acta Chir. Scand. (Suppl.) 197:1, 1954.

Friedland, G. W., and Cunningham, J.: The elusive ectopic ureteroceles. Am. J. Roentgenol., 116:792–811, 1972.

Gaddy, C. D., Gibbons, M. D., Gonzales, E. T., Jr., and Finegold, M. J.: Obstructive uropathy, renal dysplasia and nodular renal blastema: Is there a relationship to Wilms' tumor? J. Urol., 134:330–333, 1985.

Gearhart, J. P., and Jeffs, R. D.: The use of topical vasodilators as an adjunct in infant renal surgery. J. Urol., 134:298–300, 1985.

Gerridzen, R., and Schillinger, J.: Transurethral puncture in management of ectopic ureteroceles. Urology, 23:43–47, 1984.

Gibson, T. E.: A new operation of ureteral ectopia: Case report. J. Urol., 77:414, 1957.

Gill, R. D.: Triplication of the ureter and renal pelvis. J. Urol., 68:140, 1952.

Gilmore, O. J.: Unilateral triplication of the ureter. Br. J. Urol., 46:588, 1974.

Glassberg, K. I., Braren, V., Duckett, J. W., et al.: Suggested terminology for duplex systems, ectopic ureters and ureteroceles. J. Urol., 132:1153–1154, 1984.

Glenn, J. F.: Agenesis of the bladder. JAMA, 169:2016, 1959.

Golomb, J., and Ehrlich, R. M.: Bilateral ureteral triplication with crossed ectopic fused kidney associated with the VACTRL syndrome. J. Urol., 141:1398–1399, 1989.

Gotoh, T., and Koyanagi, T.: Clinicopathologic and embryologic considerations of single ectopic ureters opening into Gartner's duct cyst: A unique subtype of single vaginal ectopia. J. Urol., 137:969–972, 1987.

Gotoh, T., Koyanagi, T., and Matsuno, T.: Surgical management of ureteroceles in children: Strategy based on the classification of ureteral hiatus and the eversion of ureteroceles. J. Pediatr. Surg., 23:159–165, 1988.

Gotoh, T., Morita, H., Tokunaka, S., Koyanagi, T., and Tsuji, I.: Single ectopic ureter. J. Urol., 129:271–274, 1983.

Greene, L. F., and Ferris, D. O.: Urinary incontinence due to bilateral ectopic ureters. Surg. Gynecol. Obstet., 82:712, 1946.

Gross, R. E., and Clatworthy, H. W.: Ureterocele in infancy and childhood. Pediatrics, 5:68–77, 1950.

Heloury, Y., Bachy, B., Bawab, F., and Mitrofanoff, P.: Conservative treatment by high anastomosis in duplications with lesions of the superior pelvis. J. Urol. (Paris), 94:27–31, 1988.

Hendren, W. H., and Mitchell, M. E.: Surgical correction of ureteroceles. J. Urol., 121:590–597, 1979.

Hendren, W. H., and Monfort, G. J.: Surgical correction of ureteroceles in childhood. J. Pediatr. Surg., 6:235–244, 1971.

Hernanz-Schulman, M., Genieser, N., Ambrosino, M., and Hana, M.: Bilateral duplex ectopic ureters terminating in the seminal vesicles: Sonographic and CT diagnosis. Urol. Radiol., 11:49–52, 1989.

Huisman, T. K., Kaplan, G. W., Brock, W. A., and Packer, M. G.: Ipsilateral ureteroureterostomy and pyeloureterostomy: A review of 15 years of experience with 25 patients. J. Urol., 138:1207–1210, 1987.

Hutch, J. A., and Chishol, E. R.: Surgical repair of ureterocele. J. Urol., 96:445, 1966.

Hutton, I. M., and Green, N. A.: High dose delayed urogram in the detection of the occult ectopic ureter. Br. J. Urol., 46:289, 1974.

Johnson, D. K., and Perlmutter, A. D.: Single system ectopic ureteroceles with anomalies of the heart, testis and vas deferens. J. Urol., 123:81, 1980.

Johnston, J. H.: Urinary tract duplication in childhood. Arch. Dis. Child., 36:180, 1961.

Johnston, J. H., and Davenport, T. J.: The single ectopic ureter. Br. J. Urol., 41:428, 1969.

Johnston, J. H., and Johnson, L. M.: Experiences with ectopic ureteroceles. Br. J. Urol., 41:61–70, 1969.

Juskiewenski, S., Soulie, M., Baunin, C., Moscovici, J., and Vayss, Ph.: Ureteral triplication. Chir. Pediatr., 28:314–321, 1987.

Katzen, P., and Trachtman, B.: Diagnosis of vaginal ectopic ureter by vaginogram. J. Urol., 72:808, 1954.

Kelalis, P. P.: Ureterocele. Clin. Obstet. Gynecol., 10:155, 1967.

Koyanagi, T., Hisajima, S., Goto, T., Tokunaka, S., and Tsuji, I.: Everting ureteroceles: Radiographic and endoscopic observation and surgical management. J. Urol., 123:538, 1980.

Kroovand, R. L., and Perlmutter, A. D.: A one-stage surgical approach to ectopic ureterocele. J. Urol., 122:367–369, 1979.

Leadbetter, G. W., Jr.: Ectopic ureterocele as a cause of urinary incontinence. J. Urol., 103:222, 1970.

Leef, G. S., and Leader, S. A.: Ectopic ureter opening into the rectum: A case report. J. Urol., 87:338, 1962.

Livaditis, A., Maurseth, K., and Skog, P. A.: Unilateral triplication of the ureter and renal pelvis: Report of a case. Acta Chir. Scand., 127:181, 1964.

Mackelvie, A. A.: Triplicate ureter: Case report. Br. J. Urol., 27:124, 1955.

Mackie, G. G., Awang, H., and Stephens, F. D.: The ureteric orifice: The embryologic key to radiologic status of duplex kidneys. J. Pediatr. Surg., 10:473, 1975.

Mackie, G. G., and Stephens, F. D.: Duplex kidneys: A correlation of renal dysplasia with position of the ureteral orifice. J. Urol., 114:274, 1975.

Malek, R. S., Kelalis, P. P., Burke, E. C., and Stickler, G. B.: Simple and ectopic ureterocele in infancy and childhood. Surg. Gynecol. Obstet., 134:611–616, 1972a.

Malek, R. S., Kelalis, P. P., Stickler, G. B., et al.: Observations on ureteral ectopy in children. J. Urol., 107:308, 1972b.

Mandell, J., Bauer, S. B., Colodny, A. H., Lebowitz, R. L., and Retik, A. B.: Ureteral ectopia in infants and children. J. Urol., 126:219–222, 1981.

Mandell, J., Colodny, A. H., Lebowitz, R. L., Bauer, S. B., and Retik, A. B.: Ureteroceles in infants and children. J. Urol., 123:921–926, 1980.

Marshall, S.: Reimplantation of the dilated ectopic ureter of the duplex system as a separate unit. J. Urol., 135:574–575, 1986.

McCall, I. W., Atkinson, D. O., and Moule, N. J.: Multiple ureteral diverticula associated with bilateral ureteroceles. Br. J. Urol., 47:538, 1975.

McKay, R. W., and Baird, H. H.: Bilateral single ureteral ectopia terminating in the urethra. J. Urol., 63:1013, 1950.

Mogg, R. A.: Some observations on the ectopic ureter and ureterocele. J. Urol., 97:1003, 1967.

Mogg, R. A.: The single ectopic ureter. Br. J. Urol., 46:3, 1974.

Moussali, L., Cuevas, J. O., and Heras, M. R.: Management of ectopic ureterocele. Urology, 31:412–414, 1988.

Musselman, B. C., and Barry, J.: Varying degrees of ureteral ectopia and duplication in five siblings. J. Urol., 110:476, 1973.

Noseworthy, J., and Persky, L.: Spectrum of bilateral ureteral ectopia. Urology, 19:489–494, 1982.

Nussbaum, A. R., Dorst, J. P., Jeffs, R. D., Gearhart, J. P., and Sanders, R. C.: Ectopic ureter and ureterocele: Their varied sonographic manifestations. Radiology, 159:227–235, 1986.

Passerini-Glazel, G., Milani, C., Bassi, P., Chiozza, L., Rizzoni, G., and Pagano, F.: Bilateral single ectopic ureter. Eur. Urol., 14:454–457, 1988.

Perkins, P. J., Kroovand, R. L., and Evans, A. T.: Ureteral triplication. Radiology, 108:533, 1973.

Perrin, E. V., Persky, L., Tucker, A., et al.: Renal duplication and dysplasia. Urology, 4:660, 1974.

Politano, V. A., and Leadbetter, W. F.: An operative technique for the correction of vesicoureteral reflux. J. Urol., 79:932, 1958.

Prantl, M., and Tewes, G.: Ureteral triplication with contralateral duplication. Z. Kinderchir., 43:350–352, 1988.

Prewett, J. H., Jr., and Lebowitz, R. L.: The single ectopic ureter. Am. J. Roentgenol., 127:941, 1976.

Rajfer, J., Eggleston, J. C., Sanders, R. C., and Walsh, P. C.: Fever and a prostatic mass in a young man. J. Urol., 119:555–558, 1978.

Redman, J. F.: Unsuspected duplex ureters. Urology, 5:196, 1975.

Riba, L. W., Schmidlapp, C. J., and Bosworth, N. L.: Ectopic ureter draining into the seminal vesicle. J. Urol., 56:332, 1946.

Rich, M. A., Keating, M. A., Snyder, H. McC., III, and Duckett, J. W.: Low transurethral incision of single system intravesical ureteroceles in children. J. Urol., 144:120–121, 1990.

Ritchey, M. L., Kramer, S. A., Benson, R. C., Jr., and Kelalis, P. P.: Bilateral single ureteral ectopia. Eur. Urol., 14:41–45, 1988.

Royle, M. G., and Goodwin, W. E.: The management of ureteroceles. J. Urol., 106:42, 1971.

Scherz, H. C., Kaplan, G. W., Packer, M. G., and Brock, W. A.: Ectopic ureteroceles: Surgical management with preservation of continence: Review of 60 cases. J. Urol., 142(part 2):538–541, 1989.

Schnitzer, B.: Ectopic ureteral opening into seminal vesicle: A report of four cases. J. Urol., 93:576, 1965.

Scott, R.: Triplication of the ureter. Br. J. Urol., 42:150, 1970.

Shappley, N., and Keeton, J.: Unusual presentation of cecoureterocele. Urology, 6:605, 1975.

Share, J. C., and Lebowitz, R. L.: Ectopic ureterocele without ureteral and calyceal dilatation (ureterocele disproportion): Findings on urography and sonography. AJR, 152:567–571, 1989.

Shaw, R. E.: Ureterocele. Br. J. Surg., 60:337, 1973.

Sherwood, T., and Stevenson, J. J.: Ureteroceles in disguise. Br. J. Radiol., 42:899, 1969.

Simms, M. H., and Higgins, P. M.: Diagnosis of the occult ectopic ureter in a duplex kidney. J. Urol., 114:697, 1975.

Smith, F. L., Ritchie, E. L., Maizels, M., Zaontz, M. R., Hsueh, W., Kaplan, W. E., and Firlit, C. F.: Surgery for duplex kidneys with ectopic ureters: Ipsilateral ureteroureterostomy versus polar nephrectomy. J. Urol., 142(part 2):532–543, 1989.

Smith, I.: Triplicate ureter. Br. J. Surg., 34:182, 1946.

Spangler, E. B.: Complete triplication of the ureter. Radiology, 80:795, 1963.

Squadrito, J. F., Jr., Rifkin, M. D., and Mulholland, S. G.: Ureteral ectopia presenting as epididymitis and infertility. Urology, 30:67–69, 1987.

Srivastava, H. C.: Bilateral termination of the ureter in the uterine tube. Indian J. Med. Sci., 22:37, 1968.

Stephens, F. D.: Double ureter in the child. Aust. N. Z. J. Surg., 26:81–94, 1956.

Stephens, F. D.: Ureterocele in infants and children. Aust. N. Z. J. Surg., 27:288, 1958a.

Stephens, F. D.: Anatomical vagaries of double ureters. Aust. N. Z. J. Surg., 28:27–33, 1958b.

Stephens, F. D.: Intramural ureter and ureterocele. Postgrad. Med. J., 40:179, 1964.

Stephens, F. D.: Congenital Malformations of the Urinary Tract. New York, N.Y., Praeger, 1983.

Stephens, F. D.: Caecoureterocele and concepts on the embryology and aetiology of ureteroceles. Aust. N. Z. J. Surg., 40:239–248, 1971.

Subbiah, N., and Stephens, F. D.: Stenotic ureterocele. Aust. N. Z. J. Surg., 41:257–263, 1972.

Swenson, O., and Ratner, I. A.: Pyeloureterostomy for treatment of symptomatic ureteral duplications in children. J. Urol., 88:184, 1962.

Tanagho, E. A.: Anatomy and management of ureteroceles. J. Urol., 107:729, 1972.

Tanagho, E. A.: Embryologic basis for lower ureteral anomalies: A hypothesis. Urology, 7:451–464, 1976.

Tanagho, E. A.: Ureteroceles: Embryogenesis, pathogenesis and management. Urology, 18:13, 1979.

Tank, E.: Experience with endoscopic incision and open unroofing of ureteroceles. J. Urol., 136:241–242, 1986.

Thompson, G. J., and Greene, L. F.: Ureterocele: A clinical study and a report of thirty-seven cases. J. Urol., 47:800, 1942.

Thompson, G. J., and Kelalis, P. P.: Ureterocele: Clinical appraisal of 176 cases. J. Urol., 91:488, 1964.

Timothy, R. P., Decter, A., and Perlmutter, A.: Ureteral duplication: Clinical findings and therapy in 46 children. J. Urol., 105:445, 1971.

Tokunaka, S., Gotoh, T., Koyanagi, T., and Tsuji, I.: Morphological study of the ureterocele: A possible clue to its embryogenesis as evidenced by a locally arrested myogenesis. J. Urol., 126:726–729, 1981.

Uehling, D. T., and Bruskewitz, R. C.: Initiation of vesicoureteral reflux after heminephrectomy for ureterocele. Urology, 23:302–304, 1989.

Uson, A. C., Lattimer, J. K., and Melicow, M. M.: Ureteroceles in infants and children: A report based on 44 cases. Pediatrics, 27:971, 1961.

Uson, A. C., and Schulman, C. C.: Ectopic ureter emptying into the rectum: Report of a case. J. Urol., 108:156, 1950.

Uson, A. C., Womack, C. E., and Berdon, W. E.: Giant ectopic ureter presenting as an abdominal mass in a newborn infant. J. Pediatr., 80:473, 1972.

Vanhoutte, J. J.: Ureteral ectopia into a wolffian duct remnant (Gartner's ducts or cysts) presenting as a urethral diverticulum in two girls. Am. J. Roentgenol. Radium Ther. Nucl. Med., 110:540, 1970.

Weinstein, A. J., Bauer, S. B., Retik, A. B., Mandell, J., and Colodny, A. H.: The surgical management of megaureters in duplex systems: The efficacy of ureteral tapering and common sheath reimplantation. J. Urol., 139:328–331, 1988.

Weiss, J. P., Duckett, J. W., and Snyder, H. McC., III: Single unilateral vaginal ectopic ureter: Is it really a rarity? J. Urol., 132:1177–1179, 1984.

Weiss, R. M., and Spackman, T. J.: Everting ectopic ureteroceles. J. Urol., 111:538, 1974.

Wigglshaff, C. C., and Kiefer, J. H.: Ureteral ectopia: Diagnostic difficulties. J. Urol., 96:671, 1966.

Williams, D. I.: The ectopic ureter: Diagnostic problems. Br. J. Urol., 26:253, 1954.

Williams, D. I.: Ectopic ureterocele. Proc. R. Soc. Med., 51:783, 1958.

Williams, D. I., and Lightwood, R. G.: Bilateral single ectopic ureters. Br. J. Urol., 44:267, 1972.

Williams, D. I., and Lillie, J. G.: The functional radiology of ectopic ureterocele. Br. J. Urol., 44:417, 1972.

Williams, D. I., and Royle, M.: Ectopic ureter in the male child. Br. J. Urol., 41:421, 1969.

Williams, D. I., and Woodard, J. R.: Problems in the management of ectopic ureterocele. J. Urol., 92:635, 1964.

Willmarth, C. L.: Ectopic ureteral orifice within a urethral diverticulum: Report of a case. J. Urol., 59:47, 1948.

Wines, R. D., and O'Flynn, J. D.: Transurethral treatment of ureteroceles. Br. J. Urol., 44:207, 1972.

Winters, W. D., and Lebowitz, R. L.: Importance of prenatal detection of hydronephrosis of the upper pole. AJR, 155:125, 1990.

Wyly, J. B., and Lebowitz, R. L.: Refluxing urethral ectopic ureters: Recognition by the cyclic voiding cystourethrogram. AJR, 142:1263–1267, 1984.

Yachia, D.: An entirely endoscopic treatment for simple ureteroceles in nonduplicated systems: A preliminary report. J. Urol., 140:815–817, 1988.

Zaontz, M. R., and Kass, E. J.: Ectopic ureter opening into seminal vesicle cyst associated with ipsilateral renal agenesis. Urology, 29:523–525, 1987.

Zielinski, J.: Avoidance of vesicoureteral reflux after transurethral ureteral meatotomy for ureterocele. J. Urol., 88:386, 1962.

46

EXSTROPHY OF THE BLADDER, EPISPADIAS, AND OTHER BLADDER ANOMALIES

John P. Gearhart, M.D.
Robert D. Jeffs, M.D.

The surgical management of bladder exstrophy, cloacal exstrophy, and epispadias is emphasized in this chapter. The primary objectives in the surgical management of bladder exstrophy are to obtain the following: (1) secure abdominal wall closure, (2) urinary continence with the preservation of renal function, and (3) reconstruction of a functional and cosmetically acceptable penis in the male patient. These objectives can be achieved with primary bladder closure, bladder neck reconstruction, and epispadias repair. Although many reconstructive techniques have been described, a unified approach to the surgical management of this disorder has only currently evolved because most modalities were associated with substantial failure rates and operative morbidity.

Formerly, surgical reconstruction of cloacal exstrophy, the most severe variant of the exstrophy-epispadias complex, was considered futile. However, advances in anesthesia, neonatal care, and nutrition along with the application of the principles that have evolved in the treatment of classic bladder exstrophy have improved the outcome in this group of patients. The surgical management of epispadias, the least extensive anomaly of this complex, is fairly straightforward and involves reconstruction of the genitalia and restoration of continence in complete epispadias. In this chapter, the techniques for managing the epispadias-exstrophy variants are discussed, a detailed description of our surgical approach to these anomalies is presented, and the results of surgical intervention are summarized. Lastly, management of the exstrophy patient who does not respond to treatment and management of the small capacity bladder after initial closure are discussed.

EMBRYOLOGY OF BLADDER DEVELOPMENT

Bladder exstrophy, cloacal exstrophy, and epispadias are variants of the exstrophy-epispadias complex (Fig. 46–1). The etiology of this complex has been attributed to the failure of the cloacal membrane to be reinforced by ingrowth of mesoderm (Muecke, 1964). The cloacal membrane is a bilaminar layer situated at the caudal end of the germinal disc that occupies the infraumbilical abdominal wall. Mesenchymal ingrowth between the ectodermal and endodermal layers of the cloacal membrane results in formation of the lower abdominal muscles and the pelvic bones. The cloacal membrane is subject to premature rupture; depending on the extent of the infraumbilical defect and the stage of development when rupture occurs, bladder exstrophy, cloacal exstrophy, or epispadias results (Ambrose and O'Brien, 1974).

After mesenchymal ingrowth occurs, downgrowth of the urorectal septum divides the cloaca into a bladder anteriorly and a rectum posteriorly (Fig. 46–2). Distally, the septum meets the posterior remnant of the bilaminar membrane, which eventually perforates and forms anal and urogenital openings. The paired genital tubercles migrate medially and fuse in the midline cephalad to the dorsal membrane before perforation.

The theory of embryonic maldevelopment in exstrophy held by Marshall and Muecke (1968) is that the basic defect is an abnormal overdevelopment of the cloacal membrane, preventing medial migration of the mesenchymal tissue and proper lower abdominal wall development. The timing of the rupture of this cloacal

Types of Syndromes

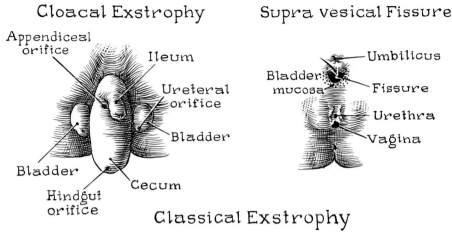

Cloacal Exstrophy

Appendiceal orifice

Ileum

Ureteral orifice

Bladder

Bladder

Cecum

Hindgut orifice

Supra vesical Fissure

Umbilicus

Bladder mucosa

Fissure

Urethra

Vagina

Figure 46–1. Various entities in the exstrophy-epispadias syndrome. (Drawing by Leon Schlossberg.)

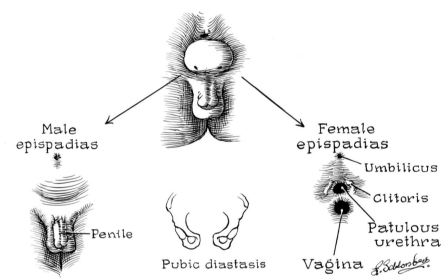

Classical Exstrophy

Male epispadias

Penile

Pubic diastasis

Female epispadias

Umbilicus

Clitoris

Patulous urethra

Vagina

defect determines the variant of the exstrophy-epispadias complex that results (Figs. 46–3 and 46–4). This theory is supported by Muecke's work in the chick embryo and by the expected high incidence of central perforations resulting in the preponderance of classic exstrophy variants. A classic exstrophy accounts for 50 per cent of the patients born with this complex (Marshall and Muecke, 1968; Muecke, 1964).

However, other plausible theories concerning the cause of the exstrophy-epispadias complex exist. One group has postulated an abnormal caudal development of the genital hillocks with fusion in the midline below rather than above the cloacal membrane, a view that has been accepted by other investigators (Ambrose and O'Brien, 1974; Patten and Barry, 1952). Another interesting hypothesis describes an abnormal caudal insertion of the body stalk, which results in failure of interposition of the mesenchymal tissue in the midline (Mildenberger et al., 1988). As a consequence of this failure, the translocation of the cloaca into the depths of the abdominal cavity does not occur. A cloacal membrane that remains in a superficial infraumbilical position represents an unstable embryonic state with a strong tendency

to disintegrate (Johnston, 1974). However, the theory of an abnormal caudal insertion of the body stalk remains controversial because the embryogenesis of the rat in this area differs in many ways from that of the human.

BLADDER EXSTROPHY

Incidence and Inheritance

The incidence of bladder exstrophy has been estimated as between one in 10,000 (Rickham, 1960) and one in 50,000 (Lattimer and Smith, 1966) live births. However, new data from the international clearinghouse for birth defects monitoring system estimated the incidence to be 3.3 cases in 100,000 live births (Lancaster, 1987). The male-to-female ratio of bladder exstrophy derived from multiple series is 2.3:1 (Bennett, 1973; Harvard and Thompson, 1951; Higgins, 1962; Jeffs et al., 1982). However, two series reported a 5:1 to 6:1 ratio of male-to-female exstrophy births (Ives et al., 1980; Lancaster, 1987).

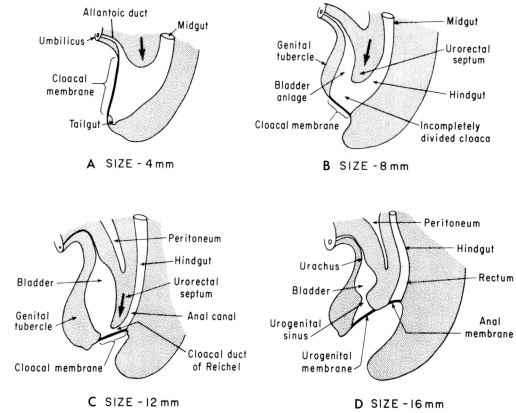

Figure 46–2. Developmental changes of the cloaca and cloacal membrane in the 4-mm to 16-mm embryo. Arrows show direction of growth of the urorectal septum. (Drawings are not to scale.)

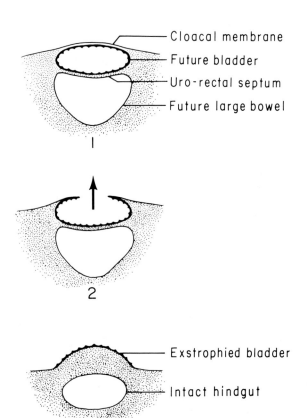

Figure 46–3. Diagram of events leading to classic exstrophy.

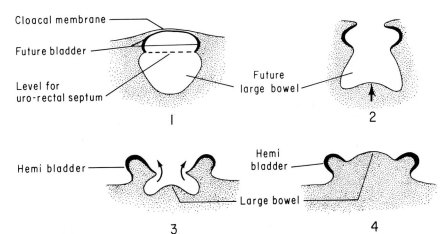

Figure 46–4. Diagram of eventration of cloaca to form cloacal exstrophy.

The risk of recurrence of bladder exstrophy in a given family is approximately one in 100 (Ives et al., 1980). Shapiro and co-workers (1984) conducted a questionnaire of pediatric urologists and surgeons in North America and Europe and identified the recurrence of exstrophy and epispadias in only nine of approximately 2500 indexed cases. Lattimer and Smith (1966) cited a set of identical twins with bladder exstrophy and another set of twins in whom only one child had exstrophy. Shapiro's series identified five sets of male and female nonidentical twins in whom only one twin was affected with exstrophy; five sets of male identical twins in whom both twins were affected; one set of identical male twins in whom only one twin was affected; and three sets of female identical twins in whom only one twin had the exstrophy anomaly (Shapiro et al., 1985).

The inheritance pattern of bladder exstrophy in a literature review by Clemetson (1958) identified 45 women with bladder exstrophy who produced 49 offspring. In no instance did any of their offspring demonstrate features of the exstrophy-epispadias complex. Bladder exstrophy or epispadias had not been reported until currently, in offspring of parents with the exstrophy-epispadias complex. Shapiro and colleagues (1985) reported two women with complete epispadias who each gave birth to sons with bladder exstrophy, and they reported another woman with bladder exstrophy who gave birth to a son with bladder exstrophy. The inheritance of these three cases of bladder exstrophy was identified in a total of 225 offspring (75 boys and 150 girls) produced by individuals with bladder exstrophy and epispadias. Shapiro determined that the risk of bladder exstrophy in the offspring of individuals with bladder exstrophy and epispadias is one in 70 live births, a 500-fold greater incidence than in the general population. In a multinational review of exstrophy patients (Lancaster, 1987), two interesting trends were found: (1) bladder exstrophy tends to occur in infants of younger mothers and (2) an increased risk at higher parity is observed for bladder exstrophy but not for epispadias.

Prenatal Diagnosis and Management

Sonographic evaluation of the fetus, especially by means of high-resolution, real-time units, allows a thorough survey of fetal anatomy, even during routine obstetric sonograms. Most studies, however, have dealt with the prenatal evaluation of hydronephrosis. However, some reports have indicated that it is indeed possible to diagnose prenatally classic bladder exstrophy (Mirk et al., 1986; Verco et al., 1986). In the quoted reviews, the absence of a normal, fluid-filled bladder on repeated examinations suggested the diagnosis, as did a mass of echogenic tissue lying on the lower abdominal wall (Verco et al., 1986). In a review of prenatal ultrasound examinations, the absence of bladder filling along with a low-set umbilicus was the key factor of note in eight exstrophy pregnancies reviewed in retrospect (Gearhart and Jeffs, 1988).

Exstrophy Complex and Variants

Because the entire exstrophy group of anomalies represents a spectrum, it is not surprising that transitions among bladder exstrophy, epispadias, and cloacal exstrophy have been reported. A close relationship exists among all forms of the exstrophy-epispadias complex because the fault in its embryogenesis is common to all; therefore, all clinical manifestations are merely variations on a theme.

Pseudoexstrophy

The presence of the characteristic musculoskeletal defect of the exstrophy anomaly with no major defect in the urinary tract has been named *pseudoexstrophy* (Marshall and Muecke, 1968). Predominant characteristics include an elongated, low-set umbilicus and divergent rectus muscles, which attach to the separated pubic bones (Fig. 46–5). In this variant, the mesodermal migration has been interrupted in its superior aspect only, and perhaps, the caudal flow of the mesoderm from the umbilical stalk alone was impeded, thus separating the musculoskeletal elements of the lower abdominal wall without obstructing the formation of the genital tubercle (Marshall and Muecke, 1968).

Superior Vesical Fissure

In this variant of the exstrophy complex, the musculature and skeletal defects are exactly as those in classic

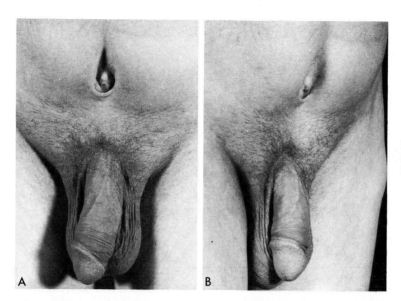

Figure 46–5. Pseudoexstrophy in an adult male patient. Musculoskeletal deformity characteristic of exstrophy is present, but the urinary tract is intact.

exstrophy; however, the persistent cloacal membrane opens only at the uppermost portion. Thus, a superior vesical fissure results. Bladder exstrusion is minimal and is present only over the abnormal umbilicus (Fig. 46–6). Both Muecke (1986) and Uson and Roberts (1958) have presented cases of superior vesical fissure and stressed the important differences between superior vesical fissure with its musculoskeletal anomalies and a patent urachus without any musculoskeletal abnormali-

ties. One of two patients whom we have seen died of total anomalous pulmonary drainage shortly after birth.

Duplicate Exstrophy

Duplicate exstrophy occurs when a superior vesical fissure opens but there is later fusion of the abdominal wall and a portion of the bladder elements (mucosa) remains outside. In a case report by Muecke (1986), the

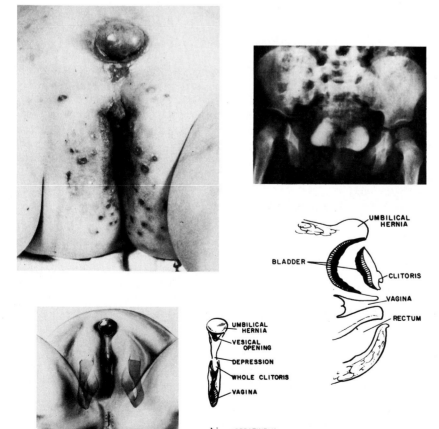

Figure 46–6. Superior vesical fissure in a girl. Musculoskeletal deformities are those typical of exstrophy of the bladder.

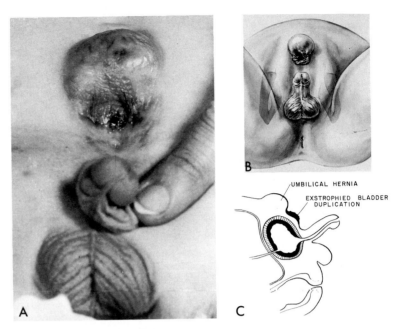

Figure 46–7. Duplicate exstrophy in a boy with an intact urinary tract.

patient had exstrophy of the mucosa but a normal bladder inside (Fig. 46–7). The patient had a very widened symphysis and a stubby, upward-pointing penis. Three additional cases have been reported by Arap and Giron (1986) in which the patients had classic musculoskeletal defects, and two of the three were continent. In the two male patients, one had an associated complete epispadias, whereas the other had a completely normal penis. Thus, the external genital manifestations of duplicate exstrophy can be quite variable.

Covered Exstrophy

Besides pseudoexstrophy, superior vesical fissure, and duplicate exstrophy, isolated occurrences of a fourth entity—covered exstrophy—have been reported (Cerniglia et al., 1989; Narasimharao et al., 1985). These anomalies have also been referred to as split symphysis variants. A common factor present in these patients is the musculoskeletal defect associated with classic exstrophy with no significant defect of the urinary tract. However, in most cases reported as covered exstrophy (Cerniglia et al., 1989; Narasimharao et al., 1985), an isolated ectopic bowel segment has been present on the inferior abdominal wall near the genital area, which can be either colon or ileum, with no connection with the underlying gastrointestinal tract and epispadias in male patients (Fig. 46–8).

Anatomic Considerations

The local anatomic abnormalities in classic exstrophy can be seen in the other variants of the complex. Anomalous development of one system in the fetus frequently results in defects in other body systems, apparently because the causal agent interferes with normal development at multiple embryonic sites. In bladder exstrophy, most anomalies are related to defects of the abdominal wall, bladder, genitalia, rectum, and anus (Fig. 46–9). In unpublished data, Charrios observed the following coexisting anomalies in 12 of 43 children with classic bladder exstrophy: two multiple skin hemangiomas, two corneal opacities, three renal

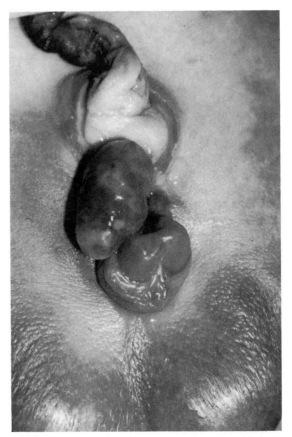

Figure 46–8. Covered exstrophy with isolated ecotpic bowel segment present on the inferior abdominal wall, just above the penis. (Courtesy of Dr. Frank Cerniglia.)

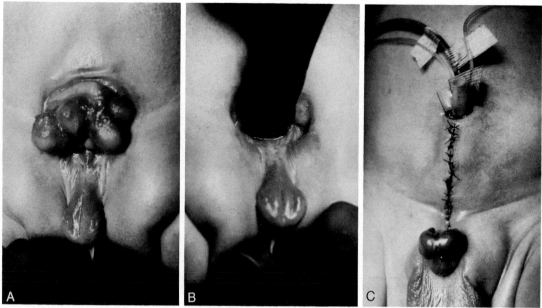

Figure 46–9. Male exstrophy. *A,* At presentation. *B,* With bladder indented. *C,* Following primary closure.

anomalies, one hemihypertrophy, one clubfoot, one pectus excavatum, one case of epilepsy, and one chylothorax. Gross and Cresson (1952) described seven cases of spina bifida, five of omphaloceles, three of rectovesical fistulas, two of rectoperineal fistulas, and three of myelomeningoceles in their series of 80 bladder exstrophy cases. It is difficult to determine whether cases of cloacal exstrophy were included in this series. This relatively high incidence of spinal cord and rectal anomalies has not been observed in our experience. Children presenting with bladder exstrophy are frequently robust, full-term babies with the anomalous development confined to structures adjacent to the cloacal membrane.

Musculoskeletal Defects

All cases of exstrophy have the characteristic widening of the symphysis pubis caused by the outward rotation of the innominate bones, in relation to the sagittal plane of the body, along both sacroiliac joints. In addition, an outward rotation or eversion of the pubic rami at their junction with the ischial and iliac bones occurs. Another component is present in more severe cases of exstrophy, namely, a lateral separation of the innominate bones inferiorly, with the fulcrum at the iliosacral joint (Fig. 46–10). It is these rotational deformities of the pelvic skeletal structures that may contribute to a short, pendular penis. The outward rotation and lateral displacement of the innominate bones also account for the increased distance between the hips, the waddling gait, and the outward rotation of lower limbs of these children, which, in itself, causes little disability.

A waddling gait develops secondary to the external rotation of the lower extremities, resulting from the posterolateral position of the acetabula (Cracchiolo and Hall, 1970). The wide and waddling gait, although noticeable when the child begins to walk, soon corrects itself and leaves no orthopedic problems. Reapproxi-

mation of the divergent pubis, therefore, does not provide any functional musculoskeletal advantage.

The triangular defect caused by the premature rupture of the abnormal cloacal membrane is occupied by the open bladder. The fascial defect is limited inferiorly by the intersymphyseal band, which represents the divergent urogenital diaphragm. The anterior sheath of the rectus muscles, seeking midline attachment, has a fanlike extension behind the urethra and bladder neck, which inserts into the intersymphyseal band.

At the upper end of the triangular defect and bladder is the umbilicus. In bladder exstrophy, the distance between the umbilicus and the anus is always foreshortened. Because the umbilicus is situated well below the horizontal line of the iliac crest, there is an unusual expanse of uninterrupted abdominal skin. Although an umbilical hernia is always present, it is usually of insignificant size. The umbilical hernia should be repaired at the time of the abdominal wall closure. Omphaloceles are rarely associated with bladder exstrophies; however, they are frequently associated with cloacal exstrophy. The omphaloceles associated with exstrophy-epispadias complex are usually small and can be closed when the bladder is closed.

Ruptured omphaloceles require immediate surgical attention. A large omphalocele may be treated conservatively by painting it with antiseptic solution, which promotes skin overgrowth, or the omphalocele can be covered with skin flaps (Haller, 1974). We have managed two large omphaloceles in cloacal exstrophy patients, which required these special considerations before the bladder exstrophy itself could be closed. The frequent occurrence of indirect inguinal hernias is attributed to persistent processus vaginalis, large internal and external inguinal rings, and lack of obliquity of the inguinal canal. An inguinal hernia should be treated at the time of presentation, and it requires both excision of the hernial sac and repair of the transversalis fascia and muscle defect to prevent recurrence or direct hernia.

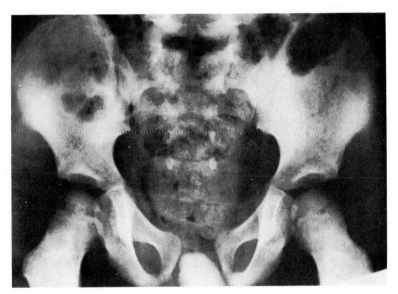

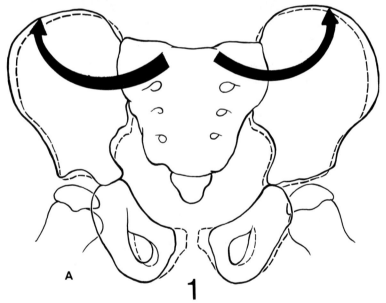

Figure 46–10. Rotational and lateral deformities of the pelvic girdle in cases of exstrophy. *A*, (1) Widening of the symphysis caused by outward rotation of the innominate bones, usually the only skeletal abnormality present in epispadias.

Illustration continued on following page

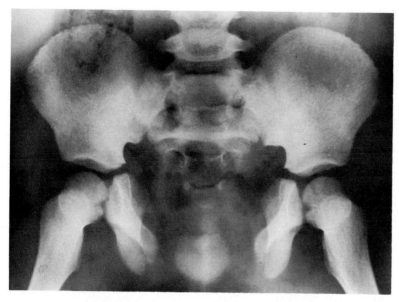

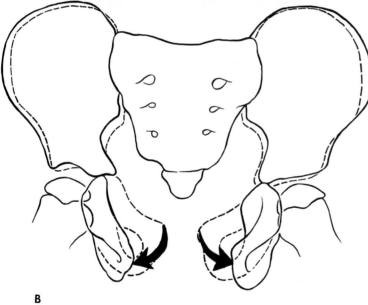

Figure 46–10 *Continued B,* (1 + 2) An additional external (outward) rotation of the pubic bones: the characteristic skeletal changes in classic forms of exstrophy.

B

1+2

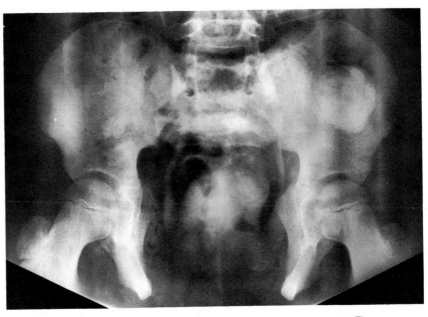

Figure 46–10 *Continued C,* (1 + 2 + 3) The final addition of lateral inferior separation of the innominate bones present in the extreme manifestation of complex cloacal exstrophy.

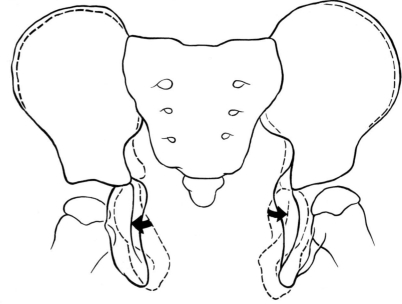

C

1+ 2+ 3

Anorectal Defects

The perineum is short and broad. The anus, situated directly behind the urogenital diaphragm, is displaced anteriorly and corresponds to the posterior limit of the triangular fascial defect. The anal canal may be stenotic and rarely ends ectopically in a rectovaginal or perineal fistula. Anal stenosis is usually treated by dilatation; however, anoplasty is required for the rare rectovaginal fistula. The anal sphincter mechanism is also anteriorly displaced, and it should be preserved intact in case internal urinary diversion should be required in future patient management.

The divergent levator ani and puborectalis muscles and the distorted anatomy of the external sphincter contribute to varying degrees of anal incontinence and rectal prolapse. Anal continence is usually imperfect at an early age. In some patients, the rectal sphincter mechanism may never be adequate to control liquid content of the bowel. Rectal prolapse frequently occurs in untreated exstrophy patients with a widely separated symphysis. It is usually transient and reduced without difficulty. Rectal prolapse is frequently exacerbated by the child's straining and crying, which causes discomfort of the irritated, exposed bladder. Prolapse virtually always disappears after bladder closure or cystectomy and urinary diversion. The appearance of prolapse is indication to proceed with definitive management of the exstrophied bladder.

Male Genital Defects

The male genital defect is severe and may be the most troublesome aspect of the surgical reconstruction, independent of the decision to treat by staged closure or by urinary diversion (Fig. 46–11). The individual corpus cavernosum in bladder exstrophy is usually of normal caliber; however, the penis appears foreshortened because of the wide separation of the crural attachments, the prominent dorsal chordee, and the shortened ure-thral groove. The urethral groove may be so short and the dorsal chordee so severe that the glans becomes located adjacent to the verumontanum. A functional and cosmetically acceptable penis can be achieved when the dorsal chordee is released, the urethral groove lengthened, and the penis is lengthened by mobilizing the crura in the midline. Duplication of the penis and unilateral hypoplasia of the glans and corpus are rare variants, which further complicate surgical management (Fig. 46–12). A patient with a very small or dystrophic penis should be considered for sex reassignment. The need for sex reassignment in classic exstrophy occurred only once in 150 cases in our experience.

The vas deferens and ejaculatory ducts are normal, provided that they are not injured iatrogenically (Hanna and Williams, 1972). Testicular function has not yet been comprehensively studied in a large series of postpubertal exstrophy patients, but it is generally believed that fertility is not impaired. The autonomic innervation of the corpus cavernosum is provided by the cavernous nerves. The cavernous nerves normally course along the posterolateral aspect of the prostate, traversing the urogenital diaphragm along or within the membranous urethra (Walsh and Donker, 1982). These autonomic nerves are displaced laterally in patients with exstrophy (Schlegel and Gearhart, 1989) because potency is preserved following functional bladder closure, penile lengthening, and dorsal chordee release. Retrograde ejaculation may occur following functional bladder closure, because the internal sphincter remains patent. The testes frequently appear undescended in their course from the widely separated pubic tubercles to the flat, wide scrotum. Most testes are retractile and have an adequate length of spermatic cord to reach the scrotum without the need for orchiopexy.

Female Genital Defects

Reconstruction of the female genitalia presents a less complex problem than reconstruction of the male geni-

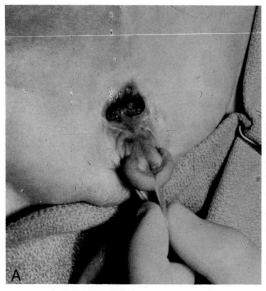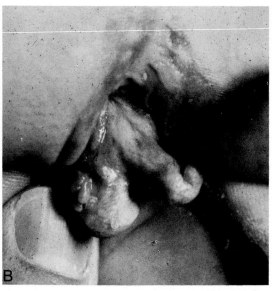

Figure 46–11. Difficult genital reconstruction. *A,* Short penis and very small bladder. *B,* Duplex penis.

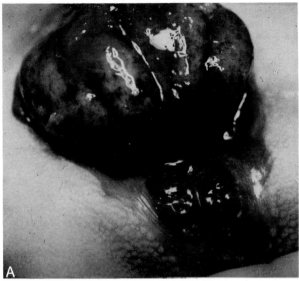

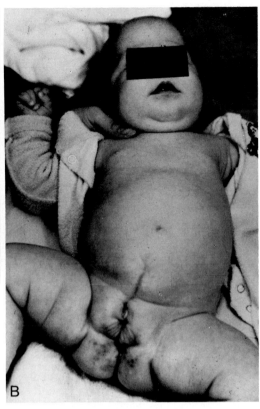

Figure 46–12. *A,* Male exstrophy with rudimentary penis. *B,* Reconstructed and raised as female.

talia (Fig. 46–13). The urethra and vagina are short; the vaginal orifice is frequently stenotic and displaced anteriorly; the clitoris is bifid; and the labia, mons pubis, and clitoris are divergent. The uterus, fallopian tubes, and ovaries are normal except for occasional uterine duplication. Approximation of the clitoral halves in the hair-bearing skin of the mons pubis provides satisfactory cosmetic restoration of the external genitalia (Dees, 1949). Vaginal dilatation or episiotomy may be required

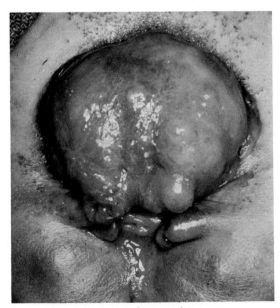

Figure 46–13. Female exstrophy.

to allow satisfactory intercourse in the mature female patient. The defective pelvic floor may predispose mature female patients to uterine prolapse, making uterine suspension necessary. Uterine prolapse does not appear to occur when osteotomy and closure of the anterior defect are performed early in life.

Urinary Defects

At birth, the bladder mucosa may appear normal; however, ectopic bowel mucosa or an isolated bowel loop may appear on the bladder surface. Abnormal histology was observed in each of 23 bladder specimens obtained from individuals between the ages of 1 month and 52 years with exstrophy. Squamous metaplasia, cystitis cystica, cystitis glandularis, and acute and chronic inflammation were commonly identified in these exstrophied bladder specimens (Culp, 1964).

Scanning and transmission electron microscopy of human exstrophied bladders have demonstrated microvilli and the absence of surface ridges on the uroepithelial cells (Clark and O'Connell, 1973). The abnormal histologic features demonstrated by both light and electron microscopy may represent chronic mucosal changes secondary to persistent infection.

The size, distensibility, and neuromuscular function of the exstrophied bladder as well as the size of the triangular fascial defect to which the bladder muscles attach affect the decision to attempt functional closure. When the bladder is small, fibrosed, and inelastic, functional closure may be impossible. The more normal bladder may be invaginated or may bulge through a small fascial defect, indicating the potential for satisfactory capacity.

The exstrophied bladder may be incapable of normal detrusor function because normal bladder function was achieved in only 22 per cent of closed exstrophies (Nisonson and Lattimer, 1972). Persistent reflux and chronic infection may account for the apparent detrusor insufficiency observed in this series. Bladder function was assessed in a group of continent closed exstrophy patients, and normal reflexive bladders and normal electromyograms were obtained in 70 per cent and 90 per cent of cases, respectively (Toguri et al., 1978). Muscarinic cholinergic drugs, such as propantheline bromide (Pro-banthine) and bethanechol chloride (Urecholine), clinically and experimentally affect bladder muscle function. Shapiro and associates (1985), using radiolig- and receptor binding techniques, demonstrated that exstrophied and normal control bladders contained similar levels of muscarinic cholinergic receptors.

The upper urinary tract is usually normal, but anomalous development does occur. Horseshoe kidney, pelvic kidney, hypoplastic kidney, solitary kidney, and dysplasia with megaureter have all been observed in these patients. The ureters have an abnormal course and termination. The peritoneal pouch of Douglas between the bladder and rectum is enlarged and unusually deep, forcing the ureter downward and laterally, in its course across the true pelvis. The distal segment of the ureter approaches the bladder from a point inferior and lateral to the orifice, entering the bladder with little or no obliquity. Therefore, reflux in the closed exstrophied bladder occurs in nearly 100 per cent of cases and requires subsequent surgery. Terminal ureteral dilatation frequently appears on pyelograms and is usually the result of edema, infection, and fibrosis of the terminal ureter acquired after birth.

Surgical Management: Historical Considerations

The first description of exstrophy of the bladder appears on an Assyrian tablet from 2000 B.C., which is preserved in the British Museum in London. No other written reference occurs until Scheuke von Grafenberg describes it in 1597, which may indicate a rather drastic treatment of newborn anomalies in ancient times. In 1849, Mackay and Syme advocated the application of an external urinary receptacle. Syme performed the first successful ureterosigmoid anastomosis in 1852; but 9 months later, the patient died of ascending pyelonephritis. Carl Thiersch covered the bladder with lateral flaps, obtaining a bladder capacity of 100 ml. Successful urinary diversion began with Karl Maydle (1874), who transplanted the trigone into the rectum. Ureterosigmoidostomy began with Coffey's method, but infection and acidosis caused severe complications until the introduction of mucosa-to-mucosa anastomosis by Nesbit in 1949 and the combined tunnel and mucosa technique of Leadbetter in 1955.

Functional Bladder Closure: Primary Bladder Neck Closure and Bladder Neck Reconstruction

Trendelenburg (1906) attempted to achieve urinary continence by sacroiliac synchondrosis and bladder closure with narrowing of the patulous urethra. Trendelenburg attributed the lack of success with this procedure to subsequent lateral displacement of the pubis. After Trendelenburg's report, sporadic successes were reported by Burns (1924) and Janssen (1933).

Young (1942) reported the first successful functional closure for bladder exstrophy in a female patient. A narrow strip of posterior urethral mucosa was selected, the mucosa lateral to the posterior urethra was excised, the posterior urethral strip was tubularized, and the neourethra was reinforced with denuded detrusor muscle. The bladder was inverted and closed, and the abdominal wall defect was closed with fascial flaps. The patient eventually developed a 3-hour continent interval; however, preservation of renal function was not mentioned. Marshall and Muecke (1970) reviewed 329 functional bladder closures reported in the literature between 1906 and 1966 and determined that urinary continence with preservation of renal function was achieved in only 16 cases (5 per cent). Dehiscence of the abdominal wall and bladder, urinary fistula, incontinence, persistent reflux, and pyelonephritis frequently resulted in subsequent urinary diversion. A report from Montagnani (1988) revealed that eight patients remained incontinent after bladder closure, osteotomy, bladder neck reconstruction with bilateral ureteral reimplantation, and single-stage urethral reconstruction. However, among this group, there were no cases of dehiscence or prolapse of the bladder. This finding is likely attributed to the fact that osteotomy was performed at the time of functional bladder closure. Over the past 20 years, modifications in the management of functional bladder closure have contributed to a dramatic increase in the success of the procedure. The most significant changes in the management of bladder exstrophy are as follows: (1) staging the reconstructive procedures, (2) performing bilateral osteotomies, (3) reconstructing a competent bladder neck, and (4) defining strict criteria for the selection of patients suitable for this approach.

Bladder Neck Reconstruction

Dees (1949) modified the Young technique for reconstructing the bladder neck for complete epispadias. A triangular wedge of tissue was removed from the roof and lateral aspect of the proximal urethra as well as adjacent bladder wall, including a portion of each lateral lobe of the prostate gland. The remaining posterior urethral mucosal strip was tubularized, and the neourethra was reinforced with adjacent denuded muscle. Leadbetter (1964) considered that the length and the tone of the muscular reinforcement of the neourethra contributed to the achievement of urinary continence. The Dees procedure was modified by tubularizing a posterior urethral strip, 3.5 cm long, which included trigonal mucosa, and the neourethra was reinforced with the trigonal muscle. Bilateral ureteroneocystostomies were performed to allow greater length of the urethral strip. A posterior urethral strip of this length may be excessive because urethral pressure profilometry in a series of continent bladder exstrophy patients demonstrated that continence can be achieved with a functional closure pressure as low as 20 cm of H_2O pressure and a continence length as low as 0.6 cm of H_2O (Toguri et al., 1978). The median functional closure pressure and continence length in this group of continent exstrophies were 40 cm of H_2O and 1.35 cm of H_2O, respectively. Gearhart and Jeffs (1987), utilizing intraoperative urodynamics, showed that a continence length of 25 to 35 mm and a closure pressure of greater than 60 cm H_2O intraoperatively were adequate for eventual postoperative continence.

Osteotomy

Schultz (1964) combined primary bladder closure with bilateral iliac osteotomies. The efficacy of iliac osteotomies is still somewhat controversial. The primary arguments against osteotomy are as follows: (1) the pubis retracts eventually, (2) the penis retracts farther, and (3) continence can be achieved without osteotomies (Marshall and Muecke, 1970). The advantages of bilateral iliac osteotomies include the following: (1) reapproximation of the symphysis diminishes the tension on the abdominal closure and eliminates the need for fascial flaps; (2) placement of the urethra within the pelvic ring reduces the excessive urethrovesical angle and permits urethral suspension after bladder neck plasty; and (3) reapproximation of the urogenital diaphragm and approximation of the levator ani may aid in eventual urinary control, and after pubic approximation with osteotomy, some patients show the ability to stop and start the urinary stream (Gearhart and Jeffs, 1989; Jeffs et al., 1982).

Ezwell and Carlson (1970) observed that urinary diversion was subsequently performed in 20 per cent of functional closures in patients who had undergone osteotomies, whereas 75 per cent of those who had not undergone osteotomies during bladder closure eventually required urinary diversion. Of patients referred to our institution following partial or complete dehiscence, 90 per cent had not undergone an osteotomy (Lowe and Jeffs, 1983). Our recommendation is to perform bilateral iliac osteotomy when primary bladder closure is performed after 72 hours of life. In addition, if the pelvis is not malleable or if the pubic bones are unduly wide at the time of the examination using anesthesia, osteotomy should be performed even if the closure is performed before 72 hours of age.

STAGED SURGICAL RECONSTRUCTION OF BLADDER EXSTROPHY

The disadvantage of performing the entire surgical reconstruction of bladder exstrophy as a single-stage procedure is that one complication jeopardizes the entire repair. Sweetser and co-workers (1952) described a staged surgical approach for bladder exstrophy. Bilateral iliac osteotomies were performed 4 to 6 days prior to bladder closure. Epispadias repair was performed as a separate procedure. The continence procedure was limited to freeing the fibrous intersymphyseal band and wrapping this band around the urethra at the time of closure. A staged approach to functional bladder closure that includes three separate stages (bladder closure, bladder neck reconstruction with an antireflux procedure, and epispadias repair) has been recommended for most cases of exstrophy reconstruction beginning in the early 1970s (Cendron, 1971; Gearhart and Jeffs, 1989; Jeffs et al., 1972; Williams and Keaton, 1973).

Patient Selection

Treatment of exstrophy by functional closure demands that the potential for success in each child be considered at birth (Fig. 46–14). Size and functional capacity of the detrusor muscle are important considerations in the eventual success of functional closure. The correlation between apparent bladder size and potential bladder capacity must not be confused. In minor grades of exstrophy that approach the condition of complete epispadias with incontinence, the bladder may be small yet may demonstrate acceptable capacity either by bulging when the baby cries or by indenting when touched by a gloved finger (Chisholm, 1962). Stimulation of the bladder by a stream of cold water will indicate the ability of the detrusor muscle to contract and relax, proving its functional integrity. Once removed from surface irritation and repeated trauma, the small bladder will enlarge and will gradually increase its capacity, even in the absence of continence or outlet resistance. The exstrophied bladder that is estimated at birth to have a capacity of 3 ml or more and that demonstrates elasticity and contractility may be expected to develop a useful size and capacity following successful closure.

Small Bladder Unsuitable for Closure

A small, fibrotic bladder patch that is stretched between the edges of a small triangular fascial defect without either elasticity or contractility cannot be selected for the usual closure procedure. Examination using anesthesia may at times be required to adquately assess the bladder, particularly if considerable edema, excoriation, and polyp formation have developed between birth and time of assessment. The elasticity of the bladder can be demonstrated in this way, and the size of the triangular fascial defect can be appreciated by simultaneous abdominal and rectal examination. A neonatal closure, even when the bladder is small, allows for later assessment of bladder potential and provides an initial step in genital reconstruction, which is helpful in gaining acceptance by the family. Other conditions that preclude primary closure include the following: penile-scrotal duplication, ectopic bowel within the ex-

Conditions Not Functional For Functional Closure

Exstrophy c̄ ectopic bowel

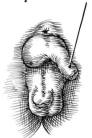

Hypoplastic left sided bladder

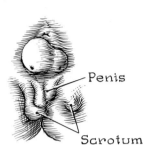

Penis

Scrotum

Small bladder patch

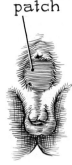

Penile-Scrotal duplication

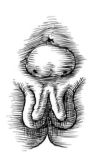

Hydroureteronephrosis

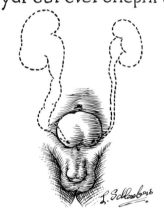

Figure 46–14. Classic exstrophy bladders that may not be suitable for functional closure. (Drawings by Leon Schlossberg.)

strophied bladder, hypoplastic bladder, and significant hydronephrosis.

A review by Oesterling and Jeffs (1987) showed that of 51 patients treated solely at one institution, only one required initial diversion instead of primary closure. However, there will be patients, for reasons mentioned previously, who cannot undergo closure primarily. In most cases, there is no need at birth for management. Later, options for the management of these patients include excision of the bladder and nonrefluxing colon conduit. Another more appealing alternative is urinary diversion and placement of the small bladder inside to be used later for a posterior urethra in an Arap-type procedure. Additionally, one could wait for several months to see if the bladder plate did increase in size. I have seen this in one patient; after 6 to 12 months, the bladder increased in size and primary closure was effected. Lastly, augmentation cystoplasty at the time of initial closure is not recommended.

Delivery Room and Nursery

The disappointment and sense of tragedy that attend the birth of any deformed child affects the obstetric staff, nursery staff, pediatrician, and most of all, the parents. Usually, the child with bladder exstrophy is the

first such patient that the obstetrician and nursing staff have seen. The family practitioner and pediatrician may have seen a case during training or during lengthy practice, but they cannot be considered experts. The counseling of the parents and decisions regarding eventual therapy should be made by surgeons with special interest and experience in managing cases of bladder exstrophy. This is especially true regarding the sex of rearing of boys with bladder exstrophy. We have worked with several families who were made even more distraught by being told that the child also needed a change in gender. The need for changing the sex of rearing is extremely rare in the male child born with bladder exstrophy.

At birth, the bladder mucosa is usually smooth, thin, and intact; it is also sensitive and easily denuded. In the delivery room, the umbilical cord should be tied with nylon or Dexon sutures relatively close to the abdominal wall so that the umbilical clamp or long cord does not traumatize the bladder mucosa and cause excoriation of the bladder surface. The bladder may be covered with a nonadherent film of Saran Wrap or other plastic film to prevent the mucosa from sticking to clothing or diapers. Standard varieties of Vaseline gauze become dry and lift off the delicate mucosa when they are removed.

At this stage, the parents need reassurance. An awareness that renal function, ambulation, sexual function, and fertility in bladder exstrophy patients can certainly approach normal will help. The parents should know that a carefully considered decision by an experienced surgeon concerning the management of urinary storage, drainage, and control will be made as soon as possible. The parents can then begin to understand the implications of the problem and help with the medical and social decisions that need to be made. They will also be relieved to learn that the expectation of bladder exstrophy recurring in future offspring is low and that patients with exstrophy rarely produce children with the exstrophy-epispadias complex (Shapiro et al., 1985).

The social services offered by the hospital can be a great help to the parents in facing the family problems resulting from prolonged hospitalization of the child and the financial strain of unexpected medical care, family separation, and home-to-hospital travel. An advantage of these patients being treated at a large medical center, where there is expertise in the treatment of bladder exstrophy, is the fact that several exstrophy support groups now exist, which help provide personal help and housing for the parents.

Early Management

Cardiopulmonary and general physical assessment can be carried out in the first few hours of life. Immediate intravenous pyelographic assessment of the kidneys in the newborn may lack clarity and detail. Radionuclide scans and ultrasound studies can provide evidence of renal function and drainage, even in the first few hours of life.

Circumstances may be less than ideal at birth; however, a neonatal assessment may have to be deferred until transportation to a children's medical center can be arranged. Generally, no child is more than a few hours away from a neonatal center with full diagnostic and consultative services. During travel, the bladder should be protected by a plastic membrane (not Vaseline gauze) to prevent contact of dressing or clothing with the delicate newborn bladder mucosa.

Operative Procedure

The primary objective in functional closure of classic bladder exstrophy is to convert the exstrophy to a complete epispadias with incontinence while preserving renal function. Secondarily, the best management for the incontinence and epispadias will be determined in a later stage or stages (Table 46–1).

Osteotomy

When patients are seen within the first 48 hours of life, the bladder and pelvic ring closure can be carried out without osteotomy because of the malleability of the pelvic ring (Ansell, 1983). However, when the separation is unduly wide or when delay in referral occurs and the patient is not seen until he or she is

several days of age or older, osteotomy will be required to achieve anterior closure of the pelvic ring. Osteotomy should be carried out at the same time as bladder closure. A well-coordinated surgical and anesthesia team can carry out osteotomy and proceed to bladder closure without undue loss of blood or risk of prolonged anesthesia. However, osteotomy along with bladder closure is a 5- to 7-hour procedure in these patients.

Two separate approaches are currently being used for osteotomy in the exstrophy group: posterior bilateral iliac osteotomy and anterior bilateral transverse innominate osteotomy. Both of these approaches, when well performed, can improve symphyseal approximation in the exstrophy patient. With appropriate approximation, distress on the midline abdominal closure is lessened. Also, in our experience, the dehiscence rate is lower if osteotomies are performed (Gearhart and Jeffs, 1990; Oesterling and Jeffs, 1987). In addition, pubic closure allows approximation of the levator and puborectile sling, inclusion of the bladder neck and urethra within the pelvic ring, and improved eventual continence rate (Gearhart and Jeffs, 1989; Oesterling and Jeffs, 1987).

Several reports have demonstrated experience with an anterior approach through the innominate bone just above the acetabulum (Gokcora et al., 1989; Montagnani, 1988; Sponseller et al., 1990). Although our experience with posterior iliac osteotomy reveals no failure of initial closures, we are disappointed with the poor mobility of the pubis, the occasional delayed union or malunion of the ilium, and most importantly the need to turn the patient from the prone to the supine position. Initially, our interest in anterior osteotomy was in those patients who had failed an initial exstrophy closure with or without prior posterior iliac osteotomy (Fig. 46–15A) (Sponseller et al., 1990). The results with that approach were so satisfactory that anterior innominate osteotomy is now being used for primary closures of bladder exstrophy. The anterior iliofemoral approach to the pelvis was performed similar to that of a Salter osteotomy. Both sides were exposed simultaneously and a horizontal innominate anterior osteotomy was performed using a Gigli saw. If the patient is younger than 6 months, an oscillating saw was used instead of a Gigli saw (Sponseller et al., 1990). The level of the osteotomy is from 5 mm above the anterior-inferior iliac spine to the most cranial part of the sciatic notch in order to leave a sizeable inferior segment for fixation. An external fixator is commonly used, and the pins are inserted before wound closure (Fig. 46–15B). A horizontal mattress suture of No. 2 nylon is placed between the fibrous cartilage of the pubic rami and tied anterior to the pubic closure at the time of bladder closure. If the suture works loose or cuts through the tissues during subsequent healing, the anterior placement of the knot in the horizontal mattress suture ensures that it will not erode into the urethra and interfere with the bladder or urethral lumen.

Posterior iliac osteotomy is still utilized in several medical institutions and is performed through bilateral incisions over the sacroiliac region. The posterior iliac osteotomy is performed vertically and close to the midline to allow the two wings of the pelvis to hinge and

Table 46–1. INITIAL PRESENTATION AND MANAGEMENT OF PATIENTS WITH EXSTROPHY OF BLADDER

Age	Problem	Possible Solution
Initial Presentation		
0–72 hours	Classic exstrophy with reasonable capacity and moderate symphyseal separation; long urethral groove; mild dorsal chordee	I: Midline closure of bladder, fascia, and symphysis to level of posterior urethra; no osteotomy
0–72 hours	Abovementioned findings with short urethra and severe dorsal chordee	II: Close as in I, adding lengthening of dorsal urethral groove by paraexstrophy skin (cautiously)
0–72 hours or late presentation	Abovementioned findings with very wide separation of symphysis or late presentation of patient (beyond 72 hours up to 1–3 years) for initial treatment	Osteotomy (posterior or anterior) and closure as in I or II
0–2 weeks	Male, penis duplex or extremely short	Consider female sex of rearing and closure as in I or II
0–2 weeks	Very small, nondistensible bladder patch	Prove by examination under anesthesia, then nonoperative expectant treatment awaiting internal or external diversion
Incontinent Period After Initial Closure		
1 month–3 years	Infection with residual resulting from outlet stenosis	Urethral dilatation, occasional meatotomy or bladder neck revision
	Infection, grade III reflux, with pliable outlet resistance	Continuous antibiotic suppression with plan for early ureteroneocystostomy
	Partial dehiscence at bladder neck or partial prolapse of bladder (both prevent bladder capacity increase)	Reclosure of bladder neck with osteotomy and epispadias repair if older than 1 year of life
Continence and Epispadias Repair		
2½–5 years	Closed bladder with incontinence, normal intravenous pyelogram, bladder capacity 60 ml or more (under anesthesia), bilateral reflux, good penile size and length of urethral groove	Plan bilateral ureteroneocystostomy, bladder neck reconstruction, epispadias repair followed by 3 weeks of suprapubic drainage; prepare 5 weeks and 2 weeks before operation with two injections of testosterone in oil, 2 mg/kg
2½–5 years	Same as abovementioned but with small bladder capacity, less than 60 ml (under anesthesia)	Epispadias repair only after preparation with testosterone; bladder capacity will improve postoperatively
	Epispadias repaired, capacity greater than 60 ml	Proceed to bladder neck plasty and ureteroneocystostomy
	Epispadiac penis, short with severe chordee, before or after bladder neck reconstruction	Correction of chordee, lengthening of urethral groove, and epispadias repair; prepare with testosterone; consider osteotomy to aid in achieving increased penile length
3 years and older	Completed repair of bladder, bladder neck, and epispadias with dry interval but wet pants	Patience, biofeedback, oxybutynin chloride (Ditropan), imipramine, and time (up to 2 years)
	Abovementioned with marked stress incontinence and good bladder capacity	Wait—may require bladder neck revision or endoscopic injection or possible artificial sphincter
	Small capacity bladder unchanged by time, epispadias repair, or attempted bladder neck reconstruction	Consider augmentation cystoplasty and bladder neck reconstruction; acceptance of intermittent catheterization with abdominal or urethral access may be necessary
3–7 years	Late presentation of untreated exstrophy, unsuitable for closure	Consider temporary diversion by colon conduit with plan to undivert to bladder using bladder to form urethra and conduit for augmentation; in patients older than 7 years, artificial sphincter or continent diversion can be considered
3–7 years	Small closed exstrophy unsuitable for bladder neck reconstruction or augmentation	Consider permanent external or internal diversion; internal diversion direct by ureterosigmoidostomy or indirect by colocolostomy; evaluate day continence of anal sphincter and nighttime seepage before surgery
5–15 years	Closed exstrophy with epispadias repaired with uncontrolled stress or dribbling incontinence	Consider (1) revision of bladder neck reconstruction, (2) endoscopic injection, (3) augmentation and bladder neck revision, (4) artificial sphincter with omental wrap, and (5) continent diversion
10–20 years	Closed exstrophy with inadequate penis	Consider penile lengthening, urethral reconstruction using free graft, pedicle grafts, and tissue transfer
10–20 years	Diverted exstrophy with inadequate penis	As abovementioned or penile lengthening without urethral reconstruction (prostatic fistula at base)

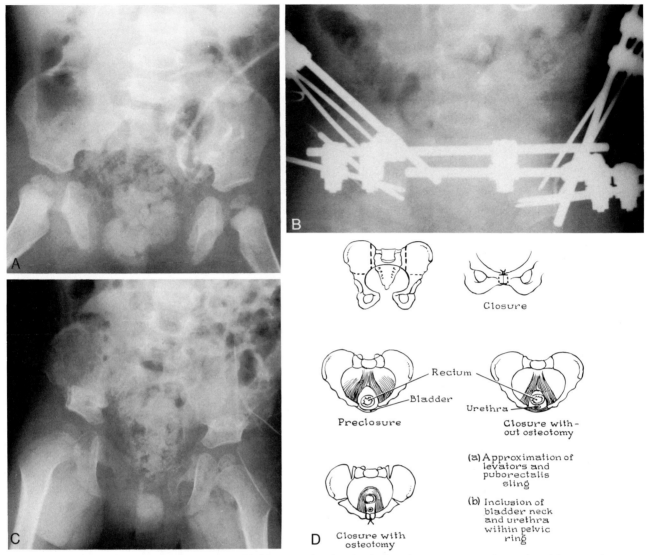

Figure 46–15. *A,* Eight-month-old patient with classic bladder exstrophy closed at birth without osteotomy with complete dehiscence first seen at 8 months. *B,* Patient after having undergone anterior innominate osteotomy with placement of intrafragmentary pins and external fixator. *C,* The same patient 4 months after removal of external fixator and infragramentary pins. No dehiscence was observed with this closure. *D,* The technique of posterior iliac osteotomy or anterior innominate osteotomy showing the incision site and advantages of either approach.

come together without anterior-to-posterior flattening of the true pelvic ring (Fig. 45–15*D*). Success of posterior osteotomy is demonstrated in the review by Andalen and co-workers (1980). Among 100 patients who underwent posterior iliac osteotomy, for those who achieved symphyseal approximation of less than 2 cm, there was a higher continence rate than for those who achieved pubic diastasis greater than 2 cm.

Whether posterior or anterior osteotomy is performed, the pelvic ring closure not only allows midline approximation of the abdominal wall structures but also allows levator ani and puborectalis muscles to lend potential support to the bladder outlet, thereby adding resistance to urinary outflow (Fig. 45–15*C,* D). Furthermore, the incontinence procedure can be carried out on the bladder neck and urethra within the closed pelvic ring at a distance from the surface and freed from independent movement of the two halves of the pubis. When the urethra and bladder neck are set more normally in the true pelvis, they represent a more natural relationship with the vertical axis of the bladder rather than having an acute angulation.

Postoperatively, both bladder exstrophy patients undergoing closure without osteotomies in the first 48 hours of life and patients receiving posterior osteotomies are immobilized by modified Bryant's traction. Adhesive skin traction is used with the patient in a position in which the hips have 90 degrees of flexion and the knees are slightly bent to protect the arterial tree. When modified Bryant's traction is chosen, the traction is left in place for 3 to 4 weeks (Fig. 46–16). If anterior osteotomy has been performed, an external fixator is applied with light Buck's traction for 2 weeks to maintain comfort and bed rest. External fixation is continued for 6 weeks, and the fixation is removed.

Bladder and Prostatic Urethra Closure

The various steps in primary bladder closure are illustrated in Figure 46–17. A strip of mucosa, 2-cm

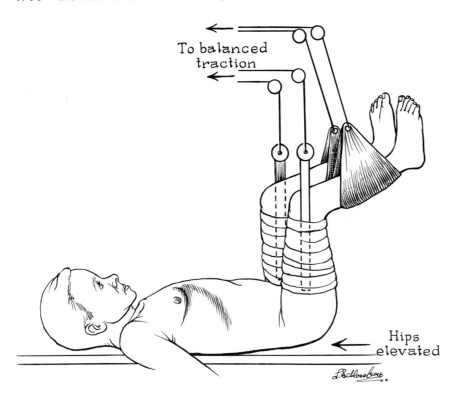

To balanced traction

Hips elevated

Figure 46–16. Modified Bryant's traction used for postoperative immobilization after osteotomy and initial bladder closure. (Drawing by Leon Schlossberg.)

wide, extending from the distal trigone to below the verumontanum in the male and to the vaginal orifice in the female, outlines prostatic and posterior urethral reconstruction. The male urethral groove length may be adequate, and no transverse incision of the urethral plate need be made for urethral length. However, when the length of the urethral groove from the verumontanum to the glans is so short that it interferes with eventual penile length, the urethral groove is elongated after the manner of Johnston (1974) or Duckett (1977).

The diagrams indicate that an incision is made outlining the bladder mucosa and the prostatic plate (Fig. 45–17C, D). The urethral groove is transected distal to the verumontanum, but continuity is maintained between the thin, mucosa-like, non–hair-bearing skin adjacent to the posterior urethra and bladder neck and the skin and mucosa of the penile shaft and glans. Flaps from the area of thin skin are subsequently moved distally and rotated to reconstitute the urethral groove, which may be lengthened by 2 to 4 cm. Further urethral lengthening can then be performed at the time of epispadias repair by the method of Cantwell (1895) and Ransley and associate (1989).

Penile lengthening is achieved by exposing the corpora cavernosum bilaterally and freeing the corpora from their attachments to the suspensory ligaments and the anterior part of the inferior pubic rami. If the mucosal plate has been transected, the partially freed corpora are joined in the midline; the bare corpora are covered with flaps of the thin paraexstrophy skin, which are rotated medially to be attached to the distal mucosa of the posterior plate (Fig. 46–17E through 46–17I). These flaps are inward rotation flaps and not long paraexstrophy skin flaps running up the lateral aspect of the exstrophied bladder. The urethra in the female patient usually does not require lengthening at the time of closure.

Bladder closure proceeds by excision of the umbilical area. The redundant skin adjacent to the superior aspect of the bladder mucosa is discarded, and the bladder muscle is freed from the fused rectus sheaths on each side. This dissection is facilitated by exposing the peritoneum above the umbilicus and carefully dissecting extraperitoneally, to enter the retropubic space on each side from above. The wide band of fibers and muscular tissue representing the urogenital diaphragm is detached subperiostally from the pubis bilaterally. The dissection must be extended onto the inferior ramus of the pubis to allow the bladder neck and posterior urethra to fall back and achieve a position deep within the pelvic ring. Reluctance to free the bladder neck and urethra well from the inferior ramus of the pubis will certainly move the neobladder opening cephalad, if any separation of the pubis occurs during healing. The mucosa and muscle of the bladder and posterior urethra are closed in the midline anteriorly. This orifice should accommodate a 14-Fr. sound comfortably. The size of the opening should allow enough resistance to aid in bladder adaption and to prevent prolapse but not enough outlet resistance to cause upper tract changes. The posterior urethra and bladder neck are buttressed with a second layer of local tissue if possible (Fig. 46–17J through 46–17M).

The bladder is drained by a suprapubic Malecot catheter for a period of 3 to 4 weeks. The urethra is *not* stented in order to avoid pressure necrosis or the accumulation of infected secretions in the neourethra. Ureteral stents provide drainage during the first 7 to 10 days when swelling or the pressure of closure of a small bladder may obstruct the ureters and give rise to obstruc-

Text continued on page 1795

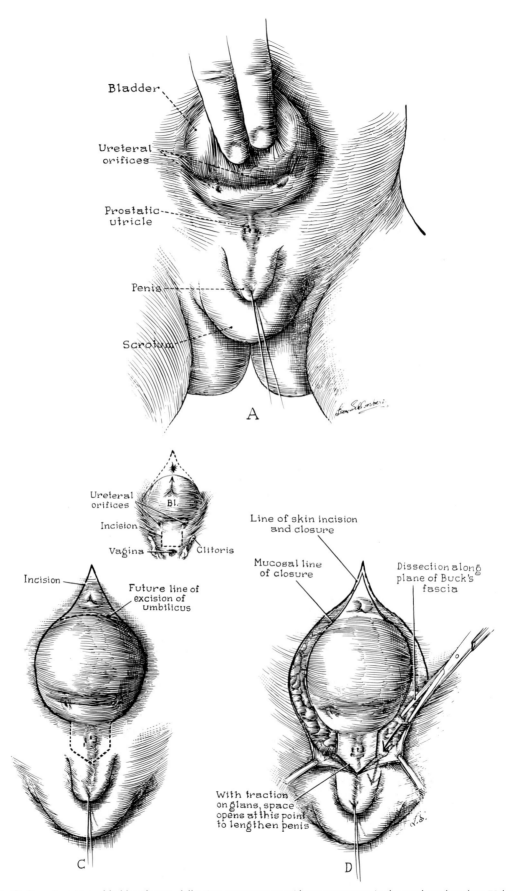

Figure 46–17. *A to O,* Steps in primary bladder closure, following osteotomy or without osteotomy, in the newborn less than 72 hours of age. *A, B, C,* and *D* depict the incision line around the umbilicus and bladder down to the urethral plate. If the male urethral groove is adequate no transverse incision is made in the urethral plate or initial urethral lengthening.

Illustration continued on following page

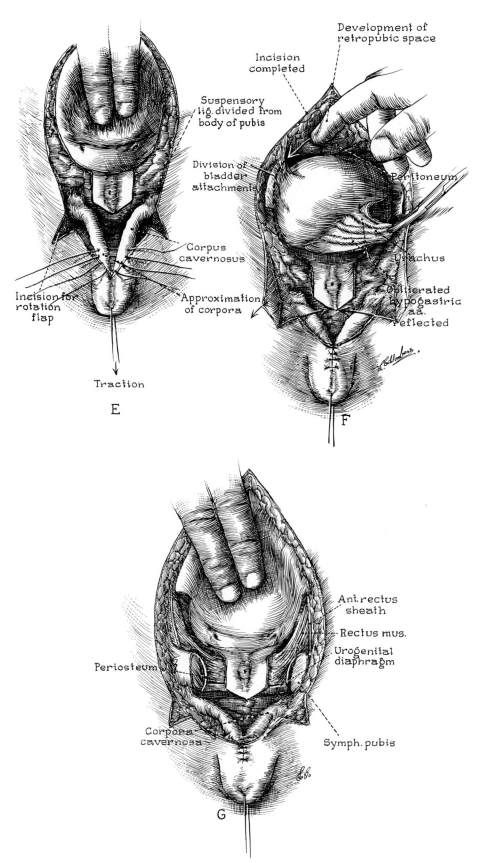

Figure 46–17 *Continued E,* Lateral skin incisions allow rotation of paraexstrophy skin to cover the elongated penis if the urethral groove has been transected. *F,* Development of the retropubic space from below the area of umbilical dissection to facilitate separation of the bladder from the rectus sheath and muscle. *G,* Medial fan of rectus muscle attaching behind the prostate to the urogenital diaphragm. The urogenital diaphragm and anterior corpus are freed from the pubis in a subperiosteal plane.

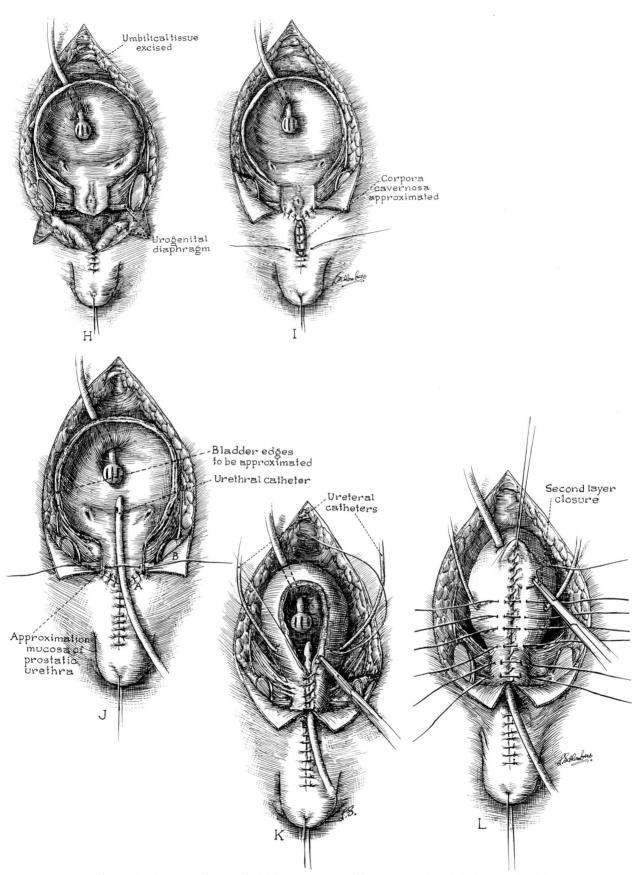

Figure 46–17 *Continued H to L depict the anastomosis of the paraexstrophy skin to the prostatic plate.*

Illustration continued on following page

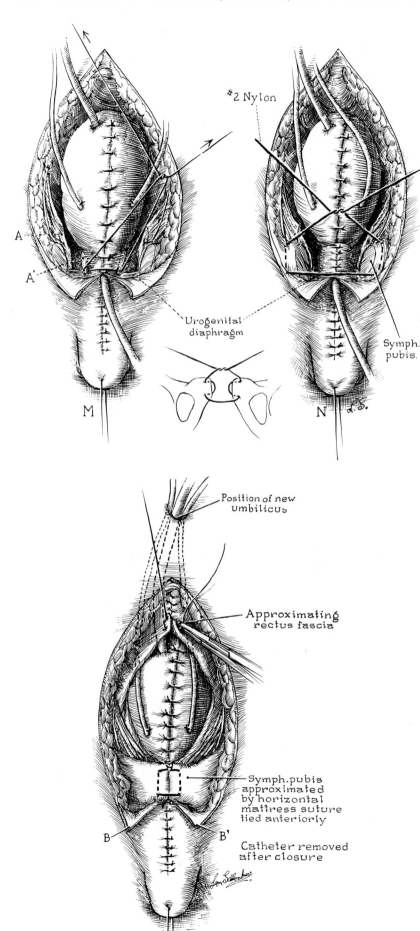

#2 Nylon

A

A'

Urogenital
diaphragm

M

N

Symph.
pubis.

Position of new
umbilicus

Approximating
rectus fascia

Symph. pubis
approximated
by horizontal
mattress suture
tied anteriorly

Catheter removed
after closure

B   B'

O

Figure 46–17 *Continued M,* Urogenital diaphragm is closed with a separate layer of sutures if possible. Oftentimes, this will not be possible. *N,* Horizontal mattress suture tied on external surface of symphysis while assistant applies medial rotation of greater trocanters. *O,* Approximation of skin point B to B1 provides an anterior step from penile closure to abdominal wall closure. (Drawings by Leon Schlossberg.)

tion and transient hypertension. If no problems with the stents occur during healing, we leave the stents in place for up to 2 weeks. When the bladder and urethra have been closed and the drainage tubes placed, pressure over the greater trocanters bilaterally allows the pubic bones to be approximated in the midline. Horizontal mattress sutures are placed in the pubis and tied with the knot away from the neourethra (Fig. 46–17N, O). Oftentimes, we are able to use another stitch or two of No. 2 nylon as the most caudal stitches in the rectus fascia, which may help add to the security of the pubic closure. A V-shaped flap of abdominal skin at a point corresponding to the normal position of the umbilicus is tacked down to the abdominal fascia, and the drainage tubes exit this orifice.

Before and during this procedure, the patient is given broad-spectrum antibiotics in an attempt to convert a contaminated field into a clean surgical wound. Nonreactive sutures of Dexon and nylon are selected to avoid undesirable reactions or abscesses.

Management After Primary Closure

The procedure described converts exstrophy into complete epispadias and incontinence. Prior to removal of the suprapubic tube 4 weeks postoperatively, the bladder outlet is calibrated by urethral catheter or urethral sound or by cystoscopy to ensure free outlet drainage. An intravenous pyelogram (IVP) is obtained to record the status of the renal pelvis and ureters, and appropriate urinary antibiotics are administered to treat any bladder contamination that may be present after removal of this suprapubic tube. Residual urine is estimated by straight catheterization, and cultures are obtained before the patient leaves the hospital and at subsequent intervals to detect infection and to ensure adequate drainage. If the initial IVP shows good drainage, upper tract imaging by ultrasound is repeated 3 months after hospital discharge. These will be repeated at intervals of 6 months to 1 year during the next 2 to 3 years to detect any upper tract changes caused by reflux or infection. Prophylactic antibiotics should be continued at least through the first 6 months and as necessary thereafter. If bladder outlet resistance is such that urine is retained within the bladder, and reflux and ureteral dilatation develop with infected urine, it may be necessary to dilate the urethra or occasionally to begin intermittent catheterization. If bladder outlet resistance persists, an antireflux procedure may be required as early as 6 months to 1 year after the initial bladder closure. If a useful continent interval has resulted from the initial closure, no further operation for incontinence may be required, but this situation is rare.

In the case converted from exstrophy to complete epispadias with incontinence, the bladder gradually increases in capacity, and inflammatory changes in the mucosa resolve. Cystograms using *anesthesia* at 2 to 3 years of age will indicate bilateral reflux in nearly 100 per cent of patients and will provide an estimate of bladder capacity. Even in the completely incontinent patient, bladder capacity gradually increases to the point at which the bladder can be distended at cystography to a capacity of 50 to 60 ml. In some patients with very small bladders, bladders may require 4 to 5 years to achieve this capacity.

A tight bladder closure, urinary tract infection, and reflux may cause uncontrollable ureteral dilatation. If severe upper tract changes occur, surgical revision of the bladder outlet by advancing skin flaps into the orifice may be necessary to prevent scarring and further obstruction. Judgment is required to know when to abort attempts at functional closure and to turn to urinary diversion as a means of preserving renal function. This change of plan is seldom necessary if an adequate outlet has been constructed at initial closure and if careful attention has been paid to details of follow-up.

Penile and Urethral Reconstruction in Exstrophy

Formerly, we performed bladder neck reconstruction prior to urethral and penile reconstruction. However, the significant increase in bladder capacity after epispadias repair in those patients with extremely small bladder capacities prompted a change in our management program (Gearhart and Jeffs, 1989). In this group of patients with small bladders, after initial closure, there was a mean increase in capacity of 55 ml after only 22 months. Construction of the neourethra, further penile lengthening, and dorsal chordee release are performed between 2 and 3 years of age. Because the majority of boys with exstrophy have a somewhat small penis and a shortage of available penile skin, most of our patients undergo testosterone stimulation prior to urethroplasty and penile reconstruction (Gearhart and Jeffs, 1988).

Many surgical techniques have been described for reconstruction of the penis and urethra in patients with classic bladder exstrophy. Four key concerns must be addressed to ensure a functional and cosmetically acceptable penis: (1) dorsal chordee, (2) urethral reconstruction, (3) glandular reconstruction, and (4) penile skin closure.

Although it is possible to achieve some penile lengthening with release of chordee at the time of initial bladder closure, it is often necessary to perform formal penile elongation with release of chordee at the time of urethroplasty in exstrophy patients (Fig. 46–18). Certainly, all remnants of the suspensory ligament and old scar tissue from the initial bladder closure must be excised. Also, further dissection of the corpora cavernosa from the inferior pubic ramus can be achieved. It is often surprising how little was done at the time of initial exstrophy closure (Gearhart and Jeffs, 1989). Lengthening of the urethral groove is also essential. Regardless of whether paraexstrophy skin flaps were used at the time of bladder closure, further lengthening will be needed. This technique can be as simple as Cantwell's (1895) original principle involving transection of the urethral plate and replacement with other genital tissues (Hendren, 1979; Horton and Devine, 1980; Monfort et al., 1987; Thomala and Mitchell, 1984; Vyas et al., 1987).

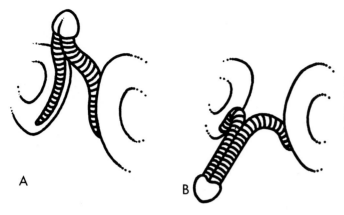

Figure 46–18. *A,* An important factor in the pathogenesis of the penile shortness is the separation of the pubes. *B,* Lengthening is obtained by partial detachment of the crura from the puboischial rami so that the extra penile parts of the corpora cavernosa can be advanced into the shaft.

Furthermore, to release dorsal chordee, one can lengthen the dorsomedial aspect of the corpora by incision and anastomosis of the corpora (Ransley et al., 1989) or placement of a dermal graft to allow lengthening of the distal aspect of the corpora (Brzezinski et al., 1986; Woodhouse and Kellett, 1984). Another technique to improve dorsal chordee prior to urethroplasty is shortening or medial rotation of the ventral corpora (Koff and Eakins, 1984). Osteotomy initially or repeated with approximation of the inferior pubis ramus may correct lateral drift of the pubis with subsequent shortening and curvature of the phallus (Schillinger and Wiley, 1984).

Urethral reconstruction is an important aspect of external genitalia reconstruction in exstrophy. This procedure can be accomplished by many previously reported methods. Tubularization of the dorsal urethral groove as a modified Young urethroplasty is currently our preference when there is sufficient penile skin for both construction and coverage of the neourethra. Nonetheless, interposition of a free graft of genital skin, extragenital skin, or even bladder mucosa can be used (Hendren, 1979; Horton and Devine et al., 1980; Vyas et al., 1987). In addition, ventral transverse island flaps and double-faced ventral island flaps have been employed with some success for urethral reconstruction in exstrophy patients (Monfort et al., 1987; Thomalla and Mitchell, 1984).

Free graft and island graft techniques have the advantage that the entire urethral reconstruction can be done in one stage, even with a limited amount of penile skin. However, the foreskin is certainly smaller in exstrophy patients than in those with hypospadias, and the complication rate can be quite high (Monfort et al., 1987). After construction, the urethra can be mobilized almost completely and transferred to the ventrum of the penis under the separated corpora. Ransley and colleagues (1989) have modified and refined this concept in exstrophy and epispadias patients with success.

Although it is not currently in common use, the two-stage method of urethral reconstruction has been utilized for epispadias associated with bladder exstrophy (Michalowski and Modelski, 1963). This method may have limited application in those patients with a significant paucity of penile skin and in those for which there is hesitation to use extragenital skin grafts or even bladder

mucosa. Also important in the reconstruction of the genitalia in exstrophy is the management of the glans penis. A ventral meatotomy is important to move the urethral meatus to a more normal position and to ensure a good urinary stream. Mucosal triangles from the inner aspect of the splayed glans are removed so that local raw surfaces will coapt over the neourethra. Vertical mattress sutures keep the coapted glans together while healing takes place and are removed in 10 days to prevent any additional glans scarring.

Skin closure remains a problem in genital reconstruction because of the paucity of skin in this condition. A Z-plasty incision and closure at the base of the penis prevent skin contraction and upward tethering of the penis. The ventral foreskin can be split in the midline and brought to the dorsum as lateral preputial flaps for coverage. If the flaps are made a bit assymetric, a staggered dorsal suture line results with less upward tethering. Also, a buttonhole can be made in the ventral foreskin and simply transferred to the dorsum for additional skin coverage. As a last resort, with minimal remaining skin for coverage, burying the penis under a bridge of scrotal skin for temporary skin coverage could be effected.

As stated, our preference for urethroplasty in the exstrophy patient when the urethral groove has adequate length is the modified Young procedure. The modified Young urethroplasty is begun by placing a nylon suture through the glans, which provides for traction of the penis (Fig. 46–19*A* through 46–19*K*). Incisions are made over two parallel lines, previously marked on the dorsum of the penis, that outline an 18-mm strip of penile skin extending from the prostatic urethral meatus to the tip of the glans. Triangular areas of the dorsal glans are excised adjacent to the urethral strip, and the glandular flaps are constructed. The lateral skin flaps are mobilized, and a Z incision over the suprapubic area permits exposure and division of the remaining suspensory ligaments and old scar tissue. The urethral strip is outlined and the edges are mobilized for closure if no further lengthening is required. The urethral strip is then closed in a linear manner from the prostatic opening to the glans over a No. 10 Silastic stent with 6-0 polyglycolic acid sutures.

A ventral meatotomy has already been made in the glans to move the urethral meatus to a more ventral

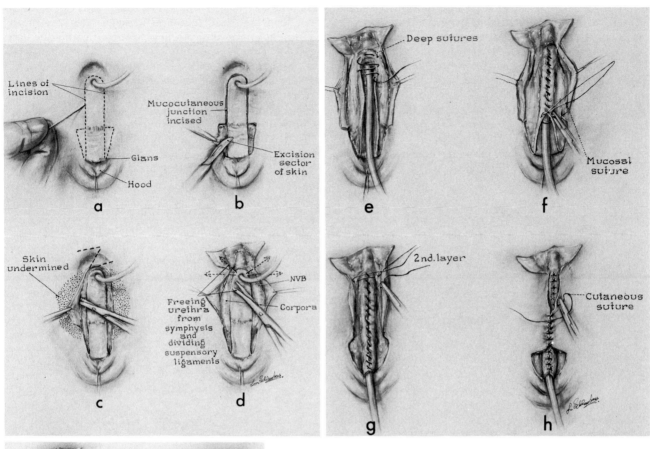

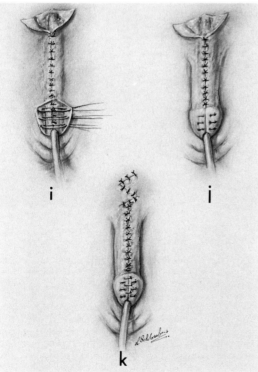

Figure 46–19. *A* to *K*, Modified Young's urethroplasty for repair of epispadias when the urethral groove is of sufficient length naturally or following a lengthening procedure. (Drawings by Leon Schlossberg.)

position. The glans is then reapproximated with vertical mattress sutures of 4-0 Prolene, and these sutures are removed in 10 days. Small pieces of a soft vessel loop are applied under both the knot and the loop of these sutures to prevent pressure necrosis of the glandular tissue and scarring secondary to edema. The Z-plasty is closed with interrupted 6-0 polyglycolic acid suture. Several 6-0 polyglycolic acid sutures are inserted between the Prolene sutures in the glans for proper skin approximation. A No. 10 Silastic stent is left indwelling in the neourethra as a stent and sewn to the glans with a Prolene stitch. Drainage occurs through the stent at low pressure and may be further ensured by a percutaneously placed suprapubic tube. If there is abundant subcutaneous tissue and the urethra is not to be trans-

ferred below the corporal bodies, the subcutaneous tissue is simply closed with two separate continuous layers of 6-0 polyglycolic acid suture. Occasionally, when there is a copacious ventral foreskin, part of this can be denuded and used as an extra layer over the urethra suture line. The skin is reapproximated with interrupted 5-0 polyglycolic acid sutures.

One problem with the Young procedure is that it may not give adequate support to the reconstructed neourethra. However, at this stage, if further lengthening or correction of dorsal chordee is required, the method of Cantwell-Ransley can be employed (Fig. 46–20A through 46–20J). The urethral strip is approached from below when one is seeking additional urethral lengthening (Fig. 46–20E). The urethral strip is mobilized,

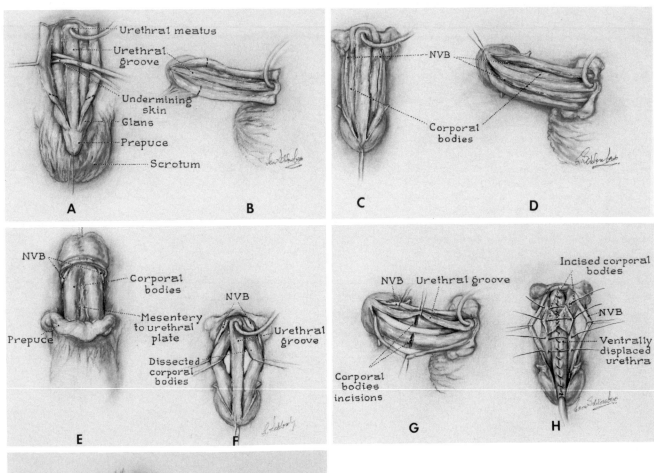

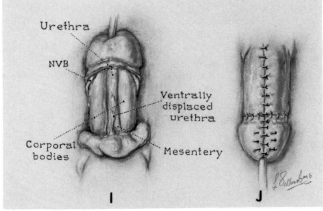

Figure 46–20. *A* to *J*, *A* and *B*, Marking an incision of the urethral groove and mobilization of the penile skin. *C* and *D*, Incision of the glans and exposure of the neurovascular bundles. *E* and *F*, Separation of the urethral groove from the corporal bodies with dissection initially started from below. *G* and *H*, Mobilization of neurovascular bundles from corporal bodies and incision in corporal bodies. Closure of urethral groove to tip of penis, closure of corporal incision displacing urethra ventrally. Further sutures placed distally to further bury urethra under corporal bodies. *I* and *J*, Completed repair with urethra below corporal bodies and skin closure of penis. (Drawings by Leon Schlossberg.)

and the neurovascular bundles are freed up bilaterally (Fig. 46–20*F*); vessel loops are utilized to retract them laterally (Fig. 46–20*G*). The urethra is then closed and transferred below the corporal bodies. Matching incisions are made in the medial aspect of the corporal bodies, and these are sewn together with 5-0 polydioxanone suture (PDS) (Fig. 46–20*G, H*). This not only causes a downward deflection of the penis but also helps bury the urethra under the corporal bodies (Fig. 46–20*I*). After transferring the urethra to the ventrum and closing the corpora above, the rest of the maneuvers proceed as the Young procedure (Fig. 46–20*J*).

Incontinence and Antireflux Procedures

The bladder capacity is measured using anesthesia, after the child reaches the 3rd year of life. If the bladder capacity is 60 ml or greater, bladder neck reconstruction can be planned. The incontinence and antireflux procedures are illustrated in Figure 46–21*A* through 46–21*I*. The bladder is originally opened through a transverse incision at the bladder neck, but a vertical extension is used (Fig. 46–21*A*). The midline closure of this incision narrows the width of the bladder neck area and enlarges the vertical dimension of the bladder, which in exstrophy is often short. The illustration depicts a Cohen (1975) type of transtrigonal advancement procedure for correcting reflux in which a new hiatus lateral to the original orifice is selected prior to advancing the ureter across the bladder above the trigone. Also, the ureter can be taken in a more cephalad direction, the cephalotrigonal reimplant (Fig. 46–21*B, C*) (Canning et al., 1989). In addition, if the ureters are low on the trigone and there is a need to move the ureteral hiatus higher on the trigone, the hiatus is simply cut in a cephalad direction and cross-trigonal reimplants are performed on the upper aspect of the trigone (Fig. 46–21*C*).

The procedure for incontinence is begun by selecting a posterior strip of mucosa 15 to 18 mm wide and 30 mm long that extends distally from the midtrigone to the prostate or posterior urethra (Fig. 46–21*D, E*). The bladder muscle lateral to this mucosal strip is denuded of mucosa. It is often helpful at this juncture to use 1:200,000 epinephrine–soaked sponges to aid in the control of bleeding and in the visualization of the denuded area. Tailoring of the denuded lateral triangles of bladder muscle is aided by multiple small incisions in the free edges bilaterally, which allow the area of reconstruction to assume a more cephalad position. The edges of the mucosa and underlying muscle are formed into a tube by interrupted sutures of 4-0 polyglycolic acid (Fig. 46–21*F*). The adjacent denuded muscle flaps are overlapped and sutured firmly in place with 3-0 polyglycolic acid sutures to provide reinforcement of the bladder neck and urethral reconstruction (Fig. 46–21*G*). An 8-Fr. urethral stent may be employed as a guide during urethral reconstruction but is removed after the bladder neck reconstruction is complete.

Somewhat radical dissection of the bladder, bladder neck, and posterior urethra is required within the pelvis and from the posterior aspect of the pubic bar to provide enough mobility for the bladder neck reconstruction. This maneuver allows for subsequent anterior suspension of the newly created posterior urethra and bladder neck. If visualization of this area is problematic, the intersymphyseal bar can simply be cut, thus providing a widened field of exposure (Peters and Hendren, 1988). This bar is simply closed again with heavy sutures of PDS. Patient mobility should be restricted postoperatively to allow proper healing of the intersymphyseal bar.

Urethral pressure profiles can be obtained intraoperatively to measure continence length and urethral closure pressures. Retrospective comparisons of these values with subsequent success or failure in producing continence serve as guidelines for reconstructing the bladder neck. Our experience with intraoperative urodynamics shows that an intraoperative continence length of 2.5 to 3.5 cm is desirable (Gearhart et al., 1986). Also, intraoperative closure pressures ranging between 70 and 100 cmH$_2$O are required to prevent leakage when the bladder pressure is raised to 50 cm H$_2$O intraoperatively (Gearhart et al., 1986). At the end of the procedure, the bladder neck reconstruction is further enhanced by suspending the urethra and bladder neck to the structures of the pubis and anterior rectus sheath in the manner of Marshall-Marchetti-Krantz (Marshall et al., 1949) (Fig. 46–21*I*). Profiles taken after this stage of the procedure indicate that additional increases in continence length and closure pressures are achieved with this suspension. The continence length increases by at least 1 cm, and the closure pressure is at least doubled in all patients (Gearhart et al., 1986). Undoubtedly, the measurements of continence length and urethral closure pressure will be considerably less in eventual follow-ups when stretching occurs and swelling and edema subside.

Ureteral stents are placed in the reimplanted ureters and the bladder is drained by a suprapubic catheter, which is left indwelling for a 3-week period. Suprapubic catheter drainage prevents stretching or pressure on the reconstructed bladder neck. No urethral stent is used, and catheterization or instrumentation through the urethra is strictly avoided for a minimum of 3 weeks. The adequacy of bladder neck reconstruction is tested by water manometer at the end of the procedure. The bladder neck should support 50 cm of H$_2$O pressure, without leakage if the bladder neck plasty and suspension are adequate. Immediate revision is advisable when this degree of resistance is not obtained. Attempts are made to reduce postoperative frequency and severity of bladder spasms by the use of propantheline bromide (Pro-banthine), oxybutynin chloride (Ditropan), diazepam (Valium), or imipramine hydrochloride (Tofranil).

Patients are given intravenous antibiotics for 7 days to prevent infection. Prophylactic antibiotics are begun and continued for the foreseeable future. Little or no leakage of urine should occur through the urethra during the 3 weeks of suprapubic drainage. Prior to removal of the suprapubic catheter, a clamp is applied to initiate voiding. The urethra is calibrated with a soft 8-Fr. catheter. Cultures are taken so that medication may be

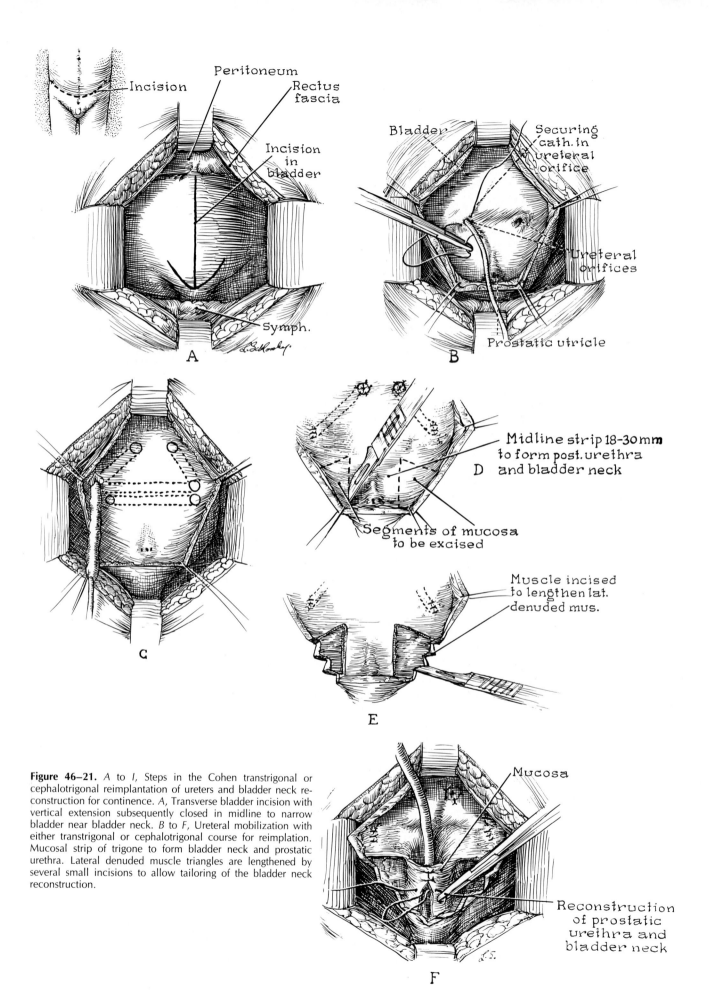

Figure 46–21. *A* to *I*, Steps in the Cohen transtrigonal or cephalotrigonal reimplantation of ureters and bladder neck reconstruction for continence. *A*, Transverse bladder incision with vertical extension subsequently closed in midline to narrow bladder near bladder neck. *B* to *F*, Ureteral mobilization with either transtrigonal or cephalotrigonal course for reimplantation. Mucosal strip of trigone to form bladder neck and prostatic urethra. Lateral denuded muscle triangles are lengthened by several small incisions to allow tailoring of the bladder neck reconstruction.

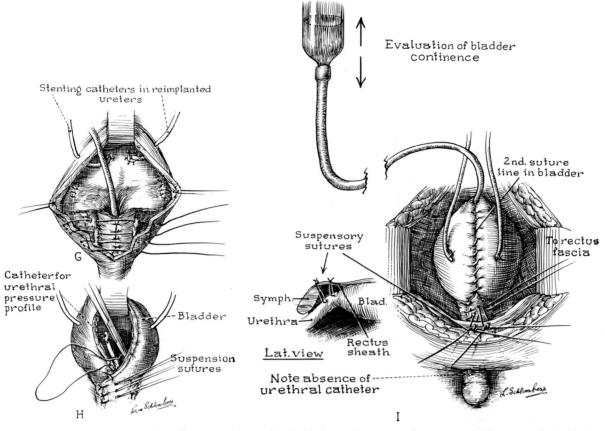

Figure 46–21 *Continued G to H,* These illustrations depict the double-breasted nature and exact suture placement of the bladder neck reconstruction. A pressure profile catheter can be left, and can be urethral pressure profile can be obtained prior to closure of the bladder dome. Suspension sutures are elevated manually to estimate the final urethral pressure profile. *I,* Bladder neck and urethra unstented. Drainage is by ureteral catheters and suprapubic tube. Bladder outlet resistance is estimated by water manometer. (Drawings by Leon Schlossberg.)

given to clear any bacterial contamination. In some patients, immediate voiding after suprapubic clamping will not occur. Occasionally, an infant cystoscope will be needed to help "find the way." Oftentimes, at this juncture, a soft 8-Fr. Foley-Dover catheter is left in place for 24 to 48 hours to help dilate the passage. It is mandatory that there be catheterizable access through the urethra and bladder neck before the suprapubic tube is removed. In some patients, a period of intermittent catheterization may be required if reasonable bladder emptying does not occur.

When the catheter is removed, a short dry interval is expected to occur. Bladder size and operative reaction may allow a capacity of no more than a few milliliters initially. Patients have to learn to recognize bladder

filling and to initiate a detrusor contraction, which they may not have previously experienced. A readjustment period occurs that may extend for many months before a useful bladder volume and long dry interval develop. Initially, the absence of stress incontinence or continuous urethral dribbling suggests that urethral resistance has been produced and that an increasing dry interval will occur. The patient learns to use this interval profitably for daytime and, later, nighttime continence.

RESULTS

Staged Functional Closure

Current reviews of functional bladder closure in bladder exstrophy have demonstrated dramatic improve-

Table 46–2. URINARY CONTINENCE FOLLOWING FUNCTIONAL BLADDER CLOSURE

Series*	No. of Closures Evaluated	Patients Who Became Continent	
		Number	%
Chisholm (1979)	95	43	45
Mollard (1980)	16	11	69
Jeffs (1982)	55	33	60
Ansell (1983)	23	10	43
Husmann and colleagues (1989a)	80	60	75
Connor and associates (1988)	40	33	82
Canning and co-workers (1989)	67	51	75

*Only personal series (one or two surgeons only) reporting continence rates greater than 40 per cent are included.

ments in the frequency of successful reconstructions. Several series (Ansell, 1983; Jeffs, 1979; Mollard, 1980; and Chisholm, 1979), have shown the success and applicability of the staged functional closure approach to bladder exstrophy. Series by Connor and co-workers (1988), Hussman and colleagues (1988), and Canning and associates (1989) have shown most acceptable continence rates with preservation of renal function in the majority of patients (Table 46–2).

Primary Bladder Closure

Of 68 consecutive patients with bladder exstrophy referred to our pediatric urology service between 1972 and 1989, 67 underwent bladder closure (Canning et al., 1989). One patient had a small bladder patch unsuitable for bladder closure and underwent primary urinary diversion. The complications following primary bladder closure and the additional surgical procedures required to correct these complications are presented in Table 46–1. The importance of a successful initial closure has been emphasized by Oesterling and Jeffs (1987) and by Hussman and co-workers (1989a), whereby the onset of eventual continence was quicker and the continence rate was higher in those who underwent a successful initial closure with or without osteotomy. Also, the importance of an early initial bladder closure is emphasized by the data of Hussman and associates (1989), which showed only 10 per cent of those patients who had bladder closure before 1 year of age needed eventual augmentation, whereas 40 per cent of those patients who underwent bladder closure after 1 year of age required eventual bladder augmentation.

Bladder Neck Reconstruction

A total of 75 patients, some of whom underwent initial closure elsewhere, underwent initial bladder neck reconstruction at our institution between 1975 and 1989 (Canning et al., 1989). Current voiding status of each patient was obtained based on parental or patient interview or direct observation by the nursing and physician staff. The patients were noted as spontaneously voiding or on intermittent catheterization and were assigned a continence number as the following: group 1, dry; group 2, dry during the day with occasional nighttime wetting; group 3, dry for greater than 3 hours during the day with occasional nighttime wetting; group 4, dry for more than 3 hours during the day but wet at nighttime; and group 5, wet. Patients in groups 1, 2, or 3 were considered continent, and patients in groups 4 and 5 were defined as intermediately continent and incontinent, respectively.

Fifty-five patients (75 per cent) are continent following bladder neck reconstruction. Twelve patients (16 per cent) are dry for 1 to 2 hours during the day and wet at nighttime, and eight patients (10 per cent) remain totally wet. The majority (84 per cent) are voiding and 12 patients (16 per cent) are on intermittent catheterization (Table 46–3). Renal units from 75 patients have been evaluated by IVP or ultrasound between 6 months and

Table 46–3. URINARY CONTINENCE FOLLOWING 75 INITIAL BLADDER NECK RECONSTRUCTIONS*

Result	Average Daytime Dry Interval (hours)	Patients	
		Number	%
Continent	3	55	75
Intermediate	1–3	12	16
Wet	1	8	10

Of these patients, 63 are voiding and 12 currently empty with intermittent catheterization.

10 years following bladder neck reconstruction to assess the preservation of renal function following the continence procedure. Only two patients have shown significant hydronephrosis and deterioration of renal function. There were 23 complications in 20 patients. Major complications included ureteral obstruction in three patients and bladder outlet obstruction requiring intermittent catheterization or prolonged suprapubic drainage in 14 patients.

Several interesting findings were noted in the bladder neck reconstruction group. Eventual continence was improved in those patients who underwent initial bladder closure before 72 hours of age or after 72 hours of age with an osteotomy, whereas those who underwent closure after 72 hours of age without osteotomy had a very low continence rate (25 per cent). These findings agree with those of Husmann and co-workers (1989), who found that those patients who underwent delayed closure without osteotomy had a significantly lower rate of eventual continence (10 per cent). The continence rate in our group of exstrophy patients compares quite favorably with the data gathered by Husmann and associates (1989) with a continence rate of 75 per cent and to that of Connor and colleagues (1988) with a continence rate of 82 per cent (see Table 46–2). Another important factor is bladder capacity at the time of bladder neck reconstruction. In our series and others, the continence rate is certainly higher in those patients who have an adequate bladder capacity at the time of bladder neck reconstruction (Hussman et al., 1989). Thus, the bladder capacity under anesthesia prior to bladder neck reconstruction is an important predictor of eventual urinary continence.

Half of our patients underwent epispadias repair prior to bladder neck reconstruction. The mean increase in bladder volume was 49.7 ml over a 2-year period. The onset of continence was an interesting time period in this group of exstrophy patients. All but four patients achieved continence within the first 2 years following bladder neck reconstruction. Of a select group of 34 patients included in the group of 75, 23 actually became continent in the 1st year after bladder neck reconstruction.

Urethroplasty

Some 55 patients with bladder exstrophy underwent initial urethral reconstruction at the Johns Hopkins Hospital between 1975 and 1989. A modified Young urethroplasty was performed in 51 patients, a distal urethral free graft in two, a bladder mucosal graft in one, and a ventral preputial pedicle flap in one. The average age at the time of urethral reconstruction was 3.5 years.

Fistulas developed in 21 patients following epispadias repair. One of the fistulas closed spontaneously and 20 required surgical closure (Table 46–4). The majority of these fistulas occurred at the junction of the corona and glans. This area is where there is not only a paucity of skin but also where the most tension lies in the skin closure. A multiple-layered closure is most difficult to achieve at the junction of the corona and glans over the neourethra. At the glans level, broad raw flaps of glans cover the neourethra; proximally, the skin is more redundant and proximal skin flaps can be maneuvered over the proximal shaft (Kramer and Jackson, 1986). However, the coronal sulcus is the weakest point in the repair. Fistulas were closed by excising a small rim of penile skin and separating the fistulous tract from the adjacent penile skin. The urethra is then closed with 6-0 Vicryl suture. Multiple layers of soft tissue are brought together over the urethra to further bolster the repair. Most of these patients have had preoperative testosterone to increase the availability of local penile skin (Gearhart and Jeffs, 1987). The fistulas were all repaired in a separate procedure.

In a review by Lepor and Jeffs (1983), five parameters were evaluated as to their effect on subsequent fistula formation: (1) osteotomy, (2) sequence of bladder neck reconstruction and epispadias repair, (3) hospital of initial treatment, (4) number of prior bladder closures performed, and (5) preoperative hormonal administration. Of 55 patients, 49 (89 per cent) had bilateral osteotomy performed prior to epispadias repair. As in the original series of Lepor and Jeffs (1983), a prior osteotomy appeared to decrease the number of fistulas requiring surgical closure. In this expanded series, more than half of the fistulas occurred in patients without prior osteotomy. The fistula rate was found to be independent of the sequence of bladder neck reconstruction and epispadias repair, the number of prior bladder closures, and the use of hormonal stimulation of the genitalia. In this group of exstrophy patients, if the initial bladder closure was performed elsewhere, the fistula rate after urethroplasty was 53.8 per cent. However, if the initial closure was performed at our institution, the fistula rate was 36 per cent.

In the original report by Lepor and Jeffs, an attempt

Table 46–5. EVALUATION OF GENITAL RECONSTRUCTION IN EXSTROPHY PATIENTS

	Number of Patients	Percentage of Patients
Parents surveyed		
Parents contacted	18	75
Parents not contacted	4	17
Too early to evaluate	2	8
Angulation of penis when standing		
Upward	3	17
Horizontal	9	50
Downward	6	33
Erections		
Documented	15	83
Not documented	3	17
Angulation of penis during erection		
Upward	7	39
Horizontal	7	39
Downward	1	1
No documented erection	3	7
Overall evaluation of penile reconstruction		
Very satisfied	18	100
Satisfied	0	0
Dissatisfied	0	0

From Lepor, H., Shapiro, E., and Jeffs, R. D.: J. Urol., 131:512, 1984.

was made to evaluate the current status of the genital reconstruction from parental interviews (Table 46–5)—49 parents were interviewed. Four parents could not be contacted, and two patients were too early in the postoperative period to be evaluated.

The angulation of the child's flaccid penis when standing was directed downward in 83 per cent of boys. This finding compares favorably with the series of Mesrobian and co-workers (1986) with 18 patients who had undergone primary closure who had a straight penis and a downward angulation in 55 per cent of cases. Erections were witnessed in 83 per cent of the youngsters in the Lepor and Jeffs series (1984). In these individuals, the erect penis was directed upward in 47 per cent, horizontally in 47 per cent, and downward in 6 per cent. Every parent was extremely satisfied with the appearance of the child's penis, although some expressed concern about whether the penis would attain adequate size for sexual intercourse after puberty. In follow-up of a group of postpubertal patients, Mesrobian and colleagues (1986) found that of those postpubertal patients with a straight penis, 86 per cent could achieve satisfactory intercourse; of those with a curved penis, fully half could also have what they quoted as satisfactory sexual intercourse.

A review of staged functional closure of bladder exstrophy at the Johns Hopkins Hospital between 1975 and 1989 clearly demonstrates that secure abdominal wall closure, urinary continence with preservation of the upper urinary tracts, and a cosmetically acceptable penis can be achieved without wound dehiscence, with infrequent deterioration of renal function, and with urethral fistulas that can be surgically repaired. Therefore, it is strongly recommended that all neonates with bladder exstrophy be considered for staged functional bladder closure.

Table 46–4. OPERATIVE COMPLICATIONS FOLLOWING 55 INITIAL URETHRAL RECONSTRUCTIONS

	Incidence	
Complication	Number	%
Fistulas	21	38
Surgical closure	20	36
Spontaneous closure	1	2
Stricture	1	2
Wound distribution	1	2

MANAGEMENT OF PATIENTS WITH TREATMENT FAILURES

Failed Initial Closure

Failure of the initial bladder closure unfortunately does occur. In a study by Lowe and Jeffs (1983), wound infection was noted in cases of dehiscence in 42 per cent of patients. In a series of exstrophy patients reported by Husmann and associates (1989), abdominal distention, bladder prolapse, and loss of diverting catheters before 7 days postoperatively were other risk factors associated with prolapse and dehiscence. In our collective experience, some degree of bladder prolapse occurred in 11 patients and a complete wound dehiscence in 3 of 75 patients (Table 46–6). In the series of Husmann and co-workers (1989), ten of 80 patients had bladder dehiscence after initial closure. In this series, no statistical correlation could be found among the development of bladder dehiscence, age of the child at the time of closure, or performance of osteotomy.

Although not highly significant, the exit site of the drainage tubes was related to dehiscence when they left through the urethra. When faced with a major degree of bladder prolapse or complete dehiscence, the surgeon has three choices: (1) excise the bladder and perform urinary diversion; (2) leave the bladder extruded and close the exstrophy in 4 to 6 months after the inflammation has settled down; and (3) divert the urine, close the small bladder as a urethra, and use the bladder later as part of an Arap procedure. Our preference is to wait an appropriate length of time and to reclose the exstrophy along with anterior iliac osteotomy, even if a prior osteotomy has been performed (Sponseller et al., 1990) (see Table 46–1). We have reclosed 15 patients referred to us with initially failed exstrophy closures in the last 3 years with anterior innominate osteotomies. No patient has suffered a dehiscence.

Failure to Gain Capacity

The staged approach to functional closure of bladder exstrophy has gained increasing popularity during the last several years. However, not all patients gain an adequate capacity for eventual bladder neck reconstruction. A small incontinent bladder with reflux is not an ideal situation for a successful Young-Dees-Leadbetter procedure. If the child does not have a bladder capacity of 60 ml on a gravity cystogram *using general anesthesia* at the time of cystoscopy, then we proceed with epispadias repair. Of 28 patients seen with an inadequate bladder capacity at 3 years of age, 25 increased capacity after epispadias repair and underwent bladder neck reconstruction. The mean interval to obtain bladder capacity was 22 months, and the mean increase in capacity was 55 ml. Similar increases have been reported in incontinent epispadias with small bladders (Peters et al., 1988). The actual mechanism of the increase in capacity without hydronephrosis is unclear. A logical explanation would be gradual bladder adaption at low

Table 46–6. COMPLICATIONS IN 75 PRIMARY BLADDER CLOSURES

	Number
Complication	
Bladder prolapse	11
Outlet obstruction (hydronephrosis)	2
Bladder calculi	2
Renal calculi	1
Wound dehiscence	3
Stitch granuloma	2
Corrective Surgical Procedure	
Repair of bladder prolapse/dehiscence	14
Cystolithopexy	2
Urethrotomy	1
Augmentation cystoplasty	2

pressure to retain increasing volumes of urine during periods of rest, particularly at night. Other methods, such as bladder cycling, have been met with very poor results because of the young age of the patient, lack of cooperation, and leakage from around the catheter. Lastly, even if bladder capacity does not increase to a satisfactory enough level to allow the child to undergo bladder neck reconstruction, any increase in capacity will make subsequent ureteral reimplantation and simultaneous bladder augmentation less difficult to perform (see Table 46–1). Distal urethral revision may increase the capacity in the female patient also.

Unfortunately, even after epispadias repair and waiting until the child is older, not all patients gain an adequate capacity for bladder neck reconstruction. In this group of patients, the main therapeutic option is augmentation cystoplasty. This can be performed as a simple augmentation if outlet resistance is adequate or combined with a bladder neck reconstruction. In a current series, Gearhart and Jeffs (1988) presented 12 patients with bladder exstrophy who required bladder augmentation. Of the 12 patients, 11 are now dry on intermittent catheterization. Only five augmentations were performed for an inadequate bladder capacity before any type of continence procedure had been performed. Most patients had a prior continence procedure and underwent augmentation along with an adjunctive procedure, such as a repeat Young-Dees-Leadbetter, an artificial urinary sphincter, or a transuretero-ureterostomy. Series by Kramer (1989) and Mitchell and Piser (1987) also show the applicability of bladder augmentation to the child with a small bladder associated with the exstrophy condition.

Failed Bladder Neck Reconstruction

Urinary continence, defined as a 3-hour dry interval, is usually achieved within 1 year following bladder neck reconstruction. Delayed achievement of urinary continence has been associated with puberty in the male patient (Kramer and Kelalis, 1982). The increasing urethral length associated with prostatic enlargement may provide additional resistance to urinary outflow. In our experience, patients who do not achieve a 3-hour dry interval within 1 to 2 years following bladder neck reconstruction seldom develop a sufficient continence mechanism. These incontinent individuals may be treated by the following means: (1) repeat Young-Dees-Leadbetter bladder neck reconstruction with or without simultaneous bladder augmentation; (2) tubularization of the remaining bladder into a neourethra and bladder augmentation by colocystoplasty (Arap et al., 1976); (3) artificial urinary sphincter device (Decter et al., 1988); (4) transection of the bladder neck, bladder augmentation, and creation of a catheterizable abdominal stoma; and (5) as a last resort, urinary diversion (see Table 46–1).

A patulous bladder neck with adequate bladder capacity is best managed by repeating the Young-Dees-Leadbetter procedure (Gearhart and Jeffs, 1989). In this series, six of seven patients who underwent repeat Young-Dees-Leadbetter procedure without augmentation are dry for greater than 3 hours and are voiding by way of the urethra. However, the majority of patients who fail initial Young-Dees-Leadbetter procedures typically need bladder augmentation along with a continence procedure (Gearhart and Jeffs, 1989).

Some workers report the use of an artificial urinary sphincter in the patient after a failed bladder neck reconstruction (Decter et al., 1988; Hanna, 1981). Although the continence rate is 90 per cent in those patients in whom the sphincter is working (Decter et al., 1988), the revision and erosion rate is significant. The compromised blood supply to the urethral and periurethral tissues from previous surgical manipulations increases the likelihood for the erosion of the device. We have inserted two artificial urinary sphincters in patients with bladder exstrophy who were referred to our institution following failed bladder neck reconstruction. In one patient, despite insertion and delayed activation of the device in two stages, erosion into the urethra occurred. In another patient, the artificial sphincter was placed around the bladder, which had been revised in the Arap manner, and success was achieved. Similar experiences have been reported with anti-incontinence devices and complete epispadias (Hanna, 1981; Kramer and Kelalis, 1982). The artificial sphincter may be useful in older children who have well-vascularized bladder neck tissues or in those who have a mature omentum that can be interposed between the cuff and the reconstructed bladder neck.

We have currently treated several exstrophy patients with multiple complications, including failed prior bladder neck reconstructions, scarred tortuous urethras, and small bladder capacities. In these patients, a successful outcome was obtained with transection of the bladder neck, augmentation of the bladder, and creation of a continent abdominal stoma (Leonard et al., 1990).

Failed Genital-Urethral Reconstruction

The most common complication in exstrophy patients after urethral reconstruction is a urethrocutaneous fistula occurring in 36 per cent in our current experience. Modern techniques of hypospadias surgery, including optical magnification, de-epithelialized skin flaps, testosterone stimulation, and so forth, can make most of these fistulas straightforward to repair. However, the three most common problems observed in these boys are as follows: (1) need for additional penile length, (2) correction of residual chordee, and (3) unsightly scars on old suture lines.

Certainly, in the young patient, extensive mobilization of the penile skin with or without further dissection of the corpora from the pubic ramus will add some length (see Table 46–1). However, in the adolescent and older patient, this technique alone may not be adequate to gain additional length (Woodhouse, 1989). Through this approach, the corpora can be mobilized more completely from the pubis, and any tethering scar tissue can be excised. We like to use rhomboid flaps (Kramer and Jackson, 1986), because this technique allows good access to the base of the phallus.

The need for additional correction of chordee varies. Mesrobian and associates (1986) found little need for additional correction of chordee in older patients because the majority of patients, even those with a curved penis, could have "satisfactory intercourse." Woodhouse (1989) has a different experience, and may simply be due to better penile lengthening at the time of initial closure and at the time of epispadias repair (Gearhart and Jeffs, 1989). However, patients will be seen who need further corrective procedures. Certainly, even several intraoperative erections may be needed to assess the true curvature of the penis. Cavernosography may also be required preoperatively in the most severe cases (Woodhouse, 1989).

In many cases, the urethra is too short and may have to be transected and replaced with a free graft (Devine and Horton, 1980). If the amount of curvature is not significant after immobilization of all the scar tissue and the corporal bodies, then a Nesbit procedure may correct any remaining upward chordee (Brezinski et al., 1986; Frank et al., 1981). Also, one may use the ventrum of the phallus and perform a Koff corporal rotation procedure to direct the phallus in a more downward manner (Koff and Eakins, 1984). If the amount of remaining chordee is significant, a transverse incision must be made on the dorsum of the penis at the point of greatest curvature. When this procedure needs to be performed, the urethra typically also has to be transected. This incision, when properly performed, will leave an elliptic defect in the tunica albuginea, which must be closed with a graft. Our experience has been only with full-thickness skin grafts or dermal grafts to cover the defect (Brezinski et al., 1986). However, Woodhouse (1986) has employed lyophilized dura mater with good results.

Some older adolescents and adults simply dislike the unsightly scars from suture lines on the phallus. The technique chosen for urethroplasty and penile elongation dictates to a large extent the type of skin coverage remaining on the penis. If there is adequate penile skin, we have simply excised the area and effected a plastic type closure. However, if there is a paucity of skin, enough usually remains to cover most of the shaft. Rhomboid skin flaps (Kramer, 1986) can be used to cover the proximal shaft and corpora. Also, full-thickness skin grafts can be utilized for penile coverage after scar excision.

OTHER TECHNIQUES

Unfortunately, not all children born with bladder exstrophy are candidates for staged functional closure, usually because of small bladder plates or significant hydronephrosis. Additional reasons for seeking other methods of treatment include failure of initial closure with a small remaining bladder and failure of incontinence surgery (see previous section). Therefore, excluding those patients with failure in initial treatment (see preceding section), this discussion deals with options available if staged functional closure is not suitable or for other reasons is not chosen by the surgeon.

Whichever diversion option is chosen, the upper tracts and renal function initially are usually normal. This occurrence will allow the reimplantation of normal-sized ureters in a reliable nonrefluxing manner into the colon or other suitable urinary reservoir. Historically, ureterosigmoidostomy was the first form of diversion to be popularized in the exstoophy patient group. Although the initial series had multiple metabolic problems, when newer techniques of reimplantation of the ureter into the colon came along, the results improved markedly (Leadbetter, 1955; Zarbo and Kay, 1986). Ureterosigmoidostomy is favored by some because of the lack of an abdominal stoma. However, this form of diversion should not be offered until one is certain that anal continence is normal and after the family has been made aware of the potential for serious complications, including pyelonephritis, hyperchloremic acidosis, rectal incontinence, ureteral obstruction, and late development of malignancy (Duckett and Gazak, 1983; Spence et al., 1979; Stockel et al., 1990).

Because of the many complications associated with ureterosigmoidostomy, several alternative techniques of urinary diversion for bladder exstrophy have been described. Maydl (1894) described a method of trigonosigmoidostomy. Boyce and Vest (1952) reviewed 23 trigonosigmoidostomy cases, followed for a mean interval of 10 years. Renal function, assessed by excretory urography, was normal in 21 cases (91 per cent); stones formed in two (9 per cent); and hypokalemic acidosis developed in approximately 50 per cent. However, only a few individuals required chronic alkalinization, and reoperation was performed in only two cases (9 per cent).

All the children achieved daytime continence; overall, 18 cases (78 per cent) were considered to have good results. Kroovand's (1988) update of Boyce's 37-year experience with this procedure shows that the majority of patients had stable upper urinary tracts, minimal leakage, and no electrolyte imbalances or malignant change in the vesicorectal reservoir. The Heitz-Boyer-Hovelaque (1912) procedure included diverting the ureters into an isolated rectal segment and pulling the sigmoid colon through the anal sphincter muscle just posterior to the rectum. Taccinoli and co-workers (1977) reviewed 21 staged Heitz-Boyer-Hovelaque procedures

for bladder exstrophy followed between 1 and 16 years. They reported 95 per cent fecal and urinary continence; no cases of urinary calculi, electrolyte abnormalities, or postoperative mortality; and three patients (14 per cent) who developed ureterorectal strictures requiring surgical revision. Isolated cases treated in North America with this approach have been subject to multiple and severe complications.

The early results following ileal conduit urinary diversions suggested that this technique might be ideal for urinary drainage in bladder exstrophy patients because fecal contamination and acidosis due to reabsorption were avoided. Unfortunately, significant long-term complications developed in children 10 to 15 years following ileal conduit diversion (Jeffs and Schwartz, 1975; Shapiro et al., 1975). Ileal conduit diversion is not acceptable for children with exstrophy, who may have a normal life expectancy (MacFarlane et al., 1979).

As an alternative method of treatment, Hendren (1976) first established an antirefluxing colonic conduit and later undiverted this conduit into the sigmoid colon. The nonrefluxing ureterointestinal anastomosis represents the primary advantage of colon conduits. The colon conduit is constructed at 1 year of age. When anal continence is achieved, and there is no reflux or upper tract deterioration, the conduit is undiverted into the colon at age 4 to 5 years. Sixteen colon conduits and 11 subsequent colocoloplasties were reported by Hendren (1976); the only reported postoperative complications were intestinal obstruction in three cases (19 per cent) and ureteral obstruction in one case (6 per cent). No cases have been reported of stomal complications, persistent reflux, pyelonephritis, or upper tract deterioration in the Hendren series. The long-term assessment of renal function and continence following colon conduit diversion and subsequent colocoloplasty requires further investigation. Despite our preference for primary functional bladder closure for bladder exstrophy, colon conduit urinary diversion represents the most attractive alternative because a nonrefluxing anastomosis is achieved and undiversion can be performed when clinically indicated.

An additional innovative approach by Rink and Retik (1987) was the creation of a nonrefluxing ileocecal segment that can be rejoined to the sigmoid colon. The proximity of the fecal and urinary streams may predispose the child to later risk of malignancy. Leonard has reported the series of Gearhart and Jeffs (1990); success was obtained in these difficult failed exstrophy reconstructions by the use of multiple reconstructive techniques, including the Mitrofanoff and Benchekroun principles along with continent urinary diversion.

Arap and colleagues (1976) managed bladder exstrophy by initially constructing a colon urinary conduit. The entire bladder was subsequently tubularized into a 5- to 6-cm neourethra, and the colon conduit was anastomosed to the urethrovesical tube. This technique may be useful for the patient with a failed Young-Dees-Leadbetter bladder neck procedure and a small contracted bladder or for the initial treatment of a bladder exstrophy when the bladder capacity is less than 3 ml.

The best method for urinary diversion currently in

children is the nonrefluxing colon conduit, which requires an external stoma and appliance. However, techniques of continent urinary diversion are rapidly improving as are the results in the treatment of the bladder exstrophy patient, especially those with an initial failure. However, we believe that the accepted form of treating bladder exstrophy today is the staged functional reconstructive approach. Those patients with small bladders unsuitable for closure, late closures, or multiple closures who do not develop an adequate bladder capacity after the first-stage reconstruction are problematic. These patients are best treated with any of the multiple reconstructive procedures mentioned previously (Leonard et al., 1990).

ASSOCIATED CONCERNS

Growth of Secondary Sex Organs

In the past, it was thought that prostatic growth at puberty would lead to eventual continence in exstrophy patients. Ritchey and associates (1988) found that this was true in those patients with complete epispadias who gained continence at puberty. However, this was not true in the exstrophy group. Gearhart and co-workers (1990) reviewed magnetic resonance imaging (MRI) scans of the prostate gland in 14 adult patients with classic bladder exstrophy. The volume and cross-sectional area of the prostate gland was the same in exstrophy patients as in normal, age-matched controls. However, the configuration of the prostate gland in exstrophy patients was very unusual and did not surround the urethra in any patient voiding through the urethra. The seminal vesicle length was normal in all exstrophy patients when compared with normal controls. Whether the prostate gland and its unusual configuration aid eventual continence is unknown, but the data of Ritchey and colleagues (1988) suggest that it does not in exstrophy patients.

Malignancy

In the 1920s, it was estimated that 50 per cent of individuals with bladder exstrophy died by 10 years of age (Mayo and Hendricks, 1926). The development of operative techniques that preserve renal function, availability of broad-spectrum antibiotics, and understanding of the metabolic disorders associated with urinary diversion have resulted in 91 per cent of patients with this disorder surviving to the age of 30 years (Lattimer et al., 1978). This extended survival has uncovered two latent malignant processes that are associated with bladder exstrophy. Of carcinomas identified in exstrophied bladders, 80 per cent are adenocarcinomas (Kandzari et al., 1974). The prevalence of adenocarcinoma in exstrophied bladders is approximately 400-fold greater than that in normal bladders (Engel and Wilkerson, 1970). According to Mostofi (1954), chronic irritation, infection, and obstruction can induce a metaplastic transformation of the urothelium to cystitis granularis,

a premalignant lesion. Adenocarcinoma may also develop from the malignant degeneration of embryonic rests of gastrointestinal tissue that is incorporated into the exstrophied bladder (Engel and Wilkerson, 1970). The inherent malignant potential of the closed exstrophy bladder has not been determined because long-term follow-up of a large number of bladder exstrophy cases without urinary tract infection, obstruction, and chronic irritation has not been done.

Bladder abnormalities, including squamous metaplasia, acute inflammation, fibrosis, and epithelial submucosal inclusions, were observed in exstrophied bladders of patients at 2 weeks of age (Culp, 1964). This observation suggests that exstrophied bladders are inherently abnormal. In comparison, consider the case of the 17-year-old boy who underwent primary exstrophy closure at age 1 year and developed normal urinary control with preservation of the upper urinary tracts. He was killed in an automobile accident, and serial section of the bladder revealed no evidence of malignant or premalignant changes (Jeffs, 1979) (Fig. 46–22). Until the malignant potential of the exstrophied bladder is determined, a high suspicion should be maintained for potential malignant degeneration. Only two epithelial malignancies have been reported in closed exstrophy patients, and these bladders were not closed at birth. Both bladder tumors were squamous in nature.

In untreated exstrophied bladders that are left everted, the patient is predisposed to develop adenocarcinoma secondary to repeated trauma. Squamous cell carcinoma accounted for only four of 57 (7 per cent) of the carcinomas reported in exstrophied bladders (Kandzari et al., 1974). Rhabdomyosarcoma has been observed in three individuals with bladder exstrophy (Engel, 1973; Jeffs, unpublished data; Semerdjian et al., 1972). Krishnansetty and co-workers (1988) found 104 cases of malignancy in untreated bladder exstrophy patients and, as previously reported, the majority are adenocarcinomas with occasional squamous cell carcinomas and rhabdomyosarcomas. In a review by Hartmann and colleagues (1984), adenocarcinoma was found in 93 per cent, squamous cell carcinoma in 3 per cent, undifferentiated carcinoma in 2 per cent and rhabdomyosarcoma in 1 per cent of 97 patients with untreated bladder exstrophy.

Adenocarcinoma of the colon adjacent to the ureterointestinal anastomosis in an exstrophy patient was initially described by Dixon and Weisman (1948). The risk of adenocarcinoma of the colon in exstrophy patients following ureterosigmoidostomy is 7000 times that of the general population 25 years of age or under (Krishnansetty et al., 1988). Spence and associates (1979) surveyed the literature to identify patients with bladder exstrophy who developed tumors following ureterosigmoid diversion. The mean latency interval from the time of ureterointestinal anastomosis to the diagnosis of intestinal tumor in these cases was 10 years, and the longest interval was 46 years. Of 35 compiled tumors, 28 were malignant and 24 were adenocarcinomas. Approximately half the adenocarcinomas had metastasized at the time of diagnosis. In a large series of cancers associated with ureterosigmoidostomy in exstrophy pa-

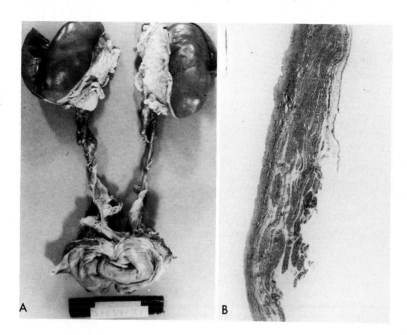

Figure 46–22. Gross *(A)* and microscopic *(B)* views of bladder of exstrophy patient who died accidentally after 17 years of normal bladder function.

tients, Krishnansetty and co-workers (1988) reported a review of the world's literature and discovered 90 cases.

Fertility/Pregnancy

Reconstruction of the male genitalia and preservation of fertility were not primary objectives of the early surgical management of bladder exstrophy. Sporadic accounts of pregnancy, or the initiation of pregnancy by men with bladder exstrophy, had been reported. In two large exstrophy series, male fertility was rarely documented. Only three of 68 men (Bennett, 1973), and four of 72 men (Woodhouse et al., 1983) had successfully fathered children. Six of 26 and seven of 27 women with bladder exstrophy in these respective series successfully delivered offspring. Shapiro's (1984) survey of 2500 exstrophy and epispadias patients identified 38 men who had fathered children and 131 women who had borne offspring.

Hanna and Williams (1972) compared semen analyses of men who had undergone primary bladder closure and ureterosigmoidostomy. A normal sperm count was found in only one of eight men following functional bladder closure and in four of eight men with urinary diversions. The difference in observed fertility potential probably was attributable to iatrogenic injury of the verumontanum during functional closure. Retrograde ejaculation may also account for the low sperm counts observed following functional bladder closure.

Libido in exstrophy patients is very high (Woodhouse et al., 1983). The erectile mechanism in patients who had undergone epispadias repair appears intact because 87 per cent of boys and young men in our series have experienced erections following epispadias repair (Lepor et al., 1984).

Clemetson's (1958) review of the literature identified 45 women with bladder exstrophy who successfully delivered 49 normal offspring. The main complication following pregnancy was cervical and uterine prolapse, which occurred in six of seven women (Krisiloff et al., 1978). A large review of 40 women ranging from 19 to 36 years of age who were treated in infancy for bladder exstrophy was performed by Burbige and co-workers (1986). There were 14 pregnancies in 11 women, which resulted in nine normal deliveries, three spontaneous abortions, and two elective abortions. Uterine prolapse occurred in seven of 11 patients, all of whom underwent previous diversions during pregnancy. The patient must be informed of the likelihood of uterine prolapse following pregnancy. Spontaneous vaginal deliveries were experienced by women who had undergone urinary diversions, and cesarean sections were performed in women who had undergone functional bladder closure to eliminate stress on the pelvic floor and to avoid traumatic injury to the delicate urinary sphincter mechanism (Krisiloff et al., 1978; Lattimer et al., 1978).

CLOACAL EXSTROPHY

Cloacal exstrophy represents one of the most severe congenital anomalies that is compatible with intrauterine viability. Fortunately, this entity is exceedingly rare, occurring in approximately one in 200,000 to 400,000 live births (Gravier, 1968). The incidence in males and females is said to be similar (Soper and Kilger, 1965); however, current reports indicate a male-to-female ratio of approximately 2:1 (Gearhart and Jeffs, 1990; Hurwitz et al., 1987). Reports have shown that this condition can be reliably diagnosed antenatally (Meizner and Bar-Ziv, 1985). The inheritance pattern of cloacal exstrophy is unknown because offspring have never been produced from individuals with this disorder.

Anatomy and Embryology

Anatomically, there is exstrophy of the foreshortened hindgut or cecum, which displays its bulging mucosa between the two hemibladders (Fig. 46–23). The orifices of the terminal ileum, the rudimentary tailgut, and a single or paired appendix are apparent on the surface of the everted cecum. The tailgut is blind-ending, and the ileum is usually prolapsed. The pubic symphysis is widely separated, the hips are externally rotated and abducted, and the phallus is separated into a right and left half with adjacent labium or scrotum (Fig. 46–24).

Schlegel and Gearhart (1989) defined the neuroanatomy of the pelvis in the child born with cloacal exstrophy (Fig. 46–25). The autonomic innervation to the hemibladders and corporal bodies arises from a pelvic plexus on the anterior surface of the rectum. The nerves to the hemibladders travel in the midline along the posterior-inferior surface of the pelvis and extend laterally to the hemibladders. The autonomic innervation to the duplicated corporal bodies arises from the sacral pelvic plexus, travels in the midline, perforates the inferior portion of the pelvic floor, and courses medially to the hemibladder. Duplication of the inferior vena cava is also seen (Schlegel and Gearhart, 1989).

During normal embryogenesis, after 4 weeks of life, the urorectal septum divides the cloaca into an anterior urogenital sinus and a posterior anorectal canal. Simultaneously, the infraumbilical abdominal wall is formed by primitive mesoderm, which migrates around the cloacal membrane. The cloacal membrane reaches its

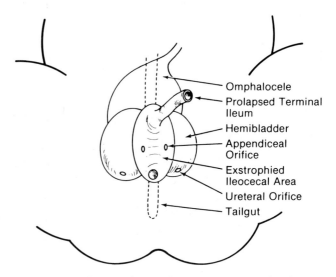

Figure 46–23. Schematic drawing showing gastrointestinal and urinary defects in children of either sex born with cloacal exstrophy. (Courtesy of Dr. Richard Hurwitz.)

greatest dimension at 5 weeks of gestation and then regresses in size. Normally, the membrane ruptures after 6 weeks, when the urorectal septum is formed, and the urethral, vaginal, and anal orifices have opened onto the perineum. According to Marshall and Muecke

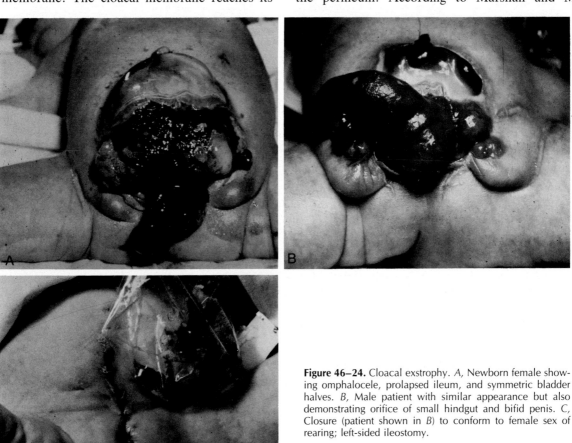

Figure 46–24. Cloacal exstrophy. *A,* Newborn female showing omphalocele, prolapsed ileum, and symmetric bladder halves. *B,* Male patient with similar appearance but also demonstrating orifice of small hindgut and bifid penis. *C,* Closure (patient shown in *B*) to conform to female sex of rearing; left-sided ileostomy.

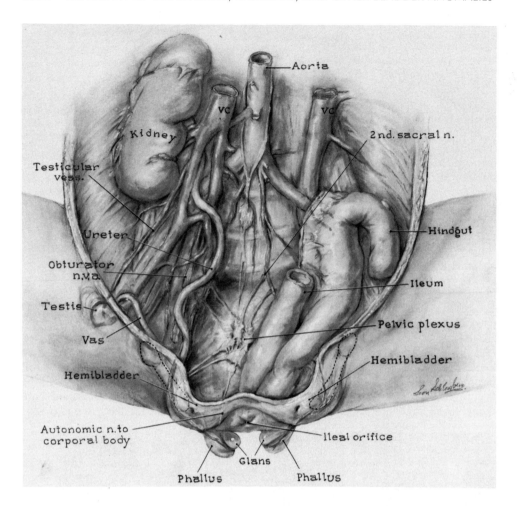

Figure 46–25. Internal view of patient with cloacal exstrophy. Pudendal vessels, nerves, as well as other vessels and autonomic innervation to the corporeal bodies are demonstrated. Internal structure of the pelvis along with duplication of the vena cava in dissected specimen is also shown.

(1968), an abnormally extensive cloacal membrane produces a wedge effect by serving as a mechanical barrier to mesodermal migration, which results in impaired development of the abdominal wall, failure of fusion of the paired genital tubercles, and diastasis pubis. Exstrophy of the cloaca results when the wedge effect occurs before formation of the urorectal septum at 6 weeks.

Hurwitz and associates (1987) have suggested a schema to describe classic cloacal exstrophy and its variants using coding grids. The grid depicted shows type I or classic cloacal exstrophy. Type IIA grids show variations of the bladder (covered bladder or hemibladder); type IIB grids show variations of distal exstrophied bowel segments (duplications); and type IIC grids show variations in which both bowel and bladder variations occur. The grid describes the penis (hemi- or unilateral) and the clitoris and vaginal status (duplications). An addition to the grid recommended by us would show the status of the tailgut (Fig. 46–26).

Associated Conditions

Soper and Kilger (1964) described the anomalies associated with cloacal exstrophy in 57 cases reviewed in the literature. Of the 74 renal units described, 44 were abnormal. The following specific renal anomalies were identified: absent kidney, 4; hydronephrosis, 6;

hydroureter, 11; multicystic kidney, 2; small kidney, 5; ptosis, 13; ureteral atresia, 6; and vascular anomalies, 4. Genital anomalies included an absent penis in eight, single in five, and bifid in 15. The clitoris was absent in 14, single in one, and bifid in seven. In all genetic males, the testes were present and undescended in 24 of 26 patients. Because of the severity of the midline defect, disorders related to nonfusion of the müllerian ducts were frequently seen. The vagina was absent in six,

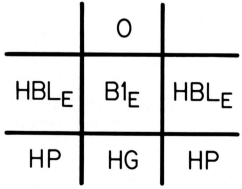

Figure 46–26. Coding grid used to describe classic cloacal exstrophy and its variants. O, Omphalocele; HBL, hemibladder; Bl_E, everted bowel; HP, hemiphallus; and HG^O, hindgut. (Modified from Hurwitz, R. S., et al.: J. Urol., 138:1060, 1987.)

single in two, and double in 14. The uterus was double in 22 of 23 described cases. In the male, the vas deferens may enter the bladder or distal ureter—the anatomic variant corresponding to a persistent mesonephric duct.

Common extragenitourinary anomalies were observed in 45 of 57 cases. The anomalies involved the extremities in ten, cardiovascular system in nine, small intestine in four, ribs in three, large intestine in two, and diaphragm in two. An omphalocele was described in 36 of 41 cases, and a myelomeningocele was described in 24 cases. In a large series of cloacal exstrophy patients, Hurwitz and co-workers (1987) found associated anomalies in 85 per cent of cases. The most common genitourinary anomalies were pelvic kidneys, unilateral renal agenesis, multicystic kidneys, and ureteral duplication, in decreasing order. Forty-eight per cent of patients had vertebral anomalies, and 46 per cent had associated gastrointestinal anomalies. Twenty-nine per cent had central nervous system anomalies (myelomeningocele, meningocele, lipomeningocele), and 26 per cent had severe anomalies of the lower extremities.

Surgical Management

Steinbuchel (1900) described the first reported surgically reconstructed cloacal exstrophy. The omphalocele was corrected at birth, and the atretic colon was pulled through to the perineum; however, the neonate died at age 5 days. Surgical reconstruction of cloacal exstrophy was considered futile, and untreated neonates usually died from prematurity, sepsis, short bowel syndrome, or renal and central nervous system deficits. Remigailo and colleagues (1976) reported the unusual case of a well-adjusted, 18-year-old patient with cloacal exstrophy, who had never undergone surgical reconstruction.

Rickham (1960) reported the first case of cloacal exstrophy to survive surgical reconstruction. The omphalocele was repaired, the intestinal strip was separated from the hemibladders, and the blind-ending colon was pulled out through the perineum. The hemibladders were then reapproximated. A ureteroileal conduit was reconstructed at age 18 months, and a cystectomy was subsequently performed. Fecal continence is rarely, if ever, achieved following perineal pull-through procedures. An alternative approach described by Fonkalsrud and Linde (1970) included terminal ileostomy at birth followed by cystectomy and ileal loop diversion at age 2 years.

Our approach to reconstruction of cloacal exstrophy is by staged surgical reconstructive procedures (Table 46–7). The child's condition at birth may be critical, and attempts to reconstruct and repair may be futile or morally or ethically unwise. The more robust infant will survive, and reparative surgery is initiated at birth. Most individuals with cloacal exstrophy should be reared as females because of the severe deformity and deficiency of the phallus (Husmann et al., 1989b). A gonadectomy is done when sex reassignment is indicated. At birth, the omphalocele is repaired and terminal ileostomy or a colostomy is performed, preserving as much of the

Table 46–7. STAGED FUNCTIONAL CLOSURE OF CLOACAL EXSTROPHY

Immediate Neonatal Assessment
Evaluate associated anomalies
Decide whether to proceed with reparative surgery

Functional Bladder Closure (immediately after neonatal assessment)
Bilateral iliac or innominate osteotomies
Gonadectomy in males with a duplicated or an absent penis
Terminal ileostomy
Closure of hemibladders

Anti-Incontinence and Antireflux Procedure (age 3–5 years)
Bladder capacity greater than 60 ml: Young-Dees-Leadbetter bladder neck plasty with Cohen ureteral reimplantations and Marshall-Marchett-Krantz bladder neck suspension
Bladder capacity less than 60 ml: tubularized bladder into a urethrovescial tube; ureters are reimplanted into a bladder or a bowel segment used to augment bladder capacity or continent diversion with/without abdominal stoma
Anti-incontinence devices: used for refractory incontinence

Vaginal Reconstruction (age 14–18 years)
Vagina constructed or augmented using rudimentary colon

hindgut as possible, including the rudimentary terminal colon (Howell et al., 1983). The exstrophied bladder is closed, and the bifid phallus is reapproximated in the midline. Both anterior and posterior innominate osteotomy have been done in the closure of cloacal exstrophy. With a large omphalocele defect, bladder closure and osteotomy may be delayed until respiratory and GI stability is achieved. Anterior osteotomy allows placement of pins for external fixation and is preferred when severe lumbosacral dysraphism is present.

An additional stage may be required to join the terminal ileum to the colon segment to form a colostomy. Figure 46–24 illustrates the surgical result following the first stage of cloacal exstrophy closure. Usually, intestinal absorption problems are resolved at approximately 3 to 4 years of age, and the most advantageous type of urinary control can be considered. Urinary continence can be achieved in these individuals in many ways. An orthotopic urethra can be constructed from local tissue, vagina, ileum, or even ureter. A catheterizable stoma can be constructed from ileum when fluid losses are stable. The bladder may be augmented with unused hindgut (in situ), ileum, or stomach (Gearhart and Jeffs, 1990; Mitchell and Rink, 1988). However, surgery to produce a continent reservoir should be delayed until a method of evacuation can be predicted and the child is old enough to participate in self-care. The choice between a catheterizable urethra and an abdominal stoma depends on the adequacy of the urethra and bladder outlet; interest and dexterity of the child; and orthopedic status regarding spine, hip joints, braces, and ambulation.

In a current series, Gearhart and Jeffs (1990) used multiple techniques to produce continence in a select group of ten cloacal exstrophy patients who underwent staged functional closure, including the following: Young-Dees-Leadbetter in four; ileal nipple in one; Kropp procedure plus augmentation in one; and continent abdominal stoma plus augmentation in four. Staged reconstruction can produce urinary continence in this complex anomaly. An innovative approach is required to find the most suitable solution for each individual patient concerning bladder size and function and mental, neurologic, and orthopedic status. With the advent of modern pediatric anesthesia and intensive care, the survival rate is high. This high survival makes reconstructive techniques applicable to a large percentage of infants born with this condition. The type II variants demand variation and innovation in the aforementioned schema of treatment.

EPISPADIAS

Epispadias varies from a glandular defect in a covered penis, to the penopubic type with complete incontinence, to the complete variety associated with exstrophy of the bladder.

Types

Epispadias in males is classified according to the position of the dorsally displaced urethral meatus. The degree of penile deformity and the occurrence of urinary incontinence are related to the extent of the dorsally displaced urethral meatus. The displaced meatus may be found in the glans, penile shaft, or penopubic region. All types of epispadias are associated with varying degrees of dorsal chordee. In penopubic or subsymphyseal epispadias, the entire penile urethra is open and the bladder outlet may be large enough to admit the examining finger, indicating obvious gross incontinence. The pubic symphysis is divergent and contributes to the deficiency of the external urinary sphincter mechanism. The divergence of the pubis symphysis and the shortened urethral plate result in prominent dorsal chordee and a penis that appears short. The penile deformity is virtually identical to that observed in bladder exstrophy. In a combined study, Dees (1949) reported the incidence of complete epispadias to be one of 117,000 males and one of 484,000 females. The reported male-to-female ratio of epispadias varies between 3:1 (Dees, 1949) and 5:1 (Kramer and Kelalis, 1982).

Kramer and Kelalis (1982) reviewed their surgical experience of 82 males with epispadias. Penopubic epispadias occurred in 49 cases, penile epispadias in 21, and glandular epispadias in 12. Urinary incontinence was observed in 46 of 49 cases of penopubic epispadias, in 15 of 21 cases of penile epispadias, and in no cases of glandular epispadias.

Epispadias in the female is characterized by a bifid clitoris, flattening of the mons, and separation of the labia. Three degrees of epispadias occur in females. In the least degree of epispadias, the urethral orifice merely appears patulous; in intermediate epispadias, the urethra is dorsally split along most of the urethra; and in the most severe degree of epispadias, the urethral cleft involves the entire length of the urethra and the sphincter mechanism is rendered incompetent.

Associated Anomalies

The anomalies associated with complete epispadias are usually confined to deformities of the external genitalia, diastasis of the pubic symphysis, and deficiency of the urinary continence mechanism. The only renal anomaly observed in 11 cases of complete epispadias was agenesis of the left kidney (Campbell, 1952). In a review by Arap and colleagues (1988), one case of unilateral renal agenesis and one ectopic pelvic kidney occurred in 38 patients. The ureterovesical junction is inherently deficient in complete epispadias, and reflux has been reported in a number of series to be around 30 to 40 per cent (Arap et al., 1988; Kramer and Kelalis, 1982).

Surgical Management

The objectives for the repair of penopubic epispadias include achievement of urinary continence with preservation of the upper urinary tract and reconstruction of functional and cosmetically acceptable genitalia. The surgical management of incontinence in penopubic epispadias is virtually identical to that of a closed bladder exstrophy.

Young (1922) reported the first cure of incontinence in a male patient with complete epispadias. Since Young reported his approach to obtain continence, results have progressively improved (Arap et al., 1988; Burkholder and Williams, 1965; Kramer and Kelalis, 1982; Peters et al., 1988). In patients with complete epispadias and good bladder capacity, epispadias and bladder neck reconstruction can be performed in a single stage. Urethroplasty formerly was performed after bladder neck reconstruction (Arap et al., 1988; Kramer and Kelalis, 1982). However, our results with the small bladder associated with exstrophy (Gearhart and Jeffs, 1989) and the small bladder associated with epispadias (Peters et al., 1988) have led us to perform urethroplasty and penile elongation prior to bladder neck reconstruction. A small incontinent bladder with reflux is hardly an ideal situation for bladder neck reconstruction and ureteral reimplantation. With urethroplasty prior to bladder neck reconstruction, there was an average increase in bladder capacity of 95 ml within 18 months in those patients with a small bladder capacity initially associated with epispadias and a continence rate overall of 87 per cent after the continence procedure (Peters et al., 1988).

In epispadias group, much as in the exstrophy group, bladder capacity is the most predominant indicator of eventual continence (Ritchey et al., 1988). Also, in a current series, Arap and co-workers (1988) obtained a much higher continence rate in those with adequate bladder capacity (71 per cent) prior to bladder neck reconstruction than in those with inadequate capacity (20 per cent). In addition, in Arap's group of complete epispadias patients, most attained continence within 2 years, much like those patients with classic bladder exstrophy (Canning et al., 1989).

A firm intersymphyseal band bridges the divergent symphysis, and an osteotomy is not usually performed.

The Young-Dees-Leadbetter bladder neck plasty, Marshall-Marchett-Krantz bladder neck suspension, and ureteral reimplantation are performed when the bladder capacity reaches approximately 60 ml, which usually occurs between 3 and 4 years of age.

The genital reconstruction and urethroplasty in epispadias and exstrophy are quite similar. The following must take place: release of dorsal chordee and division of suspensory ligaments; dissection of the corpora from their attachment to the inferior pubic ramus; lengthening of the urethral groove; and lengthening of the corpora, if needed, by incision and anastomosis or grafting, or by medial rotation of the ventral corpora in a more downward direction.

Urethral reconstruction in complete epispadias can be as simple as a modified Young urethroplasty to even a two-stage repair (Kramer and Kelalis, 1982). All modern techniques of hypospadias repair have been used to aid in the treatment of epispadias, including the use of the prepuce to the bladder mucosa and even full-thickness skin grafts. A transverse ventral island flap has been done by Monfort (1987). The urethra, once reconstructed, can be positioned between and below the corpora (Cantwell, 1895; Ransley et al., 1989). Lastly, a two-stage repair has been performed with good success in these reconstructions (Kramer and Kelalis, 1982). The glandular and skin closure is performed in a manner similar to the reconstruction of the penis in patients with bladder exstrophy (see previous section).

The achievement of urinary continence following bladder neck reconstruction in patients with epispadias is summarized in Table 46–8 (Arap et al., 1988; Burkholder and Williams, 1965; Dees, 1949; Kramer and Kelalis, 1982; Peters et al., 1988). The majority of these patients underwent reconstruction by means of a Young-Dees-Leadbetter bladder neck plasty. Urinary continence was achieved in 74 per cent of males and 85 per cent of females following bladder neck reconstruction. Urinary diversion should seldom be considered in the initial management of complete epispadias. Delayed achievement of urinary continence occurred in more than half the males with complete epispadias, who eventually became continent following the continence procedures (Kramer and Kelalis, 1982). The effect that urethral lengthening and prostatic enlargement have on increasing bladder outlet resistance is emphasized by these observations in the epispadias group. However, in a series by Arap and colleagues (1988), establishment of continence had no relationship to puberty and usually occurred within 2 years; in a majority of patients, continence preceded puberty by several years.

The results of urethroplasty for epispadias have been reviewed by Kramer and Kelalis (1988). A Thiersch-Duplay procedure (modified Young urethroplasty) was selected in 49 of 67 cases (73 per cent), and various other reconstructive techniques were selected in the remaining 18 cases. Urethral fistula requiring surgical repair occurred in 21 per cent of these urethroplasties.

Kramer and Kelalis (1988) reported the success of genital reconstruction in epispadias with a straight penis angled downward in almost 70 per cent of patients with normal erectile function. Of this group, 80 per cent has had satisfactory intercourse and of 29 married patients, 19 have fathered children. The carefully constructed and well-planned approach to the management of urinary incontinence and genital deformities associated with complete epispadias should provide a satisfactory cosmetic appearance, normal genital function, and preservation of fertility potential in most patients.

OTHER BLADDER ANOMALIES

Agenesis/Hypoplasia

Agenesis of the bladder is an extremely rare congenital anomaly with only 44 cases reported in the English literature up to 1988. Campbell (1951) reported seven

Table 46–8. URINARY CONTINENCE FOLLOWING BLADDER NECK RECONSTRUCTION IN PATIENTS WITH COMPLETE EPISPADIAS

	Kramer and Kelalis (1982)	Peters et al. (1989)	Arap et al. (1988)	Burkholder and Williams (1965)	Dees (1949)	Total
Total number of patients with complete epispadias	53	17	38	27	6	141
Number of males with complete epispadias treated with BNR	32*	11	21	17	5	86
Number of males with surgically corrected incontinence	22	11	15	8	5	61
Percentage of males with surgically corrected incontinence	69	83	71	47	100	74†
Number of females with complete epispadias treated with BNR	8	6	9	10	1	34
Number of females with surgically corrected incontinence	8	6	7	7	1	29
Percentage of females with surgically corrected incontinence	88	90	77	70	100	85†

*Male patients with penopublic epispadias and total incontinence included.
†Average value.
Abbreviation: BNR, bladder neck reconstruction.

cases in 19,046 autopsies (two were anocephalic monsters and in all seven, other severe anomalies coexisted). Glenn (1959) found only one case in 600,000 patients seen at Duke University Hospital in 28 years. Agenesis of the bladder is seldom compatible with life, and only 15 live births have been reported, all except one being females (Akdas et al., 1988; Aragona et al., 1988; Krull et al., 1988).

The cause of agenesis of the bladder is uncertain. Because the hindgut is normal in these infants, it may be assumed that embryologic division of the cloaca into the urogenital sinus and anorectum has proceeded normally. Bladder agenesis may be the result of secondary atrophy of the anterior division of the cloaca, perhaps because of a lack of distention with urine caused by the failure of incorporation of the mesonephric ducts and ureters into the trigone, thus preventing urine from accumulating in the bladder (Krull et al., 1988).

The results of this anomaly depend on the sex of the fetus. In the female with normally developed müllerian structures, the ureteral orifice may end in the uterus, anterior vaginal wall, or vestibule. In these cases with ectopic ureteral openings, there is usually some preservation of renal function (Krull et al., 1988). In the male, the only means to achieve adequate outlet drainage would be cloacal persistence with the ureters draining into the rectum or by way of patent urachus. Considering the severity of this defect, it is not surprising that other urologic anomalies, including solitary kidney, renal agenesis, dysplasia, and absence of prostate gland and seminal vesicles, exist (Aragona et al., 1983). Treatment in most reported cases of surviving infants has included urinary diversion either by ureterosigmoidostomy or external stoma (Glenn, 1959).

The small bladder may be dysplastic or hypoplastic. Dysplasia is observed in conditions such as duplicate exstrophy or hemibladder exstrophy, in which the rudiment is small, fibrotic, and nondistensible. Hypoplastic bladders have the potential to enlarge and are seen in conditions of severe incontinence, such as complete epispadias and bilateral ectopic ureters.

Duplication

Complete duplication of the bladder and urethra is rare with only 45 cases reported in the literature (Kapoor and Saha, 1987). Complete duplication of the bladder involves two bladder halves, each with a full-thickness muscular wall and each with its own ipsilateral ureter and urethra (Fig. 46–27). This anomaly is observed more commonly in males than in females. Associated congenital anomalies of other organ systems are present in the majority of cases of complete duplication of the bladder and urethra. In 40 cases reviewed by Kossow and Morales (1973), 90 per cent had some type of duplication of the external genitalia and 42 per cent had duplication of the lower gastrointestinal tract. Spinal duplication and fistulas between the rectum, vagina, and urethra were other associated abnormalities.

Incomplete bladder duplication has been reported (Abrahamson, 1965). This entity involves two full-thick-

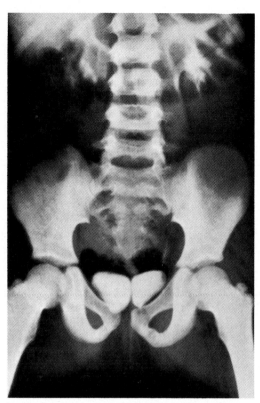

Figure 46–27. Roentgenogram of bladder duplication as reported by Nesbit and Bromme.

ness bladders, each with its own ureter; but unlike complete bladder duplication, the two communicate and drain into a common urethra.

Congenital Bladder Diverticulum

Congenital bladder diverticula unassociated with posterior urethral valves or neurogenic bladder are unusual (Barrett et al., 1976; Johnston, 1960). This entity almost always occurs in male patients. Congenital diverticula usually occur in a smooth-walled bladder, are most often solitary, and occur without evidence of outflow obstruction. The cause of these diverticula is an inherent weakness in the bladder musculature. The diverticula probably originate near the ureteral orifice but not in the hiatal area (Johnston, 1960). As the diverticulum enlarges, it may incorporate the ureteral tunnel, and the ureter may drain into the diverticulum with resulting reflux. These congenital diverticula are often larger than those associated with neurogenic bladder or lower tract obstructive anomalies. These structures may also cause outlet obstruction at the bladder neck or urethral location (Taylor et al., 1979) or ureteral obstruction (Lione and Gonzalez, 1985). These diverticula are not difficult to diagnose on a voiding cystourethrogram, especially with postvoiding images. Upper tract imaging, although important, is not believed to be the best method to diagnose a bladder diverticulum initially; this is because only two of 24 patients in Allen and Atwell's (1980) series had bladder diverticula that were seen on intravenous urography.

Currently, 11 cases of congenital bladder diverticula have been described in children with Ehlers-Danlos syndrome. This is a congenital connective tissue disorder characterized by abnormalities of collagen structure and function. However, the link between the connective tissue disorder and the occurrence of these bladder diverticula has yet to be proved. All of the reported cases of congenital bladder diverticula associated with Ehlers-Danlos syndrome have been in males (Levard, 1989).

Congenital Megacystis

Historically, congenital megacystis is an entity describing the bladder associated with massively refluxing megaureters. This term was first described with massive reflux by Williams (1957). The physiologic result of massive reflux is constant cycling of urine between the massively dilated refluxing megaureters and the bladder. The bladder contractability is normal, although a majority of each vesical contraction empties into the upper tracts. The effect of this constant recycling of urine is a progressive increase in residual urine and bladder capacity. The trigone is wide and poorly developed with laterally gaping, incompetent orifices. Correction of the reflux should lead to a resumption of normal voiding dynamics. The rarity of this condition in present urologic practice suggests an acquired causation. *Escherichia coli* infection and reflux in a normal system may cause bladder and ureteral atony with subsequent dilatation. The cause of the dilated bladder in neonates may be difficult to determine. When reflux, obstruction, and neurogenic abnormalities are excluded, a group of patients remains with large bladder and unknown etiology. Prenatal temporary obstruction, metabolic abnormality, and cerebral anoxia have been implicated.

URACHAL ABNORMALITIES

Anatomy and Histology

The urachus lies between the peritoneum and transversalis fascia and extends from the anterior dome of the bladder toward the umbilicus (Fig. 46–28). The urachus varies from 3 to 10 cm in length and from 8 to 10 mm in diameter. The urachus is encased between two layers of umbilicovesical fascia, which tend to contain the spread of urachal disease. The urachus is adjacent to the umbilical ligaments—the remnants of the umbilical arteries. When the urachus is present as a muscular tube, three distinct tissue layers are recognized: (1) an epithelial canal of cuboidal or, more typically, transitional epithelium; (2) a submucosal connective tissue layer; and (3) an outer layer of smooth muscle, which is thickest near the bladder. The central lumen is irregular and beaded and is filled with desquamated epithelial debris and epithelial islands. When the upper urachus becomes a fibrous cord, there are generally no recognizable urachal elements (Begg, 1927; Hammond et al., 1941; Hector, 1961; Steck and Helwig, 1965).

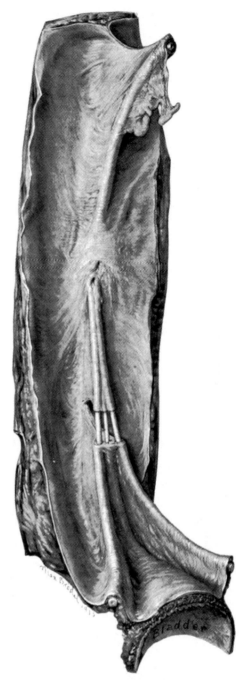

Figure 46–28. Posterior view of the umbilical region of the anterior abdominal wall showing the relation of the urachus to the umbilical ligaments, peritoneum, and bladder dome. The urachus does not extend fully to the umbilicus. The ligamentum teres is seen superior to the umbilicus. (From Cullen, T. S.: Embryology, Anatomy and Diseases of the Umbilicus. Philadelphia, W. B. Saunders Co., 1916.)

Embryology

The allantois is an extra-embryonic cavity located within the body stalk that projects onto the anterior surface of the cloaca, the future bladder. The descent of the bladder into the pelvis is associated with elongation of the urachus, a tubular structure that extends from the fibrotic allantoic duct to the anterior bladder. During the 4th and 5th months of gestation, the urachus narrows to a small-caliber epithelial tube (Nix et al.,

1958). During fetal development, as the bladder descends into the pelvis, its apical portion narrows progressively into a fibromuscular strand of urachus, which maintains continuity with the allantoic duct. As the fetus develops, the urachus loses its attachment to the umbilicus. Hammond and associates (1941) observed that continuity of the urachus with the posterior surface of the umbilicus and the apex of the bladder persisted in only 50 per cent of fetal specimens. Shortly after the embryonic stage of development, the tract apparently obliterates because patency was observed in only 2 per cent of adult specimens. The obliteration of the urachus results in different patterns of urachal termination: a well-defined urachal remnant may maintain an identifiable attachment to the umbilicus; at a variable distance above the bladder, the urachal cord may merge with one or both of the obliterated umbilical arteries, resulting in a single common ligament to the umbilicus—the medial vesicular ligament; or an atrophic extension from a short, tubular urachus may terminate within the fascia or blend into a plexus of fibrous tissue—the plexus of Luschka—formed by the urachus and the umbilical arteries (Blichert-Toft and Nielson, 1971b; Hammond et al., 1941).

Patent Urachus

Congenital patent urachus is a lesion that is usually recognized in the neonate. It is a rare anomaly occurring in only three of more than 1 million admissions to a large pediatric center (Nix et al., 1958). The two forms of congenital patent urachus are persistence of the patent urachus with a partially distended bladder; and a vesicoumbilical fistula representing failure of the bladder to descend at all (Fig. 46–29). When the bladder forms, the bladder apex never forms a true urachal tract. The more common form of a patent urachus results when there is failure of obliteration of the urachal remnant. Persistence of the urachus has been attributed to intrauterine urinary obstruction; however, only 14 per cent of neonates born with a patent urachus have evidence of urinary obstructions (Herbst, 1937). It is unlikely that urinary obstruction is directly related to the development of a patent urachus because even the most severe cases of posterior urethral valves are not associated with this anomaly. Furthermore, urethral tubularization occurs after obliteration of the urachal remnant, suggesting that urinary obstruction is not the major factor producing the patent urachus (Schreck and Campbell, 1972).

Acquired patent urachus in the adult is usually a urinary umbilical fistula that results from bladder outflow obstruction. In these cases, extravasation of infected urine into the periurachal space ultimately may result in erosion through the umbilical region, a relatively weak segment of the abdominal wall. Because the urachus can remain attached to the umbilicus in a minority of normal adults, at least some acquired umbilical urinary fistulas may drain through the existing urachal canal. A patent urachus is rarely diagnosed when there is free discharge of urine through the umbilicus. The patent urachus should be suspected when the umbilical cord is enlarged and edematous or when its normal slough is delayed. On occasion, the fistula is tiny, and the discharge of urine may be minimal or intermittent.

The diagnosis of a patent urachus is confirmed by catheterization or by probing of the urachal tract, intravesical instillation of colored dye, and analysis of the discharge fluid for blood urea nitrogen (BUN) and creatinine. Voiding cystourethrography is helpful in fully evaluating the lesion and any associated bladder outlet obstruction. Fistulography distinguishes the condition from a patent omphalomesenteric duct. Although cystoscopy is essential in an older patient, it is not in the neonate, provided that the urethra appears radiologically normal. The differential diagnosis of a wet umbilicus in the infant includes patent urachus, omphalitis (an infection of the umbilical stump), simple granulation of the healing stump, patent vitelline or omphalomesenteric duct (enteroumbilical fistula), infected umbilical vessel, and external urachal sinus. The presence of both urinary and enteric fistulas at the umbilicus is exceedingly rare (Davis and Nikhaus, 1926; Herbst, 1937;

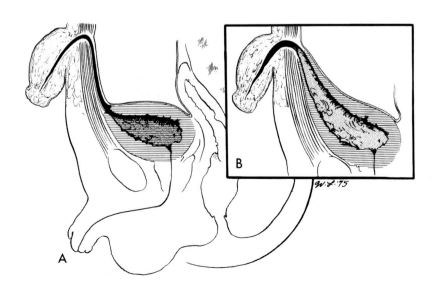

Figure 46–29. Forms of patent urachus. Note hydrops of the umbilical cord. *A,* Typical patent urachus. *B,* Vesicoumbilical fistula.

Kenigsberg, 1975; Mendoza et al., 1968; Steck and Helwig, 1965). Antenatal diagnosis of patent urachus was reported by Persutte and co-workers (1988). Not only is prenatal diagnosis helpful, but postnatal confirmation of these omphalovesical anomalies can be readily accomplished with high-resolution ultrasound imaging (Avni et al., 1988).

Urachal Cyst

A cyst may form within the isolated urachal canal if the lumen is enlarged from epithelial desquamation and degeneration. A connection frequently persists between the tract and the bladder and may permit bacterial infection, which becomes loculated (Fig. 46–30A). Infected cysts occur most commonly in adults (Blichert-Toft and Nielson, 1971a; Sterling and Goldsmith, 1953). However, they have been reported in infants (Geist, 1952; Hinman, 1961). The cyst manifests itself because infection has developed. The most common organism cultured in the cyst fluid is *Staphylococcus aureus* (MacMillan et al., 1973; Tauber and Bloom, 1951). Untreated, the infected cyst may drain into the bladder or through the umbilicus, or it may drain intermittently internally and externally, resulting in an alternating sinus (Blichert-Toft and Nielson, 1971a; Hinman, 1961; Neidhardt et al., 1968; Sterling and Goldsmith, 1953).

Serious complications of infected umbilical cysts include rupture into the preperitoneal tissues, rupture into the peritoneal cavity with significant peritonitis, and rarely inflammatory involvement of the adjacent bowel with the formation of enteric fistulas (Berman et al., 1988; Nunn, 1952). The symptoms and signs of a loculated, infected urachal cyst are lower abdominal pain; fever; voiding symptoms; midline hypogastric tenderness; often, a palpable mass; and evidence of urinary infection. Urachal cyst should be suspected whenever localized suprapubic pain and tenderness are present with disturbed micturition, even when the urine remains clear. Useful diagnostic studies include excretory urography, cystography, cystoscopy, and high-resolution ultrasound (Avni, 1988). Computed tomographic scan of the abdomen may be helpful in determining the extent of the disease and the possibility of involvement of other organ systems (Berman et al., 1988).

External Urachal Sinus

Persistence of the urachal apex alone will result in a blind external sinus that opens at the umbilicus (Fig. 46–30B). This condition may become symptomatic at any age with an infected discharge. In adults, umbilical pilonidal disease can mimic an external sinus (Steck and Helwig, 1965). Because the differential diagnosis also includes the lesions as listed in the previous section, probing and radiographic evaluation should be undertaken before surgery. A urachal sinus extends inferiorly, unlike an omphalomesenteric duct remnant, which extends inward toward the peritoneal cavity.

Urachal Diverticulum

A diverticulum of the bladder apex (Fig. 46–30C), or "blind internal sinus," may be an incidental finding on radiographic studies, which does not require treatment when it is small and minimally contractile. However, lesions of massive proportions have been reported in adults, requiring percutaneous drainage and eventual surgery (Berman et al., 1988). The large urachal diverticula, frequently seen in prune-belly syndrome (Lattimer, 1958) and occasionally associated with severe urethral obstruction, may require resection. These may be poorly contractile or may expand paradoxically during voiding. Urachal diverticula occasionally contain calculi (Bandler et al., 1942; Ney and Friedenberg, 1968).

Treatment

Adequate therapy for a patent urachus requires excision of all anomalous tissue with a cuff of bladder. Some workers advocate conservative treatment initially while reserving radical surgical excision of the urachus for persistent cases or recurrences. Similarly, simple drainage of a urachal cyst is associated with recurrent infections in 30 per cent of cases, and late occurrence of adenocarcinoma has been reported (Blichert-Toft and Nielson, 1971b; Nix et al., 1958).

In the treatment of benign urachal lesions in children, it is rarely necessary to remove the umbilicus; whenever possible, cosmetic considerations should prevail. In in-

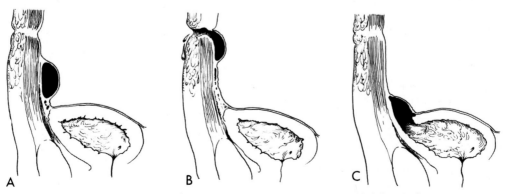

Figure 46–30. *A,* Urachal cyst. *B,* External urachal sinus. *C,* Urachal diverticulum.

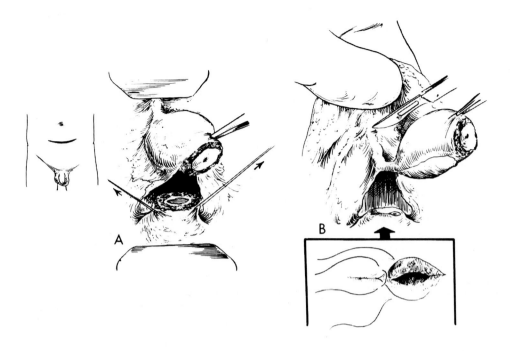

Figure 46–31. Surgical removal of a urachal cyst. Transverse midhypogastric incision. *A,* Lesion removed with a cuff of the bladder apex. *B,* Urachal stalk detached from the posterior umbilicus. A cuff of adherent peritoneum is excised with the specimen.

fants, a small, curved, subumbilical incision is usually ample, for at this age the bladder dome is still high and readily accessible through this exposure.

A transverse midhypogastric incision is adequate exposure in older children and adults and allows for both superior and inferior dissection. Surgical management of umbilical anomalies is depicted in Figure 46–31. The urachal stalk or fibrous urachal remnant should be detached from the dermis posterior to the umbilicus. A "buttonhole" in the umbilical area is of no consequence. Application of a small gauze pledget under the dressing obliterates dead space, maintains umbilical configuration, and allows the skin to close secondarily.

When peritoneum and umbilical ligaments are adherent to the inflammatory mass, these structures should be excised in continuity with the lesion. A vertical midline incision is the best approach for removal of an extensive inflammatory mass. Elliptic excision of the umbilicus may be necessary if it is involved in the inflammatory process, especially with an external urachal sinus or alternating sinus. A suppurative infection within a cyst or external sinus may require initial incision and drainage and treatment as for an abscess. After healing is complete, an internal excision of urachal tissue should be done.

REFERENCES

Abramson, J.: Double bladder and related anomalies: Clinical and embryological aspects in a case report. Br. J. Urol., 33:195, 1965.

Adams, M. C. C., Mitchell, M. E., et al.: Gastrocystoplasty: An alternate solution to the problem of urological reconstruction in severely compromised patients. J. Urol., 140:1152, 1988.

Akdas, A., Iseri, C., Ozgur, S., and Kirkali, Z.: Bladder agenesis. Int. Urol. Nephrol., 20:261, 1988.

Allen, N. H., and Atwell, J. D.: The paraureteric diverticulum in children. Br. J. Urol., 52:264, 1980.

Ambrose, S. S., and O'Brien, D. P.: Surgical embryology of the exstrophy-epispadias complex. Surg. Clin. North Am., 54:1379, 1974.

Andalen, R. M., O'Phelan, E. H., Chisholm, J. C., McFarland, F. A., and Sweetser, J. H.: Exstrophy of the bladder. Long-term results of bilateral posterior iliac osteotomies and two-stage anatomic repair. J. Clin. Orthop., 68:156–162, 1970.

Ansell, J. E.: Exstrophy and epispadias. In Glenn, J. F. (Ed.): Urologic Surgery. Philadelphia, J. B. Lippincott Co., 1983, p. 647.

Aragona, F., Passerini, G., Zarembella, P., Zorzi, C., et al.: Agenesis of the bladder: A case report and review of the literature. Urol. Radiol., 10:207, 1988.

Arap, S., and Giron, A. N.: Duplicated exstrophy: Report of three cases. Eur. Urol., 12:451, 1986.

Arap, S., Giron, A., and Degoes, G. M.: Complete reconstruction of bladder exstrophy. Urology, 7:413, 1976.

Arap, S., Nahas, W. C., Giron, A. M., Bruschini, H., and Mitra, I.: Incontinent epispadias: Surgical treatment of 38 cases. J. Urol., 140:577, 1988.

Avni, E. F., Matos, C., Diard, F., and Schuman, C. C.: Midline omphalovesical anomalies in children. Contribution of ultrasound imaging. Urol. Radiol., 2:189, 1988.

Bandler, C. G., Milbed, A. H., and Alley, J. L.: Urachal calculus. N.Y. State J. Med., 42:2203, 1942.

Barrett, D. M., Malek, R. S., and Kelalis, P. P.: Observations of vesical diverticulum in children. J. Urol., 116:234, 1976.

Begg, R. C.: The urachus and umbilical fistulae. J. Anat., 64:170, 1927.

Bennett, A. H.: Exstrophy of the bladder treated by ureterosigmoidostomies. Urology, 2:165, 1973.

Berman, S. M., et al.: Urachal remnants in adults. Urology, 31:17, 1988.

Blichert-Toft, M., and Nielson, O. V.: Diseases of the urachus simulating intra-abdominal disorders. Am. J. Surg., 112:123, 1971a.

Blichert-Toft, M., and Nielson, O. V.: Congenital patent urachus and acquired variants. Acta Chir. Scand., 137:807, 1971b.

Boyce, W. H., and Vest, S. A.: A new concept concerning treatment of exstrophy of the bladder. J. Urol., 677:503, 1952.

Brzezinski, A. E., Homsy, Y. L., and Leberg, I.: Orthoplasty in epispadias. J. Urol., 136:259, 1986.

Burbige, K. A., Hensle, T. W., Chambers, W. J., Leb, R., and Jeter, K. F.: Pregnancy and sexual function in women with bladder exstrophy. Urology, 28:12, 1986.

Burkholder, G. V., and Williams, D. I.: Epispadias and incontinence: Surgical treatment of 27 children. J. Urol., 94:674, 1965.

Burns, J. E.: A new operation for exstrophy of the bladder. JAMA, 82:1587, 1924.

Campbell, M.: Epispadias: A report of fifteen cases. J. Urol., 67:988, 1952.

Canning, D. A., Gearhart, J. P., Oesterling, J. E., and Jeffs, R. D.: A computerized review of exstrophy patients managed during the past thirteen years [Abstract 219]. Presented at the American Urological Association Annual Meeting. Dallas, Texas, May 7, 1989.

Cantwell, F. V.: Operative technique of epispadias by transplantation of the urethra. Ann. Surg., 22:689, 1895.

Cendron, J.: La reconstruction vesicale. Ann. Chir. Infant, 12:371, 1971.

Cerniglia, F. R., Roth, D. A., and Gonzalez, E. T.: Covered exstrophy and visceral sequestration in a male newborn: Case report. J. Urol., 141:903, 1989.

Chisholm, T. C.: Exstrophy of the urinary bladder. In Kiesewetter, W. B. (Ed.): Long-term follow-up in congenital anomalies. Pediatr. Surgical Symposium. Vol. 6, p. 31. Pittsburgh Children's Hospital, 1979.

Chisholm, T. C.: Pediatric Surgery, Vol. 2. Chicago, Year Book Medical Publishers, 1962, p. 933.

Clark, M., and O'Connell, K. J.: Scanning and transmission electron microscopic studies of an exstrophic human bladder. J. Urol., 110:481, 1973.

Clemetson, C. A. B.: Ectopia vesicae and split pelvis. J. Obstet. Gynaecol. Br. Monnw., 65:973, 1958.

Coffey, R. C.: Transplantation of the ureter into the large intestine in the absence of a functioning bladder. Surg. Gynecol. Obstet., 32:383, 1921.

Cohen, S. J.: Ureterozystoneostomie eine neve antirefluxtechnik. Aktuel. Urol. 6:24, 1975.

Connor, J. P., Lattimer, J. K., Hensle, T. W., and Burbige, K. A.: Primary bladder closure of bladder exstrophy: Long-term functional results in 137 patients. J. Pediatr. Surg., 23:1102, 1988.

Cracchiolo, A., III, and Hall, C. B.: Bilateral iliac osteotomy. Clin. Orthop., 68:156, 1970.

Culp, D. A.: The histology of the exstrophied bladder. J. Urol., 91:538, 1964.

Davis, H. H., and Nikhaus, F. W.: Persistent omphalomesenteric duct and urachus in the same case. JAMA, 86:685, 1926.

Decter, R. M., Roth, D. R., Fishman, I. J., Shabsigh, R., Scott, F. B., and Gonzalez, E. T.: Use of the AS 800 device in exstrophy and epispadias. J. Urol., 140:1202, 1988.

Dees, J. E.: Congenital epispadias with incontinence. J. Urol., 62:513, 1949.

Devine, C. J., Jr., Horton, C. E., and Scarff, J. E., Jr.: Epispadias: Symposium of pediatric urology. Urol. Clin. North Am., 7:465, 1980.

Dixon, C. F., and Weisman, R. E.: Polyps of the sigmoid occurring 30 years after bilateral ureterosigmoidostomies for exstrophy of the bladder. Surgery, 24:6, 1948.

Duckett, J. W.: Use of paraexstrophy skin pedicle grafts for correction of exstrophy and epispadias repair. Birth Defects, 13:171, 1977.

Duckett, J. W., and Gazak, J. M.: Complications of ureterosigmoidostomy. Urol. Clin. North Am., 10:473, 1983.

Engel, R. M.: Bladder exstrophy: Vesicoplasty or urinary diversion. Urology, 2:29, 1973.

Engel, R. M., and Wilkinson, H. A.: Bladder exstrophy. J. Urol., 104:699, 1970.

Ezwell, W. W., and Carlson, H. E.: A realistic look at exstrophy of the bladder. Br. J. Urol., 42:197, 1970.

Fonkalsrud, E. W., and Linde, L. M.: Successful management of vesicointestinal fissure: Report of 2 cases. J. Pediatr. Surg., 5:309, 1970.

Frank, J. D., Mor, S. B., and Pryor, J. P.: The surgical correction of erectile deformities of the penis of 100 men. Br. J. Urol., 53:645, 1981.

Gearhart, J. P., and Jeffs, R. D.: The use of parenteral testosterone therapy in central reconstructive surgery. J. Urol., 138:1077, 1987.

Gearhart, J. P., and Jeffs, R. D.: Augmentation cystoplasty in the failed exstrophy reconstruction. J. Urol., 139:790, 1988.

Gearhart, J. P., and Jeffs, R. D.: Bladder exstrophy: Increase in capacity following epispadias repair. J. Urol., 142:525, 1989a.

Gearhart, J. P., and Jeffs, R. D.: State of the art reconstructive surgery for bladder exstrophy at the Johns Hopkins Hospital. Am. J. Dis. Child., 143:1475, 1989b.

Gearhart, J. P., and Jeffs, R. D.: Techniques for continence in the cloacal exstrophy patient. J. Urol. (In press.)

Gearhart, J. P., Jeffs, R. D., and Saunders, R.: Prenatal diagnosis of congenital bladder exstrophy—a retrospective review for diagnostic clues. Unpublished data.

Gearhart, J. P., Williams, K. A., and Jeffs, R. D.: Intraoperative urethral pressure profilometry as an adjunct to bladder neck reconstruction. J. Urol., 136:1055, 1986.

Gearhart, J. P., Yang, A., Leonard, M. P., Jeffs, R. E., and Zirhuni, E. A.: Prostatic size and configuration in adult men with classic bladder exstrophy [Abstract 849]. Presented at the American Urological Association Meeting. New Orleans, Louisiana, May 11, 1990.

Geist, D.: Patent urachus. Am. J. Surg., 84:118, 1952.

Glenn, J. F.: Agenesis of the bladder. JAMA, 169:2016, 1959.

Gokcora, I. H., and Yazar, T.: Bilateral transverse iliac osteotomy in the correction of neonatal bladder exstrophy. Int. Surg., 74:123, 1989.

Gravier, L.: Exstrophy of the cloaca. Am. Surg., 34:387, 1968.

Gross, R. E., and Cresson, S. L.: Exstrophy of the bladder: Observations from eighty cases. JAMA, 149:1640, 1952.

Haller, J. A., Jr.: Pediatric surgery. In Schwartz, S. I., Lillehei, R. C., Shires, G. T., Spencer, F. C., and Starer, E. H. (Eds.): Surgery. New York, McGraw-Hill Book Co., 1974, p. 1513.

Hammond, G., Yglesias, L., and David, J. E.: The urachus, its anatomy and associated fasciae. Anat. Rec., 80:271, 1941.

Hanna, M. K.: Artificial urinary sphincter for incontinent children. Urology, 18:370, 1981.

Hanna, M. K., and Williams, D. J.: Genital function in males with vesical exstrophy and epispadias. Br. J. Urol., 44:1969, 1972.

Hartmann, R., Schuberg, L. G. E., and Bichler, K. H.: Bladder exstrophy and cancer. Aktuel. Urol., 15:116, 1984.

Harvard, B. M., and Thompson, G. J.: Congenital exstrophy of the urinary bladder: Late results of treatment by the Coffey-Mayo method of ureterointestinal anastomosis. J. Urol., 65:223, 1951.

Hector, A.: Les vestiges de l'ouraque et leur pathologie. J. Chir. (Paris), 81:449, 1961.

Heitz-Boyer, M., and Hovelaque, A.: Creation d'une nouvelle vessie et d'une nouvelle uretre. J. Urol., 1:237, 1912.

Hendren, W. H.: Exstrophy of the bladder: An alternative method of management. J. Urol., 115:195, 1976.

Hendren, W. H.: Penile lengthening after previous repair of epispadias. J. Urol., 12:527, 1979.

Herbst, W. P.: Patent urachus. South Med. J., 30:711, 1937.

Higgins, C. C.: Exstrophy of the bladder: Report of 158 cases. Am. Surg., 28:99, 1962.

Hinman, F., Jr.: A method of lengthening and repairing the penis in exstrophy of the bladder. J. Urol., 79:237, 1958.

Hinman, F., Jr.: Surgical disorders of the bladder and umbilicus of urachal origin. Surg. Gynecol. Obstet., 113:605, 1961.

Howell, C., Caldamone, A., Snyder, H., et al.: Optimal management of cloacal exstrophy. J. Pediatr. Surg., 18:365, 1983.

Hurwitz, R. S., Manzoni, G. A., Ransley, P. G., and Stephens, F. D.: Cloacal exstrophy: A report of 34 cases. J. Urol., 138:1060, 1987.

Husmann, D. A., McLorie, G. A., and Churchill, B. M.: A comparison of renal function in the exstrophy patient treated with staged reconstruction vs. urinary diversion. J. Urol., 140:1204, 1988.

Husmann, D. A., McLorie, G. A., and Churchill, B. M.: Closure of the exstrophic bladder: An evaluation of the factors leading to its success and its importance on urinary continence. J. Urol., 142:522, 1989a.

Husmann, D. A., McLorie, G. A., and Churchill, B. M.: Phallic reconstruction in cloacal exstrophy. J. Urol., 142:563, 1989b.

Ives, E., Coffey, R., and Carter, C. O.: A family study of bladder exstrophy. J. Med. Genet., 17:139, 1980.

Janssen, P.: Die operation der blasenektopie ohne inanspruchnahme des intestinums. Zentralbl. Chir., 60:2657, 1933.

Jeffs, R. D.: Personal communication, 1979.

Jeffs, R. D., Charrios, R., Many, M., and Juransz, A. R.: Primary closure of the exstrophied bladder. In Scott, R. (Ed.): Current Controversies in Urologic Management. Philadelphia, W. B. Saunders Co., 1972, p. 235.

Jeffs, R. D., Guice, S. L., and Oesch, I.: The factors in successful exstrophy closure. J. Urol., 127:974, 1982.

Jeffs, R. D., and Schwarz, G. R.: Ileal conduit urinary diversion in children: Computer analysis follow-up from 2 to 16 years. J. Urol., 114:285, 1975.

Johnston, J. H.: Vesical diverticula without urinary obstruction in childhood. J. Urol., 84:535, 1960.

Johnston, J. H.: Lengthening of the congenital or acquired short penis. Br. J. Urol., 46:685, 1974.

Johnston, J. H., and Kogan, S. J.: The exstrophic anomalies and their surgical reconstruction. Curr. Probl. Surg., August: 1–39, 1974.

Kandzari, S. J., Majid, A., Ortega, A. M., and Milam, D. F.: Exstrophy of the urinary bladder complicated by adenocarcinoma. Urology, 3:496, 1974.

Kapoor, R., and Saha, M. M.: Complete duplication of the bladder, common urethra and external genitalia in the neonate: A case report. J. Urol., 137:1243, 1987.

Kenigsberg, K.: Infection of umbilical artery simulating patent urachus. J. Pediatr., 86:151, 1975.

Koff, S. A., and Eakins, M.: The treatment of penile chordee using corporeal rotation. J. Urol., 131:931, 1984.

Kossow, J. H., and Morales, P. A.: Duplication of bladder and urethra and associated anomalies. Urology, 1:71, 1973.

Kramer, S. A.: Augmentation cystoplasty in patients with exstrophy-epispadias. J. Pediatr. Surg., 24:1293, 1989.

Kramer, S. A., and Jackson, I. T.: Bilateral rhomboid flaps for reconstruction of the external genitalia in epispadias-exstrophy. Plast. Reconstr. Surg., 77:621, 1986.

Kramer, S. A., and Kelalis, P. P.: Assessment of urinary continence in epispadias: A review of 94 patients. J. Urol. 128:290, 1982.

Kramer, S. A., Mesrobian, H. G., and Kelalis, P. P.: Long-term follow-up of cosmetic appearance and genital function in male epispadias. Review of 70 cases. J. Urol., 135:543, 1986.

Krishnansetty, R. M., Rao, M. K., Hines, C. R., Saikali, E. P., Corpus, R. P., and Debandi, H. O.: Adenocarcinoma in exstrophy and defunctional ureterosigmoidostomy. J. Ky. Med. Assoc., 86:409, 1988.

Krisiloff, M., Puchner, P. J., Tretter, W., MacFarlane, M. T., and Lattimer, J. K.: Pregnancy in women with bladder exstrophy. J. Urol., 119:478, 1978.

Kroovand, R. L., and Boyce, W. H.: Isolated vesicorectal internal urinary diversion: A 37-year review of the Boyce-Vest procedure. J. Urol., 140:572, 1988.

Krull, C. L., Hanes, C. F., and DeKlerk, D. P.: Agenesis of the bladder and urethra: A case report. J. Urol., 140:793, 1988.

Lancaster, P. A. L.: Epidemiology of bladder exstrophy: A communication from the international clearing house for birth defects monitoring systems. Teratology, 36:221, 1987.

Lattimer, J. K.: Congenital deficiency of the abdominal musculature and associated genitourinary anomalies: A report of 22 cases. J. Urol., 79:343, 1958.

Lattimer, J. K., Beck, L., Yeaw, S., Puchner, P. J., MacFarlane, M. T., and Krisiloff, M.: Long-term follow-up after exstrophy closure—late improvement and good quality of life. J. Urol., 119:664, 1978.

Lattimer, J. K., and Smith, M. J. K.: Exstrophy closure: A followup on 70 cases. J. Urol., 95:356, 1966a.

Leadbetter, W. F.: Consideration of problems incident to performance of ureteroenterostomy: Report of a technique. J. Urol., 73:67, 1955.

Leadbetter, W. F., Jr.: Surgical correction of total urinary incontinence. J. Urol., 91:261, 1964.

Leonard, M. P., Gearhart, J. P., and Jeffs, R. D.: Continent urinary diversion in childhood J. Urol., 144:330, 1990.

Lepor, H., and Jeffs, R. D.: Primary bladder closure and bladder neck reconstruction in classical bladder exstrophy. J. Urol., 130:1142, 1983.

Lepor, H., Shapiro, E., and Jeffs, R. D.: Urethral reconstruction in males with classical bladder exstrophy. J. Urol., 131:512, 1984.

Levard, G., Aigrain, Y., Ferkadji, L., et al.: Urinary bladder diverticula and the Ehlers-Danlos syndrome in children. J. Pediatr. Surg., 24:1184, 1989.

Lione, P. M., and Gonzales, E. T.: Congenital bladder diverticula causing ureteral obstruction. Urology, 25:273, 1985.

Lowe, F. C., and Jeffs, R. D.: Wound dehiscence in bladder exstrophy: An examination of the etiologies and factors for initial failure and subsequent closure. J. Urol., 130:312, 1983.

MacFarlane, M. T., Lattimer, J. K., and Hensle, T. W.: Improved life expectancy for children with exstrophy of the bladder. JAMA, 242:442, 1979.

MacMillan, R. W., Schulinger, J. N., and Santulli, V. T.: Pyourachus: An unusual surgical problem. J. Pediatr. Surg., 8:87, 1973.

Marshall, V. F., Marchetti, A. A., and Krantz, K. E.: The correction of stress incontinence by simple vesicourethral suspension. Surg. Gynecol. Obstet., 88:509, 1949.

Marshall, V. F., and Muecke, E. C.: Congenital abnormalities of the bladder. *In* Handbuch de Urolgie. New York, Springer-Verlag, 1968, p. 165.

Marshall, J. T., Muecke, E. C.: Functional closure of typical exstrophy of the bladder. J. Urol., 104:205, 1970.

Maydl, K.: Uber die radikaltherapie der ectopia vesical urinarie. Wien. Med. Wochenschr. 25:1113–1115, 1894.

Mayo, C. H., and Hendricks, W. A.: Exstrophy of the bladder. Surg. Gynecol. Obstet., 43:129, 1926.

Meizner, I., and Bar-Ziv, J.: In utero prenatal ultrasonic diagnosis of a rare case of cloacal exstrophy. J. Clin. Ultrasound, 13:500, 1985.

Mendoza, C. B., Jr., Cueto, J., Payan, H., and Gerwig, W. H., Jr.: Complete urachal tract associated with Meckel's diverticulum. Arch. Surg., 96:438, 1968.

Mesrobian, H. J., Kelalis, P. P., and Kramer, S. A.: Long-term follow-up of cosmetic appearance and genital function in boys with exstrophy: Review of 53 patients. J. Urol., 136:256, 1986.

Michalowski, E., and Modelski, M.: The surgical treatment of epispadias. Surg. Gynecol. Obstet., 117:476, 1963.

Mildenberger, H., Kluth, D., and Dziuba, M.: Embryology of bladder exstrophy. J. Pediatr. Surg., 23:116, 1988.

Mirk, M., Calisti, A., and Feleni, A.: Prenatal sonographic diagnosis of bladder exstrophy. J. Ultrasound Med., 5:291, 1986.

Mitchell, M. E., and Piser, J. A.: Intestinocystoplasty and total bladder replacement in children and young adults: Follow-up in 129 cases. J. Urol., 138:579, 1987.

Mollard, P.: Bladder reconstruction in exstrophy. J. Urol., 124:523, 1980.

Monfort, G., Lacombe, G. M., Guys, J. M., and Coquet, M.: Transverse island flap and double flap procedure in the treatment of congenital epispadias in 32 patients. J. Urol., 138:1069, 1987.

Montagnani, C. A.: Functional reconstruction of exstrophied bladder: Timing and technique: Follow-up of 39 cases. Kinderchirurgie, 43:322, 1988.

Mostofi, R. K.: Potentialities of bladder epithelium. J. Urol., 71:705, 1954.

Muecke, E. C.: The role of the cloacal membrane in exstrophy: The first successful experimental study. J. Urol., 92:659, 1964.

Muecke, E. C.: Exstrophy, epispadias, and other anomalies of the bladder. *In* Walsh, P. C., Gittes, R. F., Perlmutter, A. D., and Stoney, T. A. (eds.): Campbell's Urology, 5th edition. Philadelphia, W. B. Saunders Co., 1986.

Narasimharao, K. I., Chana, R. S., Mitra, S. R., and Pathak, I. C.: Covered exstrophy and visceral sequestration: A rare exstrophy variant. J. Urol., 133:274, 1985.

Neidhardt, J. H., Morin, A., Spay, G., Guelpa, G., and Chavvier, J.: Mise au oint sur les kystes suppures de l'ouraque. J. Urol. Nephrol. (Paris), 74:793, 1968.

Ney, C., and Friedenberg, R. M.: Radiographic findings in the anomalies of the urachus. J. Urol., 99:288, 1968.

Nisonson, I., and Lattimer, J. K.: How well can the exstrophied bladder work? J. Urol., 107:668, 1972.

Nix, J. T., Menville, J. G., Albert, M., and Wendt, D. L.: Congenital patent urachus. J. Urol., 79:264, 1958.

Nunn, L. L.: Urachal cysts and their complications. Am. J. Surg., 84:252, 1952.

Oesterling, J. E., and Jeffs, R. D.: The importance of a successful initial bladder closure in the surgical management of classical bladder exstrophy: Analysis of 144 patients treated at the Johns Hopkins Hospital between 1975 and 1985. J. Urol., 137:258, 1987.

Patton, B. M., and Barry, A.: The genesis of exstrophy of the bladder and epispadias. Am. J. Anat., 90:35, 1952.

Persutte, W. H., Lenke, R. R., Kropp, K., and Ghareb, C.: Antenatal diagnosis of fetal patent urachus. J. Ultrasound Med., 7:399, 1988.

Peters, C. A., Gearhart, J. P., and Jeffs, R. D.: Epispadias and incontinence: The challenge of the small bladder. J. Urol., 140:1199, 1988.

Peters, C. A., and Hendren, W. H.: Splitting the pubis for exposure in difficult reconstruction for incontinence [Abstract 23]. Presented at the American Academy of Pediatrics Urology Section. San Francisco, California, October 15, 1988.

Ransley, P. G., Duffy, P. G., and Wollin, M.: Bladder exstrophy closure and epispadias repair. *In* Operative Surgery—Paediatric Surgery, Ed. 4. Edinburgh, Butterworths, 1989, p. 620.

Remigailo, R. V., Woodard, J. R., Andrews, H. G., and Patterson, J. H.: Cloacal exstrophy: 18-year survival of an untreated case. J. Urol., 116:811, 1976.

Rickham, P. P.: Vesicointestinal fissure. Arch. Dis. Child., 35:967, 1960.

Rink, R. C., and Retik, A. B.: Ureteroileocecalsigmoidostomy and avoidance of carcinoma of the colon. *In* Bladder Reconstruction and Continent Urinary Diversion. Chicago, Year Book Medical Publishers, 1987, p. 172.

Ritchey, M. L., Kramer, S. A., and Kelalis, P. P.: Vesical neck reconstruction in patients with epispadias-exstrophy. J. Urol., 139:1278, 1988.

Schillinger, J. F., and Wiley, M. J.: Bladder exstrophy: Penile lengthening procedure. Urology, 24:434, 1984.

Schlegel, P. N., and Gearhart, J. P.: Neuroanatomy of the pelvis in an infant with cloacal exstrophy: A detailed microdissection with histology. J. Urol., 141:583, 1989.

Schreck, W. R., and Campbell, W. A.: The relationship of bladder outlet obstruction to urinary umbilical fistula. J. Urol., 108:641, 1972.

Schultz, W. G.: Plastic repair of exstrophy of the bladder combined with bilateral osteotomy of the ilia. J. Urol., 92:659, 1964.

Shapiro, E., Jeffs, R. D., Gearhart, J. P., and Lepor, H.: Muscarinic cholinergic receptors in bladder exstrophy: Insights into surgical management. J. Urol., 134:309, 1985.

Shapiro, E., Lepor, H., and Jeffs, R. D.: The inheritance of classical bladder exstrophy. J. Urol., 132:308, 1984.

Shapiro, S. R., Lebowitz, R., and Colodny, A. H.: Fate of 90 children with ileal conduit urinary diversion a decade later. J. Urol., 114:133, 1975.

Semerdjian, H. S., Texter, J. H., and Yawn, D. H.: Rhabdomyosarcoma occurrence in repaired exstrophic bladder: Case report. J. Urol., 108:354, 1972.

Soper, R. T., and Kilger, K.: Vesico-intestinal fissure. J. Urol., 92:490, 1964.

Spence, H. M., Hoffman, W. W., and Fosmire, P. P.: Tumors of the colon as a later complication of ureterosigmoidostomy of exstrophy of the bladder. Br. J. Urol., 51:466, 1979.

Spence, H. M., Hoffman, W. N., and Pate, V. A.: Exstrophy of the bladder: Long-term results in a series of 37 cases treated by ureterosigmoidostomy. J. Urol., 114:133, 1975.

Sponseller, P. D., Gearhart, J. P., and Jeffs, R. D.: Iliac osteotomies for revision of bladder exstrophy failures. J. Urol. Submitted for publication.

Steck, W. D., and Helwig, E. B.: Umbilical granulomas, pilonidal disease, and the urachus. Surg. Gynecol. Obstet., 120:1043, 1965.

Steinbuchel, W.: Ueber nabelschnurbruch and blasenbauchspalte mit codken bildung von seiten des dunndormers. Arch. Gynaeckol., 60:465, 1900.

Sterling, J. A., and Goldsmith, R.: Lesions of urachus which appear in the adult. Ann. Surg., 137:120, 1953.

Stockel, M., Becht, E., Voges, G., Riedmiuer, H., and Hohenfellner, R.: Ureterosigmoidostomy: An outdated approach to bladder exstrophy. J. Urol., 143:770, 1990.

Sweetser, T. H., Chisholm, T. C., and Thompson, W. H.: Exstrophy

of the urinary bladder: Discussion of anatomic principles applicable to its repair with a preliminary report of a case. Minn. Med., 35:654, 1952.

Taccinoli, M., Laurenti, C., and Racheli, T.: Sixteen years experience with the Heitz-Boyer Hovelacque procedure for exstrophy of the bladder. Br. J. Urol., 49:385, 1977.

Tauber, J., and Bloom, B.: Infected urachal cyst. J. Urol., 66:692, 1951.

Taylor, W. N., Alton, D., Toguri, A., et al.: Bladder diverticulum causing posterior urethral obstruction in children. J. Urol., 122:415, 1979.

Thiersch, C.: Ueber die ensstehuns weise und operative behandlung der epispadie. Arch. Heilkunde, 10:20, 1869.

Thomalla, J., and Mitchell, M. E.: Ventral preputial island flap technique for the repair of epispadias with or without exstrophy. J. Urol., 132:985, 1984.

Toguri, A. G., Churchill, B. M., Schillinger, J. F., and Jeffs, R. D.: Continence in cases of bladder exstrophy. J. Urol., 119:538, 1978.

Trendelenburg, R.: The treatment of ectopia vesicae. Ann. Surg., 44:281, 1906.

Uson, A. C., and Roberts, M. S.: Incomplete exstrophy of the urinary bladder: A report of 2 cases. J. Urol., 79:57, 1958.

Verco, P. W., Khor, B. H., Barbary, J., and Enthoven, C.: Ectopic vesicae in utero. Australas. Radiol., 30:117, 1986.

Vyas, P. R., Roth, D. P. R., and Perlmutter, A. B.: Experience with free grafts in urethral reconstruction. J. Urol., 137:471, 1987.

Walsh, P. C., and Donker, P. J.: Impotence following radical prostatectomy: Insight into etiology and prevention. J. Urol., 128:492, 1982.

Williams, D. I.: Congenital bladder neck obstruction and megaureter. Br. J. Urol., 29:389, 1957.

Williams, D. I., and Keaton, J.: Vesical exstrophy: Twenty years' experience. Br. J. Surg., 60:203, 1973.

Woodhouse, C. R. J.: The management of erectile deformity in adults with exstrophy and epispadias. J. Urol., 135:932, 1986.

Woodhouse, C. R. J.: Reconstruction in the epispadias penis in adolescence. Progr. Pediatr. Surg., 23:165, 1989.

Woodhouse, C. R. J., and Kellett, M. J.: Anatomy of the penis and its deformities in exstrophy and epispadias. J. Urol., 132:1122, 1984.

Woodhouse, C. R. J., Ransley, P. C., and Williams, D. I.: The exstrophy patient in adult life. Br. J. Urol., 55:632, 1983.

Young, H. H.: An operation for the cure of incontinence associated with exstrophy. J. Urol., 7:1, 1922.

Young, H. H.: Exstrophy of the bladder: The first case in which a normal bladder and urinary control have been obtained by plastic operation. Surg. Gynecol. Obstet., 74:729, 1942.

Zarbo, A., and Kay, R.: Uterosigmoidostomy in bladder exstrophy: A long-term follow-up. J. Urol., 136:396, 1986.

47
CLOACAL MALFORMATIONS

W. Hardy Hendren, M.D.

In the early embryo (5 weeks), the urinary, genital, and gastrointestinal tracts empty into a common chamber, the cloaca. The Latin word "cloaca" stands for sewer. At this stage, the cloaca is covered by a membrane. In the 6th week, the urorectal septum descends, dividing the cloaca into an anterior urogenital sinus and a posterior gastrointestinal canal. Simultaneously, lateral folds migrate to the midline to separate these two compartments.

The lower urorectal septum becomes the perineal body, which separates the genitourinary and anorectal tracts. The mesonephric (wolffian) ducts enter the cloaca laterally, and from them come the ureteral buds, which induce renal development. In male embryos, the lower mesonephric ducts give rise to the epididymides, vasa deferens, and seminal vesicles, but they regress in females. Paired paramesonephric (müllerian) ducts lie medial to the wolffian ducts and later fuse in the midline, becoming fallopian tubes, uterus, and upper vagina.

Many steps in this complex embryologic sequence can go awry, producing a wide spectrum of anomalies (Bremer, 1957; Gray and Skandalakis, 1972; Johnson et al., 1972; Marshall et al., 1979; Pohlman, 1911; Stephens and Smith, 1971). In males, maldevelopment can result in imperforate anus with fistula to the urinary tract and various urologic anomalies. It has become axiomatic that any child—male or female—with imperforate anus requires urologic screening, because there is a high coincidence of correctable urologic malformations (Belman and King, 1972; Hall et al., 1970; Hendren, 1988; Hoekstra et al., 1983; McLorie et al., 1987; Munn and Schullinger, 1983; Parrott, 1985; Rich et al., 1988; Smith, 1968; Wiener and Kiesewetter, 1973).

In the female embryo, the genital tract interposed between the bladder and rectum produces a wide variety of anatomic possibilities in addition to imperforate anus. Conditions within this wide spectrum are clinically termed "cloacal malformations" (Gough, 1959; Kay and Tank, 1977; Palken et al., 1972; Snyder, 1966; Williams and Bloomberg, 1976). A cloaca is normal anatomy for birds, reptiles, and some fishes; but, in humans, it can be disastrous. Nevertheless, for most patients, there is a satisfactory surgical solution.

Remarks in this chapter are based on my personal experience with 104 cases of cloacal malformations. Sixty four were primary cases—patients who had not undergone major reconstructive surgery. Forty were secondary cases—patients who had previously undergone some type of reconstructive operation, often a rectal pull-through procedure, without correction of the genital and urologic aspects of the malformation. To illustrate the serious urologic consequences seen in females with cloacas, 26 of the secondary cases had undergone a prior urinary diversion (four ileal loops, six ureterostomies, and 16 vesicostomies). Furthermore, serious vesicoureteral reflux was found in 57 patients. Many of these cases have been described previously (Hendren, 1977, 1980, 1982, 1986, 1988, 1990; Hendren et al., 1987; Hendren and Molenaar, 1987).

ANATOMY

Appearance of Perineum

The external anatomy varies widely in female infants and children with cloacal malformations. This diversity is shown to some degree in Figure 47–1. At the mild end of the developmental spectrum is an almost normal-looking vaginal introitus, with the anal opening very close to it, but not actually incorporated into the urogenital sinus. The perineal body is very thin. In the next degree of severity, the rectum is further forward, so that its actual opening is incorporated into the urogenital sinus at a low level.

The external topography when there is one perineal opening also varies greatly. The opening may resemble the normal female vaginal introitus. In the next degree of severity, the labial tissue is displaced forward with the clitoris, which may appear enlarged, and the external opening is reduced in size. In this degree of severity, the perineum can then have a completely blank-looking appearance with no opening immediately visible until one lifts the clitoris and observes the opening at its base surrounded by rudimentary labia.

In some cases, the urogenital sinus extends to the tip

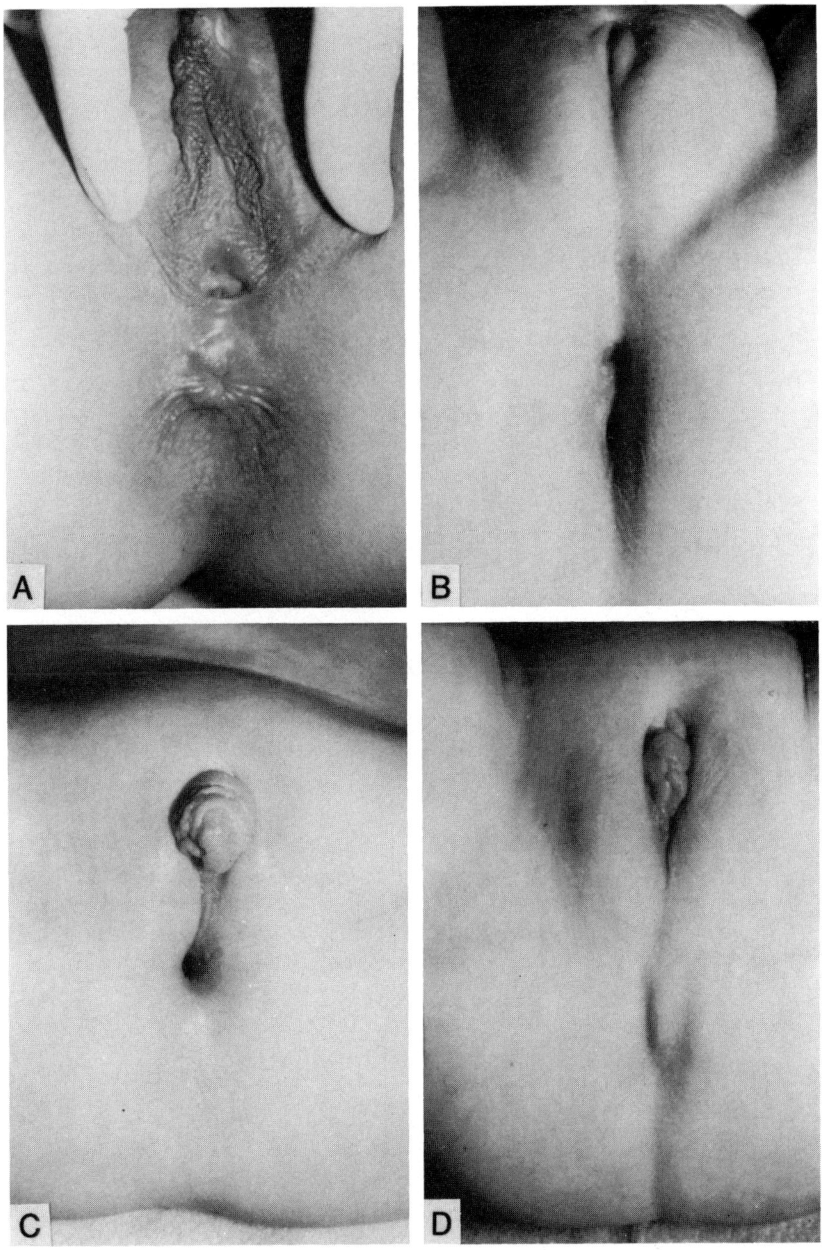

Figure 47–1. Spectrum of appearance of perineum in females with cloacal malformations. *A,* Minimal anomaly with anteriorly displaced anus, which is just short of converging with urogenital sinus. Urogenital sinus opening had been previously "cut back" but shows inadequate entry to vagina. *B,* Single opening far back in perineum. When the buttocks were spread widely, the anal opening and the urogenital sinus opening were visible close to one another. Extending forward from this cloacal chamber was a thread-like passage emerging at the tip of the clitoris. Urine passed through the perineum, not through that accessory tract. *C,* Progressing toward more severe cloacal anatomy, with single opening in perineum into which urethra, vagina, and rectum entered. Note phallic structure, which is inappropriately large for a clitoris yet not like hypospadias with chordee, because there are no scrotal structures. *D,* Typical severe cloacal anatomy with blank perineum and single opening at base of phallic structure. This patient has a well-developed gluteal cleft, which signifies good perineal muscle beneath it, in contrast to the patient shown in *C* with a poorly developed gluteal cleft, which usually denotes lack of good muscle.

of the rudimentary phallic structure (Fig. 47–2). In three of our cases in which a well-defined cloacal opening was found in the perineum, a tiny secondary accessory passage arose on its anterior wall, running up into the tip of the phallus. This finding has also been described by others (Karlin et al., 1989).

Paralleling this wide range in external topography is a wide range in the spectrum of the internal anatomy, shown in Figure 47–3. The structures may converge relatively low in the pelvis, so that there is a length of urethra between the bladder neck and the entry of the urethra into the urogenital sinus. In others, there is a high confluence, so that all three systems—bladder, vagina, and rectum—converge at the same high level. Similarly, these structures can come together in the trigone of the bladder, so that there is no bladder neck, which poses an even greater task for the reconstructive surgeon.

Vagina

Great variability is found in the vaginal anatomy (Fig. 47–4). It is important to define this anatomy preoperatively. In 50 cases, a single vagina with a single uterine cervix was found. However, in 43 cases, two vaginas were discovered, and these vaginas can vary greatly in their anatomy. Most commonly, the two vaginas lie side by side, with a midline septum between them. They can be easily converted into a single vaginal passage by incising the center of the septum with a cutting electrode, from its lower end up to the level of the two cervices, which lie on each side of the septum at the apex of the two vaginas. In some cases, the lower vaginas are adjacent, but soon diverge, one to each side of the pelvis. Rarely, two separate ostia are present, each entering separately into the side of the urogenital sinus.

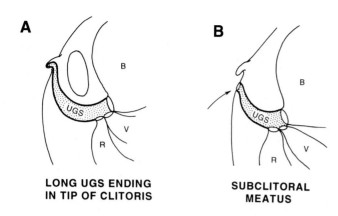

A LONG UGS ENDING IN TIP OF CLITORIS

B SUBCLITORAL MEATUS

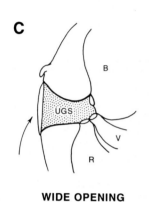

C WIDE OPENING (Like a vagina)

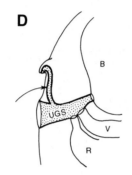

D WITH ACCESSORY TRACT

Figure 47–2. Urogenital sinus (UGS) variations, which can differ widely. *A*, A long urogenital sinus, which ends in a small aperture at the tip of the phallic structure. This finding is usually associated with a severe cloacal malformation. Cutting the UGS back a few millimeters at birth will facilitate endoscopy and intermittent catheterization to decompress the lower urinary tract. *B*, Subclitoral meatus. *C*, A wide opening of the UGS. This opening will need to be tapered to construct a urethra from it. *D*, A rare variant showing a nonfunctional accessory tract leading forward from the UGS to the tip of the phallus. It should be marsupialized at the time of a definitive reconstruction.

Figure 47–3. The spectrum of anatomy seen in urogenital sinus and cloacal malformations. *A*, The rectum in normal position. *B*, The anorectal canal clearly farther forward than normal, but not actually joining the urogenital sinus. *C*, Low cloacal malformation, which can usually be repaired through a posterior sagittal approach. *D*, High confluence of the three organ systems, which may require an abdominal approach as well.

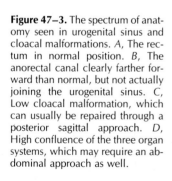

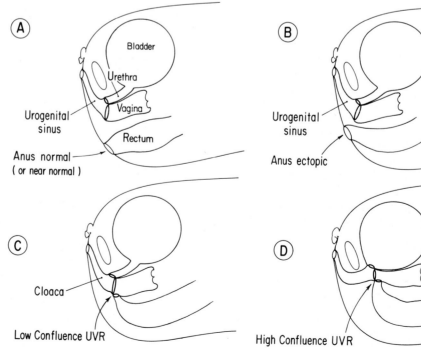

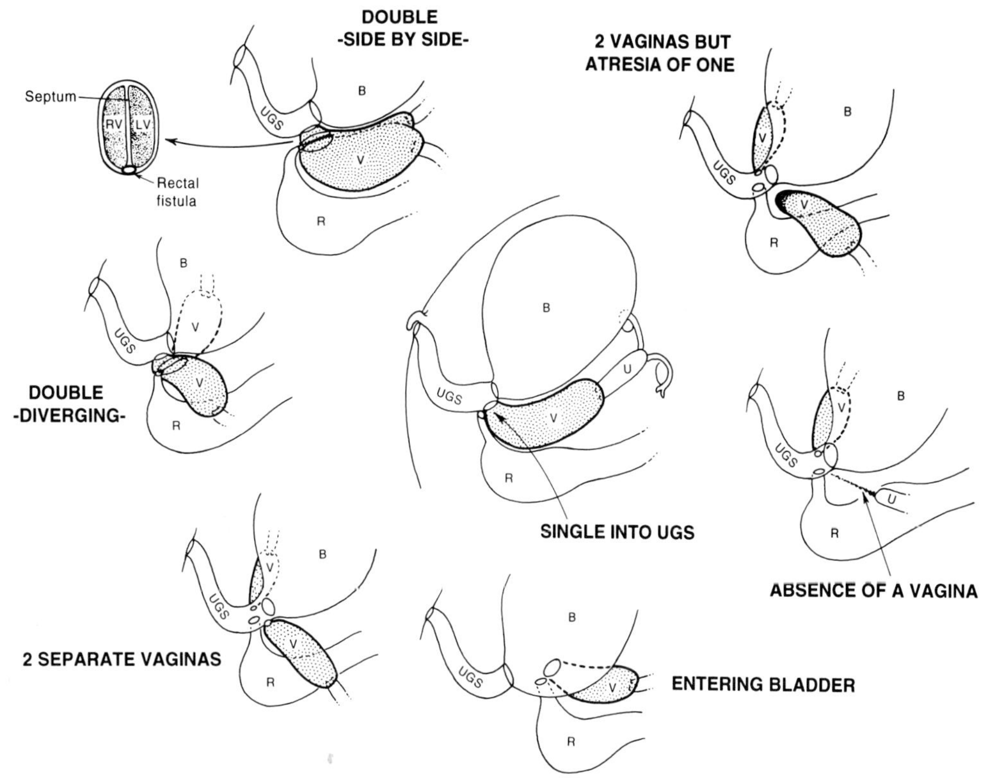

Figure 47–4. Variations in vaginal anatomy in cloacal malformations. Most commonly, there is a single vagina entering the urogenital sinus (UGS), with the rectal fistula entering at 6 o'clock adjacent to it, or just inside the vaginal opening. As shown, there can be two vaginas side by side; two vaginas that diverge laterally; two separate vaginas, each with its own opening into the UGS; atresia of a vagina; absence of a vagina, but presence of a uterus on that side; and entry of the vagina, or two vaginas, directly into the bladder. (B, bladder; V, vagina; R, rectum.)

Other variations include absence of a vagina, but presence of its uterus, and absence of the vagina and uterus. When there are two separate vaginas, they can sometimes be joined into one. In other cases, it may be better to retain one and remove the other. Sometimes, the vagina is very large. In other cases, however, it can be small, offering no chance for bringing it to the perineum except by using an extension of bowel.

The technique of creating a bowel extension for a vagina has been described previously (Hendren, 1986). The segment of bowel to be used is brought down to the perineum between the opening for the urethra and the anus, employing a combined abdominal-perineal access. When the bowel segment has been joined to the perineum, the short vagina is anastomosed to it in end-to-end or end-to-side fashion, depending on the length of the bowel segment and the size of the vagina. If colon is used for this, it may be the part that was the previously dilated terminal rectal segment, and the next higher level of bowel is used for the pull-through procedure. Conversely, if the lower colon is well-suited as rectum, a piece of sigmoid colon may be brought down as the extension for the vagina. Alternatively, an isolated segment of small bowel can be used to extend the vagina if the colon is not adaptable for that purpose.

Lower Rectum

The most common location for entry of the rectum into a cloaca is at the posterior margin of the vaginal orifice, as shown in Figure 47–5, or at the base of the vaginal septum, when one exists. Usually, the dilated terminal colon is located just above the entry site.

Occasionally, the fistula is a long tract running the full length of the vagina, so that the dilated lower colon is high in the pelvis and enters just behind the uterus. The relationship of the rectal fistula and vaginas can be transposed, so that the rectal opening lies anterior to the single or duplicated vaginal openings. Obviously, it is very important for the surgeon to work out such anatomic vagaries preoperatively to guide the operative repair of the anomaly.

Urinary Tract

Vesicoureteral reflux is common in these cases. The ureter often enters laterally, without a suitable tunnel, similar to what is seen routinely in exstrophy of the bladder after primary bladder closure. In other cases, the ureters may be ectopically located, too close to the bladder neck. A wide spectum of other associated problems has been encountered, including ureterocele, megaureter, ureteropelvic junction obstruction, and so forth. The urologic aspects of cloacal malformations are life-threatening if not properly managed.

In the past, many of these children underwent abdominal-perineal pull through of the rectum, so that they could have bowel movements from below; correction of the genitourinary problems was deferred. This practice led to disastrous consequences with the upper urinary tracts when there was massive reflux with infection. It is my firm conviction that some of these patients require a urologic procedure early in life, such as correction of reflux; the genital and gastrointestinal tracts can be dealt with later.

Occasionally, when the urologic aspects of a case have

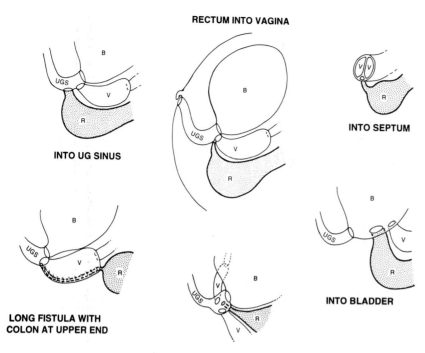

RECTUM INTO VAGINA

INTO UG SINUS

LONG FISTULA WITH
COLON AT UPPER END

RECTAL FISTULA ENTERING NEXT TO
BLADDER NECK AND ANTERIOR TO VAGINA(S)

INTO SEPTUM

INTO BLADDER

Figure 47–5. Variations in the rectal anatomy in cloacal malformations. Most commonly, the rectum enters at 6 o'clock in the vaginal orifice. When there are two vaginas, it usually enters at the base of the intervaginal septum. Rarely, the rectum opens into the urogenital sinus distal to the opening of the vagina. Occasionally, there is a long fistula, which opens in the usual location, but the actual rectal segment to be mobilized and pulled through is much higher. The rectal fistula can lie adjacent to the bladder neck, anterior to the vaginal opening(s). The bowel may enter the bladder itself, usually seen in cases with severely deranged anatomy. (B, bladder; R, rectum; UGS, urogenital sinus; V, vagina.)

been mild, we have elected to deal with the major cloacal reconstruction first, i.e., the urogenital sinus, vaginas, and colon, and with the urologic problem later. However, I am firmly convinced that there is absolutely no place today for an isolated rectal pull-through reconstruction early in life, deferring the more difficult aspects of the anomaly until later, "when the child grows up."

MANAGEMENT OF THE NEWBORN WITH CLOACAL MALFORMATION

At birth, or soon thereafter, the female infant with a severe cloacal malformation usually presents with abdominal distention and is noted to have an abnormal perineum characterized by imperforate anus and variable development of an external opening and labia. In the most severe cases, the phallus is similar to the primitive genital tubercle of the early embryo. At first, some are thought to have sexual ambiguity. However, an infant with this appearance is a genetic female with a cloacal malformation.

Plain radiographs of the abdomen will usually show a large, fluid-filled structure in the lower abdomen, as seen in Figure 47–6. In some, this structure is the bladder; but, more often, it is a very distended vagina, or vaginas, filled with urine. If diagnosis is delayed for a day or two, air may enter this large, fluid-filled structure, confusing the picture further if the clinician is not aware of the cloacal malformation.

Decompressive colostomy should be performed immediately. The location of the colostomy, in my opinion, should be in the right upper quadrant to maintain intact the blood supply of the left colon, sigmoid colon, and rectum. This approach will provide greater flexibility during a definitive reconstructive operation later. The colostomy should be divided to prevent continuing spillover of fecal material into the distal colon, which communicates with the urogenital sinus. It is tempting to perform an exploratory laparotomy simultaneously to view the pelvic organs; however, I think this procedure should be avoided to minimize the extent of the laparotomy for the distended baby and to avoid creating more postoperative bowel adhesions, which can cause intestinal obstruction.

Decompression of the Urinary Tract

In some cases with cloacal anatomy, the urogenital sinus is not obstructed, the infant empties the bladder easily, and the vagina is not dilated. In many of these cases, however, decompression of the urinary tract is needed urgently. Typically, the vagina is distended, pushing the bladder forward, and causing severe hydronephrosis, as shown in Figure 47–7.

Intermittent catheterization is begun immediately to see if it will decompress the lower urinary tract. This procedure can be done with a small plastic catheter or a small metal catheterizing sound. It may be necessary to cut back the urogenital sinus a few millimeters to facilitate catheterization. Almost invariably the catheter enters the distended vagina, not the bladder, because the passage into the bladder is angulated forward sharply, so that the catheter goes more easily into the vagina.

In some neonates, we have performed endoscopy immediately after the colostomy, introducing a 5-French plastic feeding catheter into the vagina and another into

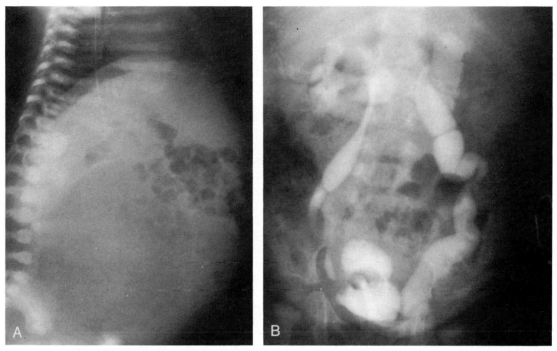

Figure 47–6. Roentgenograms from a typical cloacal case. *A*, Plain film showing large, rounded structure in lower abdomen. This structure was the vagina. *B*, Subsequent intravenous pyelogram after colostomy and decompression of the urinary tract, showing bilateral hydroureteronephrosis.

the bladder to decompress both structures. This procedure can be accomplished by passing an 8-French endoscope through the urogenital sinus into the vagina, removing the telescope, and passing the 5-French plastic catheter through it. The dilated end of the catheter is cut off so that the endoscope sheath can be withdrawn, leaving the catheter in place.

After the distended vagina is decompressed, the same maneuver can be repeated for the bladder. The two tubes are fastened in place, thereby securing good drainage for several days until the infant's course is stabilized and the colostomy begins to function. These tubes also allow introduction of contrast medium into the bladder and vagina to delineate the anatomy. The

Figure 47–7. Obstruction of the lower urinary tract by compression from vagina, which fills with urine in some cloacal malformations. At endoscopy, it may prove impossible to visualize the urethra or bladder neck until passing the endoscope into the vagina to drain it. During cystoscopy, the anterior displacement of the bladder is readily apparent. Ureteral orifices are often laterally placed and wide in caliber, consistent with reflux. Alternatively, they can be normal in appearance and location, or they can be ectopic near the bladder neck.

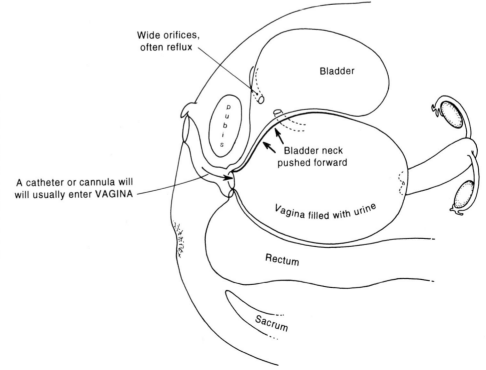

rectal anatomy can be demonstrated by introducing contrast medium into the distal limb of the colostomy.

If intermittent catheterization of the distended vagina fails to decompress the lower urinary tract, vesicostomy and/or tube vaginostomy can be considered. However, I believe these measures have possibly been used more often than needed. I treated two infants for whom vesicostomy had been performed at birth in whom it appeared that there was secondary obstruction of the urogenital sinus because it was tethered across the pubic symphysis by the vesicostomy, which had been performed high to avert prolapse of the bladder—a known complication of vesicostomy. Furthermore, I treated an infant in whom the distended vagina had been exteriorized in the anterior midline, with the mistaken idea that it was the bladder. This procedure deformed the right side of the bladder and its ureter, causing right hydronephrosis. Vesicostomy had been performed later in that patient, resulting in an unusual situation with a vaginostomy in the low anterior midline and a vesicostomy superior to it.

Diagnostic Imaging

Radiologic findings and imaging recommendations in cloacal patients have been described (Jaramillo et al., 1990). The upper urinary tract can be studied by ultrasound examination, or intravenous pyelogram if necessary. Contrast medium introduced into the urogenital sinus should disclose its anatomy and its relationship to the bladder neck, vagina(s), and rectal fistula. Contrast medium can be introduced into the distal limb of the colostomy to study the point of entry of the gastrointestinal tract into the cloaca. In a secondary case in which vesicostomy or vaginostomy has been performed, those openings can also be utilized for introduction of contrast medium.

These examinations are time consuming. The greater the experience of the radiologist, the greater the yield of information. Since the advent of magnetic resonance imaging (MRI) of the lumbosacral spine, this examination has become routine, to exclude the presence of tethering of the spinal cord. Normally, the spinal cord ends at the level of the first lumbar vertebra. If it is tethered to a lower level, sometimes with an associated lipoma of the spinal canal, it can produce neurologic deficit. Neurosurgical release of the spinal cord may prove helpful in preventing a neurologic deficit. Once a deficit is established, it is unlikely to be improved after detethering the cord.

Endoscopic Evaluation

An unhurried endoscopic examination is mandatory before embarking on the definitive correction of a cloacal malformation. If the vagina fills when the endoscope is introduced into the urogenital sinus, it can displace the bladder neck so far forward that visualization of the bladder entry is impossible. In this instance, the bladder and vagina should be emptied, and the endoscope should be passed again along the anterior wall of the urogenital sinus, looking for the opening to the bladder just anterior to the opening of the vagina. When the rectal fistula is identified, it is convenient to pass a ureteral catheter through it, turning the endoscope 180 degrees so that its beak points backward. This technique will usually allow it to enter the rectal fistula, with visualization of the interior of the colon.

If there is old fecal material or impacted mucus in the distal colon, it should be cleaned out to prevent contamination of the operative field during subsequent reconstructive surgery. Washing out impacted fecal material can be accomplished from above, through the distal limb of the colostomy, or from below, by directing the endoscope up through the rectal fistula, washing from below upward and out the colostomy. It is important to use a physiologic salt solution for such prolonged irrigation of the colon, not water, which can be absorbed and cause water intoxication.

If the patient has undergone a simple loop colostomy, there can be an enormous fecal impaction in the distal colon segment. Thorough cleansing can take several hours and a very large volume of irrigating fluid. It is better to spend this time cleansing the bowel properly, than to proceed with stool in the bowel. By adhering rigidly to this principle, wound contamination and pelvic sepsis are avoided in cloacal reconstructions.

This type of prolonged endoscopy should precede a definitive operation by several days to give the child ample time to fully recover from the anesthetic. In some particularly complex malformations, it has been helpful to invite the radiologist to the operating room to study the patient with a C-arm fluoroscopy device. As each orifice entering the urogenital sinus is visualized endoscopically, a catheter is introduced to instill contrast medium. The events are recorded radiographically and the information is correlated with the endoscopy findings.

DEFINITIVE REPAIR OF CLOACAL MALFORMATIONS

These reconstructions are usually long and difficult and should be deferred until about 1 year of age, when the infant is better able to withstand major surgery. In addition to the preliminary washout of the defunctioned distal colon, the proximal bowel is prepared with a day of clear liquids by mouth and GoLYTELY gastrointestinal lavage solution (Braintree Laboratories, Braintree, MA). Expert anesthesiology is mandatory, with complete monitoring including blood gases, acid-base balance, arterial pressure, serial hematocrit determinations, and urine output.

As shown in Figure 47–8, the patient is prepared and draped circumferentially, with the legs sterilely wrapped. The uppermost drapes in the surgical field are fastened loosely, to allow turning of the patient intraoperatively. This arrangement permits the surgeon to work on the patient in the supine position, through the abdomen; in the prone, jackknifed position, for posterior sagittal access; or in the lithotomy position. Fre-

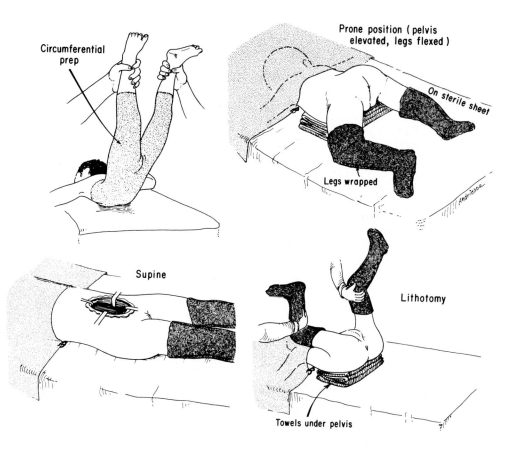

Figure 47–8. Preparation of patient to allow prone, supine, and lithotomy positions during operation. Note that the entire patient is circumferentially prepared, and the legs are sterilely wrapped. The patient is on a double thickness of sterile sheets. Beneath the sterile sheets are "lamb's wool padding" and a heating blanket. The upper sterile drape is clipped loosely enough so that the patient can be turned intraoperatively. After each turning, the exposed side is swabbed once again with povidone-iodine (Betadine) solution. A stack of sterile towels is placed beneath the patient when in prone or lithotomy positions.

quently, all three positions are used in a given case. When the patient is turned, the arms and all attached monitoring lines and tubes are brought straight up above the head, to allow turning without dislodging them. Two anesthesiologists are at the head of the table during turning.

In my initial experience with cloacal reconstructive surgery, we performed these operations using combined abdominal-perineal exposure, holding the legs upward to work in lithotomy position, and dropping them to gain access to the belly. Since 1982, after deVries and Peña (1982) emphasized the usefulness of the posterior sagittal position in correcting anorectal malformations, I have used that approach in these cases (Peña, 1990). In a straightforward case with low confluence of all structures, the entire repair can be performed through a posterior sagittal approach, separating the rectum, vagina, and urogenital sinus, and bringing each to the perineum. However, in some cases it is better to start in the abdomen if there has been a vesicostomy or vaginostomy, which tethers those structures upward, or if there is a very high entry of the rectum into the vagina or backwall of the bladder. Separation of the rectum in those circumstances may be more easily accomplished from above, later turning to the posterior sagittal approach for doing the actual reconstruction.

When commencing in the posterior sagittal position, as shown in Figure 47–9, the perineum is electrically stimulated, marking the point of maximum contraction of the sphincter muscles at which the anus will be later located. This point is marked boldly, using brilliant green dye and a toothpick or wooden applicator. Similarly, the locations for the perineal body, the vagina, and the urethra are marked.

A vertical midline incision is made in the gluteal cleft, progressing in the midline down to the underlying structures. I find it easier to stay in the exact midline holding the buttocks apart with thumb and third finger of the left hand. If two individuals each hold a buttock apart with unequal tension, it is easy to stray from the midline. It is vital to place a metal sound in the urogenital sinus, holding it upward and dissecting down in the midline to the metal sound to approach the urogenital sinus, urethra or bladder neck, vagina, and rectum.

If the urogenital sinus is wide and needs to be tapered to construct a urethra of proper size, the incision into it starts at the skin, proceeding upward from there until the openings of the other structures are identified. However, if the urogenital sinus is of normal caliber for a urethra, it is preserved, incising it at a higher level where the converging structures will be found.

The rectal fistula usually enters the back wall of the vagina at 6 o'clock, but that is not always the case. If it enters very high, well above the level of the coccyx into the apex of the vagina, it may be impossible to reach it through the posterior sagittal approach. Also, the rectal fistula can enter adjacent to the bladder neck and anterior to the entry of the vagina, especially if there are two diverging vaginas. It is for this reason that it is so important to determine the anatomy preoperatively by appropriate imaging and endoscopy.

I have encountered six cases in which no vagina was

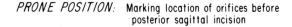

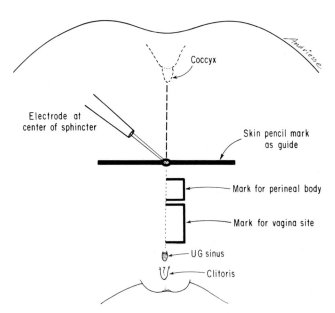

Figure 47–9. Identifying landmarks by electrical stimulation. It is helpful to mark heavily the line where anal sphincter contraction is maximal, renewing this marking intraoperatively as needed. Marks are placed also for the anticipated location of the perineal body and the vagina. These marks, together with visualization and stimulation of the muscle mass intraoperatively, are helpful in placing the three openings accurately. (UG, urogenital.)

seen by preoperative imaging, including ultrasound examination, or by endoscopic study. A vagina was indeed present, but it did not communicate with the urogenital sinus. The surgeon must maintain a high degree of suspicion that such an occult vagina may be present. In one complex urogenital sinus case, a sigmoid vaginoplasty was performed, during which the presence of a small vagina was not appreciated. At menarche, a large midline blood-filled mass appeared, which was subsequently anastomosed to the previously reconstructed sigmoid vagina! Others have also noted genital tract complications at puberty in females with imperforate anus (Fleming et al., 1986; Hall et al., 1985; Mollitt et al., 1981).

The rectum can be freed in two ways. The first is to incise the back wall of the rectum, visualizing the fistula from its interior, circumscribing it, and dissecting the rectum away from the vagina with the lower rectum open. The rectal wall should never be grasped with tooth forceps, which will do damage during its mobilization. Instead, many fine silk sutures are placed along the cut edge, to exert gentle traction. I routinely employ this approach in ordinary imperforate anus cases, in which the rectum is being mobilized from the urethra or bladder neck in the male, or from the posterior vaginal fourchette in the female.

A second way to mobilize the rectum is to place a Foley catheter in its ostium, partially filling its balloon, and securing it with a pursestring suture around the fistulous opening. The balloon catheter provides a convenient means for traction on the rectal pouch while

dissecting it from surrounding tissues. Occasionally, it is helpful to inflate the rectum with air through the Foley catheter as an aid in identifying the plane of dissection. In reoperative cases, usually in older patients, where the rectum is surrounded by scar, it is very helpful to put an index finger into the rectal lumen as a guide in this dissection.

As a further precaution against contamination of the operative field, a povidone-iodine–soaked gauze sponge is placed up into the rectal lumen to prevent possible soiling of the operative field despite a thorough bowel preparation. In reoperative anorectal surgery employing these general principles, we have been able to do the procedure without a complementary colostomy. Virtually all previously unoperated cloacal patients will have the original colostomy in place during their definitive reconstruction.

A most tedious part of cloacal surgery is separation of the vagina(s) from the bladder neck and posterior bladder wall. The vagina usually wraps halfway around the urogenital sinus and is closely related to the bladder neck. Partially opening the lower vagina and placing traction sutures on its edges is a great help in initiating this separation. It is useful to fill the bladder with saline solution or air to distend its wall to help identify this plane of cleavage. It is important not to inadvertently enter the back wall of the bladder or bladder neck, because that will predispose the patient to development of a urinary tract fistula postoperatively. Thus, if either structure is to be violated during this dissection, it is better to make holes in the vagina, not the bladder.

The lateral attachments of the vagina must be dissected quite high to gain adequate length to bring it to the perineum. Surprisingly, we have found that some vaginas, although large in size, will not come down easily to the perineum. Formerly, I used flaps of vaginal wall fashioned from above, but those passages usually require enlarging at a later time. A small amount of length can be overcome by making flaps from skin of the perineum. When there is a great gap, however, it is better to consider the use of a bowel segment to bridge the distance between the vagina and the perineum. That bowel segment can be from the lower rectum, from the sigmoid colon, or even from the terminal ileum.

I reconstructed secondarily a patient whose vagina had sloughed during a reconstruction elsewhere. Interposing a bowel segment between the pulled-through colon and the repaired urogenital sinus was difficult. When the vagina has been mobilized, its lateral walls are usually intact. Rotating the vagina to have an intact wall of vagina overlying the closure of the bladder neck and urogenital sinus will offer protection against development of a fistula, which can occur with adjacent suture lines.

Some surgeons use cautery to separate these converging structures. Although it makes a bloodless dissection, I prefer not to use cautery to avoid thermal burn of the tissues that must heal per primum if fistulization is to be avoided. Therefore, I use sharp knife or fine scissor dissection and optical magnification to do these dissections, which have been accomplished to date without occurrence of a postoperative fistula.

Closure of the bladder neck and urogenital sinus is performed in two layers. The first layer is a running, inverting continuous suture of 4–0 or 5–0 polydioxanone suture (PDS). A second layer of adjacent muscle is closed over this with interrupted horizontal mattress sutures of the same material. In some cases, the urogenital sinus is of satisfactory caliber to be used as a urethra. In that case, it is opened only at its upper end, to accomplish separation of the rectum and vagina, and then closed as described previously. However, if the urogenital sinus is a large, funnel-shaped passageway, it is opened fully. Later, its caliber is reduced by trimming mucosa on each side and fashioning it into a urethra of appropriate size. The posterior sagittal approach not only allows very accurate division of the three organ systems but also ensures accurate placement of the structures within the pelvic muscles.

A segment of bowel can be used to extend the vagina in two ways. First, one can place a large, stuffed drain of appropriate size where the bowel extension will be placed after closing the urogenital sinus and putting the bowel into its ideal location within the anorectal sphincter muscle. Turning to the abdominal approach, the bowel segment can be pulled through in the space temporarily occupied by the stuffed drain. The bowel segment is sewn to the perineum with the patient in the lithotomy position. Its upper end is anastomosed to the vagina in need of extension.

Alternatively, the bowel can be pulled down. The patient is turned once more to the prone position, and the bowel segment is sutured in place, completing the rectal pull through. Later, the patient is turned to the supine position, to expose the abdomen. When the rectal pull through is performed, dilated bowel is tapered to appropriate size. If a higher segment of bowel is used, which is not so dilated, I sometimes simply imbricate its wall, in the same manner as described by Kalicinski and co-workers (1977) for the imbrication of the wall of a megaureter.

At the end of a cloacal reconstruction, the child's face is usually edematous from having been positioned in the prone, jackknifed position. This problem is accentuated by the large fluid requirements needed to maintain satisfactory urinary output during these long cases, particularly if abdominal surgery is required. Thus, it is routine for these children to spend the next day or two postoperatively in the intensive care unit, often with ventilatory support. For several days postoperatively, they are maintained flat, not partially upright, which can increase venous pressure in the pelvis and cause edema of the pelvic organs.

Postoperatively, the urinary tract is drained by a small straight plastic catheter in the urogenital sinus. I do not use a Foley catheter for this drainage because I prefer to avoid having an inflated balloon adjacent to a repaired bladder neck and urogenital sinus. Relying on a balloon to hold the catheter in place can be risky because it may deflate. Similarly, inadvertent pulling of an inflated balloon through a repaired urogenital sinus could prove disastrous.

A straight catheter that is adequately secured is safer. If the abdomen was entered during a repair, a suprapubic tube is placed in the bladder as an additional means for drainage. Twelve days postoperatively, the urethral catheter is removed, and a "pullout urethrogram" is obtained. This study confirms an intact repair. The child is then allowed to void, and the suprapubic tube is opened every 3 to 4 hours to estimate residual urine volume. If voiding is uneventful, the suprapubic tube is soon removed. Sometimes, however, these children will be unable to void temporarily or for a longer period of time.

The parents are instructed in catheterization. When that is accomplished, the suprapubic catheter can be removed. If catheterization is not easy, parental instruction is delayed for at least another week to allow further healing of the repair. If catheterization continues to be difficult, endoscopy is performed gently to ascertain why catheterization is difficult. Sometimes a mucosal fold is blocking catheter passage and can be remedied by endoscopic incision. In some cases, a parent is brought to the operating room to observe the endoscopy on a television monitor. The parent passes the catheter while the child is asleep to become acquainted with the technique.

Cloacal surgery is long and difficult; it must be performed in meticulous fashion if satisfactory results are to be achieved. It is important that there be either a team of surgeons, who include expertise in all of the organ systems involved, working in a coordinated fashion, or a single surgeon who is thoroughly conversant with surgery of the urinary tract, the genital tract, and the gastrointestinal tract.

CASE STUDIES

The following cases illustrate most of the cardinal points in cloacal reconstruction. It is important to realize that each case will differ in some aspects from every other cloacal reconstruction case. Nevertheless, the same general principles apply in dealing with all of them. These general principles include precise delineation of anatomy, separation of the three organ systems, and the bringing of each to the perineum without tension while avoiding adjacent suture lines, which can cause fistulization from one structure to another.

Case 1

An Uncomplicated Case Repaired Solely Through the Posterior Sagittal Approach. An infant was referred at age 16 months in 1986. At birth, colostomy had been performed. Urologic investigation showed severe hydronephrosis, as shown in Figure 47–10, but this disappeared after intermittent catheterization of the vagina was begun. The anatomy, as shown in Figure 47–11, included two side-by-side vaginas and a rectal fistula opening at the base of the vaginal septum.

At operation, the intervaginal septum was incised endoscopically, converting it to a single passage. The vagina was disconnected from the urogenital sinus, which was narrowed and closed. After mobilization, the

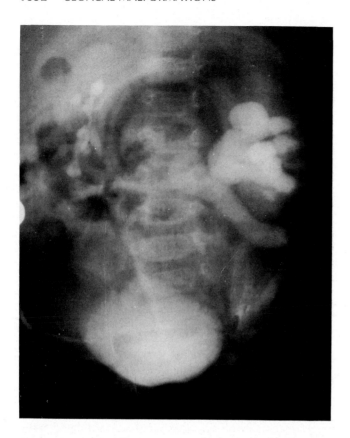

Figure 47–10. *(Case 1)* Intravenous pyelogram of patient as an infant, showing hydronephrosis. This condition disappeared after cutback of the urogenital sinus and intermittent catheterization of the vagina by the mother.

vagina was brought to the perineum, a perineal body was constructed, and the tapered rectum was pulled through to the perineum, with closing of the levators and sphincter muscles appropriately around it.

The patient was discharged from the hospital 12 days postoperatively. Her mother passed daily a 9–10 Hegar dilator into the vagina and rectum to prevent postoperative contracture. The colostomy was closed 3 months later. The patient is now 6 years old. She has normal urinary control and a normal upper urinary tract by intravenous pyelography. She required periodic soapsuds enemas initially to move her bowels, but later established completely normal bowel control. Barium study showed a normal-appearing rectum, as seen in Figure 47–12. MRI studies of the lumbosacral spine showed normal findings.

Comment. This child's anatomy was very favorable for repair, because she had no other serious problems and her hydronephrosis resolved after intermittent catheterization of the vagina. Pre- and postoperative views of the perineum are shown in Figure 47–13.

Case 2

Cloaca with Diverging Vaginas and Rectal Fistula Anterior to Them. A 3-year-old girl was referred in 1988. At birth, colostomy had been performed. No urinary decompression was required because there was no obstructive uropathy; the patient was completely incontinent.

Evaluation was performed. A solitary, normal left kidney showed compensatory hypertrophy. Cystogram showed a small-capacity bladder with incompetent blad-

der neck and grade 3 reflux. MRI of the lumbosacral spine showed normal findings. Inspection showed a large perineal opening, with the appearance of a normal vaginal introitus. Urine flowed freely from it. Endoscopically, two vaginal orifices were visible, with a septum between them. The rectal opening was not immediately apparent, but it could be seen by injecting saline solution and air into the distal colostomy limb. It lay near the bladder neck and anterior to the two vaginas.

One week later, reconstructive surgery was performed as seen in Figure 47–14. It was accomplished with the patient in the prone, jackknifed position, through a posterior sagittal approach. The two vaginas, colon, and bladder neck were separated. The coccyx and a cyst adjacent to it were removed. A urethra was constructed from the roof of the wide urogenital sinus. The two vaginas were opened, sewn together, and brought to the perineum. They were rotated 90 degrees to cover the urethra with intact vaginal wall, thereby avoiding the presence of adjacent suture lines, which might fistulize. The perineal body was constructed. The dilated lower rectum was tapered, and the rectum was placed within the sphincter and levator muscles.

The urethral catheter was removed 2 weeks postoperatively. No difficulty with urinary retention occurred. The patient was discharged 3 weeks postoperatively on a program of daily dilatation of the anorectal canal and vaginal opening with a 10 Hegar dilator. When evaluated 9 months later, the patient had developed some continence from her new urethra, but there was grade 3 reflux into the ectopic ureter in the bladder neck.

A second operation was performed to close the colostomy. There was a 4:1 discrepancy in the size of the two limbs of the colostomy. The ectopic ureter was reim-

BEFORE

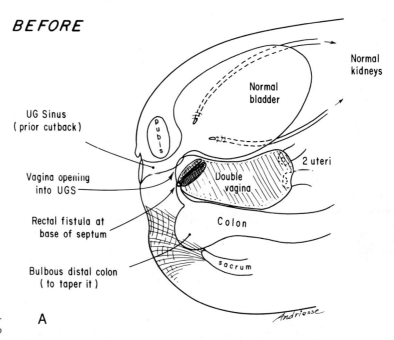

Figure 47–11. *(Case 1) A,* Preoperative anatomy showing moderately high confluence of the vaginas into urogenital sinus (UGS). *B,* After reconstruction, which was possible from a posterior sagittal approach with pull through of vagina and rectum, without need to enter abdomen.

AFTER

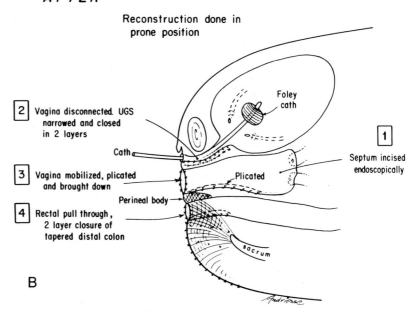

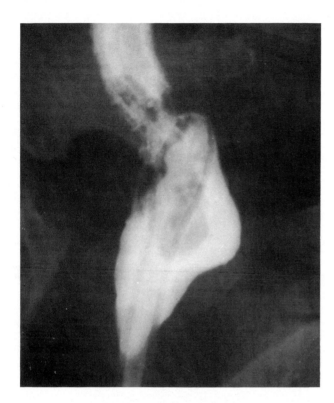

Figure 47–12. *(Case 1)* Postoperative barium enema showing normal rectum, with slight tapering of the back wall.

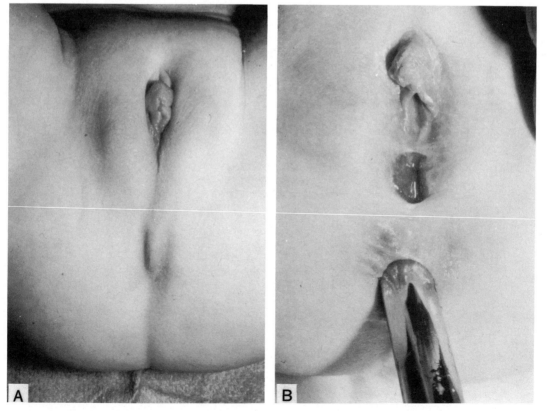

Figure 47–13. *(Case 1)* *A,* Preoperative appearance. *B,* Postoperative appearance. Note Hegar dilator in anus, perineal body between anus and pulled through vagina, and separate urethral opening beneath clitoris.

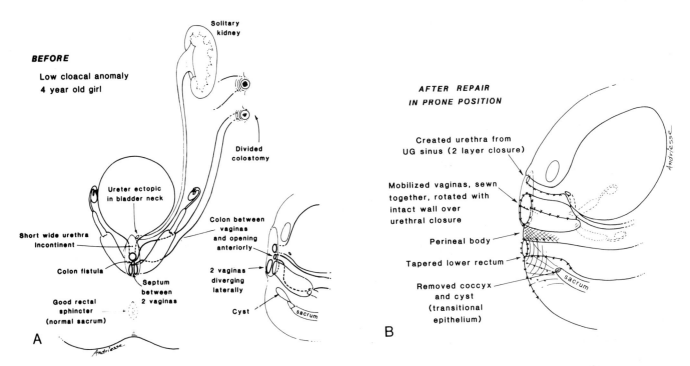

Figure 47–14. *(Case 2) A,* Preoperative anatomy. *B,* Postoperative anatomy. Note diverging vaginas, which were joined, and unusual anterior location of colonic fistula between the original vaginal openings and the bladder neck. This was a low malformation, which could be corrected entirely from a posterior sagittal approach. Not shown is the subsequent narrowing of the bladder neck and reimplantation of the ectopic ureter, performed at the time of colostomy closure. (UG, urogenital.)

planted diagonally across the back wall of the bladder together with a Young-Dees bladder neck lengthening and narrowing to gain more outlet resistance. The belly was a mass of intra-abdominal adhesions from the original exploratory laparotomy in the neonatal period. An incidental cecal duplication was resected.

When the suprapubic tube was clamped intermittently 2 weeks later, the patient was able to void only small amounts. The mother was taught how to perform clean intermittent catheterization, and the suprapubic tube was removed. The patient was discharged 4 weeks postoperatively. She was soon able to void, so intermittent catheterization was discontinued. The mother reported normal urinary and bowel control 3 months later.

Comment. This child's cloacal malformation presented an entirely different technical problem from that described in Case 1. The vaginas could not be made into one by simply incising a vaginal septum. We have encountered a case similar to this, in which the vaginas were too short to reach the perineum; thus, they were joined together and extended with a segment of bowel. Note also that this patient had essentially no effective urethra; the bladder neck emptied directly into the large urogenital sinus. The anterior position of the rectal opening is unusual but not rare. This case underscores the importance of defining the specific anatomy in each cloaca before embarking on its repair.

Case 3

Cloaca and Large Pelvic Tumor; Tube Diversion Since Birth. A 15-month-old girl was referred in 1987 with the unusual problem of a large sacrococcygeal teratoma and a cloacal malformation as seen in Figure 47–15. At birth, suprapubic cystostomy and left upper quadrant loop colostomy had been performed.

An aortogram showed displacement of the iliac vessels by the intrapelvic component of the tumor (Fig. 47–16*A*). Preoperative roentgenographic evaluation (Fig. 47–16*B*) showed high confluence of bladder, vagina, and rectum, and a wide urogenital sinus. Reconstruction was performed as shown in Figure 47–15*B*.

Beginning with the patient in the prone, jackknifed position, an elliptical incision was made around the teratoma, leaving the involved skin with it, and extending the incision forward for posterior sagittal exposure access. The coccyx was transected with the specimen during its mobilization from below. When no further tumor mobilization could be performed from below, the patient was turned to enter the abdomen. A temporary pack was placed in the posterior wound.

The colostomy was taken down because there was insufficient length of colon distal to it to perform a pull through. The tumor was freed intra-abdominally, with special attention to both ureters. The bowel was replaced into the abdomen and covered with moist gauze, and the abdominal wall was temporarily approximated with three large sutures over the gauze. The child was placed in the prone position once again, and the tumor was removed by extraction from below. Pathologic examination disclosed apparently complete removal. The urogenital sinus was then reduced in caliber to create a urethra. The vagina was mobilized, rotated somewhat, and brought to the perineum.

Turning the patient again to the supine position, the

BEFORE

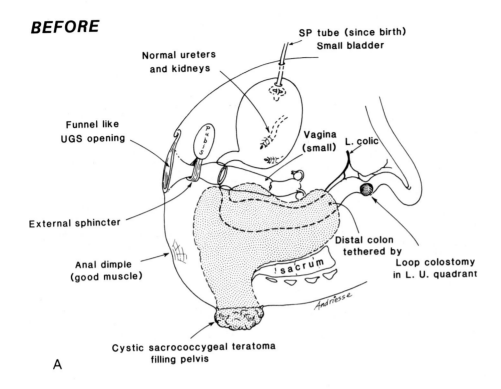

Normal ureters and kidneys

SP tube (since birth)
Small bladder

Funnel like UGS opening

Vagina (small)

L. colic

External sphincter

Anal dimple (good muscle)

Distal colon tethered by
Loop colostomy in L. U. quadrant

Andriesse

Cystic sacrococcygeal teratoma filling pelvis

A

Figure 47–15. *(Case 3) A,* Cloacal anatomy and a large intrapelvic sacrococcygeal teratoma. *B,* Scheme of operative repair, which required five positional changes. (SP, suprapubic; UGS, urogenital sinus.)

AFTER

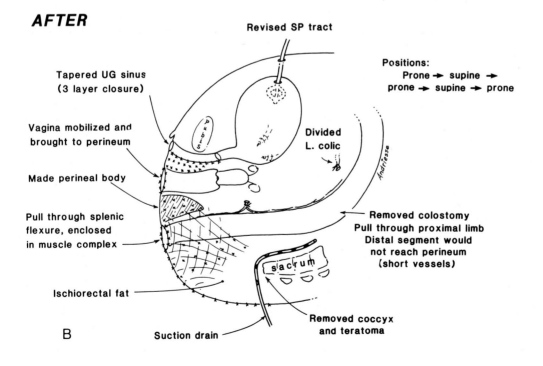

Revised SP tract

Positions:
Prone → supine →
prone → supine → prone

Tapered UG sinus (3 layer closure)

Vagina mobilized and brought to perineum

Divided L. colic

Made perineal body

Pull through splenic flexure, enclosed in muscle complex

Removed colostomy
Pull through proximal limb
Distal segment would not reach perineum (short vessels)

Ischiorectal fat

Suction drain

Removed coccyx and teratoma

B

Andriesse

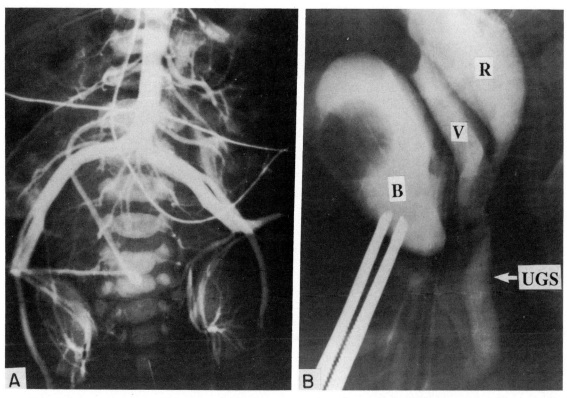

Figure 47–16. *(Case 3)* Roentgenograms. *A,* Aortogram of the patient as an infant, showing marked displacement of iliac vessels by tumor. *B,* Preoperative "cloacagram" filling through Foley catheters in the suprapubic site and distal limb of the colostomy. Note high confluence of bladder (B), vagina (V), and rectum (R), and wide urogenital sinus (UGS).

colon was mobilized further. The left colic artery was divided to obtain enough length to reach the perineum. After raising the legs of the patient, the colon was pulled through and tacked to the cul de sac peritoneum. The trap beneath its mesentery was closed, and the abdomen was closed definitively. A new suprapubic cystostomy site was established. A fresh site will close when extubated, whereas an old site might require surgical closure. The abdominal wall was closed definitively, and the patient was turned for the final time to complete the rectal repair, placing it within the muscle complex.

The patient was unable to void postoperatively 2 weeks later. A catheter could not be passed easily from below. Therefore, 1 week later, endoscopy was performed. A prominent shelf of bladder mucosa was noted at the bladder neck at 12 o'clock. It was incised with a cutting electrode, after which catheterization was accomplished using a coude-tipped catheter. The mother was instructed in the catheterization technique in the operating room. Two months later, the suprapubic tube was removed. Three years later, a slight rectal prolapse was trimmed.

Now, at age 5 years, the patient continues on intermittent catheterization five times daily. She does not move her bowels spontaneously. An enema washout of the colon each day gives satisfactory bowel emptying, and she does not soil while on that regimen. MRI of the spine showed no tethering of the cord. Urodynamic study showed urethral resistance of 100 ml of water and urethral length of 3.5 cm. Bladder volume is 300 ml.

Comment. This case demonstrates the usefulness of being able to turn the patient for various aspects of a complex case requiring all three positions—prone, supine, and lithotomy. It also demonstrates how some of these patients will require intermittent catheterization to empty the urinary tract. In this instance, this outcome may represent some denervation of the bladder secondary to removal of the huge pelvic tumor. Except for the need to catheterize and the need to empty the colon with a daily soapsuds enema, the patient leads a normal life.

Case 4

Cloaca Requiring Preliminary Urologic Operation. A female infant was referred at age 2 weeks in 1984. Transverse colostomy had been performed at birth.

Intravenous pyelogram showed severe hydronephrosis. Endoscopy showed high confluence of two vaginas just below the bladder neck. A long rectal fistula entered the base of the intervaginal septum. The ureteral orifices were each located in a bladder diverticulum. Massive vesicoureteral reflux was found (Fig. 47–17).

The urogenital sinus was cut back enough to facilitate intermittent catheterization of the vaginas (Fig. 47–18). The midline vaginal septum was incised to create a single vaginal cavity. The patient had multiple urinary tract infections despite antibiotics and frequent catheterization. Therefore, at age 7 months, bilateral ure-

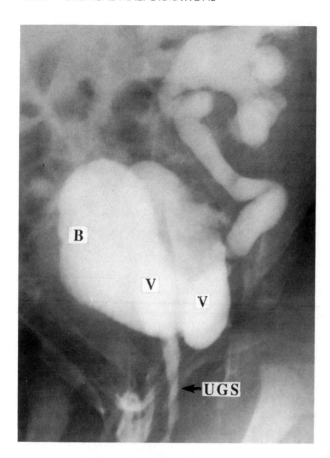

Figure 47–17. *(Case 4)* Cystogram preoperatively, showing two vaginas (V), bladder (B), urogenital sinus (UGS), and grade five vesicoureteral reflux on the left side.

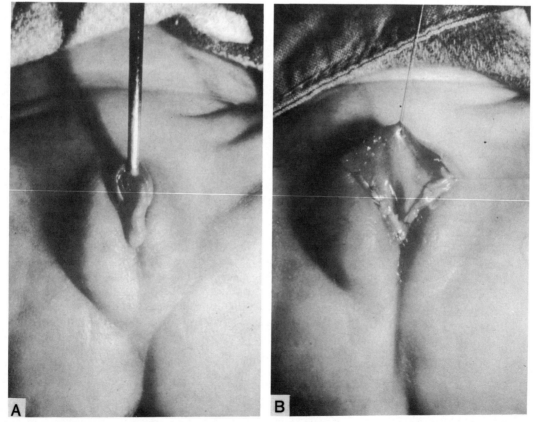

Figure 47–18. *(Case 4)* Perineum of the patient as a neonate. *A,* Sound in urogenital sinus, which came to tip of clitoris. *B,* Cutting back end of urogenital sinus to a point mappropriate for the urethral meatus later to perform cystoscopy and to facilitate intermittent catheterization of the urine-filled vagina.

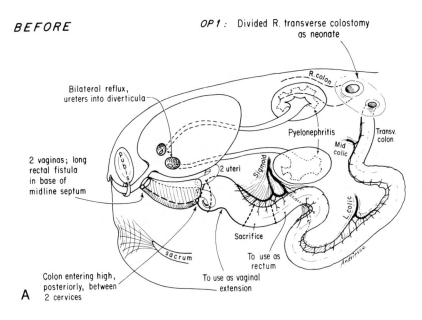

BEFORE

OP1: Divided R. transverse colostomy
as neonate

Bilateral reflux,
ureters into diverticula

2 vaginas; long
rectal fistula
in base of
midline septum

Pyelonephritis

R. colon

Transv.
colon

Mid
colic

2 uteri

Sigmoid

L. colic

Sacrifice

sacrum

To use as
rectum

To use as vaginal
extension

Colon entering high,
posteriorly, between
2 cervices

A

Figure 47–19. (Case 4) A, Preoperative anatomy. This infant required early correction of
massive reflux, deferring the rest of reconstruction until later. Note the long rectal fistula in
the base of the intervaginal septum, but high
position of rectum itself. B, The operation was
begun in the prone position, disconnecting the
vagina, and placing drains for subsequent pull
through of bowel extension of vagina and rectum. C, Completed repair in supine position.
Subsequent colostomy closure. (OP, operation;
UG, urogenital; UGS, urogenital sinus; UTI,
urinary tract infection.)

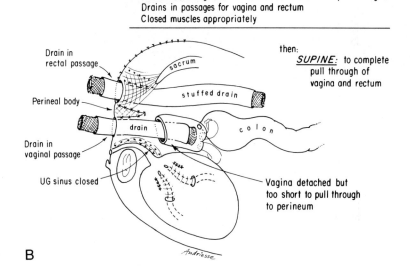

PRONE POSITION:　Defined muscle complex
Disconnected vagina from UG sinus (too short for pull through)
Drains in passages for vagina and rectum
Closed muscles appropriately

Drain in
rectal passage

sacrum

then:

SUPINE: to complete
pull through of
vagina and rectum

Perineal body

stuffed drain

drain

c o l o n

Drain in
vaginal passage

UG sinus closed

Vagina detached but
too short to pull through
to perineum

B

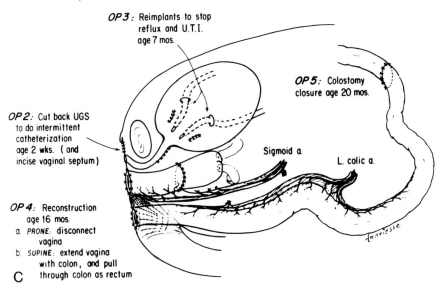

AFTER 5 operations

OP3: Reimplants to stop
reflux and U.T.I.
age 7 mos.

OP5: Colostomy
closure age 20 mos.

OP2: Cut back UGS
to do intermittent
catheterization
age 2 wks. (and
incise vaginal septum)

Sigmoid a.

L. colic a.

OP4: Reconstruction
age 16 mos.
a. PRONE: disconnect
vagina
b. SUPINE: extend vagina
with colon, and pull
through colon as rectum

C

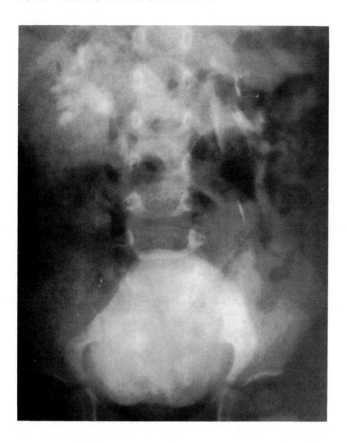

Figure 47–20. *(Case 4)* One year later, showing delicate upper tracts but scarring from the original pyelonephritis. No reflux was observed after ureteral reimplantation.

teral reimplantations were performed. Urinary infections ceased and the hydronephrosis improved. At age 16 months, reconstruction was performed (Fig. 47–19).

The distal colon was lavaged thoroughly from below through the rectovaginal fistula, with emptying through the distal limb of the colostomy. Today, this procedure is done during a separate anesthesia. Through the posterior sagittal approach, the urogenital sinus was opened, disconnecting the vaginas. The urogenital sinus was then repaired. Despite maximum mobilization, the vagina would not reach the perineum. The muscle complex was closed over two stuffed drains to allow passage of two bowel segments from above.

The patient was turned to the supine position, and work was done alternatively between the belly and the perineum by elevating the legs. The distal colon was brought down to extend the vagina. The left colon was brought down as rectum. Colostomy closure was performed 4 months later.

The patient is now 7 years old. Intravenous pyelogram shows stable, delicate upper tracts, but some scarring from the original pyelonephritis when reflux was present (Fig. 47–20). The patient is socially clean of stool with a daily enema washout of the colon. A vaginal washout is done once daily as well to remove mucus from the colon segment used to extend the vagina. She urinates normally and is free from urinary tract infection. MRI of the lumbosacral spine showed normal findings.

Comment. This case demonstrates the priority of the urinary tract in the management of some patients with cloacal malformations. If massive reflux had persisted, renal function would have deteriorated. Rather than

waiting until an age appropriate to do a definitive reconstruction, the antireflux operation was performed first. We have seen many secondary cases of patients in whom the rectal pull through was performed first with deferment of the urinary tract correction until later. This approach is incorrect because the rectal problem is not life-threatening.

Retrospective review of some cases in which the rectum had been pulled through showed deterioration of the urinary tract after an isolated pull through. The rectum and distal colostomy limb can drain urine that might otherwise accumulate in the vagina; however, after the fistula is divided and the bowel is pulled through, this mechanism cannot occur. I believe that end colostomy should be avoided in these infants at birth, in part, for the same reason.

Case 5

Complex Secondary Reconstruction. A 4-year-old patient was referred in 1986. Right transverse colostomy had been performed at birth. At age 4 months, reconstruction had been unsuccessfully attempted through the posterior sagittal approach, followed 2 days later by suprapubic cystostomy.

Radiographic evaluation through the suprapubic tube revealed confluence of the bladder, vaginas, and colon, as well as vesicoureteral reflux (Fig. 47–21). There was no communication with the perineum.

Reconstruction was begun with the patient in the prone position. The colon and the two vaginas were

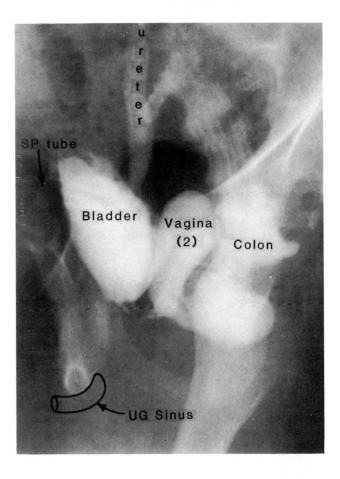

Figure 47–21. *(Case 5)* Preoperative roentgenogram, filling through suprapubic (SP) tube in bladder. Note free flow of contrast from bladder, to the vaginas, and into the colon, as well as vesicoureteral reflux. No continuity with the urogenital (UG) sinus was present.

separated from the urinary tract (Fig. 47–22). The patient was turned, and the ectopic ureters were moved to a higher level in the bladder. A bladder flap was constructed to join to the remnant of urogenital sinus. This construction was facilitated by splitting the pubic symphysis for exposure. The vaginas were converted to one, and joined to the perineum with a segment of bowel. Colon was pulled through to the perineum. The small bladder was augmented with intestine.

The patient was unable to void spontaneously. Intermittent catheterization by the mother was begun. The colostomy was closed 8 months later. The patient is now 9 years old. She is completely dry, but she must catheterize to empty the augmented bladder. She is completely continent of stool, but she requires a daily enema to empty the colon. MRI study in 1989 showed no spinal abnormality.

Comment. Although the posterior sagittal approach offers great advantages in separating the urogenital sinus, vagina, and rectum, it also poses great risk if the surgeon is not familiar with it. Somehow, the urogenital sinus was completely destroyed in the initial operation. This created a major problem to repair. In addition, the patient had a very small bladder, probably from long-term suprapubic drainage, which, in turn, required bladder augmentation. It has been our experience that an augmented bladder can usually be emptied by abdominal pressure if the patient has a normal bladder outlet, but that intermittent catheterization is usually necessary when there is a neurologic problem or a reconstructed bladder outlet (Hendren and Hendren, 1990).

Case 6

Complex Cloacal Malformation with Intravesical Communication of Vaginas and Bowel. The patient was referred as a newborn in 1987 with cloacal malformation and intestinal obstruction. A funnel-shaped vaginal introitus was the only opening on the perineum. Plain film of the abdomen was consistent with intestinal atresia. Cystogram showed multiple diverticulum-like projections from the bladder. The urachus was patent. On the 1st day of life, endoscopic examination was performed. It was possible to pass a 15-French endoscope up the introitus and out the urachus. Multiple openings were found in the bladder, no bladder neck was present, and the ureteral orifices were not readily seen.

After this brief examination, laparotomy was performed. The patient had ileal atresia, with a gap in the mesentery and a short segment of colon in the lower abdomen. The upper end of the distal bowel was blind and its lower end joined to the bladder. On each side, a uterus tube and an ovary were present. The urachus was divided and closed. Ileostomy was performed. The blind end of colon was exteriorized as a mucous fistula. Cystogram performed by filling through the mucous fistula showed the multilobulated bladder with communicating vaginas but did little to shed light on the actual anatomy (Fig. 47–23).

At age 7 months, endoscopy was performed, but the findings were unclear. At age 15 months, endoscopy was repeated with the radiologist in the operating room

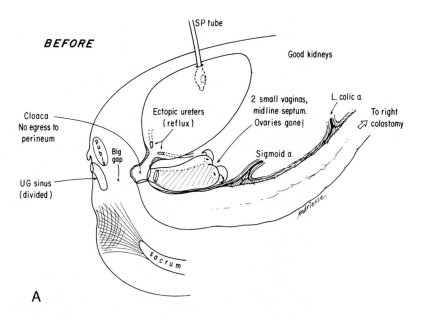

BEFORE

SP tube

Good kidneys

2 small vaginas, midline septum. Ovaries gone!

L. colic a.

To right colostomy

Ectopic ureters (reflux)

Cloaca No egress to perineum

Sigmoid a.

pubis

Big gap

UG sinus (divided)

sacrum

Andriesse

A

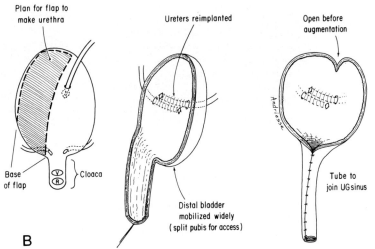

Plan for flap to make urethra

Ureters reimplanted

Open before augmentation

Base of flap

V
R

Cloaca

Distal bladder mobilized widely (split pubis for access)

Tube to join UG sinus

Andriesse

B

Figure 47–22. *(Case 5) A,* Preoperative anatomy. *B,* Scheme for bridging gap between the urinary tract and remaining distal urogenital sinus. *C,* Postoperative anatomy. (UG, urogenital; SP, suprapubic; V, vagina; R, rectum; UGS, urogenital sinus.)

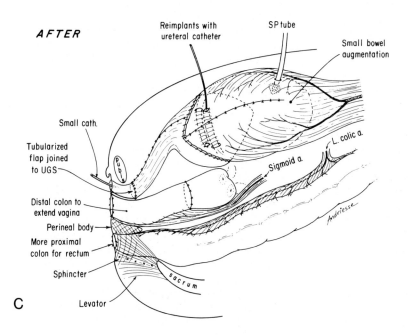

AFTER

Reimplants with ureteral catheter

SP tube

Small bowel augmentation

Small cath.

Tubularized flap joined to UGS

L. colic a.

pubis

Sigmoid a.

Distal colon to extend vagina

Perineal body

More proximal colon for rectum

Sphincter

Levator

sacrum

Andriesse

C

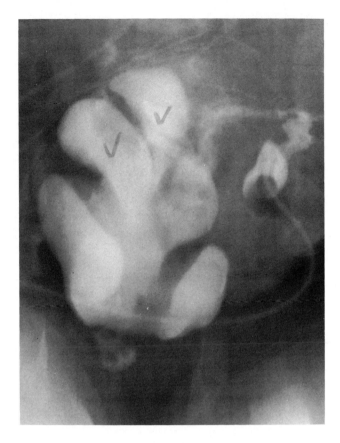

Figure 47–23. *(Case 6)* Cloacagram by filling through Foley catheter in postoperative mucous fistula, showing a multilobulated appearance. This study was not helpful in discerning the anatomy. A combined endoscopy-radiography session in the operating room was needed. (V, vagina.)

together with a fluoroscopy unit. No structures were seen distal to the bladder neck. By catheterizing and injecting contrast medium into various openings, the anatomy shown in (Fig. 47–24*A*) was appreciated. At age 23 months, the reconstructive operation was performed, beginning by way of the abdomen (Fig. 47–24*B*). Biopsies were taken of both ends of the distal bowel to determine its correct orientation in the suspicion that the blind end might be distal hind gut as occurs in cloacal exstrophy and not the next segment below an ileal atresia. Biopsy findings showed that the end attached to the bladder should be joined later to the ileum and that the originally blind end should be rectum.

The two vaginas were dissected free from the bladder, working intravesically. They were joined together. The ureters were reimplanted. The bowel segment joining the bladder was dissected free. Continuity of that mesentery with the mesentery of the ileostomy confirmed the suspicion that, embryologically, this was the forme fruste of a cloacal exstrophy. The two hemibladders were joined together, and a large diverticulum was removed at the dome.

The patient was then placed in the prone, jackknifed position. A urethra was fashioned from the roof of the urogenital sinus. The two vaginas were mobilized further and brought to the perineum; they were rotated to avoid adjacent suture lines. A perineal body was constructed. The end of distal bowel that had originally been a mucous fistula was pulled through as rectum. Appropriate muscle closure was performed. The patient was then turned to reenter the temporarily closed abdomen and reimplant the ureters. This complex operation lasted 20

hours, required 750 ml of blood transfusion, 160 ml of albumin solution, and 3150 ml of crystalloid solution intravenously.

Three weeks later, examination under anesthesia showed all structures to be healed well. A No. 12 plastic catheter could be passed up the reconstructed urethra into the bladder. The parents were taught how to catheterize the child and how to pass Hegar dilators into the new vagina and anus. One month later, on outpatient examination, the vaginal opening was found to be stenotic because the mother had not been passing the dilators. The need for this was reemphasized after a brief operation to enlarge the stenotic orifice. Three months later, bowel continuity was reestablished with anastomosis of the ileostomy to the defunctioned distal bowel. The genitourinary repair looked satisfactory.

Early in the postoperative period, the patient had many loose stools and excoriation of the perineum. Cholestyramine for 6 months cured the excoriation. Now, at age 4 years, the patient moves her bowels spontaneously five times daily, passes solid stools, and rarely soils. Enemas are not required. There is no urinary leakage. The patient voids on the toilet but empties incompletely. Therefore, the mother catheterizes her five times daily for residual urine, usually obtaining 100 ml. MRI at age 2 years was normal.

Comment. The unusual anatomy described in this case appears to be an intermediate form between the usual cloaca and cloacal exstrophy, because there were two hemibladders; two separate vaginas, which communicated with the bladders; and bowel that opened into the back wall of the bladder. The appearance of the mes-

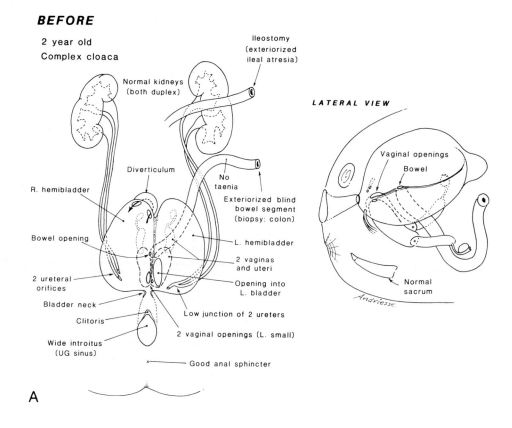

BEFORE

2 year old
Complex cloaca

Ileostomy
(exteriorized
ileal atresia)

Normal kidneys
(both duplex)

LATERAL VIEW

Diverticulum

No
taenia

R. hemibladder

Exteriorized blind
bowel segment
(biopsy: colon)

Bowel opening

L. hemibladder

2 vaginas
and uteri

2 ureteral
orifices

Opening into
L. bladder

Bladder neck

Low junction of 2 ureters

Clitoris

2 vaginal openings (L. small)

Wide introitus
(UG sinus)

Good anal sphincter

Vaginal openings
Bowel

Normal
sacrum

Andriesse

A

AFTER

Positions: Supine ← Prone ← Supine

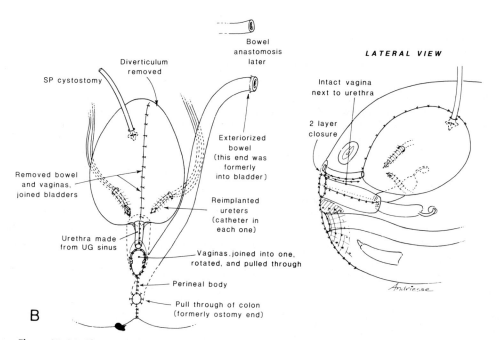

Bowel
anastomosis
later

Diverticulum
removed

SP cystostomy

LATERAL VIEW

Intact vagina
next to urethra

Exteriorized
bowel
(this end was
formerly
into bladder)

2 layer
closure

Removed bowel
and vaginas,
joined bladders

Reimplanted
ureters
(catheter in
each one)

Urethra made
from UG sinus

Vaginas joined into one,
rotated, and pulled through

Perineal body

Pull through of colon
(formerly ostomy end)

Andriesse

B

Figure 47–24. *(Case 6) A,* Preoperative anatomy. *B,* Postoperative anatomy. (UG, urogenital; SP, suprapubic.)

entery and the biopsies of both ends of that segment of bowel made it seem that the end connected to the bladder was proximal and that the blind end originally exteriorized as the mucous fistula was distal. That too is consistent with cloacal exstrophy. This case demonstrates the importance of close collaboration between the radiologist and the surgeon in sorting out such unusual anatomy. Furthermore, this case illustrates that a satisfactory surgical solution is possible even for a case with extremely complex anatomy.

Case 7

Long-Standing Diversion and Previous Pull Through of the Rectum with Fecal Incontinence. A 9-year-old girl was referred in 1985 for evaluation of the anatomy shown in Figure 47–25A. Colostomy and tube vaginostomy had been performed at birth. At age 4 months, loop cutaneous ureterostomy had been performed for one of two ureters on the left, both of which entered the vagina. Because of recurrent urinary tract infection, tube cystostomy was performed at age 2 years, together with abdominal perineal pull through of the rectum and, later, colostomy closure. There was fecal incontinence and constant dripping of urine from the urogenital sinus opening.

The patient's previous anorectal pull through had been placed too far forward in the perineum and clearly anterior to the excellent contractile muscle that was evident (Fig. 47–26). With the patient in the prone position, the rectum was mobilized, the urogenital sinus was opened, and the vagina, which despite mobilization would not reach the perineum, was disconnected. Therefore, as shown in Figure 47–25B, the urogenital sinus was closed, a drain was placed in the passage appropriate for a vaginal extension, the perineal body was constructed, the rectum was placed in an optimal position within the muscle complex, and the posterior wound was closed.

The patient was then turned for laparotomy to complete the repair. A segment of sigmoid colon was used to extend the vagina to the perineum. The right ureter was reimplanted. Both ectopic ureters were removed from the vagina. The better ureter was used for transureteroureterostomy, and the second moiety was drained into it by pyeloureterostomy. A ureteral valve was removed at the junction of the lower pole ureter with its renal pelvis. Anesthesia for this complex reconstruction lasted 19 hours. When the patient was discharged 2 weeks later, the mother was instructed in intermittent catheterization, because the patient could void but did not empty the bladder completely. Three months later, she emptied completely and so catheterization was discontinued. By then she had developed normal urinary control and normal bowel control without soiling. Now, at age 13 years, the patient is well and without urologic or bowel problems. The patient has not had an MRI examination of the spine.

Comment. This child is one of many whom we have seen who had previously undergone a rectal pull through, leaving the genitourinary problems unresolved.

Clearly, her most important problem was the urinary tract. It should be noted that, in ordinary pediatric surgical operations, fluid losses are generally 5 to 10 ml/kg/hour. An extensive reconstruction like this may require as much as 20 to 25 ml/kg/hour to maintain adequate urinary flow and metabolic homeostasis. Close monitoring of urinary output can be maintained by placing catheters in the ureters in the operative field, letting them drain into a rubber glove, and measuring the volume hourly.

Case 8

Cloaca with "Occult Vagina." A 3-year-old girl was referred in 1985 for vaginoplasty. At birth, one opening on the perineum, a vaginal introitus, had been noted. Cutback anoplasty was performed. There was a normal left kidney and no right kidney. When the patient was referred, inspection of the perineum showed the cutback anal orifice to be clearly too far forward and no perineal body between it and the urethra (Fig. 47–27). Preoperative and postoperative anatomy is shown in Figure 47–28.

On rectal examination, a small midline uterus was palpable. Ultrasound showed a probable uterus, but no vagina. The urethra looked normal endoscopically. In lithotomy position, the rectum was mobilized widely up to the cul de sac peritoneum. The rectal wall was tapered about 50 per cent to reduce its caliber. It was then positioned in the center of the perineal muscles. A perineal body was constructed. A stuffed drain was placed through the introitus up into the peritoneal cavity in the anticipation that it would be necessary to pull through a segment of bowel as vagina.

At laparotomy, dissection was carried down along the anterior aspect of the uterus. Behind the bladder, with a ureteral catheter in place for protection of the left ureter, an incision was made in the tissue distal to the cervix. This tissue proved to be the anterior wall of a blindly ending vagina, which contained no fluid or mucus. By opening its wall further and inserting a finger (Raffensperger and Ramenofsky, 1973), the vagina was mobilized and brought to the perineum. At age 8 years, the patient had some rectal prolapse, which was trimmed elsewhere. Now, at age 9 years, she has normal urinary control, and almost normal bowel control. The only residual bowel symptom is a slight tendency to soil when doing athletic activities.

Comment. This child's anatomy is at the minimal end of the cloacal spectrum. It illustrates that a blindly ending vagina can be present but be missed by radiographic imaging. In the recent past, I have seen six such "occult vaginas." In two, the vaginas had been missed during prior major pelvic surgery. They became evident at puberty when they filled with menstrual blood. Today, this child's rectal placement would be done through a posterior sagittal approach, because it permits more accurate placement of the rectum in the muscle complex. If she has significant anal soiling as she grows older, this procedure can still be offered to correct it.

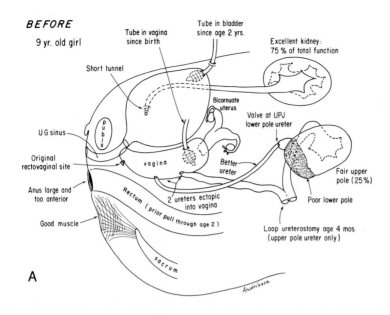

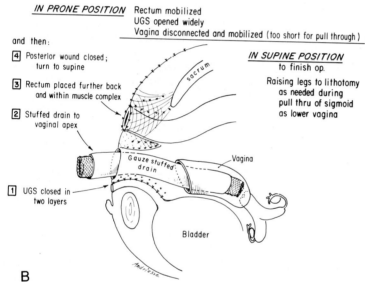

Figure 47–25. *(Case 7) A,* Preoperative anatomy showing severe urologic anomalies and long-standing tube drainage of bladder and vagina. Rectum had been pulled through previously. Note that rectal pull through was not within muscle complex, making bowel continence impossible. Note that only one of two ectopic ureters had been exteriorized during infancy. Typical urogenital (UG) sinus and ureteropelvic junction (UPJ) obstruction of lower pole of left kidney caused by a valve. *B,* Aspects of reconstruction that were possible in prone position, that is, detaching vagina from urogenital sinus (UGS), delineating passage for vaginal extension to be made, and placing rectum within muscle complex to improve bowel continence. *C,* Anatomy after completing reconstruction with patient in supine and lithotomy positions. (SP, suprapubic; TUU, transureteroureterostomy.)

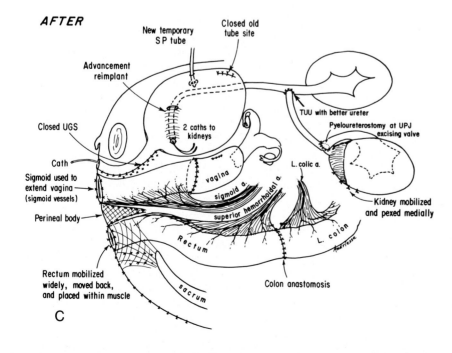

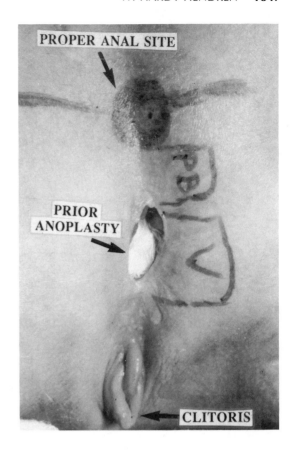

Figure 47–26. *(Case 7)* Preoperative photograph of perineum in prone position after marking perineum and before making posterior sagittal incision. Dark area is future location for anus, in center of sphincter muscle. PB is future site for perineal body. V is location for vagina, to be disconnected and pulled through. Note inappropriately anterior position of previously pulled through rectum, which has gauze in its lumen.

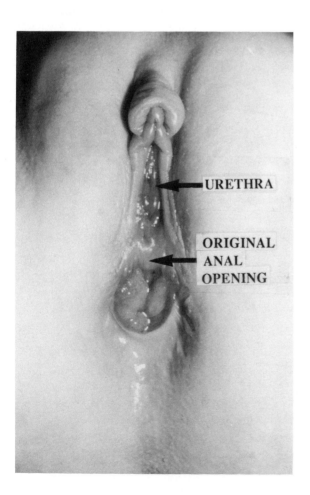

Figure 47–27. *(Case 8)* Perineum preoperatively. Note anterior location of rectum, which had been treated inappropriately by cutback procedure as neonate. It is clearly too far forward. Note proximity of urethra and anus. On rectal examination, there was no perineal body. Note phallic structure, which is larger than a normal clitoris, and rudimentary labia posterior to it.

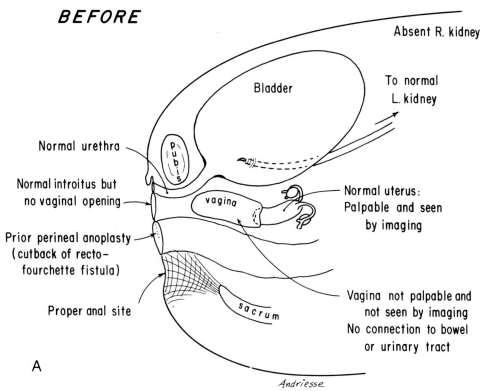

BEFORE

Absent R. kidney

Bladder

To normal
L. kidney

Normal urethra

Normal introitus but
no vaginal opening

Prior perineal anoplasty
(cutback of recto-
fourchette fistula)

Proper anal site

pubis

vagina

Normal uterus:
Palpable and seen
by imaging

Vagina not palpable and
not seen by imaging
No connection to bowel
or urinary tract

sacrum

A

Andriesse

Figure 47–28. *(Case 8) A,* Preoperative anatomy. Although the vagina was present, it was not palpable preoperatively or during the revision of the anorectal canal. Furthermore, it was not seen preoperatively by ultrasound imaging. *B,* Technique of Raffensperger and Ramenofsky for mobilizing and pushing the vagina down to the perineum from above at laparotomy. Rectum was tapered and repositioned further posteriorly in muscle complex.

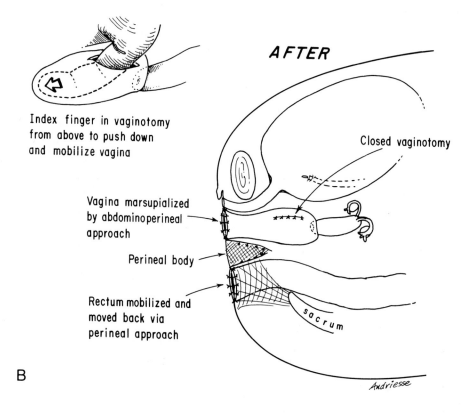

Index finger in vaginotomy
from above to push down
and mobilize vagina

AFTER

Closed vaginotomy

Vagina marsupialized
by abdominoperineal
approach

Perineal body

Rectum mobilized and
moved back via
perineal approach

sacrum

B

Andriesse

Discussion

These cases illustrate the broad spectrum seen in cloacal malformations. To plan reconstruction for an individual case requires knowledge of the wide range of anatomy that can present. Long-range plans must be made for the urinary tract, the genital tract, and the bowel. To consider one system without the other invites disaster. There must be close collaboration among specialists who can work together in treating these infants, or the surgeon must be able to manage all aspects of the problem.

Immediate treatment requires decompression of the bowel. In my experience, it is best to perform a divided loop transverse colostomy. If hydronephrosis is present, it should be decompressed by intermittent catheterization of the vagina. To do that may require a cutback procedure of the distal urogenital sinus. Only if catheterization proves ineffective should vesicostomy or vaginostomy be undertaken. Some children may need an initial urinary reconstructive operation, such as correction of massive reflux. In no case should a preliminary rectal operation take precedence. Ideally, all aspects of a cloaca can be repaired at a single operation. Occasionally, a urologic reconstructive operation should be considered later, as in Case 2. The patient underwent elective bladder neck narrowing and reimplantation of a solitary ectopic ureter at the time of colostomy closure.

All of these patients should have MRI of the lumbosacral spine to rule out neurosurgically correctable pathology (Karrer et al., 1988; Sato et al., 1988). Of 28 patients with cloacas who were screened by MRI, eight had tethered spinal cords, one had a cord syrinx, and 19 had normal findings. Vertebral anomalies and missing sacral segments are common in these children.

New vaginal and rectal passages are calibrated with Hegar dilators. The parents are instructed in passing the dilators, which are passed daily, at first, and later, with decreasing frequency. Excellent anesthesia is mandatory for these operations, some of which take many hours to accomplish. Ultimate urinary and bowel control cannot always be predicted, particularly when there are sacral or other spinal abnormalities. It is my experience that, if intermittent catheterization is required temporarily, or even long-term, it is well-tolerated and better than a urinary diversion procedure. If spontaneous normal bowel movements do not result, despite tapering the caliber of the colon and placing it accurately within the muscle complex, a daily enema will achieve bowel emptying and freedom from soiling. Long-term evaluation of these important parameters is needed, because urinary control and bowel control so often improve gradually as children grow older.

To date, two of the early patients have given birth to normal children, both by cesarean section. Long-term follow-up of sexual function and fertility will be needed, particularly in those with bowel extension for the vagina. Because the experience with sigmoid vaginoplasty in adult patients has shown that intercourse can be accomplished, it is anticipated that some of these patients should be able to become pregnant in the future. Three infants in this series died before having reconstructive surgery; one from renal dysplasia and two from severe congenital heart disease. Despite the complexity of many of the cases, there were no early or late deaths in those who had reconstructions.

These patients require long-term, continuous follow-up. Some develop prolapse of the pulled-through rectum or bowel segment used to extend the vagina, which can be trimmed. Anal stenosis at the mucocutaneous junction can be managed with two small z-plasties. Some of these girls have redundant "labioscrotal tissue" anteriorly in the perineum. Mobilizing that tissue and moving it back toward the anus may improve the appearance of the perineum. Similarly, a primitive phallic structure may have redundant labial tissue, which can be mobilized and sewn more posteriorly, thereby giving the clitoris a more normal appearance and creating labia minora. Formerly, there was high mortality and morbidity in females with cloacal anatomy. Today, a functionally satisfactory outcome can be achieved in most of these patients.

REFERENCES

Belman, B. A., and King, L. R.: Urinary tract abnormalities associated with imperforate anus. J. Urol., 108:823, 1972.
Bremer, J. L.: Congenital Anomalies of the Viscera—Their Embryological Basis. Cambridge, Harvard University, 1957.
deVries, P. A., and Peña, A.: Posterior sagittal anorectoplasty. J. Pediatr. Surg., 17:638, 1982.
Fleming, S. E., Hall, R., Gysler, M., et al.: Imperforate anus in females: Frequency of genital tract involvement, incidence of associated anomalies and functional outcome. J. Pediatr. Surg., 21:146, 1986.
Gough, M. H.: Anorectal agenesis with persistence of cloaca. Proc. R. Soc. Med., 52:886, 1959.
Gray, S. W., and Skandalakis, J. E.: The colon and rectum. In Embryology for Surgeons. Philadelphia, W. B. Saunders Co., 1972, p. 187.
Hall, J. W., Tank, E. S., and Lapides, J.: Urogenital anomalies and complications associated with imperforate anus. J. Urol., 103:810, 1970.
Hall, R., Fleming, S., Gysler, M., et al.: The genital tract in female children with imperforate anus. Surg. Gynecol. Obstet., 151:169, 1985.
Hendren, W. H.: Surgical management of urogenital sinus abnormalities. J. Pediatr. Surg., 12:339, 1977.
Hendren, W. H.: Urogenital sinus and anorectal malformation: Experience with 22 cases. J. Pediatr. Surg., 15:628, 1980.
Hendren, W. H.: Further experience in reconstructive surgery for cloacal anomalies. J. Pediatr. Surg., 17:695, 1982.
Hendren, W. H.: Repair of cloacal anomalies: Current techniques. J. Pediatr. Surg., 21:1159, 1986.
Hendren, W. H.: Urological aspects of cloacal malformations. J. Urol., 140:1207, 1988.
Hendren, W. H.: Imperforate anus and cloacal malformations. In Glenn, J. F. (Ed.): Urologic Surgery, Ed. 4. Philadelphia, J. B. Lippincott Co., 1990, p. 958.
Hendren, W. H., and Hendren, R. B.: Bladder augmentation: Experience with 129 children and young adults. J. Urol., 144:445, 1990.
Hendren, W. H., and Molenaar, J. C.: Simultaneous construction of vagina and rectum in a patient with absence of both. Z. Kinderchir., 42:112, 1987.
Hendren, W. H., Oesch, I., Tschaeppeler, H., et al.: Repair of cloacal malformation using combined posterior sagittal and abdominal perineal approaches. Z. Kinderchir., 42:115, 1987.
Hoekstra, W. J., Scholtmeijer, R. J., Molenaar, J. C., et al.: Urogenital tract abnormalities associated with congenital anorectal anomalies. J. Urol., 130:962, 1983.

Jaramillo, D., Lebowitz, R. L., and Hendren, W. H.: The cloacal malformation: Radiologic findings and imaging recommendations. Radiology, 177:441, 1990.

Johnson, R. J., Palken, M., Derrick, W., et al.: The embryology of high anorectal and associated genitourinary anomalies in the female. Surg. Gynecol. Obstet., 135:759, 1972.

Kalicinski, Z. H., Kansy, J., Kotarbinska, B., et al.: Surgery of megaureters—modification of Hendren's operation. J. Pediatr. Surg., 12:183, 1977.

Karlin, G., Brock, W., Rich, M., et al.: Persistent cloaca and phallic urethra. J. Urol., 142:1056, 1989.

Karrer, E. M., Flannery, A. M., Nelson, M. D., et al.: Anorectal malformations: Evaluation of associated spinal dysraphic syndromes. J. Pediatr. Surg., 23:45, 1988.

Kay, R., and Tank, E. S.: Principles of management of the persistent cloaca in the female newborn. J. Urol., 117:102, 1977.

Marshall, F. F., Jeffs, R. D., and Sarafyan, W. K.: Urogenital sinus abnormalities in the female patient. J. Urol., 122:568, 1979.

McLorie, G. A., Sheldon, G. A., Fleisher, M., et al.: The genitourinary system in patients with imperforate anus. J. Pediatr. Surg., 22:1100, 1987.

Mollitt, D. L., Schullinger, J. N., Santulli, T. V., et al.: Complications at menarche of urogenital sinus with associated anorectal malformations. J. Pediatr. Surg., 16:349, 1981.

Munn, R., and Schullinger, J. F.: Urologic abnormalities found with imperforate anus. Urology, 21:260, 1983.

Palken, M., Johnson, R. J., Derrick, W., et al.: Clinical aspects of female patients with high anorectal agenesis. Surg. Gynecol. Obstet., 135:411, 1972.

Parrott, T. S.: Urologic implications of anorectal malformations. Urol. Clin. North Am., 12:13, 1985.

Peña, A.: Atlas of Surgical Management of Anorectal Malformations. New York, Springer-Verlag, 1990.

Peña, A., and deVries, P. A.: Posterior sagittal anorectoplasty: Important technical considerations and new applications. J. Pediatr. Surg., 17:796, 1982.

Pohlman, A. G.: The development of the cloaca in human embryos. Am. J. Anat., 12:1, 1911.

Raffensperger, J. G., and Ramenofsky, M. L.: The management of a cloaca. J. Pediatr. Surg., 8:647, 1973.

Rich, M. A., Brock, W. A., and Peña, A.: Spectrum of genitourinary malformations in patients with imperforate anus. Pediatr. Surg. Int., 3:110, 1988.

Sato, Y., Pringle, K. C., Bergman, R. A., et al.: Congenital anorectal anomalies: MR imaging. Radiology, 168:157, 1988.

Smith, D. E.: Urinary anomalies and complications in imperforate anus and rectum. J. Pediatr. Surg., 3:337, 1968.

Snyder, W. H., Jr.: Some unusual forms of imperforate anus in female infants. Am. J. Surg., 111:319, 1966.

Stephens, F. D., and Smith, E. D.: Anorectal Malformations in Children, Vol. 4. Chicago, Year Book Medical Publishers, 1971, p. 118.

Wiener, E. S., and Kiesewetter, W. B.: Urologic abnormalities associated with imperforate anus. J. Pediatr. Surg., 8:151, 1973.

Williams, D. I., and Bloomberg, S.: Urogenital sinus in the female child. J. Pediatr. Surg., 11:51, 1976.

48
PRUNE-BELLY SYNDROME

John R. Woodard, M.D.

Prune-belly syndrome is the most common term for congenital absence, deficiency, or hypoplasia of the abdominal musculature accompanied by a large hypotonic bladder, dilated and tortuous ureters, and bilateral cryptorchidism (Osler, 1901). Known since Frolich's description in 1839, it has been of interest to urologists since 1895 when Parker described the genitourinary involvement. Because of the abdominal musculature–urinary tract–testicular involvement, the term "triad syndrome" (Stephens, 1963) is a commonly used eponym. It is also frequently referred to as the Eagle-Barrett syndrome (Eagle and Barrett, 1950).

Although prune-belly syndrome occurs almost exclusively in boys and only once in 35,000 to 50,000 live births (Garlinger and Ott, 1974), few syndromes have presented greater interest or challenge for the urologic surgeon. Historically, infants born with the full-blown syndrome have a poor prognosis for long-term survival. Of the cases reported prior to 1970, almost half were postmortem reports: 20 per cent were either stillborn or neonatal deaths, and another 30 per cent had died by 2 years of age, most commonly of urinary sepsis, renal failure, or both (Barnhouse, 1972; Burke et al., 1969; Lattimer, 1958; McGovern and Marshall, 1959). Although the prognosis for these patients has certainly improved, a controversy has arisen between those who believe a more aggressive approach toward surgical reconstruction of the urinary tract might improve the quality of life of these unfortunate infants (Fallat et al., 1989; Hendren, 1972; Jeffs et al., 1977; Randolph et al., 1981b; Woodard and Parrott, 1978a) and those who advocate limited, if any, surgical intervention (Duckett, 1980; Woodhouse et al., 1979).

Although, in rare instances, a girl is affected by absence of the abdominal muscles, it is exceptional to find the characteristic urinary tract anomaly (Aaronson and Cremin, 1980). Virtually by definition, the fully developed syndrome occurs almost exclusively in boys.

Infants with the prune-belly syndrome may be born of entirely normal pregnancies; however, oligohydramnios is more often the rule and is responsible for some of the associated and complicating conditions, especially those of the pulmonary and skeletal variety. With the increased use of diagnostic fetal ultrasound, it is no longer novel for a presumptive diagnosis of prune-belly syndrome to be made in utero. The clinical significance of such a fetal diagnosis is discussed further. The appearance of the neonate is characteristic (Fig. 48–1) and is now so well known to neonatologists and pediatricians that it is unlikely to be missed. The abdominal wall is thin and lax and, because of the sparsity of subcutaneous tissue, tends to crease and wrinkle like a wizened prune. The liver edge, spleen, intestines, and distended bladder are often quite evident on viewing the abdominal wall externally.

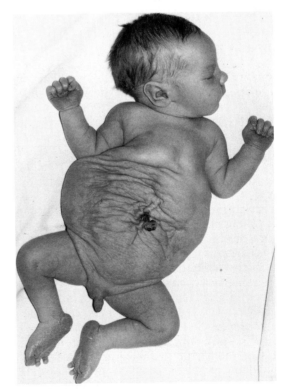

Figure 48–1. Newborn infant with the prune-belly syndrome, showing the characteristic appearance of the abdominal wall, the empty scrotum, and the talipes equinovarus.

The cause of the prune-belly syndrome remains unknown. Some have suggested that both the abdominal wall defect and the intra-abdominal cryptorchidism are secondary to distention of the urinary tract during early fetal development. Obstruction in the posterior urethra is a possible cause of this distention and would explain the predominance of male patients (Nakayama et al., 1984; Pagon et al., 1979). This theory suggests that testicular descent is blocked by a distended bladder and that the abdominal wall defect is secondary to either urinary tract distention or fetal ascites. However, other types of severe obstruction in the posterior urethra, such as posterior urethral valves, do not result in either a similar abdominal wall defect or the same type of upper urinary tract distortion. In addition, a higher instance of cryptorchidism has not been observed in the other obstructive uropathies.

Several investigators (Moerman et al., 1984; Monie and Monie, 1979) have suggested that prostatic dysgenesis and fetal ascites are key factors in the causation of the syndrome, with fetal ascites producing the abdominal wall defect. Although ascites is rarely present in patients with prune-belly syndrome (Smythe, 1981), it is speculated that ascites was transient with absorption toward the end of gestation. Another commonly quoted and, at one time, more popular theory is that a primary mesodermal error might account for both the abdominal wall defect and the genitourinary abnormalities because both arise from the paraxial intermediate and lateral plate mesoderm (Smith, 1970). Some investigators have suggested that the syndrome is caused by a complex chromosomal mutation (Riccardi and Grum, 1977).

PATHOPHYSIOLOGY

Abdominal Wall Defect

Despite the fact that most affected infants have similar appearances, the abdominal wall defect may be quite variable. It is often asymmetric and patchy in distribution. Characteristically, the abdominal muscles are absent in the lower and medial parts of the abdominal wall, although the upper rectus muscles and outer oblique muscles are developed. Some (Welch and Kearney, 1974) claim that the muscles are present but hypoplastic, whereas others (Afifi et al., 1972) find the deficiency to range from slight hypoplasia to complete absence of muscles. Secondary atrophy interspersed with some muscles that are hypertrophied (Mininberg et al., 1973) has also been reported.

The flanks often bulge markedly, with the thorax demonstrating a secondary flaring at the costal margins. This poor support for the lower chest wall interferes with an effective cough mechanism and contributes to a greater vulnerability to respiratory infections. These children also have difficulty in sitting up from the supine position. Although the wrinkled appearance is typical of the abdominal wall in the infant, the older child tends to take on a potbellied appearance (Fig. 48–2).

Surprisingly, the defective abdominal wall has caused little difficulty for the surgeon. Wound healing proceeds

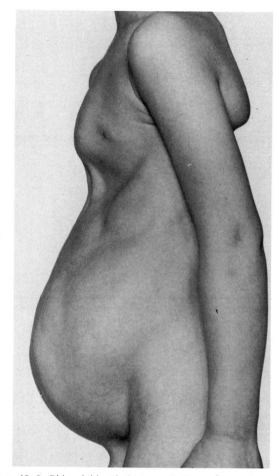

Figure 48–2. Older child with the prune-belly syndrome, showing the absence of wrinkling, the "potbelly" appearance, and the consequent deformity of the lower ribs.

satisfactorily despite the absence of layers for suturing. Wound dehiscence and other wound complications are rare.

Kidney

Although the kidneys may be normal, renal dysplasia and hydronephrosis are the two renal abnormalities typically associated with the syndrome. Often the prognosis is actually determined by the degree of dysplasia, which seems to be more severe in patients who have urethral stenosis, megalourethra, or imperforate anus (Potter, 1972). The spectrum may vary widely from marked dysplasia to a totally normal histologic appearance, and the findings are often asymmetric. For example, a completely dysplastic, multicystic kidney may be present on one side with normal renal histologic characteristics on the other.

Most patients with prune-belly syndrome have some degree of hydronephrosis, which may vary from mild to severe and does not appear to be related to the degree of abdominal deficiency. The degree of hydronephrosis is often less than what is anticipated from the degree of dilatation of the ureter. It is also common to find the renal parenchyma to be thicker and of better quality than might be expected from the degree of distortion in the drainage system. Although these findings have prognostic importance, they also suggest that the mechanism for the hydronephrosis might differ from that of other obstructive uropathies.

The infundibula are often long and narrow, whereas the renal pelves may vary from small to large. Occasional patients might also have ureteropelvic junction obstructions, and this possibility must not be overlooked in deciding on a plan of management. The function in these hydronephrotic kidneys is often surprisingly good, and it appears to be infection rather than obstruction per se that leads to their deterioration.

Ureter

The ureters are characterized by various degrees of tortuosity and dilatation. Both the tortuosity and dilatation are segmental, however, with the lower end of the ureter being the most severely affected whereas the upper ureter, in many cases, is actually surprisingly small in caliber (Fig. 48–3). Histologically, the ureteral wall demonstrates fibrosis and a scarcity of muscle bundles (Palmer and Tesluk, 1974). Some have also found a decrease in nerve plexuses (Ehrlich and Brown, 1977). The ureterovesical junction is markedly abnormal in most patients with vesicoureteral reflux being present in most but not all of these ureters. Fluoroscopic studies may reveal poor ureteral peristalsis. This finding may be reversible because function does seem to improve after surgical straightening and tapering or, in some patients, simply after growth and elongation have occurred.

The difference in functional and morphologic quality of the upper and lower ureters is an important consideration in planning corrective surgery. It may explain some of the failures observed when the distal ureter was used in reconstructive procedures.

Bladder and Urachus

Current studies suggest that detrusor hypertrophy occurs in some fetuses having the phenotypic appearance of the prune-belly syndrome, a finding not yet confirmed in postnatal studies (Massad and Kogan, 1990).

The role of bladder function in the clinical course of patients with prune-belly syndrome may be greater than previously suspected. That is, the function of the prune bladder has a significant impact on the status of the upper urinary tract, whether or not surgical remodeling has been carried out. Urodynamic pressure/flow data show that the typical prune bladder is compatible with "normal" function. That is, outflow resistance and maximum urinary flow rate may very well be within the normal range. Urodynamic studies have also shown, however, that a significant percentage of patients will have an unbalanced voiding mechanism with a disproportion between intravesical voiding pressure and outflow resistance; upper urinary tract status has been correlated with quality of bladder function (Woodard, 1990a).

The prune-belly bladder is typically very large and irregular in outline and has a thick wall. This does not represent true bladder wall hypertrophy, however, and actual trabeculation (with the exception of Massad and Kogan's current findings in the fetus) is seldom if ever seen. The apex of the bladder is attached to the abdom-

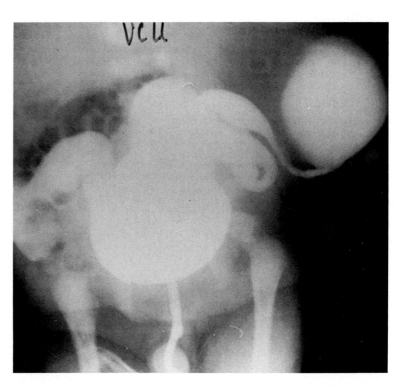

Figure 48–3. Cystogram showing massive bilateral vesicoureteral reflux. Note the marked difference in caliber of the left upper ureter as compared with the lower ureter.

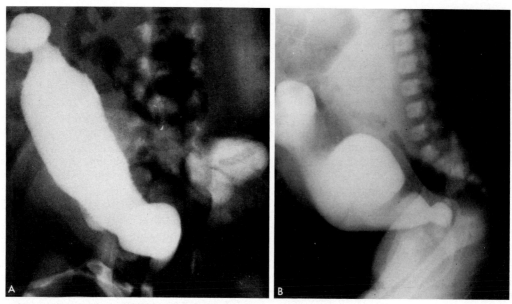

Figure 48–4. *A* and *B*. Voiding cystograms in two patients, showing the pseudodiverticulum configuration of the dome of the bladder. Note the wide, triangular prostatic urethra in both cystograms and the small utricular diverticulum in *B*.

inal wall at the umbilicus. Often, the dome of the bladder will bulge to resemble a pseudodiverticulum (Fig. 48–4). The trigone is very large, at times enormous, with ureteral orifices posteriorly placed and quite wide apart. Vesicoureteral reflux is commonly present (Fig. 48–5) although, surprisingly, it is not demonstrable in some patients. The bladder neck tends to be wide, relaxed, and ill-defined. In many patients, voiding pressures and urine flow rates are normal, and some are capable of emptying their bladders completely. Others, however, have significant volumes of postvoid residual urine because of unbalanced voiding mechanisms (Snyder et al., 1976). Interestingly, some investigators have reported improved voiding patterns with increasing age (Lee, 1977), whereas others (Williams, 1979) have seen the residual urine volume increase with age in some patients.

The urachus may be patent. This is likely with urethral atresia but may also occur in some patients without definite urethral obstruction.

Prostate

Below the wide bladder neck, the prostatic urethra has a dilated and somewhat triangular configuration (Fig. 48–6). It tapers to a relatively narrow point in the membranous portion of the urethra at the urogenital diaphragm. This may produce a configuration on the voiding cystourethrogram that resembles posterior urethral valves. The coincidental occurrence of a true posterior urethral valve in a patient with prune-belly syndrome must, however, be quite rare. In most cases, there is no clearly defined obstruction at this point, even though some obstructive element, perhaps occurring in utero, must be postulated. In addition, this relative narrowing may contribute to unbalanced voiding and, hence, the apparent effectiveness of internal urethrotomy in some patients. In a few cases, complete atresia of the membranous area of the urethra is present, with consequent destruction of the upper urinary tract. A tubular diverticulum, assumed to be of utricular origin (Kroovand et al., 1982), commonly arises from the level of the verumontanum (Fig. 48–6). During voiding urethrography, reflux of contrast material into the ejaculatory ducts is also occasionally seen.

Histologic studies of autopsy specimens have revealed a lack of development of the epithelial elements of the prostate gland (Deklerk and Scott, 1978; Moerman et al., 1984). This prostatic hypoplasia or dysgenesis may

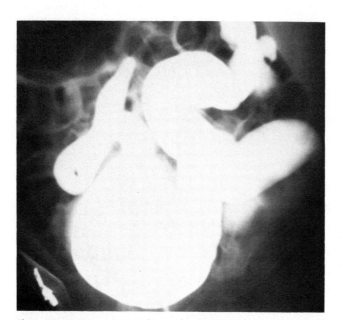

Figure 48–5. Cystogram in a boy with prune-belly syndrome, showing massive bilateral reflux. The upper ureter has an abrupt upper termination without any filling of the renal pelvis, an appearance that is characteristic of the multicystic kidney.

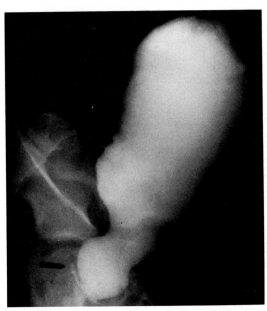

Figure 48–6. Voiding cystogram in a boy, showing the abrupt narrowing of urethra and apex of the wide, triangular prostatic portion. Note the utricular diverticulum *(arrow).*

be an etiologic factor (Hoagland and Hutchins, 1987; Monie and Monie, 1979), and it appears to explain the configuration of the prostatic urethra as seen radiographically.

Little information is available regarding ejaculation or sexual function in men with prune-belly syndrome, but no cases of fertility have been documented. Current data suggest that erection and orgasm are normal in these patients, but that retrograde ejaculation is common (Woodhouse and Snyder, 1984).

Urethra

The anterior urethra and the penis are normal in most prune-belly patients. However, it is well known that congenital megalourethra (scaphoid) is occasionally associated with the syndrome (Sellars et al., 1976; Shrom et al., 1981). In one patient series (Kroovand et al., 1982), this association was rather prominent; other coexisting abnormalities of the penis, including dorsal chordee, ventral chordee, hypospadias, and absence of the corporal bodies, were noted.

Testis

Bilateral cryptorchidism is characteristic of the syndrome and, in most patients, both testes lie intraabdominally, usually overlying the ureters at the pelvic brim near the sacroiliac level. The etiology of cryptorchidism in this particular circumstance is not known, but it is reasonable to speculate that it might be different from cryptorchidism seen in otherwise normal children. Some workers have suggested that the failure of

testicular descent in these patients is the result of the absence of abdominal muscles or gubernaculum or an intrinsic abnormality of the testis itself (Nunn and Stephens, 1961; Williams and Burkholder, 1967). Although some observers have noted the testicular histologic appearance to be normal for the age of the patient when the testis is biopsied (Nunn and Stephens, 1961), current observations suggest an absence of spermatogonia in some of these patients (Hadziselimovic, 1984; Uehling, 1982).

Gastrointestinal Anomalies

Most individuals with this syndrome have intestinal malrotation secondary to a universal mesentery with an unattached cecum (Silverman and Huang, 1950). Much less frequent is imperforate anus, which is more likely to occur in association with urethral atresia and renal dysplasia (Morgan et al., 1978). Gastroschisis and Hirschsprung's disease have also been reported in these patients (Cawthern et al., 1979; Willert et al., 1978). Constipation also appears to be a problem that is secondary to deficiency of the abdominal musculature, and it may lead to an acquired megacolon. Splenic torsion has also been reported (Heydenrych and DuToit, 1978).

Orthopedic Deformities

Various orthopedic anomalies of the limbs are commonly associated with and are probably the direct result of fetal compression secondary to oligohydramnios. The most frequent and benign finding is a dimple on the outer aspect of the knee or elbow at which point the skin is adherent to the underlying joint structures (Fig. 48–7). This finding is of no great clinical significance. However, more severe limb deficiencies have been reported in as many as 3 per cent of the patients (Carey et al., 1982). Because there are no reported cases of upper extremity deficiency with this syndrome, the lower limb abnormalities are thought to be due to compression of the iliac vessels from a markedly distended bladder (Ralis and Forbes, 1971). Club foot deformity and, less commonly, congenital hip dislocation are other orthopedic anomalies found with some frequency (Tuck and Smith, 1978). More than half of the patients reported since 1958 have had some musculoskeletal deformity and, as survival improves, the orthopedic surgeon will undoubtedly play a greater role in the future management of these patients.

Cardiac Anomalies

Ventricular septal defect, atrial septal defect, and tetrology of Fallot occur with increased frequency in this patient population. The incidence of cardiac abnormalities in these patients is approximately 10 per cent (Adebonojo, 1973).

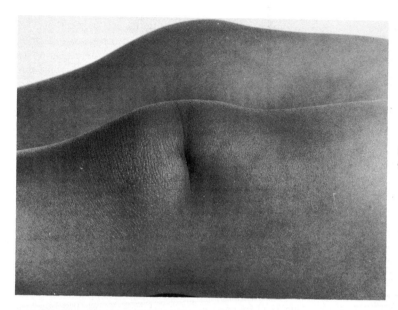

Figure 48–7. The dimple on the outer aspect of the knee characteristic of the prune-belly syndrome.

CLINICAL PRESENTATION AND NATURAL HISTORY

Prenatal Diagnosis

An ultrasound examination at some stage during pregnancy is now common practice. Indeed, interval ultrasound examinations during pregnancy are a standard part of prenatal care in some countries (Hellstrom et al., 1984). In the United States, obstructed kidneys and other urinary tract anomalies are most often found by chance during a routine ultrasound examination being performed to check for gestational age or number of fetuses. The sonographic findings consistent with prune-belly syndrome include markedly dilated ureters, enlarged bladder, and flaccid-appearing abdominal wall (Bovicelli et al., 1980; Christopher et al., 1982; Shih et al., 1982). Fetal ascites also has been detected (Monie and Monie, 1979). The diagnosis seems to be most readily made at about the 30th week of gestation but can be detected as early as the 20th week (Okulski, 1977). In clinical practice, it has proved difficult to accurately distinguish the fetus with prune-belly syndrome from one with primary vesicoureteral reflux or posterior urethral valves (Kramer, 1983). An instance in which fetal intervention was proved of benefit to a baby born with prune-belly syndrome has not been found. Therefore, the widespread use of fetal/maternal ultrasound and its increased frequency of fetal diagnosis of prune-belly syndrome does not appear to have altered either the incidence of the syndrome or its clinical management at this time (Woodard, 1990b).

Neonate

Although all cases should be recognized by the pediatrician/neonatologist on routine postnatal examination, there is a considerable variability in the severity of the disorder and in the urgency with which urologic advice is sought. This is obviously a syndrome with a wide spectrum. Patients can be placed in groups according to severity. The classification shown in Table 48–1 is simple and clinically useful.

Category I includes neonates with severe pulmonary difficulty or marked renal dysplasia, either of which precludes survival beyond the first days of life. In some of these infants, there will be a patent urachus and complete urethral obstruction. These patients are not subject to successful treatment. The more severely affected babies in this category might be stillborn. Because of severe oligohydramnios, others may have some of the features described in cases of renal agenesis, such as Potter's facies. The serum creatinine level is normal at birth but rises steadily thereafter. If these babies do not die quickly from pulmonary hypoplasia, they succumb only slightly later from renal failure. Drainage procedures result in a very scanty flow of dilute urine. In a few of these cases, in which there appears to be a chance for survival, a simple drainage procedure, such as vesicostomy, may be justified.

Patients in category II have the potential to survive

Table 48–1. THE SPECTRUM OF THE PRUNE-BELLY SYNDROME

Distinguishing Characteristics	Category Classification
Oligohydramnios, pulmonary hypoplasia, or pneumothorax. May have urethral obstruction or patent urachus and club foot.	I
Typical external features and uropathy of the full blown syndrome but no immediate problem with survival. May have mild or unilateral renal dysplasia. May or may not develop urosepsis or gradual azotemia.	II
External features may be mild or incomplete. Uropathy is less severe and renal function stable.	III

the neonatal period. They have the typical, full-blown uropathy with diffuse dilatation of the urinary tract and hydronephrosis. Renal dysplasia may exist, but it is unilateral or less severe than that found in patients in category I. Most of these infants are able to void urine from the bladder and often do so with apparent ease. Others suffer a general failure to thrive with enormous abdominal distention. All such infants should be transferred to medical centers with pediatric nephrologists, urologists, and other neonatal experts before any instrumentation is permitted.

Included in category III are infants with definite but relatively mild or incomplete features of the syndrome. Some uropathy is present, but the renal parenchyma is apparently of high quality, and urinary stasis is generally less marked. General agreement exists that patients in category III may require little if any urologic reconstructive surgery. However, they may later show signs of progressive upper tract deterioration, particularly if they are prone to urinary infection. They will also be candidates for treatment of cryptorchidism. All surviving patients require surveillance.

Pulmonary Aspects

Although infants born with prune-belly syndrome are subject to a variety of pulmonary complications, they fall into two major categories. The first group includes those with pulmonary hypoplasia (Fig. 48–8) secondary to oligohydramnios. The relationship between oligohydramnios and pulmonary hypoplasia is now well documented. Although renal factors, such as proline production, may play a role in fetal pulmonary development, the pulmonary hypoplasia associated with obstruction of the fetal urinary tract appears to be due to the oligohydramnios per se and the lack of intraluminal stenting fluid for the developing fetal lung (Docimo et al., 1989). It no longer appears that external uterine pressure on the fetal thorax, causing an arrest in the growth of the lung, is the cause of pulmonary hypoplasia. Pneumomediastinum or pneumothorax are common occurrences in patients with hypoplastic lungs. Neonates in this category commonly die from respiratory failure. If the patient does survive the neonatal period, the lungs grow and eventually attain adequate capacity. As the patient becomes older, however, he still may have respiratory problems secondary to the deficiency of accessory respiratory muscles in the abdominal wall.

The second major category of pulmonary complications includes patients who are prone to lobar atelectasis or pneumonia. Because the abdominal walls are important in powerful expiration, patients with prune-belly syndrome have a decreased ability to cough effectively, thus making them more vulnerable to complications during periods of excess mucus production. A number of anesthetic complications have been reported (Hannington-Kiff, 1970; Karamanian et al., 1974). Sedatives and analgesics must be used judiciously so that respiratory depression may be avoided. Apnea monitors play an important role in the neonatal surveillance of these patients.

Adult Presentation

Diagnosis of prune-belly syndrome is usually made in the neonatal period and almost always during early infancy. However, an occasional, rare patient will escape diagnosis until adulthood. Such patients have been known to present with hypertension and renal insufficiency (Lee, 1977). Others have been observed in middle life with renal insufficiency but no hypertension (Asplund and Laska, 1975). One would expect such a patient to have renal insufficiency, although not all patients who have presented as adults have had diminished kidney function. Texter and Koontz (1980) reported a 33-year-old man with prune-belly syndrome who presented with decreased libido but had normal renal function. Other patients have been reported who seem to do well with little or no treatment during their younger years only to succumb to urinary sepsis as adults (Culp and Flocks, 1954).

Female Syndrome

In the strictest sense, only a male patient may harbor the complete syndrome. Yet, about 3 per cent of the reported cases occur in genetic females. When less strict criteria of diagnosis are applied, the percentage quoted is sometimes higher. The affected female patient appears to have no urethral abnormality. The defect involves the abdominal wall, bladder, and upper urinary tract (Rabinowitz and Schillinger, 1977). Actually, fewer than 20 cases of the female syndrome have been reported, and the principles of management are essentially the same as for the male. Many of the female patients have had incomplete forms of the syndrome with normal upper urinary tracts. The syndrome has also been reported in a patient with Turner's syndrome (XO karyotype) (Lubinsky et al., 1980).

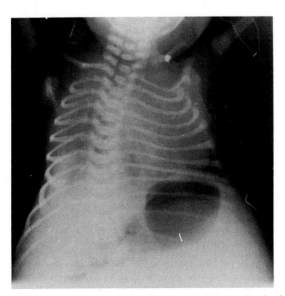

Figure 48–8. Chest radiograph of an infant who died shortly after birth from pulmonary hypoplasia.

Incomplete Syndrome

Although it is exceptionally rare to encounter a normal urinary tract in association with the characteristic abdominal wall defect in a male, the converse is not unusual. Some patients ("pseudo–prune-belly syndrome") with a normal or relatively normal abdominal wall exhibit many or all of the internal urologic features, usually in a less severe form. These may include dysplastic or dysmorphic kidneys; dilated, tortuous ureters; large-capacity bladder; and the typical configuration of the bladder neck and prostatic urethra.

GENETIC ASPECTS

The genetic basis of the prune-belly syndrome is still the subject of controversy and speculation. Some suspect that a single-gene defect might be responsible (Garlinger and Ott, 1974), whereas others propose that it might result from different genes producing identical results (Riccardi and Grum, 1977). The last theory suggests that the anomaly might represent a superficial X-linkage mimicry. In fact, other evidence supports a sex-linked inheritance (Adenyokunnu et al., 1975; Adenyokunnu and Familusi, 1982; Lockhart et al., 1979; Woodard, 1978), and the occurrence of prune-belly syndrome in siblings has now been reported several times. When counseling parents of infants with prune-belly syndrome, it is important to make them aware of a possibility of occurrence in a subsequent sibling although the degree of risk is, at present, unknown.

Of great interest is the association between twinning and the prune-belly syndrome. Among all pregnancies, the incidence of twinning is about 1 in 80, whereas the incidence of twinning among patients with prune-belly syndrome is about 1 in 23, or four times greater than normal (Ives, 1974). All reported pairs of twins are discordant for the syndrome. The possibility of a normal monozygotic twin must be kept in mind if a kidney donor should be needed for a patient with prune-belly syndrome who develops chronic renal failure.

The karyotype is normal in most prune-belly patients. Only a few cases of chromosomal abnormalities have been reported, including one with a minute additional chromosome (Halbrecht et al., 1972). Reports have been made of two siblings with prune-belly syndrome who had mosaicism (Harley et al., 1972) and others who had the syndrome in association with Turner's syndrome (Lubinsky et al., 1980).

TREATMENT

Theoretically, at least, treatment might now begin with in utero intervention following a fetal diagnosis by ultrasound. However, at this time, there is no evidence that potential for renal or pulmonary function can be altered by such a procedure. Perhaps further laboratory and clinical investigation will open new horizons in this area. At present, treatment of the infant with prune-belly syndrome begins with the initial neonatal evaluation.

Initial Diagnostic Evaluation

The syndrome is now well known and, because of the typical external features, the diagnosis of prune-belly syndrome and the presence of prune-belly uropathy are seldom in doubt. Although the urologist is usually notified immediately, the affected neonate rarely represents a true urologic emergency. The most urgent matters are actually those concerned with cardiopulmonary function. Pulmonary hypoplasia, pneumomediastinum, pneumothorax, and cardiac abnormalities, which are perhaps less evident from external inspection, may demand immediate attention. These matters must not be overlooked. It should be noted whether a patent urachus is present and whether the infant can void. An orthopedic examination should also be done initially.

Early urologic assessment of each patient is necessary to individualize treatment (Jeffs et al., 1977). However, some compromises must be made because of the risks inherent in diagnostic procedures requiring instrumentation of the urinary tract. Clearly, radiographic examination of the chest, evaluation of pulmonary and cardiac function, and serial blood studies to estimate the level of renal function are first-priority procedures. An abdominal ultrasound examination provides considerable useful information and avoids the disadvantage of either instrumentation or additional x-ray exposure (Fig. 48–9). Because urinary infection may occur even in the absence of instrumentation, urine cultures must be done and the patient should be placed on antimicrobial prophylaxis.

If the baby is in stable condition and the serum creatinine level remains normal, one may wait for several days before obtaining a radioisotope renal scan or an excretory urogram. However, these studies should be done and the remainder of the diagnostic evaluation must then be tailored to one's attitude toward definitive management (Fig. 48–10). It is perhaps better initially to simply assume that reflux is present rather than to prove it. If the pyelographic findings and renal functional parameters are such that early reconstruction to correct obstruction or reflux, or both, might be considered, a voiding cystogram may be indicated. Any instrumentation of the urinary tract in these patients, however, may result in bacterial contamination that might be both hazardous to the patient and difficult to eradicate.

By following the serum creatinine levels, urine bacteriology, and pyelographic and sonographic findings, it is possible to formulate a reasonable plan of clinical management. Evidence of infection or deteriorating renal function is usually an indication for surgical intervention. In the absence of such complications, one should monitor the respiratory function closely for 2 to 3 months, at which time a more thorough urologic evaluation might be appropriate. Many different approaches have been advocated for the management of prune-belly uropathy, each with its rationale and each with its own proponents. All methods have the same

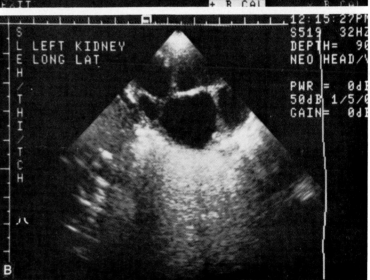

Figure 48–9. Right *(A)* and left *(B)* kidneys in a 1-day-old infant with typical prune-belly syndrome. The infant was seen at birth, placed on antibiotics, and followed closely with urine cultures, serum creatinine determinations, and renal ultrasound imaging. (From Woodard, J. R., and Zucker, I.: Current management of the dilated urinary tract in prune-belly syndrome. Urol. Clin. North Am., 17(2):412, 1990.)

ultimate aim of maintaining renal function and preventing urinary infection.

Vesicoureteral Dysfunction

In the typical patient, the bladder is large, thick-walled, and flabby, and it tends to empty slowly and, perhaps, incompletely. Usually, but not always, vesicoureteral reflux is found. The ureter is long, redundant, irregularly dilated, and tortuous. Some degree of hydronephrosis usually exists. Considerable controversy has arisen concerning the proper management of this aspect of the syndrome.

Nonoperative Treatment

Although successful results are possible with aggressive reconstructive operations, many investigators (Burke et al., 1969; Duckett, 1976; Rogers and Ostrow, 1973; Williams and Burkholder, 1967) contend that extensive reconstructive operations may fail to improve

the ultimate fate of these patients. As a result, a "hands-off" attitude or nonsurgical approach has been adopted by many. Despite rather gross urographic abnormalities, many newborns seem to do quite well (Fig. 48–11).

Woodhouse and co-workers (1979) reviewed a series of prune-belly patients who had been managed conservatively. A total of nine of 11 patients, followed from infancy, had remained well except for a few urinary tract infections for periods up to 24 years. These patients were reported to have normal voiding patterns and normal renal function. Certainly, patients in category III are candidates for this type of management. Unfortunately, in the more severe category II patient, long-term follow-up data from a larger number of patients are necessary to evaluate the results of either medical management or extensive surgical reconstruction; such data are not yet available. Many patients with prune-belly syndrome have ultimately required renal transplantation (Reinberg et al., 1989). Others have seemed to do well for years only to succumb to urologic complications later (Culp and Flocks, 1954).

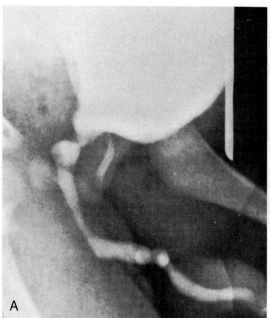

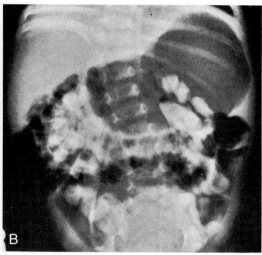

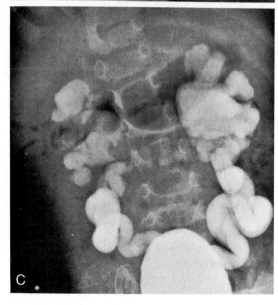

Figure 48–10. Same infant as shown in Figure 48–9 when he was re-evaluated at the age of 1 month with voiding cystourethrogram *(A)*. Note reflux posterior to bladder and typical wide bladder neck with long triangular prostatic urethra. *(B)*, Film from intravenous urogram also at 1 month of age. *(C)*, Film from voiding cystogram made as part of his re-evaluation 7 months later. Note grade V bilateral vesicoureteral reflux with marked ureteral tortuosity. Patient underwent major reconstructive surgery following this study. (From Woodard, J. R., and Zucker, I.: Current management of the dilated urinary tract in prune-belly syndrome. Urol. Clin. North Am., 17(2):413, 1990.)

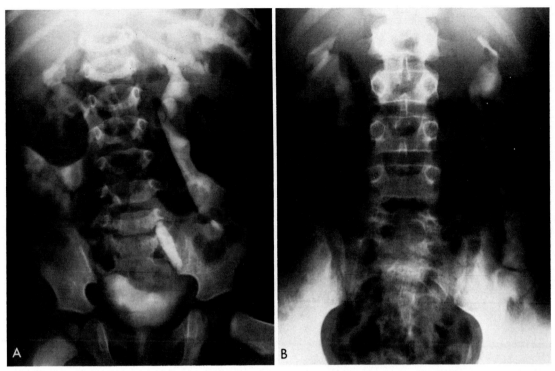

Figure 48–11. Intravenous urograms in a boy with prune-belly syndrome. *A,* At age 2 years, showing classic appearance of tortuous, dilated ureters with relatively well preserved kidneys. *B,* At age 19 years, showing improvement in ureteric dilatation without surgical treatment and no deterioration in renal function.

Temporary Diversion

When urinary infection becomes a problem, or it appears that renal function is deteriorating, a urinary drainage procedure must be considered. Advantages exist in selecting a tubeless type of diversion, and the simplest of these is *cutaneous vesicostomy* (Duckett, 1976). Vesicostomy provides expedient and effective bladder drainage and is an operation that is tolerated by most of these patients (Fig. 48–12). The procedure is performed through a small transverse incision midway between the umbilicus and the symphysis pubis. A small ellipse of skin and rectus fascia is excised. The dome of the bladder is mobilized and delivered into the incision, at which point it is sutured to the rectus fascia and skin, and a small bladder stoma is fashioned. The urine is allowed to drain freely into a diaper, using no collection device or tubes. Subsequent closure of the vesicostomy is also simple. Vesicostomy is useful either as a primary temporary drainage procedure or as a preliminary drainage procedure prior to a more extensive reconstructive operation at some later date. It might be argued that, in some instances, it fails to provide optimal drainage to the upper urinary tract in patients with markedly redundant and tortuous ureters, in which case one might wonder whether a more proximal drainage procedure would be superior. In addition, there is the occasional patient in whom obstruction exists at the ureteropelvic junction.

For patients who have urosepsis or progressive deterioration of renal function, *high loop cutaneous ureterostomy* or *pyelostomy* has been advocated (Williams and Parker, 1974). Although not as simple as vesicostomy, it is still an expedient procedure and has the advantage of providing good proximal drainage to each kidney while permitting inspection and biopsy of the kidney at the time of operation. By allowing for a subsequent evaluation of differential kidney function, it may also aid in the planning of subsequent reconstructive operations. The main disadvantage of this procedure is that it may hinder an eventual reconstructive procedure by damaging the upper ureter, which is an important consideration in these patients because that may be the only portion of ureter which is nearly normal in caliber and function. Although this procedure may have some merit in a few selected cases, its popularity has, with good reason, decreased.

Extensive Ureteral Reconstruction

The role of extensive surgical remodeling of the urinary tract in patients with prune-belly syndrome is understandably controversial because some patients appear to do well without major reconstruction and others seem to have been harmed by unsuccessful surgical attempts. There is little question, however, that the urinary tract in patients with prune-belly syndrome is characterized by stasis and that this stasis predisposes to bacteriuria, which may lead to deterioration of renal function as well as to troublesome clinical symptoms. Therefore, it is likely that many surgeons will continue their efforts at remodeling these distorted urinary tracts.

Success in these surgical reconstructions depends to a great extent on the use of the upper few centimeters of

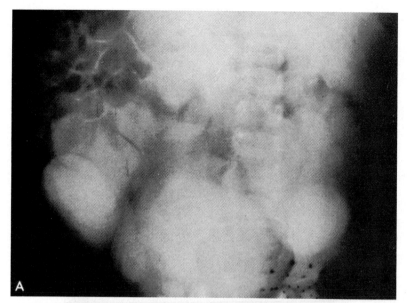

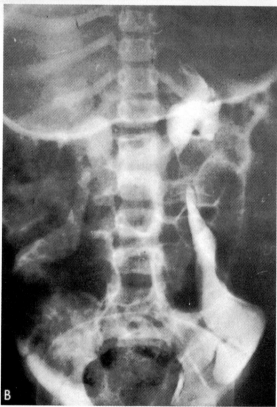

Figure 48–12. Vesicostomy drainage. *A,* Intravenous pyelogram in an 18-month-old boy with prune-belly syndrome. *B,* Intravenous pyelogram 10 years later with cutaneous vesicostomy alone.

ureter, which are usually less dilated, less tortuous, and morphologically better than the distal ureter. Meticulous surgical technique with adherence to established principles of ureteral tailoring and reimplantation surgery is required (Fig. 48–13). Unfortunately, both the bladder and the ureter, by the very nature of this bizarre uropathy, are difficult structures with which to work. Despite these inherent difficulties, in experienced hands, a reasonably high degree of success is possible with this extensive reconstructive surgery, both in the neonate as a primary procedure (Figs. 48–14 and 48–15) and in the older infant or child (Fig. 48–16) as a primary or staged procedure (Woodard and Parrott, 1978a; Woodard, 1990a).

Vesicourethral Dysfunction

Little question exists that poor bladder emptying, with resulting recurrent and chronic urinary tract infection, leads to upper tract deterioration in many of these patients (Woodard, 1990b). The large bladder capacity, abnormal bladder wall, and relative narrowing of the membranous urethra may all play some role. Although some efforts have been made to delineate this problem urodynamically (Snyder et al., 1976), such data is still sparse. Efforts have, however, been made toward improving detrusor function and reducing outflow resistance.

Reduction Cystoplasty

As noted, the bladders in most of these patients are large and tend to bulge in pseudodiverticulum–like fashion at the dome. Fluoroscopic studies indicate that the dilated dome portion of the bladder may hinder micturition (Perlmutter, 1976). Reduction cystoplasty is a useful procedure in treating such a large, poorly functioning bladder and can be employed alone or as part of a major upper tract reconstructive procedure (see Fig. 48–13*B*, *D*).

The technique involves generous resection of the bladder dome with a significant reduction in bladder capacity. This appears to improve bladder function by creating a more spherical detrusor. Plication of the bladder dome has also proved successful in some instances (Williams and Parker, 1974), and Hanna (1982) has reported improvement in detrusor function by "remodeling" the bladder.

Internal Urethrotomy

Although prune-belly uropathy is compatible with normal voiding dynamics, pressure–flow studies in some patients demonstrate an unbalanced voiding mechanism, and the condition of these patients may be improved by internal urethrotomy (Cukier, 1977; Snyder et al., 1976; Woodhouse et al., 1979). This procedure may be useful for children who develop difficulty in voiding or who develop increased residual urine volume. A child with residual urine, a dilated posterior urethra, reflux, or ureteral dilation may be considered a suitable candidate.

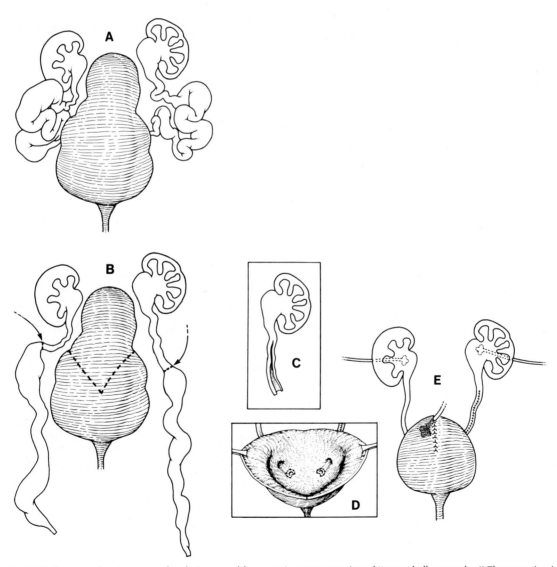

Figure 48–13. Artist's drawings showing surgical technique used for extensive reconstruction of "prune-belly uropathy." The operation is performed transperitoneally. No attempt is made to straighten the lower ureter because only the upper portion is needed for reestablishing continuity. The ureter may or may not require tapering. Dome of bladder is excised *(dotted line)* in most patients. Ureteral stents (not shown) are employed, and nephrostomy tubes are frequently used.

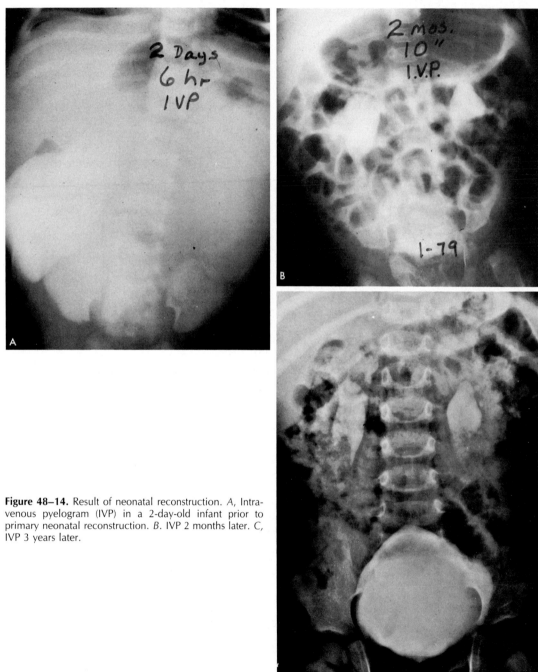

Figure 48–14. Result of neonatal reconstruction. *A,* Intravenous pyelogram (IVP) in a 2-day-old infant prior to primary neonatal reconstruction. *B.* IVP 2 months later. *C,* IVP 3 years later.

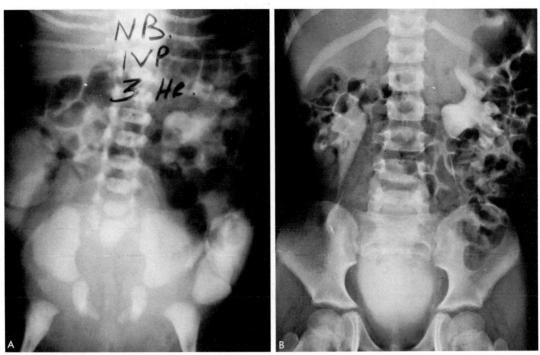

Figure 48–15. Results of neonatal reconstruction. *A,* Intravenous pyelogram during first week of life, just prior to reconstruction. *B,* Ten years later after a single primary reconstructive procedure.

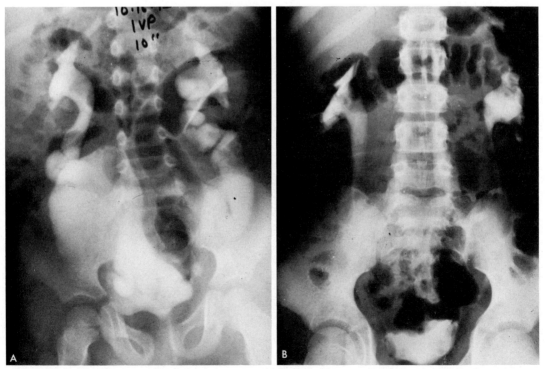

Figure 48–16. *A,* Intravenous pyelogram in a 2½-year-old boy who had worn a suprapubic catheter since birth. Extensive reconstruction was done. *B,* The pyelographic result seen 7 years later.

Internal urethrotomy appears to be an easy method of improving bladder emptying in these circumstances. Unfortunately, it might also be an easy method for producing urinary incontinence, although its advocates suggest that this may be temporary (Williams, 1979). Incontinence would seem to be less of a risk in the unbalanced voiding situation that exists in some of these patients. However, it would perhaps be wise to limit its use to patients in whom urodynamic evaluation confirms this imbalance. Clearly, urethrotomy has some role to play in the management of many patients with prune-belly uropathy.

Urethrotomy may be performed with the Otis urethrotome or an endoscope. Williams (1979) advocates making one or two cuts anteriorly or anterolaterally to size 24 or 30 Fr followed by a period of catheter drainage. A visual urethrotomy would seem preferable to the Otis procedure and should be made through the narrowed area in the urethra, which is typically at the end of the prostatic portion. Because the bladder neck appears wide in these individuals, a cut in that area does not appear warranted. In some patients, urethrotomy alone produces notable improvement in the radiographic appearance of the upper urinary tract (Fig. 48–17).

Megaurethra Repair

In the rare child in whom the anterior urethra is grossly dilated, surgery is required to reduce it to a normal caliber. Usually only the penile urethra is involved, and the meatus and the glanular portion are normal. In such a case, a circumferential incision around the coronal sulcus with stripping back of the penile skin provides the best approach. The redundant wall of the urethra is excised, and the lumen is reconstructed over a catheter. The penile skin is then drawn forward and sutured. In more severe cases, it may be necessary to cut back from the meatus, excising both redundant skin and urethra, with reconstruction based on the methods of hypospadias repair.

Cryptorchidism

Fertility in patients with prune-belly syndrome is, at best, doubtful. Whether the wide bladder neck will allow for normal ejaculation and whether germ cells are present in the testicles of some of these patients has been questioned (Hadziselimovic, 1984; Uehling, 1982; Woodhouse and Snyder, 1984). Nonetheless, the testes do have good hormonal function and orchiopexy is attempted in most of these patients.

Rarely, if ever, is the standard surgical technique for inguinal orchiopexy successful in these circumstances. Staged procedures of the classic type have also been less than satisfactory. At present, three alternatives are available for the management of cryptorchidism in these patients.

Early Transabdominal Orchiopexy

In the neonate and in patients up to at least 6 months of age, transabdominal complete mobilization of the spermatic cord almost always allows the testis to be

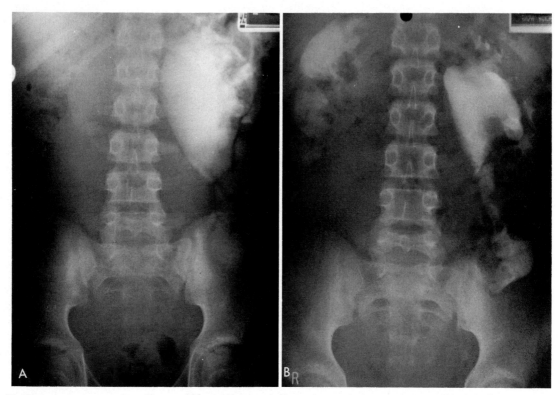

Figure 48–17. Intravenous urograms in a 12-year-old boy with prune-belly syndrome. *A*, At presentation with residual urine volume of 2 L. *B*, Following Otis urethrotomy.

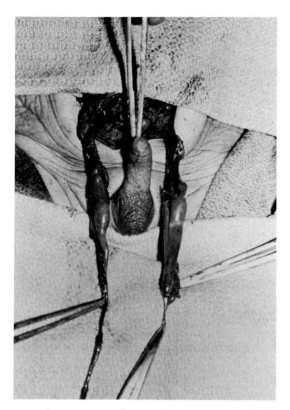

Figure 48–18. Operative photograph showing the ease with which the testes reach the scrotum following neonatal transabdominal mobilization of the spermatic cords.

positioned in the dependent portion of the scrotum without tension and without dividing the vascular portion of the spermatic cord (Fig. 48–18) (Woodard and Parrott, 1978b). This procedure was found to be partic-

ularly applicable to infants undergoing extensive ureteral reconstructive procedures during the neonatal period because it could be done simultaneously. Currently, with patients having reconstructive surgery done later, the technique has been found to be equally applicable to older infants (Fallat et al., 1989; Woodard, 1990a). In patients who do not require reconstructive ureteral surgery, one might wait until 3 to 6 months of age to ensure stability of the upper urinary tract as well as the status of cardiopulmonary function before performing this operation.

Fowler-Stephens (Long Loop Vas) Technique

The Fowler-Stephens technique for performing orchiopexy in patients with intra-abdominal testes has become part of the standard urologic armamentarium (Fowler and Stephens, 1963). The operation involves division of the spermatic vessels above the level of the internal ring with preservation of the anastomotic connections between the vessels of the vas deferens and the distal spermatic vessels. A layer of peritoneum should be left over the vas to preserve these collaterals.

In patients with prune-belly syndrome, the operation is done transperitoneally with wider-than-usual exposure; the success rate has been reported as approximately 75 per cent (Gibbons et al., 1979). This procedure, therefore, represents a reasonable approach to the intra-abdominal testis in the patient with prune-belly syndrome and may allow for greater flexibility in the timing of the procedure.

Enthusiasm has been generated for the so-called staged Fowler-Stephens operation, in which the spermatic vessels are ligated several months prior to the

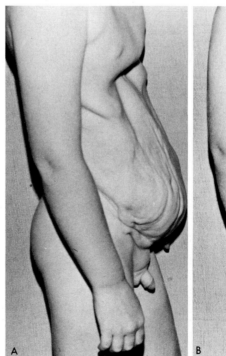
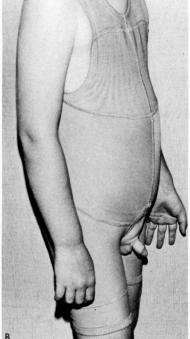

Figure 48–19. Photograph of a 4-year-old boy without (A) and with (B) his elasticized corset.

orchiopexy operation itself. The rationale of this modification is to allow the development of increased collateral circulation between the vasal and distal testicular arteries, which may improve the success rate of the Fowler-Stephens procedure in these patients.

Microvascular Autotransplantation

It is technically feasible to perform autotransplantation of the abdominal testis to the scrotum with microvascular anastomosis of the spermatic vessels to the inferior epigastric vessels. Although enthusiasm is limited for this procedure, the technique has been applied successfully in patients of various ages with prune-belly syndrome (MacMahon et al., 1976; Wacksman et al., 1980). Although there is no evidence of offspring from fathers with prune-belly syndrome, androgenic function

in these testes appears to be good, and it is likely that orchiopexy will continue to be part of the treatment for these individuals. Current reports of testicular tumors arising in several patients with prune-belly syndrome add importance to the treatment of this aspect of the problem.

Abdominal Wall Defect

The most obvious external feature of the prune-belly syndrome is the abdominal wall defect itself. Although it clearly offers a cosmetic disadvantage to the patient, the role this deficiency might play in either pulmonary or bladder function has been difficult to document with accuracy. Consequently, some controversy has existed in the past regarding the need for surgical procedures

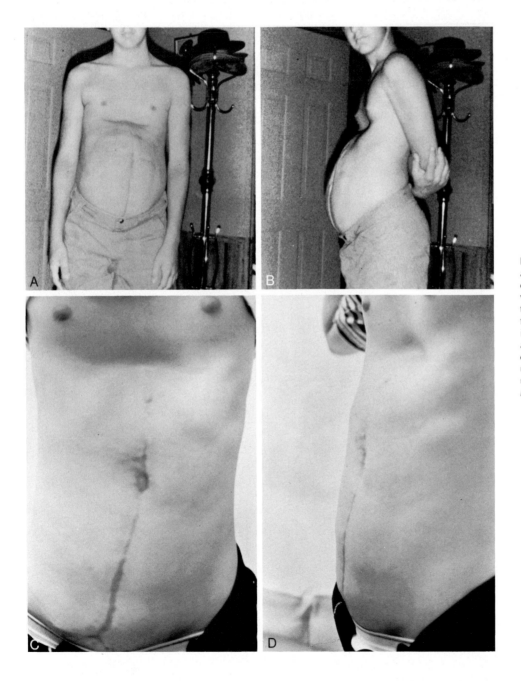

Figure 48–20. A and B, Anterior and lateral views of the abdomen of a 14-year-old boy who underwent major surgical remodeling of the urinary tract during early infancy with good results. Note typical abdominal configuration. C and D, Anterior and lateral views of the same boy 1 month after undergoing abdominal wall–plasty using the technique described by Monfort.

to improve the abdominal wall. Enthusiasm for this seems to wax and wane. Many patients have been treated simply with abdominal supports or corset devices (Fig. 48–19). At the present time, however, there appears to be renewed interest in abdominal wall reconstruction. Some of the new techniques appear promising.

Abdominal Wall Reconstruction

Electromyographic studies have demonstrated that the major functioning or recoverable muscle exists in the lateral and upper section of the abdomen; usually, little or no useful muscle is present in the more central and lower portion of the abdomen. Based on this information, the technique of abdominal wall plication—involving excision of a transverse elliptic portion of the lower abdominal wall—as described by Randolph and colleagues (1981a) has produced good results and is a procedure worthy of consideration, at least in selected patients (Duckett, 1980).

This procedure reduces the abdominal protuberance and allows for the wearing of normal trousers when this might otherwise not be possible. However, Randolph reports satisfactory results after the first procedure in only about half of his patients, with some requiring repeat operation (Fallat et al., 1989). This procedure involves removing the full thickness of the abdominal wall in such a way as to spare potentially functioning musculature and corresponding motor nerves.

Two currently described techniques for vertical abdominal wall–plasty have met with early enthusiastic support (Ehrlich et al., 1986; Monfort, personal communication, 1990). These operations seem to produce a more normal physique and provide more consistently satisfactory results. Unlike the technique of Randolph, these operations add increased thickness to the anterior abdominal wall and produce a more definite waist (Fig. 48–20).

External Support Devices

The parents of most children with prune-belly syndrome, if left to their own devices, will provide their children with some type of corset or external support device. When properly designed, such a corset will give the child a fairly normal appearing physique while clothed (see Fig. 48–19). The corsets can be worn with ease and comfort and are relatively inexpensive. Because the abdominal wall deformity in some patients seems to improve slightly with age, external support devices may have a practical advantage over major surgical abdominal wall plication procedures in some patients, at least initially.

Outlook

The considerable improvements in the medical, surgical, and urodynamic management of patients born with the prune-belly syndrome will certainly result in a prognosis far better than that previously reported, both for survival and for the quality of life. The syndrome is clearly a disorder with a wide spectrum. Some patients may benefit from major urologic reconstruction, but others require little if any such surgery. All of the patients need careful evaluation and individualized management and, because urodynamics may change with age, long-term surveillance and periodic reappraisal are necessary.

REFERENCES

Aaronson, I. A., and Cremin, B. J.: Prune-belly syndrome in young females. Urol. Radiol., 1:151, 1980.

Adebonojo, F. O.: Dysplasia of the abdominal musculature with multiple congenital anomalies; prune-belly or triad syndrome. J. Natl. Med. Assoc., 65:327, 1973.

Adenyokunnu, A. A., Adeniyi, T. M., Kolawole, T. M., et al.: Prune-belly syndrome: A study of ten cases in Nigerian children with common and uncommon manifestations. East Afr. Med. J., 52:438, 1975.

Adenyokunnu, A. A., and Familusi, J. B.: Prune belly syndrome in two siblings and a first cousin. Am. J. Dis. Child., 136:23, 1982.

Afifi, A. K., Rebiez, J. M., Andonian, S. J., et al.: The myopathy of the prune-belly syndrome. Neurol. Sci., 15:153, 1972.

Asplund, J., and Laska, J.: Prune-belly syndrome at the age of 37. Scand. J. Urol. Nephrol., 9:297, 1975.

Barnhouse, D. H.: Prune-belly syndrome. Br. J. Urol., 44:356, 1972.

Bovicelli, L., Rizzo, N., Orsini, L. F., et al.: Prenatal diagnosis of the prune-belly syndrome. Clin. Genet., 18:79, 1980.

Burke, E. C., Shin, M. H., and Kelalis, P. P.: Prune-belly syndrome. Am. J. Dis. Child., 117:668, 1969.

Carey, J. C., Eggert, L., and Curry, C. J. R.: Lower limb deficiency and the urethral obstruction sequence. Birth Defects, 18:19, 1982.

Cawthern, T. H., Bottene, C. A., and Grant, D.: Prune-belly syndrome associated with Hirschsprung's disease. Am. J. Dis. Child., 133:652, 1979.

Christopher, C. R., Spinelli, A., and Severt, D.: Ultrasonic diagnosis of prune-belly syndrome. Obstet. Gynecol., 59:391, 1982.

Cukier, J.: Resection of the urethra in the prune-belly syndrome. Birth Defects, 13:95, 1977.

Culp, D. A., and Flocks, R. H.: Congenital absence of abdominal musculature. J. Iowa State Med. Soc., 44:155, 1954.

Deklerk, D. P., and Scott, W. W.: Prostatic maldevelopment in prune-belly syndrome: A defect in prostatic stromal-epithelial interaction. J. Urol., 120:241, 1978.

Docimo, S. G., Luetic, T., Crone, R. K., et al.: Pulmonary development in the fetal lamb with severe bladder outlet obstruction and oligohydramnios: A morphometric study. J. Urol., 142:657, 1989.

Duckett, J. W., Jr.: The prune-belly syndrome. In Kelalis, P. P., King, L. R., and Belman, A. B. (Eds.): Clinical Pediatric Urology. Philadelphia, W. B. Saunders Co., 1976, p. 615.

Duckett, J. W., Jr.: The prune-belly syndrome. In Holder, T. M., and Ashcroft, K. W. (Eds.): The Surgery of Infants and Children. Philadelphia, W. B. Saunders Co., 1980, pp. 802–815.

Eagle, J. F., and Barrett, G. S.: Congenital deficiency of abdominal musculature with associated genitourinary anomalies: A syndrome: Reports of 9 cases. Pediatrics, 6:721, 1950.

Ehrlich, R. M., and Brown, W. J.: Ultrastructural anatomic observations of the ureter in the prune-belly syndrome. Birth Defects, 13:101, 1977.

Ehrlich, R. M., Lesavoy, M. A., and Fine, R. N.: Total abdominal wall reconstruction in the prune belly syndrome. J. Urol., 136:282, 1986.

Fallat, M. E., Skoog, S. J., Bellman, A. B., Eng, G., and Randolph, J. G.: The prune-belly syndrome: A comprehensive approach to management. J. Urol., 142:802, 1989.

Fowler, R., Jr., and Stephens, F. D.: The role of testicular vascular anatomy in the salvage of high undescended testes. In Stephen, F. D. (Ed.): Congenital Malformations of the Rectum, Anus, and Genitourinary Tract. Baltimore, Williams & Wilkins Co., 1963.

Frolich, F.: Der Mangel der Muskeln, insbesondere der Seitenbauchmuskeln. Dissertation, Wurzberg, C. A. Zurn, 1839.

Garlinger, P., and Ott, J.: Prune-belly syndrome—possible genetic implications. Birth Defects, 10:173, 1974.

Geary, D. F., MacLusky, I. B., Churchill, B. M., et al.: A broader spectrum of abnormalities in the prune-belly syndrome. J. Urol., 135:324, 1986.

Gibbons, M. D., Cromie, W. J., and Duckett, J. W., Jr.: Management of the abdominal undescended testis. J. Urol., 122:76, 1979.

Greskovich, F. J., and Nyberg, L. N., Jr.: The prune-belly syndrome: A review of its etiology, defects, treatment and prognosis. J. Urol., 140:707, 1988.

Hadziselimovic, F.: Personal communication, July 1984.

Halbrecht, I., Komlos, L., and Shabtal, F.: Prune-belly syndrome with chromosomal fragment. Am. J. Dis. Child., 123:518, 1972.

Hanna, M. D.: New concept in bladder remodeling. Urology, 19:6, 1982.

Hannington-Kiff, J. G.: Prune-belly syndrome and general anesthesia. Br. J. Anaesthesiol., 42:649, 1970.

Harley, L. M., Chen, Y., and Rattner, W. H.: Prune-belly syndrome. J. Urol., 108:174, 1972.

Hellstrom, W. J. G., Kogan, B. A., Jeffrey, R. B., and McAninch, J. W.: The natural history of prenatal hydronephrosis with normal amounts of amniotic fluid. J. Urol., 132:947, 1984.

Hendren, W. H.: Restoration of function in the severely decompensated ureter. In Johnston, J. H., and Scholtmeijer, R. J. (Eds.): Problems in Paediatric Urology. Amsterdam, Excerpta Medica, 1972, pp. 1–56.

Heydenrych, J., and DuToit, P. E.: Torsion of the spleen and associated prune-belly syndrome—case report and review of the literature. S. Afr. Med. J., 53:637, 1978.

Hoagland, M. H., and Hutchins, G. M.: Obstructive lesions of the lower urinary tract in prune-belly syndrome. Arch. Pathol. Lab. Med., 111:154, 1987.

Ives, E. J.: The abdominal muscle deficiency triad syndrome—experience with ten cases. Birth Defects, 10:127, 1974.

Jeffs, R. D., Comisarow, R. H., and Hanna, M. K.: The early assessment for individualized treatment in the prune-belly syndrome. Br. J. Birth Defects, 13:97, 1977.

Karamanian, A., Kravath, R., Nagashima, H., et al.: Anesthetic management of prune-belly syndrome. Br. J. Anaesthesiol., 46:897, 1974.

Kramer, S. A.: Current status of fetal intervention for hydronephrosis. J. Urol., 130:641, 1983.

Kroovand, R. L., Al-Ansari, R. M., and Perlmutter, A. D.: Urethral and genital malformations in prune-belly syndrome. J. Urol., 127:94, 1982.

Lattimer, J. K.: Congenital deficiency of the abdominal musculature and associated genitourinary abnormalities: A report of 22 cases. J. Urol., 79:343, 1958.

Lee, M. L.: Prune-belly syndrome in a 54-year-old man. JAMA, 237:2216, 1977.

Lockhart, J. L., Reeve, H. R., Bredael, J. J., et al.: Siblings with prune-belly syndrome and associated pulmonic stenosis, mental retardation and deafness. Urology, 14:140, 1979.

Lubinsky, M., Koyle, K., and Trunca, C.: The association of prune-belly with Turner's syndrome. Am. J. Dis. Child., 134:1171, 1980.

MacMahon, R. A., O'Brien, M. C., and Cussen, L. J.: The use of microsurgery in the treatment of the undescended testis. J. Pediatr. Surg., 11:521, 1976.

Massad, C., and Kogan, B. A.: Prune-belly syndrome: Bladder histology. Dialog. Pediatr. Urol., 13(8):8, 1990.

McGovern, J. H., and Marshall, V. F: Congenital deficiency of the abdominal musculature and obstructive uropathy. Surg. Gynecol. Obstet., 108:289, 1959.

Mininberg, D. T., Montoya, F., Okada, K., et al.: Subcellular muscle studies in the prune-belly syndrome. J. Urol., 109:524, 1973.

Moerman, P., Fryns, J., Goddeeris, P., and Lauweryns, J. M.: Pathogenesis of the prune-belly syndrome: A functional urethral obstruction caused by prostatic hypoplasia. Pediatrics, 73:470, 1984.

Monfort, G.: Personal communication, 1990.

Monie, I. W., and Monie, B. J.: Prune-belly syndrome and fetal ascites. Teratology, 19:111, 1979.

Morgan, C. L., Jr., Grossman, H., and Novak, R.: Imperforate anus and colon calcification in association with the prune belly syndrome. Pediatr. Radiol., 7:19, 1978.

Nakayama, D. K., Harrison, M. R., Chinn, D. H., and deLorimier,

A. A.: The pathogenesis of prune-belly. Am. J. Dis. Child., 138:834, 1984.

Nunn, I. N., and Stephens, F. D.: The triad syndrome: A composite anomaly of the abdominal wall, urinary system and testes. J. Urol., 86:782, 1961.

Okulski, T. A.: The prenatal diagnosis of lower urinary tract obstruction using B scan ultrasound: A case report. J. Clin. Ultrasound, 5:268, 1977.

Osler, W.: Congenital absence of the abdominal musculature, with distended and hypertrophied urinary bladder. Bull. Johns Hopkins Hosp., 12:331, 1901.

Pagon, R. A., Smith, D. W., and Shepard, T. H.: Urethral obstruction malformation complex: A cause of abdominal muscle deficiency and the "prune belly". J. Pediatr., 94:900, 1979.

Palmer, J. M., and Tesluk, H.: Ureteral pathology in the prune-belly syndrome. J. Urol., 111:701, 1974.

Parker, R. W.: Case of an infant in whom some of the abdominal wall muscles were absent. Trans. Clin. Soc. Lond., 28:201, 1985.

Perlmutter, A. D.: Reduction cystoplasty in prune-belly syndrome. J. Urol., 115:456, 1976.

Potter, E. L.: Abnormal development of the kidney. In Potter, E. L. (Ed.): Normal and Abnormal Development of the Kidney. Chicago, Year Book Medical Publishers, 1972, pp. 154–220.

Rabinowitz, R., and Schillinger, J. F.: Prune-belly syndrome in the female subject. J. Urol., 118:454, 1977.

Ralis, Z., and Forbes, M.: Intrauterine atrophy and gangrene of the lower extremity of the fetus caused by megacystis due to urethral atresia. J. Pathol., 104:31, 1971.

Randolph, J., Cavett, C., and Eng, G.: Abdominal wall reconstruction in the prune-belly syndrome. J. Pediatr. Surg., 16:960, 1981a.

Randolph, J., Cavett, C., and Eng, G.: Surgical correction and rehabilitation for children with "prune-belly" syndrome. Ann. Surg., 193:757, 1981b.

Reinberg, Y., Manivel, J. C., Fryd, D., Najarian, J. S., and Gonzalez, R.: The outcome of renal transplantation in children with the prune-belly syndrome. J. Urol., 142:1541, 1989.

Riccardi, V. M., and Grum, C. M.: The prune-belly anomaly: Heterogeneity and superficial X-linkage mimicry. J. Med. Genet., 14:266, 1977.

Rogers, L. W., and Ostrow, P. T.: The prune-belly syndrome: Report of 20 cases and description of a lethal variant. J. Pediatr., 83:786, 1973.

Sellers, B. B., McNeil, R., Smith, R. V., et al.: Congenital megalourethra associated with prune-belly syndrome. J. Urol., 16:814, 1976.

Shih, W., Greenbaum, L. D., and Baro, C.: In utero sonogram in prune-belly syndrome. Urology, 20:102, 1982.

Shrom, S. H., Cromie, W. J., and Duckett, J. W.: Megalourethra. Urology, 17:152, 1981.

Silverman, F. M., and Huang, N.: Congenital absence of the abdominal muscle associated with malformation of the genitourinary and alimentary tracts: Report of cases and review of literature. Am. J. Dis. Child., 80:9, 1950.

Smith, D. W.: Recognizable Patterns of Human Malformation. Philadelphia, W. B. Saunders Co., 1970, p. 5.

Smythe, A. R.: Ultrasonic detection of fetal ascites and bladder dilation with resulting prune-belly. J. Pediatr., 98:978, 1981.

Snyder, H. M., Harrison, N. W., Whitfield, H. N., et al.: Urodynamics in the prune-belly syndrome. Br. J. Urol., 48:663, 1976.

Stephens, F. D.: Congenital malformations of the rectum, anus, and genito-urinary tracts. London and Edinburgh, Livingstone, 1963, pp. 149, 186, 187.

Texter, J. H., and Koontz, W. W.: Prune-belly syndrome seen in the adult. Soc. Pediatr. Urol. Newsletter, February 6, 1980.

Tuck, B. A., and Smith, T. K.: Prune-belly syndrome: A report of 12 cases and review of the literature. J. Bone Joint Surg., 60:109, 1978.

Uehling, D. T.: Testicular histology in triad syndrome. Soc. Pediatr. Urol. Newsletter, December 30, 1982.

Wacksman, J., Dinner, M., and Staffon, R. A.: Technique of testicular autotransplantation using a microvascular anastomosis. Surg. Gynecol. Obstet., 150:399, 1980.

Welch, K. J., and Kearney, G. P.: Abdominal musculature deficiency syndrome: Prune-belly. J. Urol., 111:693, 1974.

Willert, C., Cohen, H., Yu, Y. T., et al.: Association of prune-belly syndrome and gastroschisis. Am. J. Dis. Child., 132:526, 1978.

Williams, D. I.: Prune-belly syndrome. *In* Harrison, J. H., Gittes, R. F., Perlmutter, A. D., et al. (Eds.): Campbell's Urology, ed. 4. Philadelphia, W. B. Saunders Co., 1979, pp. 1743–1755.

Williams, D. I., and Burkholder, G. V.: The prune-belly syndrome. J. Urol., 98:244, 1967.

Williams, D. I., and Parker, R. M.: The role of surgery in the prune-belly syndrome. *In* Johnston, J. H., and Goodwin, W. F. (Eds.): Reviews of Pediatric Urology. Amsterdam, Excerpta Medica, 1974, pp. 315–331.

Woodard, J. R.: The prune-belly syndrome. Urol. Clin. North Am., 5:73, 1978.

Woodard, J. R.: The bladder in prune-belly syndrome. Dialog. Pediatr. Urol., 13(8):6, 1990a.

Woodard, J. R.: The impact of fetal diagnosis on the management of obstructive uropathy. Postgrad. Med. J., 66(Suppl. 1):37, 1990b.

Woodard, J. R., and Parrott, T. S.: Reconstruction of the urinary tract in prune-belly uropathy. J. Urol., 119:824, 1978a.

Woodard, J. R., and Parrott, T. S.: Orchiopexy in prune-belly syndrome. Br. J. Urol., 50:348, 1978b.

Woodhouse, C. R. J., Kellett, M. J., and Williams, D. I.: Minimal surgical interference in prune-belly syndrome. Br. J. Urol., 51:475, 1979.

Woodhouse, C. R. J., and Snyder, H. M.: Testicular and sexual function in adults with prune-belly syndrome. Submitted for publication, 1984.

49

POSTERIOR URETHRAL VALVES AND OTHER URETHRAL ANOMALIES

Edmond T. Gonzales, Jr., M.D.

The embryology of the male urethra is complex and is not completely understood. Development of the urethra can be considered in two separate phases: differentiation of the cloacal (urogenital sinus) portion, the posterior urethra; and tubularization of the urethral plate, the anterior urethra. The mature male urethra is generally divided into four segments: (1) the prostatic urethra—from the bladder neck to the proximal margin of the urogenital diaphragm; (2) the membranous urethra—the segment that traverses the urogenital diaphragm (the striated sphincter); (3) the bulbous urethra—the portion from the distal margin of the membranous urethra to the penoscrotal angle; and (4) the penile urethra—the segment that traverses the length of the penile shaft, including the glans.

The prostatic and membranous portions of the urethra are not entirely androgen-dependent, because these segments of the urethra also develop in the female. However, it is obvious that androgen action on the tissues of the prostate gland and the mesonephric ducts (the embryologic anlage of the male genital ducts) has a significant impact on final differentiation of these segments of the male urethra. The bulbous and penile urethra are uniquely male and are entirely dependent on androgen action for differentiation. The presence of androgen insensitivity in peripheral tissues, as a result of abnormal androgen receptor number or function, 5-alpha-reductase deficiency, or inadequate androgenic steroid production by the testes, will result in incomplete tubularization of the anterior segments of the male urethra.

These multiple disorders represent the various syndromes of incomplete virilization that can be seen in genotypic (XY) males, spanning the anatomic spectrum from mild degrees of hypospadias to complete phenotypic females (testicular feminization syndrome) (Griffin and Wilson, 1989). This chapter, however, is concerned with anomalies of the male urethra not known or be-

lieved to result as a consequence of androgen deficiency and includes the following topics: (1) posterior urethral valves, (2) anterior urethral obstruction, (3) megalourethra, and (4) urethral duplications. Normal urethral embryology is described elsewhere. This chapter emphasizes the abnormal embryology, as it is generally understood, to explain the individual anomalies discussed here.

POSTERIOR URETHRAL VALVES

Dr. H. Hampton Young is generally given credit for the first clear description and classification of posterior urethral valves. He recognized three distinct varieties of congenital proximal urethral obstruction and classified these as type I, II, and III urethral valves (Fig. 49–1) (Young et al., 1919). Type II urethral valves were initially described as folds radiating in a cranial direction from the verumontanum to the posterolateral aspect of the bladder neck. It is now generally accepted that these folds are not obstructive and, in fact, that type II valves as a clinical entity do not exist. These folds represent hypertrophy of the strip of superficial muscle that runs from the ureteral orifice to the verumontanum (muscle derived from the tissue of the mesonephric ducts which forms the layer of bladder muscle known as the superficial trigone). In response to increased resistance to voiding, hypertrophy of these muscle bands occurs.

This finding can be detected when true mechanical obstruction is present, but it may also be seen in cases of functional obstruction (neuropathic bladder, detrusor-sphincter dyssynergia). Although it is generally accepted that type II valves do not exist, the traditional classification scheme is so ingrained in the urologic vernacular that the usual congenital obstructions of the proximal urethra continue to be described as type I and

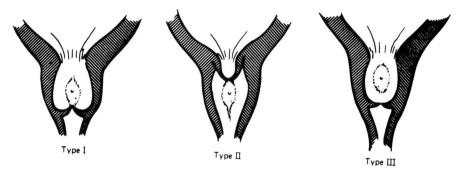

Figure 49–1. The original classification and diagrammatic depiction of urethral valves as presented by Young and co-workers. (Adapted from Young, H. H., et al.: J. Urol., 3:289, 1919.)

Type I   Type II   Type III

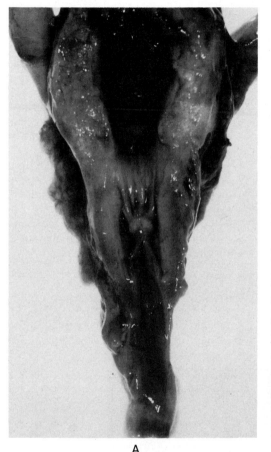

A

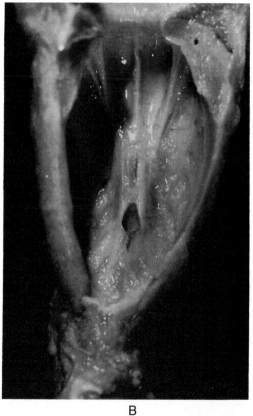

B

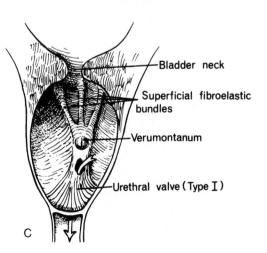

C

Figure 49–2. *A,* A posterior urethral valve specimen unfolded after an anterior urethra midline incision gives the impression of two folds coapting in the midline. *B,* Another specimen opened by unrooting rather than incising anterior urethral wall shows the folds to be an oblique diaphragm fused anteriorly. Note also the proximal folds confused as type II valves. (From Robertson, W. B., and Hayes, J. A.: Br. J. Urol., 41:592, 1969.) *C,* Drawing of typical appearance of type I urethral valve.

type III. This accepted classification will be continued for this chapter.

Stephens (1983) suggested the existence of an additional type of proximal urethral obstruction, which he has dubbed a type IV valve. Seen most often in the prune-belly syndrome, these obstructions occur when a flabby, poorly supported prostate folds on itself and causes relative outlet obstruction.

Type I Urethral Valves

A type I urethral valve is an obstructing membrane that radiates in a distal direction from the verumontanum posteriorly toward the membranous urethra anteriorly. Although it is usually represented in line sketches as two coapting folds, a type I urethral valve is actually a single membranous structure with the opening in the membrane positioned posteriorly near the verumontanum (Fig. 49–2) (Robertson and Hayes, 1969). During voiding, the fused anterior portion of the membrane bulges into the membranous urethra and possibly into the bulbous urethra, leaving only a narrow opening along the dorsal wall of the urethra. This predictable anatomy gives type I urethral valves a characteristic radiologic appearance (Fig. 49–3).

The embryology of type I valves is not completely understood, but it is generally believed that they represent the end result of anomalous insertion of the mesonephric ducts into the primitive fetal cloaca. Normally, the mesonephric ducts insert laterally on the cloaca. As the cloaca folds inward in its midportion to separate the anorectal canal from the urogenital sinus, the ostium of each mesonephric duct migrates posteromedially and cranially to assume a final position at the verumontanum. In the normal male urethra, this pathway of migration persists as the plicae colliculi—delicate mucosal folds that emanate from the verumontanum in a distal and slightly lateral direction along the dorsal floor of the urethra. Type I posterior urethral valves are thought to develop when the mesonephric ducts enter the cloaca more anteriorly than normal. During infolding and separation of the cloaca, their migration is impeded and they may fuse anterolaterally (Stephens, 1983). Children with classic type I valves do not have plicae colliculi (Fig. 49–4).

Type III Posterior Urethral Valves

Type III valves are believed to represent incomplete dissolution of the urogenital membrane. The obstructing membranes are situated distal to the verumontanum, at the level of the membranous urethra (Fig. 49–5). Classically described as a discrete ring-like membrane with a central aperture, these lesions can assume the most bizarre configuration, depending on the elasticity of the membrane and the location of the perforation in the membrane (Fig. 49–6). Long, willowy folds may prolapse well down into the urethra during voiding and suggest more of a bulbar urethral obstruction—the classic wind-sock valve described by Field and Stephens (1974) (Fig. 49–7).

Overall, type I urethral valves make up more than 95 per cent of the lesions in large series; type III valves make up the remainder. However, despite their different embryology, there is no clear difference in the clinical presentation, pathophysiology, management, or prognosis of children with either anomaly, and the following discussion applies to both anomalies.

Clinical Presentation

Children with congenital posterior urethral obstruction present in a variety of ways depending primarily on

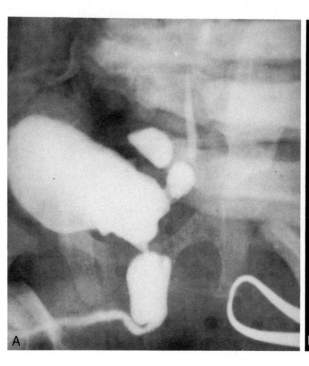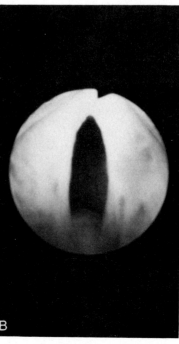

Figure 49–3. *A,* Radiologic appearance of type I urethral valve. Note the bulging anterior membrane, the posteriorly positioned perforation in the valve, the dilated prostatic urethra, and the narrowed and thickened bladder neck. These findings are typical of type I valves when the urethra is viewed in an oblique position. *B,* Cystoscopic picture of type I valve. The verumontanum is the small nodule at the 6 o'clock position.

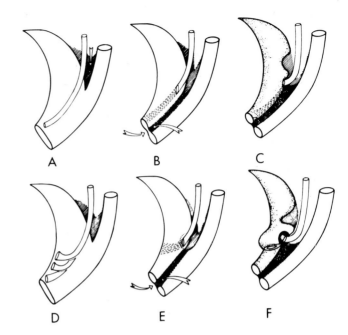

Figure 49–4. Development of type I valves.

A to *C*, Development of the normal urethral crest. Migration of the orifice of the wolffian duct from its anterolateral position in the cloaca to the site of the Müller tubercle on the posterior wall of the anorectal septum occurs synchronously with cloacal division. (Dots denote pathway of migration.) This wolffian remnant is more lateral and posterior and remains as the normal inferior crest and the plicae colliculi.

D, Abnormal anterior positions of the wolffian duct orifices.

E, Abnormal migration of the terminal ends of the ducts.

F, Circumferential obliquely oriented ridges that compose the valve. (From Kelalis, P. P., and King, L. R. (Eds.): Clinical Pediatric Urology. Philadelphia, W. B. Saunders Co., 1976.)

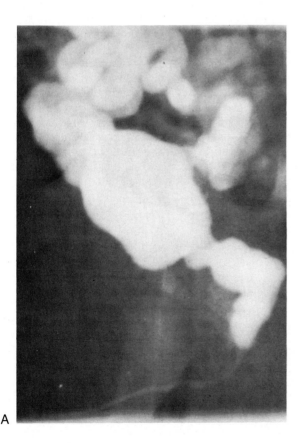

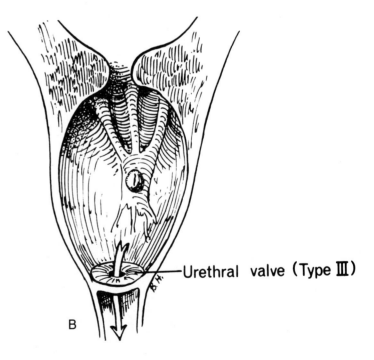

—Urethral valve (Type III)

Figure 49–5. *A*, Congenital urethral membrane (Young's type III urethral valve) causing severe obstruction with bilateral renal dysplasia; a retrograde catheter could not be passed. *B*, Drawing of typical appearance of type III urethral valve.

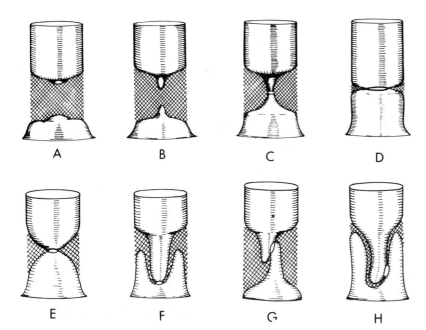

Figure 49–6. Development of congenital urethral membranes (type III valves).

A to *D*, Normal canalization of the urogenital membrane. *D* shows normal slight constriction at the level of the perineal membrane.

E, Stricture formation.

F, Canalization by central downgrowth and circumferential ingrowth resulting in bulging membrane with a central stenotic orifice.

G and *H*, Side openings creating valvular "wind sock" membranes. (Drawings and descriptions supplied through the courtesy of Dr. F. D. Stephens. From Kelalis, P. P., and King, L. R. (Eds.): Clinical Pediatric Urology. Philadelphia, W. B. Saunders Co., 1976.)

the degree of obstruction. Classically, presenting symptoms are age-dependent. In the newborn, palpable abdominal masses (distended bladder, hydronephrosis), ascites, or respiratory distress from pulmonary hypoplasia suggest the possibility of severe bladder outlet obstruction. Other features may include an obstetric history of oligohydramnios (the bulk of the amniotic fluid is made of fetal urine) and findings in the neonate consistent with Potter's syndrome (dysmorphic facial features, fetal growth retardation, positional limb deformations, pulmonary hypoplasia). The neonate with severely obstructing valves has a very thick-walled bladder that is easily palpable through the flaccid abdomen of this age group—even when the bladder empties completely. The dilated renal pelves and large, tortuous, tense ureters are often easily felt on abdominal examination.

Neonatal ascites results from many diverse etiologies, but nearly 40 per cent of patients with ascites have

urinary ascites secondary to obstructive uropathy—most often infravesical in location (Fig. 49–8) (Adzick et al., 1985). The ascites actually represents a transudation of retroperitoneal urine across the thin and permeable peritoneum of the neonate. Extravasation may develop at any number of sites, but most often is seen at the renal fornix (Fig. 49–9). Although newborns with urinary ascites may develop severe electrolyte abnormalities and life-threatening abnormal fluid shifts shortly after birth, the presence of ascites actually bodes a more favorable prognosis regarding ultimate renal function than for a similar group of children without ascites (Rittenberg et al., 1988).

Pulmonary hypoplasia is frequently associated with severe obstructive uropathy, especially when oligohydramnios is present also. Whereas several theories have been proposed to explain the etiology of pulmonary hypoplasia, the most accepted one proposes that oligohydramnios prevents normal chest mobility and lung

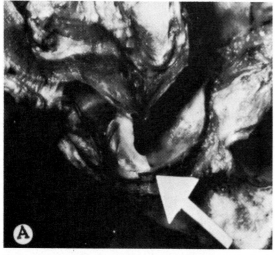
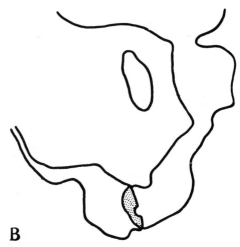

Figure 49–7. Wind sock membrane. *A*, Obstructing membrane attached in membranous urethra and ballooned like wind sock into expanded bulbous urethra (autopsy specimen). *B*, Diagram of the anatomic findings. (From Field, P. L., and Stephens, F. D.: J. Urol., 111:250, 1974.)

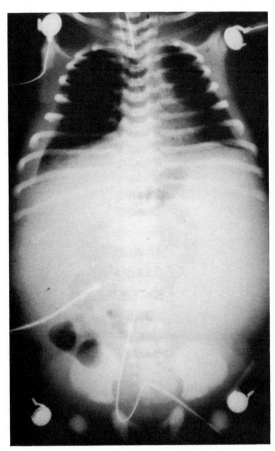

Figure 49–8. Typical radiographic findings of urinary ascites in a neonate, showing the centrally positioned bowel loops, ground glass appearance of the abdomen, and bulging flanks.

Today, the majority of infants with bladder outlet obstruction are recognized on prenatal ultrasound examination and are promptly evaluated and managed before continuing obstruction or infection does further renal parenchymal damage (Fig. 49–10). Our current ability to diagnose this problem before birth also raises the possibility that intervention before birth (percutaneous placement of vesicoamniotic shunts or primary fetal surgery) may better preserve renal and pulmonary function in some babies than if we electively wait to initiate treatment at birth. A discussion of the issues surrounding fetal intervention follows the section on the clinical management of urethral valves.

Pathophysiology

Congenital urethral obstruction causes a broad array of abnormalities in the urinary tract, including damage to the renal parenchyma as well as to the smooth muscle function of the ureter and bladder. These changes may persist despite successful relief of the primary obstruction. Because urethral valves are present during the earliest phase of fetal development, primitive tissues mature in an abnormal environment of high intraluminal pressures. Increasingly, studies are demonstrating that this situation results in permanent maldevelopment and long-lasting functional abnormalities (McConnell, 1989). The pathophysiology of the urinary tract associated with congenital urethral obstruction is discussed under five

expansion in utero (Landers and Hanson, 1990). At birth, these infants are cyanotic and have low Apgar scores. They require immediate pulmonary resuscitation with endotracheal intubation and positive-pressure ventilation, and they may develop pneumothorax or pneumomediastinum, which necessitates placement of chest tubes. Some centers are employing the technique of extracorporeal membrane oxygenation (ECMO) to assist the severely affected infant during the early postnatal period (Detjer and Gibbons, 1990). Today, most neonates who die as a result of posterior urethral valves die from respiratory causes—not from renal or infectious causes. Indeed, infants with urethral valves and significant pulmonary hypoplasia still have a mortality rate as high as 50 per cent (Nakayama et al., 1986).

Severely affected neonates who are not diagnosed at birth most commonly present within a few weeks with urosepsis, dehydration, and electrolyte abnormalities. Some infants may have only failure to thrive from renal insufficiency. Less commonly, a dribbling urinary stream may call attention to the problem.

Patients presenting during the toddler years are more likely to have somewhat better renal function and generally present because of urinary infection or voiding dysfunction. School-aged boys—the least common age for presentation—more often will have voiding dysfunction as their primary complaint, which is generally recognized as urinary incontinence.

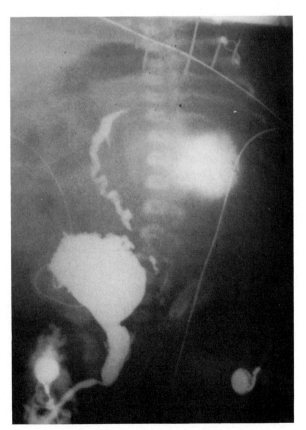

Figure 49–9. Voiding cystourethrogram in the patient with ascites shown in Figure 49–8. On this study, reflux occurred on the left, demonstrating the site of urinary extravasation to be at the renal fornix.

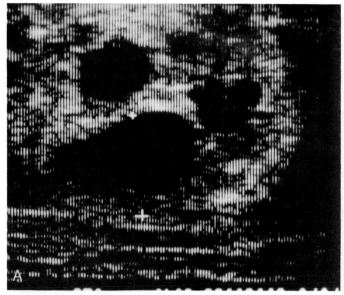

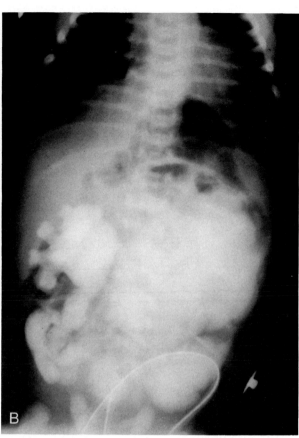

Figure 49-10. *A,* Typical findings of a urethral valve on prenatal ultrasound (bilateral hydronephrosis; distended, thickened bladder). *B,* Postnatal intravenous pyelogram of same patient.

categories: reduced glomerular filtration, abnormal renal tubular function, hydronephrosis (luminal dilatation), vesicoureteral reflux, and detrusor dysfunction.

Glomerular Filtration

The ultimate goal of management of posterior urethral valves is to maximize and preserve glomerular filtration. Although this issue has always been the area of primary concern, it is especially acute now because of our ability to make the diagnosis of urethral valves with substantial accuracy in the fetus. Today, our decisions regarding management for the unborn, both timing and technique, may have significant impact on ultimate renal function. The data relative to patient survival as well as the anticipated levels of renal function are gradually being rewritten.

Two decades ago, 25 per cent of children with urethral valves died within the 1st year of life, 25 per cent died later in childhood, and the remaining half survived into the young adult years with varying degrees of renal insufficiency (Churchill et al., 1983). Today, a neonatal death from renal insufficiency or sepsis is rare. Dialysis and, ultimately, renal transplantation are available to the youngest babies. Neonatologic and nephrologic support are universally available, and overall outlook is greatly improved. Children who die within the neonatal period generally die a respiratory death from pulmonary hypoplasia (Churchill et al., 1990). Nonetheless, children with valves may have severe renal insufficiency at birth, are at risk of infection even after relief of the obstruction because of stasis of urine or reflux, may develop hypertension with its deleterious effects on renal function, and in some cases, demonstrate a tendency toward gradually deteriorating renal function over time—the cause for which often remains elusive (Burbige and Hensle, 1987). Decreasing renal function may be a result of renal parenchymal dysplasia, hydronephrotic damage, infectious atrophy, and, perhaps, progressive glomerulosclerosis from hyperfiltration.

Renal parenchymal dysplasia is commonly associated with urethral valves. The renal dysplasia seen in association with urethral valves tends to be microcystic in nature and develops most severely in the peripheral cortical zone. It has long been suspected that this dysplasia is a result of the primitive metanephric blastema maturing in the presence of high intraluminal pressures. Experimental data suggest that this factor probably does play a role. Beck first reported the development of cystic, dysplastic changes in the kidneys of fetal sheep that underwent ureteral obstruction created in the midtrimester (Beck, 1971). Subsequent experimental studies by Glick and co-workers (1984) in lambs and by McVary and Maizels (1989) in the chick embryo have also demonstrated the development of dysplastic changes in normal fetal kidneys after creation of fetal ureteral obstruction.

Henneberry and Stephens (1980), however, have argued that the dysplasia seen with urethral valves may also be a primary embryologic abnormality resulting from abnormal positioning of the primitive ureteral bud along the mesonephric duct. In a careful anatomic dissection of the trigone in 11 cases of urethral valves (22 renal units), they noted that, in 11 instances, the ureters were very laterally ectopic (D position), and that these kidneys were more dysplastic than those associated with more normally positioned ureters. Hoover and Duckett (1982) observed that a relationship exists between nonfunction of a kidney (severe dysplasia) and the presence of ipsilateral massive vesicoureteral reflux in patients with urethral valves. Commonly known as the VURD syndrome (*v*alves, *u*nilateral *r*eflux, *d*ysplasia), this finding is thought to be another clinical manifestation of abnormal ureteral budding.

Regardless of the mechanism that initiates abnormal parenchymal histology, it is clear that the development of dysplasia is an early embryologic event. The presence of renal dysplasia is the single most significant abnormality that will determine ultimate renal function, and it is perhaps the only aspect of this congenital disorder over which the clinician has no impact.

Satisfactory relief of the high intravesical and intraureteral pressures associated with urethral obstruction should prevent progressive renal parenchymal damage from the obstruction. What is not clearly known is which therapeutic approach for managing valves (primary ablation, temporary diversion, and so forth) is most likely to prevent further damage as well as possibly allow for some recovery of renal function. In the newborn and very young infant, in particular, data suggest that satisfactory relief of obstruction allows for the growth of new renal tissue along with an absolute measurable increase in glomerular filtration (Mayor et al., 1975). This item is discussed in greater detail under specifics of management, but controversy exists regarding the optimal approach to therapy in relation to ultimate renal function.

Other causes for progressive renal failure are recurrent urinary tract infection and, perhaps, glomerulosclerosis associated with hyperfiltration. Although the child who has had a urethral valve is at risk of recurrent urinary infection because of the presence of vesicoureteral reflux, ureteral stasis, or incomplete bladder emptying, careful selected surgical intervention and the use of long-term chemoprophylaxis, when necessary, should prevent significant, progressive damage from infection. The significance of hyperfiltration remains controversial (Brenner et al., 1982). When experimental animals with a significant reduction in renal mass are fed diets that result in a high renal solute load, thereby requiring significant renal work to excrete the metabolic byproducts, progressive deterioration of renal function occurs much faster than in a similar group fed a diet with a low renal solute load. Whether this phenomenon might play a role in the child who has had valves and who now has moderate renal insufficiency remains unclear. Of the major food groups, protein provides a higher renal solute load by weight than either fats or carbohydrates. Experimentally, diets high in protein are most often associated with progressive renal functional deterioration. At this time, however, it is not entirely clear what effect severe limitation of protein intake in children will have on satisfactory somatic and central nervous system growth, and there is not yet great enthusiasm for embracing a severely protein-restricted diet in an infant with significant renal insufficiency (Klahr, 1989).

Several anatomic conditions seen in association with urethral valves appear to be associated with generally improved renal function, presumably by allowing lower intraluminal pressures during fetal development (Conner et al., 1988; Rittenberg et al., 1988). These conditions include the following: (1) massive unilateral vesicoureteral reflux, (2) large bladder diverticula, and (3) urinary ascites. In each situation, there is a "pop-off valve," which potentially absorbs high intraluminal pressures and thereby allows the fetal renal parenchyma to develop in a more normal environment.

Renal Tubular Function

Because high ureteral pressures always affect the most distal aspect of the nephron first, some patients with urinary obstruction will encounter more abnormalities with urinary concentrating ability than with reduction in glomerular filtration. This abnormality (an acquired form of nephrogenic diabetes insipidus) results in persistently high urinary flow rates regardless of the fluid intake or the state of dehydration. This phenomenon has two significant consequences.

The newborn or infant with fixed high urinary flow rates is particularly prone to development of severe episodes of dehydration and electrolyte imbalance whenever there is increased fluid loss elsewhere, such as excessive gastrointestinal losses (vomiting, diarrhea), high fever, or third space fluid sequestration. As long as adequate fluid and electrolytes are able to be taken orally, the high urinary output is of limited significance. If the infant is unable to maintain adequate oral intake, he or she will rapidly dehydrate because of the persistently high urinary output despite significant total body water depletion.

The second major consequence of high urinary flows involves ureteral and vesical dysfunction. Significantly high ureteral flow rates may cause persistent ureteral dilation that would otherwise seem less significant with a lower urinary flow rate. In addition, high urinary flow rates rapidly fill the bladder. In situations in which poor bladder compliance is present, this means that higher resting bladder pressures are achieved much more quickly. High urinary flow rates can be controlled to some extent with the use of lower solute diets. Hormonal therapy with antidiuretic hormone is generally not successful because this renal diabetes insipidus results from damage to the collecting ducts.

Hydronephrosis

In the presence of significant urethral obstruction, ureteral dilatation of varying, but usually considerable, degree is expected. After satisfactory relief of the obstruction, either by endoscopic destruction of the valve or by vesicostomy, gradual but substantial reduction in the degree of hydronephrosis will generally occur (Fig. 49–11). When this does not happen, several questions must be raised. Is the persisting dilatation a result of

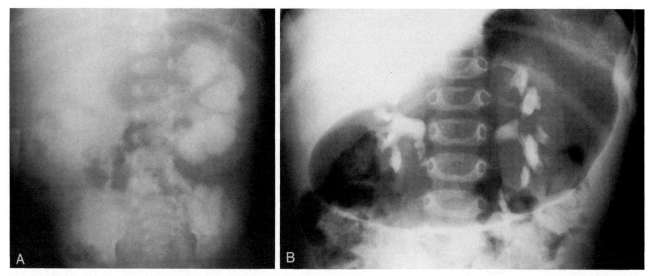

Figure 49–11. *A,* Initial intravenous pyelogram (IVP) at the time of diagnosis of urethral valves. *B,* IVP 3 months after valve ablation alone, showing marked improvement in the degree of hydronephrosis.

true ureterovesical junction obstruction? Is the ureteral musculature faulty and unable to generate effective peristalsis? In this situation, the dilatation of the ureters may be a permanent facet of the child's disorder. Could these changes be the result of high intravesical pressures or be secondary to high urinary flow rates? Each of these factors may play a role in an individual case.

Johnston and Kulatilako (1971) demonstrated many years ago that it may take years after primary valve ablation for final improvement in ureteral caliber to occur. They suggested that the responsible physician should not be anxious to proceed with further surgical therapy on the ureter in young infants as long as renal function is stable and urinary infection is controlled. When it is evident that substantial recovery is not going to occur, then it becomes necessary to address the role of each of the issues noted previously (Fig. 49–12).

Properly performed vesical urodynamic tests are essential. If the child has a noncompliant bladder associated with high intravesical pressures, this condition must be corrected before any attempt at surgical remodeling of the ureter is considered. Dynamic flow studies of the upper urinary tract may be necessary to differentiate nonobstructive ureteral dilatation from true ureterovesical junction obstruction (Whitaker, 1973). The diuretic-enhanced renogram is less invasive but difficult to interpret in the presence of relatively poor renal function; dilute, high-volume urine flow; and dilated ureters. Percutaneous pressure-flow studies of the upper urinary tract (Whitaker test) will often be necessary to differentiate nonobstructive ureteral dilatation from true ureterovesical junction obstruction.

When investigators looked critically at this issue, they discovered that true ureterovesical junction obstruction is rare. In Whitaker's series (1973), only 4 of 17 ureters in children with urethral valves with suspected secondary ureterovesical junction obstruction were found to actually have criteria consistent with obstruction when both pressures and flow were considered. In the Whitaker test, flow is constant and pressure varies. Wood-

bury (1989) described an upper tract urodynamic test in which pressure is stable but flow may vary. Whether this additional diagnostic tool will offer a reassessment of older data remains unknown at this time.

An accurate assessment of a timed urinary volume is also an important factor in this evaluation. As noted previously, many children who have had urethral valves have significant hyposthenuria and excrete very large urinary volumes. As in children who have primary diabetes insipidus, this excessive, high-flow state may also contribute to persisting ureteral dilatation.

Vesicoureteral Reflux

Vesicoureteral reflux is commonly found in association with posterior urethral valves. Between one third and one half of children with valves will have reflux at the time of initial diagnosis. Most often, this probably represents secondary vesicoureteral reflux resulting from high intravesical pressures, development of paraureteral diverticula, and loss of ureterovesical valvular competence. In some instances, however, the reflux may be primary and may be due to a ureteral bud anomaly. As noted previously, Henneberry and Stephens (1980), in their study of fetuses and newborn infants with severe posterior urethral valves, reported a significant incidence of lateral ectopia of the ureteral orifice.

The presence of vesicoureteral reflux should not in itself influence the initial management of children with posterior urethral valves (Johnston, 1979). In about one third of cases, the reflux will resolve spontaneously after obstruction is eliminated. In another one third of the cases, the reflux may persist but will be no problem as long as the child is maintained on chemoprophylaxis. Decisions regarding reimplantation then should be made after a period of observation following initial valve ablation, as long as urinary infection is able to be controlled with maintenance chemoprophylaxis. Even if reflux persists, dilated ureters will generally decrease in caliber over time. If reimplantation is ultimately neces-

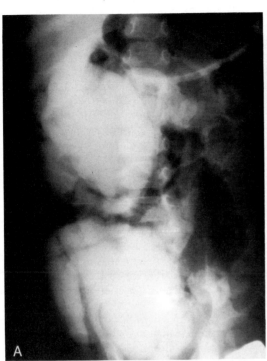

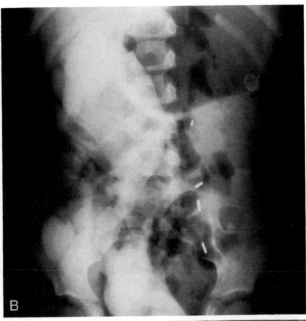

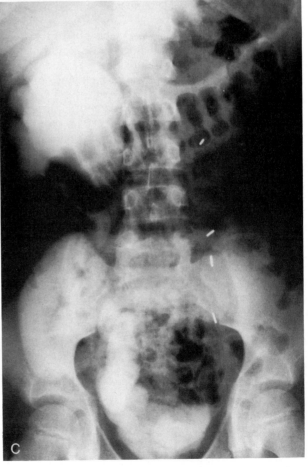

Figure 49–12. Series of intravenous pyelogram (IVP) films in a child with urethral valves, a functioning right kidney, and a nonfunctioning left kidney.

A, IVP at diagnosis.

B, IVP 1 year after valve ablation and left nephroureterectomy. The voiding urethrogram appeared normal, and no vesicoureteral reflux was present. Little or no improvement in the degree of hydronephrosis is apparent.

C, IVP 4 years later. The degree of hydronephrosis remains essentially unchanged. Urodynamic studies revealed a compliant bladder, which emptied satisfactorily, and a Whitaker study was thought to be normal. Renal function has been stable at a serum creatinine level of 0.6 mg/dl for all of these years.

sary, this surgery likely will be able to be accomplished without extensive tailoring or remodeling of the ureter. About one third of the patients will have problems associated with their reflux during follow-up and are best managed by earlier reimplantation.

Vesical Dysfunction

For many years, it has been recognized that some children with urethral valves (as many as 25 per cent) have varying degrees of abnormal bladder function. Most often, this abnormality presents as urinary incontinence. Many years ago, investigators assumed that this incontinence was primarily due to incompetent sphincter function as a result of either primary maldevelopment of the membranous urethra and bladder neck (because of the anatomic location of the valve at the level of the voluntary sphincter, causing distention and dilatation of that region of the urethra during embryogenesis) or as a result of direct injury to the sphincter at the time of endoscopic valve ablation. However, with the application of modern urodynamics to pediatric urology, it has become increasingly obvious that primary vesical dysfunction is commonly present in association with urethral valves, that this vesical dysfunction does not necessarily abate after relief of the obstruction, and that, ultimately, this abnormal bladder function has a significant impact on prognosis.

Tanagho (1974) and Lome and associates (1972) first brought to our attention the difficulties encountered in establishing adequate bladder volume after a period of bladder defunctionalization (usually after high loop urinary diversion). Review of these data from the 1960s and 1970s shows that many children included in these series had also had previous bladder surgery or placement of indwelling suprapubic tubes for initial management of the urethral valves. How much impact this previous bladder surgery had on final bladder function was not clearly defined. Glassberg and colleagues (1982) and Bauer and colleagues (1979) studied a series of children who had urethral valves and reported several abnormalities of detrusor function, including primary myogenic failure, uninhibited bladder activity, and findings consistent with a noncompliant detrusor muscle. Campaiola and co-workers (1985) reported similar observations.

Vesical dysfunction not only contributes to problems of urinary incontinence but may also be a primary factor in persisting ureterectasis and high intravesical and intraureteral pressures that ultimately may cause renal function to deteriorate. Parkhouse and associates (1988) followed a series of children with urethral valves into adolescence. They observed that those children who were incontinent during childhood ultimately developed more severe degrees of renal insufficiency during adolescence than did children who had demonstrated normal urinary control. They proposed that children who were incontinent had more severe bladder dysfunction than did those children who had normal urinary control. Presumably, at puberty, the development of the prostate may have increased outlet resistance, improving continence but raising intravesical pressures and producing

unfavorable effects on renal function. Unfortunately, routine urodynamic studies were not consistently performed in all of these children to unquestionably support these observations and conclusions.

Depending on the extent and nature of bladder dysfunction and the ability of the bladder to empty, management may consist of anticholinergic therapy, to reduce uninhibited detrusor contractions; clean, intermittent catheterization, to afford satisfactory bladder emptying; or bladder augmentation, to improve bladder volume and compliance (Glassberg, 1985). In older, cooperative boys, a program of planned, timed voidings might keep bladder volumes sufficiently low so that intravesical pressures remain acceptable.

Management

Management of the child with posterior urethral valves is entirely dependent on the degree of renal insufficiency as well as the age of the child. Older children who present with voiding dysfunction but satisfactory renal function are easily and effectively treated initially by endoscopic destruction of the urethral valve alone. Decisions concerning selective surgery for persisting vesicoureteral reflux, lingering ureterovesical junction obstruction (uncommon), or detrusor dysfunction are made on an individual basis.

The main issues related to treatment of urethral valves involve the very young infant. In these situations, the potential for maximal recoverability of renal function is at its greatest. In addition, the increasing recognition of urethral valves in the fetus raises ongoing questions about timing for intervention and offers the responsible physician an opportunity to perform procedures that will decompress the urinary tract and allow for maximal recoverability of renal function during the period when maximal growth of renal tissue is thought to be possible.

In the past, most infants with urethral valves presented because of urosepsis. These infants were often dehydrated and had severe acidosis and electrolyte abnormalities. The next most common presentation was failure to thrive in the first several weeks after birth. Once again, in this situation, significant chronic renal insufficiency was usually present. In both cases, management was usually begun with placement of a small transurethral catheter to provide unobstructed vesical drainage as well as the initiation of appropriate antibiotics and parenteral fluid administration. Initiation of these measures allows for immediate improvement of renal function in most cases. In general, 5 to 7 days of catheter drainage should allow one to adequately assess the existent level of glomerular filtration.

Currently, more patients with posterior urethral valves are being recognized by observation of hydronephrosis on prenatal ultrasound than by one of the more traditional histories as described. At birth, these children will have renal functional variables equivalent to maternal renal function. The placement of a urethral catheter and initiation of prophylactic antibiotic management allow for assessment of the baseline level of renal function during the first few days after birth. In each of these situations, further management will be dictated by the level of renal function.

In the presence of normal or near-normal renal function (most often described as a serum creatinine of less than 1.0 mg/dl in the newborn after several days of catheter drainage, although a healthy neonate at 4 weeks of age may have a serum creatinine of 0.2 to 0.4 mg/dl), endoscopic destruction of the valves would be considered. Today, endoscopes with excellent optics are available in sufficiently small caliber for even the tiniest newborn. Most of the systems today accept small operating cautery electrodes sufficient for destruction of the valve. For the child whose urethra is too small to accept the available endoscopes, antegrade destruction of the valve by percutaneous access to the bladder has been described by Zaontz and Firlit (1985). MacAninch (personal communication) has suggested that this technique is made easier by using the rigid ureteroscope. The longer instrument allows the endoscopist increased maneuverability—one of the limiting factors in this technique when the short cystoscope is used. Other techniques employed for primary destruction of urethral valves include the neodymium-yttrium-aluminum-garnet laser (Ehrlich and Shanberg, 1988), the cautery hook as originally described by Williams and improved by Deane and co-workers (1988), and antegrade extraction of a balloon catheter (Kolicinski, 1988). None of these techniques has yet achieved generalized acceptance, although the use of the laser for valve destruction seems especially promising.

Valve ablation must be done carefully. Only a single wire (not a loop) or a small electrode should be used. The current on the electrosurgical unit should be set at a level just sufficient to incise the valve, but not so high as to diffuse thermal injury to surrounding urethral tissues. I prefer to incise the valve at 4 o'clock, 8 o'clock, and 12 o'clock; but I believe that the 12 o'clock incision is most important, because it is the one that separates the anteriorly fused membrane. A small, transurethral catheter may be left in place for 1 or 2 days, but it is generally not necessary.

After satisfactory destruction of the valve is accomplished, one should follow the child expectantly with regular estimates of renal function as well as imaging studies that assess improvement in the degree of hydronephrosis or the presence of vesicoureteral reflux. A follow-up voiding cystourethogram is generally done 2 months after the valve destruction to be sure that the obstruction was satisfactorily relieved. If renal function remains stable and infection is avoided (chemoprophylaxis is generally recommended), improvement in the anatomy of the urinary tract and continued stabilization of renal function are expected. The improvement in ureteral dilatation can be gradual and may take months or, occasionally, years.

Careful endoscopic destruction of valves, even in the newborn, has not been associated with a significant incidence of urethral stricture. In the unusual situation in which the newborn urethra seems too small to accommodate the available endoscopes, an elective vesicostomy is appropriate and safe. Indeed, Walker has preferred a vesicostomy rather than endoscopic ablation in the neonate, believing that this technique may be safer and may reduce the incidence of urethral strictures. However, a review of his approach did not suggest any benefit in overall improvement of renal function as compared with endoscopic management of valves only (Walker and Padron, 1990).

The major area of continuing controversy involves the most appropriate approach to treating the infant who has significant renal insufficiency. The options for managing this group of children include endoscopic destruction of the urethral valves only, elective vesicostomy, or high loop, temporizing ureteral diversion. The issue of concern is which therapeutic approach maximizes recoverability of renal function and brings hydrodynamics of the upper urinary tract most nearly to normal (Gonzales, 1990).

During the 1960s, high loop ureterostomy was a commonly performed, generally accepted approach for the initial management of infants with urethral valves (Johnston, 1963). After ureterostomy, renal function appeared to improve and generally remained stable, ureteral diameter decreased, and the infant was healthy. Reconstruction was then done electively within 1 to 2 years in a larger, healthier infant.

During this same interval, a few investigators experimented with different techniques to destroy valves transurethrally. Johnston (1966) demonstrated that many infants treated in this manner also showed stabilization or improved renal function and gradual, but progressive, reduction in the degree of hydronephrosis. When better endoscopes became available in the 1970s, most pediatric urologists switched to primary endoscopic destruction as their preferred form of management.

Krueger and associates, in 1980, published a provocative article that compared two series of children with posterior urethral valves: one group treated by high loop ureterostomy and a second group treated by endoscopic ablation only. Their data suggested that children who presented with renal insufficiency and who were managed by high loop cutaneous ureterostomy ultimately showed improved glomerular filtration rate and somatic growth potential when compared with a group of children presenting with renal function of similar degree who were managed by endoscopic destruction of valves only. They proposed that high loop diversion probably lowered ureteral luminal pressures more and thereby allowed the renal parenchyma to recover in an environment more nearly normal than when the management was by valve ablation only. This report has been challenged by Duckett and Norris (1989) and others on the basis that it is not a controlled study, but it remains an area of ongoing controversy.

The decision to proceed with a high loop ureterostomy is a significant one, because it commits the child to a major reconstructive procedure later with its attendant complications, and therefore, the indications for high loop ureteral diversion are limited. Severe urosepsis that does not respond to appropriate chemotherapy would be one indication, but similar results today can usually be achieved by placing percutaneous nephrostomy tubes—a less morbid procedure often able to be done without general anesthesia.

Most often, whether to do a loop ureterostomy revolves around the question of whether this procedure is likely to offer the child overall improved renal function. The study by Krueger and associates (1980) has certain experimental design flaws, especially when one considers that two separate groups collected at different times and managed arbitrarily by two different techniques are compared. Considering all these variables and the concepts of transitional nephrology—whereby one expects that within the first few months after birth, the kidney continues to grow new cells (increased DNA content) (Hayslett, 1983), I believe there is still a place for occasional use of loop ureterostomy in these infants. My own criterion is a nadir serum creatinine of 1.8 mg/dl or greater after several days of transurethral catheter drainage. Infants who have a nadir creatinine of 1.5 to 1.8 mg/dl are a difficult group, and I generally offer parents either endoscopic management or loop ureterostomy. I manage most infants with a serum creatinine less than 1.5 mg/dl by primary valve ablation with a "wait-and-see" approach.

The decision regarding appropriate management in this schema demands satisfactory vesical drainage for several days after the diagnosis is established. The "valve bladder" may be very irritable and placement of an indwelling catheter can induce severe detrusor spasm with secondary ureteral obstruction. Noe and Jerkins (1983) observed an infant who was anuric during the period of transurethral catheterization but had normal renal function after loop ureterostomy. A similar observation was reported by Jordan and Hoover (1985). The infant who has a high nadir creatinine on catheter drainage that falls to near-normal levels immediately after ureterostomy likely represents the same phenomenon. The purpose in considering loop ureterostomy is long-term, gradual improvement in renal function by maximizing renal growth potential, not immediate improvement in renal function. It is prudent during the period of catheter drainage, if renal function does not improve to satisfactory levels, to consider placing the infant on anticholinergic therapy to reduce detrusor spasm.

Several techniques have been described to perform loop ureterostomies (Fig. 49–13). I prefer a single-loop procedure (Novak and Gonzales, 1978). The more complex procedures require more operative time and incur a greater risk of immediate surgical complications (Sober, 1972; Williams and Cromie, 1975). These procedures are being done in the sickest infants, and I recognize no significant benefit from making the procedure more complex.

Prenatal Considerations

Today, many, probably most, patients with urethral valves are recognized on prenatal ultrasound. If one accepts that renal parenchymal damage associated with

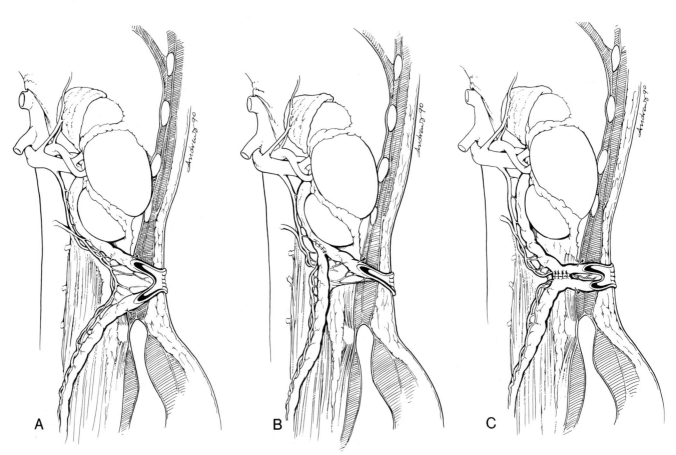

Figure 49–13. Techniques of high cutaneous ureterostomy. *A,* Loop ureterostomy. *B,* Sober ureterostomy. *C,* Ring ureterostomy.

urethral valves is progressive, then it is reasonable to ask how soon after recognition should appropriate relief of obstruction be accomplished. Initial enthusiasm for prenatal intervention, however, waned when it became evident that certain inherent problems existed: (1) inability to make the diagnosis of urethral valves with absolute certainty on prenatal ultrasound; (2) difficulty in assuring placement and patency of vesicoamniotic shunt catheters; (3) fetal and maternal risks directly related to the procedure (hemorrhage, infection, initiation of early labor); and (4) lack of objective data supporting that any benefit was provided by prenatal intervention which was greater than what would have occurred had the infant been treated promptly and appropriately at birth.

Modern ultrasound technology offers much improved imaging, and the diagnostic accuracy of prenatal ultrasound is substantially improved over what was present 10 years ago. The characteristic findings in a fetus with posterior urethral valves are bilateral hydronephrosis, a distended and *thickened* bladder, a dilated prostatic urethra (seen occasionally), and varying degrees of amniotic fluid abnormality. The renal parenchyma can often be described as normal or echodense (the latter suggesting dysplasia). However, similar findings can be described for the prune-belly syndrome—a disorder not generally thought to be primarily obstructive in nature. An infant with massive bilateral vesicoureteral reflux might have marked hydronephrosis and a distended (although usually not thickened) bladder. Either of these two problems might be thought to be urethral valves on prenatal evaluation, yet prenatal drainage would not be indicated. Diagnostic inaccuracies are still present in the technique (Skolder et al., 1988).

Any technically oriented procedure will incur certain risks, which should gradually lessen as individuals become more familiar with the procedure and its technology. The most serious complications are those that risk both mother and fetus and include severe hemorrhage, infection, and induction of premature labor. In the selected cases done to date, these risks have been felt to be acceptable. However, the incidence is directly related to the experience of the center and the personnel involved. It is still prudent that these prenatal procedures be done in a limited number of medical centers with the most experience.

The greatest deterrent to more frequent use of prenatal intervention has been the lack of any objective data to measure whether prenatal intervention is beneficial as far as ultimate renal function is concerned. It is generally believed that dysplasia is an early gestational event and that it occurs before the fetus is large enough to even be considered for prenatal manipulation. Absolutely no data are available indicating that dysplasia will improve after relief of obstruction. In comparison, the spectrum of severity of obstruction from urethral valves is very wide, and the level of glomerular filtration does not correlate directly with the severity of ureteral dilation. Because of this, some children would undergo diversion who did not really require urgent drainage, increasing the risks associated with prenatal intervention.

Certain parameters can be used to suggest the degree of renal functional compromise. First, as noted previously, dysplastic renal parenchyma is echodense when compared with normal renal parenchyma. Second, the majority of the amniotic fluid is made from urine. Severe oligohydramnios suggests poor renal function, but normal volumes of amniotic fluid do not mean normal renal function. Lastly, Glick and associates (1985) have developed a technique of percutaneous urine sampling with measurement of certain urinary parameters (Table 49–1). Fetal urine is normally low in sodium and is dilute relative to serum. High sodium losses and isosthenuria suggest poor overall renal function. A fetus with unfavorable urine parameters would likely not benefit from prenatal drainage.

Unfortunately, none of these observations directly relates to whether prenatal intervention or early postnatal management makes any difference regarding long-term renal outlook. Thus, decisions regarding prenatal intervention should be highly selective and should be made with full knowledge of the potential risks involved. Perhaps the most objective finding today that suggests that prenatal intervention should be considered is when a fetus with ultrasound findings of infravesical obstruction initially is judged to have normal amounts of amniotic fluid but then is noted on follow-up ultrasound examinations to develop oligohydramnios.

Additional considerations that influence decisions regarding fetal intervention involve the possible benefits of protecting the fetus from developing pulmonary hypoplasia. Just as the degree of urinary obstruction associated with urethral valves varies widely, the pathophysiology of the pulmonary hypoplasia that may also develop is very variable. The presence of oligohydramnios is associated with an increased risk of pulmonary hypoplasia; but some infants with severe oligohydramnios have good pulmonary function, and some with normal amniotic fluid volume have pulmonary insufficiency. The development of pulmonary hypoplasia may be multifaceted, and factors other than amniotic fluid volume alone undoubtedly play a role (Landers and

Table 49–1. PROGNOSTIC VARIABLES FOR THE FETUS WITH POSTERIOR URETHRAL VALVES

Variable	Predicted Postnatal Renal Function	
	Good	*Poor*
Amniotic fluid volume	Normal to moderately decreased	Moderate to severely decreased
Sonographic appearance of renal parenchyma	Normal to slightly increased echogenicity	Definite increased echogenicity to frankly cystic
Fetal urinary chemistries		
Sodium (mEq/L)	<100	>100
Chloride (mEq/L)	<90	>90
Osmolarity (mOsm)	<210	>210
Urinary output (ml/hour)	>2	<2

Adapted from Glick, P. L., Harrison, M. R., Golbus, M. S., et al.: J. Pediatr. Surg., 20:376, 1985.

Hanson, 1990). Current clinical and experimental evidence suggests that increasing the amniotic fluid volume, when it is initially reduced, lowers the overall risk of severe pulmonary insufficiency (Harrison et al., 1982). Within the broad spectrum of offering the parents of a newborn with severe renal insufficiency the option of continuous peritoneal dialysis and eventual transplantation, the prevention of pulmonary hyperplasia is another possible indication for considering prenatal intervention in selected cases.

Prognosis

The prognosis for children with urethral valves is improving, and current management is gradually rewriting the historical data. In most modern, large series, neonatal deaths make up only 2 to 3 per cent of the series (Churchill et al., 1990). Early (prenatal) recognition, control of infection, appropriate and selective surgery, recognition of harmful urodynamic abnormalities, modern nephrologic management, and eventual dialysis and transplantation all combine to increase survival now to an extent unheard of in the recent past. The original series reported total mortality as high as 50 per cent by the end of the adolescent period (Johnston and Kulatilake, 1972). Certainly, those statistics no longer hold true today. In all series, prognosis relates closely to nadir serum creatinine. Warshaw and associates (1985) noted that infants with a serum creatinine level less than 1.0 mg/dl at 1 year of age generally fared well, although a serum creatinine at this level does not insure long-term satisfactory renal function. The fact remains that many children with urethral valves have significant degrees of parenchymal dysplasia and will demonstrate gradual, but progressive loss of renal function during their lifetime (Burbige and Hensle, 1987; Parkhouse et al., 1988; Tejani et al., 1986). It is important that parents be aware that the diagnosis of urethral valves means a long-term commitment to surveillance and care and that even today the eventual outcome is unclear in many instances.

ANTERIOR URETHRAL OBSTRUCTION

Congenital obstruction of the more distal urethra is much less common than obstruction of the proximal urethra. Congenital obstruction of the anterior urethra is varied and can include anterior urethral valves (congenital diverticulum of the urethra), valvular obstruction of the fossa navicularis, and cystic dilatation of the ducts of Cowper's glands (syringoceles). Of these, the most common abnormality is anterior urethral valves.

An anterior urethral valve, in nearly all cases, is actually a congenital urethral diverticulum (Fig. 49–14) (Tank, 1987). During voiding, the diverticulum expands, ballooning ventrally and distally beneath the thinned corpus spongiosum. The flap-like dorsal margin of the diverticulum then extends into the urethral lumen, occluding urinary flow (an obstructing valve). Anterior

urethral valves have been described in every portion of the anterior urethra in nearly equal incidence. They may be small, minimally obstructive, and of limited clinical concern (Fig. 49–15). Often, though, they are severely obstructing and result in all of the findings seen with posterior urethral valves.

The diagnosis of anterior urethral valves is confirmed on voiding cystourethrography. At times, difficulty with catheterization may be encountered because the catheter preferentially slips into the diverticulum. However, this occurs less often than one might suspect because the proximal wall of the diverticulum is often not hollowed out nearly as extensively as the distal wall. Because the diverticula nearly always are placed in the midline ventrally, a dorsally oriented coudé-tipped catheter can usually be negotiated without difficulties into the more proximal urethra. The entire penile urethra must be included in the voiding phase of the study or more distally located lesions will be missed.

The etiology of these anomalies is not entirely clear, but they seem to represent incomplete fusion of a segment of the urethral plate. Another possible cause might be a focally incomplete development of the corpus spongiosum with ballooning of the urethral mucosa due to inadequate support. Small, nonobstructing diverticula often appear stable for many years and do not show continuous enlargement and progressively worsening obstruction.

Initial management of the child with a congenital anterior urethral valve parallels the management for the more commonly seen posterior urethral valve. Initial imaging studies will assess the extent of hydronephrosis, thickness and quality of renal parenchyma (echogenicity on renal ultrasound, uptake on renal scan), and the presence or absence of vesicoureteral reflux. Infants presenting with urosepsis and/or severe renal insufficiency require a period of transurethral or suprapubic (by percutaneous route) catheter drainage for stabilization, antibiotics, electrolyte management, and assessment of renal functional improvement. As with infants with posterior urethral valves, a temporizing, tubeless diversion (vesicostomy, loop ureterostomy) might be chosen on an individual basis (Rushton et al., 1987).

Management of the urethral anomaly may be endoscopic or open. A hooked, single-wire, electrocautery "knife" can engage the distal margin of the diverticulum and incise it in the midline. When performing this procedure, the surgeon must be very careful not to place the tip of the wire too close to the floor of the diverticulum. At this location, the wall of the urethra can be very thin and thermal injury might result in the development of a urethrocutaneous fistula. Even after satisfactory destruction of the leaflet, postoperative urethrography is often disappointing, because the appearance of the diverticulum may be unchanged. One must carefully assess the quality of flow (a flow rate if the child is old enough) and the extent of filling of the distal urethra to evaluate the results of the procedure.

Some surgeons have advocated open resection and reconstruction of the diverticulum (Tank, 1987). This technique allows one to completely excise the distal lip and to provide a more homogeneous caliber to the

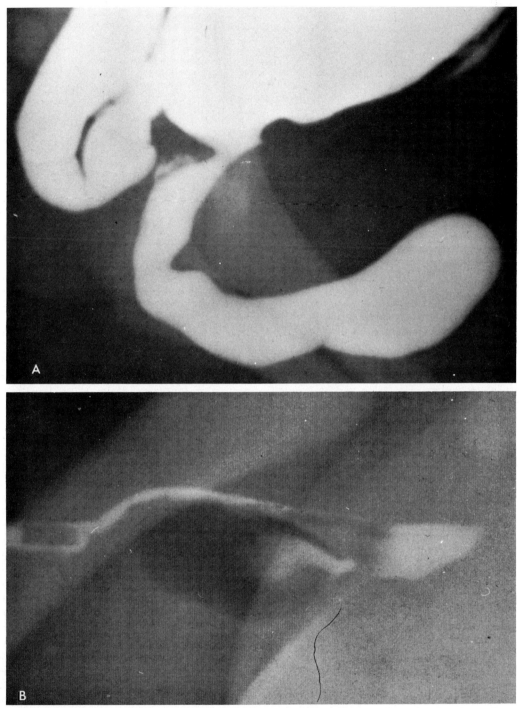

Figure 49–14. *A*, Anterior urethral diverticulum (valve). This voiding cystourethrogram in a newborn boy shows severe obstruction associated with reflux into a dysplastic left kidney and compromised right renal function. *B*, Demonstration of anterior diverticulum, using air injected retrograde with compression of urethra in perineum, followed by contrast injection, showing neck of diverticulum and mechanism of obstruction.

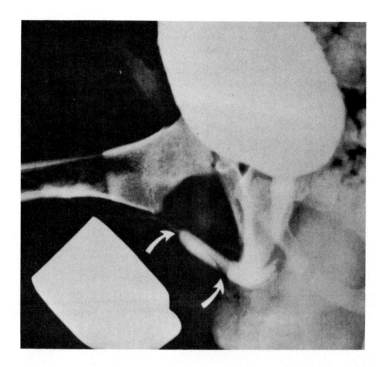

Figure 49–15. Anterior urethral diverticulum (valve) demonstrated by voiding cystourethrogram in 4-year-old boy with symptoms of straining to void and a fine stream.

urethra. In most cases, a patch graft urethroplasty is the preferred procedure. If the diverticulum is on the penile shaft, a sleeve dissection of the penile shaft skin from the corona to the penoscrotal angle will allow the urethroplasty to be completed without ending up with overlapping suture lines.

Some anterior urethral valves may not be associated with a urethral diverticulum. DeCastro and colleagues (1987) described three children who had anterior urethral membranes without the associated diverticulum. Scherz and associates (1987) described valvular obstruction in the region of the fossa navicularis in three children. Whether these isolated variations represent a portion of the spectrum described previously is unclear.

Syringoceles are cystic dilations of the duct of Cowper's gland within the bulbous urethra (Maizels et al., 1983). They are generally small, inconsequential lesions; but, rarely, they can be of sufficient size to cause varying degrees of outlet obstruction. Management, when necessary, is generally by endoscopic unroofing. After unroofing, a diverticulum-like defect may result on the posterolateral wall of the bulbous urethra. However, these defects are rarely obstructing and do not need further management.

MEGALOURETHRA

Nonobstructive urethral dilatation (megalourethra) is a rare entity that is associated with abnormal development of the corpus spongiosum and, occasionally, with abnormal development of the corpus cavernosum. Traditionally, megalourethra has been divided into two varieties: scaphoid megalourethra and fusiform megalourethra. In the scaphoid variety, the corpus spongiosum is generally thought to be the only abnormal segment, whereas the fusiform variety is associated with defects of the corpus cavernosum also. However, this distinction is arbitrary and is not based on any recognized embryologic difference between the two varieties (Appel et al., 1986). Although megalourethra may be an isolated event, it is often associated with upper tract abnormalities. Appropriate imaging of the urinary tract is indicated in every case. Megalourethra is especially common in association with the prune-belly syndrome and may represent a defect in development of the mesoderm, one of the proposed etiologies for the prune-belly anomaly (Mortensen et al., 1985).

Management of the megalourethra itself is primarily cosmetic if the upper tracts are satisfactorily normal (Fig. 49–16). The large, bulbous urethra can be trimmed and tailored for a more homogeneous and normal urethral caliber. If the corpora cavernosa are severely deficient, consideration of a change of the sex of rearing in the newborn is appropriate.

An interesting subset of boys with megalourethra are often classified as having a variant of hypospadias. These anomalies have been described by Duckett and Keating (1989) as the "megameatus, intact prepuce." The patients present with a coronally positioned, wide-mouthed meatus and a fully formed foreskin. The urethra for a centimeter or so is often very large, and the corpus spongiosum is very thin. Ventral chordee is not present. This anomaly contrasts with the more usual variety of hypospadias thought to represent a fetal androgen deficiency, in which the meatus is often small, the distal urethra is narrowed and inelastic, the foreskin is unfused ventrally, and ventral chordee is expected.

URETHRAL DUPLICATION

Duplication of the urethra is an uncommon anomaly. Urethral duplications are complex anomalies, and different embryologic abnormalities are thought to be responsible for the many variations seen. A universally

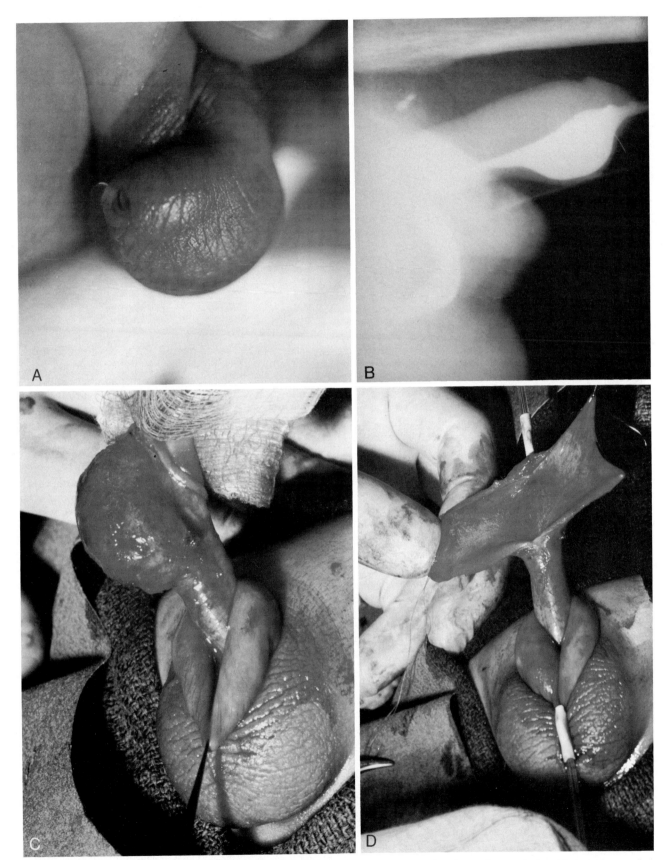

Figure 49–16. *A,* Photograph of a newborn male with megalourethra. This photograph was taken during the act of micturition.
B, Voiding urethrogram of same patient.
C, Appearance of the urethra after degloving of the penis.
D, The dilated segment of the urethra opened. Excess urethral tissue is excised, leaving just enough to reconstruct a urethra of normal caliber.

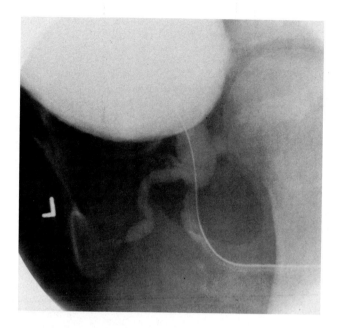

Figure 49–17. Voiding cystourethrogram in a 17-year-old male with ventral urethral duplication with one meatus at the anus. The catheter is passed up the perineal opening. The penile urethra was very atretic.

accepted classification has not yet been described (Ortolano and Nasaralloh, 1986). Urethral duplications are conveniently divided into dorsal duplications and ventral duplications. Most duplications occur in the same sagittal plane, that is, they occur one on top of the other. Less commonly, duplex urethras lie side by side. This is the usual finding in children with a completely duplicated phallus, but occasionally it can occur when the phallus is fused, but widened. This anatomic appearance is also more common when the bladder is completely duplicated.

In the dorsal variety, the normal urethra is the ventrally positioned channel that generally ends in a normal meatus on the glans. The accessory (abnormal) channel opens on the shaft in an epispadiac position anywhere from the glans to the base of the penis. Often, dorsal penile chordee is present, and the foreskin may be unfused dorsally. The abnormal dorsal segment extends proximally beneath the symphysis pubis for a varying length. Many end blindly before reaching the bladder. If these abnormal urethras do reach the bladder, the patient will usually be incontinent. Widening of the symphysis pubis may also be found. These findings suggest a relationship of this anomaly to the exstrophy/epispadias complex (Campbell et al., 1987; Sharma et al., 1987). Cases have been described in which this accessory channel never entered the bladder but continued along the ventral surface and joined with the urachus, suggesting that this might represent more of an abortive duplication of the bladder rather than of the urethra.

Because the normally positioned urethra has a normal bladder neck and sphincter mechanism, excision of the abnormal, epispadiac urethra will usually cure any incontinence affecting the patient. Significant penile chordee may also have to be repaired.

Ventral duplications of the urethra are less clearly understood embryologically. These anomalies may be complete, in which two separate urethras come off the bladder. Other cases are incomplete, in which the urethra bifurcates somewhere distal to the bladder neck. Patients may present with a hypospadiac meatus on the penile shaft. However, the most serious variation occurs when the ventral meatus is present at the anterior anal margin. The dorsal, penile urethra is often narrowed and inelastic. The two urethras may have separate origins from the bladder, but more often they bifurcate at the level of the prostatic urethra (Fig. 49–17). Urinary flow is preferentially through the anal opening, and the ventral urethra is generally considered the more normal urethra, because it traverses the sphincter mechanism.

Urethral duplication may not always require surgical management, and some cases are noted incidentally during voiding cystourethrography (Hoekstra and Jones, 1985). Management of the more severe perianal duplication has generally involved advancement of the ventral channel to the perineum as the initial procedure, followed by a formal urethroplasty. Usually, this was accomplished by excising the existing dorsal urethra and then performing a standard urethroplasty. The more normally positioned dorsal channel is often very narrowed with focal areas of atresia and has generally not been used in the reconstruction (Holst and Peterson, 1988). However, Passerini-Glazel and co-workers (1988) demonstrated that, if the dorsal urethra can be catheterized—even if the lumen is very tiny—gentle, gradual, prolonged dilatation in situ may allow for eventual use of this urethra.

REFERENCES

Adzick, N. S., Harrison, M. R., Flake, A. W., and de Lorimier, A. A.: Urinary extravasation in the fetus with obstructive uropathy. J. Pediatr. Surg., 20:608, 1985.

Appel, R. A., Kaplan, G. W., Brock, W. A., and Streit, D.: Megalourethra. J. Urol., 135:747, 1986.

Bauer, S. B., Dieppa, R. A., Labib, K., et al.: The bladder in boys with posterior urethral valves: A urodynamic assessment. J. Urol., 121:769, 1979.

Beck, A. D.: The effect of intra-uterine urinary obstruction upon the development of the fetal kidney. J. Urol., 105:784, 1971.

Brenner, B. M., Meyer, T. W., and Hosteller, T. H.: Dietary protein intake and the progressive nature of kidney disease. N. Engl. J. Med., 307:652, 1982.

Burbige, K. A., and Hensle, T. W.: Posterior urethral valves in the newborn: Treatment and functional results. J. Pediatr. Surg., 22:165, 1987.

Campaiola, J. M., Perlmutter, A. P., and Steinhardt, G. F.: Noncompliant bladder resulting from posterior urethral valves. J. Urol., 134:708, 1985.

Campbell, J., Beasley, S., McMullin, N., and Hutson, J. M.: Congenital prepubic sinus: Possible variant of dorsal urethral duplication. J. Urol., 137:505, 1987.

Churchill, B. M., Krueger, R. P., Fleisher, M. H., et al.: Complications of posterior urethral valve surgery. Urol. Clin. North Am., 10:519, 1983.

Churchill, B. M., McLorie, G. A., Khoury, A. E., et al.: Emergency treatment and long-term follow-up of posterior urethral valves. Urol. Clin. North Am., 17:343, 1990.

Conner, J. P., Hensle, T. W., Berdon, W., and Burbige, K. A.: Contained neonatal urinoma: Management and functional results. J. Urol., 140:1319, 1988

Deane, A. M., Whitaker, R. H., and Sherwood, T.: Diathermy hook ablation of posterior urethral valves in neonates and infants. Br. J. Urol., 62:593, 1988.

DeCastro, R., Battaglino, F., Casolari, E., et al.: Valves of the anterior urethra without diverticulum: Description of three cases. Pediatr. Med. Chir., 9:211, 1987.

Dejter, S., and Gibbons, D.: The newborn valve. In Gonzales, E. T., and Roth, D. R. (Eds.): Common Problems in Pediatric Urology, Chap. 8. Houston, Mosby-Year Book, 1990, p. 76.

Duckett, J. W., and Keating, M. A.: Technical challenge of the megameatus intact prepuce hypospadias variant: The pyramid procedure. J. Urol., 141:1407, 1989.

Duckett, J. W., and Norris, M.: The management of neonatal valves with advanced hydronephrosis and azotemia. In Carlton, C. E. (Ed.): Controversies in Urology. Chicago, Year Book Medical Publishers, 1989, p. 2.

Ehrlich, R. M., and Shanberg, A.: Neodymium-YAG laser ablation of posterior urethral valves. Dialogues Pediatr. Urol., 11:29, 1988.

Field, P. L., and Stephens, F. D.: Congenital urethral membranes causing urethral obstruction. J. Urol., 111:250, 1974.

Glassberg, K. I.: Current issues regarding posterior urethral valves. Urol. Clin. North Am., 12:175, 1985.

Glassberg, K. L., Schneider, M., Haller, J. O., et al.: Observations on persistently dilated ureter after posterior urethral valve ablation. Urology, 20:20, 1982.

Glick, P. L., Harrison, M. R., Adzick, N. S., et al.: Correction of congenital hydronephrosis in utero: IV. In utero decompression prevents renal dysplasia. J. Pediatr. Surg., 19:649, 1984.

Glick, P. L., Harrison, M. R., Golbus, M. S., et al.: Management of the fetus with congenital hydronephrosis: II. Prognostic criteria and selection for treatment. J. Pediatr. Surg., 20:376, 1985.

Gonzales, E. T.: Alternatives in the management of posterior urethral valves. Urol. Clin. North Am., 17:335, 1990.

Griffin, J. E., and Wilson, J. D.: The androgen resistance syndromes: 5α-Reductase deficiency, testicular feminization, and related syndromes. In Scriner, C. R., Beaudet, A. L., Sly, W. S., and Valle, D. (Eds.): The Metabolic Basis of Inherited Disease. New York, McGraw-Hill, 1989, pp. 1919–1944.

Harrison, M. R., Nakayama, D. K., and Rooll, R.: Correction of congenital hydronephrosis in utero: II. Decompression versus the effects of obstruction on the fetal lung and urinary tract. J. Pediatr. Surg., 17:965, 1982.

Hayslett, J. P.: Effect of age on compensatory renal growth. Kidney Int., 23:599, 1983.

Henneberry, M. O., and Stephens, F. A.: Renal hypoplasia and dysplasia in infants with posterior urethral valves. J. Urol., 123:912, 1980.

Hoekstra, I., and Jones, B.: Duplication of the male urethra: Report of three cases. Clin. Radiol., 36:529, 1985.

Holst, S., and Peterson, N. E.: Fulguration-ablation of atypical accessory urethra. J. Urol., 140:347, 1988.

Hoover, D. L., and Duckett, J. W.: Posterior urethral valves, unilateral reflux, and renal dysplasia: A syndrome. J. Urol., 128:994, 1982.

Johnston, J. H.: Temporary cutaneous ureterostomy in the management of advanced congenital urinary obstruction. Arch. Dis. Child., 38:161, 1963.

Johnston, J. H.: Posterior urethral valves: An operative technique using an electric auriscope. J. Pediatr. Surg., 1:583, 1966.

Johnston, J. H.: Vesicoureteric reflux with urethral valves. Br. J. Urol., 51:100, 1979.

Johnston, J. H., and Kulatilake, A. E.: The sequelae of posterior urethral valves. Br. J. Urol., 43:743, 1971.

Johnston, J. H., and Kulatilake, A. E.: Posterior urethral valves: Results and sequelae. In Johnston, J. H., and Scholtmeyer, R. Y. (Eds.): Problems in Pediatric Urology. Amsterdam, Excerpta Medica, 1972, p. 161.

Jordan, G. H., and Hoover, D. L.: Inadequate decompression of the upper tracts using a Foley catheter in the valve bladder. J. Urol., 134:137, 1985.

Klahr, S.: The modification of diet in renal disease study. N. Engl. J. Med., 320:864, 1989.

Kolicinski, Z. H.: Foley balloon procedure in posterior urethral valves. Dialogues Pediatr. Urol., 11:7, 1988.

Krueger, R. P., Hardy, B. E., and Churchill, B. M.: Growth in boys with posterior urethral valves. Urol. Clin. North Am., 7:265, 1980.

Landers, S., and Hanson, T. N.: Pulmonary problems associated with congenital renal malformations. In Gonzales, E. T., and Roth, D. R. (Eds.): Common Problems in Pediatric Urology, Chap. 9. Houston, Mosby-Year Book, 1990, p. 85.

Lome, L. G., Howat, J. M., and Williams, D. I.: The temporarily defunctionalized bladder in children. J. Urol., 107:469, 1972.

Maizels, M., Stephens, F. D., King, L. R., and Firlit, C. F.: Cowper's syringocele—a classification of dilatations of Cowper's duct based upon clinical characteristics of 8 boys. J. Urol., 129:111, 1983.

Mayor, G., Genton, R., Torrado, A., and Geirgnard, J.: Renal function in obstructive nephropathy: Long-term effects of reconstructive surgery. Pediatrics, 58:740, 1975.

McConnell, J. D.: Detrusor smooth muscle development. In Husmann, D., and McConnell, J. D. (Eds.): Dialogues in Pediatric Urology, Vol. 12, December 1989.

McVary, K. T., and Maizels, M.: Urinary obstruction reduces glomerulogenesis in the developing kidney: A model in the rabbit. J. Urol., 142:646, 1989.

Mortensen, P. H., Johnson, H. W., Coleman, G. U., et al.: Megalourethra. J. Urol., 134:358, 1985.

Nakayama, D. K., Harrison, M. R., and de Lorimier, A. A.: Prognosis of posterior urethral valves presenting at birth. J. Pediatr. Surg., 21:43, 1986.

Noe, H. N., and Jerkins, G. R.: Oliguria and renal failure following decompression of the bladder in children with posterior urethral valves. J. Urol., 129:595, 1983.

Novak, M. E., and Gonzales, E. T.: Single stage reconstruction of urinary tract after loop cutaneous ureterostomy. Urology, 11:134, 1978.

Ortolano, V., and Nasaralloh, P. F.: Urethral duplication. J. Urol., 136:909, 1986.

Parkhouse, H. F., Barratt, T. M., Dillon, M. J., et al.: Long-term outcome of boys with posterior urethral valves. Br. J. Urol., 62:59, 1988.

Passerini-Glazel, G., Araguna, F., Chiozza, L., et al.: The PADUA (progressive augmentation by dilating the urethra anterior) procedure for the treatment of severe urethral hypoplasia. J. Urol., 140:1247, 1988.

Rittenberg, M. H., Hulbert, W. C., Snyder, H. M., Duckett, J. W.: Protective factors in posterior urethral valves. J. Urol., 140:993, 1988.

Robertson, W. B., and Hayes, J. A.: Congenital diaphragmatic obstruction of the male posterior urethra. Br. J. Urol., 41:592, 1969.

Rushton, H. G., Parrott, T. S., Woodard, J. R., and Walther, M.: The role of vesicostomy in the management of anterior urethral valves in neonates and infants. J. Urol., 138:107, 1987.

Scherz, H. C., Kaplan, G. W., and Packer, M. G.: Anterior urethral valves in the fossa navicularis in children. J. Urol., 138:1211, 1987.

Sharma, S. K., Kapoor, R., Kumar, A., and Mandal, A. K.: Incomplete epispadiac urethral duplication with dorsal penile curvature. J. Urol., 138:585, 1987.

Skolder, A. J., Maizels, M., Depp, R., Firlit, C. F., et al.: Caution in antenatal intervention. J. Urol., 139:1026, 1988.

Sober, I.: Pelvioureterostomy-en-Y. Urology, 107:473, 1972.

Stephens, F. D.: Congenital Malformations of the Urinary Tract. New York, Praeger Publishers, 1983, pp. 96, 103.

Tanagho, E. A.: Congenitally obstructed bladders: Fate after prolonged defunctionalization. J. Urol., 111:102, 1974.

Tank, E. S.: Anterior urethral valves resulting from congenital urethral diverticula. Urology, 30:467, 1987.

Tejani, A., Butt, K., Glassberg, K., et al.: Predictors of eventual end stage renal disease in children with posterior urethral valves. J. Urol., 136:857, 1986.

Walker, R. D., and Padron, M.: Management of posterior urethral valves by initial vesicostomy and delayed valve ablation. J. Urol., 144:1212, 1990.

Warshaw, B. L., Hymes, L. C., Trulock, T. S., et al.: Prognostic features in infants with obstructive uropathy due to posterior urethral valves. J. Urol., 133:240, 1985.

Whitaker, R. H.: The ureter in posterior urethral valves. Br. J. Urol., 45:395, 1973.

Williams, P. I., and Cromie, W. J.: Ring ureterostomy. Br. J. Urol., 47:789, 1975.

Woodbury, P. W.: Constant pressure perfusion: A method to determine obstruction in the upper urinary tract. J. Urol., 142:632, 1989.

Young, H. H., Frontz, W. A., and Baldwin, J. C.: Congenital obstruction of the posterior urethra. J. Urol., 3:289, 1919.

Zaontz, M. R., and Firlit, C. F.: Percutaneous antegrade ablation of posterior urethral valves in premature or underweight term neonates: An alternative to primary vesicostomy. J. Urol., 134:139, 1985.

50
HYPOSPADIAS

John W. Duckett, M.D.

Hypospadias is a congenital defect of the penis resulting in the incomplete development of the anterior urethra. The abnormal urethral opening may be anywhere along the shaft of the penis or into the perineum. The more proximal the meatus, the more likely will ventral curvature (chordee) appear to be shortened.

The normal anatomy of the penis consists of paired corpora cavernosa covered by a thick fibrous tunica albuginea with a midline septum. The urethra traverses the penis within the corpus spongiosum, which lies ventral in the groove between the two corpora cavernosa. The urethra emerges at the distal end of the conical glans penis. The spermatic fascia or dartos fascia is the loose layer of connective tissue immediately beneath the skin. Superficial lymphatics and the dorsal veins of the penis are located in this fascia. Beneath the dartos fascia is Buck's fascia, which surrounds the corpora cavernosa and splits to contain the corpora spongiosum separately. The dorsal neurovascular bundle lies deep to Buck's fascia in the groove between the corpora cavernosa.

Hypospadias results in various degrees of urethral and corpus spongiosum deficiency. The fibrous tissue found with chordee replaces Buck's fascia and the dartos fascia. The skin on the ventral surface is thin. The prepuce is deficient ventrally and forms a dorsal hood over the glans.

CLASSIFICATION

The most commonly used classification of hypospadias (Browne, 1936) relates to the location of the meatus (glanular, distal penile, proximal penile, penoscrotal junction, and perineal). However, the severity of hypospadias cannot always be defined by the original site of the meatus. The meatus may be close to the tip of the glans yet have significant chordee. We, therefore, prefer classification not according to the original site but rather according to the new location after correction of the associated chordee (orthoplasty*) as proposed by Barcat (1973).

Welch (1979) estimated that 62 per cent of the openings were subcoronal or penile, 22 per cent were at the penoscrotal angle, and 16 per cent opened in the scrotum or perineum. Using the Barcat classification, Juskiewenski and colleagues (1983) reported 536 patients with hypospadias as 71 per cent anterior, 16 per cent middle, and 13 per cent posterior. Of the anterior group (383 patients), 13 per cent were classified as balantic, 43 per cent as subcoronal, and 38 per cent as distal shaft; 6 per cent had the prepuce intact (megameatus intact prepuce).

Our own experience at The Children's Hospital of Philadelphia corresponds to these reports: 65 per cent anterior, 15 per cent middle or midpenile, and 20 per cent in a posterior location (Duckett, 1991) (Fig. 50–1). The anterior group was further classified as 19 per cent glanular, 47 per cent coronal, and 34 per cent distal shaft.

EMBRYOLOGY

The location of the cloacal membrane at the caudal end of the primitive streak provides the surrounding mesoderm with vast developmental potential. During the 4th week, paired swellings anterolateral to the membrane appear, which fuse into the midline *genital tubercle* by the 6th week. Simultaneously, the posterolateral anal tubercles form and the lateral mesoderm heaps up to form the urethral and *genital folds*. All of these mesodermal components retain the capacity to convert testosterone to dihydrotestosterone, thus heralding the first signs of sexual differentiation.

As the urorectal septum completes its descent and fuses with the cloacal membrane, the perineal body is formed. The urogenital sinus then begins to elongate onto the ventral surface of the phallus to the level of the corona, forming the urethral groove, which is

---

*Orthoplasty (Greek *orthus*, straighten) is a term used in Europe referring to chordee excision and penile straightening.

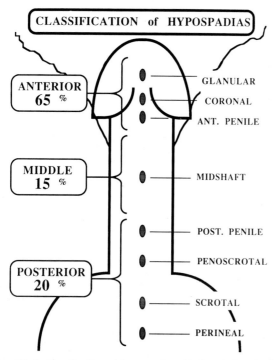

Figure 50–1. Classification of hypospadias. Urethroplasty selection is based on meatal location after correction of penile curvature. (From Keating, M. A., and Duckett, J. W.: Recent advances in the repair of hypospadias. *In* Nyhus, L. (Ed.): Surgery Annuals, vol. 22. Norwalk, CT, Appleton–Century–Crofts, 1991. In press.)

flanked laterally by mesoderm. Conversion of the anterior walls of the urogenital sinus results in the formation of an *endodermal urethral plate* on the floor of the urethral groove. This soon disintegrates, deepening the groove and facilitating the formation of the anterior urethra. At this time, the urethral and cloacal membranes rupture.

From the indifferent state, the external genital structures develop a typically male configuration under the influence of testosterone. As the phallus elongates, the urethral groove extends to the level of the corona. Gradually, the urethral folds coalesce in the midline, closing the urethra and forming the median raphe of the scrotum and penis. Dorsal to the urethra, mesenchyme coalesces to form the corporal bodies, vascular channels, and nerves.

The glanular urethra may form by an identical mechanism, although there is controversy surrounding this premise. Glenister (1954) believes that the distal glans channel, most likely induced by hormonal and local factors, forms a solid core that tunnels to join the proximal urethra, which is created by closure of the urethral groove. This core later undergoes canalization, forming a complete urethra. Because this is the last step in the formation of the normal urethra, there is a higher incidence of hypospadias with the meatal opening at the subcoronal region (Sommer and Stephens, 1980) (Fig. 50–2).

The prepuce forms as a ridge of skin from the corona that gradually grows to enclose the glans circumferentially with fusion to the glans epithelium. The preputial defect associated with hypospadias has a deficient ven-

tral segment and resultant dorsal hood. The normal scrotal and penile raphe divides in hypospadias into a Y running onto the dorsal preputial hood around the glans in varying configurations. Even with the severe scrotal meatus, this defect of the raphe is apparent, fusing the penis into a vulviform appearance; even a penoscrotal transformation may occur. A glanular cleft may exist with a normal intact foreskin (Kumar, 1986). We have designated this variant as *megameatus intact prepuce* (MIP) (Duckett and Keating, 1989).

Chordee is the abnormal ventral curvature of the penis, an entity that is poorly understood. Apparently, the mesenchyme, which is deficient, would normally form the corpus spongiosum and fascial layers distal to the hypospadiac meatus in the normal urethra and persist as fibrous tissue (Kaplan and Brock, 1981; Kaplan and Lamm, 1975; Mettauer, 1842). Thus, the abnormal disintegration of the urethral plate and the missing mesenchymal ingrowth distal to the hypospadiac opening give rise to fibrous tissue, which causes the downward curvature. The mere presence of this tissue is not responsible for all cases of penile curvature. Rather, during penile development, a growth differen-

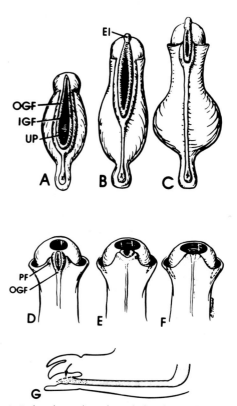

Figure 50–2. Embryology of penile and glanular urethra.

A through *C*, The inner and outer genital folds cover the urethral plate (UP) and form the raphe. The glanular urethra is a compound of ectodermal pit at tip of glans and open end of the urethral groove.

D through *F*, Further closure of the groove by outer genital and preputial folds, and orifice of the intervening septum to create one orifice, the fossa navicularis and the lacuna magna.

G, Arrow indicates site of "anastomosis" between the ectodermal pit and the urethral groove. (OGF, outer genital folds; IGF, inner genital folds; PF, preputial folds; UP, urethral plate; EI, ectodermal tag marking site of ectodermal ingrowth.) (From Sommer, J. T., and Stephens, F. D.: Dorsal urethral diverticulum of the fossa navicularis: Symptoms, diagnosis and treatment. J. Urol., 124:94, 1980.)

tial between the normally formed dorsal tissue of the corporal bodies and deficient ventral tissue and urethra may result in the curvature in some cases (Bellinger, 1981).

INCIDENCE AND GENETICS

The incidence of hypospadias has been calculated to be 3.2 per 1000 live male births or one in 300 (Sweet et al., 1974). Sorenson (1953) as well as Avellan (1975) in Sweden—where very accurate birth defect data are kept—estimated an incidence of one in 300. In the United States, about 6000 boys with hypospadias are born each year (Duckett, 1991).

Familial tendencies indicate some polygenic factors. Fathers have hypospadias in 8 per cent of patients, whereas 14 per cent of male siblings are affected (Bauer et al., 1981). The condition is more common in whites than in blacks, and it is more common in Italians and Jews (Welch, 1979). The higher incidence in monozygotic twins (8.5 times) (Roberts and Lloyd, 1973) might be explained by the demand of two male fetuses on the placental production of human chorionic gonadotropin (hCG) in phase 3 organogenesis.

ASSOCIATED ANOMALIES

The most common anomalies associated with hypospadias are undescended testes and inguinal hernia. Khuri and co-workers (1981) found a 9.3 per cent incidence of undescended testes in patients with hypospadias. Third-degree hypospadias was associated with a 31.6 per cent incidence of undescended testes; second-degree hypospadias, 6.2 per cent; and first-degree hypospadias, 4.8 per cent. They also found the incidence of inguinal hernia to be 9.1 per cent in the total group, with an incidence of 17 per cent in third-degree hypospadias; 8.5 per cent in second-degree; and 7.1 per cent in first-degree. Ross and colleagues (1959) reported a similar incidence of either cryptorchidism or hernia in 16 per cent, whereas Cerasaro and co-workers (1986) found an incidence of 18 per cent.

Conflicting reports have been made as to the significance of anomalies of the upper urinary tract associated with hypospadias, and the question of obtaining routine intravenous urography or voiding cystography has been debated (Shelton and Noe, 1985). McArdle and Lebowitz (1975) found a 3 per cent incidence; Cerasaro and colleagues (1986), 1.7 per cent; and Avellan (1975), only 1 per cent. Khuri and co-workers (1981) grouped the patients according to the degree of hypospadias and subdivided them as to whether there was isolated hypospadias, hypospadias associated with cryptorchidism, or hypospadias associated with other system anomalies. The incidence was low (5.5 per cent) unless other system anomalies were associated. If one other system was present, the incidence was 12.2 per cent; two other systems, 16.7 per cent; whereas three other system anomalies increased the incidence to 50 per cent. With imperforate anus, the incidence was 46 per cent. With

myelomeningocele, the incidence was 33 per cent. They concluded that all patients with hypospadias of any degree who had associated anomalies should have the urinary tract screened, whereas screening was not indicated for those with hypospadias alone with or without undescended testes or hernia.

UTRICLES

Utriculus masculinus (utricle) is a residual prostatic urethral outgrowth that may persist in severe forms of hypospadias. The incidence of utricles may be as high as 10 to 15 per cent with perineal or penoscrotal hypospadias (Devine et al., 1980; Shima et al., 1979). These represent either incomplete müllerian duct regression or incomplete masculinization of the urogenital sinus. There are no uterine elements. The vasa course in the lateral walls must be divided if the utricle is removed. Few situations exist where removal is required. Stone formation and infection may result from obstruction (Ritchey et al., 1988).

INTERSEX

The presence of hypospadias is thought by some to be a form of intersex. Certainly, the diagnosis of intersex must be ruled out in the more severe forms of hypospadias, especially with cryptorchidism (Rajfer and Walsh, 1976). However, in general, the majority of hypospadias cases should not be considered as an intersex condition. The intersex states that must be ruled out in a child with hypospadias include the following:

1. *Adrenogenital syndrome (AGS).* Clearly, if a baby has undescended testes, she is a girl until proved otherwise, no matter how masculinized.

2. *Mixed gonadal dysgenesis (MGD).* This is the second most frequent cause of ambiguous genitalia in the neonate. With a testis on one side and a streak gonad on the other, the most frequent karyotype is 45,XO/46,XY (Davidoff and Federman, 1973). Many of these MGD patients (60 per cent) are severely undervirilized with micropenis at birth (phallus less than 2.5 cm). After inadequate response to testosterone stimulation, gender conversion may be appropriate.

3. *Incomplete male pseudohermaphroditism, type I; Reifenstein syndrome.* These boys have perineal scrotal hypospadias with azoospermia, infertility, incomplete virilization at puberty, and gynecomastia that develops at or after puberty. Severe manifestations may involve a vagina with small testes, which are cryptorchid. The etiology of this syndrome can be demonstrated by fibroblast culture to be a defect in androgen binding to a varying degree. The severe cases, if detected early, should be gender converted to female whereas the milder forms, in the majority of cases, are phenotypic and physiologic males, and the hypospadias can be repaired. Supplemental testosterone, unfortunately, is not effective.

4. *Incomplete male pseudohermaphroditism, type II; pseudovaginal-perineal-scrotal hypospadias–5-alpha-re-*

ductase deficiency. These very rare patients have a blind vaginal pouch of variable size opening either into the urogenital sinus or, more frequently, into the urethra immediately behind the urethral orifice (Opitz et al., 1972; Walsh et al., 1974). Unlike type I patients, they have well-developed and histologically normal testes as well as normal epididymis, vasa, and seminal vesicles, which terminate in the blind-ending vagina. Most patients are raised as females. Because of an enlarged clitoris, they are diagnosed early and castration is performed early. If the natural history is allowed, they will develop profound masculinization at puberty with muscle development, phallomegaly, ejaculation, and erections. In some, the sperm count has even been normal. Such a population has been studied in the Dominican Republic (Peterson et al., 1977).

5. *True hermaphroditism.* In these rare cases, both an ovary and a testis or an ovotestis is present. The external genitalia display all gradations from male to female, but most are masculinized to some degree. For that reason, 75 per cent of patients have been reared as males. Twenty-five per cent of the patients have bilateral ovotestes; 35 per cent, unilateral; 25 per cent, a testis on one side and an ovary on the other; and 10 per cent, indeterminant (Butler et al., 1969). Fifty per cent have a 46,XX karyotype, 20 per cent have an XY karyotype, and 30 per cent are mosaics. Abdominal exploration with biopsy of both gonads is appropriate in these cases and, in one sufficiently virilized to warrant male gender assignment, inappropriate ovarian tissue and müllerian structures should be removed. Repair of the hypospadias is indicated.

6. *Micropenis.* Micropenis is a miniature penis unaffected with hypospadias. Most often, this is due to central defect of gonadotropin deficiency, but some are idiopathic.

Allen and Griffin (1984) presented evidence in support of the concept that hypospadias is not just a local dysmorphic problem but rather a local manifestation of a systemic endocrinopathy. A variety of endocrine abnormalities were seen. They failed to confirm the impression that the principal defect lies in the inability of the target tissues to respond to androgen, either because of the numbers of androgen receptors or because of the inability to convert testosterone to dihydrotestosterone (Gearhart et al., 1988; Gearhart et al., 1989).

HISTORY OF SURGICAL PROCEDURES

The first account of hypospadias surgery was by Heliodorus and Antyllus (100–200 A.D.). The repair consisted of amputation of the shaft distal to the existing meatus. Dieffenbach (1838) pierced the glans to the normal urethral meatus, allowing a cannula to remain in position until the channel became lined with epithelium—an unsuccessful procedure. Mettauer (1842) suggested that the "organ be liberated by multiple subcutaneous incisions," whereas Bouisson (1861) was the first to suggest a transverse incision at the point of greatest curvature. He also reported the use of scrotal tissue to reconstruct the urethra. Thiersch (1869) described local tissue flaps to repair epispadias, a technique he later used in hypospadias. Thiersch suggested that perineal urinary diversion be done to temporarily divert the urine away from the urethral reconstruction. He also did the first buttonhole flap in the prepuce to allow resurfacing of the ventrum of the penis with the prepuce.

Duplay (1874) utilized Bouisson's technique to release chordee and, as a later stage, formed a central flap, which was tubed and then covered with lateral penile flaps. He also stated that it did not matter if the central tube was incompletely formed because he believed epithelialization would occur to form a channel if the tube was buried under lateral flaps; this technique was later popularized by Denis Browne (1950). Wood (1875) described a meatal-based flap to form the urethral channel and combined this with the Thiersch-type buttonhole flap to cover the raw surface—a technique quite similar to that of Ombredanne (1932) and of Mathieu (1932).

Rosenberger (1891), Landerer (1891), Bidder (1892), and Bucknall (1907) all used scrotal tissue for urethroplasty and described burying the penis in the scrotum to obtain skin coverage, similar to the techniques of Leveuf (1936) and Cecil-Culp (1951).

Hook (1896) described a vascularized preputial flap for urethroplasty, similar to the Davis procedure (1950). Hook further suggested the lateral oblique flap from the side of the penis, later popularized by Broadbent (1951).

Beck and Hacker (1897) undermined and advanced the urethra onto the glans for subcoronal cases, similar to the technique of Waterhouse and Glassberg (1981). Beck (1897) and White and Martin (1917) employed adjacent rotation flaps from the scrotum for resurfacing after a Duplay-type urethroplasty, similar to those of Marberger and Pauer (1981) and Turner-Warwick (1979). Nove-Josserand (1897 and 1914) reported attempts to repair hypospadias with split-thickness grafts, similar to the technique of McIndoe (1937). Rochet (1899) chose a large, distally based scrotal flap for urethroplasty and buried this in a tunnel on the ventral surface of the penis. Edmunds (1913) was the first to transfer the skin of the prepuce to the ventral surface of the penis at the time of release of chordee. This abundant ventral skin was then used in a Duplay-type urethroplasty at a later stage, similar to techniques by Blair (1933) and, later, Byars (1955). Bevan (1917) utilized a urethral meatal-based flap channeled through the glans for distal repair, similar to the procedure by Mustarde (1965). References for the aforementioned review are found in Horton, Devine, and Baran (1973).

Multi-Staged Repairs

In the standard two-stage repair, the chordee release (orthoplasty) was accomplished by dividing the urethral plate distal to the meatus, straightening the penis, and allowing the meatus to retract to a more proximal position. Skin cover of the ventrum was achieved by mobilizing the dorsal preputial and penile skin around to the ventrum to be available in a later urethroplasty. Because the modern technique of artificial erection (Gittes and McLaughlin, 1974) was not used, residual chordee was not an unusual result of this urethroplasty. Secondary chordee releases were required before proceeding to form the urethra.

Denis Browne (1953) was very influential in promoting the "buried strip" principle for hypospadias repair. A ventral strip of skin was covered by generous mobilized skin flaps brought together in the midline with "beads and stops." The channel under the skin flaps would epithelialize around a stenting catheter left in place for 3 to 6 weeks. Results were never very satisfactory until Van der Meulen (1964) demonstrated that a rotated skin cover from the dorsum with an eccentric suture line would offer more successful healing. In fact, he avoids stenting and diversion of urine and has the patient void through the repair, leaving only subcutaneous drains for several days. The lifetime results are dramatic—no fistulas (Van der Muelen, 1982)!

Byars (1955) further developed the two-stage method by extending the foreskin onto the glans in the first stage and rolling a complete tube in the second. Durham Smith (1973, 1990) refined the Byars approach by denuding the epithelium on one skin edge to allow "double-breasting" of raw surfaces. Smith's review (1990) of 503 repairs with only 1.8 per cent fistulas, 7.6 per cent meatal stenoses, and 1 per cent incomplete chordee correction is commendable.

In 1955, Elmer Belt devised a technique that he never published but which gained acclaim after Fuqua (1971) published his series. Hendren (1981) had the largest series with excellent results.

Numerous other methods have been introduced to repair hypospadias. Creevy (1958) and Backus and DeFelice (1960) provide excellent reviews of the multistaged procedures performed up to 1960. A complete review up to 1970 is reported by Horton, Devine, and Baran (1973). All of these methods must be studied to understand the pitfalls of this difficult surgery. However, emphasis in this chapter is placed on the one-stage methods that are currently popular.

One-Stage Repairs

In the late 1950s, when surgeons were more confident of their ability to remove chordee tissue in its entirety, one-stage hypospadias procedures became popular. In 1900, Russell described a procedure for one-stage repair of hypospadias, using a urethral tube constructed from a flap that was developed on the ventral surface of the penis. This flap extended around the entire circumference of the corona to include a cuff of the prepuce. This new urethra was placed through a tunnel in the glans and secured to the tip of the glans. Broadbent, Woolf, and Toksu (1961) created a urethral tube from the skin of the penis and prepuce and laid this tube into the split glans. Des Prez, Persky, and Kiehn (1961) developed a one-stage procedure similar to that of Broadbent and associates (1961). In 1954, McCormack reported a two-

stage procedure in which a full-thickness tube graft urethroplasty was placed at the first procedure, but the proximal anastomosis closure was delayed. In 1955, Devine and Horton developed this technique further by using a free graft of preputial skin to replace the urethra after release of chordee; they then completed this McCormack procedure in one stage (1961). In 1970 and 1972, Hodgson described three different procedures that utilized vascularized flaps from the dorsal prepuce as well as penile skin. This urethral flap was brought to the ventral aspect with a buttonhole transposition (Hodgson, 1975).

One-stage hypospadias repair has withstood the test of time, supporting the feasibility of this type of surgery. Besides the desirability of completing the reconstruction in one operation, a one-stage procedure has the additional advantage of using skin that is unscarred from previous surgical procedures, the normal blood supply of which has not been disrupted. The main impediment to the success of this procedure, inadequate chordee release, has been nearly eliminated since the introduction of the artificial erection technique (Gittes and McLaughlin, 1974).

TREATMENT OF HYPOSPADIAS

The object of therapy is to construct a straight penis with the meatus as close as possible to the normal site to allow a forward-directed stream and normal coitus. Culp and McRoberts (1968) stated, "It is the inalienable right of every boy to be a pointer instead of a sitter by the time he starts school and to write his name legibly in the snow."

"Hypospadiology" is liberally sprinkled with eponyms, each representing a symbol for a technique or principle. It seems appropriate to continue this descriptive method so entrenched in surgery today. There have likely been over 200 reported original methods of urethral reconstruction, and they continue today as modifications of modifications. Although certain surgeons have arrived at perfection, their success has not been accepted or at least transferable to colleagues. David M. Davis wrote in 1951, "I would like to say that I believe the time has arrived to state that the surgical repair of hypospadias is no longer dubious, unreliable, or extremely difficult. If tried and proven methods are scrupulously followed, a good result should be obtained in every case. Anything less than this suggests that the surgeon is not temperamentally fitted for this kind of surgery." So much depends on experience, but even more so, a familiarity with all the options available. Indeed, with this familiarity as a prerequisite, hypospadiology would be an appropriate term for this discipline (Duckett, 1981a).

The phases of surgical repair include (1) meatoplasty and glanuloplasty, (2) orthoplasty (straightening), (3) urethroplasty, (4) skin cover, and (5) scrotoplasty. These various elements of surgical technique can be applied sequentially or in various combinations to achieve a surgical success.

Meatoplasty and Glanuloplasty

For many years, the two-staged techniques (e.g., Byars, 1955; Denis Browne, 1953) left the meatus just beneath the glans. Currently, an effort has been made to move the meatus to the tip, particularly in the more extensive one-stage repairs (e.g., Devine and Horton, 1961; Duckett, 1980a). Even with distal hypospadias, the trend is to achieve the same goal in patients with relatively minor defects. The meatal advancement and glanuloplasty (MAGPI) procedure (Duckett, 1981b) have come under considerable scrutiny in this regard. Using electronic video photography, MacMillan and co-workers (1985) recorded high-speed pictures of urinary streams after the MAGPI repair and concluded that the excellent cosmetic results are achieved with preservation of normal voiding.

Several differing techniques are known with which to achieve an apical meatus, depending on the variation of the proximal meatus (Gibbons and Gonzales, 1983). The *triangularized glans* (Devine and Horton, 1961) achieves a flap meatoplasty and avoids a circumferential meatal closure. Glans wings are developed, which wrap around the neourethra on the ventrum. Although this maneuver avoids meatal stenosis, the glans is flattened with distortion of the normal configuration. *Extension of the meatus onto the ventral glans* may be done with either a meatal-based flap (Mathieu) or onlay vascularized flap as described later. In this case, a strip of urethral plate remains in between the glans wings onto which a roof of urethra is placed with a glans wrap closure. The *glans split* (Barcat, 1973; Redman, 1987) permits the urethral extension to be placed deeper in the glans tissue. The *glans fillet* described by Turner-Warwick (1979) and Cronin and Guthrie (1973) is a two-stage procedure that lays preputial skin onto the ventrum of the spatulated glans. The meatus can later be tubularized and the glans closed over it to achieve a quite normal-appearing glans with an apical meatus. This technique is more applicable to the adult penis requiring redo.

The *glans channel* technique to deliver the urethra to the apex is another method. Bevan (1917) devised a technique that created a proximal penile flap, which was converted into a urethral tube and pulled through a tunnel in the glans. Mays (1951) employed a staged technique that straightened the penis, bringing the prepuce over the glans to cover the ventral defect and constructing a preputial flap for a glanular urethra that was carried through a tunnel to the tip of the glans. Davis (1940, 1951) developed a similar procedure. Both Ricketson (1958) and Hendren (1981) have channeled a full-thickness skin tube through the glans. Hinderer (1971) employs a trocar to tunnel, entering the glans at the tip and emerging a few millimeters below the coronal sulcus through a "trap-door" flap of albuginea. Duckett (1980a, b, and c) combined the glans channel with a transverse preputial island flap.

In the more distal cases of hypospadias, the configuration of the glans may dictate the type of meatoplasty. If the glans furrow is deep, a Mathieu procedure may be preferred. In contrast, if the glans is broad and flat, an onlay island flap technique will allow rolling of the glans around the glanular vascularized two-faced tube.

Orthoplasty

Curvature (Chordee)

The curvature of the penis is caused by a deficiency of the normal structures on the ventrum of the penis. Factors contributing include skin deficiency, dartos fascia fibrosis, and true fibrous chordee with tethering of the ventral shaft or corpora cavernosa disproportion.

The role played by skin deficiency is especially striking in manipulation of the penis without artificial erection, which creates an apparent curvature of the tip. The skin and fibrous dartos fascia beneath will together contribute to curvature with artificial erection, which is relieved after skin drop back (Allen and Spence, 1968).

Fibrous Chordee

When associated with hypospadias, chordee has commonly been attributed to hypoplasia of the corpus spongiosum distal to the hypospadiac meatus. This situation results in a midline fibrous band or fan-shaped area of fibrosis, tethering the penis ventrally. When this tissue is excised *(orthoplasty)*, the penis straightens. This simplified explanation is not altogether applicable to the variety of expressions of hypospadias or pure chordee without hypospadias. Certainly, the concept of a "bowstring" tethering that requires a simple incision is not true.

Kaplan and Lamm (1975) put forth a convincing case that chordee may indeed be an arrest of normal embryologic development analogous to failure of testicular descent. Thus, fibrosis is conspicuously absent in some clinical cases of chordee. Chordee may also result from differential growth of the dorsal and ventral aspect of the corpora (Bellinger, 1981), best corrected by shortening the dorsal tunica albuginea.

Devine and Horton (1973) proposed three types of chordee, but this distinction has not been widely accepted.

Artificial Erection

Introduced in 1974 by Gittes and McLaughlin, artificial erection has been a very significant contribution to orthoplasty. By placing a tourniquet at the base of the penis and injecting a corpus cavernosum with saline, both corporal bodies fill and it is possible to determine the extent of chordee and the success of chordee correction. The assurance of complete correction is essential to proceed to a one-stage repair with urethroplasty. So far there has been no report of damage to the cavernous tissue by this technique. It has also been used extensively in adults with no untoward effects. Care must be taken to assure that normal saline is used. Penile necrosis occurred when 50 per cent saline was injected inadvertently. Injecting through the glans on the side of the shaft avoids hematoma formation.

Technique for Orthoplasty

For true fibrous chordee, the penis is curved ventrally with only a short distance between the location of the meatus and the glans. An incision is made around the corona, and carried well below the glans cap just distal to the urethral meatus and down to the tunica albuginea of the corpora cavernosa. Proximal dissection is then achieved, freeing the fibrous plaque of tissue closely adherent to the tunica albuginea with sharp dissection, moving from side to side as the ventral curvature is released. The urethra is elevated from the corpora in this en bloc dissection. In most cases, the chordee tissue surrounds the urethral meatus and extends proximally along the urethra for a distance. This tissue should all be freed well down to the penoscrotal junction and many times into the scrotoperineal area. Once this urethral mobilization is accomplished, the shaft of the penis should be stripped of any fibrous tissue, extending out to the lateral shaft of the penis and distally below the glans. Artificial erection tests the success of this excision.

Several further "tricks" have been offered for releasing the last bit of bend. A midline incision along the septum between the two corpora cavernosa has, in some cases, been effective (Devine, 1983). Lateral incisions in a stepwise manner may be effective in the groove between the dorsal corpora and the ventral aspect.

If, after adequate excision of all abnormal fibrous tissue, artificial erection continues to demonstrate curvature, corporal disproportion is present. This should be corrected by *dorsal plication*. Buck's fascia is elevated on either side of the midline (10 o'clock and 2 o'clock) to avoid the neurovascular bundle. Parallel incisions are made through the tunica albuginea about 8 mm long and 5 to 8 mm apart. The outer edges of the incisions are sutured together with permanent interrupted sutures (5-0 Prolene). This symmetrically tucks the dorsum to correct the ventral bend.

In the rare case, there is so much deficiency of the tunica albuginea on the ventrum that excision of the tunica albuginea is required with replacement by dermal graft or with tunica vaginalis (Hendren and Keating, 1988). Tunica vaginalis is obtained by exposing the testis and removing a patch of the tunica from around the testis.

Once the chordee has been released, a urethroplasty may proceed in the one-stage repair if a vascularized neourethra is used. If a dermal graft has been placed on the ventrum, a free full-thickness skin neourethra will likely not succeed.

Congenital Curvature of the Penis (Chordee Without Hypospadias)

Congenital curvature of the penis without hypospadias is quite rare. Much more common in adults are the secondary curvatures associated with Peyronie's disease, or periurethral sclerosis associated with urethral stricture. There are two kinds of primary curvature: those associated with a normal urethral spongiosum and those with a hypoplastic urethra.

Primary curvature with a normal corpus spongiosum comprises two thirds of congenital curvatures. The penis when flaccid looks normal with a circular prepuce. During erection, the penis is usually curved downward but may have a lateral curvature of as much as 90 degrees. An upward curvature (without epispadias) is exceptional (Udall, 1980). This deformity becomes noticeable to the adolescent or young adult. However, many find little difficulty with intercourse with this condition. The lateral deviations seen in about one third of cases are almost always to the left. With erection, disproportion of the corpora cavernosa is usually apparent.

Physiologic ventral curvature of the penis in the fetus has been noted at different stages of development (Kaplan and Brock, 1981; Kaplan and Lamm, 1975). It usually disappears by birth yet may be found in premature infants more commonly. Within the first several years of life, this curvature slowly disappears (Cendron and Mclin, 1981).

In cases in which the urethra is normal, treatment varies with the direction of the deviation and whether one believes that true chordee tissue is responsible for the ventral bend (Devine and Horton, 1975). Good results have been reported by Devine and Horton with resection of fibrous dartos fascia beneath and beside the mobilized normal urethra. However, this rather extensive dissection does not offer consistent results (Kramer et al., 1982).

More accepted has been the concept Nesbit described in 1965 of taking tucks or plicating the disproportionally large tunica albuginea. This technique was first described by Philip Syng Physick, the "Father of American Surgery," in the early 19th century. He treated chordee by shortening the dorsal tunica albuginea (Pancoast, 1844). When the arc of maximum curvature is located with artificial erection, wedges of tunica albuginea are excised in a stepwise fashion. These diamond-shaped wedges are closed transversely with permanent suture until the penis is straight. It is possible to plicate the fascia without cutting the tunica by placing several rows of sutures at the maximum convex side. Nesbit (1966), however, reported long-term follow-up with this method as disappointing. Exposure for the surgical approach is achieved by retracting the penile skin toward the base as a sleeve.

The age at which this defect should be corrected is important. Cendron believes it should not be done too early for two reasons: the curvature may spontaneously improve with age, and there is risk of disturbing the growth of the phallus by altering the tunica of the corpora. Both of these reasons suggest that it is better to do the repair after puberty.

Primary curvature with a hypoplastic urethra comprises about one third of these congenital curvature cases (Cendron and Melin, 1981). In this type, the urethral meatus is well situated on the glans, but the foreskin is incomplete and the ventral penis is not normal. The skin covering the urethra is very thin, and there is no spongiosal tissue for a long portion. Chordee is present with erection. Lengthening the frenulum and eliminating the penoscrotal web does not alter the curvature. Because the segment of urethra is hypoplastic, it may be considered a "concealed" hypospadias. Congenitally short urethra is another term for this condition.

For the hypospastic urethra or short urethra variant of congenital curvature, a chordee release with division of the midportion of the hypoplastic urethra is required. Urethroplasty employing the same techniques applicable to the usual hypospadias anomaly will follow. I prefer to replace the midurethral segment with an island flap from the ventral prepuce, making two oblique anastomoses with the remaining good proximal and distal urethral segments, and leaving the meatus naturally on the glans.

Urethroplasty

After orthoplasty, when the proximal meatus retracts near or below the penoscrotal junction, there are three basic categories for urethroplasty techniques: (1) adjacent skin flaps, (2) free skin grafts, and (3) mobilized vascular flaps.

Skin adjacent to the meatus may be tubularized for the neourethra similar to techniques of Broadbent and colleagues (1961) and Des Prez and co-workers (1961) in their one-stage procedures.

Free skin grafts should be full-thickness rather than split-thickness. Devine (1983) has had a successful experience for more than 25 years using the inner preputial skin detached and defatted as a thin full-thickness graft to form the neourethra. His good results have not been reproducible in uniform manner in the hands of others (Filmer et al., 1977; Rober et al., 1990; Redman, 1983; Woodard and Cleveland, 1982). Because the free graft must be revascularized, the key element to success is perfect skin cover of the graft with well-vascularized dorsal preputial and penile skin. Humby (1941) described full-thickness graft taken from the inner surface of the arm or groin as a urethroplasty done in one stage.

Vascularized flaps of preputial or penile skin may be mobilized to the ventrum for the urethroplasty. Hodgson (1970) chose the inner face prepuce in a vertical orientation with a tumble flap technique (Hodgson I). He later added the vertically oriented dorsal penile skin urethra (Hodgson II and III techniques), which were transposed to the ventrum with a buttonhole maneuver (Hodgson, 1972 and 1975).

Asopa and co-workers (1971) employed a vascularized flap attached to the outer prepuce but not freed as an island flap. In this Asopa technique, the ventral preputial skin is rolled into a tube, left attached to the penile skin, and spiraled around to the ventrum. The results were asymmetric and bulky.

Skin Cover

Once the urethroplasty has been accomplished, the ventral surface of the penis must be resurfaced with skin. Because of the abundant dorsal foreskin, coverage may be achieved by mobilizing the penile and preputial

skin to the ventrum, in most cases. The skin may be transferred by one of several techniques.

The preputial tissue may be transposed by opening a small *buttonhole* in the midline, spreading the vasculature laterally and bringing the glans penis through the buttonhole. Transposition in this manner is first credited to Thiersch (1869). However, Ombredanne (1932), Nesbit (1941), and Mustarde (1965) also selected this method. The well-vascularized dorsal preputial tissue will resurface the ventrum. The major drawback, however, is the lateral edges, which are difficult to fashion without leaving bulky wedges of skin. One must be cautious not to trim these lateral pedicles too much at this stage and risk devascularizing the flap. I have abandoned this technique.

The prepuce may be split vertically taking care not to disturb the vertically oriented vessels. The bipedicled preputial skin may be brought around to the ventrum for resurfacing (see Fig. 50–12). If this is done in a symmetric fashion for the first stage of a two-stage procedure (as in the Blair-Byars technique), redundant preputial skin is relocated on the distal shaft and glans (Smith, 1981 and 1990). If, however, this technique is utilized to cover a urethroplasty in a one-stage technique, there is sometimes difficulty in overlapping these flaps to make the symmetry acceptable. The "bear-hug" arrangement of the two flaps above and below each other avoids a midline suture (Fig. 50–3) (Devine, 1983). Likewise, an eccentric preputial split, which is transposed to the ventrum, will avoid a midline suture line, as described by King (1981) and by Marberger and Pauer (1981). When a well-vascularized neourethra is created, the concern for a midline closure is nullified. We, therefore, fashion a split dorsal prepuce/penile flap, which frees the ventral skin for a midline closure, excising the distal preputial skin edges (see Fig. 50–12).

Ventral skin cover may also be achieved by rotation of the entire penile and preputial skin in a spiral method around to the ventrum. Van der Meulen (1971, 1982), Asopa and colleagues (1971), and Hodgson (1981) (see Figs. 50–10 and 50–11) use this technique. In the Hodgson XX and the Asopa techniques, the neourethra is attached to the dorsal preputial or penile skin (see Fig. 50–13).

Fortunately, the healing of the penile skin and preputial layers is generally quite satisfactory without unsightly scarring or hypertrophic thickening. The scars usually blend in with the coloring of the penile skin and are quite unnoticeable. It is possible, for instance, as Denis Browne (1953) has demonstrated, to incise the dorsal penile skin down the midline, relaxing the tension on the ventral skin. This dorsal defect will epithelialize with very little scarring. Although this technique is rarely needed, the results have been helpful in understanding penile scarring. Skin graft of such a defect is not needed.

When an inner preputial island flap is developed, the lateral tips of the outer preputial skin may be devascularized to a certain degree. Although the edges of these flaps are discarded in most cases, sometimes the poor vascularization extends farther than anticipated. There may be a slough of this ventrally positioned preputial skin, and in our experience, the neourethra is well vascularized and does not suffer. When the eschar is

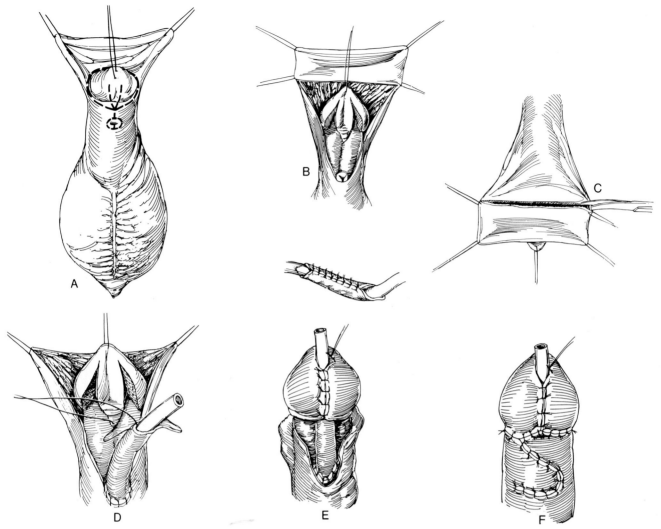

Figure 50–3. Horton-Devine free skin graft. *A,* A circumferential incision is made around the corona, and a dart of glans is developed. *B,* Triangularized glans wings are mobilized and chordee is released, dropping the meatus proximally. The inner preputial skin is outlined. *C,* The inner preputial skin is dissected free of its blood supply and defatted to make a full-thickness free skin graft (see inset). *D,* The proximal meatus is spatulated and fixed to the tunica albuginea. The glans wings are further developed. The free graft is anastomosed to the proximal urethra in an oblique fashion and distally to the triangularized glans flaps, as depicted. *E,* Glans wings are brought around the distal urethral extension onto the glans. *F,* Byars flaps are brought around the ventrum to cover the skin defect. (From Hinman, F., Jr.: Atlas of Urologic Surgery. Philadelphia, W.B. Saunders Co., 1989, pp. 58–60.)

removed, this area epithelializes, similar to the Denis Browne experience on the dorsum. Hinman (1991) has warned of this and recommends leaving the outer and inner preputial edges attached.

Using the double-faced preputial island flap technique provides symmetric skin cover with the pedicle undisturbed (see Fig. 50–13). The outer preputial skin, the distal edges of which may have a precarious blood supply in the island flap technique, is left attached to the joint blood supply to the inner prepuce. Thus, when transposed to the ventrum, the thicker outer preputial skin serves as a skin cover of the ventral midportion of penile shaft, and the dorsal penile skin covers the rest. Unfortunately, our results with the double-faced island flap procedure have not been as optimal as anticipated.

The older technique of burying the ventral penis in the scrotum for skin coverage, as exemplified by the Culp (1959) technique, is helpful on occasion. A midline incision is made into the scrotum. The subcutaneous

tissue of the dartos fascia of the scrotum is fixed to the dartos fascia on the penis in one layer. The skin edges are closed. Two layers must be closed to prevent the penis from pulling on the skin edges too much. At a later time (3 to 6 months), the penis is lifted from the scrotal trough. The penile skin is sufficiently mobile to bring together on the penile surface in the midline. No scrotal skin is transposed to the penis in this fashion. It is used only when penile skin is deficient. Marberger and Pauer (1981) and Turner-Warwick (1972) have both employed scrotal flaps to cover penile deficiencies, but these are mainly in adults and for secondary procedures. Marberger and Pauer showed the usefulness of asymmetric rotational scrotal flaps (1981).

Scrotoplasty

The final element to complete the hypospadias repair is needed only rarely. Penoscrotal transposition needs

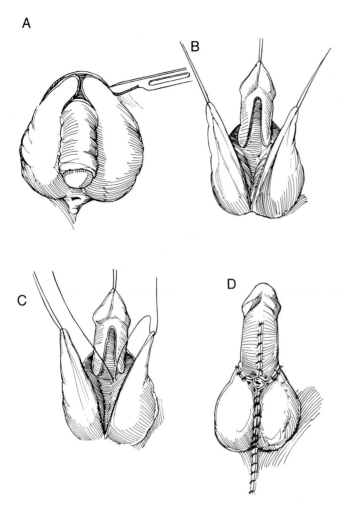

Figure 50–4. Scrotoplasty. *A,* Flaps of scrotal skin above and lateral to the penis are incised. *B,* Generous mobilization of these flaps will transpose them to beneath the penis. *C,* The bifid scrotum is freed so the midline will be flat. *D,* Chromic closure is done excising excess flaps to improve cosmesis. (From Hinman, F., Jr.: Atlas of Urologic Surgery. Philadelphia, W.B. Saunders Co., 1990, pp. 62–64.)

to be corrected when the penis is engulfed between the two scrotal halves. Because this phase is dependent on rotational skin flaps adjacent to the penile skin, it is best to perform a second stage after the urethroplasty and orthoplasty have healed. The lateral scrotal extension above the penile shaft is rotated beneath the penis, and the lateral skin edges are moved medially toward the penis (Ehrlich and Scardino, 1982; Koyanagi et al., 1984; Marshall et al., 1979; Nonomura et al., 1988) (Fig. 50–4).

TECHNIQUES FOR ANTERIOR HYPOSPADIAS

Anterior hypospadias comprises approximately 65 per cent of cases of hypospadias. The most common lesion appears with a proximal glanular or subcoronal meatus, a glanular distal groove, and a transverse web resulting in deflection of the urethral stream at 30 to 40 degrees downward. Meatal stenosis and penile torsion may also be present. In many instances, the ventral skin is somewhat deficient, causing superficial tethering and apparent chordee. After this is released and its glanular extensions are freed, the majority of these cases will be straight. If chordee persists, of course, division of the urethral plate distal to the meatus would drop the meatus more proximally and thereby change the anterior hypospadias classification.

Meatal Advancement and Glanuloplasty

Most of the more distal cases (glanular and subcoronal meatuses) can be managed with the meatal advancement and glanuloplasty (MAGPI) procedure. The decision to use this standard MAGPI procedure depends on the mobility of the urethra. This is tested with fine forceps and distal traction on the lateral lifts of the meatus. If immobile, a proper advancement cannot be achieved because the distal glans must then be brought proximally to meet the meatus, giving the glans a depressed or flattened appearance (MacMillan et al., 1985).

MAGPI Technique (Fig. 50–5)

It is helpful to instill 1:100,000 of epinephrine in 1 per cent lidocaine (Xylocaine), particularly in the glans tissue, to assist in hemostasis. For the meatal advancement, a generous longitudinal incision is made from inside the dorsal edge of the meatus to the distal glans groove. Sometimes this tissue is thickened, and a wedge is removed instead of a vertical incision. This step effectively obliterates the bridge of tissue that deflects the urinary stream ventrally. The dorsal meatal edge is left with a "V" configuration that enlarges it, correcting any stenosis. The dorsal wall of the urethra is advanced to the apex of the glanular groove in a transverse fashion and closed with 6-0 chromic suture. This procedure effects a Heineke-Mikulicz transverse closure of the vertical incision. The dorsal meatal edge is now flattened

Figure 50–5. Meatoplasty and glanuloplasty repair (MAGPI). *A,* Circumferential subcoronal incision 5 to 8 mm below corona. *B,* Dissection of dartos fascia fibrosis causing tethering of the ventral glans. *C,* Vertical incision in the glanular groove out to the tip and down into the stenotic meatus. *D,* Transverse advancement of the dorsal meatal wall into the apical extent of the diamond-shaped defect. *E,* Glanuloplasty. Conical reconfiguration of the glans is made by ventral rotation of the glanular wings. Excess ventral skin is excised up to glanular margin, and deep Vicryl sutures are placed in glanular tissue to bring deep glans together in the midline. *F,* Superficial horizontal mattress sutures finish the glans approximation with 7–0 chromic sutures. *G,* Sleeve re-approximation of the penile skin with excision of excess foreskin is the usual case. *H,* Alternative rotation of dorsal skin around to the ventrum for midline closure (Byars technique with dorsal preputial midline split). *I,* Rotation of dorsal skin around to ventrum. *J,* Excision of excess skin. *K,* Midline closure and circumferential closure. (From Hinman, F., Jr.: Atlas of Urologic Surgery. Philadelphia, W.B. Saunders Co., 1990, pp. 37–40.)

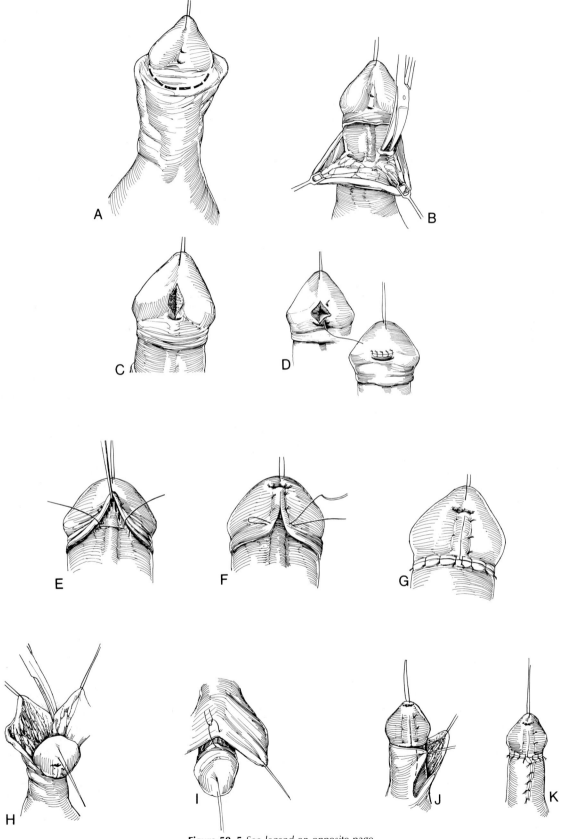

Figure 50–5 *See legend on opposite page*

into the glanular groove so that the stream is not deflected, and the meatus is advanced and enlarged.

A circumferential incision is made approximately 6 to 8 mm from the coronal edge and proximal to the meatus. Extreme care must be taken in dissecting the thin skin over the urethra because it is not difficult to injure the urethra. A "drop back" of the penile skin is accomplished by dissecting in a sleeve-like fashion between the dartos fascia and the layer of subcutaneous tissue of the prepuce. Torsion may be corrected by carrying this drop back to the base of the penis.

The *glanuloplasty* portion of the procedure is accomplished by placing a small holding stitch on the ventral meatal edge and retracting this toward the glans. The lateral edges of the glans form an inverted "V" in this fashion and can be brought together in the midline, bringing glanular tissue beneath the meatus to advance and support it. The redundant skin on these lateral glans edges is removed. The glanular tissue is approximated with deep polyglycolic sutures and a more superficial chromic layer for the skin edges. Sleeve re-approximation of the skin is usually accomplished. Sometimes, a limited rotation of preputial skin to the ventrum may be necessary to cover a ventral skin defect.

No diversion is required for the MAGPI procedure nor is an elaborate dressing. The penis is wrapped with a petroleum jelly (Vaseline) gauze for 48 hours.

In 1990 (Duckett), we reported a total of 1111 MAGPI procedures with a complication rate of 1.2 per cent. This is a secondary surgery rate. In four cases, fistulas occurred. The main complication is glanular breakdown with retraction of the meatus. This can be avoided by placing the deep stitches of glanular tissue in the glanuloplasty.

Preservation of the foreskin is requested by parents, more commonly among Europeans. Preservation is possible in combination with the MAGPI procedure. Polus and Lotte (1965) also demonstrated foreskin preservation in a combined procedure similar to the Mathieu procedure.

The Arap Modification of the MAGPI
(Fig. 50–6)

The Arap modification of the MAGPI procedure was designed for a more proximal meatus that requires some urethral extension (Arap et al., 1984). Two ventral skin wings are brought together in the midline as an "M" configuration and used as the floor of the urethra. A glanuloplasty is then brought around this. We have not been very satisfied with this modification because it leaves a very large meatus and a glans configuration that is not as normal as possible. We would prefer a Mathieu or an onlay procedure in these situations.

Urethral Mobilization

Another method of dealing with the subcoronal meatus is by distal urethral mobilization. Reported almost 100 years ago by Beck and Hacker (1897) and Beck (1917), urethral mobilization was revived by Belman (1977), Waterhouse and Glassberg (1981), Koff (1981), Nasrallah and Minott (1984), DeSy and Oosterlinck (1985), and Spencer and Perlmutter (1990). This technique requires mobilization of the penile urethra to obtain an extensive enough mobilization to advance this to the tip of the penis. The meatal stenosis rate is significant.

Parameatal-Based Flap (Mathieu Procedure) (Fig. 50–7)

When the meatus is too proximal on the shaft to achieve a MAGPI procedure, and there is no chordee by artificial erection, the meatus may be advanced onto the glans as described by Mathieu (1932) and as reported by Hoffman and Hall (1973), Kim and Hendren (1981), Wacksman (1981), Gonzales and co-workers (1983), Devine (1983), Brueziere (1987), and Kass and Bolong (1990).

A strip of urethral plate is left on the glanular groove with glans wings developed on either side. This midline strip is about 5 mm in width. A flap of parameatal skin is raised proximal to the meatus, taking care to preserve the vascular subcutaneous tissue. The proximal flap closes into the glans groove as do the leaves of a book, and two suture closures are made on either side of the flap, extending the meatus to the tip of the glans. Preserving the vasculature of the flap is important. The lateral glans wings will come together for closure over the urethral advancement, and deep and superficial sutures are required. Appropriate skin cover is achieved. We use urinary diversion for 5 to 7 days, but others have shown that no diversion is needed (Rabinowitz, 1987). Results with the Mathieu procedure are quite successful. We have a 6 per cent complication rate (Elder et al., 1987).

Redman (1987) has revived the Barcat (1973) modification of the Mathieu by mobilizing a glans flap in addition to the parameatal flap, and splitting the glans dorsally to bury the urethral extension farther to the apex of the glans.

Megameatus Intact Prepuce (MIP)

In 6 per cent of cases of anterior hypospadias, the prepuce is intact and a megameatus exists under the normal foreskin with a wide glanular defect (Duckett and Keating, 1989). These anomalies may be recognized only after circumcision is performed. The correction, therefore, is more complex.

We have reported a technique that we call the Pyramid dissection (Fig. 50–8), indicating that the distal megameatus needs to be mobilized carefully down into the shaft of the penis and the distal urethra reduced in caliber to a more normal size. In doing this, an extension of the urethra can be made onto the glans; glanular wings are developed and brought around this repair. A very normal-appearing glans can be achieved. Urinary diversion is in place for 5 days. The success with this

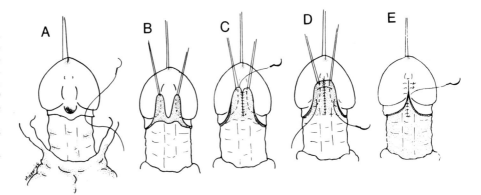

Figure 50–6. Modified MAGPI (Arap) procedure. *A,* Meatal advancement may be unnecessary. Two traction sutures are placed on perimeatal cuff after circumferential incision. *B* and *C,* Distal traction allows re-approximation in the midline. *D* and *E,* Glans re-approximated over the neourethra in two layers. (From Keating, M. A., and Duckett, J. W.: Recent advances in the repair of hypospadias. *In* Nyhus, L. (Ed.): Surgery Annuals, vol. 22. East Norwalk, CT, Appleton and Lange. In press.)

technique has been quite satisfactory with two fistulas in 47 repairs.

Onlay Island Flap Urethral Extension
(Fig. 50–9)

If there is no chordee, but the meatus is too proximal for a Mathieu procedure or the ventral skin is too thin for a flap, a procedure to replace the ventral urethra is required. The urethral plate in this situation may be left intact. A strip of urethral plate onto the glans will serve as the dorsal urethral wall, whereas the ventral urethral wall is created by a vascularized island flap of tissue from the inner prepuce. A U-shaped closure extends the meatus to the glans tip. Glanular tissue is wrapped around the new urethral tube in such a way that a suitable conical glans can be obtained (Duckett, 1986; Elder et al., 1987).

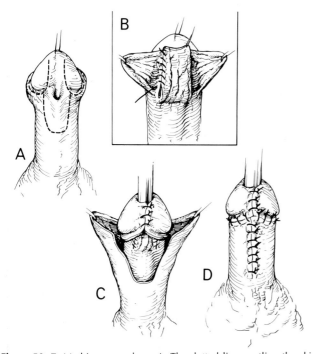

Figure 50–7. Mathieu procedure. *A,* The dotted lines outline the skin flaps. *B,* The proximal flap is rotated, and the lateral glans flaps are developed. *C,* The glans flaps cover the neourethra, and preputial skin is moved if necessary. *D,* Completed repair.

Such a technique will cover a rather long strip on the ventrum if the proximal urethra is deficient (Hollowell et al., 1990). Even though the proximal meatus may be located near the corona, the urethra should be opened back to good spongiosum tissue, discarding the thin ventral urethra. This method can be chosen only when there is no chordee.

Our current results with this onlay flap technique have been satisfactory with the secondary surgical rate of 5 to 6 per cent. In most of these cases, the urethral meatus is in the middle third of the shaft (Elder et al., 1987; Hollowell et al., 1990). Other techniques to extend the distal meatus with hypospadias include tubularization of the distal urethral plate into a full tube with skin cover by various means (Belman and King, 1979). Nesbit (1966) described this method, as did King (1970 and 1981), and Perlmutter and Vatz (1975).

We have found the versatility of the onlay island flap procedure quite useful and have employed this technique more often. The results are excellent, with a 5 to 6 per cent complication rate even with the more proximal technique. The ability to take some dorsal tucks in the tunica albuginea to correct residual chordee makes this procedure versatile.

The Devine-Horton Flip-Flap Procedure

This technique with triangularization of the glans was quite popular in the past, but it has not been used even by its originators (Devine, 1983). It is of historic interest only.

The Mustarde Procedure

This procedure should more appropriately be called the Bevan (1917) procedure, but it carries the eponym of Mustarde (1965) because he popularized the technique. This technique is a more extensive Mathieu procedure with tubularization of the proximal parameatal-based flap. This procedure is chosen in cases in which chordee is present distal to the meatus, permitting the tubularized flap to be hinged forward and channeled through the glans. The main criticism of the technique is in the viability of the pedicle flap, which is likely to be compromised as it goes through the glans channel. Distal meatal stenosis is a common problem. We have

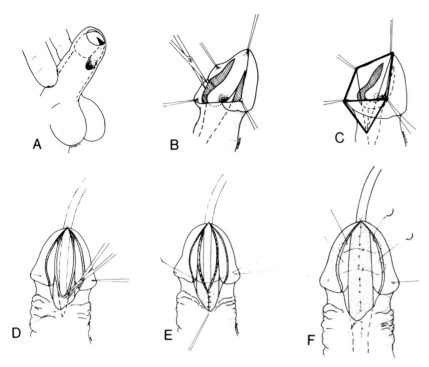

Figure 50–8. Pyramid procedure. *A*, Megameatus intact prepuce (MIP) variant. Intact prepuce conceals an often impressive anomaly. *B* and *C*, Traction sutures define the megameatus and pyramid base. *D*, Sharp dissection to the apex of the pyramid mobilizes urethra and glans wings. Widened distal urethra is tapered. *E*, Neourethra created by tubularizing the urethral plate. *F*, Repair completed by two-layer glans re-approximation. (From Duckett, J. W., and Keating, M. A.: Technical challenge of the megameatus intact prepuce hypospadias (MIP) variant: The pyramid procedure. J. Urol., 141:1407–1409, 1989.)

found the Mustarde technique appropriate for some secondary cases combining resection of residual chordee and retrusive meatus.

TECHNIQUES FOR MIDDLE HYPOSPADIAS

A surprising number of cases have no chordee, and urethral extension can be done with the onlay island flap technique. Other procedures for this situation are described by King (1970 and 1981), and Perlmutter and Vatz (1975). Nesbit (1966) also described a urethral extension. The Hodgson II procedure is an onlay flap employing preputial skin in a vertically oriented fashion, sometimes called the tumble-tube (Hodgson, 1972).

TECHNIQUES FOR POSTERIOR HYPOSPADIAS

Posterior hypospadias represent approximately 20 per cent of all cases of hypospadias and certainly are the most challenging to repair. These reconstructions have a higher complication rate compared with correction of the less severe forms. Adjacent skin flaps were used in the early 1960s and 1970s (Broadbent et al., 1961; Des Prez et al., 1961; Hinderer, 1971). Skin adjacent to the meatus and in the axis of the shaft of the penis was tubularized in continuity with the meatus, making a new urethra out of penile skin and continuous preputial skin on the lateral aspect. Less than optimal vascularity of these thin rotational flaps makes results with these methods more prone to complications. In the 1960s and 1970s, importance was placed on keeping the native urethra and meatus intact while extending the urethra

with adjacent skin to prevent proximal strictures. This principle has since been disproved.

Free skin graft should be full thickness rather than split thickness. Devine (1983) has had successful experience for more than 30 years utilizing the inner preputial skin detached and defatted as a thin full-thickness graft to form the neourethra. Their good results have not been reproducible in a uniform manner in the hands of others, however (Filmer et al., 1977; Redman, 1983; Rober et al., 1990; Woodard and Cleveland, 1982). Because the free graft must be revascularized, the key element to success is perfect skin cover of the graft with well-vascularized dorsal preputial and penile skin (Hendren and Horton, 1988; Kaplan, 1988).

Vascularized flaps of the preputial and penile skin may be mobilized to the ventrum for urethroplasty by attaching them to the outer face of the prepuce or as an island flap unrestricted by the limitations of the skin of the outer face. Hodgson (1970) used the inner face prepuce in a vertical orientation with the tumble-flap technique (Hodgson I). He later added the vertically oriented dorsal penile skin neourethra (Hodgson II and III), which was transposed to the ventrum with a buttonhole maneuver (Hodgson, 1972, 1975, 1978, and 1981).

Asopa and colleagues (Asopa et al., 1971; Asopa and Asopa, 1984) employed the vascularized flap attached to the outer prepuce (Fig. 50–10). The ventral preputial skin is used for the new urethra but is left attached to the penile skin and is spiraled around to the ventrum. The result was asymmetric and bulky, but modifications have made the cosmetic results much better (Duckett, 1991).

A similar procedure is now preferred by Hodgson (1986) (Fig. 50–11), that is, the inner preputial-tangential tube. Standoli (1982) has reported an island flap

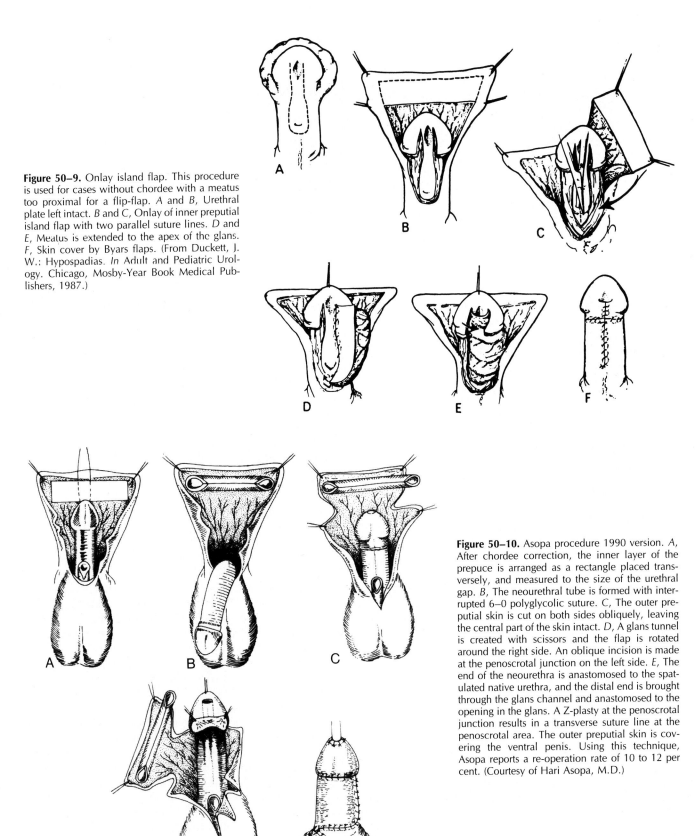

Figure 50–9. Onlay island flap. This procedure is used for cases without chordee with a meatus too proximal for a flip-flap. *A* and *B*, Urethral plate left intact. *B* and *C*, Onlay of inner preputial island flap with two parallel suture lines. *D* and *E*, Meatus is extended to the apex of the glans. *F*, Skin cover by Byars flaps. (From Duckett, J. W.: Hypospadias. *In* Adult and Pediatric Urology. Chicago, Mosby-Year Book Medical Publishers, 1987.)

Figure 50–10. Asopa procedure 1990 version. *A*, After chordee correction, the inner layer of the prepuce is arranged as a rectangle placed transversely, and measured to the size of the urethral gap. *B*, The neourethral tube is formed with interrupted 6–0 polyglycolic suture. *C*, The outer preputial skin is cut on both sides obliquely, leaving the central part of the skin intact. *D*, A glans tunnel is created with scissors and the flap is rotated around the right side. An oblique incision is made at the penoscrotal junction on the left side. *E*, The end of the neourethra is anastomosed to the spatulated native urethra, and the distal end is brought through the glans channel and anastomosed to the opening in the glans. A Z-plasty at the penoscrotal junction results in a transverse suture line at the penoscrotal area. The outer preputial skin is covering the ventral penis. Using this technique, Asopa reports a re-operation rate of 10 to 12 per cent. (Courtesy of Hari Asopa, M.D.)

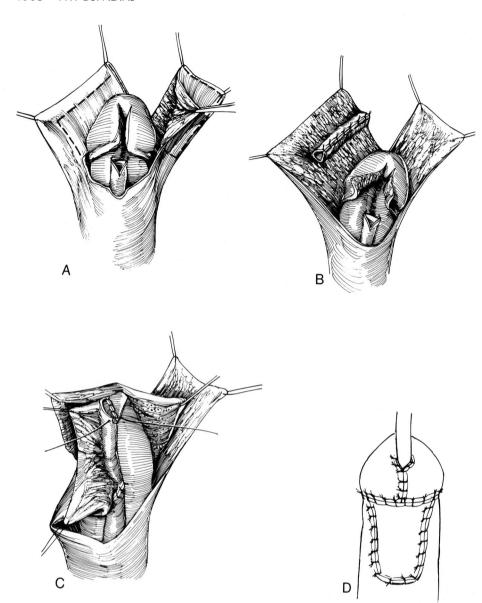

Figure 50–11. Hodgson XX. This procedure is similar to the Asopa procedure. A, The dorsal and ventral preputial flaps are, however, split eccentrically. B, The inner preputial skin is left attached to the outer foreskin and tubularized. C, This is rolled around to the ventrum and anastomosed in an oblique way to a glans dart. Glans wings are developed and cover the distal anastomosis. D, The outer preputial skin is used to cover the ventral defect. (From Hinman, F., Jr.: Atlas of Urologic Surgery. Philadelphia, W.B. Saunders Co., 1989, pp. 53–54.)

procedure using the outer preputial skin to form the neourethra (Duckett, 1987).

Healing of these neourethras from vascularized tissue is better than from the free graft techniques.

Transverse Preputial Island Flap and Glans Channel (Fig. 50–12)

We have developed this technique over the last 10 years as a modification of the Hodgson III and Asopa procedures. We firmly believe that a vascularized urethral tube is more preferable than a free graft. The blood supply to the inner preputial transverse island flap is abundant with vascularization oriented in a longitudinal fashion (Quartey, 1983). This tissue is dissected free from the penile skin and outer preputial skin, leaving the major vasculature to the island flap. Devascularization of the penile and preputial outer skin is in

practice not as much a problem as theoretically supposed (Hinman, 1991). Certainly, the outer extents of the preputial skin are not well vascularized and will slough if used in the ventral cover. This excess skin is excised during the skin cover phase.

As the transverse preputial island flap is developed, a broad extension is mobilized. This is trimmed to fit a template of 12-Fr. caliber so that the neourethra does not bulge and form diverticula with redundancy (Aigen et al., 1987). It is surprising how well an island flap can be developed in length, if the skin of the prepuce is splayed out transversely. A length of 5 to 6 cm can be obtained. The inner portion of the tube is closed with running 7–0 Vicryl, and the ends are interrupted so that they may be excised to fit the proper length. An additional layer may be more secure (Kass and Bolong, 1990). For a long tube, the meatus is attached first and the tube is stretched down into the perineum for the appropriate distance. Very rarely, a proximal extension

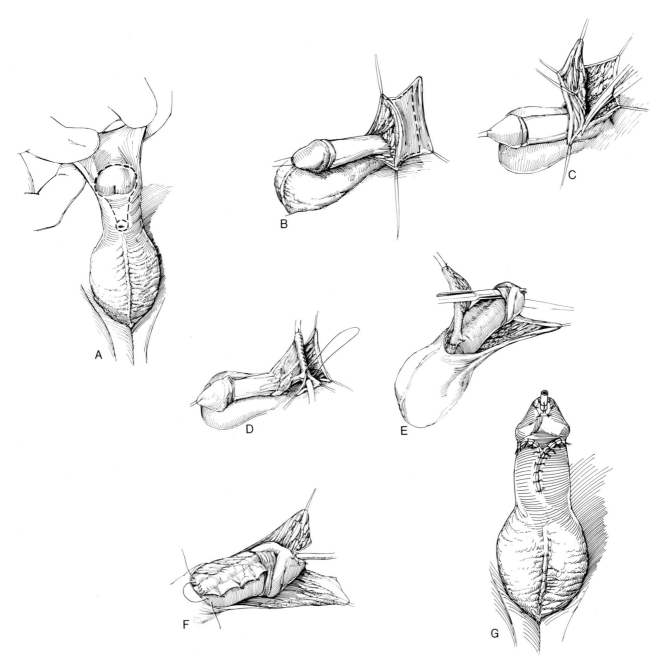

Figure 50–12. Transverse preputial island flap (Duckett). *A,* Circumferential incision is made around the corona and carried down proximal to the meatus. A strip of urethral plate is left intact for an onlay procedure if the penis is straight on erection. *B,* The inner preputial skin is splayed out with holding sutures in a rectangular fashion. *C,* The inner layer of the prepuce is dissected free from the outer prepuce and penile skin down to the base of the penis. The majority of the visible axially oriented vessels are left with the flap of tissue. *D,* The inner preputial tube is trimmed to roll the transverse surface into a neourethra. This tube is calibrated at 12 French. The edges are inverted with running sutures in the midportion and interrupted sutures on the distal ends so that they may be trimmed accordingly. *E,* A glans channel is made, staying next to the corporal bodies. A generous channel of 14 to 18 French is dissected. A proximal anastomosis is made in an oblique fashion, fixing the proximal anastomosis to the tunica albuginea. *F,* Subcutaneous flap tissue is splayed out to cover the anastomosis. Care is taken not to permit the rotated flap to create torsion in the shaft of the penis. *G,* The outer preputial skin is split and brought around to the ventrum in the midline for a closure up to the glans cap. A urethral drainage is established with a 6 French Silastic tube passed into the bladder and sutured to the glans with a permanent suture. This is left in place for 10 to 14 days. (From Hinman, F., Jr.: Atlas of Urologic Surgery. Philadelphia, W.B. Saunders Co., 1989, pp. 50–52.)

of the urethra may be required for perineal openings (Duckett, 1987), but this, in modern experience, is rarely needed.

An oblique anastomosis is made fixing the native urethra to the tunica albuginea. All of the skin edges of the native urethra are excised so that good spongiosum

is available. Fixation of the neourethra to the tunica albuginea also prevents overlapping and kinking of the proximal anastomosis.

Once the neourethra is in place, bougienage with a bougie à boule of 10 to 12 Fr. is done routinely to make sure there are no bumps, kinks, or lips. The urethra is filled with saline with an indwelling 8-Fr. catheter to check for leaks after the repair is intact. These are oversewn with Vicryl.

The glans channel is made by sharp dissection against the corporal bodies out to the tip of the glanular groove. A button of glans epithelium is removed, and dissection is carried down into the glanular tissue with removal of enough to permit a broad channel through the glans. The neourethra and its vasculature must traverse this area without compression. The most common error is making the glans channel too small. Interrupted fine chromic sutures are placed in a circumferential way to the glans meatus.

The skin cover for the transverse preputial flap is made by splitting the dorsal outer prepuce and stretching the lateral wings around to the ventrum so that a midline closure is made with horizontal mattress 7–0 chromic sutures up to the glans. These preputial flaps are *not* rotated in a "huggy-bear" transposition. Excess skin is excised, leaving good viable penile and preputial skin for cover.

A 6-Fr. Silastic stent is placed into the bladder approximately 2 cm from the bladder neck and sutured to the glans and meatus with a 5–0 Prolene interrupted suture. Extra length (4 to 5 cm) is permitted to drip urine into the diaper. The patient does not void through the tube.

A sandwich-like dressing is applied using benzoin on the skin, a Telfa to keep the penis from sticking to the skin, a Telfa on the ventral repair, a 4-×-4 folded four times for pressure onto the abdomen, and a bio-occlusive dressing (Tagaderm), compressing the penis against the abdomen. This dressing is removed in 48 hours after the bleeding is controlled. The penis is cared for with Polysporin ointment placed on the wound without a dressing in the diaper.

Onlay Island Flap Technique
(see Fig. 50–9)

This procedure has become our most employed technique for middle and posterior hypospadias over the past 3 to 5 years. A higher percentage than we had previously recognized of hypospadias patients have intact urethral plates. When this urethral plate is long enough to extend out to the glanular area, there is often very little curvature. We, therefore, make every attempt to maintain this urethral strip in cases as we make our initial incisions. As the circumferential incision is made around the corona, it is carried up to the urethral plate where parallel markings are made out to the glans tip. The incision is then brought proximal around the meatus, and the skin and dartos fascia are dissected, freeing fibrous tethering. Once this skin drop back is made, an artificial erection is done to see the extent of curvature. Often, there is very little curvature after this skin drop back. If mild to moderate curvature exists, a dorsal plication will be used. Otherwise, the urethral plate is divided, the proximal urethra is dropped back into the scrotal location, and formal ventral chordee resection undertaken. It is surprising how many cases still have

curvature after this maneuver, and dorsal plicating stitches are still required. A full tubularized island flap with glans channel is done.

With the urethral plate outlined with parallel incisions about 4 to 6 mm in width, a strip is made all the way to the tip of the glanular groove developing glanular wings very similar to a Mathieu-type repair. The proximal urethra is cut back to good spongiosum, and the excess skin edge is excised, making the urethral plate uniform.

Once this maneuver is accomplished, a ventral preputial island flap is developed without making any attempt to measure the appropriate size. This is mobilized to the ventrum and placed alongside the urethral plate. A running 7–0 Vicryl suture closes one side of the onlay.

A marking pen outlines the amount of onlay flap. With a 4- to 6-mm strip, the onlay need be no more than 6 to 8 mm wide for a 12-Fr. caliber neourethra. The epithelium is excised from the onlay and the pedicle is kept intact, supplying this strip of epithelium. The onlay is rotated over the urethral plate, and interrupted sutures are made around the horseshoe shape of the proximal urethra. A running suture is closed on the lateral side, completing the repair out to the tip of the glans. Throughout this onlay process, bougie à boules calibrate the urethra to make sure it is not too wide. A diverticulum might form if too much redundancy is used. A urethral distention with saline is done to check for leaks.

The lateral glans wings are brought around the ventrum of the urethral onlay, excising any excess mucosa, and an interrupted meatoplasty is made. The glanular wings are brought over the onlay with deep Vicryl stitches and a superficial running chromic suture stitch. This completes the glansplasty and the meatoplasty.

The pedicle is splayed over the anastomosis and tacked to the tunica albuginea so that it is flattened out. Excess tissue is excised from the flap to avoid any bulkiness.

Skin cover is achieved in the usual manner of dividing the dorsal preputial skin and stretching the skin around to the ventrum for a midline closure up to the glans. Horizontal chromic suture is used for this part of the procedure. A urethral stent described previously is placed, dripping into the diaper.

We have employed this onlay island technique, to 3.5 cm in length, in conjunction with dorsal plicating stitches to make a straight penis. The results have been quite satisfactory with a complication rate of 5 per cent for secondary surgeries. The cosmetic results are excellent (Duckett, 1986, 1990, and 1991; Hollowell et al., 1990).

Double-Faced Island Flap

If the inner and outer preputial layers are left intact, an island flap vascular pedicle is left supplying both layers; this permits excellent mobility of the two surfaces to the ventrum. If the inner preputial layer is tubularized in a longitudinal fashion, this can act as the neourethra for the urethroplasty. The outer layer of preputial skin remains as a ventral penile skin cover oriented longitu-

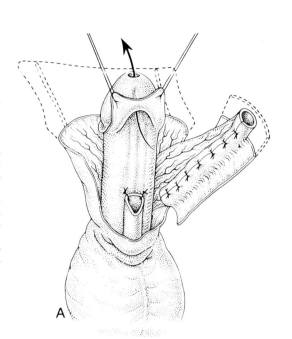

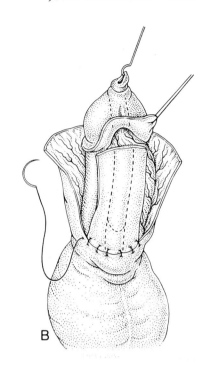

Figure 50–13. Double-faced island flap. *A*, The outer and inner preputial layers are mobilized together as an island flap. The inner layer is tubularized for the neourethra but remains attached to the pedicle. *B*, The urethra is channeled through the glans, discarding some of the outer skin. The outer prepuce is then fashioned to cover the ventral one third of the penis, while the remaining penile skin covers the dorsal two thirds. (From Duckett, J. W.: Hypospadias repair. *In* Frank, J. D., and Johnston, J. H.: Operative Paediatric Urology, Chap. 17. London, Churchill-Livingstone, 1990, pp. 197–208.)

dinally, acting as a surface of the ventral one third. The penile skin remains as the other two thirds of the cylinder. We described this technique in the previous issue of *Campbell's Urology* (Duckett, 1986) (Fig. 50–13). Over the subsequent 6 years, however, our results with this method carry with it a higher secondary surgical rate, mostly due to fistula formation. We theorize that the extra abundant skin layers are taxing the vascular supply of the single pedicle, and diminishing the excellent healing results that we have obtained with the single-faced island flap.

Hinman (1991) describes the theoretic advantage of leaving both layers attached. We have, however, not found this to be the case in practice. The double-faced island flap is an extension of the Asopa procedure (Asopa and Asopa, 1984) (see Fig. 50–10) and the Hodgson (1986) inner preputial tangential tube (see Fig. 50–11).

TECHNICAL ASPECTS

Instruments

Principles of plastic surgery regarding fine instruments and fine suture material along with precise, delicate tissue handling have advanced the principles of hypospadiology over the years. Instruments consist of fine iris scissors, delicate tooth forceps (0.5 mm), and Castroviejo needle holders for the very fine maneuvers (Monfort et al., 1983). Skin hooks may prevent overhandling of the tissues although we prefer fine chromic stay sutures.

Suture Material

Removal of permanent sutures usually mandates an anesthetic. Therefore, most surgeons select absorbable material. Chromic catgut suture is a favorite for the skin because it absorbs rapidly and will be gone in 10 to 20 days. Polyglycolic sutures remain a longer time and are ill-advised for skin closure. The 6–0 or 7–0 polyglycolic material is quite satisfactory for constructing the neourethra and for buried sutures. Polydioxanone (PDS) remains for a much longer period of time. Pull-out nylon sutures (4-0) are used by some to close the urethra and also for the skin suture lines in several layers (Belman, 1982). By cutting one end of the suture, the other may be wrapped around a hemostat and removed easily.

Hemostasis

Hemostasis may be achieved in a number of ways. A tourniquet at the base of the penis should be removed every 20 to 30 minutes (Ossandon and Ransley, 1982). We prefer the injection of 1:100,000 epinephrine in 1 per cent lidocaine (Xylocaine) using a 26-gauge needle. Infiltration around the proximal urethra, into the chordee tissue, and into the glans for creation of a glans channel is helpful. Usually only 1.5 to 2.0 ml is required. There is a wide range of safety before epinephrine will sensitize the myocardium to arrhythmias with inhalational anesthetics. At least 10 mg per kg of epinephrine may be given safely for cutaneous infiltration (Karl et al., 1983). At no time have we thought that epinephrine compromised the vasculature of these flaps. Gunter and co-workers (1990) claim that caudal epidural anesthesia reduces blood loss with hypospadias repair. Various methods of coagulation have been recommended; we prefer a low-current Bovie. Bipolar electrodes stick to the tissue too much. With epinephrine, the need for electrocoagulation is diminished.

Magnification

Optical magnification has been demonstrated to be a significant advance. The better loupes are generally supplied in 3.5 to 6.5 power. They give a narrow field of vision. When one is familiar with their use, they are indispensable. We prefer an Optivisor, which allows a broader field of vision but a lower magnification at 1.5 to 2.5. The focal length is 14 to 20 inches, which is quite satisfactory for this type of surgery. The major drawback is the bulk of the Optivisor and the likelihood of contaminating instruments and sutures. Some operating room microscopes will have 3.5 power, but most have 10 power, which is too great a magnification (Wacksman, 1987). Each surgeon must try all of these forms of magnification and select the one best suited.

Dressing

The most significant factor contributed by the proper dressing is to provide immobilization with prevention of hematoma and edema. Protection of the suture lines from contamination is the least important factor. It is unlikely that dressings contribute to skin slough or subsequent fistula formation (Cromie and Bellinger, 1981). Many dressings have been used, such as a polyurethane foam (DeSy and Oosterlinck, 1980) and an adhesive membrane (Vordermark, 1982). In some cases, after fistula closure, "super glue" is applied for cover (Duckett et al., 1982). We prefer a sandwich-like dressing, consisting of Telfa and a gauze folded four times, laid on top of the penis followed by a bio-occlusive (Tagaderm), which compresses the layers and the penis against the abdominal wall. This is removed in 48 hours with Polysporin ointment application thereafter.

Diversions

Although percutaneous suprapubic cystotomy drainage has been the most common diversion in the past, we prefer a Silastic tubing of 6 Fr., placed through the urethra and sutured to the glans. The free end drips constantly into the diaper (Duckett and Snyder, 1985; Montagnino et al., 1988). Any tubing connected to drainage bags is likely to get caught, exerting traction on the meatus. A perfect glanuloplasty can be destroyed with one careless moment. We thus advise open drainage into diapers when possible, using chemoprophylaxis to control infection (Sugar and Firlit, 1989). The simplest forms of dressing and diversion work the best.

Bladder Spasms

Bladder spasms are most aggravating to the patient and his family. Because they occur without warning, medication as needed will not likely help. We use Banthine (methantheline bromide) and opium suppositories (B and O), cut into thirds, for immediate relief.

Oral Pro-Banthine (propantheline bromide) or oxybutynin also may help.

Analgesia

A supplemental local block (Jensen, 1981) with bupivacaine (Marcaine) at the beginning of the procedure is most helpful. A caudal block and penile block in two groups of children were found to be equal in duration and degree of analgesia. However, 30 per cent of those with caudal blocks were unable to walk at 6 hours (Yeoman et al., 1983). A penile block seems the better choice and should be a supplement to hypospadias surgery. Gunter and associates (1990) report better hemostasis with caudal anesthesia.

Age of Repair

Comparison of normal penile size with age indicates some growth in the first 2 years followed by a relative plateau until puberty. Thus, 2 to 5 years was usually the age selected for staged repairs. However, the adverse psychologic effects of maternal-child separation with hospitalization at this age became apparent. Schultz and colleagues (1983) pointed out that an ideal time might be age 6 to 18 months to minimize the emotional effect of this traumatic insult. The advantage of improved optical magnification has made surgical correction at an earlier age more successful. Thus, many surgeons, using a one-stage repair, chose 6 to 18 months as the optimal time (Belman, 1982; Manley and Epstein, 1981). Anesthesia risks are minimized after 3 months of age, when the chance of sudden infant death syndrome (SIDS) is diminished. Day surgical cases may be performed after the patient reaches 3 months of age. If younger, the patient should remain hospitalized overnight. Generally, the penis with hypospadias is of sufficient size at 3 months to accomplish this delicate surgery with the aid of optical magnification.

Testosterone Stimulation

Enlargement of the infant penis is possible by testosterone stimulation. A 5 per cent testosterone cream rubbed on the genitals daily for 3 weeks works by local absorption. Blood levels of testosterone reach pubertal levels quickly. Dihydrotestosterone (DHT) is also given (Monfort and Lucas, 1982). Equally as effective is testosterone proprionate, 25 mg intramuscularly (IM) once a week for 3 weeks (Gearhart and Jeffs, 1987). The IM dosage is better controlled and is preferable to asking the parents to rub cream on the baby's penis to make it bigger. We have not found testosterone stimulation to be beneficial.

Outpatient Surgery

With the continued escalation of health care costs, maximal hospital benefit has become a concept of economic necessity today. The postoperative management of hypospadias surgery is concerned mainly with the difficulties associated with diversion and dressings. Candidates for elective surgery require little in the way of medication or wound care that cannot be offered by the parents. Therefore, the surgeon is obligated to coordinate postoperative care by adequate preoperative education, simplification of instructions, and ready accessibility to the telephone in order to accomplish most of the care on an outpatient basis. A day surgical procedure or an overnight hospital stay should be the goal.

Psychosocial Support

Psychosocial support should be offered by the surgeon or well-trained nurse to alleviate the parent's guilt that frequently accompanies this genital anomaly. Unexpressed anxieties as to the cause for hypospadias and the later sexual capabilities of the patient must be anticipated and discussed. The child's future positive body image may well depend on his parents' thorough understanding of his condition. The surgeon must be certain that these issues are made clear to the parents.

Follow-Up Care

Follow-up care depends on the complexity of the procedure required. Dressing changes, catheter or tube removals, and wound care may be done in the office or outpatient clinic without the need for general anesthetic support. Bougienage of the meatus or urethra may be accomplished deftly and with minimal discomfort if small-caliber, straight sounds or bougie à boules are employed. Care should be taken not to force through a narrowing. A kink at the proximal anastomosis is more likely than a stricture in the early postoperative period. Probing of the meatus with the nozzle tip of an ophthalmic ointment tube prevents the meatus from crusting. Follow-up visits are at 2- and 6-week intervals and, thereafter, as needed.

COMPLICATIONS

Acute Complications

Attention to the details that will avoid complications is paramount (Duckett et al., 1980; Retik et al., 1988). Diversion of urine by either suprapubic or urethral tube is intended to allow sealing of the suture lines and sufficient healing to avoid leakage of urine into the tissues outside the neourethra. A few squirts of urine out the new urethra with bladder spasms will cause little harm, as long as the meatus is patent. Therefore, meatal probing to dislodge crusting is required periodically. A stent for 5 to 7 days accomplishes the same goal.

To avoid *wound infection*, well-prepared skin should be ensured. Separation of the foreskin adherence with removal of the desquamated epithelial debris should be done utilizing anesthesia prior to application of a satis-

factory skin preparation. In the postpubertal male, cleansing should commence several days before surgery. Infection seems more of a problem in this age group. Prophylactic antibiotics have little value in avoiding wound infection. Sulfonamide or nitrofurantoin suppression may prevent cystitis, particularly if the tube is left to drain in the diaper.

Poor wound healing is primarily due to ischemic flaps. If a technique is selected in which preputial skin and its arterial pedicle are separated from the penile skin, it may be more likely that the covering tissue will be less vascularized. If, however, the neourethra is well vascularized, healing should occur per primam in this layer, and the sloughed covering skin will granulate and re-epithelialize without a noticeable scar.

Edema occurs to some degree in most hypospadias repairs. A compression dressing has been the standard method in an attempt to diminish this effect on healing. It is, of course, difficult to obtain a diffuse compression effect, and many different dressing methods have been attempted. A compression dressing left for 2 to 3 days seems effective, not only for controlling edema formation but also hematoma formation.

Drain tubes applied as wicks underneath the repair are important if a free full-thickness graft or bladder mucosa is used. The interface between the graft and the overlying skin should be perfectly approximated. A vacuum suction on the tubing can be created with a mini-Hemovac using vacuum tubes and scalp vein needles (Devine, 1983). Firm compression should be applied at the end of the procedure to evacuate all subcutaneous blood clots and to control the immediate postoperative ooze.

Postoperative *erections* are a problem in the postpubertal patient. Various medications have been administered but without much success. The best medication is probably amylnitrate pulvules.

Chronic Complications

Urethrocutaneous fistulas are likely to remain an inherent risk of hypospadias repair for years to come. The fistula rate after a particular procedure is often cited as a measure of the effectiveness of that surgical repair. Currently, an expected complication rate of 5 to 10 per cent (mostly fistulas) exists for one-stage hypospadias surgery.

The second procedure required to close a hypospadias fistula may unfortunately carry a rather significant failure rate of up to 40 per cent (Walker, 1981). Details of various techniques of fistula closure in the literature emphasize wide mobilization; adjacent skin flaps; multilayered closures; and urinary diversion by urethral catheter or suprapubic cystotomy, including several days to weeks in the hospital (Horton et al., 1980).

We recommend a microtechnique involving magnification and delicate instruments (Carmignani et al., 1982; Duckett et al., 1982). A properly sized lacrimal duct probe placed in the fistulous tract assists in the identification of the epithelial-lined tract, while careful dissection is made down to the urethra. Fine catgut closes the urethral edge in Lembert-type sutures. A watertight closure is ensured by distending the distal urethra with saline, while compressing the bulbar urethra in the perineum. The skin is approximated loosely with vertical mattress sutures. No diversion of urine is needed. The patient is allowed to void by the fistula repair and goes home the same day. We have a 10 per cent fistula recurrence with this method (Duckett, 1986).

The most common error in fistula closure is failure to recognize a concomitant diverticulum or distal stricture. A *diverticulum* can be demonstrated by probing either with a bougie à boule or with a urethrogram prior to fistula closure. Diverticula should be excised along with the fistula to ensure adequate repair. Meatal stenosis may also need enlarging with the fistula repair.

Residual chordee is another complication, particularly in those cases that were repaired many years ago prior to artificial erection techniques. The residual chordee may be resolved with a circumferential incision around the corona, dissecting the urethral meatus and urethra along with the sleeve of skin cover down to the penoscrotal junction. Residual chordee tissue is excised, and artificial erection is used to ascertain proper correction. The sleeve of penile skin and urethra is brought back as far as possible and is fixed onto the tunica albuginea. A further extension of the urethroplasty is usually required and may be done by mobilizing a flap of skin on the ventrum in a manner similar to a Mustarde procedure. When done, a glans channel can be created, placing the meatus on the tip. Otherwise, innovative techniques for a more extensive urethroplasty may be required (Stecker et al., 1981). If slight ventral chordee remains, dorsal plication with permanent sutures may achieve adequate penile straightening (Duckett, 1986).

Rarely, extensive scarring on the ventrum of the penis or ventral tunical deficiency requires excision of a patch of the tunica albuginea with replacement with a strip of tunica vaginalis obtained from the paratesticular tunica (Duckett, 1981a). Dermal grafts have also been chosen for this tunica albuginea replacement (Devine and Horton, 1975). If dermal grafts are applied, care must be taken that all the epithelial elements are removed. Otherwise, dermal cysts develop. Woodhouse and Ransley (1984) have successfully replaced the tunica with lyophilized dura mater.

Urethroplasty problems may occur with a *stricture* at the proximal anastomosis (Scherz et al., 1988). This may be due to "angulation" of the anastomosis and may be avoided by lateral fixation of the anastomosis to the tunica albuginea so that the back wall will not overlap the front. Strictures may be repaired by excision and reanastomosis. Optical cold-knife urethrotomy is not effective usually.

The neourethra may inadvertently be made too wide, resulting in *diffuse diverticulum* formation (Aigen et al., 1987). If meatal stenosis occurs, further dilatation may occur. Reduction of such a diverticulum in a longitudinal fashion is necessary. Anastomotic urinary extravasation may epithelialize in such a way that a bulbous diverticulum results at the penoscrotal junction that must be excised. A diverticulum and fistula may occur simultaneously, and excision of both is necessary.

Use of *hair-bearing skin* for urethroplasty has been criticized for many years. If scrotal tissue is incorporated, a hairy urethra may occur after puberty with stone formation and encrustation. Excision of the hairy urethra may be required with replacement with non–hair-bearing skin.

Persistent hypospadias with a *retrusive meatus* that deflects the stream downward is a common complaint with the older procedures. This condition may be improved using a Mustarde-type flap and a glans channel, or a Mathieu flip-flap technique. Occasionally, mobilization of the urethra for several centimeters will permit an advancement into the glans.

If persistent chordee along with the proximal meatus is present, a vascularized flap from some of the remaining dorsal penile skin may be an option. Adjacent skin with its vasculature may be used or, most commonly now, an onlay island flap is used.

Meatal stenosis should be avoided by a generous channel through the glans, excising tissue to lay the neourethra and pedicle in place without compromising blood supply. If flap loss should occur through the glans, a dense intraglanular stricture may appear. This effect generally requires excision and reconstruction. Occasionally, a V-flap meatoplasty may widen the more restricted distal meatal stenosis (Brannen, 1976).

Balanitis xerotica obliterans (BXO) is a later complication resulting from chronic inflammation (Bale et al., 1987). Short-term diminution of the inflammation may be achieved with steroid injection, but we have not been able to control this process for more than several years. Excision of the BXO lesion is required with a meatoplasty as indicated. The Brannen meatoplasty in adults is useful (Brannen, 1976). The DeSy meatoplasty may be applicable in the future (DeSy, 1984).

Scars of the penile skin are rarely a problem. Excision with Z-plasties or scrotal flaps, or replacement with a free split-thickness graft is an option.

Complex Hypospadias

Those patients with multiple repairs that have failed have been in the past branded as "hypospadias cripples," an unfortunate designation that should be abandoned. It is usually necessary to discard the problem-plagued urethra created previously and start anew. This occurs in the free grafts of preputial skin but more commonly in extragenital skin free full-thickness grafts (inner arm or inguinal skin donor sites) years later. There appears to be a delay of many years of a chronic inflammation similar to BXO, which affects the entire graft (Hendren and Crooks, 1980). Bladder mucosal grafts are currently in vogue for the reconstruction of these urethral replacements.

Bladder Mucosa Graft (Fig. 50–14)

Memmelaar (1947) first described the bladder mucosa in a one-stage hypospadias repair. Marshall and Spellman (1955) were initially enthusiastic about bladder mucosa, but they did this repair in a two-stage procedure. Coleman and associates (1981) and Li and associates (1981) revived interest in the bladder mucosa

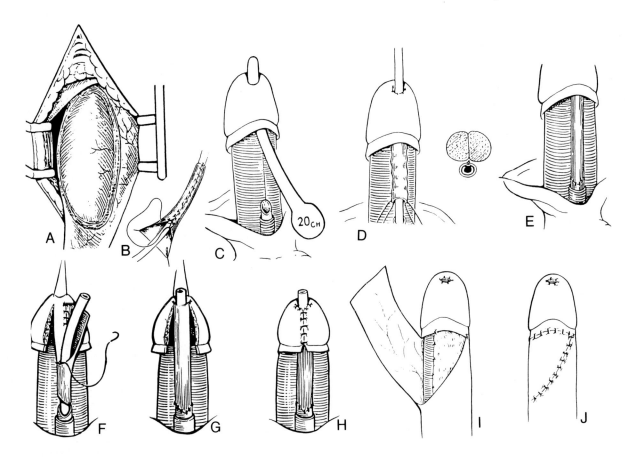

Figure 50–14. Composite of bladder mucosa graft (Mollard, et al. 1989).

A, Bladder is filled with saline and exposed with a transverse skin incision and a vertical fascial incision. The muscle is incised down to the underlying muscle and dissected off to expose the bladder mucosa.

B, For a 1- to 2-year-old patient, a mucosal strip is rolled loosely over a 14-Fr. stent with running, locking, and inverting 7–0 absorbable suture.

C, A 20-Fr. channel is made through the glans. The proximal native urethra is exposed with an inner cuff of mucosa and an outer cuff of spongiosum.

D, An apical glans meatus is created by excising a piece of glans. The graft is anastomosed to the meatus first, permitting exact approximation of the tissues without eversion of the graft. *Inset,* The graft is placed with the suture line against the corpora.

E, A proximal anastomosis is made to mucosa alone in an elliptic anastomosis, with 7–0 interrupted sutures. The graft is covered with two layers of well-vascularized tissue.

F, G, and *H,* An alternative use of bladder mucosa is an onlay onto a urethral strip, developing glans wings brought together in the midline.

I and *J,* The dorsal preputial skin is divided in the midline. Both are swung around to the ventral surface. The epithelium of the smaller flap is trimmed, and the subcutaneous tissue is used to cover the graft with an inner layer sewn to the corpus cavernosum. The other skin flap is sutured similar to that in a double-breasted coat. (Courtesy of Pierre Mollard, M.D.).

graft. Others have reported good results (Hendren and Reda, 1986; Keating and Duckett, 1990; Koyle and Ehrlich, 1987; Mollard et al., 1989; Ransley et al., 1987; Song et al., 1982). This technique is mainly chosen for secondary cases in our country, whereas Mollard in France and Chinese physicians have chosen it for primary cases.

The bladder is exposed with either a transverse or horizontal incision. The muscle of the fluid-filled bladder is split in a vertical fashion down to the mucosa, and the muscle is separated from the mucosa. A distance sufficient to harvest the needed graft is outlined on the anterior portion of the bladder. Once the bladder is entered and the graft is taken, it may be extended over the dome of the bladder all the way to the posterior wall for a distance as long as 15 to 20 cm from inside the bladder. When the graft is taken, it is placed in saline and kept wet throughout its manipulation. The bladder closure need not be concerned with mucosal approximations because this tissue regenerates very rapidly. Only the muscle is closed. A suprapubic tube is used for diversion purposes as well as bladder healing.

The graft is tubularized over an 18- to 22-Fr. template, taking a width of about 2 cm of bladder mucosa. The graft is laid in the bed of the previously removed urethra, and a proximal anastomosis to the native urethra is made in an oblique fashion. Care is taken to cover the anastomosis with subcutaneous tissue. The distal graft is channeled through the glans and anastomosed to the glanular epithelium in a circumferential manner. Similar care is needed to extend the graft to its fullest extent so it is not redundant. Leaving it on a catheter stent is appropriate for this maneuver.

Skin cover is achieved by re-approximating a cylinder of skin back to the corona of the glans or by bringing penile flaps over the graft. If at all possible, a dorsal pedicle of previous preputial subcutaneous tissue can be mobilized and brought over the bladder mucosal graft.

A tunica vaginalis pedicle is an alternative (Snow, 1986). It is appropriate to leave a suction drainage tube beside the graft to make sure that the skin cover seals well to the graft. This is essential to avoid a hematoma and to assure the rapid revascularization of the graft.

The main complication of this technique is surprisingly not the proximal anastomosis as much as the meatal problem. The mucosa does not withstand the irritation at the skin surface and eversion occurs. Revision of the meatus is common. Meatal dilation on a daily basis may help avoid this complication.

ADULT FOLLOW-UP

Long-term follow-up is available on patients undergoing previous repair (Berg et al., 1981; Berg and Berg, 1983; Svensson and Berg, 1983). Discouraging outcomes reported by some may reflect the difficulty of hypospadias surgery in the past as well as the older ages at which repair was carried out; therefore, these outcomes may not be a true reflection of our modern methods (Kenawi, 1975).

Cosmetic and functional results are far better today than in the past. The concept of one-stage hypospadias repair accomplished at an early age, coupled with low complication potential, reinforces the current positive approach to this problem. Correction of chordee is extremely important and is crucial for assuring satisfactory sexual function. There appears to be no increase in infertility unless cryptorchidism or another testiculopathy coexists. Evidence supports the fact that urethral growth with vascular flaps occurs. Psychologically, early hypospadias repair avoids castration anxiety as well as separation anxiety (Kaplan et al., 1989). It is comforting to be able to counsel parents that there is optimism in striving for an excellent cosmetic and functional result in boys with all degrees of hypospadias.

CONCLUSION

"Hypospadias is a grievous deformity which must ever move as to the highest surgical endeavor. The refashioning of the urethra offers a problem as formidable as any in the wide field of our art" (Humby, 1941). Hypospadiology requires an in-depth study of the contributions of our predecessors as well as a thorough knowledge of the methods and maneuvers of current experts. To study at a medical center where large numbers of hypospadias cases are managed proves more beneficial than the anguish of learning through one's mistakes. The minor complications of a properly executed one-stage procedure in a fresh case are far less difficult to manage to a successful outcome than poorly conceived failures. It is to be hoped that the hypospadias cripple (Stecker et al., 1981) will eventually be of historical interest only.

It is difficult to be truly objective, therefore I have not tried to restrain my bias. Clearly, some of my colleagues have differing opinions. Hypospadiology will continue to produce innovative new methods as we refine the old ones. Dramatic improvements have been made over the past 25 years. Much of our current success should be attributed to the delicate and precise methods of tissue handling, as well as to the principles of flaps and grafts learned in conjunction with plastic surgery. The delicate ophthalmic instruments and optical magnification are also significant improvements. Although we have made great advances, more may be anticipated in this fascinating, challenging field of hypospadiology.

REFERENCES

Aigen, A. B., Khawand, N., Skoog, S. J., et al.: Acquired megalourethra: An uncommon complication of the transverse preputial island flap urethroplasty. J. Urol., 137:712–713, 1987.
Allen, T. D., and Griffin, J. E.: Endocrine studies in patients with advanced hypospadias. J. Urol., 131:310–314, 1984.
Allen, T. D., and Spence, H. M.: The surgical treatment of coronal hypospadias and related problems. J. Urol., 100:504–508, 1968.
Arap, S., Mitre, A. I., and DeGoes, G. M.: Modified meatal advancement and glanuloplasty repair of distal hypospadias. J. Urol., 131:1140, 1984.
Asopa, H. S., Elhence, E. P., Atria, S. P., et al.: One-stage correction of penile hypospadias using a foreskin tube: A preliminary report. Int. Surg., 55:435–448, 1971.
Asopa, R., and Asopa, H. S.: One-stage repair of hypospadias using double island preputial skin tube. Indian J. Urol., 1:41–43, 1984.
Avellan, L.: The incidence of hypospadias in Sweden. Scand. J. Plast. Reconstr. Surg., 9:129–138, 1975.
Backus, L. H., and DeFelice, C. A.: Hypospadias: Then and now. Plast. Reconstr. Surg., 25:146–168, 1960.
Bale, P. M., Lochhead, A., Martin, H. C., et al.: Balanitis xerotica obliterans in children. Pediatr. Pathol., 7:617–627, 1987.
Barcat, J.: Current concepts of treatment. In Horton, C. E. (Ed.): Plastic and Reconstructive Surgery of the Genital Area. Boston, Little, Brown & Co., 1973, pp. 249–263.
Bauer, S. B., Retik, A. B., and Colodny, A. H.: Genetic aspects of hypospadias. Urol. Clin. North Am., 8:559–564, 1981.
Beck, C.: Hypospadias and its treatment. Surg. Gynecol. Obstet., 24:511–532, 1917.
Beck and Hacker, 1897, as quoted in Horton, C. E. (Ed.): Plastic and Reconstructive Surgery of the Genital Area. Boston, Little, Brown & Co., 1973.
Bellinger, M. F.: Embryology of the male external genitalia. Urol. Clin. North Am., 8:375–382, 1981.
Belman, A. B.: Urethroplasty. Soc. Pediatr. Urol. Newsletter, December 1977.
Belman, A. B.: The Broadbent hypospadias repair. Urol. Clin. North Am., 8:483, 1981.
Belman, A. B.: The modified Mustarde hypospadias repair. J. Urol., 127:88–90, 1982.
Belman, A. B., and Kass, E. J.: Hypospadias repair in children less than one year old. J. Urol., 128:1273–1274, 1982.
Belman, A. B., and King, L. R.: The urethra. In Kelalis, P. P., King, L. R. (Eds.): Clinical Pediatric Urology. Philadelphia, W.B. Saunders Co., 1979, pp. 576–594.
Berg, R., and Berg, G.: Penile malformation, gender identity and sexual orientation. Acta Psychiatr. Scand., 68:154–166, 1983.
Berg, R., Svensson, J., and Astrom, G.: Social and sexual adjustment of men operated on for hypospadias during childhood: A controlled study. J. Urol., 125:313–317, 1981.
Bevan, A. D.: A new operation for hypospadias. JAMA, 68:1032–1033, 1917.
Brannen, G. E.: Meatal reconstruction. J. Urol., 116:319–321, 1976.
Broadbent, T. R., Woolf, R. M., and Toksu, E.: Hypospadias: One-stage repair. Plast. Reconstr. Surg., 27:154–157, 1961.
Browne, D.: An operation for hypospadias. Lancet, 1:141, 1936.
Browne, D.: A comparison of the Duplay and Denis Browne techniques for hypospadias operation. Surgery, 34:787–793, 1953.
Brueziere, J.: How I perform the Mathieu technic in the treatment of anterior penile hypospadias. Ann. Urol. (Paris), 21:277–280, 1987.
Butler, L. J., Snodgrass, G. J. A., France, N. E., Russell, A., and

Swain, V. A. J.: True hermaphroditism or gonadal intersexuality. Arch. Dis. Child., 44:666, 1969.

Byars, L. T.: Technique of consistently satisfactory repair of hypospadias. Surg. Gynecol. Obstet., 100:184–190, 1955.

Carmignani, G., Belgrande, E., Gabardi, F., et al.: Microsurgical one-stage repair of hypospadias with a rectangular transverse dorsal preputial vascularized skin flap. J. Microsurg., 3:222–227, 1982.

Cendron, J., and Melin, Y.: Congenital curvature of the penis without hypospadias. Urol. Clin. North Am., 8:389–395, 1981.

Cerasaro, T. S., Brock, W. A., and Kaplan, G. W.: Upper urinary tract anomalies associated with congenital hypospadias: Is screening necessary? J. Urol., 135:537–542, 1986.

Coleman, J. W., McGovern, J. H., and Marshall, V. F.: The bladder mucosal graft technique for hypospadias repair. Urol. Clin. North Am., 8:457–462, 1981.

Creevy, C. D.: The correction of hypospadias: A review. Urol. Surv., 8:2–68, 1958.

Cromie, W. J., and Bellinger, M. F.: Hypospadias dressing and diversions. Urol. Clin. North Am., 8:545–558, 1981.

Cronin, T. D., and Guthrie, T. H.: Method of Cronin and Guthrie for hypospadias repair. In Horton, C. E. (Ed.): Plastic and Reconstructive Surgery of the Genital Area. Boston, Little, Brown & Co., 1973, pp. 302–314.

Culp, O. S.: Experience with 200 hypospadias: Evaluation of therapeutic plans. Surg. Clin. North Am., 39:1007–1010, 1959.

Culp, O. S., and McRoberts, J. W.: Hypospadias. In Alken, C. E., Dix, V. W., Goodwin, W. E., et al. (Eds.): Encyclopedia of Urology. New York, Springer-Verlag, 1968, pp. 11307–11344.

Davidoff, F., and Federman, D. D.: Mixed gonadal dysgenesis. Pediatrics 52:727–747, 1973.

Davis, D. M.: Pedicle tube graft in surgical management of hypospadias, male, with new method of closing small urethral fistulas. Surg. Gynecol. Obstet., 71:790–796, 1940.

Davis, D. M.: Surgical treatment of hypospadias, especially scrotal and perineal. J. Urol., 65:595–602, 1951.

Des Prez, J. D., Persky, L., and Kiehn, C. L.: A one-stage repair of hypospadias by island flap technique. Plast. Reconstr. Surg., 28:405–410, 1961.

DeSy, W. A.: Aesthetic repair of meatal stricture. J. Urol., 132:678–679, 1984.

DeSy, W. A., and Oosterlinck, W.: Silicone foam elastomer: Significant improvement in postoperative penile dressing. J. Urol., 128:39–41, 1980.

DeSy, W. A., and Oosterlinck, W.: Urethral Advancement of Hypospadias Repair. Film presented at the International Congress of Urology, Vienna, 1985.

Devine, C. J., Jr.: Chordee and hypospadias. In Glenn, J. F., and Boyce, W. H. (Eds.): Urologic Surgery, ed. 3. Philadelphia, J.B. Lippincott Co., 1983, pp. 775–797.

Devine, C. J., Gonzales-Serva, L., Stecker, J. F., Jr., et al.: Utricular configuration in hypospadias and intersex. J. Urol., 123:407–411, 1980.

Devine, C. J., Jr., and Horton, C. E.: A one-stage hypospadias repair. J. Urol., 85:166–172, 1961.

Devine, C. J., Jr., and Horton, C. E.: Chordee without hypospadias. J. Urol., 110:264–267, 1973.

Devine, C. J., Jr., and Horton, C. E.: Use of dermal graft to correct chordee. J. Urol., 113:56–58, 1975.

Duckett, J. W.: Transverse preputial island flap technique for repair of severe hypospadias. Urol. Clin. North Am., 7:423–431, 1980a.

Duckett, J. W.: Hypospadias. Clin. Plast. Surg., 7:149–160, 1980b.

Duckett, J. W.: Repair of hypospadias. In Hendry, W. F. (Ed.): Recent Advances in Urology/Andrology, vol. 3. New York, Churchill-Livingstone, 1980c, pp. 279–290.

Duckett, J. W.: Forward: Symposium on Hypospadias. Urol. Clin. North Am., 8:371–373, 1981a.

Duckett, J. W.: MAGPI (meatal advancement and glanuloplasty): A procedure for subcoronal hypospadias. Urol. Clin. North Am., 8:513–520, 1981b.

Duckett, J. W.: The island flap technique for hypospadias repair. Urol. Clin. North Am., 8:503–511, 1981c.

Duckett, J. W.: Hypospadias. In Walsh, P. C., Gittes, R. F., Perlmutter, A. D., and Stamey, T. A. (Eds.): Campbell's Urology, ed. 5, Chap. 47. Philadelphia, W.B. Saunders Co., 1986, pp. 1969–1999.

Duckett, J. W.: Hypospadias. In Gillenwater, J. Y., Grayhack, J. T.,

Howards, S. S., and Duckett, J. W. (Eds.): Adult and Pediatric Urology, vol. 2, Chap. 57. Chicago, Year Book Medical Publishers, 1987, pp. 1880–1915.

Duckett, J. W.: Advances in Hypospadias Repair. Festschrift honoring Sir David I. Williams. Postgrad. Med. J. (London, England), 66:S62–S71, 1990.

Duckett, J. W.: Hypospadias repair. In O'Donnell, B. (Ed.): Paediatric Urology, ed. 3. Surrey, England, Butterworth Co., 1991. In press.

Duckett, J. W., Caldamone, A. A., and Snyder, H. M.: Hypospadias fistula repair without diversion [abstract 11]. In Programs and Abstracts of the AAP Annual Meeting, New York, October 23–28, 1982.

Duckett, J. W., Kaplan, G. W., Woodard, J. R., et al.: Panel: Complications of hypospadias repair. Urol. Clin. North Am., 7:443–452, 1980.

Duckett, J. W., and Keating, M. A.: Technical challenge of the megameatus intact prepuce hypospadias (MIP) variant: The pyramid procedure. J. Urol., 141:1407–1408, 1989.

Duckett, J. W., and Snyder, H. M.: Hypospadias "pearls." Soc. Pediatr. Urol. Newsletter, 7:4, 1985.

Duckett, J. W., and Snyder, H. M.: The MAGPI hypospadias repair after 1,000 cases: Avoidance of meatal stenosis and regression. J. Urol. In press.

Ehrlich, R. M., and Scardino, P. T.: Surgical correction of scrotal transposition and perineal hypospadias. J. Pediatr. Surg., 17:175–177, 1982.

Elder, J. S., Duckett, J. W., and Snyder, H. M.: Onlay island flap in the repair of mid and distal penile hypospadias without chordee. J. Urol., 138:376–379, 1987.

Filmer, R. B., Duckett, J. W., and Sowden, R.: One-stage correction of hypospadias/chordee. Birth Defects, 13:267–270, 1977.

Fuqua, F.: Renaissance of a urethroplasty: The Belt technique of hypospadias repair. J. Urol., 106:782, 1971.

Gearhart, J. P., Donohou, P. A., Brown, T. R., et al.: Long-term endocrine follow-up of patients with hypospadias [abstract 10]. J. Urol., 141:45-A, 1989.

Gearhart, J. P., and Jeffs, R. D.: The use of parenteral testosterone therapy in genital reconstructive surgery. J. Urol., 138:1077–1078, 1987.

Gearhart, J. P., Linhard, H. R., Berkovitz, G. D., et al.: Androgen receptor levels and 5-alpha-reductase activities in preputial skin and chordee tissue of boys with isolated hypospadias. J. Urol., 140:1243–1246, 1988.

Gibbons, A. D., and Gonzales, E. T., Jr.: The subcoronal meatus. J. Urol., 130:739–742, 1983.

Gittes, R. F., and McLaughlin, A. P., III: Injection technique to induce penile erection. Urology, 4:473–475, 1974.

Glenister, J. W.: The origin and fate of the urethral plate in man. J. Anat., 288:413–418, 1954.

Gonzales, E. T., Jr., Veeraraghavan, K. A., and Delaune, J.: The management of distal hypospadias with meatal-based, vascularized flaps. J. Urol., 129:119–120, 1983.

Gunter, J. B., Forestner, J. E., and Manley, C. B.: Caudal epidural anesthesia reduces blood loss during hypospadias repair. J. Urol., 144:517–519, 1990.

Hendren, W. H.: The Belt-Fuqua for repair of hypospadias. Urol. Clin. North Am., 8:431–450, 1981.

Hendren, W. H., and Crooks, K. K.: Tubed free skin graft for construction of male urethra. J. Urol., 123:858–862, 1980.

Hendren, W. H., and Horton, C. E., Jr.: Experience with one-stage repair of hypospadias and chordee using free graft of prepuce. J. Urol., 140:1259–1264, 1988.

Hendren, W. H., and Keating, M. A.: Use of dermal graft and free urethral graft in penile reconstruction. J. Urol., 140:1265–1269, 1988.

Hendren, W. H., and Reda, E. F.: Bladder mucosa graft for construction of male urethra. J. Pediatr. Surg., 21:189–192, 1986.

Higgins, C. C.: Hypospadias. Cleve. Clin. Q., 14:176, 1947.

Hinderer, U.: New one-stage repair of hypospadias (technique of penis tunnelization). In Hueston, J. T. (Ed.): Transactions of the 5th International Congress of Plastic and Reconstructive Surgery. Stoneham, MA, Butterworth Co., 1971, pp. 283–305.

Hinman, F., Jr.: The blood supply to preputial island flaps. J. Urol., 145:1232, 1991.

Hodgson, N. B.: A one-stage hypospadias repair. J. Urol., 104:281–284, 1970.

Hodgson, N. B.: In defense of the one-stage hypospadias repair. *In* Scott, R., Jr., Gordon, H. L., Scott, F. B., et al. (Eds.): Current Controversies in Urologic Management. Philadelphia, W.B. Saunders Co., 1972, pp. 263–271.

Hodgson, N. B.: Hypospadias. *In* Glenn, J. F., and Boyce, W. H. (Eds.): Urologic Surgery, ed. 2. New York, Harper & Row, 1975, pp. 656–667.

Hodgson, N. B.: Hypospadias and urethral duplication. *In* Harrison, J. H. (Ed.): Campbell's Urology, ed. 4. Philadelphia, W.B. Saunders Co., 1978, pp. 1566–1595.

Hodgson, N. B.: Use of vascularized flaps in hypospadias repair. Urol. Clin. North Am., 8:471–482, 1981.

Hodgson, N. B.: Personal communication, 1986.

Hoffman, W. W., and Hall, W. V.: A modification of Spence's hood for one-stage surgical correction of distal shaft penile hypospadias. J. Urol., 109:1017–1018, 1973.

Hollowell, J. G., Keating, M. A., Snyder, H. M., et al.: Preservation of urethral plate in hypospadias repair: Extended applications and further experience with the onlay island flap urethroplasty. J. Urol., 143:98–101, 1990.

Horton, C. E., Devine, C. J., and Baran, N.: Pictorial history of hypospadias repair techniques. *In* Horton, C. E. (Ed.): Plastic and Reconstructive Surgery of the Genital Area. Boston, Little, Brown & Co., 1973, pp. 237–248.

Horton, C. E., Devine, C. J., and Graham, J. K.: Fistulas of the penile urethra. Plast. Reconstr. Surg., 66:407–418, 1980.

Humby, G.: A one-stage operation for hypospadias. Br. J. Surg., 29:84–92, 1941.

Jensen, B. H.: Caudal block for postoperative pain relief in children after genital operations: A comparison between bupivacaine and morphine. Acta Anesthesiol. Scand., 25:373–375, 1981.

Juskiewenski, S., Vaysse, P., Guitard, J., et al.: Traitement des hypospadias anterieurs. Chir. Pediatr., 24:75–79, 1983.

Juskiewenski, S., Vaysse, P., Moscovici, J., et al.: A study of the arterial blood supply to the penis. Anat. Clin., 4:101–107, 1982.

Kaplan, G. W.: Repair of proximal hypospadias using a preputial free graft for neourethral construction and a preputial pedicle flap for ventral skin coverage. J. Urol., 140:1270–1272, 1988.

Kaplan, G. W., and Brock, W. A.: The etiology of chordee. Urol. Clin. North Am., 8:383–387, 1981.

Kaplan, S. D., Hensle, T. W., Burbige, K. A., et al.: Hypospadias: Associated behavior problems and male gender role development [abstract 11]. J. Urol., 141:45A, 1989.

Kaplan, G. W., and Lamm, D. L.: Embryogenesis of chordee. J. Urol., 114:769–773, 1975.

Karl, G. W., Swedlon, D. B., Lee, K. W., et al.: Epinephrine-halothane interaction in children. Anesthesiology, 58:142–145, 1983.

Kass, E. J., and Bolong, D.: Single-stage hypospadias reconstruction without fistula. J. Urol., 144:520–522, 1990.

Keating, M. A., and Duckett, J. W.: Bladder mucosa in urethral reconstructions. J. Urol., 144:827–834, 1990.

Kenawi, M. M.: Sexual function in hypospadias. Br. J. Urol., 47:883–890, 1975.

Khuri, F. J., Hardy, B. E., and Churchill, B. M.: Urologic anomalies associated with hypospadias. Urol. Clin. North Am., 8:565–571, 1981.

Kim, S. H., and Hendren, W. H.: Repair of mild hypospadias. J. Pediatr. Surg., 16:806–811, 1981.

King, L. R.: One-stage repair without skin graft based on a new principle: Chordee is sometimes produced by skin alone. J. Urol., 103:660–662, 1970.

King, L. R.: Cutaneous chordee and its implications in hypospadias repair. Urol. Clin. North Am., 8:397–403, 1981.

Koff, S. A.: Mobilization of the urethra in the surgical treatment of hypospadias. J. Urol., 125:394–397, 1981.

Koyanagi, T., Nonomura, K., Gotoh, T., et al.: One-stage repair of perineal hypospadias and scrotal transposition. Eur. Urol., 10:364–367, 1984.

Koyle, M. A., and Ehrlich, R. M.: The bladder mucosal graft for urethral reconstruction. J. Urol., 138:1093–1095, 1987.

Kramer, S. A., Aydin, G., and Kelalis, P. P.: Chordee without hypospadias in children. J. Urol., 128:559–561, 1982.

Kumar, S.: Hypospadias with normal prepuce. J. Urol., 136:1056–1057, 1986.

Li, Z. C., Zheng, Z. H., Shen, Y. X., et al.: One-stage urethroplasty for hypospadias using a tube constructed with bladder mucosa—a new procedure. Urol. Clin. North Am., 8:463–470, 1981.

MacMillan, R. D. H., Churchill, B. M., and Gilmore, R. F.: Assessment of urinary stream after repair of anterior hypospadias by meatoplasty and glanuloplasty. J. Urol., 134:100–102, 1985.

Manley, C. B., and Epstein, E. S.: Early hypospadias repair. J. Urol., 125:698–700, 1981.

Marberger, H., and Pauer, W.: Experience in hypospadias repair. Urol. Clin. North Am., 8:403–419, 1981.

Marshall, M., Johnson, S. H., Price, S. E., et al.: Cecil urethroplasty with concurrent scrotoplasty for repair of hypospadias. J. Urol., 121:335–339, 1979.

Marshall, V. F., and Spellman, R. M.: Construction of urethra in hypospadias using vesical mucosal graft. J. Urol., 73:335–342, 1955.

Mathieu, P.: Traitement en un temps de l'hypospadias balanique et juxta-balanique. J. Chir. (Paris), 39:481–484, 1932.

Mays, H. B.: Hypospadias: A concept of treatment. J. Urol., 65:279–287, 1951.

McArdle, F., and Lebowitz, R.: Uncomplicated hypospadias and anomalies of upper urinary tract: Need for screening? Urology, 5:712–716, 1975.

McCormack, R. M.: Simultaneous chordee repair and urethral reconstruction for hypospadias. Plast. Reconstr. Surg., 13:257, 1954.

Memmelaar, J.: Use of bladder mucosa in a one-stage repair of hypospadias. J. Urol., 58:68–73, 1947.

Mettauer, J. P.: Practical observations on those malformations of the male urethra and penis, termed hypospadias and epispadias, with an anomalous case. Am. J. Med. Sci., 4:43, 1842.

Mollard, P., Mouriquand, P., Bringeon, G., and Bugmann, P.: Repair of hypospadias using a bladder mucosal graft in 76 patients. J. Urol., 142:1548–1551, 1989.

Monfort, G., Jean, P., and Lacoste, M.: One-stage correction of posterior hypospadias using a transverse pedicle flap (Duckett's operation). Chir. Pediatr., 24:71–74, 1983.

Monfort, G., and Lucas, C.: Dihydrotestosterone penile stimulation in hypospadias surgery. Eur. Urol., 8:201–203, 1982.

Montagnino, B.A., Gonzales, E. T., Jr., and Roth, D. R.: Open catheter drainage after urethral surgery. J. Urol., 140:1250–1252, 1988.

Mustarde, J. C.: One-stage correction of distal hypospadias and other people's fistulae. Br. J. Plast. Surg., 18:413–420, 1965.

Nasrallah, P. F., and Minott, H. B.: Distal hypospadias repair. J. Urol., 131:928–930, 1984.

Nesbit, R. M.: Plastic procedure for correction of hypospadias. J. Urol., 45:699–702, 1941.

Nesbit, R. M.: Congenital curvature of the phallus: Report of three cases with description of corrective operation. J. Urol., 93:230–232, 1965.

Nesbit, R. M.: Operation for correction of distal penile ventral curvature with and without hypospadias. Trans. Am. Assoc. Genitourin. Surg., 58:12–14, 1966.

Nonomura, K., Koyanagi, T., Imanaka, K., et al.: One-stage total repair of severe hypospadias with scrotal transposition: Experience in 18 cases. J. Pediatr. Surg., 23:177–180, 1988.

Ombredanne, L.: Precis Clinique et Operation de Chirurgie Infantile. Paris, Masson, 1932, p. 851.

Opitz, J. M., Simpson, J. L., Sarto, G. E., Summitt, R. L., New, M., and German, J.: Pseudovaginal perineoscrotal hypospadias. Clin. Genet., 3:1, 1972.

Ossandon, F., and Ransley, P. G.: Lasso tourniquet for artificial erection in hypospadias. Urology, 19:656–657, 1982.

Pancoast, J. A.: Treatise on Operative Surgery. Philadelphia, Carrey and Hart, 1844, pp. 317–318.

Perlmutter, A. D., and Vatz, A. D.: Meatal advancement for distal hypospadias without chordee. J. Urol., 113:850–852, 1975.

Peterson, R. E., Imperato-McGinley, J., Gautier, T., and Sturla, E.: Male pseudohermaphroditism due to steroid 5-alpha-reductase deficiency. Am. J. Med., 62:170, 1977.

Polus, J., and Lotte, S.: Chirurgie des hypospades: Une nouvelle technique esthetique et fonctionnelle. Ann. Chir. Plast., 10:3–9, 1965.

Quartey, J. K. M.: One-stage penile/preputial cutaneous island flap urethroplasty for urethral stricture: A preliminary report. J. Urol., 129:284–287, 1983.

Rabinowitz, R.: Outpatient catheterless modified Mathieu hypospadias repair. J. Urol., 138:1074–1076, 1987.

Rajfer, J., and Walsh, P. C.: The incidence of intersexuality in patients with hypospadias and cryptorchidism. J. Urol., 116:769–770, 1976.

Ransley, P. G., Duffy, P. G., Oesch, I. L., et al.: The use of bladder mucosa and combined bladder mucosa/preputial skin grafts for urethral reconstruction. J. Urol., 138:1096–1098, 1987.

Redman, J. F.: Experience with 60 consecutive hypospadias repairs using the Horton-Devine techniques. J. Urol., 129:115–118, 1983.

Redman, J. F.: The balanic groove technique of Barcat. J. Urol., 137:83–85, 1987.

Retik, A. B., Keating, M. A., and Mandel, J.: Complications of hypospadias repair. Urol. Clin. North Am., 15:223–236, 1988.

Rich, M. A., Keating, M. A., Snyder, H. M., et al.: "Hinging" the urethral plate in hypospadias meatoplasty. J. Urol., 142:1551–1553, 1989.

Ricketson, G.: A method of repair for hypospadias. Am. J. Surg., 95:279–283, 1958.

Ritchey, M. L., Benson, R. C., Jr., Kramer, S. A., et al.: Management of mullerian duct remnants in the male patient. J. Urol., 140:795–799, 1988.

Rober, P. E., Perlmutter, A. D., and Reitelman, C.: Experience with 81 one-stage hypospadias/chordee repairs using free graft urethroplasties. J. Urol., 144:526–529, 1990.

Roberts, C. J., and Lloyd, S.: Observations on the epidemiology of simple hypospadias. Br. Med. J. [Clin. Res.], 1:768–770, 1973.

Ross, F., Farmer, A. W., and Lindsay, W. K.: Hypospadias—a review of 230 cases. Plast. Reconstr. Surg., 24:357–368, 1959.

Russell, R. H.: Operation for severe hypospadias. Br. J. Med. [Clin. Res.], 2:1432, 1900.

Sauvage, P., Rougeron, G., Bientz, J., et al.: Use of the pedicled transverse preputial flap in the surgery of hypospadias: Apropos of 100 cases. Chir. Pediatr., 28:220–223, 1987.

Scherz, H. C., Kaplan, G. W., Packer, M. G., et al.: Post-hypospadias repair of urethral strictures: A review of 30 cases. J. Urol., 140:1253–1255, 1988.

Schultz, J. R., Klykylo, W. M., and Wacksman, J.: Timing of elective hypospadias repair in children. Pediatrics, 71:342–351, 1983.

Shelton, T. B., and Noe, H. N.: The role of excretory urography in patients with hypospadias. J. Urol., 135:97–100, 1985.

Shima, H., Ikoma, F., Terakawa, T., et al.: Developmental anomalies associated with hypospadias. J. Urol., 122:619–621, 1979.

Smith, E. D.: A de-epithelialized overlap flap technique in the repair of hypospadias. Br. J. Plast. Surg., 26:106–109, 1973.

Smith, E. D.: Durham-Smith repair of hypospadias. Urol. Clin. North Am., 8:451–455, 1981.

Smith, E. D.: Hypospadias. In Ashcraft, K. (Ed.): Pediatric Urology. Philadelphia, W.B. Saunders Co., 1990.

Snow, B. W.: Use of tunica vaginalis to prevent fistulas in hypospadias surgery. J. Urol., 136:861–863, 1986.

Snyder, H. M., and Duckett, J. W.: Hypospadias "pearls." Soc. Pediatr. Urol. Newsletter, May 1984.

Sommer, J. T., and Stephens, F. D.: Dorsal ureteral diverticulum of the fossa navicularis: Symptoms, diagnosis and treatment. J. Urol., 124:94–98, 1980.

Song, R., Wang, X., and Zuo, Z.: Hypospadias repair. Clin. Plast. Surg., 9:91–95, 1982.

Sorenson, R.: Hypospadias with special reference to etiology. Op. Dom. Biol. Hered. Hum., 31:1, 1953.

Spencer, J. R., and Perlmutter, A. D.: Sleeve advancement distal hypospadias repair. J. Urol., 144:523–525, 1990.

Standoli, L.: Correzione dell'ipospadias con tempo ad isola prepuziale. Rass. Italia Chir. Pediatr., 21:82–91, 1979.

Standoli, L.: One-stage repair of hypospadias: Preputial island flap technique. Ann. Plast. Surg., 9:81–88, 1982.

Stecker, J. F., Horton, C. E., Devine, C. J., et al.: Hypospadias cripples. Urol. Clin. North Am., 8:539–544, 1981.

Sugar, E. C., and Firlit, C. F.: Urinary prophylaxis and postoperative care of children at home with an indwelling catheter after hypospadias repair. Urology, 32:418–420, 1989.

Svensson, J., and Berg, R.: Micturition studies and sexual function in operated hypospadias. Br. J. Urol., 55:422–426, 1983.

Sweet, R. A., Schrott, H. G., Kurland, R., et al.: Study of the incidence of hypospadias in Rochester, Minnesota, 1940–1970, and a case-control comparison of possible etiologic factors. Mayo Clin. Proc., 49:52–59, 1974.

Thiersch, C.: Ueber die Entstehungsweise und operative Behandlung der Epispadie. Arch. Heitkunde, 10:20, 1869.

Turner-Warwick, R.: The use of pedicle grafts in the repair of urinary tract fistulae. Br. J. Urol., 44:644–656, 1972.

Turner-Warwick, R.: Observations upon techniques for reconstruction of the urethral meatus, the hypospadiac glans deformity and the penile urethra. Urol. Clin. North Am., 6:643–655, 1979.

Udall, D. A.: A correction of three types of congenital curvatures of the penis including the first reported case of dorsal curvature. J. Urol., 124:50–54, 1980.

Van der Meulen, J. C.: Hypospadias Monograph. Leiden, The Netherlands, A. G. Stenfert, Kroese, NV, 1964.

Van der Meulen, J. C.: Hypospadias and cryptospadias. Br. J. Plast. Surg., 24:101–108, 1971.

Van der Meulen, J. C.: Correction of hypospadias: Types I and II. Ann. Plast. Surg., 8:403–411, 1982.

Vordermark, J. S.: Adhesive membrane: A new dressing for hypospadias. Urology, 20:86, 1982.

Wacksman, J.: Modification of the one-stage flip-flap procedure to repair distal penile hypospadias. Urol. Clin. North Am., 8:527–530, 1981.

Wacksman, J.: Repair of hypospadias using new mouth-controlled microscope. Urology, 29:276–278, 1987.

Walker, R. D.: Outpatient repair of urethral fistulae. Urol. Clin. North Am., 8:582–583, 1981.

Walsh, P. C., Madden, J. D., Harrod, M. J., Goldstein, J. L., MacDonald, P. C., and Wilson, J. D.: Familial incomplete male pseudohermaphroditism, Type 2. Decreased dihydrotestosterone formation in pseudovaginal perineoscrotal hypospadias. N. Engl. J. Med., 291:18,944, 1974.

Waterhouse, K., and Glassberg, K. I.: Mobilization of the anterior urethra as an aid in the one-stage repair of hypospadias. Urol. Clin. North Am., 8:521–525, 1981.

Welch, K. J.: Hypospadias. In Ravitch, M. M., Welch, K. J., Benson, C. D., et al. (Eds.): Pediatric Surgery, ed. 3. Chicago, Year Book Medical Publishers, 1979, pp. 1353–1376.

Wilson, J. D.: Familial incomplete male pseudohermaphroditism, type 1. Evidence for androgen resistance and variable clinical manifestations in a family with Reifenstein syndrome. N. Engl. J. Med., 290:1097–1103, 1974.

Woodard, J. R., and Cleveland, R.: Application of Horton-Devine principles to the repair of hypospadias. J. Urol., 127:1155–1158, 1982.

Woodhouse, C., and Ransley, P. R.: Personal communication, 1984.

Yeoman, D. M., Cooke, R., and Hain, W. R.: Penile block for circumcision? A comparison with caudal block. Anesthesia, 38:862–866, 1983.

51
CONGENITAL ANOMALIES OF THE GENITALIA

Jack S. Elder, M.D.

Neonatal genital anomalies are common and may result from a disorder in sexual differentiation, genital differentiation, and/or genital growth. Many genital anomalies are associated with developmental abnormalities of other organ systems.

Recognition of normal embryology is essential to understanding the pathogenesis of genital anomalies. In the male embryo, differentiation of the external genitalia occurs between weeks 9 and 13 of gestation and requires production of testosterone by the testis as well as conversion of testosterone into dihydrotestosterone (DHT) under the enzymatic influence of 5α-reductase in the genital anlagen. Under the influence of DHT, the genital tubercle differentiates into the glans penis; the genital folds become the shaft of the penis; and the genital swellings migrate inferomedially, fusing in the midline to become the scrotum. In the female, and in the male with an abnormality in fetal testosterone production, 5α-reductase deficiency, or androgen receptor defect, the genital tubercle develops passively into the clitoris, the genital folds become labia minora, and the genital swellings become labia majora.

NORMAL GENITALIA

In a normal term male neonate, the penis is 3.5 ± 0.7 cm in stretched length and 1.1 ± 0.2 cm in diameter (Table 51–1). At birth, the inhibitory effect of maternal estrogens on the fetal pituitary is removed; this causes a rebound surge in gonadotropins that results in an early transient surge in testosterone production by the Leydig cells, stimulating penile growth during the first 6 months of life. During the remainder of childhood, the penis grows much more slowly. Normally, the penis has a fully developed foreskin and a median raphe on the shaft of the penis. However, in 10 per cent of males, there is deviation of the raphe, usually to the left side (Ben-Ari et al., 1985). Although deviation of the raphe

may be associated with penile torsion or chordee without hypospadias, it is usually an insignificant finding. However, in the newborn male with deviation of the raphe, careful inspection of the glans is important.

The appearance of the normal female genitalia is much less variable. The clitoris, urethral meatus, and hymen may be visualized when the labia minora are separated. Approximately 3 per cent of females have hymenal variants, such as tags or transverse bands (Jenny et al., 1987). In the neonate, the vulva may be hyperpigmented and enlarged as a consequence of circulating maternal estrogens. The breadth of the newborn clitoris ranges from 2 to 6 mm, with a mean of 3.7 to 3.9 mm (Riley and Rosenbloom, 1980). Huffman (1976) reported a "clitoral index" obtained by multiplying the breadth of the glans by its length, with an index of 4.35 being the upper limit of normal. Generally, infants with a clitoral breadth greater than 6 mm or clitoral index greater than 10 mm should be evaluated. The clitoris does not change in size during the first year of life.

Table 51–1. STRETCHED PENILE LENGTH IN NORMAL MALES

Age	Mean (cm)	Tenth Percentile (cm)
Newborn, 30 weeks	2.5 ± 0.4	
Newborn, 34 weeks	3.0 ± 0.4	
Newborn, term	3.5 ± 0.4	
0–5 months	3.75	2.7 (0–12 months)
6–12 months	4.3	
1–2 years	4.8	3.6
2–3 years	5.2	
3–4 years	5.6	4.1
4–5 years	5.85	
5–8 years	6.1	4.7
8–11 years	6.4	4.8
Adult	13.1	11.3

Adapted from Feldman, K. W., and Smith, D. W.: Fetal phallic growth and penile standards for newborn male infants. J. Pediatr., 86;395, 1975 and Schonfeld, W. A., and Beebe, G. W.: Normal growth and variation in the male genitalia from birth to maturity. J. Urol., 48:759, 1942.

GENITAL ANOMALIES AND ASSOCIATION WITH OTHER ABNORMALITIES

Congenital anomalies of the genitalia often are associated with abnormalities of other organ systems or are part of recognized syndromes (Table 51–2). As many as 50 per cent of children with congenital anorectal malformation also have an associated urologic malformation (Hoekstra et al., 1983), and frequently, the external genitalia are involved. For example, in a series of boys with high imperforate anus, 29 per cent had an abnormality of the external genitalia, including hypospadias, penile duplication, micropenis, or scrotal deformity, whereas hypospadias was the primary genital abnormality in those with low imperforate anus (Hoekstra et al., 1983). Among girls with imperforate anus, genital anomalies occur in 35 per cent, including bicornuate uterus, uterus didelphys, hypoplastic uterus, vaginal septum, vaginal agenesis, imperforate hymen, and absence of the lower third of the vagina (Fleming et al., 1986; Hoekstra et al., 1983). Among boys with esophageal atresia and/or tracheoesophageal fistula, genital deformities also are common, including hypospadias (6 per cent) and penile agenesis, penoscrotal transposition, scrotal malformation, and scrotal agenesis (1.5 per cent each) (Berkhoff et al., 1989). Consequently, involvement of the urologist in the initial evaluation and long-term management of these patients is important.

Table 51–2. GENITAL ANOMALIES COMMONLY OCCURRING IN VARIOUS SYNDROMES

Male	Female
Microphallus/Ambiguous Genitalia/ Bifid Scrotum	***Hypoplastic Labia Majora***
Anencephaly	Escobar syndrome
Aniridia-Wilms' tumor association	Popliteal pterygium syndrome
Bladder exstrophy	Robinow syndrome
Borjeson-Forssman-Lehman syndrome	Trisomy 18
Carpenter syndrome	9p–, 18q–
CHARGE association	***Double Vagina and/or Bicornuate Uterus***
Cloacal exstrophy	Cloacal exstrophy
Fraser syndrome	Fraser syndrome
Johanson-Blizzard syndrome	Johanson-Blizzard syndrome
Meckel-Gruber syndrome	Rokitansky sequence
Noonan syndrome	Trisomy 13
Opitz syndrome	***Vaginal Atresia***
Pallister-Hall syndrome	Cloacal exstrophy
Popliteal pterygium syndrome	MURCS association
Prader-Willi syndrome	Rokitansky sequence
Rapp-Hodgkin ectodermal dysplasia syndrome	Sirenomelia sequence
Rieger syndrome	
Robinow syndrome	
Schinzel-Giedian syndrome	
Short rib–polydactyly	
Smith-Lemil-Opitz syndrome	
Triploidy syndrome	
Trisomy 4p, 9, 20p	
XXY, XXXXY	

Adapted from Jones, K. L.: Smith's Recognizable Patterns of Human Malformation, ed. 4. Philadelphia, W. B. Saunders Co., 1988.

MALE GENITAL ANOMALIES

Penile Anomalies

Phimosis

At birth, there is a physiologic phimosis or inability to retract the foreskin in the majority of neonates because of natural adhesions between the prepuce and the glans. During the first 3 to 4 years of life, as the penis grows, epithelial debris (smegma) accumulates under the prepuce, gradually separating the foreskin from the glans. Intermittent penile erections aid in allowing the foreskin to eventually become retractable. By 3 years of age, 90 per cent of foreskins are retractable, and less than 1 per cent of males have phimosis by 17 years of age (Oster, 1968).

Early forceful retraction of the foreskin generally is not recommended because recurrent adhesions between the de-epithelialized glans may occur and a cicatricial preputial ring may form, causing secondary phimosis. However, in some boys with phimosis who develop balanitis or balanoposthitis, manual retraction of the foreskin with lysis of adhesions should be considered. This may be done during an office visit. It may be helpful to apply lidocaine cream topically prior to the procedure (MacKinley, 1988). In uncircumcised boys in whom the tip of the foreskin remains tight beyond the age of 4 to 5 years, as well as in young boys with phimosis causing ballooning of the foreskin or recurrent balanitis, strong consideration should be given to performing a circumcision or dorsal slit.

Circumcision

In pediatrics, few topics generate as much controversy as whether the newborn male should undergo circumcision, perhaps because it is the most common surgical procedure in the United States and because it is usually performed for social reasons. In 1975, the American Academy of Pediatrics declared: "There is no absolute medical indication for routine circumcision of the newborn" (Thompson et al., 1975). This stance was supported by the American College of Obstetricians and Gynecologists.

Reasons given supporting circumcision included prevention of penile cancer, sexually transmitted diseases, and phimosis; and lessening of the risk of balanitis. Although carcinoma of the penis develops primarily in uncircumcised men, in Scandinavian countries, where few men are circumcised and there is excellent genital hygiene, the incidence of penile cancer is exceedingly low.

It has become apparent that the uncircumcised newborn is predisposed to urinary tract infection (UTI) in the neonatal period. For example, in a study of 100 neonates with UTI, Ginsburg and McCracken (1982) found that only three of the 62 males (5 per cent) who developed a UTI were circumcised. More currently, Wiswell and colleagues (1985) studied more than 2500 male infants and found that 41 had symptomatic UTI, of whom 88 per cent were uncircumcised. In that study, uncircumcised males were nearly 20 times more likely to develop UTI than circumcised neonates. Other studies of larger groups of infants have corroborated these reports (Wiswell et al., 1986). Presumably, UTIs result from colonization of the prepuce by urinary pathogens (Fussell et al., 1988; Wiswell et al., 1988). In view of these findings, the American Academy of Pediatrics reviewed their policy and published an updated scholarly report on neonatal circumcision (AAP Task Force on Circumcision, 1989). The report reviews penile hygiene, cancer of the penis, UTI, sexually transmitted diseases, cervical carcinoma, pain, local anesthesia, contraindications, and complications, and concludes: "Newborn circumcision has potential medical benefits and advantages as well as disadvantages and risks. When circumcision is being considered, the benefits and risks should be explained to the parents and informed consent obtained." The report is very readable and should be given to families who are undecided regarding the issue.

Penile Cysts

The most common cystic lesion of the penis is accumulation of epithelial debris, or smegma, under the unretractable foreskin. In young boys, because the foreskin eventually will retract, the foreskin should not be retracted unless there is associated infection or inflammation.

At times, epidermal inclusion cysts may form following circumcision or other forms of penile surgery. In addition, epidermal cysts may rarely form along the median penile raphe. These cystic lesions may be treated with simple excision.

Webbed Penis

Webbed penis is a condition in which the scrotal skin extends onto the ventrum of the penis (Fig. 51–1). When this is a congenital condition, the underlying urethra and the remainder of the scrotum, in most cases,

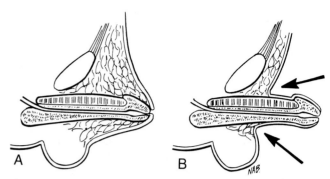

Figure 51–2. Concealed penis (A), which may be visualized by retracting skin lateral to penile shaft (B).

are normal. At other times, this condition is iatrogenic following circumcision or other penile surgery and results from excessive removal of ventral penile skin.

Although the webbed penis is usually asymptomatic, the cosmetic appearance often is unacceptable. This condition may be corrected by incising the web transversely, which separates the penis from the scrotum, and closing the skin vertically (Kenawi, 1973; Perlmutter and Chamberlain, 1972). In other cases, however, the distal urethra may be hypoplastic, and correction of the anomaly in this situation requires urethral reconstruction.

Concealed (Buried) Penis

A concealed penis is a normally developed penis that becomes camouflaged by the suprapubic fat pad; this anomaly may be congenital or iatrogenic following circumcision (Fig. 51–2). In infants and young children, the congenital condition has been speculated to result because of inelasticity of the dartos fascia (which normally allows the penile skin to slide freely on the deep layers of the shaft), restricting extension of the penis (Devine, 1989), and because the penile skin is not anchored to the deep fascia. In older children and adolescents with obesity, the abundant fat on the abdominal wall may hide the contour of the penile shaft. A concealed or buried penis also may result following neonatal circumcision in a baby with significant scrotal swelling from a hydrocele or hernia, or following routine circumcision in a baby with a webbed penis. In some neonates, the penile shaft seems to retract naturally into the scrotum, and if circumcision is performed in this situation, the skin at the base of the penis may form a cicatrix over the retracted phallus (Fig. 51–3). In its most severe form, this complication can predispose the child to UTIs and may cause urinary retention.

On inspection, the contour of the penile shaft and the glans cannot be seen. However, careful palpation allows one to determine that the penile shaft actually is concealed and normal in size rather than a microphallus or a penis that has undergone circumcision injury. It is important to determine whether the glans can be exposed simply by retracting the skin covering the glans. If so, it remains the surgeon's judgment whether correction is warranted. In a child who has undergone previous circumcision and in whom a cicatrix is present that

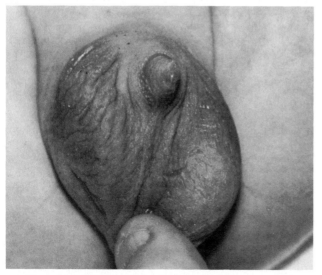

Figure 51–1. Webbed penis. Penile shaft is normal in length.

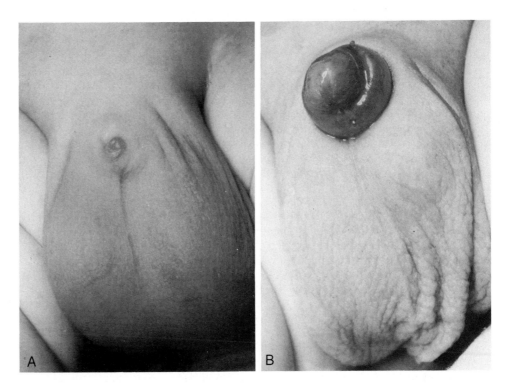

Figure 51–3. *A,* Concealed penis resulting from circumcision. *B,* Same patient following revision of circumcision.

prevents visualization of the glans, however, repair is recommended.

Several techniques have been described to correct the concealed penis (Donahoe and Keating, 1986; Maizels et al., 1986; Redman, 1985; Shapiro, 1987; Shiraki and Shirai, 1975). The indications for this type of surgery as well as the timing of reconstruction are controversial. In moderately severe cases, the dysgenic bands of tissue, which are located primarily on the dorsal surface of the shaft of the penis, must be removed. In addition, the subcutaneous tissue on the dorsal aspect of the penis should be fixed to the pubic fascia, and the subcutaneous tissue of the scrotum should be fixed to the ventral aspect of the base of the penile shaft. In the most severe

cases, the suspensory ligament of the penis must be divided, suprapubic fat must be excised, and spermatic cords must be protected. Liposuction has been reported to be helpful in severe cases (Maizels et al., 1986). In some cases, an island pedicle of ventral preputial skin may be used to cover the penis and aid in reconstruction.

Penile Torsion

Penile torsion refers to a rotational defect of the penile shaft (Fig. 51–4). Almost always, it occurs in a counterclockwise direction, that is, to the left side. In most cases, penile development is normal, and the condition is unrecognized until circumcision or until

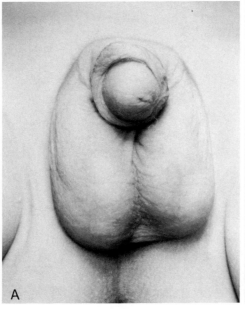
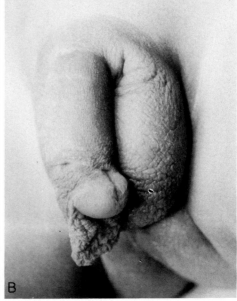

Figure 51–4. Penile torsion in a 1-year-old *(A)*, and 9-year-old *(B)*.

foreskin is retracted. In some cases, however, penile torsion is associated with mild forms of hypospadias or a hooded prepuce. In most cases of penile torsion, the median raphe spirals obliquely around the shaft. In general, the defect has primarily cosmetic significance and correction is unnecessary if the rotation is less than 60 degrees to 90 degrees from the midline.

Although the glans may be directed greater than 90 degrees from the midline, the orientation of the corporeal bodies and the corpus spongiosum at the base of the penis is normal. In the milder forms of penile torsion, the penile skin may be degloved and simply reoriented such that the median raphe is restored to its normal position (Pomerantz et al., 1978). However, in boys with penile torsion greater than or equal to 90 degrees, simply rearranging the skin on the shaft of the penis is insufficient. In these more severe forms of the disorder, the base of the penis must be mobilized so that dysgenic bands of tissue may be identified and incised. If the penis still remains rotated, correction may be accomplished by placing a nonabsorbable suture through the lateral aspect of the base of the corpora cavernosa on the side opposite the direction of the abnormal rotation (i.e., on the right corporeal body) and fixing it to the pubic symphysis dorsal to the penile shaft.

Lateral Curvature of the Penis

Lateral penile curvature usually is caused by overgrowth or hypoplasia of one corporeal body (Fitzpatrick, 1976). Lateral penile curvature usually is congenital; however, it is often unrecognized until later in childhood because the penis is normal when flaccid, and the disparity in corporeal size becomes apparent only during an erection. Surgical repair of this lesion involves degloving the penis and performing a modified Nesbit procedure, in which ellipses of tunica albuginea are excised from the site of maximum curvature to allow

straightening of the penis (Gavrell, 1974). The intraoperative technique of artifical erection is critical to the procedure's success (Gittes and McLaughlin, 1974). During correction, one must be careful to avoid injury to the neurovascular bundles.

Micropenis

Micropenis is defined as a normally formed penis with a size greater than 2 standard deviations below the mean (Fig. 51–5A). Generally, the ratio of the length of the penile shaft to its circumference is normal. In a few cases, the corpora cavernosa are severely hypoplastic. The scrotum generally is fused but often is diminutive. The testes usually are small and frequently are undescended.

The assessment of length is made by measuring the penis from its attachment to the pubic symphysis to the tip of the glans (Fig. 51–5B). In an obese infant or child, one must be careful to depress the suprapubic fat pad completely to obtain an accurate measurement. Stretched penile length is used because it correlates more closely with erectile length than the relaxed length of the penis. The measurements should be compared with standards for penile length (see Table 51–1). In general, the penis of a term newborn should be at least 2.5 cm in length. A webbed or concealed penis often resembles micropenis, but examination shows a normal penile shaft.

Knowledge of the endocrinologic regulation of penile development allows one to understand how micropenis occurs. Differentiation of the male external genitalia is complete by the 12th week of gestation and requires a normal testis producing testosterone, stimulated by maternal chorionic gonadotropin. During the 2nd and 3rd trimesters, growth of the penis occurs under the direction of fetal androgen, which is controlled by the secretion of fetal luteinizing hormone (LH). An abnormality in the production or utilization of testosterone results

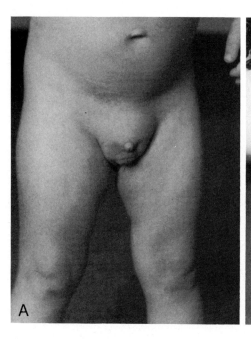
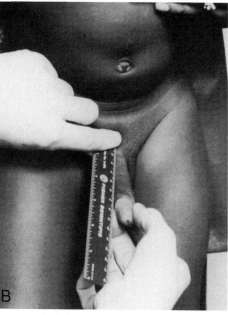

Figure 51–5. *A*, Microphallus. *B*, Technique of measuring stretched penile length.

not only in a small penis but usually in hypospadias also, whereas a true micropenis often seems to be a consequence of a deficiency of gonadotropic hormones.

There are numerous causes of micropenis, including isolated gonadotropin defects without involvement of other organ systems and generalized endocrinopathies that may be associated with central nervous system defects. The most common etiologies of micropenis include (1) hypogonadotropic hypogonadism, (2) hypergonadotropic hypogonadism (primary testicular failure), and (3) idiopathic micropenis (Gonzales, 1983; Lee et al., 1980b).

Hypogonadotropic hypogonadism may result from hypothalamic dysfunction, such as Kallmann's syndrome or Prader-Willi syndrome, and is a common cause of micropenis (Danish et al., 1980; Walsh et al., 1978). In other cases, there is an associated growth hormone deficiency (Burstein et al., 1979) or neonatal hypoglycemia secondary to congenital hypopituitarism (Lovinger et al., 1975). Micropenis secondary to hypergonadotropic hypogonadism may result from gonadal dysgenesis, or rudimentary testes syndrome, and occurs in Robinow syndrome (Lee et al., 1980b). Failure of serum testosterone to rise appropriately following human chorionic gonadotropin (hCG) stimulation has been the test most frequently utilized to identify this subgroup. However, in patients with Kallmann's syndrome and undescended testes, the serum testosterone level may not increase following hCG administration. Rarely, a patient with partial androgen insensitivity syndrome has micropenis; more commonly, however, the patient has sexual ambiguity. Some patients may have an idiopathic form of micropenis, and endocrine studies demonstrate a normal hypothalamic-pituitary-testicular axis. In these cases, micropenis may result from improper timing or delayed onset of gonadotropin stimulation in the fetus (Lee et al., 1980a).

All patients with micropenis should have a karyotype performed. Consultation generally is obtained from the pediatric endocrinology service to help determine the etiology of the micropenis as well as to assess whether other abnormalities are also present. Several issues need to be addressed, the most important of which is the growth potential of the penis. In addition, the endocrine abnormality needs to be defined. Testicular function may be assessed by measuring serum testosterone levels before and after hCG stimulation. Primary testicular failure would show an absent response and elevated basal LH and follicle-stimulating hormone levels. In some cases, a gonadotropin-releasing hormone stimulation test is done also. The endocrine evaluation of patients with micropenis is not standardized.

Prior to extensive evaluation of the hypothalamic-pituitary-testicular axis, androgen therapy should be administered to determine end organ response. In general, testosterone enanthate, 25 mg monthly for 3 months, is given. Although prolonged treatment might advance skeletal maturation, short courses of treatment do not affect height (Burstein et al., 1979). If the penis does not respond to testosterone, gender reassignment probably should be performed.

In the neonate with a micropenis who undergoes androgen therapy, if the treatment increases the size of the penis such that it falls within the normal range, what will happen at puberty? This is an unanswered question, but most think that the response of the penis to the increase in serum testosterone levels at puberty probably will not be striking. Reilly and Woodhouse (1989) have studied this issue. They reported on 20 patients with a primary diagnosis of micropenis in infancy. Of these, 8 patients were prepubertal and 12 were postpubertal; nearly all had received androgen therapy during childhood. Only one child in the prepubertal group had a stretched penile length above the 10th percentile. None of the adults had a penis in the satisfactory range. In the prepubertal group, all parents considered their children as normal boys and thought that the penile appearance was satisfactory, but expressed concern about the size of the penis and wondered whether sexual function in adulthood would be a problem. All boys stood to urinate. In the adult group, nine of the 12 patients had a normal male appearance, and three appeared eunuchoid despite regular testosterone therapy. All of the patients had a strong male identity, although half had experienced teasing because of their genital appearance. Nine of the 12 patients were sexually active. This important study demonstrated that, although the ultimate penile size in these patients may not fall within what would be considered a normal range, the majority can still function satisfactorily. Another option that may be beneficial for some of these patients is insertion of a penile prosthesis (Burkholder and Newell, 1983).

Aphallia

Penile agenesis results from failure of development of the genital tubercle. The disorder is rare with an estimated incidence of one in 10,000,000 births; approximately 70 cases have been reported. In these cases, the karyotype almost always is 46,XY, and the usual appearance is that of a well-developed scrotum with descended testes and absent penile shaft (Fig. 51–6). The anus generally is displaced anteriorly. The urethra often opens at the anal verge, adjacent to a small skin tag, and in other cases, opens into the rectum.

Associated malformations are common, including cryptorchidism, vesicoureteral reflux, horseshoe kidney, renal agenesis, imperforate anus, and musculoskeletal and cardiopulmonary abnormalities (Oesch et al., 1987; Skoog and Belman, 1989). The connection between the genitourinary and gastrointestinal tract is variable (Gilbert et al., 1990). Skoog and Belman (1989) reviewed 60 reports of aphallia and found that the more proximal the urethral meatus, the higher the incidence of other anomalies and the greater the percentage of neonatal deaths. At least 60 per cent had a postsphincteric meatus located on a peculiar appendage at the anal verge (Fig. 51–6B). There was an average of 1.2 associated anomalies, and mortality was 13 per cent. Of the 28 per cent who had a presphincteric urethral communication (prostatorectal fistula), mortality was 36 per cent. In the 12 per cent with a vesicorectal fistula and urethral atresia, there was an average of four anomalies per patient, and mortality was 100 per cent.

Children with this lesion should be evaluated imme-

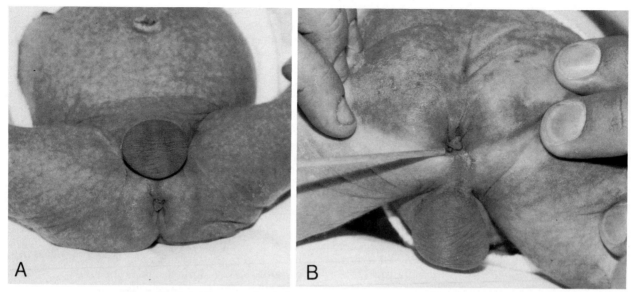

Figure 51–6. *A,* Neonate with aphallia. *B,* Urethral meatus at skin tag on anal verge.

diately with a karyotype and other appropriate studies to determine whether there are associated malformations of the urinary tract or other organ systems. Gender reassignment is recommended in the newborn, with orchiectomy and feminizing genitoplasty. At a later age, construction of a neovagina is necessary. Because of the proximity of the urethra to the rectum, this reconstruction can be formidable. Construction of an intestinal neovagina through a posterior sagittal and abdominal approach in two patients with penile agenesis has been described (Stolar et al., 1987).

Diphallia

Duplication of the penis is a rare anomaly and has a spectrum from a small accessory penis (Fig. 51–7) to a complete duplication (Hollowell et al., 1977). In some cases, each phallus has only one corporeal body and urethra, whereas others seem to be a variant of twinning with each phallus having two corpora cavernosa and a urethra. The penes usually are unequal in size and lie side by side. Associated anomalies are common, including hypospadias, bifid scrotum, duplication of the bladder, renal agenesis or ectopia, and diastasis of the pubic symphysis (Kapoor and Saha, 1987; Rao and Chandrasekharam, 1980). Anal and cardiac anomalies also are common. Evaluation should include imaging of the entire urinary tract. Sonography has been reported to aid in assessment of the extent of phallic development (Marti-Bonmati et al., 1989). Treatment must be individualized to attain a satisfactory functional and cosmetic result.

Meatal Stenosis

Meatal stenosis is a condition that almost always results following neonatal circumcision. Following disruption of the normal adhesions between the prepuce

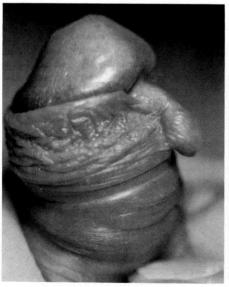

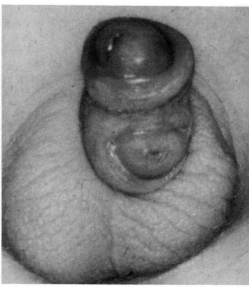

Figure 51–7. *A,* Diphallia. (Courtesy of Dr. Richard Hurwitz.) Urethra in diminutive phallic structure. *B,* Second example of diphallia.

and glans and removal of the foreskin, a significant inflammatory reaction results, which can cause meatitis and cicatrix formation, resulting in an extremely narrow meatus, a membranous web across the ventral aspect of the meatus, or an eccentric healing resulting in a prominent lip of ventral meatal tissue. Symptoms of meatal stenosis vary with the appearance. In most cases, meatal stenosis does not become apparent until after the child is toilet trained. If the meatus is pinpoint, boys are noted to void with a forceful, fine stream with a great casting distance. Some boys have a deflected stream and prolonged voiding times. Dysuria, frequency, terminal hematuria, and incontinence are symptoms that may lead to the discovery of meatal stenosis but generally are not attributable to the finding. Other boys with meatal stenosis simply have deflection of the urinary stream. These concepts regarding meatal stenosis, reflect the philosophy espoused by the Urology Section of the American Academy of Pediatrics (Committee from the Urology Section, 1978).

In a boy with suspected meatal stenosis, the meatus should be calibrated with a bougie à boule (Table 51–3) or assessed with infant sounds. Not infrequently, an asymptomatic boy with suspected meatal stenosis actually has a compliant meatus of normal caliber. If the meatus is diminished in size, or if the child has abnormal voiding symptoms, a renal and bladder ultrasound is indicated. Furthermore, if the child has a history of UTI, a voiding cystourethrogram should be done also. However, meatal stenosis rarely causes obstructive changes in the urinary tract. In boys with UTI, often it is uncertain whether the infection was the result of meatal stenosis. In a series of 280 children with meatal stenosis, 5 per cent of the patients had surgically significant lesions on voiding cystourethrogram (VCUG), and only 1 per cent had upper tract abnormalities (Noe and Dale, 1975). All of the patients with radiologic findings had experienced UTIs.

In selected cases, meatotomy can be accomplished in the physician's office using 1 per cent lidocaine with 1:100,000 epinephrine as an anesthetic infiltrated into the ventral web with a 26-gauge needle. In most cases, however, general anesthesia is necessary. An incision is made toward the frenulum sufficiently to give a normal-caliber meatus, which can be checked with the bougie. The urethral mucosa is sutured to the skin with fine chromic catgut sutures. Cystoscopy is unnecessary unless the child has symptoms of obstruction and has not had a VCUG.

In the rare case, a boy with suspected meatal stenosis and obstructive symptoms may have an anterior urethral valve in the fossa navicularis (Scherz et al., 1987). In some neonates with hypospadias, the meatus may appear extremely stenotic. However, obstruction in these cases is unusual and meatotomy rarely is needed. Another form of meatal stenosis that can result in urinary retention is balanitis xerotica obliterans. In these cases, application of cloquinal hydrocortisone cream may be effective in reducing the risk of recurrent meatal stenosis.

Parameatal Urethral Cysts

Another rare anomaly is the parameatal urethral cyst. Shiraki (1975) suggested that these cysts result from occlusion of paraurethral ducts, whereas in other cases, they may result from faulty preputial separation from the glans along the coronal sulcus. The cyst wall has been reported to consist of transitional and squamous as well as columnar epithelium (Hill and Ashken, 1977).

Scrotal Anomalies

Penoscrotal Transposition (Scrotal Engulfment)

Penoscrotal transposition may be complete or partial (Fig. 51–8). Its less severe forms have been termed bifid scrotum, doughnut scrotum, prepenile scrotum, and shawl scrotum. Frequently, the condition occurs in conjunction with perineal, scrotal, or penoscrotal hypospadias with chordee. The condition also has been reported in association with caudal regression (Lage et al., 1987), Aarskog syndrome (Shinkawa et al., 1983), and sex chromosome abnormalities (Cohen-Addad et al., 1985; Yamaguchi et al., 1989). Presumably, this anomaly results from incomplete, or failure of, inferomedial migration of the labioscrotal swellings.

When the abnormality is associated with severe hypospadias, the hypospadias repair is generally accomplished with a transverse preputial island flap in conjunction with Thiersch-Duplay tubularization of the proximal urethra. To minimize the possibility of devascularizing the preputial flap, correction of the scrotal engulfment generally is done as a second stage, 6 months later (Elder and Duckett, 1990). If the penis is normal, scrotoplasty can be accomplished when the child is 6 to 12 months of age.

Scrotoplasty is begun by circumscribing the superior aspects of each half of the vertical aspect of the scrotum and extending these incisions laterally to include at least half of the scrotum (Fig. 51–9). The medial aspects of the incision are joined on the ventral aspect of the penis, and the incision is carried down the midline along the median raphe for 4 or 5 cm. Prior to making the incision, it is helpful to infiltrate the skin with 1 per cent lidocaine with 1:100,000 epinephrine to diminish bleeding. Trac-

Table 51–3. NORMAL MEATAL SIZE IN BOYS

Age	Size (Fr.)	Number (%)	Size (Fr.)	Number (%)
6 weeks–3 years	<8	62/425 (15)	10	363/425 (85)
4–10 years	tight 8	41/508 (8)	12	384/508 (76)
11–12 years	<10	4/85 (5)	14	64/85 (75)

Adapted from Litvak, A. S., Morris, J. A., Jr., and McRoberts, J. W.: Normal size of the urethral meatus in boys. J. Urol., 115:736, 1976 and Morton (1963).

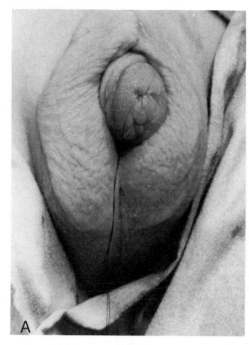 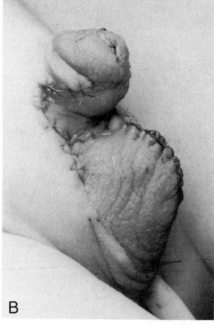

Figure 51–8. *A,* Scrotal engulfment in child with penoscrotal hypospadias following transverse preputial island flap urethroplasty. *B,* Same patient following scrotoplasty.

tion sutures are placed on the superior aspect of the scrotal flaps, and these are dissected out in the areolar layer. Deeper dissection may result in cutting the tunica vaginalis, which is unnecessary and may injure the spermatic cord. The scrotal wings are rotated medially under the penis and are sutured together in the midline in an everted manner. During this dissection, there frequently is moderate oozing from the areolar tissue, and it may be necessary to leave a small dependent drain for 24 to 48 hours. In many cases, the bare area

on either side of the penis can be closed. However, in more severe cases of penoscrotal transposition, dorsal interposition flaps may be necessary, allowing caudal advancement of the skin of the abdominal wall (Dresner, 1982). Usually, scrotoplasty can be accomplished as an outpatient procedure.

Ectopic Scrotum

Ectopic scrotum is rare and refers to the anomalous position of one hemiscrotum along the inguinal canal. Most commonly, it is suprainguinal (Fig. 51–10), although it also may be infrainguinal or perineal (Elder

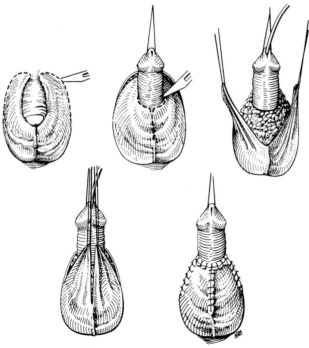

Figure 51–9. Repair of penoscrotal transposition. (See discussion in text.)

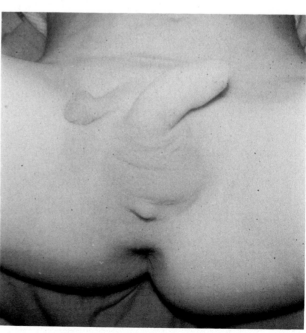

Figure 51–10. Child with ectopic scrotum.

and Jeffs, 1982; Lamm and Kaplan, 1977). This anomaly has been associated with cryptorchidism, inguinal hernia, and exstrophy, as well as the popliteal pterygium syndrome (Cunningham et al., 1989). In one review, 70 per cent of patients with a suprainguinal ectopic scrotum exhibited ipsilateral upper urinary tract anomalies, including renal agenesis, renal dysplasia, and ectopic ureter (Elder and Jeffs, 1982). Consequently, children with this anomaly should undergo upper urinary tract imaging. Because the embryology of the gubernaculum and scrotum is intimately related chronologically and anatomically, it seems likely that the ectopic scrotum results from a defect in distal gubernacular formation that prevents migration of the labioscrotal swellings. Scrotoplasty and orchiopexy may be performed at 6 to 12 months of age, or earlier if other surgical procedures are necessary.

Scrotal Hemangioma

Congenital hemangiomas are common and affect the genitalia in approximately 1 per cent of cases. Strawberry hemangiomas are the most common type and result from proliferation of immature capillary vessels. Although the lesions may undergo a period of rapid growth lasting 3 to 6 months, gradual involution is common, and most lesions require no treatment (Casale and Menashe, 1989). If ulceration develops, intervention is necessary to prevent complications from bleeding. The most popular form of therapy is oral steroids. In some cases, surgical excision is necessary. In the future, ablation with the argon laser may become the most appropriate therapy.

FEMALE GENITAL ANOMALIES

Although minor variations in the appearance of the female genitalia are common, significant abnormalities are uncommon and may represent a disorder in sexual differentiation.

The female reproductive system is derived primarily from the müllerian ducts. In the absence of androgen production by the fetal ovary, the wolffian ducts regress; and in the absence of müllerian inhibiting factor, the paired müllerian ducts, lateral to the wolffian ducts, move medially and fuse in the midline. The fused müllerian ducts join the urogenital sinus at the müllerian tubercle, and following fusion of their distal portions and absorption of the septum, the single uterovaginal canal is formed. The fused portion of the müllerian ducts forms the uterus and upper two thirds of the vagina, whereas the proximal nonfused portions form the fallopian tubes.

The presence of a normal wolffian duct contiguous with the müllerian system is important for the latter's development (Gruenwald, 1941). An abnormality in the wolffian duct may result in anomalous differentiation of the internal female genitalia. In the absence of androgen, the primitive external genital anlagen develop into female external genitalia. The genital tubercle forms the clitoris, the genital swellings fuse posteriorly to form the posterior fourchette and enlarge laterally to form the labia majora, and the genital folds develop into the labia minora.

Labial/Clitoral Anomalies

Labial Adhesion

Labial adhesion usually results from chronic inflammation of the vulva and rarely is present at birth. The condition has also been associated with sexual abuse. Labioscrotal fusion is a different entity from labial adhesion and refers to virilization of the female external genitalia. In many girls, labial adhesions are asymptomatic (Fig. 51–11). However, in some cases, the introitus is nearly completely sealed, which can result in vaginal voiding and classically results in urinary dribbling when the child stands after voiding. In addition, urinary stasis predisposes the child to UTIs. At times, the condition is not recognized until the child is to be catheterized for a VCUG.

Treatment of labial adhesions traditionally consists of application of estrogen cream to the labia three times daily for 7 to 10 days. However, the cream rarely is effective, and in most cases, the adhesion must be lysed manually with a probe, which generally can be accomplished in an office setting. Following the procedure, a small amount of bleeding often occurs. It is important to apply estrogen cream to the labial surface three times daily for 1 week following lysis of the adhesion to prevent another adhesion from forming between the raw labial surfaces.

Ectopic Labium

Ectopia of the labium majus is a rare anomaly that has been associated with renal agenesis (So et al., 1980).

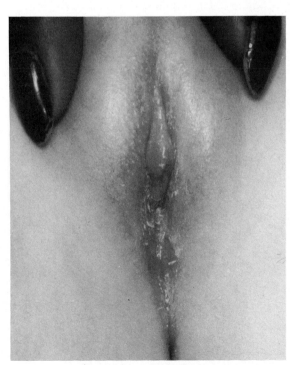

Figure 51–11. Labial adhesion.

Its etiology probably is similar to that of ectopic scrotum in the male.

Clitoral Duplication

Clitoral duplication usually occurs in association with exstrophy/epispadias anomalies. In the newborn female with bladder exstrophy, paraexstrophy flaps allow one to bring the bifid clitoris together. In girls with epispadias without exstrophy, the only visibly apparent anomalies are the urethra and bifid clitoris; these girls have total incontinence. The disorder is rare, with an incidence of one in 480,000.

Clitoral Hypertrophy

Clitoromegaly is suggestive of fetal exposure to excessive androgens, most commonly from congenital adrenal hyperplasia or other disorders of sexual differentiation, as well as from maternal progesterone use or maternal arrhenoblastoma. The presence of a gonad in the groin or labia majora should raise concern regarding the possibility of intersex.

In premature infants, the clitoris may appear large normally (Fig. 51–12), but it does not change in size and seems to regress. Female neonates with a clitoral width greater than 6 mm or a clitoral index (Huffman, 1976) greater than 10 mm should be evaluated. Other causes of clitoromegaly include chronic severe vulvovaginitis (Dershwitz et al., 1984) and neurofibromatosis (Greer and Pederson, 1981).

Another clitoral anomaly is the female phallic urethra that occurs in association with the persistent cloaca (Sotolongo et al., 1983). This anomaly affects 4 to 8 per cent of girls with persistent cloaca (Karlin et al., 1989) and has been described in association with embryologic exposure to cocaine. The management of cloacal anomalies is discussed in Chapter 47.

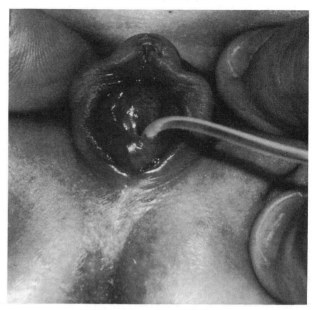

Figure 51–13. Paraurethral cyst.

Interlabial Masses

The detection of an interlabial mass in a neonate or young girl often is of tremendous concern to the child's family and referring physician. However, careful evaluation and knowledge of the causes of interlabial masses generally allow one to make the diagnosis promptly (Nussbaum and Lebowitz, 1983).

In the neonate, a *paraurethral cyst* results from retained secretions in Skene's glands, secondary to ductal obstruction (Klein et al., 1986) (Fig. 51–13). The cyst displaces the meatus in an eccentric manner. However, urethral obstruction and infection of the cyst are rare. Most paraurethral cysts regress in size during the first 4 to 8 weeks, although occasionally it is necessary to incise them.

Urethral prolapse has an appearance of erythematous, inflamed protruding mucosa surrounding the urethral meatus; it occurs almost exclusively in black girls between 1 and 9 years of age with an average age of 4 years (Fig. 51–14) (Jerkins et al., 1984). The most common signs are bloody spotting on the underwear or diaper, although dysuria or perineal discomfort also may occur. The prolapsed appearance represents eversion of the urethral mucosa. It has been proposed that urethral prolapse results from poor attachment between the smooth muscle layers of the urethra in association with episodic increases in intra-abdominal pressure because a cleavage plane between the inner longitudinal and outer circular/oblique smooth muscle layers of urethra has been identified (Lowe et al., 1986). The lesion is not obstructive. For obvious reasons, sexual abuse is suspected in many of these cases until the diagnosis of urethral prolapse is made. No known relationship exists between external genital trauma and urethral prolapse.

After the diagnosis is made, the usual therapy includes application of estrogen cream two to three times daily to the prolapsed urethra for 1 to 2 weeks as well as sitz baths (Richardson et al., 1982). If the prolapsed urethra

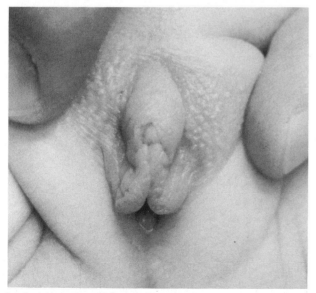

Figure 51–12. Clitoral hypertrophy in premature infant with gonad in left labium majorum; karyotype 46,XX. Labial mass was normal ovary with inguinal hernia.

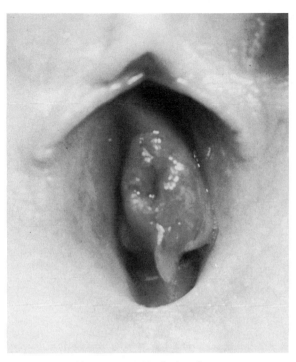

Figure 51–14. Urethral prolapse.

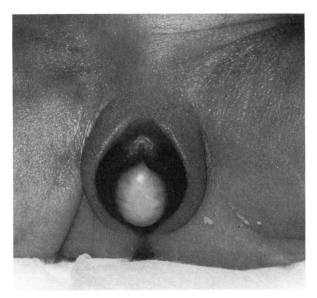

Figure 51–15. Imperforate hymen with hydrocolpos.

persists for several months, it usually results in bloody spotting and formal excision is necessary. The preferred method of excision is a circumscribing incision with removal of the everted mucosa and closure of normal urethral mucosa to introital mucosa with interrupted absorbable sutures. Catheterization is unnecessary, and the procedure can be performed on an outpatient basis. If the child is undergoing examination for suspected sexual abuse and is under general anesthesia, excision of the prolapsed urethra at that time is recommended.

An *imperforate hymen* appears as a bulging interlabial mass in the newborn with retained vaginal secretions that result from stimulation by maternal estrogens (Fig. 51–15). Because of its elasticity, the vagina may contain as much as 1 L of mucus (Rock and Azziz, 1987). In general, simple incision (hymenotomy) allows satisfactory drainage of the imperforate hymen. Related entities are covered further in this chapter. Preoperatively, these neonates should undergo upper urinary tract evaluation with ultrasonography, which not only demonstrates the extent of vaginal distention but also determines whether there are secondary obstructive effects on the upper urinary tracts (Wilson et al., 1978). Usually, signs of upper urinary tract obstruction resolve following decompression of the hydrocolpos.

Uterovaginal prolapse is a rare cause of an interlabial mass. It generally occurs in the newborn and has been associated with meningomyelocele (Rock and Azziz, 1987). The anomaly may result from partial or complete denervation of the levator ani, which supports the uterus and vagina. Spontaneous resolution may occur, but in other cases, temporary mechanical support with a rubber nipple or pessary restores the uterus to its normal position (Carpenter and Rock, 1987).

A *prolapsed ectopic ureterocele* appears as a cystic mass arising from the urethra (Fig. 51–16) and is a

presenting symptom in approximately 10 per cent of girls with ureteroceles (Caldamone et al., 1984). It may be erythematous or, if ischemic, purplish or even black. The typical age of presentation is between 1 month and 3 years. When it is protruding, the child typically is extremely irritable. The urethra is difficult to identify, but the hymen and vagina generally can be determined to be in a normal position, although it may be difficult to visualize them if the prolapsed ureterocele is quite large. The ureterocele may reduce spontaneously and occasionally can be reduced manually. Nearly all of these ureteroceles are associated with an obstructed upper pole ureter of a complete duplex system.

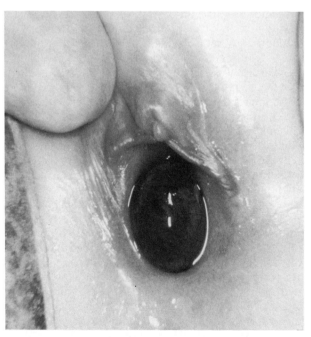

Figure 51–16. Prolapsed ectopic ureterocele. Intravenous pyelogram (IVP) demonstrated obstructed upper pole of right kidney.

Ultrasonography should be performed to visualize the upper urinary tracts, to determine the side of the ureterocele, and to demonstrate the ureterocele in the bladder. In addition, a VCUG and an intravenous pyelogram (IVP) or renal scan should be done. It is uncommon for the prolapsed ureterocele to cause bladder outlet obstruction. Because the obstructed upper pole nearly always is dysplastic, upper pole heminephrectomy with removal of the obstructed upper pole segment and as much ureter as possible through a flank incision or dorsal lumbotomy allows decompression of the ureterocele (Caldamone et al., 1984). Routine transurethral incision of the ureterocele is not recommended because it may result in postoperative reflux into the ureterocele, but the procedure may be necessary if the prolapsed ureterocele recurs following upper pole heminephrectomy.

Sarcoma botryoides (rhabdomyosarcoma) is another cause of interlabial mass. The lesion may be visible as a firm grape-like mass protruding from the introitus, may result in vaginal bleeding or the passage of sloughed tissue fragments from the vagina, and may be detected by palpating a vaginal mass on bimanual examination. The pelvis and abdomen should be evaluated with sonography and computed tomography scan (McHenry et al., 1988). The diagnosis and histologic type (usually embryonal) are established by biopsy.

Urethral Anomalies

Distal Urethral Stenosis

The concept of the relationship among female urethral pathology, recurrent UTIs, and voiding dysfunction has changed over the past 30 to 40 years. Previously, when a VCUG demonstrated narrowing of the bladder neck and a wide distal urethra in a girl with recurrent UTIs, it was assumed that bladder neck obstruction was the cause and that the urethra was wide because of poststenotic dilatation. The urethral finding was termed the "spinning top urethra" (Fig. 51–17). One of the disconcerting features of this diagnosis was that the bladder musculature was not hypertrophied as expected. Although cure rates as high as 50 per cent with Y-V-plasty of the bladder neck or internal urethrotomy were reported, the majority of urologists agreed with D.I. Williams (1958), who commented, "The clinical and the pathological diagnosis has been made by the process of exclusion." Subsequently, Lyon (1974) compared the preoperative and postoperative voiding patterns in three patients undergoing Y-V-plasty and found that the intermittent stream persisted and the residual urine remained high. At that time, it became apparent that the bladder neck probably was not the source of "obstruction," and the concept of distal urethral stenosis evolved. Investigators reported that 70 per cent of girls with recurrent UTIs seemed to have a fibrous ring in the distal third of the urethra, and that in all cases, the bougie à boule passed easily through the bladder neck. Furthermore, vigorous overdilation of the urethra (28 Fr. to 32 Fr.) reportedly often resulted in restoration of a normal voiding pattern and elimination of recurrent

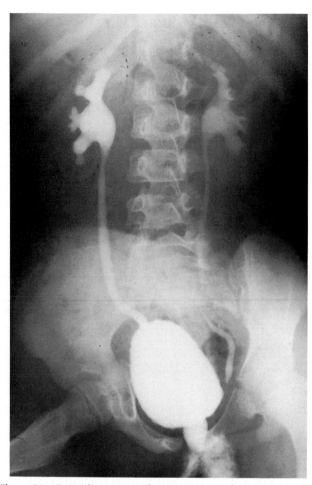

Figure 51–17. Voiding cystourethrogram (VCUG) demonstrating spinning top urethra and bilateral vesicoureteral reflux.

UTIs (Lyon and Smith, 1963). The site of distal urethral narrowing came to be known as Lyon's ring.

At birth, no apparent evidence exists of the distal urethral ring (Fisher et al., 1969). However, during the first few months, the ring was reported to develop as a normal anatomic structure that calibrated at 14 Fr. at 2 years of age and at 16 Fr. between the ages of 4 and 10 (Lyon and Tanagho, 1965). At puberty, the ring was noted to disappear. Thus, it was speculated that absence of estrogens leads to the development of the lesion.

Tanagho and Smith (1966) reported that the inner longitudinal detrusor muscle fibers continue as the inner longitudinal fibers of the urethra, the outer longitudinal detrusor fibers continue into the urethra as the outer circular coat of fibers, and the middle circular fibers of the detrusor do not enter the urethra. The striated external sphincter surrounds the two layers of urethral musculature, and the inner and outer layers of urethral musculature appear to insert into a dense collagenous tissue ring situated in the distal urethra. The overabundance of collagen was thought to encroach upon and indent the lumen of the distal urethral segment, which was the anatomic basis of the ring (Lyon, 1974). It was thought that rupture of the ring was accomplished by urethral dilation. Lyon (1974) noted that adequate urethral dilation should result in urethral bleeding and that

Table 51–4. CALIBER OF NORMAL FEMALE URETHRA

Age (years)	Median (Fr.)
2–4	14
6–10	16
12	20
≥14	24

Adapted from Immergut, M., Culp, D., and Flocks, R. H.: The urethral caliber in normal female children. J. Urol., 97:693, 1967.

a large catheter should be placed for 30 to 60 minutes as a tamponade. Lyon and Marshall (1971) reported that in the 15 to 20 per cent of children who continued to experience chronic bacilluria, repeat calibration disclosed a persistent "ring" between 26 Fr. and 30 Fr. that did not require dilation. Subsequently, internal urethrotomy also became a popular method of dealing with the obstructing ring, and several modifications were developed (Halverstadt and Leadbetter, 1968).

At that time, however, Immergut and co-workers (1967) reported the mean size of the urethral meatus and distal urethra in 136 girls undergoing tonsillectomy (Table 51–4), and it became apparent that these measurements were not dissimilar from those previously reported by Lyon in girls with recurrent UTIs. Subsequently, Immergut and Wahman (1968) demonstrated that the urethral caliber in 77 girls with recurrent UTIs was larger than the urethral size of normal uninfected girls. Graham and colleagues (1967) reported that dilation of a urethra that calibrated at 14 Fr. or less was most likely to result in improvement in symptoms; however, they also noted that, often, the narrow caliber probably was coincidental and actually normal in the majority of girls in whom it was found. Later, Kaplan and co-workers (1973) compared urethral dilation, internal urethrotomy, and antimicrobial therapy in girls with UTIs and found no differences in treatment results.

What, then, accounts for the abnormal urethral appearance? Many of these girls have interrupted, staccato streams consistent with obstruction. Johnston and associates (1978) speculated that the finding is more likely due to differing degrees of distensibility of various parts of the urethra and that the spinning top is normal in girls with high voiding rates. The spinning top urethra probably is related more to detrusor instability and/or detrusor-sphincter dyssynergia (Saxton et al., 1988). In such girls, urge incontinence and squatting to prevent loss of urine are common symptoms. Many of these girls also have recurrent UTIs, and combined therapy with anticholinergic medication and antimicrobial suppression is indicated.

Currently, most girls with UTIs and/or incontinence respond to medical management and do not require cystoscopic evaluation. Consequently, urethral calibration and dilation is performed infrequently, at present. However, if a girl is undergoing endoscopic evaluation for these problems and the urethra is less than 14 Fr. to 16 Fr., dilation to these sizes often is performed. Internal urethrotomy should be avoided because overvigorous incision of the bladder neck in these girls can result in incontinence (Kessler and Constantinou, 1986).

Hypospadias

Hypospadias in an otherwise normal girl is a rare condition, and when present, it is usually not symptomatic. Generally, it becomes significant only as a result of difficulty with urethral catheterization. Although one might suspect that it could result in symptoms of vaginal voiding (i.e., postmicturition incontinence), girls who experience vaginal voiding almost always have normal external genital anatomy. A form of hypospadias may occur in girls with urogenital sinus abnormalities.

Vaginal Anomalies

Hydrocolpos refers to the accumulation of secretions in the vagina caused by excessive intrauterine stimulation of the infant's cervical mucous glands by maternal estrogen in association with obstruction of the genital tract by an intact hymen, vaginal membrane, or vaginal atresia. Hydrometrocolpos refers to the accumulation of secretions in the vagina and uterus. These two conditions generally result in a lower midline abdominal or bulging perineal mass in the newborn or infant. Hematometrocolpos refers to the accumulation of menstrual products caused by an imperforate hymen or other obstruction at menarche. These terms do not define the cause of the obstruction.

Vaginal anomalies may be organized with regard to their etiology (Table 51–5). Disorders of vertical fusion result either from an abnormality in caudal development of the müllerian duct and/or canalization of the vaginal plate, whereas disorders of medial fusion result from failure of medial fusion of the two müllerian ducts. Internal genital anomalies occur in one third of girls with anorectal anomalies (Fleming et al., 1986) and are common in girls with urogenital sinus and cloacal anomalies also. Because differentiation of the müllerian duct is intimately associated with development of the wolffian duct, females with vaginal agenesis or disorders of medial fusion often have associated congenital upper urinary tract anomalies. In contrast, obstructive disorders of vertical fusion often cause secondary obstructive effects on the urinary tract that resolve following treatment, but congenital urinary tract anomalies are uncommon. The Mayer-Rokitansky syndrome generally has referred to vaginal agenesis. However, it has been

Table 51–5. CONGENITAL VAGINAL ANOMALIES

Disorders of Vertical Fusion
Obstructive
   Vaginal agenesis
   Transverse vaginal septum
   Imperforate hymen
Nonobstructive
   Incomplete transverse vaginal septum

Disorders of Medial Fusion
Obstructive
   Unilateral obstructing vaginal septum
Nonobstructive
   Longitudinal vaginal septum
   Vaginal duplication

proposed that the syndrome be applied to the entire spectrum of müllerian anomalies in genotypic and phenotypic females with normal endocrine status, specifically excluding those with associated anorectal or cloacal malformations (Tarry et al., 1986).

Disorders of Vertical Fusion

Vaginal agenesis occurs in one of every 4000 to 5000 females and is the second most common cause of primary infertility in women after gonadal dysgenesis (Rock and Azziz, 1987). Vaginal agenesis probably results from incomplete or absent canalization of the vaginal plate, which begins at the 11th week of gestation and is completed by the 20th week. Characteristically, the uterus in these patients is rudimentary without a lumen, although normal fallopian tubes are present, and ovarian function is normal (Fraser et al., 1973). Approximately one third of these women have renal anomalies (Griffin et al., 1976), most commonly renal agenesis or ectopia. In addition, renal fusion anomalies, such as horseshoe kidney, are common. Furthermore, skeletal anomalies have been reported in 12 per cent of these patients (Chitayat et al., 1987; Griffin et al., 1976), with two thirds having anomalies of the spine, ribs, or limbs, including polydactyly. The MURCS association of anomalies refers to *m*üllerian duct aplasia, *r*enal agenesis, and *c*ervicothoracic *s*omite abnormalities (Duncan et al., 1979).

Vaginal agenesis usually is diagnosed at puberty in girls with amenorrhea. The external genitalia are normal in appearance, and the vagina is absent or there may be a shallow pouch of 2 to 3 cm in depth. However, the diagnosis also should be suspected in any female child with an absent or a blind vagina.

Timing of vaginoplasty is variable, although it is generally performed late in the teenage years. It is generally accomplished with either a full-thickness skin graft or an isolated segment of sigmoid colon.

Another disorder of vertical fusion is the *transverse vaginal septum,* which can be high, in the middle third of the vagina, or in the lower third of the vagina (Fig. 51–18), affecting one in 80,000 females. High transverse septa are the most common, occurring in 46 per cent of cases, whereas obstruction in the middle and lower third of the vagina is found in 35 per cent and 19 per cent of cases, respectively (Rock et al., 1982). These anomalies result from abnormal canalization of the vaginal plate. Septa in the upper part of the vagina frequently are incomplete, whereas in the lower third of the vagina, the septa are usually obstructive (Rock and Azziz, 1987).

The diagnosis of transverse vaginal septum generally is made following the development of hydrocolpos, which is detectable on bimanual examination. At times, the mass may be large enough to obstruct venous return from the lower extremities, resulting in lymphedema (Tran et al., 1987). Abdominal ultrasonography demonstrates the large midline sonolucent mass with debris. Upper urinary tract obstruction is common, and an IVP or computed tomography scan may demonstrate hydronephrosis, whereas a VCUG may show anterior displacement of the bladder (Fig. 51–19). At times, percutaneous needle aspiration and injection of contrast

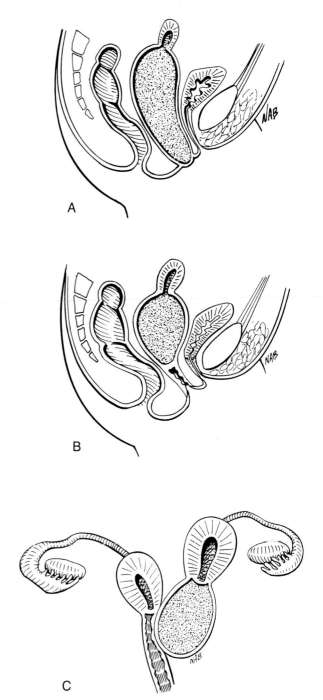

Figure 51–18. *A,* Hydrocolpos secondary to imperforate hymen. *B,* Hydrocolpos secondary to high transverse vaginal septum. *C,* Obstructed hemivagina in patient with uterus didelphys.

material may aid in the diagnosis. In the infant who does not develop an abdominal mass, the transverse septum is not detected until adolescence, when the patient develops amenorrhea, cyclic abdominal pain, and an abdominal mass secondary to hematocolpos.

The treatment of the obstructing transverse vaginal septum is variable, depending on the anatomy, and often an exploratory laparotomy is necessary (Rock and Azziz, 1987). Prompt therapy of an obstructing transverse vaginal septum is important, because ultimate fertility is decreased and is believed to be caused by a

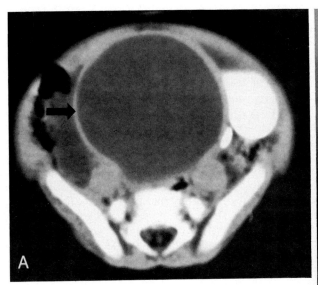

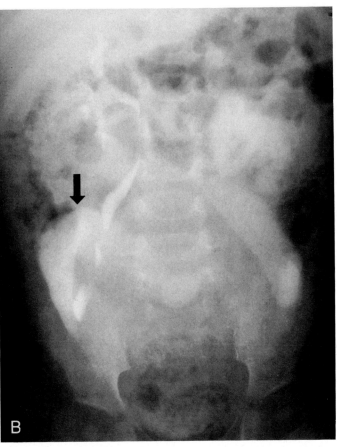

Figure 51–19. *A,* Computed tomography scan in an infant with hydrocolpos *(arrow)* secondary to transverse vaginal septum. *B,* Intravenous pyelogram (IVP) showing left hydroureteronephrosis and bilateral ureteral deviation. Arrow points to displaced bladder.

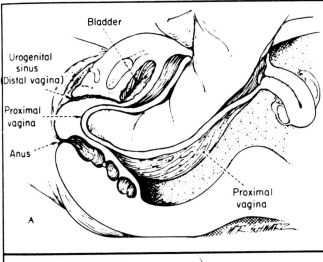

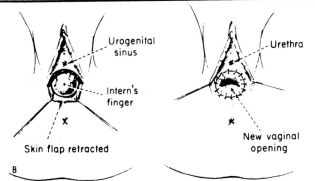

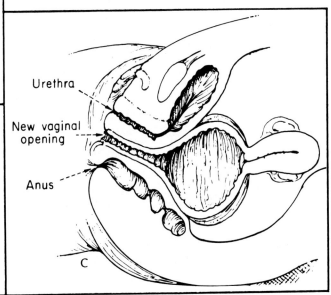

Figure 51–20. Ramenofsky-Raffensperger abdominoperineal pull-through vaginoplasty. (From Ramenofsky, M. L., and Raffensperger, J. G.: An abdomino-perineal-vaginal pull-through for definitive treatment of hydrometrocolpos. J. Pediatr. Surg., 6:381, 1971.)

high incidence of endometriosis, resulting from prolonged obstruction of menses (Rock et al., 1982). In a female with a high transverse vaginal septum or vaginal obstruction associated with a urogenital sinus abnormality, the Ramenofsky-Raffensperger abdominoperineal pull-through vaginoplasty (Ramenofsky and Raffensperger, 1971; Fig. 51–20) may be indicated.

In the neonate, hydrocolpos secondary to an *imperforate hymen* usually appears as a bulging cystic interlabial mass (see Fig. 51–15). In addition, a suprapubic abdominal mass may be evident. An imperforate hymen usually is not associated with other congenital anomalies. Preoperatively, sonographic assessment of the urinary tract should be done, and if hydronephrosis is present, it should be monitored until it resolves following definitive therapy. Treatment of an imperforate hymen is hymenotomy, using a cruciate incision and oversewing the cut edges with absorbable sutures. A small drain should be inserted through the introitus to prevent adhesion of the raw edges, and antibiotics are administered to prevent infection.

Disorders of Medial Fusion

The process of fusion of the paired müllerian structures can be arrested at any stage of development. If there is partial fusion of the müllerian structures, a *bicornuate uterus* with a single vagina results (Sayer and O'Reilly, 1986). If they are completely separated, *uterus didelphys* with *vaginal duplication* results. Often, one side of the duplex vagina is obstructed (see Fig. 51–18C; Burbige and Hensle, 1984), whereas in other cases, there is a nonobstructing longitudinal septum. The obstructed hemivagina and bicornuate uterus are almost always associated with ipsilateral renal agenesis (Gilsanz

and Cleveland, 1982; Woolf and Allen, 1953). Consequently, women with unilateral renal agenesis should be evaluated radiologically for an anomaly of the female genital system. In the rare patient, the vaginal duplication may extend through the lower third of the vagina and hymen (Fig. 51–21) and probably is secondary to incomplete caudal twinning.

The obstructed hemivagina may be detected in the neonate following detection of an abdominal mass on physical examination or ultrasound. However, it may not be detected until puberty in girls who experience cyclic abdominal pain and develop an abdominal mass. In these patients, one horn of the uterus functions normally and, thus, menstrual flow is not affected (Foglia et al., 1987; Tolete-Velcek et al., 1989). The internal genital anatomy must be evaluated carefully prior to definitive treatment, and the urinary tract should be evaluated. Often, the finding of unilateral agenesis helps provide the diagnosis. In some cases, the distended chamber may be incised by a vaginal approach, whereas in other cases, a pull-through vaginoplasty may be necessary. If one of the duplex uterine chambers is infected, it may need to be excised.

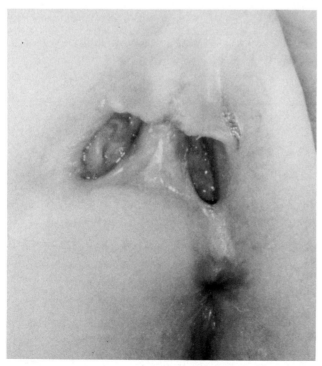

Figure 51–21. Infant with vaginal duplication.

REFERENCES

Anomalies of the Male Genitalia

AAP Task Force on Circumcision: Report of the Task Force on Circumcision. Pediatrics, 84:388, 1989.

Ben-Ari, J., Merlob, P., Mimouni, F., and Reisner, S. H.: Characteristics of the male genitalia in the newborn: Penis. J. Urol., 134:521, 1985.

Berkhoff, W. B. C., Scholtmeyer, R. J., Tibboel, D., and Molenaar, J. C.: Urogenital tract abnormalities associated with esophageal atresia and tracheoesophageal fistula. J. Urol., 141:362, 1989.

Burkholder, G. V., and Newell, M. E.: New surgical treatment for micropenis. J. Urol., 129:832, 1983.

Burstein, S., Grumbach, M. M., and Kaplan, S. L.: Early determination of androgen-responsiveness is important in the management of microphallus. Lancet 2:193, 1979.

Casale, A. J., and Menashe, D. S.: Massive strawberry hemangioma of the male genitalia. J. Urol., 141:593, 1989.

Cohen-Addad, N., Zarafu, I. W., and Hanna, M. K.: Complete penoscrotal transposition. Urology, 26:149, 1985.

Committee from the Urology Section: Urethral meatal stenosis in males. Pediatrics, 61:778, 1978.

Cunningham, L. N., Keating, M. A., Snyder, H. M., and Duckett, J. W.: Urological manifestations of the popliteal pterygium syndrome. J. Urol., 141:910, 1989.

Danish, R. K., Lee, P. A., Mazur, T., Amrhein, J. A., and Migeon, C. J.: Micropenis: II. Hypogonadotropic hypogonadism. Johns Hopkins Med. J., 146:177, 1980.

Devine, C. J., Jr.: Comment. In Hinman, F., Jr.: Atlas of Urologic Surgery. Philadelphia, W. B. Saunders Co., 1989, p. 67.

Donahoe, P. J., and Keating, M. A.: Preputial unfurling to correct the buried penis. J. Pediatr. Surg., 21:1055, 1986.

Dresner, M. L.: Surgical revision of scrotal engulfment. Urol. Clin. North Am., 9:305, 1982.

Elder, J. S., and Duckett, J. W.: Complications of hypospadias surgery. In Smith, R. B., and Ehrlich, R. M. (Eds.): Complications of Urologic Surgery. Philadelphia, W. B. Saunders Co., 1990, p. 549.

Elder, J. S., and Jeffs, R. D.: Suprainguinal ectopic scrotum and associated anomalies. J. Urol., 127:336, 1982.

Feldman, K. W., and Smith, D. W.: Fetal phallic growth and penile standards for newborn male infants. J. Pediatr., 86:395, 1975.

Fitzpatrick, T. J.: Hemihypertrophy of the human corpus cavernosum. J. Urol., 115:560, 1976.

Fussell, E. N., Kaack, M. B., Cherry, R., and Roberts, J. A.: Adherence of bacteria to human foreskins. J. Urol., 140:997, 1988.

Gavrell, G. J.: Congenital curvature of the penis. J. Urol., 112:489, 1974.

Gilbert, J., Clark, R. D., and Koyle, M. A.: Penile agenesis: A fatal variation of an uncommon lesion. J. Urol., 143:338, 1990.

Ginsburg, C. M., and McCracken, G. H., Jr.: Urinary tract infections in young infants. Pediatrics, 69:409, 1982.

Gittes, R. F., and McLaughlin, A. P., III: Injection technique to induce penile erection. Urology, 4:473, 1974.

Gonzales, J. R.: Micropenis. AUA Update Series, 2(39):1, 1983.

Hill, J. T., and Ashken, M. H.: Parameatal urethral cysts: A review of 6 cases. Br. J. Urol., 49:323, 1977.

Hoekstra, W. J., Scholtmeijer, R. J., Molenaar, J. C., Schreeve, R. H., and Schroeder, F. H.: Urogenital tract abnormalities associated with congenital anorectal anomalies. J. Urol., 130:962, 1983.

Hollowell, J. G., Jr., Witherington, R., Ballagas, A. J., and Burt, J. N.: Embryologic consideration of diphallus and associated anomalies. J. Urol., 117:728, 1977.

Kapoor, R., and Saha, M. M.: Complete duplication of the bladder, urethra and external genitalia in a neonate—a case report. J. Urol., 137:1243, 1987.

Kenawi, M. M.: Webbed penis. Br. J. Urol., 45:569, 1973.

Lage, J. M., Driscoll, S. G., and Bieber, F. R.: Transposition of the external genitalia associated with caudal regression. J. Urol., 138:387, 1987.

Lamm, D. L., and Kaplan, G. W.: Accessory and ectopic scrota. Urology, 9:149, 1977.

Lee, P. A., Danish, R. K., Mazur, T., and Migeon, C. J.: Micropenis: III. Primary hypogonadism, partial androgen insensitivity syndrome, and idiopathic disorders. Johns Hopkins Med. J., 147:175, 1980a.

Lee, P. A., Mazur, T., Danish, R., Amrhein, J., Blizzard, R. M., Money, J., and Migeon, C. J.: Micropenis: I. Criteria, etiologies and classification. Johns Hopkins Med. J., 146:156, 1980b.

Litvak, A. S., Morris, J. A., Jr., and McRoberts, J. W.: Normal size of the urethral meatus in boys. J. Urol., 115:736, 1976.

Lovinger, R. D., Kaplan, S. L., and Grumbach, M. M.: Congenital hypopituitarism associated with neonatal hypoglycemia and microphallus: Four cases secondary to hypothalamic hormone deficiencies. J. Pediatr., 87:1171, 1975.

MacKinley, G. A.: Save the prepuce: Painless separation of preputial adhesions in the outpatient clinic. Br. Med. J., 297:590, 1988.

Maizels, M., Zaontz, M., Donovan, J., Bushnick, P. N., and Firlit, C. F.: Surgical correction of the buried penis: Description of a classification system and a technique to correct the disorder. J. Urol., 136:268, 1986.

Marti-Bonmati, L., Menor, F., Gomez, J., Cortina, H., and Ibarra, F. G.: Value of sonography in true complete diphallia. J. Urol., 142:356, 1989.

Morton, H. G.: Meatus size in 1,000 circumcised children from two weeks to sixteen years of age. J. Fla. Med. Assoc., 50:137, 1986.

Noe, H. N., and Dale, G. A.: Evaluation of children with meatal stenosis. J. Urol., 114:455, 1975.

Oesch, I. L., Pinter, A., and Ransley, P. G.: Penile agenesis: A report of six cases. J. Pediatr. Surg., 22:172, 1987.

Oster, J.: Further fate of the foreskin: Incidence of preputial adhesions, phimosis, and smegma among Danish schoolboys. Arch. Dis. Child., 43:200, 1968.

Perlmutter, A. D., and Chamberlain, J. W.: Webbed penis without chordee. J. Urol., 107:320, 1972.

Pomerantz, P., Hanna, M., Levitt, S., and Kogan, S.: Isolated torsion of penis: Report of 6 cases. Urology, 11:37, 1978.

Rao, T. V., and Chandrasekharam, V.: Diphallus with duplication of cloacal derivatives: Report of a rare case. J. Urol., 124:555, 1980.

Redman, J. F.: A technique for the correction of penoscrotal fusion. J. Urol., 133:432, 1985.

Reilly, J. M., and Woodhouse, C. R. J.: Small penis and the male sexual role. J. Urol., 142:569, 1989.

Scherz, H. C., Kaplan, G. W., and Packer, M. G.: Anterior urethral valves in the fossa navicularis in children. J. Urol., 138:1211, 1987.

Schonfeld, W. A., and Beebe, G. W.: Normal growth and variation in the male genitalia from birth to maturity. J. Urol., 48:759, 1942.

Shapiro, S. R.: Surgical treatment of the "buried" penis. Urology, 30:554, 1987.

Shinkawa, T., Yamauchi, Y., Osada, Y., and Ishisawa, N.: Aarskog syndrome. Urology, 22:624, 1983.

Shiraki, I. W.: Parameatal cysts of the glans penis: a report of 9 cases. J. Urol., 114:544, 1975.

Shiraki, I. W., and Shirai, R. S.: Congenital micropenile skin sleeve. J. Urol., 114:469, 1975.

Skoog, S. J., and Belman, A. B.: Aphallia: Its classification and management. J. Urol., 141:589, 1989.

Stolar, C. J. H., Wiener, E. S., Hensle, T. W., Silien, M. L., Sukarochana, K., Sieber, W. K., Goldstein, H. R., and Pettit, J.: Reconstruction of penile agenesis by a posterior sagittal approach. J. Pediatr. Surg., 22:1076, 1987.

Thompson, H. C., King, L. R., Knox, E., and Keanes, S. B.: Report of the ad hoc task force on circumcision. Pediatrics, 56:610, 1975.

Walsh, P. C., Wilson, J. D., Allen, T. D., Madden, J. D., Porter, J. C., Neaves, W. B., Griffin, J. E., and Goodwin, W. E.: Clinical and endocrinological evaluation of patients with congenital microphallus. J. Urol., 120:90, 1978.

Wiswell, T. E., Miller, G. M., Gelston, H. M., Jr., Jones, S. K., Clemmings, A. F., et al.: Effect of circumcision status on periurethral bacterial flora during the first year of life. J. Pediatr., 113:442, 1988.

Wiswell, T. E., and Roscelli, J. D.: Corroborative evidence for the decreased incidence of urinary tract infections in circumcised male infants. Pediatrics, 78:96, 1986.

Wiswell, T. E., Smith, F. R., and Bass, J. W.: Decreased incidence of urinary tract infections in circumcised male infants. Pediatrics, 75:901, 1985.

Yamaguchi, T., Hamasuna, R., Hasui, Y., Kitida, S., and Osada, Y.: 47,XXY/48,XXY,+21 chromosomal mosaicism presenting as hypospadias with scrotal transposition. J. Urol., 142:797, 1989.

Anomalies of the Female Genitalia

Burbige, K. A., and Hensle, T. W.: Uterus didelphys and vaginal duplication with unilateral obstruction presenting as a newborn abdominal mass. J. Urol., 132:1195, 1984.

Caldamone, A. A., Snyder, H. McC., III, and Duckett, J. W.: Ureteroceles in children: Follow-up of management with upper tract approach. J. Urol., 131:1130, 1984.

Carpenter, S. E., and Rock, J. A.: Procidentia in the newborn. Int. J. Obstet. Gynecol., 25:151, 1987.

Chitayat, D., Hahm, S. Y. E., Marion, R. W., Sachs, G. S., Goldman, D., Hutcheon, R. G., Weiss, R., Cho, S., and Nitowsky, H. M.: Further delineation of the McKusick-Kaufman hydrometrocolpos-polydactyly syndrome. Am. J. Dis. Child., 141:1133, 1987.

Dershwitz, R. A., Levitsky, L. L., and Feingold, M.: Vulvovaginitis: A cause of clitoromegaly. Am. J. Dis. Child., 138:887, 1984.

Duncan, P. A., Shapiro, L. R., Stangel, J. J., Klein, R. M., and Addonizio, J. C.: The MURCS association: Mullerian duct aplasia, renal aplasia, and cervicothoracic somite dysplasia. J. Pediatr., 95:399, 1979.

Fisher, R. E., Tanagho, E. A., Lyon, R. P., and Tooley, W. H.: Urethral calibration in newborn girls. J. Urol., 102:67, 1969.

Fleming, S. E., Hall, R., Gysler, M., and McLorie, G. A.: Imperforate anus in females: Frequency of genital tract involvement, incidence of associated anomalies, and functional outcome. J. Pediatr. Surg., 21:146, 1986.

Foglia, R. P., Kim, S. H., Cleveland, R. H., and Donahoe, P. K.: Complications of vaginal atresia in association with a duplicated müllerian duct. J. Pediatr. Surg., 22:653, 1987.

Fraser, I. S., Baird, D. T., Hobson, B. M., Mitchie, E. A., and Hunter, W.: Cyclical ovarian function in women with congenital absence of the uterus and vagina. J. Clin. Endocrinol. Metab., 36:634, 1973.

Gilsanz, V., and Cleveland, R. H.: Duplication of the müllerian ducts and genitourinary malformation, parts I and II. Radiology, 144:793, 1982.

Graham, J. B., King, L. R., Kropp, K. A., and Uehling, D. T.: The significance of distal urethral narrowing in young girls. J. Urol., 97:1045, 1967.

Greer, D. M., Jr., and Pederson, W. C.: Pseudo-masculinization of the phallus. Plast. Reconstr. Surg., 68:787, 1981.

Griffin, J. E., Edwards, C., Madden, J. D., Harrod, M. J., and Wilson, J. D.: Congenital absence of the vagina: The Mayer-Rokitansky-Kuster-Hauser syndrome. Ann. Intern. Med., 85:224, 1976.

Gruenwald, P.: The relation of the growing müllerian duct to the wolffian duct and its importance for the genesis of malformations. Anat. Rec., 81:1, 1941.

Halverstadt, D. B., and Leadbetter, G. W., Jr.: Internal urethrotomy and recurrent urinary tract infection in female children: I. Results in the management of infection. J. Urol., 100:297, 1968.

Huffman, J. W.: Some facts about the clitoris. Postgrad. Med., 60 (November): 245, 1976.

Immergut, M., Culp, D., and Flocks, R. H.: The urethral caliber in normal female children. J. Urol., 97:693, 1967.

Immergut, M. A., and Wahman, G. E.: The urethral caliber of female children with recurrent urinary tract infections. J. Urol., 99:189, 1968.

Jenny, C., Kuhns, M. L. D., and Arakawa, F.: Hymens in normal female infants. Pediatrics, 80:399, 1987.

Jerkins, G. R., Verheeck, K., and Noe, H. N.: Treatment of girls with urethral prolapse. J. Urol., 132:732, 1984.

Johnston, J. H., Koff, S. A., and Glassberg, K. I.: The pseudo-obstructed bladder in enuretic children. Br. J. Urol., 50:505, 1978.

Kaplan, G. W., Sammons, T. A., and King, L. R.: A blind comparison of dilatation, urethrotomy and medication alone in the treatment of urinary tract infection in girls. J. Urol., 109:917, 1973.

Karlin, G., Brock, W., Rich, M., and Pena, A.: Persistent cloaca and phallic urethra. J. Urol., 142:1056, 1989.

Kessler, R., and Constantinou, C. E.: Internal urethrotomy in girls and its impact on the intrinsic and extrinsic continence mechanisms. J. Urol., 136:1248, 1968.

Klein, F. A., Vick, C. W., III, and Broecker, B. H.: Neonatal vaginal cysts: Diagnosis and management. J. Urol., 135:371, 1986.

Lowe, F. C., Hill, G. S., Jeffs, R. D., and Brendler, C. B.: Urethral prolapse in children: Insights into etiology and management. J. Urol., 135:100, 1986.

Lyon, R. P.: Distal urethral stenosis. In Johnston, J. H., and Goodwin, W. E. (Eds.): Reviews in Paediatric Urology. Amsterdam, Excerpta Medica, 1974, p. 1.

Lyon, R. P., and Marshall, S.: Urinary tract infections and difficult urination in girls: Long-term follow-up. J. Urol., 105:314, 1971.

Lyon, R. P., and Smith, D. R.: Distal urethral stenosis. J. Urol., 89:414, 1963.

Lyon, R. P., and Tanagho, E. A.: Distal urethral stenosis in little girls. J. Urol., 93:379, 1965.

McHenry, C. R., Reynolds, M., and Raffensperger, J. G.: Vaginal neoplasms in infancy: The combined role of chemotherapy and conservative surgical resection. J. Pediatr. Surg., 23:842, 1988.

Nussbaum, A. R., and Lebowitz, R. L.: Interlabial masses in little girls: Review and imaging considerations. AJR, 141:65, 1983.

Ramenofsky, M. L., and Raffensperger, J. G.: An abdomino-perineal-vaginal pull-through for definitive treatment of hydrometrocolpos. J. Pediatr. Surg., 6:381, 1971.

Richardson, D. A., Hajj, S. N., and Herbst, A. J.: Medical treatment of urethral prolapse in children. Obstet. Gynecol., 59:69, 1982.

Riley, W. J., and Rosenbloom, A. L.: Clitoral size in infancy. J. Pediatr., 96:918, 1980.

Rock, J. A., and Azziz, R.: Genital anomalies in childhood. Clin. Obstet. Gynecol., 30:682, 1987.

Rock, J. A., Zacur, H. A., Dlugi, A. M., Jones, H. W., and TeLinde, R. W.: Pregnancy success following surgical correction of inperforate hymen and complete transverse vaginal septum. Obstet. Gynecol., 59:448, 1982.

Saxton, H. M., Borzyskowski, M., Mundy, A. R., and Vivian, G. C.: Spinning top urethra: Not a normal variant. Radiology, 168:147, 1988.

Sayer, T., and O'Reilly, P. H.: Bicornuate and unicornuate uterus associated with unilateral renal aplasia and abnormal solitary kidneys: Report of 3 cases. J. Urol., 135:110, 1986.

So, E. P., Brock, W., and Kaplan, G. W.: Ectopic labium and VATER association in a newborn. J. Urol., 124:156, 1980.

Sotolongo, J. R., Jr., Gribetz, M. E., Saphir, R. L., and Begun, G. R.: Female phallic urethra and persistent cloaca. J. Urol., 130:1186, 1983.

Tanagho, E. A., and Smith, D. R.: The anatomy and function of the bladder neck. Br. J. Urol., 38:54, 1966.

Tarry, W. F., Duckett, J. W., and Stephens, F. D.: The Mayer-Rokitansky syndrome: Pathogenesis, classification and management. J. Urol., 136:648, 1986.

Tolete-Velcek, F., Hansbrough, F., Kugaczewski, J., Coren, C. V., Klotz, D. H., Price, A. F., Laungani, G., and Kottmeier, P. K.: Uterovaginal malformations: A trap for the unsuspecting surgeon. J. Pediatr. Surg., 24:736, 1989.

Tran, A. T. B., Arensman, R. M., Falterman, K. W.: Diagnosis and management of hydrohematometrocolpos syndromes. Am. J. Dis. Child., 141:632, 1987.

Williams, D. I.: Urology in Childhood. Berlin, Springer-Verlag, 1958, p. 73.

Wilson, D. A., Stacy, T. M., and Smith, E. I.: Ultrasound diagnosis of hydrocolpos and hydrometrocolpos. Radiology, 128:451, 1978.

Woolf, R. B., and Allen, W. M.: Concomitant malformations. Obstet. Gynecol., 2:236, 1953.

52
SURGERY OF THE SCROTUM AND TESTIS IN CHILDHOOD

Stuart S. Howards, M.D.

The surgical treatment of disorders of the testis and scrotum is described in this chapter. The reader should refer to Chapter 38 for a discussion of the pathophysiology, diagnosis, and medical therapy of these conditions. The operative treatment of penile scrotal transposition is covered in Chapter 51. In general, only one surgical approach is illustrated, although for most conditions several satisfactory alternatives exist.

ORCHIOPEXY

The diagnosis of undescended testis is made by physical examinations as outlined in Chapter 38. The infant should be examined in a warm room with the cremasteric reflex neutralized by flexing the hips. If the testis can be brought well down into the scrotum and remains there, the boy has a retractile testis and, with rare exceptions, will not require orchiopexy. I do not usually treat patients who have unilateral undescended testis with human chorionic gonadotropin (hCG) or gonadotropin-releasing hormone (GnRH) analogues because of the low success rate, particularly in the very young child. If the parents wish a trial of endocrine treatment, this is not harmful; indeed, in the boy with bilateral undescended testis, it may be useful. The indications for surgery, including possible preservation of fertility, simpler diagnosis of malignancy, cosmesis, and psychologic benefits, are explained to the parents. The procedure is done between the ages of 9 and 14 months. No unequivocal proof exists that earlier intervention is advantageous.

A skin-crease incision along one of Langer's lines is made (Fig. 52-1) and deepened through Scarpa's fascia to the external oblique fascia. The external oblique fascia is carefully exposed, including its lateral edge, so that the external ring can be defined (Fig. 52-2). Care is taken not to injure the ilioinguinal nerve. Then, the external oblique muscle is incised in the direction of its fibers. At this point, the testis, covered by tunica vagi-

nalis, is usually evident. The distal attachment of the gubernaculum is then divided, taking care not to injure the vas deferens, which occasionally loops well below the testis ("long-looped vas"). The vas deferens should not be handled with a forceps because pressure necrosis can result. A fine holding suture is then passed through the residual gubernaculum. If the tunica vaginalis has been incised, the suture may be passed through the testis itself and the spermatic vessels and the vas deferens are dissected to the internal ring (Fig. 52-3).

The principles originally emphasized by Bevan (1899)—mobilization of the spermatic cord, repair of the associated hernia, and adequate scrotal fixation without tension—should be followed. Very early in the dissection, the decision must be made as to whether it will be necessary to transect the spermatic vesicles. If this is the case, great care must be taken to preserve the blood supply to the vas deferens and to dissect it without removing the adjacent peritoneum.

After the dissection has been completed, one should see how much length has been obtained. If the testis will reach into the scrotum without difficulty, conventional orchiopexy can be performed. The hernia sac or peritoneal attachment, which lies anteromedial, must be dissected off the spermatic vessels and vas deferens. This dissection can be difficult for the novice and is facilitated by the wearing of optical loupes. The hernia sac is ligated and, if it has been adequately mobilized, should rise out of the operative field.

Next, the internal oblique muscle is retracted, and the lateral spermatic fascia is incised (Fig. 52-4). If the length is inadequate at this point, it may help to incise the internal oblique muscle to allow a higher dissection. Also, the floor of the inguinal canal and inferior epigastric vessels may be incised (Prentiss et al., 1962), or the testis and its cord may be passed under the inferior epigastric vessels. I believe that this technique infrequently gains significant length.

The testis should be securely fixed in the scrotum. Although it is certainly correct that the main factor in

1939

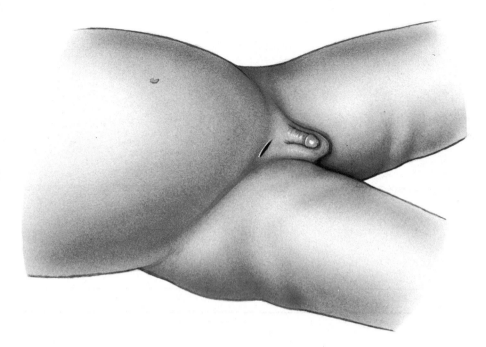

Figure 52–1. A transverse incision is made for orchiopexy, hernia repair, or hydrocele repair in a naturally occurring skin crease in the inguinal area.

preventing a retraction is adequate length, nevertheless, great care should be taken to secure the testis in the scrotum. Several techniques can be utilized to keep the testis in the scrotum. I prefer the dartos pouch technique to which I often add a permanent suture between the testis and the scrotal septum. Any sutures in the testis should penetrate the tunica albuginea on the medial aspect of the upper pole, because this area is least likely to contain major superficial arteries (Jarrow, 1990). The surgeon's finger is passed from the inguinal incision down to the scrotum, and a transverse skin incision is made near the bottom of the scrotum (Fig. 52–5). A pouch is then made between the skin and the dartos muscle, and a long delicate clamp is passed to the

inguinal incision through the scrotal incision puncturing the dartos. The testis or its holding suture is grasped and pulled down (Fig. 52–6). I believe it is important to close the opening in the dartos so that the testis cannot retract through the dartos muscle (see Fig. 52–6) and to place one or two permanent sutures from the tunica albuginea to the scrotal septum. The testis is placed in the subdartos pouch, and the incisions are closed.

If the testis won't go into the scrotum without undue tension, the surgeon has four options: orchiectomy, staged orchiopexy, vessel transection as described by Fowler and Stephens (1959), and autotransplantation. If the testis is small, dysgenetic, or atrophic, and if a normal contralateral testis is present, orchiectomy is a reasonable option. A prosthesis may be placed in the

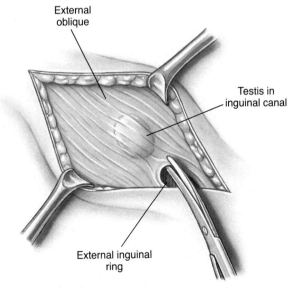

Figure 52–2. The skin and subcutaneous tissue are retracted. The external ring has been identified. The fibers of the external oblique can be visualized. The testis is in the inguinal canal under the external oblique muscle.

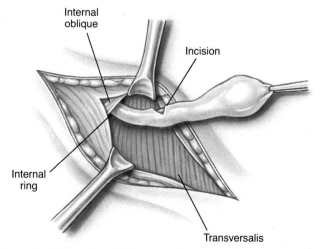

Figure 52–3. The external oblique muscle has been divided. The testis is still covered by peritoneum. The internal oblique muscle is in the upper corner of the incision, and the peritoneum or the hernia sac has been incised.

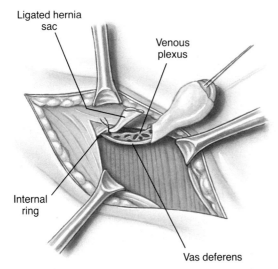

Figure 52–4. The ligated hernia sac, the freed vas deferens, the testicular vessels, and the internal ring are shown.

Table 52–1. STAGED ORCHIOPEXY RESULTS

Author	No. of Cases	No. (%) of Successes
Snyder and Chaffin (1955)	7	6 (86)
Gross and Replogle (1963)	24	24 (100)
Persky and Albert (1971)	13	9 (70)
Firor (1971)	32	30 (94)
Corkery (1975)	5	5 (100)
Zer et al. (1975)	62	48 (77)
Kiesewetter et al. (1981)	60	56 (93)

Adapted from Woodard, J. R., and Trulock, T. S.: Surgical treatment of cryptorchidism. *In* Hadziselimovic, F. (Ed.): Cryptorchidism: Management and Implications. New York, Springer-Verlag, 1983, p. 178.

Orchiopexy Using the Fowler-Stephens Principle

The testicular artery is not an end artery, as Fowler and Stephens (1959) pointed out in their review of the anatomy of the testicular blood supply. The clinical application of this principle allows transection of the testicular artery in difficult orchiopexies. The arteries actually entering the testes are end arteries and have no anastomoses from the vessels of the epididymis. However, there are numerous investigations, including the testicular angiography studies of Fowler and Stephens (1959), which document many proximal anastomoses among the three major arterial supplies to the testis and epididymis—the cremasteric vessels, the artery of the vas deferens, and the testicular or internal spermatic artery. Thus, the basic principle of the Fowler and Stephens orchiopexy is that, if these anastomotic connections are maintained, the testis will remain viable.

To do this, one should avoid dissecting the vas def-

scrotum at this time if that option has been discussed with the family, or it may be placed at a later date. Staged orchiopexy has been recommended by Persky and Albert (1971). They sutured the testis to the external inguinal ring or the pubis and did a second-stage repair 8 to 18 months later. The procedure resulted in failure in one third of the boys. Other workers have reported success rates from 70 to 100 per cent (Table 52–1). Corkery, in 1975, recommended wrapping the cord in silastic at the time of the first procedure to simplify the second stage (Fig. 52–7). Steinhardt and co-workers, in 1985, reported that this technique is useful, but that it is far from being a panacea.

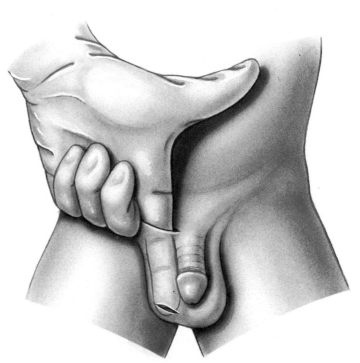

Figure 52–5. Surgeon's finger passing through the incision down into the scrotum to facilitate the incision.

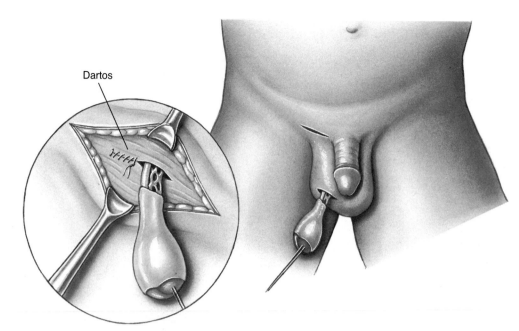

Dartos

Figure 52–6. The testis is pulled through the opening that has been created in the scrotal skin in the dartos muscle. *Inset,* The dartos opening is closed snugly but not too tightly around the cord.

erens and the distal spermatic artery as much as possible. The procedure is particularly applicable to the long-looped vas variety of undescended testis. The first reports of this type of procedure were by Mignon in 1902 and Bevan in 1903. The procedure was reported to be highly successful by Moschowitz, but not nearly as successful by Mixter in 1924. Fowler and Stephens popularized the operation with their publication in 1959, in which they reported on 12 cases.

If the dissection is carried high enough, particularly in normal testis, ligation of the internal spermatic artery does not result in testicular atrophy. The proof of this is from the experience of the surgeons who have purposely taken the testicular artery in repairing a varicocele in hundreds of cases without the development of atrophy.

Once the spermatic vessels, the vas deferens preserving its adjacent peritoneum, and the testis have been carefully dissected out, the surgeon contemplating the use of the Fowler-Stephens principle should place a

bulldog clamp on the testicular arteries at a very high level. A small biopsy of the testis is performed, and the site is observed for several minutes to determine whether arterial bleeding is present (Fig. 52–8). Another option is to inject fluorescein dye after clamping the artery (see Fig. 52–8). The scrotal procedures are carried out as described previously.

Some investigators suggest, without documentation, that the success rate of the Fowler-Stephens orchiopexy could be improved if the procedure were staged with an initial high ligation of the internal spermatic artery and a subsequent orchiopexy (Bloom et al., 1988; Ransley et al., 1984). Pascual and associates (1989) have shown that high ligation of the testicular artery in rats results in an initial decrease in testicular blood flow followed in 1 month by a return to normal blood flow. Half of the testes did exhibit some necroses of seminiferous tubules. This work gives some support to the staged approach but should be viewed with caution because of species differences.

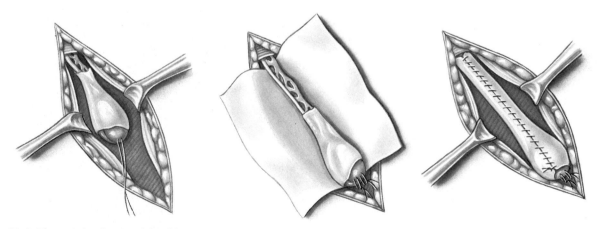

Figure 52–7. The testis has been mobilized but will not reach into the scrotum. It is wrapped in a sheet of Silastic in order to facilitate dissection at the time of the second-stage orchiopexy.

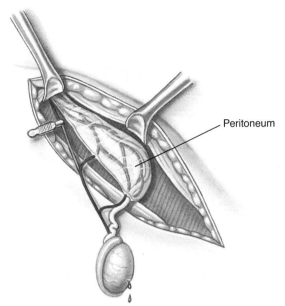

Peritoneum

Figure 52–8. The testis has been dissected, the internal spermatic artery clamped, and the vas deferens and venous plexus are preserved with a strip of peritoneum in order to ensure collateral blood supply. The testis is biopsied and observed for bleeding after the clamp has been applied.

Autotransplantation

The final option is autotransplantation of the testis. This procedure takes advantage of some of the principles outlined previously. Therefore, in dissecting out the vessels, great care should be taken to preserve the collateral circulation. In 1976, Silber and Kelley first described an autotransplantation in a patient with undescended testis. Since that time, several other workers have reported small series of similar procedures. A Boston Children's Hospital group published a paper describing ten autotransplantations in seven patients. Results were that four testes were normal, four became atrophied, and two were intermediate in size. The investigators in the study thought that autotransplantation should not be done in a patient with a normal testis.

Autotransplantation requires special equipment and surgical skills. Logistically, the procedure takes several hours longer than a routine orchiopexy. Therefore, sufficient operating room time must be available. It is often not practical to make a decision in the operating room to do an autotransplant. Certainly, it is preferable to have contemplated this option preoperatively and worked out the logistics in advance. Although I do not routinely provide hormone therapy before orchiopexy, a strong argument could be made for the preoperative preparation of the patient with hCG or testosterone in hope of enlarging the vessels to facilitate the anastomosis.

Microsurgical equipment necessary to perform such an operation includes a good operating microscope. I prefer a Zeiss microscope, but several other instruments are adequate. It is very important to have foot control for focus, zoom, and positioning of the microscope. It is also necessary to have microforceps, microvascular clamps, microneedle holder, microscissors, and 10-0 nylon sutures with fine microneedles.

The testicular artery may well be less than 1 mm in size. Anastomosis of vessels of this caliber was not possible until the preliminary work of Buncke, who in 1967 documented that a microscope could be utilized to obtain predictably good results with vessels of 1 mm in diameter. Acland (1972) further advanced the field when he demonstrated that with the appropriate microneedles, one could do satisfactory anastomoses of vessels of 0.5 mm in diameter.

The initial step in a testicular artery transplantation is mobilization of the recipient and donor vessels. A testicular artery should be mobilized as high as possible through an intraperitoneal exposure. The donor vessels usually are the inferior epigastric artery and vein. Giuliani and Carmignani (1985) believe that it is important to save the common trunk of the epigastric vein in order to have a large-caliber vessel. Some disagreement exists as to whether topical agents, such as lidocaine and papaverine, should be applied to the vessels and whether systemic anticoagulation and heparin should be used. Topical lidocaine and systemic heparinization are certainly reasonable techniques, but the most critical factor in obtaining a patent anastomosis is the surgical technique.

The vessels should be dissected out with a microscope at low magnification, usually 5 × to 10 ×. Branches of the vessels should be coagulated approximately 2 mm away from the donor vessel. It is important to have 1 to 3 cm of the vessel dissected free of the surrounding tissue. The next step is to remove perivascular connective tissue from the vessel. This vessel tends to undergo spasm at this point, which can be relieved by applying 1 per cent lidocaine. The vessels should be kept moist with warmed saline. Once the vessels are isolated, the clamp approximator should be applied. Enough space must be available between the end of the vessel and the clamp to allow proper suturing, and the clamp must be placed so that it can be flipped without difficulty. After the clamp is placed, loose tissue must be removed. The vessel is then transected. The adventitia is pulled over the lumen at several points, after which it is pulled forward and cut flush with the lumen. This lumen is irrigated with heparinized saline to remove any clots and debris, and then stretched with a small jeweler's forceps. The clamp is adjusted to leave an appropriate distance between the two vessel ends, so that suturing can be done without tension.

Several techniques are satisfactory for vessel anastomosis. One recommended by Daniel and Terzis (1977) is outlined as follows (Fig. 52–9). In this method, similar to that described by Carrel in 1902, three guide sutures are placed to triangulate the vessel. It is important that the sutures be placed with full-thickness bites that are symmetric (see Fig. 52–9). Two guide sutures are placed, and a suture is passed between them. It is helpful to place a smooth jeweler's forceps in the lumen to guide the suture. Gentle traction is placed on the first guide suture while the second suture is being placed. Some surgeons prefer two guide sutures 180 degrees apart. After the guide sutures are placed, one can fill in the

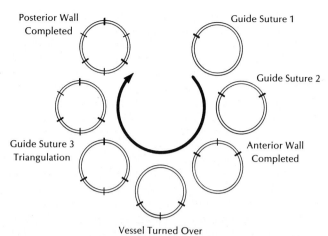

Figure 52–9. The steps involved in a microvascular anastomoses are schematically represented according to the principles of Daniel and Terzis.

anterior wall between them and flip the vessel to proceed with the posterior wall.

After the anastomosis is completed, it is wrapped in clear plastic or a silicone cuff can be placed. The clamps are removed, and the anastomosis is observed. The distal clamp is removed initially, and the surgeon watches for backflow. Then, the proximal clamp is removed. If the anastomosis is patent, the surgeon will observe expansile pulsations and wriggling distal to the anastomosis.

If there is vessel size discrepancy, a smaller vessel can be transected in a somewhat oblique fashion in an attempt to make the anastomosis more proportional. The surgical technique for vascular anastomosis outlined here is that of Daniel and Terzis. Obviously, each surgeon will develop an appropriate technique. Microsurgery should be done only by someone who is skilled in the method. I do a considerable amount of microsurgery but not vascular microsurgery. Therefore, when I plan an autotransplantation, I do it in collaboration with a plastic surgeon, who is more familiar with the microsurgery of small vessels.

Fixation of the testis in the scrotum is not as critical a factor in prevented retraction as is prevention of tension. Nevertheless, the fixation should be done carefully. Many methods have been recommended. I prefer a dartos pouch, usually with the addition of one or two permanent sutures between the scrotal septum and the tunica albuginea of the testis (see preceding discussion).

Repeat Orchiectomy

A repeat orchiopexy for a failed primary repair or the second stage of a two-staged orchiectomy should be done at least 6 months after the original procedure. The family should be advised that an atrophic testis may be found or that it may not be possible to get the testis into the scrotum.

I usually use the old incision for repeat operations, but I do not hesitate to extend it or even to make a separate incision in selected cases. Obviously, great care

must be taken to avoid injury. The ilioinguinal nerve is often extremely difficult to see and, indeed, occasionally must be sacrificed. The most critical factor, in addition to the principles outlined, is to carry the dissection above the level of the previous procedure, which usually results in adequate length.

Nonpalpable Testis

Unilateral nonpalpable testis can be approached in the same manner as the palpable testis. Sonography, computed tomography, and angiography may be utilized to determine whether a testis is present. Because false-negative findings are common with the first two techniques and angiography is invasive, indeed dangerous in the infant, I do not perform these tests.

Laparoscopy can be employed to determine whether a testis is present and to aid in planning the surgical approach (see following discussion) (Weiss and Seashore, 1987). I do not routinely use this technique for unilateral nonpalpable testis. Instead, I explore the inguinal and retroperitoneal areas as described previously. If a testis or a blind-ending vas deferens *and* blind-ending gonadal vessel are found, the procedure is terminated. If not, the incision is extended medially and the peritoneal cavity is explored. Small Deaver retractors obtain good exposure. A very careful search is conducted to find the testis or the blind-ending vessels. If a testis is located, it is often necessary to implement one of the four aforementioned alternatives to a standard orchiopexy, because it is frequently not possible to place the testis in the scrotum without undue tension.

If bilateral nonpalpable testes are found, an hCG stimulation test should be performed. When the gonadotropin levels are normal and an elevation in serum testosterone level occurs in response to the hCG, testicular tissue is present on at least one side. If there is no elevation of the testosterone level but the gonadotropin levels are normal, nonfunctioning testicular tissue is present. However, if the gonadotropin levels are elevated for age and there is no response in the testosterone level, there is no testicular tissue and exploration can be avoided.

Many believe that laparoscopy is useful in patients with bilateral nonpalpable testes. Laparoscopy is done through a small infraumbilical incision. A Verres needle is inserted, and the peritoneal cavity is distended with carbon dioxide at a pressure of less than 20 mm Hg. A pediatric laparoscope is introduced with a trocar. The patient is placed in the Trendelenburg position, and the pelvis is examined. The normal vas deferens can be seen crossing the lateral umbilical ligament and terminating at the internal ring. The spermatic vessels enter the ring laterally. If this anatomy is seen, the gonad is in the canal, in the superficial inguinal pouch, or absent. When the testis is seen, the gonad is high and, although retroperitoneal, must be approached through the peritoneum. With blind-ending vas and spermatic vessels cephalad to the internal ring, the testis is absent.

Proponents of laparoscopy think that these findings can void unnecessary surgical exploration and help plan the surgical approach when the testis is present. For example, if the testis is high above the ring, a midline incision can be made or an autotransplantation can be planned in advance. However, other investigators believe that any situation can be handled through bilateral extended inguinal incisions and that it is not safe to rely on laparoscopy to rule out the presence of a testis.

TORSION OF THE SPERMATIC CORD

The testis that has undergone antenatal torsion appears as a hard, often blue, mass, which does not transilluminate. I usually wait until the infant is 1 to 2 months old before performing an inguinal orchiectomy. Some surgeons place an infant prosthesis at this time, but I find that most parents prefer to wait until the child can participate in the decision and a larger prosthesis can be accommodated. Whether the contralateral testis should be fixed is controversial. Opponents cite the fact

that antenatal torsion is usually an extravaginal event and, thus, unlikely to be bilateral. Bilateral antenatal torsion has rarely been reported and there is concern regarding possible injury to the small normal testis. Proponents state that synchronous antenatal torsion or asynchronous neonatal torsion is more common than previously thought (LaQuaglia et al., 1987).

Any time acute torsion of the spermatic cord is suspected and cannot be ruled out (see Chapter 38), emergency surgical exploration is indicated. A transverse scrotal incision is made, and the testis is exposed. The incision is carried through the tunica vaginalis (Fig. 52–10), and the cord is untwisted. The testis is observed, and if normal color returns, it is anchored by three nonabsorbable sutures through the tunics and into the scrotal wall (see Fig. 52–10). The sutures through the tunica albuginea should be placed on the medial aspect of the upper pole, if the testis is pexed to the septum, or the lateral aspect of the upper pole, if the testis is

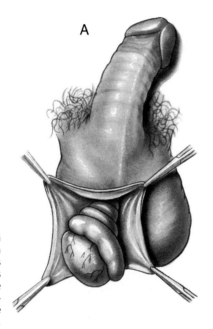
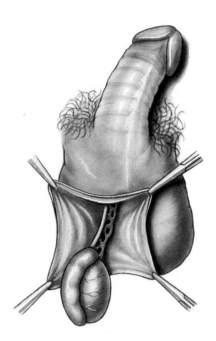

A

Figure 52–10. *A,* The scrotum and tunica vaginalis have been opened. The spermatic cord is twisted. On the left, the epididymis and testis are elevated; on the right, after untwisting, the vas deferens and spermatic cord can be identified. The testis is now lower. *B,* On the left, the pexis sutures have been placed through the tunica albuginea of the testis and the tunica vaginalis as well as the scrotal septum. They will be tied, and the tunica vaginalis will be closed. On the right, the bilateral scrotal incision has been closed after pexis of the contralateral testis.

B

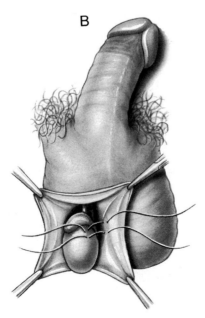
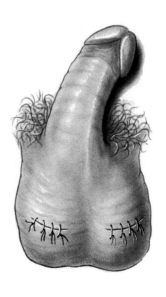

pexed to the lateral scrotal wall. In humans, these areas are least likely to have major superficial arteries, whereas the medial, anterior, and lateral aspects of the lower pole are most likely to contain major superficial arteries (Jarrow, 1990). I prefer to place these sutures through the median septum, but sometimes the scrotal wall is more convenient.

Delayed torsion has been described after orchiopexy with reabsorbable sutures. If extravaginal torsion is present, a more extensive dissection of the cord structures is necessary to ensure that detorsion is complete and that normal circulation is restored to the testis.

If obvious and complete necrosis of the testis has occurred, orchiectomy is advisable. However, with reasonable doubt regarding the future viability of the testis, it should be left in situ. Testes with apparently irreversible ischemia may remain viable and support Leydig's cell function. Sepsis and abscess formation are rare, even if a totally infarcted testis is left in place.

Upon completion of detorsion and fixation of the ipsilateral testis, the contralateral scrotal compartment must be opened. The testis should be firmly affixed to surrounding structures to prevent future torsion on this unaffected side, which does occur and can result in anorchia.

TORSION OF THE APPENDIX TESTIS OR EPIDIDYMIS

When the diagnosis of torsion of the appendix testis or epididymis is unequivocal, surgical intervention is not required. I recommend bed rest for 48 hours. If the pain has not resolved, I operate. A transverse scrotal incision is made, the tunica vaginalis is incised, and the affected appendix is removed (Fig. 52–11). Of course, if there is any possibility that the patient may have torsion of the spermatic cord rather than the appendix, emergency surgical exploration is indicated.

HERNIA AND HYDROCELE

Hernia

The nonincarcerated infant hernia should be repaired on an urgent, but nonemergent, basis. A very small transverse incision is made in a skin fold in the inguinal region (see Fig. 52–1). The subcutaneous fat and Scarpa's fascia are divided. The external oblique and the external ring are identified. It is usually not necessary to incise the external oblique fascia. The sack is located anteriomedially on the cord. It is separated by blunt dissection free of the cord (Fig. 52–12), twisted, and sutured. Great care must be taken not to injure the vas deferens, the ilioinguinal nerve, and the spermatic vessels. Before closing the incision, the surgeon should check to be certain that the testis is in the scrotum. A subcuticular closure is done. Unless the patient is very young (under 3 months of age), the repair is an outpatient procedure. Disagreement exists regarding contralateral repair. I perform bilateral surgery in the patient with a history of a bulge or a silk-glove sign.

Repair of hydroceles should be delayed until the age of 9 to 12 months, because many of these will spontaneously resolve in that time period. The incision and the initial steps in the repair are the same as those described previously for a hernia. I then deliver the testis and incise the tunica vaginalis. I replace the testis in the scrotum without performing a bottle or similar procedure, because interruption of the patent tunica vaginalis should resolve the hydrocele. The closure is as described previously. In an older boy, a secondary noncongenital hydrocele may be repaired through a scrotal incision (Fig. 52–13), because there will not be an associated hernia. In boys presenting with secondary hydroceles, a testis tumor must be ruled out. The surgeon may wish to do a bottle closure of the tunica vaginalis (Fig. 52–14A to C).

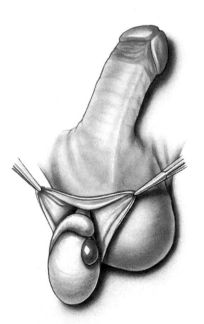 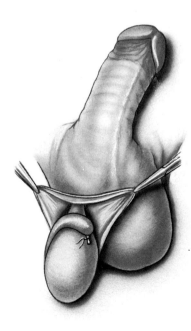

Figure 52–11. On the left, the swollen appendix testis is identified. On the right, it has been removed.

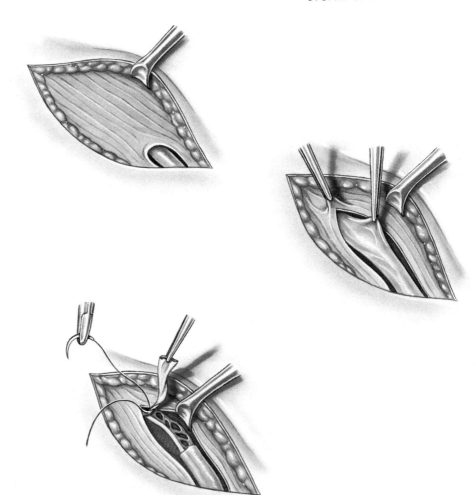

Figure 52–12. *Top left,* The skin and subcutaneous skin have been incised. *Middle right,* The hernial sac is elevated at the external ring. *Lower left,* Hernial sac has been dissected off the cord and suture ligated.

Varicocele

The diagnosis of varicocele is made by physical examination. The concept of subclinical varicocele is not applicable to the pediatric age group. The indications for operative correction are controversial. I believe that the massive size, persistent pain, and ipsilateral growth retardation are indications for surgery. The first two indications are rare, whereas the third is not uncommon. The varicocele can be repaired through an incision at the level of the internal ring or the external ring (Fig. 52–15A).

High Ligation

While under suitable anesthesia, the patient is prepared, draped, and then placed in the reverse Trendelenberg position to fill the veins. A short transverse incision is made just medial to the anterior superior iliac spine, approximately at the level of the internal ring (Fig. 52–15A). The external oblique fascia is incised in the direction of its fibers (Fig. 52–15B). The internal oblique muscle is retracted caudad with an abdominal retractor (Fig. 52–15C). The dilated vein is usually identified without any further dissection. The vein is freed from the surrounding fat by blunt or, preferably, sharp dissection. The dissection is continued toward the renal vein to as high a level as is convenient to look for anastomosing collateral vessels. The vein is ligated, and a segment is removed (Fig. 52–15D). The area is inspected for additional veins. At this level, there are usually only one or two veins, although multiple veins are occasionally encountered.

Care is taken to avoid dividing the artery or lymphatic channels. Optical loupes and a Doppler probe make identification of the artery simpler and I routinely employ both. Although interruption of the internal spermatic artery at this level probably does not significantly injure the testis, I nevertheless preserve the vessel. The vas deferens can be seen at the lower medial aspect of the incision as it curves into the pelvis (Fig. 52–15D). The internal oblique muscle is tacked back into position, and the external oblique is closed with nonabsorbable sutures. A subcuticular skin closure is used for aesthetic reasons and to eliminate the need for suture removal. The procedure is done on an "in-and-out" or day-surgery basis. Performed in the manner described, this technique is simple and does not, as has been asserted, convert simple procedure into a major operation.

Low Ligation

The incision for the inguinal approach is indicated by the dashed line in Figure 52–15A. The spermatic cord is delivered as it exits the external ring and is isolated with a Penrose drain. Any perforating veins can be

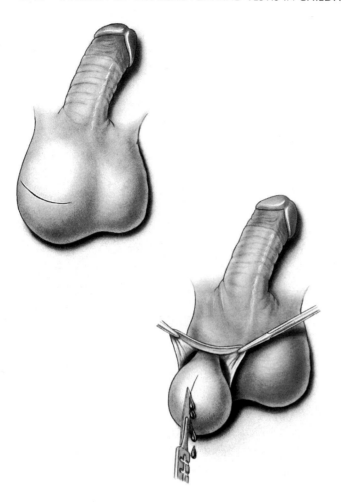

Figure 52–13. For a secondary hydrocele in an older boy, a scrotal incision is made. The hydrocele sac is incised as shown in the lower right.

divided at this point. With the aid of optical loupes and a Doppler probe, the cord can be inspected and all of the veins ligated with preservation of the spermatic artery and some lymphatics to avoid hydrocele formation. Some workers believe, without proof, that this approach reduces the incidence of persistent or recurrent varicoceles. Intraoperative venography has also been recommended to reduce the failure rate. The closure is

similar to that described previously. Recurrent varicoceles should be repaired percutaneously at the time of venography.

Orchiectomy

A boy with a testis tumor or an infarcted testis requires an orchiectomy. The inguinal approach is in-

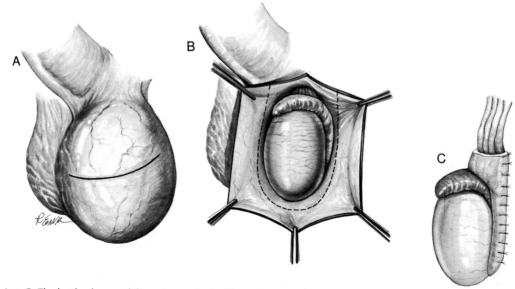

Figure 52–14. A to C, The bottle closure of the tunica vaginalis. The tunica vaginalis is incised and sutured behind the epididymis and spermatic cord.

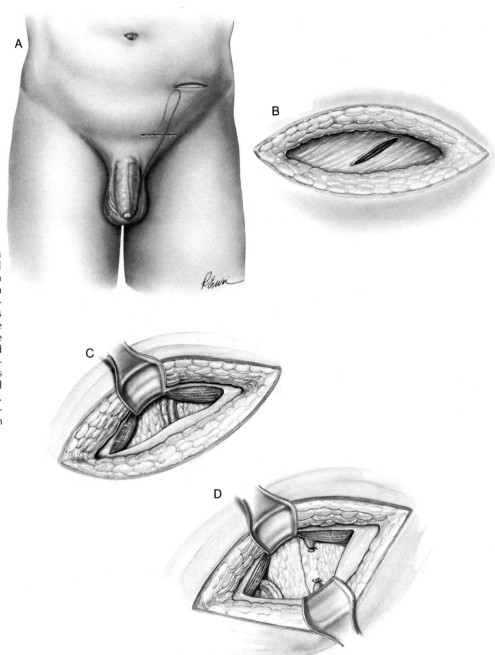

Figure 52–15. *A,* Incisions for a high (internal ring) or low (external ring) approach. *B,* After the skin and subcutaneous tissue have been incised, the external oblique muscle is opened in the direction of its fibers. *C,* The external oblique muscle has been incised, and the internal oblique muscle is retracted upward, revealing the dilated spermatic vein on the right and the vas deferens on the left. *D,* The internal spermatic vein has been ligated. The vas deferens is toward the pelvis on the left. The artery has been preserved.

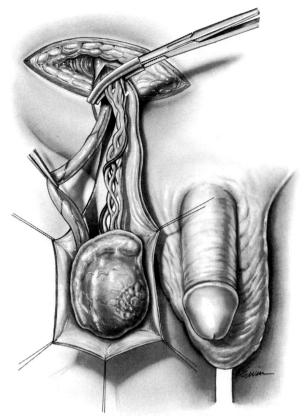

Figure 52–16. After the inguinal incision has been made, the spermatic cord is clamped with a vascular clamp or rubber shod clamp. The testis is delivered and inspected. If malignancy is present, the testis is removed along with its cord, and a high ligation is performed.

dicated when malignancy of the scrotal contents has not been ruled out. I prefer a transverse incision in the skin fold above the inguinal ligament rather than the standard inguinal incision (see Fig. 52–1). The fascia of the external oblique muscle is incised in the direction of its fibers, upward from the external ring; the ilioinguinal nerve is identified; and the cord is isolated. If the diagnosis is in doubt, a rubber shod or vascular clamp is placed across the vascular pedicle before the testis is delivered from the scrotum (Fig. 52–16). If an intratesticular mass is present, immediate orchiectomy rather than biopsy is usually indicated. The vessels and the vas deferens are clamped individually at points as high as possible, and the cord structures are divided between clamps. I prefer suture ligations and one long, permanent suture so that the end of the spermatic cord can be identified during retroperitoneal lymphadenectomy,

if indicated. The operative specimen is draped out of the area of the incision, particularly if a biopsy is performed.

REFERENCES

Acland, R. D.: Prevention of thrombosis in microvascular surgery. Br. J. Plast. Surg., 25:292, 1972.

Bevan, A. D.: Operation for undescended testicle and congenital inguinal hernia. J. Am. Med. Assoc., 33:773, 1899.

Bloom, D. A., Ayers, J. W. T., and McGuire, E. J.: The role of laparoscopy in management of nonpalpable testes. J. Clin. Urol., 94:465, 1988.

Buncke, H.: The suture repair of 1 millimeter vessels. In Donaghy, R. M. P., and Yasargil, M. C. (Eds.): Micro-Vascular Surgery. Stuttgart, Thieme, 1967.

Carrel, A.: The operative technique of vascular anastomoses and the transplantation of viscera. Med. Lyon., 98:859, 1902 (English Translation, Clin. Orthop., 29:3, 1963).

Corkery, J. J.: Staged orchiopexy—a new technique. J. Pediatr. Surg. 10:515, 1975.

Daniel, R. L., and Terzis, J. K.: Reconstructive Microsurgery. Boston, Little, Brown & Co., 1977.

Firor, H. V.: Two-staged orchidopexy. Arch. Surg., 102:598, 1971.

Fowler, R., Jr., and Stephens, F. D.: The role of testicular vascular anatomy in the salvage of high undescended testes. Aust. N. Z. J. Surg., 29:92, 1959.

Giuliani, L., and Carmignani, G.: Autotransplantation of the testicle. In Wagenknect, L. V. (Ed.): Microsurgery in Urology. New York, Georg Thieme Verlag, 1985, pp. 203–206.

Gross, R. E., and Replogle, R. L.: Treatment of undescended testes. Postgrad. Med. J., 34:266, 1963.

Jarrow, J. P.: Intratesticular arterial anatomy. J. Androl., 11:255, 1990.

Kiesewetter, W. B., Mammen, K., and Kalyglov, M.: The rationale and results in two-stage orchiopexies. J. Pediatr. Surg., 16:631, 1981.

LaQuaglia, M. P., Bauer, S. B., Eraklis, A., Feins, N., and Mandell, J.: Bilateral neonatal torsion. J. Urol., 138:1051, 1987.

Pascual, J. A., Villanveva-Meyer, J., and Salido, E.: Recovery of testicular blood flow following ligation of testicular vessels. J. Urol., 142:549, 1989.

Persky, L., and Albert, D. J.: Staged orchiopexy. Surg. Gynecol. Obstet., 132:43, 1971.

Prentiss, R. J., et al.: Surgical repair of undescended testicle. Calif. Med., 96:401, 1962.

Ransley, P. G., Vordermark, J. S., and Caldamone, A. A.: Preliminary ligation of gonadal vessels prior to orchidopexy for the intraabdominal testicle. World J. Urol., 2:266, 1984.

Silber, S. J., and Kelley, J.: Successful autotransplantation of an intraabdominal testis. J. Urol., 115:452, 1976.

Snyder, W. H., and Chaffin, L.: Surgical management of undescended testes. JAMA, 157:129, 1955.

Steinhardt, G. F., Kroovand, R. L., and Perlmutter, A. D.: Orchiopexy: Planned 2-stage technique. J. Urol., 133:434, 1985.

Weiss, R. M., and Seashore, J. H.: Laparoscopy in the management of the nonpalpable testis. J. Urol., 138:382, 1987.

Zer, M., Wollochi, Y., and Dintsman, M.: Staged orchiorrhaphy. Arch. Surg., 110:387, 1975.

53
SURGICAL MANAGEMENT OF INTERSEXUALITY

Alan D. Perlmutter, M.D.
Claude Reitelman, M.D.

Ambiguity of the external genitalia is an urgent neonatal problem that must be treated as a medical and social emergency requiring a thoughtful and systematic approach. Of the many complex decisions that are essential to the evaluation and management of these so-affected infants and their families, the most important is the appropriate assignment of gender as soon as possible after birth. Undue procrastination, a temporary choice, and an inappropriate gender assignment at birth are unacceptable. These may lead to disturbances in psychosexual development and lifetime repercussions for both the family and child.

This chapter describes the surgical approaches to genital reconstruction in the intersex patient. A summary of the embryology of normal and disordered sexual differentiation provides essential background. In addition, a useful classification of and diagnostic approach to patients with ambiguous genitalia are presented.

NORMAL SEXUAL DIFFERENTIATION

Normal sexual differentiation results from an orderly sequential process: chromosomal sex directs gonadal sex, which in turn directs phenotypic sex (internal genital ducts and external genitalia). Interference with this sequential process may result in genital ambiguity. To appreciate the pathophysiology of disordered sexual differentiation, one must first have a clear understanding of normal sexual differentiation.

Gonads

The chromosomal sex directs the development of the paired bipotential gonads into either testes or ovaries (Jost et al., 1973; Kim et al., 1979). Each gonad develops independently. For development of a testis, factors located on the Y chromosome, on the X chromosome,

and possibly on the autosomal chromosomes are necessary (Wachtel et al., 1976). The most important of these factors, the testis determining factor (TDF), is located on the Y chromosome (Page et al., 1987). In the absence of this factor, testicular differentiation does not occur and an ovary is formed 11 to 12 weeks after conception.

Internal Genital Ducts

Two sets of paired primordial internal duct systems are present in both male and female fetuses: the mesonephric and the paramesonephric. In the male, regression of the paramesonephric ducts and development of the mesonephric ducts require hormonal action. Sertoli cells of the seminiferous tubules of the fetal testis produce a nonsteroidal hormone called müllerian inhibitory substance (MIS)—a specific fetal regressor glycoprotein—which acts locally to cause regression of the paramesonephric ducts (Blanchard and Josso, 1974; Josso, 1971). Slightly later, testosterone secreted by the Leydig cells of the fetal testis, also acting locally, causes the ipsilateral mesonephric duct to differentiate into the epididymis, vas deferens, and seminal vesicle (Siiteri and Wilson, 1974). Both of these events require a normal fetal testis. If secretion of MIS is impaired or absent, paramesonephric duct regression is incomplete or does not occur, and to varying degrees a fallopian tube, hemiuterus or uterus, and vagina may develop on the side of the abnormal testis. If secretion of testosterone is impaired or absent, differentiation of the mesonephric duct into the epididymis, vas deferens, and seminal vesicle is incomplete or does not occur.

In the female, the paramesonephric ducts normally persist, differentiating into the fallopian tubes, uterus, cervix, and upper vagina. The mesonephric ducts regress, after giving rise to the ureteral bud. Because these changes do not depend on gonadal or hormonal stimulation, paramesonephric duct differentiation and mesonephric duct regression similarly occur in the absence of a gonad.

External Genitalia

The primordia of the external genitalia are bipotential, consisting of genital tubercle, urethral folds, genital swellings, and urogenital sinus (Fig. 53–1). In the male, virilization of the genital tubercle, fusion of the urethral folds, and scrotalization of the genital swellings are dependent on the conversion of fetal testosterone to dihydrotestosterone by the enzyme 5-alpha reductase, which is present in the cells of the external genitalia and urogenital sinus. Dihydrotestosterone, in turn, binds with an intracellular androgen receptor to effect molecular changes that result in virilization. The genital tubercle enlarges to form the glans penis. The urethral folds fuse to encompass the anterior urethra, and the genital swellings migrate dorsally and fuse to form the scrotum. The prostate develops from the urogenital sinus. With absent or deficient testosterone or 5-alpha reductase or with abnormal androgen-receptor binding or action, the differentiating external genitalia develop along female lines to form the clitoris, labia minora and majora, and lower vagina, or degrees of incomplete virilization result (Barinka et al., 1968).

In the female and in the absence of androgen influence, the genital tubercle forms the clitoris, the urethral folds form the labia minora, and the genital swellings form the labia majora. The lower vagina arises from the urogenital sinus.

In correlating the clinical presentations of genital ambiguity with normal sexual development, certain concepts are important and are summarized as follows:

1. Initially, the gonad is bipotential in all fetuses and its differentiation into a testis or an ovary is dependent on its chromosomal composition.

2. Initially, two sets of paired internal (mesonephric and paramesonephric) ducts are present in all fetuses.

3. Differentiation of the internal ducts along female lines is autonomous.

4. Virilization of the internal ducts requires specific direction from the fetal testis, with the elaboration of

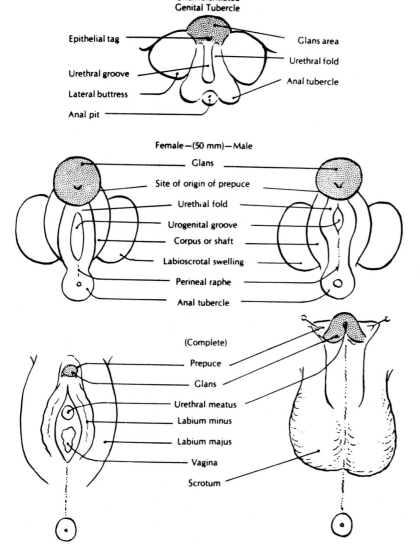

Figure 53–1. Differentiation of the external genitalia.

hormones, MIS, and testosterone. The effect of these hormones is local and limited to the ipsilateral internal ducts.

5. Differentiation of the external genitalia along female lines is autonomous.

6. Virilization of the external genitalia requires the presence of testosterone, its conversion to 5-dihydrotestosterone, and normal androgen receptor activity.

CLASSIFICATION OF AMBIGUOUS GENITALIA

The common causes of ambiguous genitalia are the following: chromosomal anomalies resulting in abnormal gonadal differentiation (e.g., true hermaphroditism, mixed gonadal dysgenesis); excessive androgen in a genetic female resulting in virilization of the external genitalia (e.g., female pseudohermaphroditism); and defective androgen production or action in a genetic male resulting in incomplete virilization or feminization of the external genitalia (e.g., male pseudohermaphroditism).

The four categories into which ambiguous genitalia in the neonate are classified in terms of their relative frequency are considered: female pseudohermaphroditism, mixed gonadal dysgenesis, male pseudohermaphroditism, and true hermaphroditism (Fig. 53–2) (Allen, 1976).

Female Pseudohermaphroditism (Adrenogenital Syndrome)

Female pseudohermaphroditism results when a chromatin-positive 46XX female is exposed to endogenous or exogenous androgen in utero. The most common etiology for female pseudohermaphroditism is congenital adrenal hyperplasia (CAH), which accounts for more than 60 per cent of children with ambiguous genitalia (Perlmutter, 1979). The autosomal recessive form of the disorder, called the adrenogenital syndrome, is caused by a deficiency in one of the several enzymes necessary for adrenal steroidogenesis. This deficiency leads to defective cortisol biosynthesis, common to all forms of CAH. As a result, adrenocorticotropic hormone (ACTH) secretion is elevated, causing increased levels of various cortisol precursors.

Several forms of CAH with different clinical manifestations have been described, depending on the particular enzyme defect in the cortisol biosynthetic pathway. For some forms, accumulation of these precursors results in excessive androgen production and fetal virilization (Fig. 53–3). A review of CAH by Mininberg and co-workers (1979) provides excellent and detailed descriptions of its several clinical and biochemical manifestations, which are beyond the scope of this presentation. This chapter considers those forms of CAH associated with genital ambiguity and likely to be encountered by urologists.

The majority of patients (95 per cent) with female

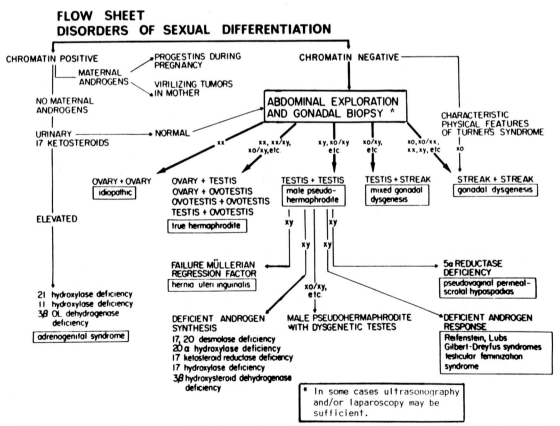

Figure 53–2. Flow chart depicts disorders of sexual differentiation. (From Allen, T. D.: Disorders of sexual differentiation. Urology (Suppl), 7:1, 1976.)

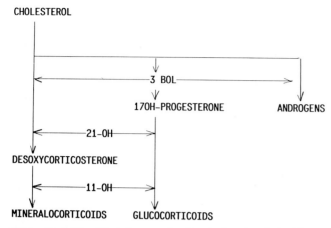

Figure 53–3. Simplified diagram of pathways for adrenal steroid synthesis (BOL, 3-beta-hydroxysteroid dehydrogenase).

virilization from CAH have 21-hydroxylase deficiency, which exists in two forms, mild and severe. In the mild form, the enzyme activity is reduced, resulting in a partial decrease in cortisol synthesis. Despite virilization, signs of adrenal insufficiency are uncommon. In the severe form, the marked deficiency of 21-hydroxylase activity results in greater degrees of cortisol and aldosterone deficiency, with associated salt wasting and more extreme virilization. Untreated, this severe degree of cortisol and aldosterone deficiency can result in clinical signs and symptoms of marked adrenal insufficiency within 1 to 2 weeks after birth. These consist of anorexia, vomiting, dehydration, and ultimately, if untreated, circulatory collapse.

With 11-beta-hydroxylase deficiency, by contrast, salt and water retention occurs and hypertension can result. Increased secretion of desoxycorticosterone, a sodium-retaining steroid, is responsible.

Two earlier blocks in the adrenal steroidal pathways—3-beta-hydroxysteroid dehydrogenase (3-beta-OL) and

17-hydroxylase deficiency—are also rare causes of genital ambiguity.

Embryology of Virilizing Congenital Adrenal Hyperplasia

The significant embryology of girls with virilizing CAH is as follows: They are genetically normal except for the hereditary adrenal enzyme deficiency. The internal (paramesonephric) ductal and ovarian development is normal. In the absence of fetal testicular tissue, there is no müllerian inhibitory factor to prevent the paramesonephric ducts from differentiating normally into the fallopian tubes, uterus, and upper vagina. The mesonephric ducts appropriately regress because this event occurs before adrenal function begins. However, the later onset of embryonic adrenal function is in time to cause virilization of the urogenital sinus and the external genitalia. The abnormal, virilizing, adrenal steroidogenesis provokes varying degrees of urogenital sinus fusion, hypoplasia of the lower vagina, and clitorimegaly (Fig. 53–4).

Mixed Gonadal Dysgenesis

Mixed gonadal dysgenesis (MGD) is second only to CAH in frequency as a cause of ambiguous genitalia in the neonate. Most patients with MGD have the mosaic karyotype 45X/46XY. Infants with MGD usually have a streak gonad on one side and a testis on the other (Davidoff and Federman, 1973). All have infantile uterus or hemiuterus, cervix, and at least one fallopian tube. Mesonephric duct–derived structures may be present on the side of the testis.

The appearance of the external genitalia is quite variable; however, the majority are poorly virilized and therefore raised as females (Kim et al., 1979). Un-

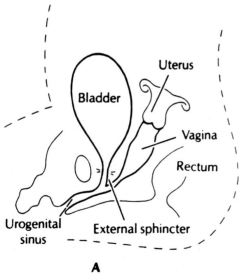

A

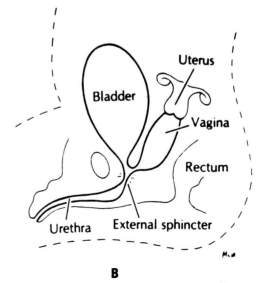

B

Figure 53–4. Anatomic variations of the urogenital sinus in girls with adrenogenital syndrome. A, In the most common form, the vagina enters the urogenital sinus distal to the external urethral sphincter. B, The vagina enters the posterior urethra at the site of the verumontanum in a patient with complete phallic urethra. This is a rare type that is present in some patients with complete 21-hydroxylase deficiency (salt losing).

treated, most tend to virilize at puberty. Although some have a phallus adequate for a hypospadias reconstruction, short adult stature is common for these children, with ultimate height rarely above 148 cm. Therefore, when a male gender assignment is considered, this outcome should be kept in mind. Because of the marked tendency for malignant degeneration of undescended gonadal tissue in this condition (Aarskog, 1970), occasionally occurring in early childhood (gonadoblastoma and seminoma dysgerminoma), early gonadectomy is recommended for intra-abdominal gonads.

Male Pseudohermaphroditism

Male pseudohermaphrodites are genetic males with testis tissue and incomplete virilization of the external genitalia. This disorder may be the result of deficient testosterone synthesis, decreased testosterone action due to deficient 5-alpha reductase, or decreased androgen receptor binding in the target tissues. Cryptorchidism and defective paramesonephric duct regression may also be associated with some forms of male pseudohermaphroditism.

Deficient testosterone synthesis is an uncommon cause for male pseudohermaphroditism and is characteristic of dysgenetic testes. Defective testosterone action is a more common cause of male pseudohermaphroditism, with decreased or absent virilization, pseudovaginal perineoscrotal hypospadias (PPH), or testicular feminization syndrome (TFS) (Walsh et al., 1974).

The individual with TFS has the appearance of a phenotypically normal female with a short or absent vagina. TFS is caused by deficient androgen receptor binding and is most often diagnosed at puberty, when amenorrhea despite appropriate feminization is investigated, or earlier, when a childhood inguinal hernia repair is made. Strictly speaking, *complete* TFS is not an intersex state, as it is associated with a normal female phenotype. PPH is associated with 5-alpha reductase deficiency. Defective paramesonephric duct regression (hernia uteri inguinale) is a condition in which phenotypic males, usually with cryptorchidism, are found to have a rudimentary uterus and fallopian tubes with variable development of the vasa deferentia. Hypospadias may also be present.

Owing to similar therapeutic considerations, several additional disorders of sexual differentiation in genetic males with normal gonads but diminutive although not ambiguous genitalia or absent phallus are included in the category of male pseudohermaphroditism (micropenis and penile agenesis). Those genetic males with severe exstrophy of the bladder and extremely small epispadiac penis and those with cloacal exstrophy and hypoplastic bifid penis generally should be considered for female gender assignment and appropriately feminized (see Chapter 46).

True Hermaphroditism

True hermaphroditism is defined as genital ambiguity with gonadal tissue of both sexes present. It is a rare cause of ambiguous genitalia in newborn infants. These infants may have a testis on one side and an ovary on the other (lateral type), a unilateral ovotestis in combination with a contralateral ovary or testis (unilateral type), or bilateral ovotestes (bilateral type). In most true hermaphrodites a uterus or hemiuterus is present. On each side, the genital duct tends to conform to the sex of the ipsilateral gonad—a fallopian tube on the side of an ovary and a vas deferens on the side of a testicle. The degree of virilization of the external genitalia in true hermaphrodites is quite variable, although most have a large phallus with chordee and varying degrees of labioscrotal fusion. Through the years most of these infants have been assigned a male gender because of phallic size. Gonadal tissue is often palpable in the labioscrotal fold or groin on one or both sides and most often represents testicular tissue, although ovotestes or ovaries may also descend into the labioscrotal folds.

The majority of true hermaphrodites have a 46XX karyotype; however, 46XY and various mosaic patterns also occur (Wachtel et al., 1976). Fertility is unusual but has been reported in both sex roles (Edmonds and Dewhurst, 1986), supporting the concept of preservation of concordant gonadal tissue once sex assignment is made (Nihoul-Fekete et al., 1984).

DIFFERENTIAL DIAGNOSIS AND GENDER ASSIGNMENT

Because of the serious psychosocial consequences that can result if the sex of rearing is changed after the age of 18 months, it is very important to assign the proper sex of rearing as soon as possible after birth (Rosenfield et al., 1980). A multidisciplinary team approach, typically including a pediatrician or a neonatologist, a psychiatrist, an endocrinologist, and a reconstructive surgeon, is required not only in arriving at the diagnosis and the proper gender assignment but also in developing an appropriate plan of management (Walsh, 1978).

As part of the initial discussion with the family of a child born with ambiguous genitalia, the family should be told that the external genitalia are underdeveloped or incompletely formed and that further tests are necessary to establish the sex and the direction for future development. The assigning of a neuter name for the child should be avoided because this admits ambivalence and casts doubt on the final decision that is made. Generally, gender choice should be based on the infant's functional anatomic potential and not on the karyotype or the prospects for fertility, except for girls with CAH who are potentially fertile regardless of the severity of virilization. Because it is simpler to construct a vagina than a satisfactory penis, only the infant with a phallus of adequate size should be considered for a male gender assignment.

In addition to a complete history and physical examination, critical diagnostic tests include biochemical assays, buccal smear for Barr bodies, fluorescent Y staining, karyotyping, pelvic ultrasound, and contrast studies of the urogenital sinus (Federman, 1968; Gale, 1983; Haller et al., 1977). Based on the results of these studies, proper assignment to one of the four categories of ambiguous genitalia is usually possible. Early laparotomy is rarely necessary except when gonadal biopsy might influence the sex of rearing, as with true hermaphroditism, or when gonadectomy might be appropriate, as with mixed gonadal dysgenesis and removal of discordant gonadal tissue.

SURGICAL MANAGEMENT: FEMALE PSEUDOHERMAPHRODITISM

For females typically virilized with CAH, the surgical considerations are both functional and cosmetic. Establishment of an adequate vaginal inlet will allow later sexual intercourse and, because these girls are potentially fertile, will even allow pregnancy. A reduction clitoroplasty provides a suitable feminine appearance.

The optimal timing of surgery remains controversial. Arguments exist for initiating reconstruction in infancy, even as early as the neonatal period. Certainly, the surgery should be done before the age of 3 or 3 1/2 years, when sexual awareness is appearing (Lewis and Money, 1977). On one hand, in favor of surgery in early infancy, correction of conspicuous ambiguity may reduce the parents' anxiety about the infant's sex and ease their acceptance of a female sexual assignment. On the other hand, any corrective surgery in the neonatal period will not allow for maximum spontaneous diminution of clitorimegaly after institution of steroid replacement therapy. Furthermore, the chance of vaginal injury or stenosis is greater with early surgery. If the surgery is done late in the first year of life, at a time of physiologic obesity, the ability to establish the proper vestibular size and appropriate anatomic clitoral-vaginal relationships may be compromised. An alternative is early clitoroplasty with delay of the vaginoplasty until later childhood or even puberty. Although this procedure corrects the gross ambiguity and avoids the risks of a vaginal stricture, it has the disadvantage of not positioning the clitoris in a known relationship to the remainder of the vulva.

It is our personal preference to perform a vaginoplasty before the clitoroplasty, with plans to complete both steps during the same operation whenever feasible. This practice allows the clitoral reduction to be accomplished readily in appropriate relation to the vestibular anatomy, even if staged. The reconstruction is accomplished without great difficulty at 15 to 18 months of age, although we have been willing to operate in the first 6 months for more severe ambiguity or when parental anxiety requires it. Most parents, however, adjust surprisingly well after working with the multidisciplinary intersex team, and are willing to delay the infant's surgery until the time recommended as most suitable.

SURGICAL TECHNIQUES

Vaginoplasty

The principles of vaginoplasty include some form of incision of the urogenital sinus to expose the vulva and

an inlay flap of perineal skin to enlarge the outer vaginal barrel (Fortunoff et al., 1964; Perlmutter, 1979). For a minimal degree of urogenital sinus fusion, a simple midline cutback in the form of an episiotomy may be sufficient. However, with the more usual degrees of virilization, the lower, urogenital sinus–derived portion of the vagina is narrow and underdeveloped. Here, the insertion of a well-vascularized perineal skin flap creates an adequate vaginal lumen and minimizes the likelihood of significant secondary stenosis from contracture of overlapping suture lines.

Although the flap can be eccentric, based laterally or posterolaterally, we prefer a short, midline, posteriorly based U-shaped flap with a fairly broad base just within the ischial tuberosities (Perlmutter, 1979). After mobilizing the flap and incising midline perineal and perivaginal tissues, the posterior vaginal midline is exposed, mobilized, and incised to the level of normal vaginal tissue with its normal lumen. Because the flap is elastic and hinged and drops into the posteriorly incised and separated perivaginal space, and because the posterior wall of the vagina has been mobilized, flap length in the infant or very young child need not exceed 2.5 cm or, at most, 3 cm (Fig. 53–5).

Suprasphincteric Vaginoplasty

Rarely, complete virilization is encountered in virilizing adrenogenital syndrome, and the genitalia have a totally male appearance. In this patient, the distal vaginal segment is often no larger than a narrow fistula and enters the urogenital sinus through, or proximal to, the external urethral sphincter (Fig. 53–4B). In this case, the type of vaginoplasty described earlier may result in urinary incontinence from urethral sphincter disruption, if the true (proximal) urethra is very short. The alternative is a procedure that involves endoscopic insertion of a Fogarty balloon catheter into the vagina (Fig. 53–6A), followed by detachment of the lower vaginal segment from the urethral wall (urogenital sinus), using a perineal approach (Fig. 53–6B to F).

The transverse perineal muscles are left attached to the perineal body between the urethra and the future vaginal outlet instead of being located rectovaginally. Extensive lateral and posterior skin flaps are required to exteriorize the detached vaginal cuff (Fig. 53–6G to H). Readers should consult the literature for details of repair in this situation (Hendren and Crawford, 1969 and 1972; Hendren and Donahue, 1980). When an adequate length of posterior urethra is present between the bladder neck and junction with the vagina, however, a flap vaginoplasty as described is still possible. A balloon catheter should be placed endoscopically in the vaginal opening to assist in the dissection, which will be more difficult in this situation because of the high position of the short vagina.

Vaginal Substitution

Rarely, an intersex patient requires the creation of a vagina. In addition, genotypic males who undergo gen-

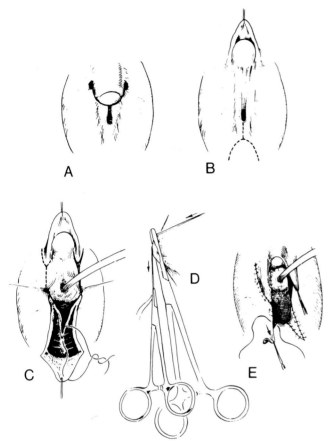

Figure 53–5. Technique of flap vaginoplasty.

A, Preoperative appearance of genitalia.

B, Outline of skin incisions to open midline planes and to develop short, broad-based U flap.

C, Posterior wall of congenitally narrow, lower vagina has been exposed. At times, it is surrounded by corpus spongiosum that, after division, requires hemostasis by cautery or by oversewing with fine catgut suture. A midline incision has been made in the narrow vaginal segment, which should be carried into the wider, thicker, müllerian-derived portion of the vagina, after blunt dissection and exposure of the posterior wall in the midline. This diagram also shows the incision around the ventral preputial folds, which will be advanced inferiorly to create labia minora.

D, A heavy clamp on the perineal drape, lateral to the genitalia, is shown as a hook over which sutures can be placed to provide lateral traction for symmetric exposure during dissection and repair.

E, Details of labial advancement and vaginal flap suturing. If labioscrotal skin is redundant, this tissue can be pulled downward as diagrammed and trimmed if necessary to flatten the rugae and to give the labia majora a more appropriate appearance.

der reassignment, i.e., males with microphallus, penile agenesis, or cloacal exstrophy, may also need such procedures. Treatment options include nonsurgical dilation of a small vaginal pit (e.g., TFS), full- or split-thickness skin graft, or intestinal substitution. Nonsurgical dilation, first described by Frank (1938), essentially involves progressive self-dilation of the perineum. Although a small series of patients was reported with acceptable results using this technique (Wabeek et al., 1971), nonsurgical dilation has not been met with widespread acceptance. This technique is best suited for a highly compliant patient with a rudimentary introital pouch or cavity.

Free skin graft vaginoplasty was popularized by Mc-Indoe and Bannister in 1938. The technique involves harvesting a suitable full- or split-thickness piece of skin, fashioning it into a cavity over a mold, and inserting the mold and skin graft into a previously prepared perineal space. After the free skin graft has had time to take, the mold is removed. Despite long-term problems with contracture and occasional early sloughing of the graft (Cali and Pratt, 1968), the procedure remains a mainstay of the treatment of vaginal atresia and aplasia.

Intestinal substitution was introduced in 1902 by Baldwin (1904). As originally described, the operation involved isolating a piece of ileum on its mesentery and anastomosizing it to the perineum. Subsequently, numerous modifications of the procedure have been described, including the utilization of sigmoid and ileocecal segments (Cali and Pratt, 1968; Pratt, 1972; Pratt and Smith, 1966). A well-vascularized intestinal substitution has the advantage of less risk of contraction. Mucus discharge, unfortunately, has been a frequent and annoying problem.

Our preference is to perform an intestinal substitution when the adjacent perineal structures are thought to be hypoplastic, e.g., the posterior urethral wall. Free skin graft techniques under such circumstances are more likely to result in fistula formation into adjacent structures and are more likely to contract, owing to a poor vascular bed.

Clitoroplasty

Because the clitoris will reduce in size to a definite, although limited, degree after the infant has been placed on an appropriate and adequate regimen of steroid replacement, a decision about the type of clitoroplasty for clitorimegaly should not be made at the initial neonatal evaluation.

Clitorectomy

Clitorectomy is mentioned only to be condemned. Historically, clitorectomy was the procedure of choice for clitoral hypertrophy. Currently, however, because of a better understanding of the anatomy of the clitoris and a realization that progressive enlargement does not occur with adequate steroid replacement, the clitoris is preserved. Newer techniques result in an improved cosmetic result while, more importantly, preserving clitoral sensation.

Clitoral Recession

Current procedures emphasize the preservation of clitoral sensation by reducing and relocating the clitoris, using techniques designed to conceal it or make it less conspicuous. With recession of a very large, penis-sized phallus, however, bulging of the shaft under the mons pubis can occur during erections, causing pain and making the clitoris fairly conspicuous. This problem

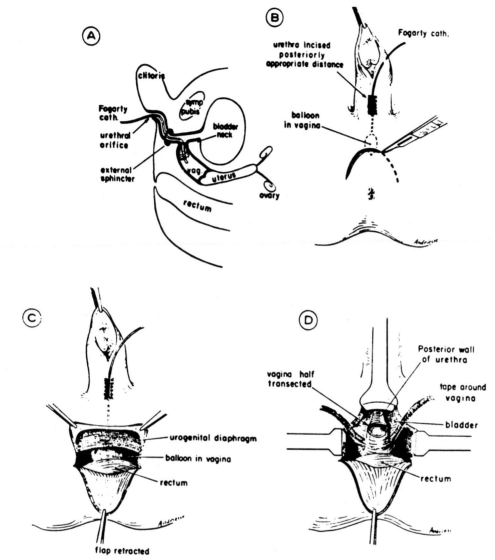

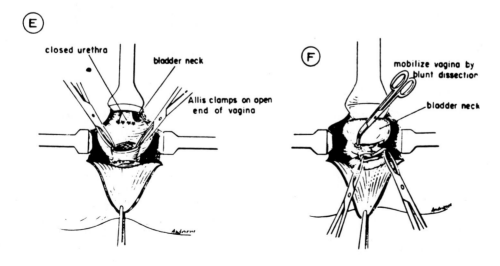

Figure 53–6. A to H, Operative technique of "pull-through" vaginoplasty for an infant in whom the vagina enters the proximal urethra. (From Hendren, W. H., and Crawford, J. D.: Adrenogenital syndrome: The anatomy of the anomaly and its repair. Some new concepts. J. Pediatr. Surg., 4:49, 1969.)

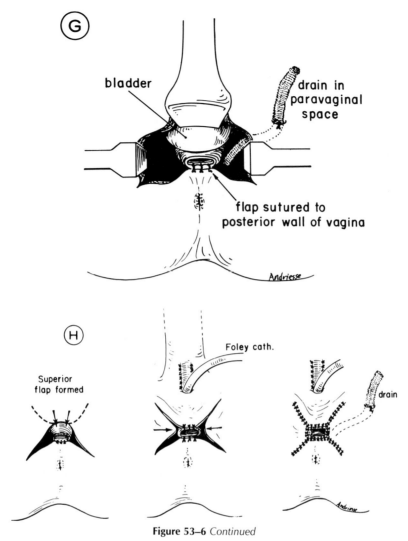

Figure 53–6 *Continued*

limits the choice of recession to a phallus that is not too large to be adequately concealed.

If clitoral hypertrophy is minimal but yet sufficient to warrant correction, Ansell and Rajfer (1981) described a procedure of clitoral concealment, whereby the labia majora are approximated over the clitoris. The procedure has the advantage of simplicity (Fig. 53–7). These workers have employed the procedure along with other clitoroplasty techniques to enhance cosmetic results.

With the exception of Lattimer's technique (1966) for relocation of the shaft and glans, most recession-based procedures provide for relocation of the phallic body by attaching it more cephalad on the anterior periosteum of the symphysis and then closing the mons tissues over the shaft (Randolph and Hung, 1970). This maneuver is often combined with a reduction of glans size by trimming the lateral coronal margins and adjacent glans (Hendren and Crawford, 1972). For any form of clitoral recession or reduction, the glans can be made a more suitable size by a variety of trimming and wedging techniques (Fig. 53–8).

Corporal Plication

Plication of the shaft is particularly suited to mild or moderate clitorimegaly. Heavy longitudinal through-and-through sutures on each side of the shaft, avoiding the neurovascular bundles, will shorten the shaft and partially obliterate the erectile spaces (Fig. 53–9) (Stefan, 1967). Excision of multiple wedges of tunica vaginalis is an alternative to corporal plication for shortening the shaft (Glassberg and Laungani, 1981), but this procedure does not diminish corporal width or control bulging erections.

In any form of clitoral revision involving a vaginoplasty, more than one stage may be required to complete the clitoroplasty, especially the monsplasty and deeper mons dissection necessary for recession. This is because marked lymphedema may follow the extensive flap procedures employed in the earlier steps of the operation. In such a situation, it is better to complete the procedure at another time than to jeopardize tissue viability. A female with congenital adrenal hyperplasia who under-

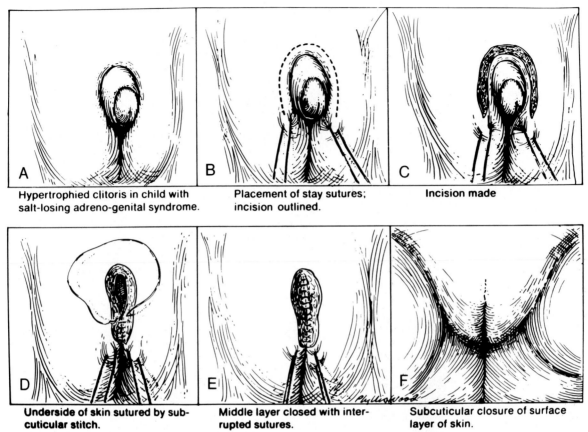

A Hypertrophied clitoris in child with salt-losing adreno-genital syndrome.

B Placement of stay sutures; incision outlined.

C Incision made

D Underside of skin sutured by sub-cuticular stitch.

E Middle layer closed with interrupted sutures.

F Subcuticular closure of surface layer of skin.

Figure 53–7. *A* to *F,* Surgical method of concealing the hypertrophied clitoris. (From Ansell, J. S., and Rajfer, J.: A new and simplified method for concealing the hypertrophied clitoris. J. Pediatr. Surg., 16:681, 1981.)

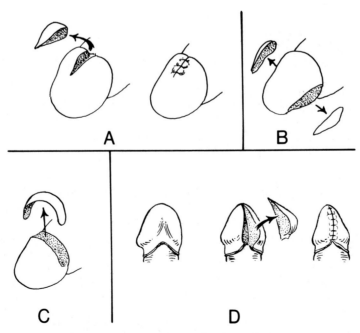

Figure 53–8. *A* to *D,* Options for glans reduction.

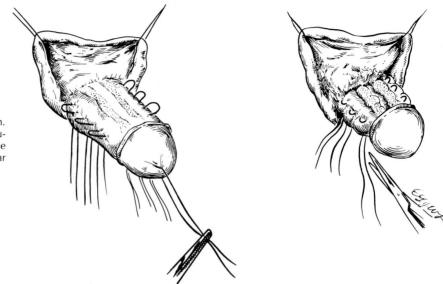

Figure 53–9. Technique for corporal plication. Heavy longitudinal through-and-through sutures shorten the phallus and obliterate the corporal cavities. The dorsal neurovascular bundles should be avoided.

went a flap vaginoplasty and a clitoroplasty by corporal plication is shown in Figure 53–10.

Corporal Reduction (Resection)

To deal with a large phallic shaft, several investigators have proposed shaft excision with preservation of the glans. Spence and Allen (1973) proposed total removal of the shaft and crura through a dorsal shaft degloving incision (a dorsal circumcision incision) or, alternatively, after an elliptic transverse excision of excess dorsal midshaft skin. The glans is left attached to the midline vulval mucosa and is sutured to the pubic periosteum. Although the cosmetic results appear to be satisfactory, these workers did not describe preservation of the dorsal glans innervation.

Others have proposed excision of the shaft while identifying and preserving the dorsal neurovascular bundles. The glans is reattached to the proximal stump (Fig. 53–11) (Barinka et al., 1968; Kumar et al., 1974; Schmid, 1961; Snyder et al., 1983). The shaft and prepuce skin can be handled in a variety of ways for appropriate redistribution and creation of labia minora. When the midline mucosal strip is elongated, it can be detached from the glans, shortened, and reattached to the ventral edge of the glans, provided the dorsal neurovascular bundle has not been compromised. Goodwin (1981) describes resection of the corpora from a ventral approach (Fig. 53–12).

Allen and colleagues (1982) have also performed dorsal shaft resection and dorsal glans wedging without regard to the dorsal nerves, relying on innervation to the residual glans tissue through an intact ventral mucosal strip. They report postoperative clitoral sensation, as tested by bioelectrical stimulation, and the ability of older patients to experience erotic gratification.

A modification of corporal resection for clitoral reduction has been described by Kogan and associates (1983). It involves subtunical resection of a segment of the erectile tissue within each corporal body. The midline ventral mucosa is intentionally divided to mobilize the shaft, and it can be shortened, as appropriate, during reconstruction. The technique has the advantages of simplicity and added safety. There is little risk of glans necrosis or of superficial epithelial slough of the glans from trauma to the dorsal neurovascular tissue, which can occur with corporal resection. Kogan's technique is now our treatment of choice for management of the large phallus. Our version of the procedure is diagrammed in Figure 53–13.

Vulvoplasty

Male pseudohermaphrodites with ambiguous genitalia consisting of a micropenis with a fused perineum are best assigned a female gender role. The smallest size of a miniature penis that can develop into a sexually adequate adult penis is not known with certainty, but the responsiveness to growth of such an organ can be tested in early infancy with systemic testosterone administration. A phallus originally less than 2.5 cm in the full-term neonate is likely to be inadequate (Kogan, 1981). In making decisions about altering sex assignment, it is helpful to have standards for normal ranges of penile size at all ages, including the newborn. Nomograms are available for this purpose (Feldman and Smith, 1975; Schonfeld and Beebe, 1942).

In the patient with micropenis, simple exteriorization of the penile and bulbar urethra (extended external urethrostomy) will simulate the appearance of a vulva. Lateral preputial or shaft skin flaps can be advanced inferiorly on either side of the opened urethra to form labia minora. As in flap vaginoplasty, a small flap can be turned into the deep bulbar urethra to avoid perineal contracture during healing (Fig. 53–14). When a short vaginal pouch from incomplete müllerian duct inhibition

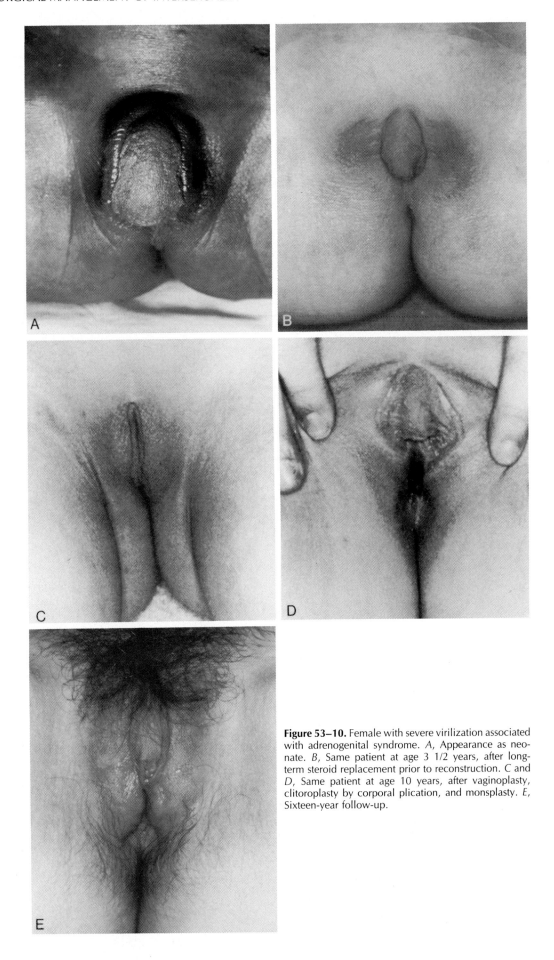

Figure 53–10. Female with severe virilization associated with adrenogenital syndrome. *A*, Appearance as neonate. *B*, Same patient at age 3 1/2 years, after long-term steroid replacement prior to reconstruction. *C* and *D*, Same patient at age 10 years, after vaginoplasty, clitoroplasty by corporal plication, and monsplasty. *E*, Sixteen-year follow-up.

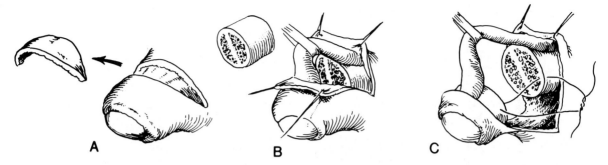

Figure 53–11. Technique for corporal resection with preservation of glans and its innervation. *A,* One method for approaching the phallic shaft and simultaneously trimming back the shaft skin by excising a transverse dorsal wedge. The shaft can also be exposed by dorsal degloving. *B,* Diagrammatic view of corporal excision with neurovascular preservation. *C,* Attachment of glans to phallic stump.

is also present, the flap can be turned into the vagina at the time of the urethral exteriorization. Orchiectomy, of course, should be done (Fig. 53–15).

POSTOPERATIVE MANAGEMENT

Immediate postoperative management, aside from appropriate steroid replacement in cases of adrenogenital syndrome, consists primarily of wound care. It is usually possible to remove the urethral catheter inserted at surgery on the 2nd or 3rd postoperative day. When excessive edema is present, the tube is best left a few more days. At the completion of the vaginoplasty, the vaginal outlet is loosely packed with a strip of 1-inch petroleum jelly (Vaseline)–coated gauze, which keeps the suture lines apart and contributes to local hemostasis. This packing should be removed after 24 hours to avoid tissue maceration and to allow for drainage of serosanguineous intravaginal fluid.

The genitoplasty should be bandaged with a fluffy gauze dressing, utilizing gentle compression to limit local edema. Dressings can generally be discontinued on the 2nd or 3rd day, before or at the time of catheter removal. Topical conjugated estrogen cream can be started after dressings are discontinued and applied twice daily for a period of up to 1 week at a time. This regimen causes temporary local pubertal changes that

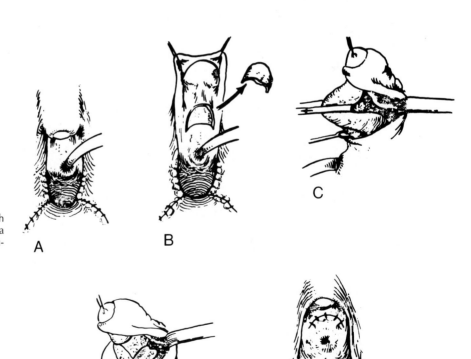

Figure 53–12. *A* to *E,* Corporal resection with preservation of neurovascular bundle, from a ventral approach. The midline ventral mucosal strip can be shortened, if necessary.

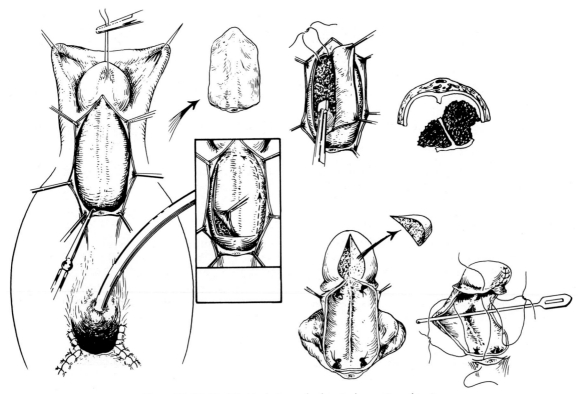

Figure 53–13. Modified technique of subtunical resection of tunica.

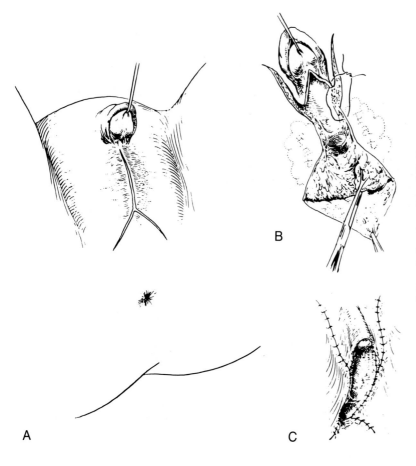

Figure 53–14. Technique for creating vulva (vulvoplasty) in the male pseudohermaphrodite with ambiguous genitalia or micropenis.

A, Urethrotomy. Dorsal urethra becomes mucosa of created vestibule.

B, Defatting of perineal portion of labia majora creates a flatter, more feminine contour of the genitalia. Development of V flaps for labia minora. Advancement of these flaps posteriorly on either side of new vestibule also pulls phallus downward.

C, Completed repair. Flap plasty into deep bulb, or into small vaginal pouch when present, minimizes contracture of created vestibule during healing.

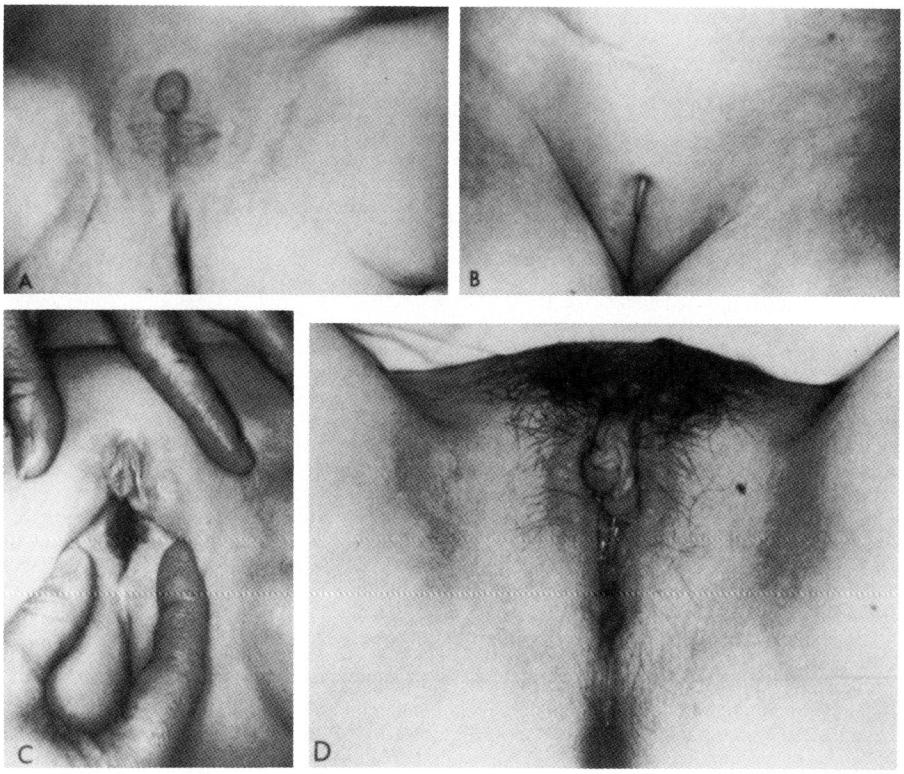

Figure 53–15. Male pseudohermaphrodite treated by vulvoplasty and vaginoplasty. *A,* One-year-old infant male—XY with dysgenetic testes. Phallus is tiny. Scrotum is underdeveloped and empty. The infant was treated as in Figure 53–14. A small vaginal pouch was present. *B* and *C,* Appearance at age 5 years. *D,* Appearance at age 12 years, 11 years postoperatively, after beginning exogenous estrogen therapy. Hymen and vaginal orifice are visible. Appearance is appropriately female.

are beneficial during healing. During the first few weeks postoperatively, gentle passage of a catheter or sound into the distal vagina may be helpful, when focal vaginal outlet narrowing is suspected. However, overdilation can injure the repair and result in a dense scar.

Long-term results from multiple large series of children undergoing genital reconstruction for management of intersexuality by current techniques are not yet available. Details about adult sexual functioning are still scanty. Several series have emphasized the generally good results obtained following vaginoplasty for adrenogenital syndrome, although two thirds or more of patients may require a revisional vaginoplasty for stenosis (Azziz et al., 1986; Jones et al., 1976; Mulaikal et al., 1987; Nihoul-Fekete et al., 1982; Sotiropoalous et al., 1976).

Azziz and associates (1986) reported that revisional vaginoplasty was nearly twice as likely to be required in salt-losing than in non–salt-losing patients. Such differences in surgical results between the two patient groups could be due to the variety of medical regimens and compliance levels, as suggested by these workers, as well as to the inherent variety of the anatomy of the patients (e.g., hypoplastic lower vagina segment in salt-losing cases). Revisional vaginoplasty is best delayed until after puberty when the patient's menarche, maturity, and compliance are well established. Similarly, complex vaginoplasties may best be delayed until after puberty unless urinary obstruction or infection or menstrual obstruction mandates early intervention.

Clitoroplasty, with or without resection of the shaft, has also had generally favorable results, although an occasional revision is necessary. With regard to fertility, Jones and co-workers (1976) reported that fertility cor-

related with sexual activity, which in turn was primarily related to the adequacy of the vaginal introitus. A confounding factor in all these long-term studies is the issue of patient compliance with glucocorticoid replacement therapy. Many patients with CAH on long-term follow-up demonstrate noncompliance as evidenced by hirsutism. The effects of noncompliance with medications and the resultant increase in androgenic precursors on the physical and psychosocial well-being of the patient remain uncertain.

One interesting observation of patients with CAH who have become pregnant to term is the high incidence of cesarean sections for alleged cephalopelvic disproportion (Edmonds and Dewhurst, 1986). This may be due to premature closure of the ephiphyses or to an android pelvis.

Despite some tendency toward tomboyish behavior during childhood, early sex assignment to a female gender role for girls with the adrenogenital syndrome, plus appropriate steroidal replacement, has resulted in favorable outcome, and patients have made satisfactory adjustments in the sex of assignment (Money and Schwartz, 1977). As Money (1973) has pointed out, "They experience romance, erotic attraction and marriage, usually concordantly with the sex of assignment and rearing. They experience genito-pelvic pleasure, not necessarily losing the orgasm even after extensive genital excision and reconstruction."

REFERENCES

Aarskog, D.: Clinical and cytogenetic studies of hypospadias. Acta Paediatr. Scand. (Suppl.), 203:7, 1970.

Allen, L. E., Hardy, B. E., and Churchill, B. M.: The surgical management of the enlarged clitoris. J. Urol., 128:351, 1982.

Allen, T. D.: Disorders of sexual differentiation. Urology (Suppl. 4), 7:24, 1976.

Ansell, J. S., and Rajfer, J.: A new and simplified method for concealing the hypertrophied clitoris. J. Pediatr. Surg., 16:681, 1981.

Azziz, R., Mulaikas, R. M., Migeon, C. J., Jones, H. W., and Rock, J. A.: Congenital adrenal hyperplasia: Long-term results following vagina reconstruction. Fertil. Steril., 46:1011, 1986.

Baldwin, A. F.: Ann. Surg., 40:398, 1904.

Barinka, L., Stavratjev, M., and Toman, M.: Plastic adjustment of female genitals in adrenogenital syndrome. Acta Chir. Plast., 10:99, 1968.

Bengmark, S., and Forsberg, J. G.: On the development of the rat vagina. Acta Anat. (Basel), 37:106, 1959.

Blanchard, M. D., and Josso, N.: Source of the anti-müllerian hormone synthesized by the fetal tests: Müllerian-inhibiting activity of fetal bovine Sertoli cells in tissue culture. Pediatr. Res., 8:968, 1974.

Cali, R. W., and Pratt, J. H.: Congenital absence of the vagina: Long-term results of vaginal reconstruction in 175 cases. Am. J. Obstet. Gynecol., 100:752, 1968.

Davidoff, F., and Federman, D. D.: Mixed gonadal dysgenesis. Pediatrics, 92:725, 1973.

Edmonds, D. K., and Dewhurst, J.: Reproductive potential in adolescent girls with ambiguous genitalia. Pediatr. Ann. 15:530, 1986.

Federman, D. D.: Abnormal Sexual Development: A Genetic and Endocrine Approach to Differential Diagnosis. Philadelphia, W. B. Saunders Co., 1968.

Feldman, K. W., and Smith, D. W.: Fetal phallic growth and penile standards for newborn male infants. J. Pediatr., 80:395, 1975.

Fortunoff, S., Lattimer, J. K., and Edson, M. M.: Vaginoplasty technique for female pseudohermaphrodites. Surg. Gynecol. Obstet., 118:545, 1964.

Frank, R. T.: The formation of an artificial vagina without operation. Am. J. Obstet. Gynecol., 35:1053, 1938.

Gale, M. E.: Hermaphroditism demonstrated by computed tomography. AJR, 141:99, 1983.

Glassberg, K. I., and Laungani, G.: Reduction clitoroplasty. Urology, 17:604, 1981.

Goodwin, W. E.: Partial (segmental) amputation of the clitoris for female pseudohermaphroditism. Soc. Pediatr. Urol. Newsletter, Jan. 21, 1981.

Haller, J. O., Schneider, M., Kassner, E. G., et al.: Ultrasonography in pediatric gynecology and obstetrics. Am. J. Roentgenol., 128:423, 1977.

Hendren, W. H., and Crawford, J. D.: Adrenogenital syndrome: The anatomy of the anomaly and its repair. Some new concepts. J. Pediatr. Surg., 4:49, 1969.

Hendren, W. H., and Crawford, J. D.: The child with ambiguous genitalia. Curr. Probl. Surg., Nov.:1–64, 1972.

Hendren, W. H., and Donahue, P. K.: Correction of congenital abnormalities of the vagina and perineum. J. Pediatr. Surg., 15:751, 1980.

Jones, H. W., Garcia, S. C., and Klingensmith, G. J.: Secondary surgical treatment of the masculinized external genitalia of patients with virilizing adrenal hyperplasia. Obstet. Gynecol., 48:73, 1976.

Josso, N.: Interspecific character of müllerian inhibiting substance: Action of the human fetal testis, ovary, and adrenal on the fetal rat. J. Clin. Endocrinol. Metab., 32:404, 1971.

Jost, A.: Problems of fetal endocrinology: The gonadal and hypophyseal hormones. Recent Prog. Horm. Res., 8:379, 1953.

Jost, A., Vigier, B., Prepin, J., et al.: Studies sex differentiation in mammals. Recent Prog. Horm. Res., 29:1, 1973.

Kim, M. H., Gumpel, J. A., and Gruff, P.: Pregnancy in a true hermaphrodite. Obstet. Gynecol. (Suppl.), 53:415, 1979.

Kogan, S. J.: Micropenis. Etiologic and management considerations. In Kogan, S. J., Hafel, E. S. (Eds.): Clinics in Andrology—Pediatric Andrology. Boston, Martinus Nijhoff, 1981.

Kogan, S. J., Smey, P., and Levitt, S. B.: Subtunical total reduction clitoroplasty: A safe modification of existing techniques. J. Urology, 130:746, 1983.

Kumar, H., Kiefer, J. H., Rosenthal, I. E., and Clark, S. S.: Clitoroplasty: Experience during a 19-year period. J. Urology, 111:81, 1974.

Lattimer, J. K.: Relocation and recession of the enlarged clitoris with preservation of the glans: An alternative to amputation. J. Urology, 86:113, 1966.

Lewis, V. G., and Money, J.: Adrenogenital syndrome: The need for early surgical feminization in girls. In Lee, P. A., Plotnick, L. P., Kowarski, A. V., et al. (Eds.): Congenital Adrenal Hyperplasia. Baltimore, University Park Press, 1977, p. 463.

McIndoe, A. H., and Bannister, J. B.: An operation for the cure of congenital absence of vagina. J. Obstet. Gynecol. Br. Emp., 45:490, 1938.

Mininberg, D. T., Levine, L. S., and New, M. I.: Current concepts in congenital adrenal hyperplasia. Invest. Urol., 17:169, 1979.

Money, J.: Intersexual problems. Clin. Obstet. Gynecol., 16:169, 1973.

Money, J., and Schwartz, M.: Dating, romantic and non-romantic friendships and sexuality in 17 early treated adrenogenital females, aged 16-25. In Lee, P. A., Plotwick, J. P., Konarski, A. V., and Migeon, C. J. (Eds.): Congenital Adrenal Hyperplasia. Baltimore, University Park Press, 1977, pp. 419–431.

Mulaikal, R. M., Migeon, C. J., and Rock, J. A.: Fertility rates in female patients with congenital adrenal hyperplasia due to 21-hydrolase deficiency. N. Engl. J. Med., 316:178, 1987.

Nihoul-Fekete, C. N., Philippe, F., Thiband, E., Rappaport, K., and Pellerin, D.: Resultants a moyen et long terme de a chirurgie reparatice des organcs gcnitaux chez les filles aheintes d'hyperplasie congenitale viriusante des surrenales. Arch. Fr. Pediatr., 39:13, 1982.

Nihoul-Fekete, C., Lortat-Jacob, S., Cachin, O., and Josso, N.: Preservation of gonadal function in true hermaphroditism. J Pediatr. Surg., 19:50, 1984.

Page, D. C., Mosher, R., Simpson, E. M., et al.: The sex-determining region of the human Y chromosome encodes a finger region. Cell SI:1091, 1987.

Perlmutter, A. D.: Management of intersexuality. In Harrison, J. H., Gittes, R. F., Perlmutter, A. D., et al. (Eds.): Campbell's Urology. Philadelphia, W. B. Saunders Co., 1979, p. 1535.

Pratt, J. H.: Vaginal atresia corrected by use of small and large bowel. Clin. Obstet. Gynecol. 15:639, 1972.

Pratt, J. H., and Smith, G. R.: Vaginal reconstruction with a sigmoid loop. Am. J. Obstet. Gynecol., 96:31, 1966.

Randolph, J. G., and Hung, W.: Reduction clitoroplasty in females with hypertrophied clitoris. J. Pediatr. Surg., 5:224, 1970.

Rosenfield, R. L., Lucky, A. W., and Allen, T. D.: The diagnosis and management of intersex. In Gluck, L. (Ed.): Current Problems in Pediatrics. Chicago, Year Book Medical Publishers, 1980.

Schmid, M. A.: Plastiche Korrektur des ausseren Genitales bei einem mannlichen Scheinzwitter. Arch. Klin. Chir., 298:977, 1961.

Schonfeld, W. A., and Beebe, G. W.: Normal growth and variation in the male genitalia from birth to maturity. J. Urology, 48:759, 1942.

Siiteri, P. K., and Wilson, J. D.: Testosterone formation and metabolism during male sexual differentiation in the human embryo. J. Clin. Endocrinol. Metab., 38:113, 1974.

Snyder, H. M., Retik, A. B., Bauer, S. B., and Colodny, A. H.: Feminizing genitoplasty: A synthesis. J. Urol., 129:1024, 1983.

Sotiropoalous, A., Morishimg, A., Homsy, Y., and Lattimer, J. K.: Long-term assessment of genital reconstruction in female pseudohermaphrodites. J. Urology, 115:599, 1976.

Spence, H. M., and Allen, T. D.: Genital reconstruction in the female with the adrenogenital syndrome. Br. J. Urology, 45:126, 1973.

Stefan, H.: Surgical reconstruction of the external genitalia in female pseudohermaphrodites. Br. J. Urology, 39:347, 1967.

Wabeek, A. J., Millard, P. R., Wilson, W. B., and Pion, R. J.: Creation of a neovagina by the Frank nonoperative method. Obstet. Gynecol., 37:408, 1971.

Wachtel, S., Koo, G. C., Breg, W., et al.: Serologic detection of a Y-linked gene in XX males and XX true hermaphrodites. N. Engl. J. Med., 295:750, 1976.

Walsh, P. C.: The differential diagnosis of ambiguous genitalia in the newborn. Symposium in congenital anomalies of the lower genitourinary tract. Urol. Clin. North Am., 5:213, 1978.

Walsh, P. C., Madden, J. D., Harros, M. S., et al.: Familial incomplete male pseudohermaphroditism, type 2: Decreased dihydrotestosterone formation in pseudovaginal perineoscrotal hypospadias. N. Engl. J. Med., 291:944, 1974.

54
PEDIATRIC ONCOLOGY

Howard M. Snyder III, M.D.
Giulio J. D'Angio, M.D.
Audrey E. Evans, M.D.
R. Beverly Raney, M.D.

WILMS' TUMOR AND OTHER RENAL TUMORS OF CHILDHOOD

History

Rance, in 1814, apparently was the first to describe the tumor; Max Wilms, in 1899, better characterized the tumor that has become associated with his name. Other more descriptive terms commonly used include mixed tumor of the kidney, embryoma of the kidney, and nephroblastoma.

These neoplasms often are massive in size before becoming clinically evident; thus, only rare efforts were made to excise them, and most children died. By the 1930s, better surgical techniques, especially improvements in anesthesia, and better understanding of pediatric surgical care led to a lowering of the operative mortality rates, and survival rates of 25 per cent had been achieved by the 1940s (Gross and Neuhauser, 1950).

The multimodal approach to the management of pediatric solid tumors originated with the treatment of Wilms' tumor, because it was learned that this tumor was responsive to radiation therapy. With this addition, survivals rose to the 50 per cent range, where they remained until the advent of chemotherapy.

The introduction of aminopterin in the 1940s for the treatment of leukemia opened the era of chemotherapy for pediatric cancers. Sidney Farber and co-workers at the Boston Children's Hospital reported actinomycin D to be an effective treatment for Wilms' tumor in 1956. This marked the first successful treatment of a pediatric solid neoplasm by chemotherapy. By 1966, Farber reported a survival rate of 81 per cent for children with Wilms' tumor treated by surgery, radiotherapy, and chemotherapy with actinomycin D at the Boston Children's Hospital compared with a 40 per cent survival rate for children treated by surgery and radiotherapy only. Wolff and associates (1968) reported that multiple courses of chemotherapy were more effective than a single course.

At about the same time, the *Vinca* alkaloids were found to be effective oncolytic agents. Sutow and Sullivan reported in 1965 the successful use of vincristine as a single agent in the treatment of Wilms' tumor. Vincristine was also shown to be effective in patients who had previously been treated with actinomycin D (Sutow et al., 1963). Subsequently, high-dose cyclophosphamide (Finkelstein et al., 1969) and doxorubicin (Adriamycin; Adria, Columbus, OH) (Wang et al., 1971) were demonstrated to be helpful in the treatment of Wilms' tumor.

The evolution of modern treatment of Wilms' tumor owes much to the cooperative studies carried out in many medical centers to compare different modes of treatment. The intergroup National Wilms' Tumor Study (NWTS) in the United States and trials conducted by the International Society of Pediatric Oncology (SIOP) and the United Kingdom Medical Research Council helped guide the development of current treatment.

Incidence

Wilms' tumor is the most common malignant neoplasm of the urinary tract in children and is responsible for 8 per cent of all solid tumors in children. It makes up more than 80 per cent of genitourinary cancers in children younger than 15 years (Young et al., 1978). Approximately seven new cases occur per million children per year in the United States, resulting in about 350 new cases per year. In about 75 per cent of cases, the diagnosis is made between 1 and 5 years of age. Of all patients, 90 per cent are seen before age 7 years with a peak incidence between ages 3 and 4 years. The male-to-female ratio is almost equal (.97/1.0). Occasionally, the tumor occurs in adults (Olsenn and Bischoff, 1970). Familial cases are rare (1 per cent).

Etiology and Embryology

Wilms' tumor is thought to be the result of an abnormal proliferation of metanephric blastema without normal differentiation into tubules and glomeruli. The median age incidence of 3½ years makes it unlikely that Wilms' tumor is a truly congenital neoplasm, although there clearly is a hereditary component. Evidence (Bove and McAdams, 1976; Machin, 1980a and b) suggests that the lesions of the nephroblastomatosis complex may function as a carrier state, bringing blastemal tissue to a point at which a subsequent change leads to the development of clinical Wilms' tumor. The two-stage mutational model of Knudson and Strong (1972) suggests separation of Wilms' tumors into two classes: hereditary and nonhereditary, depending on whether or not the initial tumor mutational event occurred in a germ cell. Patients with familial or bilateral tumors and those associated with aniridia or genitourinary anomalies present at a younger age and appear to represent hereditary cases.

In the etiology of Wilms' tumor, the loss of allelic heterozygosity on the distal portion of 11p (seen in a third of sporadic cases) suggests that the loss of function of a recessive tumor suppressor gene in the 11p13 region is important (Hoffman, 1989; Koufos et al., 1984). Mutational events at other gene loci may also be involved. In some cases, the allelic heterozygosity is distal to 11p13 and may involve the distal portion of 11p15 as seen with Wilms' tumor in the Beckwith-Wiedemann syndrome (Manners et al., 1988; Reeve et al., 1989). Thus it appears that during tumor formation, maternal chromosome 11 alleles are preferentially lost (Schroeder et al., 1987; Williams et al., 1989).

The association of pseudohermaphroditism, nephron disorders, and Wilms' tumor raises the question of whether an embryologic event might be occurring before the differentiation of renal and genital structures, and, therefore, affecting both (Drash et al., 1970). Teratogens in animal models have also produced Wilms' tumor as well as other neoplasms. Expression of a transforming gene on the maternal chromosome may be muted by genomic imprinting (Wilkins, 1989), raising the possibility of parental occupational exposures as possible risk factors. Children of machinists have been identified at higher risk of Wilms' tumor (Bunin et al., 1989; Olshan et al., 1990), although the exact exposure remains to be identified.

Associated Anomalies

About 15 per cent of children with Wilms' tumor have other congenital abnormalities (Miller, 1968; Miller et al., 1964; Pendergrass, 1976). *Aniridia* was found in 1.1 per cent of the children in the first NWTS. Whereas the occurrence of aniridia in the general population is one in 50,000 persons, it is present in about one in 70 patients with Wilms' tumor. The sporadic form of aniridia, rather than the familial form, is associated with Wilms' tumor. In sporadic aniridia, especially when associated with the 11p deletion, there is an approximate 33 per cent risk of Wilms' tumor. The full syndrome, in addition to the tumor and congenital eye lesions, includes presentation generally before 3 years of age; genitourinary anomalies; deformities of the external ear; mental retardation; and, less frequently, facial or skull dysmorphism; inguinal and umbilical hernias; and hypotonia (Haicken and Miller, 1971). This has become known as the WAGR syndrome—Wilms' tumor, aniridia, genitourinary anomalies, and retardation (Narahara et al., 1984).

Hemihypertrophy, characterized by an asymmetry of the body, has been found in 2.9 per cent of cases of Wilms' tumor, not necessarily lateralized to the side of the tumor. It may even become evident after the Wilms' tumor has appeared (Janik and Seeler, 1976). The incidence of hemihypertrophy in the general population is one in 14,300; whereas, in Wilms' tumor, it is found in 1 of 32 cases. An increased incidence of other cancers is associated with hemihypertrophy, e.g., embryonal carcinomas, especially adrenal cortical carcinomas and hepatoblastomas. The patients often manifest multiple pigmented nevi, hemangiomas, and genitourinary anomalies (Meadows and Jarrett, 1978).

The *Beckwith-Wiedemann syndrome* (Fig. 54–1) consists of visceromegaly involving the adrenal cortex, kidney, liver, pancreas, and gonads. Additionally, omphalocele, hemihypertrophy, microcephaly, mental retardation, and macroglossia may be found. Approximately one in ten children with this syndrome develops a neoplasm (Sotelo-Avila et al., 1980). The malignancies affect the liver, adrenal cortex, and kidney; the same organs are at risk in children with hemihypertrophy. Many cases listed as hemihypertrophy may represent incomplete forms of the Beckwith-Wiedemann syndrome.

Musculoskeletal anomalies have been found in 2.9 per cent of patients with Wilms' tumor who demonstrate a 7.9 per cent incidence of hamartomas, including hemangiomas, multiple nevi, and café au lait spots. A 30-fold increase in the incidence of *neurofibromatosis* is found in patients with Wilms' tumor (Stay and Vawter, 1977).

Genitourinary anomalies are found in 4.4 per cent of cases. Most often seen are renal hypoplasia, ectopia, fusions, duplications, cystic disease, hypospadias, cryptorchidism, and pseudohermaphroditism. As mentioned, this finding suggests that the primary event in the genesis of this tumor occurs before the differentiation of renal and genital structures has taken place and accordingly affects both.

A number of associated *second malignant neoplasms* have been reported in long-term survivors of Wilms' tumor. The incidence of these neoplasms is up to 15 per cent and has included sarcomas, adenocarcinomas, and leukemias. Most of the sarcomas, generally osteogenic, and carcinomas have been found within previous fields of radiation therapy. Such tumors may be induced by previous treatment or may result from a genetic predisposition to the second tumor. Perhaps others are a result of a combination of these factors.

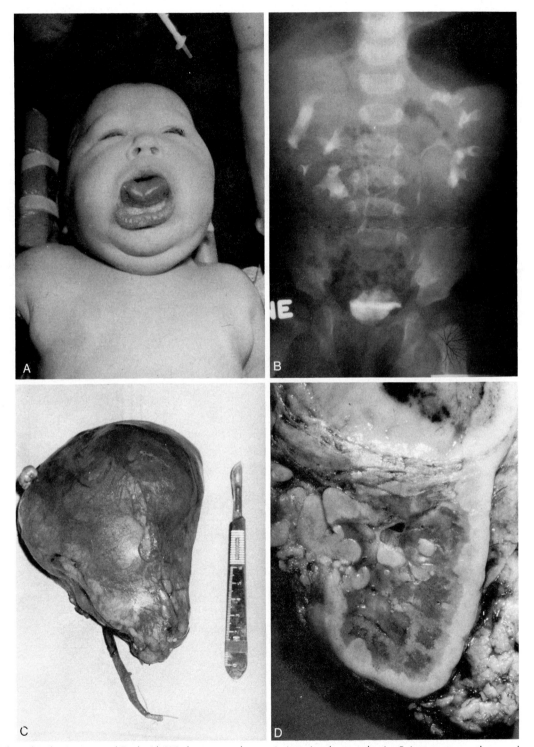

Figure 54–1. Bilateral Wilms' tumor and Beckwith-Wiedemann syndrome. *A,* Associated macroglossia. *B,* Intravenous pyelogram showing calyceal distortion in both kidneys. *C,* Right kidney with large upper pole Wilms' tumor. *D,* Cut specimen showing Wilms' tumor and inferior rim of nephroblastomatosis and Wilms' tumorlets.

Pathology

Gross Features

Classic Wilms' tumor is a sharply demarcated and usually encapsulated solitary tumor occurring in any part of the kidney (Fig. 54–2). The cut tumor bulges with a fleshy tan surface. Necrosis is frequent. It may lead to hemorrhage or the appearance of cyst formation. True cysts are seen occasionally. The tumor distorts the calyceal anatomy, accounting for the typical radiographic picture. Uncommonly, the tumor grows into the renal pelvis, where it may lead to hematuria or obstruction. Renal venous invasion occurs in 20 per cent of cases (Fig. 54–3). Although lymph node metastases often appear to be present at surgery, histologic examination frequently proves this to be a false impression, making gross assessment of nodal involvement unreliable (Martin et al., 1979).

It may be possible from gross examination to distinguish Wilms' tumor from some other renal tumors. Congenital mesoblastic nephroma on examination of the cut surface has a typical interlacing pattern, which is similar to a uterine fibroid (Fig. 54–4). If multiple small lesions are present, they suggest the diagnosis of nephroblastomatosis with or without Wilms' tumor.

Rarely, extrarenal Wilms' tumors have been found (Aterman et al., 1979) in the retroperitoneum and

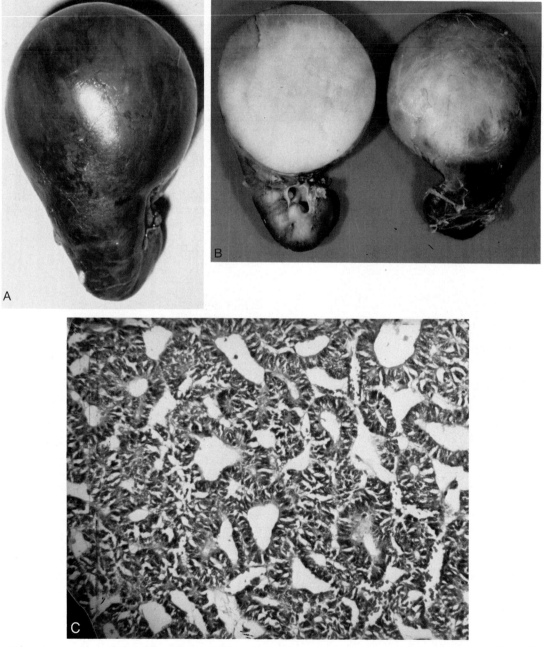

Figure 54–2. Wilms' tumor with epithelial differentiation. *A,* Kidney with large upper pole tumor. *B,* Cut specimen showing well-encapsulated tumor. *C,* Well-differentiated Wilms' tumor with epithelial component forming tubules (favorable histology) (× 320).

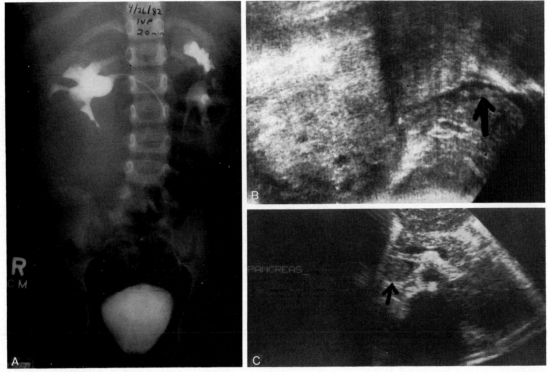

Figure 54–3. Wilms' tumor with caval invasion. *A,* Intravenous pyelogram showing a large right lower pole intrarenal tumor displacing the collecting system upward. Note course of ureter coursing over tumor. Abdominal ultrasound study showing tumor *(arrow)* in inferior cava on sagittal *(B)* and transverse *(C)* views.

inguinal regions, or as part of complex teratomas. Other sites include the posterior mediastinum, retroperitoneum, posterior pelvis, inguinal canal, and sacrococcygeal area (Coppes et al., 1991; McCauley et al., 1979).

Microscopic Features

It is difficult to describe a "typical" Wilms' tumor, because the neoplasm can exhibit a wide spectrum of the structures of the metanephros and mesoderm from which it takes its origin. The tumor is triphasic. The most diagnostic feature is a swirl of "nephrogenic" cells having a tubuloglomerular pattern against a background of "stromagenic" cells (Fig. 54–5). These cells are undifferentiated and generally compact, but they may have a mixoid appearance. The stromal component may occasionally differentiate into striated muscle (frequent), cartilage or fat (rare), or bone (very rare). The epithelial component of Wilms' tumor can be well differentiated, with characteristic mature tubules, or it may be very primitive.

Experience with the pathologic examination of large numbers of specimens has suggested histologic characteristics that tend to be associated with a favorable or an ominous prognosis. Chatten (1976) recognized that epithelial predominance may indicate a better prognosis (Lawler et al., 1977). Although data from the Medical Research Council Nephroblastoma Trial supported this concept, data from the NWTS did not (Beckwith and

Palmer, 1978). The reason for this difference may be that overall survival for Wilms' tumor is now so high (approaching 90 per cent) that it may be impossible to separate histologic features that confer a particularly favorable prognosis. Although the poor outlook predicted for those with tumors having unfavorable histologic features may be confirmed by the clinical course, it may be that especially favorable histologic variants cannot be recognized because the overall success with treatment prevents singling out these cases.

UNFAVORABLE HISTOLOGIC TYPES

One of the first important pathologic correlations to come from the NWTS was the recognition of three particularly unfavorable histologic types. Although these three categories made up only about 10 per cent of the cases studied, they accounted for at least 60 per cent of the deaths.

Anaplasia is strictly defined as a threefold variation in nuclear size with hyperchromatism and abnormal mitotic figures. These features may be found in any of the various elements of a Wilms' tumor. When anaplasia is diffuse rather than focal, the prognosis is more unfavorable. This type has a greater incidence in older children.

The second unfavorable category, which is no longer believed to be a form of Wilms' tumor, is the *rhabdoid* tumor which, while making up only 2 per cent of the renal tumors entered in the NWTS, is and continues to

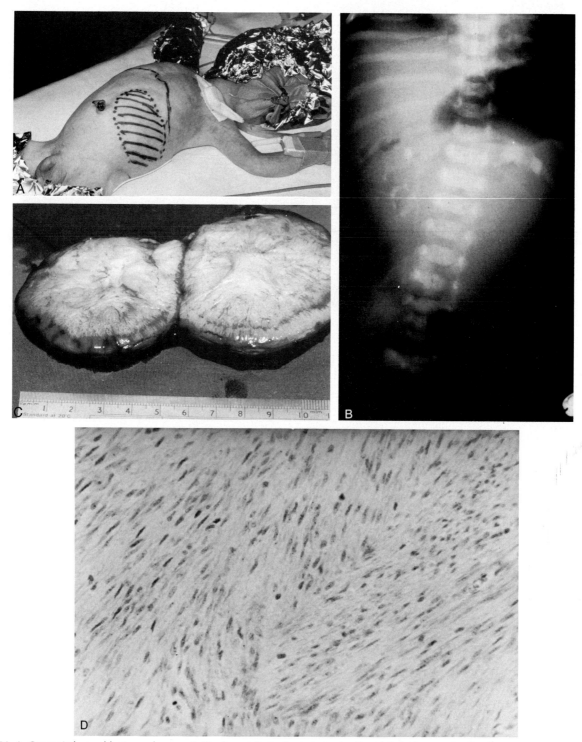

Figure 54–4. Congenital mesoblastic nephroma. *A,* Newborn infant who presented with a left flank mass (outlined). *B,* Intravenous pyelogram showing large left lower pole renal tumor displacing collecting system superiorly. *C,* Gross specimen shows characteristic dense, pale tumor composed of interlacing bundles grossly resembling a leiomyoma. *D,* Histology is tumor composed of sheets of uniform spindle-shaped cells with no capsule.

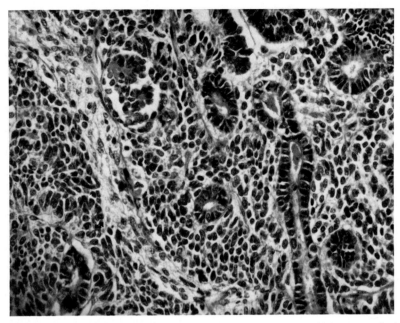

Figure 54–5. Wilms' tumor pathology: Classic triphasic histology showing swirls of primitive renal blastema and tubules against a background of undifferentiated stroma.

be the most lethal (82 per cent died from tumor) (Fig. 54–6) (Sotelo-Avila et al., 1986; Weeks et al., 1987). Histologically, the cells are uniform and large with large nuclei and very prominent nucleoli. The cytoplasm contains eosinophilic inclusions, which, by electron microscopy, can be shown to be fibrils. These large cells are suggestive of rhabdomyoblasts and gave the tumor its name, but neither light nor electron microscopy actually confirms the presence of muscle. Indeed, if striated muscle can be identified, as in conventional Wilms' tumor, it excludes the diagnosis of a rhabdoid tumor and the outlook is not bad. In fact, these neoplasms may not be a form of Wilms' tumor at all. They are now considered by many to be a distinct sarcoma of childhood not of metanephric origin. They tend to metastasize to the brain and have a high association

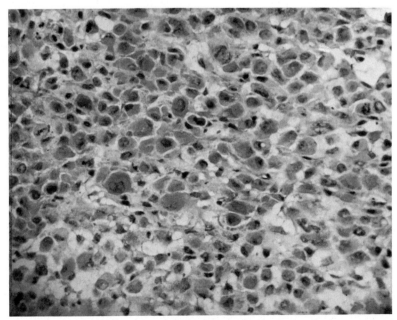

Figure 54–6. Rhabdoid Wilms' tumor: unfavorable histology. Uniform cells with large nuclei and prominent nucleoli. The cytoplasm contains eosinophilic inclusions, which by electron microscopy can be shown to be fibrils.

with independent primary central nervous system tumors (Palmer and Beckwith, 1981).

The third unfavorable variant has been referred to as *clear cell sarcoma* of the kidney and seems to be the same as the "bone metastasizing renal tumor of childhood" described by Marsden and Lawler (1980). In NWTS-III, this tumor formed 3 per cent of entered renal tumors and was equal to anaplastic Wilms' tumor in frequency. It also is now identified as a separate tumor from Wilms' tumor. Histologically, the tumors are characterized by a spindle cell pattern with a vasocentric arrangement. The nucleoli are not prominent, and the cytoplasm is scanty with variably eosinophilic characteristics. Because tubules may be seen in the primary tumor but are not seen in metastatic sites, it is possible that tubules are merely being trapped by the tumor. The tumor characteristically metastasizes to bone (Morgan and Kidd, 1978) and is frequent in males.

Opinion is building to classify this tumor as a distinct entity rather than as a variant of Wilms' tumor (Carcassonne et al., 1981). Some ultrastructural studies have suggested that the tumor may be derived from blastemal cells (Novak et al., 1980). Clear cell sarcoma may reflect a malignant phase of the normally benign congenital mesoblastic nephroma. In NWTS-III, a better prognosis was achieved for clear cell sarcoma cases with the addition of doxorubicin (Adriamycin) to treatment protocols (D'Angio et al., 1989).

FAVORABLE HISTOLOGIC TYPES

Several other renal lesions are found in children that have a characteristic morphology and that tend to have a relatively benign course. Their exact relationship to classic Wilms' tumor continues to be debated, but perhaps they are best considered as variants rather than as distinct pathologic entities (Ganick et al., 1981).

MULTILOCULAR CYST. The characteristic aspect of a multilocular cyst (MLC) is its gross appearance. Typically, the lesion is round and smooth on its external border. It consists of a localized cluster of cysts within the kidney and is almost always unilateral. Two peaks occur in the age incidence of MLC (Banner et al., 1981; Coleman, 1980). The first peak occurs in the pediatric age group and is characterized by the presence of blastema in the septae of the cyst. Although this lesion may have the potential for eventually developing into a classic Wilms' tumor (Fig. 54–7), the MLC itself has a benign course. Local excision constitutes adequate treatment.

The second peak incidence occurs in the adult, and the tumor is seen more commonly in females than in males. Histologically, more mature fibrous tissue is found in the wall. Again, this is a benign tumor. Unfortunately, not all cystic localized lesions of the kidney fall into such a straightforward classification (Cho et al., 1979). Joshi (1979) and Joshi and Beckwith (1989) defined another entity in the spectrum of these cyst tumors—the cystic, partially differentiated nephroblastoma (CPDN)—in which typical elements of Wilms' tumor are seen in the septae. Here, a simple nephrectomy, but not a partial one, appears curative. Because of such cases, it is wise to have a frozen-section analysis before deciding to carry out a partial nephrectomy.

CONGENITAL MESOBLASTIC NEPHROMA. The patient with this renal tumor typically presents in early infancy before the age peak for classic Wilms' tumor (Howell et al., 1982). A frequent association with polyhydramnios has been reported (Blank et al., 1978). A male predominance has been noted. Grossly, this is a massive, firm tumor, which on cut surface demonstrates interlacing bundles of whitish tissue grossly resembling a leiomyoma (see Fig. 54–4). Microscopically, the tumor consists of sheets of spindle-shaped uniform cells (Bolande, 1973, 1974), and ultramicroscopically, the cells appear to be fibroblasts or myofibroblasts (Wockel et al., 1979). The margin of the tumor tends to show local infiltration rather than the pseudocapsule of classic Wilms' tumor. Cartilaginous tissue may appear at the tumor margin, a characteristic suggesting dysplasia.

When completely excised, classic congenital mesoblastic nephroma (CMN) has a uniformly benign course

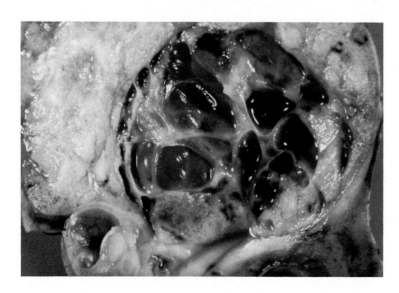

Figure 54–7. Wilms' tumor containing a multilocular cyst that demonstrates a typical characteristic series of adjacent cysts with an overall round configuration.

(Snyder et al., 1981). Greater morbidity has arisen from the treatment of small infants with radiation therapy and chemotherapy than from the tumor itself in the belief that CMN was a true Wilms' tumor. Wigger (1969) argued that this tumor is a hamartoma and not a form of Wilms' tumor.

Occasionally, a "cellular variant" of CMN is seen. This tumor has a higher mitotic index and a more sarcomatous appearance. The distinction between this variant and clear cell sarcoma of the kidney may be difficult. Indeed, the age and sex incidence, spindle morphology, prominent vascularity, and trapping of mature renal elements may suggest that the clear cell sarcoma is the malignant counterpart of the normally benign classic CMN (Hartman, 1981).

RHABDOMYOSARCOMA TUMOR. This is a rare but favorable Wilms' tumor variant characterized by the presence of fetal striated muscle. It should not be confused with unfavorable rhabdoid tumor, which does not contain muscle (Harms et al., 1980).

When any high grade of differentiation is recognized in pediatric renal tumors, it tends to impart a better patient prognosis in the various lesions that are grouped together under the term "nephroblastoma."

Nephrogenic Rests, Nephroblastomatosis, and Relation to Wilms' Tumor

In the 1970s, our understanding of the pathogenesis of Wilms' tumor improved considerably with the description of what was then called the nephroblastomatosis complex of lesions (Bove and McAdams, 1976; Machin, 1980a and b). This complex of pathologic entities has been reexamined by Beckwith and co-workers (1990). A new classification and terminology has been suggested, which has the potential to simplify what was previously quite a confusing topic. As an embryonic tumor, Wilms' tumor has a rather late presentation at 3 years, suggesting it is not a truly congenital tumor. It has been speculated that lesions that are precursors of Wilms' tumor are present, which may undergo a second "hit" in the two-step process of oncologic induction (Knudson and Strong, 1972). It was postulated that these previously noted pathologic entities representing the persistence of nephrogenic elements beyond the end of nephrogenesis at 36 weeks might be such a carrier state, permitting the persistence into childhood of embryologic tissue capable of completing evolution into Wilms' tumor.

Such potential embryologic precursors for Wilms' tumor have been found in approximately 1 per cent of infant postmortem examinations (Bennington and Beckwith, 1975). Such lesions have been found in 30 to 44 per cent of kidneys removed for Wilms' tumor (Bove and McAdams, 1976).

Beckwith's recommendation is to define a *nephrogenic rest* as a focus of abnormally persistent nephrogenic cells, which retains cells that can be induced to form a Wilms' tumor. *Nephroblastomatosis* is defined as the diffuse or multifocal presence of nephrogenic rests or their recognized derivatives. The term also is applied to cases in which the prior presence of rests can be inferred (i.e., multicentric or bilateral cases of Wilms' tumor). The major categorization of nephrogenic rests is into *intralobar* (ILNR) and *perilobar* nephrogenic rests (PLNR). This categorization stresses the relationship between renal lobar topography and the chronology of renal development.

The medullary pyramid is the earliest portion of the renal lobe to form. The juxtamedullary nephrons are, thus, the oldest, and the ones nearest the lobar surface are the youngest. Theoretically, by seeing the location of a nephrogenic rest, one might obtain an important clue as to the timing of the teratogenic event that led to its formation. Events occurring late in fetal life would be at the lobar periphery. This would include lesions along the columns of Bertin within the kidney, which are at the periphery. Earlier events would be manifest deeper in the cortex or medullary areas. A very early disturbance could produce a total disruption of lobar organization.

The intralobar position of ILNRs implies an earlier developmental event leading to their creation than would be postulated for PLNRs. The two categories are not absolute and overlapping cases are probable. A number of morphologic differences are found between PLNRs and ILNRs (Table 54–1).

The patterns of nephrogenic rest distribution can be unifocal, multifocal, and diffuse. The diffuse patterns are what have been previously referred to as nephroblastomatosis. In an effort to help clarify the fate of nephrogenic rests, Beckwith and associates (1990) suggested a subclassification of PLNRs and ILNRs (Table 54–2). Most commonly, rests undergo retrogressive changes with time (sclerosing, regressing, and obsolescent nephrogenic rests). Those rests that do not involute may show progressive changes in two patterns: (1) growth of the rest as a whole (hyperplastic nephrogenic rests) and (2) localized cell proliferation within the rest (neoplastic

Table 54–1. MORPHOLOGIC DIFFERENCES BETWEEN PLNRs AND ILNRs

Feature	PLNRs	ILNRs
Position in lobe	Peripheral	Random
Rest margin	Well-defined, usually smooth	Irregular, often indistinct
Composition	Blastemal predominant in early lesions; epithelial and sclerosing changes in older lesions	Stroma usually predominant; blastemal and epithelial cells usually present
Distribution	Usually numerous, sometimes diffuse at lobar periphery	Usually single, rarely numerous

Abbreviations: ILNR, intralobar nephrogenic rest; PLNR, perilobar nephrogenic rest.

Table 54–2. SUBCLASSIFICATION OF NEPHROGENIC RESTS*

Rest Subtype	Description
I. Nascent or dormant rests	Microscopic size; composed of blastemal or other embryonal cell types
II. Maturing, sclerosing, and obsolescent rests	Few or no blastemal cells; differentiating epithelial or stromal cells in maturing rests; stromal hyalinization in sclerosing and obsolescent rests
III. Hyperplastic rests	Grossly visible lesions of same shape as original dormant rests; blastemal or embryonal cells during growth phase, but sclerosing hyperplastic rests are often observed.
IV. Neoplastic rests	Any of the above three rest types containing one or more spherical, expanding nodular lesions; compressed remnants of rest around the nodules
A. Adenomatous rests	Neoplastic nodules contain only well-differentiated cells, with few to absent mitoses.
B. Nephroblastomatous rests	Neoplastic nodules of any size are composed of crowded embryonal cells identical to Wilms' tumors; mitoses numerous.

*Applies to perilobar and intralobar nephrogenic rests.
Data from Beckwith, J. B., Kiviat, N. B., and Bonadio, J. F.: Nephrogenic rests, nephroblastomatosis, and the pathogenesis of Wilms' tumor. Pediatr. Pathol. 10(1–2):1–36, 1990.

nephrogenic rests). This last category of neoplastic neph-rogenic rests may be either benign appearing (adenom-atous) or early Wilms' tumors, and both types may coexist. Several of these different subclassifications may occur in the same rest.

As the incidence of nephrogenic rests on routine autopsies is about 100 times the incidence of clinical Wilms' tumor, it is evident that most rests do involute without tumor formation. In Beckwith's reviews, most of the rests were PLNRs—ILNRs are rare. Interestingly, the Wilms' tumors that arise in association with ILNRs appear in a younger age group (Breslow et al., 1988). The Wilms' tumors associated with PLNRs exhibit purely blastemal or epithelial cells with scanty stroma and only rare heterogeneous elements, such as muscle. In contrast, Wilms' tumors arising in association with ILNRs have more variation and exhibit more stroma. They may replicate early nephrogenesis. More hetero-genic cell types, such as muscle, are seen.

Beckwith and co-workers (1990) report a 22 per cent incidence of ILNRs with Wilms' tumor, a 17 per cent incidence of PLNRs, and a 3 per cent incidence of both types of nephrogenic rests, giving a total incidence of 41 per cent of Wilms' tumors in association with neph-rogenic rests. In bilateral synchronous Wilms' tumors, there is almost a 100 per cent incidence of nephrogenic rests with the incidence of PLNRs being twice that of ILNRs. Both types exist together in six per cent of cases. When an ILNR is seen in association with a unilateral Wilms' tumor, there appears to be an in-creased risk for a later metachronous contralateral Wilms' tumor. The implications are that ILNRs are less often multifocal; but, as stated earlier, such rests may have a greater likelihood than PLNRs to undergo trans-formation into a Wilms' tumor.

The association of nephrogenic rests with Wilms' tumor syndromes is interesting. In the WAGR syn-drome, one sees that aniridia and the 11p13 deletion are associated with a high incidence of ILNRs. A younger age at presentation is characteristic. In the Drash syndrome, again, ILNRs are commonly seen. In contrast, in hemihypertrophy and in the Beckwith-Wie-demann syndrome, there is prevalence of PLNRs; how-ever, there is a moderate frequency of ILNRs, which may coexist, producing combined nephroblastomatosis.

The mean age for presentation of patients with this group of Wilms' tumors is similar to that for the overall incidence of the tumor.

A number of important clinical implications can be drawn from experience with nephrogenic rests. One of the most important is that the microscopic appearances of Wilms' tumor and nephrogenic rests can be indistin-guishable. Accordingly, the growth characteristics of the lesion as manifested on serially repeated imaging studies may be more important in revealing the biologic nature of the lesion than its histology. Indeed, because of this feature, repeated imaging with computed tomographic (CT) scans, ultrasound, or, perhaps, magnetic resonance may provide more clinically useful information than a second-look procedure and biopsy.

Further emphasis on the importance of imaging lies in the fact that ILNRs may occur deep in the paren-chyma, as can PLNRs in association with the column of Bertin. Because most of these precursor nephrogenic rests do not seem to be headed for the development of a frank Wilms' tumor, their routine removal need not be advocated. However, careful imaging to detect growth of a tumor, which might indicate the need for early intervention, is required for this approach. When nephrogenic rests are bilateral or multiple, the key is to preserve nephrons. Because chemotherapy tends to obliterate only proliferating cells, nephrogenic rests with a malignant potential may well be the ones most likely to be affected. The more benign ones, such as sclerosing rests and those with extensively differentiated elements, may not disappear after chemotherapy. Accordingly, serial imaging is important in planning appropriate in-tervention and in avoiding the unnecessary removal of benign rests.

Wilms' Tumor Presentation

Discovery of an abdominal mass and increasing ab-dominal girth are the most frequent presenting signs leading to the diagnosis of Wilms' tumor. They are seen in more than three quarters of cases. Usually, the child is well without a history of worrisome symptoms. About one third of patients present with abdominal pain. This pain may range from vague, poorly localized discomfort to acute flank pain reflecting hemorrhage into the tumor. A history of acute onset of pain with fever, abdominal mass, anemia, and hypertension suggests Wilms' tumor with sudden subcapsular hemorrhage (Ramsey et al., 1977). Rarely, a child may present with the signs of an acute abdomen secondary to intraperitoneal rupture of the tumor (Thompson et al., 1973). Although gross hematuria is uncommon, microscopic blood may be found in up to 25 per cent of cases. A history of minor renal trauma is often elicited.

On physical examination, a firm, nontender, smooth, unilateral abdominal mass is most common. Very large tumors may cross the midline, but most do not. This finding is in contradistinction to neuroblastoma, which often appears with a more nodular irregular tumor growing across the midline. The child with neuroblastoma also usually looks sick.

Hypertension may be found in Wilms' tumor patients if the blood pressure is carefully checked—a practice not common in the past. The incidence of hypertension has been reported from 25 per cent to as high as 63 per cent. Hypertension may result from compression of normal renal tissue (renal ischemia) or from direct production of renin by the tumor itself (Ganguly et al., 1973; Marosvari et al., 1972).

Rare cases of Wilms' tumor associated with polycythemia secondary to erythropoietin production by the tumor have been reported (Shalet et al., 1967). Occasionally, a patient with Wilms' tumor is found to have an associated nephrotic syndrome leading to the term "Wilms' nephritis." This may be a chance association because neither problem is rare; however, it has been proposed that both conditions may result from a common embryologic renal misadventure and, thus, the relationship may not be due to chance alone (Drash et al., 1970).

Even more rare presentations of Wilms' tumor have included varicocele, hernia, enlarged testis, congestive failure from propagation of tumor into the heart or from intrarenal arteriovenous fistula, hypoglycemia, Cushing's syndrome, hydrocephalus from a brain metastasis, and acute renal failure (Sanyal et al., 1976). Occasionally, pulmonary metastases may lead to an initial presentation with cough, pleural effusion, or pleural pain.

Differential Diagnosis

The differential diagnosis for Wilms' tumor is the same as that for any abdominal mass (Table 54–3).

Renal tumors can usually be distinguished from nonrenal ones by a combination of intravenous pyelography and ultrasonography. Neuroblastoma may cause diagnostic problems even after these two tests, particularly if the tumor arises intrarenally (Shende et al., 1979); but a bone marrow aspiration with positive results for neuroblastoma cells or an elevation of the urinary catecholamine levels is conclusive. The diagnosis of the other malignant tumors is usually not difficult once the origin of the abdominal mass is identified correctly. Most benign abdominal masses can be distinguished from a Wilms' tumor by intravenous pyelography or ultrasonography. An intrarenal abscess may be confus-

Table 54–3. DIFFERENTIAL DIAGNOSIS FOR WILMS' TUMOR

Malignant Tumors
Renal: renal cell carcinoma
Neuroblastoma
Rhabdomyosarcoma
Hepatoblastoma
Lymphoma, lymphosarcoma

Benign Abdominal Masses
Renal: renal abscess, multicystic dysplastic kidney, hydronephrosis, polycystic kidney, congenital mesoblastic nephroma
Mesenteric cysts
Choledochal cysts
Intestinal duplication cysts
Splenomegaly

ing if signs of sepsis are not prominent (Simonowitz and Reyes, 1976). Splenomegaly is occasionally confused with a left-sided Wilms' tumor.

Age is of importance in the differential diagnosis; in the newborn period, a renal mass is most likely a ureteropelvic junction obstruction or multicystic dysplastic kidney. Infantile polycystic disease usually appears with bilateral nephromegaly. The rare congenital mesoblastic nephroma, found early in life, requires histopathologic examination for accurate diagnosis. In the first NWTS, 5 per cent of the patients were misdiagnosed preoperatively (Ehrlich et al., 1979). The most common errors were a diagnosis of neuroblastoma or renal cystic disease.

Diagnostic Imaging

In spite of the rapid development of ultrasound, CT, and magnetic resonance imaging (MRI), which have assumed dominant roles in the imaging of Wilms' tumor, the conventional intravenous pyelogram continues to be a commonly used study in the diagnosis of this tumor. The characteristic radiographic appearance is deformation and distortion of the calyceal morphology by an intrarenal mass (see Figs. 54–1B and 54–3A). Radiolucent areas may be produced by hemorrhage or necrosis in the tumor. The initial plain film of the abdomen should be examined carefully. Calcification is rarely present but, when found, it has a characteristic peripheral, "egg-shell" pattern resulting from old hemorrhage. If a stippled pattern is found, the diagnosis of neuroblastoma is probable. The intravenous pyelogram also permits an assessment of the kidney opposite the side of the clinical mass. It is important to make certain that a contralateral renal anomaly is not present before removing the tumor. About 10 per cent of Wilms' tumors are bilateral.

Nonvisualization of the affected kidney on the intravenous pyelogram occurs in about 10 per cent of cases (Nakayama et al., 1988). This finding may suggest complete blockage of the urinary outflow tracts (pelvis and/or ureter) or, less commonly, severe obstruction of the renal vein or massive parenchymal replacement by tumor. Ultrasound is particularly valuable in the evaluation of a nonvisualizing kidney.

Modern real-time ultrasonography has eliminated

much of the diagnostic doubt that occasionally surrounded renal masses in the past. Renal agenesis, hydronephrosis, and multicystic kidneys can be rapidly distinguished from Wilms' tumor, which has a characteristic echogenic pattern distinct from that of a number of other infiltrative renal diseases (Hunig and Kinser, 1973). Although Wilms' tumor may be completely solid or predominantly cystic, the tumor characteristically exhibits a heterogeneous echo pattern, reflecting necrosis and hemorrhage in the tumor, as well as the varied tissues that may be present (Jaffe et al., 1981). Another benefit of ultrasound is that, when used to follow a Wilms' tumor in a patient receiving chemotherapy, the appearance of new anechoic areas may indicate a response even when the overall size of the tumor does not change (Shimizu et al., 1987).

Ultrasound also permits an assessment of the renal vein and inferior vena cava for intraluminal tumor (see Fig. 54–3*B, C*) (Green et al., 1979). When a tumor thrombus is identified in the cava, extension into the right atrium can be determined. Given the increased morbidity associated with resecting a tumor of this extent through a thorocoabdominal approach, preoperative chemotherapy is increasingly being elected. Retroperitoneal nodes and possible liver metastases may be ascertained. By observing movement of the tumor in relation to the liver during breathing, it may be possible to determine if there is direct involvement of the liver. Assessment of the contralateral kidney may detect small tumors missed by intravenous pyelography and may show a pattern suggestive of nephroblastomatosis. This is of importance in directing attention to specific areas of the opposite kidney for biopsy. In the majority of cases, ultrasonography and intravenous pyelography will establish the diagnosis and extent of disease accurately and obviate the need for other time-consuming and costly examinations.

MRI has assumed an increasing role in the evaluation of abdominal masses in children and is becoming increasingly important in the imaging of Wilms' tumor (Belt et al., 1986; Hricak et al., 1988). The extent and size of tumor is accurately assessed by MRI. The signal intensity of the tumor is variable in most cases. On T1-weighted pulse sequences, areas of hemorrhage show increased signal intensity, whereas areas of necrosis show a decreased signal. Both areas show increased signal intensity on T2-weighted pulse sequences. Unfortunately, MRI is not able to differentiate Wilms' tumor from other renal tumors by relaxation times. On postoperative follow-up, MRI studies may be the most cost-effective single imaging technique.

Arteriography, which carries a significant morbidity in childhood, is recommended by the NWTS only in cases for which (1) the mass is not clearly intrarenal; (2) the mass is so small that it cannot be assessed by other modalities; (3) the tumors are suspected to be bilateral, especially if heminephrectomy is being considered; and (4) the nonvisualization of the kidney is present and cannot be adequately assessed by other means. In practice, angiography is rarely needed. Inferior vena cavography to evaluate renal vein or caval involvement is subject to false-positive studies caused by blood shunting from the Valsalva effect during crying. The opaque column is forced into the paravertebral plexus of veins, suggesting inferior vena caval obstruction. Ultrasound is the more reliable study.

CT provides precise anatomic delineation of renal and retroperitoneal anatomy, but it requires a general anesthetic in the small child and is usually not necessary in Wilms' tumor. This study may have a greater role in the evaluation of neuroblastoma. Renal scans are usually needed only in the evaluation of a possible renal pseudotumor. In this situation a ^{99m}Tc–dimercaptosuccinic acid (DMSA) or glucoheptonate renal scan is useful (Katz and Landau, 1979). A renal pseudotumor exhibits normal function, whereas a Wilms' tumor is cold.

A retrograde ureteropyelogram is rarely needed today. It is indicated in the presence of hematuria, especially when the kidney is not visualized by intravenous pyelography. Ureteral metastases from calyceal invasion (Stevens and Eckstein, 1976) and direct ureteral invasion by Wilms' tumor have occasionally been reported and are important to diagnose, to permit an en bloc resection.

Evaluation for metastatic disease in children with Wilms' tumor routinely involves careful imaging of the chest because the lungs are the most frequent sites for metastases. At the Children's Hospital of Philadelphia, we obtain chest radiographs in frontal, lateral, and both oblique views. CT scan may be helpful to evaluate suspicious-looking areas.

Other imaging studies are generally not carried out until the pathology has been examined. If a rhabdoid tumor is found, imaging of the brain by radionuclear scan or CT is indicated because of the high incidence of central nervous system (CNS) involvement with either metastases or second independent brain tumors. The finding of a clear cell sarcoma should lead to a skeletal survey or radionuclide bone scan because of the high incidence of bony metastases with this tumor. These studies are complementary (Feusner et al., 1990).

Laboratory Studies

Standard laboratory evaluations of a child with a retroperitoneal mass include a complete blood count and urinalysis. To help rule out neuroblastoma in questionable cases, the LaBrosse spot test for urinary catecholamines is of assistance (Evans et al., 1971). Bone marrow aspiration and biopsy usually are not carried out unless the diagnosis of neuroblastoma is suspected. Wilms' tumor rarely infiltrates the marrow in the absence of bone metastases, if then. A blood urea nitrogen (BUN) and serum creatinine level, as well as liver enzymes, are usually determined to provide baseline comparisons. Although formal creatinine clearances are seldom needed before surgery, they may be useful to assess renal function following treatment. Glomerular filtration rate calculations by nuclear medicine techniques can provide similar follow-up information.

Surgical Treatment

Until the introduction of radiotherapy, increased survival in patients with Wilms' tumor experienced in this century correlated with improved surgical and anesthetic techniques. The hallmark of success with Wilms' tumor continues to be the complete removal of the tumor. Although surgery is no longer regarded as the emergency it once was, exploration of the abdomen should be undertaken as soon as the child can be completely evaluated diagnostically and his or her condition stabilized appropriately.

We usually position the child with rolls beneath the back to hyperextend the back with the involved side elevated approximately 30 degrees. A very generous incision is made from below the tip of the 12th rib on the involved side to the lateral margin of the opposite rectus muscle. This incision generally affords excellent exposure and, today, we rarely find a need to resort to the thoracoabdominal approach. The extent of the tumor is first evaluated. The liver should be inspected and palpated, as well as the para-aortic and hilar lymph nodes and cava. Although node assessment can be frustratingly inaccurate at surgery, the presence of large node masses should certainly lead to biopsy (Othersen et al., 1990).

Exploration of the contralateral kidney should be carried out before beginning efforts to remove the tumor. The colon is reflected and Gerotas's capsule is entered with mobilization of the uninvolved kidney that is adequate to permit a careful palpation and visual study of its entire surface. The presence of nephrogenic rests may be suggested by an abnormal-looking cleft or discoloration on the surface of the kidney. In spite of the better ability of newer diagnostic imaging techniques, it continues to be the responsibility of the surgeon to adequately visualize both surfaces of the contralateral kidney. Biopsy should be done for any suspicious-looking lesion.

The resectability of the tumor must then be determined. It is not unusual for Wilms' tumor to invade through the renal capsule and to be adherent to or invade adjacent organs, such as the adrenal, duodenum, liver, pancreas, spleen, diaphragm, colon, or muscles of the abdominal wall. Although it may be appropriate to do a limited resection of these involved organs to permit primary extirpation of the tumor, a heroic initial undertaking is not justified. Pretreatment with chemotherapy with or without radiation therapy will shrink the size of a tumor and allow its removal.

The approach to the tumor begins with the reflection of the colon on the involved side. If the mesocolon appears to be adherent, it may be left with the tumor, because the bowel will generally be adequately vascularized through the marginal vessel (Williams and Martin, 1982). When approaching a large left-sided tumor, it may be helpful to reflect the cecum and the base of the mesentery to permit exposure of the infrarenal vena cava. This maneuver quickly may permit exposure of the left renal vein and artery, which can thus be ligated from a right-sided approach (Todani et al., 1976). We usually begin the tumor mobilization by establishing a plane of dissection against the posterior abdominal wall inferiorly and along the great vessels medially. The ureter is divided early, below the level of the iliac vessels and along with the gonadal vessels. The advantage of establishing these planes of dissection is that they are as far away from the tumor as possible, thus helping to avoid rupture of the tumor. The dissection along the great vessels leads to the early identification of the renal vessels.

It is appropriate to the basic principles of cancer surgery to always try to ligate the renal artery and vein before mobilization of the tumor to avoid hematogenous spread. With renal tumors, division of the renal artery before the vein has been advocated to avoid venous engorgement of the tumor. Although we do try to adhere to this principle, we have not hesitated to divide the renal vein first when exposure of the artery was difficult. We have not been impressed that this approach has materially affected the tumor or the difficulty of the operation.

Major efforts should be made to avoid tumor rupture and spillage of viable cells into the peritoneal cavity. This event has been shown to be associated with an increased incidence of relapse in the abdomen (Breslow et al., 1985; Cassady et al., 1973). Occasionally, there will be a limited rupture, which can be contained by the judicious application of surgical sponges or suction. Keeping the tumor from diffusely spilling may avoid the need for total abdominal irradiation.

The adrenal gland is taken with the tumor if it involves the upper pole. However, the adrenal gland may be spared when the upper pole of a kidney is normal.

It is important to establish by careful palpation whether the renal vein and cava contain tumor, because renal vein ligation when a tumor thrombus is present may lead to the separation of a tumor embolus (Shurin et al., 1982). Engorged retroperitoneal venous collaterals indicate obstruction of the renal vein. Surgical management requires cross-clamping of the cava above the neoplastic plug and opening of the renal vein and cava, if necessary, to extract the thrombus. The tumor is usually free and may be extracted with surprising ease. If a right-sided mass has grown into the wall of the cava, the vessel can be resected up to the level of the hepatic veins. The left kidney has adequate venous collaterals through gonadal and adrenal veins to survive caval resection (Duckett et al, 1973). Preliminary chemotherapy is advocated for major caval involvement, especially if the tumor extends to the atrium, in order to avoid the morbidity of a major vascular procedure and/or cardiopulmonary bypass (Nakayama et al., 1986; Ritchey et al., 1988). The preoperative embolization of Wilms' tumor to facilitate removal has been reported (Danis et al., 1979); however, we have not found this procedure necessary.

Although some have advocated a formal radical lymph node dissection for Wilms' tumor (Martin and Reyes, 1969), no improvement in survival was achieved by radical dissection when the nodes were positive (Jereb et al., 1980). With Wilms' tumor, there are often enlarged hilar or para-aortic nodes, which are reactive and do not contain tumor. Nonetheless, biopsies of these nodes should always be performed, and the site of large masses of matted nodes marked with metal clips. The presence of positive nodes has important prognostic implications. When tumor excision has been incomplete, it is advisable to utilize a limited number of metal clips to mark the extent of tumor. This approach assists the radiation specialist in designing the treatment. Many clips are inadvisable because they interfere with CT scanning of the area postoperatively if it becomes necessary.

When a tumor seems unresectable, consideration should be given to pretreatment with chemotherapy, radiation therapy, or both, with a subsequent surgical attempt at tumor removal. This approach to pretreatment has become popular in Europe and is being considered more often in the United States, primarily to lower intraoperative morbidity (Keating and D'Angio, 1988). Radiation therapy, as well as actinomycin D and vincristine, has been shown to produce good preoperative shrinkage of tumors (Bracken et al., 1982; Lemerle et al., 1976, 1983; Waggert and Koop, 1970). The NWTS has shown that, in the United States, preoperative diagnostic error is on the order of 5 per cent. Because of this rate of error and concerns that treatment might change the pathologic findings, making it more difficult to ascertain the need for subsequent treatment, pretreatment before surgical exploration of a tumor has not been popular (D'Angio, 1983). No evidence indicates that pretreatment with radiotherapy (Lemerle et al., 1976) or chemotherapy (D'Angio et al., 1976; Lemerle et al., 1983) influences long-term survival. However, the incidence of surgical rupture of the tumor has been shown by SIOP to be decreased by preoperative radiation or chemotherapy (Lemerle et al., 1976 and 1983). SIOP data have also shown that preoperative actinomycin D and vincristine produce results at least as good as those for preoperative radiotherapy (Lemerle et al., 1983).

Staging

A number of different staging systems have been advocated for Wilms' tumor, notably that of Garcia as modified by others (Cassady et al., 1973). The clinical-pathologic staging system created by the NWTS has been the one most widely adopted (Table 54–4).

One problem that emerged from NWTS-I and NWTS-II was that there was not adequate discrimination between groups II and III. In NWTS-II, the 2-year relapse-free survival rates for patients in groups II and III were 80 per cent and 72 per cent, with survival rates of 86 per cent and 84 per cent, respectively. Lymph node involvement was associated with a poor prognosis (Jereb and Eklund, 1973). The previous NWTS grouping system was therefore changed to the current staging system. All patients with positive lymph nodes were assigned to stage III. Analyses based on NWTS-II experience showed relapse-free survival rates for NWTS-II patients of 85 per cent and 69 per cent for stages II and III, and survival rates of 94 per cent and 79 per cent, respectively. Better discrimination between these two forms of localized but extensive disease promises to be useful.

Results and Conclusions from National Wilms' Tumor Studies I–III

NWTS-I, which ran from 1969 to 1974, began the opening of new vistas for the treatment of this common tumor. The adverse prognostic effect of anaplasia was clear. It was shown that there was no advantage to routine radiotherapy for stage I tumors in patients younger than 2 years if actinomycin D were given for 15 months. Vincristine and actinomycin D together were better than either drug alone. The treatment of stage IV patients with preoperative vincristine confirmed no advantage in those treated postoperatively with radiation therapy, actinomycin D, and vincristine.

Delays of greater than 10 days in starting radiation therapy had a deleterious effect on outcome. In patients who underwent tumor biopsy or who had local spillage, whole abdomen irradiation was not demonstrated to confer any advantage over localized flank irradiation. Thus, it was realized that a confined spill of tumor or tumor biopsy was not an indication to upstage the tumor. When the tumor was completely excised, the extension of Wilms' tumor into the renal vein or local direct

---

Table 54–4. NATIONAL WILMS' TUMOR STAGING SYSTEM*

Stage I:	Tumor limited to kidney and completely excised. The surface of the renal capsule is intact. Tumor was not ruptured before or during removal. There is no residual tumor apparent beyond the margins of resection.
Stage II:	Tumor extends beyond the kidney but is completely removed. There is regional extension of the tumor, i.e., penetration through the outer surface of the renal capsule into perirenal soft tissues. Vessels outside the kidney substance are infiltrated or contain tumor thrombus. The tumor may have undergone biopsy or there has been local spillage of tumor confined to the flank. There is no residual tumor apparent at or beyond the margins of excision.
Stage III:	Residual nonhematogenous tumor confined to abdomen. Any one or more of the following occur: a. Lymph nodes on biopsy are found to be involved in the hilus, the periaortic chains, or beyond. b. There has been diffuse peritoneal contamination by tumor, such as by spillage of tumor beyond the flank before or during surgery, or by tumor growth that has penetrated through the peritoneal surface. c. Implants are found on the peritoneal surfaces. d. The tumor extends beyond the surgical margins either microscopically or grossly. e. The tumor is not completely resectable because of local infiltration into vital structures.
Stage IV:	Hematogenous metastases. Deposits beyond stage III, e.g., lung, liver, bone, and brain.
Stage V:	Bilateral renal involvement at diagnosis. An attempt should be made to stage each side according to the above criteria on the basis of extent of disease before biopsy.

*Staging, which is on the basis of gross and microscopic tumor distribution, is the same for tumors with favorable and with unfavorable histologic features. The patient should be characterized, however, by a statement of both criteria, e.g., stage II, favorable histologic features or stage III, unfavorable histologic features. Tumors of unfavorable type are those with focal or diffuse anaplasia, or those with sarcomatous histology (D'Angio et al., 1989).

Data from D'Angio, G. J., Breslow, W., Beckwith, J.B., Evans, A., et al.: Treatment of Wilms' tumor: Results of the Third National Wilms' Tumor Study. Cancer, 64:349–360, 1989.

extension beyond the kidney itself posed no adverse effect on outcome (D'Angio et al., 1976a, 1978, 1980).

NWTS-II was conducted from 1974 to 1979 and was more revealing. For stage I tumors, 6 months of actinomycin D and vincristine were shown to be as effective as 15 months of therapy (D'Angio et al., 1981). Stage II, III, and IV tumors did better when doxorubicin was added to actinomycin D and vincristine. With improvements in chemotherapy, age over 2 years or tumor size more than 250 g no longer appeared to be important prognostic variables. An adverse effect was shown from the presence of local nodal disease in the abdomen (Breslow et al., 1985; Thomas et al., 1984).

NWTS-III was conducted from 1979 to 1985 and provided further important information. In patients with stage II tumors, radiotherapy conferred no additional benefit. In patients with stage III tumors, 1000 cGy provided as good an outcome as 2000 cGy. In patients with stage II and III tumors, no benefit was obtained from adding doxorubicin to vincristine and actinomycin D. Patients with stage I favorable histology tumors appeared to do as well with vincristine and actinomycin D for 10 weeks as for 6 months. However, subset analysis showed a slight benefit for the 6-month course, providing the rationale for this standard for NWTS-IV.

For patients with stage I anaplastic tumors, it was recognized that they did as well as their stage I favorable histology counterparts and, thus, did not require more intensive treatment. Unfortunately, cyclophosphamide showed only a marginal improvement in high-risk patients and will be continued to be studied in NWTS-IV. Clear cell sarcoma was recognized to be responsive to doxorubicin, and patients responded almost as well at 2 years with three-drug therapy as those with comparative stages of favorable histology Wilms' tumor. Four-year rates were not as good, however. Rhabdoid sarcoma continued to be an enigma with no therapeutic regimens improving its dismal outcome. The current survival data for NWTS-III are given in Table 54–5 (D'Angio et al., 1989).

Prognostic Factors

From all the knowledge gained from the first three NWTS, four important prognostic aspects of the tumor have emerged. Most important has been *histology*. An-

Table 54–5. RESULTS OF THE NATIONAL WILMS' TUMOR STUDY III

Stage	Histology	4-Year Postnephrectomy Survival (%)
I	Favorable	97
II	Favorable	92
III	Favorable	84
IV	Favorable	83
I–III	Unfavorable	68
IV	Unfavorable	55
All patients	Unfavorable	89
Clear cell sarcoma		75
Rhabdoid sarcoma		26

Adapted from D'Angio, G. J., et al.: Cancer, 64:349–360, 1989.

aplasia is characterized by the presence of mitotic figures, a threefold enlargement in the nuclei, and a hyperchromatic pattern. Flow cytometry may now be enabling us to identify these cases more simply (Rainwater et al., 1987). Anaplasia increases with age (Bonadio et al., 1985). Patients with anaplasia make up approximately 5 per cent of all Wilms' tumor cases. In this group, the relapse rate is four times higher and the death rate nine times greater than when anaplasia is absent (Zuppan et al., 1988).

The second unfavorable prognostic determinant is the presence of *hematogenous metastases,* whether they involve the lung (most common), liver, bone, or brain. Aggressive chemotherapy has improved the patient's prognosis in this group dramatically.

The third prognostic factor is the presence of *lymph node involvement.* In NWTS-III, patients with positive lymph nodes were placed in stage III because it was recognized from NWTS-II that there was an 82 per cent overall survival for those with negative nodes versus a 54 per cent survival for those with positive nodes. This fact emphasizes the importance of careful node sampling to accurately stage Wilms' tumor.

The fourth prognostic area relates to *tumor extension at the site of the primary tumor* (Weeks et al., 1987). The presence of an inflammatory pseudocapsule or invasion of the tumor into the capsule or the intrarenal veins was associated with an increased risk of local relapse. The tumor tends to spread into the renal sinus initially, and tumor in this area has also been associated with increased local relapse. One or more of these features were seen in 100 per cent of relapsed stage I favorable histology Wilms' tumors.

By careful study of NWTS-II and NWTS-III, a subgroup of patients with relapsed tumors was identified in which the postrelapse survival for 3 years exceeded 40 per cent and thus constituted a favorable group (Grundy et al., 1989). The five favorable characteristics in this patient group were as follows: (1) favorable histology tumors that recurred only in the lung, (2) local relapse in the abdomen when radiation therapy had not been previously given, (3) originally stage I tumors, (4) tumors originally treated with only two drugs, and (5) tumors that recurred 12 or more months after diagnosis. The recognition of this subgroup permitted salvage with aggressive conventional therapy. Those without these favorable characteristics needed a more aggressive approach to therapy based on experimental protocols.

With the addition of doxorubicin, clear cell sarcoma of the kidney no longer has an unfavorable prognosis. Unfortunately, for patients with renal rhabdoid sarcoma, the prognosis continues to be grim.

National Wilms' Tumor Study IV

The goals of NWTS-IV are to strive to limit therapy for patients with favorable prognoses while improving the outcome for those with unfavorable prognoses (Table 54–6).

Stage I favorable histology tumors or stage I anaplastic tumors should receive no radiation therapy or cyclo-

Table 54–6. NATIONAL WILMS' TUMOR STUDY IV: PROCEDURES AND STUDY DESIGN AT A GLANCE

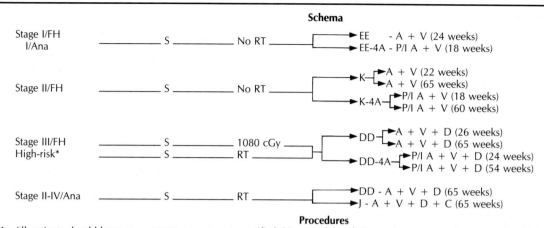

Procedures

1. All patients should have an excretory urogram or opacified CT scan of the abdomen for accurate placement of radiation therapy portals.
2. The initial randomization to standard or pulsed, intensive chemotherapy *need not await final determination of stage or histology* because the initial randomization is the same for virtually all patients.† Randomization is to take place within 72 hours of nephrectomy; *which will be considered day zero,* but not later than 5 calendar days thereafter. If a patient must be randomized during the weekend or on a holiday to remain eligible, the Data and Statistical Center (DSC) should be called ahead of time and special arrangements will be made.

*High risk = clear cell sarcoma of kidney (CCSK) (all stages) and stage IV/FH. CCSK patients receive RT (1080 cGy), and stage IV/FH patients receive RT (1080 cGy) if the primary tumor would qualify as stage III were there no metastases.
†Re-randomization will be offered should the tumor qualify later as stage II–IV/Ana.
Abbreviations: S, surgery; A, actinomycin D; D, doxorubicin (Adriamycin); V, vincristine; C, cyclophosphamide; Ana, anaplastic tumors; P/I, pulsed, intensive; FH, favorable histology; RT, radiation therapy.

phosphamide. Six months will continue to be the standard for chemotherapy because of the slight benefit produced. Pulsed, intensive actinomycin D and vincristine are being studied to see if this can increase the convenience of chemotherapy administration without adverse effect on outcome. Liver toxicity has been an initial problem with this approach.

Stage II favorable histology tumors are also treated without radiation therapy or doxorubicin. Again, pulsed, intensive actinomycin D and vincristine are being studied, as well as the overall length of chemotherapy.

For treatment of stage III favorable histology tumors, flank irradiation to only 1000 cGy is used. Doxorubicin is continued as a third drug because it appears to "cover" the lower dose of radiation. The decision to continue this program was made because of the fewer number of abdominal relapses and the hope that a lower radiation dose might lead to less musculoskeletal growth disturbance. Additionally, in spite of chemotherapy with doxorubicin, no increase in cardiac problems has been demonstrated in NWTS patients who have survived 5 or more years (Evans et al., 1991).

For stage IV favorable histology tumors, triple chemotherapy continues to be the standard with pulmonary irradiation to 1200 cGy. The good results in this group are thought to be due to a combination of chemotherapy and radiation therapy, based on a less satisfactory outcome for a similar group treated in Britain with chemotherapy only (Pritchard et al., 1988). For children who have anaplastic tumors, except those with stage I tumors, aggressive chemotherapy with three drugs will be continued, randomizing the addition of cyclophosphamide, which has not yet been conclusively evaluated in this high-risk group. For clear cell sarcoma, three-drug chemotherapy will be continued with the addition of flank radiotherapy to prevent local recurrence. Un-

fortunately, prospects for improved chemotherapy for rhabdoid sarcoma of the kidney appear poor.

Radiation Therapy

Radiation therapy generally is begun 1 to 3 days after surgery. A dose of 2000 cGy is delivered to the flank of all children with unfavorable histology because they have been shown to be at high risk for abdominal relapse (D'Angio et al., 1978). No children with stage I or II tumors of favorable histology are irradiated, nor are those with stage I anaplastic neoplasms. Stage III favorable histology patients are given 1000 cGy to the tumor bed, and to the whole abdomen when there is abdominal dissemination. This approach helps protect against infradiaphragmatic relapses, which have been shown to be associated with poor outcomes (Sutow et al., 1982). Supplemental doses of 500 to 1000 cGy are delivered to regions of residual bulky disease, including portions of the liver if necessary.

Portals similar to those described are given for anaplastic stage II, III, and IV tumors, but higher doses (1200 to 4000 cGy) are given to the tumor bed, modulated according to age. This practice is based on the recognition that growth deformities are more pronounced in the smaller child with the same dose of radiation therapy (Neuhauser et al., 1952).

Chemotherapy

Chemotherapy is usually commenced after surgery once bowel function has been regained. The administration of prolonged courses of chemotherapy in small children has been greatly facilitated by the advent of the Broviac central venous lines, which can be placed

Table 54–7. NWTS IV CHEMOTHERAPEUTIC
DRUG REGIMENS

Actinomycin D
  15 µg/kg/day for 5 consecutive days; repeat at 6 weeks, at 3
  months, and thereafter at 12- to 13-week intervals

Vincristine*
  1.5 mg/m² weekly for 8–10 weeks initially; thereafter, at beginning
  and end of each course of actinomycin D

Doxorubicin
  20 mg/m² per day for 3 days every 12 weeks; beginning 6 weeks
  after the first course of actinomycin D

---

*Vincristine is given more intensively for stage II/FH. (See D'Angio, G. J., et al., 1989 for details.)

and maintained for prolonged periods to facilitate the administration of chemotherapy. The doses and schedule followed for the three most commonly used drugs are outlined in Table 54–7. Patients with stage I favorable histology are treated for 24 weeks. All others are treated for 65 weeks.

Blood counts should be carefully monitored, and it is appropriate to withhold radiation therapy as well as chemotherapy when the total neutrophil count is less than 1000/ml³ and the platelet count less than 75,000/ml³. The recommendation of the NWTS is to reduce the dose of all drugs to one-half standard for a child less than 13 months of age because of increased toxicity in this group.

Inanition may be encountered in children receiving combination chemotherapy, especially when wide-field radiation therapy is also employed. Hyperalimentation by way of an enteral feeding tube or by an intravenous route may permit the completion of a successful course of chemotherapy in this situation (Donaldson et al., 1982).

Doxorubicin is cardiotoxic, especially when combined with cardiac irradiation, and has occasionally resulted in death. Careful monitoring is important, particularly by cardiac echogram, if this drug is administered.

Treatment of Metastatic and Recurrent Tumor

The lungs are the most common location for hematogenous metastases of Wilms' tumor. If pulmonary metastases are present, both lungs should be irradiated, regardless of the number or location of the metastases. A dose of 1200 cGy is appropriate.

The second most common site of metastasis is the liver. Liver scans may show focal defects secondary to irradiation, which can be misinterpreted as metastases. Regenerating liver can produce identical confusion for the therapist. Thus, it is wise to have tissue confirmation before irradiating the liver. A dose of 2000 cGy for favorable histology and 3000 cGY for anaplastic histology to liver metastases is delivered over 2½ to 4 weeks.

If a significant hepatic resection for metastatic disease is undertaken, it must be kept in mind that radiation therapy begun during the period of liver regeneration can abort the process and lead to severe chronic hepatic impairment (Filler et al., 1969). If a significant hepatic resection is part of the initial tumor removal, it is recommended that both actinomycin D and radiation therapy be delayed until liver regeneration is well established, and only vincristine be given during that interval. Cases are documented of patients with both pulmonary and hepatic metastases who have experienced long-term cures by judicious combinations of radiation therapy, chemotherapy, and selective surgery (Smith et al., 1974; Wedemeyer et al., 1968; White and Krivit, 1962). Those patients with liver metastasis at diagnosis do no worse than those with pulmonary metastases (Grundy et al., 1989).

Wilms' tumor can metastasize to such unlikely sites as the salivary glands and tonsils (Movassaghi et al., 1974), but those instances are rare. Sarcomatous clear cell tumors tend to metastasize to bone and brain, and rhabdoid lesions tend to metastasize to the brain. Involvement of those organs by favorable-histology tumor is uncommon. An occasional patient with cerebral metastases will survive after radiation therapy and chemotherapy with or without surgical removal of the tumor (Mohammad et al., 1977; Traggis et al., 1975).

Chemotherapy for metastatic or locally recurrent Wilms' tumor depends on the drugs used before that event. Doxorubicin is the mainstay of treatment for children who have received only actinomycin D and vincristine, and it is added to those two drugs. No well-established regimen can be recommended for those who experience relapse after therapy with actinomycin D, vincristine, and doxorubicin. The addition of cyclophosphamide plus actinomycin D and vincristine was employed by Ortega and associates (1980) to "retrieve" patients who developed metastatic disease while on vincristine and actinomycin D. The regimen utilized vincristine more intensively than as shown in Table 54–7. The UK Medical Research Council has shown that aggressive doses and schedule of vincristine are more effective than the usual doses and schedule. Contrariwise, NWTS-III did not demonstrate any major gain when cyclophosphamide was added to actinomycin D and vincristine for either favorable-histology or unfavorable-histology tumors. Those clinicians wishing to provide these three drugs to children who experience relapse should therefore follow the specific recommendations of Ortega and co-workers (1980). Dimethyltriazeno-imidazole-carboxamide (DTIC) (Cangir et al., 1976) and cis-platinum (Baum and Gaynon, 1981) may also be helpful. Combinations of etoposide and ifosfamide or carboplatinum are also useful (Miser et al., 1987).

Complications of Chemotherapy and Radiation Therapy

Considerable acute and chronic morbidity and, indeed, mortality may result from the treatment of Wilms' tumor (Jaffe et al., 1980; Mathe and Oldham, 1974). The problem is compounded by the potential of actinomycin D and doxorubicin to potentiate the toxicity of radiotherapy. Infants are at particular risk (Siegel and Moran, 1981). Li and colleagues (1975a) reported 14 deaths among 140 patients with Wilms' tumor who survived 36 months after diagnosis. Nine died as a result of treatment-associated problems without evidence of any residual cancer. In the second NWTS, 2 per cent of the children treated died of causes directly attributable to complications of therapy (D'Angio et al., 1981). In a later review of the NWTS, toxicity and infection accounted for 15 per cent of all the deaths among NWTS children usually attributed to more intensive salvage treatments (D'Angio et al., 1989).

Acute hematologic toxicity due to the effects of chemotherapy on bone marrow is very common and well known, and it is not discussed further in this chapter. Acute gastrointestinal toxicity from chemotherapy, in the form of nausea, vomiting, and diarrhea, is common in the postoperative period, especially in patients who are young or who require total abdominal irradiation. A syndrome of delayed radiation enteritis may appear within a couple of months of completion of radiotherapy. Symptoms include the secondary onset of vomiting and diarrhea with a distended abdomen. It has been reported by Donaldson and co-workers (1975) that a diet free of lactose, gluten, and bovine protein along with limited dietary fat and residue may improve the malabsorption that is produced by radiation enteritis. Over a longer course, intestinal obstruction may result from intussusception, fibrosis, or postoperative adhesions (Kuffer et al., 1968).

Hepatic toxicity may be acute, long-term, or both. This complication occurs primarily in children with right-sided tumors in whom the radiation field includes a portion of the right lobe of the liver or in whom the liver is irradiated as part of total abdominal irradiation. In the first NWTS, liver dysfunction was noted in 6 per cent of children who underwent irradiation. Initially, there may be transient hepatic enlargement, abnormal liver function, and thrombocytopenia with hypoproteinemia and ascites (Jayabose and Lanzkowsky, 1976; McVeagh and Eckert, 1975; Samuels et al., 1971). Selective thrombocytopenia may be a particularly prominent aspect of hepatotoxicity. It is probably the result of platelet entrapment from radiation-induced hyperemia with hepatic congestion and secondary portal hypertension, or the result of a consumption coagulopathy in the congested liver (Tefft, 1977). Symptoms of liver toxicity may reappear during subsequent treatment with actinomycin D (Tefft, 1971) or doxorubicin. This complication is being encountered more frequently, even in children not receiving radiation and even after adjustments of drug dosage, for reasons that are not yet clear (Green et al., 1990).

Late orthopedic complications were distressingly frequent, with up to 30 per cent of children who had undergone irradiation sustaining clinically appreciable sequelae (Katzman et al., 1969; Riseborough et al., 1976). Orthopedic changes were most severe when children younger than 2 years of age were treated with high-dose radiation therapy (Neuhauser et al., 1952). Vertebral hypoplasia and scoliosis were produced by the direct effect of radiation therapy despite care taken to treat the entire width of the vertebral bodies. Because, even when spinal irradiation is evenly administered, soft tissue fibrosis in an asymmetric fashion may produce tethering with resulting scoliosis (Evans et al., 1986).

Now far fewer patients are being irradiated, and those given radiation therapy receive much lower doses. The proportion of survivors showing pronounced musculoskeletal changes has dropped dramatically (Evans et al., 1991).

Renal problems may also follow radiation of the kidney. Acute changes occur beginning 1 to 2 months after completion of radiotherapy. Potentiating chemotherapeutic agents make the kidney more susceptible (Tefft, 1977). Acutely, the patient may demonstrate microscopic hematuria, azotemia, and edema. It is also possible for chronic nephritis to develop without acute changes having been manifest. Long-term follow-up has indicated that normal renal function usually results after unilateral nephrectomy and combination chemotherapy/radiotherapy if the opposite kidney is not irradiated with a dose greater than 1200 cGy (Mitus et al., 1969). The long-term follow-up of NWTS has not identified many patients with renal problems after more modern methods of management (Evans et al., 1991).

Pulmonary complications are related to the amount of treated lung, the concomitant chemotherapy, and complicating factors, such as infection (Wara et al., 1973). An acute interstitial radiation pneumonitis may begin 1 to 3 months after radiotherapy. No symptoms or a mild cough and fever may be present. Generally, symptoms resolve in less than a month. The long-term effects of pulmonary radiation therapy in children may be an eventual decrease in both lung and chest wall size (Wohl et al., 1975). Fortunately, today these problems are less common than they once were (Littman et al., 1976). However, in the most recent review of the NWTS experience, 18 (12 per cent) of 153 stage IV patients who received bilateral pulmonary irradiation developed clinical and radiographic signs of pulmonary toxicity. Three patients with *Pneumocystis carinii* pneumonitis survived. Of the remaining 15 patients with interstitial pneumonitis, 11 died (Green et al., 1989).

Myocardial damage may occur with doxorubicin, with or without thoracic radiotherapy. The clinical picture is that of congestive heart failure with cardiomegaly. Fortunately, this complication is rare with the doses employed in the NWTS.

The *ovary* is unfortunately quite sensitive to the effects of radiation therapy. Following whole abdomen radiation, ovarian failure may be noted in the postpubertal period (Scott, 1981). This condition usually manifests with poor development of secondary sexual characteristics and primary amenorrhea. Follicle-stimulating hormone (FSH) and luteinizing hormone (LH) levels are elevated. Hormonal replacement therapy may be required. Of those women with preserved fertility, abdominal orthovoltage radiotherapy may predispose them to low-birthweight infants (Green, 1982). The scatter dose of radiation therapy to the *testis* may be sufficient to produce oligospermia (Shalet and Beardwell, 1979). Drugs, especially cyclophosphamide, may contribute to these effects on the ovary and testis (Shalet, 1982).

Numerous reports describe the occurrence of *secondary neoplasms* in patients treated previously for Wilms' tumor. The exostosis is the most common of the benign tumors. Malignant neoplasms include soft tissue sarcomas, bone tumors, especially osteosarcomas (Tucker et al., 1987), hepatomas, thyroid carcinomas, and leukemias (Li et al., 1975b). Colon cancer has also been reported (Opitz, 1980). Most of these secondary malignancies have developed in fields of prior radiation therapy.

The cumulative probability of a second cancer in long-term survivors of Wilms' tumor who were treated with radiotherapy has been calculated to be 17 per cent over 5 to 25 years with a peak incidence at 15 to 19 years after initial diagnosis (Li et al., 1975b). Mike and colleagues (1982) found a lower incidence of secondary neoplasms (3 per cent) among 20-year survivors of Wilms' tumor. The risk of developing a secondary neoplasm may be decreased in patients who received actinomycin D in addition to radiation therapy (D'Angio et al., 1976b). Lifelong surveillance is nonetheless important for those cured of Wilms' tumor.

Bilateral Wilms' Tumor

In the NWTS, the incidence of synchronous bilateral Wilms' tumor was reported to be approximately 4.2 per cent (Breslow and Beckwith, 1982). Bilateral Wilms' tumors exhibit a number of features distinct from those of unilateral tumors (Table 54–8) (Blute et al., 1987; Bond, 1975a, 1975b).

Mothers of children with bilateral Wilms' tumor tend to be older. The children tend to present at a younger age. A positive family history for cancer was found in 42 per cent with a 21 per cent incidence of genitourinary malignancy. Associated anomalies are more frequent in patients with bilateral Wilms' tumor. The incidence of genitourinary anomalies is four times that for patients with unilateral Wilms' tumor, and hemihypertrophy is twice as common. The incidence of aniridia and hypertension is similar in unilateral and bilateral Wilms' tumor cases.

A pathologic examination with multicentric involvement showing nephrogenic rests was identified in 61 per cent. Beckwith and co-workers (1990) believe this may be an underreporting because samplings from the tumor were restricted, in many cases, at initial biopsy. The fact that many of these children present with very large tumors and do very well in spite of that may be related to the fact that these tumors are often compound neoplasms made up of the confluence of a number of low-stage tumors. Unfavorable histology was seen in 10 per cent (15 patients), an incidence similar to that for unilateral tumors. Of the 15 children, 12 were females, indicating a dominance of anaplasia in girls. Discordant histology between the tumors found in opposite kidneys was seen in six of the 145 bilateral cases presented by Blute and associates (1987). This figure represented 4 per cent of the series as a whole but 40 per cent of the unfavorable histology subset. Of the 15, 11 had stage III or IV disease in the more advanced neoplasm, and ten died during the follow-up.

Beckwith and colleagues (1990) believe that bilateral Wilms' tumors exhibit nephrogenic rests in 100 per cent of cases. In their review, they report a prevalence of PLNRs in synchronous Wilms' tumor. This figure contrasts with the approximately equal prevalence of the two types of rests in unilateral Wilms' tumor cases. Beckwith postulates that PLNRs are more likely to be seen in both kidneys, accounting for this finding. ILNRs are less frequently seen in bilateral cases. When a metachronous bilateral Wilms' tumor is seen, it more characteristically is associated with an ILNR. Beckwith attributes this to the fact that ILNRs may tend to be less often multifocal; however, when this type of rest is present, it has a high incidence of eventually developing into a Wilms' tumor. Metachronous bilateral Wilms' tumors were reported in only 0.6 per cent of NWTS patients (Jones, 1982). However, the prognosis for these patients is poor with only 39 per cent free from disease 2 or more years after developing the second Wilms' tumor.

The overall survival for synchronous bilateral Wilms' tumor is excellent, with a 76 per cent 3-year survival. Bilateral Wilms' tumor clearly responds as well to chemotherapy as do unilateral cases. In the review by Blute and co-workers (1987), several interesting characteristics of this tumor were revealed. Outcome did not appear to be influenced by whether an initial tumor resection or merely a biopsy was carried out. The presence of residual disease did not influence outcome and, indeed, only 38 per cent of the patients had all tumor resected at one or more operations. The outcome was not influenced by whether a nephrectomy was ever carried out. Additionally, survival was not influenced by salvage radiotherapy. This finding suggests that residual disease after more intensive initial chemotherapy does not tend to be responsive to radiation therapy. Aggressive chemotherapy appears to be the mainstay in the care of synchronous bilateral Wilms' tumor.

From analysis of the experience of Blute and associates (1987) and Asch and colleagues (1985), a number of prognostic variables have been revealed to be important. The age at diagnosis is important in children younger than 3 years of age with favorable histology who exhibit an 86 per cent survival, compared with those older than 3 years of age, who exhibit a 57 per cent survival. The majority of young patients presented with stage I disease; older children more commonly presented with advanced stage tumors. Anaplasia was observed infrequently in children younger than 2 years

Table 54–8. FEATURES OF UNILATERAL AND BILATERAL WILMS' TUMOR

	Unilateral	Bilateral
Distribution	Unifocal (usual)	Multifocal (nephroblastomatosis)
Patient age (average)	42 mo	15 mo
Mother's age (average)	28 yr	34 yr
Associated anomalies	4%	45%
Inheritance	sporadic	?dominant

Adapted from Bond, J. V.: Lancet, 2:721, 1975 and Blute, M. L., et al.: J. Urol., 138:968–973, 1987.

of age, also helping to explain this age-related variable. Histology was also pivotal as in unilateral Wilms' tumor. In the NWTS series, 16 per cent with unfavorable histology survived compared with 84 per cent with favorable histology. Stage of the most advanced lesion and histology thus were the most important prognostic variables.

Additionally, positive lymph nodes were important. If lymph node biopsies showed positive results, survival was only 56 per cent compared with a survival of 85 per cent when node biopsies showed negative results. Overall, the survival of more than 75 per cent of NWTS patients with synchronous bilateral Wilms' tumor indicates the favorable prognosis for patients with this tumor. The results in this series are similar to those reported by Bishop and co-workers (1977) (87 per cent) and by Wikstrom and co-workers (1982) (83 per cent).

In surgical management, the importance of initial exploration of the contralateral tumor when disease appears to be unilateral is emphasized by the fact that a preoperative diagnosis of bilateral Wilms' tumor in Blute's series (1987) was only 64 per cent. Thus, more than one third of bilateral cases were detected by a careful inspection of both surfaces of the contralateral kidney. This failure of diagnostic imaging to detect contralateral disease is supported by the radiologic review of Kirks and associates (1981).

In the past, the traditional initial surgical approach to bilateral Wilms' tumor was to carry out a nephrectomy for the larger tumor and to perform a biopsy for the smaller one. This approach has now changed to an official recommendation from the NWTS (Kelalis, 1985) for a renal-sparing approach. The official NWTS surgical recommendation is for an initial transabdominal transperitoneal staging laparotomy without nephrectomy. Careful tumor biopsy and sampling of the nodes are needed. An excisional biopsy is carried out only if two thirds of total renal parenchyma may be spared.

Chemotherapy is undertaken for a period of 6 weeks to a maximum of 6 months following the standard Wilms' tumor chemotherapy protocols based on the stage of the more advanced tumor. At second-look surgery, a partial nephrectomy or excisional biopsy is carried out only if all tumor can be removed. If this appears impossible, then the recommendation is to close and continue with more chemotherapy and the addition of focal radiotherapy.

A third-look operation would then be carried out in less than 6 months, with surgery at this time continuing to be focused on the maximal preservation of renal parenchyma. In patients with stage II or III unfavorable histology at initial biopsy, a more aggressive surgical approach is appropriate. Because of the poor prognosis for these patients, renal-preservative approaches are of secondary importance. After initial biopsy, three-drug chemotherapy and radiation therapy are recommended, followed by a more radical second surgical look. Unfortunately, to date, survival in this group has been poor.

Special techniques, such as bench surgery, have been used in bilateral cases (Altman et al., 1977), and it is important to keep such techniques in mind while making efforts to spare renal parenchyma. Bilateral nephrectomy and renal transplantation may be rarely required in bilateral tumors but may be more appropriate when anaplasia is encountered (deLorimier et al., 1971). If transplantation is contemplated, some investigators advocate a waiting period of 2 years to be certain that no metastatic disease is present (Penn, 1979).

Future Considerations

The history of the treatment of Wilms' tumor has been one of the success stories of pediatric oncology, and the future offers hope for further advances. The experience with bilateral Wilms' tumor suggests that, in the future, surgery focused on the preservation of renal parenchyma may become an important consideration even in children with unilateral disease. The goal of NWTS-IV is to continue the effort to minimize the morbidity of chemotherapy and radiation therapy for patients with a favorable prognosis. Conversely, patients with poor prognostic characteristics are continuing to be treated more intensively with new therapeutic regimens in an effort to salvage more of these difficult cases. Epidemiologic studies are underway to seek possible environmental and genetic causes for Wilms' tumor. The long-term effects of successful therapy on the gonads, lungs, and other treated organs are also being studied with the goal of prevention of some of these problems in the future.

Other Renal Tumors of Childhood

Primary renal neoplasms of childhood other than Wilms' tumor are rare; *renal cell carcinoma* is the most common of them. Although it is the most frequent malignant tumor of the kidney in adults, it accounts for less than 7 per cent of all renal tumors in those younger than 21 years. Most children with renal cell carcinoma are 5 years of age or older at the time of diagnosis, but cases have been reported in patients in the 1st year of life (Castellanos et al., 1974). The signs and symptoms are the same in the adult: hematuria, abdominal or flank pain, an abdominal mass, or nonspecific symptoms, such as weight loss, anorexia, and fever. Intravenous pyelography reveals calyceal deformation resembling Wilms' tumor, but calcifications are more common. The metastatic spread of renal cell carcinoma is to regional lymph nodes, bones, lungs, and liver. Renal vascular invasion or the absence of a pseudocapsule around the tumor are ominous anatomic features (Dehner et al., 1970).

Most renal cell carcinomas in children appear to be sporadic cases, similar to adults, but some families with an increased incidence have been reported. The tumor, in one family with 10 involved members, appeared to be passed as an autosomal dominant trait with a characteristic chromosomal translocation (Cohen et al., 1979). An increased incidence of renal cell carcinoma has also been reported in patients with von Hippel-Lindau disease and polycystic kidney disease (Kantor, 1977).

Reviews of renal cell carcinoma in childhood by Raney and co-workers (1983), Castellanos and co-workers (1974), and Dehner and co-workers (1970) reveal an overall survival rate of about 50 per cent. The outlook seems best in children under 11 years of age, and in those with stage I lesions. All six children under age 11 and all five with stage I lesions survived in the series reported by Raney and colleagues (1983). Radiation therapy, chemotherapy, and hormonal therapy did little, if anything, to improve survival over that produced by nephrectomy alone. At present, the most effective treatment continues to be a radical nephrectomy with regional lymph node dissection.

In 1980, Chatten and associates reported two male infants with what was termed *ossifying tumor of the infantile kidney*. The infants presented with hematuria and were found to have small calcified renal masses, which appeared to be calculi. At histologic examination, dense cores of bone were found surrounded by a periphery of undifferentiated cells that were firmly adherent to the renal parenchyma. These investigators postulate that these tumors were derived from urothelium rather than from metanephric blastema. They also postulated that the tumors were separate benign pediatric renal tumors, distinct from Wilms' tumors.

Additional very rare primary intrarenal tumors are found in children including the following: neuroblastoma, rhabdomyosarcoma, leiomyosarcoma, fibroma, hemangiopericytoma, cholesteatoma, lymphangioma, and hamartoma. The diagnosis of these tumors is rarely made before histologic examination. The renal *angiomyolipoma* is a form of hamartoma usually seen in adulthood but rarely observed in childhood (Bennington and Beckwith, 1975). This tumor is very common in patients with tuberous sclerosis and may be bilateral. Diagnostic and therapeutic measures are similar to those used in adults. Although more commonly found in the pararenal retroperitoneal space, *teratomas* may rarely occur as intrarenal tumors.

By far the most common *secondary tumor* seen in the kidney is involvement produced by non-Hodgkin's lymphoma or leukemia. Tumor involvement is generally diffuse. Unlike the other non-Wilms' renal tumors discussed previously, therapy consists of radiation therapy, chemotherapy, or both.

Although rare, both benign and malignant tumors of the renal pelvis and ureter have also been reported. Ureteral lesions are most commonly benign fibrous polyps located in the upper third of the ureter. Symptoms usually consist of intermittent pain from obstruction. Treatment is by local excision with a ureteroureterostomy or ureteral pyelostomy (Colgan et al., 1973). Rarely, a transitional epithelial cancer of the renal pelvis will be seen in infancy or childhood (Koyanagi et al., 1975.)

NEUROBLASTOMA

History

In 1864, Virchow was the first to characterize neuroblastoma, which he labeled glioma. Marchand, in 1891, commented on the histologic similarities between neuroblastoma and developing sympathetic ganglia. Herxheimer (1914), using a specific neural silver stain, showed that fibrils in neuroblastoma shared staining characteristics with nervous tissue. This finding contributed to the establishment of the tissue of origin of this tumor.

The biochemical aspects of neuroblastoma began to be understood as Mason and co-workers, in 1957, reported the presence of pressor amines in the urine of a child with neuroblastoma. Subsequently, we have come to recognize elevated levels of norepinephrine, its precursors, and metabolites in the urine of patients with this tumor.

Another early landmark in our understanding of neuroblastoma came in 1927 when Cushing and Wolbach reported for the first time a transformation of neuroblastoma into benign ganglioneuroma. Everson and Cole (1966) noted that this event generally occurred in infants under the age of 6 months. That spontaneous regression of neuroblastoma may be more common than is clinically evident was suggested by Beckwith and Perrin (1963), who noted microscopic clusters of neuroblastoma cells in the adrenal glands in a number of infants under 3 months of age who had died of other causes. They called these foci of tumor cells "neuroblastoma in situ." They estimated neuroblastoma in situ to occur about 40 times more frequently than the number of cases of neuroblastoma that were clinically diagnosed. Under normal circumstances, recession appeared usually to be complete after 3 months of age.

Etiology

Although the cause of neuroblastoma, as for most other carcinomas, is unknown, it arises from cells of the neural crest that form the sympathetic ganglia and adrenal medulla. Bolande (1979) has termed this tumor a type of "neurocristopathy." Other neurocristopathies include pheochromocytoma, paraganglioma, medullary carcinoma of the thyroid, carcinoid melanoma, neurocutaneous melanosis, neurofibramotosis, and multiple endocrine neoplasia. Sympathetic nervous system tumors can apparently differentiate along two lines: the pheochromocytoma line and the sympathoblastoma line. The sympathoblastoma line includes the neuroblastoma, ganglioneuroblastoma, and ganglioneuroma forms.

A genetic influence is apparent in this tumor. Knudson and Strong (1972) suggested that approximately 20 per cent of cases arise in children predisposed to the tumor by a dominant transmittable mutation. Knudson and Meadows (1976) suggested that familial cases result from a prezygotic mutation and that nonfamilial ones result from a postzygotic somatic mutation. Rare families have been described with more than one member affected with this tumor (Arenson et al., 1976; Chatten and Voorhees, 1967).

Incidence

Neuroblastoma is the most common malignant tumor of infancy and, after brain tumors, the most common malignant solid tumor of childhood (Young and Miller, 1975). Neuroblastoma accounts for 6 to 8 per cent of all childhood malignancies. In the United States, the incidence is 9.6 per million in white children and 7.0 per million in black children per year. There is a slight male predominance of 1.1 to 1 (Miller et al., 1968). The actual incidence is much higher than the reported incidence because of the proclivity for spontaneous regression of neuroblastoma in situ.

Although neuroblastoma may occur throughout childhood and occasionally in adulthood, the tumor predominantly develops early in life. Of all cases, 50 per cent occur in children under the age of 2, and more than 75 per cent of cases have been encountered by the 4th year of life (Fortner et al., 1968; Peterson et al., 1969). This is a younger age of presentation than that for Wilms' tumor. Unlike Wilms' tumor, there is a low incidence of associated congenital anomalies. One exception is an increased incidence of brain and skull defects approaching 2 per cent in children with neuroblastoma (Miller et al., 1968). An association with neurofibromatosis and Hirschprung's disease has been noted (Hope et al., 1965; Knudson and Amromin, 1966).

Pathology

Neuroblastoma

On gross examination, small tumors usually are well encapsulated and firm. On cut surface, the tumor is fairly soft and lobulated with a grayish-to-pink color. The tumor has a tendency to break through its pseudocapsule and infiltrate surrounding tissues. When it does, it is found to be friable and soft with hemorrhage and necrosis. Cystic areas may be present.

Histologically, neuroblastoma is one of the small round cell tumors of childhood. Light microscopy shows a similarity between neuroblasts, lymphocytes, and the cells of lymphomas, embryonal myosarcomas, and Ewing's sarcomas. When the tumor cells can be seen to form themselves into rosettes, and neurofibrals are evident, the degree of differentiation is quite good and the tumor is recognizable as a neuroblastoma. Unfortunately, these signs are often absent. Ewing's sarcoma and rhabdomyosarcoma usually contain glycogen, which can be seen by periodic acid–Schiff (PAS) staining.

Neuroblastoma lacks glycogen. Neuroblastoma cells may be recognized by the use of a rapid fluorescence assay for intracellular catecholamines or a tissue culture assay for neurite outgrowth (Reynolds et al., 1981). Neuron-specific enolase staining of tumor has also been reported to be fairly specific for neuroblastoma (Odelstad et al., 1982). This test is useful to distinguish neuroblastoma from poorly differentiated Wilms' tumor. The importance of this distinction lies in the different responses to chemotherapy of these neoplasms.

The ultrastructure of neuroblastoma is quite distinctive and reflects the neural crest derivation of neuroblasts. Characteristic peripheral dendritic processes that contain longitudinally oriented microtubules are seen. Small, spherical, membrane-coated granules with electron-dense cores representing cytoplasmic accumulations of catecholamines are seen. The larger number of granules seen in some tumors reflects a higher degree of differentiation and has been reported by Romansky and colleagues (1978) to be a favorable prognostic factor. Conventional microscopy, occasionally supplemented by electron microscopy, will usually enable a bone marrow aspirate to be identified and then diagnosed as neuroblastoma, avoiding the need for an open biopsy in a child with disseminated disease.

Efforts have been made for a number of years to correlate the histologic characteristics of neuroblastoma with the biologic behavior of this tumor. A grading system was devised by Shimada and associates (1984), which examines the number of mitotic cells per high-power field, the tumor stroma, the distribution of immature cells, and the age of the patient to identify patients with a favorable versus an unfavorable prognosis. This histologic grading is now recognized as a pivotal factor in selecting patients for a less or more intensive therapeutic approach (Silber et al., 1991).

Ganglioneuroma

At the other end of the spectrum of neuroblastoma lies the benign counterpart—the ganglioneuroma. By definition, these tumors do not metastasize, but they can recur following resection. They can become quite large with projections that envelop adjacent structures and occasionally extend through intervertebral foramina and produce neurologic symptoms by way of cord compression. On cut surface, they tend to be more firm and better encapsulated than neuroblastoma. Histologically, they are composed of large, mature ganglion cells with abundant cytoplasm and a large nucleus. They are scattered throughout a collagen-rich background with bundles of neurofibrils.

Ganglioneuroblastoma

This tumor is intermediate between neuroblastoma and the ganglioneuroma. Histologically, there are grades of ganglioneuroblastoma exhibiting the full spectrum from benign ganglioneuroma to malignant neuroblastoma. The outcome is varied.

Location, Presentation, and Differential Diagnosis

Because neuroblastomas and their more benign variants may occur anywhere along the sympathetic chain from the head to the pelvis, their presentation and differential diagnosis will vary with the site of tumor origin (Fig. 54–8). More than half of neuroblastomas have their origin in the abdomen, and two thirds of these arise in the *adrenal gland*. When a tumor has its origin in the adrenal gland, there is less likelihood of metastasis than from nonadrenal abdominal paravertebral sites. A mass is the most common presenting symptom. This is characteristically an irregular, firm,

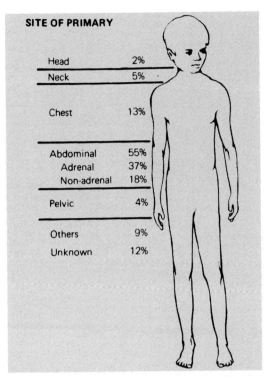

SITE OF PRIMARY

Head	2%
Neck	5%
Chest	13%
Abdominal	55%
Adrenal	37%
Non-adrenal	18%
Pelvic	4%
Others	9%
Unknown	12%

Figure 54–8. Neuroblastoma: Site of primary tumor. Composite data from the literature. (From Williams, T. E., and Donaldson, M. H.: Neuroblastoma. *In* Sutow, W. W., Vietti, T. J., and Fernback, D. J. (Eds.): Clinical Pediatric Oncology. St. Louis, C. V. Mosby Co., 1973, p. 388.)

nontender, fixed mass, often extending beyond the midline. In comparison, Wilms' tumor usually occurs with a smooth flank mass that does not cross the midline.

Neuroblastoma that arises from an *abdominal paravertebral sympathetic ganglion* has a greater likelihood of growing through an intervertebral foramen to form a dumbbell-shaped tumor compressing the spinal cord (Akwari et al., 1978; Traggis et al., 1977). In about 40 per cent of these cases, the intraspinal component will be asymptomatic. Paravertebral tumors always warrant evaluation for possible intraspinal extension. Prompt recognition may prevent permanent neurologic sequelae. Early intervention is warranted, because patients with these dumbbell neuroblastomas generally have an excellent prognosis. Chemotherapy can be as effective as neurosurgery and avoids the late orthopedic complications. These tumors may be more mature or even completely benign within the spinal canal and less mature in the abdominal extension. They must be differentiated from primary intraspinal tumors.

Neuroblastoma may also arise in the *presacral* region, presumably from the organ impar, or along the aorta from organs of Zuckerkandl. In the pelvis, the tumor may lead to urinary frequency or retention from extrinsic pressure on the bladder (Hepler, 1976). Constipation may also result. These tumors are quite rare, constituting only 4 per cent of neuroblastomas. The differential diagnosis of abdominal and pelvic neuroblastoma involves other abdominal and retroperitoneal tumors, such as Wilms' tumors, teratomas, and rarer primary neoplasms in the pancreas or liver.

One of the rarest primary sites for a neuroblastoma is the *olfactory bulb* (esthesioneuroblastoma). This tumor usually presents with unilateral nasal obstruction and epistaxis. It tends to occur later in life than the typical neuroblastoma arising in other sites (Homzie and Elkon, 1980) and is now considered a peripheral neuroectodermal tumor rather than a true neuroblastoma.

Neuroblastomas having their origin in the *cervical sympathetic ganglion* account for approximately 5 per cent of these tumors. A Horner's syndrome may result with inward sinking of the eyeball, ptosis of the upper eyelid, elevation of the lower eyelid, pupillary constriction, narrowing of the palpebral fissure, and anhidrosis. Because the sympathetic nervous system is involved with the development of pigmentation in the iris, neuroblastoma affecting the ophthalmic sympathetic nerves can lead to heterochromia iridis, an unequal color between the two irises. Both syndromes may occur together (Jaffe et al., 1975). Hoarseness may indicate compression of the recurrent laryngeal nerve by tumor. Cervical neuroblastoma may appear as a neck mass and must be differentiated from branchial cleft cysts, benign adenopathy, lymphoma, and leukemia, and other malignant tumors found in the neck.

Thoracic neuroblastoma, accounting for 13 per cent of tumors, may become massive before becoming clinically evident. More often, these lesions are discovered by radiographs taken for the diagnosis of an unrelated disease. The patient may have cough, dyspnea, or pulmonary infection from tracheal or bronchial compression. The superior vena cava may be compressed. Weakness of an upper extremity may indicate brachial plexus involvement. Pain in the neck, back, abdomen, or pelvis may be caused by a dumbbell extension of the tumor to produce spinal cord compression. In the posterior mediastinum, neuroblastoma must be differentiated from teratomas, esophageal duplications, and bronchogenic cysts.

In its early stages, neuroblastoma is usually a silent tumor. *Metastatic* dissemination of the tumor may occur early and does not appear to be related to the size of the primary tumor. Up to 70 per cent of patients have metastatic disease at the time of diagnosis (Gross et al., 1959). In the young, metastases tend to go to the liver; in older children, bony metastases are more common. Unexplained fever, general malaise, anorexia, weight loss, irritability, bone pain, and pallor secondary to anemia are all common manifestations of widespread disease. Occasionally, such symptoms may be noted without evidence of dissemination. The high incidence of disseminated disease with neuroblastoma accounts for the more frequent presentation of a generally unwell child in contradistinction to the presentation of a child with Wilms' tumor, who usually seems well and robust.

The *liver* suffers the brunt of metastatic dissemination, especially in the infant (Fig. 54–9A). The tumor may appear as a rapidly growing hepatic neoplasm, which may embarrass respiration (Bond, 1976). Primary hepatoblastoma must be differentiated.

Often, the first symptoms of neuroblastoma reflect *bony* involvement. The skull and long bones are most commonly involved. Metastatic disease usually occurs

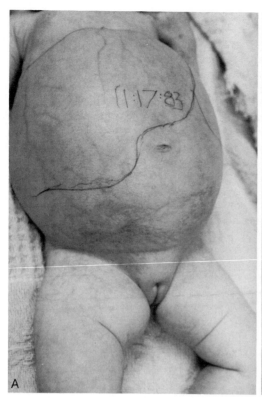
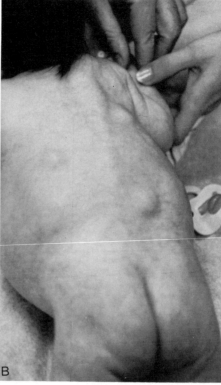

Figure 54–9. Neuroblastoma: Stage IV-S. *A,* Liver metastases causing abdominal distention. *B,* Skin metastases on back.

in the diaphysis and may be bilaterally symmetric. On radiographs, metastases appear as lytic defects with an irregular margin and some periosteal reaction. Symptoms may include local bone pain or a limp. Metastatic bone lesions must be differentiated from primary bone tumors, lymphoreticular malignancies, or infectious processes.

More than 50 per cent of children with neuroblastoma have *bone marrow* involvement, even in the absence of radiographic evidence of change in the bone (Finklestein et al., 1970). Bone marrow replacement with depletion of one or more cell lines in the peripheral blood may lead to the incorrect diagnosis of aplastic anemia or other diseases that may cause thrombocytopenia or anemia (Quinn and Altman, 1979). Neuroblastoma cells in the bone marrow can usually be distinguished from leukemic infiltration, because neuroblastoma cells appear in small clusters and may exhibit rosettes and neurofibrils. Electron microscopy, as mentioned earlier, may occasionally be useful in distinguishing neuroblastoma from other malignancies that invade the bone marrow. The recognition of neuroblastoma may also be assisted by appropriate monoclonal antibodies and fluorescence microscopy (Cheung et al., 1985; Horne et al., 1985; Kemshed and Coakham, 1983).

Subcutaneous nodules (Fig. 54–9B) are also a common metastatic pattern for neuroblastoma in infants. They often have a bluish color, and the infants have been likened in appearance to blueberry muffins. Such subcutaneous nodules have been reported in up to one third of neonates with neuroblastoma (Schneider et al., 1965). These skin lesions may become erythematous for several minutes after palpation and then blanch, presum-

ably as a result of vasoconstriction attributable to catecholamine release from the tumor cells. When present, this reaction may be a diagnostic sign of neuroblastoma (Hawthorne et al., 1970). These nodules must be differentiated from leukemic infiltrates of the skin.

Periorbital metastatic disease is also common in children with neuroblastoma (Fig. 54–10). Retrobulbar soft

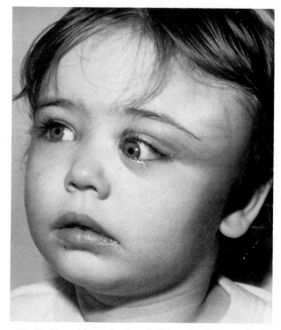

Figure 54–10. Neuroblastoma. Retrobulbar metastases producing proptosis.

tissue involvement may cause periorbital edema and proptosis. Periorbital ecchymoses may give a "raccoon-like" appearance to the child. Ecchymosis typically occurs in the upper eyelid. This is in contradistinction to lower eyelid ecchymosis, which is more common with trauma.

Some organs are rarely the site of metastases; these include the heart, lungs, brain, and spinal cord. Pulmonary metastases are occasionally seen in very advanced disease secondary to extensive lymphatic spread or direct growth through the diaphragm.

Occasionally, children are seen whose symptoms are produced by the biochemical activity of the tumor. As neural crest tumors, neuroblastomas usually secrete *catecholamines*. Occasional children are seen with paroxysmal attacks of sweating, pallor, headaches, hypertension, palpitations, and flushing. Voute and co-workers (1970) reported six mothers who had these symptoms in the 8th and 9th months of pregnancy and who subsequently delivered infants diagnosed as having neuroblastoma during the first few months of life. The mothers' symptoms presumably were caused by fetal catecholamines entering the maternal circulation. When symptoms of catecholamine release are prominent, neuroblastoma may simulate pheochromocytoma.

Children have also presented with intractable watery diarrhea and hypokalemia. This presentation was found to be due to tumor secretion of an enterohormone known as *vasoactive intestinal peptide* (VIP) (El Shafie et al., 1983; Mitchell et al., 1976). A variety of other tumors besides neuroblastoma, including pancreatic tumors and bronchiogenic carcinoma, have been shown to secrete VIP. Pearse (1978) suggested that these tumors share a common ancestor cell in the neural crest. The tumors have cytochemical characteristics that are shared. The most important characteristic is the ability to absorb amines from the environment and convert them into hormones or hormone-like products. This ability is referred to as APUD—amine precursor uptake and decarboxylation—and these tumors are thus termed APUDomas.

One of the most interesting systemic manifestations of neuroblastoma is *acute myoclonic encephalopathy*. This condition is seen in approximately 2 per cent of children with neuroblastoma. The syndrome consists of rapid multidirectional eye movements (opsoclonus), myoclonus, and truncal ataxia in the absence of increased intracranial pressure (Senelick et al., 1973). Although it was initially thought that the encephalopathy was caused by a toxic neurologic effect of circulating catecholamine catabolites, at least one child has been reported who developed this neurologic symptom 7 months after removal of a primary tumor and return to normal of previously elevated levels of urinary catecholamines (Delalieux et al., 1975). An alternate explanation may be the existence of an autoimmune factor, perhaps an antibody directed against a neuroblastoma antigen, which is cross-reacting with a common antigen in the cells of the cerebellum, resulting in damage (Bray et al., 1969). Tumors associated with this syndrome are often well differentiated, located in the thorax, and

associated with a good prognosis (Altman and Baehner, 1976).

On rare occasions, a neonate will present with a syndrome that may mimic *erythroblastosis*. Massive metastasis to the liver and bone marrow may produce jaundice, anemia, and hepatosplenomegaly. This syndrome may mimic hemolytic disease in the newborn. Two cases with congenital neuroblastoma were reported by Anders and colleagues (1973); these patients had congenital neuroblastoma that was metastatic to the liver and placenta and were thought to have hydrops fetalis.

From these descriptions of the multiple possible sites and presentations for neuroblastoma, it should be evident why this tumor has been referred to as the "great mimicker." A prepared mind is requisite to make a proper diagnosis in many of these enigmatic cases (Jaffe, 1976).

Diagnostic Evaluation

Hematologic Studies

The complete blood count (CBC) is usually normal in a child with neuroblastoma until the disease becomes disseminated. With dissemination, anemia may be present because of bone marrow involvement by tumor or resulting from hemorrhage into the tumor. Rarely, thrombocytopenia may be seen because of bone marrow involvement or because of platelet trapping in the tumor. Liver involvement may cause a bleeding diathesis through disseminated intravascular coagulopathy. The erythrocyte sedimentation rate is usually raised in the child with systemic disease.

Bone marrow aspiration is indicated in every suspected case of neuroblastoma. As many as 70 per cent of bone marrow aspirates in patients with neuroblastoma have been reported to be positive (Finklestein et al., 1970). Although it is not unusual to find tumor cells in the bone marrow aspirate with no evidence of skeletal metastases, occasionally a patient may demonstrate widespread bony metastases with no cells in the marrow. As discussed previously, neuroblastoma will frequently form pseudorosettes in the bone marrow. This feature helps distinguish neuroblastoma in the marrow from leukemia and metastatic carcinomas, such as lymphosarcoma, retinoblastoma, Ewing's sarcoma, and other small round cell tumors that have a proclivity to metastasize to bone. In the child with disseminated disease, careful evaluation of the bone marrow may obviate the need for an open biopsy of the tumor.

Catecholamine Excretion

Since the first report of urinary catecholamine excretion in neuroblastoma was made by Mason and associates in 1957, much attention has been given to the biochemical products of this tumor. The two major metabolites of catecholamine production by neuroblastoma are vanillylmandelic acid (VMA) and homovanillic acid (HVA). Williams and Greer (1963) reported that 95 per cent of patients with neuroblastoma have an elevated urinary excretion of VMA, HVA, or both. Occasional patients are seen with no elevation of catecholamine excretion (Voorhees, 1971). These tumors are most commonly found in the thorax and probably arise from dorsal spinal nerve roots and ganglia, which are nonsecretors of catecholamines. No correlation has been found between the pattern of catecholamine excretion and the age of patients, symptomatology, or histologic pattern.

Because hypertension is not common in neuroblastoma, it is interesting to speculate why elevated catecholamine production does not lead to clinical symptoms in most cases. It may be that norepinephrine is catabolized within the tumor and, thus, does not become systemically active (LaBrosse and Karon, 1962). Also, it is possible that the initial enzyme in catecholamine synthesis, tyrosine hydrolase, is subject to normal "feedback" inhibition by norephinephrine, dopamine, and dopa (Imashuku et al., 1971). These factors may help explain why high levels of serum norepinephrine and hypertension are uncommon in neuroblastoma; in comparison, in pheochromocytoma, excessive amounts of tyrosine hydrolase are present because of lack of normal feedback inhibition.

Although quantitative determination of all catecholamines and their metabolites in a 24-hour urine collection is clearly the most accurate method of biochemical diagnosis of neuroblastoma, the collection of 24-hour urine specimens in infants and small children is difficult. This problem led Gitlow and co-workers (1970) to propose the simultaneous assay of VMA, HVA, and creatinine in a single spot urine specimen. The upper limits of normal have been found to be 20 μg/mg of creatinine for VMA and 40 μg/mg of creatinine for HVA. Although this test provides an accurate diagnostic approach, it is quite cumbersome.

In 1968, LaBrosse developed a filter paper spot test for VMA in the urine. This test has approximately a 75 per cent positivity when used in the diagnosis and follow-up of patients with neuroblastoma (Evans et al., 1971a). It is, however, generally agreed that VMA screening tests, although useful, lack total reliability and that confirmation by specific quantitative assays is important (Johnsonbaugh and Cahill, 1975).

Cystathionine and carcinoembryonic antigen levels have also been reported to be elevated in patients with neuroblastomas. The lack of specificity of these products for neuroblastoma, however, has limited the clinical usefulness of urinary assays.

Imaging

Appropriate roentgenographic and nuclear medicine diagnostic studies can localize the site of primary disease as well as define the presence and extent of metastatic spread. For abdominal tumors, an *intravenous pyelogram* (IVP) should be routinely carried out. With a suprarenal neuroblastoma, the kidney is characteristically displaced inferiorly and laterally with the maintenance of a normal calyceal pattern. In comparison, an

intrarenal Wilms' tumor distorts the calyceal pattern (Figs. 54–11 and 54–12). Very rarely, intrarenal neuroblastoma (Gibbons and Duckett, 1979) will closely mimic Wilms' tumor.

An abdominal paravertebral neuroblastoma may displace the ureter laterally. Occasionally, there will be delayed visualization or nonvisualization of the kidney if ureteral obstruction is present. Calcification in a characteristically speckled pattern can be seen in 50 per cent of cases on plain films (Fig. 54–12). CT can distinguish calcification in an additional 30 per cent. This speckled pattern contrasts with the less frequent calcification seen with Wilms' tumor, which tends to be curvilinear.

Ultrasonography may be very helpful in determining the exact location of an intra-abdominal primary tumor. The ability of ultrasound to evaluate the retroperitoneum may give evidence of direct spread or nodal involvement. The cava is well visualized by ultrasound and is often anteriorly displaced. Complete obstruction or tumor invasion of the cava is rare. The liver can be examined, often making a liver scan unnecessary. CT can add useful diagnostic information, although it does have the disadvantage of usually requiring sedation. An IVP and abdominal ultrasound continue to suffice in many situations.

A new diagnostic agent, [131]I-*meta*-iodobenzylguanidine (MIBG) has been introduced to image both primary and metastatic neuroblastoma (Geatti et al., 1985; Haefnagel et al., 1985; Horne et al., 1985). MIBG competes with norepinephrine and is taken up by adrenergic secretory vesicles in neuroblastoma, thus permitting imaging of the tumor.

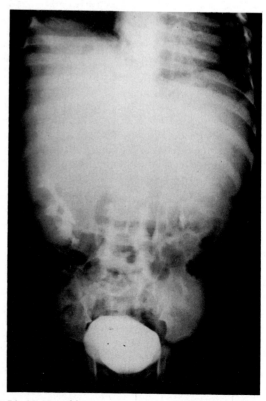

Figure 54–11. Neuroblastoma: Intravenous pyelogram showing inferior and lateral displacement of right kidney by adrenal neuroblastoma.

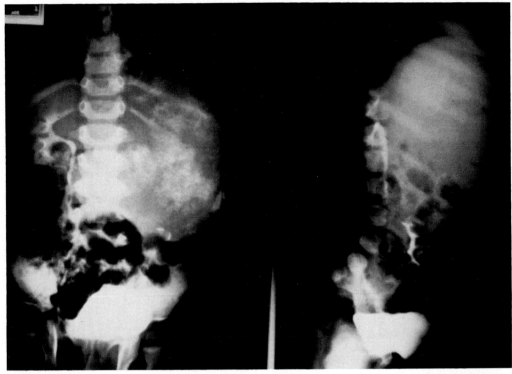

Figure 54–12. Neuroblastoma: Left suprarenal tumor with characteristic speckled calcification. Intravenous pyelogram (posteroanterior and lateral) shows inferior and lateral displacement of kidney.

A *chest radiograph* should be routinely carried out. Careful examination of the posterior mediastinum in patients with abdominal tumors is important, because extension can take place through the diaphragm. Next to abdominal tumors, thoracic neuroblastomas are second in frequency. Usually, the tumor is in the posterior mediastinum. Both sides of the thorax are affected equally, and calcification is seen in about half of the cases. Oblique views, as well as anterior and posterior ones, are important to detect dumbbell tumors with invasion of the neural foramina. The posterior portion of the ribs may be separated, and the ribs themselves narrowed by erosion.

Because metastatic involvement of the skeleton is so common, a *skeletal survey* should be routine in the evaluation of a patient with neuroblastoma. Bony metastases occur most commonly in the skull and in the diaphyses of the distal tubular bones, femur, and humerus. Metastatic spread is rare distal to the elbow and knee. Metastases may also be seen in the ribs, scapula, vertebral bodies, and pelvis. The distribution of metastases is often both bilateral and symmetric, but it rarely involves epiphyses. The lesions are usually lytic and irregular with periosteal reaction. Occasionally, a pathologic fracture occurs. The degree of involvement varies from barely perceptible to massive. A radionuclear *bone scan* may be useful in detecting disease not detected by radiographic bone survey (D'Angio et al., 1969).

Arteriography and venography are not generally required in the evaluation of neuroblastoma.

Table 54–9. STAGING OF NEUROBLASTOMA

Stage 0:	Neuroblastoma in situ
Stage I:	Tumors confined to the organ or structure of origin
Stage II:	Tumors extending in continuity beyond the organ or structure of origin but not crossing the midline. The regional lymph nodes on the ipsilateral side may be involved.
Stage III:	Tumors extending in continuity beyond the midline. Regional lymph nodes may be involved bilaterally.
Stage IV:	Distant metastases involving bones, bone marrow, brain, skin, liver, lung, soft tissues, or distant lymph node groups*
Stage IV-S:	Patients who would otherwise be classified with stage I or II disease but who have remote spread of tumor confined to one or more of the following sites: liver, skin, or bone marrow (without roentgenographic evidence of bond metastases on complete skeletal survey)†

*These patients usually have elevated ferritin levels and E-rosette inhibitory factor, which help distinguish them from patients who have stage IV-S disease.
†Inclusion of bone marrow disease in this stage may not be justifiable. If the marrow is extensively involved the prognosis is probably poor.
Adapted from Evans, A. E., et al.: Cancer, 27:374, 1971.

Staging

Accurate staging of patients with neuroblastoma is of critical importance because of the information this provides regarding prognosis and the determination of the extent of treatment. Although, in the 1960s, a number of staging systems for neuroblastoma were proposed, the one advocated by Evans, D'Angio, and Randolph in 1971 is most widespread clinically (Table 54–9).

For tumors that arise in midline structures, such as the sympathetic tissue at the origin of the inferior mesenteric artery (organs of Zuckerkandl), extension beyond the capsule with involvement of lymph nodes on the same side is considered stage II disease. Bilateral extension of any type is considered stage III.

Stage IV-S neuroblastoma (see Fig. 54–9) is a unique form of disseminated disease, which occurs most commonly in infancy. In contradistinction to stage IV neuroblastoma, which has an approximate 10 per cent survival rate, stage IV-S disease has a survival rate on the order of 80 per cent (D'Angio et al., 1971). Children with this condition usually appear to have robust good health and lack the malaise, weight loss, fever, and often anemia that is seen in those with typical stage IV disseminated disease. Disease in children with IV-S neuroblastoma is limited to the liver, skin, or bone marrow. No radiographic evidence of bony metastases is found. Although local tumor growth may rarely cause serious problems, generally, the tumor regresses spontaneously without treatment. The infants have an excellent prognosis.

The Evans' classification continues to be the most widely used classification today because of its clinical applicability. A variation of this schema has been adopted for international use (Brodeur et al., 1988). Other factors (see following discussion) are critical to the prognosis of neuroblastoma, but a staging system incorporating them would become so unwieldy as to be impractical. Instead, Silber and co-workers (1991) have developed a formula taking these many factors into account.

Prognostic Factors and Survival

A number of variables determine the prognosis for neuroblastoma. In general, survival for 2 years with no evidence of disease is usually equivalent to cure (de-Lorimier et al., 1969; Gross et al., 1959). Occasional later deaths have been reported, and chemotherapy may have prolonged somewhat the lives of some children with disease without influencing overall survival. Bone marrow transplantation can be followed at times by a rather late disease relapse.

The *site of origin* is a factor of prognostic significance. Coldman and co-workers (1980) reported that nonadrenal abdominal tumors are associated with a greater likelihood of survival than are adrenal primary tumors. This characteristic appears to be independent of age and stage of disease. Mediastinal neuroblastoma, even when there is node involvement, Horner's syndrome, bony erosion, or cord compression, also has an improved prognosis (Filler et al., 1972). This finding may be due to the fact that tumors above the diaphragm are usually less disseminated at presentation (Evans et al., 1976). Five-year actuarial survival rates for posterior mediastinal tumors have been reported to be as high as 88 per cent (Adam and Hochholzer, 1981). Patients with neuroblastomas that take origin in the neck or pelvis also have an improved prognosis, perhaps because these tumors become symptomatic early in their course and are diagnosed before dissemination.

The DNA content of tumor cells compared with that of normal cells (DNA Index) is important. This index can be determined by flow cytometry (Look et al.,

1984). An index of 1 rarely occurs in low-stage disease. In disseminated disease, an index of 1 is associated with a poorer response to cyclophosphamide and doxorubicin (Gansler et al., 1986). Kaneko and associates (1987) found pseudodiploidy associated with higher stage disease also. The N-*myc* oncogene has been found to be amplified in neuroblastoma cells (Phillips et al., 1991; Schwab et al., 1983). Rarely is the N-*myc* oncogene amplified in patients with localized neuroblastoma, but it is amplified in about half of the patients with disseminated disease (Brodeur and Seeger, 1986). Amplification tends to be homogeneous within any given tumor and, thus, is reflective of the intrinsic biologic property of the tumor. Gangliosides (sialic acid–containing glycosphingolipids) are found on the membranes of neuroblastoma cells, and from there they are shed into the circulation. They are not present or are present only in small amounts in the more differentiated forms of neuroblastoma. The serum levels may be a prognostic factor (Cheung et al., 1985).

Disagreement exists regarding the prognostic significance of positive nodes and surgical resectability. In stage II disease, Ninane and colleagues (1982) reported that, for patients with negative nodes, all survived, whereas among patients with positive nodes, 6 of 13 died of the tumor. In patients with stage II and III disease, Hayes and colleagues (1983) reported an 83 per cent survival if nodes were negative versus 31 per cent survival with positive nodes. Surgical resectability also appears to have a favorable prognosis (Hayes et al., 1983). The problem with these studies is that the tumors that are resectable or have negative nodes may be the biologically more favorable tumors. Thus, the actual surgical procedure may not be positively influencing the outcome but merely serving as a marker of a favorable form of neuroblastoma.

Although the aforementioned factors may be important in the prognosis of neuroblastoma, the four major indices are age, stage of disease, serum ferritin level, and the Shimada index (Shimada et al., 1984). The use of these indices is most critical in determining where therapeutic efforts must be directed in neuroblastoma, and each of these prognostic factors deserves comment.

In patients with neuroblastomas, survival is inversely correlated with *age at diagnosis* (Sutow, 1958). In the review by Breslow and McCann (1971), children under 1 year of age had a survival rate of 74 per cent. Between 12 and 23 months, survival was 26 per cent, and in those over 2 years of age, it was only 12 per cent. Spontaneous remission of neuroblastoma appears to be most likely in children under 6 months of age. Interestingly, data are now accumulating to suggest that survival expectancy improves for children who present over the age of 6 years (Evans, 1980; Sather et al., 1981). Nonetheless, only about one child in four with neuroblastoma in this age group survives.

The *stage of disease* is an important prognostic factor and appears to be independent of age at diagnosis and site of tumor (Coldman et al., 1980). When the disease is localized (stage I and II), survival rates of 80 per cent can be expected. Disseminated disease of the IV-S type has a similar survival rate. In contrast, stage III disease has a survival of approximately 37 per cent and stage IV disease, 5 to 7 per cent (Breslow and McCann, 1971; Grosfeld, 1983). In recent years, these figures have changed little.

Serum *ferritin* level has emerged as a critical prognostic index. Neuroblastoma excretes elevated levels of this serum protein (Hann et al., 1979). The serum ferritin level is elevated in disseminated disease; it is elevated in 40 to 50 per cent of stage III or IV cases. In stage III disease, if the serum ferritin is not elevated, patients do better (76 per cent versus 23 per cent survival without disease at 2 years). For stage IV disease, there is not such a marked difference (27 per cent versus 3 per cent) (Hann et al., 1985). Neuroblastoma patients, like others with malignant disease, may have reduced E-rosette formation by T lymphocytes (Fuks et al., 1976). It has been speculated that ferritin may be responsible for this. Thus, indirectly, E-rosette formation may be of prognostic significance also. The report by Hann and colleagues (1981) suggested that the majority of children with stage IV disease and elevated serum ferritin levels have E-rosette inhibition but that ferritin levels were not elevated and E-rosette formation was not inhibited in patients with stage IV-S disease. Neurone-specific enolase is a comparable marker to ferritin as an adverse marker for disseminated disease (Zelter et al., 1983). However, neurone-specific enolase is more difficult to assay, giving the clinical edge to the utilization of serum ferritin levels.

The last critical prognostic variable is the *Shimada index*. For low-stage disease (I, II, and IV-S), the histology by the Shimada index appears to be the most important prognostic variable. For disseminated disease (stage III and IV), ferritin alone appears to be the most important prognostic variable. Using these four prognostic indices, it is possible to divide patients with neuroblastoma into two groups: those with a favorable tumor and those with an unfavorable tumor (Silber et al., 1991). For the favorable group, therapy can be limited; in the unfavorable group, a more aggressive approach is indeed justified.

Treatment of Favorable Disease

In any discussion of the management of neuroblastoma, it must be emphasized that this tumor continues to be a most frustrating pediatric malignancy to treat. In spite of extensive efforts to improve outcome, little has changed in the prognosis of these children over the past 20 years. What we now face is the recognition that we must identify patients who will do well almost in spite of whatever therapy is undertaken and reduce care for these patients, while focusing our attention on a more aggressive approach in the unfavorable group.

Surgery

In the treatment of well-localized favorable disease, simple surgical extirpation of the primary tumor continues to be the main mode of treatment. Complete surgical removal often is accomplished in stage I and II disease but may not be possible once the midline has been crossed in stage III disease, when the aorta and inferior vena cava are frequently involved. In general, although total excision is the goal, en bloc removal of major organs in continuity with the tumor is not justified. An exception to this is the adjacent kidney for adrenal tumors. In clinical practice, tumors either tend to be localized enough to permit excision or to be so extensive that even heroic operations would be impossible. Today, we recognize that this factor is probably more of a reflection of the biologic character of the tumor than anything else.

A second important role for surgery is to stage the neoplasm. It should be determined if a tumor infiltrates across the midline or involves contralateral lymph nodes. This is only a staging maneuver and there is no evidence that radical node dissection is of value in neuroblastoma. Accurate staging is helpful because, with the good prognosis for stage II disease, therapy can be limited to surgical excision alone.

Previously it has been thought that second-look procedures had a role with stage III and, occasionally, stage II inoperable tumors. It was believed that through chemotherapy and radiation therapy, it might be possible to permit a curative operation (Smith et al., 1980). However, with further follow-up data, it is becoming evident that second surgical procedures have their greatest value as part of an aggressive chemotherapy and radiation therapy program intended to move toward bone marrow transplantation (Evans et al., 1987). It is now well recognized that operations to "debulk" tumor have little to contribute to improved long-term survival (Sitarz et al., 1983).

Chemotherapy

Neuroblastoma in stage I and II has an 80 per cent survival rate; no evidence indicates that chemotherapy improves survival (Evans et al., 1984). Thus, in the patient group with favorable neuroblastoma, little treatment further than surgical removal is needed.

Radiotherapy

Although neuroblastoma is a radiosensitive tumor, in the favorable group radiation therapy does not appear to improve prognosis in what is already a disease with a good prognosis (Evans et al., 1984); accordingly, radiotherapy is usually not employed.

Treatment of Unfavorable Disease

Surgery

Other than perhaps performing a biopsy of the tumor, there appears to be little the surgeon is able to contribute to patients in the unfavorable group. For a period, there was enthusiasm for an "assault" on the tumor in the belief that this might affect outcome; unfortunately, this approach has not resulted in any improvement in the dismal prognosis for the unfavorable type of neuroblastoma. Indeed, the results of the Children's Cancer Study Group (CCSG) suggest that initial surgery may worsen the outcome (Sitarz et al., 1983). Although previously it was thought that second-look procedures might have a role in stage III and occasionally in stage II inoperable tumors, it is now becoming clear that they contribute little to outcome. Second-look procedures perhaps may be useful as part of an aggressive chemotherapy and total body radiotherapy effort that is part of a bone marrow transplant program.

Radiation Therapy

Radiation therapy has a primary role in the palliation of painful or unsightly metastases. Relatively short treatment to produce doses in the range of 1000 to 2000 cGy generally suffices, although higher doses may be useful if the patient is anticipated to have a longer period of time remaining before death from the tumor. A more aggressive radiation therapy in stage IV disease appears to have little to contribute to improved survival (Evans, 1982).

Chemotherapy

Neuroblastoma is definitely a chemotherapy-responsive tumor, and a multitude of different agents have been shown to be effective (Table 54–10). Most major medical centers have four- to six-drug programs; however, no clear advantage has been shown for any particular combination therapies. Indeed, it can be debated whether combination chemotherapy is actually much more effective than any one agent alone. Unfortunately, aggressive chemotherapy has done little to increase the long-term cure of unfavorable neuroblastoma.

Two new therapeutic approaches deserve emphasis. Targeted radiation therapy with labeled MIBG or monoclonal antibodies is done early in the development phase but perhaps offers some help for the group with unfavorable disease (Cheung et al., 1985; Haefnagel et al., 1985; Horne et al., 1985). To date, this new approach has been chosen primarily for the treatment of relapse, although some medical centers in Europe are beginning to utilize this for an initial approach.

Bone marrow transplant for salvage of patients with unfavorable disease following a lethal combination of chemotherapy and total body irradiation continues to offer some hope (Hartmann et al., 1985; Philip et al., 1987). We reported a 40 per cent 2-year actuarial

Table 54–10. SINGLE–AGENT RESPONSES WITH CHEMOTHERAPY FOR NEUROBLASTOMA

	%
Cyclosphosphamide	59
Doxorubicin	41
Cisplatin	46
Epipodophyllotoxins	30
Vincristine	24
Dicarbazine	14
Peptichemio	67

survival in 10 patients with recurrent stage IV neuroblastoma (August et al., 1984). Although the transplant itself can have a lethal outcome, to have any survivors following the recurrence of metastatic neuroblastoma is a major advance. Variations on bone marrow transplant protocols continue to be developed within the CCSG in efforts to improve the dismal prognosis for this group.

Treatment of IV-S Disease

Patients with IV-S neuroblastoma and disease confined to the liver, skin, and bone marrow usually are infants. Because the likelihood of spontaneous tumor regression is high, it is usually recommended that these children be observed for a period of time before initiating any form of therapy (Evans, 1980). Occasionally, infants with massive hepatic involvement develop respiratory difficulty or vascular compression from increasing hepatomegaly. In this situation, low-dose radiation or chemotherapy may halt the growth and initiate tumor regression. Radiotherapy administered as 150 cGy daily for 3 days through lateral portals angled 15 degrees above the horizontal to avoid the ovaries and spine is recommended by Evans and co-workers (1980).

If inadequate reversal of the process is produced, low-dose chemotherapy may be instituted. For example, cyclophosphamide plus vincristine may be used. Chemotherapy must be administered in reduced doses because of the increased toxicity in the very young. If radiation therapy and chemotherapy are unsuccessful, a ventral hernia with a Silastic pouch may be effective to temporarily relieve the problem until spontaneous tumor regression ensues (Schnaufer and Koop, 1975).

Future Treatment Expectations

In closing this section, we would like to emphasize the developments in treatment of neuroblastoma that hinge on recognition of the importance of the patient's immune response to this tumor. Lauder and Aherne (1972) early recognized a better prognosis for patients whose tumors were infiltrated with lymphocytes. Altman and Baehner (1976) proposed that opsoclonus may be associated with a good prognosis, because the symptom may be due to an antibody formed to the neuroblastoma that cross reacts with cerebellar cells to produce the neurologic symptom.

Hellstrom and Hellstrom (1972) demonstrated that lymphocytes from children with neuroblastoma are capable of specific inhibition of neuroblastoma cells. This was the beginning of data suggesting immunotherapy for neuroblastoma (Bernstein, 1980). Sawada and associates (1981) reported on early work utilizing interferon as an immune enhancer. Biologic response modifiers, such as interleukin-2, may have a role. Cytotoxic and radiation-conjugated antibodies, as mentioned earlier, may also have a future role. Immunotherapy is the forefront in the future treatment of neuroblastoma.

RHABDOMYOSARCOMA AND OTHER PELVIC TUMORS OF CHILDHOOD

Incidence

Sarcomas rising in soft tissues are the fifth most common solid tumor of childhood after CNS tumors, lymphomas, neuroblastomas, and Wilms' tumor. Rhabdomyosarcoma, a malignancy rising from the same embryonal mesenchyme that gives rise to striated skeletal muscle, is the most common soft tissue sarcoma, accounting for about 50 per cent of all soft tissue sarcomas of childhood. It accounts for 5 to 15 per cent of all solid malignant tumors and 4 to 8 per cent of all malignant disease in children under 15 years of age (Young and Miller, 1975). In the United States, the annual incidence is approximately 4.4 per million white children and 1.3 per million black children per year. The ratio of males to females is 1.4:1 (Maurer et al., 1977). Two age peaks occur, the first between 2 and 6 years, and the second between 15 and 19 years (Maurer et al., 1977; Sutow et al., 1970). About 70 per cent of cases occur before the age of 10 years.

A genetic component has been found in rhabdomyosarcoma. Familial aggregations of rhabdomyosarcoma with other sarcomas, breast carcinomas, and brain tumors have been reported (Li and Fraumeni, 1969). An increased incidence of rhabdomyosarcoma has been reported in patients with neurofibromatosis (McKeen et al., 1978). Associated congenital anomalies are otherwise not common with rhabdomyosarcoma. Of seven associated congenital anomalies detected in 43 autopsies carried out as part of the Intergroup Rhabdomyosarcoma Study (IRS), there were four malformations of the CNS (Ruymann et al., 1977).

Rhabdomyosarcomas may arise from any part of the body that contains embryonal mesenchyme, whether striated muscle tissue is present concomitantly or not. In the collected experience of the first IRS (Maurer et al., 1981), tumors arising in the genitourinary region made up approximately 20 per cent of the total. Only head and neck rhabdomyosarcomas occur more commonly. The most common genitourinary sites involve the prostate, the bladder (most frequently in the area of the trigone), and the vagina, where tumors tend most frequently to involve the anterior vaginal wall contiguous to the bladder. Paratesticular rhabdomyosarcomas, which arise in the mesenchyme of the spermatic cord, are discussed with other testis tumors. Rhabdomyosarcomas arising in the pelvis outside of the bladder or prostate also often come to urologic consideration. These tumors may reach large size before becoming symptomatic. Such patients have a worse prognosis than their counterparts with tumors in the bladder, prostate, vagina, or paratesticular region (Crist et al., 1985; Raney et al., 1981, 1986).

The natural history of rhabdomyosarcoma involves rapid growth with invasion of adjacent tissue. The tumor tends to be unencapsulated and infiltrative, making total surgical excision of the tumor often difficult. The tumor may both spread into the regional lymphatic areas of drainage and invade the bloodstream. When metastases occur, three quarters will manifest themselves within 6 months of diagnosis, and more than 80 per cent will manifest by 1 year (Heyn et al., 1974). Before the development of effective chemotherapy, patients with rhabdomyosarcoma usually died with widespread metastases in spite of local surgical removal, radiotherapy, or both in 70 to 80 per cent of cases (Mahour et al., 1967; Sutow et al., 1970).

Pathology

On gross examination, rhabdomyosarcomas tend to be nodular and firm. When viewed at operation, they are often deceptively well circumscribed while actually infiltrating extensively into adjacent tissue. There are no remarkable gross features of rhabdomyosarcoma, except *sarcoma botryoides* (Figs. 54-13 and 54-14), which looks like a cluster of grapes and tends to arise in hollow organs, such as the bladder or vagina.

The histologic classification of rhabdomyosarcoma reflects the wide range of mesenchymal differentiation that may be seen. *Embryonal* rhabdomyosarcoma is the most common type in childhood. Morphologically, it resembles developing skeletal muscle as observed in the 7- to 10-week fetus (Patton and Horn, 1962). This type is composed mainly of spindle-shaped cells with a central nucleus and abundant eosinophilic cystoplasm. About 30 per cent demonstrate cross striations. This type accounts for approximately two thirds of the rhabdomyosarcomas of the genitourinary tract and for 50 to 60 per cent of all rhabdomyosarcomas in children (Maurer et al., 1977). Sarcoma botryoides is a polypoid form of embryonal rhabdomyosarcoma.

The *alveolar* form of rhabdomyosarcoma histologically resembles skeletal muscle in the 10- to 21-week

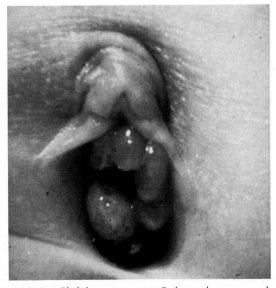

Figure 54–13. Rhabdomyosarcoma. Embryonal tumor prolapsing through urethra in female infant.

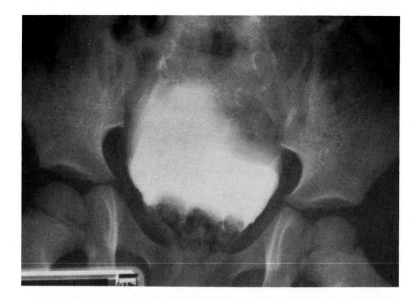

Figure 54–14. Rhabdomyosarcoma. Embryonal tumor—sarcoma botryoides—of bladder base showing characteristic polypoid configuration on cystogram.

fetus. The tumor is often more firm and less myxoid than the embryonal type. Histologically, there are clusters of small round cells with scanty eosinophilic cytoplasm. Cross striations are rarely present. This type is more commonly seen in adolescents and young adults and is more commonly associated with tumors occurring in the extremities and trunk than the genitourinary tract.

The *pleomorphic* type of rhabdomyosarcoma makes up only about 1 per cent of all childhood cases and is the form usually found in adults. As with the alveolar type, it is more common in the extremities and trunk than in the genitourinary tract. As its name implies, the histologic appearance of the tumor cells varies from racket-shaped to large, round cells with giant or multiple nuclei to strap-shaped cells with multiple nuclei in tandem.

One can also encounter histologically *mixed* rhabdomyosarcoma. In addition, there is a group of 10 to 20 per cent of cases that are so undifferentiated that they do not fit into the standard classification. Histologically, they are primitive small round cell tumors approximately half of which strongly resemble Ewing's sarcoma. The primary difference is that, unlike Ewing's, they arise from soft tissue rather than bone. Thus, many histologic patterns are possible with rhabdomyosarcoma. Mierau and Favara (1980) have suggested that all childhood rhabdomyosarcomas are basically embryonal tumors, which vary only in the degree to which they have differentiated and responded to microenvironmental factors.

Presentation

The signs and symptoms of nonparatesticular rhabdomyosarcoma of the genitourinary tract depend on the site of origin and the size of the tumor (Hays, 1980). If the bladder or prostate is involved, the child may present with strangury caused by lower urinary tract obstruction. This condition may lead to urinary retention and secondary incontinence or infection. Hematuria may occur if tumor breaks through the lining of the genitourinary tract. If the tumor arises in the vagina, a bloody, foul-smelling discharge may be present. In the child with a sarcoma botryoides type of tumor, the tumor may prolapse through the urethra (Fig. 54–13) or be seen in the vagina. Occasionally, a child may void a fragment of tumor tissue. Pelvic rhabdomyosarcomas may grow to large size before they impinge sufficiently upon the rectum or genitourinary tract to produce symptoms. Indeed, a large palpable mass is the single most common presentation for rhabdomyosarcoma.

Diagnostic Evaluation

Although the children may present with a large abdominal mass with a primary site that is difficult to determine, the diagnostic effort is important because of the different prognosis for patients with tumors arising in different sites. These tumors may undergo both hematogenous and lymphatic dissemination, and a careful search for metastatic deposits is needed to stage the disease accurately.

Diagnostic imaging is usually satisfactorily accomplished with the intravenous urogram, CT scan, and ultrasound examination. Filling the bladder or rectum with water may permit better ultrasound imaging. If the tumor has a botryoid configuration, these imaging techniques may strongly suggest the diagnosis (see Fig. 54–14). A combination of cystoscopy and vaginoscopy is often helpful in delineating the site of the tumor. If the mucosa of the bladder or prostatic urethra is clearly abnormal and an endoscopic biopsy confirms the presence of tumor, the site of origin is most likely in the bladder wall or prostate. Similarly, a tumor that can undergo biopsy on vaginoscopy confirms the probable origin of the tumor from that structure. Often, however, these children present with a large pelvic mass which, while displacing the bladder and urethra or vagina, does not appear to involve the mucosal surfaces of these structures. In this situation, establishing the site of the primary is much more difficult. Careful bimanual examination with a cystoscope or catheter in the urethra may be useful. A large tumor may so completely fill the pelvis that its exact site of origin may not become evident until significant tumor shrinkage has been produced by chemotherapy, radiotherapy, or both.

The histologic diagnosis of rhabdomyosarcoma is established by biopsy. In obtaining an endoscopic biopsy with the pediatric resectoscope, it is important to be aware that the use of a resectoscope loop electrode may result in a sufficient degree of coagulation of the specimen to make it uninterpretable. The cold cup biopsy forceps are generally more satisfactory. These may be passed through a 13-Fr. resectoscope. The 10-Fr. resectoscope can be used with a Collings knife electrode to remove a polypoid specimen by cutting through its base and thus avoiding coagulation artifact in the rest of the specimen.

If, as is often the case, the child presents with a large abdominal mass displacing the bladder, prostate, or vagina but without evidence of mucosal abnormality, a needle biopsy may be useful. Perineal or extraperitoneal suprapubic biopsies may be obtained with needles of the Vim-Silverman type. We have found that the Tru-Cut needle usually produces an excellent core of tissue that is adequate for diagnosis. If the tumor is not able to be approached percutaneously, a laparotomy is required. A careful effort should be made to establish the origin of the tumor. Because approximately 20 per cent of genitourinary rhabdomyosarcoma will have spread to the retroperitoneal lymph nodes by the time of diagnosis (Lawrence et al., 1977), careful inspection and appropriate sampling of these nodes are important to accurately stage the tumor.

Extensive deposits may also be evident on CT scan examination of the chest, which is more successful in detecting metastatic lesions than plain film radiography. A technetium bone scan and a bone marrow aspirate or a biopsy or both are also indicated. Precision of clinical staging is warranted because of the prognostic importance of stage and the varying intensity of treatment programs.

Clinical Staging

Staging systems for rhabdomyosarcoma have largely depended on the resectability of the primary tumor and the status of the draining lymph nodes. Although there have been a number of different systems, the one most commonly employed today is that developed by the major collaborative study of rhabdomyosarcoma in the United States—the IRS (Maurer et al., 1977).

The IRS clinical grouping classification is as follows:

GROUP I
Localized disease, completely removed, regional nodes not involved.

A. Confined to muscle or organ of origin.

B. Contiguous involvement with infiltration outside the muscle or organ of origin, as through fascial planes; inclusion in this group includes both gross impression of complete removal and microscopic confirmation of complete removal.

GROUP II
A. Grossly removed tumor with microscopic residual disease; no evidence of gross residual tumor; no evidence of regional node involvement.

B. Regional disease, completely removed (regional nodes involved and/or extension of tumor into an adjacent organ; no microscopic residual disease).

C. Regional disease with involved nodes, grossly removed, but with evidence of microscopic residual disease.

GROUP III
Incomplete removal or biopsy with gross residual disease.

GROUP IV
Distant metastatic disease present at onset.

One problem with this staging system is that the stage is dependent on the type of surgical resection carried out before initiation of chemotherapy. This arrangement may produce a situation wherein equivalent pathologic stages are considered as different clinical stages. In the report of the first IRS, 118 patients with genitourinary tumors were staged as follows: group I, 36 patients; group II, 28 patients; group III, 27 patients; and group IV, 27 patients (Maurer et al., 1977). As can be seen, more than half of patients have disseminated disease (groups III, IV) when diagnosed.

Currently, the IRS is exploring a presurgical staging system and will compare that with the clinical grouping system described here.

Treatment

Historical Approach

Surgical excision of the primary tumor was the first successful form of treatment of rhabdomyosarcoma. Often, this required a radical excision, which, for genitourinary rhabdomyosarcoma, meant an anterior or total pelvic exenteration. Long-term survival for patients with vaginal tumors treated by surgery alone was 40 per cent and for patients with bladder/prostate rhabdomyosarcoma, 73 per cent (Green and Jaffe, 1978). These surgical results were considerably better than what was achieved for rhabdomyosarcoma elsewhere in the body. The improved prognosis for bladder/prostate rhabdomyosarcoma when compared with that for vaginal rhabdomyosarcoma may be related to the fact that these tumors become symptomatic sooner and thus have less opportunity to become disseminated. Ghazali (1973) found that botyroid-type embryonal tumors of the bladder had a better outlook compared with solid embryonal tumors, perhaps because botryoid tumors are more superficial and are discovered sooner.

Ancillary treatment of rhabdomyosarcoma with radiation therapy began to emerge following the 1950 report by Stobbe and Dargeon that at least some rhabdomyosarcomas are radiosensitive. Experience indicated that persistent local control of tumor often required a high dose of radiation therapy, in excess of 4500 cGy (Edland, 1965; Sagerman et al., 1972). D'Angio and colleagues (1959) recognized the favorable synergism that actinomycin D had with radiation therapy for rhabdomyosarcoma.

Chemotherapy for rhabdomyosarcoma developed with single agents employed for the treatment of metastatic disease. The following drugs have been recognized to be effective: vincristine, actinomycin D, cyclophosphamide, mitomycin C, doxorubicin, imidazole carboxamide, cisplatin, and eptoposide (Baum et al., 1981; Green and Jaffe, 1978). Later, these drugs were combined in various protocols for the treatment of metastatic disease.

In 1961, Pinkel and Pickren suggested coordinating aggressive initial surgery with postoperative radiotherapy and "prophylactic" chemotherapy following what appeared to be grossly complete tumor removal, to try to eliminate microscopic residual disease. The effectiveness of this approach was confirmed by Heyn and associates in 1974. These investigators reported the results in children with localized rhabdomyosarcoma who were rendered grossly free of tumor by radical surgery. They were then treated with postoperative radiation therapy with or without actinomycin D and vincristine administered for 1 year. Of 28 patients, 24 (85.8 per cent) survived relapse-free for 2 years after initial treatment if chemotherapy had been administered, compared with only 7 of 15 (47 per cent) of those children who received no chemotherapy. The difference was statistically significant. This finding indicated the importance of administration of multiple-agent chemotherapy to all children with rhabdomyosarcoma. An extension of the role of chemotherapy was suggested by Wilbur (1974) to make even the advanced lesions amenable to surgical treatment.

As more therapeutic alternatives began to become available for the treatment of rhabdomyosarcoma, it became evident that the limited clinical experience of individual institutions would not permit an evaluation of the available options. Thus, in 1972, the IRS was born. This group has carried out prospective multidisciplinary studies of rhabdomyosarcoma.

The first IRS trial, which ran from 1972 to 1978, adhered to the prevailing approach to management at that time. An effort was made surgically to resect the tumor with follow-up radiation therapy and chemotherapy (Hays et al., 1981, 1982a). Of the 62 patients with sarcoma arising in the bladder, prostate, or vagina, 34 (55 per cent) had all gross tumor removed at the primary operation. Chemotherapy consisted of vincristine, actinomycin D, and cyclophosphamide (VAC) for 2 years in most cases.

Of the 54 patients with bladder and prostate rhabdomyosarcoma, 47 (87 per cent) were treated with radiation therapy with doses varying from 2000 to 5500 cGy. Of these 54 patients, 41 (76 per cent) are alive and relapse-free at a median of 4.5 years. Of these 41, 16 (39 per cent) have avoided exenterative surgery and retain the bladder. Eight patients had vaginal rhabdomyosarcoma, half of whom were treated with radiation therapy as well as chemotherapy. Seven of the eight

patients (88 per cent) are alive and relapse-free for 4 or more years, and six of the seven (86 per cent) have retained the bladder. The overall survival rate for IRS-I was 50 of 62 patients (81 per cent). This is a substantial improvement over the historical series of patients treated by surgery alone.

Recurrence of tumor in IRS-I, whether local or distant, occurred within 2 years of initiation of treatment in all but two children. These two late recurrences were successfully treated and represent the only survivors of recurrent rhabdomyosarcoma. Thus, relapse is particularly ominous with this tumor with only 2 of 13 patients (15 per cent) being long-term survivors. One patient died of treatment-related causes.

Current Therapeutic Approach

After the demonstration that chemotherapy and radiation therapy were clearly effective for rhabdomyosarcoma, a widespread interest developed in the possible utilization of primary chemotherapy and radiation therapy to avoid the exenterative surgery so often previously required for genitourinary rhabdomyosarcoma (Maurer, 1980; Ortega, 1979; Rivard et al., 1975). This approach was studied in IRS-II (Hays et al., 1982b; Raney et al., 1983). Primary surgical treatment was restricted to tumor biopsy only. Subsequent management was as presented in Figure 54–15.

Intense chemotherapy with repetitive monthly courses of VAC (pulse-VAC) followed. After 8 weeks of treatment, the patient underwent clinical and radiologic re-evaluation. If there was a complete or partial response, chemotherapy was continued until week 16. At this time, a similar re-evaluation was followed by surgical exploration, to determine the extent of residual disease. If there was gross or microscopic residual disease after surgical resection, the patient had radiotherapy added to the program and then continued on pulse-VAC therapy for a total of 2 years. If there was no residual tumor present after surgery, the radiotherapy was omitted, but the patient continued on pulse-VAC chemotherapy for 2 years.

IRS-II is now closed and some conclusions can be drawn from the information thus far accrued (Raney et al., 1983). The hope that primary chemotherapy would avoid the need for radiation therapy and radical surgery has not been realized. Only about 10 per cent of patients have achieved relapse-free survival with chemotherapy alone. Three quarters of patients with bladder/prostate tumors required radiotherapy. Approximately two thirds of these patients are alive and relapse-free with a median follow-up of 2.7 years. Although the IRS-II design led to a higher rate of bladder salvage early, by 3 years after beginning treatment, only one fourth of the survivors still retained the bladder (Raney, B., Jr., Personal Communication, 1989). Of the patients with vaginal rhabdomyosarcomas, all are surviving, but two thirds required partial vaginectomy to remove residual tumor. The overall survival rate for IRS-II thus far is 80 per cent, which is virtually identical to the survival rate in IRS-I.

The IRS-III trial, just undergoing analysis now, in-

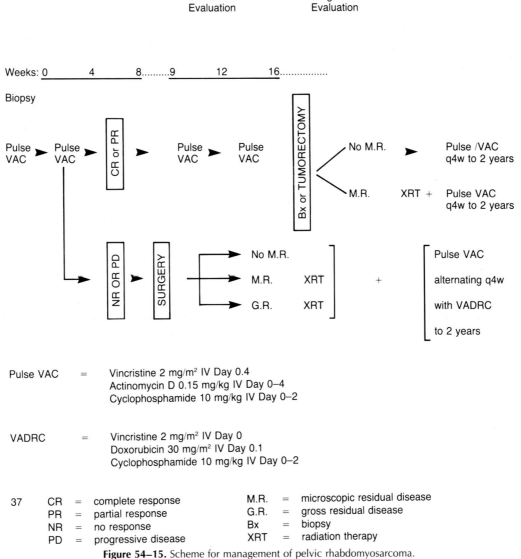

Pulse VAC   =   Vincristine 2 mg/m² IV Day 0.4
                Actinomycin D 0.15 mg/kg IV Day 0–4
                Cyclophosphamide 10 mg/kg IV Day 0–2

VADRC   =   Vincristine 2 mg/m² IV Day 0
                Doxorubicin 30 mg/m² IV Day 0.1
                Cyclophosphamide 10 mg/kg IV Day 0–2

37 CR = complete response   M.R. = microscopic residual disease
    PR = partial response   G.R. = gross residual disease
    NR = no response   Bx   = biopsy
    PD = progressive disease   XRT   = radiation therapy

Figure 54–15. Scheme for management of pelvic rhabdomyosarcoma.

corporated the addition of doxorubicin and cisplatin to the VAC regimen. Also, radiotherapy was given to patients with prostate and bladder neck tumors beginning at 6 weeks after diagnosis. The results should be available in the near future.

Optimal therapy for rhabdomyosarcoma has yet to be completely defined. Perhaps a more intense chemotherapy program as advocated by Voute and Vos (1977) and Voute and colleagues (1984) will be more effective. With respect to radiotherapy, it has now been recognized that moderately high doses of radiation, in the range of 4000 to 5500 cGy, are required to prevent an increased incidence of local recurrence (Tefft, 1981). It may be that altering the timing of radiotherapy will improve results. The timing and nature of surgical intervention may be altered to improve survival. Procedures including total cystectomy will still be required in a sizable number of cases. It is hoped that, in the future, a combination of treatments will evolve that will permit a high rate of survival without requiring extensive mutilative surgical procedures (Donaldson, 1989).

IRS-IV is being launched now; it is based on the results of IRS-II, because the results of IRS-III are too preliminary. An important change is a plan to evaluate the validity of a treatment based on the pretreatment (tumor, node, metastasis; TNM) stage.* Staging will follow this format:

- *Stage I:* All favorable sites, nonmetastatic (Ta, Tb; N0, N1; M0)
- *Stage II:* All favorable sites, primary tumor less than 5 cm in diameter, nodes negative, nonmetastatic (Ta; N0; M0)
- *Stage III:* All unfavorable sites with primary tumor greater than 5 cm in diameter and/or nodes positive (Ta; N1; M0 or Tb; N0; M0 or Tb; N1; M0)
- *Stage IV:* All metastatic disease

*Ta, tumor less than 5 cm in greatest diameter; Tb, tumor is 5 cm or larger; N0, regional lymph nodes are not clinically involved; N1, regional nodes are clinically involved by tumor; M0, no distant metastases; and M1, metastases are present.

Chemotherapy is based on the stage, with stages I, II, and III being randomized to one of three regimens: A = VAC, B = VAI, and C = VIE (V, vincristine; A, actinomycin D; I, ifosfamide; and E, etoposide).

Local radiotherapy is given starting at week 9 and is based on the old IRS grouping system (resulting from the initial surgical procedure). Hyperfractionation of radiotherapy will be randomized in group 3 to see if effect can be improved while morbidity is reduced. Thus, radiation therapy will entail: group 1, no radiation therapy; group 2, standard radiation therapy of 5040 cGy (180 cGy for 28 days); and group 3, randomized between standard radiotherapy and hyperfractionated therapy of 5940 cGy (110 cGy b.i.d. for 54 days).

Other Pelvic Tumors

Transitional cell carcinoma of the bladder is very rare before puberty (Benson et al., 1983; Ray et al., 1973). Most such tumors in children are of low grade and stage. Almost all can be managed by endoscopic resection fulguration, or both. Random bladder biopsies rarely detect any further abnormality. When the bladder appears to be free from tumor at the initial follow-up cystoscopy a few months later, it is rare to see a recurrence. It appears likely that transitional cell carcinomas in children are not part of a field defect as is more likely in adults. When the cancer is invasive in children, it is managed in a fashion similar to that for adults.

Leiomyosarcoma of the bladder is a very rare soft tissue sarcoma in children (MacKenzie et al., 1968). Biologically, the tumor is less aggressive than rhabdomyosarcoma, and local excision usually provides adequate therapy.

Adenocarcinoma of the exstrophied bladder or that arising from the urachus tends to be seen in adults rather than children (Engle and Wilkinson, 1970). Although endoscopic surveillance of adults with a closed bladder exstrophy appears to be warranted, the risk of cancer is not sufficiently high to discourage attempts at functional reconstruction of bladder exstrophy.

Neurofibroma of the bladder may occur in a patient with neurofibromatosis. A case has been reported in which neurofibroma caused such bilateral ureteral obstruction that local excision required bladder augmentation by ileocecal cystoplasty (Schoenberg and Murphy, 1961).

Lymphohemangioma may occur in the pelvis and invade the bladder and ureters. Although it is a benign hamartomatous tumor, we have seen a case involving incontinence caused by invasion of the tumor and compression of the bladder; the patient was satisfactorily treated with restoration of continence by bladder augmentation using ileocecal cystoplasty.

Clear cell adenocarcinoma may occur in either the vagina or the cervix. Maternal diethylstilbestrol (DES) during pregnancy has been strongly implicated in the etiology of this tumor (Herbst et al., 1976; Ulfelder, 1976). DES-related adenocarcinoma is very rare before age 14 years. The peak incidence is at age 19, and the tumor rarely develops after age 24 years. Although much emphasized in the press, the actual risk is quite low (1/1000) (Herbst et al., 1977).

Benign adenosis, also caused by DES, is more common than clear cell carcinoma. Adenosis appears as ridges or folds in the vagina or cervix and, because it contains no glycogen, it does not stain with Schiller's iodine. Adenosis, which may be the precursor to adenocarcinoma, appears to heal with time, probably accounting for the incidence of this tumor mainly in young women. These tumors are equally divided between the cervix and the vagina, and survival for clear cell adenocarcinoma is directly related to the size of the primary tumor and the depth of invasion. The larger the tumor, the more likely it is to be symptomatic; thus, a patient with symptoms tends to have a worse prognosis. Radical surgical excision is still advocated, although radiotherapy may also produce a good outcome. Overall 5-year survival is about 80 per cent (Herbst, 1980).

Adenocarcinoma of the infant vagina is a rare, highly malignant tumor, which histologically resembles the embryonal cell carcinoma that is seen in the infant testis (Chu et al., 1978; Norris et al., 1970). Hinman and Perez-Mesa (1958) speculated that this tumor may arise in mesonephric remnants, although an endodermal diverticulum of the yolk-sac or extraembryonic membranes could also be a possible source. The mesonephric papilloma, a form of hamartoma, is occasionally found in the infant vagina and may be the benign form of this tumor.

Squamous cell carcinoma of the cervix (Pollack and Taylor, 1979) and *adenocarcinoma of the uterus* (Lockhart, 1935) are both exceedingly rare tumors in children.

TESTIS TUMORS IN CHILDREN

Testicular tumors in children are not uncommon, accounting for about 1 to 2 per cent of all pediatric solid tumors (Ise et al., 1976). Pediatric testicular tumors represent roughly 2 per cent of all testicular tumors (Manger, 1973). The peak age incidence occurs at roughly 2 years (Li and Fraumeni, 1972).

In contradistinction to adults, in whom germ cell tumors represent about 95 per cent of all testis tumors, germ cell tumors represent only 60 to 75 per cent of testis tumors occurring in children. Another distinction between adults and children is the higher incidence of benign tumors in the pediatric population when compared with the adult population (Hopkins et al., 1978). Whereas only a small number of adult testis tumors are benign, between one fourth and one third of pediatric testis tumors are not malignant. However, there is no doubt that some of these tumors in children do result in death. From 1960 to 1967, the death rate from testis tumors for children in the United States has been calculated at just under 1 death per 10,000,000 population per year. Roughly half the deaths occur in patients with yolk-sac tumors (Li and Fraumeni, 1972).

Classification of Prepubertal Testis Tumors

No universally accepted system has been developed for classification of prepubertal testis tumors. Seminomas and choriocarcinomas are extremely rare in children, so adult classifications are not entirely appropriate. With this in mind, the Section on Urology of the American Academy of Pediatrics has proposed the classification shown in Table 54–11. The distribution of tumor types is shown in Table 54–12, which is taken from the data of Houser and co-workers (1965).

Presentation

As in adults, the most common presentation is a painless scrotal swelling. Testis tumors may be mistaken for epididymitis, testicular torsion, inguinal hernia, or hydrocele. The last is not surprising, because 10 to 25 per cent of malignant testis tumors are associated with a hydrocele (Karamehmedovic et al., 1975). Aside from an occasionally painful paratesticular rhabdomyosarcoma or hormonally active nongerminal cell tumor, most testis tumors are asymptomatic in children. Thus, it is no surprise that there is often a significant delay between noticing a mass and presenting for evaluation.

On physical examination, a hard mass may be readily evident. Conversely, some patients who have hormonally active tumors may have such small lesions that the testis feels normal on palpation. A normal physical examination is not sufficient to exclude a tumor. An ultrasound examination may be particularly helpful in this situation (Ilondo et al., 1981). Transillumination of a hydrocele may permit identification of an enlarged testis; however, ultrasonography is generally more reliable (Leopold et al., 1979). If there has been lymphatic

Table 54–11. CLASSIFICATION OF PREPUBERTAL TESTIS TUMORS

I. Germ cell tumors
  Yolk-sac tumor
  Teratoma
  Teratocarcinoma
  Seminoma
II. Gonadal stromal tumors
  Leydig cell
  Sertoli cell
  Intermediate forms
III. Gonadoblastoma
IV. Tumors of supporting tissues
  Fibroma
  Leiomyoma
  Hemangioma
V. Lymphomas and leukemias
VI. Tumor-like lesions
  Epidermoid cyst
  Hyperplastic nodule attributable to congenital adrenal
    hyperplasia
VII. Secondary tumors
VIII. Tumors of adnexa

Data from Kaplan G. W.: Testicular tumors in children. AUA Update Series, Lesson 12, Vol 2, 1983.

Table 54–12. DISTRIBUTION OF TESTIS TUMOR TYPES IN CHILDREN

	%
Yolk sac	47
Leydig cell	18
Teratoma	14
Sertoli cell	10
Rhabdomyosarcoma	4
Lymphoma	2
Fibrosarcoma	1
Other sarcomas	1
Hemangioma	0.5
Fibroma	0.5
Other	2

Adapted from Houser, R., et al.: Am. J. Surg., 110:876, 1965.

dissemination, an abdominal mass or a supraclavicular node may be palpable.

Germ Cell Tumors

The most common germ cell tumor, indeed, the most common prepubertal testis tumor overall, is the *yolk-sac carcinoma* (Pierce et al., 1970; Weissbach et al., 1984). This tumor has been known by a plethora of terms, including endodermal sinus tumor, orchidoblastoma, embryonal adenocarcinoma, embryonal carcinoma, infantile adenocarcinoma of the testis, and testicular adenocarcinoma with clear cells. Most of these terms reflect the confusion concerning the exact origin of the tumor.

Current opinion supports Teilum's (1959) concept that these tumors originate from yolk-sac elements that were present early in the life of the embryo. The histologic hallmark of yolk-sac tumors is the presence of eosinophilic, PAS-positive inclusions in the cytoplasm of the clear cells, which by specific staining techniques can be shown to consist of alpha-fetoprotein (AFP) (Kurman et al., 1977). AFP is made by yolk-sac cells in the embryo but has usually disappeared from the serum by 3 months of age. AFP levels are usually elevated in children with yolk-sac carcinoma and thus provide a biologic marker for the tumor. The half-life of AFP is 5 days so that, after successful removal of a yolk-sac tumor, levels should be normal (less than 20 ng/ml), usually within 1 month.

Although these tumors may bear some histologic resemblance to adult embryonal tumors (Brown, 1976), their clinical behavior is quite different; this has led to controversy concerning management. The tumor tends to occur in infancy, usually in children under the age of 2 years. It tends to remain localized for a relatively long period of time. When spread occurs, it is predominantly hematogenous spread to the lungs (20 per cent) and much less commonly spread by the lymphatics to the retroperitoneal nodes (4 to 5 per cent) (Brosman, 1979). This tendency for nodal spread is much less common than that with embryonal carcinoma in the adult. In a young child, the prognosis is excellent. Brosman (1979) reported a 2-year tumor-free survival rate of 89 per cent in children younger than 2 years of age, but only 23 per cent for those older than 2 years. The series of Jeffs (1972), Exelby (1979), and Drago and associates (1978) confirm the favorable prognosis for the young child.

Controversy has centered on management. Although retroperitoneal metastases are not frequent, Staubitz and colleagues (1965) demonstrated that patients with retroperitoneal disease can be cured by orchiectomy and retroperitoneal node dissection alone. In most series, the retroperitoneal node dissection did not demonstrate tumor; however, microscopic metastases may have been missed. Because of possible long-term morbidity of retroperitoneal node dissection and the presence of a good marker (i.e., AFP) for the tumor, the advisability of routine node dissection has been raised. Additionally, combination chemotherapy with vincristine, actinomycin D, and cyclophosphamide (i.e., VAC) with or without doxorubicin has been effective with this tumor (Colodny and Hopkins, 1977; Exelby, 1979; Griffin et al., 1987). Kramer (1981) pointed out the ability of chemotherapy to salvage patients who experience relapse. Radiotherapy is not indicated unless retroperitoneal nodes are demonstrated to contain tumor (Tefft et al., 1967).

Based on these facts, our current practice is as follows: A radical inguinal orchiectomy is carried out with initial AFP level determination. CT and ultrasound are used to evaluate the retroperitoneum and chest for evidence of dissemination. If a child younger than 1 year of age has an AFP level that rapidly falls to normal and has no evidence of metastatic spread, he is observed for 2 years with chest radiographs and serum AFP levels. If the chest examination findings are negative but the retroperitoneum is suspicious looking, especially if the AFP level remains elevated after orchiectomy, laparatomy and retroperitoneal node sampling are carried out. All resectable tumor is removed. If the chest examination findings are negative but retroperitoneal disease is present, chemotherapy is begun with VAC, with or without doxorubicin, as for rhabdomyosarcoma. Radiation therapy is usually not employed. If pulmonary metastases are present, surgical removal may be indicated. If multiple metastases are present, chemotherapy is begun, and the child is watched closely for response. If there is not a prompt decrease in tumor, bilateral pulmonary radiotherapy is added. Because children over 1 year of age are at increased risk for pulmonary metastases, we generally give a course of vincristine and actinomycin D for a total of six courses over 1 year. Kramer's (1981) report of salvage chemotherapy may call this approach into question. Additionally, vinblastine, bleomycin and cisplatin, which have been given in the treatment of adult testicular carcinoma, may help salvage cases of recurrent yolk-sac carcinoma (Chu et al., 1978; Holbrook et al., 1980). The management of this tumor will continue to evolve in the future.

Other germ cell tumors of childhood are the *teratoma and teratocarcinoma*. These tumors contain elements derived from more than one of the three germ tissues: ectoderm, endoderm, and mesoderm. The lesions are often cystic and may transilluminate. The lesions can be bilateral (Carney et al., 1973). On cut section, there may be skin and sebum, hair, neural tissue, bone, and even teeth. Testicular teratomas in infancy and childhood are usually mature with well-differentiated tissue. Pure immature teratoma with primitive endoderm, neuroectoderm, and mesoderm is extremely rare. About 15 per cent of teratomas contain areas of dedifferentiation with a malignant appearance. In spite of this, testicular teratomas found in children younger than 24 months of age are consistently benign. Orchiectomy or the simple removal of the tumor with salvage of the remaining testicular tissue will provide a cure.

The older patient with testicular teratocarcinoma is managed similarly to the adult with germ cell tumor. The prognosis for these patients has been much improved using chemotherapy regimens that employ cisplatin, bleomycin, and vinblastine. More than 80 per cent of patients with disseminated disease can be expected to be long-term survivors (Einhorn and Donohue, 1979).

Seminoma is extremely rare before puberty (Viprakasit et al., 1977). It is seen in boys in whom puberty and spermatogenesis occur early and should in essence be considered a postpubertal tumor. Management is the same as that in the adult.

Gonadal stromal tumors are the most common nongerminal testicular tumors in children. *Leydig cell tumors* are the most common gonadal stromal tumor, both in children and in adults. The peak incidence is in children 4 to 5 years of age. Leydig cells, normally producers of testosterone, may continue testosterone synthesis when they undergo neoplastic transformation, and consequently, Leydig cell tumors may produce precocious puberty (Pomer et al., 1954). Rapid somatic growth, increased bone age, deepening voice, phallic growth, and pubic hair development may precede the appearance of a palpable mass. The hallmark of the diagnosis is the triad of precocious puberty, testicular mass, and elevated urinary 17-ketosteroid level. Leydig cell tumors account for about 10 per cent of cases of precocious puberty in boys (Urban et al., 1978). The differentiation from pituitary lesions, which may also cause precocious puberty, is made by finding LH and FSH at low prepubertal levels with an elevated serum testosterone level.

Leydig cell tumors may also be associated with gynecomastia. Johnstone (1967) reported gynecomastia in five of 39 reviewed cases of Leydig cell tumor. Although estrogen levels are usually elevated with these tumors, gynecomastia is more pronounced when the progesterone level is elevated. The estrogen increase is thought to produce an alteration in the normal androgen-to-estrogen ratio and, thus, lead to an overproduction of growth hormone. This change results in an advancement of bone age, which may not completely regress following removal of the tumor (Ilondo et al., 1981).

Leydig cell tumors must be differentiated from the hyperplastic nodules that often develop in the testis of boys with poorly controlled congenital adrenal hyperplasia (CAH). Because CAH is genetically transmitted, a family history may be useful. Moderate elevation of the urinary 17-ketosteroid level may occur in both conditions. However, a major elevation is characteristic of the 17-hydroxylase deficiency type of CAH. Urinary pregnanetriol levels are absent with Leydig cell tumors but significantly elevated with 21-hydroxylase deficiency–type CAH. When CAH is brought under control with replacement glucocorticoids, the hyperplastic testicular nodules will regress, whereas a Leydig cell tumor remains unchanged.

Treatment for Leydig cell tumors is simple orchiectomy, because they are very rarely malignant (Mostofi and Price, 1973). Simple enucleation of the tumor has been suggested when the diagnosis has been made preoperatively (Urban et al., 1978).

Sertoli cell tumors are the next most common gonadal stromal tumors of childhood. They appear earlier than Leydig cell tumors, usually as a painless mass in a boy under 6 months of age. Histologically, the tumor resembles the fetal testis (Brosman, 1979). They generally produce no endocrinologic effect on the child. Although several malignant tumors have been found in adults, only one with documented retroperitoneal metastases has been found in a child (Rosvoll and Woodard, 1968). Orchiectomy alone is sufficient treatment, but careful follow-up for possible retroperitoneal spread is appropriate.

The *gonadoblastoma* is believed to recapitulate gonadal development more completely than any other tumor. It is a neoplasm containing an intimate mixture of germ cells and germinal stromal cells (Scully, 1970). Usually, the germ cells overgrow the other elements, and the tumor resembles a dysgerminoma (seminoma) and is not hormonally active. In less than 10 per cent of cases, more malignant germ cell tumors may be also present. The tumor is bilateral in one third of cases.

The tumor develops almost exclusively in abnormal gonads in children whose karyotype contains a Y chromosome. The most common karyotypes are 46XY and 45XO/46XY. All of these children have sexual abnormalities. Eighty per cent are phenotypic females with intra-abdominal testes (testicular feminization syndrome) or female phenotypes with intra-abdominal streak gonads and a karyotype with a Y (pure gonadal dysgenesis, XY type). Of gonadoblastomas, 20 per cent arise in patients whose phenotypes are tending more to the male line, but which often exhibit ambiguity. The gonads may be bilaterally dysgenetic cryptorchid testes or a streak associated with a contralateral testis (mixed gonadal dysgenesis).

The likelihood of gonadoblastoma arises significantly at puberty in these intersex states, all of which have a Y chromosome in the karyotype (Manuel et al., 1976; Mulvihill et al., 1975). Although metastatic spread of gonadoblastoma is not common, appropriate treatment is by gonadectomy before the development of the tumor.

Tumor-Like Lesions of the Testis

The hyperplastic testicular nodules associated with CAH were discussed previously in the section about Leydig cell tumors. *Epidermoid cysts* of the testis may present as a painless mass. The cysts are usually single and lined by squamous epithelium, and they contain keratinized debris. No teratomatous elements are present. These lesions make up less than 1 per cent of all testis tumors (Price, 1969). These tumors are benign and could be removed with testicular preservation; however, an orchiectomy is usually carried out.

Secondary Tumors

The most common malignancies to secondarily involve the testis are lymphomas and leukemias. About 4 per cent of male patients with *Burkitt's lymphoma* will have a tumor involving the testis, and this may be the main presenting symptom (Lamm and Kaplan, 1974). The testis may also be involved by acute lymphoblastic leukemia (ALL) (Oakhill et al., 1980). Because the testis appears to act as a sanctuary site, perhaps secondary to the blood-testis barrier, it has become apparent that as patients with ALL are increasingly controlled by chemotherapy, the testis may come to harbor residual tumor. In many centers, it has been routine to obtain bilateral testicular biopsies before discontinuing treatment in patients who are apparently cured of the leukemia. About 10 per cent will have positive results and about two thirds of these patients may eventually be salvaged by further chemotherapy and radiation therapy to the testes (Byrd, 1981; Wong et al., 1980). Although enough stromal elements may survive to avoid a need for hormonal replacement, fertility is unlikely.

Rarely, *Wilms' tumor* and *neuroblastoma* may spread to the testis via the processus vaginalis and confused with a primary testis tumor (deCamargo et al., 1988).

Tumors of the Adnexa

Although it is not actually a testis tumor, *paratesticular rhabdomyosarcoma* must be considered because it arises in the mesenchymal tissue of the spermatic cord and appears as a scrotal mass, which is occasionally tender. These tumors may grow rapidly, and a hydrocele may be present.

Most paratesticular rhabdomyosarcomas are of the embryonal type. As with other genitourinary rhabdomyosarcomas, early metastasis to lymph nodes or by hematogenous spread is common, and long-term survival was less than 50 per cent before the advent of effective chemotherapy and radiotherapy. Current experience suggests that about 90 per cent of these boys should be long-term survivors (Raney et al., 1987).

Paratesticular rhabdomyosarcoma has a higher incidence of retroperitoneal spread than other genitourinary malignancies. Raney and colleagues (1978), in their initial review of the IRS experience, found 40 per cent positive retroperitoneal node dissections and confirmed this percentage by a review of the literature. Although most of these cases can be salvaged by radiotherapy and chemotherapy, this is not without significant morbidity, such as bowel obstruction, intestinal fistula, and myelosuppression (Tefft et al., 1976). A routine retroperitoneal node dissection is indicated to stage the disease (Banowsky and Shultz, 1970; Olney et al., 1979). Because there is no convincing evidence that it is the node dissection itself which improves salvage, the dissection is usually a unilateral one on the side of the tumor with sampling of any suspicious contralateral nodes. By avoiding bilateral node dissection, later problems with ejaculation may be prevented (Bracken and Johnson, 1976).

A mention must be made of the approach to a group of patients (Olive et al., 1984; Olive-Sommelet, 1989) in which staging retroperitoneal node dissection was not performed; instead, the investigators relied on lymphangiography, ultrasound, and CT. Between 1971 and 1988, 46 boys, representing 65 per cent of those presenting with paratesticular rhabdomyosarcoma, had a negative evaluation and thus were thought to have, at most, micrometastasis in the retroperitoneum. All have received only intensive chemotherapy, and all 46 are surviving disease-free with a follow-up of at least 3 years in 34. Although this approach is interesting, it should be noted that many boys were treated with doxorubicin, with its known effect of long-term cardiomyotoxicity. It is the belief of the IRS investigators that there is more potential morbidity from this chemotherapy than from the staging retroperitoneal dissection described previously.

Our current recommendations for treatment of patients with paratesticular rhabdomyosarcoma are as follows (Cromie et al., 1979; Raney et al., 1987): After the diagnosis is confirmed following an inguinal orchiectomy, all patients without distant metastasis should undergo retroperitoneal lymph node biopsy. If the results of the biopsies are negative, chemotherapy is carried out as described for rhabdomyosarcoma, and radiation therapy is omitted. If the biopsies of the nodes show positive results, radiotherapy to the retroperitoneal node area is advised, along with chemotherapy. If a transscrotal procedure has been carried out to establish the diagnosis, then either hemiscrotectomy or radiotherapy of the scrotum is indicated. To protect the contralateral testis from radiotherapy, it may be relocated to the thigh (D'Angio et al., 1974).

Tumors Arising in the Undescended Testis

One clearly identifiable risk factor associated with testicular malignancy is the presence of an undescended testis. About 10 per cent of all germinal tumors of the testis develop in an undescended testis (Fonkalsrud, 1970; Gallager, 1976). The risk of malignancy in an undescended testis is about 35 times greater than that in a descended testis. A testis in the inguinal canal has an approximate 1 per cent risk compared with an approximate 5 per cent risk for the intra-abdominal testis (Campbell, 1942, 1959). The 15 per cent of cryptorchid testes that are intra-abdominal contribute almost 50 per cent of the malignancies. The degree of seminiferous tubule dysgenesis appears to correlate directly with the likelihood of malignant degeneration. Boys with cryptorchidism have a higher incidence of dysgenesis in the contralateral descended testis, and along with that an increased risk of tumor formation in that testis. Campbell's review (1942) indicated that, with bilateral cryptorchidism associated with testicular tumors, there was a 25 per cent incidence of bilateral tumors.

The most common tumor that arises in an undescended testis is the seminoma. However, if the testis is brought down into the scrotum, the incidence of embryonal carcinoma rises (Batata et al., 1980). Although it has been always assumed that there would be a higher incidence of inguinal metastases in an undescended testis that had been surgically placed into the scrotum because of the disturbance in lymphatic drainage, at least one review has found this not to be so (Batata et al., 1980). The prognosis for an individual who develops a malignancy in a surgically treated undescended testis parallels that of an individual with normally descended gonads who develops a malignancy.

Orchidopexy early in life has become common only in recent years. At present, it is rare to see a testis tumor develop in a boy who had an orchidopexy before age 5. However, our period of follow-up is not adequate yet to establish this fact firmly. An orchidopexy carried out after puberty does nothing to diminish the risk of malignancy. The current recommendation is for orchiectomy and placement of a testicular prosthesis if the other testis is satisfactorily in the scrotum (Martin, 1979). Hinman (1979) suggested the removal of all intra-abdominal testes if the contralateral one appears to be satisfactorily positioned and normal. We continue to carry out orchidopexy for these testes, often using the Fowler-Stephens technique (Gibbons et al., 1979).

Because spontaneous testicular descent ceases after 1 year of age, our current recommendation is to carry out orchidopexy soon after 1 year of age, once the diagnosis can be clearly established. Because the average age for the development of a tumor in a formerly undescended testis appears to be age 40, it is clear that prolonged awareness of an increased tumor risk is important. We instruct the families of our patients to ensure that the boys are instructed in testicular self-examination beginning after puberty. This issue seems particularly relevant because testicular tumors are now the leading cause of death from solid tumors in all men between the ages of 15 and 34 years (Grabstald, 1975).

REFERENCES

Wilms' Tumor

Altman, R. P., Anderson, K. D., Matlak, M. E., et al.: Evolution of surgical treatment of bilateral Wilms' tumor. Surgery, 82:760, 1977.

Asch, M. J., Siegel, S., White, L., Fonkalsrud, E., Hays, D., and Isaacs, H.: Prognostic factors and outcome in bilateral Wilms' tumor. Cancer, 56:2524, 1985.

Aterman, K., Grantmyre, E., and Gillis, D. A.: Extrarenal Wilms' tumor: A review and case report. Invest. Cell Pathol., 2:309, 1979.

Banner, M. P., Pollack, H. M., Chatten, J., and Witzleben, C.: Multilocular renal cysts: Radiologic-pathologic correlation. AJR, 136:239, 1981.

Baum, E. S., and Gaynon, P. S.: Phase II, Trial of cis-dichlorodiammine-platinum II in refractory childhood cancer: Children's Cancer Study Group Report. Cancer Treat. Rep., 65:815, 1981.

Beckwith, J. B., Kiviat, N. B., and Bonadio, J. F.: Nephrogenic rests, nephroblastomatosis, and the pathogenesis of Wilms' tumor. Pediatr. Pathol., 10(1–2):1–36, 1990.

Beckwith, J. B., Norkool, P., Breslow, N., and D'Angio, G. J.:

Clinical observations in children with clear-cell sarcoma of the kidney [Abstract]. Proc. Am. Assoc. Cancer Res., 27:200, 1986.

Beckwith, J. B., and Palmer, N. F.: Histopathology and prognosis of Wilms' tumor. Cancer, 41:1937, 1978.

Belt, T. G., Cohen, M. D., Smith, J. A., et al.: MRI of Wilms' tumor: Promise as the primary imaging method. AJR, 146:955–961, 1986.

Bennington, J. L., and Beckwith, J. B.: Tumors of the kidney, renal pelvis, and ureter. In Atlas of Tumor Pathology, Second Series, Fascicle 12. Bethesda, Armed Forces Institute of Pathology, 1975.

Bishop, H. C., Tefft, M., Evans, A. E., and D'Angio, G. J.: Survival in bilateral Wilms' tumor—review of 30 National Wilms' Tumor Study cases. J. Pediatr. Surg., 12:631, 1977.

Blank, E., Neerhout, R. C., and Burry, K. A.: Congenital mesoblastic nephroma and polyhydramnios. JAMA, 240:1504, 1978.

Blute, M. L., Kelalis, P. P., Offord, K. P., Breslow, N., Beckwith, J. B., and D'Angio, G. J.: Bilateral Wilms' tumor. J. Urol., 138:968–973, 1987.

Bolande, R. P.: Congenital mesoblastic nephroma of infancy. In Perspectives in Pediatric Pathology, Vol. 1. Chicago, Year Book Medical Publishers, 1973.

Bolande, R. P.: Congenital and infantile neoplasia of the kidney. Lancet, 2:1497, 1974.

Bonadio, J. F., Storer, B., Norkool, P., Farewell, V. T., Beckwith, J. B., and D'Angio, G. J.: Anaplastic Wilms' tumor: Clinical and pathological studies. J. Clin. Oncol., 3:513–520, 1985.

Bond, J. V.: Bilateral Wilms' tumour and urinary tract anomalies. Lancet, 2:721, 1975a.

Bond, J. V.: Bilateral Wilms' tumour: Age at diagnosis, associated congenital anomalies and possible pattern of inheritance. Lancet, 2:482, 1975b.

Bove, K. E., and McAdams, A. J.: The nephroblastomatosis complex and relationship to Wilms' tumor: A clinico-pathologic treatise. Perspect. Pediatr. Pathol., 3:185, 1976.

Bracken, R. B., Sutow, W. W., Jaffe, N., et al.: Preoperative chemotherapy for Wilms' tumor. Urology, 19:55, 1982.

Breslow, N. E., and Beckwith, J. B.: Epidemiological features of Wilms' tumor. JNCI, 68:429, 1982.

Breslow, N. E., Beckwith, J. B., Ciol, M., and Sharples, K.: Age distribution of Wilms' tumor: Report from the National Wilms' Tumor Study. Cancer Res., 48:1653–1657, 1988.

Breslow, N., Churchill, G., Beckwith, J. B., et al.: Prognosis for Wilms' tumor patients with non-metastatic disease at diagnosis: Results of the Second National Wilms' Tumor Study. J. Clin. Oncol., 3:521–531, 1985.

Bunin, G. R., Nass, C. C., Kramer, S., et al.: Parental occupation and Wilms' tumor: Results of a case-control study. Cancer Res. 49:725–729, 1989.

Cangir, A., et al.: Combination chemotherapy with Adriamycin (NSC-123127) and dimethyl tirazeno imidazole carboxamide (DTIC) (NSC-45388) in children with metastatic solid tumors. Med. Pediatr. Oncol., 2:183, 1976.

Carcassone, M., Raybaird, C., and Lebrenil, G.: Clear cell sarcoma of the kidney in children: A distinct entity. J. Pediatr. Surg., 16:645, 1981.

Cassady, J. R., Tefft, M., Filler, R. M., et al.: Considerations in the radiation therapy of Wilms' tumor. Cancer, 32:598–608, 1973.

Castellanos, R. D., Aron, B. S., and Evans, A. T.: Renal adenocarcinoma in children: Incidence, therapy and prognosis. J. Urol., 111:534, 1974.

Chatten, J.: Epithelial differentiation in Wilms' tumor: A clinicopathologic appraisal. Perspect. Pediatr. Pathol., 3:225, 1976.

Chatten, J., Cromie, W. J., and Duckett, J. W.: Ossifying tumor of infantile kidney: Report of two cases. Cancer, 45:609, 1980.

Cho, K. J., Thornbury, J. R., Bernstein, J., Heidelberg, K. P., and Walter, J. F.: Localized cystic disease of the kidney: Angiographic-pathologic correlation. AJR, 132:891, 1979.

Cohen, A. J., Li, F. P., Berg, S., et al.: Hereditary renal-cell carcinoma associated with a chromosomal translocation. N. Engl. J. Med., 301:592, 1979.

Coleman, M.: Multilocular renal cyst: Case report: Ultrastructure and review of the literature. Virchows Arch. [A], 387:207, 1980.

Colgan, J. R., III, Skaist, L., and Morrow, J. W.: Benign ureteral tumors in childhood: A case report and a plea for conservative management. J. Urol., 109:308–310, 1973.

Coppes, M. J., Wilson, P. C. G., and Weitzman, S.: Extrarenal

Wilms' tumor: Staging, treatment and prognosis. J. Clin. Oncol., 9:167–174, 1991.

D'Angio, G. J., et al.: Management of children with Wilms' tumor: Defining the risk-benefit ratio. In Childhood Cancer: Triumph over Tragedy. Frontiers of Radiation Therapy and Oncology, Vol. 16. Basel, S. Karger, 1982.

D'Angio, G. J.: SIOP and the Management of Wilms' Tumor [Editorial]. J. Clin. Oncol., 1:595, 1983.

D'Angio, G. J., Beckwith, J. B., Breslow, N. E., et al.: Wilms' tumor: An update. Cancer, 45:1791, 1980.

D'Angio, G. J., Breslow, W., Beckwith, J. B., Evans, A., et al.: Treatment of Wilms' tumor: Results of the Third National Wilms' Tumor Study. Cancer, 64:349–360, 1989.

D'Angio, G. J., Evans, A. E., Breslow, N., et al.: The treatment of Wilms' tumor: Results of the National Wilms' Tumor Study. Cancer, 38:633, 1976a.

D'Angio, G. J., Evans, A. E., Breslow, N., et al.: The treatment of Wilms' tumor: Results of the Second National Wilms' Tumor Study. Cancer, 47:2302, 1981.

D'Angio, G. J., Evans, A. E., Breslow, N., et al.: Results of the Third National Wilms' Tumor Study (NWTS-3): A preliminary report [Abstract 723]. Proc. Am. Assoc. Cancer Res., 25:183, 1984.

D'Angio, G. J., Meadows, A., Mike, V., et al.: Decreased risk of radiation associated second malignant neoplasms in actinomycin-D treated patients. Cancer, 37 (Suppl):1177–1185, 1976b.

D'Angio, G. J., Tefft, M., Breslow, N., et al.: Radiation therapy of Wilms' tumor: Results according to dose, field, post-operative timing and histology. Int. J. Radiat. Oncol. Biol. Phys., 4:769, 1978.

Danis, R. K., Wolverson, M. K., Graviss, E. R., O'Connor, D. M., Joyce, P. F., and Cradock, T. V.: Preoperative embolization of Wilms' tumors. Am. J. Dis. Child., 133:503, 1979.

Dehner, L. P., Leestma, J. E., and Price, E. B., Jr.: Renal cell carcinoma in children: A clinicopathologic study of 15 cases and review of the literature. J. Pediatr., 76:358, 1970.

deLorimier, A. A., Belzer, F. O., Kountz, S. L., and Kushner, J. O.: Treatment of bilateral Wilms' tumor. Am. J. Surg., 122:275, 1971.

Donaldson, S. S., et al.: Radiation enteritis in children: A retrospective review, clinicopathologic correlation and dietary management. Cancer, 35:1167, 1975.

Donaldson, S. S., Wesley, M. N., Ghavimi, F., et al.: A prospective randomized clinical trial of total parenteral nutrition in children with cancer. Med. Pediatr. Oncol., 10:129, 1982.

Drash, A., Sherman, F., Hartmann, W. H., et al.: A syndrome of pseudohermaphroditism, Wilms' tumor, hypertension and degenerative renal disease. J. Pediatr., 76:585, 1970.

Duckett, J. W., Lifland, J. J., and Peters, P. C.: Resection of the inferior vena cava for adjacent malignant disease. Surg. Gynecol. Obstet., 136:711–716, 1973.

Ehrlich, R. M., Bloomberg, S. D., Gyepes, M. T., Levitt, S. B., Kogan, S., Hanna, M., and Goodwin, W. E.: Wilms' tumor, misdiagnosed preoperatively: A review of 19 National Wilms' Tumor Study I cases. J. Urol., 122:790, 1979.

Ehrlich, R. M., Freedman, A., Goldsobel, A. B., and Stiehn, E. R.: The use of sodium 2-mercaptoethane sulfonate to prevent cyclophosphamide cystitis. J. Urol., 131:960, 1984.

Evans, A. E., Blore, J., Hadley, R., and Tanindi, S.: The LaBrosse spot test: A practical aid in the diagnosis and management of children with neuroblastoma. Pediatrics, 47:913, 1971.

Evans, A. E., Norkool, P., Evans, M. S., et al.: Late effects of treatment for Wilms' tumor. A report from the national Wilms' Tumor Study Group. Cancer, 67:331–336, 1991.

Farber, S.: Chemotherapy in the treatment of leukemia and Wilms' tumor. JAMA, 198:826, 1966.

Farber, S., Toch, R., Sears, E. M., and Pinkel, D.: Advances in chemotherapy of cancer in man. Adv. Cancer Res., 4:1, 1956.

Farewell, V. T., D'Angio, G. J., Breslow, N., and Norkool, P.: Retrospective validation of a new staging system for Wilms' tumor: A report from the National Wilms' Tumor Study. Cancer Clin. Trials, 4:167, 1981.

Feusner, J. H., Beckwith, J. B., and D'Angio, G. J.: Clear cell sarcoma of the kidney: Accuracy of imaging methods for detecting bone metastases. Report from the National Wilms' Tumor Study. Med. Pediatr. Oncol., 18:225–227, 1990.

Filler, R. M., Tefft, M., Vawter, G. F., et al.: Hepatic lobectomy in childhood: Effects of x-ray and chemotherapy. J. Pediatr. Surg., 4:31, 1969.

Finklestein, J. Z., Hittle, R. E., and Hammond, G. D.: Evaluation of a high dose cyclophosphamide regimen in childhood tumors. Cancer, 23:1239, 1969.

Ganguly, A., Gribble, J., Tune, B., Kempson, R. L., and Luetscher, J. A.: Renin-secreting Wilms' tumor with severe hypertension. Ann. Intern. Med., 79:835, 1973.

Ganick, D. J., Gilbert, E. F., Beckwith, J. B., and Kiviat, N.: Congenital cystic mesoblastic nephroma. Hum. Pathol., 12:1039, 1981.

Green, B., Goldstein, H. M., and Weaver, R. M.: Abdominal pansonography in the evaluation of renal cancer. Radiology, 132:421, 1979.

Green, D. M.: Offspring of patients treated for unilateral Wilms' tumor in childhood. Cancer, 49:2285, 1982.

Green, D. M., Finklestein, J. Z., Beckwith, J. B., and Norkool, P.: Diffuse interstitial pneumonitis after pulmonary irradiation for metastatic Wilms' tumor: A report from the National Wilms' Tumor Study. Cancer, 63:450–453, 1989.

Green, D. M., Norkool, P., Breslow, N. E., et al.: Severe hepatic toxicity after treatment with vincristine and dactinomycin using single-dose or divided dose schedules: A report from the National Wilms' Tumor Study. J. Clin. Oncol., 8:1525–1530, 1990.

Gross, R. E., and Neuhauser, E. B. D.: Treatment of mixed tumors of the kidney in childhood. Pediatrics, 6:843, 1950.

Grundy, P., Breslow, N., Green, D. M., Sharples, K., Evans, A., and D'Angio, G. J.: Prognostic factors for children with recurrent Wilms' tumor: Results from the Second and Third National Wilms' Tumor Study. J. Clin. Oncol., 7:638–647, 1989.

Haicken, B. N., and Miller, D. R.: Simultaneous occurrence of congenital aniridia, hamartoma and Wilms' tumor. J. Pediatr., 78:497, 1971.

Harms, D., Gutjahr, P., Hohenfellner, R., and Willke, E.: Fetal rhabdomyomatous nephroblastoma: Pathologic histology and special clinical and biological features. Eur. J. Pediatr., 133:167, 1980.

Hartman, D. S., Lesar, M. S. L., Madewell, J. E., Lichtenstein, J. E., and Davis, C. J., Jr.: Mesoblastic nephroma: Radiologic-pathologic correlation of 20 cases. Am. J. Roentgenol., 136:69, 1981.

Hoffman, M.: One Wilms' tumor gene is cloned; Are there more? Science, 246:1387, 1989.

Howell, C. G., Othersen, H. B., Kiviat, N. E., et al.: Therapy and outcome in 51 children with mesoblastic nephroma: A report of the National Wilms' Tumor Study. J. Pediatr. Surg., 17:826, 1982.

Hricak, H., Thoeni, R. F., Carroll, P. R., et al.: Detection and staging of renal neoplasms: A reassessment of MR imaging. Radiology, 166:643–649, 1988.

Hunig, R., and Kinser, J.: Ultrasonic diagnosis of Wilms' tumor. AJR, 117:119, 1973.

Jaffe, M. H., White, S. J., Silver, T. M., et al.: Wilms' tumor: Ultrasonic features, pathologic correlation and diagnostic pitfalls. Radiology, 140:147–152, 1981.

Jaffe, N., McNeese, M., Kayfield, J. K., and Riseborough, E. J.: Childhood urologic cancer therapy, related sequelae and their impact on management. Cancer, 45:1815, 1980.

Janik, J. S., and Seeler, R. A.: Delayed onset of hemihypertrophy in Wilms' tumor. J. Pediatr. Surg., 11:581, 1976.

Jayabose, S., and Lanzkowsky, P.: Hepatotoxicity of chemotherapy following nephrectomy and radiation therapy for right-sided Wilms' tumor. J. Pediatr., 88:898, 1976.

Jereb, B., and Eklund, G.: Factors influencing the cure rate in nephroblastoma. Acta Radiol. Ther., 12:84–106, 1973.

Jereb, B., Tournade, M. F., Lemerle, J., et al.: Lymph node invasion and prognosis in nephroblastoma. Cancer, 45:1632, 1980.

Jones, B.: Metachronous bilateral Wilms' tumor. Am. J. Clin. Oncol., 5:545, 1982.

Joshi, V. V.: Cystic, partially differentiated nephroblastoma: An entity in the spectrum of infantile renal neoplasia. Perspect. Pediatr. Pathol., 5:217, 1979.

Joshi, V. V., and Beckwith, J. B.: Multilocular cyst of the kidney (cystic nephroma) and cystic, partially differentiated nephroblastoma. Terminology and criteria for diagnosis. Cancer, 64:466–479, 1989.

Kantor, A. F.: Current concepts in the epidemiology and etiology of primary renal carcinoma. J. Urol., 117:415, 1977.

Katz, A. S., and Landau, S. J.: Pseudotumor of kidney. Urology, 13:450, 1979.

Katzman, H., Haugh, T., and Berdon, W.: Skeletal changes following irradiation of childhood tumors. J. Bone Joint Surg., 51A: 825, 1969.

Keating, M. A., and D'Angio, G. J.: Wilms' tumor update: Current issues in management. Dialogues Pediatr. Urol., 11:1–8, 1988.

Kelalis, P. P.: Surgical treatment: NWTS recommendations. Dialogues Pediatr. Urol., 8:6, 1985.

Kirks, D. R., Merten, D. F., Grossman, H., and Bowie, J. D.: Diagnostic imaging of pediatric abdominal masses: An overview. Radiol. Clin. North Am., 19:527, 1981.

Knudson, A. G., Jr., and Strong, L. C.: Mutation and cancer: A model for Wilms' tumor of the kidney. JNCI, 48:313, 1972.

Koufos, A., Hansen, M. F., Lampkin, B. C., et al.: Loss of alleles at loci on human chromosome 11 during genesis of Wilms' tumor. Nature, 309:170–172, 1984.

Koyanagi, T., Sasaki, K., Arikado, K., et al.: Transitional cell carcinoma of renal pelvis in an infant. J. Urol., 113:114–117, 1975.

Kuffer, F., Fortner, J., and Murphy, M. I.: Surgical complications of children undergoing cancer therapy. Ann. Surg., 167:21, 1968.

Lawler, W., Marsden, H. B., and Palmer, M. K.: Histopathological study of the first Medical Research Council nephroblastoma trial. Cancer, 40:1519, 1977.

Lemerle, J., Voute, P. A., Tournade, M. F., et al.: Preoperative versus postoperative radiotherapy, single versus multiple courses of actinomycin D, in the treatment of Wilms' tumor: Preliminary results of a controlled clinical trial conducted by the International Society of Pediatric Oncology (SIOP). Cancer, 38:647, 1976.

Lemerle, J., Voute, P. A., Tournade, M. F., et al.: Effectiveness of preoperative chemotherapy in Wilms' tumor: Results of an International Society of Pediatric Oncology (SIOP) clinical trial. J. Clin. Oncol., 1:604, 1983.

Li, F. P., Bishop, Y., and Katsioules, C.: Survival in Wilms' tumour. Lancet, 1:41, 1975a.

Li, F. P., Cassady, J. R., and Jaffe, N.: Risk of second tumors in survivors of childhood cancer. Cancer, 35:1230, 1975b.

Littman, P., Meadows, A. T., Polgar, G., et al.: Pulmonary function in survivors of Wilms' tumor. Cancer, 37:2773, 1976.

Machin, G. A.: Persistent renal blastema (nephroblastomatosis) as a frequent precursor of Wilms' tumor: A pathological and clinical review. Part 1: Nephroblastomatosis in context of embryology and genetics. Am. J. Pediatr. Hematol. Oncol., 2:165, 1980a.

Machin, G. A.: Persistent renal blastema (nephroblastomatosis) as a frequent precursor of Wilms' tumor: A pathological and clinical review. Part 3: Clinical aspects of nephroblastomatosis. Am. J. Pediatr. Hematol. Oncol., 2:353, 1980b.

Malcolm, A. W., Jaffe, J., Folkman, M. J., and Cassady, J. R.: Bilateral Wilms' tumor. Int. J. Radiat. Oncol. Biol. Phys., 6:167, 1980.

Manners, M., Slater, R. M., Heyting, C., et al.: Molecular nature of genetic changes resulting in loss of heterozygosity of chromosome 11 in Wilms' tumors. Human Genetics, 81:41–48, 1988.

Marosvari, I., Kontor, F., and Kallay, K.: Renin-secreting Wilms' tumour. Lancet, 1:1180, 1972.

Marsden, H. B., and Lawler, W.: Bone metastasizing renal tumour of childhood: Histopathological and clinical review of 38 cases. Virchows Arch. [A], 387:341, 1980.

Martin, L. W., and Reyes, P. M.: An evaluation of 10 years' experience with retroperitoneal lymph node dissection for Wilms' tumor. J. Pediatr. Surg., 4:683, 1969.

Martin, L. W., Schaffner, D. P., Cox, J. A., et al.: Retroperitoneal lymph node dissection for Wilms' tumor. J. Pediatr. Surg., 14:704, 1979.

Mathe, G., and Oldham, R. K.: Complications of cancer chemotherapy, recent results. Cancer Res., 49:1, 1974.

McCauley, R. G. K., Safaii, H., Crowley, C. A., and Pinn, V. W.: Extrarenal Wilms' tumor. Am. J. Dis. Med., 133:1174, 1979.

McVeagh, P., and Ekert, H.: Hepatotoxicity of chemotherapy following nephrectomy and radiation therapy for right-sided Wilms' tumor. J. Pediatr., 87:627, 1975.

Meadows, A. T., and Jarrett, P.: Pigmented nevi, Wilms' tumor, and second malignant neoplasms. J. Pediatr., 93:889, 1978.

Mike, V., Meadows, A. T., and D'Angio, G. J.: Incidence of second malignant neoplasms in children: Results of an international study. Lancet, II: 1326–1331, 1982.

Miller, R. W.: Relation between cancer and congenital defects: An epidemiologic evaluation. JNCI, 40:1079, 1968.

Miller, R. W., Fraumeni, J. F., and Manning, M. D.: Association of Wilms' tumor with aniridia, hemihypertrophy and other congenital malformation. N. Engl. J. Med., 270:922, 1964.

Miser, J. S., Kinsella, T. J., Triche, T. J., et al.: Ifosfamide with mesna uroprotection and etoposide: An effective regimen in the treatment of recurrent sarcomas and other tumors of children and young adults. J. Clin. Oncol., 5:1191–1198, 1987.

Mitus, A., Tefft, M., and Fellers, F. X.: Long-term follow-up of renal function of 108 children who underwent nephrectomy for malignant disease. Pediatrics, 44:912, 1969.

Mohammad, A. M., Meyer, J., and Hakami, N.: Long-term survival following brain metastasis of Wilms' tumor. J. Pediatr., 90:660, 1977.

Morgan, E., and Kidd, J. M.: Undifferentiated sarcoma of the kidney: A tumor of childhood with histopathologic and clinical characteristics distinct from Wilms' tumor. Cancer, 42:1916, 1978.

Movassaghi, N., Leiken, S., and Chandra, R.: Wilms' tumor metastasis to uncommon sites. J. Pediatr., 84:416, 1974.

Nakayama, D. K., DeLormier, A. A., O'Neill, J. A., et al.: Intracardiac extension of Wilms' tumor. A report of the National Wilms' Tumor Study. Ann. Surg., 204:693–697, 1986.

Nakayama, D. K., Ortega, W., D'Angio, G. J., and O'Neill, J. A.: The nonopacified kidney with Wilms' tumor. J. Pediatr. Surg., 23:152–155, 1988.

Narahara, K., Kikkawa, K., Kimira, S., et al.: Regional mapping of catalase and Wilms' tumor: Aniridia, genitourinary abnormalities, and mental retardation triad loci to the chromosome segment 11p1305 p1306. Hum. Genet., 66:181, 1984.

Neuhauser, R. B. D., Wittenborg, M. H., Berman, C. Z., and Cohen, J.: Irradiation effects of roentgen therapy on the growing spine. Radiology, 59:637, 1952.

Novak, R. W., Caces, J. N., and Johnson, W. W.: Sarcomatous renal tumor of childhood: An electron microscopic study. Am. J. Clin. Pathol., 73:622, 1980.

Olsen, B., and Bischoff, A.: Wilms' tumor in adults. Cancer, 25:2, 1970.

Olshan, A. F., Breslow, N. E., Daling, J. R., et al.: Wilms' tumor and parental occupation. Cancer Res., 50:3212–3217, 1990.

Opitz, J. M.: Adenocarcinoma of the colon following Wilms' tumor. J. Pediatr., 96:775, 1980.

Ortega, J. A., et al.: Vincristine, dactinomycin and cyclophosphamide (VAC) chemotherapy for recurrent metastatic Wilms' tumor in previously treated children. J. Pediatr., 96:502, 1980.

Othersen, H. B., DeLorimer, A., Hrabovsky, E., et al.: Surgical evaluation of lymph node metastases in Wilms' tumor. J. Pediatr. Surg., 25:330–331, 1990.

Palmer, N. F., and Beckwith, J. B.: Multiple primary tumor syndrome in children with rhabdoid tumors of the kidney (RTK) [Abstract C-288]. ASCO, 1981.

Pendergrass, T. W.: Congenital anomalies in children with Wilms' tumor. Cancer, 37:403, 1976.

Penn, I.: Renal transplantation for Wilms' tumor: Report of 20 cases. J. Urol., 122:793, 1979.

Pritchard, J., Barnes, J. M., Gough, D., et al.: Preliminary results of the first United Kingdom Children's Cancer Study Group (UKCCSG) Wilms' tumour study [Abstract]. Med. Pediatr. Oncol., 16:413, 1988.

Rainwater, L. M., Hosaka, Y., Farrow, G. M., Kramer, S. A., Kelalis, P. P., and Lieber, M. M.: Wilms' tumors: Relationship of nuclear deoxyribonucleic acid ploidy to patient survival. J. Urol., 138:974, 1987.

Ramsey, N., Dehner, L., Coccia, P., D'Angio, G. J., and Nesbit, M.: Acute hemorrhage into Wilms' tumor. Pediatrics, 91:763, 1977.

Rance, T. F.: Case of fungus haematodes of the kidneys. Med. Phys. J., 32:19, 1814.

Raney, R. B., Palmer, N., Sutow, W. W., Baum, E., and Ayala, A.: Renal cell carcinoma in children. Med. Pediatr. Oncol., 11:91, 1983.

Reeve, A. E., Sih, S. A., Raizis, A. M., et al.: Loss of allelic heterozygosity at a second locus on chromosome 11 in sporadic Wilms' tumor. Mol. Cell Biol., 9:1799–1803, 1989.

Riccardi, V. M.: Genetics of pediatric genitourinary tumors. In Broecker, B. H., and Klein, F. A. (Eds.): Pediatric Tumors of the Genitourinary Tract. New York, Alan R. Liss, Inc., 1988.

Riseborough, E. J., Gravias, S. L., Burton, R. I., and Jaffe, N.: Skeletal alterations following irradiation for Wilms' tumor. J. Bone Joint Surg., 5A:526, 1976.

Ritchey, M. L., Kelalis, P. P., Breslow, N., et al.: Intracaval and atrial involvement with nephroblastoma: review of National Wilms' Tumor Study. J. Urol., 140:1113–1118, 1988.

Samuels, L. D., Grosfeld, J. L., and Kartha, M.: Radiation hepatitis in children. J. Pediatr., 78:68, 1971.

Sanyal, S. K., Saldivar, V., Coburn, T. P., et al.: Hyperdynamic heart failure due to A-V fistula associated with Wilms' tumor. Pediatrics, 57:564, 1976.

Scott, J. E. S.: Pubertal development in children treated for nephroblastoma. J. Pediatr. Surg., 16:122, 1981.

Schroeder, W. T., Chao, L. Y., Dao, D. D., et al.: Nonrandom loss of maternal chromosome 11 alleles in Wilms' tumors. Am. J. Hum. Genet., 40:413–420, 1987.

Shalet, M. F., Holder, T. M., and Walters, T. R.: Erythropoietin-producing Wilms' tumor. J. Pediatr., 70:615, 1967.

Shalet, S. M.: Abnormalities of growth and gonadal function in children treated for malignant disease: a review. J. R. Soc. Med., 75:641, 1982.

Shalet, S. M., and Beardwell, C. G.: Endocrine consequences of treatment of malignant disease in childhood: A review. J. Roy. Soc. Med. 72:39–41, 1979.

Shende, A., Wind, E., and Lanzkowsky, P.: Intrarenal neuroblastoma mimicking Wilms' tumor. N.Y. State J. Med., 79:93, 1979.

Shimizu, H., Jaffe, N., Eftekhari, F.: Massive Wilms' tumor: Sonographic demonstration of therapeutic response without alteration in size. Pediatr. Radiol., 17:493–494, 1987.

Shurin, S. B., Ganderer, M. W. L., et al.: Fatal intraoperative pulmonary embolization of Wilms' tumor. J. Pediatr., 101:559, 1982.

Siegel, S. E., and Moran, R. G.: Problems in the chemotherapy of cancer in the neonate. Am. J. Pediatr. Hematol. Oncol., 3:287, 1981.

Simonowitz, D. A., and Reyes, H. M.: Renal abscess mimicking a Wilms' tumor. J. Pediatr. Surg., 11:269, 1976.

Smith, W. B., Wara, W. M., Margoli, L.W., et al.: Partial hepatectomy in metastatic Wilms' tumor. J. Pediatr., 84:259, 1974.

Snyder, H. S., Lack, E. E., Chetty-Baktavizian, A., Bauer, S. B., Colodny, A. H., and Retik, A. B.: Congenital mesoblastic nephroma: Relationship to other renal tumors of infancy. J. Urol., 126:513, 1981.

Sotelo-Avila, C., Gonzalez-Crussi, F., deMello, D., et al.: Renal and extrarenal rhabdoid tumors in children: A clinicopathologic study of 14 patients. Semin. Diagn. Pathol., 3:151, 1986.

Sotelo-Avila, C., Gonzalez-Crussi, F., and Fowler, J. W.: Complete and incomplete forms of Beckwith-Wiedemann syndrome: Their oncogenic potential. J. Pediatr., 96:47, 1980.

Stay, E. J., and Vawter, G.: The relationship between nephroblastoma and neurofibromatosis (Von Recklinghausen's disease). Cancer, 39:2550, 1977.

Stevens, P. S., and Eckstein, H. B.: Ureteral metastases from Wilms' tumor. J. Urol., 115:467, 1976.

Sullivan, M. P., Sutow, W. W., Cangir, A., et al.: Vincristine sulfate in the management of Wilms' tumor: Replacement of preoperative irradiation by chemotherapy. JAMA, 202:381, 1967.

Sutow, W. W., Breslow, N. E., and Palmer, N. F.: Prognosis in children with Wilms' tumor metastases prior to or following primary treatment: Results from the First National Wilms' Tumor Study (NWTS-1). Am. J. Clin. Oncol., 5:339, 1982.

Sutow, W. W., and Sullivan, M. P.: Vincristine in primary treatment of Wilms' tumor. Tex. State J. Med., 61:794, 1965.

Sutow, W. W., Thurman, W. C., and Windmiller, J.: Vincristine (leurocristine) sulfate in the treatment of children with metastatic Wilms' tumor. Pediatrics, 32:880, 1963.

Tefft, M.: Radiation related toxicities in National Wilms' Tumor Study Number I. Int. J. Radiat. Oncol. Biol. Phys., 2:455, 1977.

Tefft, M., D'Angio, G. J., and Grant, W.: Postoperative radiation therapy for residual Wilms' tumor: Review of group III patients in the National Wilms' Tumor Study. Cancer, 37:2768, 1976.

Tefft, M., Mitus, A., and Jaffe, N.: Irradiation of the liver in children: Acute effects enhanced by concomitant chemotherapeutic administration? Am. J. Roentgenol. Radium Ther. Nucl. Med., 111:165, 1971.

Thomas, P. R. M., Tefft, M., Farewell, V. T., Norkool, P., Storer, B., and D'Angio, G. J.: Abdominal relapses in irradiated Second

National Wilms' Tumor Study patients. J. Clin. Oncol., 2:1098–1101, 1984.

Thompson, M. R., et al.: Extrarenal Wilms' tumors. J. Pediatr. Surg., 8:37, 1973.

Todani, T., Tabucki, K., and Watanabe, Y.: No touch isolation technique for left-sided Wilms' tumor. Z. Kinderchir., 19:93, 1976.

Traggis, D., Jaffe, N., Tefft, M., et al.: Successful treatment of Wilms' tumor with intracranial metastases. Pediatrics, 56:472, 1975.

Tucker, M. A., Meadows, A. T., Boice, J. D., D'Angio, G. J., et al.: Bone sarcomas linked to radiotherapy in children. N. Engl. J. Med., 17:588, 1987.

Waggert, J., and Koop, C. E.: Wilms' tumor: Preoperative radiotherapy and chemotherapy in the management of massive tumors. Cancer, 26:338, 1970.

Wang, J. J., Cortes, F., Sinks, L. F., et al.: Therapeutic effect and toxicity of Adriamycin in patients with neoplastic disease. Cancer, 28:837, 1971.

Wara, W. M., Philips, T. L., Margolis, I. W., et al.: Radiation pneumonitis: A new approach to the derivation of time-dose factors. Cancer, 32:547, 1973.

Wasiljew, B. K., Besser, A., and Raffensperger, J.: Treatment of bilateral Wilms' tumors: A 22-year experience. J. Pediatr. Surg., 17:265, 1982.

Wedemeyer, P. P., White, J. G., Nesbit, M. E., et al.: Resection of metastases in Wilms' tumor: A report of three cases cured of pulmonary and hepatic metastases. Pediatrics, 41:446, 1968.

Weeks, D. A., Beckwith, B., and Luckey, D. W.: Relapse-associated variables in Stage I favorable histology Wilms' tumor: A report of the National Wilms' Tumor Study. Cancer, 60:1204, 1987.

White, J. C., and Krivit, W.: Surgical excision of pulmonary metastases. Pediatrics, 29:927, 1962.

Wigger, H. J.: Fetal hamartoma of kidney: A benign symptomatic congenital tumor, not a form of Wilms' tumor. Am. J. Clin. Pathol., 51:323, 1969.

Wikstrom, S., Parkkulainen, K. V., and Louhimo, I.: Bilateral Wilms' tumor and secondary malignancies. J. Pediatr. Surg., 17:269, 1982.

Wilkins, R. J.: Genomic imprinting and carcinogenesis. Lancet, 1:328–331, 1989.

Williams, D. I., and Martin, J.: Renal tumors. In Pediatric Urology, Ed. 2. London, Butterworths, 1982.

Williams, J. C., Brown, K. W., Mott, M. G., et al.: Maternal allele loss in Wilms' tumor. Lancet, 1:283–284, 1989.

Wockel, W., Lagerman, A., and Scheber, K.: Konnatales mesoblastisches nephron und nodulares renales blastem bei einem sangling. Zentralbl. Allg. Pathol., 123:222, 1979.

Wohl, M. E. B., Griscom, N. T., Traggis, D. G., et al.: Effects of therapeutic irradiation delivered in early childhood upon subsequent lung function. Pediatrics, 55:507, 1975.

Wolff, J. A., Krivit, W., Newton, W. A., Jr., et al.: Single versus multiple dose dactinomycin therapy of Wilms' tumor. N. Engl. J. Med., 279:290, 1968.

Young, J. L. J., Heise, H. W., Silverberg, E., and Myers, M. H.: Cancer incidence, survival and mortality for children under 15 years of age. American Cancer Society Professional Education Publication, September, 1978.

Zuppan, C., Beckwith, J. B., and Luckey, D.: Anaplasia in unilateral Wilms' tumor: A report from the National Wilms' Tumor Study Pathology Center. Hum. Pathol., 19:1199–1209, 1988.

Neuroblastoma

Adam, A., and Hochholzer, L.: Ganglioneuroblastoma of the posterior mediastinum: A clinicopathologic review of 80 cases. Cancer, 47:373, 1981.

Akwari, O. E., Payne, W. S., Onofrio, B. M., et al.: Dumbbell neurogenic tumors of the mediastinum: Diagnosis and management. Mayo Clin. Proc., 54:353, 1978.

Altman, A. J., and Baehner, R. I.: Favorable prognosis for survival in children with coincident opsomyoclonus and neuroblastoma. Cancer, 37:846, 1976.

Anders, D., Kindermann, G., and Pfeifer, U.: Metastasizing fetal neuroblastoma with involvement of the placenta simulating fetal erythroblastosis. J. Pediatr., 82:50, 1973.

Arenson, E. B., Hutter, J. J., Jr., Restuccia, R. D., and Holton, C. P.: Neuroblastoma in father and son. JAMA, 235:727–729, 1976.

August, C., et al.: Treatment of advanced neuroblastoma with the supralethal chemotherapy, radiation and allogeneic or autologous marrow reconstitution. J. Clin. Oncol., 2:609–616, 1984.

Beckwich, J. B., and Perrin, E. V.: In situ neuroblastoma: A contribution to the natural history of neural crest tumors. Am. J. Pathol., 43:1089, 1963.

Bernstein, I. D.: Prospects for immunotherapy of neuroblastoma. In Evans, A. E. (Ed.): Advances in Neuroblastoma Research. New York, Raven Press, 1980, p. 243.

Bolande, R. P.: Developmental Pathology. New York, Harper & Row Publishers, Inc., 1979.

Bond, J. V.: Neuroblastoma metastatic to the liver in infants. Arch. Dis. Child., 51:879, 1976.

Bray, P. F., Ziter, F. A., Lahey, M. E., et. al.: The coincidence of neuroblastoma and acute cerebellar encephalopathy. J. Pediatr., 76:9833, 1969.

Breslow, N., and McCann, B.: Statistical estimation of prognosis for children with neuroblastoma. Cancer Res., 31:2098, 1971.

Brodeur, G., and Seeger, R.: Gene amplification in human neuroblastomas: Basic mechanisms and clinical implications. Cancer Genet. Cytogenet., 19:101–111, 1986.

Brodeur, G. M., Seeger, R. C., Barrett, A., et al.: International criteria for diagnosis, staging and response to treatment in patients with neuroblastoma. J. Clin. Oncol., 6:1874–1881, 1988.

Brodeur, G. M., Seeger, R. C., Schwab, M., Varmus, H. E., and Bishop, J. M.: Amplification of N-myc in untreated human neuroblastomas correlates with advanced disease stage. Science, 224:1121–1124, 1984.

Chatten, J., and Voorhees, M. L.: Familial neuroblastoma: Report of a kindred with multiple disorders, including neuroblastomas in four siblings. N. Engl. J. Med., 277:1230, 1967.

Cheung, N. K., Saarinen, U., Neely, J., Landmeier, B., Donovan, D., and Coccia, P.: Monoclonal antibodies to a glycolipid antigen on human neuroblastoma cells. Cancer Res., 45:2642–2649, 1985.

Coldman, A. J., Fryer, C. J. H., Elwood, J. M., and Sonley, M. J.: Neuroblastoma: Influence of age at diagnosis, stage, tumor site and sex on prognosis. Cancer, 46:1896, 1980.

Cushing, H., and Wolbach, S. B.: The transformation of a malignant paravertebral sympathicoblastoma into a benign ganglioneuroma. Am. J. Pathol., 3:203, 1927.

D'Angio, G. J., Evans, A. E., and Koop, C. E.: Special pattern of widespread neuroblastoma with a favorable prognosis. Lancet, 1:1046, 1971.

D'Angio, G. J., Loken, M., and Nesbit, M.: Radionuclear (75 Se) identification of tumor in children with neuroblastoma. Radiology, 93:615, 1969.

Delalieux, C., Ebinger, G., Maurus, R., et al.: Myoclonic encephalopathy and neuroblastoma. N. Engl. J. Med., 292:46, 1975.

deLorimier, A. A., Bragg, K. V., and Linden, G.: Neuroblastoma in childhood. Am. J. Dis. Child., 118:441, 1969.

El Shafie, M., Samuel, D., Klippel, C. H., et al.: Intractable diarrhea in children with VIP-secreting ganglioneuroblastomas. J. Pediatr. Surg., 18:34, 1983.

Evans, A. E.: Staging and treatment of neuroblastoma. Cancer, 65:1799, 1980.

Evans, A. E.: Neuroblastoma: Diagnosis and management. Curr. Concepts Oncol., 4:10, 1982.

Evans, A. E., Albo, V., D'Angio, G. J., et al.: Factors influencing survival of children with non-metastatic neuroblastoma. Cancer, 38:661, 1976.

Evans, A. E., Blore, J., Hadley, R., and Tanindi, S.: The LaBrosse spot test: A practical aid in the diagnosis and management of children with neuroblastoma. Pediatrics, 47:913, 1971a.

Evans, A. E., Chatten, J., D'Angio, G. J., et al.: A review of 17 IV-S neuroblastoma patients at the Children's Hospital of Philadelphia. Cancer, 45:833, 1980.

Evans, A. E., D'Angio, G. J., and Koop, C. E.: The role of multimodal therapy in patients with local and regional neuroblastoma. J. Pediatr. Surg., 19:77, 1984.

Evans, A. E., D'Angio, G. J., Propert, K., Anderson, J., Hann, H. W.: Prognostic factors in neuroblastoma. Cancer, 59:1853–1859, 1987.

Evans, A. E., D'Angio, G. J., and Randolph, J.: A proposed staging for children with neuroblastoma. Cancer, 27:374, 1971b.

Everson, I. C., and Cole, W. H.: Spontaneous Regression of Cancer: A Study and Abstract of Reports in the World Medical Literature and of Personal Communications Concerning Spontaneous Regression of Malignant Disease. Philadelphia, W. B. Saunders Co., 1966, p. 88.

Filler, R. M., Traggis, D. G., Jaffe, N., et al.: Favorable outlook for children with mediastinal neuroblastoma. J. Pediatr. Surg., 7:136, 1972.

Finklestein, J. Z., Eckert, H., Isaacs, H., and Higgens, G.: Bone marrow metastases in children with solid tumors. Am. J. Dis. Child., 119:49, 1970.

Fortner, J., Nicastri, A., and Murphy, M. L.: Neuroblastoma: Natural history and results of treating 133 cases. Ann. Surg., 167:132, 1968.

Fuks, Z., Strober, S., and Kaplan, H. S.: Interaction between serum factors and T-lymphocytes in Hodgkin's disease. N. Engl. J. Med., 295:1273, 1976.

Gansler, T., Chatten, J., Varello, M., Bunin, G., and Atkinson, B.: Flow cytometric DNA analysis of neuroblastoma. Cancer, 58:2453–2458, 1986.

Geatti, O., Shapiro, B., Sisson, J., Hutchison, R., Mallette, S., Eyre, P., and Beierwaltes, W. H.: Iodine-131 metaiodobenzylguanidine scintigraphy for the location of neuroblastoma: Preliminary experience in ten cases. J. Nucl. Med., 26:736–742, 1985.

Gibbons, M. D., and Duckett, J. W.: Neuroblastoma masquerading as congenital ureteropelvic junction obstruction. J. Pediatr. Surg., 14:420, 1979.

Gitlow, S. E., Bertani, L. M., Rausen, A., Gribetz, D., and Dziedzic, S. W.: Diagnosis of neuroblastoma by qualitative and quantitative determination of catecholamine metabolites in urine. Cancer, 25:1377, 1970.

Grosfeld, J. L.: Management of solid tumors in infancy and childhood: The Indiana experience. Jpn. J. Pediatr. Surg., 19:256, 1983.

Gross, R. E., Farber, S., and Martin, L. W.: Neuroblastoma sympatheticum: A study and report of 217 cases. Pediatrics, 23:1179, 1959.

Haefnagel, C., Voute, P., DeKraker, J., and Marcuse, H.: Total body scintigraphy with ^{131}I-metaiodobenzylguanidine for detection of neuroblastoma. Diagn. Imaging Clin. Med., 54:21–27, 1985.

Hann, H. L., Evans, A. E., Cohen, I. J., et al.: Biologic differences between neuroblastoma Stages IV-S and IV. N. Engl. J. Med., 305:425, 1981.

Hann, H., Evans, A., Siegel, S., Wong, K., Sather, H., Dalton, A., Hammond, D., and Seeger, R.: Prognostic importance of serum ferritin in patients with Stage III and IV neuroblastoma: The CCSG experience. Cancer Res., 45:2843–2848, 1985.

Hann, H. L., Levy, H. M., Evans, A. E., and Drysdale, J. W.: Serum ferritin and neuroblastoma [Abstract 509]. Proc. Am. Assoc. Cancer Res. Soc. Clin. Oncol., 20:126, 1979.

Harlow, P. J., Siegel, M. M., Siegel, S. E., et al.: Antitumor activity of chemotherapeutic agents alone or in combination using a human neuroblastoma model system. *In* Evans, A. E. (Ed.): Advances in Neuroblastoma Research. New York, Raven Press, 1980, p. 319.

Hartmann, O., Kalifa, C., Benhamou, E., Beaujean, F., Patte, C., and Lemerle, J.: High-dose chemotherapy and ABMT as consolidation therapy in metastatic neuroblastoma. Proc. Am. Soc. Clin. Oncol., 4:236, 1985.

Hawthorne, H. C., Nelson, J. S., Witzleben, C. L., et al.: Blanching subcutaneous nodules in neonatal neuroblastoma. J. Pediatr., 77:297, 1970.

Hayes, F. A., Green, A., Hustu, H. O., and Kumar, M.: Surgicopathologic staging of neuroblastoma: Prognostic significance of regional lymph node metastases. J. Pediatr., 102:59–62, 1983.

Hellstrom, K. E., and Hellstrom, I.: Immunity to neuroblastoma and melanomas. Ann. Rev. Med., 23:19, 1972.

Hepler, A. B.: Presacral sympathicoblastoma in an infant causing urinary obstruction. J. Urol., 39:777, 1976.

Herxheimer, G.: Ueber Tumoren des Nebennierenmarkes, insbesondere das Neuroblastoma sympaticum. Beitr. Pathol. Anat., 57:112, 1914.

Homzie, M. J., and Elkon, D.: Olfactory esthesioneuroblastoma—variables predictive of tumor control and recurrence. Cancer, 46:2509, 1980.

Hope, J. W., Borns, P. F., and Berg, P. K.: Roentgenologic manifestations of Hirschsprung's disease in infancy. Am. J. Roentgenol. Radium Ther. Nucl. Med., 95:217, 1965.

Horne, T., Granowska, M., Dicks-Mireaux, C., Hawkins, L., Britton, K., Mather, S., Bomanji, J., Kemshead, J., Kingston, J., Malpas, J.: Neuroblastoma imaged with ^{123}I-metaoidobenzylguanidine and with ^{123}I-labelled monoclonal antibody, UJI3A, against neural tissue. Br. J. Radiol., 58:476–480, 1985.

Imashuku, S., LaBrosse, E. H., Johnson, E. M., Jr., Morgenroth, V. H., and Zenker, N.: Tyrosine hydroxylase in neuroblastoma. Biochem. Med., 5:2229, 1971.

Jaffe, N.: Neuroblastoma: Review of the literature and an examination of factors contributing to its enigmatic character. Cancer Treat. Rev., 3:61, 1976.

Jaffe, N., Cassady, R., Filler, R. M., et al.: Heterochromia and Horner syndrome associated with cervical and mediastinal neuroblastomas. J. Pediatr., 87:75, 1975.

Johnsonbaugh, R. E., and Cahill, R.: Screening procedures for neuroblastoma: False-negative results. Pediatrics, 56:267, 1975.

Kaneko, Y., Kanada, N., Maseki, N., Sakurai, M., Tsuchida, Y., Takida, T., Okabe, I., and Sakurai, M.: Different karyotypic patterns in early and advanced stage neuroblastoma. Cancer Res., 47:311–318, 1987.

Kemshed, J., and Coakham, H.: The use of monoclonal antibodies for the diagnosis of intracranial tumors and the small round cell tumors of childhood. J. Pathol., 141:249–257, 1983.

Knudson, A. G., and Amromin, G. D.: Neuroblastoma and ganglioneuroma in a child with multiple neurofibromatosis. Cancer, 19:1032, 1966.

Knudson, A. G., Jr., and Meadows, A. T.: Developmental genetics of neuroblastoma. JNCI, 57:675, 1976.

Knudson, A. G., Jr., and Strong, L. C.: Mutation and cancer: Neuroblastoma and pheochromocytoma. Man. J. Hum. Genet., 24:514, 1972.

LaBrosse, E. H.: Biochemical diagnosis of neuroblastoma: Use of a urine spot test. Proc. Am. Assoc. Cancer Res., 9:39, 1968.

LaBrosse, E. H., and Karon, M.: Catechol-O-methyltransferase activity in neuroblastoma tumour. Nature, 196:1222, 1962.

Lauder, I., and Aherne, W.: The significance of lymphocytic infiltration in neuroblastoma. Br. J. Cancer, 26:321, 1972.

Look, A. T., Hayes, F. A., Nitschke, R., McWilliams, N. B., and Green, A. A.: Cellular DNA content as a predictor of response to chemotherapy in infants with unresectable neuroblastoma. N. Engl. J. Med., 311:231–235, 1984.

Marchand, F.: Beitrage zur Kenntniss der normalen und pathologischen Anatomie der Glandula carotica und der Nebennieren: Festschrift fur Rudolph. Virchows Arch., 5:578, 1891.

Mason, G. H., Hart-Nercer, J., Miller, E. J., et al.: Adrenalinsecreting neuroblastoma in an infant. Lancet, 2:322, 1957.

Miller, R. W., Fraumeni, J. F., and Hill, J. A.: Neuroblastoma: Epidemiologic approach to its origin. Am. J. Dis. Child., 115:253, 1968.

Mitchell, C. H., Sinatra, F. R., Crast, F. W., et al.: Intractable watery diarrhea, ganglioneuroblastoma and vasoconstrictive intestinal peptide. J. Pediatr., 89:593, 1976.

Ninane, J., Pritchad, J., Morris-Jones, P. H., et al.: Stage II neuroblastoma: Adverse prognostic significance of lymph node involvement. Arch. Dis. Child., 57:438–442, 1982.

Odelstad, L., Pahlma, S., Lackgren, G., Grotte, G., and Nilsson, K.: Neuron specific enolase: A marker for differential diagnosis of neuroblastoma and Wilms' tumor. J. Pediatr. Surg., 17:381, 1982.

Pearse, A. G. E.: The APUD concept: Embryology, cytochemistry and ultrastructure of the diffuse neuroendocrine system. *In* Friesen, S. R., and Bolinger, R. E. (Eds.): Surgical Endocrinology: Clinical Syndromes. Philadelphia, J. B. Lippincott Co., 1978, pp. 18–34.

Peterson, D. R., Bill, A. H., Jr., and Kirkland, I. S.: Neuroblastoma trends in time. J. Pediatr. Surg., 4:244, 1969.

Philip, T., Bernard, J., Zucker, J., Pinkerton, R., Lutz, P., Bordigoni, P., Plouvier, E., Robert, A., Carton, R., Philippe, N., Philip, I., Chauvin, F., and Favrot, M.: High-dose chemoradiotherapy with bone marrow transplantation as consolidation treatment in neuroblastoma: An unselected group of Stage IV patients over 1 year of age. J. Clin. Oncol., 5:266–271, 1987.

Phillips, W. S., Stafford, P. W., Duvol-Arnold, B., and Ghosh, B. C.: Neuroblastoma and the clinical significance of N-myc oncogene amplification. Surg. Cynecol. Obstet., 172:73–80, 1991.

Quinn, J. J., and Altman, A. J.: The multiple-hematologic manifestations of neuroblastoma. Am. J. Pediatr. Hematol. Oncol., 1:201, 1979.

Reynolds, C. P., Smith, R. G., and Frenkel, E. P.: The diagnostic dilemma of the "small round cell neoplasm": Catecholamine fluorescence and tissue culture morphology as markers for neuroblastoma. Cancer, 18:2088, 1981.

Romansky, S. G., Crocker, D. W., and Shaw, K. N. F.: Ultrastructural studies on neuroblastoma: Evaluation of cytodifferentiation and correlation of morphology and biochemical survival data. Cancer, 42:2392, 1978.

Sather, H., Siegel, S., Finkelstein, J., et al.: The relationship of age at diagnosis to outcome for children with metastatic neuroblastoma [Abstract]. Proc. Am. Soc. Clin. Oncol., 22:409, 1981.

Sawada, T., Takamatsu, T., Tanaka, T., et al.: Effects of intralesional interferon on neuroblastoma: Changes in histology and DNA content distribution of tumor masses. Cancer, 48:2143, 1981.

Schnaufer, L., and Koop, C. E.: Silastic abdominal patch for temporary hepatomegaly in Stage IV-S neuroblastoma. J. Pediatr. Surg., 10:73, 1975.

Schneider, K. M., Becker, J. M., and Krasna, I. H.: Neonatal neuroblastoma. Pediatrics, 36:359, 1965.

Schwab, M., Alitalo, K., Klempnauer, K.-H., Varmus, H. E., Bishop, J. M., Gilbert, F., Brodeur, G., Goldstein, M., and Trent, J.: Amplified DNA with limited homology to myc cellular oncogene is shared by human neuroblastoma cell lines and a neuroblastoma tumour. Nature, 305:1245–1248, 1983.

Senelick, R. C., Bray, P. F., Lahey, M. E., et al.: Neuroblastomas and myoclonic encephalopathy: Two cases and a review of the literature. J. Pediatr. Surg., 8:623, 1973.

Shimada, H., Chatten, J., Newton, W. A., et al.: Histopathologic prognostic factors in neuroblastic tumors. JNCI, 73:405–416, 1984.

Silber, J. H., Evans, A. E., and Fridman, M.: Models to predict outcome from childhood neuroblastoma: The role of serum ferritin and tumor histology. Cancer Res., 51:1426–1433, 1991.

Sitarz, A., Finklestein, J., Grosfeld, S., et al.: An evaluation of the role of surgery in disseminated neuroblastoma: A report from the Children's Cancer Study Group. J. Pediatr. Surg., 18:147, 1983.

Smith, E. I., Krous, H. F., Tunell, W. P., and Hitch, D. C.: The impact of chemotherapy and radiation therapy on secondary operations for neuroblastoma. Ann. Surg., 191:561, 1980.

Sutow, W. W.: Prognosis in neuroblastoma of childhood. Am. J. Dis. Child., 96:299, 1958.

Traggis, D. G., Filler, R. M., Druckman, H., et al.: Prognosis for children with neuroblastoma presenting with paralysis. J. Pediatr. Surg., 12:119, 1977.

Virchow, R.: Hyperplasie der Zirbel und der Nebennieren. In Die krankhaften Geschwulste, Vol. 2. Berlin, A. Hirschwald, 1864–1865.

Voorhees, M. I.: Neuroblastoma with normal urinary catecholamine excretion. J. Pediatr., 78:680, 1971.

Voute, P. A., Jr., Wadman, S. K., and van Putten, W. J.: Congenital neuroblastoma: Symptoms of the mother during pregnancy. Clin. Pediatr., 9:206, 1970.

Williams, C., and Greer, M.: Homovanillic acid and vanillylmandelic acid in diagnosis of neuroblastoma. JAMA, 183:836, 1963.

Wong, K. Y., Hanenson, I. B., and Lampkin, B. C.: Familial neuroblastoma. Am. J. Dis. Child., 121:415, 1971.

Young, J. L., and Miller, R. W.: Incidence of malignant tumors in U.S. children. J. Pediatr., 86:254, 1975.

Zelter, P., Marganos, P., Parma, A., et al.: Raised neuron-specific enolase in serum of children with metastatic neuroblastoma. Lancet, 2:361–363, 1983.

Rhabdomyosarcoma and Other Pelvic Tumors of Childhood

Baum, E. S., Gaynon, P., Greenberg, L., et al.: Phase II trial of cis-dichlorodiammine-platinum II in refractory childhood cancer: Children's Cancer Study Group Report. Cancer Treat. Rep., 65:815–822, 1981.

Benson, R. C., Tomera, K. M., and Kelalis, P. P.: Transitional cell carcinoma of the bladder in children and adults. J. Urol., 130:54, 1983.

Chu, J. Y., O'Connor, D. M., DeMello, D., Razek, A. A., and McElfresh, A. E.: Childhood embryonal carcinoma of testis: Report of two unusual cases and the implication on clinical management. Med. Pediatr. Oncol., 4:175, 1978.

Crist, W. M., Raney, R. B., Tefft, M., Heyn, R., Hays, D. M., Newton, W., Beltangady, M., and Maurer, H. M.: Soft tissue sarcomas arising in the retroperitoneal space in children: A report from the Intergroup Rhabdomyosarcoma Study (IRS) Committee. Cancer, 56:2125–2132, 1985.

D'Angio, G. J., Farber, S., and Maddock, C. L.: Potentiation of x-ray effects by actinomycin D. Radiology, 73:175, 1959.

Donaldson, S. S.: Rhabdomyosarcoma: Contemporary status and future directions. Arch. Surg., 124:1015–1020, 1989.

Edland, R. W.: Embryonal rhabdomyosarcoma. Am. J. Roentgenol. Radium Ther. Nucl. Med., 93:67, 1965.

Engle, R. M., and Wilkinson, H. A.: Bladder exstrophy. J. Urol., 104:699, 1970.

Ghazali, S.: Embryonic rhabdomyosarcoma of the urogenital tract. Br. J. Surg., 60:124, 1973.

Green, D. M., and Jaffe, N.: Progress and controversy in the treatment of childhood rhabdomyosarcoma. Cancer Treat. Rev., 5:7, 1978.

Hays, D. M.: Pelvic rhabdomyosarcoma in childhood: Diagnosis and concepts of management reviewed. Cancer, 45:1811, 1980.

Hays, D. M., Raney, R. B., Jr., Lawrence, W., Jr., et al.: Rhabdomyosarcoma of female urogenital tract. J. Pediatr. Surg., 16:828, 1981.

Hays, D. M., Raney, R. B., Jr., Lawrence, W., Jr., et al.: Bladder and prostatic tumors in the Intergroup Rhabdomyosarcoma Study (IRS-I): Results of therapy. Cancer, 50:1472, 1982a.

Hays, D. M., Raney, R. B., Jr., Lawrence, W., Jr., et al.: Primary chemotherapy in the treatment of children with bladder-prostate tumors in the Intergroup Rhabdomyosarcoma Study (IRS-II). J. Pediatr. Surg., 17:812, 1982b.

Herbst, A. L.: DES update. Cancer, 30:326, 1980.

Herbst, A. L., Cole, P., Colton, T., et al.: Age-incidence and risk of diethylstilbestrol related clear cell adenocarcinoma of the vagina and cervix. Am. J. Obstet. Gynecol., 128:43, 1977.

Herbst, A. L., Sculby, R. E., Welch, W. R., and Robboy, J.: Registry of clear cell adenocarcinoma of the genital tract in young females, 1976 report.

Heyn, R. M., Holland, R., Newton, W. A., Jr., et al.: The role of combined chemotherapy in the treatment of rhabdomyosarcoma in children. Cancer, 34:2128, 1974.

Hinman, F., and Perez-Mesa, C.: Infantile carcinoma: A clinicopathological study and classification of 39 cases. Cancer, 11:181, 1958.

Lawrence, W., Jr., Hays, D. M., and Moon, T. M.: Lymphatic metastases with childhood rhabdomyosarcoma. Cancer, 39:556, 1977.

Li, F. P., and Fraumeni, J. F.: Soft tissue sarcomas, breast cancer and other neoplasms: A familial syndrome. Ann. Intern. Med., 71:747, 1969.

Lockhart, H.: Cancer of the uterus in childhood. Am. J. Obstet. Gynecol., 30:76, 1935.

MacKenzie, A. R., Whitmore, W. F., and Melamed, M. R.: Myosarcomas of the bladder and prostate. Cancer, 22:833, 1968.

Mahour, G. H., Soule, E. H., Mills, S. D., and Lynn, H. B.: Rhabdomyosarcoma in infants and children: A clinicopathologic study of 75 cases. J. Pediatr. Surg., 2:402, 1967.

Maurer, H. M.: The Intergroup Rhabdomyosarcoma Study II: Objectives and study design. J. Pediatr. Surg., 15:371, 1980.

Maurer, H. M., Donaldson, M., Gehan, E. A., et al.: The Intergroup Rhabdomyosarcoma Study: Update, November 1978. NCI Monogr., 56:61, 1981.

Maurer, H. M., Moon, T., Donaldson, M., et al.: The Intergroup Rhabdomyosarcoma Study: A preliminary report. Cancer, 40:2015, 1977.

McKeen, E. A., Bodurtha, J., Meadows, A. T., et al.: Rhabdomyosarcoma complicating multiple neurofibromatosis. J. Pediatr., 93:992, 1978.

Mierau, G. W., and Favara, B. E.: Rhabdomyosarcoma in children: Ultrastructural study of 31 cases. Cancer, 46:2035, 1980.

Norris, H. J., Bagley, G. P., and Taylor, H. B.: Carcinoma of the infant vagina: A distinctive tumor. Arch. Pathol., 90:473, 1970.

Ortega, J. A.: A therapeutic approach to childhood pelvic rhabdomyosarcoma without pelvic exenteration. J. Pediatr., 94:205, 1979.

Patton, R. B., and Horn, R. C., Jr.: Rhabdomyosarcoma: Clinical and pathological features and comparison with human fetal and embryonal skeletal muscle. Surgery, 52:572, 1962.

Pinkel, D., and Pickren, J.: Rhabdomyosarcoma in children. JAMA, 175:293, 1961.

Pollack, R. S., and Taylor, H. C.: Carcinoma of the cervix during the first two decades of life. Am. J. Obstet. Gynecol., 53:135, 1979.

Raney, B., Jr., Carey, A., Snyder, H. M., Duckett, J. W., Schnaufer, L., Rosenberg, H. K., Mahboubi, S., Chatten, J., and Littman, P.: Primary site as a prognostic variable for children with pelvic soft tissue sarcomas. J. Urol., 136:874–878, 1986.

Raney, R. B., Jr., Donaldson, M. H., Sutow, W. W., Lindberg, R. D., Maurer, H. M., and Tefft, M.: Special considerations related to primary site in rhabdomyosarcoma: Experience of the Intergroup Rhabdomyosarcoma Study, 1972–1976. NCI Monogr., 56:69–74, 1981.

Raney, R. B., Jr., Gehan, E. A., Hays, D. M., et al.: Primary chemotherapy with or without radiation therapy and/or surgery for children with localized sarcoma of the bladder, prostate, vagina, uterus and cervix. Cancer, 66:2072–2081, 1990.

Ranson, J. L., et al.: Retroperitoneal rhabdomyosarcoma in children: Results of multimodality therapy. Cancer, 45:845, 1980.

Ray, B., Grabstald, H., Exelby, P. R., and Whitmore, W. W., Jr.: Bladder tumors in children. Urology, 11:426, 1973.

Rivard, G., Ortega, J., Hittle, R., et al.: Intensive chemotherapy as primary treatment for rhabdomyosarcoma of the pelvis. Cancer, 36:1593, 1975.

Ruymann, F. B., Gaiger, A. M., and Newton, W.: Congenital anomalies in rhabdomyosarcoma. In Programs and Abstracts of the Conference on Congenital Birth Defects, Memphis, June 9–11, 1977.

Sagerman, R. H., Tretter, P., and Ellsworth, R. M.: The treatment of orbital rhabdomyosarcoma of children with primary radiation therapy. Am. J. Roentgenol. Radium. Ther. Nucl. Med., 114:31, 1972.

Schoenberg, H. S., and Murphy, J. J.: Neurofibroma of the bladder. J. Urol., 85:899, 1961.

Stobbe, G. C., and Dargeon, H. W.: Embryonal rhabdomyosarcoma of the head and neck in children and adolescents. Cancer, 3:826, 1950.

Sutow, W. W., et al.: Prognosis in childhood rhabdomyosarcoma. Cancer, 25:1384, 1970.

Tefft, M.: Radiation of rhabdomyosarcoma in children: Local control in patients enrolled into the Intergroup Rhabdomyosarcoma Study. NCI Monogr., 56:75, 1981.

Ulfelder, H.: The stilbestrol-adenosis-carcinoma syndrome. Cancer, 38:426, 1976.

Voute, P. A., and Vos, A.: Combination chemotherapy as primary treatment of children with rhabdomyosarcoma to avoid mutilating surgery or radiotherapy Proc. A. A. C. R., 18:327, 1977.

Voute, P. A., Vos, A., and deKraker, J.: Chemotherapy at initial treatment in rhabdomyosarcoma [Abstract C-341]. Proc. Am. Soc. Clin. Oncol., 3:87, 1984.

Wilbur, J. R.: Combination chemotherapy of embryonal rhabdomyosarcoma. Cancer Chemother. Rep., 58:281, 1974.

Young, J. L., and Miller, R. W.: Incidence of malignant tumors in U.S. children. J. Pediatr., 86:254, 1975.

Testis Tumors

Banowsky, L. H., and Shultz, G. N.: Sarcoma of the spermatic cord and tunics: Review of the literature, case report and discussion of the role of retroperitoneal lymph node dissection. J. Urol., 103:628, 1970.

Batata, M. S., Whitmore, W. F., Jr., Chu, F. C. H., et al.: Cryptorchidism and testicular cancer. J. Urol., 124:382, 1980.

Bracken, R. B., and Johnson, D. E.: Sexual function and fecundity after treatment for testicular tumors. Urology, 7:35, 1976.

Brosman, S. A.: Testicular tumors in prepubertal children. Urology, 18:581, 1979.

Brown, N. J.: Teratomas and yolk-sac tumors. J. Clin. Pathol., 29:1021, 1976.

Byrd, R. L.: Testicular leukemia: Incidence and management results. Med. Pediatr. Oncol., 9:493–500, 1981.

Campbell, H. E.: Incidence of malignant growth of the undescended testicle: A critical and statistical study. Arch. Surg., 44:353, 1942.

Campbell, H. E.: The incidence of malignant growth of the undescended testicle: A reply and re-evaluation. J. Urol., 81:663, 1959.

Carney, J. A., Kelalis, P. P., and Lynn, H. B.: Bilateral teratoma of testis in an infant. J. Pediatr. Surg., 8:49, 1973.

Chu, J. Y., O'Connor, D. M., DeMello, D., Razek, A. A., and McElfresh, A. E.: Childhood embryonal carcinoma of testis: Report of two unusual cases and the implication on clinical management. Med. Pediatr. Oncol., 4:175, 1978.

Colodny, A., and Hopkins, T. B.: Testicular tumors in infants and children. Urol. Clin. North Am. 4:347, 1977.

Cromie, W. J., Raney, R. B., Jr., and Duckett, J. W.: Paratesticular rhabdomyosarcoma in children. J. Urol., 122:80, 1979.

D'Angio, G. J., Exelby, P. R., Ghavimi, F., Cham, W. C., and Tefft, M.: Protection of certain structures from high doses of irradiation. Am. J. Roentgonol. Radium Ther. Nucl. Med., 122:103, 1974.

DeCamargo, B., Pinus, J., Lederman, H., and Saba, L.: Intrascrotal metastasis from Wilms' tumor. Med. Pediatr. Oncol., 16:381–383, 1988.

Drago, J. R., Nelson, R. P., and Palmer, J. M.: Childhood embryonal carcinoma of testes. Urology, 12:499, 1978.

Einhorn, L. H., and Donohue, J. P.: Combination chemotherapy in disseminated testicular cancer: The Indiana University experience. Semin. Oncol., 6:87, 1979.

Exelby, P. R.: Testis cancer in children. Semin. Oncol., 6:116, 1979.

Fonkalsrud, E. W.: Current concepts in the management of the undescended testis. Surg. Clin. North Am., 50:847, 1970.

Gallager, H. S.: Pathology of testicular and paratesticular neoplasms. In Johnson, D. E. (Ed.): Testicular Tumors, Ed 2. Flushing, NY, Medical Examination Publishing Co., 1976.

Gibbons, M. D., Cromie, W. J., and Duckett, J. W., Jr.: Management of the abdominal undescended testicle. J. Urol., 122:76, 1979.

Grabstald, H.: Germinal tumors of the testis. CA, 25:82, 1975.

Griffin, G. C., Raney, R. B., Tefft, M., Heyn, R., Hays, D. M., Newton, W., Beltangady, M., and Maurer, H. M.: Soft tissue sarcomas arising in the retroperitoneal space in children: A report from the Intergroup Rhabdomyosarcoma Study (IRS) Committee. Cancer, 56:2125–2132, 1985.

Hinman, F., Jr.: Unilateral abdominal cryptorchidism. J. Urol., 122:71, 1979.

Hinman, F., and Perez-Mesa, C.: Infantile carcinoma: A clinicopathological study and classification of 39 cases. Cancer, 11:181, 1958.

Holbrook, C. T., Crist, W. M., Cain, W., and Bueschen, A.: Successful chemotherapy for childhood metastatic embryonal cell carcinoma of the testicle: A preliminary report. Med. Pediatr. Oncol., 8:75, 1980.

Hopkins, G. B., Jaffe, N., Colodny, A., Cassady, J. R., and Filler, R. M.: The management of testicular tumors in children. J. Urol., 120:96, 1978.

Houser, R., Izant, R. J., and Persky, L.: Testicular tumors in children. Am. J. Surg., 110:876, 1965.

Ilondo, M. M., Van der Mooter, F., Marchal, G., Vereecken, A., Wynants, P., Lauweryns, J. M., Eeckels, R., and Van de Schueren-Looe Weycky, M.: A boy with Leydig cell tumor and precocious puberty: Ultrasonography as a diagnostic aid. Eur. J. Pediatr., 137:221, 1981.

Ise, T., Ohtsuki, H., Matsumoto, K., and Sano, R.: Management of malignant testicular tumors in children. Cancer, 37:1539, 1976.

Jeffs, R. D.: Management of embryonal adenocarcinoma of the testis in childhood: An analysis of 164 cases. In Gooden, J. A. (Ed.): Cancer in Childhood. Toronto, The Ontario Cancer Treatment and Research Foundation, 1972.

Johnstone, G.: Prepubertal gynecomastia in association with an interstitial cell tumor of the testis. Br. J. Urol., 39:211, 1967.

Kaplan, G. W.: Testicular tumors in children. AUA Update Series, Lesson 12, Vol. 2, 1983.

Karamehmedovic, O., Woodtli, W., and Pluss, H. J.: Testicular tumors in childhood. J. Pediatr. Surg., 10:109, 1975.

Kramer, S. A.: Embryonal cell carcinoma in children. Pediatr. Urol. Letter Club, October 21, 1981.

Kurman, R. J., Scardino, P. T., McIntire, K. R., Waldmann, T. A., and Javadpour, N.: Cellular localization of alpha-feto-protein and human chorionic gonadotrophin in germ cell tumors of the testis using an indirect immunoperoxidase technique: A new approach to classification utilizing tumor markers. Cancer, 40:2136, 1977.

Lamm, D. L., and Kaplan, G. W.: Urological manifestation of Burkitt's lymphoma. J. Urol., 112:402, 1974.

Leopold, G. R., Woo, V. L., Scheible, F. W., Nachtsheim, D., and Grosink, B. B.: High-resolution ultrasonography of scrotal pathology. Radiology, 131:719, 1979.

Li, F. P., and Fraumeni, J. F., Jr.: Testicular cancers in children: Epidemiologic characteristics. JNCI, 48:1575, 1972.

Manger, D.: Pathology of tumors of the testis in children. *In* Gooden, J. O. (Ed.): Cancer in Childhood. New York, Plenum Press, 1973, p. 60.

Manuel, M., Katayama, K. P., and Jones, H. W., Jr.: The age of occurrence of gonadal tumors in intersex patients with a Y chromosome. Am. J. Obstet. Gynecol., 124:293, 1976.

Martin, D. C.: Germinal cell tumors of the testis after orchiopexy. J. Urol., 121:422, 1979.

Mostofi, F. K., and Price, E. B.: AFIP Fascile #8, 2nd Series, Tumors of the Male Genital System, 1973, p. 99.

Mulvihill, J. J., Wade, W. M., and Miller, R. M.: Gonadoblastoma in dysgenetic gonads with a Y chromosome. Lancet, 1:863, 1975.

Oakhill, A., Mainwaring, D., Hill, F. G. H., Gornall, P., Cudmore, R. E., Banks, A. J., Brock, J. E. S., Martay, J., and Mann, J. R.: Management of leukemic infiltration of the testis. Arch. Dis. Child., 55:564, 1980.

Olive, D., Flamant, F., Zucker, J. M., Voute, P., Brunat-Mentigny, M., Otten, J., and Dutou, L.: Para-aortic lymphadenectomy is not necessary in the treatment of localized paratesticular rhabdomyosarcoma. Cancer, 54:1283–1287, 1984.

Olive-Sommelet, D.: Paratesticular rhabdomyosarcoma. Dialog. Pediatr. Urol., 12(11):1–8, 1989.

Olney, L. E., et al.: Intrascrotal rhabdomyosarcoma. Urology, 14:113, 1979.

Pierce, G. B., Bullock, W. K., and Huntington, R. W., Jr.: Yolk-sac tumors of the testis. Cancer, 25:644, 1970.

Pomer, F. A., Stiles, R. E., and Graham, J. H.: Interstitial cell tumors of the testis in children: Report of a case and review of the literature. N. Engl. J. Med., 250:233, 1954.

Price, E. B.: Epidermoid cysts of the testis: A clinical and pathologic analysis of 69 cases from the testicular tumor registry. Urology, 102:708, 1969.

Raney, R. B., Jr., Hays, D. M., Lawrence, W., Jr., Soule, E. H.,

Tefft, M., and Donaldson, M. H.: Paratesticular rhabdomyosarcoma in childhood. Cancer, 42:729, 1978.

Raney, R. B., Jr., Tefft, M., Lawrence, W., Jr., Ragab, A. H., Soule, E. H., Beltangady, M., and Gehan, E. A.: Paratesticular sarcoma in childhood and adolescence: A report from the Intergroup Rhabdomyosarcoma Sarcoma Studies I and II, 1973–1983. Cancer, 60:2337–2343, 1987.

Rosvoll, R. V., and Woodard, J. R.: Malignant Sertoli cell tumor of the testis. Cancer, 22:8, 1968.

Scully, R. E.: Gonadoblastoma: A review of 74 cases. Cancer, 25:1340, 1970.

Staubitz, W. J., Jewett, T. C., Jr., Magoss, I. V., Schenk, W. L., Jr., and Phalakornkulf, S.: Management of testicular tumors in children. J. Urol., 94:683, 1965.

Tefft, M., Lattin, P. B., Jereb, B., et al.: Acute and late effects on normal tissues following combined chemo- and radiotherapy for childhood rhabdomyosarcoma and Ewing's sarcoma. Cancer, 37:1201, 1976.

Tefft, M., Vawter, G. F., and Mitus, A.: Radiotherapeutic management of testicular neoplasms in children. Radiology, 88:457, 1967.

Teilum, G.: Endodermal sinus tumors of ovary and testis: Comparative morphogenesis of the so-called mesonephroma ovarii (Schiller) and extraembryonic (yolk sac-allantoic) structures of the rat's placenta. Cancer, 23:1092, 1959.

Urban, M. D., Lee, P. A., Plotnick, L. P., and Migeon, C. J.: The diagnosis of Leydig cell tumors in childhood. Am. J. Dis. Child., 132:494, 1978.

Viprakasit, D., Navarro, G., Guarin, U. K., and Garnes, H.: Seminoma in children. Urology, 9:568, 1977.

Weissbach, L., Altwein, J. E., and Stiens, R.: Germinal testicular tumors in childhood. Eur. Urol., 10:73, 1984.

Wong, K. Y., Ballard, E. T., Strayer, F. H., Kisker, C. T., and Lampkin, B. C.: Clinical and occult testicular leukemia in long-term survivors of acute lymphoblastic leukemia. J. Pediatr., 96:569, 1980.

XII
RENAL DISEASES OF UROLOGIC SIGNIFICANCE

55
RENOVASCULAR HYPERTENSION

E. Darracott Vaughan, Jr., M.D.
R. Ernest Sosa, M.D.

Renovascular disease is one of the most common causes of secondary hypertension. A rising rate of detection is being experienced as more definitive diagnostic tests are developed. The need for identification of this entity is apparent because this type of hypertension is difficult to manage with medical therapy (Hunt and Strong, 1973), and many renal lesions are progressive (Schreiber et al., 1984), leading to renal damage.

Fortunately, newer diagnostic tests to identify these patients, which often do not require hospitalization (Sosa and Vaughan, 1983, 1989), have reduced the high cost of evaluation (McNeil and Adelstein, 1975; McNeil et al., 1975), resulting in a more aggressive approach. In this chapter, we review the current strategies that are useful in identifying patients with renovascular hypertension, with emphasis on renin determinations and angiotensin-converting enzyme inhibitors for diagnostic purposes.

In addition, progressive renal arterial disease can lead to loss of renal function, another indication for intervention (Novick, 1989). We also discuss the identification and selection of patients for renal reconstruction to preserve renal function (Jacobson, 1988).

HISTORICAL BACKGROUND

Richard Bright (1827), Physician Extraordinary to the Queen of England, was the first to associate proteinuria, fullness and hardness of the pulse, and dropsy with "hardening of the kidneys." In 1856, Traube, from an analysis of pulse tracings, suggested that the abnormality might be high blood pressure. Mohomed (1874) demonstrated "high tension in the arterial system" in association with renal disease.

The critical experimental work was the discovery of renin by Tigerstedt and Bergmann (1898), who noted an increase in arterial blood pressure in rabbits injected with a saline renal extract. They reasoned that the renal extract contained a pressor substance and coined the term "renin." However, the significance of their work was not recognized until the critical experiments by Goldblatt and co-workers (1934). They produced diastolic hypertension in dogs by clamping the main renal arteries and corrected the hypertension by unclamping these arteries.

Soon thereafter, Butler (1937) reported the first reversal of hypertension following nephrectomy in a patient with a small "pyelonephritic kidney." One year later, Leadbetter and Burkland (1938) reported another cure of hypertension in a child with pathology demonstrating a renal arterial lesion.

These clinical observations were paralleled by laboratory investigation, and in 1940, Page and Helmer and Braun-Menendez and colleagues independently reported that renin itself was not a pressor substance but acted as an enzyme to release a pressor peptide, now called angiotensin, from a circulating plasma globulin. Goormaghtigh and Grimson (1939), who had previously described the juxtaglomerular cells, then described increased granularity of these cells in both animals and humans with renal hypertension and postulated that these cells were secreting excessive amounts of renin.

There followed an aggressive yet disappointing clinical experience with nephrectomy for cure of hypertension in patients with unilateral renal disease. This experience led to the search for a method of proving that a renal lesion was actually causing the hypertension. Homer Smith (1948), in a review of the literature, reported relief of hypertension in only 38 (19 per cent) of 200 patients whose elevated blood pressure was thought to result from unilateral renal disease. Thus, it became apparent that even if pressor mechanisms did underlie some forms of renal hypertension, they could not be measured.

This challenge led to studies of the effect of renal artery constriction on renal function. In dogs, renal artery constriction resulted in a marked decrease in sodium and water excretion from the affected kidney (Blake et al., 1950; Pitts and Duggan, 1950). In 1954, Howard and Conner used these observations to develop a differential renal function test based on bilateral ureteral catheterization to identify the "ischemic kidney." Another major advance was the development of translumbar aortography and the demonstration of its value in visualizing renal arterial lesions (Smith et al., 1952). By 1957, the first large series of patients with renal arterial lesions was reported (Poutasse and Dustan, 1957).

In addition, interest in what would become the renin-angiotensin-aldosterone system was also emerging as new discoveries were made. Accordingly, it was determined that there were two forms of angiotensin (Skeggs et al., 1954), and angiotensin was sequenced (Skeggs et al., 1956) and synthesized (Bumpus et al., 1957). These critical advancements have led to accurate radioimmunoassay for angiotensin, development of angiotensin analogues, and angiotensin-converting enzyme inhibitors—all major tools now used to identify the patient with renovascular hypertension. Moreover, it is recognized that the renin-angiotensin-aldosterone system is a critical integrated system regulating not only blood pressure and sodium and potassium balance but also regional blood flow and, in particular, glomerular filtration rate (Laragh and Sealey, 1991; Sealey et al., 1988a).

DEFINITIONS

Hypertension

It has been difficult to establish a precise definition of hypertension. The problem was best stated by Sir George Pickering, who wrote that "there is no dividing line. The relationship between arterial blood pressure and mortality is quantitative; the higher the pressure, the worse the prognosis" (Pickering, 1990b). Indeed, cumulative data obtained from insurance companies have validated this point. Untreated blood pressure in excess of 140/90 mm Hg is associated with an excessive mortality rate, and diastolic pressure below 70 mm Hg is optimal (Lew, 1973). For operational purposes, the World Health Organization has defined hypertension in adults as a systolic pressure greater than 160 mm Hg and/or a diastolic pressure greater than 95 mm Hg. However, the benefit of treating mild hypertension remains controversial (Pickering, 1990b). In addition, consistent elevation of blood pressure should be established with repeated readings before further evaluation is instituted. In our survey of hypertension detection in Charlottesville, Virginia, we found that half the patients identified as hypertensive in a house-to-house survey were normotensive on a repeat blood pressure measurement (Carey et al., 1976).

In children, a rise in blood pressure occurs with age, with an upper limit of normal reaching 130/80 by age 12 to 15 years. The most accurate evaluation, utilizing an appropriately small cuff, requires comparison of the measured blood pressure with a standard nomogram showing blood pressure related to age (Fig. 55–1) (Sinaiko and Wells, 1990).

Renal Arterial Disease Versus Renovascular Hypertension

The development of arteriography provided an accurate means of identifying renal arterial disease and

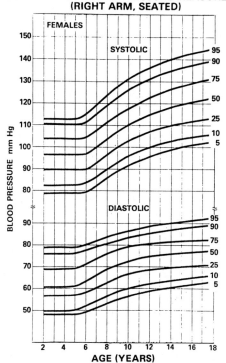

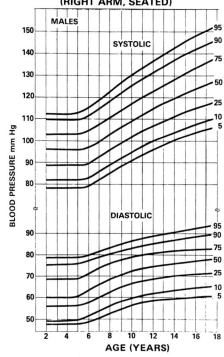

Figure 55–1. Distribution curves for seated blood pressure readings in male and female children from ages 2 to 18 years. (From Loggie, J. H.: In Brunner, H. F., et al. (Eds.): Hypertension in the Child and Adolescent. New York, Marcel Dekker, 1982.)

heralded the advent of renal arterial vascular repair (Freeman et al., 1954), which led to renewed enthusiasm for surgical management. However, it soon became apparent that normotensive patients undergoing arteriography for other reasons often had renal arterial disease (Eyler et al., 1962), especially those with arteriosclerotic disease (Wilms et al., 1990). Autopsy data support the radiologic findings (Holley et al., 1964). Accordingly, the finding of renal arterial disease alone is not sufficient justification to warrant correction in a hypertensive patient. The lesion must be functionally significant, i.e., it must reduce blood flow by an amount sufficient to activate renin release, initiating renovascular hypertension. Hence, a practical definition of renovascular hypertension is hypertension resulting from a renal arterial lesion that is relieved by correction of the offending lesion or removal of the kidney.

All renal arterial lesions do not cause renovascular hypertension. Mann and co-workers (1938) showed that the internal diameter of the carotid artery could be reduced 70 per cent before a significant fall in blood flow occurred (Fig. 55–2). Similarly, Goldblatt and associates (1934) realized that a critical degree of renal arterial stenosis had to be reached before sufficient pressure gradient and flow reduction occurred to initiate hypertension. This observation was carried further by Selkurt (1951), who showed that a 40 mm Hg gradient across a renal artery stenosis was required before there was a change in renal plasma flow, glomerular filtration, sodium excretion, or urinary flow rate. The renal vascular anatomy is important as a guide for choice of transluminal angioplasty or surgical repair, but the demonstration of a renal vascular lesion alone is inadequate to predict the blood pressure response following correction of the obstructing lesion.

Cure Following Correction of Renal Artery Stenosis

Inherent in the care of patients with renovascular hypertension is close and continuing postoperative blood pressure recording. In fact, sustained blood pressure response at least 1 year after surgical correction or angioplasty is mandatory before the diagnosis of renovascular hypertension is validated. In the past, the definition of "successful" revascularization was often arbitrary, especially in terms of the category "improvement," defined as a 15 per cent decrease in diastolic pressure or "blood pressure easier to control with antihypertensive medications" (Foster et al., 1975).

The definition of a surgical response now should be based on reversal of the pathophysiologic abnormalities underlying renovascular hypertension. Hence, patients with inadequate blood pressure responses to surgical intervention require repeat plasma renin activity (PRA) determinations and repeat testing with captopril. Persistence of the criteria characteristic of renovascular hypertension postoperatively signifies technical failure of renal revascularization (Vaughan et al., 1979). In contrast, following successful renal angioplasty and normalization of blood pressure, the peripheral plasma renin activity (PRA) indexed to sodium excretion usu-

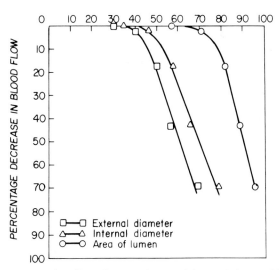

PERCENTAGE DECREASE IN DIAMETER, AND AREA OF LUMEN

Figure 55–2. The effect of progressive arterial constriction on blood flow distal to the stenotic area. (From Mann, F. C., et al.: Surgery, 4:249, 1938.)

ally returns to normal, and bilateral symmetric renal renin secretion returns (Pickering et al., 1984).

PATHOLOGY

The two major pathologic entities that cause renal arterial disease are atherosclerosis and fibromuscular disease. The Cleveland Clinic group has emphasized the importance of the various distinct histologic patterns, identifiable by angiographic techniques, that have predictable natural histories (Harrison and McCormack, 1971; Schreiber et al., 1984, 1989; Stewart et al., 1970). Their classification is shown in Table 55–1.

Atherosclerosis

Atheromatous lesions of the renal artery are common and account for about 60 to 70 per cent of the lesions that cause renovascular hypertension. They usually occur in the proximal 2 cm of the renal artery including the aorta (ostial lesions) but can involve the distal artery or branches (Fig. 55–3). The natural history of this disease has been described, and the stage of the disease may prove to be a major factor in the response to transluminal renal angioplasty (Ratliff, 1985).

Atherosclerosis begins as a proliferation of smooth muscle or myointimal cells in the intima. As they proliferate, the cells form a rounded, eccentric mound that protrudes into the lumen. The fully formed initial lesion consists of a mass of smooth muscle cells with a varying amount of connective tissue. Subsequently, lipid deposition occurs, with necrosis, inflammation, and formation of an atherosclerotic plaque. Local complications of hemorrhage, calcification, or surface erosion with secondary thrombus formation may ensue (Fig. 55–4).

Accordingly, the early lesion may be amenable to percutaneous angioplasty, whereas the mature lesion is

Table 55–1. CLASSIFICATION AND NATURAL HISTORY OF RENOVASCULAR DISEASE

Atherosclerosis: Proximal intimal plaques. Seen predominantly in males and usually in older age groups. Progressive in about 40 per cent of patients; may dissect or thrombose. May involve renal arteries only or may involve carotid and coronary arteries, aorta, and other vessels.

Intimal Fibroplasia: Collagenous disease involving intima; seen in children and young male adults. Progressive; may dissect. May involve other vessels.

True Fibromuscular Hyperplasia: Diffusely involves media. Seen in children and young adults. Progressive. Radiographically indistinguishable from intimal fibroplasia. Very rare.

Medial Fibroplasia: Series of collagenous rings involving media of main renal artery, often extending into branches. Usually seen in women in the thirties and forties. Produces typical "string of beads" pattern in angiography. Does not dissect, thrombose, or rupture and seldom progresses after age 40. May involve other vessels.

Perimedial (Subadventitial) Fibroplasia: Dense collagenous collar involving outer media, just beneath adventitia of vessel. Tightly stenotic, with extensive collateral circulation on angiography. Seen mostly in young women ("girlie disease"). Progressive. Involves renal arteries only.

Miscellaneous: Renal artery aneurysms, middle aortic syndrome, periarterial fibrosis, and post-traumatic intimal or medial disease. Variable in location and obstruction; occurs in diverse clinical settings.

From Stewart, B. H., Dustan, H. P., Kiser, W. S., et al.: J. Urol., 104:231, 1970.

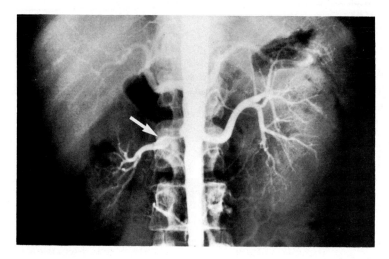

Figure 55–3. Severe atherosclerotic stenosis of the proximal right renal artery in an elderly man. Note the poststenotic arterial dilatation *(arrow)*. (From Walter, J. F., and Bookstein, J. J.: *In* Stanley, J. C., et al. (Eds.): Renovascular Hypertension. Philadelphia, W. B. Saunders Co., 1984.)

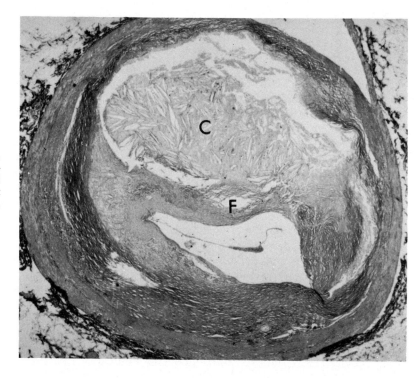

Figure 55–4. Atheromatous plaque. F, fibrous cap; C, central lipid core with typical cholesterol clefts. (Courtesy of Dr. C. Haudenschild, Boston University Medical Center. From Robbins, S. L., et al. (Eds.): Pathologic Basis of Disease. Philadelphia, W. B. Saunders Co., 1984.)

more difficult to traverse, more rigid, and more likely to shed atheromatous emboli (Ratliff, 1985). Total reversal of hypertension following correction of atherosclerotic lesions is less common than in patients with fibromuscular disease. These patients often have diffuse atherosclerotic disease and underlying essential hypertension. In a cooperative study of renovascular hypertension, patients with bilateral atherosclerotic disease had the lowest cure rate and the highest morbidity of the various groups operated upon (Foster et al., 1975). However, attention to concurrent carotid and coronary disease prior to renal revascularization and avoidance of a severely diseased aorta have markedly reduced the morbidity of reconstructive surgery in this group (Novick et al., 1981; Novick, 1989).

Intimal Fibroplasia

This lesion is characterized by circumferential accumulation of collagen, which compromises the lumen inside the internal elastic membrane (Fig. 55–5). It

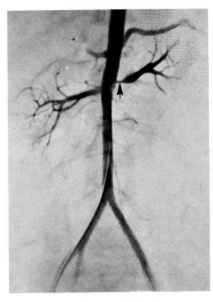

Figure 55–6. Aortogram of a 6-year-old boy demonstrates proximal left renal artery stenosis *(arrow)* from intimal fibroplasia. (From Novick, A. C.: *In* Kelalis, P. P., King, L. R., and Belman, A. B. (Eds.): Clinical Pediatric Urology. Philadelphia, W. B. Saunders Co., 1984.)

occurs in children and young adults, is almost always progressive, may be complicated by dissection, and accounts for 10 per cent of the total number of fibrous lesions. Angiography reveals a smooth, fairly focal stenosis usually involving the midportion of the vessel or its branches (Fig. 55–6). Because of progression and dissection, the lesion should be corrected when identified.

Fibromuscular Hyperplasia

This rare lesion, composing only 2 to 3 per cent of the total, is the only one in which true hyperplasia of the smooth muscle and fibrous tissue are present. The angiographic picture may be indistinguishable from that of intimal fibroplasia. It also occurs in children and young adults, and, because it is progressive, intervention is warranted.

Medial Fibroplasia

This lesion is usually referred to as fibromuscular hyperplasia—a misnomer because it does not consist of true muscle hyperplasia. It gives the typical "string of beads" pattern (Fig. 55–7) on angiography, which is caused by the presence of a series of fibrous rings interspersed with aneurysmal dilatations. The aneurysms themselves are greater in diameter than the normal renal artery, and the actual degree of stenosis is difficult to assess. It is the most common fibrous lesion, constituting 75 to 80 per cent of the total, and characteristically occurs in women between the ages of 20 and 50 years. The lesion does not hemorrhage or dissect but may progress (Schreiber et al., 1984, 1989). Intervention is indicated in the younger patient. The older patient probably can be treated with antihypertensive agents if renal function and size are carefully monitored.

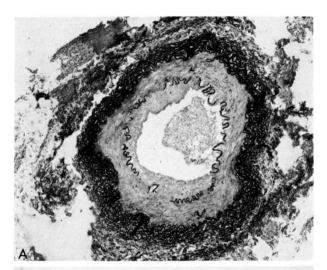

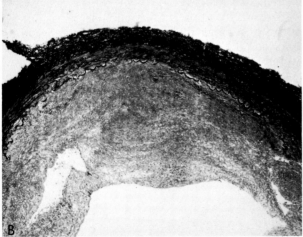

Figure 55–5. *A,* Photomicrograph cross section demonstrating intimal fibroplasia with focal fragmentation and partial absence of the elastica interna. *B,* Photomicrograph cross section demonstrating severe renal arterial intimal fibroplasia with a dense cuff of intimal collagen apposed to the luminal surface of a partially disrupted elastica interna. A small recannulized channel is noted in the lower left. (From Novick, A. C.: *In* Kelalis, P. P., King, L. R., and Belman, A. B. (Eds.): Clinical Pediatric Urology. Philadelphia, W. B. Saunders Co., 1984.)

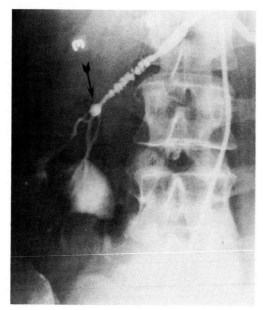

Figure 55–7. Selective right renal arteriogram reveals medial fibroplasia involving the main renal artery with typical "string of beads" appearance. (From Novick, A. C.: *In* Kelalis, P. P., and King, L. R. (Eds.): Clinical Pediatric Urology. Philadelphia, W. B. Saunders Co., 1984.)

Perimedial (Subadventitial) Fibroplasia

This is a tightly stenotic lesion with dense collagen within intact adventitia (Fig. 55–8). In this case, the arterial beading is due to constriction, and the beads are smaller than the diameter of the normal artery (Fig. 55–9). The lesion, accounting for 10 to 15 per cent of the fibrous disorders, is progressive and is seen primarily in young females. It occurs only in the renal artery and predominantly involves the right side. Repair of the lesion is indicated because of progression and severe hypertension that usually accompanies the disease.

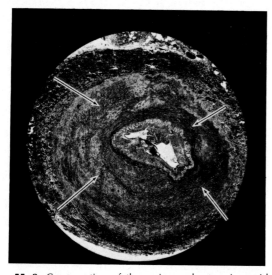

Figure 55–8. Cross section of the main renal artery in a girl with perimedial fibroplasia, demonstrating a dense collagenous collar involving the outer media of the vessel, which causes a severe progressive stenosis. (From Novick, A. C.: *In* Kelalis, P. P., King, L. R., and Belman, A. B. (Eds.): Clinical Pediatric Urology. Philadelphia, W. B. Saunders Co., 1984.)

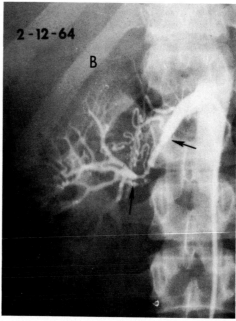

Figure 55–9. Renal arteriogram in patient with perimedial fibroplasia, showing slightly irregular yet severe stenosis of the midrenal artery associated with extensive collateral circulation to the kidney. The small size of the arterial irregularities and the presence of collateral circulation distinguishes this lesion radiographically from medial fibroplasia. (From Novick, A. C.: *In* Kelalis, P. P., King, L. R., and Belman, A. B. (Eds.): Clinical Pediatric Urology. Philadelphia, W. B. Saunders Co., 1984.)

Miscellaneous Lesions

Saccular renal artery aneurysms not associated with coexisting renal arterial vascular disease rarely cause hypertension and usually have a benign natural history (Tham et al., 1983). Although these lesions can be repaired with a high degree of success (Ortenberg et al., 1983), the current trend favors a conservative approach. If hypertension is present, the etiologic role of the aneurysm should be proved before resection is advised.

Takayasu's aortitis is a chronic sclerosing aortitis of unknown etiology that may involve the renal arteries (Rose and Sinclair-Smith, 1980). The disease is progressive and difficult to manage but has been treated with angioplasty (Kumar et al., 1990).

Renal vascular lesions can also occur following irradiation (McGill et al., 1979), in association with neurofibromatosis (Halpern and Currarino, 1965) or in association with a variety of other diseases (Gephardt and McCormack, 1982) (Table 55–2). Moreover, hypertension can be caused by a number of unilateral renal parenchymal diseases (Sosa and Vaughan, 1989).

NATURAL HISTORY

Relatively few reports have been published about the natural history of renal artery lesions. However, in an important current study, Cragg and co-workers (1989) reviewed the results of 1862 renal arteriograms obtained from potential renal donors. Fibromuscular dysplasia

Table 55–2. OTHER VASCULAR LESIONS OR DISEASES ASSOCIATED WITH HYPERTENSION

Intrinsic Lesions
Vascular
Aneurysm (Perry: Arch. Surg., 102:216, 1971)
Emboli (Arakawa: Arch. Intern. Med., 129:958, 1972)
Arteritis
    Polyarteritis nodosa (Dornfield: JAMA, 215:1950, 1971)
    Takayasu's (Kirschbaum: Am. Heart J., 80:811, 1970)
Arteriovenous fistula (Bennet: Am. J. Roentgenol. Radium Ther. Nucl. Med., 95:372, 1965)
Angioma (Farreras-Valenti: Am. J. Med., 34:735, 1973)
Neurofibromatosis (Halpern: N. Engl. J. Med., 273:248, 1965)
Tumor thrombus (Jennings: Br. Med. J., 2:1053, 1964)
Renal transplant rejection (Gunnels: N. Engl. J. Med., 274:543, 1966)
Renal Parenchymal
Vesicoureteral reflux and renal scarring (Savage: Lancet, 1:441, 1978)
Renal tuberculosis (Stockigt: Aust. N.Z. J. Med., 6:229, 1976)
Ask-Upmark kidney (Amat: Virchows Arch., 390:193, 1981)
"Page kidney" (Sufrin: J.Urol., 113:450, 1975)
Solitary cyst (Kala: J. Urol., 116:710, 1976)
Polycystic kidney disease (Nash: Arch. Intern. Med., 137:1571, 1977)
Radiation nephritis (Shapiro: Arch. Intern. Med., 137:848, 1977)
Renal cell carcinoma (Hollifield: Arch. Intern. Med., 135:859, 1975)
Wilms' tumor (Mitchell: Arch. Dis. Child., 45:376, 1970)
Reninoma (Robertson: Am. J. Med., 43:963, 1967)
Unilateral hydronephrosis (Riehle: J. Urol., 126:243, 1981)
Bilateral hydronephrosis (Vaughan: J. Urol., 109:286, 1973)

Extrinsic Lesions
Vascular
Stenosis of celiac axis with "steal of renal blood flow" (Alfidi: Radiology, 102:545, 1972)
Congenital fibrous band (Lampe: Angiology, 16:677, 1965)
Hypoplastic aorta (Kaufman: J. Urol. 109:711, 1973)
Postradiation arteritis (McGill: J. Pediatr. Surg., 14:831,1979)
Traumatic occlusion (Cornell: JAMA, 219:1754, 1972)
Coarctation (Shumaker: N. Engl. J. Med., 295:148, 1976)
Other Lesions
Pheochromocytoma (Rosenheim: Am. J. Med., 34:735, 1963)
Metastatic tumors (Weidemann: Am. J. Med., 47:528, 1969)
Ptosis (Derrick: Am. J. Surg., 106:673, 1963)

was present in 71 patients (3.8 per cent). Of 30 normotensive patients who did not undergo nephrectomy, 8 (26.6 per cent) developed hypertension over a mean follow-up of 7.5 years. This information in normotensive patients complements data from several longitudinal angiographic studies of hypertensive patients, which showed progression in about 40 per cent. Thus, the limited data available suggest that many patients with both atherosclerotic disease (Dean, 1989; Wollenweber et al., 1968) and fibromuscular disease (Meaney et al., 1968) will have progressive disease. However, it has been difficult to predict which lesions would undergo progression from the initial arteriogram (Stewart et al., 1970). The important question of progression has been addressed by Schreiber and co-workers (1984, 1989), and more precise information is now available.

Serial angiographic studies over a mean interval of 52 months in 85 patients with atherosclerotic disease revealed progressive vascular obstruction in 37 patients (44 per cent). Total arterial occlusion occurred in 14 patients, most commonly in those with a greater than 75 per cent stenosis on the initial arteriogram. Decline in renal function was more common in patients with progressive disease. Accordingly, these investigators suggested that renal revascularization might be indicated for preservation of renal function in individuals whose advanced atherosclerotic disease was a major threat to overall renal function. These patients are characterized by azotemia and high-grade renal artery stenosis (greater than 75 per cent), bilateral high-grade stenosis, and stenosis involving a solitary kidney (Novick, 1989; Schreiber et al., 1984, 1989).

Sixty patients with medial fibroplasia were also followed for a mean interval of 45 months. Progressive renal arterial obstruction was observed in 22 of 66 patients (33 per cent); however, there were no cases of progression to total occlusion. Of particular interest was the similar development of progressive disease in patients older than 40 years of age (15 of 46). Previously, it was thought that the disease was stable in this age group (Meaney et al., 1968). Despite the angiographic progression demonstrated, increases in serum creatinine value or reduction in renal size seldom occurred. Accordingly, the investigators did not suggest renal revascularization or angioplasty for preservation of renal function alone in this group.

NORMAL PHYSIOLOGY OF THE RENIN-ANGIOTENSIN-ALDOSTERONE SYSTEM

The renin-angiotensin-aldosterone system (RAAS) (Fig. 55–10) is the major renal hormonal system involved in the regulation of systemic blood pressure, sodium and potassium balance, and regional blood flow.

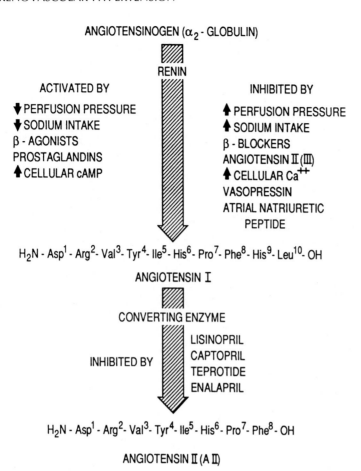

ANGIOTENSINOGEN (α_2 - GLOBULIN)

RENIN

ACTIVATED BY

↓ PERFUSION PRESSURE
↓ SODIUM INTAKE
β - AGONISTS
PROSTAGLANDINS
↑ CELLULAR cAMP

INHIBITED BY

↑ PERFUSION PRESSURE
↑ SODIUM INTAKE
β - BLOCKERS
ANGIOTENSIN II (III)
↑ CELLULAR Ca^{++}
VASOPRESSIN
ATRIAL NATRIURETIC
PEPTIDE

H_2N - Asp^1 - Arg^2- Val^3- Tyr^4- Ile^5- His^6- Pro^7- Phe^8- His^9- Leu^{10}- OH

ANGIOTENSIN I

CONVERTING ENZYME

INHIBITED BY

LISINOPRIL
CAPTOPRIL
TEPROTIDE
ENALAPRIL

H_2N - Asp^1 - Arg^2- Val^3- Tyr^4- Ile^5- His^6- Pro^7- Phe^8- OH

ANGIOTENSIN II (A II)

A II RECEPTOR

ACTIVATION OF RECEPTOR
RESULTS IN:

1. VASOCONSTRICTION
2. SODIUM RETENTION
3. RELEASE OF ALDOSTERONE
4. RELEASE OF CATECHOLAMINES

A II RECEPTOR BLOCKED BY
A II ANALOGUES: PROTOTYPE

(Sarcosine^1, Valine^5,
Alanine^8) A II (Saralasin)

Figure 55–10. The renin-angiotensin-aldosterone system.

Its main components are renin; angiotensin II (AII), an octapeptide that is a pressor agent; and aldosterone, a mineralocorticoid released from the adrenal cortex. The system is thus involved in both the vasoconstriction and the volume/sodium components of blood pressure control (Laragh and Sealey, 1991).

Prorenin is the biosynthetic precursor molecule of renin (Inagami and Murakami, 1980). The amino acid sequence of prorenin has been determined from the nucleotide sequence of the human renin gene, thus establishing prorenin as an inactive precursor of renin (Imai et al., 1983; Soubrier et al., 1983). It is believed that prorenin acts through active renin. However, there may be an independent second prorenin system functioning at a local level in the kidney, ovary, testis, and other organs where it is found; for example, prorenin may play a role in reproductive function (Sealey et al., 1980, 1986, 1988b).

Renin is an aspartyl protease with a molecular weight of 37,200 daltons containing 340 amino acids; a single human renin gene has been determined (Imai et al., 1983; Soubrier et al., 1983). The major source of active renin in humans is the juxtaglomerular (JG) apparatus in the kidney, which secretes renin in response to well-defined stimuli (Fig. 55–11) (Barajas et al., 1990). The half-life of plasma renin is usually reported as between 15 and 20 minutes, and its major site of metabolism is in the liver. Release of renin from the JG cells is regulated by several factors to be discussed.

Once in the plasma, renin acts on its substrate, angiotensinogen. Angiotensinogen is a glycoprotein of molecular weight 56,800 daltons, which is produced by the liver. The complementary DNA (cDNA) sequence for rat angiotensinogen has been determined (Ohkubo et al., 1983). Human renin splits a leucyl-valine peptide bond and causes release of the decapeptide angiotensin I (AI). AI itself is basically an inactive species, and its biologic activity results from its conversion to the active species, AII. Angiotensin-converting enzyme (ACE) a peptidyl dipeptide hydrolase, also known as kininase II, is a carboxydipeptidase that splits the terminal histidyl-leucine from AI, yielding the octapeptide AII, which is the active peptide in the system (Soffer, 1981). Angiotensin-converting enzyme is found in lung (Ng and Vane, 1967), plasma, and endothelium of vascular beds, including the kidney. It is the discovery of converting enzyme inhibitors that has contributed much to the understanding of the RAAS. However, with the broad substrate specificity of ACE, it may be unwise to attribute all the effects of ACE inhibitors to ablation of the RAAS. In summary, angiotensinogen is split into AI by the action of renin. Converting enzyme converts AI to AII. Because all the components of the system are present in the kidney, AII may function as an intrarenal as well as an extrarenal hormone (Levens et al., 1981).

AII is a compound with a wide range of biologic activity. Most of its actions are directed toward maintenance or increase of blood pressure. This control is accomplished through both its direct effect as a vasoconstrictor and its effect on sodium and volume. The data suggest that the RAAS is activated by sodium depletion to maintain sodium balance and blood pressure by direct vasoconstriction, aldosterone biosynthesis, and renal conservation of salt and water (see Chapters 2 and 3). In 1960, Laragh and colleagues demonstrated that AII infusion caused a rise in plasma aldosterone levels. This is a direct effect of AII on the adrenals, because AII increases aldosterone release from isolated adrenal slices and adrenal zona glomerulosa cell suspensions. AII acts by stimulating the conversion of cholesterol to pregnenolone, an early step in aldosterone biosynthesis; and at a later step, corticosterone to aldosterone. Aldosterone, an 18-aldehyde steroid, is secreted in nanogram amounts, but it is a potent regulator of sodium and potassium balance (Carey and Sen, 1986). Aldosterone acts primarily on the renal tubule to promote the reabsorption of sodium and the excretion of potassium. Both plasma and urinary levels of aldosterone can be measured by precise radioimmunoassay (see Chapter 64).

AII also has been shown to have a direct sodium-retaining effect, acting at the ascending limb of the loop of Henle (Munday et al., 1971). Mechanisms that serve to dampen the system are feedback-inhibiting loops. The "long" loop involves inhibition of renin release mediated by aldosterone-induced sodium retention, volume expansion, and increased blood pressure. There is also a "short" intrarenal loop, in which AII directly inhibits renin release (Ayers et al., 1969, 1977).

Renin release from the JG cells is controlled indirectly by at least three separate mechanisms—baroreceptor, macula densa, and beta-adrenergic—and directly by various hormones acting at the level of the JG cells (Keeton and Campbell, 1980). The baroreceptor mechanism involves changes in renin release in response to changes in pressure at the afferent arteriole (Tobian et al., 1959). Increased pressure decreases renin release, and decreased pressure increases renin release (see Fig. 55–10).

The macula densa mechanism involves changes in electrolyte composition detected at the macula densa, a segment of the distal tubule that is in very close proximity to the vascular pole of the glomerulus (Barajas and Latta, 1964; Barajas et al., 1990). For many years, it was believed that sodium was the ion controlling reactivity of the macula densa. It was known that, with decreased salt intake, the filtered fraction of sodium reabsorbed in the proximal tubule increased, and less sodium reached the distal tubule. Decreased salt intake is associated with increased PRA. The opposite is true of increased sodium intake. This observation led to the conclusion that renin secretion is inversely related to

Figure 55–11. Diagram of the juxtaglomerular apparatus. The two intrarenal receptors, the vascular receptor and the macula densa, are depicted in their close physical relationship. According to current theory, the vascular receptor includes the juxtaglomerular cells and adjacent renal afferent arteriole, and this receptor responds to changes in wall tension. A change in renal tubular sodium appears to give the signal for stimulation of the macula densa, with a resulting influence on renin release. The juxtaglomerular cells secrete renin into the lumen of the renal afferent arteriole and into the renal lymph. The renal nerves are shown ending in both the juxtaglomerular cells and the smooth muscle cells of the renal afferent arteriole. Attention is also called to the intimate relationship of the efferent arteriole and the macula densa; granular cells have been observed, but rarely, in the efferent arteriole. (From Davis, J. O.: In Laragh, J. H. (Ed.): Hypertension Manual. New York, Yorke Medical Books, 1973.)

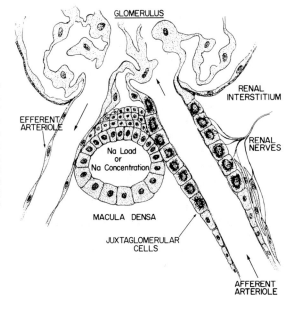

sodium load. Data also have been obtained concerning the role of chloride in regulating the macula densa response. Kotchen and co-workers (1978) maintained animals on diets containing identical sodium concentrations but differing chloride compositions; chloride delivery was measured by micropuncture. Increased chloride consumption decreased PRA (Kotchen et al., 1978).

The JG cells of rats, dogs, and humans are innervated by sympathetic fibers. Vander (1965) demonstrated that electrical stimulation of the renal artery and its associated sympathetics causes renin release. Because these studies did not control for other changes in renal function, they did not establish that a specific adrenergic receptor was involved. However, later studies established that, in dogs with a single nonfiltering kidney, renal nerve stimulation increased renin secretion (Johnson et al., 1971).

Several groups have studied this phenomenon to characterize this response pharmacologically. In general, this receptor appears to have the properties of a beta-adrenergic receptor. For example, changes in renin release caused by nerve stimulation are blocked by 1-propranolol, a beta-blocker, but not by its inactive stereoisomer, D-propranolol. In addition, beta-adrenergic antagonists suppress basal renin release, and these drugs appear to act on the beta-receptors of the JG cells (Buhler et al., 1972).

Changes in renin secretion induced by all these stimuli are mediated by changes in intracellular calcium or complementary adenosine monophosphate (cAMP) within JG cells (Churchill, 1985, 1990). Thus, an increase in cytosolic calcium suppresses renin release, and an increase in cAMP increases renin release. Converse relationships also pertain.

The hierarchy of control of renin release remains under study; however, it appears that the signals are often interdependent (Briggs and Schnermann, 1986).

Mechanisms of Experimental Goldblatt Hypertension

The initial work of Goldblatt stimulated a search for a clearer understanding of the relationship between the renin system and renovascular hypertension. The first advancement was the realization that two models of experimental Goldblatt hypertension can be produced. In one model, a renal artery is clamped and the opposite kidney is left in place. In the other, a renal artery is clamped, but the other kidney is removed. Although animals are equally hypertensive in both models, in the two-kidney, one-clip model, PRA and renin content are increased in the kidney with the stenosed artery and decreased in the opposite kidney (Gross, 1971; Mohring et al., 1975). In the one-kidney, one-clip model, Goldblatt hypertension is characterized by volume expansion and normal or suppressed PRA (Liard et al., 1974).

A second advance in exposing the role of AII in these experimental models was the administration of compounds that either block the conversion of AI to AII or are specific AII-receptor antagonists (Brunner et al., 1971; Miller et al., 1972). These drugs have been im-

portant in their elucidation of the role of the RAAS in the normal and abnormal state and, in the case of converting enzyme inhibitors, in their clinical use in renovascular hypertension.

Knowledge of the structure of AII and improved methods of peptide synthesis have led to the synthesis of many AII analogues of modified amino acid sequence. In the process, analogues were discovered with differing biologic potencies, which led to an understanding of the contribution of each of the amino acid residues to the action of AII (Peach, 1979). Further modifications led to the synthesis of the [sarcosine[1], Val[5], Ala[8]] AII derivative, saralasin (Pals et al., 1971). The substitution of alanine at position 8 resulted in severe reduction of biologic activity without a loss of affinity for the receptor. The presence of sarcosine at the amino terminus allowed for resistance to hydrolysis by peptidases. These characteristics made saralasin a prototype of AII-receptor antagonist with a significant duration of action. Because saralasin is not completely devoid of biologic activity (thus, it is a partial agonist), studies in which it is used require careful evaluation (Case et al., 1976b).

Captopril (SQ 14225; D-3-mercapto-2-methylpropanoyl-L-proline) is a clinical antihypertensive drug, which is an ACE inhibitor (Rubin et al., 1978). Its synthesis followed, by approximately 10 years, the discovery of several naturally occurring converting enzyme inhibitors (CEIs) found in snake venom (Bakhle, 1968). The active components of snake venom that were CEIs were small peptides. Synthesis of large numbers of peptide analogues resulted in synthesis of a nonapeptide CEI (SQ 20881, teprotide), the first CEI used in humans (Cheung and Cushman, 1973). Although useful, SQ 20881 was limited in its effectiveness, owing to a lack of oral activity. Further modifications led to the synthesis of captopril.

Typically, a CEI blocks the pressor response that occurs following injection of AI, which is due to conversion of AI to AII. Blockade of the pressor response to AI occurs without simultaneous blockade of the pressor response to AII or other pressor agents. In addition, because ACE also participates in the metabolism of bradykinin, the depressor effect of bradykinin is potentiated in the presence of a CEI (Rubin et al., 1978).

The animal model with hypertension that is most analogous to human renovascular hypertension is the two-kidney, one-clip Goldblatt preparation. The hypertension in this model is initially dependent on increased renin secretion from the kidney with the clipped vessel, leading to AII formation and arteriolar vasoconstriction. The administration of an AII analogue (saralasin) (Brunner et al., 1971) or an AI-converting enzyme inhibitor (captopril) (Anderson et al., 1990; Weed et al., 1979) can prevent or reverse the hypertension. This early state of two-kidney, one-clip Goldblatt hypertension exhibits four characteristics (Fig. 55–12): (1) increased renin secretion from the damaged kidney, (2) absence of renin secretion from the opposite kidney, (3) decreased renal blood flow to the damaged kidney, and (4) elevated blood pressure secondary to AII-induced vasoconstriction. The identification of these character-

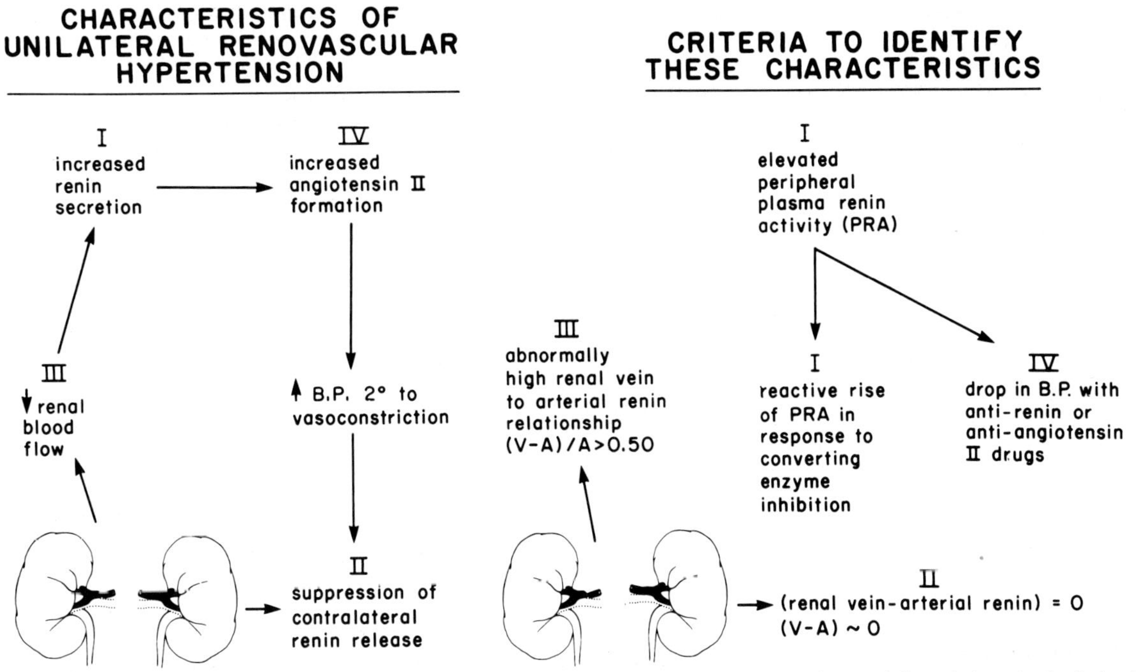

CHARACTERISTICS OF UNILATERAL RENOVASCULAR HYPERTENSION

CRITERIA TO IDENTIFY THESE CHARACTERISTICS

I increased renin secretion

IV increased angiotensin II formation

III ↓ renal blood flow

↑ B.P. 2° to vasoconstriction

III abnormally high renal vein to arterial renin relationship (V–A)/A>0.50

II suppression of contralateral renin release

I elevated peripheral plasma renin activity (PRA)

I reactive rise of PRA in response to converting enzyme inhibition

IV drop in B.P. with anti-renin or anti-angiotensin II drugs

II (renal vein – arterial renin) = 0 (V–A) ~ 0

Figure 55–12. Characteristics of the early phase of two-kidney one-clip Goldblatt hypertension in the rat (*left*) and the criteria derived from the animal model that identify the patient with correctable renal hypertension. (From Vaughan, E. D., Jr., et al.: Urol. Clin. North Am., 11:393, 1984.)

istics has permitted the development of a rational approach to the use of plasma renin determinations (PRA) and angiotensin blockade in the diagnosis of renovascular hypertension (Sosa and Vaughan, 1989; Vaughan et al., 1973, 1984).

In contrast, the one-kidney, one-clip Goldblatt model rapidly establishes hypertension unresponsive to AII antagonists (Brunner et al., 1971) or converting enzyme inhibition unless the animal is sodium-depleted (Gavras et al., 1973). In addition, it is apparent that the early phase of experimental two-kidney, one-clip Goldblatt hypertension is transitory (Gavras et al., 1975; Weed et al., 1979). The blood pressure in these animals subsequently becomes resistant to acute AII blockade unless the animals are subjected to a restriction in dietary sodium. The animals now resemble the one-kidney, one-clip model. However, failure of a blood pressure response to acute AII blockade does not eliminate totally an action of AII in blood pressure maintenance. In fact, long-term administration of captopril (Bengis et al., 1978) leads to a decrease in blood pressure accompanied by natriuresis and diuresis in "saralasin-resistant" one-kidney, one-clip Goldblatt hypertensive rats.

With animal data as the bases, the patient most likely to be cured following successful correction of a renal arterial lesion will exhibit the characteristics of the early-phase two-kidney, one-clip Goldblatt model. The information gained from the one-kidney model suggests that, in any clinical series, there will be patients who do not meet defined preoperative criteria predicting curability, who will have reversal of the hypertension following successful revascularization. It is not known whether these patients are analogous to the chronic two-kidney, one-clip model. Blood pressure control could be due to restoration of renal blood flow (RBF), glomerular filtra-

tion rate (GFR), and sodium excretion, or to reversal of an ill-defined role of AII in the presence of normal PRA. It is estimated that 20 per cent of patients with renal artery stenosis whose hypertension is cured by renal angioplasty will have normal peripheral PRA (Pickering et al., 1984).

IDENTIFYING THE PATIENT WITH RENOVASCULAR HYPERTENSION

Clinical means by which patients with functionally significant renal artery stenosis can be identified have proved to be more elusive than might have been predicted. Certainly, there are no pathognomonic clinical characteristics that lead to a reliable diagnosis (Simon et al., 1972). However, a number of clinical features should arouse suspicion that renovascular hypertension may be present. These are summarized in Table 55–3. Factors implicated as being of importance in patients with fibromuscular dysplasia are cigarette smoking and genetic predisposition (Sang et al., 1989). Ptosis and oral contraceptive use were not found to be causal factors.

The only laboratory finding of importance is hypokalemia. The low potassium level is due to secondary hyperaldosteronism. However, a low serum potassium level is found in less than 20 per cent of patients with renovascular hypertension.

In many patients, none of the usual clinical clues is present to prompt a definitive evaluation. Thus, the unreliability of clinical information led to the development of a variety of approaches to screen for the patient with renovascular hypertension.

Table 55–3. CLINICAL CLUES SUGGESTIVE OF RENOVASCULAR HYPERTENSION

History	Comment
Hypertension in the absence of any family history of hypertensive disease	Suspect if family history is negative; however, about one third of patients with renovascular hypertension will have a positive family history.
Age of onset of hypertension: less than 25 years or greater than 45 years	The average age of onset for essential hypertension is 31 ± 10 (SD) years. Children and young adults usually will have fibromuscular disease, whereas adults over 45 years are more likely to have atherosclerotic narrowing of arteries.
Abrupt onset of moderate to severe hypertension	Whereas essential hypertension usually begins with a "labile" phase before mild hypertension becomes established, renovascular hypertension usually has a more telescoped natural history, often first appearing as moderate hypertension of recent onset.
Development of severe or malignant hypertension	Renovascular hypertension often becomes moderately severe and is prone to produce acceleration or malignant phase hypertension; both forms of hypertension involve markedly increased renin release.
Headaches	Essential hypertension is usually asymptomatic. There seem to be more headaches with renovascular hypertension, possibly related to its severity or high levels of angiotensin II, a potent cerebrovascular vasoconstrictor.
Cigarette smoking	In a recent survey, 74 per cent of patients with fibromuscular renal artery stenosis were smokers; 88 per cent of those with atherosclerotic disease smoke (Nicholson et al., 1983).
White race	Renovascular hypertension is uncommon in the black population.
Resistance to or escape from blood pressure control with standard diuretic therapy or antiadrenergic agents	Probably the most typical feature of renovascular hypertension is that it responds poorly to diuretics and often only transiently to antiadrenergic drugs.
Excellent antihypertensive response to converting enzyme inhibitors, e.g., captopril	Converting enzyme inhibitors block the renin-angiotensin system most effectively and are, therefore, highly specified agents.

Physical Examination and Routine Laboratory Tests	Comment
Retinopathy	Hemorrhages, exudates, or papilledema indicate acceleration or malignant phase.
Abdominal or flank bruit	A helpful clue, but bruits are commonly present in elderly individuals and occasionally present in younger patients who have no apparent vascular stenosis.
Carotid bruits or other evidence of large vessel disease	Commonly, the vascular pathology is not limited to the renal bed.
Hypokalemia—in the untreated state or in response to a thiazide diuretic	Increased aldosterone stimulation by the renin-angiotensin system tends to reduce the serum potassium level. In untreated essential hypertension, this does not occur. Thiazide diuretics accentuate this phenomenon in renovascular hypertension.

From Vaughan, E. D., Jr., Case, D. B., Pickering, T. G., et al.: Urol. Clin. North Am., 11:393, 1984.

An additional clue to the presence of bilateral renal artery stenosis is rapid renal deterioration after treatment with ACE inhibitors; this phenomenon, although less dramatic, can occur in patients with unilateral renal artery stenosis (Hricik et al., 1983).

Differential Renal Function Studies

As previously discussed, the observation in animals that partial occlusion of the renal artery resulted in increased fractional reabsorption of sodium and water (Blake et al., 1950) and increased urinary concentration of nonreabsorbable solute led to the development of differential renal function studies (Howard et al., 1954). The initial criterion for a positive test finding was a 50 per cent decrease in urine flow and a 15 per cent or greater decrease in sodium concentration from the affected kidney. The test underwent numerous modifications (Stamey, 1963); the most popular version included the infusion of inulin, para-aminohippuric acid (PAH), and antidiuretic hormone during a urea-saline diuresis to accentuate the disparity in salt and water reabsorption between the two kidneys (Stamey et al., 1961). However, the complexity involved in performing differential split renal function studies coupled with the

development of more accurate methods to measure activity of the RAAS has almost eliminated this technique. Generally, at this time, differential renal function studies are performed only if renin studies are equivocal or if the patient has unilateral parenchymal disease. In contrast, the Vanderbilt group still believes that, in many cases, renin studies and split renal function studies are complementary and that the omission of either will increase the false-negative rate (Dean, 1989). In the setting of unilateral parenchymal disease, differential function studies are most useful. The treatment choice is nephrectomy or antihypertensive medical management. Medical management is preferable when the affected kidney is contributing substantially to total renal function. Hence, the technique is used to measure the GFR of the involved kidney. If the kidney has sufficient function to sustain life, medical treatment should be the first management strategy.

Intravenous Urogram

The rapid-sequence intravenous urogram is actually a radiographic differential renal function study using the contrast material as the indicator. Reduced RBF is indicated by decreased renal mass or size; decreased

GFR by delayed calyceal appearance time of contrast agent; and hyperreabsorption of water by delayed hyperconcentration of nonreabsorbable solute, the iodinated contrast material. The most reliable abnormality seen in patients with proven unilateral renovascular hypertension is delayed calyceal appearance time on the side of the offending lesion (Bookstein et al., 1972). Accordingly, the rapid-sequence series of 1- to 4-minute films after injection is critical if this test is to be used.

However, the incidence of renovascular hypertension is 5 to 15 per cent and essential hypertension, 85 to 95 per cent; thus, a false-positive rate of about 13 per cent and a false-negative rate of 22 per cent makes the test unreliable (Maxwell and Lupu, 1968; Thornburg et al., 1982) (Table 55–4).

Moreover, the presence of a positive urogram in a patient with renal arterial disease does not predict the blood pressure response to surgery. In the Cooperative Study of Renovascular Hypertension, abnormal urograms were found in 80 per cent of both the cured patients and those patients whose blood pressure failed to respond to surgical repair (Bookstein et al., 1972). Similarly, the radionuclide renogram, despite numerous modifications, has been plagued with variability that has led to even less specificity. In fact, review of a variety of techniques disclosed a false-positive rate of 25 per cent (Maxwell et al., 1968), whereas a later study using a refined technique reduced the false-positive rate to 10 per cent—still no better than the urogram (Franklin and Maxwell, 1975). In summary, both the intravenous urogram and the nuclide studies have failed to achieve suitable sensitivity and specificity to be reliable screening tests for renovascular hypertension. Captopril renography is discussed later, following definition of the captopril test.

Digital Subtraction Angiography

The introduction of computer-assisted digital subtraction angiography (DSA) was a major advance, which allows outpatient definition of the anatomic renal anatomy at the time of renal venous sampling for renin (Buonocure et al., 1981; Hillman et al., 1982).

However, with further experience, major disadvantages of DSA have been revealed. Two studies have compared DSA with conventional angiography; to accurately identify anatomic renal artery stenosis, the sensitivity was 83 to 87 per cent and the specificity was only 79 to 87 per cent (Buonocure et al., 1981; Smith et al., 1982). In addition, 5 to 20 per cent of studies are uninterpretable; good patient compliance is necessary; central catheter placement is required; and a large volume of contrast is given, raising the risk of contrast-induced renal dysfunction.

Doppler Ultrasound Angiography

Duplex ultrasound scanning combines B-mode ultrasound imaging with pulsed Doppler ultrasound to provide imaging and velocity information along vessels. The

Table 55–4. PREDICTIVE VALUE OF SCREENING TESTS FOR RENOVASCULAR HYPERTENSION*

	IVP†	DIVA†	PRA‡§	Single-Dose Captopril‖
Sensitivity (%)	75	88	80	100
Specificity (%)	86	89	84	95
False Positive (%)	14	11	16	5
False Negative (%)	25	12	20	0
Predictive Value (%) Prevalence (%)				
2	9.9	14.6	9.3	29
5	22.1	30.5	20.8	51.3
10	37.5	48.1	35.7	69
Exclusion Value (%) Prevalence (%)				
2	99.4	99.7	99.5	100
5	98.5	99.3	99.8	100
10	96.7	98.5	97.4	100

*Calculations:

$$\text{Predictive value} = \frac{\text{sensitivity} \times \text{prevalence}}{(\text{sensitivity} \times \text{prevalence}) + \text{false-positive} \times (100 - \text{prevalence})} \times 100$$

$$\text{Exclusive value} = \frac{\text{specificity} \times (100 - \text{prevalence})}{\text{specificity} \times (100 - \text{prevalence}) + (\text{false-negative rate} \times \text{prevalence})} \times 100$$

Abbreviations: IVP, intravenous pyelogram; DIVA, digital intravenous angiography; PRA, plasma renin activity.
†From Harvey, R. J., Krumlovsky, F., DelGroco, F., et al.: Screening for renovascular hypertension. JAMA, 254:388, 1985.
‡From Pickering, T. G. Sos, T. A., Vaughan, E. D. Jr., et al.: Predictive value and changes of renin secretion in hypertensive patients with unilateral renovascular disease undergoing successful renal angioplasty. Am. J. Med., 76:398, 1984.
§From Brunner, H. R., Gavras, C., Laragh, J. H., et al.: Angiotensin II blockade in man by SAR¹-Ala⁸-angiotensin II for understanding and treatment of high blood pressure. Lancet, 2:1045, 1973.
‖From Muller, F. B. Sealey, J. E., Case, D. B., et al.: The captopril test for identifying renovascular disease in hypertensive patients. Am. J. Med., 80:633, 1986.
Sosa, R. E., and Vaughan, E. D., Jr.: Renovascular hypertension, chapter 25. *In* J. Y. Gillenwater, J. J. Grayhack, S. S. Howard, and J. W. Duckett (Eds.): Adult and Pediatric Urology. St. Louis, Mosby Year Book, 1991.

technique has gained wide acceptance in peripheral vessels and is now being used to detect renal artery stenosis (Handa et al., 1988; Hawkins et al., 1989; Kohler et al., 1986; Strandness, 1990). A number of different parameters have been utilized including peak systolic velocity, renal aortic ratio, and the renal artery resistive index. Despite enthusiasm for a noninvasive test, a considerable number of patients are unsuitable candidates, the test is technically arduous, and segmental disease cannot be detected. At present, Doppler ultrasound does not appear to be an adequate screening test for renovascular hypertension (Desberg et al., in press). However, additional information is needed before a final determination of the test's usefulness can be made.

Accordingly, attention has been directed toward tests that determine the functional effects of renal artery stenosis.

Increased Renin Secretion: Peripheral Plasma Renin

After the initial work of Goldblatt, it was assumed that excess renin secretion, leading to excess AII formation, was the underlying derangement in renovascular hypertension. Unfortunately, this possibility was soon

challenged when circulating PRA was found to be normal in both animal models (Ayers et al., 1969) and a fraction of patients with renovascular hypertension (Marks and Maxwell, 1975). This review of the literature found the peripheral PRA to be elevated in only 109 of 196 patients (56 per cent) with verified cases of correctable renovascular hypertension. However, upon careful review of the primary studies, it is apparent that these samples were often obtained under conditions that are now recognized to invalidate or limit accurate interpretation of the values obtained. For example, it is known that PRA is inversely related to sodium intake and must be indexed in some fashion to the state of sodium balance (Fig. 55–13). Moreover, all antihypertensive drugs influence PRA and must be stopped 2 weeks before blood sampling for PRA. Aids to increase the accuracy of determinations of peripheral PRA are shown in Table 55–5.

The peripheral PRA is emphasized because it represents an index of renin secretion (Sealey et al., 1973). A common misconception is that increased renin secretion is determined from differential renal vein renin measurements. Actual renin secretion (renal vein renin concentration minus arterial renin concentration multiplied by renal blood flow) is rarely determined. Accordingly, a high renal venous renin concentration may reflect increased secretion with a normal renal blood or, alternatively, a normal amount of renin secreted into

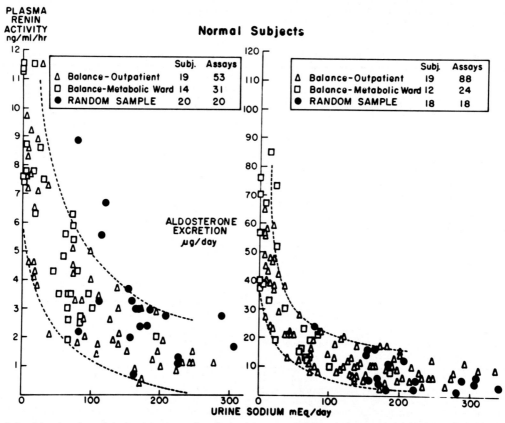

Figure 55–13. Relationship of renin activity in plasma samples obtained at noon and the corresponding 24-hour urinary excretion of aldosterone to the concurrent daily rate of sodium excretion. For these normal subjects, the data describe a similar dynamic hyperbolic relationship between each hormone and sodium excretion. Of note is the fact that subjects studied on random diets outside the hospital exhibited similar relationships, a finding that validates the use of this nomogram in studying outpatients or subjects not receiving constant diets. (From Laragh, J. H., et al.: *In* Laragh, J. H. (Ed.): Hypertension Manual. New York, Yorke Medical Books, 1973.)

Table 55–5. AIDS TO INCREASE THE ACCURACY OF DETERMINATIONS OF PERIPHERAL PLASMA RENIN ACTIVITY (PRA)

Problems	Solution
The "normal" value for PRA varies from laboratory to laboratory.	Clearly understand the factors that affect "normal" values in your laboratory: time of sampling, state of ambulation (upright posture influences PRA), state of sodium intake.
The method of collection of blood samples from patients may vary from that used to collect samples designed to establish normal range.	Use identical conditions for sampling.
All antihypertensive and diuretic drugs alter PRA.	Stop all treatment 2 weeks prior to blood sampling for PRA.
PRA is inversely related to sodium intake/excretion.	Collect a 24-hr urine for sodium determinations at the time that you collect blood for PRA; use the sodium intake level that your laboratory uses to define their normal range.*
Inferior vena cava renin used as "peripheral."	Obtain peripheral blood for PRA as described on a day separate from renal vein sampling.

*If a new methodology is being established, suggest the development of a renal/sodium index.
Adapted from Vaughan, E. D., Jr.: Urol. Clin. North Am., 6:485, 1979.

reduced renal blood flow (i.e., secretion = concentration × flow).

Increased secretion of renin is characteristic of renovascular hypertension and should, therefore, be reflected by elevated peripheral PRA compared with PRA values obtained from normotensive controls that are collected and analyzed under exactly the same conditions. Peripheral PRA (determined in blood collected at noon after 4 hours of patient ambulation), when indexed against the rate of urinary sodium excretion, is an excellent tool for identifying abnormally high renin secretion. In a study of patients who subsequently had successful transluminal angioplasties, the peripheral PRA was elevated in 80 per cent (Fig. 55–14). Moreover, the PRA always decreased and usually returned to normal following successful renal angioplasty, thereby confirming the hypothesis that the peripheral PRA is an indicator of increased renin secretion, which is corrected following relief of the offending stenotic lesion (Pickering et al., 1984).

Measurement of PRA in this manner as a screening test for renovascular hypertension has important limitations (see Table 55–4). In addition to a 20 per cent false-negative rate (i.e., a normal PRA indexed against sodium excretion) in patients with proven renovascular hypertension, there is a technical problem. Many patients with renovascular hypertension have severe life-threatening hypertension or coexistent heart disease that precludes cessation of antihypertensive medication prior to collecting blood for peripheral PRA determinations. Thus, sampling blood while patients are on drugs invalidates the accuracy of peripheral PRA as a practical screening tool. In addition, 16 per cent of the large population of patients with essential hypertension have high PRA (Brunner et al., 1972). Taken altogether, these problems have led to the search for an additional test to screen for renovascular hypertension.

Stimulation with Angiotensin-Blocking Drugs to Enhance Accuracy of Peripheral Plasma Renin Activity

The first angiotensin-blocking agent used for testing in human hypertension was saralasin. The initial results demonstrated that the compound did, as predicted, lower blood pressure in high-renin forms of hypertension, including renovascular hypertension (Brunner et al., 1973). In a second generation of studies in humans with saralasin, the partial agonist activity of the drug was exposed (Carey et al., 1978; Case et al., 1976a). Thus, in clinical settings in which PRA was low, the drug actually increased blood pressure. Moreover, the blood pressure–lowering effect of the drug was found to be inversely proportional to the sodium intake. Thus, the test was limited because of the need for intravenous

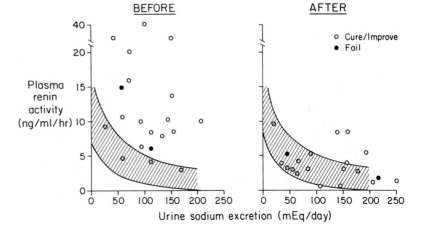

Figure 55–14. Effect of angioplasty on peripheral plasma renin activity indexed against 24-hour sodium excretion. *Left,* Before angioplasty; *right,* 6 months after angioplasty. Hatched area shows normal range. (From Pickering, T. G., et al.: Am. J. Med., 76:398, 1984.)

infusion, the agonist effect of the drug, and the influence of sodium balance on the blood pressure response to the agent.

A second approach to the use of angiotensin blockade to expose renovascular hypertension came from experience following the development of CEIs that block AII formation. A nonapeptide obtained from the venom of the *Bothrops jararaca* viper, teprotide or SQ 20881, was shown to block the vasopressor effect of AI; it was possible to demonstrate a close direct correlation between the pretreatment level of PRA and the magnitude of the depressor response (Case et al., 1976b). Moreover, in untreated hypertensive patients on the same normal sodium intake, intravenous teprotide lowered blood pressure to the greatest extent in the group profiled as high-renin by the renin-sodium index but did not lower blood pressure significantly in the low-renin subgroup. From these studies, it was possible to predict that inhibition of converting enzyme might be a helpful diagnostic approach for detecting angiotensin-dependent forms of hypertension.

The success of the intravenous CEI was a potent stimulus to the development of an orally active form—the first of which to be used in humans was captopril (SQ 14225). Captopril has the potential for use as a diagnostic probe, like teprotide, because it has a rapid onset of action (within 10 to 15 minutes), reaching a peak effect by 90 minutes (Case et al., 1978). Initial studies showed a close relationship between the pretreatment PRA and the magnitude of the depressor response induced after the first dose of captopril (Case et al., 1978).

During the early studies of the effect of these agents on blood pressure in hypertensive patients, it was noted that angiotensin blockade resulted in a marked rise in PRA in selected patients.

With the availability of the oral CEI, captopril, we began providing single oral test doses instead of intravenous infusions. Results very similar to those obtained with the intravenous competitive antagonist, saralasin, or the CEI, teprotide, were found (Case et al., 1978–1982). An additional advantage was the observation that renovascular hypertensive patients being treated with a beta-adrenergic blocker still responded to oral administration of captopril with a fall in blood pressure and a rise in PRA (Fig. 55–15) (Case et al., 1982).

The protocol for a single oral doses of captopril to screen for renovascular hypertension is shown in Table 55–6. Our current criteria for a positive test finding to identify a patient with renovascular hypertension are a post-captopril PRA of ≥ 12 ng/ml/hour and an increase in renin of ≥ 10 ng/ml/hour, plus a per cent increase in renin of greater than 400 per cent if the baseline PRA was <3 ng/ml/hour, and greater than 150 per cent if the baseline renin was >3 ng/ml/hour (Muller et al., 1986). In summary, single-dose captopril appears to accurately distinguish patients with renovascular or renal hypertension from those with essential hypertension. Moreover, a 24-hour urine collection is not necessary, and the patient can remain on beta-blockade if the baseline PRA is >1 ng/ml/hour. The test is not valid if the PRA is <1 ng/ml/hour. Hence, the test is complementary to the renin-sodium index to identify renin hypersecretion (see Table 55–4).

Numerous other studies now have confirmed the usefulness of converting enzyme inhibition in the identification of renovascular hypertension (Derkx et al., 1987; Gosse et al., 1989; Wilcox et al., 1988) in adults and in children (Willems et al., 1989). In contrast, others (Idrissi et al., 1988; Salvetti et al., 1987) have found the test less helpful as a prospective screening test. Addressing these differences, Gaul and co-workers (1989) reviewed 16 studies involving 805 patients. They found numerous differences in the studies, including documen-

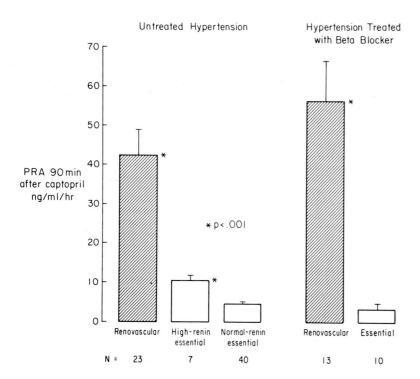

Figure 55–15. Levels of plasma renin activity in renovascular and essential hypertension 90 minutes after a single dose of captopril. A marked reactive hyperreninemia was found in the group with renovascular hypertension whether they were already receiving betablocker therapy or not. (From Case, D. B., et al.: In Laragh, J. H., et al. (Eds.): Frontiers in Hypertension Research. New York, Springer-Verlag, 1982.)

Table 55–6. SINGLE-DOSE CAPTOPRIL TEST

Drugs
The patient should not receive any medications for at least 2 weeks, if possible. Otherwise, the patient may be given a beta-blocker, but omit all diuretics, converting enzyme inhibitors, or nonsteroidal anti-inflammatory drugs for at least 1 week (ideally, 2 weeks).

Diet
A diet with normal or high salt or sodium content is needed. Too low a sodium intake will produce falsely positive results. If there is a question about diet, a 24-hour urine collection for sodium will closely reflect the intake.

Procedure
The patient may be supine, semirecumbent, or seated for the test, but measurements must be made with the patient in the same position.
After measurements of blood pressure are stable (this usually takes about 10 to 20 minutes), a blood sample for plasma renin activity is drawn in a lavender-topped Vacutainer kept at room temperature.
Crush a 25-mg tablet of captopril (to ensure that it dissolves) and pour in water to produce a suspension of about 30 ml. Instruct the patient to drink the suspension, wash the contents out twice, and drink those also.
Remeasure blood pressure and plasma renin activity after 1 hour.

From Vaughan, E. D., Jr., Case, D. B., Pickering, T. G., et al.: Urol. Clin. North Am., 11:393, 1984.

tation of renovascular hypertension, methodology of captopril administration, and different definitions of a positive test.

In conclusion, the captopril test or the use of other CEIs (Ideishi et al., 1989) appears to be useful in identifying patients with renovascular hypertension and is safe and simple to perform. However, there is a need for standardization of the test and more precise definition of a positive test as well as more prospective study.

Captopril Renogram

The study of CEIs in both the diagnosis and treatment of renovascular hypertension led to the finding of decreased renal function in some patients (Hricik et al., 1983). The response of RBF and GFR to converting enzyme inhibition in the two-kidney, one-clip dog model established in our laboratories is shown in Figure 55–16 (Sosa, 1987). Infusion of enalapril produces a dramatic fall in RBF and GFR in the kidney with renal artery

stenosis, whereas RBF is increased in the opposite kidney despite a dramatic fall in blood pressure. These results, coupled with physiologic studies (Laragh and Sealey, 1991), show that AII plays a major role in preserving GFR in kidneys with renal artery stenosis by causing efferent arteriolar constriction and increasing filtration fraction (London and Safar, 1989). Inhibition of AII by a CEI results in a fall in efferent resistance and GFR (Pederson et al., 1989), an effect that is the physiologic basis for the captopril renogram (Meier et al., 1990).

As previously stated, the isotopic renogram has not proven to be an accurate test to identify patients with renovascular hypertension (Maxwell et al., 1968). However, performing the renogram before and after the administration of captopril can induce dramatic falls of GFR and RBF in the involved kidney as well as a fall in blood pressure and reactive rise in renin (Ritter et al., 1990). In theory, the test not only screens for renovascular hypertension but also identifies the involved kidney, perhaps obviating the need for renal vein renin determinations (Geyskes et al., 1987; Meier et al., 1990; Nally, 1989; Nally et al., 1986). Wilcox and coworkers (1989) reviewed the results of three series (Geyskes et al., 1987; Sfakianakis et al., 1987; Wentig et al., 1984) and concluded that the predictive value of the test did not yet approach that of renal vein renin determinations (Pickering et al., 1984).

Later advancements include determination of both RBF and GFR, employment of new agents, single-day study, and re-evaluation of response criteria. The final role of this relatively complex test in the evaluation of hypertensive patients remains to be determined. Differential renal vein renin determinations remain the gold standard in identifying which kidney is the cause of abnormal renin secretion in a patient with renovascular hypertension.

Contralateral Suppression of Renin Secretion and an Elevated Renal Vein to Arterial Renin Relationship—Use of Differential Renal Vein Renin Determinations

Since the development of the technique (Judson and Helmer, 1965), differential renal vein renin determina-

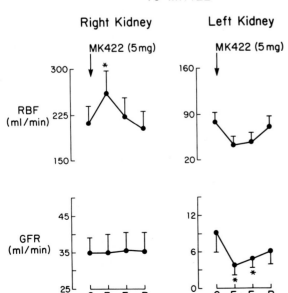

Figure 55–16. Effect of angiotensin-converting enzyme inhibition on renal blood flow (RBF) and glomerular filtration rate (GFR), showing a marked fall in GFR in the kidney with renal artery stenosis. (C, control; E, experimental periods, R, recovery.)

tions have emerged as the most useful tools in identifying correctable renovascular hypertension. The most common approach has been to calculate the renal vein renin ratio, that is, stenotic side PRA values divided by normal side PRA values with some arbitrary "positive" ratio (usually 1.5:1). The major difficulty with this method is in selecting a ratio that has the accuracy to distinguish precisely patients with renovascular hypertension from those with essential hypertension (Marks and Maxwell, 1975). Generally, a positive renal vein ratio predicts a fall in blood pressure following correction of the vascular lesion in more than 90 per cent of cases. However, a negative ratio does not preclude a successful response to revascularization. In the review by Marks and Maxwell (1975), 49 per cent of patients with a negative ratio were cured by appropriate surgical intervention. However, these patients were a minority of the total patients studied, and the actual false-negative rate was 15 per cent (62 of 412 patients).

In addition, the collection of renal vein blood alone for PRA is subject to the risk of a sampling error caused either by incorrect catheter placement or by sampling from a renal vein that does not subtend the renal area supplied by the stenotic artery. Sampling from the inferior vena cava below the renal veins is a safeguard against this source of error, and the absence of a 50 per cent renin increment from both kidneys together identifies an inadequate differential renal vein renin study (Vaughan et al., 1973).

A positive renal vein ratio does not exclude bilateral, albeit asymmetric, renin secretion, which would indicate bilateral renal disease. In this setting, correction of a unilateral lesion may not totally eliminate the underlying pathology, with subsequent failure of total blood pressure control.

In view of these limitations of the traditional renal vein ratio analysis, another method for analysis of renin values has been devised. It is based on the characteristics of the experimental two-kidney, one-clip Goldblatt hypertension, as detailed in Table 55–7 (also see Fig. 55–12).

Hypersecretion of renin, as determined by the renin-sodium index or captopril stimulation, serves as the primary criterion for the diagnosis of renovascular hypertension. A second criterion is the demonstration of the absence of renin secretion from the contralateral or noninvolved kidney. Suppression of renin secretion from this kidney can be determined by subtracting the arterial plasma renin activity (A) from the renal venous renin activity (V). Because the inferior vena caval (IVC) renin and aortic renin are the same, the IVC renin value can be substituted for (A) in this equation (Fig. 55–17) (Sealey et al., 1973). Hence, a patient with curable renovascular hypertension exhibits an absence of renin secretion from the opposite kidney, i.e., (V − A) = 0, also termed contralateral suppression of renin (Stockigt et al., 1972; Vaughan et al., 1973). Contralateral suppression of renin indicates that the noninvolved kidney is responding in an appropriately "normal" fashion to the elevated blood pressure, increased circulating AII levels, and increased sodium chloride at the macula densa by shutting off renin secretion. This phenomenon is at times present not only in patients with unilateral renal arterial lesions but also in patients with bilateral disease demonstrated by arteriograms, who have a dominant lesion on one side (Gittes and McLaughlin, 1974; Pickering et al., 1986).

A third criterion is based on studies of renal vein and arterial renin relationships in patients with essential hypertension. The mean renal venous renin level has been determined to be about 25 per cent higher than arterial PRA (Fig. 55–18) (Sealey et al., 1973). Hence, a total renin increment (both kidneys) of approximately 50 per cent is necessary to maintain a given peripheral renin level $(V − A)/A = 50$ per cent. However, a reduction in RBF also influences the renal venous renin level. In this setting, the renal venous renin concentration will be misleadingly high, shifting the renal

---

Table 55–7. RENIN VALUES FOR PREDICTING CURABILITY OF RENOVASCULAR HYPERTENSION

Collection of Samples
(moderate sodium intake ± 100 mEq/day)

1. Ambulatory peripheral renin and 24-hour urine sodium excretion under steady-state conditions (i.e., not on day of arteriography)
2. Collection of blood for PRA before and after converting enzyme blockade
3. Collection of supine
   a. Renal vein renin from suspect kidney (V1) and inferior vena cava renin (A1)
   b. Renal vein from contralateral kidney (V2) and inferior vena cava renin (A2)
4. Enhancement of renin secretion by converting enzyme blockade if initial renin sampling is inconclusive

Criteria for Predicting Cure	
High PRA in relation to $U_{Na}V$	Measurement of hypersecretion of renin
Contralateral kidney: (V2 − A2) = 0	An indicator of absent renin secretion from the contralateral kidney
Suspect kidney: (V1 − A1)/A1 ≧ 0.50	As indicator of unilateral renin secretion
	Measurement of reduced renal blood flow
$\dfrac{(V − A)}{A} + \dfrac{(V − A)}{A} < 0.50$ In patients with high PRA Means: a. Incorrect sampling b. Segmental disease	Repeat with segmental sampling

From Vaughan, E. D., Jr., In Brenner, B. M., and Stein, J. M. (Eds.): Hypertension. New York, Churchill Livingstone, 1981.

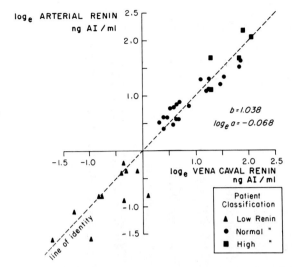

Figure 55–17. Relationship of renin activity in blood collected from the aorta to that found in vena caval blood. The two values do not differ in patients with essential hypertension. (From Sealey, J. E., et al.: Am. J. Med., 55:391, 1973.)

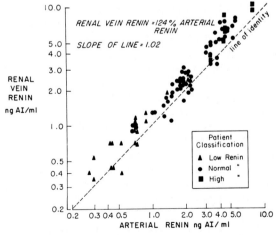

Figure 55–18. Relationship of renal vein renin to arterial (or venous) renin in patients with essential hypertension. The slope of the line does not differ from the line of identity, indicating that the relationship of renal vein renin to arterial renin is constant at all levels of plasma renin activity found in essential hypertension. The intercept of 1.24 indicates that the renal vein renin is 124 per cent of arterial renin. (From Sealey, J. E., et al.: Am. J. Med., 55:391, 1973.)

vein:arterial renin relationships upward. The elevation of the increment above approximately 50 per cent becomes an index of the severity of the reduction in blood flow consequent to the obstructing vascular lesion (Fig. 55–19). The combination of these criteria found in a group of patients managed by renal revascularization is shown in Figure 55–20 (Vaughan et al., 1979).

In a group of 46 hypertensive patients with arteriographically proven unilateral renal artery stenosis who underwent successful angioplasties, 34 had technically successful sampling (Pickering et al., 1984). Of the 34 patients with technically acceptable values, there were 23 true-positive, no false-positive, three true-negative, and eight false-negative results. Of the eight false-negative findings, four had a (V − A)/A between 40 and 48 per cent, and six had contralateral suppression.

ESSENTIAL HYPERTENSION

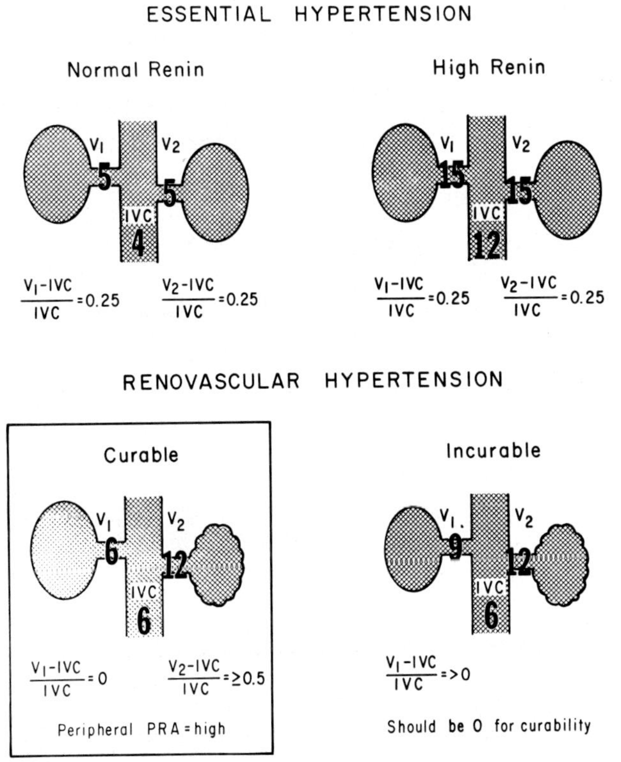

Figure 55–19. Renal vein renin diagnostic patterns. In essential hypertension *(top)* at all levels of renin secretion, the renin level in each renal vein is about 25 per cent greater than either the peripheral arterial or the venous level. In the setting of unilateral renin secretion (curable renovascular hypertension), the active kidney is solely responsible for maintaining the peripheral renin levels. Hence, the increment is 50 per cent (0.5) and becomes progressively greater as renal blood flow is reduced. Unequal bilateral renin secretion *(bottom right)* indicates bilateral disease and decreases the chance of cure following corrective unilateral surgery. (From Laragh, J. H., and Sealey, J. E.: Cardiovasc. Med., 2:1053, 1977. Reprinted with permission from the Physicians World Communications Group.)

Only two patients had symmetric renal vein renin values (Pickering et al., 1984). The present approach therefore gave a sensitivity of 74 per cent and a specificity of 100 per cent, better indices than those found by renin ratio analysis.

An additional aid to renal vein sampling is the utilization of segmental renal venous sampling (Schambelan et al., 1974), especially when sampling from the major renal veins fails to demonstrate a combined renin increment of 50 per cent from both kidneys, suggesting either a technical error or segmental disease. This approach may be particularly helpful in children with segmental parenchymal disease (Parrott et al., 1984).

Converting Enzyme Inhibition to Enhance the Accuracy of Renal Vein Renin Analysis

Following the initial report of renin stimulation by angiotensin blockade (Re et al., 1978), several groups of investigators have reported increased renin release from the ischemic kidney with converting enzyme inhibition (Lyons et al., 1983; Thibonnier et al., 1984). The magnitude of these induced changes is shown in Figure 55–21. These data were determined from 26 patients

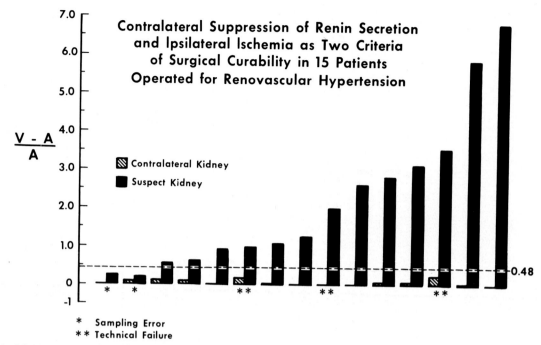

Figure 55–20. Of 15 patients with renovascular hypertension, 13 exhibited (V − A)/A in excess of 48 per cent from the suspect kidney and a suppressed value from the contralateral kidney. V is renal venous plasma renin activity (PRA); A is arterial or infrarenal inferior vena cava PRA. Asterisks denote the three patients who had values suggesting surgical curability, yet had residual or recurrent hypertension due to technical failure. (From Vaughan, E. D., Jr., et al.: Kidney Int., 15:S83, 1979.)

with unilateral renovascular hypertension. Not shown is the observation that the IVC levels (systemic or peripheral) were comparable to those values measured from the normal side, revealing the continued suppression of renin secretion from that kidney even after stimulation. Although more information is required to distinguish the subtleties (e.g., bilateral renovascular disease, branch lesions, total occlusion, coexistent renal parenchymal disease, and so forth), it is clear that stimulation adds to the analysis in certain specific situations: (1) when patients are already undergoing drug therapy,

e.g., beta-blockers, and the renin levels are generally reduced; (2) when there is a question about the reliability of the PRA measurements, particularly of low levels; (3) when experience in performing renal vein renin determinations is limited and subject to sampling errors; and (4) when equivocal values already exist.

In summary, renal vein renin sampling after captopril stimulation accentuates renin release from ischemic renal tissue, which is particularly useful when values are equivocal, when branch stenoses are present, or when renovascular disease is superimposed on coexisting hypertension or renal disease.

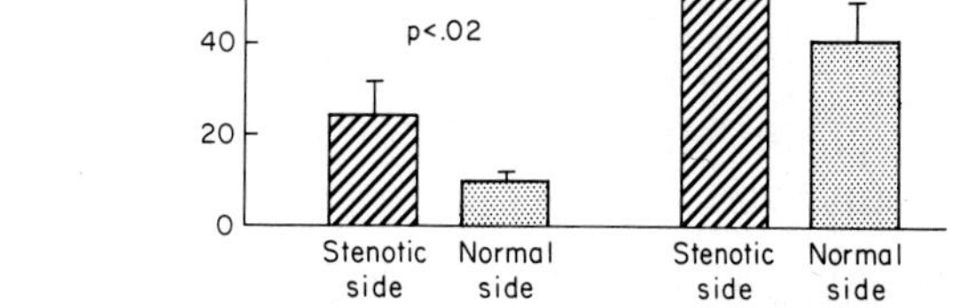

ANATOMIC CONFIRMATION OF THE FOUR CRITERIA. It should be noted that virtually the entire evaluation of the hypertensive patient can now be accomplished without hospitalization, thus avoiding much of the expense previously thought to be too great to warrant the evaluation (McNeil et al., 1975). We usually perform digital subtraction angiography (DSA) by way of a central injection at the time of renal vein sampling (Pickering, 1990). The only caveat is that, because digital intravenous angiography (DIVA) only detects anatomic vascular disease, the functional significance of the lesion must still be demonstrated.

Screening criteria have been identified to ensure both that the patient with renovascular disease will be physiologically and anatomically characterized and that the success of a corrective procedure can be predicted. When these criteria have been met, the patient is admitted to the hospital for definitive management of the offending lesion.

VALIDATION OF THE CRITERIA. In addition to a favorable clinical response to renal angioplasty, we have had the unique opportunity to study the effect of restoration of blood flow on renal vein renin concentra-

Figure 55–21. Renal vein renin determinations (renal vein levels only) in patients with documented renovascular hypertension before and after captopril stimulation. Captopril accentuates renin secretion from the ischemic kidney. Not shown are the inferior vena cava levels, which are the same as the levels measured from the normal side both before and after captopril stimulation. (From Vaughan, E. D., Jr., et al.: Urol. Clin. North Am., 11:393, 1984.)

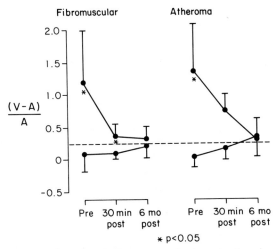

Figure 55–22. Effect of angioplasty on renal vein renin. Samples were taken immediately before angioplasty, 30 minutes after, and 6 months after. The higher values are for the ischemic kidney; the lower values are for the contralateral kidney. Asterisk indicates significant difference between the two kidneys, and the dotted line is the normal level of (V − A)/A (0.24). (From Pickering, T. G., et al.: Am. J. Med., 76:398, 1984.)

tion and renin secretion (Pickering et al., 1984; Vaughan et al., 1981). To accomplish this goal, we have monitored the immediate effect of successful angioplasty on renal renin secretion. A marked reduction in the renal vein renin from the previously stenotic side occurred 30 minutes following angioplasty (Fig. 55–22). The residual ipsilateral increment of renal vein renin was about 50 per cent above the peripheral level, while contralateral renin suppression persisted. This 50 per cent increment had been predicted to occur in the setting of unilateral renin secretion and normal RBF (Sealey et al., 1973).

Several months after angioplasty, there was a marked fall in peripheral PRA with a return to normal in most patients, indicating a reduction of renin secretion (see Fig. 55–14). Of equal interest is the restoration of a bilateral renin increment of about 25 per cent above the IVC renin level (see Fig. 55–22) (Pickering et al., 1984). Hence, contralateral renin suppression was reversed following successful angioplasty. This 25 per cent increment from both kidneys is characteristic of the renin secretory pattern found in patients with essential hypertension (Sealey et al., 1973).

The finding that the renal renin secretory characteristics of renovascular hypertension are reversed following successful angioplasty with correction of the hypertension is strong evidence that they truly reflect the abnormal secretory behavior of renin in curable renovascular hypertension.

IDENTIFYING THE POTENTIALLY CURABLE PATIENT: A COST-EFFECTIVE APPROACH

Our current approach is outlined in Figure 55–23. All patients with fixed hypertension are potential candidates for this protocol because we believe that nearly all patients with renovascular hypertension, when identified, can be best managed by angioplasty or revascular-

ization. With respect to this empirical protocol, it could be argued that patients with highly suspect findings could be screened initially with a digital angiogram or a captopril scan. However, the functional significance of an anatomic lesion with respect to ischemia-induced renin release still must be established as well as the predictive value of the captopril scan, so we routinely begin with a peripheral PRA.

In our experience, a low PRA is rarely found in untreated patients with nonazotemic renal arterial disease, and we therefore do not usually continue this evaluation in these patients unless they demonstrate refractoriness to treatment. Patients with high or normal PRA undergo a peripheral captopril test. The test cannot be performed if the patient has been taking captopril for a long period. If the test finding is positive, the differential renal vein sampling and digital angiography are performed together. The sampling procedure ideally is done first, and the catheter is advanced into the superior vena cava for injection of contrast material. This combined study is performed in the radiology suite. The patient lies quietly after the study in the hypertension unit for 2 to 4 hours before returning home. After the diagnostic criteria have been established, the patient is briefly hospitalized for selective arteriography, and percutaneous transluminal angioplasty or renal revascularization is required.

We continue to believe that the functional significance of a renal artery lesion must be identified before the therapeutic decision is directed toward intervention.

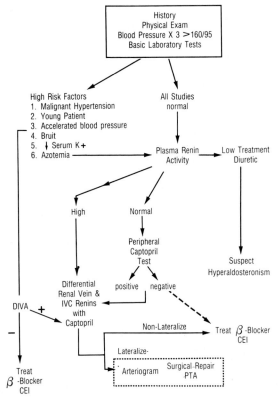

Figure 55–23. Evaluation plan to identify patients with renovascular hypertension. (From Sosa, R. E., and Vaughan, E. D., Jr.: AUA Update Series 2: Lesson 31, 1983.)

TAILORED THERAPY FOR RENOVASCULAR HYPERTENSION

The rationale for identifying patients with renovascular hypertension is that their management will differ from that offered to patients with essential hypertension. Indeed, hypertension of renal origin is difficult to manage with conventional antihypertensive drugs. In a randomized study (Hunt and Strong, 1973), morbidity and mortality were greater in patients with renal hypertension who were treated in the medical group in contrast to the surgical group. In addition, as previously discussed, most renovascular lesions are progressive with time, and there is little evidence to suggest that successful control of hypertension influences the natural history of the various pathologic entities (Goncharenko et al., 1981; McCormack et al., 1966; Schreiber et al., 1984). Accordingly, for properly selected cases, surgical management has been the preferable choice.

Medical Management

With the development of more specific antihypertensives, such as CEIs, beta-adrenergic blockers, and calcium-channel blockers, it is now possible to treat renovascular hypertension effectively. Medical management is used in those patients awaiting angioplasty or revascularization, those who refuse or who are too ill for intervention, and those who have failed to respond following intervention (Pickering, 1989, 1990).

The major concern of medical management is the demonstrated progressive deterioration of renal function found in some patients despite adequate blood pressure control (Dean et al., 1981). As previously described during the discussion of the captopril renogram, a major compensatory mechanism to maintain glomerular filtration pressure is efferent arteriolar constriction induced by AII (London and Safar, 1989; Rosivall et al., 1990). Accordingly, the administration of CEIs to patients with renovascular hypertension can lead to either renal deterioration (Burnier et al., 1989; Chrysant et al., 1983; Dominiczak et al., 1988; Mason and Hilton, 1983; Ying et al., 1984) or total renal artery occlusion (Postma et al., 1989).

Loss of renal function following chronic CEI treatment of the two-kidney, one-clip Goldblatt model of hypertension in rats (Jackson and Johnson, 1989) despite good blood pressure control supports this concept. However, upon review of the world experience of CEI therapy for renovascular hypertension, progressive renal failure sufficient to discontinue treatment occurred in only 5 per cent of patients, whereas there was good blood pressure control in 74 per cent (Hollenberg, 1988). In summary, converting enzyme inhibition is effective in controlling blood pressure in these patients; it is most dangerous in patients with bilateral disease or solitary kidneys and, in all patients on medical therapy, careful follow-up, including serial tests of renal function and size, must be scheduled. The role of calcium-channel blockers, which induce afferent arteriolar dilatation, to prevent the potential of renal deterioration is being explored (Ribstein et al., 1988).

Percutaneous Transluminal Renal Artery Angioplasty

Percutaneous transluminal angioplasty (PTA) was first introduced by Dotter and Judkins in 1964 for the treatment of peripheral vascular stenoses. The difficulties associated with the technique were overcome by the introduction of a flexible, double-lumen balloon catheter by Gruntzig and Hopff (1974), permitting the development of percutaneous balloon angioplasty of renal artery stenosis. The original concept of Dotter was that the atherosclerotic material would be compressed by the balloon; subsequently, it has been shown that there is actual disruption of the plaque at the junction of the intima and media with the creation of a cleft in the intima and media. During dilatation, the media and adventitia are, in fact, stretched beyond the normal caliber (Castenada-Zuniga et al., 1980; Fogarty and Chen, 1981). The fibromuscular dysplasias and unilateral, nonosteal, nonoccluded atherosclerotic renal artery stenoses are the most suitable lesions for treatment with PTA. In addition, PTA has been used in patients with arteritis (Kumar et al., 1990; Martin et al., 1980), in patients with recurrent stenosis following initially successful PTA, and in patients with anastomotic strictures of the renal artery following surgical correction.

The major groups who do not respond to PTA include patients with diffuse atherosclerotic disease primarily involving the aorta, which gives rise to a secondary occlusion of the renal artery ostium. Therefore, in ostial stenosis, the success rate of PTA is poor although an occasional patient will have long-term success (Cicuto et al., 1981; Sos et al., 1983). Patients with total occlusion of the renal artery are also poor candidates for the technique, although new laser techniques may make the procedure more feasible. The management of patients with total renal artery occlusion is discussed in Chapter 67. Patients with multiple branch lesions, particularly at vessel bifurcation, are less likely to respond to angioplasty. This situation is only a relative contraindication to PTA and pertains primarily to cases involving atherosclerotic disease.

The ideal patient for PTA, therefore, is one with unilateral disease, positive renin indices, and fibromuscular dysplasia or nonosteal, nonoccluded atherosclerotic renal artery stenosis. Another indication, which is discussed later, is angioplasty for preservation of renal function.

One of the advantages of transluminal angioplasty is the ability to avoid a general anesthetic, the relatively low morbidity of the procedure, and the short hospitalization. It is critical that this be a team approach involving not only the radiologist but also medical and surgical teams who are familiar with the management of patients with hypotension and any potential surgical complication. Patients are often volume-depleted due to AII-induced vasoconstriction prior to angioplasty and often require vigorous hydration to avoid postangioplasty hypotension, electrolyte imbalance, and contrast-induced injury (Katzen et al., 1979; Schwarten, 1987). Some of these complications can be avoided if the patients who are on long-term therapy with CEIs are allowed restoration of vascular volume prior to angio-

Table 55–8. SUMMARY OF OUTCOME AFTER ANGIOPLASTY IN TEN PUBLISHED SERIES OF HYPERTENSIVE PATIENTS ACCORDING TO INDICATION FOR ANGIOPLASTY—ATHEROMATOUS OR FIBROMUSCULAR RENAL ARTERY STENOSIS*

| | Atheromatous Renal Artery Stenosis | | | | Fibromuscular Renal Artery Stenosis | | | |
| | *Technically Successful Angioplasty* | *Blood Pressure Response* | | | *Technically Successful Angioplasty* | *Blood Pressure Response* | | |
Reference		Cured	Improved	Failed†		Cured	Improved	Failed†
Martin et al., 1981	13	2 (15)	4 (31)	7 (54)	8	5 (63)	1 (13)	2 (25)
Colapinto et al., 1982	44	8 (18)	29 (66)	7 (16)	9	4 (44)	5 (56)	0 (0)
Geyskes et al., 1983	44	4 (9)	19 (43)	21 (48)	21	10 (48)	10 (48)	1 (5)
Sos et al., 1983	34	7 (21)	10 (29)	17 (50)	27	16 (59)	9 (33)	2 (7)
Tegtmeyer et al., 1984	61	15 (25)	46 (75)	0 (0)	27	10 (37)	17 (63)	0 (0)
Miller et al., 1985	34	5 (15)	15 (44)	14 (41)	13	11 (85)	2 (15)	0 (0)
Martin et al., 1985	60	9 (15)	30 (50)	21 (35)	20	5 (25)	12 (60)	3 (15)
Kaplan-Pavlobcic et al., 1985	48	11 (23)	21 (44)	16 (33)	21	10 (48)	8 (38)	3 (14)
Kuhlmann et al., 1985	31	9 (29)	15 (48)	7 (23)	22	11 (50)	7 (32)	4 (18)
Bell et al., 1987	22	3 (14)	13 (59)	6 (27)	7	5 (71)	2 (29)	0 (0)
Totals	391	73 (19)	202 (52)	116 (30)	175	87 (50)	73 (42)	15 (9)
Range (%)		9–29	29–75	0–54		25–85	13–63	

*Results are expressed as numbers (percentages) of patients.
†Excludes technical failures.
From Ramsay, L. E., and Waller, P. C.: Blood pressure response to percutaneous transluminal angioplasty for renovascular hypertension. An overview of published series. Br. Med. J., 300:569, 1990.

plasty. In contrast, patients also may have increased blood pressure requiring medical management postangioplasty or may simply maintain their pre-existing pressure for some period before resolution occurs. Accordingly, these patients need to be in the hospital for careful blood pressure monitoring and fluid replacement.

Conflict exists concerning systemic anticoagulation during or after angioplasty. Although some clinicians use systemic heparinization, a majority believe that aspirin administration is sufficient.

In summary, a general consensus exists at the present time that PTA is the treatment of choice for patients with medial fibroplasia (Tack and Sos, 1989; Vaughan and Sosa, 1989). As shown in Table 55–8, combined results from ten series reveal a success of greater than 90 per cent (Ramsay and Waller, 1990). Considerably more controversy concerning treatment of patients with atherosclerotic disease exist. The technical success rate is lower (70 to 80 per cent), and the blood pressure benefit is considerably more variable (see Table 55–8) and less than that found following surgical revascularization (see Chapter 67). Patient selection remains critical and undoubtedly influences whether results are good (Canzanello et al., 1989) or disappointing (Beebe et al., 1988). Newer techniques employing lasers, stents, and fibrolytic agents will undoubtedly influence future success (Olin et al., 1989; Sanborn et al., 1989).

Angioplasty has also been successfully incorporated into the treatment strategy of children with renovascular hypertension (Guzzetta et al., 1989; Simunic et al., 1990). The success rate using both PTA and revascularization in children is now excellent.

Thus, PTA has assumed a major role in the treatment of renovascular hypertension. In addition, successful surgical correction can be performed without added morbidity in patients who have failed PTA (Martinez et al., 1991). The critical information still lacking is long-term follow-up, which is now available following renal revascularization and shows effective long-term benefit (Lawrie et al., 1989; van Bockel et al., 1988, 1989; Von Knorring et al., 1989).

Angioinfarction

Rarely, a patient is too ill for any form of intervention, the kidney has minimal function, and medical management is inadequate. In this unusual setting, percutaneous renal ablation with ethanol can be performed and has been reported to be successful (Iaccarino et al., 1989; Klimberg et al., 1989).

Renal Reconstruction or Angioplasty for Preservation of Renal Function

The work of Schreiber (discussed earlier) has called attention to the threat of atherosclerotic renal artery disease to overall renal function. This observation is now recognized as an important clinical issue separate from the problem of renovascular hypertension. In addition, the Schreiber study suggested that progression occurred primarily within the first 2 years of angiographic follow-up in patients with greater than 50 per cent stenosis on the initial angiogram. Moreover, loss of renal parenchyma could not be attributed to poor blood pressure control. In a separate study, Novick and co-workers (1984) reviewed patients undergoing dialysis over a 10-year period and identified 25 patients with end-stage renal disease as a consequence of atherosclerotic renal artery disease.

Therefore, a second indication for intervention with angioplasty or revascularization is to preserve renal function whether or not there is associated renovascular hypertension.

Novick and colleagues (1984) established the following criteria for angiographic screening of atherosclerotic renal arterial disease: (1) evidence of generalized atherosclerosis, (2) unilateral small kidney, (3) mild to moderate azotemia (serum creatinine level greater than 1.5 mg/dl), and (4) hypertension. If the patient is subsequently found to have a high-grade (greater than 75 per cent) arterial stenosis affecting the entire renal mass (namely, in cases in which such a stenosis is present bilaterally or involves a solitary kidney), then intervention is recommended.

An additional indicator for intervention is a marked drop in effective renal plasma value and glomerular filtration rate when the patient is challenged with the vasodilator sodium nitroprusside (Texter et al., 1985). The mechanism of the fall in blood pressure was discussed previously.

In a 10-year review of patients at the Cleveland Clinic, 161 of 241 with atherosclerotic disease underwent surgical revascularization to achieve preservation of renal function. Within this group, renal function was improved in 93 patients (57.7 per cent), stable in 50 patients (31.1 per cent), and deteriorated in 10 patients (6 per cent) (Bedoya et al., 1989).

Based on the earlier observations of Novick (Casarella, 1986), Schwarten (1987) began in 1983 to perform transluminal angioplasty on a similar group of patients. He currently reported on 32 patients with mild to moderate renal insufficiency. All patients had a serum creatinine level in the range of 2 to 3.1 mg/dl and kidneys greater than 9 cm in size. Fifteen patients had bilateral renal artery stenoses of greater than 75 per cent, and 17 patients had greater than 75 per cent unilateral renal artery stenosis in a single functioning kidney. Angioplasty was performed using dilute contrast material and low volume. In follow-up, 23 patients were improved, seven patients exhibited no change, and two patients were worse. Therefore, the early results of angioplasty appear to be similar to those reported for surgical intervention.

This topic is discussed further in Chapter 67. However, it is clear that we always should suspect renal arterial disease in any azotemic patient without a clearly documented cause of renal impairment. Renal vascular disease should be excluded before the patient is provided medical treatment for renal insufficiency. Moreover, renin determinations and blood pressure response to converting enzyme inhibition are inaccurate and often falsely negative in azotemic patients. In this setting, PTA or renal revascularization is based on the finding of renal artery disease not on establishing the kidney as the cause of coexisting hypertension as described in this chapter.

REFERENCES

Anderson, W. P., Ramsey, D. E., and Takata, M.: Development of hypertension from unilateral renal artery stenosis in conscious dogs. Hypertension, 16:441, 1990.

Ayers, C. R., Harris, R. H., and Lefer, L. G.: Control of renin release in experimental hypertension. Circ. Res., 24/25(Suppl. 1):103, 1969.

Ayers, C. R., Katholi, R. E., Vaughan, E. D., Jr., Carey, R. M., Kimbrough, H. M., Jr., Yancey, M. S., and Morton, C. L.: Intrarenal renin-angiotensin-sodium interdependent mechanism controlling post clamp renal artery pressure and renin release in the conscious dog with chronic one-kidney Goldblatt hypertension. Circ. Res., 40:238, 1977.

Bakhle, Y. S.: Conversion of angiotensin I to angiotensin II by cell-free extracts of dog lung. Nature, 220:919, 1968.

Barajas, L., and Latta, H.: The innervation of the juxtaglomerular apparatus: An electron microscopic study of the innervation of the glomerular arterioles. Lab. Invest., 13:916, 1964.

Barajas, L., Salido, E. C., and Powers, K. V.: The juxtaglomerular apparatus: A morphologic perspective, chap. 67. In Laragh, J. H., and Brenner, B. M. (Eds.): Hypertension Pathophysiology, Diagnosis and Management. New York, Raven Press, 1990.

Bedoya, L., Ziegelbaum, M., Vidt, D. G., et al.: The effect of baseline renal function on the outcome following renal revascularization. Cleve. Clin. J. Med., 56:415, 1989.

Beebe, H. G., Chesebro, K., Merchant, F., and Bush, W.: Results of renal artery balloon angioplasty limit its indications. J. Vasc. Surg., 8:300, 1988.

Bell, G. M., Reid, J., and Buist, T. A. S.: Percutaneous transluminal angioplasty improves blood pressure and renal function in renovascular hypertension. Q. J. Med., 63:393, 1987.

Bengis, R. G., Coleman, T. G., Young, D. B., and McCaa, R. E.: Long-term blockade of angiotensin formation in various normotensive and hypertensive rat models using converting enzyme inhibitor (SQ 14225). Circ. Res., 43(Suppl. 1):145, 1978.

Blake, W. D., Wegria, R., Ward, H. P., and Frank, C. W.: Effect of renal arterial constriction on excretion of sodium and water. Am. J. Physiol., 163:422, 1950.

Bookstein, J. J., Abrams, H. L., Buenger, R. E., Lecky, J., Franklin, S. S., Reiss, N. D., Bleifer, K. H., Klatte, E. C., Varady, P. D., and Maxwell, M. H.: Radiologic aspects of renovascular hypertension: Part II. The role of urography in unilateral renovascular disease. JAMA, 220:1225, 1972.

Braun-Menendez, E., Fasciolo, J. C., Leloir, L. R., and Munoz, J. M.: The substance causing renal hypertension. J. Physiol., 98:283, 1940.

Briggs, J. P., and Schnermann, J.: Macula densa control of renin secretion and glomerular vascular tone: Evidence for common cellular mechanisms. Renal Physiol. Basel., 9:193, 1986.

Bright, R.: Reports of medical cases, selected with a view of illustrating symptoms and cure of disease by reference to morbid anatomy. London, Longman Group, Ltd., 1827.

Brunner, H. R., Gavras, H., Laragh, J. H., and Keenan, R.: Angiotensin II blockade in man by SAR¹-Ala⁸-angiotensin II for understanding and treatment of high blood pressure. Lancet, 2:1045, 1973.

Brunner, H. R., Kirshmann, J. D., Sealey, J. E., and Laragh, J. H.: Hypertension of renal origin: Evidence for two different mechanisms. Science, 174:1344, 1971.

Brunner, H. R., Laragh, J. H., Baer, L., Newton, M. A., Goodwin, F. T., Krakoff, L. R., Bard, R. M., and Buhler, F. R.: Essential hypertension: Renin and aldosterone, heart attack, and stroke. N. Engl. J. Med., 286:441, 1972.

Buhler, F. R., Laragh, J. H., Baer, L., Vaughan, E. D., Jr., and Brunner, H. R.: Propranolol inhibition of renin secretion. N. Engl. J. Med., 287:1209, 1972.

Bumpus, F. M., Schwarz, H., and Page, I. H.: Synthesis and pharmacology of the octapeptide angiotensin. Science, 125:886, 1957.

Buonocore, E., Meaney, P. F., Borkowsky, G. P., Pavlicek, W., and Gallagher, J.: Digital subtraction angiography of the abdominal aorta and renal arteries. Radiology, 139:281, 1981.

Burnier, M., Waeber, B., Nussberger, J., and Brunner, H. R.: Effect of angiotensin converting enzyme inhibition in renovascular hypertension. J. Hypertens., 7(7):S27, 1989.

Butler, A. M.: Chronic pyelonephritis and arterial hypertension. J. Clin. Invest., 16:889, 1937.

Canzanello, V. J., Millin, V. G., Spiegel, J. E., Ponce, S. P., Kopelman, R. I., and Madias, N. E.: Percutaneous transluminal renal angioplasty in management of atherosclerotic renovascular hypertension: Results in 100 patients. Hypertension, 13:1639, 1989.

Carey, R. M., Reid, R. A., Ayers, C. R., Lynch, S. S., McLain, W. L., III, and Vaughan, E. D., Jr.: The Charlottesville blood pressure survey: Value of repeat blood pressure measurement to define the prevalence of labile and sustained hypertension. JAMA, 236:847, 1976.

Carey, R. M., and Sen, S.: Recent progress in the control of aldosterone secretion. Recent Prog. Horm. Res., 242:251, 1986.

Carey, R. M., Vaughan, E. D., Jr., Ackerly, J. A., Peach, M. J., and Ayers, C. R.: The immediate pressor effect of saralasin in man. J. Clin. Endocrinol. Metab., 46:36, 1978.

Casarella, W. J.: Non-coronary angioplasty. Curr. Probl. Cardiol., 11:3, 1986.

Case, D. B., Atlas, S. A., and Laragh, J. H.: Physiologic effects and blockade. In Laragh, J. H., Buhler, F. R., and Seldin, D. W.

(Eds.): Frontiers in Hypertension Research. New York, Springer-Verlag, 1982, pp. 541–550.

Case, D. B., Atlas, S. A., Laragh, J. H., Sealey, J. E., Sullivan, P. A., and McKinstry, D. N.: Clinical experience with blockade of the renin-angiotensin-aldosterone system by oral converting enzyme inhibitor (SQ 14225, captopril) in hypertensive patients. Prog. Cardiovasc. Dis., 21:195, 1978.

Case, D. B., Wallace, J. M., Keim, H. J., Sealey, J. E., and Laragh, J. H.: Usefulness and limitations of saralasin, a weak competitive agonist for angiotensin II, for evaluating the renin and sodium factor in hypertensive patients. Am. J. Med., 60:825, 1976a.

Case, D. B., Wallace, J. M., Keim, H. J., Weber, M. A., Drayer, J. I. M., White, R. P., Sealey, J. E., and Laragh, J. H.: Estimating renin participation in hypertension: Superiority of converting enzyme inhibitor over saralasin. Am. J. Med., 61:790, 1976b.

Castenada-Zuniga, W. R., Formanek, A., and Tadavarthy, M.: The mechanism of angioplasty. Radiology, 135:565, 1980.

Cheung, H. S., and Cushman, D. W.: Inhibition of homogenous angiotensin-converting enzyme of rabbit lung by synthetic venom peptides of *Bothrops jararaca*. Biochim. Biophys. Acta, 293:451, 1973.

Chrysant, S. G., Dunn, M., and Marples, D.: Severe reversible azotemia from captopril therapy. Arch. Intern. Med., 143:437, 1983.

Churchill, P. C.: Second messengers in renin secretion. Am. J. Physiol., 249:F175, 1985.

Churchill, P. C.: First and second messengers in renin secretion, Chap. 77. In Laragh, J. H., and Brenner, B. M. (Eds.): Hypertension: Pathophysiology, Diagnosis and Management. New York, Raven Press, 1990, p. 1233.

Cicuto, K. P., McLean, G. K., and Oleaga, J. A.: Renal artery stenosis: Anatomic classification for percutaneous transluminal angioplasty. Am. J. Roentgenol., 137:599, 1981.

Colapinto, R. F., Stronell, R. D., Harries-Jones, E. P., et al.: Percutaneous transluminal dilatation of the renal artery: Follow-up studies on renovascular hypertension. AJR, 139:722, 1982.

Cragg, A. H., Smith, T. P., Thompson, D. H., Maroney, T. P., Stanson, A. W., Shaw, G. T., Hunter, D. W., and Cochran, S. T.: Incidental fibromuscular dysplasia in potential renal donors: Long-term clinical follow-up. Radiology, 172:145, 1989.

Dean, R. H.: Renovascular hypertension: An overview, chap. 108. In Rutherford, R. B. (Ed.): Vascular Surgery. Philadelphia, W. B. Saunders Co., 1989.

Dean, R. H., Kieffer, R. W., Smith, B. M., Oates, J. A., Nadeau, J. H. J., Hollifield, J. U., and DuPont, W. D.: Renovascular hypertension: Anatomic and functional changes during drug therapy. Arch. Surg., 116:1408, 1981.

Derkx, F. H. M., Tan-Tjiong, H. L., Wentig, G. J., Man, In'T., Yeld, A. J., Yanseyen, A. J., and Schalekamp, M. A. D. H.: Captopril test for diagnosis of renal artery stenosis. In Glorioso, M. (Ed.): Renovascular Hypertension. New York, Raven Press, 1987, p. 295.

Desberg, A. L., Paushter, D. M., Limmert, G. K., Hale, J. C., Troy, R. B., Novick, A. C., Nally, J. V., Weltevreden, A. M.: Renal artery stenosis: Evaluation with color flow doppler. In press.

Dominiczak, A., Isles, C., Gillen, G., and Brown, J. J.: Angiotensin converting enzyme inhibition and renal insufficiency in patients with bilateral renovascular disease. J. Hum. Hypertens., 2:53, 1988.

Dotter, C. T., and Judkins, M. P.: Transluminal treatment of arteriosclerotic obstruction. Circulation, 30:654, 1964.

Eyler, W. R., Clark, M. D., Garman, J. E., Rian, R. L., and Meininger, D. E.: Angiography of the renal areas including a comparative study of renal arterial stenosis in patients with and without hypertension. Radiology, 78:879, 1962.

Fogarty, T. J., and Chen, K. A.: Adjunctive intraoperative arterial dilatation: Simplified instrumentation and technique. Arch. Surg., 116:1391, 1981.

Foster, J. H., Maxwell, M. H., Franklin, S. S., Bleifer, K. H., Trippel, O. H., Julian, O. C., DeCamp, P. T., and Varady, P. Y.: Renovascular occlusive disease: Results of operative treatment. JAMA, 231:1043, 1975.

Franklin, S. S., and Maxwell, M. H.: Clinical workup for renovascular hypertension. Urol. Clin. North Am., 2:301, 1975.

Freeman, N. E., Leeds, F. M., and Elliot, W.: Thromboendarterectomy for hypertension due to renal artery occlusion. JAMA, 156:1077, 1954.

Gaul, M. K., Linn, W. D., and Mulrow, C. D.: Captopril-stimulated renin secretion in the diagnosis of renovascular hypertension. Am. J. Hyperten., 2:335, 1989.

Gavras, H., Brunner, H. R., Thurston, H., and Laragh, J. H.: Reciprocation of renin dependency with sodium volume dependency in renal hypertension. Science, 188:1316, 1975.

Gavras, H., Brunner, H. R., Vaughan, E. D., Jr., and Laragh, J. H.: Angiotensin-sodium interaction in blood pressure maintenance of renal hypertensive and normotensive rats. Science, 180:1369, 1973.

Gephardt, G. N., and McCormack, L. J.: Pathology of the renal artery in hypertension. In Breslin, D. J., Swinton, N. W., Jr., Libertino, J. A., and Zinman, L. (Eds.): Renovascular Hypertension. Baltimore, Williams & Wilkins Co., 1982, pp. 63–72.

Geyskes, G. G., Puylaert, C. B. A., Oei, H. Y., Mees, E. J.: Follow-up study of 70 patients with renal artery stenosis treated by percutaneous transluminal dilatation. Br. Med. J., 287:333, 1983.

Geyskes, G. G., Oei, H. Y., Puylaert, C. B. A. J., Mees, E. J.: Renovascular hypertension identified by captopril-induced changes in the renogram. Hypertension, 9:451, 1987.

Gittes, R. F., and McLaughlin, A. P.: Unilateral operation for bilateral renovascular disease. J Urol., 111:292, 1974.

Goldblatt, H., Lynch, J., Hanzal, R. F., and Summerville, W. W.: Studies on experimental hypertension: I. The production of persistent elevation of systolic blood pressure by means of renal ischemia. J. Exp. Med., 59:347, 1934.

Goncharenko, V., Gerlock, A. J., Shaff, M. I., and Hollifield, S. W.: Progression of renal artery fibromuscular dysplasia in 42 patients as seen on angiography. Radiology, 139:45, 1981.

Goormaghtigh, N., and Grimson, K. S.: Vascular changes in renal ischemia, cell mitosis in the media of arteries. Proc. Soc. Exp. Biol. Med., 42:227, 1939.

Gosse, P., Dupas, J. Y., Reynaud, P., Jullien, E., and Dallocchio, M.: Am. J. Hypertens. 2:191, 1989.

Gross, F.: The renin-angiotensin system in hypertension. Ann. Intern. Med., 75:777, 1971.

Gruntzig, A., and Hopff, M.: Perkutane rekanalisation chronischer arterieller ver schlusse mit einem neuen dilatations katheter: Modifikation der Dotter technik. Dtsch. Med. Wochenschr., 99:2505, 1974.

Guzzetta, P. C., Potter, B. M., Ruley, J., Majd, M., and Bock, G. W.: Renovascular hypertension in children: Current concepts and evaluation and treatment. J. Pediatr. Surg., 24:1236, 1989.

Halpern, M., and Currarino, M.: Vascular lesions causing hypertension in neurofibromatosis. N. Engl. J. Med., 73:248, 1965.

Handa, N., Fuganaga, R., Ogawa, S., Matsumoto, M., Kimura, K., and Kamada, T.: A new accurate and non-invasive screening method for renovascular hypertension: The renal artery doppler technique. J. Hypertens., 6:S458, 1988.

Harrison, E. G., Jr., and McCormack, L. J.: Pathologic classification of renal arterial disease in renovascular hypertension. Mayo. Clin. Proc., 46:161, 1971.

Hawkins, P. G., McKnoulty, L. M., Gordon, R. D., Klemm, S. A., and Tunny, P. J.: Renal artery duplex ultrasonography: A reliable new screening test for functionally significant renal artery stenosis. Clin. Exp. Pharmacol. Physiol., 16:293, 1989.

Hillman, B. J., Ovitt, P. W., Capp, M. D., Prosnitz, E. H., Osborne, R. W., Goldstone, J., Gutowski, C. F., and Mallone, J. M.: The potential impact of digital video subtractions angiography on screening for renovascular hypertension. Radiology, 142:577, 1982.

Hollenberg, N. K.: Medical therapy for renovascular hypertension: A review. Am. J. Hypertens., 1:338S, 1988.

Holley, K. E., Hunt, J. C., Brown, A. L., Kincaid, O. W., and Sheps, S. G.: Renal artery stenosis: A clinical-pathologic study in normotensive patients. Am. J. Med., 37:14, 1964.

Howard, J. E., Berthrong, N., Gould, D., and Yendt, E. R.: Hypertension resulting from unilateral renovascular disease and its relief by nephrectomy. Bull. Johns Hopkins Hosp., 94:51, 1954.

Howard, J. E., and Conner, T. B.: Use of differential renal function studies in the diagnosis of renovascular hypertension. Am. J. Surg., 107:58, 1954.

Hricik, D. E., Browning, P. J., Kopelman, R., Goorno, W. E., Madias, N. V., and Zau, V. J.: Captopril induced functional renal insufficiency in patients with bilateral renal artery stenosis or renal artery stenosis in a solitary kidney. N. Engl. J. Med., 308:373, 1983.

Hunt, J. C., and Strong, C. S.: Renovascular hypertension: Mechanism, natural history and treatment. Am. J. Cardiol., 32:562, 1973.

Iaccarino, V., Russo, D., Niola, R., Muto, R., Testa, A., Andreucci, V. E., and Porta, A. E.: Total or partial percutaneous renal ablation in the treatment of renovascular hypertension: Radiological and clinical aspects. Br. J. Radiol., 62:593, 1989.

Ideishi, M., Sasaguri, M., Ikeda, M., and Arakawa, K.: Effective angiotensin converting enzyme inhibitors captopril, rentiapril and alacepril in patients with essential and renovascular hypertension. Clin. Ther., 11:441, 1989.

Idrissi, A., Fournier, A., Renaud, H., Voudailliez, B., El Esper, N., Fievet, P., Westeel, P. F., Makdassi, R., and Redmond, A.: The captopril challenge test as a screening test for renovascular hypertension. Kidney Int., 34:S138, 1988.

Imai, T., Miyazaki, H., Hirosc, S., Hori, H., Hayashi, T., Kageyame, R., Ohkubo, H., Nakanishi, S., and Murakami, K.: Cloning and sequence analysis of the cDNA for human renin precursor. Proc. Natl. Acad. Sci. USA, 80:7405, 1983.

Inagami, P., and Murakami, K.: Prorenin. Biomed. Res., 1:456, 1980.

Jackson, B., and Johnston, C. I.: Angiotensin-converting enzyme inhibition in renal disease: Contrasting effects on renal function in renal artery stenosis and progressive renal injury. J. Hum. Hypertens., 3:107, 1989.

Jacobson, H. R.: Ischemic renal disease: An overlooked clinical entity? Kidney Int., 34:729, 1988.

Johnson, J. A., Davis, J. O., and Witty, R. T.: Effects of catecholamines and renal nerve stimulation on renin release in the nonfiltering kidney. Circ. Res., 29:646, 1971.

Judson, W. E., and Helmer, O. M.: Diagnostic and prognostic values of renin activity in renal venous plasma in renovascular hypertension. Hypertension, 13:79, 1965.

Kaplan-Pavlobcic, S., Koselj, M., Obrez, I., et al.: Percutaneous transluminal renal angioplasty: Follow-up studies in renovascular hypertension. Przegl. Lek., 43:342, 1985.

Katzen, B. T., Chang, J., Lukowsky, G. H., et al.: Percutaneous transluminal angioplasty for the treatment of renovascular hypertension. Radiology, 131:53, 1979.

Keeton, T. K., and Campbell, W. B.: The pharmacologic alteration of renin release. Pharmacol. Rev., 32:81, 1980.

Klimberg, I. W., Locke, D. R., Hawkins, I. F., and Drylie, T. M.: Absolute ethanol renal autoinfarction for control of hypertension. Urology, 33:153, 1989.

Kohler, T. R., Zierler, R. E., and Martin, R. L.: Non-invasive diagnosis of renal artery stenosis by ultrasound duplex scanning. J. Vasc. Surg., 4:450, 1986.

Kotchen, T. A., Galla, J. H., and Luke, R. G.: Contribution of chloride to the inhibition of plasma renin by sodium chloride in the rat. Kidney Int., 13:201, 1978.

Kuhlmann, U., Greminger, P., Gruntzig, A., et al.: Long-term experience in percutaneous transluminal dilatation of renal artery stenosis. Am. J. Med., 79:692, 1985.

Kumar, S., Mandalim, R., Raovr, K., Subramanyan, R., Gupta, A. K., Joseph, S., Unni, M., and Rao, A. S.: Percutaneous transluminal angioplasty in non-specific aortoarthritis (Takayasu's disease): Experience in 16 cases. Cardiovasc. Intervent. Radiol., 12:321, 1990.

Laragh, J. H., Angers, M., Kelly, W. G., et al.: The effect of epinephrine, norepinephrine, angiotensin II, and others on the secretory rate of aldosterone in man. JAMA, 174:234, 1960.

Laragh, J. H., and Sealey, J. E.: The renin-angiotensin-aldosterone system and the renal regulation of sodium, potassium, and blood pressure regulation. *In* Windhager, E. E. (Ed.) Handbook of Physiology. New York, Oxford University Press, 1991.

Lawrie, G. M., Morris, G. C., Gleaser, D. H., and deBakey, M. E.: Renovascular reconstruction: Factors affecting long-term prognosis in 919 patients followed up to 31 years. Am. J. Cardiol., 63:1085, 1989.

Leadbetter, W. F., and Burkland, C. F.: Hypertension in unilateral renal disease. J. Urol., 39:611, 1938.

Levens, N. R., Peach, M. J., and Carey, R. M.: Role of the intrarenal renin-angiotensin system in the control of renal function. Circ. Res., 48:157, 1981.

Lew, E. A.: High blood pressure, other risk factors and longevity. *In* Laragh, J. H. (Ed.): The Insurance Viewpoint in Hypertension Manual. New York, Yorke Medical Books, 1973.

Liard, J. F., Cowley, A. W., McCaa, R. E., McCae, C. S., and Guyton, A. C.: Renin, aldosterone, body fluid volumes, and the baroreceptor reflex in the development and reversal of Goldblatt hypertension in conscious dogs. Circ. Res., 34:549, 1974.

London, G. M., and Safar, M. E.: Renal hemodynamics in patients with sustained essential hypertension and in patients with unilateral stenosis of the renal artery. Am. J. Hypertens., 2:244, 1989.

Lyons, D. F., Streck, W. F., Kem, D. C., et al.: Captopril stimulation of differential renins in renovascular hypertension. Hypertension, 5:65, 1983.

Mann, F. C., Herrick, J. F., Essex, H. E., and Baldes, E. J.: The effect on the blood flow of decreasing lumen of a blood vessel. Surgery, 4:249, 1938.

Marks, L. S., and Maxwell, M. H.: Renal vein renin value and limitations in the prediction of operative results. Urol. Clin. North Am., 2:311, 1975.

Martin, E. C., Diamond, N. G., and Casarella, W. J.: Percutaneous transluminal angioplasty in non-atherosclerotic disease. Radiology, 135:27, 1980.

Martin, E. C., Mattern, R. F., Baer, L., Fankuchen, E. I., and Casarella, W. J.: Renal angioplasty for hypertension: Predictive factors for long-term success. AJR, 137:921, 1981.

Martin, L. G., Price, R. B., Casarella, W. J., et al.: Percutaneous angioplasty in clinical management of renovascular hypertension: Initial and long-term results. Radiology, 155:629, 1985.

Martinez, A. G., Novick, A. C., and Hayes, J. M.: Surgical treatment of renal artery disease following failed percutaneous transluminal angioplasty. J. Urol. In press.

Mason, J. C., and Hilton, P. J.: Reversible renal failure due to captopril in a patient with transplant artery stenosis. Hypertension, 5:623, 1983.

Maxwell, M.H., and Lupu, A. N.: Excretory urogram in renal arterial hypertension. J. Urol., 100:395, 1968.

Maxwell, M. H., Lupu, A. N., and Taplin, G. V.: Radioisotope renogram in renal arterial hypertension. J. Urol., 100:376, 1968.

McCormack, L. J., Poutasse, E. F., Meaney, T. F., Noto, T. J., and Dustan, H. P.: A pathologic arteriographic correlation of renal arterial disease. Am. Heart J., 72:188, 1966.

McGill, C. W., Holder, T. M., and Smith, T. H.: Post-radiation renovascular hypertension. J. Pediatr. Surg., 14:831, 1979.

McNeil, B. J., and Adelstein, S. J.: Measures of clinical efficacy: The value of case finding in hypertensive renovascular disease. N. Engl. J. Med., 293:221, 1975.

McNeil, B. J., Varady, P. D., and Burrows, B. A.: Measures of clinical efficacy: Cost-effectiveness calculations in the diagnosis and treatment of hypertensive renovascular disease. N. Engl. J. Med., 293:216, 1975.

Meaney, T. F., Dustan, H. P., and Gilmore, J. P.: Angiotensin I conversion in the kidney and its modulation by sodium balance. Am. J. Physiol., 224:1104, 1973.

Meaney, T. F., Dustan, H. P., McCormack, L. J.: Natural history of renal arterial disease. Radiology, 9:877, 1968.

Meier, G. H., Sumpio, B., Black, H. R., and Gusberg, R. J.: Captopril renal scintigraphy—an advance in the detection and treatment of renovascular hypertension. J. Vasc. Surg., 11(6):770, 1990.

Miller, E. D., Jr., Samuels, A. I., and Haber, E.: Inhibition of angiotensin conversion in experimental renovascular hypertension. Science, 177:1108, 1972.

Miller, G. A., Ford, K. K., Braun, S. D., et al.: Percutaneous transluminal angioplasty vs. surgery for renovascular hypertension. AJR, 144:447, 1985.

Mohomed, F. A.: The etiology of Bright's disease and the prealbuminuric stage. Med. Chir. Trans., 57:197, 1874.

Mohring, J., Mohring, B., Naumann, J. H., Dauda, G., Kazda, S., Gross, F., Philippi, A., Homsy, E., and Orth, H.: Salt and water balance and renin activity in renal hypertension of rats. Am. J. Physiol., 228:1847, 1975.

Muller F. B., Sealey, J. E., Case, D. B., et al.: The captopril test for identifying renovascular disease in hypertensive patients. Am. J. Med., 80:633, 1986.

Munday, K. A., Parsons, B. J., and Post, J. A.: The effect of angiotensin on cation transport in rat kidney cortex slices. J. Physiol. (Lond.), 215:269, 1971.

Nally, J. V.: Use of captopril renography for the diagnosis of renovascular hypertension. World J. Urol., 7:72, 1989.

Nally, J. V., Clark, A. H. S., Grecos, G. P., Saunders, M., Gross,

M. L., Potvin, W. J., and Windham, J. P.: Effective captopril ^{99}Tc-diethylenetriaminepentaacetic acid renograms in 2-kidney, 1-clip hypertension. Hypertension, 8:685, 1986.

Ng, K. K. F., and Vane, J. R.: Conversion of angiotensin I to angiotensin II. Nature, 215:762, 1967.

Nicholson, J. P., Alderman, M. H., Pickering, T. G., Teishman, S. L., Sos, T. A., and Laragh, J. H.: Cigarette smoking in renovascular hypertension. Lancet, 2:765, 1983.

Novick, A. C.: Selection of patients with atherosclerosis for renal reconstruction to preserve renal function. World J. Urol., 7:98, 1989.

Novick, A. C., Straffon, R. A., Stewart, B. H., Gifford, R. W., and Vidt, D.: Diminished operative morbidity and mortality in renal revascularization. JAMA, 246:749, 1981.

Novick, A. C., Textor, S. C., Bodie, B., and Khauli, R. B.: Revascularization to preserve renal function in patients with atherosclerotic renovascular disease. Urol. Clin. North Am., 11:477, 1984.

Ohkubo, H., Kageyama, R., Uhihara, M., Hirosc, T., Inayama, S., and Nakashini, S.: Cloning and sequence analysis of cDNA for rat angiotensinogen. Proc. Natl. Acad. Sci. USA, 80:2196, 1983.

Olin, J. W., Graor, R. A., and Young, J. R.: Thrombolytic therapy for renal artery occlusions: A preliminary report. Cleve. Clin. J. Med., 56:434, 1989.

Ortenberg, J., Novick, A. C., Straffon, R. A., and Stewart, B. H.: Surgical treatment of renal artery aneurysm. Br. J. Urol., 55:341, 1983.

Page, I. H., and Helmer, O. M.: A crystalline pressor substance (angiotonin) resulting from the reaction between renin and renin activator. J. Exp. Med., 71:29, 1940.

Pals, D. T., Masucci, F. D., Denning, G. S., Jr., et al.: Role of the pressor action of angiotensin II in experimental hypertension. Circ. Res., 29:673, 1971.

Parrott, T. S., Woodard, J. R., Trulock, T. S., and Glenn, J. F: Segmental renal vein renins and partial nephrectomy for hypertension. J. Urol., 131:736, 1984.

Peach, M. J.: Structural features of angiotensin II which are important for biologic activity. Kidney Int., 15:S3, 1979.

Pederson, E. B., Sorensen, S. S., Amdisen, A., Danielsen, H., Eiskjaer, H., Hansen, H. H., Jensen, F. T., Jespersen, B., Madsen, B., and Nielsen, H. K.: Abnormal glomerular and tubular function during angiotensin converting enzyme inhibition in renovascular hypertension evaluated by the lithium clearance method. Eur. J. Clin. Invest., 19:135, 1989.

Pickering, T. G.: Medical management of renovascular hypertension. World J. Urol., 7:77, 1989.

Pickering, T. G.: Renovascular hypertension: Medical evaluation and non-surgical treatment, chap. 95. In Laragh, J. H., and Brenner, B. M. (Eds.): Hypertension: Pathophysiology, Diagnosis and Management. New York, Raven Press, Ltd., 1990a, p. 1539.

Pickering, T. G.: Hypertension: Definitions, natural histories and consequences, chap. 1. In Laragh, J. H., and Brenner, B. M. (Eds.): Hypertension: Pathophysiology, Diagnosis, and Management. New York, Raven Press, Ltd., 1990b.

Pickering, T. G., Sos, T. A., Vaughan, E. D., Jr., et al.: Predictive value and changes of renin secretion in hypertensive patients with unilateral renovascular disease undergoing successful renal angioplasty. Am. J. Med., 76:398, 1984.

Pickering, T. G., Sos, T. A., Vaughan, E. D., Jr., and Laragh, J. H.: Differing patterns of renal vein renin secretion in patients with renovascular hypertension, and their role in predicting the response to angioplasty. Nephron 44 (Suppl. 1):8–11, 1986.

Pitts, R. F., and Duggan, J. J.: Studies on diuretics: II. The relationship between glomerular filtration rate, proximal tubular absorption of sodium, and diuretic efficacy of mercurials. J. Clin. Invest., 29:372, 1950.

Postma, C. T., Hoefnagels, W. H. L., Barentsz, J. O., Deboo, T. H., and Thein, T. H.: Occlusion of unilateral stenosed renal arteries—relation to medical treatment. J. Hum. Hypertens., 3:185, 1989.

Poutasse, E. F., and Dustan, H. P.: Arteriosclerosis and renal hypertension: Indications for aortography in hypertensive patients and results of surgical treatment of obstructive lesions of renal artery. JAMA, 165:1521, 1957.

Ramsay, L. E., and Waller, P. C.: Blood pressure response to percutaneous transluminal angioplasty for renovascular hypertension: An overview of published series. Br. Med. J., 300:569, 1990.

Ratliff, N. B.: Renal vascular disease: Pathology of large blood vessel disease. In Porush, J. G. (Ed.): Hypertension and the Kidney. New York, Grune & Stratton, 1985.

Re, R., Noveline, R., Escourrou, M. -T., Athanasoulis, C., Burton, J., and Haber, E.: Inhibition of angiotensin-converting enzyme for diagnosis of renal-artery stenosis. N. Engl. J. Med., 298:582, 1978.

Ribstein, J., Mourad, G., and Mimran, A.: Contrasting effects of captopril and nifedipine on renal function in renovascular hypertension. Am. J. Hypertens., 1:239, 1988.

Ritter, S. G., Bentley, M. D., Fiksen-Olsen, M. J., Brown, M. L., Romero, J. C., and Zachariah, P. K.: Effect of captopril on renal function in hypertensive dogs with unilateral renal artery stenosis, studied with radionuclide dynamic scintigraphy. Am. J. Hypertens., 3:591, 1990.

Rose, A. G., and Sinclair-Smith, C. C.: Takayasu's arteritis: A study of sixteen autopsy patients. Arch. Pathol. Lab. Med., 104:231, 1980.

Rosivall, L., Blantz, R. C., and Navar, L. G.: Guest editors: Renovascular effects of angiotensin II. Kidney Int. (Suppl. 30), 1990.

Rubin, B., Laffan, R. J., Kotler, D. G., et al.: SQ 14225 (D-3-mercapto-2-methylpropanoyl-L-proline), a novel orally active inhibitor of angiotensin I-converting enzyme. J. Pharmacol. Exp. Ther., 204:271, 1978.

Salvetti, A., Arzilli, P., Nuccorini, A., Maura, M., and Gilvanetti, R.: Does humoral and hemodynamic response to acute ACE inhibition identify true renovascular hypertension? In Glorioso, M. (Ed.): Renovascular Hypertension. New York, Raven Press, 1987, p. 305.

Sanborn, T. A., Cumberland, D. C., Greenfield, A. J., Motarjeme, A., Schwarten, D. E., Leachman, R., Ferris, E. J., Myler, R. K., McCowan, T. C., Tatpati, D., Ginsburg, R., and White, R. I.: Peripheral laser-assisted balloon angioplasty. Arch. Surg., 124:1099, 1989.

Sang, C. N., Whelton, P. K., Hamper, U. M., Connolly, M., Kidir, S., White, R. I., Saunders, R., Liang, K. -Y., and Bias, W.: Etiologic factors in renovascular fibromuscular dysplasia: A case-control study. Hypertension, 14:472, 1989.

Schambelan, M., Glickman, M., Stockigt, J. R., and Biglieri, E. G.: The selective renal vein renin sampling in hypertensive patients with segmental renal lesions. N. Engl. J. Med., 290:1153, 1974.

Schreiber, M. J., Jr., Novick, A. C., and Pohl, M. A.: The natural history of atherosclerotic and fibrous renal artery disease. World J. Urol., 7:59, 1989.

Schreiber, M. J., Pohl, M. A., and Novick, A. C.: The natural history of atherosclerotic and fibrous renal artery disease. Urol. Clin. North Am., 11:383, 1984.

Schwarten, D. E.: Percutaneous transluminal renal artery angioplasty. In Kaplan, N. M., Brunner, B. M., and Laragh, J. H. (Eds.): The Kidney and Hypertension. New York, Raven Press, 1987.

Sealey, J. E., Atlas, S. A., and Laragh, J. H.: Prorenin and other large molecular weight forms of renin. Endocr. Rev., 1:365, 1980.

Sealey, J. E., Blumenfeld, J. D., Bell, G. M., Pecker, M. S., Sommers, S. C., and Laragh, J. H.: On the renal basis for essential hypertension: Nephron heterogeneity with discordant renin secretion and sodium excretion causing a hypertensive vasoconstriction-volume relationship. J. Hypertens. 6:763, 1988a.

Sealey, J. E., Buhler, F. R., Laragh, J. H., and Vaughan, E. D., Jr.: The physiology of renin secretion in essential hypertension: Estimation of renin secretion rate and renal plasma flow from peripheral and renal vein renin levels. Am. J. Med., 55:391, 1973.

Sealey, J. E., Glorioso, N., Itskovitz, J., and Laragh, J. H.: Prorenin as a reproductive hormone: New form of the renin system. Am. J. Med., 81:1041, 1986.

Sealey, J. E., Goldstein, M., Pitarresi, T. M., Kudlak, T., Glorioso, N., Fiamengo, S. A., and Laragh, J. H.: Prorenin secretion from human testis: No evidence for secretion of active renin or angiotensinogen. J. Clin. Endocrinol. Metab., 66:974, 1988b.

Selkurt, E. E.: The effect of pulse pressure and mean arterial pressure modification of renal hemodynamics and electrolyte and water excretion. Circulation, 4:541, 1951.

Sfakianakis, G. N., Bourgoignie, J. J., Jaffe, D., Kyriakides, G., Perez-Stable, E., and Duncan, R. C.: Single-dose captopril scintigraphy in the diagnosis of renovascular hypertension. J. Nucl. Med., 28:1383, 1987.

Simon, N., Franklin, S. S., Bleifer, K. H., and Maxwell, M. H.: Clinical characteristics of renovascular hypertension. JAMA, 220:1209, 1972.

Simunic, S., Winter-Fuduric, I., Radanovic, B., Bradic, I., Marinovic,

B., Marinkovic, M., Cavka, K., Batinica, S., Batinic, D., and Roglic, M.: Percutaneous transluminal renal angioplasty (PTRA) as a method of treatment for renovascular hypertension in children. Eur. J. Radiol., 10:143, 1990.

Sinaiko, A. R., and Wells, T. G.: Childhood hypertension, chap. 115. In Laragh, J. M., and Brenner, B. M. (Eds.): Hypertension: Pathophysiology, Diagnosis, and Management. New York, Raven Press, Ltd., 1990, p. 1853.

Skeggs, L. T., Jr., Lentz, K. E., Kahn, J. R., Shumway, N. P., and Woods, K. R.: Amino acid sequence of hypertension II. J. Exp. Med., 104:193, 1956.

Skeggs, L. T., Marsh, W. H., Kahn, J. R., and Shumway, N. P.: The existence of two forms of hypertension. J. Exp. Med., 99:275, 1954.

Smith, C. W., Winfield, A. C., and Price, R. R.: Evaluation of digital venous angiography for the diagnosis of renovascular hypertension. Radiology, 144:51, 1982.

Smith, H. W.: Hypertension and urologic disease. Am. J. Med., 4:724, 1948.

Smith, P., Rush, T. W., and Evans, A. T.: The technique of translumbar arteriography. JAMA, 148:255, 1952.

Soffer, R. L.: Angiotensin converting enzyme. In Soffer, R. L. (Ed.): Biochemical Regulation of Blood Pressure. New York, John Wiley & Sons, 1981, p. 123.

Sos, T. A., Pickering, T. G., Sniderman, K. W., et al.: Percutaneous transluminal renal angioplasty in renovascular hypertension due to atheroma or fibromuscular dysplasia. N. Engl. J. Med., 309:274, 1983.

Sosa, R. E.: Effects of converting enzyme inhibition on renal function in chronic 2-kidney, 1-clip hypertensive dogs. J. Urol., 137:209A, 1987.

Sosa, R. E., and Vaughan, E. D., Jr.: Evaluation for surgically curable hypertension. AUA Update Series, 2:Lesson 31, 1983.

Sosa, R. E., and Vaughan, E. D., Jr.: Hypertension of renal origin. World J. Urol., 7:64, 1989.

Soubrier, F., Panthier, J. J., Corvol, P., and Rougeon, F.: Molecular cloning and nucleotide sequence of the human renin cDNA fragment. Nucleic Acids Res., 11:7181, 1983.

Stamey, T. A.: Renovascular Hypertension. Baltimore, Williams & Wilkins Co., 1963.

Stamey, T. A., Nudelman, I. J., Good, T. H., Schwentker, E. N., and Hendricks, F.: Functional characteristics of renovascular hypertension. Medicine, 40:347, 1961.

Stewart, B. H., and Dustan, H. P., Kiser, W. S., Meaney, T. F., Straffon, R. A., and McCormack, L. J.: Correlation of angiography and natural history in evaluation of patients with renovascular hypertension. J. Urol., 104:231, 1970.

Stockigt, J. R., Noakes, C. A., Collins, R. D., Schambelan, M., and Biglieri, E. G.: Renal-vein renin in various forms of renal hypertension. Lancet, 1:1194, 1972.

Strandness, D. L., Jr.: Duplex scanning in diagnosis of renovascular hypertension. Surg. Clin. North Am., 70:109, 1990.

Tack, C., and Sos, T. A.: Percutaneous transluminal renal angioplasty. World J. Urol., 7:82, 1989.

Tegtmeyer, C. J., Kellum, C. D., and Ayers, C.: Percutaneous transluminal angioplasty of the renal artery. Radiology, 153:77, 1984.

Textor, S. C., Novick, A. C., Tarazi, R. C., et al.: Critical perfusion pressure for renal function in patients with bilateral atherosclerotic renovascular disease. Ann. Intern. Med., 102:308, 1985.

Tham, G., Ekelund, L., Herrlin, K., Lindstedt, E. L., Olin, T., and Bergentz, S. -E.: Renal artery aneurysms: Natural history and prognosis. Ann. Surg., 197:348, 1983.

Thibonnier, M., Joseph, A., Sassano, P., Guyenne, T. T., Corvol, P., Raynaud, A., Seurot, M., and Gaux, J. C.: Improved diagnosis of unilateral renal artery lesions after captopril administration. JAMA, 251:56, 1984.

Thornbury, J. R., Stanley, F. C., and Freyback, D. G.: Hypertensive urogram: A non-discriminatory test for renovascular hypertension. AJR, 138:43, 1982.

Tigerstedt, R., and Bergmann, T. G.: Niere und kreislauf. Skand. Arch. Physiol., 8:233, 1898.

Tobian, L., Tomboulian, A., and Janecek, J.: Effect of high perfusion pressure on the granulation of juxtaglomerular cells in an isolated kidney. J. Clin. Invest., 38:605, 1959.

Traube, L.: Uber den Zusammenhang von Herz- und Nieren-Krankheiten. In Gesammelte Beitraege zur Pathologie und Physiologie, Vol. II, Part I, Clinical Investigations. Berlin, A. Hirschwalt, 1856.

van Bockel, J. H., van Schilfgaard, R., van Brummelen, P., and Terpstra, J. L.: Long-term results of renal artery reconstruction with autogenous artery in patients with renovascular hypertension. Eur. J. Vasc. Surg., 3:515, 1989.

van Bockel, J. H., van Schilfgaarde, R., Felthuis, W., van Brummelen, P., Terpstra, J. L.: Reconstructive surgery for renovascular hypertension secondary to arteriosclerosis and fibrodysplasia: III. The early and late effects of surgery on hypertensive target organ damage. Neth. J. Med., 32:159, 1988.

Vander, A. J.: Effect of catecholamines and the renal nerves on renin secretion in anesthetized dogs. Am. J. Physiol., 209:659, 1965.

Vaughan, E. D., Jr., Buhler, F. R., Laragh, J. H., Sealey, J. E., Baer, L., and Bard, R. H.: Renovascular hypertension; renin measurements to indicate hypersecretion and contralateral suppression, estimate renal plasma flow and score for surgical curability. Am. J. Med., 55:402, 1973.

Vaughan, E. D., Jr., Carey, R. M., Ayers, C. R., Peach, M. J., Tegtmeyer, C. J., and Wellons, M. A., Jr.: A physiologic definition of blood pressure response to renal revascularization in patients with renovascular hypertension. Kidney Int., 15:S83, 1979.

Vaughan, E. D., Jr., Case, D. B., Pickering, T. G., Sosa, R. E., Sos, T. A., and Laragh, J. H.: Clinical evaluation for renovascular hypertension and therapeutic decisions. Urol. Clin. North Am., 11:393, 1984.

Vaughan, E. D., Jr., Sos, T. A., Sniderman, K. W., Pickering, T. G., Case, D. B., Sealey, J. E., and Laragh, J. H.: Renal venous renin secretory patterns before and after percutaneous transluminal angioplasty: Verification of analytic criteria. In Laragh, J. H. (Ed.): Frontiers in Hypertension Research. New York, Springer-Verlag, 1981.

Vaughan, E. D., Jr., and Sosa, R. E.: Renovascular hypertension: Treatment Options. AUA Update Series, 8: Lesson 36, 1989.

Von Knorring, J., Lepantalo, M., and Fyhrquist, F.: Long-term prognosis of surgical treatment of renovascular hypertension. J. Intern. Med., 225:303, 1989.

Weed, W. C., Vaughan, E. D., Jr., and Peach, M. J.: Prolongation of the saralasin responsive state of two-kidney, one-clip hypertension in the rat by the orally administered converting enzyme inhibitor captopril (SQ 14225). Hypertension, 1:8, 1979.

Wenting, G. J., Tan-Tjiong, H. L., Derkx, F. H. M., de Bruyn, J. H. B., manin't Veld, A. J., Schalekamp, M. A.: Split renal function after captopril in unilateral renal artery stenosis. Br. Med. J., 288:886, 1984.

Wilcox, C. S., Williams, C. M., Smith, T. B., Fredrickson, E. D., Wingo, C., and Bucci, C. M.: Diagnostic uses of angiotensin-converting enzyme inhibitors in renovascular hypertension. Am. J. Hypertens., 1:344S, 1988.

Wilcox, G. S., Smith, T. P., Fredrickson, E. D., Wingo, C. D., Phillips, M. I., and Williams, C. M.: The captopril glomerular filtration rate renogram in renovascular hypertension. Clin. Nucl. Med., 14:1, 1989.

Willems, C. E. D., Shah, V., Uchiyama, M., and Dillon, M. J.: Arch. Dis. Child., 64:229, 1989.

Wilms, G., Marchal, G., Peene, P., and Baert, A. L.: The angiographic incidence of renal artery stenosis in the arteriosclerotic population. Eur. J. Radiol., 10(3):195, 1990.

Wollenweber, J., Sheps, S. G., and David, D. G.: Clinical course of atherosclerotic renovascular disease. Am. J. Cardiol., 21:60, 1968.

Ying, C. Y., Tifft, C. P., Gavras, H., et al.: Renal revascularization in the azotemic hypertensive patient resistant to therapy. N. Engl. J. Med., 311:1070, 1984.

56
ETIOLOGY, PATHOGENESIS, AND MANAGEMENT OF RENAL FAILURE

Joseph I. Shapiro, M.D.
Robert W. Schrier, M.D.

RENAL FUNCTION

The kidney serves a number of important physiologic and hormonal functions. It plays a central role in maintaining acid-base, water, and electrolyte homeostasis as well as regulating extracellular volume and blood pressure. The kidney is also involved in erythropoiesis and bone metabolism, and, of course, is the normal route for excreting nitrogenous and other waste products derived from intermediary metabolism. Thus, the kidney has a number of functions in addition to preventing azotemia.

Many of the renal functions can be quantitated clinically. Urinary concentrating or diluting ability may be assessed with a water deprivation or a water load test, respectively. Urine acidification may be assessed with a wide range of tests. Urine electrolyte concentrations may also be monitored to determine if tubular handling of these electrolytes is normal (Shapiro and Schrier, 1988). However, the most important tests of renal function are those that assess the glomerular filtration rate (GFR).

Laboratory Assessment

Most arterial blood delivered to the kidney passes through glomerular capillaries where a portion, known as the filtration fraction, is filtered. Under normal circumstances, this filtrate is without blood cells and contains only small amounts of protein. This filtered fluid is modified by tubular reabsorption and secretion to regulate the quality and quantity of body fluids as previously discussed. The rate at which fluid is filtered by the glomerulus is an important clinical parameter of renal function, which can be measured (Brenner et al., 1986).

Measurement of GFR is accomplished by measuring the renal clearance of a substance that is freely filtered by the glomerulus, is not reabsorbed or degraded, and is not secreted by any tubular segment. The renal clearance of such a substance, X (Cl_X), can be calculated as

$$Cl_X = (U_X \times V)/P_X$$

where U_X is the urine concentration of X, V is the urine flow rate, and P_X is the plasma concentration of X. No endogenous compound that can be easily measured fits this description perfectly. For experimental work, inulin, a polysaccharide not normally found in humans, is infused to achieve a steady-state plasma concentration. Subsequent determination of its clearance by the kidney is the gold standard for GFR measurement (Brenner et al., 1986). Iodothalamate is a compound that can be radiolabeled with ^{125}I and can also be used for GFR determinations (Gagnon et al., 1971).

However, neither of these two measurements is practical on a routine clinical basis. The plasma concentration of urea has been used in the past to assess renal function. Urea is a breakdown product of protein catabolism; its plasma levels generally have an inverse correlation with GFR. Unfortunately, urea production rate is variable and depends on dietary intake and the rate of catabolism as well as liver function. Moreover, urea is not only filtered by the glomerulus but is also absorbed by the tubules to a significant and variable degree, depending on volume status and urine flow rate. Therefore, neither urea clearance nor plasma urea concentrations provide an accurate estimation of GFR.

In comparison, creatinine, an important compound in

energy metabolism, is another nitrogenous compound that is a breakdown product of creatine. Creatinine is produced at a relatively constant rate, which is dependent on the amount of total creatine in the body, an index of total body muscle mass. Therefore, for a given individual, daily creatinine production is relatively constant. Creatinine is freely filtered at the level of the glomerulus and is not reabsorbed, but it is secreted to some extent. Although, in patients with normal renal function, creatinine secretion accounts for only 10 per cent of total creatinine excretion, tubular creatinine secretion may represent a greater proportion in some patients with renal disease, particularly those with large amounts of proteinuria.

Despite this drawback, plasma creatinine values and renal creatinine clearance measurements are used to estimate GFR (Brenner et al., 1986). The measurement of creatinine clearance when tubular creatinine secretion is inhibited with cimetidine or trimethoprim has been shown to correlate quite well with iodothalamate clearance measurements in patients with normal and abnormal renal function (Roubenoff et al., 1990). Thus, in the future, this approach will be used more routinely in the clinical setting.

GFR is not constant throughout the day and is influenced greatly by dietary protein intake. In patients with normal renal function, a marked increase in GFR occurs rapidly and persists for several hours following ingestion of a large protein meal. This increase in GFR following protein ingestion may be blunted or absent in patients with chronic renal failure. This ability to increase GFR with protein ingestion, referred to as the "renal reserve," might be a sensitive measurement of renal function (Losito et al., 1988; Notghi and Anderton, 1988; ter-Wee et al., 1987; von-Herrath et al., 1988). Further studies are needed to demonstrate the clinical utility of this measurement.

ACUTE RENAL FAILURE

Definition and Clinical Description

Acute renal failure (ARF) is probably best understood as an acute deterioration in renal functions resulting in a buildup of nitrogenous wastes in the plasma (i.e., azotemia) and a failure of the kidney to regulate extracellular fluid volume and composition. Although this definition offers a reasonable understanding of the concept, it is vague and ill-suited for reporting precise clinical data. For example, in clinical reports, definitions of ARF range from a need for dialysis therapy to 0.5-mg/dl increases in plasma creatinine concentrations. Thus, the criterion to define patient selection with ARF will greatly influence estimations of incidence and mortality.

Because the most obvious evidence of renal function is the production of urine, the first descriptions of ARF were limited to patients who developed marked reductions in urine flow rate. Maximal urine osmolality is about 1000 mOsm/kg and obligate solute excretion is about 500 mOsm/day (for a 70-kg man). Reductions of

urine flow rate to values below 500 ml/day are not compatible with the maintenance of solute balance. In the oliguric patient, azotemia invariably occurs. Reduction of urine flow rate to values below 500 ml/day is referred to as oliguria. Virtual cessation of urine flow is called anuria. Although oliguria and anuria are certainly concerning, their absence does not exclude ARF. The acute accumulation of nitrogenous solutes in the blood as daily urine flow exceeds 500 ml/day is referred to as nonoliguric ARF.

ARF is still common, especially in hospitalized patients. The most common cause of ARF is prerenal azotemia, but acute tubular necrosis (ATN) and urinary obstruction (postrenal azotemia) also occur frequently (vida infra) (Hou et al., 1983). Because ARF is associated with marked increases in morbidity and mortality, avoidance of and prompt therapy for ARF are important. This approach requires an understanding of the different causes of ARF, the differential diagnosis, and the appropriate therapy.

Etiology

ARF may be associated with a variety of insults. Often, more than one insult may be implicated (Rasmussen and Ibels, 1982).

Classification

Clinically, it is helpful to distinguish prerenal, intrarenal, and postrenal causes of ARF. Assignment of a patient to one of these groups usually requires a combination of clinical and laboratory evaluation and may occasionally require imaging studies or invasive measurements of central hemodynamics. Because the clinical management of ARF may be very different in patients with prerenal, intrarenal, and postrenal ARF, this diagnostic determination is of critical importance (Schrier and Conger, 1986).

PRERENAL ACUTE RENAL FAILURE

Prerenal ARF occurs because of inadequate renal perfusion pressure to maintain GFR. Under normal circumstances, the kidney can maintain normal renal blood flow and GFR down to a mean arterial pressure of 60 mm Hg. This phenomenon is known as autoregulation and requires a complex interplay of physiologic factors for its maintenance. In many patients, these physiologic factors are not all intact, and decreases in renal blood flow and GFR occur with modest or even no discernible reductions in blood pressure.

In the setting of decreased renal perfusion pressure, angiotensin II, which has selectively greater vasoconstrictive effects on the efferent arterioles than on the afferent arterioles, and vasodilatory prostaglandins, which cause afferent arteriolar vasodilatation, are important in maintaining glomerular hydrostatic pressure and GFR (Brenner et al., 1986). Drugs that selectively block angiotensin II synthesis or action or that inhibit prostaglandin synthesis may therefore cause ARF in some clinical situations.

The common causes of prerenal azotemia, which is also called prerenal ARF, are listed in Table 56–1. Of these, the most common is probably simple dehydration. It must be stressed, however, that gross extracellular volume expansion with edema formation, as observed with liver failure, nephrotic syndrome, and heart failure, may be associated with prerenal azotemia. Prerenal azotemia due to fluid or blood loss can be treated quite simply by volume expansion. However, prerenal ARF related to heart failure may require careful titration of diuretics, afterload reduction, and use of inotropic agents to improve renal perfusion. The prerenal ARF associated with liver failure is particularly difficult to treat because these patients are particularly susceptible to develop ATN or hepatorenal syndrome (HRS) with overaggressive diuresis.

HRS is a severe form of prerenal azotemia in which renal vasoconstriction apparently cannot be reversed by manipulation of cardiac filling pressure and total peripheral resistance. Interestingly, this renal vasoconstriction can be reversed by transplanting the kidney from the patient with HRS into a patient with a well-functioning liver. HRS can also be reversed by liver transplantation (Arroyo et al., 1988).

PARENCHYMAL CAUSES OF ACUTE RENAL FAILURE

ARF may result from a variety of parenchymal causes. The more important causes of ARF are listed in Table 56–2. Clinically, it is helpful to separate these causes into those secondary to systemic diseases, primary glomerular renal diseases, and primary tubulointerstitial renal diseases.

Although a variety of systemic diseases are associated with renal manifestations, relatively few of these commonly cause ARF. Of note are the systemic vasculitides, in particular, polyarteritis nodosa, essential mixed cryoglobulinemia, and systemic lupus erythematosus as well as multiple myeloma (Ballard et al., 1970; Hecht et al., 1976; Martinez-Maldonado et al., 1971; Shapiro and Schrier, 1988). Although diabetes is not a typical cause

Table 56–1. MAJOR CAUSES OF PRERENAL AZOTEMIA

| Decreased cardiac output |
| Decreased intravascular volume |
| Dehydration |
| Hemorrhage |
| Anaphylactic shock |
| Decreased venous tone |
| Autonomic neuropathy |
| Spinal injury |
| Decreased contractile function |
| Ischemic heart disease |
| Cardiomyopathy |
| Pericardial tamponade or constriction |
| Normal or increased cardiac output |
| Systemic disorders |
| Liver disease |
| Sepsis |
| Local renal disease |
| Renal artery stenosis |

Table 56–2. MAJOR PARENCHYMAL CAUSES OF ACUTE RENAL FAILURE

| Primary renal disease |
| Glomerular |
| Primary acute glomerulonephritis |
| Tubulointerstitial |
| Acute interstitial nephritis |
| Acute tubular necrosis |
| Pyelonephritis |
| Transplant allograft rejection |
| Nephrolithiasis |
| Radiation nephritis |
| Systemic disease |
| Glomerular |
| Vasculitis |
| Goodpasture's syndrome |
| Secondary acute glomerulonephritis (e.g., bacterial endocarditis) |
| Tubulointerstitial |
| Tumor lysis syndrome |
| Infiltration of kidney with tumor (rare) |

for ARF on its own, it is a significant predisposing factor for ARF from other causes, in particular, ARF caused by radiocontrast (Schrier and Shapiro, 1985b). ARF may complicate the hemolytic uremic syndrome (HUS) or the syndrome of thrombotic thrombocytopenic purpura (TTP) (Glassock and Babcock, 1990). Distinction of these syndromes from that of preeclampsia or of renal cortical necrosis in pregnancy-associated ARF may be difficult. ARF in the setting of pregnancy has a very guarded prognosis for renal recovery, perhaps because it may involve cortical necrosis (Kelleher and Berl, 1981).

Primary glomerular diseases most commonly associated with ARF are those caused by anti–glomerular basement membrane antibody either with pulmonary hemorrhage (Goodpasture's syndrome) or without pulmonary hemorrhage. ARF may also occur in association with nephrotic syndrome and nil disease. Other forms of primary glomerular disease, such as membranous glomerulopathy and membranoproliferative glomerulonephritis, may have accelerated courses (Shapiro and Schrier, 1988).

Of the primary tubulointerstitial diseases causing ARF, the most important is ATN. ATN may be caused by a variety of insults. Often, ATN cannot be ascribed to any one insult but develops with multiple potential etiologies (Rasmussen and Ibels, 1982). ATN, as it was first described secondary to crush injuries, had a rather predictable course with a 10- to 14-day period of oliguria followed by a 10- to 14-day polyuric recovery phase (Swann and Merrill, 1953). We now know that nonoliguric ATN is about as frequent as oliguric ATN, and that both forms of ATN may follow variable courses. Oliguric ATN has an associated mortality of 60 to 80 per cent as compared with nonoliguric ATN, which has an associated mortality of 20 per cent (Anderson et al., 1977; Stott et al., 1972).

Renal ischemia is the most common predisposing cause of ATN. It can, in fact, result from virtually any of the causes of prerenal azotemia. Renal ischemia leading to ATN is most often related to prolonged hypotension or surgical interruption of renal blood flow, such as during aortic aneurysm resection or in the course of renal transplantation (Morris, 1986). Some drugs, such as nonsteroidal anti-inflammatory agents (NSAIAs), angiotensin-converting enzyme inhibitors (CEIs), and cyclosporine A, may cause ARF by hemodynamic means, especially in settings of reduced renal perfusion pressure. In most cases, these drugs simply cause prerenal azotemia, but they can, in some cases, cause frank ATN (Bakris and Kern, 1989; Bennett and Pulliam, 1983; Paller, 1990).

Nephrotoxic antibiotics, in particular, the aminoglycosides, are a common and important cause of ATN. Aminoglycoside-associated ATN is typically nonoliguric; usually develops after 5 to 7 days of therapy; and is most often seen in patients who are older, have underlying chronic renal insufficiency, have had recent additional courses of aminoglycosides, or have had other renal insults, particularly ischemia (Appel, 1990).

Radiocontrast-induced ATN is also fairly common and is also more likely to affect patients with chronic renal insufficiency, especially due to diabetes or multiple myeloma. In contrast to aminoglycoside nephrotoxicity, radiocontrast-induced ATN is usually oliguric in nature (Schrier and Shapiro, 1985b). Despite the associated oliguria, radiocontrast nephropathy typically runs a short and benign course. Other drugs that may cause ATN include amphotericin, acyclovir, and cisplatinum, which also typically results in renal potassium and magnesium wasting that can persist for extremely long durations. Drug intoxications, especially with acetaminophen or ethylene glycol, may cause ATN (Paller, 1990).

Acute interstitial nephritis (AIN) is a relatively uncommon, but important, cause of ARF. Classically described in association with use of penicillin antibiotics, it can complicate therapy with a myriad of drugs (Table 56–3). The classic features of AIN include fever, eosinophilia, rash, and eosinophiluria. In many cases, several if not all of these features may be absent, and in some cases, renal biopsy is the only way to make the diagnosis (Neilson, 1989). In particular, NSAIAs may be associated with AIN in concert with heavy proteinuria but without associated fever, eosinophiluria, eosinophilia, or rash (Bakris and Kern, 1989; Porile et al., 1990).

Table 56–3. DRUGS COMMONLY ASSOCIATED WITH ACUTE INTERSTITIAL NEPHRITIS

Antibiotics	Seizure medications
Penicillins*	Phenytoin
Cephalosporins	Carbamazepine
Trimethoprim	Phenobarbital
Sulfa derivatives	Nonsteroidal anti-inflammatory agents
Rifampicin	Fenoprofen†
Diuretics	Miscellaneous
Furosemide	Cimetidine
Thiazides	Allopurinol
Triamterene	Azathoprine
Antihypertensives	Penicillamine
Captopril	
Alpha methyldopa	

*Most often seen with methicillin.
†Virtually all nonsteroidal anti-inflammatory agents have been reported to cause acute interstitial nephritis, but the association is strongest with fenoprofen use.

Finding eosinophils in the urine of patients with AIN may be difficult. Nolan and colleagues (1986) demonstrated that Hansel's stain is superior to the more traditional Wright's stain in evaluating the urine for eosinophils. These investigators point out that eosinophils in the urine may also be observed with other causes of renal failure, in particular, acute glomerulonephritis (Nolan et al., 1986; Nolan and Kelleher, 1988). Although gross and microscopic hematuria may be seen in both AIN and acute glomerulonephritis, the presence of red blood cell casts strongly suggests the latter diagnosis.

Acute pyelonephritis does not typically cause ARF, perhaps because most patients with this disease have unilateral involvement and a normally functioning contralateral kidney. However, in patients with a solitary native kidney or a transplant kidney, acute pyelonephritis can cause ARF. In renal transplant patients, the major differential diagnosis of ARF includes cyclosporine nephrotoxicity, allograft rejection, and ischemic ARF; occasionally, however, acute pyelonephritis will cause ARF with a similar presentation to allograft rejection (Morris, 1986).

POSTRENAL ACUTE RENAL FAILURE

Obstruction to the flow of urine may occur, at any site, from microscopic obstruction to tubular fluid flow to the urethra. The different causes of urinary obstruction are discussed in much detail in other chapters in this textbook. The diagnosis of urinary tract obstruction should be considered in every patient who presents with ARF (Schrier and Conger, 1986).

Pathogenesis of Acute Tubular Necrosis

ATN is a major form of ARF. Awareness of the pathogenetic factors involved in its initiation, maintenance, and recovery is important in approaching its prevention and therapy.

The ischemic form of ATN has been best studied and is discussed primarily. Reductions in GFR during ATN are generally due to both vascular and tubular factors. The vascular factors include reductions in glomerular perfusion pressure and decreases in the ultrafiltration coefficient of the glomerulus. Reductions in glomerular perfusion pressure might result from either decrease in renal plasma flow or, in the setting of decreased renal plasma flow, dilatation of the efferent arteriole, as might be observed with a CEI that removes the efferent constrictive effects of angiotensin II. In most cases of ischemic ATN, reduction in renal perfusion pressure from decreased renal plasma flow is a factor in the initiation of but not the maintenance of ARF. In experimental models as well as in patients, renal plasma flow increases toward normal 24 to 48 hours following the ischemic insult without functional recovery, and efforts to increase renal plasma flow with renal vasodilators in the postischemic period generally do not ameliorate the course of ARF. Thus, maintenance factors in ischemic ATN are primarily tubular (Levinsky, 1977).

Tubular factors may involve two separate processes, namely, backleak of glomerular filtrate and tubular obstruction. Although it is clear that backleak may occur in some experimental models of ARF, tubular obstruction appears to be the most important maintenance factor in ATN. Sloughed brush border membranes, cellular debris, Tamm-Horsfall protein, and decreased filtration pressure may all contribute to tubular obstruction after an ischemic insult (Burke et al., 1980).

Because of the contribution of cell necrosis in the formation of this obstructing debris, most research in this area has focused on the cellular events occurring during ischemic ATN (Schrier and Conger, 1986). Decreases in substrate supply lead to decreases in cellular adenosine triphosphate (ATP) concentrations, failure to regulate cell volume, increases in cytosolic calcium, and activation of phospholipases. Further metabolism of adenine nucleotides to purine breakdown products as well as release of free iron into the cytosol from ferroproteins facilitates one electron transfers and oxygen radical formation. These free radicals may lead to protein and lipid peroxidation and further membrane injury.

The net effect of these alterations may be to increase membrane permeability to calcium, which will accelerate the process. Because the mitochondrial calcium buffering competes with mitochondrial oxidative phosphorylation and ATP synthesis, ATP synthesis may be further impaired. During reflow, increases in calcium delivery to renal tissue, intracellular alkalinization, and a burst of respiratory activity may worsen cellular injury (Schieppati and Schrier, 1990; Schrier and Shapiro, 1985a). Lesser degrees of injury may be complicated by a loss of epithelial cell polarity, which may alter renal sodium handling (Molitoris et al., 1989a). However, more severe injury results in epithelial cell necrosis with cellular debris, tubular obstruction, and perhaps, backleak of glomerular filtrate, which maintain decreased GFR and ARF (Schrier and Conger, 1986).

In most experimental models of ischemic ATN, the major site of injury is the S3 segment of the proximal tubule (Venkatachalam et al., 1978). Brezis and coworkers (1984b) suggested that the more common form of renal ischemia encountered clinically is less complete, and that the thick ascending limb of Henle, which normally lives on the edge of anoxia, may be the segment at greatest risk. In experimental preparations, this segment clearly can show transport-related injury, which these workers believe may be operant in the development of clinical ischemic ATN (Brezis et al., 1984a, 1984b). Morphologic abnormalities of ATN in humans, however, occur primarily in the proximal tubule rather than the thick ascending limb of Henle.

The experimental manipulations with the best efficacy in ameliorating ischemic ATN are directed at these pathogenetic steps. Loop diuretics and osmotic diuretics, when given before the ischemic insult, appear to ameliorate experimental ischemic ATN (Burke et al., 1980, 1983; Patak et al., 1979). This effect may be due to increased tubular pressures and flows, which alleviate tubular obstruction, but some direct beneficial cellular effects may also be involved (Brezis et al., 1984a). Supplementation of the adenine nucleotide pool with ATP-$MgCl_2$ has been demonstrated to ameliorate ischemic ATN, even when given after the insult (Siegel et al., 1983). Diminished cytosolic calcium overload with calcium-channel blockers has also been found to be efficacious when these agents are administered before or after the ischemic insult (Burke et al., 1984; Shapiro et al., 1985). Administration of the hormone, atrial natriuretic factor (ANF), which may also have some calcium-channel blocking cellular effects, affords protection in experimental ARF (Nakamoto et al., 1987; Shaw et al., 1987). Administration of oxygen radical scavengers has also been effective in some models of ARF (Linas et al., 1987). Clinical trials using these agents are currently underway.

One of the more interesting observations made many years ago was that patients who died with ATN of prolonged duration were noted to have fresh ischemic lesions of the kidney on autopsy. Although reductions in renal plasma flow are not necessary to maintain the low GFR seen with ATN, recurrent ischemic insults may lead to a delay and possibly failure of recovery mechanisms. This finding led to experimental studies of the renal vasculature after an ischemic insult. Conger and colleagues (1989) demonstrated that autoregulation of blood flow is significantly impaired in experimental ARF. After an ischemic renal insult in experimental animals, modest reductions in systemic blood pressure are accompanied by major reductions in renal plasma flow. This renal ischemia with modest hypotension may be ameliorated by renal denervation. Of potential therapeutic significance is the observation that calcium-channel blockers may actually restore autoregulation of renal blood flow in this model (Conger et al., 1989).

From these experimental data, several clinical points seem clear. First, avoidance of renal ischemia is of paramount importance. In settings where renal ischemia is likely to be encountered, agents such as osmotic or loop diuretics should be used prophylactically to increase urinary solute excretion. Second, although the data is still not clear for calcium-channel blockers in all settings, reports suggest that they may be advantageous in the setting of cadaveric renal transplantation to prevent ischemic ATN (Wagner et al., 1988). Lastly, avoidance of even mild hypotension in the setting of ischemic ATN may be important in shortening the course of the renal failure. Our therapeutic approach to established ATN that cannot be managed conservatively may be altered by this approach (see following discussion). Certainly, further clinical studies regarding the use of pharmacologic agents to ameliorate ATN will be of value.

Approach to the Differential Diagnosis of Acute Renal Failure

As discussed, differentiation among causes of ARF is a key step in clinical management. This objective is accomplished primarily with a thorough history and physical examination, although laboratory evaluation, examination of the urine, and in some cases, imaging studies and invasive hemodynamic measurements are necessary.

The history source in ARF includes the hospital chart as well as the interview with the patient. A detailed history must include specific attention to possible hypotensive episodes, blood transfusions (especially with hemolytic reactions), intravenous radiocontrast administered during radiographic studies, and other medications received. The meticulous listing of medications is important to detect possible direct renal toxins, like cisplatinum, or possible causes of AIN, such as penicillin antibiotics.

Medications that are normally excreted by the kidney must have their dosage adjusted for the current level of renal function. In the intensive care unit (ICU) setting, it is quite common for a nephrology consultant to detect (1) continued administration of magnesium-containing antacids, which may cause magnesium intoxication; (2) cimetidine or other H$_2$ blockers at full dose, which may result in central nervous system (CNS) depression; and (3) nephrotoxic antibiotics, such as aminoglycosides, being given without appropriate dosage reduction.

The history is also useful in establishing how much weight the patient has gained or lost during the hospitalization or during the patient's experience outside the hospital. Rapid reductions in weight are most consistent with dehydration, whereas rapid increases in weight are seen with parenchymal ARF and urinary obstruction as well as heart failure, liver failure, and cirrhosis.

The physical examination helps one to evaluate the volume status of the patient. Examination of the neck veins to noninvasively estimate the central venous pressure, auscultation of the lungs and heart to evaluate for signs of heart failure, and examination of the extremities and presacral area to evaluate for edema are all important in directing the physician to the cause of ARF. Cutaneous evidence for vasculitis or other rashes may also provide important clues. Evaluating the bladder size by percussion after voiding may also provide an important clue to the cause of ARF.

It cannot be overstated how important dipstick evaluation and microscopic examination of the urine are in the differential diagnosis of ARF. Prerenal azotemia is usually associated with a concentrated urine, which has a relatively high specific gravity. Although some hyaline casts may be noted, few cellular components should be noted. Urinary obstruction may be associated with dilute or isotonic urine, which upon microscopy either appears completely benign or shows white blood cells or red blood cells if infection is superimposed.

ATN is usually associated with an isotonic urine. Microscopic examination of urine from a patient with ATN shows tubular-epithelial cells with coarsely granular casts (renal failure casts) and possibly tubular epithelial cell casts. AIN is usually accompanied by pyuria and white blood cell casts. White blood cell casts strongly suggest AIN, acute pyelonephritis, or acute glomerulonephritis. Acute glomerulonephritis typically is associated with high urine protein concentrations as well as hematuria and red blood cell casts. In the setting of oliguria, however, high urine concentrations of protein are rather nonspecific and may be observed with other types of ARF (Schrier and Conger, 1986).

Blood tests may be of some help in the differential diagnosis of ARF. As discussed previously, marked eosinophilia should suggest the possibility of AIN but may also occur with the cholesterol emboli syndrome. Other types of leukocytosis should suggest infection, possibly pyelonephritis, but are relatively nonspecific. Increases of blood urea nitrogen (BUN) levels out of proportion to increases in serum creatinine (Cr) levels so that BUN/serum Cr > 20 suggest prerenal azotemia, urinary obstruction, or increased rates of catabolism as seen with sepsis, burns, and patients receiving large doses of corticosteroids. The evaluation of renal sodium handling using urine chemistries may be particularly helpful.

In some settings, clinical evaluation of volume status using history, physical examination, and laboratory tests (see following discussion) is simply not adequate to differentiate among adequate and inadequate left ventricular filling pressures. In these settings, which are typically encountered in patients with severe liver, pulmonary, or cardiac disease, invasive measurements of cardiac output and left ventricular end diastolic pressure are necessary for optimal clinical management.

Imaging modalities may be necessary in the differential diagnosis of ARF. In transplant patients, renal scans that measure renal perfusion may help differentiate between rejection, which is usually associated with early decreases in renal perfusion, and ATN or cyclosporine toxicity, which shows less severe decreases in renal blood flow. HRS, with its marked renal vasoconstriction, should also be associated with marked reductions in renal blood flow. These perfusion studies may also be helpful in identifying acute renal arterial thrombosis or dissection. In nuclear studies that measure tubular secretion and GFR, all causes of ARF should show delayed excretion of these radioactive compounds. However, urinary obstruction may be associated with a characteristic sustained increase in counts derived from the kidney, reflecting marked delays in collecting system transit. Gallium scans may detect inflammation present with AIN or allograft rejection; however, these changes are relatively nonspecific.

Renal ultrasound has become extremely important in the evaluation of ARF. Dilatation of the collecting system detected by ultrasonography is a sensitive test for obstruction to urine flow. A 20 per cent false-positive incidence has been reported. With bilaterally small, shrunken kidneys, false-negative results may occur. With the use of Doppler techniques, ultrasound may also measure renal blood flow in different vessels within the kidney. Because this test is noninvasive, it is a very reasonable screening test to rule out urinary obstruction. Magnetic resonance imaging yields information similar to that from ultrasound with better anatomic definition; however, its increased cost negates this potential advantage. Experimental data, however, suggest that magnetic resonance spectroscopy using the P-31 nucleus may someday be useful in the differential diagnosis of ARF (Chan and Shapiro, 1987).

Radiocontrast studies, such as intravenous pyelogram (IVP), are rarely useful in the setting of ARF and may further complicate this condition with superimposed radiocontrast toxicity. However, for anatomic localization within the urinary tract, retrograde pyelography or antegrade pyelography from a percutaneous nephrostomy may be helpful.

Tests of Renal Sodium Handling

Our physiologic understanding of the different causes of ARF has led to the incorporation of tests of renal sodium handling into the clinical approach. With decreased renal perfusion pressure, tubular sodium and water reabsorption increases to preserve intravascular volume and to restore renal perfusion pressure. The result of this avid sodium reabsorption is a low urine concentration of sodium. The effect of the avid water reabsorption is to increase the urine osmolarity and the concentration of creatinine. In contrast, with ATN, both sodium and water reabsorption will be impaired. The relative clearance of sodium to the clearance of creatinine, i.e., the fraction excretion of sodium (FE_{Na}), is calculated as follows (Espinel, 1976):

$$FE_{Na} = (U_{Na}/P_{Na}) \times (P_{Cr}/U_{Cr}) \times 100$$
(expressed in per cent)

The renal failure index (RFI), which was proposed earlier (Handa and Madin, 1967), is calculated in a similar fashion, except the P_{Na} term is dropped and there is no multiplication by 100:

$$RFI = U_{Na} \times (P_{Cr}/U_{Cr})^*$$

The FE_{Na} and RFI are conceptually and quantitatively quite similar (Shapiro and Anderson, 1984).

Miller and colleagues (1978) observed that, in patients with ARF, a low FE_{Na} or RFI (<1) predicted prerenal azotemia quite well, especially in patients with oliguria. In comparison, other causes of ARF, especially ATN, were associated with a higher FE_{Na} or RFI (>2). These tests may be somewhat less useful in the setting of nonoliguria; however, an FE_{Na} or RFI > 2 is still suggestive of ATN, even when urine flow rates exceed 500 ml/day (Miller et al., 1978).

ATN secondary to radiocontrast or sepsis is typically associated with a low FE_{Na} and RFI, suggesting an important vascular component in its pathogenesis. Moreover, pigment nephropathy, i.e., ATN caused by rhabdomyolysis or hemolysis, may also be associated with a low FE_{Na} and RFI. Also, patients with early acute urinary tract obstruction, acute glomerulonephritis, and transplant allograft rejection may have a low FE_{Na} and RFI (Shapiro and Anderson, 1984). Conversely, patients with marked elevations in serum bicarbonate levels and resultant bicarbonaturia may have a relatively high FE_{Na} or RFI in the setting of prerenal azotemia, because sodium ions accompany the bicarbonate in the urine as obligate cations. Anderson and co-workers (1984) found that a fractional excretion of chloride (FE_{Cl}) less than 1 suggests prerenal azotemia in this setting.

*U_{Na}, urinary Na concentration; P_{Na}, plasma Na concentration; U_{Cr}, urinary Cr concentration; and P_{Cr}, plasma Cr concentration.

Conservative Approach to Acute Renal Failure

The first approach to ARF is to diagnose its cause. Therapy is, of course, directed toward the cause of ARF. Regarding the entity of ATN, prevention is the best therapy. Prevention of ARF may be accomplished by avoiding or minimizing insults that can cause ATN as discussed previously. Although more clinical work needs to be done in this area, some data support the prophylactic use of osmotic diuretics and calcium-channel blockers to avoid ARF in the settings of high-risk surgery, radiocontrast administration to high-risk individuals, and cadaveric renal transplantation (Old and Lehrener, 1980; Wagner et al., 1988).

In terms of therapy for established ATN, there is no proven therapy for improving renal function or shortening the course of ARF. About 15 years ago, Abel and co-workers (1973) reported that administration of "renal failure fluid," a combination of essential amino acids and dextrose, improved renal recovery and lessened the need for dialysis in patients with ARF. These results were extremely provocative but have simply not been confirmed in subsequent trials (Leonard et al., 1975). Therefore, at present, aggressive hyperalimentation cannot be recommended in the hope of improving renal recovery by nutritional mechanisms.

As already discussed, treatment with osmotic diuretics, such as mannitol; infusion of $ATP-MgCl_2$; calcium-channel blockers, such as verapamil, nifedipine, and diltiazem; and ANF has been shown to ameliorate established ARF in experimental models. Unfortunately, there are as yet no clinical trials that have established the utility of these agents, either alone or in combination, for treatment of established ARF. Such trials are currently being performed, and it is likely that, when the next edition of this text is printed, we will be able to make such recommendations. At the present time, therapy of ATN is directed at prophylaxis and treatment of the complications of ARF, which are summarized in Table 56–4.

Management of Fluid Disturbances

Patients with ATN may be oliguric. Such patients, if administered large volumes of intravenous fluids, as is

Table 56–4. COMPLICATIONS OF ACUTE RENAL FAILURE

Fluid overload	Uremic signs and symptoms
Electrolyte imbalance	*(Continued)*
Hyperkalemia	Cardiac
Hypermagnesemia	Pericarditis
Hyperphosphatemia	Uremic cardiomyopathy
Hypocalcemia	Pulmonary
Acidosis	Pleuritis
Uremic signs and symptoms	Uremic pneumonitis
Gastrointestinal	Hematologic
Nausea	Bleeding
Vomiting	Anemia
Neurologic	Immunologic
Mental status changes	Impaired granulocyte function
Seizures	Impaired lymphocyte function
Coma	
Peripheral neuropathy	

typical for hyperalimentation regimens, or if allowed free access to oral fluids are at risk for developing fluid overload. At the current time, data support the use of high doses of loop diuretics (1 to 3 g/day) to convert oliguric to nonoliguric ATN in some patients (Bailey et al., 1973; Cantarovich et al., 1970, 1971). It appears that patients who respond to such therapy have a lower FE_{Na} than patients who do not respond, suggesting that responders have less severe tubular injury (Anderson et al., 1977). Uncontrolled studies suggest that addition of dopamine in renal doses (2.5 μg/kg/minute) will increase the number of patients who respond to loop diuretics (Graziani et al., 1984; Lindner, 1983). Because patients with a reasonable urine output have less problems with hyperkalemia and volume overload and are, therefore, less likely to require dialysis therapy, we advocate such an approach.

It has not been established, however, that conversion of the patient from an oliguric state to a nonoliguric state decreases mortality or hastens renal recovery. Patients who remain oliguric following such therapy should either have their fluids limited to insensible losses and titrated to maintain an appropriate left ventricular filling pressure, or have early institution of nonconservative therapy (see following discussion).

If fluid overload in ARF presents an acute emergency, it must be remembered that nonconservative therapy, e.g., dialysis or continuous arteriovenous hemofiltration (CAVH), requires some finite time to be initiated. Valuable time may be gained by the administration of oxygen, venodilators, such as nitroglycerin, and arterial vasodilators to control hypertension while such nonconservative therapy is undergoing implementation. In such patients, loop diuretics may provide transient benefit by dilating veins and decreasing pulmonary congestion.

Careful attention to fluid intake must be maintained in patients with ARF, either oliguric or nonoliguric. Attempts should be made to maintain patients in a euvolemic state by restricting total fluids to no more than urine output plus insensible losses. If invasive monitoring is being used, the pulmonary capillary wedge pressure is the best guideline for volume status; however, it will be normal in states of noncardiogenic pulmonary edema.

Management of Electrolyte Disturbances

Patients with ARF, especially secondary to ATN, are prone to develop electrolyte abnormalities, such as acidosis, hyperkalemia, hypermagnesemia, hyperphosphatemia, and hypocalcemia. To some degree, these problems can be minimized by the prophylactic institution of a low-potassium, low-protein diet accompanied by fluid restriction and oral phosphate binders. Despite these precautions, electrolyte disturbances, especially in patients with oliguric ARF, are quite possible.

We discuss these abnormalities in some detail here; however, although refractory electrolyte disturbances and refractory fluid overload are indications for nonconservative therapy of ARF, the conservative maneuvers must not be overlooked. Even after it is decided to provide nonconservative therapy, these conservative maneuvers may provide valuable time, and, in fact, may be lifesaving while nonconservative therapy for these abnormalities is pending.

Hyperkalemia is probably the most common and most dangerous electrolyte abnormality seen with ARF. A serum potassium value greater than 6.0 mEq/L is an indication for performing an electrocardiogram (ECG), and subsequent therapy should be based on the ECG changes. With hyperkalemia, the earliest changes of the ECG consist of peaking of the T waves. This ECG finding is followed by a decrease in the amplitude of the P wave, various conduction disturbances, and finally, widening of the QRS complex. With severe hyperkalemia, the ECG tracing may resemble a sine wave.

We believe that any of the ECG alterations of hyperkalemia warrant some form of intravenous therapy for the patient. Calcium, administered as the chloride or gluconate salt, will ameliorate the effects of hyperkalemia on the cardiac electrical potential and provide valuable time for methods of potassium removal, such as hemodialysis, to be employed. Generally, one ampule of calcium chloride or two ampules of calcium gluconate (9.6 mEq of calcium) is administered in this setting and has immediate effects. This therapy does not affect the serum potassium concentration and is only effective for 20 to 30 minutes.

Intravenous insulin, administered with glucose to avoid hypoglycemia, causes a shift of potassium from the extracellular to intracellular compartment. Alkalinization with bicarbonate also causes such a shift. These approaches have a rapid onset of action but the effect persists for a relatively short period of time. Repeated doses of bicarbonate, either as boluses or as an infusion, will be accompanied by volume expansion, which may lead to fluid overload. Also, respiratory compensation for metabolic alkalosis may limit the effectiveness of bicarbonate therapy. Bicarbonate is therefore only recommended as an acute intervention to gain time. In contrast, an insulin infusion will continue to shift potassium into cells and may be useful over a prolonged period of time.

Administration of potassium-binding resins, such as sodium polystyrene sulfonate (Kayexalate; Winthrop-Breon, New York, NY), effectively removes potassium, but several hours are needed for the onset of action. Potassium-binding resins may be sufficient therapy alone when hyperkalemia is less severe and is not accompanied by ECG changes. However, this approach is simply not an adequate approach to hyperkalemia accompanied by ECG changes. In this setting, emergent therapy with intravenous calcium and/or insulin and bicarbonate, is appropriate. Hyperkalemia is a medical emergency, and although it may eventually mandate nonconservative therapy of ARF, every physician must know how to evaluate and treat this entity acutely while such therapy is being considered (Shapiro and Schrier, 1988).

Hyperphosphatemia almost always accompanies ARF. Although some experimental data suggest that it may worsen the course of ARF, this issue is controversial. Hyperphosphatemia is usually treated with oral phosphate binders, especially because clearance of phosphate with hemodialysis or peritoneal dialysis is limited.

Extremely severe hyperphosphatemia may be accompanied by symptomatic hypocalcemia, and as such, must be considered an indication for hemodialysis. Less severe hypocalcemia is usually best treated by oral phosphate binders, which control the serum phosphate level. Magnesium-containing antacids or cathartics should be avoided in ARF to avoid the risk of dangerous hypermagnesemia (Shapiro and Schrier, 1985).

Acidosis attributable to ARF does not generally constitute an emergency because it is relatively slow to develop and is accompanied by respiratory compensation. However, it is possible that acidosis in the patient with ARF is caused by another disturbance, such as lactic acidosis due to circulatory insufficiency, and in the setting of ARF, may rapidly become quite severe. This is a very difficult therapeutic situation. The acute infusion of sodium bicarbonate in the setting of lactic acidosis may, in fact, be deleterious to hemodynamic stability and is extremely controversial (Narrins and Cohen, 1987; Stacpoole, 1986).

Even if the physician elects to administer bicarbonate, it is possible that it will be difficult to administer a sufficient amount for correction of the acidosis without causing volume overload. Complicating this issue, nonconservative therapy, such as hemodialysis, may be difficult to institute because of circulatory instability. Because it has less hemodynamic effects, CAVH may be the best therapeutic intervention in this setting (Maguire and Anderson, 1986). When acidosis develops at a slower pace, it may be treated conservatively with oral or slow intravenous infusions of sodium bicarbonate, or it may be addressed by institution of nonconservative therapy.

Nonconservative Approach to Acute Renal Failure

Conservative therapy is often inadequate for the management of ARF due to ATN. Indications for nonconservative therapy include fluid and electrolyte disturbances that are refractory to conservative management, and the development of uremic signs and symptoms. The uremic signs and symptoms observed in ARF are summarized in Table 56–4. Nausea and vomiting, mental status changes, a bleeding tendency, and decreased ability to defend against infection are characteristic of ARF. Less commonly, pleural effusions, uremic pneumonitis, pericarditis (symptoms of pericarditis, development of a pericardial effusion, or an asymptomatic friction rub), and uremic seizures occur as complications of ARF. Uremia is discussed in greater detail in the section of this chapter devoted to chronic renal failure.

In addition to fluid and electrolyte abnormalities and signs and symptoms of uremia, it has become the standard of care to provide nonconservative therapy to maintain a BUN level less than 100 mg/dl and a serum creatinine level less than 10 mg/dl. The choice of nonconservative therapy is predicated on the experience of the physician and the medical center as much as on the relative advantages and disadvantages of the treatment modalities available. These aspects must be considered in the implementation of nonconservative treatment of uremia.

Basically, nonconservative therapies for ARF are limited to hemodialysis, peritoneal dialysis, and a relatively new technique, CAVH, and its modifications—slow, continuous hemodialysis (SCH) and continuous arteriovenous hemofiltration and hemodialysis (CAFHD). We discuss the relative merits and disadvantages of these techniques in the next section (Table 56–5).

Hemodialysis, Peritoneal Dialysis, and Continuous Arteriovenous Hemofiltration

The most widely employed method to treat ARF is hemodialysis. In this technique, blood is removed from the patient by a blood pump and sent to a dialyzer (i.e., artificial kidney) where it comes into close proximity with dialysate, which is separated by a semipermeable membrane. This contact with the dialysate allows the removal of solutes by the process of diffusion, which is driven by a concentration gradient from blood to dialysate. Fluid and some solute may also be removed by the process of ultrafiltration, which is driven by a pressure gradient across the dialyzer. The dialyzed blood is then returned to the patient.

To perform this procedure, access to the circulation is essential. Most commonly, a venous catheter is placed percutaneously into the subclavian or internal jugular vein, although, occasionally, femoral venous catheterization, and, rarely, placement of a Scribner arteriovenous shunt are performed. Hemodialysis allows for more rapid removal of fluid and solutes relative to peritoneal dialysis or CAVH.

Hemodialysis treatments, however, are quite stressful hemodynamically and may be complicated by hypotension, hypoxia, bleeding related to the anticoagulant administered (usually heparin) as well as the dialysis dysequilibrium syndrome with its manifestations ranging from cramps and headache to seizures and coma. Al-

Table 56–5. NONCONSERVATIVE APPROACHES TO ACUTE RENAL FAILURE

Modality	Advantages	Disadvantages
Hemodialysis	Rapid correction of electrolyte and fluid abnormalities	Expensive and hemodynamically stressful; anticoagulation necessary; vascular access necessary
Peritoneal dialysis	Inexpensive and hemodynamically well tolerated; no anticoagulation or vascular access needed	Relatively slow correction of fluid and electrolyte disturbances; may have associated leaks and infection
CAVH (or CAVHD)	Intermediate expense; moderately rapid correction of fluid overload	Need arterial vascular access and anticoagulation; less rapid correction of electrolyte abnormalities

Abbreviations: CAVH, continuous arteriovenous hemofiltration; CAVHD, continuous arteriovenous hemofiltration and hemodialysis.

though controversial, it is possible that recurrent hypotension suffered during the dialysis treatment for ARF may actually prolong the course of this disease. Clinical studies are underway to test this hypothesis. An additional drawback of hemodialysis is the expense of the procedure, which is related to the special equipment as well as the trained personnel required to perform the treatment (Schetz et al., 1989).

Hemodialysis treatments are generally instituted for the indications discussed previously, then continued until evidence for renal recovery is apparent. In a small prospective study, it was shown that intensive daily dialysis treatment was not superior to more conservative, every other day treatments (Conger, 1975). The dialysis prescription is generally tailored to maintain a BUN level less than 100 mg/dl while maintaining normal electrolyte, acid-base, and volume status and preventing uremic symptoms and signs (Schrier and Conger, 1986).

Peritoneal dialysis allows the removal of solutes using the peritoneal membrane as the dialyzer. It does not require access to the circulation, and, in general, is hemodynamically less stressful than hemodialysis. With this approach, dialysate is instilled into the peritoneal space by means of a percutaneously placed catheter, allowed to dwell for a period of time, and then removed with the uremic solutes, which have diffused across the peritoneal membrane. Ultrafiltration of fluid is performed using an osmotic pressure gradient induced by the addition of relatively high concentrations of glucose to the peritoneal dialysate. For noncatabolic ARF patients, peritoneal dialysis generally allows the physician to maintain fluid and electrolyte homeostasis as well as to prevent uremic symptoms and signs.

The peritoneal dialysis method offers relatively slower correction of electrolyte imbalance or fluid overload than hemodialysis. Therefore, it is best used before indications for dialysis are urgent. Although safe and generally well tolerated, the procedure may be complicated by peritonitis, leaking of peritoneal dialysate, and occasionally, hydrothorax. In general, peritoneal dialysis is best avoided following recent abdominal surgery. The major advantages of peritoneal dialysis are its relatively inexpensive nature, the absence of need for anticoagulants, and the absence of major hemodynamic stress. Disadvantages of this method are related to the relatively slow correction of fluid and electrolyte disturbances (Nolph, 1978).

CAVH was first reported by Kramer and co-workers (1977) in the late 1970s. This technique uses the patient's own blood pressure to send blood to a hemofilter where fluids and solutes are removed by ultrafiltration. The blood is then returned to the patient accompanied by replacement fluid. This replacement fluid must be sterile because it is instilled directly into the patient's vein. With good arterial and venous access, usually accomplished by cannulation of the femoral artery and vein, ultrafiltration rates of 10 to 12 ml/minute are achievable with this technique. If one applies suction on the ultrafiltration compartment, one can further increase the ultrafiltration rate. Perhaps more efficient is the administration of dialysate, driven by a pump, to allow dialysis to occur with ultrafiltration. Generally, dialysate is run at a rate of approximately 15 ml/minute, a process that

dramatically increases net solute removal. When combined with dialysis, this process is called CAVHD.

Other variants of this method are slow, continuous ultrafiltration (SCUF) and slow, continuous dialysis (SCD). Although CAVH and its variants are used infrequently, they offer some potential advantages over hemodialysis: hemodynamic stability is quite good, and expensive equipment and trained hemodialysis technicians are not necessary. CAVH is superior to peritoneal dialysis in the volume-overloaded patient because fluid may be more rapidly removed. The major disadvantages of CAVH and its variants are that arterial access is necessary and anticoagulation must be continuous (Maguire and Anderson, 1986).

Other Complications

Despite continued improvements in nonconservative therapy of ARF, mortality remains high. Because of the availability of dialysis and its alternatives as well as awareness of electrolyte and fluid disturbances and uremic symptomatology, patients generally die with rather than of ARF. Death in patients with ARF usually results from either uncontrolled hemorrhage or infection, and both of these complications may be due to the effects of uremia on the immune and coagulation systems. Specifically, bleeding disturbances associated with renal failure may be related to accumulation of nitrogenous wastes, such as phenols and guanidosuccinic acid, but the finding that best correlates with uremic bleeding is a deficiency of von Willebrand factor multimers. When dialysis does not adequately correct an abnormal bleeding time, administration of desmopressin acetate (DDAVP), which causes the release of von Willebrand factor multimers from endothelial cells, and infusion of cryoprecipitate, which contains these multimers, may be useful to acutely correct the bleeding time. If more prolonged therapy is necessary to correct a bleeding tendency, administration of conjugated estrogens appears to increase the synthesis and release of von Willebrand factor multimers. ARF is also associated with impaired immune responses and granulocyte function, factors that may contribute to the increased incidence of infections in ARF patients. Thus, despite the availability of dialytic therapy, ARF is still an extremely adverse condition, and all possible efforts to avoid ARF should be made (Schrier and Conger, 1986).

CHRONIC RENAL FAILURE

Definition and Clinical Description

In an analogous fashion to ARF, chronic renal failure (CRF) can be considered a chronic deterioration in renal functions, resulting in a buildup of nitrogenous wastes in the plasma and a failure of the kidney to regulate extracellular fluid volume or composition. CRF is differentiated from ARF by the time it takes to develop but also by its generally irreversible and, in fact, progressive nature.

CRF develops insidiously. Patients often do not know they have CRF until blood assays of BUN and serum creatinine are obtained, either as part of a routine chemical screen or as directed by complaints of fatigue, sleep disturbances, nausea and vomiting, or pruritus. Proteinuria or microscopic evidence of blood in the urine usually precedes development of CRF from most causes. The urinalysis, therefore, remains an important screening test for patients during periodic health evaluations. The military as well as insurance companies appreciate the relevance of proteinuria to subsequent morbidity and mortality.

Etiology

CRF may result from diseases involving the blood supply to the kidney, the urinary collecting system, and the parenchyma of the kidney. We review the most important of these diseases in the following discussion.

Parenchymal Renal Disease

Parenchymal causes of CRF can best be understood based on the pathologic features. Our ability to accurately assign a pathologic diagnosis has, in fact, dramatically improved in the past 20 years with the widespread availability of electron microscopy (EM) and immunofluorescence (IF) methods to complement standard light microscopy (LM). Renal diseases are often classified based on their histologic characteristics; however, this morphologic approach may, in fact, lump a number of pathogenetic processes together if the appearance of the tissue reaction to these processes is similar.

GLOMERULAR VERSUS TUBULOINTERSTITIAL RENAL DISEASE

It is useful to divide parenchymal diseases of the kidney into those that primarily affect the glomeruli and those that primarily involve the tubulointerstitial area of the kidney. However, the pathologic processes affect both glomeruli and tubules in virtually all forms of kidney disease. The amount of tubulointerstitial disease observed histologically, in general, correlates better with the functional derangement (i.e., decreased GFR) of the kidney than does the extent of pathologic glomerular changes.

Besides pathologic examination, the causes of CRF may often be differentiated as glomerular versus tubulointerstitial based on the degree of proteinuria. Generally, proteinuria exceeding 3.5 g/day (normalized per 1.73 m^2 body surface area) suggests glomerular disease, whereas more modest degrees of proteinuria (i.e., 1 to 2 g/day) suggest tubulointerstitial disease. Unfortunately, many milder cases of glomerular disease show modest degrees of proteinuria, and some forms of tubulointerstitial disease may show considerable degrees of proteinuria, particularly when complicated by glomerulosclerosis. In patients who are not candidates for renal biopsy, however, this approach to classification may be useful.

PRIMARY RENAL DISEASE

Primary renal diseases that cause CRF may be classified as glomerular and tubulointerstitial as discussed previously (Table 56–6). These histologic appearances may also be associated with systemic diseases involving the kidney.

Minimal change disease (MCD), also called nil disease, is a common cause of nephrotic syndrome. It most often affects children, although it has been reported in virtually all age groups. Commonly, the patient presents with nephrotic syndrome featuring massive proteinuria and anasarca. Hypertension is usually absent. Microscopic examination of the urine may demonstrate fat but, generally, neither red nor white blood cells are found. Histologic evaluation reveals essentially no changes on LM or IF, and only epithelial foot process fusion on EM.

The pathogenesis of nil disease is unknown, although alterations in cell-mediated immunity are believed to be involved. Nil disease frequently undergoes spontaneous remission and is often responsive to corticosteroid therapy. This disease almost never progresses to CRF (Glassock and Babcock, 1990). When progression to CRF does occur, it is likely that the disease process was actually focal and segmental glomerulosclerosis rather than nil disease.

Focal and segmental glomerulosclerosis (FSGS) is also a common cause of nephrotic syndrome, and in contrast to nil disease, often progresses to CRF. This disease typically affects older children and young adults, although it can occur at any age. Afflicted patients are typically nephrotic and may also be hypertensive. The histologic entity of FSGS has been associated with patients who abuse intravenous drugs as well as patients who have acquired immunodeficiency syndrome (AIDS). The pathologic evaluation of biopsy specimens from afflicted patients generally demonstrates focal and segmental scarring of glomeruli on LM and EM. IF may show IgM, IgG, and complement as well as fibrin in these scars. The pathogenesis of this disease is also

Table 56–6. MAJOR PRIMARY RENAL DISEASES THAT CAN CAUSE CHRONIC RENAL FAILURE

Classification	Progression to CRF
Glomerular	
Nil disease	Rare
Focal segmental glomerulosclerosis	Very common
Membranous glomerulopathy	Variable
Berger's disease	Uncommon
Poststreptococcal glomerulonephritis	Rare
Membranoproliferative glomerulonephritis	Common
Rapidly progressive glomerulonephritis	Very common
Chronic glomerulonephritis	Very common
Tubulointerstitial	
Autosomal dominant polycystic kidney	Very common
Juvenile polycystic kidney	Common
Medullary cystic disease	Rare
Reflux nephropathy	Variable
Analgesic nephropathy	Variable

Abbreviations: CRF, chronic renal failure.

poorly understood, although it is probably safe to say that it is not caused by immune complexes.

In animal models of CRF, reductions of renal mass may lead to this histologic appearance. Based on research with these models, a hemodynamic cause involving increases in glomerular capillary hydrostatic pressure (Brenner, 1985; Brenner et al., 1982). At the present time, there is no effective therapy for this disease, although it appears rational to treat any associated hypertension aggressively.

Membranous glomerulopathy (MGN) also usually appears with the nephrotic syndrome. MGN affects adults in middle age but can occur at any age. Microscopic examination of the urine may show fat and, often, also demonstrates microscopic hematuria. Generally, this disease either undergoes spontaneous remission or progresses to end-stage renal disease (ESRD). Massive proteinuria, presence of hypertension, impaired renal function on presentation, and male sex are all poor prognostic signs. The pathogenesis of MGN is believed to involve in situ formation of immune complexes.

Research with animal models has demonstrated the importance of complement and leukocytes in the expression of this disease. On LM, glomeruli are noted to have widened glomerular capillary loops without increased numbers of glomerular cells. On EM, dense deposits are observed in an epimembranous position, i.e., on the epithelial side of the basement membrane. Reaction to these deposits involving synthesis of new basement membrane adjacent to these deposits (spiking) or encircling these deposits may be noted. Using special LM stains (e.g., silver or trichrome), these deposits and the basement membrane reaction can be detected. IF will demonstrate IgG and complement staining in capillary loops in a "lumpy bumpy" pattern. Treatment of this entity with corticosteroids may be efficacious, although this issue is currently debated (Glassock and Babcock, 1990). An approach using alternate months of corticosteroids and cytotoxic agents has also been advocated (Ponticelli et al., 1984).

Focal proliferative glomerulonephritis (FPGN) features microscopic hematuria or recurrent episodes of gross hematuria. Urinalysis may demonstrate the presence of red blood cells (RBCs) and RBC casts. Typically, FPGN affects older children and adolescents. On LM, FPGN is characterized by predominantly mesangial proliferation and expansion. On IF, deposits of IgG, IgM and/or IgA, and complement are noted within the mesangium.

If the deposits are primarily IgA, the disease is called Berger's disease or IgA nephropathy. Berger's disease is closely related to the systemic vasculitis, Henoch-Schönlein purpura, which is discussed later. EM analysis of FPGN generally demonstrates electron-dense deposits within the mesangium. Marked proteinuria, hypertension, and renal insufficiency are ominous prognostic signs. If these features are absent, progression to CRF is uncommon. No known therapy definitely affects the natural history of Berger's disease. In extremely progressive cases, immunosuppression with corticosteroids or cytotoxic agents may be considered, although their efficacy is unproved. Some investigators believe that

anticoagulation may be beneficial; however, this approach is also unproved (Glassock and Babcock, 1990).

Acute glomerulonephritis (AGN) is a clinical diagnosis based on clinical features and urinary sediment findings. Patients present with dark urine, oliguria, and hypertension, and other evidence of circulatory overload, including edema in the legs and periorbital regions and, sometimes, pulmonary edema. Urinalysis by dipstick shows positive findings for hemoglobin and protein, and, on microscopy, RBCs and RBC casts as well as white blood cells (WBCs) and, occasionally, WBC casts may be found. This collection of findings is called the nephritic syndrome. Elevations in serum creatinine levels generally are part of the initial presentation.

Diffuse proliferative glomerulonephritis (DPGN) is the typical histologic appearance of renal disease that manifests with the acute nephritic syndrome. The most well characterized cause of AGN is a reaction to nephritogenic group A streptococci, hence, its synonym, poststreptococcal glomerulonephritis. DPGN usually occurs 2 to 4 weeks following skin infection. On examination of biopsy material in the acute phase, LM demonstrates swollen, congested glomeruli with proliferation and exudation. Cellular crescents may be present and, if extensive, may confer a more guarded prognosis. On IF, a "lumpy bumpy" distribution of IgM, IgG, and C3 is noted. In the acute stages of poststreptococcal DPGN, EM will demonstrate massive subepithelial deposits called "humps," which are composed of electron-dense material. During recovery, these subepithelial deposits are eliminated, and any remaining deposits tend to be mesangial in location.

No known therapy exists for DPGN. DPGN due to streptococcal disease progresses to CRF in a very small percentage of afflicted patients. Because of its good prognosis when left untreated, no therapy is usually advocated for poststreptococcal DPGN. However, because of the high frequency of poststreptococcal DPGN, it may be an important cause of ESRD.

Membranoproliferative glomerulonephritis (MPGN) most commonly occurs in children, but it can occur at any age. Patients present with a mixture of nephritic and nephrotic symptoms. This disease is really two diseases: MPGN type I, which is believed to be an immune complex disease; and MPGN type II, also called dense deposit disease (DDD), which is not believed to be caused by immune complex deposition. Type I and type II MPGN are both associated with reductions in the serum levels of complement component 3 (C3) as well as CH50, hence, the synonym, hypocomplementemic glomerulonephritis. In type I MPGN, parallel reductions in complement component 4 (C4) are usually found; in type II, C4 levels are usually normal. In patients with type II MPGN, evidence for alternate complement pathway activation is present. Both type I and type II MPGN are progressive diseases that gradually, but inexorably, progress to CRF in most patients.

On LM, both MPGN type I and type II show expansion of the mesangium, endocapillary and mesangial proliferation, and compression of capillary loops. Characteristically, deposition of new basement membrane material occurs around interpolating mesangial cells and mesangium and creates a "tram track" appearance on silver stain. Using IF, with type I disease, deposits that stain for IgG and complement are noted in a mesangial and subendothelial location and, rarely, in subepithelial and intramembranous locations. This latter appearance is called type III MPGN by some workers, although it is almost certainly a variant of typical type I MPGN. IF shows negative results with type II disease. For type I MPGN, EM demonstrates the immune complexes noted on IF. For type II MPGN, electron-dense deposits within the basement membrane of both glomeruli and tubules are noted. Although immunosuppression is of doubtful efficacy for MPGN, antiplatelet agents may be effective treatment for these diseases (Glassock and Babcock, 1990).

Rapidly progressive glomerulonephritis (RPGN) is another clinical syndrome characterized by a similar presentation as AGN but with progressive and inexorable development of CRF over weeks to months. The pathophysiology of this syndrome may be secondary to vasculitis, but it is also seen with anti–glomerular basement membrane (anti–GBM) antibody formation. When associated with pulmonary hemorrhage, anti–GBM antibody disease is called Goodpasture's syndrome. Renal biopsy of these patients will demonstrate a proliferative and exudative histopathology with numerous epithelial crescents on LM. EM will confirm these findings. IF will demonstrate linear deposition of IgG and C3 along the GBM. Prognosis in patients with anti–GBM antibody disease is related to their renal function on presentation as well as the number of crescents and chronicity of the changes noted on renal biopsy. Plasma exchange along with cytotoxic agents and corticosteroids is thought to be helpful in these patients (Kincaid-Smith, 1978).

Chronic glomerulonephritis (CGN) is a stage in the progression of renal diseases that involves a chronic scarring process of glomeruli. Unfortunately, patients who present with significant degrees of CRF will most often show this chronic scarring process on renal biopsy, which does not allow a diagnosis of the true underlying disorder. For this reason, renal biopsy is rarely performed in patients with bilaterally shrunken kidneys and significant degrees of CRF. Although CGN is the leading diagnosis of patients with CRF who develop ESRD, it is generally unclear which primary disease actually results in CGN in these patients.

Tubulointerstitial diseases that commonly cause CRF are summarized in Table 56–6. The most important causes are now discussed.

Polycystic kidney disease (PKD) is an important cause of CRF. PKD can occur as an adult-onset disease, which displays autosomal dominant genetics (ADPKD), or as juvenile-onset disease (JPKD), which is usually autosomal recessive. ADPKD is much more common that JPKD and typically presents in the 4th or 5th decade; however, considerable variability may exist. ADPKD is associated with a 50 to 70 per cent incidence of hypertension, which occurs at an early age and is related to activation of the renin-angiotensin-aldosterone system. Although no known therapy has been proven efficacious, some data suggest that aggressive control of blood pressure may slow the progression of this disease.

ADPKD is a systemic disease. Cystic involvement is not limited to the kidney but may also involve liver, pancreas, and spleen. In addition, cardiac malformations and cerebral berry aneurysms are associated with ADPKD.

JPKD usually presents in infants or small children. This disease is associated with hepatic fibrosis, which is often fatal. In addition to ADPKD and JPKD, other cystic diseases of the kidney occur; these include medullary cystic disease, which presents in adults and may progress to CRF, as well as medullary sponge kidney, a nondestructive hereditary cystic disorder of the renal papillary collecting ducts, which is often complicated by distal renal tubular acidosis and nephrocalcinosis but usually does not progress to CRF.

Reflux nephropathy or chronic pyelonephritis is another important tubulointerstitial cause of CRF. As discussed elsewhere in this text, reflux and associated parenchymal infections in childhood may be associated with progressive loss of renal parenchyma and may lead to CRF. Unfortunately, once substantial proteinuria is established, repair of the reflux does not appear to ameliorate the progression of CRF. The glomerular lesion of FSGS may be seen in association with reflux nephropathy and CRF.

Analgesic nephropathy may also lead to CRF; however, the incidence of this disease in the United States is debated. The absence of specific diagnostic criteria to define this entity makes it impossible to accurately estimate its incidence and prevalence. It appears that heavy use of phenacetin and aspirin in combination is most likely to cause analgesic nephropathy with associated papillary necrosis and CRF. Avoidance of further analgesic use is the only recommended therapy (Paller, 1990).

Metal intoxications with lead or cadmium may also lead to CRF. Balkan nephropathy, a rare tubulointerstitial form of renal disease of unknown etiology may also lead to CRF. The CRF associated with gout, so-called gouty nephropathy, may, in fact, be related to chronic lead intoxication rather than elevations in serum uric acid levels. CRF may, of course, complicate prolonged obstructive uropathy. Causes of urinary tract obstruction and the pathophysiology of this disease are discussed elsewhere in this text.

Chronic hypokalemia and hypercalcemia may rarely be associated with progressive tubulointerstitial nephritis and CRF. It is still debated if chronic lithium therapy is a direct cause of tubulointerstitial nephritis that leads to CRF (Paller, 1990).

SYSTEMIC DISEASES

Systemic diseases often affect the kidney. The most important systemic diseases that may cause CRF are listed in Table 56–7. Diabetes mellitus is rapidly becoming the most common cause of CRF in the United States. Patients with type I diabetes mellitus typically present with proteinuria after 10 to 15 years of diabetes, which is followed in 2 to 3 years by progressive renal insufficiency. However, only about 50 per cent of patients afflicted with type I diabetes develop kidney disease. Evidence suggests that patients with type I

Table 56–7. MAJOR SYSTEMIC DISEASES THAT MAY CAUSE CHRONIC RENAL FAILURE

Disease	Progression to CRF
Diabetes mellitus	Common
Systemic lupus erythematosus	Common
Vasculitis	
Henoch-Schönlein purpura	Uncommon
Polyarteritis nodosa	Common
Hypersensitivity angiitis	Variable
Wegener's granulomatosis	Common
Lymphomatoid granulomatosis	Variable
Sickle cell anemia	Common*
Multiple myeloma	Common
Amyloidosis	Common
Essential hypertension	Uncommon†

*If patients with sickle cell anemia live long enough (i.e., into 3rd decade), CRF is quite common.

†Although CRF is an uncommon complication of essential hypertension, episodes of accelerated hypertension may lead to CRF.

Abbreviation: CRF, chronic renal failure.

diabetes who develop kidney disease have microalbuminuria, i.e., albumin in the urine exceeding the normal range, detected with a sensitive radioimmunoassay (Shapiro and Schrier, 1988). The total urine protein concentration is still within normal limits, and GFR is supernormal in the first several years following the onset of diabetes.

Tight control of blood glucose levels does not appear to ameliorate the progression of the diabetic nephropathy to CRF once it is accompanied by overt proteinuria. Aggressive control of blood pressure, especially with agents that may decrease glomerular capillary pressure, such as CEI, may slow the rate of progression of renal failure. Clinical trials to test this hypothesis are currently underway. Although the progression of kidney disease in type II diabetes is less well understood than that in type I diabetes, it is likely that type II diabetes may ultimately be a more important cause of CRF than type I because of its greater prevalence. Specifically, 90 per cent of all diabetic patients have type II diabetes (Shapiro and Schrier, 1988).

Systemic lupus erythematosus (SLE) is another important systemic disease that affects the kidney. As for diabetes, approximately 50 per cent of patients with SLE will develop symptomatic renal disease. The renal manifestations of SLE are varied. In mesangial lupus nephropathy, renal function is usually normal, urinary abnormalities are minimal, and renal biopsy findings are limited to mesangial expansion and mesangial immune complex deposits.

In the most severe forms of lupus nephritis, where histology is either diffuse proliferative or membranoproliferative, renal function may be impaired, proteinuria is marked, and the renal sediment is extremely active. In this setting, the renal biopsy demonstrates cellular proliferation and exudation with immune complex deposits in subendothelial as well as mesangial locations. Other patients with lupus nephritis may demonstrate a histologic pattern of focal proliferative or membranous glomerulopathy and have a more benign clinical course than patients with diffuse proliferative or membranoproliferative lupus nephritis. Rarely, SLE will affect the kidney in a predominantly tubulointerstitial pattern.

The diagnosis of SLE is usually based on clinical and laboratory data, although renal biopsy may be useful in assessing prognosis and determining therapy. Corticosteroids and cytotoxic agents are useful in the management of SLE with renal involvement (Shapiro and Schrier, 1988).

A number of vasculitides affect the kidney. Many of these will have similar pathologic presentations to the primary renal diseases already discussed.

Henoch-Schönlein purpura is a leukocytoclastic vasculitis involving small arteries and venules, which manifests with lower intestinal bleeding, palpable purpura, and arthralgias in addition to renal manifestations of gross or microscopic hematuria, proteinuria, and occasionally, renal failure. On renal biopsy, mesangial IgA deposits are noted, suggesting a common link with Berger's disease. Progression to CRF is uncommon but does occur. No known therapy is effective.

Polyarteritis nodosa (PAN) in its classic or macroscopic form occurs in males in the 6th decade. Patients present with arthralgias, peripheral neuropathy, fever, and hemolytic anemia. Hypertension may be prominent and life threatening. PAN involves predominantly middle-sized muscular arteries. The classic form of this disease spares the pulmonary system and is not associated with eosinophilia; however, variants of PAN exist that may involve pulmonary manifestations, eosinophilia, or both. Liver involvement is frequent.

The diagnosis of PAN is based on clinical features and detection of microaneurysms of medium-sized arteries, usually in vessels supplying abdominal viscera. Renal involvement occurs in 80 to 90 per cent of afflicted patients and ranges from microscopic hematuria to rapid loss of renal function. The renal biopsy may demonstrate focal proliferative and necrotizing glomerulonephritis with crescent formation.

If disease is limited to the medium-sized muscular arteries, glomerular abnormalities may only include some focal collapse of glomeruli, indicating glomerular ischemia. This biopsy picture may, in fact, be difficult to differentiate from FSGS. Thus, the diagnosis of PAN is best made by clinical features and arteriographic evidence of microaneurysms in the splanchnic and renal circulations. Hepatitis B antigen is present in the serum of about 50 per cent of these patients, suggesting an immune complex etiology. PAN may cause progressive renal failure.

Hypersensitivity angiitis or microscopic PAN is a leukocytoclastic vasculitis, which involves arterioles and venules. Peripheral eosinophilia, urticaria, arthralgias, and fever are common symptoms. Renal manifestations may include proteinuria, microscopic or macroscopic hematuria, and RBC casts. Renal biopsy most often demonstrates FPGN. Rapid deterioration of renal function with extensive crescent formation on renal biopsy is generally treated with cytotoxic agents and corticosteroids. Plasmapheresis is used in some cases, although its use is not supported by controlled prospective studies.

Wegener's granulomatosis (WG) is another form of vasculitis that can cause CRF. WG is a granulomatous vasculitis that affects small arteries and venules predominantly in upper and lower airways and the kidney. The clinical presentation of WG often involves pulmonary infiltrates or sinusitis. Rarely, patients present with an active renal sediment or evidence of deteriorating renal function. Renal biopsy usually demonstrates a focal necrotizing glomerulonephritis. Crescent formation is not unusual, and if extensive, confers a poor prognosis. Treatment with cytotoxic agents and corticosteroids is often efficacious. Lymphomatoid granulomatosis is a rare form of vasculitis that has histologic similarities to WG. Many patients afflicted with lymphatoid granulomatosis eventually develop a lymphoproliferative disease.

Sickle cell anemia (SCA) is associated with several types of renal disease. Patients afflicted with either the heterozygous (trait) or the homozygous (disease) form of SCA develop progressive infarction of medullary renal tissue with age and concomitant renal concentrating and diluting defects. In patients with SCA, progressive renal insufficiency may develop later in life. Renal biopsy in such patients may demonstrate histologic evidence of FSGS, MGN, or MPGN.

Other Causes

Multiple myeloma may cause renal failure by a variety of mechanisms, including tubular precipitation of paraproteins, also called myeloma kidney; urinary obstruction secondary to uric acid or calcium-containing stones; hypercalcemia, which typically causes acute and reversible renal failure; and renal amyloidosis. Primary amyloidosis or amyloidosis secondary to inflammatory diseases may cause CRF. Ischemic nephropathy attributable to atherosclerosis or fibromuscular dysplasia of the renal arteries may also cause CRF. Therapy with surgical revascularization or angioplasty may sometimes salvage renal function.

Cholesterol emboli syndrome, which typically causes ARF, may also cause CRF. This syndrome usually occurs in the older patient with generalized atherosclerotic disease after an invasive procedure, such as aortic angiography. Fabry's disease, which is an inherited abnormality in lipid metabolism, may be complicated by renal disease and CRF. Alport's syndrome, also called hereditary nephritis, is a disorder of type IV collagen synthesis that obeys complex and varied genetic patterns in different affected families and is a fairly common form of kidney disease. Patients with Alport's syndrome are more often males and may develop deafness or ocular abnormalities. Cryoglobulinemia and other paraproteinemias may also be associated with CRF.

Numerous infections may be complicated by renal involvement. The leading cause of CRF worldwide is infection with *Schistosoma haematobium*, which causes strictures of the collecting system and obstructive uropathy. Many nonbacterial infections, including hepatitis B, *Schistosoma mansoni*, and malaria as well as more chronic bacterial infections, such as those observed with endocarditis, ventriculoperitoneal shunt infections, and deep-seeded abscesses, may be complicated by immune complex glomerulonephritis, which may progress to CRF. Treatment of the underlying infection is generally associated with improvement in renal function.

Pathogenetic Factors in the Progression of Chronic Renal Failure

It has been known for some time that chronic renal disease, once present, tends to be progressive in nature. Considerable interest in the progressive nature of renal disease has resulted in the following concepts.

Reduction of functional renal mass necessitates that the remaining nephron units "work harder" to maintain body fluid, electrolyte, and acid-base homeostasis. This idea has led to the formulation of the "surviving nephron hypothesis." Basically, this hypothesis proposes that these adaptive mechanisms, which allow the remaining nephrons to preserve the internal milieu, may ultimately be maladaptive for renal survival (Bricker, 1972).

In several experimental models of CRF, specifically the "5/6th nephrectomy" model, and in streptozocin-induced diabetes mellitus, glomerular capillary hydrostatic pressure and single-nephron GFRs have been shown to be elevated (Brenner, 1985). Reduction of the glomerular capillary hydrostatic pressure with a CEI as well as a low-protein diet ameliorates the progression of renal failure in these models (Anderson et al., 1976; Brenner et al., 1982). Our group has shown that maneuvers that reduce the increased metabolic rate of remaining tubular cells, including hypothyroidism, low-phosphate diet, and administration of calcium-channel blockers, may also ameliorate the rate of progression of CRF in experimental models (Harris et al., 1987, 1988; Jarusipipat et al., 1988; Karlinsky et al., 1980; Lumlertgul et al., 1986). Of interest, reductions of protein in the diet appear to attenuate tubular hypermetabolism as well as reduce glomerular capillary pressure (Jarusipipat et al., 1988). It is quite possible that glomerular and tubular mechanisms are synergistic in the progression of CRF. These concepts have been reviewed in some detail (Schrier et al., 1988).

Clinical Approach

Diagnostic Strategies

In the patient who presents with CRF, efforts should be made to assign a diagnosis of the primary disease. Knowledge of the primary disease, in fact, may have important implications regarding other complications that must be anticipated as considerations for possible transplantation. Careful review of the history, detailed physical examination, and directed laboratory investigations and imaging methods may yield a diagnosis. Differentiation of the disease entities into primary versus systemic and glomerular versus tubulointerstitial will narrow the differential diagnosis. If renal failure has not advanced to end stage and the kidneys are not small, renal biopsy may be undertaken in an effort to find a treatable form of kidney disease.

In all patients who present with CRF, efforts should be made to search for reversible insults to renal function. Virtually any cause of ARF may be applicable to patients with CRF. Moreover, patients with CRF are more sensitive to many of these insults. Specifically, patients with CRF are more sensitive to all forms of prerenal azotemia; to many causes of ATN, such as radiocontrast agent and aminoglycoside nephrotoxicity; and to urinary tract obstruction. Reversal of these acute insults may delay the need for renal replacement therapy, including chronic dialysis and transplantation.

Conservative Management

The conservative management of CRF includes avoidance of any additional insults to renal function, treatment of complications of CRF, and attempts to slow the progression of CRF. Specifically, in patients with CRF, prerenal azotemia from volume depletion and nephrotoxic drugs must be avoided.

Complications of CRF include the signs and symptoms of the uremic syndrome as well as acute fluid and electrolyte disorders. Electrolyte disturbances to which CRF patients are more susceptible include hyperkalemia, hyperphosphatemia, hypocalcemia, and hypermagnesemia. Metabolic acidosis may also result from CRF. Although many patients do not develop problems with hyperkalemia until CRF has reached end stage, some patients manifest difficulties in potassium homeostasis with relatively minor impairments in GFR. Most of these patients have what is referred to as a type 4 renal tubular acidosis and have difficulties in excreting a potassium load in the urine. This abnormality may result from a deficiency of aldosterone, which is common in diabetic patients, or from an inherent tubular defect seen commonly in patients with obstructive uropathy.

Other patients with CRF who are more susceptible to hyperkalemia include patients taking medications that impair potassium excretion or the shift of potassium into the intracellular compartment. Specifically, distal potassium-sparing diuretics, such as amiloride, triamterene, and spironolactone; beta-blockers; and CEIs cause hyperkalemia in CRF patients, and thus must be used with caution (Shapiro et al., 1990).

Hyperphosphatemia is the direct result of impaired renal phosphate excretion. Even with relatively mild CRF, phosphate homeostasis is preserved only at the expense of relatively high concentrations of parathyroid hormone (PTH). With more severe CRF, even extremely high concentrations of PTH cannot increase phosphate excretion enough to maintain serum phosphate levels in the normal range.

Because of increases in serum phosphate levels as well as impaired production of 1,25-dihydroxycholecalciferol with progressive kidney damage, serum calcium levels may fall. Calcium-containing phosphate binders, such as calcium carbonate, taken with meals may be used to treat the hyperphosphatemia of CRF. In patients who become hypercalcemic on such medications, aluminum hydroxide may be substituted. Administration of 1,25-dihydroxycholecalciferol is generally avoided in patients before beginning dialysis because of concerns about accelerating the progression of CRF.

Hypermagnesemia generally results from ingestion of magnesium-based antacids or magnesium-containing cathartics. These agents, therefore, should be avoided in all patients with significant renal impairment. The progressive metabolic acidosis that occurs with CRF may be exacerbated by hyperkalemia, which impairs ammoniagenesis (Halperin, 1989). Dietary protein restriction and administration of oral sodium bicarbonate may be effective in treating the metabolic acidosis, including the resultant complications of bone calcium and skeletal muscle wasting. Citrate, which is readily metabolized to bicarbonate, should be avoided in patients with significant CRF because it may increase aluminum absorption, especially if administered with aluminum-containing antacids, and thus accelerate the development of aluminum intoxication (Froment et al., 1989; Molitoris et al., 1989b).

Both clinical and basic science investigations are underway in an effort to develop approaches to slow the progression of CRF. Effective maneuvers in experimental animals include low-protein diet, low-phosphate diet, and control of blood pressure with CEIs and calcium-channel blockers. Whereas adherence to a very low protein diet is extremely difficult, the administration of calcium-containing phosphate binders to reduce phosphate intake and tight control of blood pressure with regimens containing a CEI, a calcium-channel blocker, or both, are not. Therefore, while awaiting the results of definitive clinical studies, we advocate the use of phosphate binders and tight blood pressure control in patients with CRF.

Complications of Chronic Renal Failure

In addition to the electrolyte disturbances that we have discussed, a large number of disturbances to normal bodily functions accompany CRF. Taken together, the symptoms of these dysfunctions are called the uremic syndrome. The major manifestations of uremia are summarized in Table 56–4. Virtually all organ systems of the body are involved.

Specifically, gastrointestinal function is disturbed with the development of nausea, vomiting, and occasionally, gastrointestinal bleeding. Neurologic abnormalities include peripheral neuropathy as well as mental status changes ranging from sleep and mood disturbances to seizures and coma. Hematopoietic function is impaired with decreased production of RBCs and decreases in RBC survival times combining to cause anemia. Blood clotting is abnormal with platelet dysfunction resulting from a deficiency of von Willebrand factor multimers and the presence of small molecules that impair platelet function.

Other features of the uremic syndrome include autonomic neuropathy, development of pericardial effusions, and hypertensive and uremic cardiomyopathies. Bone development and mineralization may be impaired by the presence of hyperparathyroidism, aluminum-associated osteomalacia, demineralization associated with acidosis, and deposition of beta$_2$-microglobulin in bone cysts. Beta$_2$-microglobulin deposition may also lead to compression of nerves as occurs with median nerve entrapment in carpal tunnel syndrome (Alfrey et al., 1968, 1989). As previously discussed, immune function is also impaired. Pruritus is extremely common in uremic patients and is attributable to PTH excess, increases in serum levels of phosphate, or dryness.

The pathogenesis of these uremic complications is still poorly understood. Three major theories have been proposed to describe the pathogenesis of uremic symptoms and signs: (1) small solute theory, (2) middle molecule theory, and (3) trade-off hypothesis. The small solute theory suggests that increases in small molecules, such as urea and creatinine, that arise from the breakdown of nitrogenous compounds produce the uremic syndrome. To date, however, no well-characterized small solute accounts for the majority of uremic signs and symptoms.

The middle molecule theory suggests that uremia is caused by molecules in a "middle range" of molecular weight, i.e., between 1000 and 10,000 daltons. However, no such "middle molecules" that cause the uremic syndrome have been found. Studies of the adequacy of dialysis have attempted to differentiate between the middle molecule and the small molecule theories. Although both theories have merit, operationally, smaller molecular weight solutes appear to be more important.

The trade-off hypothesis proposes that hormones which accumulate in supernormal plasma concentrations in CRF may maintain homeostasis of electrolytes and fluid balance; however, in these high concentrations, they are toxic to cellular and organ functions. At present, PTH is the most likely hormone that contributes to the uremic syndrome. All of these hypotheses have some merit, and the uremic syndrome is most likely multifactorial in its pathogenesis.

Clues to the pathogenesis of some features of uremia may emerge from the results of different therapies. Hemodialysis and peritoneal dialysis are both quite successful in improving gastrointestinal signs and symptoms, neurologic alterations, pericardial effusions, and hypertension. Peritoneal dialysis may be more successful in reversing peripheral neuropathy. Neither modality alone is successful in preventing uremic bone disease from aluminum toxicity or PTH excess or in normalizing the hematocrit in patients with CRF. The addition of phosphate binders, preferably those not containing aluminum hydroxide, the judicious use of 1,25-dihydroxycholecalciferol (Tzamaloukas, 1990), and the recent availability of erythropoietin (Eschbach and Adamson, 1988) dramatically improve the management of dialysis. Despite these quantitative improvements in dialytic therapy, renal transplantation is the preferred mode of renal replacement in appropriate candidates.

Dialysis and Transplantation

Indications

Development of uremic signs and symptoms should result in rapid institution of renal replacement therapy. Pericardial effusion may rapidly progress to life-threatening tamponade. Also, sensory neuropathy may rapidly progress to combined motor and sensory neuropathy. Motor neuropathy does not usually reverse with dialytic therapy; therefore, prevention is paramount (Raskin and Fishman, 1976a, 1976b).

Initiation of dialysis therapy or the performance of renal transplantation has been recommended at a stage before the development of uremic signs and symptoms. This practice is generally done when the creatinine clearance falls below 10 ml/minute, a state that usually corresponds to a BUN level greater than 100 mg/dl or a serum creatinine level greater than 10 mg/dl. However, we stress that, in patients on a low-protein diet and in patients who possess relatively little muscle mass, renal clearances of urea and creatinine will be much lower for any BUN or serum creatinine value.

Hemodialysis

Hemodialysis is the most widely employed modality for renal replacement. In contrast to the setting of ARF, vascular access in CRF is usually accomplished by an arteriovenous fistula or a Gortex graft placed surgically, employing the radial or ulnar artery and the cephalic vein. In situations where this form of access cannot be placed or has recently clotted, temporary access may be accomplished with a Shaldon catheter, which is placed percutaneously into the subclavian, internal jugular, or femoral vein, or a Scribner arteriovenous shunt, which is generally placed in the radial artery and cephalic vein.

Conventional hemodialysis treatment is usually performed with Cuprophane or cellulose acetate membranes with a surface area of approximately 1 m², blood flows of 250 ml/minute, and dialysate flows of 500 ml/minute. Dialysate composition may be acetate or bicarbonate based. With such therapy, the dialysis prescription is generally for about 4 hours, three times per week. More efficient hemodialysis using larger surface area (1.5 to 2.0 m²) Cuprophane or cellulose acetate dialyzers or using standard-sized dialyzers made of very porous material (polysulfone or polyacrylynitrile) with relatively high blood flow rates (350 to 500 ml/minute) and faster dialysate flow rates (600 to 750 ml/minute) has been employed in an effort to shorten the hemodialysis treatment time.

Generally, shorter dialysis times are prescribed based on the dialyzer clearance for urea, normalized for the patient's lean body mass. Such prescription dialysis based on urea kinetics has not been studied with long-term clinical investigation, but it is preferable to simply shortening dialysis times in a random manner (Tolchin et al., 1978). Because of the importance of dietary factors along with dialyzer clearance of urea in determining the predialysis BUN level, the predialysis BUN level cannot be used by itself for prescription dialysis (Shapiro et al., 1983).

Water used to mix with dialysate must be purified with either reverse osmosis or deionization methods to avoid intoxication with copper, nickel, or aluminum (Simon, 1989). Most dialysis units prescribe phosphate binders to normalize the serum phosphate level. Calcium carbonate is the preferred phosphate binder; however, some patients become hypercalcemic with this agent and, thus, must receive aluminum hydroxide to normalize serum phosphate concentrations. 1,25-Dihydroxycholecalciferol is used with many dialysis units to reduce parathyroid hyperactivity and to normalize serum calcium levels. Erythropoietin has been used in most dialysis patients to improve hematocrit to 30–35 per cent (Adamson and Eschbach, 1989; Eschbach and Adamson, 1988).

Although hemodialysis methods have been improved, and life expectancies on hemodialysis may exceed 10 to 15 years, the quality of life for the patient on hemodialysis tends to be suboptimal, primarily because of the time commitment, generalized malaise, beta$_2$-microglobulin deposition, and uremic bone disease. Vascular access infections, clotting, and other complications occur in patients on hemodialysis. The development of erythropoietin therapy and the use of porous kidneys, which may prevent beta$_2$-microglobulin accumulation and shorten dialysis times, may result in better patient satisfaction with hemodialysis.

Peritoneal Dialysis

Peritoneal dialysis is less widely used as long-term therapy in the United States than hemodialysis; however, because of its reduced cost, it is popular in many other places, particularly developing countries. With this modality, access is generally accomplished with a Tenkoff catheter placed either surgically or percutaneously into the midline of the abdomen into the right or left posterior aspect of the peritoneum. The external end is tunneled subcutaneously to exit in the lateral aspect of the lower abdomen. Sterile dialysate is infused into the abdomen, allowed to dwell, and then drained at prescribed intervals. When these intervals are evenly spaced throughout the day, this technique is known as chronic ambulatory peritoneal dialysis (CAPD). When most exchanges occur at night, with a machine performing the procedure, it is called chronic cycling peritoneal dialysis (CCPD) (Nolph, 1978).

Dialysis prescription in peritoneal dialysis is also based on solute clearance. In terms of dialysis effectiveness, peritoneal dialysis clears smaller molecules slightly poorer than does hemodialysis, but larger or middle molecules are cleared somewhat better. A peritoneal dialysis clearance of creatinine in excess of 40 liters per week is generally considered acceptable therapy. Avoidance of uremic symptoms is generally accomplished with such a clearance. Failure to achieve adequate clearance of creatinine may be due to either extremely high or low permeability of the peritoneal membrane to small solutes. If permeability is low, larger exchanges with longer dwell times may be effective in improving clearances. If permeability is too high, shorter and more rapid exchanges may be efficacious. Failure to remove fluid with hydro-osmotic gradients induced by glucose in the dialysate is generally due to high peritoneal permeability or to excessive lymphatic reabsorption of peritoneal fluid. Both of these conditions are best addressed by shorter, more frequent exchanges (Penzotti and Mattocks, 1971).

Peritoneal dialysis is generally effective and well tolerated, and it is less expensive than hemodialysis. Negative aspects of this therapy are the relatively high rates of peritonitis (approximately one episode every 1 to 2 years per patient), the ongoing protein losses in the dialysate (as much as 10 to 20 g per day), and the considerable responsibility that patients must assume for their own care. Bone disease and anemia are treated in a similar fashion as in hemodialysis patients. Although peritoneal dialysis has some advantages over hemodialysis, in general, patient satisfaction is low with this method. The conversion from peritoneal dialysis to hemodialysis is quite common in patients.

Renal Transplantation

Renal transplantation is the preferred mode of renal replacement for most patients. Absolute contraindications to a renal transplant are limited to documented failure to comply with therapy, and critical coronary or cerebral arterial lesions not amenable to therapy. Virtually all other patients on hemodialysis or peritoneal dialysis or patients with CRF about to require such therapy should be considered for renal transplantation. The surgical and medical aspects of renal transplantation are discussed in detail elsewhere in this text.

REFERENCES

Abel, R. M., Beck, C. H., Abbott, W. M., Ryan, J. A., Barnett, G. O., and Fischer, J. E.: Improved survival from acute renal failure after treatment with intravenous essential L-aminoacids and glucose. N. Engl. J. Med., 288:695, 1973.

Adamson, J. W., and Eschbach, J. W.: Management of the anemia of chronic renal failure with recombinant erythropoietin. Q. J. Med., 73:1093, 1989.

Alfrey, A. C., Froment, D. H., and Hammond, W. S.: Beta$_2$-microglobulin amyloidosis. Am. Kidney Found. Nephrol. Lett., 6:1, 1989.

Alfrey, A. C., Jenkins, D., and Groth, C. G.: Resolution of hyperparathyroidism, renal osteodystrophy and metastatic calcification with transplantation. N. Engl. J. Med., 279:1358, 1968.

Anderson, R. J., Gabow, P. A., and Gross, P. A.: Urinary chloride concentration in acute renal failure. Miner. Electrolyte Metab., 10:92, 1984.

Anderson, R. J., Linas, S. L., Berns, A. S., et al.: Nonoliguric acute renal failure. N. Engl. J. Med., 296:1134, 1977.

Anderson, S., Rennke, H. G., and Brenner, B. M.: Therapeutic advantage of converting enzyme inhibitors in arresting progressive renal disease associated with systemic hypertension in the rat. J. Clin. Invest., 77:612, 1986.

Appel, B. B.: Aminoglycoside nephrotoxicity. Am. J. Med., 159:427, 1990.

Arroyo, V., Bernadi, M., Epstein, M., Henriksen, J. H., Schrier, R. W., and Rodes, J.: Pathophysiology of ascites and functional renal failure in cirrhosis. J. Hepatol., 6:239, 1988.

Bailey, R. R., Natale, R., Turnbull, I., and Linton, A. L.: Protective effect of furosemide in acute tubular necrosis and acute renal failure. Clin. Sci. Mol. Med., 45:1, 1973.

Bakris, G. L., and Kern, S. R.: Renal dysfunction resulting from NSAIDs. Am. Fam. Physician, 40:199, 1989.

Ballard, H. S., Eisinger, R. P., and Gallo, G.: Renal manifestations of the Henoch Schoenlein syndrome in adults. Am. J. Med., 49:328, 1970.

Bennett, W. M., and Pulliam, J. P.: Cyclosporine nephrotoxicity. Ann. Intern. Med., 305:267, 1983.

Brenner, B. M.: Nephron adaptation to renal injury of ablation. Am. J. Physiol., 249:F324, 1985.

Brenner, B. M., Dworkin, L. D., and Ichikawa, I.: Glomerular filtration. In Brenner, B. M., and Rector, F. C. (Eds.): The Kidney. Philadelphia, W. B. Saunders Co., 1986, p. 93.

Brenner, B. M., Meyer, T. W., and Hostetter, T. H.: Dietary protein intake and the progressive nature of renal disease: The role of hemodynamically-mediated injury in the pathogenesis of progressive glomerulosclerosis in aging, renal ablation and intrinsic renal disease. N. Engl. J. Med., 303:652, 1982.

Brezis, M., Rosen, S., Silva, P., and Epstein, F. H.: Transport activity modifies thick ascending limb damage in the isolated perfused kidney. Kidney Int., 25:65, 1984a.

Brezis, M., Rosen, S., Silva, P., and Epstein, F. H.: Renal ischemia: A new perspective. Kidney Int., 26:375, 1984b.

Bricker, N. S.: On the pathogenesis of the uremic state: An exposition of the "trade-off." N. Engl. J. Med., 286:109, 1972.

Burke, T. J., Arnold, P. E., Gordon, J. A., Bulger, R. E., Dobyan, D. C., and Schrier, R. W.: Protective effect of intrarenal calcium membrane blockers before or after ischemia. J. Clin. Invest., 74:1830, 1984.

Burke, T. J., Arnold, P. E., and Schrier, R. W.: Prevention of ischemic acute renal failure with impermeant solutes. Am. J. Physiol., 244:F646, 1983.

Burke, T. J., Cronin, R. E., Duchin, K. L., Peterson, L. N., and Schrier, R. W.: Ischemia and tubule obstruction during acute renal failure in dogs: Mannitol in protection. Am. J. Physiol., 238:F305, 1980.

Cantarovich, F., Galli, C., Benedetti, L., et al.: High dose furosemide in established acute renal failure. Br. Med. J., 4:449, 1970.

Cantarovich, F., Locatelli, A., Fernandez, J. C., Loredo, J. P., and Cristhot, J.: Furosemide in high doses in the treatment of acute renal failure. Postgrad. Med. J., 47:13, 1971.

Chan, L., and Shapiro, J. I.: NMR in the investigation and differential diagnosis of acute renal failure. Ann. NY Acad. Sci., 508:420, 1987.

Conger, J. D.: A controlled evaluation of prophylactic dialysis in post-traumatic acute renal failure. J. Trauma, 15:1056, 1975.

Conger, J. D., Robinette, J. B., and Schrier, R. W.: Smooth muscle calcium and endothelium-derived relaxing factor in the abnormal vascular responses of acute renal failure. J. Clin. Invest., 82:532, 1989.

Eschbach, J. W., and Adamson, J. W.: Recombinant human erythropoietin: Implications for nephrology. Am. J. Kidney Dis., 11:203, 1988.

Espinel, C. H.: The FENa test. JAMA, 236:579, 1976.

Froment, D. P. H., Molitoris, B. A., Buddington, B., Miller, N., and Alfrey, A. C.: Site and mechanism of enhanced gastrointestinal absorption of aluminum by citrate. Kidney Int., 36:978, 1989.

Gagnon, J. A., Schrier, R. W., Weis, T. P., Kokotis, W., and Mailloux, L. U.: Clearance of iothalamate-I-125 as a measure of glomerular filtration rate in the dog. J. Appl. Physiol., 30:774, 1971.

Glassock, R., and Babcock, S.: Glomerular diseases of the kidney. In Schrier, R. W. (Ed.): Renal and Electrolyte Disorders. Boston, Little, Brown & Co., 1990.

Graziani, G., Cantaluppi, A., Casati, S., et al.: Dopamine and furosemide in oliguric acute renal failure. Nephron, 37:39, 1984.

Halperin, M. L.: How much new bicarbonate is formed in the distal nephron in the process of net acid excretion. Kidney Int., 35:1277, 1989.

Handa, S. P., and Madin, P. A.: Diagnostic indices in acute renal failure. Can. Med. Assoc. J., 96:78, 1967.

Harris, D. C. H., Chan, L., and Schrier, R. W.: Remnant kidney hypermetabolism and the progression of chronic renal failure. Am. J. Physiol., 23:F267, 1988.

Harris, D. C. H., Hammond, W. S., Burke, T. J., and Schrier, R. W.: Verapamil protects against progression of experimental chronic renal failure. Kidney Int., 33:41, 1987.

Hecht, B., Siegel, N., Adler, M., Kashgarian, M., and Hayslett, J. P.: Prognostic indices in lupus nephritis. Medicine, 55:163, 1976.

Hou, S. H., Bushinsky, D. A., Wish, J. B., Cohen, J. J., and Harrington, J. T.: Hospital acquired renal insufficiency: A prospective study. Am. J. Med., 74:243, 1983.

Jarusipipat, C., Shapiro, J. I., Schrier, R. W., and Chan, L.: Reduction of remnant kidney hypermetabolism by protein restriction: A survival, perfusion and P-31 NMR study to examine the potential protective mechanism in chronic renal failure. Clin. Res., 36:520A, 1988.

Karlinsky, M. L., Haut, L., Buddington, B., Schrier, N. A., and Alfrey, A. C.: Preservation of renal function in experimental glomerulonephritis. Kidney Int., 17:293, 1980.

Kelleher, S. P., and Berl, T.: Acute renal failure in pregnancy. Semin. Nephrol., 1:61, 1981.

Kincaid-Smith, P.: Plasmapheresis in rapidly progressive glomerulonephritis. Am. J. Med., 65:564, 1978.

Kramer, P., Wigger, W., Reiger, J., et al.: Arteriovenous hemofiltration: A new and simple method for treatment of overhydrated patients resistent to diuretics. Klin. Wochenschr., 55:1121, 1977.

Leonard, C. D., Luke, R. G., and Siegel, R. R.: Parenteral essential amino acids in acute renal failure. Urology, 6:154, 1975.

Levinsky, N. G.: Pathophysiology of acute renal failure. N. Engl. J. Med., 296:1453, 1977.

Linas, S. L., Whittenberg, D., and Repine, J. E.: O_2 metabolites cause reperfusion injury after short but not prolonged renal ischemia. Am. J. Physiol., 253:F685, 1987.

Lindner, A.: Synergism of dopamine and furosemide in diuretic-resistant oliguric acute renal failure. Nephron, 33:121, 1983.

Losito, A., Fortunati, F., Zampi, I., and Del-Favero, A.: Impaired renal functional reserve and albuminuria in essential hypertension. Br. Med. J. Clin. Res., 296:1562, 1988.

Lumlertgul, D., Burke, T. J., Gillum, D. M., et al.: Phosphate depletion arrests progression of chronic renal failure independent of protein intake. Kidney Int., 29:658, 1986.

Maguire, W. C., and Anderson, R. J.: Continuous arteriovenous hemofiltration in the intensive care unit. J. Crit. Care, 1:54, 1986.

Martinez-Maldonado, M., Yium, J., Suki, W. N., and Eknoyan, G.: Renal complications in multiple myeloma: Pathophysiology and some aspects of clinical management. J. Chronic Dis., 24:221, 1971.

Miller, T. R., Anderson, R. J., Linas, S. L., et al.: Urinary diagnostic indices in acute renal failure. Ann. Intern. Med., 89:47, 1978.

Molitoris, B. A., Chan, L., Shapiro, J. I., Conger, J. D., and Falk, S. A.: Loss of epithelial polarity: A novel hypothesis for reduced proximal tubule Na^+ transport following ischemic injury. J. Membr. Biol., 107:119, 1989a.

Molitoris, B. A., Froment, D. H., Mackenzie, T. A., Huffer, W. H., and Alfrey, A. C.: Citrate: A major factor in the toxicity of orally administered aluminum compounds. Kidney Int., 36:949, 1989b.

Morris, P. J.: Renal transplantation: Current status. In Robinson, R. R. (Ed.): Organ Transplantation. New York, Springer-Verlag, 1986, p. 1627.

Nakamoto, M., Shapiro, J. I., Chan, L., and Schrier, R. W.: The in vitro and in vivo protective effect of atriopeptin III in ischemic acute renal failure in the rat. J. Clin. Invest., 80:698, 1987.

Narrins, R. G., and Cohen, J. J.: Bicarbonate therapy for organic acidosis: The case for its continued use. Ann. Intern. Med., 106:615, 1987.

Neilson, E. G.: Pathogenesis and therapy of interstitial nephritis. Kidney Int., 35:1257, 1989.

Nolan, C. R., Anger, M. S., and Kelleher, S. P.: Eosinophiluria—a new method of detection and definition of the clinical spectrum. N. Engl. J. Med., 315:1516, 1986.

Nolan, C. R., and Kelleher, S. P.: Eosinophiluria. Clin. Lab. Med., 8:555, 1988.

Nolph, K. D.: Peritoneal dialysis. In Drukker, W., Parsons, F. M., and Maher, J. F. (Eds.): Replacement of Renal Function by Dialysis. Boston, Martinus Nijhoff Publishers (Kluwer), 1978, p. 2770.

Notghi, A., and Anderton, J. L.: Effect of nifedipine and mefruside on renal reserve in hypertensive patients. Postgrad. Med. J., 64:856, 1988.

Old, C. W., and Lehrener, L. M.: Prevention of radiocontrast-induced acute renal failure with mannitol. Lancet, 1:885, 1980.

Paller, M. S.: Drug-induced nephropathies. Med. Clin. North Am., 74:909, 1990.

Patak, R. V., Fadem, S. Z., Lifschitz, M. D., and Stein, J. H.: Study of factors which modify the development of norepinephrine-induced acute renal failure in the dog. Kidney Int., 15:227, 1979.

Penzotti, S. C., and Mattocks, A. M.: Effects of dwell time, volume of dialysis fluid and added accelerators on peritoneal dialysis of urea. J. Pharm. Sci., 60:1520, 1971.

Ponticelli, C., Zucchelli, P., Imbarciati, E., et al.: Controlled trial of methylprednisolone and chlorambucil in idiopathic membranous nephropathy. N. Engl. J. Med., 310:946, 1984.

Porile, J. L., Bakris, G. L., and Garella, S.: Acute interstitial nephritis with glomerulopathy due to nonsteroidal anti-inflammatory agents: A review of its clinical spectrum and effects of steroid therapy. J. Clin. Pharmacol., 30:468, 1990.

Raskin, N. H., and Fishman, R. A.: Neurologic disorders in renal failure (Part 1 of 2). N. Engl. J. Med., 294:143, 1976a.

Raskin, N. H., and Fishman, R. A.: Neurological disorders in renal failure (Part 2 of 2). N. Engl. J. Med., 294:204, 1976b.

Rasmussen, H. H., and Ibels, L. S.: Acute renal failure: Multivariate analysis of causes and risk factors. Am. J. Med., 73:211, 1982.

Roubenoff, R., Drew, H., Moyer, M., Petri, M., Whiting, O. K. Q., and Hellmann, D. B.: Oral cimetidine improves the accuracy and precision of creatinine clearance in lupus nephritis. Ann. Intern. Med., 113:501, 1990.

Schetz, M., Lauwers, P. M., and Ferdinande, P.: Extracorporeal treatment of acute renal failure in the intensive care unit: A critical view. Intensive Care Med., 15:349, 1989.

Schieppati, A., and Schrier, R. W.: Cellular calcium in the pathogenesis of ischemic acute renal failure. Contrib. Nephrol., 77:123, 1990.

Schrier, R. W., and Conger, J. D.: Acute renal failure: Pathogenesis, diagnosis, and management. *In* Schrier, R. W. (Ed.): Renal and Electrolyte Disorders. Boston, Little, Brown & Co., 1986, p. 423.

Schrier, R. W., Harris, D. C. H., Shapiro, J. I., Chan, L., and Carmelo, C.: Tubular hypermetabolism as a factor in the progression of chronic renal failure. Am. J. Kidney Dis., 12:243, 1988.

Schrier, R. W., and Shapiro, J. I.: Cellular events in ischemic acute renal failure. *In* Serono Symposium on Acute Renal Failure. New York, Raven Press, 1985a, p. 22.

Schrier, R. W., and Shapiro, J. I.: Drug-induced acute renal failure. *In* Serono Symposium on Acute Renal Failure. New York, Raven Press, 1985b, p. 242.

Shapiro, J. I., and Anderson, R. J.: Urinary diagnostic indices in acute renal failure. Am. Kidney Found. Nephrol. Lett., 1:13, 1984.

Shapiro, J. I., Argy, W., Rakowski, T., Chester, A., Siemens, A., and Schreiner, G. E.: The unsuitability of BUN as a criterion for prescription dialysis. Trans. Am. Soc. Art. Intern. Org., 29:129, 1983.

Shapiro, J. I., Cheung, C., Itabashi, A., Chan, L., and Schrier, R. W.: The protective effect of verapamil on renal function after warm and cold ischemia in the isolated perfused rat kidney. Transplantation, 40:596, 1985.

Shapiro, J. I., Mathew, A., Whalen, M., et al.: Different effects of sodium bicarbonate and an alternate buffer [Carbicarb] in normal volunteers. J. Crit. Care, 1990. In press.

Shapiro, J. I., and Schrier, R. W.: Clinical aspects of acute renal failure. *In* Serono Symposium on Acute Renal Failure. New York, Raven Press, 1985, p. 45.

Shapiro, J. I., and Schrier, R. W.: Renal and electrolyte disorders. *In* Schrier, R. W. (Ed.): Clinical Internal Medicine. Boston/Toronto, Little, Brown & Co., 1988, p. 125.

Shaw, S. G., Weidmann, P., Holder, J., Zimmerman, A., and Paternostro, A.: Atrial natriuretic peptide protects against acute ischemic renal failure in the rat. J. Clin. Invest., 80:1232, 1987.

Siegel, N. J., Avison, M. J., Reilly, H. F., Alger, J. R., and Shulman, R. G.: Enhanced recovery of renal ATP with post ischemic infusion of ATP-MgCl₂ determined by P-31 NMR. Am. J. Physiol., 245:F530, 1983.

Simon, P.: Evolution of dialytic therapy. Contrib. Nephrol., 71:10, 1989.

Stacpoole, D. W.: Lactic acidosis: The case against bicarbonate therapy. Ann. Intern. Med., 105:276, 1986.

Stott, R. B., Cameron, J. S., Ogg, C. S., Bewick, M.: Why the persistently high mortality in acute renal failure. Lancet, 2:75, 1972.

Swann, R. C., and Merrill, J. P.: The clinical course of acute renal failure. Medicine, 32:215, 1953.

ter-Wee, P. M., van-Ballegooie, E., Rosman, J. B., Meijer, S., and Donker, A. J.: Renal reserve filtration capacity in patients with type 1 (insulin-dependent) diabetes mellitus. Nephrol. Dial. Transplant., 2:504, 1987.

Tolchin, N., Roberts, J. L., Hayashi, J., and Lewis, E. J.: Metabolic consequences of high mass-transfer hemodialysis. Kidney Int., 11:366, 1978.

Tzamaloukas, A. H.: Diagnosis and management of bone disorders in chronic renal failure and dialyzer patients. Med. Clin. North Am., 74:961, 1990.

Venkatachalam, M. A., Bernard, D. B., Donohoe, J. F., and Levinsky, N. G.: Ischemic damage and repair in the rat proximal tubule: Differences among the S1, S2 and S3 segments. Kidney Int., 14:31, 1978.

von-Herrath, D., Saupe, J., Hirschberg, R., Rottka, H., Schaefer, K.: Glomerular filtration rate in response to an acute protein load. Blood Purif., 6:264, 1988.

Wagner, K., Albrecht, S., Neumayer, H. H.: Prevention of delayed graft function in cadaveric kidney transplantation by a calcium antagonist: Preliminary results of two prospective randomized trials. Transplant. Proc., 18:510, 1988.

57
OTHER RENAL DISEASES OF UROLOGIC SIGNIFICANCE

Anthony J. Schaeffer, M.D.
Francesco Del Greco, M.D.

Urologists are frequently asked to see patients whose presenting symptoms or signs may be expressions of renal rather than urologic disorders. It is therefore imperative that urologists be familiar with those primary renal diseases that they will frequently treat in daily practice. Although the clinical presentation of primary renal disease may include hematuria, flank pain, or polyuria, the majority of patients have no obvious symptoms and signs, and the underlying pathology will be revealed by routine screening of urine, blood pressure, and blood chemistries. Important clues to underlying primary renal diseases include microscopic hematuria, cylinduria, proteinuria, glycosuria, elevated serum creatinine levels, decreased serum bicarbonate levels, and hypertension. Other renal diseases should be suspected because of their association with systemic conditions that directly or indirectly affect renal function and thus produce clinical features of primary renal disease.

This chapter focuses on the major manifestations of primary renal disease—that is, hematuria, proteinuria, and rising or elevated serum creatinine levels—that urologists might encounter most frequently. Urologic conditions such as tumors, stones, or infection, which might also precipitate these signs and symptoms, are discussed in Sections VII, VIII, XI, and XIII.

HEMATURIA

Hematuria is defined as the excretion of abnormal quantities of erythrocytes in the urine. Red blood cells can readily be identified by their color (yellow to red) and their shape (biconcave in isotonic urine and swollen spheres in hypotonic urine). *Candida* spores in the urine mimic red blood cells, but they are usually larger and can be readily distinguished if mycelial forms or buds are appreciated.

For routine urinalysis, a dipstick is often used. He-moglobin from red blood cells will catalyze the conversion of the indicator by hydrogen peroxide and change the color of the stick. The test detects intact red blood cells, free hemoglobin, and myoglobin. Oxidizing agents, such as hypochlorite, may lead to false-positive results; large amounts of reducing agents, such as vitamin C, may cause false-negative results. Although dipsticks are widely used for screening, they are not sufficiently sensitive from a urologist's point of view because they miss approximately 10 per cent of patients with microscopic hematuria (Messing et al., 1987).

Detection and quantitation of red blood cells is best accomplished by microscopic examination of a freshly voided, concentrated urine specimen. A first-voided overnight urine specimen is ideal. Moderate exercise prior to urine collection frequently will accentuate hematuria associated with glomerular disease. When gross bleeding is present, examination of unspun urine may be helpful to identify other formed elements, such as casts, white blood cells, and bacteria. In all other instances, examination of unspun urine is not advantageous because of reduced sensitivity. The urine specimen should be centrifuged for 3 to 5 minutes at 2000 to 3000 rpm and the sediment examined by low-power ($\times$ 10) and high-power ($\times$ 40) light microscopy. Approximately 3 per cent of normal individuals will excrete more than 3 erythrocytes per high-power field. Although this value is commonly accepted as the upper limit of normal, in our opinion, identification of any number of erythrocytes on several repeated urine specimens from the same individual should be considered abnormal.

Localization of Hematuria

Hematuria may herald either significant nephrologic or urologic disease. Nephrologic disease is frequently indicated by the presence of concomitant casts and is nearly always indicated by the presence of heavy proteinuria. Even heavy bleeding into the urinary tract will generally not elevate the protein concentration into the range of 100 to 300 mg/dl or 2 + to 3 + proteinuria by the dipstick method; this finding is commonly observed in patients with glomerular diseases. Thus, hematuria associated with 2 + to 3 + proteinuria should always be assumed to be of glomerular or interstitial origin.

Morphologic evaluation of the red blood cells provides further localization of their origin. Erythrocytes originating from glomerular and, probably, tubulointerstitial diseases are commonly disfigured (dysmorphic) and show a wide range of morphologic alterations. In contrast, hematuria originating from a nonglomerular lesion will usually be associated with two morphologic types, most being undamaged circular (isomorphic) cells with normal hemoglobin content and the remainder being red cell "ghosts," which have lost their hemoglobin. Red blood cells present in the urine of apparently healthy persons invariably exhibit the morphologic changes characteristic of glomerular bleeding, but they are present in very small numbers. Dysmorphic cells are best recognized with phase-contrast microscopy, but after some experience, they also can be distinguished by light microscopy (Fassett et al., 1982, Schramek et al., 1989). Because the dysmorphic cells are smaller than the isomorphic cells, Coulter counter analysis of freshly voided urine with estimation of mean corpuscular diameters and the dispersion of these values can also be used as an automated method to detect and quantify the dysmorphism of urinary erythrocytes.

Glomerular Hematuria

The most common glomerular disorders in 151 patients with glomerular hematuria are listed in Table 57–1. Of these patients with glomerulonephritis of various types proven by renal biopsy, 24 (21 per cent) had glomerular hematuria not accompanied by red blood cell casts or proteinuria (Fassett et al., 1982). Assess-

Table 57–1. GLOMERULAR DISORDERS IN 115 PATIENTS WITH GLOMERULAR HEMATURIA

Disorder	Percentage of Patients	Percentage of Patients with Hematuria Alone*
IgA nephropathy (Berger disease)	30	23
Mesangioproliferative GN	14	31
Focal segmental proliferative GN	13	27
Familial nephritis (e.g., Alport syndrome)	11	23
Membranous GN	7	0
Mesangiocapillary GN	6	0
Focal segmental sclerosis	4	0
Unclassifiable	4	0
Systemic lupus erythematosus	3	0
Postinfectious GN	2	100
Subacute bacterial endocarditis	2	100
Others	4	0
Total	100	21

Adapted from Fassett, R. G., et al.: Lancet, 1:1432, 1982.
*Patients with glomerular hematuria not accompanied by red blood cell casts or proteinuria. GN, glomerulonephritis.

ment of possible glomerular hematuria should begin with a thorough history to elicit symptoms and signs associated with hematuria of glomerular or tubulointerstitial disease (Table 57–2). Poststreptococcal glomerulonephritis should be suspected in a child with recent streptococcal upper respiratory or skin infection. Associated symptoms of rash and arthritis might suggest systemic lupus erythematosus nephritis. Hemoptysis and bleeding tendencies accompanied by microcytic anemia are characteristic of the Goodpasture syndrome. A family history of renal disease, hematuria, or deafness may suggest familial hematuria or familial (Alport) nephropathy. Screening laboratory tests should initially include serum creatinine level and creatinine clearance. When proteinuria of 2 + or greater accompanies hematuria, 24-hour urine protein should be measured. Additional screening laboratory tests include complete blood count, erythrocyte sedimentation rate, chest radiograph, and screening blood chemistries (SMA 20 or equivalent).

Because glomerular hematuria is a manifestation of a variety of glomerular abnormalities, additional studies are needed to establish the diagnosis. Such additional studies will clarify whether immune or nonimmune mechanisms are involved, whether a blood dyscrasia is present, or whether other causative factors are involved. Securing specimens of tissues, such as skin and rectal mucosa, is the appropriate procedure in some cases. In others, kidney biopsy may be required, especially if the definitive diagnosis and prognosis cannot be established otherwise and if it is likely that the management of the patient will be different as a result of the biopsy (Earle, 1982). It should be emphasized that kidney biopsies are very informative if the tissue is studied by an experienced pathologist using light, immunofluorescent, and electron microscopy.

IgA Nephropathy (Berger's Disease)

Recurrent gross hematuria after an upper respiratory tract infection or exercise is the typical presentation of IgA glomerulonephritis. The condition is most common in children and young adults with predominance in males. Back pain and renal colic due to clots in the urinary tract may be associated with the hematuria. Low-grade fever and an erythematous skin rash may also be present in some patients, although there are no systemic symptoms in the majority of cases. Hematuria may persist for days or weeks, or it may subside promptly to recur later. Between attacks, microscopic hematuria may be a constant finding in some patients. The course is chronic. A young patient with IgA nephropathy generally has a good prognosis. Kidney function remains normal in the majority, although they may continue to have hematuria. Renal insufficiency develops in about 25 per cent of the patients. Old age at onset; heavy, consistent proteinuria; abnormal renal function at presentation; and hypertension are indicators of a poor prognosis (D'Amico, 1988).

The underlying pathology of IgA glomerulonephritis is limited either to some glomeruli or to lobular segments of a glomerulus. The changes are usually proliferative

Table 57–2. ASSESSMENT OF GLOMERULAR AND NONGLOMERULAR HEMATURIA

Presentation	Studies	Diagnosis
Glomerular		
Dysmorphic erythrocytes and/or erythrocyte casts; ± proteinuria		
Infection?		
Recent upper respiratory or skin infection?	ASO titer Serum C3 level	Poststreptococcal GN
Multisystem diseases?		
Rash, arthritis?	C3, C4, ANA	Systemic lupus erythematosus nephritis
Hemoptysis?	Microcytic anemia	Goodpasture syndrome
Bleeding tendencies?	Anti–double-stranded DNA	Schönlein-Henoch purpura Paraproteinemic disorders (e.g., multiple myeloma)
Hereditary?	Urinalyses in family members	Familial hematuria
Glomerular	Deafness? Audiogram	Familial (Alport) nephritis
	Serum creatinine	Minimal change disease
Other glomerulopathies?	Creatinine clearance	Focal glomerulosclerosis IgA nephropathy (Berger disease)
	Quantitative urine protein	Membranous glomerulopathy Proliferative glomerulonephritis
	ANA C3, C4 Hb, Hct Immunoglobulin level Cryoglobulins Skin, rectal, or renal biopsy	Hemolytic uremic syndrome
	Tests negative	Early glomerulonephritis Benign "idiopathic" hematuria
Nonglomerular		
Tubulointerstial, renovascular, or systemic disorder		
Circular erythrocytes; no erythrocyte casts; ± proteinuria		
Exercise?		
Prolonged running?		Runner's hematuria
Systemic coagulation disturbance?		
Hematuria-causing drug?	Stop drug	Drug-induced hematuria
Anticoagulant?	Platelet values	Hemophilia
Familial history of bleeding disorder?	PT, PTT	Thrombocytopenia
	Bleeding time	Disseminated intravascular coagulopathy Thrombotic thrombocytopenic purpura
Familial urolithiasis?	Urine calcium Urine uric acid	Hypercalciuria Hyperuricosuria
Gross hematuria?		
Hereditary?	IVU	Medullary sponge kidney
Parenchymal	Renal ultrasound	Polycystic kidney Papillary necrosis due to
Papillary necrosis?		
Black?	Sickle cell screening	Sickle cell disease or trait
Analgesic abuse?	IVU	Analgesic nephropathy
Diabetes mellitus?		
Infection?	Culture; PPD skin test	Urinary tract infection, tuberculosis
Urinary tract abnormality?	IVU; cystoscopy	Tumor, obstructive or reflux nephropathy
Malignant hypertension?	Renal ultrasound	Malignant hypertensive nephropathy
Vascular?		
Atrial fibrillation?	IVU; renal ultrasound	
Recent myocardial infarct?	Renogram	Renal artery embolism and thrombosis
Umbilical catheter?	Renal angiography	
Trauma?		
Dehydration?	IVU; renal ultrasound	
	CT scan	Renal vein thrombosis
Bruit?	Renal angiography	Arteriovenous fistula
Renal biopsy?		

Abbreviations: ANA, antinuclear antibody titer; ASO, antistreptolysin O; C3, C4, complement; CT, computerized tomography; GN, glomerulonephritis; Hb, hemoglobin; HCt, hematocrit; IVU, intravenous urography; PPD, purified protein derivative; PT, prothrombin time; PTT, partial thromboplastin time.

and confined mostly to mesangial cells. Deposits of IgA, IgG, and β_1c-globulin were first described by Berger in patients with gross hematuria and focal glomerulonephritis, hence the eponym Berger's disease (Berger and Hinglais, 1968). It should be noted, however, that IgA and IgG mesangial deposits are found in other forms of glomerulonephritis as well. Hence, the presence of IgA deposits is not truly pathognomonic of the disease. What role IgA plays is still unknown, although its deposits in mesangial cells may presumably trigger the glomerular reaction (van den Wall Bake, et al., 1989). Because gross hematuria frequently follows an upper respiratory tract infection, viral antigens have been implicated in some cases. Why hematuria is so prominent and why it so frequently follows exercise is yet to be clarified.

There is no evidence of any beneficial effect of therapy. However, because the clinical presentation of IgA glomerulonephritis may be alarming and similar to that of certain systemic diseases (e.g., Schönlein-Henoch purpura, systemic lupus erythematosus, hypersensitivity angiitis, bacterial endocarditis, Wegener's granulomatosis, Goodpasture's syndrome), careful clinical and laboratory evaluation is essential. The presence of red blood cell casts in the sediment confirms the renal origin of the hematuria. In the absence of such casts, urologic examination should be performed to exclude the urinary tract as the source of bleeding and to confirm that the hematuria is from both kidneys. Once these questions have been resolved, repeated urologic evaluation is not necessary with recurrent episodes of hematuria. Finally, the diagnosis should be validated by kidney biopsy and appropriate pathologic and immunofluorescent studies.

Benign Idiopathic Hematuria

Benign idiopathic hematuria has been recognized by pediatricians for many years. Affected children have focal glomerulonephritis of unknown cause with normal blood pressure and glomerular filtration rate (GFR). A similar syndrome appears to occur in adults and consists of recurrent or persistent gross or microscopic hematuria, normal blood pressure, normal serum creatinine level and creatinine clearance, and 24-hour urine protein excretion not exceeding 1 g. In addition, known causes of glomerulonephritis or nonglomerular causes of hematuria are absent, and renal biopsy shows focal, local glomerular cellularity (Labovitz et al., 1972). Follow-up for 10 years after initial diagnosis in children and in adults usually shows no clinical progression of disease. The syndrome of idiopathic hematuria is best considered as a multifactorial rather than a single disease, with various underlying renal changes in which both immunologic and nonimmunologic mechanisms may be involved. Careful and extended follow-up of patients with idiopathic renal hematuria through several decades is required to determine the exact prognosis.

Nonglomerular Hematuria

Nonglomerular renal hematuria is associated with tubulointerstitial, renovascular, and systemic disorders (see Table 57–2). A pattern of hematuria in relation to recent concomitant medications or exercise might suggest drug-induced or exercise-induced hematuria. Exercise-induced hematuria may be associated with stressful activities, such as running or marching for an extended period of time. Young men and women who participate in such activities may present with gross or microscopic hematuria. If physical examination and initial screening laboratory tests are within normal limits, a more extensive evaluation may be avoided as long as subsequent urinalyses show no hematuria.

A family history of hematuria or bleeding tendency may suggest a blood dyscrasia detectable by appropriate hematologic studies. A family history of urolithiasis or episodes of gross hematuria warrant 24-hour urine chemistries to detect hypercalciuria or hyperuricosuria, definable and potentially reversible causes of hematuria in adults (Andres et al., 1989). A family history of cystic renal disease should prompt radiologic evaluation for unsuspected medullary sponge or polycystic kidney disease. Papillary necrosis should be suspected in diabetic persons, in blacks (owing to sickle cell disease or trait), and in compound analgesic abusers. Vascular abnormalities should be suspected if physical examination reveals severe or accelerated hypertension, atrial fibrillation, or flank bruit. Initial screening laboratory tests should include hematocrit, hemoglobin, erythrocyte sedimentation rate, serum creatinine, chest radiograph, and screening blood chemistries. Further studies to establish the diagnosis are listed in Table 57–2.

Sickle-Cell Nephropathy

Sickle-cell trait occurs in approximately 8 per cent of blacks, whereas sickle-cell disease affects approximately 1 in 600. Most of the symptoms of sickle-cell trait or disease are related to the presence of hemoglobin S. When sickle erythrocytes become physically trapped in smaller vessels, a vicious circle develops, leading to stasis, deoxygenation, decreased pH, increased sickling and thrombosis, and infarction. The major renal disturbances are hematuria, polyuria, renal failure, and thrombotic complications that may lead to the nephrotic syndrome (Strom et al., 1972) or priapism (Schmidt and Flocks, 1971). Although the true frequency of hematuria is not known, sickle-cell hemoglobinopathy accounts for approximately one third of cases of gross hematuria in blacks. Hematuria occurs more regularly in hemoglobin SS disease than in hemoglobin SA trait, but urologists more frequently see patients with hemoglobin SA trait because of the relative frequency of the two disorders. Although the mechanism of hematuria is not clear, it presumably results from increased sickling and sludging of blood in the medulla and papillae, leading to extravasation of red blood cells, ischemia, and papillary necrosis. Hemoglobin electrophoresis readily permits identification of sickle hemoglobin and differentiation of sickle-cell trait from sickle-cell disease. Cystoscopy and intravenous urography should be performed to localize the site of bleeding, which is usually from the left, and to rule out other disorders (Buckalew and Someren, 1974).

Treatment of hematuria should begin with rest and hydration. In addition, hematuria has been treated with a variety of techniques including intravenous distilled water, sodium bicarbonate, mannitol, and loop diuretics (Knochel, 1969; Vega et al., 1971). ε-Aminocaproic acid (which inhibits urokinase), administered intravenously in small doses of 1 g at 4- to 6-hour intervals, appears to be effective and causes few or no side effects. However, this agent should be used only for severe and intractable bleeding because clotting of the blood inhibits urokinase and can produce intrapelvic or ureteral clots. If life-threatening hematuria occurs and conservative treatment fails, arteriography with arterial embolization of selected vessels should be considered. If this fails, pyeloscopy and segmental or total nephrectomy may be required. Recurrent episodes of hematuria may be diminished by regular administration of oral furosemide.

Papillary necrosis is a common complication of sickle-cell nephropathy but usually affects one papilla at a time and rarely results in serious deterioration of renal function (Vaamonde, 1984). The loss of concentrating ability is perhaps the most characteristic renal functional lesion in individuals with hemoglobin S gene. Although the degree of concentration defect is not sufficient to cause symptoms under normal conditions, affected persons may develop manifestations of early sickle-cell crisis (malaise, anorexia, joint pain) with only moderate restriction of fluid intake.

Renal Artery Embolism and Thrombosis

Thrombosis or embolism of the renal arterial vasculature can result in varied clinical, functional, and morphologic changes depending on the size of vessels involved, rate and degree of development of obstruction, and extent of renal parenchymal involvement. Because intrarenal arteries are end arteries, complete occlusion of a main renal artery or one of its branches leads to wedge-shaped infarction with coagulation necrosis and extensive parenchymal damage.

Occlusion of the main renal arteries most commonly results from emboli associated with mitral stenosis and atrial fibrillation, artificial heart valves, subacute bacterial endocarditis, or mural thrombi associated with myocardial infarct. The most important noncardiac source of renal emboli is a ruptured aortic atheromatous plaque. Although spontaneous rupture is common, manipulation of vessels during arteriography or surgery or anticoagulation with bleeding into an ulcerated plaque with subsequent rupture are more frequently implicated. Following rupture, the plaques discharge crystalline and amorphous cholesterol emboli into the small vessels of the kidneys and other organs (see following discussion of atheroembolic renal disease).

Thrombosis of major renal arteries is unusual, though it may occur following blunt abdominal trauma, manipulation of the aorta during angiography or surgery, or renal arterioplasty. Spontaneous thrombosis may occasionally occur in association with atherosclerotic or dissecting aneurysms of the aorta or with inflammatory vascular disorders, such as polyarteritis. Renal infarction occurs when a main or segmental renal artery is completely and suddenly occluded.

The clinical sequelae of major renal artery occlusion are extremely varied and may include sudden, sharp, persistent pain in the flank or upper abdomen, nausea, vomiting, and fever. However, most patients will be symptom-free.

Urinary findings of microscopic or gross hematuria accompanied by mild proteinuria are present in only about half of the cases. Leukocytosis may be present. Renal infarction characteristically causes a rapid rise in the serum level of aspartate aminotransferase, which returns to normal within 3 to 4 days followed by a striking elevation of lactate dehydrogenase, which remains elevated for as long as 2 weeks. Serum alkaline phosphatase levels may be slightly increased. If the contralateral kidney is normal, renal functional impairment may not be recognized. However, if pre-existing renal functional impairment or a solitary kidney is present, marked or complete renal failure will occur. Partial thrombotic or embolic occlusion of the major renal artery may cause sudden development of hypertension due to activation of the renin-angiotensin system.

The key to diagnosis is a high index of suspicion in the proper setting. The first clue to renal infarction is usually provided by intravenous urography, which will show absence of visualization in all or part of the kidney. Radionuclide imaging demonstrating nonperfusion of the kidney and selective renal arteriography are required to confirm the diagnosis (Fig. 57–1). Early management of renal artery thromboembolism is determined by degree of renal involvement, duration of involvement, and cause of the occlusion. Early determination of complete occlusion of the main renal artery or arteries in patients

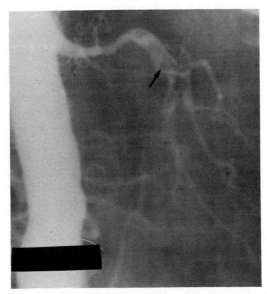

Figure 57–1. Renal artery embolus in a 68-year-old man with a history of atrial fibrillation, left flank pain, hematuria, and acute elevation in serum creatinine concentration. Abdominal aortogram demonstrates conical tapering of the left main renal artery from atherosclerosis. A large intraluminal filling defect *(arrow)* in the main renal artery extends into the proximal interlobar arteries.

with bilateral renal artery thrombi or unilateral renal artery thrombus of a single functioning kidney has been managed successfully by surgical thrombectomy or embolectomy. The best results have been reported when surgery was performed a few hours after the occlusion, but significant return of renal function has been documented in patients operated on as long as 15 to 43 days following occlusion. This finding is probably because of the gradual development of collateral circulation prior to total occlusion (Besarab et al., 1976; Perkins et al., 1967). Reports indicate that transluminal recanalization (Beraud et al., 1989) or dissolution with intra-arterial fibrinolytics (Campieri et al., 1989; Skinner et al., 1989) can result in significant recovery of renal function.

Unilateral thrombosis or embolism warrants a conservative approach because the contralateral kidney will continue to function, and recovery of function on the ischemic side has been reported. Treatment of embolic disease caused by a cardiac source is usually nonsurgical because persons thus affected often have serious underlying cardiac disease and a high surgical mortality. Anticoagulants should be instituted promptly to prevent further propagation of the clot into the renal artery or embolization of other organs. Incomplete occlusion may lead to renal ischemia, increased renin production, and hypertension, which is best managed by nephrectomy.

Arteriovenous Fistulas

Renal arteriovenous fistulas are described as either congenital or acquired, based on angiographic criteria. Congenital fistulas present as distinct, tortuous, coiled vascular channels grouped in clusters, with multiple communications between arteries and veins. They are considered to be congenital because the angiographic appearance is typical of other known congenital arteriovenous fistulas. These congenital fistulas account for approximately one quarter of all arteriovenous fistulas, are usually present in adults, and have an equal sex incidence (Messing et al., 1976). Acquired arteriovenous fistulas usually appear as solitary communications between artery and vein, account for almost three quarters of all renal arteriovenous fistulas, and are post-traumatic in origin. Percutaneous needle biopsy accounts for over 40 per cent of acquired fistulas, particularly in patients with nephrosclerosis and arterial hypertension (O'Brien et al., 1974; Wickre and Golper, 1982). Acquired renal arteriovenous fistulas also occur following penetrating or blunt abdominal trauma, partial nephrectomies, nephrolithotomies, or spontaneously, owing to tumor invasion into adjacent veins (Bosniak, 1965).

The clinical manifestations of renal arteriovenous fistulas depend primarily on their size and location. Although frequently silent, fistulas may be associated with hematuria, cardiac failure due to increased cardiac output, and hypertension due to renal ischemia distal to the fistula (Gomes and Bernatz, 1970). Almost three quarters of affected persons have a continuous abdominal or flank bruit. Intravenous urography shows no abnormalities in about one half of sufferers; the remainder manifest space-occupying lesions or nonvisualization of the kidney. Radionuclide angiography is a simple, noninvasive, and valuable screening test for arteriovenous fistulas (Lisbona et al., 1980). Although reliable when large arteriovenous communications are present, this technique may not detect small intraparenchymal fistulas, such as those seen following renal biopsy. Color Doppler ultrasound has proved effective in the identification of renal transplant arteriovenous fistulas (Middleton et al., 1989).

Contrast angiography remains the definitive diagnostic study for arteriovenous fistulas (Fig. 57–2). The arteriovenous communication usually shows as an immediate intense arterial blush, which disappears rapidly. Early visualization of the inferior vena cava is further evidence of shunting and is usually seen with high-flow shunts.

Management of arteriovenous fistulas should be based on the cause and associated symptoms. Most congenital fistulas are small, asymptomatic, and of little clinical importance. Spontaneous closure has been demonstrated (Cho and Stanley, 1978). Similarly, approximately 95 per cent of postbiopsy arteriovenous fistulas heal spontaneously in 1 to 18 months (Iloreta and Blaufox, 1979). Surgical intervention is generally indicated in patients who have symptomatic fistulas not secondary to renal biopsy. Persistent microscopic or massive hematuria or frank rupture provide clear indications for therapeutic intervention, as do high-output cardiac failure and hypertension, which can frequently be controlled or cured once the fistula is removed.

Partial or total nephrectomy as well as arterial reconstructive procedures have been utilized traditionally to treat symptomatic renal arteriovenous fistulas (Nelson et al., 1973). Large congenital arteriovenous fistulas or tumors are best treated by nephrectomy; small congenital fistulas can be managed by partial nephrectomy. Acquired types of arteriovenous fistulas generally warrant a renal-sparing procedure, traditionally by extrarenal or intrarenal vascular ligation or repair.

Transcatheter arteriographically directed embolization has gained acceptance for the treatment of both congenital and acquired arteriovenous fistulas (Cho and Stanley, 1978; Clark et al., 1983). Small arteriovenous fistulas may be managed using autogenous clots because lysis of this embolized material within a few hours may prevent renal infarction. If the fistulas are large, gelatin sponge emboli, coils, balloons, or bucrylate may be effective. Extensive embolization necessitating repeated catheterization may be required for arteriovenous malformations in which multiple vessels contribute to the lesion. Potential complications include remote venous embolization, hypertension secondary to renal ischemia, and renal infarction and refistulization in the infarcted areas.

Renal Vein Thrombosis

Renal vein thrombosis may occur in a variety of clinical conditions. Intralobular or arcuate vein thrombosis in infants may arise bilaterally in association with severe dehydration due to diarrhea or vomiting or with severe plasma hyperosmolarity related to angiography (Arneil et al., 1973). In adults, it is frequently unilateral and is usually associated with the nephrotic syndrome

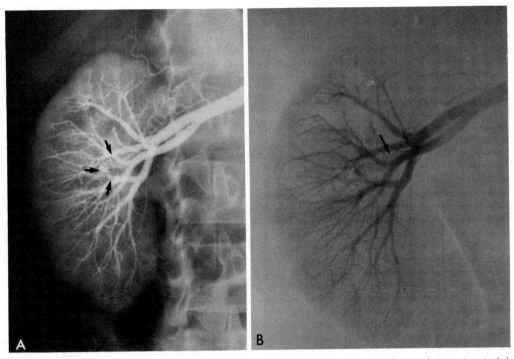

Figure 57–2. Renal arteriovenous fistulas in a 28-year-old woman with recurrent microscopic and gross hematuria. *A,* Selective right renal arteriography demonstrates a cluster of small abnormal vessels in the peripelvic region *(arrows). B,* Subtraction view demonstrates this abnormal collection of vessels as well as an early draining vein *(arrow).*

or invasion of renal veins by tumor or retroperitoneal disease. Whether renal vein thrombosis is the cause or consequence of the nephrotic syndrome is debatable. Increased renal venous pressure in association with congestive heart failure or after surgical ligation of the renal vein can produce proteinuria. However, animal experiments have shown that the contralateral kidney must be removed before the constriction leads to heavy proteinuria. In humans, obstruction of the vena cava above the renal veins or even renal vein thrombosis may not be associated with nephrotic syndrome. In comparison, the nephrotic syndrome is a hypercoagulable state, and thrombotic events occur in various vessels. For example, pulmonary embolism with or without renal vein thrombosis is a relatively common complication. An increase in clotting factors and a decrease in antithrombin III, an inhibitor of coagulation, have been demonstrated. According to some investigators, the incidence of renal vein thrombosis appears to be much higher (greater than 30 per cent) in patients with nephrotic syndrome due to membranous glomerulonephritis than to other causes (Llach et al., 1980).

The clinical presentation and course of renal vein thrombosis are dependent upon degree of occlusion and rate at which it develops. Acute thrombosis occurs more often in young children and is associated with severe flank pain, hypertension, and shock. Kidney size is frequently increased, and renal blood flow may be decreased to 25 per cent. Gross or microscopic hematuria due to focal renal infarction, proteinuria, and reduced renal function is common. Progressive thrombosis of the renal vein occurs most often in adults and may present with flank pain, hematuria, and fever or as the nephrotic syndrome. Renal failure rarely develops

if collateral venous drainage develops rapidly enough. Patients with acute or long-standing renal vein thrombosis may be asymptomatic or may present with clinical manifestations due to other thrombolic events, the most serious of which is pulmonary embolism.

Intravenous urography may show an enlarged kidney, which usually though not always excretes contrast material (Fig. 57–3). Ultrasonography during the acute phase shows an enlarged, hypoechoic kidney and thrombus in the renal vein. After 1 week, the size may diminish and echogenicity may increase owing to fibrosis and cellular infiltration. On longer follow-up, the kidney may be hypoplastic or, if the thrombus resolves, may appear normal. Computed tomographic (CT) scanning and magnetic resonance imaging (MRI) have been used to demonstrate an enlarged kidney and thrombosis of the renal vein. The definitive diagnostic study, however, is renal venography. Care should be exercised in performing this study because dislodgement and embolization may occur.

The management of renal vein thrombosis depends on the age of the patient. In infancy, thrombosis associated with dehydration is frequently fatal, and the best results have been achieved with rehydration. Emergency thrombectomy and fibrinolytic agents, such as urokinase and streptokinase, have also been favorable (Bromberg and Firlit, 1990; Thompson et al., 1975). In adults, anticoagulation should be initiated as soon as renal vein thrombosis has been diagnosed and if thromboembolic phenomena have been demonstrated. The role of prophylaxis with anticoagulation in patients with nephrotic syndrome and without renal vein thrombosis or other thromboembolic complications is not established. Surgical removal of the clots from the renal veins is not

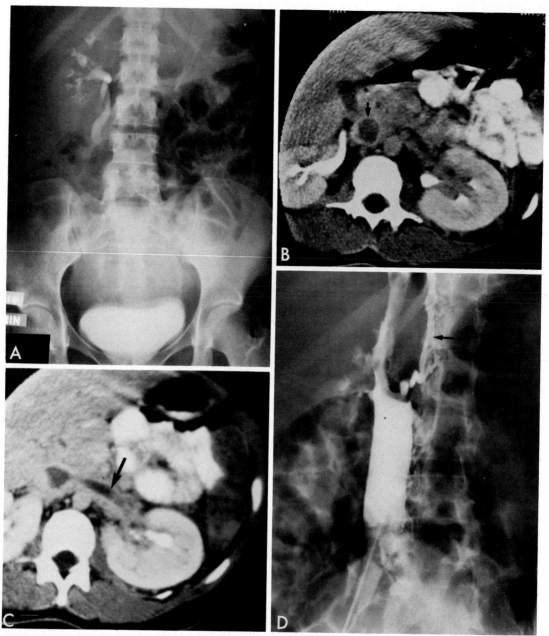

Figure 57–3. Renal vein thrombosis. A 40-year-old woman presented with pulmonary embolus, hematuria, and proteinuria.
A, Intravenous urogram demonstrates a very poorly visualizing left kidney and no abnormality of the right kidney. Note contrast material in the distal left ureter.
B, Computed tomography following an infusion of contrast material demonstrates a low-density area in the inferior vena cava *(arrow)* surrounded by a contrast-filled rim.
C, Similar findings are noted in the left renal vein *(large arrow).*
D, Inferior vena cavography demonstrates filling of the inferior vena cava below the level of the renal veins. A large intraluminal thrombus extends from the level of the renal veins to the diaphragm. A small amount of contrast traverses the thrombus and wall of the vena cava. Filling of lumbar veins *(arrow)* is demonstrated. These serve as collateral channels.

advisable or helpful because thrombosis of intrarenal channels is most likely present.

PROTEINURIA

The qualitative detection of proteinuria, particularly in patients who appear to be healthy, always raises the question of renal disease. Proteinuria may be the first indication of an underlying renal glomerular, vascular, or tubulointerstitial disease or an early presentation of overflow of abnormal protein into the urine. However, proteinuria is also found in nonrenal disorders and various physiologic states.

Protein in Normal Urine

Healthy adults excrete approximately 80 to 150 mg of protein daily. The maximum level in small children is

140 mg/m² of body surface area per day. Protein excretion up to 300 mg per day occurs transiently following severe exercise and is generally found in adolescents between the ages of 10 and 18. For any given rate of protein excretion, the concentration of protein in a single voided sample of urine will vary inversely with urine flow. The concentration of protein in normal urine usually does not exceed 10 to 20 mg/dl; thus, higher concentrations imply the existence of proteinuria. However, in persons with dilute urine, significant proteinuria may be present with concentrations well below 20 mg/dl.

The normal composition of urine protein is about 30 to 40 per cent serum albumin, 30 per cent serum globulins, and 40 per cent tissue proteins (e.g., Tamm-Horsfall). This profile can be altered by both physiologic and pathologic conditions that affect filtration, reabsorption, or excretion of urine protein. It has been proposed that determination of the urine protein profile can assist in determining the source of proteinuria.

Detection of Proteinuria

Proteinuria can be detected by either turbidimetric (protein precipitation) or colorimetric (dipstick) methods. Turbidimetric methods rely on the detection of turbidity after proteins in solution have been precipitated by strong acids (e.g., 3 per cent sulfosalicyclic acid). These methods are sensitive for total protein concentrations as low as 10 mg/dl and react with all classes of proteins. The turbidimetric test has largely been replaced by the simpler colorimetric test. The dipstick consists of bibulous paper impregnated with tetrabromphenol blue, which changes color in the presence of albumin and to the lesser extent in the presence of other proteins. The intensity of the shade of green is proportional to the concentration of protein in the urine. The reagent strips are generally sensitive to total protein concentrations as low as 20 mg/dl. Because of difficulties in the discrimination of colors, the correlation between color change and actual protein concentrations may be only approximate (Rennie and Keen, 1967).

False-positive or false-negative test results can occur with either method. Highly concentrated urine in a dehydrated but otherwise healthy person may give a positive test result. In patients with gross hematuria, contamination of the urine with plasma proteins may cause false-positive proteinuria. However, rather massive bleeding is required to elevate the protein concentration into the 100 to 300 mg/dl (2 + to 3 +) range and to the values greater than 1.0 g/24 hours commonly observed in patients with glomerular disease. Milder degrees of macroscopic or microscopic hematuria accompanied by heavy proteinuria (> 300 mg/dl, or 3 +) should always be assumed to have a glomerular or interstitial cause (Glassock, 1983). The other causes of false-positive reactions affect either the turbidimetric or colorimetric test but not both. Thus, false-positive reactions are suggested by discrepancies between the two tests. False-positive turbidimetric reactions can be caused by the presence in the urine of radiographic contrast material, high concentrations of penicillin or cephalosporin analogues, or sulfonamide or tolbutamide metabolites. False-positive colorimetric tests can occur when urine is highly alkaline (pH > 8) (e.g., as seen in urinary tract infections with urea-splitting bacteria) or following contamination with antiseptics, such as chlorhexidine or benzalkonium chloride.

False-negative results may occur with dilute urine specimens because even increased amounts of protein are diluted to below the level of detection of the method used. Highly buffered alkaline urine may give a false-negative turbidimetric test and so must be titered to a pH of between 5 and 6 before testing. Because the colorimetric strips react preferentially with albumin and are relatively insensitive to globulins and Bence Jones protein, urine that is sulfosalicylic acid–positive and dipstick-negative should be tested for light chains (Bence Jones proteinuria) to assess the patient for multiple myeloma.

Pathophysiology of Proteinuria

Proteins may enter the urine by filtration across the glomerular capillary membrane or by decreased tubular reabsorption of normally filtered protein. Increased plasma concentration of a protein with molecular features conducive to transglomerular passage (low molecular weight, cationic charge, and high deformability) will also cause proteinuria.

Glomerular proteinuria, the most common type of proteinuria, usually is caused by increased glomerular capillary permeability to proteins, especially albumin. Glomerular proteinuria may be due to any primary glomerular disease, such as lipoid nephrosis, as well as any glomerulopathy associated with a systemic illness, such as systemic lupus erythematosus or diabetes mellitus. A transient increase in protein excretion may even occur in various physiologic settings in the absence of renal disease. For example, increased protein excretion, such as may accompany standing or exercise in healthy subjects, has been attributed to some alteration in renal hemodynamics plus simultaneous changes in filtration of normal protein. The likelihood of glomerular disease is high if protein excretion exceeds 1 to 2 g/day, and proteinuria in excess of 3 to 5 g/day (nephrotic range proteinuria) invariably indicates glomerular disease. The determination of a protein/creatinine ratio in a single urine sample obtained during normal daytime activity can support the 24-hour urine collection in the clinical quantitation of proteinuria (Ginsberg et al., 1983). In the presence of stable renal function, a protein/creatinine ratio of more than 3.5 (mg/mg) suggests nephrotic range proteinuria, and a ratio of less than 0.2 is within normal limits.

Tubular proteinuria is defined as the appearance in the urine of normally filtered protein as a result of impaired tubular reabsorption. Normally, the majority of filtered proteins of low molecular weight (< 40,000 daltons), such as β_2-microglobulin, immunoglobulin light chains, zinc-binding protein, and lysozyme, are reabsorbed by the proximal tubules; but in patients with interstitial or tubular disorders, they escape tubular reabsorption. In tubular proteinuria, less than 2 to 3 g/day are excreted and low–molecular-weight proteins predominate over albumin. Examples of tubular proteinuria include Fanconi's syndrome and cadmium, lead, or mercury poisoning.

Overflow proteinuria occurs in the absence of any glomerular or tubular abnormality. Increased plasma concentrations of abnormal immunoproteins and other low–molecular-weight proteins with molecular features conducive to transglomerular passage lead to an excessive filtered load, which exceeds the reabsorptive capacity of the proximal tubules. Protein excretion may vary from 100 mg to 10 g/day. The most common example of overflow proteinuria is seen in myeloma patients, who excrete immunoglobulin light chains (Bence Jones proteins). Other examples of overflow proteinuria include lysozymuria in patients with monocytic and monomyelocytic leukemia, hemoglobinuria, and myoglobinuria. Both hemoglobinuria and myoglobinuria will yield positive results for occult blood in the urine because both compounds contain a heme group. Hemoglobinuria is suspected when the urine is red or dark brown, the dipstick is positive for blood, but erythrocytes are not seen in the sediment. The plasma of patients with hemoglobinuria is reddish brown. Myoglobinuria, in contrast, is characterized by dark urine and normal-appearing plasma. Acute renal failure coinciding with overflow proteinuria has been well documented (Baker and Dodds, 1925; Rowland and Penn, 1972).

Evaluation of Proteinuria

Patients with a result of 1 + or greater on dipstick test should have repeat dipstick tests and, if possible, turbidimetric tests on one or two additional urine samples. Proteinuria can be transient, intermittent, or persistent. A large proportion of patients, as many as 100 per cent in some pediatric series (Randolph and Greenfield, 1967; Wagner et al., 1968), will have *transient* proteinuria that disappears within days of the initial positive specimen (King and Gronbeck, 1952; Larsen and Thysell, 1969). These patients and those with functional proteinuria associated with, for example, fever, exercise, emotional stress, or congestive heart failure, require no further evaluation when urine protein excretion returns to normal. However, if repeat tests for protein remain positive, 24-hour urine protein values should be determined.

The probability of an underlying renal disease may be predicted by the pattern and amount of proteinuria and identification of associated abnormalities. In general, persistent proteinuria is most likely to be associated with renal impairment than is intermittent proteinuria (Robinson, 1985). If proteinuria is *intermittent*, it may be associated with postural change. Proteinuria that occurs only in the upright position (*orthostatic*) is a common cause for mild proteinuria that affects young men. Although total daily protein excretion may be 500 mg to 1 g, urinary protein excretion is normal when the patient is recumbent. Proteinuria eventually ceases in about half of the patients. In the remainder, fixed orthostatic proteinuria does not seem to have any impact on morbidity or mortality. If renal function is normal, no further evaluation or management is indicated, but repeat urinalysis should be performed every 1 to 2 years to monitor for evidence of progression of renal disease. Orthostatic proteinuria is usually less significant than constant proteinuria during both recumbency and quiet upright ambulation.

The likelihood of renal disease is also high if quantitative determination of protein excretion exceeds 1 to 2 g/day. Proteinuria in excess of 3 to 5 g/day (nephrotic range proteinuria) almost invariably indicates a glomerular disease (Cameron and Glassock, 1988). Proteinuria due to overflow should be suspected if the proteins in the urine are not normal constituents of plasma but rather abnormal immunoproteins. The probability of underlying renal disease is also increased if proteinuria is associated with hypertension, diabetes mellitus, gout, elevated serum creatinine levels, edema, or other abnormalities of the urine sediment, such as hematuria or casts. Conversely, when proteinuria is detected by chance in patients who have no evidence of systemic disease, renal functional impairment, or abnormal urine sediment, the probability of significant underlying renal disease is small.

Persistent Proteinuria

Persistent proteinuria is described as an increase in protein excretion above normal in all samples on repeated testing, regardless of the patient's posture. The most common causes of persistent proteinuria are listed in Table 57–3. The major renal causes of proteinuria without hematuria are diabetes mellitus, amyloidosis, multiple myeloma, arteriolar nephrosclerosis, pregnancy, and drug and heavy-metal intoxication. Patients with proteinuria and either gross or microscopic hematuria are likely to have a form of glomerulonephritis even if there is no renal functional impairment. These patients should be evaluated as noted in Table 57–2.

Diabetes Mellitus

Proteinuria is the hallmark of diabetic nephropathy and may be the first manifestation of diabetes mellitus. Diabetic patients with proteinuria generally have a poorer prognosis than those without. In some patients, the glomerular disease is severe enough that heavy proteinuria of greater than 6 g/24 hours and nephrotic syndrome result. Hypertension and decreased GFR are also usually present. Hematuria is usually absent in patients with diabetic nephropathy. When hematuria is present, other disorders, such as papillary necrosis or immune complex glomerulonephritis, should be considered.

Multiple Myeloma

Multiple myeloma is a neoplastic transformation of plasma cells leading to the production and secretion of abnormal and unique immunoglobulin proteins (para-

Table 57–3. CAUSES OF PERSISTENT PROTEINURIA

Primary glomerular disease
  Minimal change disease (lipoid nephrosis)
  Focal glomerulosclerosis
  Membranous glomerulopathy
  Proliferative glomerulonephritis
Infectious disease
  Poststreptococcal glomerulonephritis
  Infectious endocarditis
  Syphilis
Drugs and chemicals*
  Mercury
  Gold
  Penicillamine
  Probenecid
  Heroin
Neoplastic disease and paraproteinemia
  Multiple myeloma*
  Lymphoma and leukemia
  Carcinoma
Multisystem and connective tissue diseases
  Systemic lupus erythematosus
  Rheumatoid arthritis
  Amyloidosis*
  Scleroderma
  Polyarteritis
  Wegener's granulomatosis
  Cryoglobulinemia
  Goodpasture syndrome
  Sarcoidosis*
  Vasculitides
Metabolic disease
  Diabetes mellitus*
Heredofamilial diseases
  Alport syndrome
  Fabry's disease*
  Sickle cell disease
Miscellaneous
  Arteriolar nephrosclerosis*
  Pregnancy-associated*
  Renal vein thrombosis
  Reflux nephropathy
  Analgesic nephropathy

*Major causes of proteinuria without hematuria.

proteins). This disorder is characterized clinically by bone pain, anemia, hypercalcemia, and renal failure. The renal dysfunction may take a variety of forms (acute renal failure, chronic renal failure, tubular disorders) related to the type of myeloma. IgG myeloma, which accounts for approximately 60 per cent of all myelomas, has the best prognosis. The IgA form causes 20 per cent of myelomas and is more likely to be associated with hypercalcemia and amyloidosis. Light chain disease (Bence Jones proteinuria) accounts for approximately 20 per cent of myeloma cases and has the highest frequency of renal involvement and the poorest prognosis. Renal tubular disorders are most common in this group due in part to the toxic effects of the light chains on tubular cells.

Acute renal failure occurs in 5 to 10 per cent of myeloma patients and is frequently associated with or precipitated by intravenous or retrograde urography, dehydration, hypercalcemia, hyperuricemia, or pyelonephritis. Regardless of the cause of the acute renal failure in myeloma patients, the prognosis is poor, with a 60 to 75 per cent mortality. Fluid restriction should be avoided in preparing patients with multiple myeloma

for intravenous urography. Mild hypercalcemia (approximately 11 to 13 mg/dl) is a frequent complication in patients with multiple myeloma, and severe hypercalcemia (> 13 mg/dl) is also encountered in as many as 25 per cent of patients. Prompt treatment by oral or parenteral hydration and diuretics, resulting in an output of at least 3 L/day, may be adequate to prevent renal failure. Hyperuricosemia is not uncommon in patients with multiple myeloma as a result of nucleic acid turnover, which arises spontaneously or following chemotherapy. Prevention of acute uric acid nephropathy should include reduction of uric acid production by allopurinol, a maintenance of the urine output of approximately 3 L/day, and maintenance of a urine pH of 6.0 or greater by administration of sodium bicarbonate. Multiple myeloma sufferers are also very susceptible to infections, and the most frequent portal of entry is the urinary tract. Instrumentation of the lower urinary tract should be avoided.

Chronic renal failure occurs in 40 to 50 per cent of myeloma patients and may be exacerbated by obstructive nephropathy due to ureteral amyloid deposits, nephrolithiasis, papillary necrosis, or proteinaceous renal pelvic cast formation. Both hemodialysis and renal transplantation have been performed successfully in patients with multiple myeloma.

Intermittent or Orthostatic Proteinuria

Most patients with intermittent proteinuria will be free of proteinuria after a few years (Larsen and Thysell, 1969). Those younger than 30 years have mortality rates similar to age-matched controls, and death due to renal disease is very uncommon. Intermittent proteinuria is less common after the age of 50; but when present, it is associated with an excess death rate that increases with age (Gajewski et al., 1976). When intermittent excretion exceeds 1 g/day, blood pressure, urinalysis, and serum creatinine levels should be determined at 6- to 12-month intervals until the proteinuria disappears.

If an individual has evidence of orthostatic proteinuria that is transient, the likelihood of renal disease is rare. Patients with fixed orthostatic proteinuria rarely develop chronic renal disease, and a 10-year prognosis is excellent. Although renal biopsy is the only means of determining alterations in renal histology, it should be noted that the broad spectrum of histologic findings by light microscopy does not necessarily provide insight into the actual clinical significance or subsequent morbidity of the lesion. For these reasons, when proteinuria is less than 1 g/day, emphasis should be placed on follow-up, and biopsies should be deferred until there is evidence of progression of proteinuria, development of other abnormalities in the urine sediment, or other changes of the clinical course, such as development of hypertension, impaired renal function, or an abnormal urine sediment. When proteinuria initially is greater than 1 g/day, there is an increased merit to renal biopsy, and biopsy is almost surely indicated if the proteinuria is in the nephrotic range—that is, greater than 3 g/day.

ELEVATED OR RISING SERUM CREATININE LEVEL

The creatinine clearance provides a simple and reliable means for estimating GFR and, thus, the status of renal function. Creatinine is produced at a constant rate by muscle cells from the breakdown of creatine at a rate of approximately 20 mg per kg per day. If lean body mass does not change appreciably, the plasma concentration and daily urine creatinine excretion remain relatively constant. When indicated, creatinine clearance should be performed to establish baseline data. Once the clearance has been determined, measurement of creatinine levels, which closely reflect creatinine clearance, is usually sufficient to monitor renal function serially. Figure 57–4 shows the relation between GFR and serum creatinine level. For every 50 per cent reduction in GFR, the serum creatinine concentration approximately doubles. From this diagram, it is apparent that, in early stages of renal insufficiency, relatively large decreases in clearance are reflected by small changes in serum creatinine levels. In contrast, in advanced renal failure, relatively small changes in clearance result in large changes in the serum creatinine levels. Blood urea nitrogen is a less reliable indicator of renal function because factors other than the GFR, such as protein intake, the degree of hydration, anabolic or antianabolic agents (tetracycline and corticosteroids), fever, and infection, can cause changes in blood urea nitrogen in the absence of changes in renal function (Schrier, 1980).

An important consideration when evaluating renal function is the role of age. The mean serum creatinine level gradually increases between the ages of 1 and 20 years (Fig. 57–5). After the age of 50, the GFR gradually decreases in approximately half the population without hypertension or known renal disease (Fig. 57–6).

Impaired renal function as evidenced by abnormally elevated serum creatinine levels is usually associated with other features, such as hematuria, shock, hypertension, obstructive nephropathy, infection, and nephrotoxins. Current evidence has shown the important role played by atheromatous cholesterol emboli, analgesics, and radiologic contrast media in causing chronic and acute deterioration of renal function. A few comments about these causes of renal failure, therefore, seem to be appropriate.

Atheroembolic Renal Disease

Atheromatous emboli of small arteries and arterioles should be suspected in patients 50 years of age and older with known atherosclerosis or abdominal aneurysms and unexplained renal failure. Atheromatous plaques on the wall of the abdominal aorta may spontaneously rupture or erode through, permitting their contents, including cholesterol crystals and amorphous debris, to occlude the lumina of multiple small renal arteries (arcuate, intralobular, terminal). Atheromatous emboli of the renal arteries have been identified in 15 to 30 per cent of patients with severe erosive atherosclerotic lesions of the aorta and 1 per cent of patients with slight-to-moderate erosions (Humphreys, 1981). Emboli also frequently follow aortic surgery, renal or cardiac angiography, and external cardiac massage. Spotty ischemic atrophy of the parenchyma in a wedge-shaped pattern predominates over acute infarction. Recanalization of the vessels may occur, or a fibrotic reaction may lead to reduction of renal function. The diagnosis is difficult because the clinical manifestations and signs are not dramatic. Hypertension or elevated serum creatinine levels may be the only clinical findings. Acute renal failure is not unusual. Embolization of other organs occurs frequently and may lead to visual disturbances, including sudden blindness (cholesterol retinal emboli); gastrointestinal bleeding; splenic infarcts; and livedo reticularis of the skin of the lower extremities or distal extremity gangrene. Laboratory findings are nonspecific. Proteinuria is usually mild, except in the presence of malignant hypertension, when heavy proteinuria may occur. Urinalysis may reveal hematuria or leukocyturia. The diagnosis can be established with certainty only by renal biopsy showing typical elongated clefts in the small intralobular and interlobular vessels. Cholesterol emboli can also be demonstrated in muscle biopsy of the lower extremities and occasionally can be seen by ophthalmoscopy. Renal angiography is not advisable because the results are usually nonspecific and traumatic rupture of additional atheromatous plaques may occur (Kassirer, 1987).

Management of atheroembolic renal disease is difficult and usually unsatisfactory. No reported cases have regained normal renal function, and the mortality is very high as a consequence of associated widespread atheromatous disease and complicating events, such as pancreatitis, gastrointestinal bleeding, and uremia. The best treatment is prevention. Patients with widespread atheromatous disease of the aorta should not undergo angiography if at all possible or be treated with anticoagulants before angiography. During surgery, the atheromatous aorta should be handled very carefully. Once the embolic event has occurred, there is no evidence that anticoagulation therapy is effective.

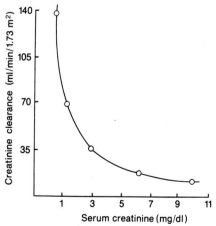

Figure 57–4. Relationship between creatinine clearance and serum creatinine. (From Earle, D. P.: Cardiovasc. Med., 3:1257, 1978. Reprinted with permission from the Physicians World Communications Group.)

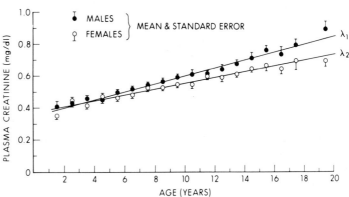

Figure 57–5. Mean plasma creatinine value plotted against age for both sexes, with the regression lines derived from 1398 values (772 males, 626 females) superimposed. Standard error limits for estimate of the mean are shown—λ_1 (males): $y = 0.35 + 0.025$ x, $r = 0.53$, $P<.0001$; λ_2 (females): $y = 0.37 + 0.018$ x, $r = 0.49$, $P<.0001$. (From Schwartz, G. J., et al.: J. Pediatr., 88:828, 1976.)

Analgesic Nephropathy

Correlation between chronic analgesic abuse, interstitial nephritis, papillary necrosis, and chronic renal failure was noted more than 30 years ago in Switzerland and is now widely recognized. Analgesic nephropathy is the cause of chronic renal failure in 20 per cent of dialysis patients in Australia and in 3 to 7 per cent of those in Europe and the United States. Large doses of phenacetin and aspirin, especially in combination, may cause renal papillary necrosis and chronic interstitial nephritis. The total amount of analgesic consumed is directly related to the degree of renal function impairment. One gram of phenacetin per day in combination with other analgesics for 1 to 3 years or a total of 2 kg of phenacetin alone is considered the minimal amount that will cause nephropathy (Pommer et al., 1989; Sandler et al., 1989).

Analgesic nephropathy is predominantly seen in women between the ages of 30 and 50. The patient is typically depressed, complains of headaches and abdominal and musculoskeletal disorders, and gives a history of years of daily ingestion of analgesics containing caffeine, aspirin, and phenacetin. Alcoholism is common. Analgesic nephropathy is usually asymptomatic and does not manifest until an elevated serum creatinine level is detected. The patient commonly presents with recurrent urinary tract infections. Proteinuria is usually less than 1 g/day. Impaired urine concentrating ability also occurs

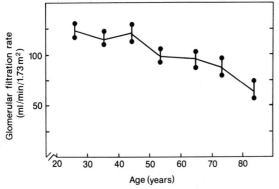

Figure 57–6. Age and glomerular filtration rate; — = mean values; ⫯ = standard deviation of the mean. (From Earle, D. P.: Cardiovasc. Med., 3:1257, 1978. Reprinted with permission from the Physicians World Communications Group.)

early, and sterile pyuria is seen in more than half of the patients with papillary necrosis. Occasionally, sloughed renal papillary tissue will cause ureteral colic and microscopic or gross hematuria. Gastric ulcer and anemia associated with secondary gastrointestinal bleeding are frequent.

The diagnosis is based on history of significant analgesic abuse and the demonstration of renal papillary necrosis by intravenous urography or retrograde pyelography. Papillary necrosis is usually bilateral and involves all the calyceal groups. Effective treatment is not available. Persons who continue to take even small amounts of analgesics will have progressive deterioration, and conversely, more than 80 per cent of patients who stop abusing analgesics will frequently show an improvement or at least a slowing of deterioration in renal function. Fluid intake should be generous to maintain urine output of at least 2 L/day. The prognosis is poorest in patients who present with small kidneys or a GFR of less than 20 ml/minute, hypertension, or persistent proteinuria. The presence of hematuria should be carefully investigated and cytologic studies performed regularly because of an increased incidence of transitional cell carcinoma.

Nonsteroidal anti-inflammatory drugs (NSAIDs) have the potential for significant nephrotoxicity and can produce a wide spectrum of nephrotoxic syndromes. The mechanisms by which NSAIDs can affect renal function include the following: (1) decreased synthesis of renal vasodilatory prostaglandins, (2) allergic interstitial nephritis, (3) impaired renin secretion, and (4) enhanced tubular water and sodium reabsorption (Cooper and Bennett, 1987; Kincaid-Smith, 1986). Oliguric renal failure occurs in patients with conditions (e.g., congestive heart failure, chronic renal insufficiency, cirrhosis and ascites, the elderly patient on diuretics) that may be associated with a decrease in renal perfusion and activation of the renin-angiotensin pathway. Angiotensin II is a potent stimulus for renal synthesis of prostaglandin E2, which through its vasodilatory effect, augments renal perfusion. NSAIDs inhibit synthesis of prostaglandins, especially prostaglandin E2, and thus lead to an acute decline in renal blood flow and GFR.

Patients recover baseline renal function within several days of discontinuing therapy with NSAIDs. Although all NSAIDs have been implicated as causes of acute renal failure, sulindac may have less deleterious effects and, thus, may be the agent of choice for patients at risk of renal insufficiency. Susceptible individuals should be persuaded to avoid NSAIDs. The other syndromes listed in Table 57–4 that are associated with NSAIDs may be caused by altered prostaglandin synthesis; are more common in high-risk patients, such as those characterized by pre-existent renal insufficiency, vascular disease or diabetes mellitus; and usually resolve after discontinuation of the NSAID.

Radiographic Contrast Media Nephropathy

Contrast media nephropathy is defined as an acute deterioration in renal function causally associated with intravascular exposure to these agents. It is the most common cause of hospital-acquired nephrotoxic acute renal failure. Radiographic contrast nephropathy rarely occurs in individuals with normal renal function. Among hospitalized patients with normal renal function, the incidence of nephrotoxicity (defined as a rise in serum creatinine level of > 1 mg/dl) from intravenous pyelography is 0.6 per cent (Abraham et al., 1983) and 2 per cent following major angiography. The major predisposing factors to contrast nephropathy are pre-existing renal insufficiency and diabetes mellitus. Approximately 5 per cent of patients with nondiabetic renal insufficiency (mean serum creatinine level of 4 mg/dl) develop nephrotoxicity, and the risk of toxicity reaches 9 per cent in diabetic persons with serum creatinine levels of 5 mg/dl (Parfrey et al., 1989). Additional factors contributing to increased risk of contrast nephropathy are age (older than 55 years), dehydration, hypertension, atherosclerotic peripheral vascular disease, hyperuricemia, proteinuria, and recent nephrotoxic drug exposure. It is apparent, therefore, that many of the patients frequently evaluated for urologic disease are at high risk of developing contrast nephropathy.

The onset of renal failure is usually abrupt and may range in severity from transient undetected deterioration in renal function to acute renal failure requiring dialysis. The diagnosis is usually based on a thorough history of possible contributing events. The clinical diagnosis is supported by nonspecific findings of tubular epithelial casts and amorphous urates in the urine sediment and a persistent nephrogram on 24-hour delayed radiographs. The clinical course is characterized in 50 per cent of patients by oliguria, which begins shortly after the contrast injection and persists for 2 to 4 days. Diuretics and osmotic agents are not effective, and the severity of renal failure correlates with the severity of pre-existing renal insufficiency. Although renal failure is

Table 57–4. RENAL SYNDROMES INDUCED BY NONSTEROIDAL/ANTI-INFLAMMATORY DRUGS

Acute renal failure
  Reversible—hemodynamically mediated (prerenal)
  Irreversible
Interstitial nephritis with or without nephrotic syndrome
Papillary necrosis
Hypertension
Sodium chloride and water retention
Hyperkalemic/hyporeninemic hypoaldosteronism

reversible in most patients, dialysis may be required, and permanent renal failure may occur in some patients with severe pre-existing renal insufficiency (Cramer et al., 1985).

Contrast nephropathy can be reduced by the cautious use of contrast materials in patients at high risk. The use of ultrasonography, isotope renogram, or retrograde pyelography in lieu of intravenous contrast studies will prevent many episodes of acute contrast nephropathy. If contrast media must be utilized, the risk of nephrotoxicity may be reduced by avoiding dehydration and by scheduling contrast studies at long intervals to avoid cumulative toxic effects. The use of the new nonionic, less hyperosmolar contrast agents may also reduce the risk of contrast nephropathy in high-risk patients. These agents decrease systemic and renal hemodynamic effects as well as urinary albumin and enzyme excretion. However, decreased renal function after infusion of nonionic contrast media has been observed, and reduced nephrotoxicity remains to be demonstrated (Schwab et al., 1989). The dose of contrast material should be small, and diuretics plus osmotic agents should be administered before and after the study. The use of other potentially nephrotoxic drugs should be avoided (Byrd and Sherman, 1970; Schwartz et al., 1963; Teruel et al., 1981).

POLYURIA

Polyuria is generally defined as a urine volume of 2500 ml or more per day. It is invariably accompanied by nocturia. Polyuria can be caused by (1) compulsive water drinking due to psychogenic factors, (2) inadequate vasopressin secretion (neurogenic diabetes insipidus), (3) diminished response of the renal tubule to vasopressin (nephrogenic diabetes insipidis), or (4) osmotic diuresis owing to excessive endogenous or exogenous solute load. Because polyuria can lead to a negative water balance and polydipsia (increased water intake), the clinician is frequently presented with the dilemma of determining whether polyuria or polydipsia is the initial event. Patients with water diuresis (psychogenic polydipsia or neurogenic or nephrogenic diabetes insipidus) typically excrete hypotonic urine with a urine osmolality as low as 50 mOsm/kg of water. Patients with polyuria due to osmotic diuresis characteristically show isotonic or slightly hypertonic urine osmolality.

Psychogenic Polydipsia

Affected individuals frequently are women with psychoneurotic disorders manifested by hypochondriac complaints and a pattern of a gradual onset of excessive daytime polydipsia. Urine osmolality is generally hypotonic to the plasma osmolality, which is usually normal. The plasma levels of antidiuretic hormone (ADH) are undetectable. Management includes gradual reduction of fluid intake, which must proceed with care because the individual is unable to concentrate urine, owing to urea washout from the renal medulla.

Neurogenic Diabetes Insipidus

Pituitary diabetes insipidus is sometimes seen as a consequence of brain tumor, after head trauma, or following pituitary ablation for acromegaly. The defect in antidiuretic hormone release is frequently transient because only 10 per cent of normal hypothalamic nuclei, which produce antidiuretic hormone, are necessary to avoid diabetes insipidus. The disease usually starts abruptly with the sudden onset of polyuria and polydipsia. Nocturia is almost invariably present, as is continuous thirst. Because, in these patients, polyuria causes polydipsia, the plasma osmolality is in the high-normal range. The plasma levels of ADH are undetectable. The treatment of neurogenic diabetes insipidus is primary replacement therapy with exogenous antidiuretic hormone.

Nephrogenic Diabetes Insipidus

Nephrogenic diabetes insipidus may be idiopathic or acquired. The idiopathic form is commonly genetic and more frequently affects males than females. During infancy, the disorder may present with dehydration, vomiting, lethargy, fever, hypernatremia, and hypertonic urine. The hypernatremia may be severe enough to cause permanent brain damage and the associated mental retardation frequently seen in this disorder. Older children may present with enuresis. Intravenous urograms often show marked hydronephrosis, dilated ureters, and megacystis presumably secondary to increased urine flow rates (Ramsey et al., 1974; Streitz and Streitz, 1988). The plasma osmolality is usually high-normal, and the ADH level is greatly elevated. An acquired form of nephrogenic diabetes insipidus may be caused by a variety of conditions (e.g., obstructive uropathy, sickle-cell disease, potassium depletion, hypercalcemia, chronic pyelonephritis, analgesic nephritis) and drugs (e.g., lithium, amphotericin B).

Unexplained hypernatremia (hyperosmolality) is often an important clue that suggests nephrogenic diabetes insipidus. The diagnosis is established by demonstrating inability to concentrate urine despite an appropriate osmotic stimulus (water deprivation), followed by the administration of exogenous ADH. In neurogenic diabetes insipidus, vasopressin administration corrects the concentrating defect, whereas in nephrogenic diabetes insipidus, vasopressin does not increase urine osmolality above 300 mOsm/kg (total unresponsiveness to antidiuretic hormone) or 800 mOsm/kg (partial nephrogenic diabetes insipidus) (Milles et al., 1983).

Treatment consists of correcting the underlying cause if possible. The diuretic chlorothiazide coupled with a low-sodium diet (2 g/day for an adult) has often been useful in reducing urine volume in patients with nephrogenic diabetes insipidus (Schotland et al., 1963). It acts by initially depleting total body sodium, which secondarily augments proximal tubular reabsorption and presumably results in increased water reabsorption and reduced urine volume. Untreated nephrogenic diabetes insipidus can result in severe dehydration, especially in an infant who is unable to respond to thirst by increasing water intake. Correction of dehydration should be with 3 per cent dextrose in water because 5 per cent dextrose alone or in saline solution may provoke an osmotic diuresis, increase water losses, and aggravate the condition. Partial nephrogenic diabetes insipidus, which is usually seen in females, may respond to chlorpropamide, which appears to sensitize the remaining functioning distal renal tubule to circulating endogenous vasopressin.

Osmotic Diuresis

Increased solute excretion per nephron decreases urine osmolality irrespective of the presence or absence of antidiuretic hormone. Polyuria due to osmotic diuresis is seen in glycosuria associated with diabetes mellitus, after relief of obstructive uropathy, with high-protein feeding, and transiently with mannitol or radiographic contrast media infusion. Diuresis after relief of urinary tract obstruction may be due to physiologic excretion of excess salt and water or osmotic diuresis due to retained urea. In addition, inappropriate losses of sodium and water may be due to an intrinsic defect in tubular reabsorption of sodium or impaired renal concentrating capacity. Postobstructive diuresis may require intravenous fluid administration, but urinary losses should be replaced only to the extent necessary to prevent hypovolemia, hypotension, hyponatremia, and hypokalemia. Orthostatic hypotension and tachycardia are excellent indicators for fluid replacement. Daily weights and electrolyte and fluid balance should be monitored. To distinguish between inappropriate diuresis and appropriate excretion of retained fluids, the rate of intravenous fluid administration can be gradually reduced and a corresponding reduction in urine volume watched for.

RADIOLOGIC DIAGNOSES

Radiologic studies may reveal unsuspected nephrologic disorders that have acute or chronic urologic significance.

Papillary Necrosis

The renal medulla and papilla are particularly vulnerable to ischemic necrosis, owing to the peculiar arrangement of its blood supply and the hypertonic environment. Even when healthy, it exists in a state of relative hypoxia because of the slow rate of blood flow in the vasa recta. Conditions that further reduce blood flow may therefore produce frank ischemic necrosis. The most common conditions among these in adults are diabetes, with its associated vascular disease and infection; urinary obstruction, which may reduce blood flow within the kidney; pyelonephritis; and sickle-cell disease, in which sickling is intensified by the hypertonic and relatively hypoxic renal medulla. The high concentration of drugs such as phenacetin in these regions probably contributes to papillary necrosis characteristic of analgesic abuse.

Papillary necrosis is a pathologic description frequently diagnosed by radiologic criteria and is not a clinical entity; therefore, the clinical manifestations may be quite varied. It may present as an acute episode of severe sepsis associated with systemic toxicity and ureteral obstruction owing to a sloughed papilla. This form most frequently occurs in patients with diabetes and pyelonephritis. Patients may also present with colicky flank pain and hematuria. Latent papillary necrosis is diagnosed during pyelography and is probably the most common presentation of papillary necrosis. It should be expected in patients with sterile pyuria and impaired concentrating abilities. The calyceal deformities of renal papillary necrosis may be divided into two forms, medullary and papillary. In the medullary form, there is central necrosis of the tip of the pyramid. Detachment of the necrotic papilla starts in the central region of the calyx, and a round or oval cavity occurs. In the papillary form, there is necrosis of the larger portion of the entire papilla. Detachment of the necrotic papilla usually begins in the region of the calyceal fornices, and the resulting defect is triangular in shape. Various stages of this process may be seen on the same radiographic examination. With poor renal function, retrograde pyelography may be required to demonstrate the calyceal changes.

Patients presenting with papillary slough and ureteral obstruction are probably best managed by ureteral catheterization or basket extraction if possible. Long-term remission may follow nephrectomy or partial nephrectomy because exacerbations are usually unilateral. As papillary necrosis proceeds, decreased GFR and kidney size may be minimized by careful management of infection, diabetes, and hydration.

MEDULLARY SPONGE KIDNEY

Medullary sponge kidney is characterized by dilatation of the collecting tubules, particularly in the papillary region. Intravenous urography characteristically demonstrates kidneys of normal size and shape, with ectatic distal collecting tubules containing clusters of calcifications. The calyceal blush may be distributed bilaterally or may involve only a few calyces. The medullary sponge kidney is asymptomatic, but it may be associated with nephrolithiasis or recurrent urinary tract infections. In the absence of complications, no therapy is required and the prognosis is excellent. Efforts to control the progression of nephrocalcinosis have not been assessed.

Table 57–5. PEDIATRIC RENAL DISEASES OF UROLOGIC SIGNIFICANCE

Hereditary nephritis and deafness (Alport syndrome)
Medullary cystic disease
Hemolytic uremic syndrome
Thrombotic thrombocytopenic purpura
Sickle cell nephropathy
Renal vein thrombosis

PEDIATRIC DISEASES OF UROLOGIC SIGNIFICANCE

The preceding discussion focused primarily on adult renal diseases of urologic significance. Renal disorders that are characteristically identified in a pediatric population are listed in Table 57–5.

REFERENCES

Abraham, P., Harkmen, S., and Kjellstrand, C.: Contrast nephropathy. *In* Massry, S. G., and Glassock, R. J. (Eds.): Textbook of Nephrology. Baltimore, Williams & Wilkins Co., 1983, p. 6.206.

Andres A., Praga, M., Bello, I., Diaz-Rolon, J. A., Gutierrez-Millet, V., Morales, J. M., and Rodicio, J. L.: Hematuria due to hypercalciuria and hyperuricosuria in adult patients. Kidney Int. 36:96, 1989.

Arneil, G. C., MacDonald, A. M., Murphy, A. V., and Sweet, E. M.: Renal venous thrombosis. Clin. Nephrol., 1:119, 1973.

Baker, S. L., and Dodds, E. C.: Obstruction of renal tubules during the excretion of haemoglobin. Br. J. Exp. Pathol., 6:247, 1925.

Beraud, J. J., Calvet, B., Durand, A., and Mimran, A.: Reversal of acute renal failure following percutaneous transluminal recanalization of an atherosclerotic renal artery occlusion. J. Hypertens., 7:909, 1989.

Berger, J., and Hinglais, N.: Les dépots intercapillaires d'IgA-IgG. J. Urol. Nephrol. (Paris), 74:694, 1968.

Besarab, A., Brown, R. S., Rubin, N. T., Salzman, E., Wirthlin, L., Steinman, T., Atlia, R. R., and Skillman, J. J.: Reversible renal failure following bilateral renal artery occlusive disease: Clinical features, pathology, and the role of surgical revascularization. JAMA, 235:28–38, 1976.

Bosniak, M. A.: Radiographic manifestations of massive arteriovenous fistula in renal carcinoma. Radiology, 85:454, 1965.

Bromberg, W. D., and Firlit, C. F.: Fibrinolytic therapy for renal vein thrombosis in the child. J. Urol., 143:86, 1990.

Buckalew, V. M., and Someren, A.: Renal manifestations of sickle cell disease. Arch. Intern. Med., 133:660, 1974.

Byrd, L., and Sherman, R. L.: Radiocontrast-induced acute renal failure: A clinical and pathophysiologic review. Medicine, 58:270, 1970.

Cameron, J. S., Glassock, R. J. (Eds.): The Nephrotic Syndrome. New York, Marcel Dekker, 1988.

Campieri, C., Raimondi, C., Fatone, F., Mignani, R., Di Luca, M., Todeschini, P., Stacchiotti, L., Boccadoro, R., Sanguinetti, M., Cacciari, M., et al.: Normalization of renal function and blood pressure after dissolution with intra-arterial fibrinolytics of a massive renal artery embolism to a solitary functioning kidney. Nephron, 51:399, 1989.

Cho, K. J., and Stanley, J. C.: Non-neoplastic congenital and acquired renal arteriovenous malformations and fistulas. Radiology, 129:333, 1978.

Clark, R. A., Gallant, T. E., and Alexander, E. S.: Angiographic management of traumatic arteriovenous fistulas: Clinical results. Radiology, 147:9, 1983.

Cooper, K., and Bennett, W. M.: Nephrotoxicity of common drugs used in clinical practice. Arch. Intern. Med., 147:1213–1218, 1987.

Cramer, B. C., Parfrey, P. S., Hutchinson, T. A., Baran, D., Melanson, D. M., Ethier, R. E., and Seely, J. F.: Renal function following infusion of radiologic contrast material: A prospective controlled study. Arch. Intern. Med., 145:87–89, 1985.

D'Amico, G.: Clinical features and natural history in adults with IgA nephropathy. Am. J. Kidney Dis., 12:353–357, 1988.

Earle, D. P. (Ed.): Manual of Clinical Nephrology. Philadelphia, W. B. Saunders Co., 1982, pp. 29–30, 71–72.

Fassett, R. G., Horgan, B. A., and Mathew, T. H.: Detection of glomerular bleeding by phase-contrast microscopy. Lancet, 1:1432, 1982.

Gajewski, J., Gonzales, C. I., and Rich, M.: Genitourinary diseases. *In* Singer, R. B., and Levinson, L. (Eds.): Medical Risks. Lexington, D. C. Health and Co., 1976, pp. 151–156.

Ginsberg, J. M., Chang, B. S., Matarese, R. A., and Garella, S.: Use of single voided urine samples to estimate quantitative proteinuria. N. Engl. J. Med., 309:1543, 1983.

Glassock, R. J.: Hematuria and pigmenturia. *In* Massry, S. B., and Glassock, R. J. (Eds.): Textbook of Nephrology. Baltimore, Williams & Wilkins Co., 1983, p. 414.

Gomes, M. M. R., and Bernatz, P. E.: Arteriovenous fistulas: A review and ten year experience at the Mayo Clinic. Mayo Clin. Proc., 45:81, 1970.

Humphreys, M. H.: Thromboembolic disorders of the major renal vessels. *In* Brenner, B. M., and Rector, F. C. (Eds.): The Kidney. Philadelphia, W. B. Saunders Co., 1981, pp. 742–750.

Iloreta, A. T., and Blaufox, M. D.: Natural history of postbiopsy renal arteriovenous fistula: A 10-year follow-up. Nephron, 24:250, 1979.

Kassirer, J. P.: Atheroembolic renal disease. *In* Glassock, R. J. (Ed.): Current Therapy of Nephrology and Hypertension. ed. 2. Toronto, B. C. Decker, 1987, pp. 229–234.

Kincaid-Smith, P.: Effects of non-narcotic analgesics on the kidney. Drugs, 32:109, 1986.

King, S. E., and Gronbeck, C.: Benign and pathological albuminuria: A study of 600 hospitalized cases. Ann. Intern. Med., 36:765, 1952.

Knochel, J. P.: Hematuria in sickle trait: The effect of intravenous distilled water, urinary alkalinization, and diuresis. Arch. Intern. Med., 123:160, 1969.

Labovitz, E. D., Steinmuller, S. R., Henderson, L. W., McCurdy, D. K., and Goldberg, M.: "Benign" hematuria with focal glomerulitis in adults. Ann. Intern. Med., 77:723, 1972.

Larsen, S. O., and Thysell, H.: Four years follow-up of asymptomatic isolated proteinuria diagnosed in a general health survey. Acta Med. Scand., 186:375, 1969.

Lisbona, R., Palayew, M. J., Satin, R., and Hyams, B. B.: Radionuclide detection of iatrogenic arteriovenous fistulas of the genitourinary system. Radiology, 134:201, 1980.

Llach, F., Papper, S., and Massry, S. G.: The clinical spectrum of renal vein thrombosis: Acute and chronic. Am. J. Med., 69:819, 1980.

Messing, E., Kessler, R., and Kavaney, P. B.: Renal arteriovenous fistulas. Urology, 8:101, 1976.

Messing, E. M., Young, T. B., Hunt, V. B., Emoto, S. E., and Wehbie, J. M.: The significance of asymptomatic microhematuria in men 50 or more years old: Findings of a home screening study using urinary dipsticks. J. Urol., 137:919, 1987.

Middleton, W. D., Kellman, G. M., Melson, G. L., and Madrazo, B. L.: Postbiopsy renal transplant arteriovenous fistulas: Color Doppler US characteristics. Radiology, 171:253, 1989.

Milles, J. J., Spruce, B., and Baylis, P. H.: A comparison of diagnostic methods to differentiate diabetes insipidus from primary polydipsia. Acta. Endocrinol., 104:410–416, 1983.

Nelson, B. D., Brosman, S. A., and Goodwin, W. E.: Renal arteriovenous fistulas. J. Urol., 109:779, 1973.

O'Brien, D. P., III, Parrott, T. S., Walton, K. N., and Lewis, E. L.: Renal arteriovenous fistulas. Surg. Gynecol. Obstet., 139:739, 1974.

Parfrey, P. S., Griffiths, S. M., Barrett, B. J., Paul, M. D., Genge, M., Withers, J., Farid, N., and McManamon, P. J.: Contrast material–induced renal failure in patients with diabetes mellitus, renal insufficiency, or both: A prospective controlled study. N. Engl. J. Med., 320:143, 1989.

Perkins, R. P., Jacobsen, D. S., Feder, F. P., Lipchik, E. O., and Fine, P. H.: Return of renal function after late embolectomy. N. Engl. J. Med., 276:1194, 1967.

Pommer, W., Bronder, E., Greiser, E., Helmert, U., Jesdinsky, H. J., Klimpel, A., Borner, K., and Molzahn, M.: Regular analgesic intake and the risk of end-stage renal failure. Am. J. Nephrol., 9:403, 1989.

Ramsey, E. W., Morrin, P. A. F., and Bruce, A. W.: Nephrogenic diabetes insipidus associated with massive hydronephrosis and bladder neck obstruction. J. Urol., 111:225, 1974.

Randolph, M. F., and Greenfield, M.: Proteinuria: A six-year study of normal infants, preschool, and school-age populations previously screened for urinary tract diseases. Am. J. Dis. Child., 114:631, 1967.

Rennie, I. D. B., and Keen, H.: Evaluation of clinical methods for detecting proteinuria. Lancet, 2:489, 1967.

Robinson, R. R.: Clinical significance of isolated proteinuria. *In* Avram, M. M. (Ed.): Proteinuria. New York and London, Plenum Medical Book Company, 1985, pp. 67–82.

Rowland, L. P., and Penn, A. S.: Myoglobinuria. Med. Clin. North Am., 56:1233, 1972.

Sandler, D. P., Smith, J. C., Weinberg, C. R., Buckalew, V. M., Jr., Dennis, V. W., Blythe, W. B., and Burgess, W. P.: Analgesic use and chronic renal disease. N. Engl. J. Med., 320:1238, 1989.

Schmidt, J. D., and Flocks, R. H.: Urologic aspects of sickle-cell hemoglobin. J. Urol., 106:740, 1971.

Schotland, M. G., Grumbach, M. M., and Strauss, J.: The effects of chlorothiazides in nephrogenic diabetes insipidus. Pediatrics, 31:741, 1963.

Schramek, P., Schuster, F. X., Georgopoulos, M., Porpaczy, P., and Maier, M.: Value of urinary erythrocyte morphology in assessment of symptomless microhaematuria. Lancet, 2:1316, 1989.

Schrier, R. W. (Ed.): Renal and Electrolyte Disorders, ed. 2. Boston, Little, Brown & Co., 1980, p. 417.

Schwab, S. J., Hlatky, M. A., Pieper, K. S., Davidson, C. J., Morris, K. G., Skelton, T. N., and Bashore, T. M.: Contrast nephrotoxicity: A randomized controlled trial of a nonionic and an ionic radiographic contrast agent. N. Engl. J. Med., 320:149, 1989.

Schwartz, G. J., Haycock, G. B., and Spitzer, A.: Plasma creatinine and urea concentration in children: Normal values for age and sex. J. Pediatr., 88:828, 1976.

Schwartz, W. B., Hurwit, A., and Ettinger, A.: Intravenous urography in the patient with renal insufficiency. N. Engl. J. Med., 269:277, 1963.

Skinner, R. E., Hefty, T., Long, T. D., Rosch, J., and Forsyth, M.: Recovery of function in a solitary kidney after intra-arterial thrombolytic therapy. J. Urol., 141:108, 1989.

Streitz, J. M., Jr., and Streitz, J. M.: Polyuric urinary tract dilatation with renal damage. J. Urol., 139:784, 1988.

Strom, T., Muehrcke, R. C., and Smith, R. D.: Sickle cell anemia with the nephrotic syndrome and renal vein obstruction. Arch. Intern. Med., 129:104, 1972.

Teruel, J. L., Marcen, R., Onaindia, J. M., Serrano, A., Quereda, C., and Ortuno, J.: Renal function impairment caused by intravenous urography, a prospective study. Arch. Intern. Med., 141:1271, 1981.

Thompson, I. M., Schneider, R., and Lababidi, Z.: Thrombectomy of neonatal renal vein thrombosis. J. Urol., 113:396, 1975.

Vaamonde, C. A.: Renal papillary necrosis in sickle cell hemoglobinopathies. Semin. Nephrol., 4:48–64, 1984.

van den Wall Bake, A. W., Daha, M. R., and van Es, L. A.: Immunopathogenetic aspects of IgA nephropathy. Nephrologie, 10:141, 1989.

Vega, R., Shanberg, A. M., and Malloy, T. R.: The use of epsilon-aminocaproic acid in sickle cell trait hematuria. J. Urol., 105:552, 1971.

Wagner, M. G., Smith, F. G., Jr., Tinglof, B. O., and Cornberg, E.: Epidemiology of proteinuria: A study of 4807 school children. J. Pediatr., 73:825, 1968.

Wickre, C. G., and Golper, T. A.: Complications of percutaneous needle biopsy of the kidney. Am. J. Nephrol., 2:173, 1982.

INDEX

Note: Page numbers in *italics* refer to illustrations;
page numbers followed by t refer to tables.

A

Abdomen, computed tomography of,
  attenuation values in, 482, 483t
  plain film radiographs of, in cloacal mal-
    formation, 1826, *1827*
  in excretory urography, 412–413, *413*,
    442, *442*
  in neonatal abdominal mass evaluation,
    1596, *1600*
  in unilateral renal agenesis, 1363, *1363*
  in urinary lithiasis, 2103, *2103*
  in urinary schistosomiasis, 895, *896*
  in urinary tract infection, 749
  stab wounds to, during pregnancy, 2593,
    2593
Abdominal incision(s), in renal surgery,
  2423, *2425–2428*, 2427
  in renovascular surgery, 2528, *2529*
Abdominal mass, neonatal, 1595–1599
  bilateral, 1596, *1597*
  excretory urography in, 1596, *1600*
  frequency of causes of, 1596, 1596t
  midline, 1596, *1598–1599*
  physical examination in, 1596
  plain abdominal radiography in, 1596
  radionuclide renal scan in, 1597
  solid or mixed density, 1598–1599
  transillumination in, 1596
  ultrasonography in, 1596t, 1596–1597,
    1598t
Abdominal musculature, congenital
  hypoplasia of, 1593, *1593*, 1605. See also
  Prune-belly syndrome
Abdominal paravertebral sympathetic
  ganglion, neuroblastoma of, 1989
Abdominal quadrant, upper, auscultation of,
  312
Abdominal stoma(s), 2608–2610
  circular incision for, 2609
  flush stoma, 2609
  loop end ileostomy, 2609–2610, *2610*
  nipple stoma ("rosebud"), 2609, *2609*

Abdominal stoma(s) *(Continued)*
  site of, 2608–2609
Abdominal wall, anterolateral, anatomy of,
  3, *10–13*, 12
  in prune-belly syndrome, 1852, *1852*,
    1867–1868, 1868–1869
  posterior, anatomy of, 3, *10–13*, 12
Abscess. See also individual types
  of appendix ureteral obstruction due to,
    549
  of kidney. See *Renal abscess*
  of prostate, 819–820
  of psoas muscle, ureteral obstruction due
    to, 557, *557*
  of retroperitoneum, ureteral obstruction
    due to, 557
  of Skene's gland, vs. urethral diverticula,
    2816
  of tubo-ovarian structures, ureteral ob-
    struction due to, 543–544
  of urethral diverticula, 2820
  perinephric. See *Perinephric abscess*
  renal. See *Renal abscess*
Absent testes syndrome, 1518–1519
Absorbent products, for detrusor
  overactivity, 654–655
  for neuromuscular voiding dysfunction,
    628
  for stress incontinence, 655
Acetazolamide, for uric acid lithiasis, 2116
Acetrizoate, chemical structure of, *402*
Acetylcholine, as neurotransmitter, 166
  for bladder emptying, 629
  in erection, 715
  ureteral effects of, 133
Acid-base balance, 79–80, *81*
  in neonate, 1346
  in renal insufficiency, 2332
  net acid excretion in, 80
  proximal bicarbonate reabsorption in,
    80
Acidosis, in acute renal failure, 2053
  metabolic. See *Metabolic acidosis*

Acquired immunodeficiency syndrome
  (AIDS), 846–859. See also *Human
  immunodeficiency virus (HIV); Human
  immunodeficiency virus infection*
  as epidemic, 853–854
  bacille Calmette-Guérin immunization and,
    954
  deficient cell-mediated immunity in, 851–852
  definition of, 852t
  nephropathy in, 857
  progression in, 852
  prostate in transmission of, 222, 222t
  seminal vesicles in transmission of, 222, 222t
Acrosome, of spermatozoon, male infertility
  and, 670, 685–686
ACTH. See *Adrenocorticotropic hormone
  (ACTH)*
Actin, in smooth muscle contractility, 116–
  117, *116–117*, 145–146
Actinomycin D, in Wilms' tumor, 1983t
Action potentials, 113–114, *113–114*
  motor unit, 591
Activity product ratio (APR), in estimation
  of calcium stone-forming activity, 2131
Acupuncture, for bladder contractility
  inhibition, 620–621
Addison's disease, due to histoplasmosis, 932
  signs and symptoms of, 2381t, 2381–2382
  test for, 2382–2383
  treatment of, 2383
Adenocarcinoma, of bladder. See *Bladder
  cancer, adenocarcinoma*
  of cervix, DES-related, 2002
  of exstrophied bladder, 2002
  of prostate, 1159–1214. See also *Prostatic
  cancer, adenocarcinoma*
  of rete testis, 1253–1254
  of seminal vesicles, characteristics of, 2948
    management of, 2948–2949
  of upper urinary tract, 1139
  of vagina, DES-related, 2002
    in infant, 2002
Adenofibroma, of testis, 1254

Adenofibromyoma, of testis, 1254
Adenoma. See also anatomic site
  adrenal, 2373, *2373*, 2379, *2379*, 2386t
  Leydig cell, 2379
  nephrogenic, of bladder, 1100, *1101*
  pituitary, 679–680, 2374
  renal cortical, 1056
  testicular, 1254
Adenomatoid tumor, of testicular adnexa, 1256
  of testis, 1254
3',5'-Adenosine monophosphate (AMP), 2125
Adenosine triphosphate (ATP), in kidney preservation, 2506
ADH. See *Antidiuretic hormone (ADH)*
Adrenal adenoma, 2379, *2379*
  causing hyperaldosteronism, age distribution of, 2386t
  computed tomography of, 2373, *2373*
  site distribution of, 2386t
  weights of, 2386t
Adrenal artery(ies), anatomy of, 13, *15*, 22
Adrenal carcinoma, 2376–2381
  aldosterone-secreting, 2380
  causing hyperaldosteronism, age distribution of, 2386t
  classification of, 2376, 2376t
  computed tomography of, 2373, *2374*
  Cushing's syndrome and, 2379
  ganglioneuroma as, *2378*
  in children, 2380
  incidentally discovered, 2376–2377, 2377t, *2377–2378*
  medical management of, 2380–2381
  metastatic, 2378, *2378*
  myelolipoma as, 2377–2378, *2378*
  surgical management of, 2380
  weights of, 2386t
Adrenal cortex, aldosterone-secreting tumors of, 2380, 2385
  diagnostic studies of, 2387–2388, 2388t
  treatment of, 2388–2389
  embryology of, 2362–2363
  estrogen-secreting tumors of, 2379–2380
  functional anatomy of, 21, *22*
  growth of, 2361, *2361*
  hormones of, 2364, *2364*. See also named hormone
    excess of, 2364–2365
    metabolism of, 2367–2368
    regulation of release of, *2365*, 2365–2366
  hyperfunction of, 2360
  malignant tumors of. See *Adrenal carcinoma*
  mature, microscopic anatomy of, 2363, *2363*
  physiology of, 2364–2368
  testosterone-secreting tumors of, 2379
  zona fasciculata of, 21, *22*
  zona glomerulosa of, 21, *22*
  zona reticularis of, 21, *22*
Adrenal cyst(s), 2381, *2382*
Adrenal gland(s), 2360–2406
  anatomic location of, 20–21, 2362, *2362*
  anatomy of, 20–22, 2360–2364, *2361–2363*
  androgens of. See *Androgen(s), adrenal*; specific hormone
  anterior anatomic relation(s) of, 21, *21*
  arteries of, 22
  blood supply to, 2362, *2362*
  carcinoma of. See *Adrenal carcinoma*
  embryology of, 2361
  histology of, *2363*, 2363–2364
  historical background of, 2360
  in newborn infant, size of, 21, *21*

Adrenal gland(s) *(Continued)*
  in unilateral renal agenesis, 1362
  injury to, 2571
  lymphatic(s) of, 22
  magnetic resonance imaging of, 488, 490
  physiology of, 2364–2369, *2364–2369*
  posterior anatomic relation(s) of, 21, *22*
  size and shape of, 21, *21*
  surgery of, 2398–2406
    flank approach in, 2401, *2401–2403*, 2403
    modified posterior approach in, 2399–2401, *2400*
    options in, 2398, 2398t
    posterior approach in, 2399, *2399*
    results of, 2405
    techniques in, 2398–2405
    thoracoabdominal approach in, 2403, *2403*
    transabdominal approach in, 2403–2405, *2404–2406*
  venous drainage of, 22, 2362, *2363*
Adrenal hemorrhage, neonatal, 1610–1613, *1611–1612*, 2361, 2361
  clinical features of, 1611
  etiologic factors in, 1611
  neuroblastoma vs., 1612–1613
  treatment of, 1613
  ultrasonography in, 1611–1612, *1612*
Adrenal hyperplasia, congenital, 1519–1522, 1953–1954, *1954*
  as neonatal emergency, 1602, *1603*
  clinical features of, 1519–1521, 1520t, *1521*, 1953–1954, *1954*
  computed tomography of, 2373, *2373*
  due to 11β-hydroxylase deficiency, 1520t, 1521, 1954
  due to 21-hydroxylase deficiency, 1519–1521, 1520t, *1521*, 1954, *1954*
  embryology of virilization of, 1954, *1954*
  male infertility due to, 665, 679
  management of, 1521–1522
  pathophysiology of, 1521
  prenatal diagnosis of, 1570
  radiography in, 1602, *1603*
  lipoid, 1520t, 1523
Adrenal insufficiency, 2381–2384
  in surgical patient, 2343, 2343t
  selective, 2383–2384
  signs and symptoms of, 2381t, 2381–2382
  treatment of, 2383
Adrenal mass, incidentally discovered, 2376–2377, 2377t, *2377–2378*
Adrenal medulla, embryology of, 2363
  functional anatomy of, 21, *22*
  neuroanatomy of, 22
  physiology of, 2368–2369
Adrenal myelolipoma, ultrasonography in, 462, *463*
  speed propagation artifact in, 462, *463*
Adrenal rest tumor, of testis, 1254
Adrenal vein(s), anatomy of, *15*, 16, 22
  left, anatomy of, *15*, 16, 22
  right, anatomy of, *15*, 16, 22
Adrenalectomy, bilateral, for Cushing's disease, 2374
Adrenergic agonists. See also *Alpha-adrenergic agonists*
  ureteral effects of, 134
Adrenergic antagonists. See also *Alpha-adrenergic antagonists; Beta-adrenergic antagonists*
  ureteral effects of, 134
Adrenergic neurotransmitters, 152t, 152–154
Adrenocorticotropic hormone (ACTH), ectopic secretion of, 2369, 2370t

Adrenocorticotropic hormone (ACTH) *(Continued)*
  treatment of, 2374, *2375*
  measurement of, in Cushing's syndrome, 2372
  regulation of release of, 2365, *2365*
Adrenocorticotropic hormone (ACTH) stimulation test, 2343
  for adrenal insufficiency, 2383, *2383*
Adrenogenital syndrome, 1953–1954, *1954*. See also *Adrenal hyperplasia, congenital*
  hypospadias vs., 1895
  neonatal hypertension due to, 1601
Adrenoreceptors, 2369t
Adriamycin. See *Doxorubicin*
African river blindness, 916
Aggregation, of crystals, 2096
Aging, in urinary lithiasis, 2087–2088, *2088*, 2140
  incontinence and, 644
  male, estradiol levels in, 235
    hypothalamic-pituitary-testicular axis in, 185, *185*
    impotence due to, 721
    prostatic change(s) due to, 57
    steroids in, differential effects of, 230, *231*
  nocturia and, 644
  perioperative pulmonary care and, 2322
  renal blood flow in, 73
  renal function and, 70–71
  residual urine volume and, 644
  ureteral function and, 130, *130–131*
  urinary tract infection in, 795–797
    bacteriology in, 796, *797*
    clinical presentation in, 795–796
    epidemiology of, 795t, 795–797, *796*
    pathophysiology of, 796
    significance of, 796–797
    treatment of, 797
Agonadism, male, 1518–1519
AIDS. See *Acquired immunodeficiency syndrome (AIDS)*
Albarran's procedure, 2272
Albright's solution, for renal tubular acidosis, 2129
Albumin, free, binding protein properties of, 235
  in surgical patient, 2344
Alcock's canal, anatomy of, 66
Alcohol ingestion, impotence due to, 717
  male infertility due to, 684–685
Aldosterone, action of, 2367
  renal physiologic effects of, 88
  renal secretion of, 104–105
  secretion of, control of, 2366, *2366*
  synthesis of, *2364*
Aldosterone-secreting tumor(s), of adrenal cortex. See under *Adrenal cortex*
Aldosteronism, primary. See *Hyperaldosteronism*
Alexandrite laser, 2924
Alkalization therapy, for uric acid lithiasis, 2116
Alkalosis, respiratory, as complication of mechanical ventilation, 2325
Alleles, definition of, 267
Allen clamp, 2602, *2603*, 2604
Allen stirrups, 3001, *3001*
Allergic reactions, to blood transfusion, 2337
Allergy, food, in enuresis, 1625
Allograft rejection, crisis treatment for, 2515t
  renal, 2512–2517
    accelerated, 2512
    acute, 2512–2513, *2513*
    blood transfusions and, 2515

Anesthesia *(Continued)*
  pulmonary effects of, 2323
  priapism due to, 723–724
  regional, to prevent thromboembolic disease, 2329
Aneuploidy, in tumor progression, 1041–1042
Aneurysm, of abdominal aorta, ureteral obstruction due to, *536*, 536–537
  of iliac artery, ureteral obstruction due to, 537, *537*
  of renal artery, 1386–1387, 2522–2524, *2523–2524*
    as complication of renal revascularization, 2547
  saccular, 2022
Angiitis, hypersensitivity, chronic renal failure due to, 2058
Angiogenesis, tumor, 1044–1045
  angiogenin in, 1045
  copper in, 1045
  fibroblast growth factor in, 1044–1045
  transforming growth factor-α in, 1045
Angiogenin, in tumor angiogenesis, 1045
Angiography, digital subtraction, in renovascular hypertension, 2029
  Doppler ultrasound, in renovascular hypertension, 2029t, 2029–2030
Angioinfarction, in upper urinary tract urothelial tumors, 1146
Angiokeratoma, in Fabry's disease, 880
Angiokeratoma of Fordyce, *869*, 880
Angioma, of penis, 1264
Angiomatoid tumor, of testis, 1254
Angiomyolipoma, renal, *1058–1060*, 1058–1061
  in children, 1987
  in tuberous sclerosis, 1462
  ultrasonography in, 462, *463*
  speed propagation artifact in, 462, *463*
Angioplasty, percutaneous transluminal, of renal artery, in atherosclerotic renal artery disease, 2039–2040
  in renovascular hypertension, 2038–2039, 2039t
Angiosarcoma, of bladder, 1136
  renal, 1085
Angiotensin II, 93–94, 2025
  physiologic actions of, *93*, 93–94, 2025
  physiologic effects of, 92
  receptors of, 94
  renal metabolism of, 104
Angiotensin-converting enzyme, 93, 2025
Angiotensinogen, 93, 2024–2025
Anion gap, definition of, 82–83
  in renal tubular acidosis, 1347
  urinary, in renal tubular acidosis, 1348
Aniridia, in Wilms' tumor, 1968
Anorchia, 1518–1519
  bilateral, cryptorchidism vs., 1549
  infertility due to, 681
Anosmia, in Kallmann's syndrome, 677
Antiandrogens, for benign prostatic hyperplasia, 1023
  for prostatic cancer, 1212–1213
Antibiotic(s), for perinephric abscess, 2257
  perioperative, for transurethral surgery, 2905
  preoperative, radical cystectomy and, 2751
  use of, in vesicovaginal fistula repair, 2822
Antibiotic bowel preparation, complications of, 2600–2601
  in urinary intestinal diversion, 2600, 2600t
Antibody toxin targeting, in cancer therapy, 1047

Anticholinergic agent(s), for bladder contractility inhibition, 614–615
  atropine as, 614–615
  methantheline as, 615
  propantheline as, 615
  for enuresis, 1627
  transient incontinence due to, 645, 645t
Anticholinesterases, ureteral effects of, 133
Anticodon, *273*, 274
Antidepressants, tricyclic, for bladder contractility inhibition, 617–619
  doxepin as, 618
  imipramine as, 618
  impotence due to, 717
Antidiuretic hormone (ADH), in fetus and newborn, 1351
  intracellular actions of, 78, *79*
  nocturnal, bladder control and, 1622
  receptor mechanisms for, 105–106, *106*
  renal metabolism of, 103
  renal physiologic effects of, 86
Antidiuretic hormone-like agents, for nocturnal bladder storage problems, 626
Antigen(s), HLA, in renal transplantation, 2508, 2513, 2514t
  in vesicoureteral reflux, 1692
  inheritance patterns of, 2514
  MHC, incompatibility with, 2513, *2513*, 2514t
  prostate-specific. See *Prostate-specific antigen*
  stone-specific, in urine, 2098
Antihypertensives, impotence due to, 717, 3036
Anti-inflammatory agents, for urinary lithiasis, 2108
Antimetastatic genes, 1043–1044
Anti-oncogenes, 1040–1041
  in familial cancer patterns, 292
  in malignant transformation, 292–293
  in retinoblastoma, 292–293
  in testicular teratocarcinoma, 293
  in Wilms' tumor, 293
Antiplatelet therapy, for thromboembolic disease, 2329
Antireflux valve(s), intestinal, 2616–2618
  intussuscepted ileal, *2617*, 2617–2618
  intussuscepted ileocecal, 2617, *2617*
  nipple, 2618, *2618*
Antispasmodic agents, for urinary lithiasis, 2108
Antisperm antibody(ies), laboratory findings in, 672–673
  ELISA for, 672
  Immunobead Assay for, 672
  indications for, 673
  Sperm-Mar test for, 672
  male infertility due to, 686–687
  steroid therapy for, 686–687, 687t
Anuria, in bilateral renal agenesis, 1360
  neonatal, 1601–1602
  reflex, in ureteral obstruction, 525–526
Anus, imperforate, 1650–1652
  anomalies associated with, 1605
  EMG studies in, 1652
  high, embryology of, 1320, *1323*
  imaging studies in, 1652, *1653*
  prenatal diagnosis of, 1570, *1570*
  spinal cord abnormality in, 1650, 1652
  urodynamic studies in, 1652
  physical examination of, 314
Aorta, abdominal, anatomy of, 12–13
  aneurysm of, ureteral obstruction due to, *536*, 536–537
  coarctation of, neonatal hypertension due to, 1601

Aorta *(Continued)*
  thrombosis of, as complication of revascularization, 2548
Aortic stenosis, perioperative management of, 2318
Aortitis, Takayasu's, 2022
Aortorenal bypass graft, 2538–2541, *2539*
  saphenous vein insertion in, 2540–2541, *2541–2542*
  saphenous vein procurement in, 2539–2540, *2540–2541*
Aphallia, 1925–1926, *1926*
Apomorphine, for erectile dysfunction, 3053
Apoptosis, 251
Appendectomy, for orthotopic Mainz pouch, 2694, *2694*
Appendiceal continence mechanisms, in self-catheterizing pouches, 2699–2700, *2700*
Appendiceal tunneling techniques, in self-catheterizing pouches, 2699, *2699*
Appendix, abscess of, ureteral obstruction due to, 549
  mucocele of, ureteral obstruction due to, 549
  schistosomiasis of, 906
Appendix epididymis, 1222, 1223
  embryology of, 58, 1334, 1500
Appendix testis, 1222, 1223
  embryology of, 58, 1500
  torsion of, 1557–1558
  surgical management of, 1946, *1946*
APUDomas, 1991
Arachidonic acid, in eicosanoid synthesis, 98, *98*
Arcus tendineus, anatomic relationships of, 64, *65*
Arginine, renal reabsorption of, 85
Argon laser, 2924
Armillifera armillatus, 919
Aromatase inhibitors, for male infertility, 688, 690t
Arrhythmias, intraoperative, 2318
  postoperative, 2318
  preoperative, 2317–2318
  treatment of, 2318t
Arterial pressure monitoring, in perioperative cardiac care, complications of, 2320
  indications for, 2319–2320
  techniques of, 2320
Arteriography, renal, in malacoplakia, 767, *768*
  in renal cell carcinoma, 1072, *1072*
  in Wilms' tumor, 1978
Arteriovenous fistula, acquired, 2524
  congenital, 2524
  idiopathic, 2524
  renal, 2524–2525, *2525*
  hematuria in, 2070, *2071*
Arteriovenous hemofiltration, continuous, in acute renal failure, 2053t, 2054
Arteritis (Takayasu's disease), 2526–2527, *2527*
Artificial sweeteners, bladder cancer due to, 1097
AS-721 urinary prosthesis, 2645, *2646*
AS-742 urinary prosthesis, 2647
AS-761 urinary prosthesis, 2645, *2647*
AS-800 urinary prosthesis, 2647, *2647*
Ascites, urinary, in newborn, 1602–1605, *1604*, 1876, *1877–1878*
  due to hydronephrosis, 1603
  due to posterior urethral valves, 1603, 1876, *1877–1878*
  evaluation in, 1603, *1604*
  treatment in, 1603, 1605

Candidal infection *(Continued)*
    regional therapy in, 942
        surgical, 943
        systemic therapy in, 942–943
    urine microscopy in, 323, *323, 325, 940,*
        940–941
    pyelonephritis due to, 939
    tinea cruris vs., 876
    vaginitis due to, 833–834, 938–939
        etiology and diagnosis of, 833–834, 938–
            939
        treatment of, 834, 939
Candiduria, microscopy in, 323, *323, 325,*
    940, 940–941
Capnography, in perioperative cardiac care,
    2321
Captopril, in Goldblatt hypertension model,
    2026
    peripheral plasma renin and, 2032, *2032,*
        2033t
Captopril renogram, in renovascular
    hypertension, 2033, *2033*
Caput epididymis, 203, *204.* See also
    Epididymis
Carbenicillin, serum vs. urinary levels of,
    743t
Carbon dioxide laser, 2924
    for condyloma acuminatum of genitalia,
        2924–2925
    for penile cancer, 2925, *2926*
Carcinoid, of testis, 1254
Carcinoma. See under anatomic site or
    histologic type
Carcinosarcoma, bladder, 1134, *1135*
    renal, 1085
Cardiac anomalies, in prune-belly syndrome,
    1855
Cardiac glycoside, ureteral effects of, 135
Cardiac morbidity, anesthesia and, 2326
Cardiac output, decreased, as complication
    of mechanical ventilation, 2324–2325
    in perioperative cardiac care, measurement
        of, 2321
Cardiac patient, perioperative care of, 2315–
    2321. See also *Perioperative care, of*
    cardiac patient
Cardinal ligaments, anatomy of, 2784, *2785,*
    2788
Cardiorespiratory system, evaluation of,
    prior to renal surgery, 2414–2415
Cardiovascular system, complications of,
    following radical nephrectomy, 2447
C-arm fluoroscopy unit, percutaneous
    nephrostomy utilizing, 2238, *2239–2240*
Casts, in urinary sediment microscopy, 322,
    324
Catecholamine(s), actions of, 2369, 2369t
    elevated, in neuroblastoma, 1991
        in pheochromocytoma, 2393, 2393t
    metabolism of, 2368–2369, *2369*
    renal physiologic effects of, 88
    storage of, 2368
    synthesis of, 2368, *2368*
Catecholamine receptors, 2369t
Cathepsin D, properties of, 249
Catheter. See specific type, e.g., *Councill*
    catheter
Catheterization, umbilical artery, renal artery
    thrombosis due to, 1601, 1614
    ureteral. See *Ureteral catheterization*
    urethral. See *Urethral catheter; Urethral*
        catheterization
Catheterizing pouch(es), for urinary
    diversion, 2698–2717. See also *Self-*
    catheterizing pouch(es); named pouch

Cauda epididymis, 203, *204.* See also
    Epididymis
Cavernosal injection, of vasoactive agents,
    for impotence, 3055–3057, *3056,* 3056t
Cavernosography, in impotence, 718
Cavernotomy, for genitourinary tuberculosis,
    976
Cavernous artery, anatomy of, 709, *710,*
    2963, *2964*
    laceration of, priapism due to, 724
    occlusion of, revascularization procedures
        in, 3063, *3064,* 3065
    perfusion pressure of, determination of,
        3043, *3043*
    new studies of, 3044
Cavernous nerve(s), anatomic distribution of,
    2963–2964
    anatomic relationship of, 714, *714*
        urethrectomy and, 2774
    autonomic, testing of, in impotent male,
        3038, *3039*
Cavernous tissue, biopsy of, 3052
Cavernous vein, anatomy of, 2962, *2962*
Cecoureterocele, 1423, 1757, *1759*
Cecum, for augmentation cystoplasty, 2636,
    2638, *2639–2641*
Celiac arterial trunk, anatomy of, 13, *15*
Celiac plexus, anatomy of, 17
Cell(s), interaction of, in renal transplant
    rejection, 2513, *2513*
    stem, 1031
Cell cycle, 1034–1036
    mitotic index for, 1035, 1035t
    phases of, 1034, *1035*
    thymidine-labeling index for, 1035–1036,
        1036t
Cell transfection, in cancer therapy, 1047–
    1048
Cellular cast, in urine, *324*
Cellular death, genetically programmed, 298
Cellular growth factors, 236, 236–237
    autocrine, 236, *236*
    cell-cell interactions and, *236,* 237
    endocrine, 236, *236*
    extracellular matrix factors and, *236,* 237
    intracrine, *236,* 237
    neuroendocrine, 236, *236*
    paracrine, 236, *236*
Cellulitis, *867,* 875
Cellulose phosphate, for calcium stone
    disease, 2133, 2133t
Central nervous system, schistosomiasis of,
    906–907
Central venous pressure monitoring, in
    perioperative cardiac care, 2320
Cephalexin, for urinary tract infection
    prophylaxis, 787
    for vesicoureteral reflux in children, 1681
    plasma vs. prostatic fluid levels of, 813t
    serum vs. urinary levels of, 743t
Cephalothin, plasma vs. prostatic fluid levels
    of, 813t
Cerebellar ataxia, voiding dysfunction due
    to, 602
Cerebral palsy, 1652–1654
    clinical findings in, 1652, 1654, *1654,* 1654t
    diagnosis of, 1652
    electromyography in, 1654, *1654*
    etiology of, 1652
    perinatal risk factors for, 1654, 1654t
    recommendations in, 1654
    urodynamic studies in, 1654, 1654t
    voiding dysfunction due to, 602–603
Cerebrovascular disease, voiding dysfunction
    due to, 601–602

Cervical sympathetic ganglion,
    neuroblastoma of, 1989
Cervicitis, schistosomal, 899–900
Cervix, adenosis of, DES-related, 2002
    clear cell adenocarcinoma of, DES-related,
        2002
    embryology of, 1502
Chancroid, 839–840
    diagnosis of, 835t, 840
    etiology of, 839–840
    treatment of, 838t, 840
Chemolysis, post-shock wave lithotripsy,
    2165
Chemotherapy, 1045–1047. See also
    individual drugs
    antibody toxin targeting in, 1047
    basic principles of, 1045
    combination, 1046–1047
    cytotoxic, 1046
    growth factor receptor targeting in, 1047–
        1048
    host toxicity to, 1047
    male infertility due to, 662, 684
Chest physiotherapy, in perioperative
    pulmonary care, 2324
Chest radiography, in bladder cancer staging,
    1118
    in germ cell tumors of testis, 1231
    in neuroblastoma, 1993
    in perioperative cardiac care, 2316
Chevron incision, in adrenal surgery, 2404,
    2404
Chiba needle, in localization of
    hydronephrotic system, 2236
Child(ren). See also individual topics;
    Infant(s)
    adrenal cortical carcinoma in, 2380
    artificial urethral spincter placement in, ap-
        propriate age for, 2647–2648
    bladder capacity in, 1622
    bladder control development and, 1621–
        1622
    candidal infection of urinary tract in, 940
    endopyelotomy in, for ureteropelvic junc-
        tion obstruction, 2280
    excretory urography in, 434–435
    genitourinary tuberculosis in, 962
    glomerular filtration rate in, 1682
    hypertension in, definition of, 2018, *2018*
    neurogenic bladder in, 1634–1664. See also
        individual disorders; *Bladder, neuro-*
        genic
    oncology for, 1967–2006. See also individ-
        ual tumor types, e.g., *Wilms' tumor*
    organ radiation dose in, for 1–R entrance
        skin exposure, 398t
    pheochromocytoma in, 2392
    renal diseases of urologic significance in,
        2080t
    renal function in, estimation of, 1682,
        1682t–1683t
    testicular tumors in, 2002–2006
    transurethral procedures in, antimicrobial
        prophalyxis for, 745
    ureteroscopy in, 2205
    urinary concentration disorders in, 1349
    urinary lithiasis in, 2135–2136
        diagnosis of, 2136
        male:female ratio of, 2136
        treatment of, 2136
    urinary tract infection in, 1669–1683
    urine output in, 1621–1622
    urodynamic studies in, 1634–1637, *1635–*
        1636
    voiding cystourethrography in, 436, 440–
        441

Chlamydia trachomatis, culture of, technique
for, 828
lymphogranuloma venereum due to, 839
nonbacterial prostatitis due to, 817
nongonococcal urethritis in males due to,
827
of male genital tract, infertility and, 671
sexual transmission of, diseases associated
with, 826t
Chloramphenicol, contraindicated in
pregnancy, 793
plasma vs. prostatic fluid levels of, 813t
Chlordiazepoxide, impotence due to, 718
Chlorpromazine, for hyperchloremic
metabolic acidosis, 2621
Cholecystectomy, for gallstone management,
2171
Cholelithiasis, lithotripsy for, 2170–2171
Cholesterol, conversion of, to pregnenolone,
1519, *1520, 2364*
in seminal fluid, 253
in steroid hormone biosynthesis, 1519,
1520, 1954
in testosterone synthesis, 193–194, *194*
Cholesterol emboli disease, chronic renal
failure due to, 2059
Cholinergic agonists, ureteral effects of, 133
Cholinergic neurotransmitters, 150–152, *151,*
152t
Chordee, acquired, 3010–3011
assessment of, artificial erection in, *2967,*
2967–2968
congenital, 3006–3007
associated with hypospadias, 3006–3007,
3007
without hypospadias, in young men,
3007–3010, *3008–3009*
surgical correction of, *3008–3009,*
3008–3010
types of, 3007, *3007*
embryology of, 1894–1895
fibrous, surgical management of, 1898–
1899
in infertility workup, 663
residual, in hypospadias repair, 1914
surgical correction of, 2976–2977, *2976–
2977*
penile skin coverage in, 2978–2979
surgical management of, 1898–1899
with hypoplastic urethra, 1899–1900
with normal corpus spongiosum, 1899
without hypospadias, surgical management
of, 1899–1900
Choriocarcinoma. See also *Nonseminoma*
of bladder, 1136
of testis, 1240
Chorioepithelioma, classification systems for,
1224t
Chorionic villus sampling, in congenital
urologic abnormality(ies), 1564
Chromaffin cell(s), of adrenal medulla, 2368,
2368
Chromosomal abnormalities, in bladder
cancer, 1096, 1112
in renal cell carcinoma, 1062
male infertility due to, 680
Chromosomal sex, 1496–1497, 1951
Chromosomal walking, in genetic analysis,
282, *283*
Chromosome(s), aneuploid, 294
banding techniques for, 294, *295*
crossing over of, 267, *268*
diploid, 294
haploid, 294
historical discovery of, 294
in malignant transformation, 295–296

Chromosome(s) *(Continued)*
karyotypic analysis of, 294, *295,* 1533
marker, 295
morphologic alterations of, 294–295
ploidy of, 294
tetraploid, 294
triploid, 294
Chyluria, definition of, 311
in lymphatic filariasis, 914
Cicatricial pemphigoid, 878
Cigarette smoking, as risk factor, in
perioperative pulmonary care, 2322
bladder cancer due to, 1096
impotence due to, 717
male infertility due to, 663, 685
upper urinary tract urothelial tumors and,
1137
Cinecystourethrography, 435
Ciprofloxacin, serum vs. urinary levels of,
743t
Circadian rhythm, loss of, in Cushing's
syndrome, 2371–2372, *2372*
of plasma cortisol, 2365, *2365*
Circular stapling device, in urinary intestinal
diversion, 2605, *2605*
Circumcaval ureter(s), 540–541, *541*
ureteral obstruction due to, 540–541, *541*
Circumcision, 1921–1922, 2972–2973
American Academy of Pediatrics policy
on, 1922
complications of, 2972, 2973
controversy over, 1921–1922
for physical examination of penis, 313
Gomco clamp used in, 2972
in patient with phimosis, 2972–2973, *2974*
preputial bacterial colonization and, 1678
ritual, 2972
sleeve, in older boys, 2972, *2973*
squamous cell carcinoma of penis and,
1270–1271, 1921
urinary tract infection and, 1922
Circumflex vein(s), anatomy of, 2962, *2962*
Cirrhosis, male infertility due to, 685
Cisterna chyli, anatomy of, 16
Citrate, for calcium stone disease, 2133t
renal reabsorption of, 85
renal secretion of, 85
Citric acid, in seminal plasma, 251–252
prostatic formation of, 251–252
Climate, role of, in urinary lithiasis, 2089–
2091, *2090*
Clindamycin, plasma vs. prostatic fluid levels
of, 813t
Clitoral index, 1920
Clitoral recession, in female pseudohermaphroditism, 1957, 1959, *1960*
Clitorectomy, in female pseudohermaphroditism, 1957
Clitoris, duplication of, 1930
hypertrophy of, 1930, *1930*
Clitoroplasty, in female pseudohermaphroditism, 1957
Cloaca, 1317–1323
embryology of, 1822, 1893
persistent, 1605
septation of, 1318, *1320–1322*
Cloacal exstrophy, 1339, 1605, 1808–1812
anatomy and embryology of, 1808–1810,
1809–1810
associated conditions in, 1810–1811
embryology of, 1772–1773, *1773, 1775*
incidence of, 1808
surgical management of, 1811t, 1811–1812
Cloacal malformations, 1822–1849
anatomic spectrum in, 1822–1823, *1823–
1824*

Cloacal malformations *(Continued)*
case studies of, 1831–1849
cloaca and large pelvic tumor with tube
diversion, 1835–1837, *1836–1837*
cloaca requiring preliminary urologic operation, 1837–1840, *1838–1840*
cloaca with diverging vaginas and anterior rectal fistula, 1832, 1835, *1835*
cloaca with occult vagina, 1845, *1847–
1848*
complex cloaca with intravesical vaginal
and bowel communication, 1841–
1845, *1843–1844*
complex secondary reconstruction in,
1840–1841, *1841–1842*
discussion of, 1849
long-standing diversion with pull through
of rectum and fecal incontinence,
1845, *1846–1847*
postoperative care and outcome in, 1849
uncomplicated case repaired through
posterior saggital approach, 1831–
1832, *1832–1834*
definitive repair of, 1828–1831, *1829–1830*
approach options in, 1829
closure of bladder neck and urogenital
sinus in, 1831
mobilization of rectum in, 1830
mobilization of vagina in, 1830
patient prep in, 1828–1829, *1829*
posterior sagittal position for, 1829,
1830
postoperative care in, 1831
rectal fistula location in, 1829
vagina in, 1829–1830
management of newborn with, 1826–1828
abdominal radiography in, 1826, *1827*
decompressive colostomy in, 1826
diagnostic imaging in, 1828
endoscopic evaluation in, 1828
urinary tract decompression in, 1826–
1828, *1827*
perineum in, 1822–1823, *1823–1824*
rectum in, 1825, *1826*
urinary tract in, 1825–1826
vagina in, 1823, 1825, *1825*
Cloacal membrane, 40, 1317, 1772, *1774*
genital tubercle and, 1318, *1318*
labioscrotal swelling and, 1317, *1318*
Clofibrate, impotence due to, 718
Clomiphene, for male infertility, 688, 689t
Clonidine, impotence due to, 717
Clonidine suppression test, for
pheochromocytoma, 2393
Clorpactin WCS-90, for interstitial cystitis,
991t, 993, 995–996
Clusterin, 251
in hydronephrosis, 500
Coagulating gland, in mice, 248, 257
Coagulation mechanisms, 2338–2340
disorders of, 2339–2340
early events in, 2338
hemostatic competence of, 2339
pathways in, 2338–2339, *2339*
Coagulopathy(ies), acquired, 2340
inherited, 2339–2340
Cocaine, impotence due to, 717
male infertility due to, 685
Coccidioides immitis, 930
Coccidioidomycosis, 930–931
epidemiology of, 930
genitourinary, 930–931, *931*
diagnosis of, 931, *931*
treatment of, 931, 944t
in renal transplantation, 930
Coccygeus muscles, anatomy of, 2783

Enemas, preoperative, radical cystectomy and, 2751
Energy, for crystal nucleation, 2095
of lasers, 2923–2924
Enflurane, as anesthetic, for pheochromocytoma patient, 2397–2398
Enkephalinergic neurotransmitters, 166–167, *167*
Enteral nutrition, 2345
Enteric infections, sexual transmission of, 841–842, 842t
Enteritis, radiation, due to Wilms' tumor therapy, 1984
Enterobiasis, pelvic, 916–917
Enterobius vermicularis, 916–917
in enuresis, 1625
Enterocele, 2809–2811
abdominal repair of, 2811
acquired, 2809
congenital, 2809
diagnosis of, 2810
pathophysiology of, 2809–2810, *2810*
physical examination for, 651
surgical treatment of, 2810
postoperative care following, 2811
vaginal repair of, 2810–2811, *2810–2811*
Enterocolitis, pseudomembranous, following antibiotic bowel preparation, 2600–2601
Enteroenterostomy, by single-layer suture anastomosis, 2602–2603, *2603*
by two-layer suture anastomosis, 2602, *2602*
Enterovesical fistula, 2771–2773
causes of, 2771, 2772t
diagnosis of, 2772
etiology of, 2771–2772
surgical treatment of, preoperative preparation in, 2772
technique in, 2772–2773, *2772–2773*
Enucleation, in retropubic prostatectomy, 2857–2868, *2860–2862, 2863*
simple, in partial nephrectomy, 2448, *2449*, 2450
Enuresis, 1621–1630, 1655–1656. See also *Bladder control; Incontinence; Voiding dysfunction*
adult, 612, 1630
definition of, 310, 1621, 1655
diurnal, definition of, 1621
etiology of, 1622–1625
developmental delay and, 1623–1624
Enterobius vermicularis infestation in, 1625
food allergy in, 1625
genetic factors in, 1625
miscellaneous factors in, 1625
organic urinary tract disease in, 1625
psychological factors in, 1625
reduced bladder capacity in, 1622
sleep factors in, 1624
stress and, 1623–1624
uninhibited bladder contractions in, 1622–1623
urinary tract infection in, 1625
urodynamic factors in, 1622–1623
evaluation in, 1626, 1655, *1655*
nocturnal, definition of, 1621
orthotopic voiding procedures and, 2685
primary, 1621, 1623–1624
secondary, 1621, 1623–1624
treatment of, 1626–1630
agents affecting urinary output in, 1627
anticholinergic therapy in, 1627
autonomic agents in, 1627
behavior modification in, 1628–1629
bladder training in, 1628–1629

Enuresis *(Continued)*
conditioning therapy in, 1629
desmopressin in, 1627
imipramine in, 1627–1628
miscellaneous, 1630
pharmacotherapy in, 1627–1628
responsibility reinforcement in, 1629
Eosinophilia, in acute interstitial nephritis, 2048
tropical pulmonary, 914
Ephedrine, for bladder outlet resistance increase, 623
for continence in meningocele, 1644, *1645*
for neuropathic bladder dysfunction, 1637t
Epidermal growth factor, properties of, 249t
prostatic effects of, 248
Epidermal growth factor receptors, in bladder cancer prognosis, 1112
in tumor molecular biology, 1039
Epidermal inclusion cyst, of penis, 1922
Epidermoid cysts, *867*, 877–878
clinical findings in, *867*, 877
of testis, 1253
in children, 2005
treatment of, 877–878
Epididymal fluid, 211
Epididymectomy, *3131*, 3131–3132
for genitourinary tuberculosis, 976
Epididymis, 202–212
adenomatoid tumors of, 1256
anatomy of, *59*, 59–60
gross, 203, *204*
arterial supply of, 204–205, *205*
contractile tissues of, 203–204
cyst of, excision of, 3132
ultrasonography of, 377, *378*
cystadenoma of, 1256–1257
embryology of, 58, 1334, *1335*, 1500
epithelium of, 205–206, *207*
functions of, 206–210
control of, 211–212
androgens in, 211
sympathetic nervous system in, 211–212
temperature in, 211
factors involved in, 211
histology of, 206
in cryptorchidism, 1552
in infertility workup, 663
in sperm maturation, 208–210, *209–210*
in sperm storage, 206, 208
in sperm transport, 206
innervation of, 204
lymphatic drainage of, 205
obstruction of, infertility due to, 692
physical examination of, 313, 314
torsion of, surgical management of, 1946, *1946*
tuberculosis of, 958, 960
tumor of, excision of, 3132
ultrasonography of, 376–377, *377*
venous drainage of, 205
Epididymitis, 830–832
acute, 830
testicular torsion vs., 1556–1557, *1557*
chronic, 830
diagnosis of, 831, *832*
etiology of, 829t, 830–831
histoplasmal, 932
idiopathic, 830–831
infertility due to, 692
schistosomal, 899
testicular torsion vs., 831
treatment of, 831–832, 832t
ultrasonography for, 379, *379*

Epidural analgesia, in perioperative care, 2327
Epidural anesthesia, for retropubic prostatectomy, 2857, 2869
Epinephrine, preprocedural administration of, in percutaneous nephrostomy, 2245
Epispadias, 1812–1813
associated anomalies in, 1812
definition of, 315
embryology of, 1772–1773, *1773*
physical examination in, 313
surgical management of, 1812–1813
types of, 1812
urinary continence after bladder neck reconstruction in, 1813, 1813t
Epitaxy, in crystallization, 2096
Epithelial cells, in urinary sediment, *327–329*, 328–329
Epithelial hyperplasia, definition of, 1098
Epithelium. See under anatomic locations
Epsilon amino caproic acid, for essential hematuria, 2268
erb A, in tumor molecular biology, 1040
erb B, in tumor molecular biology, 1039
Erectile dysfunction. See also *Detumescence; Erection; Penis; Priapism*
arteriogenic, 720
as complication of perineal prostatectomy, 2899
as complication of retropubic prostatectomy, 2884t, 2884–2885
as complication of transurethral resection of prostate, 2914
cavernosography in, 718
diagnosis of, 3033–3052
cavernous biopsy in, 3052
corporal veno-occlusive function testing in, 3044–3052
Doppler studies in, 386, 718, *719*
duplex ultrasonography in, 386–389, *387–388*, 718, *719*
gravity pharmacocavernosometry testing in, 3050, *3052*
hormonal testing in, 3041
initial examination in, 3034–3036
laboratory tests in, 3036
medical history in, 3035t, 3035–3036
neurologic testing in, 3038, *3039–3040*, 3040t
nocturnal penile tumescence testing in, 3036–3037, *3037*
pharmacocavernosometry and pharmacocavernosography in, 3044, 3046, *3047–3051*, 3050
physical examination in, 3036
psychologic testing in, 3038, 3040–3041
psychosocial history in, 3035
pudendal arteriography in, selective, 718
radioisotope measurement of venous outflow in, 3050, 3052
radiologic, 718, *719*
sexual history in, 3034
ultrasonography in, *385–388*, 385–389, 718, *719*
vascular testing in, 3041–3044
dynamic state in, 3042–3044, *3043–3045*
flaccid state in, 3041–3042
visual sexual stimulation in, 3037
due to aging, 721
due to androgen deficiency, 720–721
due to diabetes mellitus, 720
due to drug use, 717–718
due to end-stage renal disease, 2503
due to erectile tissue dysfunction, 721
due to hyperprolactinemia, 721

Fertility, male. See also *Infertility, male*
   after retroperitoneal lymph node dissection, 1241–1243
   in exstrophy of bladder, 1808
Fertilization, facilitated, oocyte micromanipulation techniques for, 3138–3139
   in vitro, for male infertility, 694
      with microsurgically aspirated epididymal sperm, 3137–3138, *3137–3138*
Fibrinogen I-125 scanning, in diagnosis of thromboembolic disease, 2328
Fibroblast growth factor, acidic, 247
   basic, 247
   in tumor angiogenesis, 1044–1045
   in tumor molecular biology, 1039
   properties of, 249t
   prostatic effects of, 247–248
   receptor for, 248
Fibroid(s), of uterus, ureteral obstruction due to, 542–543, *543*
Fibroma, renal, 1061
Fibromuscular hyperplasia, of renal artery(ies), 2021
Fibroplasia, of renal artery, intimal, 2522, *2522*
   medial, 2522, *2522–2523*
   subadventitial, 2522, *2523*
Fibrosarcoma, renal, 1085
Fibrosis, retroperitoneal. See *Retroperitoneal fibrosis*
Fibrous histiocytoma, malignant, renal, 1085
Filariasis, lymphatic, 907–916
   Brugia malayi in, 907, 908
   Brugia timori in, 907, 908
   clinical manifestation(s) of, 912–914
      asymptomatic microfilaremia as, 913
      chyluria as, 914
      endemic normals in, 912–913
      filarial fever and chronic pathology in, 913–914
      funiculoepididymitis as, 913–914
      hydrocele as, 914
      lymph scrotum as, 914
      orchitis as, 914
      scrotal and penile elephantiasis as, *913*, 914
      tropical pulmonary eosinophilia as, 914
   diagnosis of, 914–915
      amicrofilaremic state and, 915
      filarial state and, 915
      infection and, 915
   distribution and epidemiology in, 908–909
   pathology and pathogenesis of, 909–912
      hydrocele and scrotal elephantiasis in, 912, *912–913*
      immune response in, 909
      in early established infection, *909–911*, 910–911
      in late infection, 911–912, *912–913*
      in prepatent period, 909–910
   prevention and control in, 916
   prognosis in, 916
   treatment of, 915
      diethylcarbamazine for, 915
      ivermectin for, 915
      medical, 915
      surgical, 915
   Wuchereria bancrofti in, 907–908, *908–909*
Finochietto retractor, 2422
Fistula(s), as complication of surgery for stone disease, 2473, 2475
   as complication of vaginal surgery, 2806

Fistula(s) *(Continued)*
   enterovesical. See *Enterovesical fistula*
   following urinary intestinal diversion, 2607
   pancreatic, as complication of radical nephrectomy, 2447
   renal arteriovenous, 2524–2525, *2525*
   urethrovaginal, management of, 2982
   urinary. See *Urinary fistula*
   vesicocutaneous. See *Vesicocutaneous fistula*
      endosurgical management of, 2293–2295, 2295t
   vesicoumbilical, 1816, *1816*
   vesicovaginal. See *Vesicovaginal fistula*
Fixed particle theory, of crystal nucleation, 2095
   intranephronic, 2100
FK 506, 2517
   mechanism of action of, 2516t
Flank incision(s), in renal surgery, 2419, *2420–2421*, 2422, *2422*
   in simple nephrectomy, 2430–2432, *2431–2432*
Flank pain, differential diagnosis in, 312
   in bacteriuria localization, 740
Flap(s). See also named flap, e.g., *Orandi flap*
   classification of, 2958–2959, *2958–2959*
   definition of, 2958
   for ureteropelvic junction obstruction, Culp-DeWeerd technique in, 2485, *2486*
      renal capsular technique in, 2488, *2488*
      Scardino-Prince vertical technique in, 2485, *2486*, 2487
   skin, W-shaped, for penile release and lengthening, 2974, *2975*
Flavoxate, for bladder contractility inhibition, 616
   in neuropathic bladder dysfunction, 1637t
Flow cytometry, in bladder cancer, 1113–1114
   in multicystic kidney disease, 1469
Flow resectoscope, constant, 2915, *2915*
Flowmetry, 583–584, *584–585*
   in bladder outlet obstruction, 584, *585*
   technique for, 584
   volume rate nomograms in, 584
Flucytosine, 945–946
   adverse effects of, 946
   dosage for, 946
   pharmacokinetics of, 945–946
Fluid, balance of, renal insufficiency and, 2332
   collection of, post-transplant, 2517
   for renal insufficiency, intraoperative use of, 2334–2335
      preoperative use of, 2332
   increased, for cystine urinary lithiasis, 2117
      for uric acid lithiasis, 2116
   intake of, urinary lithiasis and, 2090–2091
   intravenous, after transplantation, 2511
   renal tubular reabsorption of, 76, *76–77*
Fluorohydrocortisone, for Addison's disease, 2383
Fluoroquinolone, for urinary tract infection prophylaxis, 787–788
Fluoroscopy, with percutaneous nephrostomy, 2238, *2239*
   with shock wave lithotripsy, 2163
Flush stoma, 2609
Flushing solutions, hypothermic, in kidney preservation, 2506, 2508, 2508t
Flutamide, for benign prostatic hyperplasia, 1023
   for prostatic cancer, 1212–1213

Focal point F_1, in lithotripsy, 2157, *2157*
Focal point F_2, efficacy of stone fragmentation and, 2164
   in lithotripsy, 2157, *2157*
Foley catheter, 332, *332*, 2242
   in radical cystectomy, 2757, *2757*, 2759, *2759*, 2760, 2765
Foley Y-V plasty, in ureteropelvic junction obstruction repair, 2483–2484, *2485*
Folic acid, 2337
Folic acid deficiency, 2336–2337
Follicle-stimulating hormone (FSH), male, 181–183
   bilateral orchiectomy effects on, *182*
   chemical structure of, 181
   feedback control of, *182*, 182–183
   inhibin in, 183
   GnRH in secretion of, 180, *180*
   in hypogonadotropic vs. hypergonadotropic hypogonadism, 186
   in infertility, 664
   in old age, 185, *185*
   in sexual maturation, 184, *184*
   in spermatogenesis, 183–184, 201
   isolated deficiency in, infertility due to, 679
   measurement of, 181
   prolactin and, 181–182
   secretion of, 181
Folliculitis, bacterial, 873–874
   differential diagnosis of, 874
   infectious causes of, 874
   staphylococcal, 873–874
Food(s), containing oxalates, 2130t
Food allergy, in enuresis, 1625
Forearm flap(s), radial, in penile reconstruction, 3022, *3023–3024*, 3025
   disadvantages of, 3022
   modifications of, *3024*, 3025
Foreign body(ies), retrieval of, ureteroscopy in, 2205
Foreskin. See also *Prepuce; Preputial*
   anatomy of, 61, 2961
Formalin, intravesical, for metastatic bladder cancer, 1133
Formation product ratio (FPR), in estimation of calcium stone-forming activity, 2131
Fossa navicularis, strictures of, 2994–2998, *2995–2996*
   staged repair of, 2995–2998
      unmeshed split-thickness graft urethroplasty in, 2995, *2997–2998*, 2998
Fourchette, posterior, embryology of, 1502
Fournier's gangrene, 875
Fowler-Stephens orchiectomy, 1941–1942, *1943*
Fowler-Stephens (long loop vas) technique, in prune-belly syndrome, 1867–1868
Fracture, Malgaigne, urethral rupture with, 2583, *2584*
   pelvic, urethral distraction injury associated with, 2999–3000, *2999–3000*
   penile, management of, 2979–2980
Fraley's syndrome, 2270
Free particle theory, of crystal nucleation, 2095
   extranephronic, 2100
Free water clearance, calculation of, 78
Frequency, definition of, 649
   in females, flow chart for management of, 830, *830*
   in neurourologic evaluation, 577
Fresh frozen plasma, administration of, 2340
Fructose, absent from seminal plasma, 257
   in semen analysis, 667

Megaureter *(Continued)*
    Whitaker test in, *1714,* 1715–1716
    pathology in, 1413–1414
    secondary, 1718
    prenatally diagnosed, postnatal follow-up
      of, 1575, *1576*
    radiography in, 1711–1713, *1712*
    reflux, 1413, 1711
    terminology in, 1708
    ureteral valve in, 1712
Melanoma, malignant, of bladder, 1136
    of genitalia, 870, 879
    of penis, 1291–1292
Melanosis, of penis, 1264
Melatonin, hypothalamic-pituitary-testicular
    axis and, 178–179
Mendel, Gregor, 267
Meningocele, bowel function and, 1646
    continence in, 1644–1645, *1645*
      alpha-sympathomimetic agents for, 1644,
        1645
      ephedrine for, 1644, *1645*
      oxybutynin for, 1644, *1645*
      pharmacologic therapy for, 1644, *1645*
      surgical therapy for, 1644–1645
    definition of, 1637
    electromyography in, 1639, *1639*
    guidelines for surveillance in, 1642, 1642t
    lower urinary tract denervation in, 1639,
      1639
    lower urinary tract dyssynergy in, 1639,
      1639
    lower urinary tract synergy in, 1639, *1639*
    neurologic findings and recommendations
      in, 1641–1642, *1642*
    neurologic lesion in, 1638
    newborn assessment in, 1638
    outlet obstruction and lower tract deterio-
      ration in, 1639, *1640,* 1641
    pontine-sacral reflex and sacral reflex arc
      in, 1642, *1643*
    recommendations for prophylactic treat-
      ment in, 1641, *1641*
    sexuality and, 1646
    spinal level of, 1637, 1637t
    tethered spinal cord in, 1641, *1641*
    urinary diversion and undiversion in,
      1645–1646
    urodynamic findings in, 1638–1641, *1639–
      1640*
    vesicoureteral reflux in, 1642–1644
      antireflux surgery for, 1643–1644
      Credé voiding and, 1642, *1644*
      management based on grade in, 1642
      vesicostomy drainage for, 1642–1643
Mental status evaluation, in neurourologic
    evaluation, 578
Meperidine, for pain relief, in urinary
    lithiasis, 2107
Meprobamate, impotence due to, 718
Mercier's bar, anatomy of, 47, 1689
Mesangial sclerosis, diffuse, 1461
Mesenteric artery, inferior, anatomy of, 15,
    15
    superior, anatomy of, 13, *15*
Mesenteric-to-renal artery bypass graft, with
    saphenous vein, 2545, *2545*
Mesoblastic nephroma, congenital, Wilms'
    tumor and, 1970, *1972,* 1974–1975
Mesonephros, embryology of, 70, 1304,
    1305, 1344, *1345,* 1499, *1499,* 1951–1952
Mesothelioma, of testicular adnexa, 1256
    of testis, 1254
Metabolic acidosis, hyperchloremic, as
    complication of cystoplasty, 2643,
    2645

Metabolic acidosis *(Continued)*
    treatment of, 2621
Metachlorophenylpiperazine, for erectile
    dysfunction, 3053
Metaiodobenzylguanidine (MIBG) scan, of
    pheochromocytoma, 2393, 2396, *2396*
Metal bougies, cone-shaped, acute ureteral
    dilation with, 2209, *2209–2210*
Metal intoxication, chronic renal failure due
    to, 2057
Metanephros, embryology of, 70, 1344, *1345,*
    1697, *1697*
Metastasis, 1042–1044
    antimetastatic genes and, 1043–1044
    biologic processes of, 1042–1043
Methantheline, for bladder contractility
    inhibition, 615
Methionine, restriction of, for cystine urinary
    lithiasis, 2117–2118
Methyl methacrylate, ureteral obstruction
    due to, 555, *555*
Methyldopa, impotence due to, 717, 718
Methylprednisolone, for bacteremic shock,
    772t
Methysergide, retroperitoneal fibrosis due to,
    551
Metoclopramide, for bladder emptying, 630
Metrifonate, for urinary schistosomiasis,
    897–898
Metrizamide, chemical structure of, *403*
Metronidazole, plus neomycin, as bowel
    preparation, 2600t
Metyrapone, for ectopic ACTH, 2374
Meyers-Kouvenaar syndrome, 914
Michaelis-Gutmann bodies, in malacoplakia,
    767–768
Miconazole, 946
    adverse reactions to, 946
    dosage for, 946
Microexplosive generator, 2159
Micropenis, 1531–1532, *1531–1532,* 1924–
    1925
    androgen therapy in, 1925
    causes of, 1925
    due to hypergonadotropic hypogonadism,
      1925
    due to hypogonadotropic hypogonadism,
      1925
    endocrine factors in, 1924–1925
    evaluation in, 1925
    hypospadias vs., 1896
    idiopathic, 1925
    length assessment in, 1924
    outcome after puberty in, 1925
Microvascular anastomosis, in testis
    autotransplantation, 1943, *1944*
Microwave hyperthermia, transurethral, of
    prostate, 2918, *2918*
Micturition. See *Voiding*
Micturition reflex pathway, 576
    spinal, 160, *160*
    supraspinal, 160, *160*
Mid-stream urine specimen, technique for,
    741, 741–742
Milk, human, antituberculous drugs in, 974
Mineralocorticoids, renal excretion of, 104–
    105
Minerals, daily requirement of, 2344
    in water, urinary lithiasis and, 2090
Minimal change (nil) disease, chronic renal
    failure due to, 2055
Minnesota antilymphocyte globulin
    (MALG), 2502
    for allograft rejection, 2515t
    mechanism of action of, 2516t
    preparation of, 2516

Minnesota Multiphasic Personality Inventory,
    3040
Minocycline, plasma vs. prostatic fluid levels
    of, 813t
Mitomycin C, intravesical, for superficial
    bladder cancer, 1121
Mitotane, for adrenal carcinoma, 2380–2381
Mitotic index, 1035, 1035t
Mohs micrographic surgery, in squamous cell
    carcinoma of penis, 1278, *1280–1281,*
    3075
Morbidity and mortality, of radical
    cystectomy, 2671–2672, 2761t
    of transurethral prostatectomy, 2911
Morphine, for pain relief, in urinary lithiasis,
    2107
    ureteral effects of, 134–135
Mortality, anesthesia and, 2326
    following shock wave lithotripsy, 2170
Motor activity, of intestinal segments, *2625,*
    2625–2626
Motor unit action potential, 591
MRI. See *Magnetic resonance imaging (MRI)*
Mucocele, of appendix, ureteral obstruction
    due to, 549
Mucormycosis, 933–934, *934*
Mulberry stone. See *Calcium oxalate
    calculus(i)*
Müllerian agenesis, 1522
    clinical features of, 1522, *1523*
    management of, 1522
    pathophysiology of, 1522
Müllerian duct(s), embryology of, 1333,
    1334, 1499, *1500*
    incomplete fusion of, 1339
    persistent, 1503, 1530–1531
    regression of, *1337,* 1337–1338, 1498,
      1499–1500, *1501,* 1544, 1951
      anatomic considerations in, 1337, *1337*
      molecular biology of, 1337–1338
      testicular hormones in, 1503
Müllerian inhibiting substance, 1337, 1498,
    1544, 1951
    mechanisms of action of, 1503
    properties of, 248, 249t
Müllerian tubercle, embryology of, 1333–
    1334
Multicystic kidney disease, 1465–1469. See
    also *Polycystic kidney disease; Renal
    cyst(s)*
    clinical features of, 1466–1467
      contralateral upper tract and, 1466
      involution in, 1466
    dysplasia in, 1465, *1465–1466,* 1607–1608,
      1608
      ultrasonography in, 1596t
    etiology of, 1465–1466
    evaluation in, 1467, *1468*
    flow cytometric analysis in, 1469
    histopathology in, 1467
    hydronephrosis vs., 1467
    hydronephrotic, 1467
    hypertension in, 1469
    malignant degeneration in, 1468–1469
    multilocular renal cyst vs., 1469t
    prenatal diagnosis of, 1568, *1569*
    prophylactic nephrectomy in, 1468–1469
    radionuclide scan in, 1608, *1608*
    treatment and prognosis in, 1467–1469
    ultrasonography in, 1467, *1468,* 1608, *1608*
    Wilms tumor and, 1469
Multiple endocrine adenopathy (MEA), 2391
Multiple myeloma, chronic renal failure due
    to, 2059
    proteinuria in, 2074–2075

Oncology, pediatric, 1967–2006. See also individual cancers, e.g., *Wilms' tumor*
Onuf's nucleus, 150, 715
Oocyte micromanipulation techniques, 3138–3139
    partial zona dissection in, 3139
    sub-zonal insertion in, 3139
Opiate(s), as neurotransmitters, 166–167
Opioid antagonists, for bladder emptying, 630
Oral contraceptives, rifampicin and, 973
Orandi flap, in urethral reconstruction, 2991, *2992*
Orchiectomy, 1948, 1950, *1950*
    bilateral, for prostatic cancer, 1212
    delayed, for testicular cancer, 3093
    Fowler-Stephens, 1941–1942, *1943*
    radical, for testicular cancer, 3090–3092, *3091–3092*
    scrotal, for testicular cancer, 3092–3093
Orchiopexy, 1939–1945, 2006
    scrotal, for retractable testis, in adult, 3147
    surgical technique in, 1939–1941, *1940–1942*
        autotransplantation in, 1943–1944, *1944*
        dartos pouch technique in, 1940, *1941–1942*
        external inguinal ring in, 1939, *1940*
        Fowler-Stephens orchiectomy in, 1941–1942, *1943*
        hernia sac incision in, 1939, *1940*
        in nonpalpable testis, 1944–1945
            hCG stimulation test in, 1944
            laparoscopy in, 1944–1945
        repeat orchiopexy and, 1944
        skin incision in, 1939, *1940*
        staged, 1941, 1941t, *1942*
        testis wrapped in Silastic in, 1941, *1942*
Orchitis. See also *Testis(es)*
    due to lymphatic filariasis, 914
    male infertility due to, 686
    mumps, infertility due to, 662
    tuberculous, 958
Organ(s), adjacent, shock wave damage to, 2169–2170, 2170t
    effect of shock wave lithotripsy on, 2161–2163
Organ donation, HIV infection and, 855
Orgasm, male, loss of, 311
Ormond's disease, 2556
Ornithine, renal reabsorption of, 85
Orofaciodigital syndrome type I, renal cysts in, 1464
Orthopedic complications, due to Wilms' tumor therapy, 1984
Orthopedic deformities, in prune-belly syndrome, 1855, *1856*
Orthotopic voiding diversions, 2683, 2685–2698. See also specific procedure, e.g., *Camey II operation*
Osmotic diuresis, 2079
Ossifying tumor of kidney, infantile, 1987
Osteogenic sarcoma, renal, 1084–1085
Osteomalacia, in urinary intestinal diversion, 2622
Otis bulb, urethral calibration with, 2905, *2905*
Otis urethrotome, 2905, *2906*, 2987
Ouabain, ureteral effects of, 135
Outlet, bladder. See *Bladder outlet*
Ovarian artery(ies), anatomy of, 15, *15*
Ovarian failure, due to Wilms' tumor therapy, 1984
Ovarian remnant, ureteral obstruction due to, 543

Ovarian vein(s), anatomic relationships of, 539
    postpartum thrombophlebitis of, ureteral obstruction due to, 540
Ovarian vein syndrome, ureteral obstruction due to, *539*, 539–540
Ovary(ies), cyst of, ureteral obstruction due to, 541–543
    effect of shock wave lithotripsy on, 2162
    embryology of, 1502
    fetal, endocrine differentiation of, 1498, *1498*
    in bilateral renal agenesis, 1360
    radiation dose to, for 1000–mR entrance skin exposure, 398t
        for 1–R entrance skin exposure, 399t
        typical, 396t–397t, 397–398
Oxalate, sources of, 2130, 2130t
Oxalate diet, low, for urinary lithiasis, 2147
Oximetry, pulse, in perioperative cardiac care, 2321
Oxybutynin, for bladder contractility inhibition, 615–616
    for continence in meningocele, 1644, *1645*
    for neuropathic bladder dysfunction, 1637t
    for postoperative incontinence, 2899
Oxygen saturation, venous, in perioperative cardiac care, measurement of, 2321
Oxytetracycline, plasma vs. prostatic fluid levels of, 813t

P

Pacemaker(s), perioperative management of patients with, 2319
Pacemaker potentials, *114*, 114–115
Paecilomyces infection, 933
Pagano ureterocolonic anastomosis, 2614, *2614*
    complications of, 2613t
Paget's disease, extramammary, 870
    of penis, 1292–1293
Pain, as complication of vaginal surgery, 2806
    genital, chronic, 881
    in medical history, 308–309
    prostate, 308, 807, 817–819
    referred somatic, from lower urinary tract, 40, *40*
Palsy, ulnar nerve, postoperative, 2353
Pampiniform plexus, heat exchange in, 191–192
Pancreas, carcinoma of, ureteral obstruction due to, 550
    pseudocyst of, ureteral obstruction due to, 550
    retroperitoneal position of, 19
Pancreatic fistula, as complication of radical nephrectomy, 2447
Pancreatitis, acute, ureteral obstruction due to, 550
    following shock wave lithotripsy, 2163, 2170
Pancuronium, use of, for patients with renal insufficiency, 2335
Papaverine, intracavernosal injection of, for impotence, 3055, 3056t
    priapism due to, 723
Papilla(e), renal. See *Renal papilla(e)*
Papilloma, as complication of cystoplasty, 2643
    inverted, of bladder, 1100, *1101*
    of upper urinary tract, 1139
    transitional cell, of bladder, *1104*, 1106
Papulosquamous disease, exudative, 864

Para-aminohippurate extraction method, for renal blood flow, 72
Para-aortic lymph nodes, left, anatomy of, 16
Paracaval lymph nodes, right, anatomy of, 16–17
Paracoccidioidomycosis, 933
Paracrine growth factors, *1041*
Paradidymis, 1223
    embryology of, 58, 1334
Parameatal urethral cyst, 1927
Parameatal-based flap (Mathieu procedure), in anterior hypospadias, 1904, *1905*
Parametritis, ureteral obstruction due to, IUD use and, 545
Paraneoplastic syndromes, in bladder cancer, 1112
    in renal cell carcinoma, 1067, 1067t
Parapelvic cyst(s), 1485
Paraphimosis, 2972
    definition of, 315
    pain due to, 308–309
Paraplegia, voiding cystourethrography in, 437, *438*
Pararenal fat, anatomic relationship(s) of, 26
Parasitic disease, 883–920. See also individual types; *Filariasis; Schistosomiasis*
    urologists and, 883
Parasitic prostatitis, 819
Parasternal hernia, as complication of ileal conduit urinary diversion, 2669–2670
Parasympathetic blocking agents, ureteral effects of, 133–134
Parasympathetic decentralization, voiding dysfunction due to, 610–611
Parasympathomimetic agent(s), for bladder emptying, 629–630
    acetylcholine as, 629
    bethanechol chloride as, 629–630
    metoclopramide as, 630
Paratesticular rhabdomyosarcoma, in children, 2005–2006
Paratesticular tumors, 1257–1259
    chemotherapy in, 1257–1258
    management of, 1257–1258
    radiotherapy in, 1257
Parathyroid crisis, 2127–2128
Parathyroid hormone, control of serum calcium by, 2125, *2126*
    1,25–dihydroxyvitamin D_3 and, 97
    receptor mechanisms for, 105–106, *106*
    renal metabolism of, *102*, 102–103
    renal physiologic effects of, 86–87
Paraurethral cyst(s), female, 1930, *1930*
Parenteral nutrition, effects of, on postoperative outcome, 2345
Parkinson's disease, voiding dysfunction due to, 603
Patch graft(s), in resurfacing of fossa navicularis, 2995, *2995*
    in urethral reconstruction, 2989–2991, *2990–2991*
Patient counseling, for continent urinary diversion, 2675
Patient evaluation, 307–341. See also individual parts
    medical history in, 307–311
    physical examination in, 311–317
    urinalysis in, 317–329
Patient position, for perineal prostatectomy, 2888, *2889*
    for radical cystectomy, 2752, *2752*
    for radical cystoprostatectomy, 2775, *2775*
    for urethrectomy, *2775*
Pearly penile plaques, *867*, 879–880
Pediatric cystoscope, 2206

Pediatric disorders. See *Child(ren)*;
    individual disorders; *Infant(s)*
Pediculosis pubis infection, 841, 861
Pelvic abscess, following urinary intestinal
    diversion, 2607
Pelvic diaphragm, anatomy of, 2782–2783,
    2782–2783
Pelvic enterobiasis, 916–917
Pelvic examination, 314–315
Pelvic exenteration, anterior, 2762. See also
    Cystectomy, radical, in females
Pelvic fascia, 63–65, *64–65*, *2867–2868*, 2868
    intermediate stratum of, 63
        dorsal lamina of, 63
        ventral lamina of, 63
    lateral, anatomy of, 2868, *2868*
        excision of, in retropubic prostatectomy,
            2876, 2878t, 2878, *2878–2879*
    parietal, 64
    strata of, 63
Pelvic floor muscle exercises, for stress
    incontinence, 655, 2793–2794
Pelvic floor relaxation, 2787, *2787*
Pelvic inflammatory disease, due to
    gonococcal and nongonococcal
    urethritis, 829
Pelvic lipomatosis, 563–565
    cystitis glandularis in, 565
    diagnostic imaging in, *564*, 564–565
    epidemiology and incidence of, 563
    etiology of, 563–564
    pathologic and clinical manifestations of,
        564
    pear-shaped bladder in, 564, *564*
    treatment of, 565
    ultrasonography in, 472, *472*
Pelvic lymph nodes, ultrasonography for,
    472, *472*
Pelvic lymphadenectomy, extent of, in
    radical cystectomy, 2752, *2755*
Pelvic lymphoceles, 2352
Pelvic mass, ultrasonography of, bladder vs.,
    472
    ureteral obstruction due to, 541–543, *542–
        543*
Pelvic muscle laxity, in incontinence, 651
Pelvic plexus, *2867*, 2867–2868
    anatomic distribution of, 63, 149, *149*
    anatomy of, 2964
Pelvic radiation therapy, bladder cancer due
    to, 1097
Pelvic support, anatomy of, 2782–2784,
    2782–2785
Pelvic surgery, radical, vaginal construction
    after, 3028–3029
    voiding dysfunction due to, 610–611
Pelvis, neuroanatomy of, 62–63, 149, *149–
    150*
    renal. See *Renal pelvis*
Pemphigoid, cicatricial, 878
Pemphigus, familial benign chronic, *865*, 870
Pemphigus vulgaris, 878
Penectomy, modified partial, 3076
    partial, 3076, *3076*
        reconstruction after, 1290
    total, 3076–3077
        reconstruction after, 1290–1291
D-Penicillamine, for cystine urinary lithiasis,
    2118
Penicillin G, plasma vs. prostatic fluid levels
    of, 813t
    serum vs. urinary levels of, 743t
Penicillium infection, 934
Penile artery, anatomy of, 709, *710*, 2963,
    2963
    flaccid state of, 3041–3042

Penile biothesiometry, test of afferent
    somatic dorsal nerve pathway by, 3038,
    3040, 3040t
Penile brachial index, 386, 3041
Penile prosthesis, 3057–3061
    infected, removal of, 3061
    insertion of, complications during, 3060
        surgical technique in, 3060
    postoperative complications of, 3060–3061
    types of, 3057t, 3058, *3058–3059*
Penile raphe, embryology of, 1500, 1894
Penile revascularization procedures, arterial,
    3061, *3062–3064*, 3063, 3065
    venous, 3065–3066, *3065–3066*
Penile tumescence testing, nocturnal, 3036–
    3037, *3037*
Peninsula flap(s), 2959
Penis, 60–62. See also *Detumesence; Erectile
    dysfunction; Erection;* individual
    disorders; *Priapism*
    acquired inclusion cysts of, 1264
    agenesis of, 1925–1926, *1926*
    anatomy of, 60–61, *61*, 1893, 2959–2965
    angioma of, 1264
    appliances for, in erectile dysfunction,
        3054, 3054–3055
    arterial supply of, *61*, 61–62, 709, *710–711*,
        2963, *2963–2964*
    balanitis xerotica obliterans of, *1265*,
        1265–1266
    basal cell carcinoma of, 1291
    benign cutaneous lesions of, 1264–1265
    benign noncutaneous lesions of, 1264,
        1264
    Bowenoid papulosis of, 1267–1268
    Bowen's disease of, 1269–1270, *1270*
    burns to, management of, 2980–2981
    Buschke-Löwenstein tumor of, 1268–1269
    carcinoma in situ of, 1269–1270, *1270*
    concealed (buried), 1922–1923, *1922–1923*
    condyloma acuminatum of, 1266–1267
        carginogenesis and, 1267
        human papilloma virus in, 1266
        pathologic findings in, 1266
        recurrence in, 1267
        sites involved in, 1266
        treatment of, 1267
    congenital anomalies of, 1921–1927
    congenital inclusion cysts of, 1264
    coronal papillae of, 1265
    curvature of, 3006. See also *Chordee*
        lateral, surgical correction of, 3010, *3010*
    cutaneous horns of, 1265, *1265*
    cysts of, 1922
    degloving injuries of, management of, 2980
    duplication of, 1926, *1926*
    embryology of, 60, 1328, *1328*
    erectile tissues of, 2959
    erythroplasia of Queyrat of, 1269–1270,
        1270
    fetal development of, 3006
    fracture of, management of, 2979–2980
    giant condyloma acuminatum of, 1268–
        1269
    hirsute papilloma of, 1265
    in bilateral renal agenesis, 1360
    in prune-belly syndrome, 1855
    incomplete development of, 2967. See also
        Hypospadias
    injuries of, 2589–2591
        degloving, 2590–2591, *2591*
    innervation of, *2963*, 2963–2964
    Kaposi's sarcoma of, 1268
    lateral curvature of, 1924
    leukoplakia of, 1266
    lichen planus of, 864, *865*

Penis *(Continued)*
    ligaments of, 61, 2960
    lymphatic drainage of, 62, 2963
    lymphatics of, 3073
    lymphoreticular malignancy of, 1293
    melanoma of, 1291–1292
    melanosis of, 1264
    metastatic lesions of, 1293
    neuroanatomy of, 62, *714*, 714–716
    nevi of, 1264, *1265*
    Paget's disease of, 1292–1293
    painful, in medical history, 308–309
    pearly papules of, *868*, 879–880, 1265
    penetrating injury to, management of,
        2980
    physical examination of, 313
        in infertility workup, 663
        inspection in, 313
        palpation in, 313
    premalignant cutaneous lesions of, 1265–
        1266
    pseudotumors of, 1264
    psoriasis of, 863, *865*
    radiation injury to, management of, 2981
    reconstruction of, 3022–3027
        following trauma, 3027–3028
        lateral upper arm flap in, *3025*, 3025–
            3026
            disadvantage of, 3026
        radial forearm flap in, 3022, *3023–3024*,
            3025
            disadvantages of, 3022
            modifications of, *3024*, 3025, 3026
        surgical technique for, 3026–3027
    retention cysts of, 1264, *1264*
    sarcoma of, 1292
    skin lesions on, surgical treatment of,
        2967
    squamous cell carcinoma of, 315, 1269–
        1291
        diagnosis in, 1273–1276
            biopsy in, 1274
            delay in, 1273
            grading in, 1274
            histology in, 1274
            laboratory studies in, 1274–1275
            minimal criteria for, 1277t
            physical examination in, 1273
            radiologic studies in, 1275–1276
            staging in, 1276, 1276t–1277t, *1277*
        differential diagnosis in, 1276
        etiology of, 1270–1271
            circumcision and, 1270–1271, 1921
            human papilloma virus and, 1271
            smegma and, 1270–1271
            trauma and, 1271
        incidence of, 1270
        inguinal metastasis in, 1282–1290
            chemotherapy in, 1289–1290
            radiation therapy in, 1288–1289
            surgical treatment in, 1282–1287,
                3078–3084
                anatomic considerations in, 3077–
                    3078
                aspiration cytology and, 1285–1286
                bilateral vs. unilateral, 1286–1287
                clinical correlates of, 3078
                complications of, 1283, *1284*, 3078,
                    3079t
                five-year survival rates and, 1284–
                    1285
                general considerations in, 3078–3079
                iliac node dissection and, 1287
                in stage any T, any N, M1, T4, in-
                    operable N (IV) disease, 1288

Succinylcholine, for pheochromocytoma patient, 2398
  use of, for patients with renal insufficiency, 2335
Sulfa preparations, contraindicated in pregnancy, 793–794
Sulfamethizole, serum vs. urinary levels of, 743t
Sulfamethoxazole, plasma vs. prostatic fluid levels of, 813t
Sulfisoxazole, plasma vs. prostatic fluid levels of, 813t
Sulfosalicylic acid test, Kingsbury-Clark, 318
Sunlight theory, in urinary lithiasis, 2090, *2090*
Supersaturation theory, of crystallization, 2094, *2094*, 2099
Suprapubic needle aspiration, of bladder, technique for, 740, *740*
  ultrasonography in, 470
Surgery, renal. See *Renal surgery*; specific procedure, e.g., *Nephrectomy*
  ureteral. See *Ureteral surgery*
Suture carrier, double-pronged, used in Raz transvaginal needle bladder neck suspension, 2799, *2799*
Sweeteners, artificial, bladder cancer due to, 1097
Swimmer's itch, 893. See also *Schistosomiasis*
Symphysis pubis, position of, in relation to bladder neck, radiologic determination of, 2834–2838, *2835–2838*
Syndecan, in nephrogenesis, 1309–1310
Syphilis, primary, 839
  clinical features of, 835t
  diagnosis of, 835t, 839
  etiology of, 839
  treatment of, 838t, 839
Syringocele, 1888
SZ-1 microexplosive lithotriptor, 2159

T

Tabes dorsalis, voiding dysfunction due to, 609–610
Takayasu's aortitis, 2022
Takayasu's disease (arteritis), 2526–2527, *2527*
Tamm-Horsfall protein, in Bowman's space, due to ureteral obstruction, 501
  in urine, 322
    due to contrast media, 405
    due to reflux nephropathy in children, 1677
    in interstitial cystitis, 989
Tamoxifen, for male infertility, 688, 689t–690t
Tandem repeat sequences, in genetic linkage analysis, 282
Tasker patch, in ileal cystoplasty, 2636, *2636*
TATA box, in DNA transcription, 270
TCC. See *Transitional cell carcinoma*
TCT (thyrocalcitonin), 2125
Tea drinking, bladder cancer due to, 1096–1097
Technetium-99 scan, of genitourinary injury, 2572
  of ureteropelvic junction obstruction, 2478
  prior to nephrectomy, 2473, *2474*
Tendinous arc, anatomy of, 2783, *2783*
"Tennis-racket" technique, for bladder neck closure, 2879, *2881*
Teprotide, peripheral plasma renin and, 2032
Teratocarcinoma. See also *Nonseminoma*
  classification systems for, 1224t

Teratocarcinoma *(Continued)*
  experimental models of, 1224–1225
  histology in, 1240
  of testis, in children, 2004
Teratoma. See also *Nonseminoma*
  classification systems for, 1224t
  experimental models of, 1224–1225
  histology of, 1240
  renal, in children, 1987
  testicular, in children, 2004
Terbutaline, for bladder contractility inhibition, 617
Terodiline, for bladder contractility inhibition, 616–617
Testicular adnexa, adenomatoid tumors of, 1256
  cystadenoma of, 1256–1257
  epithelial tumors of, 1255–1256
  mesothelioma of, 1256
  tumors of, 1255–1259
Testicular artery(ies), anatomy of, 13, 59, 191–192, 1223
Testicular failure, primary, infertility due to, endocrine evaluation in, 664, 664t
Testicular feminization, androgen receptor gene point mutation in, 286
  complete, 1527, *1529*
  distal vs. proximal vaginal formation in, 1338
  incomplete, 1528, *1528–1529*
  inguinal hernia and, 1555
  inheritance of, 286
Testicular intertubular capillary(ies), 192
Testicular peritubular capillary(ies), 192
Testicular venography, in cryptorchidism, 1549, *1550*
Testis(es), 59. See also individual anatomic parts; *Orchitis*
  absent, syndrome of, 1518–1519
  acute lymphoblastic leukemia of, in children, 2005
  adenofibroma of, 1254
  adenofibromyoma of, 1254
  adenoma of, 1254
  adenomatoid tumor of, 1254
  adrenal rest tumor of, 1254
  anatomy of, 59, *59*, 190–192, *191*, 1222–1223
    ultrasonography in, 476–477, *478*
  angiomatoid tumor of, 1254
  biopsy of, 3115–3116
    aspiration cytology and flow cytometry in, 3116
    complications of, 3116
    in infertility evaluation, 674–676
      end-stage testes in, 676
      germinal aplasia in, 675, 675–676
      hypospermatogenesis in, 674–675, *675*
      in hypogonadotropic hypogonadism, 676
      indications for, 674
      maturation arrest in, 675, *675*
      normal findings in, 674, *675*
      Sertoli cell–only syndrome in, *675*, 675–676
    indications for, 3115
    open, *3115*, 3115–3116
    percutaneous, 3116
  blood flow in, 190, 192, 1223
  Burkitt's lymphoma of, in children, 2005
  capsule of, contraction of, 190
  carcinoid of, 1254
  carcinoma in situ of, 1223–1224
    in cryptorchidism, 1550–1551
  carcinoma of, 315–316. See also *Nonseminoma; Seminoma*

Testis(es) *(Continued)*
  diagnosis of, 3090
  pathologic findings in, 3093–3094
  positive node distribution in, by disease stage, 3096, *3097*
  staging of, 3094t, 3094–3095
  surgical management of, 3090–3092, 3095–3111. See also *Retroperitoneal lymph node dissection*
    delayed orchiectomy in, 3093
    radical orchiectomy in, 3090–3092, *3091–3092*
    scrotal orchiectomy in, 3092–3093
  cyst of, ultrasonography of, 377, *378*
  descent of, 1543–1546. See also *Cryptorchidism*
    age effects on, 1544t, 1544–1545
    differential growth theory of, 1546
    endocrine regulation of, 1546
    epididymal theory of, 1546
    fetal, 1335, *1336*, 1501, *1501*, 1543–1544
    in other species, 1543
    in preterm infant, 1544, 1544t
    intra-abdominal theory of, 1546
    mechanism of, 1545t, 1545–1546
    traction theory of, 1545
  dimension and volume of, 663t
  ectopic, 1548, *1548*
  embryology of, 58, 198–199, 1500, 1544
  end-stage, biopsy of, 676
  epidermoid cysts of, 1253
    in children, 2005
  estrogen synthesis in, 234
  fetal, endocrine differentiation of, *1498*, 1498–1499
  fine needle aspiration cytology of, in infertility evaluation, 676
  germ cell tumors of, 1225–1235
    classification systems for, 1224t
    clinical manifestations of, 1228–1229
    clinical staging of, 1229–1234
      abdominal CT in, 1231
      chest CT in, 1231
      chest radiography in, 1231
      imaging in, 1231
      metastatic sites in, 1229–1230
      orchiectomy specimen in, 1231
      systems for, 1230t, 1230–1231
      tumor markers in, 1231–1234
    differential diagnosis of, 1228
    epidemiology of, 1225–1226
      age in, 1225
      genetics in, 1225
      histologic type and, 1226
      incidence in, 1225
      laterality and bilaterality in, 1225–1226
      race in, 1225
    etiology of, 1226–1227
      acquired causes of, 1226–1227
      atrophy in, 1227
      congenital causes in, 1226
      cryptorchidism in, 1226
      hormones in, 1226–1227
      trauma in, 1226
    imaging studies in, 1228
    in children, 2003–2005
    nonseminoma, 1239–1248. See also *Nonseminoma*
    pathogenesis and natural history of, 1227–1228
      extranodal distant metastasis and, 1227–1228
      growth rate and, 1228
      location and, 1227
      lymphatic metastasis and, 1227

Urinary tract (Continued)
  symptoms referable to, 309–310
    dysuria as, 309
    hesitancy as, 310
    intermittency as, 310
    irritative, 309
    nocturia as, 309
    obstructive, 309–310
    post-void dribbling as, 310
    urgency as, 309
  ultrasonography of, 462–477
  obstruction of, associated with lithiasis,
    pathophysiology of, 2108–2109
  perioperative infections of, 2347–2348
  pretransplant urologic evaluation of, 2503
  upper. See also individual anatomic parts
    anomalies of, 1357–1429
    deterioration of, in ileal conduit urinary
      diversion, 2669
    lesion of, biopsy of, 2254, 2254–2255
    nonurothelial tumors of, 1139
    passage of flexible ureteroscope into,
      2216
    radiolucent filling defects in, differential
      diagnosis of, 2251t
      evaluation of, 2252t
    referred somatic pain from, 40, 40
    transitional cell carcinoma of. See Tran-
      sitional cell carcinoma, of upper uri-
      nary tract
    urothelial tumors of, 1137–1146. See
      also Urothelial tumors, of upper uri-
      nary tract
  use of intestinal segments in. See Urinary
    diversion, intestinal
Urinary tract infection, 731–797. See also
  Bacteriuria; Cystitis; Pyelonephritis
  anaerobic, 768–769
  bacterial adherence in, 777–783
    adhesins in, 780–781, 781t, 782
    epithelial cells in, 778–780, 779–780
    epithelial receptors in, 780–781, 781t,
      782
    mannose-resistant hemagglutination in,
      780
    menstrual cycle day and, 779–780, 780
    pili in, 777, 777–778
      in vivo studies of, 781, 783, 783
      mannose-resistant (P pili) in, 778
      mannose-sensitive (type 1), 778, 780
    therapeutic implications of, 783
      competitive inhibitors and, 783
      receptor blockade and, 783
      vaccination and, 783
  bacterial persistence in, 735, 735t
  calculi due to, 2118–2122
    classification of, 2120, 2120t
    etiology of, 2118–2119, 2118–2119
    evaluation of patients with, 2120
    treatment of, 2120–2122
  catheter-associated, 747–748
    etiology of, 747
    incidence of, 747
    management of, 748
    methods for decreasing, 747–748
    morbidity due to, 747
    prophylaxis against, 736
  chronic, definition of, 732–733
  circumcision and, 1922
  classification of, 733–734
  complicated, definition of, 732
  definitions in, 732–733
  diabetes mellitus and, 757–758
  diagnosis of, 735–737
    bacteria counts and, 735
    improved accuracy of, 735–736

Urinary tract infection (Continued)
    tissue and stone culture in, 742, 742
    urethral and mid-stream cultures for,
      741, 741–742
    urethral catheterization of females for,
      736
  urinalysis in, 736–737
    false-negative results in, 736
    false-positive results in, 736
    pyuria in, 736–737
    white blood cells in, 736–737
  urine culture in, 737, 737–738
  vaginal vestibule culture for, 741, 741
  due to candida, 937–943. See also Candi-
    dal infection, of urinary tract
  due to congenital anomalies, 756
  due to gram-negative bacteria, 769–771,
    770t–771t
    bacteriology in, 769
    clinical presentation in, 769
    diagnosis and treatment of, 769–771
    factors affecting etiologic agents in, 770t
    management of shock in, 771t–772t
    pathophysiology in, 769
    treatment of, 770, 772t
  due to Mycobacterium tuberculosis. See
    Tuberculosis, genitourinary
  due to Proteus mirabilis, struvite stone for-
    mation in, 752–756, 754–755
    fragments remaining after treatment
      and, 754–755
    lithotripsy or surgery for, 754
    radiographic imaging in, 756
    renal damage due to, 753–754, 754–
      755
  due to schistosomiasis, 893–894
  due to streptococcal infection, microscopy
    in, 323, 325
  first, 734
  host defense mechanisms in, 783
  immunologic responses in, 750–752
    antibody titers in, 752
    direct agglutination tests for, 750
    ELISA for, 751
    fluorescent antibody-coated bacteria for,
      750–751
    passive agglutination tests for, 750
    RIA for, 751
  in children, 1669–1683
    acute hemorrhagic cystitis and, 1679
    bacterial factors in, 1670–1671
    bacteriuria in, 1670
    classification of, 1670
    clinical symptoms in, 1669, 1669t
    complications of, 1674–1679
      acute hemorrhagic cystitis as, 1679
      reflux nephropathy as, 1674–1675,
        1674–1679. See also Reflux
        nephropathy, in children
    diagnosis of, 1669–1670
    host factors in, 1671t, 1671–1672
      age as, 1671–1672
      anatomic abnormalities as, 1671
      blood group antigens as, 1671
    incidence of, 1670
    lower vs. upper tract infection in, 1672
    management of, 1679–1683
      pharmacologic, 1679
      radiologic evaluation and follow-up in,
        1679–1680
      voiding cystourethrogram in, 1679–
        1680
    recurrent, management of, 1681–1682
    renal damage risks in, 1677–1679
      elevated bladder pressure and, 1677
      peripubertal girls and, 1677–1678

Urinary tract infection (Continued)
    preputial bacterial colonization and,
      1678–1679
    vesicoureteral reflux and, 1677
    surgically correctable causes of bacterial
      persistence in, 1670t
    uninhibited bladder contraction in,
      1673–1674
    urinalysis in, 1669–1670
    urine culture in, 1669–1670
    vesicoureteral reflux in, 1672–1674, 1673
  in elderly, 795–797
    bacteriology in, 796, 797
    clinical presentation in, 795–796
    epidemiology of, 795t, 795–797, 796
    pathophysiology of, 796
    significance of, 796–797
    treatment of, 797
  in enuresis, 1625
  in females, natural history of, 771–773,
    772–774
  in pregnancy, 789–795. See also Bacteri-
    uria, in pregnancy; Pyelonephritis, in
    pregnancy
  localization of, 737–742
    bladder in, 740–741
      kidney vs., 741
      suprapubic needle aspiration for, 740,
        740
      urethral catheterization in female for,
        740–741
    kidney in, 737–740
      antibody-coated bacteria for, 739
      bladder vs., 741
      C-reactive protein for, 739–740
      Fairley bladder washout test for, 738–
        739
      fever and flank pain and, 740
      ureteral catheter localization for, 737–
        738, 738t–739t
  neurourologic evaluation and, 579
  preoperative antibiotics for, 2416
  prophylaxis against, 745–747
    antibiotics in, 733
    in transrectal prostatic needle biopsy,
      746–747
    in transurethral procedures, 745–746
      with endocarditis risk, 745
      without endocarditis risk, 745–746
  radiographic imaging in, 748–750
    abdominal plain film in, 749
    computed tomography in, 750
    excretory urogram in, 749
    indications for, 748–749, 749t
    radionuclide studies in, 750
    renal tomogram plain film in, 749
    renal ultrasound in, 749–750
    voiding cystourethrogram in, 749
  recurrent, causes of, 773–783
    definition of, 733–734
    due to benign prostatic hyperplasia, 1021
    E. coli in, virulence factors of, 777
    in children, small capacity hypertonic
      bladder and, 1656–1657, 1656–1657
    in posterior urethral valve(s), 1879
    management of, 786–789
    prophylaxis in, 786–788, 788t
      cephalexin for, 787
      efficacy of, 788
      fluoroquinolones for, 787–788
      intermittent self-start, 788–789
      introital and fecal flora and, 786
      nitrofurantoin for, 787
      post-intercourse, 789
      trimethoprim for, 786–787